Nursing Practice

Graphic illustrations: Hardlines

For Elsevier:

Senior Commissioning Editor: Ninette Premdas
Development Editor: Mairi McCubbin
Project Manager: Andrew Palfreyman
Senior Designer: Sarah Russell
Illustrations Manager: Bruce Hogarth

Nursing Practice

THIRD EDITION

Hospital and Home

The Adult

Edited by

Margaret F. Alexander BSc PhD RN RM RNT CBE FRCN

Emeritus Professor, School of Nursing, Midwifery and Community Health, Glasgow Caledonian University, Glasgow, UK

Josephine (Tonks) N. Fawcett BSc (Hons) MSc RN RNT ILTM

Head of Nursing Studies, School of Health in Social Science, University of Edinburgh, Edinburgh, UK

Phyllis J. Runciman BSc MSc MPhil RN RM RHV RNT

Formerly Senior Research Fellow, Caledonian Nursing and Midwifery Research Centre, School of Nursing, Midwifery and Community Health, Glasgow Caledonian University, Glasgow, UK

Illustrations by

Ethan Danielson

CHURCHILL LIVINGSTONE

ELSEVIER

EDINBURGH LONDON NEW YORK OXFORD PHILADELPHIA ST LOUIS SYDNEY TORONTO 2006

CHURCHILL
LIVINGSTONE
ELSEVIER

CHURCHILL LIVINGSTONE, an imprint of Elsevier Ltd

First published 1994
Second edition 2000
Third edition 2006

ISBN 10: 0443074577
ISBN 13: 978-0-443-07457-8

British Library Cataloguing in Publication Data
A catalogue record for this book is available from the British Library

Library of Congress Cataloging in Publication Data
A catalog record for this book is available from the Library of Congress

Notice
Knowledge and best practice in this field are constantly changing. As new research and experience broaden our knowledge, changes in practice, treatment and drug therapy may become necessary or appropriate. Readers are advised to check the most current information provided (i) on procedures featured or (ii) by the manufacturer of each product to be administered, to verify the recommended dose or formula, the method and duration of administration, and contraindications. It is the responsibility of the practitioner, relying on their own experience and knowledge of the patient, to make diagnoses, to determine dosages and the best treatment for each individual patient, and to take all appropriate safety precautions. To the fullest extent of the law, neither the Publisher nor the Editors assumes any liability for any injury and/or damage to persons or property arising out of or related to any use of the material contained in this book.

The Publisher

Printed in China

CONTENTS

CONTRIBUTORS

Erica S. Alabaster MSc PhD DipN RN RNT DANS RCNT WNBCert ITEC MIFA ILTM
Lecturer, School of Nursing and Midwifery Studies, Wales College of Medicine, Biology, Life and Health Sciences, Cardiff, University

32 The chronically ill person

Douglas Allan MN BEd RN RMN RNT
Programme Organiser, School of Nursing, Midwifery and Community Health, Glasgow Caledonian University, Glasgow, UK

9 Disorders of the nervous system

Joan Allwinkle DipDiab RN
Lead Diabetes Specialist Nurse, Department of Diabetes, Royal Infirmary of Edinburgh, Edinburgh, UK

5 Part 2: Diabetes mellitus

Dorothy J. Armstrong BSc PGCert RN MN RNT ILTM
Programme Director, NHS Education for Scotland, Edinburgh, UK and Visiting Lecturer, NHS Lothian

18 Shock

John Atkinson BA PhD NDNCert DipEd RN DNT
Professor, Associate Dean, Research and Commercialisation, School of Health, Nursing and Midwifery, University of Paisley, Paisley, UK

37 The person with HIV/AIDS

Sue Bale BA PhD PGDip DipN RN NDN RHV FRCN
Associate Director of Nursing, Gwent Healthcare NHS Trust, South Wales, Cardiff, UK

23 Wound healing

Karen Burnet BSc MSc OncCert RN
Lead Breast Cancer Nurse, Cambridge Breast Unit, Addenbrooke's NHS Trust, Cambridge, UK

7 Part 2: The breast

Bernadette Byrne BSc MSc ClinOnc OncCert RN
Centre Head Maggie's London, Maggie Keswick Jencks Cancer Caring Centres, Hammersmith Hospitals NHS Trust, London, UK

31 The patient with cancer

Joyce Campbell BSc RN
CNS, Familial Breast Screening Clinic, Department of Clinical Genetics, Western General Hospital, Edinburgh, UK

6 Genetic disorders

Maggie Carson BNurs (Hons) MSc RN
Endocrine Specialist Nurse, Endocrine Unit, Royal Infirmary, Edinburgh, UK

5 Part 1: Endocrine and metabolic disorders

Roseanne Cetnarskyj BSc PhD RGN SPQGenetics
Department of Clinical Genetics, Molecular Medicine Centre, Western General Hospital, Edinburgh, UK

6 Genetic disorders

Charmaine Childs BNurs MPhil PhD RN HVCert NDNCert
Senior Research Fellow, University of Manchester, Division of Medicine and Neurosciences, Hope Hospital, Salford, UK

22 Temperature control

Margaret Colquhoun MA MN PGCertTLHE RNT RN RM
Senior Nurse Lecturer, St Columba's Hospice, Edinburgh, UK

33 The patient receiving palliative care

Philip D. Cooper AdvDipDD RN
Senior Community Mental Health Nurse, Bury Community Mental Health Team, Bury St Edmunds, UK

36 Substance use

Michelle Cowen BEd(Hons) MSc DipNurs RN RNT RCNT SpLD
Lecturer in Critical Care Nursing, School of Nursing and Midwifery, University of Southampton, Southampton, UK

20 Fluid and electrolyte balance

Alison Crawshaw BSc ENB216 RN
Clinical Nurse Specialist, Department of Colorectal Surgery, Western General Hospital, Edinburgh, UK

4 Disorders of the gastrointestinal system, liver and biliary tract

---

Helen Dougan BEd DipCNE RN RCNT RNT
Formerly Senior Nurse Lecturer, St Columba's Hospice, Edinburgh, UK

33 The patient receiving palliative care

Sarah Drummond BSc RN RSCN SPQGenetics
Genetic Nurse, Department of Clinical Genetics, Western General Hospital, Edinburgh, UK

6 Genetic disorders

Fiona Duke BSc MSc DipOnc RN RMN RNT
Formerly Nurse Lecturer, Napier University, Department of Adult Physical Health, Canaan Lane Campus, Edinburgh, UK
11 Blood disorders

Sue Duke BSc MSc DipOnc RN RNT
Consultant Practitioner in Cancer Care Education, School of Nursing and Midwifery, University of Southampton, Southampton, UK
19 *Pain*

Cynthia Edmond BA MSc PhD GradDipEd RN RNT RM (Austr.) FRCNA
Formerly Lecturer, Health Occupations, University of Newcastle, NSW, Australia
3 Disorders of the respiratory system

Josephine (Tonks) N. Fawcett BSc(Hons) MSc RN RNT ILTM
Head of Nursing Studies, School of Health in Social Science, University of Edinburgh, Edinburgh, UK
17 Stress

Caroline Gibson BSc(Hons) MSc RN
Lecturer in Nursing, Queen Margaret University College, Edinburgh, UK
26 The patient facing surgery

Mary Gobbi MA PhD DipN DipNEd RN
Senior Lecturer, School of Nursing and Midwifery, University of Southampton, Southampton, UK
20 Fluid and electrolyte balance

Sue M. Green BSc MMedSci PhD RN RPHNutr IC
Senior Lecturer, School of Nursing and Midwifery, University of Southampton, Southampton, UK
21 Nutrition

Angela J. Griggs BA(Hons) PGDip ENB338, 870, 998 RN
Lecturer Practitioner, ENT Nursing, Royal Free Hampstead NHS Trust and City University, London, UK
14 Disorders of the ear, nose and throat

Mary Henry MPH AdDipN RN
Professor, Consultant Nurse Epidemiologist, Health Protection Scotland, Glasgow, UK
16 Disorders of the immune system, infection control and infectious diseases

Susan Hook DipH&SW ENBU01 RN
Haemophilia and Thrombosis Clinical Nurse Specialist, Royal Infirmary of Edinburgh, Edinburgh, UK
6 Genetic disorders

Pam Jackson BSc(Hons) MPhil RN RHV RCNT RNT
Senior Lecturer, School of Nursing and Midwifery, University of Southampton, Southampton, UK
21 Nutrition

Rosemary Kelly RN RM
Formerly Head and Neck Clinical Nurse Specialist, Canniesburn Plastic Surgery Unit, Glasgow Royal Infirmary, Glasgow, UK
15 Disorders of the mouth

Claire Kilpatrick MSc PGDipN RN
Nurse Consultant Infection Control, Health Protection Scotland, Glasgow, UK
16 Disorders of the immune system, infection control and infectious diseases

Lorrie Lawton BSc(Hons) BA MSc RN RN(child) ENB199, A33
Lecturer Practitioner, Emergency Care, Emergency Department, John Radcliffe Hospital, Oxford Brookes University, Oxford, UK
27 The patient who experiences trauma

Andrée le May BSc(Hons) PhD RN PGCEA
Professor, School of Nursing and Midwifery, University of Southampton, Southampton, UK
25 Sleep

Lesley A. Logan BSc(Hons) DipN CritCareCert CertHP ENB15 RN
Regional Manager, Donor Care and Co-ordination, UK Transplant, UK
4 Disorders of the gastrointestinal system, liver and biliary tract

Brian Lucas BA(Hons) MSc PGDipHE ENB219 RN
Orthopaedic Advanced Practice Nurse, Orthopaedic Department, Whipps Cross University Hospital NHS Trust, London, UK
10 Disorders of the musculoskeletal system

Kathleen MacDonald MSc DipAdNurs CritCareCert PGCE RN
Lecturer in Nursing, Queen Margaret University College, Edinburgh, UK
6 Genetic disorders

Kay Malloch BSc RN
Formerly Diabetes Specialist Nurse, Royal Infirmary of Edinburgh, Edinburgh, UK
5 Part 2: Diabetes mellitus

Breeda McCahill BSc PGDip NBSDip RN
Nurse Practitioner, Burns Unit, Glasgow Royal Infirmary, Glasgow, UK
30 The patient with burns

Jan McClean MPH RN RM
Acute Services Planning Manager, NHS Greater Glasgow Health Board, Glasgow, UK
3 Disorders of the respiratory system

Paula McFadyen BSR DipSocWork MSW DipCouns
Huntington's Advisor, Scottish Huntington's Association, Elderslie, UK
6 Genetic disorders

Janice McGlone BSc DipProfSt RN
Clinical Nurse Specialist, Department of Respiratory Medicine, Glasgow Royal Infirmary, Glasgow, UK
3 Disorders of the respiratory system

Marie McGill BSc(Hons) DipSocPol ENBHealthPromotion RN
Services Director, Scottish Huntington's Association, Elderslie, UK
6 Genetic disorders

Anne C. H. McQueen BA MSc MPhil DipCNE RN RM RCNT NT ILTM
Senior Lecturer, Nursing Studies, School of Health in Social Science, University of Edinburgh, Edinburgh, UK

7 Part 1: Disorders of the reproductive system

Margot Miller BSc(SPQ/GI) RN RCNT
Clinical Nurse Practitioner, Centre for Liver and Digestive Disorders, Royal Infirmary of Edinburgh, Edinburgh, UK

4 Disorders of the gastrointestinal system, liver and biliary tract

Linda Morrow BSc MSc PGCert DipDN RN RM
Professional Advisor, Continence Management, Scottish Commission for the Regulation of Care, Edinburgh, UK

24 Continence

Barbara E. Page BNurs DipN ENB25 RN
Dermatology Liaison Nurse Specialist, Queen Margaret Hospital, Dunfermline, UK

12 Skin disorders

Catherine Paton BSc(Hons) RN
Formerly Haematology Team Leader, Fife Acute Hospitals NHS and formerly Honorary Teaching Fellow, Faculty of Health and Life Sciences, Napier University Edinburgh

11 Blood disorders

Rosemary Paterson BSc(SPQ/GI) RN
Gastrointestinal Nurse Practitioner, Wishaw General Hospital, UK

4 Disorders of the gastrointestinal system, liver and biliary tract

Pauline Pearson BSc SPQGenetics PGDipCouns RN RNMD RegGenCouns
Clinical Nurse Specialist, Department of Clinical Genetics, Molecular Medicines Centre, Western General Hospital, Edinburgh, UK

6 Genetic disorders

Glynis Collis Pellatt BA(Hons) MA PhD DipN(Lond) DipNursEd RN
Senior Lecturer, Faculty of Health and Social Sciences, University of Luton, Aylesbury, UK

34 The patient in need of rehabilitation

Lesley Pemberton MEd RCNT RNT DipN FETC ENBN17 RN
Formerly Senior Lecturer in Nursing, University of Central Lancashire, Preston, UK

28 The unconscious patient

Yvonne Robb RN RM
Family Care Officer, South East of Scotland Clinical Genetic Services, Western General Hospital, Edinburgh, UK

6 Genetic disorders

Allyson Sanderson MA ENB998 DipMan PS11 RN
Emergency Care Practitioner, County Durham and Darlington Primary Care Trust, Darlington, UK

13 Disorders of the eye

Lesley Selfe BSc(Hons) MSc PhD PGDipEd RN
Director of Nursing, Emirates Hospital, Dubai, United Arab Emirates

8 Disorders of the urinary system

Anna M. Serra MSc ENTNursCert RN RNT
Senior Lecturer, Education Department, Marie Curie Hospice, Hampstead, London, UK

14 Disorders of the ear, nose and throat

Sheila Slater BSc(Hons) RMN RN
Clinical Nurse Specialist, Genetics, South East of Scotland Clinical Genetics Service, Western General Hospital, Edinburgh, UK

6 Genetic disorders

Catriona Smith BSc MSc RN
Staff Nurse, Intensive Care Unit, Royal Infirmary of Edinburgh, Edinburgh, UK

29 The critically ill patient

Graeme D. Smith BA PhD RN
Lecturer Nursing Studies, University of Edinburgh, Edinburgh, UK

17 Stress

Diane Stirling BSc RegGenCouns SPQGenetics
Macmillan Clinical Nurse Specialist in Genetics, South East of Scotland Clinical Genetics Service, Western General Hospital, Edinburgh, UK

6 Genetic disorders

Christina Thom MA OND RN
Ophthalmic Nurse Practitioner, Ophthalmology Department, St John's Hospital, Livingston, UK

13 Disorders of the eye

David Thompson BSc MA MBA PhD RN FRCN FESC
Professor of Nursing and Director, The Nethersole School of Nursing, The Chinese University of Hong Kong, Hong Kong

2 Disorders of the cardiovascular system

Alison Tonner BA RMN RN
Huntington's Advisor, Scottish Huntington's Association, Elderslie, UK

6 Genetic disorders

Debra Ugboma BN MPhil ENB134 RN
Lecturer Practitioner in Renal Nursing, School of Nursing and Midwifery, University of Southampton and Wessex Renal and Transplant Service, Queen Alexandra Hospital, Portsmouth, UK

20 Fluid and electrolyte balance

Catheryne Waterhouse BA(Hons) MSc PGCE RN
Lecturer Practitioner, Neuroscience, Neurosciences Unit, Royal Hallamshire Hospital, Sheffield, UK

28 The unconscious patient

Roger Watson BSc PhD CBiol FIBiol ILTM FRSA RN
Professor of Nursing and Director, Graduate School of Nursing and Midwifery, The University of Sheffield, Sheffield, UK;
UK Editor, Journal of Clinical Nursing

35 The older person

Rosemary Webster BSc MSc RN
Education and Practice Development Lead, Cardio-Respiratory Directorate, Glenfield Hospital, Leicester, UK

2 Disorders of the cardiovascular system

Catriona Whyte BSc RN SPQGenetics
Clinical Nurse Specialist – Genetics, Department of Clinical Genetics, Western General Hospital, Edinburgh, UK

6 Genetic disorders

Laura M. Wilson BSc RN
Ward Manager, Glasgow Royal Infirmary, Glasgow, UK

3 Disorders of the respiratory system

PREFACE

While no single text can encompass the wealth of knowledge that underpins the practice of nursing, we believe that this significantly updated third edition will continue to be an invaluable resource, not only for student nurses, but also for qualified nurses, including those returning to practice and those coming to nurse in the UK from other parts of the world, and for nurse educators. All face the challenge of new knowledge.

The structure of the book

As in the first two editions, the book is divided into three sections which are progressive in nature, encouraging the reader to move from the broad approach of Section 1 to a more in-depth appreciation of specific patient concerns and nursing issues in Sections 2 and 3. There is sufficient cross-referencing to encourage readers to make links and pursue lines of enquiry.

Section 1 — Care of patients with common disorders

Our existing confidence in the decision to adopt the systems approach for this section has been strengthened in light of the new developments in the skills and expertise that nurses may attain. They must have a thorough grounding in anatomy, physiology and disease pathology, therefore the structure of this chapter remains that of:

- anatomy and physiology
- pathophysiology
- medical management
- nursing priorities and management.

Essential anatomy and physiology have been presented. Recommendations for further reading and web addresses are given where more detail can be gained. We have been selective about the disorders chosen, concentrating on those commonly encountered by nurses in hospital and the community. Clearly, the nursing priorities and management content is the most important part of each chapter of Section 1; the wording of the heading reminds the student of the need to make appropriate clinical judgments and decisions, according to the individual's unique needs and circumstances.

Section 2 — Common patient problems and related nursing care

This section presents another way of examining nursing and builds on the foundations laid in Section 1. The focus is on common patient problems, which are not merely physiological in origin, but also arise from the subtle, complex interplay of social, psychological and economic factors. Some of these problems have a high profile, such as stress and pain. Others, such as nutrition and sleep, are often relatively neglected, but are very much the concern of nurses. These problems are not confined to, or only evident in, hospital care. They are part of life and may be experienced in many settings and at any time. Throughout the section, both the nurse's and the patient's perspectives have been considered and the basis for all interventions is that of best available evidence.

Section 3 — Nursing patients with special challenges

Some of the most challenging areas of nursing are explored in this section. By addressing these, the broad spectrum and contrasts of adult nursing are revealed. Such challenges, some long-term in nature, often make the greatest demands on the nurse's clinical and interpersonal skills. Section 3 addresses stereotypes and examines values and beliefs, raising awareness of the moral decision-making that underlies so much of day-to-day nursing practice.

Key features

In harmony with our commitment to exploring the different ways of knowing about nursing, a variety of features have been used throughout the book. These include:

- self-assessment questions STOP THINK
- further reading suggestions
- illustrations
- care plans and pathways, which are both educational and useful practice tools
- case histories, including accounts of personal 'lived experience'
- boxes highlighting key information
- research abstracts
- references
- useful addresses and websites.

The contributors and advisors

We owe a sincere debt of gratitude to the many authors and advisors who have contributed to the significant updating of this text. The authors represent many areas of adult nursing, and advisors include nursing and medical colleagues and members of the allied health professions. We pay sincere tribute here to their knowledge, experience and skills and thank them all for their key contributions to this text. We also greatly appreciated the informal advice received from academic and clinical colleagues.

As editors we have been delighted by the value placed on this book by readers, particularly the students, who are our future.

Whether you read this book, therefore, as a student nurse, a novice nurse, an expert practitioner, a preceptor/mentor or as an educator, it will provide a wealth of knowledge, derived from many sources: from professional nursing practice, from research and from the experiences of countless patients, clients and carers.

Edinburgh, 2006

Margaret F. Alexander
Josephine (Tonks) N. Fawcett
Phyllis J. Runciman

ACKNOWLEDGEMENTS

The editors would like to thank all who kindly granted permission to borrow material such as illustrations and tables from existing publications.

The editors would like to thank Roseanne Cetnarskyj for acting as coordinator for chapter 6. The editors also wish to record their thanks to those authors who contributed to the previous edition and whose work has provided the foundation for the current volume. These are:

Joyce M. Brown
S. Jose Closs
David B. Cooper
Aileen E. Crosbie
Claire Dibbs
Frances M. Davidson
Christine Docherty
Elizabeth S. Farmer
Ruth F. M. Gardner
Margaret Harris
Rhoda Hodgson
Evelyn Howie
Liz Jamieson
Vivian Leefarr
Cath M. McFarlane
Rosemary McIntyre
Mary B. Murchie
Marie-Noelle Orzel
Muriel E. Reffin
Billie Reynolds
Sheila E. Rodgers
Marion C. Stewart
Kathy Strachan
Margaret A. Studley
Jean Swaffield
Colin Torrance

Specific thanks are also expressed to the following:

For Chapter 5 Part 2, the authors wish to thank Gillian Aitken (Project Manager, Queen Margaret University College, Edinburgh) and Florence Brown (Diabetes Specialist Nurse, Gartnavel General Hospital, Glasgow).

For Chapter 9, the author wishes to thank Sarah Canning, Student Nurse, University of Edinburgh, for her contribution of Case History 9.2.

For Chapter 16, the authors wish to thank Marion Bennie, J. Claire Cameron, Beth Cullen, Simon Fallows, Jim McMenamin, Clare Mitchell, Jacqui Reilly and Vivienne Simpson for assistance with the chapter, and Hannah O'Regan, Student Nurse, University of Edinburgh, for her contribution to Figure 16.5.

For Chapter 21, the authors wish to thank Zillah Leach (Nutrition Support Nurse, Southampton University Hospitals Trust) and Peter Austin (Senior Pharmacist, Nutrition Support Team, Southampton University Hospitals Trust) for their advice and assistance on the sections on enteral and parenteral nutrition and the role of the Nutrition Support Team and the Clinical Nurse Specialist in nutrition.

For Chapter 33, the authors wish to thank Dr T. F. Benton (Medical Director) and Dorothy McArthur (Clinical Pharmacist), as well as many other members of staff at St Columba's Hospice, Edinburgh.

For chapter 37, the author wishes to thank Laura Mathers, Blood Borne Viruses Specialist Nurse, North Glasgow University Hospitals Division, for reviewing the chapter.

NURSING PRACTICE: AN INTRODUCTION

1

Margaret F. Alexander
Josephine (Tonks) N. Fawcett
Phyllis J. Runciman

Unless we are making progress in our nursing every year, every month, every week, take my word for it we are going back.
Florence Nightingale, cited in Skeet (1980, p. 100).

Introduction

Welcome to the third edition of *Nursing Practice*. The main purpose of this book is, and has been since its inception, to present knowledge about nursing, knowledge which comes to life when applied in the actual practice of nursing care. The education and practice of nursing inform each other and this book makes its contribution to both of these integral elements. Nursing is continually and rightly informed by new knowledge, new technologies and new research, much of which is incorporated in this new edition, an edition which comes at a time when nursing, its relationship with other professionals and with patients and carers, and its approaches to education and learning are undergoing significant transformation. Within a changing health care system, it is a time of rapid growth in the range and type of nursing roles and skills and nurse-led initiatives. For example, there is an increase in the number of nurse consultants and nurse endoscopists, and the prospect of nurses carrying out procedures such as angioplasty and minor surgery. A wide range of nurse-led clinics exist for prevention, treatment and rehabilitation in conditions such as heart attack, diabetes mellitus, chronic obstructive airways disease and asthma. This book reflects these changes. However, it particularly seeks to demonstrate the enduring essence of nursing care in helping individuals to maintain good health, recover from episodes of ill-health, cope day by day with chronic illness and experience dignity and comfort at life's end. So, in response to Florence Nightingale's exhortation, we are indeed making progress in our nursing; however, while welcoming the new, we are also acutely aware that the 'heart' of nursing beats on, in timeless rhythm. The nurse's sensitive communication skills, the eye contact, the listening ear, the informed and gentle hands-on care are the essential foundation for all of the complex nursing procedures and highly technical skills which nurses today are competent to carry out. Countless patients will testify to that.

Therefore, as editors, we have certain goals for this text:

- to present the knowledge and skills required for competent, evidence-based practice in the variety of settings in which nurses work, e.g. in hospitals, the community and in patients' own homes
- to value the individual 'lived experience' of health and illness, and the importance of listening carefully to the voices of patient and carers
- to illustrate the changing context and dynamic nature of health care
- to develop ways of thinking, learning and exploring critically the nature of nursing
- to encourage constructive reflection and analysis of care, the bases of sound clinical judgement
- to demonstrate the essential contribution of research in practice.

The current challenges for health care

Although the focus of this book is on health care in the United Kingdom (UK) and the context in which nursing takes place, its content has much wider relevance. As the World Health Organization points out (WHO 1996, 2003), 'health care does not take place in isolation from political, economic and cultural realities' within a country. Nurses, who constitute a major proportion of the health care workforce in many countries, and certainly in the countries of the WHO European Region, of which the UK is a part, do provide nursing care in environments which are touched by these realities. Many of the challenges which face nurses here in UK are not dissimilar to those facing nurses in other countries (WHO 2000, 2003).

Changing demography

Populations are ageing. Within the next 25 years or so, there will be a marked increase in the proportion of the population who are over 65 years of age, i.e. 1 in 4, with 1 in 12 over 80 (Scottish Executive 2005). Nurses will therefore contribute increasingly to health care for the older sector of the population and will need to acquire sound understanding of older people's perspectives and of their experiences of illness and disability. Also significant will be nursing's contribution to active ageing and to maintaining health in old age, both for older people who remain fit, and for those who must cope with health-related problems (Audit Commission 2004, WHO 2005).

Changing patterns of disease

Older people are more likely to have long-term illness, more likely to have a combination of such illnesses, e.g. cancer and cardiovascular disease, more likely to be admitted to hospital or require long-term care within the community, i.e. in care homes and at home (Scottish Executive 2005). Affecting the wider age range, there is a resurgence of diseases thought to have been eradicated, such as tuberculosis, the challenge of hospital acquired infection (HAI) and the enduring concern posed by HIV.

Changing care provision

There are tensions in current approaches to health care delivery, all of which affect nursing practice. For example, there is a mismatch between the need for proactive, integrated and preventive care for people with chronic conditions and a health care system which is perceived as prioritising specialised, episodic care for acute conditions. There are major technological and medical advances, from which arise both ethical concerns and issues of cost containment.

There are challenges associated with the integration of health and social care and with the provision of increasingly complex technical care to support patients who experience early supported discharge schemes and outreach care initiatives.

Changing expectations

Within this climate of change, there are also greater expectations from patients and carers for clear information and understanding of their health, illness and health care experience, and an increasing expectation of participation in decision making about their care (DH 2001). Effective communication underpins good care.

These challenges suggest a future in which the role of the nurse may be less hospital and medically dominated. They also may presage new opportunities for nurses to extend their knowledge and skills in many settings.

Partnerships

Partnership is a key issue in both policy and practice, here in the UK and further afield. In 1998, the World Health Organization stressed the need for partnerships and the importance of the contribution of nurses at the forefront of change in health care (WHO 1998). Partnership is essential, not only with other health and social care professionals, but also with patients and carers. In the coming decades, the consumer's voice will increasingly be sought and heard in the development and evaluation of health and social care. The emphasis on partnership means that nurses in hospital and in the community must find new ways of working with colleagues in the NHS and in a wider range of service sectors and agencies. Partnership also implies a need for strong clinical leadership. Effective partnerships are fundamental to the aims of clinical governance, with its emphasis on creating an environment in which clinical excellence will flourish. There are references throughout the text which reflect the importance of clinical judgement, decision making and risk management, all of which require clinical leadership.

Health, illness and disease

As our understanding of health grows, questions emerge:

- Why does disease develop in some healthy individuals and not in others?
- How is it possible that people manage to feel healthy in the face of coexisting disease?
- Why do such stark inequalities of health status persist between people and within communities?

Health and ill-health are now known to be influenced by a wide range of factors in people's life circumstances — economic, social, cultural, educational, psychological and genetic. Promoting health is a complex process. Nurses should be aware of the broader concepts of health currently being debated and at the same time be ready to respond in practical ways to patients' growing desire for more health-related information.

A useful distinction can be drawn between 'illness' and 'disease'. An 'illness' is what the patient experiences; a 'disease' is a description of pathological abnormality, made from the clinician's point of view. As long ago as 1977, Eisenberg drew this distinction between the personal and professional views, stating, 'Illnesses are experiences of changes in one's state of being and social function; diseases are abnormalities in the structure and function of the body organs and systems' (Eisenberg 1977). The concept of 'illness' therefore embraces all the experiential aspects of a disorder: what that patient *lives through*. The text reflects the emphasis on all three concepts — health, illness and disease — and the 'lived experience' of illness is clearly illustrated by the voices of a number of patients, 'heard' in many of the chapters of the text.

Hospital and home

The shift towards community care has had far-reaching implications for the traditional views of health, illness and disease, and for the way in which the patient's role is conceptualised. The image of the helpless person in a hospital bed — a passive recipient of paternalistic beneficence from the medical and nursing professions — has, wherever feasible, been replaced with the concept, referred to above but as yet not fully realised, of patients as partners.

The blurring of boundaries between hospital and home has made it essential for nurses to gain and interpret their knowledge and skills in a range of settings. For many people, a hospital stay may be a very brief life episode; for others, periodic visits to hospital or to/from the primary care team will become a regular, routine part of life. For some, a care home or hospital may replace their own home.

Reflection and the patient's experience

Some of the most sensitive insights of experienced nurses come from their careful, thoughtful analysis of daily work. Much can be learned from patient narratives and the telling of nursing stories, for example 'critical incidents'. Throughout this text, as noted above, we have incorporated narratives and stories which illustrate richly, in people's own words, the lived experience of health and illness at home and in hospital. Working closely with people in health and illness can be immensely satisfying, but also profoundly distressing; telling the stories of the day to those who have had similar work experiences and who share the same code of patient confidentiality can be immensely therapeutic and provide a meaningful learning experience.

In conclusion ...

The poet William Blake (1757–1827) wrote that 'art and science cannot exist but in minutely organised particulars'. This book strives to illuminate many of the particulars of nursing, but in the context of the whole. It responds to the current challenges within health care, and the need to find a meeting point between professional knowledge and expertise and the patient's lived experience.

Nursing must never be seen as 'a given', but as always developing. Practice must never be viewed complacently; its rationale must always be sought. The ways of thinking and learning, implicit in the whole approach of this book, are ways intended to encourage in the reader a love of learning, of questioning, of searching for 'the best available knowledge' which will inform nursing practice.

The knowledge needed for nursing can never be static and those who, as professional nurses, pursue such knowledge will undertake a journey of life-long learning, a journey of discovery and challenge.

To all our readers, enjoy your journey as a nurse, never lose the urge to explore, to discover or to face a challenge and, above all, never lose the gift of curiosity!

REFERENCES

Audit Commission 2004 Older people – independence and well-being: the challenge for public services. Audit Commission, London

Department of Health 2001 The expert patient: a new approach to chronic disease management for the 21st century. DH, London

Eisenberg L 1977 Disease and illness: distinction between professional and popular ideas of sickness. Culture, Medicine and Psychiatry 1(1): 9–23

Scottish Executive 2005 Framework for the future of the NHS. Scottish Executive, Edinburgh

Skeet M 1980 Notes on nursing: the science and the art. Churchill Livingstone, Edinburgh

World Health Organization (WHO) 1996 Nursing practice: report of a WHO Expert Committee. WHO Technical Report Series No. 860. WHO, Geneva

World Health Organization (WHO) 1998 HEALTH21: health for all in the 21st century. European Health for All Series, No. 6. WHO Regional Office for Europe, Copenhagen

World Health Organization (WHO) 2000 Nurses and midwives for health: a WHO European strategy for nursing and midwifery education. WHO Regional Office for Europe, Copenhagen

World Health Organization (WHO) 2003 Nurses and midwives: a force for health. WHO European strategy for continuing education for nurses and midwives. WHO Regional Office for Europe, Copenhagen

World Health Organization (WHO) 2005 Towards age-friendly primary health care. WHO, Geneva

CARE OF PATIENTS WITH COMMON DISORDERS

SECTION ONE

DISORDERS OF THE CARDIOVASCULAR SYSTEM

2

Rosemary A. Webster
David R. Thompson

INTRODUCTION

The cardiovascular system consists of the heart and blood vessels. It is a closed circuit and is responsible for ensuring that blood flows throughout the body.

Heart and circulatory disease, cardiovascular disease (CVD), includes all the diseases of the heart and blood vessels. The two main diseases in this category are coronary heart disease (CHD) and stroke, but CVD also includes congenital heart disease and a range of other diseases of the heart and blood vessels.

CVD is the greatest cause of death in the United Kingdom (UK), accounting for 39% of the deaths in 2002, a total of just under 238 000 people. Coronary heart disease is the most common cause of death in the UK, accounting for 1 in 5 deaths in men and 1 in 6 deaths in women (British Heart Foundation 2004).

Because CVD is so prevalent in Western industrial societies, it is likely to be encountered by all nurses, whether hospital- or community-based. This is particularly true now that an increasing percentage of the population is over 60 years old, an age group in which CVD is very common. However, CVD also affects the younger population, being the main cause of premature death and disability in the UK. There are marked regional variations in death rates. East Anglia, the south-east and the south-west of England have the fewest deaths from heart disease; Northern Ireland, the north of England and Scotland have the most (British Heart Foundation 2004). There is also a clear difference between socioeconomic groups in the prevalence of CVD, with the lowest incidence among the professional groups and the highest among the unskilled manual group. Ethnic background is also a significant factor. For example, a high mortality from CHD has been found in immigrants from the Indian subcontinent (Khunti & Samani 2004) and a high mortality from hypertension and stroke in immigrants from the Caribbean and Africa (Townsend et al 1992).

The burden imposed by CVD on the National Health Service (NHS) is substantial. The annual cost of health service resources for treating CHD is at least £1700 million (Liu et al 2002). In 1999, production losses and informal care associated with CHD cost the UK economy approximately £5300 million. Of the total cost of CHD to the UK, 25% was due to direct health care costs, 41% to productivity losses, and 34% to the informal care of people with CHD (British Heart Foundation 2004). CVD also has an immense impact on society in human terms. Bereavement, disability, changing roles within the family and society, and fear are some examples of its consequences.

Many cardiovascular diseases take the form of progressive debilitating illness, often becoming chronic with intermittent acute episodes. Individuals are faced with the prospect of a lifelong problem. In contrast, a heart attack (myocardial infarction, MI) is often sudden and unexpected, arousing acute distress in the individual and family as they confront a life-threatening crisis. Nurses, as one of the largest groups of health professionals, must inevitably bear some responsibility for helping to reduce the mortality, morbidity and personal suffering caused by CVD. Over a decade ago, Ashworth (1992) identified ways in which nurses can intervene to contribute to such a reduction:

- facilitating lifestyle adjustment to enable people to attain and maintain a level of health compatible with their personal goals
- assisting people to modify the demands of their activities of living, to balance with their capacity to meet them
- modifying the environment to achieve for each person the optimum possible environment within available resources
- providing physical treatment and monitoring for pathophysiological conditions
- reassuring, supporting and comforting patients and their families.

In addition, nurses are also increasingly in roles where they are able to assess and monitor the individual and make appropriate decisions about management priorities and treatment programmes. This should afford optimal care for each individual, thereby limiting symptoms, reducing the impact of the disease process and reducing the risk of adverse events and side-effects of treatment.

This chapter is based upon a nursing framework of activities of living. This framework reflects Roper et al's (2000) activities of daily living model of nursing, which has traditionally been used by many UK nurses caring for people with cardiovascular disorders. Whilst such models have been criticised for being too simplistic and not placing enough emphasis on psychosocial aspects of care, they continue to be a helpful basis for nursing assessment and care planning, even in environments where there is increased emphasis on nursing documentation as part of a critical care pathway, multidisciplinary care plan, clinical algorithms or guidelines.

Cardiovascular nursing is evolving as nurses move on from practising the skills of advanced life support, cannulation and phlebotomy, to taking greater responsibility for decisions which influence patient care management. Government frameworks and standards of care, such as the *National Service Framework for Coronary Heart Disease* (DH 2000) have resulted in opportunities for nurses to lead and develop services in and between primary, secondary and tertiary care environments. Increasingly, experienced nurses are part of the multidisciplinary team, admitting and discharging patients from specialist units via triage and fast-tracking; others are now prescribing thrombolytic therapy for patients with acute myocardial infarction (Caunt 1996), coordinating specialised clinics and leading rehabilitation and health promotion programmes (Quinn & Morse 2003).

The specialised nature of much cardiovascular nursing with established continuing educational opportunities, coupled with lower nurse–patient ratios, are other factors in the ongoing development of nursing roles in these areas. There is often the potential for therapeutic nurse–patient relationships to develop which can be used effectively in health promotion and psychological support (Broomfield 1996a). There is an increased focus on examining, from a multiprofessional perspective, the patient's experience, from onset of symptoms at home to discharge and follow-up, in an attempt to provide seamless, high-quality, evidence-based care. 'Process management', 'case management' and 'managed care' are terms which refer to this method of coordinating care. The pivotal tool for these approaches is the 'critical pathway' or 'integrated care pathway', used by medical, nursing and other professionals to provide standards for treatment plans, record progress against and monitor deviations from these standards, and document care (Kegel 1996). Despite concerns that this might limit individualised care, reduce nursing to a series of tick boxes and limit effective communication, care pathways have been developed for several cardiovascular diseases and procedures and have been shown to help in treatment decisions (Scott 2002, Kamineni & Alpert 2004). For an example of a critical pathway, see Figure 2.11 (p. 29).

The chronic nature of a large proportion of cardiovascular disease means that health professionals within the hospital see only certain episodes within the total spectrum of care. Much care is carried out in the community by the primary care team, with a focus on health education, promoting lifestyle adaptation and coping, and monitoring responses to treatment and disease progression. It is important that when people with cardiovascular problems are admitted to hospital, an emphasis is placed on a holistic multidisciplinary assessment so that staff have an understanding of the individual's home, family and work circumstances. Preparing a patient for return to their own environment with an optimum level of independence, together with any necessary support, requires good liaison between the hospital and community health care teams.

ANATOMY AND PHYSIOLOGY OF THE HEART

The heart is a muscular pump that generates pressure changes resulting in the propulsion of blood around the vascular system. The right side of the heart pumps blood around the pulmonary system where gaseous exchange takes place and then on to the left side of the heart. The left side of the heart operates under much greater pressure to enable it to pump blood around the systemic circulation. The various chambers of the heart are illustrated in Figure 2.1.

The heart is composed of three layers:

- *Pericardium* — a thick fibrous outer layer that protects the heart from injury and infection.
- *Myocardium* — a muscular layer that varies in thickness throughout the heart. The atria, which act as filling chambers, have a thin layer of myocardium as they do not, in the fit individual, have to generate high pressures. In the ventricles, the muscular layer is better developed, particularly on the left side, which is larger and thicker than in the right side, as a more forceful contraction is required to pump blood through the systemic circulation.
- *Endocardium* — a thin layer of endothelium and connective tissue that lines the inner chambers of the heart and coats the valves, which open and close to ensure a forward flow of blood at all times.

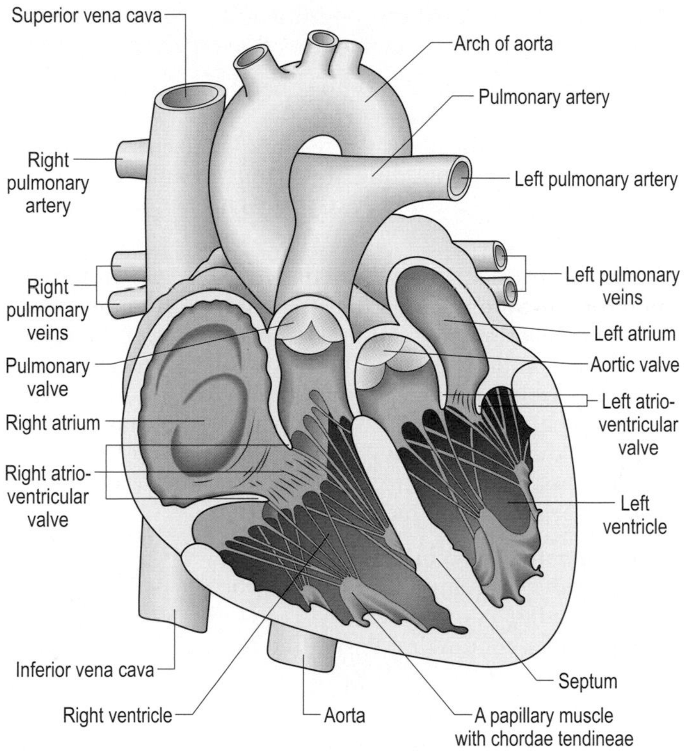

Fig. 2.1 The internal anatomy of the heart.

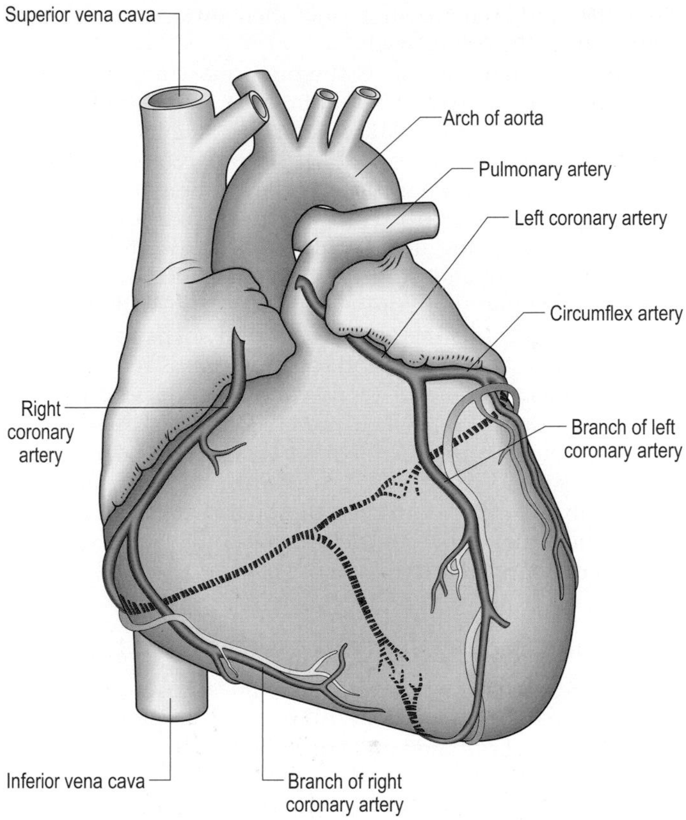

Fig. 2.2 The coronary circulation.

Coronary blood supply

Like all major organs, the heart requires blood flow to maintain cellular activity. The myocardium cannot derive oxygen and nutrients from the blood within the chambers. It receives its blood supply from the right and left coronary arteries which arise from the aorta just beyond the aortic valve (see Fig. 2.2).

The left coronary artery runs towards the left side of the heart and divides into two major branches: the left anterior interventricular branch or left anterior descending artery (LAD) and the circumflex artery (CX). The LAD follows the anterior ventricular sulcus and supplies blood to the interventricular septum and the anterior walls of both ventricles. The CX follows the coronary sulcus and supplies blood to the lateral and posterior regions of the left atrium and left ventricle. The right coronary artery (RCA) runs to the right side of the heart and divides into two branches: the posterior interventricular artery and the marginal artery. The more important posterior interventricular artery follows the posterior interventricular sulcus to the apex of the heart and supplies blood to the posterior ventricular walls. It is near the apex of the heart that the posterior and anterior interventricular arteries merge. The marginal artery follows the coronary sulcus and supplies the right ventricle. It is the RCA that normally supplies the sinoatrial (SA) and atrioventricular (AV) nodes (see Fig. 2.3).

After passing through the cardiac capillary bed, the blood drains into the cardiac veins. These join to form the coronary sinus on the posterior surface of the heart from where venous blood drains into the right atrium.

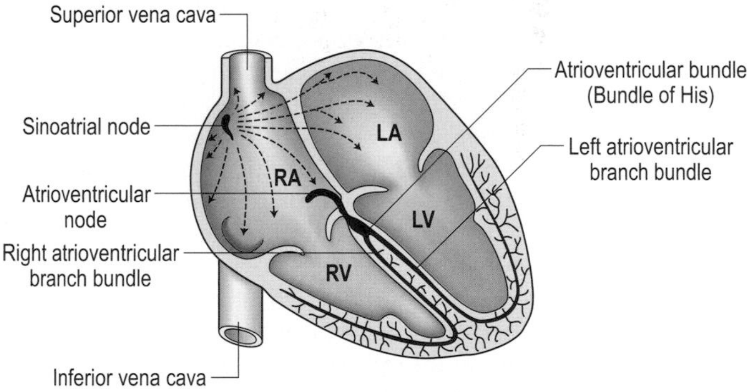

Fig. 2.3 The conducting tissues of the heart.

Structure and function of cardiac valves

The atrioventricular valves, i.e. the tricuspid and the mitral, function in a similar manner. During ventricular diastole (relaxation), they act as a funnel to promote rapid filling of the ventricles. Most of ventricular filling is passive. During ventricular systole (contraction), intraventricular pressure rises, pushing the cusps, which are restrained by the chordae tendineae, back and up towards the atria, thus preventing back-flow of blood during systole. These valves can withstand high pressure, since their surface area is much greater than the orifice itself.

The semilunar valves, i.e. the pulmonary and the aortic, have three cusps each. They are closed during ventricular diastole. Once ventricular contraction begins, the intraventricular pressure rises, and when it exceeds that in the aorta and the pulmonary artery, the semilunar valves are forced open and blood is ejected. After ventricular systole, the pressures in the aorta and pulmonary artery exceed those in the left and right ventricles, respectively. Retrograde blood flow therefore occurs due to the difference in pressure, which fills the valve cusps and snaps them home. The closure of the valves produces the sounds referred to as heart sounds. Mitral and aortic valve closure produces the first heart sound (S1) which precedes that of the tricuspid and pulmonary valves known as the second heart sound (S2). The second heart sound is normally split because the aortic valve closes before the pulmonary valve, on inspiration, when the right ventricle takes longer to expel the increased venous return.

The conducting system of the heart

It is important that the contraction of the atria and ventricles is organised to ensure that filling and emptying of the chambers is coordinated and controlled.

Cardiac cells contract and relax as a result of a stimulus response system. The heart consists of two major types of cardiac cells: unspecialised myocardial cells, which are designed for contraction, and automatic cells, which specialise in impulse formation.

The main bulk of the atria and ventricles consists of unspecialised myocardial cells. Adjacent myocardial cells are held together by a complex system of projections known as intercalated discs with relatively low electrical resistance. These permit the movement of ions (electrically charged particles) which facilitates the propagation of action potentials from one myocardial cell to another. The main ions involved in the generation of a cardiac action potential are sodium (Na^+), potassium (K^+) and calcium (Ca^{2+}). In the normal resting state, the myocardial cell is said to be polarised and, due to the distribution of ions across its cell membrane, it is negatively charged on the inside (intracellular) and positively charged on the outside (extracellular). When electrical activation of the cell occurs, changes in the cell membrane permeability result in the movement of ions, with a resulting change in electrical polarity. The membrane is now said to be depolarised and has an intracellular positive charge and an extracellular negative charge. Return to the resting state for each cell is called repolarisation and involves active pumping of ions against concentration gradients.

For further details, consult Jowett & Thompson (2003).

As the myocardial cells are 'knitted' closely together, the electrical stimulation of any one single cell causes the action potential to be propagated through all adjacent cells, eventually reaching the entire lattice work of the myocardium.

The automatic cells regulate the contraction of the myocardial cells by providing the initial electrical stimulation. They do not contribute significantly to the cardiac contraction itself. These cells possess three specific properties:

- automaticity — the ability to generate action potentials, spontaneously and regularly
- excitability — the ability to respond to electrical stimulation by generating an action potential
- conductivity — the ability to propagate action potentials.

The electrical charge on the surface of an automatic cell leaks away until a certain threshold is reached, when spontaneous complete depolarisation occurs over the whole cell surface and spreads to adjacent cells, both automatic and unspecialised. The automatic cell with the most rapid leak of charge becomes the principal pacemaking cell. Normally this is located within the SA node.

The automatic cells are found in the cardiac conducting system (see Fig. 2.3), which consists of:

- the sinoatrial (SA) or sinus node
- the atrioventricular (AV) junction (the AV node and bundle)
- ventricular conducting tissue (the right and left bundle branches).

Sequence of excitation

Depolarisation begins at the SA node and spreads through both atria. The activating impulse travels at a rate of about 1 m/s and reaches the most distant portion of the atria in about 0.08 s. The atria and ventricles remain electrically separate except via the AV junction, which allows the action potential to be conducted from the atrial to the ventricular conducting system. When the impulse reaches the AV node, there is a delay of about 0.04 s to allow blood flow from the atria to the ventricles. After emerging from the AV node, the impulse enters the rapidly conducting tissue of the bundle of His and the right and left bundle branches. The rapid spread of the impulse throughout the ventricles means that the entire ventricular mass is depolarised almost simultaneously, which is necessary for efficient contraction and pumping.

Electrocardiography

Electrocardiography is the graphic recording from the body surface of potential differences resulting from electrical currents generated in the heart. This recording may be displayed on special graph paper or on an oscilloscope (monitor) and is known as an electrocardiogram (ECG). An ECG is a graphic record of electrical changes at the skin surface plotted against time. The main value of the ECG is in the detection and interpretation of cardiac arrhythmias, diagnosis of CHD and assessment of ventricular enlargement (hypertrophy).

The sequence of electrical events produced at each heartbeat has arbitrarily been labelled P, Q, R, S and T (see Fig. 2.4).

The P wave

is associated with atrial activation. The width of the P wave represents the time necessary for the atrial activation process. Following atrial depolarisation, an absence of

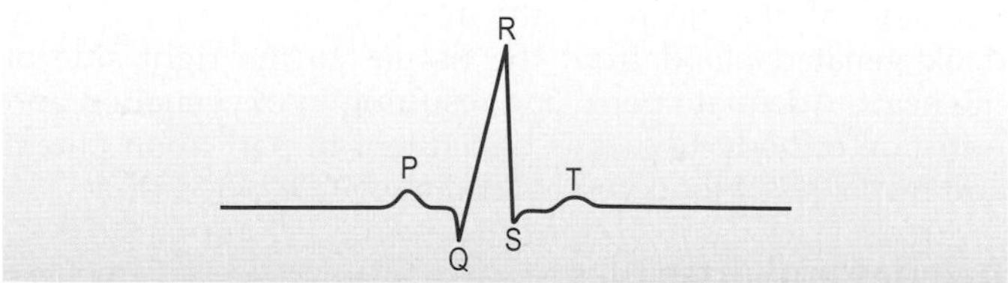

Fig. 2.4 ECG of one cardiac cycle.

electrical activity is noted on the ECG for a brief period, representing the passage of the impulse through the AV node. The PR interval, measured from the beginning of the P wave to the beginning of the QRS complex, is the time taken for the action potential to spread from the SA node, through the atrial muscle and the AV node, down the bundle of His and into the ventricular muscle mass.

The Q, R and S waves
are associated with ventricular activation. The first downward deflection after the P wave is always labelled the Q wave and the R wave is the first upward deflection. If a negative deflection follows an R wave, it is labelled an S wave. The width of the QRS complex shows how long the action potential takes to spread through the ventricles.

The ST segment,
a flat line between the S wave and the T wave, represents the early phase of ventricular muscle repolarisation, or recovery.

The T wave
represents the actual recovery of the ventricular muscle. Occasionally, a U wave can be observed following the T wave. The origin of this wave is not well understood, but it is considered significant in a state of hypokalaemia.

For more details on the ECG, see Houghton & Gray (2003).

Excitation–contraction coupling

Excitation–contraction coupling is the term used to describe the link between the electrical events and the contraction of the myocardial muscle. When an action potential passes over the cardiac muscle cell membrane, it is able to pass into the interior of each muscle cell down a series of fine branching tubules until it reaches the cell's contractile elements and stimulates the release of calcium ions. Calcium ions act as a catalyst for the chemical reaction that activates the sliding of thin muscle filaments (myofilaments) over each other to produce contraction. The strength of myocardial contraction is thus partly dependent on the intracellular concentration of free calcium ions.

Cardiac cycle

The cardiac cycle is the cyclical contraction (systole) and relaxation (diastole) of the two atria and the two ventricles. Each cycle is initiated by the spontaneous generation of an action potential in the SA node.

During diastole, each chamber fills with blood. Diastole usually lasts about 0.4 s, and during this time blood enters

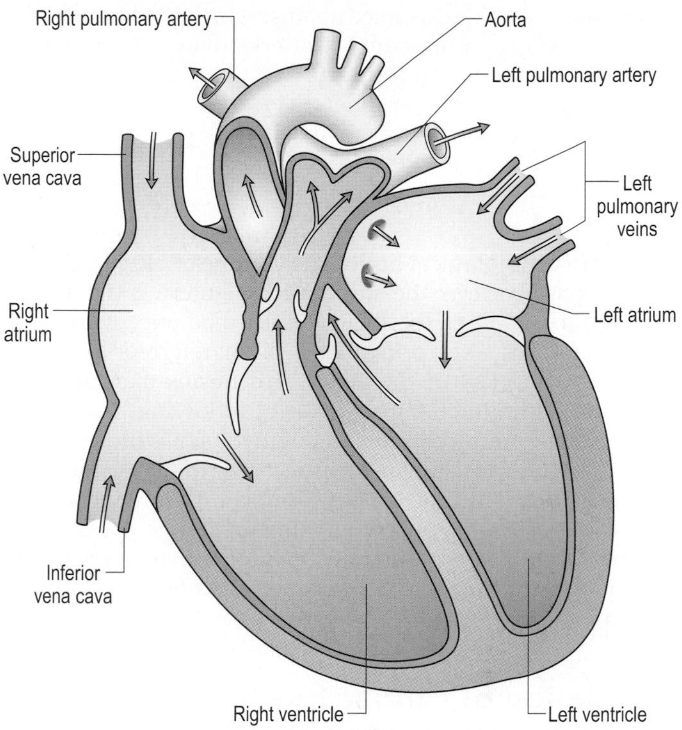

Fig. 2.5 Blood flow through the heart.

the relaxed atria and flows passively into the ventricles. During ventricular diastole, the mitral and tricuspid valves are open and the aortic and pulmonary valves are closed.

Blood is expelled from the chambers during systole. The atria contract fractionally before the ventricles and complete ventricular filling. The ventricles then begin to contract. Increasing pressure in the ventricles closes the mitral and tricuspid valves so that all four valves are closed. This is known as the isometric phase of ventricular contraction because the volume of blood in the ventricles remains constant. Ventricular pressure continues to rise until eventually the pulmonary and aortic valves are forced open and blood is ejected into the pulmonary artery and aorta. When the ventricles stop contracting, the pressure within them falls below that in the major blood vessels, the aortic and pulmonary valves close and the cycle begins again with diastole (see Fig. 2.5).

The normal heart rate is approximately 70 beats/min in the resting adult, with each cardiac cycle lasting approximately 0.8 s. With each ventricular contraction, 65–75% of the blood in the ventricle at the end of diastole is ejected. This is usually a volume of 70–80 mL of blood and is known as the stroke volume.

Cardiac output is the volume of blood ejected from one ventricle in 1 min. Although cardiac output is a traditional measure of cardiac function, it differs markedly with body size. Thus, a more informative measure is the cardiac index, which is the cardiac output per minute per metre squared of body surface area. Usually it is about 3.2 L/m^2.

The primary factors which determine cardiac output are:

- preload — the amount of tension on the ventricular muscle fibres before they contract, determined primarily by the end-diastolic volume (EDV)

- afterload — the resistance against which the heart must pump. Major components of afterload are:
  — blood pressure in the aorta
  — resistance in the peripheral vessels
  — the size of the aortic valve opening
  — left ventricular size
- contractility of the heart
- heart rate.

Within physiological limits, the volume of blood pumped out by a ventricle is the same as that entering the atrium on the same side of the heart, i.e. cardiac output matches venous return. This principle is often referred to as the Frank–Starling law of the heart. This means that the heart is able to adapt to changing loads of inflowing blood from the systemic and pulmonary circulations. Within certain limits, cardiac muscle fibres contract more forcibly the more they are stretched at the start of contraction. Once the venous return increases beyond a certain limit, the myocardium begins to fail. This regulation of the heart in response to the amount of blood to be pumped is known as intrinsic regulation.

Regulation of cardiac function by the autonomic nervous system

The autonomic nervous system alters the rate of impulse generation by the SA node, the speed of impulse conduction and the strength of cardiac contraction. It regulates the heart through both sympathetic and parasympathetic nerve fibres. The sympathetic fibres supply all areas of the atria and ventricles, and the effects on the heart include increased heart rate, increased conduction speed through the AV node and increased force of contraction. Parasympathetic impulses are conducted to the heart via the vagus nerve and affect primarily the SA node, the AV node and the atrial muscle mass. Parasympathetic stimulation produces decreased heart rate, decreased conduction rate through the AV node and decreased force of atrial contraction.

Sympathetic and parasympathetic control of the heart occurs by reflexes coordinated in the medulla oblongata of the brain. The group of neurones in the brain that affects heart activity and the blood vessels is known as the cardiovascular centre. This centre receives information from various sensory receptors. Baroreceptors, located in the atria, the aortic arch and carotid sinuses, alter their rate of impulse generation in response to changes in blood pressure; chemoreceptors, located for example in the carotid artery, respond to changes in the chemical composition of the blood.

ANATOMY AND PHYSIOLOGY OF THE BLOOD VESSELS

Systemic circulation

The systemic circulation is a high-pressure system that supplies all the tissues of the body with blood. It consists of the arteries, arterioles, capillaries, venules and veins. Blood flows through the system because of a downward pressure gradient from the aorta to the superior and inferior venae cavae. Arteries distribute oxygenated blood from the left side of the heart to the tissues, and veins convey deoxygenated blood from the tissues to the right side of the heart. Adequate perfusion resulting in oxygenation and nutrition of body tissues is dependent in part upon patent and responsive blood vessels and adequate blood flow.

Arteries and arterioles

Arteries are thick-walled structures that carry blood from the heart to the tissues. The major arteries leading from the heart branch to form smaller ones, which eventually give rise to arterioles. The walls of the arteries and arterioles are divided into three layers:

- the inner layer provides a smooth surface in contact with the flowing blood
- the middle layer, the thickest, consists of elastic fibres and muscle fibres; the elasticity of the arterial wall enables it to recoil during ventricular relaxation and maintain blood flow
- the outer layer of connective tissue anchors the vessel to its surrounding structures.

There is much less elastic tissue in the arterioles than in the arteries. The middle layer of the arteriole wall consists primarily of smooth muscle which, by contraction and relaxation, controls the vessel's diameter. Arterioles regulate the pressure in the arterial system and the blood flow to the capillaries. The arterioles respond to local conditions such as a decrease in oxygen concentration or an increase in the concentration of carbon dioxide or other waste products. This ensures that tissue that needs extra oxygen receives extra blood flow.

Arterioles will sometimes respond to changes in blood pressure. A local increase in blood pressure will cause the arterioles to constrict, in order to protect the smaller vessels in the tissue from increased pressure. If pressure in the arterioles suddenly decreases, the arterioles will dilate to ensure that the tissue receives sufficient blood flow for nutrition. This local regulatory mechanism is sometimes referred to as autoregulation and is an important factor in determining relatively constant blood flow despite alterations in arterial pressure, for example, the autoregulation ensuring glomerular filtration (see p. 358). The sympathetic nervous system will also influence the diameter of the arterioles. Increased sympathetic stimulation to blood vessels usually produces constriction, whereas decreased sympathetic stimulation results in vasodilatation.

Capillaries

The velocity of the blood is at its slowest in the capillaries, thus allowing sufficient time for exchange of materials between the blood and the interstitial space. Capillary walls lack muscle. They consist of a single layer of cells and have a large total surface area. Their thin walls allow efficient transport of nutrients to the cells and the removal of metabolic wastes. The density of capillary networks varies in different tissues.

Veins and venules

Capillaries join together to form larger vessels called venules, which in turn join to form veins. The walls of the veins are thinner and much less muscular than the arteries. This allows the veins to distend more, which permits storage of large volumes of blood in the veins under low pressure. Approximately 75% of total blood volume is contained in the veins. Some veins are equipped with valves to prevent the reflux of blood as it is propelled towards the heart. The sympathetic nervous system can stimulate venoconstriction, thereby reducing venous volume and increasing the general circulating blood volume. This adjustment of the total volume of the circulatory system to the amount of blood available to fill it contributes to the regulation of blood pressure.

Blood pressure

Blood pressure refers to the hydrostatic pressure exerted by the blood on the blood vessel walls and is a consequence of blood flow and vascular resistance. As most of the resistance to blood flow is due to the peripheral vessels, especially the arterioles, it is often described as the total peripheral resistance, as in the equation:

$$\text{mean arterial pressure} = \text{cardiac output} \times \text{total peripheral resistance}$$

Blood pressure varies in different blood vessels. However, clinically the term 'blood pressure' refers to systemic *arterial* blood pressure.

Arterial blood pressure

Arterial blood pressure fluctuates throughout the cardiac cycle. The maximum pressure occurs after ventricular systole and is known as the *systolic* pressure. Systolic pressure is dependent on the stroke volume, the force of contraction and the stiffness of the arterial walls. Systolic blood pressure normally falls a little on standing and this fall may be particularly marked in those with autonomic failure, taking vasodilator medication or in shock. The level to which arterial pressure falls before the next ventricular contraction is the minimum pressure, known as the *diastolic* pressure. Diastolic pressure varies according to the degree of vasoconstriction and is dependent on the level of the systolic pressure, the elasticity of the arteries and the viscosity of the blood. Normally the diastolic blood pressure rises a little on standing. Alterations in heart rate will also affect diastolic pressure. A slower heart rate produces a lower diastolic pressure as there is more time for the blood to flow out of the arteries. The difference between the systolic and diastolic blood pressures is known as the 'pulse pressure'. The average pressure attempting to push the blood through the circulatory system is known as the 'mean arterial pressure'.

Blood pressure values

There is no such thing as a 'normal' blood pressure, as it varies both from person to person and in individuals from moment to moment, under different circumstances. The optimal blood pressure targets are a systolic blood pressure of less than 120 mmHg and a diastolic blood pressure of less than 80 mmHg (Williams et al 2004). Factors such as age, gender and race influence blood pressure values. Pressure also varies with exercise, emotional reactions, sleep, digestion and time of day.

The predominant mechanisms that control arterial pressure within the 'normal' range are the autonomic nervous system and the renin–angiotensin–aldosterone system.

Baroreceptors respond to changes in arterial pressure and relay impulses to the cardiovascular centre in the medulla oblongata. When the arterial pressure is increased, baroreceptor endings are stretched and relay impulses that inhibit the sympathetic outflow. This results in a decreased heart rate and arteriolar dilatation and the arterial pressure returning to its former level. If the blood pressure remains chronically high, the baroreceptors are reset at a higher level and respond as though the new level were normal.

When blood flow to the kidneys decreases, with a fall in blood pressure, renin is released. Renin is an enzyme which acts on the blood protein angiotensinogen, which is converted to angiotensin I in the liver and then, by another enzyme in the kidney, to angiotensin II. Angiotensin II produces an elevation in blood pressure by direct constriction of arterioles. Angiotensin II also directly stimulates the release of the hormone aldosterone from the adrenal cortex which leads to renal retention of sodium and water in the distal convoluted tubules. This increases extracellular volume, which in turn increases the venous return to the heart, thereby raising stroke volume, cardiac output and arterial blood pressure. The kidneys respond to an increase in arterial pressure by excreting a greater volume of fluid. This decreases the extracellular fluid, resulting in a lower venous return and reduced cardiac output until arterial pressure is returned towards normal.

DISORDERS OF THE CARDIOVASCULAR SYSTEM

Atherosclerosis

Atherosclerosis is a complex disorder of the arteries characterised by the progressive accumulation of cholesterol within the intima of large and medium arteries. It is a disease with phases of stability and instability. Although the pathogenesis of atherosclerosis is still not fully understood, it is thought to involve endothelial injury, inflammatory processes and the focal distribution of lipids and fibrous tissue in the form of atheromatous plaques, particularly around branching vessels and arterial curvature. These plaques evolve over decades, a mature plaque having a soft, lipid-rich core surrounded by a hard fibrous capsule. There is thickening and hardening of the vessel walls with resultant loss of elasticity (see Figs 2.6 and 2.7).

For further details of the pathogenesis of atherosclerosis, see Jowett & Thompson (2003).

Atherosclerosis is responsible for most CHD and much peripheral and cerebrovascular disease. Emboli may arise as a result of pieces of dead tissue from the damaged arterial wall breaking off. With progression of the process, the lining of the vessel wall may become eroded and, especially if the blood pressure is elevated, the vessel may become permanently dilated and weakened, forming an aneurysm. Vessels may become blocked or stenosed or, as a result of endothelial damage and platelet adhesion, an ulcer-like site can develop, leading to thrombus formation. This thrombus may cause complete obstruction of the artery or may break down spontaneously. This dynamic process occurs over a period of hours to days, preceding an acute coronary event or spontaneous resolution.

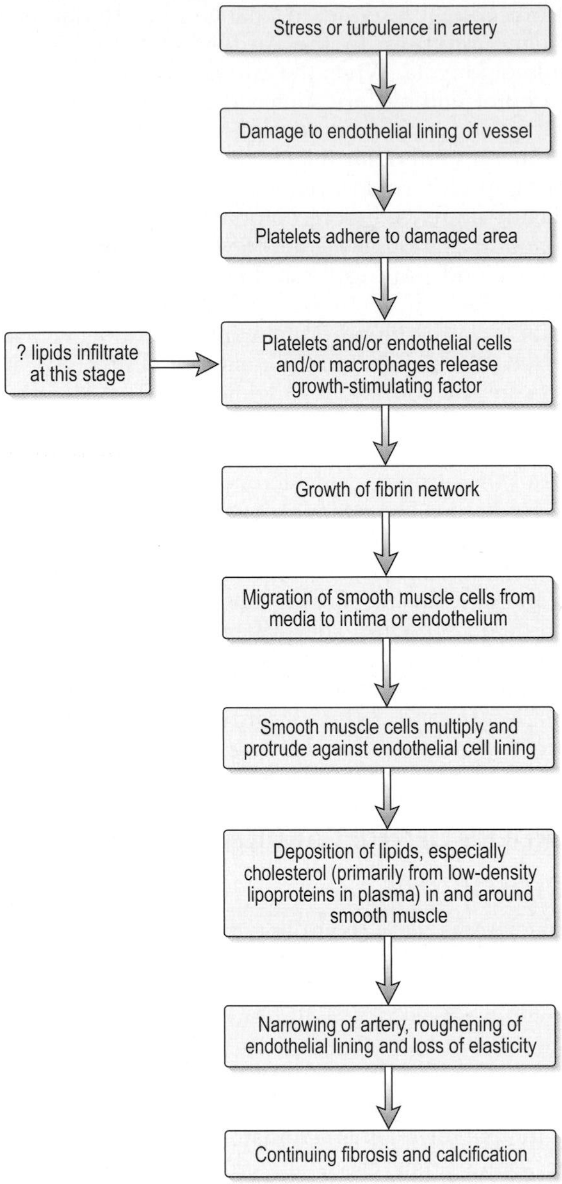

Fig. 2.6 Probable course of events in the development of atheroma.

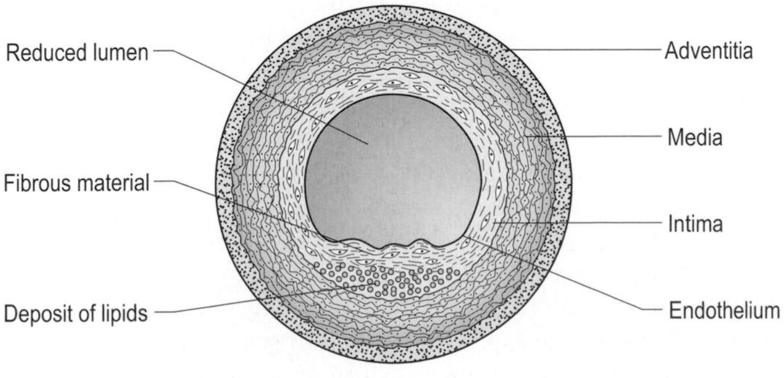

Fig. 2.7 Cross-section of an artery.

Myocardial ischaemia

Traditionally, myocardial ischaemia is defined as a condition of the heart in which there is an imbalance between oxygen supply and demand. Oxygen demand depends mainly upon heart rate, myocardial contractility and tension in the myocardial wall. Oxygen supply to the myocardium varies with coronary blood flow. The heart extracts the maximum amount of oxygen from its blood supply and is dependent upon an increased volume of blood in times of increased demand. Myocardial blood supply may be compromised by abnormalities of the vessel wall, the blood flow or in the blood itself.

Localised myocardial ischaemia may be intermittent and have reversible effects, but it inevitably causes decreased myocardial function. Ischaemia results in acidosis and the rapid accumulation of potassium in the extracellular space. Pain is usually experienced after about a minute of myocardial ischaemia.

Coronary heart disease manifests itself as:

- stable angina
- acute coronary syndrome, including unstable angina and myocardial infarction
- sudden death.

Risk factors

Epidemiological studies have sought to find associations between CHD and physical, biochemical and environmental characteristics of a population or individuals. As a result, predictive variables, termed risk factors, have been defined, which have been shown to be associated with the development of disease. These include male gender, increasing age, ethnic origin, low birth weight and a history of premature CHD. These are unavoidable risk factors; however, modifiable risk factors include:

- raised serum cholesterol levels
- cigarette smoking
- hypertension.

The known risk factors are extremely common in the UK and they tend to 'cluster' in individuals with one factor adding to the risk of another. The average level of serum cholesterol in different populations roughly predicts the risk of CHD. A raised serum blood cholesterol has been defined as being above 5.2 mmol/L, with the mean cholesterol level for men in England being 5.5 mmol/L and for women 5.6 mmol/L (British Heart Foundation 2004). The average diet in the UK is unhealthy. In particular, fat intake, especially of saturated fat, is too high and fruit and vegetable consumption is too low. More than a quarter of the population smoke cigarettes (Joint Health Surveys Unit 2001). Almost a quarter of the deaths from CHD in men are attributable to smoking (British Heart Foundation 2004) and there is a marked social class difference in smoking habits. Less than half the population take no moderate intensity physical activity in a typical week (British Heart Foundation 2004).

Individuals with blood pressure at the upper limits of the population distribution have an increased incidence of atherosclerotic, thrombotic and haemorrhagic vascular disease and an increased morbidity and mortality due to stroke, myocardial infarction and peripheral vascular disease. The systolic blood pressure is the better predictor of subsequent cardiovascular risk. The World Health Organization (WHO) has estimated that over 50% of CHD in developed countries is due to a systolic blood pressure in excess of the theoretical minimum of 115 mmHg (WHO 2002). In England, 37% of men and 34% of women have hypertension, defined as a systolic blood pressure over 140 mmHg and a diastolic blood pressure over 90 mmHg (British Heart Foundation 2004). Hypertension Society guidelines support initiation of intervention on the level of overall cardiovascular risk rather than absolute blood pressure values (Williams et al 2004).

Other risk factors are:

- obesity
- lack of physical exercise
- stress (see Ch. 17)
- diabetes mellitus and glucose intolerance.

Major geographical variations in the incidence of CHD are apparent. Mortality rates from CHD have been falling in the UK since the late 1970s; however, the rates in the UK are very close to the top of the international league table. Scotland, Northern Ireland and the north of England have the highest mortality rates; the south-east of England has the lowest. Mortality from CHD differs significantly between ethnic groups. It is highest in those born in the Indian subcontinent and is also raised in Irish- and Polish-born immigrants. Risk factors need to be viewed in conjunction with each other, as their effect is cumulative. Although, by definition, each risk factor associates positively with increased risk of CHD, it does not follow that risk factors are causal. It is also important to remember that a significant number of patients presenting with CHD do not have identifiable risk factors and that standard risk factors explain less than half the disease (see Table 2.1).

STOP THINK **2.1** Empowering people is neither simple nor easy. What might hinder people from taking greater control over their health and what might encourage them to do so?

For more information on coronary heart disease prevention, see Lindsay & Gaw (2003).

Stable angina

Angina is a symptom, rather than a disease, describing discomfort or pain resulting from a transient, reversible episode of inadequate coronary circulation occurring as a result of an imbalance between oxygen supply and demand. Similar symptoms may be caused by disorders of the oesophagus, lungs or chest wall. It is estimated that over 1.2 million people in the UK suffer from angina (British Heart Foundation 2004). Angina is regarded as stable if it has been recurring over several weeks without major deterioration, although symptoms may be variable depending on environmental temperature and emotion.

Table 2.1 Modifiable and non-modifiable risk factors for coronary heart disease

Non-modifiable risk factors	Modifiable risk factors
Age	Blood cholesterol
Gender	Tobacco smoking
Ethnicity	High blood pressure
Genetic predisposition	Overweight and obesity
Low birth weight	Diet
Diabetes mellitus	Alcohol consumption
Hormonal and biochemical factors	Social class Geographical distribution

PATHOPHYSIOLOGY

Ischaemia usually occurs as the result of reduced coronary artery blood flow following coronary artery obstruction caused by fixed atheromatous deposits in the major epicardial arteries. Spasm or thrombus may also contribute to the obstruction. There is insufficient oxygen delivery for local metabolic demand and this releases lactic acid as cells switch to anaerobic metabolism. Pain is experienced, as sensory neurones innervating the heart are richly endowed with an ion channel that is opened by the increase in lactic acid concentration. It is usually felt that a coronary artery must be narrowed by at least 50% before coronary blood fails to meet the demands of the heart during exertion. Severe anaemia and hypoxia can also produce a decreased myocardial oxygen supply. Increased demand for myocardial oxygen can occur in a variety of clinical conditions, including tachycardia, hypertension, valvular stenosis, left ventricular hypertrophy and hyperthyroidism.

Common presenting symptoms

The presentation and history may vary and initially mislead the practitioner if a thorough examination is not undertaken. The history is usually of discomfort, often related to specific events. The presenting features indicate a deficiency in the oxygen supply, such as:

- episodic pain or discomfort occurring centrally in the chest, often described as 'dull', 'aching' or a 'tight band'. This may radiate to the arms, particularly the left arm, jaw or neck. It is often induced by exercise or emotion and relieved by rest. Angina takes many forms. Typically, the duration of an attack of angina is 2–5 min
- breathlessness on exertion, e.g. walking uphill, or in cold weather
- discomfort in the epigastric region after a heavy meal.

Diagnosis

Angina is diagnosed by the nature of the symptoms, the perceived likelihood of coronary artery disease in that individual and the results of various diagnostic tests. It is recommended that all newly diagnosed cases of angina be referred to a physician with a specialist interest and training in cardiology (De Bono 1999). Where the diagnosis is in doubt, or where a positive diagnosis of angina would have significant implications, patients should have rapid access to, and be assessed by, a cardiologist within 2 weeks of referral via a rapid access chest pain clinic (DH 2000).

A good history is the most important part of the assessment as the pain of angina may be confused with the pain of oesophagitis or the pain of peptic ulceration. Patients, fearing a 'heart attack', may choose to interpret the pain as 'a little indigestion'.

MEDICAL MANAGEMENT

Investigations

are as follows:

Electrocardiogram (ECG) An abnormal ECG both supports the diagnosis and identifies those with a poor prognosis. The recording is invariably normal between attacks of angina; however, during an episode of pain, the segment between the end of the QRS complex and the beginning of the T wave may be depressed (ST depression), indicating ischaemia. The T wave may also be flattened or inverted.

Exercise tolerance test This is a means of assessing the heart's response to increased demand. It is useful for both diagnosis and assessing prognosis. The test is based on the theory that patients with ischaemic heart disease will produce marked ST segment depression on the ECG when exercising. The test is considered negative if there are no significant ECG abnormalities and the patient experiences no significant symptoms. Three common methods of exercise testing include:

- climbing stairs
- pedalling a stationary bicycle
- walking on a treadmill.

In the exercise tolerance test, the ECG, heart rate and blood pressure are recorded while the patient engages in some form of physiological stress. The principle is that coronary arteries that may be occluded will be unable to meet the heart's increased oxygen demand, resulting in chest pain, fatigue, dyspnoea, excessive heart rate (tachycardia), a fall in blood pressure or the development of arrhythmias. The test is stopped if any of these occur, or before, at the patient's request. The patient needs to have the procedure explained in detail before the test, should be advised to avoid a heavy meal prior to the test and to wear loose-fitting clothes. The term 'stress' test is best avoided as it may sound ominous and increase patient anxiety. The procedure takes about 30 min.

Holter monitoring Continuous monitoring of the ST segments of the ECG can be used to detect transient changes compatible with ischaemia.

Myocardial perfusion imaging is a non-invasive method of assessing myocardial perfusion by intravenous injection of a radioisotope, usually thallium or technetium, which is taken up by the heart and distributed throughout the myocardium in proportion to regional blood flow.

Radionuclide ventriculography is used to identify patients with poor left ventricular function.

Stress echocardiography involves the imaging of altered myocardial contractility during exercise or pharmacological stress. Using medication rather than exercise to induce stress is particularly useful if the patient is unable to exercise.

Coronary angiography involves the injection of contrast medium into the heart during cardiac catheterisation. The procedure shows the shape and size of the heart chambers and will pinpoint any stenosis or occlusion in the coronary arteries. This test is described in Box 2.1. Angiography is justifiable in all cases where the results would alter patient management. It carries a mortality of 0.1%. Elective referral for angiography is warranted for

Box 2.1

Cardiac catheterisation

Purpose

Cardiac catheterisation involves the insertion, usually under screening, of a fine, flexible, radio-opaque catheter into one or more of the heart chambers. It is increasingly being performed as a day-case procedure. The catheter is inserted via a peripheral vein or artery under sterile conditions in a cardiac catheterisation laboratory. The femoral artery/vein are the most common entry sites although the radial and brachial are also used. The right and left side of the heart may be investigated separately or together. The procedure is performed to:

- visualise the heart chambers and vessels by means of a radio-opaque substance under X-ray control (angiography), e.g. used in the diagnosis of angina
- measure pressure and record waveforms from the cavity of the heart
- obtain blood samples from the heart
- measure left ventricular function (ejection fraction).

Cardiac catheterisation will always be performed on a prospective candidate for coronary artery bypass graft surgery, valve surgery and heart transplantation. It is also used to evaluate the effect of thrombolytic agents and the patency of coronary bypass grafts.

Procedure

The patient must give written informed consent for the procedure. Cardiac catheterisation is usually carried out under local anaesthesia and the patient may be given diazepam as premedication. The patient is usually asked to fast for 4 h to prevent aspiration, should cardiac arrest occur. The groin area will be shaved. The procedure is performed by a cardiologist and takes approximately 90 min. The patient will be asked to wear a gown and should be prepared to lie flat on their back on a hard table during the procedure. A needle with a guide wire attached is inserted into the vessel and the needle then removed. A sheath is then threaded over the guide wire, the guide wire removed and the catheter inserted through the sheath. The patient is warned to expect a sudden burning sensation as the dye is injected into the heart. Angina may occur as a result of the catheter blocking the artery and may be treated with sublingual glyceryl trinitrate (GTN) spray, oxygen therapy and intracoronary isosorbide dinitrate.

Following the procedure the patient may require analgesics and should be allowed to rest. Observations are taken and the sheath removed. A pressure dressing will be applied to the wound site, which must be observed for excessive bleeding. The limb should be kept straight for 1–2 h to prevent turbulence of blood flow at the incision site. Patients usually stay in bed for 2 h and most are ready for discharge 2 h later.

Possible complications

Patients may experience transient cardiac arrhythmias and syncope. A reaction to the dye may produce symptoms ranging from a rash to anaphylaxis. There is a 0.5% risk of thrombus formation, leading to a cerebrovascular accident or myocardial infarction, and a 0.1% risk of dying from such a complication. Coronary artery dissection is a rare complication. The patient may experience pulmonary oedema whilst lying flat and this is treated with oxygen, nebuliser therapy and diuretics.

those with a positive exercise test and on maximsum medication therapy.

Treatment

The aim of treatment for angina is to:

- restore and maintain cardiac output necessary for normal living activities
- reduce the workload of the heart
- bring back into balance oxygen supply and demand
- reduce the risk of progression to acute coronary syndrome.

Treatment is achieved by:

- medication to optimise cardiac function by relieving the pain of angina and improving myocardial perfusion (see Table 2.2)
- reduction in myocardial workload
- reducing risk factors
- percutaneous coronary interventions (PCI). This describes a group of techniques that include percutaneous transluminal coronary angioplasty (PTCA), stenting, coronary artery bypass graft (CABG), athero-ablation and, more recently, transmyocardial laser revascularisation and angiogenesis. These interventions would be considered if conventional medical therapy failed to control symptoms.

STOP THINK **2.2** Read Case History 2.1(A).

(a) What is the significance of this test result?
(b) What other tests might be requested?

NURSING PRIORITIES AND MANAGEMENT: Angina

The major goals for the patient are to:

- prevent or minimise chest pain
- cope with the anginal pain and any other symptoms
- reduce anxiety
- be aware of the underlying nature of the disorder
- understand the prescribed care and be able to make informed decisions about future lifestyle in order to reduce the risk of disease progression.

Nursing input will vary according to the type of contact a person has with health care services. Practice nurses and occupational health staff may be the main source of professional information and support for those in the community. Admission to hospital is likely to occur only if the angina becomes unstable or further investigation is warranted.

Nursing assessment should pay particular attention to those activities that have been found to precede and precipitate attacks of angina pain and associated symptoms, so that a logical programme of prevention can be worked out with the patient, who needs to feel in control of their condition and to regain a realistic outlook for the future. Nurses are in a prime position to contribute to risk factor management, particularly in terms of patient education (Scholte-op-Reimer et al 2002). They also have a significant role in the care of patients with chronic angina who get limited relief from conventional medical treatment (Stewart 2003).

Maintaining a safe environment

The effect of angina on the person and on those around them needs to be considered. The patient needs to know both how to prevent attacks and how to manage them when they occur. As the nurse will not witness many of the attacks, it should be impressed upon the patient that their management lies with them and their family. As much of the nursing management involves advice about potential adaptations in lifestyle, family members will require similar information and support.

The individual needs to be advised to plan their day-to-day life around adequate rest periods. If they cannot avoid activities liable to precipitate an attack, then they should rest before and after such activity. For example, a large family gathering such as a wedding can be very stressful, with socialising, a large meal to eat and considerable preparation. As much time as possible should be spent quietly, with rest periods after dressing and after the meal. Explaining to other members of the family the reason for this is better than suffering an attack during the proceedings.

Taking glyceryl trinitrate (GTN) prophylactically is often the best way of managing situations likely to induce angina.

A change of occupation is sometimes necessary following a diagnosis of angina; it could, for example, be unsafe to drive public transport vehicles. This double blow can be very difficult for the person to accept. The occupational health nurse can help, as they will be aware of other areas to which the individual can be relocated. If retraining is required, social worker and retraining counsellors may be involved from the outset.

Mobility

Exercise is the most common cause of an attack, and patients should understand that they must stop and rest and not attempt to work through the pain. The patient should know how to use GTN, both to prevent and to treat an attack. If the patient takes GTN prior to an activity likely to cause angina, they may prevent an attack and still complete the activity. However, the patient needs to appreciate that they should not use GTN in order to over-exercise, but to maintain a reasonable quality of life and to achieve some control over the condition. They should be encouraged to keep records of the activities that induce angina. These can be reviewed with their practitioner to provide a reliable

CASE HISTORY 2.1(A)

Mr B

Mr B is a 55-year-old factory foreman who regards himself as being fit and well for his age. He plays badminton at the local sports club two or three times a week and enjoys taking his dog on regular rambles. He does not smoke and, being aware of factors leading to heart disease, has tried to reduce the fat intake in his diet over the past few years. His father died of a heart attack at the age of 73. Mr B's company offer regular medical checks to screen for health problems and on his last visit he underwent an exercise test. After 5 min of the test he felt short of breath. He was noted to have ST-segment depression.

Table 2.2 **Medications used in angina**

Medication	Use	Physiological action	Comments
Nitrates Glyceryl trinitrate (GTN) spray or tablets	Used for relief of angina Administered as spray form or tablet under the tongue to ensure rapid release into the bloodstream Can be given i.v., maintenance dose 6–10 mg/h	Venodilatation with consequent reduction in preload Also causes systemic arteriolar vasodilatation with decrease in afterload	Tablets need to be stored correctly Tablets lose potency over time and if exposed to light Tablets should not be kept for more than 2 months, should be stored in an airtight container and not be exposed to light
Suscard buccal	Slow-release form of nitrate placed in the buccal cavity	As above Used for effect for 4–5 h	
Isosorbide mononitrate (oral or i.v.)	Used for prevention of angina	As above Used as longer-term control	Patient can develop tolerance
Beta-blockers e.g. atenolol	Used in preventing angina Given once or twice daily Dose lower than when prescribed for hypertensive patients	Block sympathetic stimulation, so slowing the heart rate and reducing oxygen demand	Used with caution in patients with chronic obstructive airways disease and asthma as it may cause bronchospasm
Calcium channel blockers e.g. nifedipine	Used in preventing angina	Interfere with calcium transfer across the cell membrane, causing relaxation of arteriolar smooth muscle, thus reducing afterload Affects rate of action potential and reduces oxygen demand	
Potassium channel activators e.g. nicorandil	Have a role in unstable angina	Similar to that of nitrates May reduce transient myocardial ischaemia	
Angiotensin-converting enzyme (ACE) inhibitors e.g. captopril, enalapril, ramipril	Of particular benefit for patients with clinical signs of heart failure	Prevents the production of angiotensin II, thereby limiting vasoconstriction and decreasing aldosterone-induced sodium reabsorption in the kidney Reduces fluid load within the patient and the work of the heart	
Angiotensin-II receptor antagonists e.g. losartan	Effective alternative for patients intolerant of ACE inhibitors	Prevents the action of angiotensin II	
Anticoagulants Unfractionated heparin	Full anticoagulation with heparin is recommended in patients with increased risk of thromboembolic complications	Prevents the initiation as well as the propagation of thrombi Has a less predictable anticoagulation effect than low molecular weight heparin	Used in patients with cardiac failure, anterior MI Requires anticoagulation monitoring using the activated partial thromboplastin time (APTT)
Low molecular weight heparin, e.g. enoxaparin	Started early in unstable angina to inhibit thrombus formation	As effective and as safe as unfractionated heparin of longer duration, given once daily	The standard regimen does not require monitoring as low molecular weight heparins have a more predictable effect
Warfarin	Used for patients with arrhythmias, e.g. atrial fibrillation May also be used for anticoagulation with certain high risk MI patients	Antagonises the effect of vitamin K, essential for the formation of prothrombin	Takes 36–48 h to become effective Oral anticoagulation is monitored by the prothrombin time estimation expressed in terms of the international normalised ratio (INR)

Table 2.2 Medications used in angina *(Continued)*

Medication	Use	Physiological action	Comments
Antiplatelets Aspirin	Small dose taken daily to protect against MI	Aspirin prolongs the prothrombin time as well as decreasing platelet viscosity	Small dose should not affect the stomach lining
Clopidogrel	Used as an alternative to aspirin, particularly for medium to high risk patients	Helps prevent platelet aggregation by inhibiting the expression of the glycoprotein IIb/IIIa inhibitor	There are proven benefits of reducing MI in unstable angina if clopidogrel is used in conjunction with aspirin
Glycoprotein IIb/IIIa inhibitors, e.g. abciximab, eptifibatide, tirofiban		Inactivating the glycoprotein IIb/IIIa inhibitor blocks the final common pathway in platelet aggregation and therefore prevents clot formation	
Fibrinolytic agents Streptokinase, reteplase, tissue plasminogen activator (tPA)	Used in patients with ST elevation myocardial infarction (STEMI)	Induce dissolution of the thrombus that is blocking the coronary artery but do not affect lumen narrowing caused by atherosclerosis	Needs to be given within 12 h and, ideally, within 1 h, after the onset of chest pain in appropriate patients Contraindications include CVA, recent trauma, surgery, bleeding
Lipid regulating therapy Statins: e.g. atorvastatin, simvastatin			It is reasonable to start all cardiac patients on a statin regardless of their cholesterol level
Fibrates: e.g. bezafibrate			Fibrates are particularly useful in patients with high triglyceride levels

CVA, cerebrovascular accident; MI, myocardial infarction.

assessment of angina and of the effectiveness of therapy. Knowledge of their limitations gives the patient some feeling of control over their own life and they can then attempt to address them.

Many of the heavier household tasks induce angina, e.g. shopping, ironing and vacuuming, and often make patients feel vulnerable. A basket with wheels can be used to transport shopping, and other such simple measures are easily adapted into people's lifestyles. Help from other family members or domestic help in the home may be another solution.

Breathing

In some individuals, angina presents as, or is accompanied by, difficulty in breathing. This is often worse in cold or windy weather. Such individuals need to be advised against walking great distances in these conditions. Smokers need to be clear about the association between CHD and cigarette smoking, so that they can make informed decisions about stopping.

Cigarette smokers have a two to three times greater risk of death from CHD than non-smokers. The risk is greater in young adults and in those who smoke more than 20 cigarettes a day. Nicotine stimulation results in increased catecholamine release with an increase in heart rate, cardiac output, blood pressure and coronary blood flow. Carbon monoxide attaches itself to the haemoglobin molecule and therefore reduces its ability to transport oxygen. Oxygenation is therefore reduced, despite increased myocardial requirements. Additionally, nicotine inhibits the breakdown of fibrin and increases platelet aggregation and stickiness, making clot formation more likely.

The nursing history should include information as to whether the patient has previously tried to give up smoking and, if so, how they planned to stop, how long they were able to stop, what support they received and why they started smoking again. Any perceived benefits of smoking, e.g. stress reduction, need to be discussed and plans for stopping based on experience gained in conjunction with new information and advice given (see Ch. 3).

STOP THINK **2.3** Many strategies for giving up smoking exist and not all will suit everyone. What strategies can you identify?

Nutrition

Obese people develop CVD more frequently than others. Obesity also denotes an increased likelihood of hypertension, hyperlipidaemia and diabetes mellitus. Obese individuals also tend to take less exercise. Subjective assessments of obesity are often inaccurate and a more precise method of assessment is often made using the body mass index (BMI) that adjusts the weight for height (see Ch. 21).

However, the hip:waist ratio may be a better predictor of cardiovascular risk than the BMI as it identifies abdominal obesity which is frequently linked with impaired glucose intolerance, lipid abnormalities and hypertension.

Total serum blood cholesterol levels have been shown to be associated with CHD mortality and morbidity (see Box 2.2). However, there is a negative association between one category of lipoproteins, high-density lipoproteins (HDLs), and CHD: the risk of the disease is lower when the concentration of HDLs is raised. Dietary advice needs to take into account personal preferences and domestic, socio-economic and cultural factors. Alterations to general eating habits are preferable to restrictive diets. Sensible dietary advice includes:

- losing excess weight
- reducing fat, particularly saturated fat intake
- reducing salt intake
- increasing fibre intake
- eating five portions of fruit and vegetables a day.

Eating more fish, poultry, vegetables, grains, cereals and fruit should be encouraged. Keeping within an ideal body weight range and taking suitable physical exercise are logical recommendations (see Ch. 21).

Large meals may trigger an attack of angina, so small, frequent meals are preferable. It can be difficult to motivate people to change their diet. Involving the family is very important, particularly the person primarily responsible for buying food and preparing meals.

The patient who presents to the medical services with epigastric pain may not have a digestive problem, but have angina, particularly if the history is vague. Diagnosis requires history-taking skills and spending time with the patient.

Alcohol intake should be discussed with the individual. In small quantities, alcohol has a vasodilatory effect which is beneficial in CHD, so a small nightcap will help to relax the patient and aid sleep. However, heavy drinkers are at greater risk of cardiac events and of hepatic dysfunction.

The patient should know whether their medication should be taken before or after meals and its effect if taken alongside alcohol intake.

Work and recreation

The person with angina has to come to terms with the progressive nature of the disease. People with limited energy reserves may put all their effort into work and find they have little left for leisure pursuits. The nurse's role is to assist the individual to assess their lifestyle and make decisions about priorities and possible changes. Those with sedentary lifestyles should be advised to take regular exercise, such as walking to work, climbing the stairs, swimming and cycling. Some apparently sedentary jobs may be mentally exhausting, which can put severe strain on the compromised myocardium and lead to an anginal attack. Planning the day is important, to allow for quiet periods, particularly before and after long meetings or heavy business lunches. For certain individuals, therapy such as relaxation techniques or yoga may help. If a change of occupation, or early retirement, is proposed as the only solution, the person may resist, particularly if they are the family breadwinner.

Box 2.2

Understanding cholesterol

Definition: a steroid found in animal fats and most body tissues, especially nervous tissue.

Cholesterol has received rather bad publicity in recent years because of the role it has been found to play in the formation of atheromatous plaques, but it must be remembered that, although it is not used as an energy fuel, cholesterol is an important dietary lipid, essential in maintaining homeostatic mechanisms in the body. It is a vital constituent of cell membranes and forms the structural basis of many steroid hormones and bile salts.

The recommended daily intake of cholesterol for adults is approximately 250 mg or less. However, cholesterol is not only obtained from the diet but is synthesised in the liver, the intestinal mucosa and, to a lesser degree, other body cells. It is excreted from the body in bile salts.

Cholesterol, like fatty acids and glycerol, is insoluble in water and therefore cannot circulate freely in the bloodstream. It is transported, bound to small lipid proteins (lipoproteins), which are essentially of high-density or low-density compositions. Low-density lipoproteins (LDLs) are responsible for transporting cholesterol to the peripheral tissue so that it is available for membrane synthesis, hormone synthesis and storage, for later use. Excessive cholesterol leads to 'dumping' of the excess in the lining of the blood vessels, e.g. the coronary arteries. High-density lipoproteins (HDLs) have a different function in that they transport cholesterol from the peripheral tissue to the liver to be broken down. HDLs have been described as scavenging excess cholesterol for disposal.

High levels of total serum cholesterol have been repeatedly shown to be associated with the development of coronary artery disease and myocardial infarction. However, it is not enough merely to measure cholesterol, but rather the form in which it is being transported. HDLs can be thought of as beneficial because they promote the degradation and removal of cholesterol. On the other hand, LDLs, when excessive, can lead to a potentially serious deposition of cholesterol in the artery walls.

Although it is now regarded as important to limit our dietary cholesterol, severe restriction does not lead to a correspondingly dramatic drop in plasma cholesterol. This is because, although cholesterol production is to some extent adjusted by a feedback mechanism such that a high dietary intake will inhibit hepatic synthesis, the liver will always produce a certain amount irrespective of the diet.

It would seem that the factor that has the most significant effect on plasma cholesterol is the amount of saturated and unsaturated fat in the diet. Saturated fats, found essentially in animal produce, stimulate the hepatic synthesis of cholesterol whilst inhibiting its removal. In contrast, unsaturated fats, found in vegetable oils, enhance the excretion of cholesterol in the bile salts, thereby reducing cholesterol levels.

Other factors also appear to affect plasma cholesterol levels. Stress, coffee and smoking are thought to be implicated in increased levels of LDLs. Regular aerobic exercise has been associated with the lowering of LDLs and raising of HDLs.

If research continues to support the above findings, there are clear implications for the role of the nurse in promoting nutritional health and well-being.

Rest and sleep

Taking frequent naps throughout the day is often better than a longer sleep at night. The bedroom should be well ventilated but not cold or draughty (see Ch. 25). Certain medication, for example beta-blockers, and/or a reduction in cardiac output may make the patient feel tired and lethargic.

Sexuality

In some people with angina, sexual intercourse can trigger an anginal attack. This can be stressful for both the sufferer and their partner. Prophylactic use of GTN and some planning may help. The couple may have to adapt their usual position or the partner may have to take on a more dominant role. Touching and caressing may replace full intercourse and satisfy both. This subject needs to be approached sensitively but must be addressed, as the individual's perceived view on this aspect of daily living can affect all other aspects. A man receiving beta-blocker therapy may suffer from both weariness and impotence and the reason for this should be explained.

An important related aspect of sexuality is role reversal, e.g. if a housewife has to hand over some of her role and feels a loss of self-worth, or where the family breadwinner is forced to give up work. This may greatly affect self-esteem.

Fear of dying

People who have angina may have difficulty coming to terms with the fact that they have a progressive disease affecting their heart and probably other parts of their body. Angina can progress to myocardial infarction, which can cause death and this has to be discussed with the person to keep the situation in perspective. If they feel in control over some aspects of their condition, e.g. stopping smoking or altering their diet, they will possibly cope better than the person with a strong family history over which they have no control. Encouraging the patient to discuss their fears may help them to cope with them or alert the nurse to the fact that expert counselling is required.

Communication

Getting to know the person as an individual is important if appropriate support is to be given. The patient needs to be guided towards pinpointing aspects of lifestyle that will be affected by angina and then learning through discussion and counselling how to minimise their effect. If the person can communicate what causes pain and what relieves it, management is often simplified. Anxiety will reduce the ability to communicate, particularly when in an unfamiliar environment, such as the occupational health department or hospital. The use of a scoring table or a continuum for assessing and comparing attacks of angina may prove beneficial for monitoring the effect of therapy.

Personal hygiene and dressing

Here again, the key is living within the constraints of the condition. The person should be advised against locking the bathroom door whilst in the bath so that help can reach them if necessary. Other family members must remember this and respect privacy. Spacing activities throughout the day rather than rushing to do everything first thing in the morning may minimise the occurrence of symptoms.

CASE HISTORY 2.1(B)

Mr B — invasive treatment for angina

Mr B has now had the following investigations, all of which are normal: chest X-ray, ECG, cardiac enzymes and weight. His serum lipids are high, so, having had dietary advice, he has begun medication therapy to reduce these levels.

Cardiac catheterisation revealed that he had an 85% reduction of the lumen of the left coronary artery main stem. Mr B is advised that he should undergo percutaneous transluminal coronary angioplasty (PTCA). This is planned for the next day.

Constrictive clothing may induce breathlessness and chest tightness, and so should be avoided; however, the person should be advised to wrap up warmly in cold weather to limit increased workload on the heart for thermoregulation.

Elimination

Diuretic therapy may be indicated if a degree of cardiac failure is present (p. 45). The timing of ingestion of these medications can be controlled by the angina sufferer so that the ensuing diuresis does not disrupt daily routine.

Straining at stool should be avoided. A healthy diet will help, but the judicious use of a mild aperient may be indicated.

Cardiac catheterisation

The patient should be fully informed about the procedure (see Box 2.1, p. 16), its findings and their implications. Nurses need to be aware of the possible complications and place particular importance on pain relief.

Percutaneous transluminal coronary angioplasty (PTCA) (Box 2.3)

The patient will need to be fully aware of both the benefits and drawbacks. The importance of reporting any pain or discomfort during or following PTCA should be stressed. Pain is most likely to be experienced when the balloon is inflated over the narrowed area and the patient should be warned of this. Nitrate therapy is used for pain relief. Weight-adjusted heparin and an antiplatelet medication are also given. Increasingly, the procedure is performed in the morning and stable patients are discharged home in the evening or the next day. The patient may require assistance with various activities of living whilst mobility is temporarily limited. Discharge planning should include explaining the medication, risk factor modification and follow-up assessment. An exercise test may be performed prior to discharge, and a thallium scan, which detects myocardial perfusion, can give further information as to the achieved patency of the vessel.

If re-stenosis does occur, the procedure can be repeated.

Coronary artery stents

Coronary artery stents, a means whereby arteries can be held open, are used increasingly as an alternative to conventional angioplasty as they limit the long-term risk of

Box 2.3

Percutaneous transluminal coronary angioplasty (PTCA)

Purpose

PTCA is a technique involving the introduction of a balloon catheter into the coronary artery up to the site of a coronary stenosis, where it is inflated. This process produces compression and redistribution of the lesion and a substantial increase in the size of the lumen. PTCA may be performed to relieve the symptoms of angina if medication is ineffective, or it may be performed soon after successful thrombolysis (see p. 27) to restore perfusion to the ischaemic zone.

Procedure

PTCA is carried out under local anaesthetic in a cardiac catheterisation laboratory. If the procedure is planned, the patient will be admitted to hospital the day before and asked to fast for 4 h prior to the procedure. This is to prevent the risk of complications if bypass surgery is required. The patient will be given 300 mg aspirin prior to the procedure and the preparation is as for cardiac catheterisation.

Usually, two arterial catheters are used: a guiding catheter and a dilating catheter. The guiding catheter is inserted, usually in the leg, and advanced to the coronary artery to be dilated. The dilating catheter is then inserted and manipulated into the stenotic area of the artery. Angiography is performed and heparin administered to avoid clot formation at the catheter site. When the dilatation catheter is placed over the stenosis, it is inflated for 5–6 s and then deflated. Blood flow around the balloon is assessed by angiography. Once it has been decided that maximum dilatation has been obtained, the catheters are removed.

Following this procedure, the patient's cardiac status is usually monitored for 24 h. Peripheral pulses are checked frequently for occlusive thrombus at the insertion site. The patient is advised to rest for 4–6 h, lying as flat as is comfortably possible, to keep the leg used for catheter insertion straight in order to minimise the risk of thrombus formation at the insertion site. The introducer sheath is often left in situ for 2–3 h, until the effects of heparin have been reduced.

The patient should be encouraged to drink extra fluid to help eliminate contrast medium.

Re-stenosis occurs in 15–30% of patients, more frequently within the first few months. Repeat angioplasty may be appropriate for some patients. In an increasing number of patients, a stent is inserted at the time of angioplasty. Drug eluting stents inhibit smooth muscle migration around the stent and have a low (2–3%) re-stenosis rate. All patients will be commenced on clopidogrel and high risk patients on glycoprotein IIb/IIIa inhibitors.

Possible complications

Complications tend to be sudden and include:

- myocardial infarction
- chest pain
- vagal reaction
- intimal injury
- bleeding at the puncture site
- occlusive thrombus at the puncture site
- coronary artery spasm
- coronary artery dissection.

re-stenosis of the vessel wall. There are two main types of stent — coil and mesh — which are inserted into the widened coronary artery during cardiac catheterisation. Intravascular ultrasound is useful for accurate placement of the stent. The National Institute for Clinical Excellence (NICE) guidelines (1999) advised routine stenting during PTCA for coronary arteries between 2.5 and 3.5 mm, which should make their use appropriate for about 80–90% of procedures.

Patient management is similar to angioplasty, although more time may have to be spent in hospital in order for the patient to be stabilised on the anticoagulant warfarin. Stenosis within the stent itself can be a problem and the use of specialised stents which contain and release drugs to limit this is increasing (Gershlick 2002). Radiation emitters have also been used to reduce in-stent stenosis, a procedure known as vascular brachytherapy. Repeat PTCA is the most useful way of clearing in-stent stenosis, but laser angioplasty, which uses pulsed ultraviolet light to ablate the plaque, and atherectomy, which involves drilling into the plaque, may also be used. Levine et al (2003) provide an overview of the management of patients undergoing percutaneous coronary revascularisation.

Coronary artery bypass grafting (CABG)

This is now a routine operation performed on patients whose angina is severely limiting their lives but whose left ventricle is functioning reasonably. It is particularly appropriate for patients with triple vessel disease. It may also be carried out in the phase of myocardial infarction and for those who have experienced complications after angioplasty. The procedure is described in Box 2.4.

Bypass surgery is a potentially traumatic event, and apprehension about the procedure is common (Lyons et al 2002). Patients awaiting surgery have been found to experience a sense of dependency and impending doom (Lindsey et al 2000). Pre-admission education programmes are now offered at many centres and a visit to the operating theatre and ITU may also help. Male patients need to know that their chest will be shaved prior to the operation and all patients need to know that they may be asked to take a bath using antibacterial soap. An aperient may be required to reduce the likelihood of postoperative abdominal discomfort. Patients will be asked to fast prior to surgery and may benefit from a sedative to help them relax the night before.

The nurse should prepare the patient for what to expect on regaining consciousness, i.e. an endotracheal tube, chest drains, intravenous infusions, arterial lines, urinary catheter, cardiac monitoring and possibly a nasogastric tube. The patient should be taught breathing, coughing and leg exercises by the specialist physiotherapist.

After the operation, nursing objectives include:

- pain relief (see Chs 19 and 26)
- fluid management — patients can quickly become dehydrated
- assistance with activities of living
- psychological support — patients may become disorientated and confused and need help coming to terms with the effect of the operation (Laitinen 1996)
- preparation for discharge home.

Box 2.4

Coronary artery bypass graft surgery (CABG)

Purpose

Coronary artery bypass graft surgery is a technique in which an occluded or stenosed section of a coronary artery is bypassed using part of a vein or artery from elsewhere in the body. Most commonly, the long saphenous vein is used, although increasingly the internal mammary artery is being considered. The objectives of CABG are:

- restoration of perfusion and increased oxygenation to the ischaemic myocardium in the peri-infarction patient
- relief of angina pectoris
- improvement of functional status and quality of life
- prolongation of life.

Surgery is only feasible if the risk of the operation is less than continuing with medical therapy. The procedure tends to be offered to those who have:

- symptoms despite maximum therapy
- triple vessel disease or left main stem coronary artery stenosis
- unstable angina.

Procedure

During surgery, the heart is exposed by median sternotomy, the aorta clamped off and cardiopulmonary bypass maintained via cannulae in the descending aorta. The body temperature may be reduced to 32°C and cardiac arrest induced with a cardioplegic solution.

Revascularisation with arterial grafts is becoming more common, as they last longer (10–15 vs. 5–10 years for veins). The internal mammary artery is biologically superior for grafting compared with the saphenous vein.

The artery or vein being used is harvested whilst the chest is being opened. The distal end of the bypass graft is sutured to the required vessels. The aorta is then unclamped, the patient rewarmed if cooling has been used and normal cardiac rhythm re-established by internal defibrillation. The proximal ends of the grafts are sutured to the ascending aorta and cardiopulmonary bypass is then stopped, the cannulae removed and the chest closed. The whole operation takes up to 4 h.

The patient is normally cared for in an intensive care unit after the procedure and will be ventilated until they are haemodynamically stable. An arterial line and pulmonary artery flotation catheter will be used to monitor cardiac pressures for 24 h.

The patient will usually be able to eat a normal diet on the first or second day. Activity is increased as tolerated over the first 2 days and early mobilisation is encouraged. Patients are often fit for discharge home after about a week.

Possible complications

Complications include:

- leakage at the incision site, producing discomfort and shock
- hypertension as a result of increased sympathetic activity
- hypotension as a result of reduced cardiac output following hypothermia
- pain at both the graft and incision sites
- post-pump cardiotomy syndrome (up to 3 months)
  - — problems with coordination
  - — loss of memory
  - — loss of sense of taste
  - — disturbance of vision
- shortness of breath due to heart failure or chest infection.

Patients will be told to expect some degree of pain from the sternotomy for several weeks, discomfort on coughing or lifting the hands above the head and leg swelling (Levine et al 2003). Short-term anxiety and depression may occur if patients feel that recovery is slower than anticipated. Partners and other family members will also need ongoing information and support.

Minimally invasive cardiac surgery

This is an option for some patients with CHD. Access to the heart is made through a small thoracotomy. This procedure has the advantage of reducing patient problems associated with sternotomy, including less pain, increased mobility and a reduced hospital stay. The left internal mammary artery is grafted through an incision between the fourth and fifth intercostal spaces. Pre- and postoperative care is similar to that in conventional cardiac surgery.

Minimally invasive direct coronary artery bypass surgery (MIDCAP)

is an alternative procedure that does not require cardiopulmonary bypass. It is also termed off-pump or beating heart surgery. For selected patients, this procedure offers a less invasive approach with a faster recovery and an improved cosmetic appearance of the wound.

Fast-tracking

Patients are increasingly being 'fast-tracked' after cardiac surgery (Howard 1996). This focuses on early extubation and a move away from elective overnight ventilation following surgery. The recovery of low-risk patients can therefore be managed without overnight admission to the ITU.

The procedures outlined above unfortunately do not stop the process of atherosclerosis; they only delay it and aim to provide the sufferer with a good quality of life for a limited time. All procedures can be repeated, but ultimately the blood supply may become insufficient to sustain the ventricle so that cardiac failure ensues.

ACUTE CORONARY SYNDROME

The term acute coronary syndrome defines a continuum of manifestations of CHD. It includes all cases of unstable angina and acute myocardial infarction which have as common underlying pathology the abrupt, total or subtotal obstruction (occlusion) of a coronary artery, most often triggered following the rupture or erosion of an atheromatous plaque. This occlusion may be temporary, and often recurrent, as in unstable angina, or it may be permanent as in an acute transmural myocardial infarction. Clinical presentation of acute coronary syndrome depends predominantly

CASE HISTORY 2.1(C)
Mr B

Mr B's angioplasty has proved to be unsuccessful, as it has not been possible to enter the left coronary artery (LCA) and pass the balloon over the occlusion. Mr B is returned to the ward after 2 h in the cardiac catheterisation room. He is told that he can go home that evening but is asked to return in 2 weeks for cardiac surgery.

on whether the obstruction is abrupt or staggered in onset, the site of the occlusion, the resulting loss of blood flow to the myocardium and whether there is an alternative blood supply to the area in the form of a collateral circulation.

Unstable angina

In unstable angina, the coronary artery occlusion tends to be episodic and transient. There is often a fissuring of a plaque with the development of a thrombus, but the thrombus does not completely block the artery and subsequently breaks down with no detectable damage to the myocardium. Patients complain about angina symptoms that become progressively more frequent, more severe, triggered by less physical and/or emotional effort and unrelieved by GTN. Initial diagnosis is based on the clinical history and the standard resting ECG which may show ischaemic changes but no ST segment elevation. The lack of myocardial damage is confirmed by measurement of the highly sensitive marker troponin or other cardiac marker concentrations which will give negative results. Management for patients with unstable angina needs to be based on the risk of progressing to a totally occluded coronary artery (British Cardiac Society 2001). Low-risk patients, with a non-diagnostic ECG, negative exercise test and normal troponin marker levels, can be managed in the community with secondary prevention measures including aspirin, beta-blockers, angiotensin-converting enzyme (ACE) inhibitors and statins, plus lifestyle advice and support as discussed in the earlier section on stable angina. High-risk patients identified by history and exercise testing, who remain unstable, warrant immediate coronary angiography and revascularisation.

Myocardial infarction

Myocardial infarction, also known as a 'heart attack' or a 'coronary', refers to the death or necrosis of a portion of myocardium as a result of interruption or cessation in blood flow. Myocardial infarction is part of the spectrum of acute coronary syndromes and as a diagnosis is now divided into two categories based on ECG findings.

1. Those cases where there is some detectable myocardial injury, i.e. troponin testing will be positive, but where this damage has not affected the full thickness of the myocardium and hence there is no ST elevation on the ECG, are known as non-ST elevation myocardial infarction (NSTEMI). This condition is potentially unstable and it may be more appropriate to describe both high-risk unstable angina and NSTEMI as 'unstable coronary syndromes'. Both are high-risk conditions requiring admission to coronary care for urgent intervention to prevent progression to transmural, full thickness, myocardial infarction. Without early treatment, around 5–10% of patients will progress to more extensive myocardial damage or death within 30 days (Collinson et al 2000).
2. Those cases where there is total occlusion of a coronary artery and transmural muscle damage, i.e. troponin testing will be positive, and there is ST segment elevation on the ECG, are known as ST segment elevation myocardial infarction (STEMI). It is this group of patients who benefit from prompt reperfusion.

Nearly all the deaths from CHD are the result of myocardial infarction. In the UK, some 300 000 people suffer myocardial infarction each year, of which about 50% are fatal. In 25–30% of cases, the patient with myocardial infarction dies before reaching hospital (British Heart Foundation 2004).

PATHOPHYSIOLOGY

Myocardial cells require a constant supply of oxygen and nutrients in order to generate the high-energy phosphate compounds required for contraction. Generally, myocardial cells are irreversibly injured by 30–40 min of total ischaemia. It is now clear that the muscle damage associated with myocardial infarction almost always results from total occlusion of a coronary artery by a thrombus, usually at the site of a recently cracked or fissured atheromatous plaque. If the lumen of an artery is blocked for about 20 min, and blood supply by the small vessels of the surrounding collateral circulation is inadequate, infarction may develop. Surrounding the area of necrotic tissue there is usually a zone of injury. This tissue cannot contract but may be salvaged if an adequate blood supply can be quickly established; this is sometimes known as 'hibernating' myocardium. The ischaemic zone separates the zone of injury from undamaged tissue (see Fig. 2.8).

During the first 6 h after the onset of symptoms, the affected myocardium becomes oedematous. There is a shift in the distribution of sodium and potassium ions and an increased risk of arrhythmias. A summary of events following a myocardial infarction is given in Table 2.3. The infarcted area is replaced by fibrous scar tissue over the course of 3–6 weeks.

The site of infarction depends on which coronary artery has become occluded. The extent of infarction, and therefore the amount of muscle involved, depends on the artery involved, the previous rate of progression of the disease and

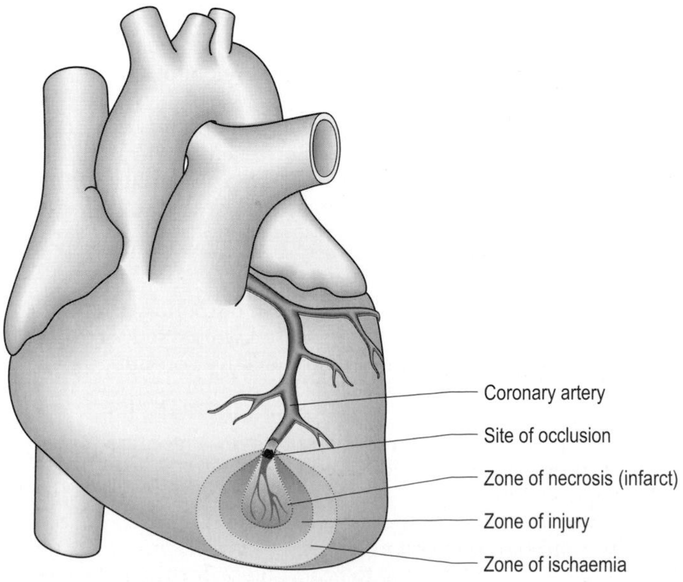

Fig. 2.8 Zones of necrosis, injury and ischaemia.

Table 2.3 Events following anterior myocardial infarction (AMI)

Length of time following AMI	Event
0–6 h	Cellular breakdown No electrical impulses conducted Necrosis occurs
24 h	Phagocytosis occurs in the infarcted area
5 days	Area infiltrated by fibroblasts, capillaries and collagen tissue Reperfusion of capillaries
2–3 weeks	Fibrosis occurs
2–3 months	Ventricular scarring

the effectiveness of the surrounding collateral circulation. In a majority of fatal myocardial infarctions, death occurs in the first hour after the attack, usually as a result of a cardiac arrhythmia.

Common presenting symptoms

Myocardial infarction can occur both in people who are known to have angina and in those who are not. Pain is usually experienced about 60 s after the onset of ischaemia and occurs in the majority of people, but is less likely to be experienced in older people or in those with diabetes mellitus. Pain typical of myocardial infarction often:

- occurs at rest
- awakens the individual from sleep
- is unrelieved by rest or nitrates
- lasts longer than 20 min
- is described as crushing, vice-like, tight or constricting in nature
- may radiate to the arms and neck.

Other signs and symptoms may include:

- shortness of breath at rest, on exertion or when lying flat
- hyperventilation as a result of anxiety
- change in cardiac rhythm or rate
- change in blood pressure
- change in level of consciousness
- increased anxiety or restlessness
- pallor
- sweaty or clammy skin
- nausea and vomiting
- cyanosis.

MEDICAL MANAGEMENT

Diagnosis may be difficult in the early stages. The ECG may be non-diagnostic and the pain difficult to quantify. Biochemical markers may also be non-specific. Therefore, high-risk patients with atypical presentations need to be observed closely.

The modern management priorities depend on whether the symptoms are thought to be the result of a thrombus occluding the coronary artery (STEMI) or an unstable coronary syndrome (NSTEMI). Management has historically been divided into three overlapping stages:

- treatment of the acute attack through:
  - — relief of symptoms by analgesics (opiates) plus antiemetic, oxygen and nitrates
  - — monitoring for and treating life-threatening complications
  - — improving blood flow to the myocardium and modification of the infarct process in STEMI
  - — thrombolysis or percutaneous coronary intervention
  - — reduction of oxygen demand by rest and beta-blockade and alteration of early physiological changes by ACE inhibition
- risk stratification (1–6 weeks)
- secondary prevention, including aspirin, or clopidogrel, beta-blocker, ACE inhibitor and a statin.

Patients should ideally be managed in a coronary care unit (CCU) and preferably be admitted there directly. In hospitals where suspected myocardial infarction patients are admitted to Emergency Departments, nurses have a role in identifying patients experiencing an acute cardiac event so that appropriate treatment can be initiated promptly and safely (Kucia et al 2001).

History and examination

The history provides subjective information about the presenting symptoms, previous patterns of health and illness, and the activities of living. A family history of ischaemic heart disease together with risk factor identification and social and psychological background adds to the picture.

It may be inappropriate to obtain a full history if the patient is in pain, acutely ill, or would benefit from prompt reperfusion therapy. An initial assessment can be enough to set early priorities, without a full physical examination or diagnostic tests.

Clinical examination includes:

- observation of general appearance, build, body posture and facial expression
- assessment of the location, nature and severity of the pain, any relieving or aggravating factors, and attempted methods of pain relief
- observation of other signs of reduced cardiac output
- observation of vital signs — arrhythmias are common; blood pressure may be low with reduced cardiac output or high due to pain and anxiety; slight pyrexia is a common response to muscle damage
- auscultation — a third heart sound is an important indicator of left ventricular dysfunction and poor outcome; it is found in 5–10% of patients with myocardial infarction
- palpation — involving a systematic examination of the chest to feel for abnormal vibrations or pulsations.

Investigations

Electrocardiogram may show characteristic changes, pinpointing the area of ventricle affected. The ECG is an imperfect diagnostic tool and, as early ECGs may appear normal, a series is necessary. The classic change is ST elevation (see Fig. 2.9).

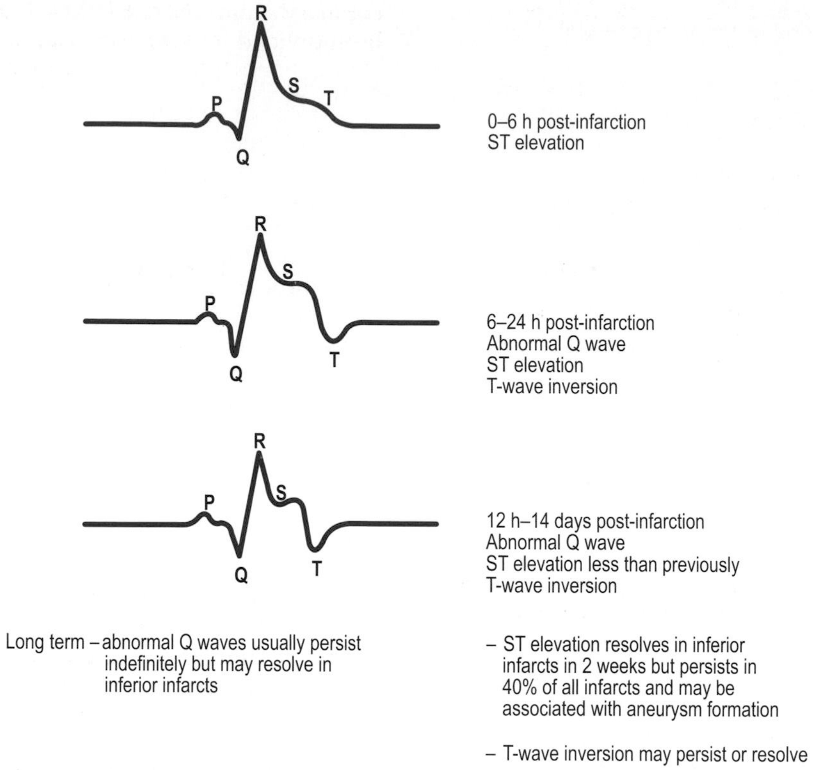

Fig. 2.9 ECG changes in myocardial infarction.

Blood tests

- *Serum cardiac markers*. Myocardial necrosis results in the release of certain molecules into the circulating blood. The rate and pattern of release are important (see Fig. 2.10). The traditional role of biochemical testing has been to provide retrospective confirmation of the presence or absence of myocardial damage through sequential measurement of serum cardiac markers on consecutive days. Modern analytical equipment now allows for certain markers, in particular the troponins, to be measured in minutes. Bedside analysis is possible, with rapid diagnosis having implications for patient triage and shortening length of hospital stay. Increasingly, measurement of cardiac troponins is allowing cardiac damage to be diagnosed with high sensitivity and specificity. Measurement of cardiac troponin T and cardiac troponin I also allows prognostic risk stratification of patients.

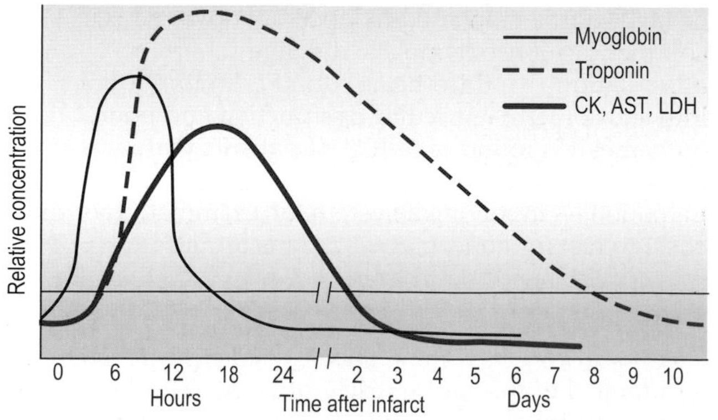

Fig. 2.10 Time–activity curves for diagnostic biochemical markers following acute myocardial infarction.

- *White cell count*. This is usually elevated for the first few days following acute myocardial infarction.
- *Erythrocyte sedimentation rate (ESR)*. This usually rises after the first few days and may remain elevated for several weeks.
- *Glucose*. Stress-related hyperglycaemia is common in the acute phase following infarction. Previously undetected diabetes is found in approximately 5% of coronary patients admitted to hospital.
- *Electrolytes*. It is important to know the serum sodium and potassium levels, as these electrolytes can have a major effect on cell excitability.
- *Lipids*. The important lipids in ischaemic heart disease are plasma cholesterol and triglycerides. Total cholesterol should be measured within the first 24 h and a full lipid profile done at 6–8 weeks.

Chest X-ray may show evidence of pulmonary oedema or hypertrophy.

Prevention of complications

Acute myocardial infarction is a very serious condition in the early stages, although the risks diminish rapidly after the first 48 h. Muscle damage will affect different areas of the heart and therefore put the patient at risk of various complications. Careful observation of the patient will help in the prevention, or at least early treatment, of these complications to prevent them becoming life threatening.

NURSING PRIORITIES AND MANAGEMENT: Thrombolytic therapy

Patients with ST elevation myocardial infarction (STEMI) will be potential candidates for thrombolytic therapy. The nurse needs to be aware of patient selection criteria and be able to assist in identifying patients who are candidates for therapy (see Box 2.5). Awareness of contraindications to therapy and of the importance of initiating therapy as soon as possible after the onset of chest pain are also necessary. Mortality in patients given thrombolytic drugs sufficiently early is one-third less than in those left untreated and the *National Service Framework for Coronary Heart Disease* (DH 2000) set specific targets for thrombolysis times. The targets are that thrombolysis should be given within 60 min from the call for help and within 20 min of the patient's arrival at hospital. Nurses in some CCUs are taking on the responsibility of initiating and/or prescribing thrombolytic therapy in accordance with agreed protocols (Rhodes 1998, Holland & Foxcroft 2000). The nurse should explain to the patient the benefits and potential problems of this therapy. It is important that the nurse is aware of possible complications so that they can monitor and observe appropriately.

On discharge, people who have been thrombolysed receive a card, indicating what medication they received and when. It may be inappropriate for them to have a second treatment with certain thrombolytics. Thrombolysis does not have any effect on the underlying cause of thrombus formation and reocclusion remains a problem. Heparin, warfarin and aspirin have been used to reduce re-thrombosis. Patients may require subsequent mechanical recanalisation with either PTCA, rescue angioplasty or surgery. Glycoprotein IIb/IIIa inhibitors which prevent platelet aggregation are recommended for use in unstable angina or NSTEMI (NICE 2002).

Primary angioplasty

Angioplasty, with or without stenting, used instead of thrombolytic therapy in acute infarction, results in better patency and causes fewer strokes. Patients most likely to gain from this procedure are those with cardiogenic shock, anterior infarcts and older people. It is also an option for patients not eligible for thrombolysis (Kastrati et al 2004). However, primary angioplasty is unlikely to become widely available because most patients with myocardial infarction are admitted directly to hospitals without intervention facilities (De Belder & Thomas 1997).

NURSING PRIORITIES AND MANAGEMENT: Acute coronary syndrome

Most unstable patients admitted to hospital are likely to benefit from admission to a CCU for monitoring and assessment for reperfusion therapy. These units were first

Box 2.5

Thrombolytic therapy

Purpose
The primary aim in limiting infarct size is the rapid recanalisation of the occluded coronary artery. Occlusion is most often caused by a thrombus at the site of a ruptured atheromatous plaque. The aim of thrombolysis is to induce dissolution of the thrombus through the administration of an intravenous drug in order to establish recanalisation and provide subsequent reperfusion to the ischaemic zone. Thrombolysis is the single most important advance in coronary care since defibrillation, resulting in increased survival and quality of life.

Action
Optimal benefit results when the thrombolytic drug is given promptly after the onset of chest pain, although it is considered worthwhile administering the treatment up to 12 h later. The main thrombolytic drugs currently available are:

- *Streptokinase* — to date, the most widely tested and used, and also the cheapest. It is a bacterial protein whose administration results in a systemic lytic state, with reduced levels of circulating fibrinogen and clotting factors V and VIII. Once given, the patient will produce antibodies to streptokinase and so the medication would be ineffective if given a second time.
- *Recombinant tissue-type plasminogen activator (tPA)* — a naturally occurring human protease that is fibrin-specific and thus works predominantly on the clot, with less risk of systemic bleeding.
- *Reteplase* — a new generation thrombolytic which appears to be as effective as streptokinase. It has the advantage that it can be given as a bolus and is non-antigenic.

Patient selection
Patients considered to be having an acute myocardial infarction, with the onset of symptoms within the previous 12 h. Contraindications include:

- active or recent bleed
- major surgery or trauma within the previous month
- cerebrovascular accident within the previous 3 months
- severe systemic hypertension.

Reperfusion
Signs and symptoms of reperfusion may include:

- abrupt cessation of chest pain
- reperfusion arrhythmias or conduction disturbances
- rapid return of the ST segment to normal
- improved left ventricular function
- an early peak in cardiac enzymes as a result of enzymes being washed out of the infarct area by the reperfused artery.

Complications
These include:

- bleeding episodes (including rarely cerebral bleeds)
- reperfusion arrhythmias
- allergic reactions
- hypotension.

established in the 1960s in order to provide surveillance from skilled personnel with electrocardiographic and resuscitation facilities in a specialised setting.

Possible patient problems include:

- pain and discomfort
- fear and anxiety
- decreased activity levels
- lack of knowledge and understanding
- misconceptions
- altered activities of living
- loss of control
- ineffective or inappropriate coping responses.

Immediate priorities

The priorities on admission to hospital include:

- cardiac monitoring (see Table 2.4); ECG
- establishment of intravenous access
- relief of pain and anxiety
- reperfusion therapy where appropriate
- decrease in the workload of the heart.

Nursing management reflects the above and is also aimed at:

- observation for signs of complications
- rehabilitation and recovery.

For a critical care pathway illustrating the management of a patient with a myocardial infarction, see Figure 2.11.

Maintaining a safe environment

The nurse is responsible for the patient's safety. This involves being aware of possible complications and how they are likely to present. The temptation to respond to monitor tracings without concurrently assessing the patient should be avoided.

Pain control

The patient must be kept free from pain. It is a sign of ongoing myocardial ischaemia and should be controlled. Patients should be told of the importance of reporting pain.

Accurate pain assessment is essential to ensure that appropriate analgesics are given. Assessment scales, where patients rate their pain numerically, can be useful (see Ch. 19). Pain can be difficult to assess and nurses have been shown to be unreliable in assessing cardiac pain (O'Connor 1995), although this can be improved with appropriate education (Thompson et al 1994). Ischaemic pain can easily be confused with pain from other sources, particularly pericarditic or pleuritic pain (see Table 2.5). Opiates are the first-line analgesics for ischaemic pain and diamorphine i.v. is the medication of choice. It is likely to produce beneficial effects through:

- decreasing anxiety through action on the central nervous system
- vasodilatation of the peripheral circulation

Table 2.4 Observing the cardiac monitor*

Parameter	Aspect to note
Rate	Is it fast/slow/normal?
Rhythm	Is it irregular/regular?
P waves	Are they present/absent?
QRST complex	Is each complex preceded by a P wave? Is each complex the same?
PR interval	Is it normal/prolonged?
Ectopics (extras)	Are there any extra P waves or extra QRST complexes?

* While observing, note whether the patient is experiencing any symptoms, such as pain, shortness of breath or light-headedness.

Table 2.5 Characteristics of chest pain*

Description	Location	Medical diagnosis
Tight, like a band around the central chest	Central chest Radiating to jaw, shoulders and arms usually on left side	Angina pectoris
Precipitated by cold, exercise, large meals, emotion Usually relieved by rest and glyceryl trinitrate (GTN)	May be associated with shortness of breath	
As above, but not relieved by GTN or other measures. Lasts longer and is more severe	As above	Myocardial infarction
Stabbing or burning pain Worse on deep inspiration, often relieved by bending forwards	Substernal and often affecting the trapezius muscle and upper abdominal area	Pericarditis
Sudden sharp pain, worsened by inspiration Dyspnoea, cough, cyanosis and possible haemoptysis	Very often lateral	Pulmonary embolus
Excruciating pain 'burning' towards the spine	Intrascapular region	Dissecting aneurysm

* Not all patients present in the manner described above. The description of chest pain to aid diagnosis should be used in conjunction with an assessment of the patient's risk of coronary heart disease and a history, physical examination and diagnostic tests.

Care categories	**Admission Day 1**	**Day 2**	**Day 3**	**Day 4/5**	**Day 5/6**
Hospital location	CCU	Ward	→	→	Home
Personnel	Appropriate specialists	Cardiac rehabilitation Dietician Social services if necessary Physiotherapy/OT	→	→	→
Tests	12-lead ECG - every 20–30 mins on admission - if pain reoccurs - 90 mins post thrombolysis Chest X-ray, 0_2 sat Cardiac enzymes x 2 FBC, U&Es, glucose on admission Cholesterol	12-lead ECG Cardiac enzymes x 1 U&Es Echocardiogram	12-lead ECG	12-lead ECG	Risk stratification via exercise, stress testing and thallium imaging Cardiac catheterisation if necessary
Activities	Bed rest and commode privileges	Sit in chair Self-care in bed/chair	Sit in chair ad lib Walk in bed area	Self-care as tolerated Walk to bathroom then walk in ward Supervised activity	Shower with supervision Walk in ward Climb stairs with supervision
Assessments	Pain assessment Vital signs/weight BMI Cardiac monitoring Intake/output	→ Echocardiogram Cardiac monitoring Intake/output	→	→	→
i.v. fluids and other medications	Oxygen Aspirin ? Thrombolytic s.c. Heparin Diamorphine with antiemetic ß-blocker	Oxygen prn Aspirin s.c. Heparin GTN prn s/l ß-blocker ?ACE inhibitor Stool softener	Oxygen prn Aspirin GTN prn s/l ß-blocker ?ACE inhibitor Stool softener	Aspirin GTN prn s/l ß-blocker ?ACE inhibitor Stool softener	Aspirin GTN prn s/l ß-blocker ?ACE inhibitor
	i.v. insulin as per protocol if blood sugar > 11 mmols	→	→	→	→
	Statin	→	→	→	→
Diet	As tolerated (may feel nauseous)	→	→	→	→
Discharge planning	Evaluate social support and living conditions for after discharge	→	Evaluate need and initiate necessary home care (nursing, social services)	Determine discharge date Discuss with family	Arrange transport Check outpatient appointment Check cardiac rehabilitation follow-up including post-discharge phone call
Teaching	Explain nature of illness and CCU environment	Explain causes of MI Explain reasons for and expected outcomes of therapy	Begin medication, diet and activity teaching	Risk factor analysis and modification/secondary prevention Recovery over next few weeks How to manage any post-discharge symptoms	Reinforce discharge teaching to accommodate transition home Provide resource options for continued support and education after discharge
Psychosocial support	Encourage patient and family to express concerns Provide appropriate information Develop therapeutic relationship	→	→	→	→

Fig. 2.11 Critical care pathway for myocardial infarction.

- central nervous system sedation and primary analgesia through stimulation of opiate receptors.

Intravenous diamorphine has immediate effect, reaches its peak effect within 20 min of administration and lasts 3–4 h. Undesirable effects include:

- nausea and vomiting, due to reduced gut motility, so it should be given with an antiemetic
- depressant effects on the central nervous system, so the antidote naloxone should be available
- hypotension, if vasodilatation occurs alongside hypovolaemia
- dry mouth and slow heart rate as a result of decreased sympathetic activity.

Patients need to know that they may experience episodes of angina after discharge. They should be aware of the importance of reducing activity if such pain occurs and feel confident to use GTN. They should also be aware of the importance of dialling 999 and summoning an ambulance if the pain has not responded to rest and GTN after 15–20 min. GTN is available in tablet or spray form, and patients need to appreciate that it is not addictive and will not mask the symptoms of a heart attack. GTN can also be taken before doing something known to produce pain. It should be taken sublingually and the person should sit down before taking it, to minimise the risk of fainting. Any pain should be resolved 5–10 min after taking the drug; if not, a further dose should be taken. Once the pain has gone, any remaining tablet should be spat out or swallowed.

GTN, particularly on initial use, can produce unpleasant side-effects such as flushing and headache due to generalised vasodilatation. Paracetamol can be taken to ease a headache.

Observation of vital signs

This is aimed at early detection of complications.

Pulse The ECG will be continuously monitored on a screen. Knowledge of the normal rhythm is vital and diagnosis of arrhythmias is part of the CCU nurse's role.

Deviations from the normal must be noted and the patient's concurrent condition assessed. Someone who is in pain or who is anxious may be tachycardic (heart rate >100 beats/min); however, the heart rate is likely to fall once analgesics have been given.

Blood pressure Recording the patient's blood pressure is a means of assessing how effectively blood is being pumped from the left ventricle. Frequency of recordings needs to be balanced against the patient's need for undisturbed rest. A fall in blood pressure may indicate that further damage or complications are occurring and that there is a reduced supply to the vital organs. Cardiac output can also be assessed by examining perfusion in the peripheries.

Temperature Pyrexia as a response to muscle damage is normal in the first 48 h, following which it should settle. Continued pyrexia may indicate pericarditis.

Respiration Changes in respiratory rate can be the first sign of patient deterioration. The patient with an acute coronary syndrome is frequently given oxygen therapy in conjunction with analgesics on admission. However, there is little evidence to support this practice in terms of evidence that oxygen reduces acute myocardial ischaemia (Nicholson 2004). Dyspnoea may indicate hypoxia or the onset of pulmonary oedema, which is a serious complication. It can also be induced by anxiety. Raised anxiety levels in coronary patients admitted to hospital have been well documented, with serial measurements generally showing that anxiety is highest on admission to the CCU (Mayou et al 2000). To exclude anxiety from masking more serious complications, the patient may benefit from the use of anxiolytics for a short period, particularly at night.

Ongoing care

The majority of life-threatening problems develop within the first 36 h, and once the patient is stable they will be transferred to the ward. The move is likely to induce anxiety and the patient will be aware that the nurse:patient ratio has been reduced. Explaining that the immediate danger period is over and that they are now beginning to recover will help to convey optimism to the patient and family. Ideally, the transfer can be planned well in advance and the nursing staff on the ward should take time to discuss natural fears and vulnerability.

These same feelings are likely to resurface as the time of discharge from hospital approaches and again nursing staff must prepare both the patient and the family to resume their life as an integral unit.

Any restrictions, such as not smoking and limiting activity, should be fully explained. Although certain activities should ideally be avoided, the patient may feel less stress if permitted a low level of involvement; for example, the business person who requires to continue working may rest more easily if they have some contact with their staff.

Communicating

Someone who has suffered an acute cardiac event is likely to be worried about the eventual outcome. Some people are able to express their feelings openly, but others find this difficult. The nurse should try to probe beneath outward signs such as hostility, withdrawal and denial to ensure the patient is not masking fear. The nurse should keep the patient informed of their progress and how it will affect their stay in hospital. Communication skills are important and answers to questions should be honest and supportive. The hospital chaplain or the patient's own spiritual advisor may be of help in this area.

Communication must also extend to the family members. They experience shock and anxiety on seeing their loved one in such an environment. Involving family members, particularly the partner, in information-giving and support can significantly reduce distress at this time (Moser & Dracup 2004). Spending time with the relatives, both when they are visiting and when they are alone, may allow fears and worries to be expressed. Frequent and adequate information about the equipment and the patient's progress is vital. The family member whose trust is gained can be a source of information to the nurse and an ally in helping to reduce anxiety in the patient. Unrestricted visiting for designated close family members is also useful in reducing anxiety.

Appropriate advice for the patient and family in hospital may include:

- explaining the structure and function of the heart as a pump, where it lies in the body and how it works

- explaining narrowing of the coronary arteries, obstruction and heart muscle damage
- describing symptoms and explaining terminology
- outlining the reasons for admission and treatment
- explaining possible angina and shortness of breath that may be experienced after discharge
- explaining the recovery process, e.g. muscle damage, swelling, scar formation and the healing period for those with myocardial infarction
- discussing the outlook for the future and the need to accept the illness
- describing the likely activity level
- explaining the reasons for stopping smoking
- explaining how to recognise possible limiting factors in physical activity
- giving advice on diet, social activities and sexual life
- giving advice on resuming work
- being prepared for changes in mood, e.g. anxiety and depression, as these can be predictors of outcome after myocardial infarction (Mayou et al 2000)
- preparation of the partner and family.

Preparation for discharge

Patients and their families need to be prepared for rehabilitation and recovery. Patients' needs for information and support should be assessed individually as people cope differently. For example, women have been found to have different concerns from men after a heart attack (Radley et al 1998).

Issues to be addressed may include:

- concerns about resumption of activities, including return to work and sexual activity
- overprotectiveness by the family
- use of medication, including GTN
- lifestyle changes
- uncertainty about informing the insurance company and Department of Social Security
- the need for definite guidelines about the amount of weight to lose and how to stop smoking.

Both community and hospital nurses have a role in tackling many of the above issues, so that the sufferer and family are equipped to cope with recovery and future lifestyle (Murchie et al 2003). Conflicting information needs to be avoided. Advice needs to be realistic, practical and accurate (Thompson & Lewin 2000). There is an increasing number of coronary rehabilitation nurses who visit both in hospital and at home. The first 2 or 3 weeks at home can be the most stressful for the person and the family, particularly the partner, as they attempt to come to terms with a frightening and often unexpected event (Thompson et al 1995). Coronary rehabilitation programmes that offer individualised packages of information, support and secondary prevention strategies on both a one-to-one and group-session basis, in addition to a graduated programme of exercises, have the potential to restore the individual to an optimum level of recovery (physical, emotional, economic and vocational) and to minimise the risk of the underlying disease progressing (NHS Centre for Reviews and Dissemination 1998). It is now recommended that every major district hospital treating people with heart disease should provide such a cardiac rehabilitation service (Thompson et al 1996, DH 2000). This programme should ideally begin from the time of admission and diagnosis and encourage long-term adherence to therapy, regular exercise and a healthy lifestyle. Home-based programmes involving cassette tapes and a manual have been shown to be effective for myocardial infarction patients not able to access a group programme (Linden 1995). The patient is likely to leave hospital having been prescribed medication they need to take long term, including aspirin, beta-blockers, a statin and an ACE inhibitor and they may need support in order to continue with this regimen. Nurses working in primary care are potential sources of support, particularly in the area of secondary prevention (Fullard 1998, Scholte-op-Reimer et al 2002; see also Research Abstract 2.1).

STOP THINK **2.4** Find out about cardiac rehabilitation services offered locally. Is there any selection process or are there exclusion criteria? Are there any outcome measures in place to measure the effectiveness of taking part in the programme?

For further information on the effectiveness of cardiac rehabilitation, see Dinnes et al (1999) and Jolliffe et al (2005).

Mobility

In hospital

While experiencing symptoms such as pain and dyspnoea, the patient should remain in bed and receive analgesics and oxygen therapy. The reasons for limiting activity should be explained. As symptoms resolve, activity levels can increase.

In recent years, the trend has been towards early resumption of activity. This allows the patient to carry out activities such as washing and going to the toilet and to progress from passive to active limb exercises when they are symptom free. Periods of gentle activity should be followed by rest periods and all activity should be stopped if the patient experiences pain, dyspnoea or palpitations. The ability to increase activity gradually is a positive reinforcement for recovery and the patient's family will also experience relief at seeing the patient regain independence. By the time of discharge, usually after 5 or 6 days, the person should be fully independent in the activities of living.

Some centres have programmes in which the patient can chart their progress towards specific goals (see Box 2.6). In other centres, activity is increased on a much less formal basis and the nurse can point out to the patient that they are making progress. Realistic aims, both pre- and post-discharge, are important.

The patient should be prepared to have good and bad days and be aware of symptoms that suggest they are doing too much, such as pain, palpitations, dyspnoea, fatigue and dizziness.

At home

Graduated physical activity should permit a return to previous daily activities over a 2–12 week period after myocardial infarction and, if applicable, return to work after 6–8 weeks. The ultimate aim should be to take some exercise at least three times a week. Recommended exercise, after 6–8 weeks, includes walking, swimming and cycling, for 15–20 min at a time.

RESEARCH ABSTRACT 2.1

Secondary prevention for coronary heart disease: How can the service be improved? Do nurses have a significant role?

People with pre-existing coronary heart disease are at particularly high risk of coronary events and death, but effective secondary prevention strategies can reduce admissions to hospital and improve quality of life and the processes of care delivery in the short term. Effective secondary prevention comprises several elements, including pharmaceutical interventions, using antiplatelet agents, statins and beta-blockers, and interventions to change behaviour and modify lifestyle, relating to smoking cessation, regular exercise and healthy eating. Most people with coronary heart disease are cared for in the primary care setting and general practitioners have been encouraged to target them for secondary prevention. This has proved difficult and surveys of baseline provision consistently show that secondary prevention is suboptimal.

This research project aimed to evaluate the effects of nurse-led clinics in primary care on secondary prevention, total mortality and coronary event rates after 4 years. It involved 1343 randomly selected patients with a diagnosis of coronary heart disease from 19 general practices in north-east Scotland. Patients in the intervention group were invited to attend nurse-led secondary prevention clinics at their general practice during which their symptoms and treatment were reviewed. The use of aspirin was promoted, lipid management reviewed, lifestyle factors such as exercise assessed and, if appropriate, behavioural changes negotiated. Patients were followed up every 2–6 months. Patients in the control group received the usual care.

Subjects were followed up over a 4-year period by postal questionnaires and review of their case notes. Significant improvements were shown at 1 year in key components of secondary prevention (aspirin, blood pressure management, lipid management, healthy diet), except smoking. These improvements were sustained at 4 years except for exercise. The authors of the report conclude that the improved medical and lifestyle components of secondary prevention produced by nurse-led clinics seem to lead to fewer total deaths and coronary events. They also conclude that nurse-led clinics should be started sooner rather than later.

Murchie P, Campbell N C, Ritchie L D et al 2003 Secondary prevention clinics for coronary heart disease: four year follow up of a randomized controlled trial in primary care. British Medical Journal 326: 84–87

The activity plan for convalescence should be based on a knowledge of the person's functional capacity, interests, previous lifestyle, needs for the future and home environment. Any inhibiting factors such as arthritis also need to be acknowledged. Many hospitals now offer formal structured exercise programmes as part of a coronary rehabilitation programme and exercise-based cardiac rehabilitation has been shown to reduce both cardiac and total mortality (Taylor et al 2004). However, such programmes might not begin for 3–6 weeks after discharge and the patient needs specific advice to prepare for the first few weeks at home. For example, most patients would be able to walk 2 miles a day at the end of 4 weeks. Patients can resume driving 4 weeks after an uncomplicated myocardial infarction although HGV drivers have to show evidence of a negative exercise test. Return to work provides increased self-satisfaction, restored self-respect and relief from financial worries, although early retirement may be a more realistic

Box 2.6

A typical activity programme for a patient following acute myocardial infarction

Phase 1 (in the coronary care unit)

Step 1
- Rest in bed. Out to chair for short periods
- 2-hourly passive range of motion exercises
- Twice-daily breathing exercises
- Independent with personal cleansing at bedside, i.e. wash hands and face
- Use bedside commode

Step 2
- Up to sit unlimited by bedside
- Walk around bed area

Phase 2 (in the ward area)

Step 3
- Walk to bathroom/toilet
- Personal cleansing in bathroom on chair

Step 4
- Unrestricted walking in ward area
- Sit in day room if desired
- Shower/bath unaided

Step 5
- Climb one flight of stairs
- Increase exercises, e.g. use of exercise bike

Phase 3 (early days at home)

Step 6 (first week at home)
- Stay within own home/garden
- Use the stairs two to three times daily
- Undertake any activity that involves standing for short periods, e.g. washing up, dusting, shaving
- Keep as active as possible and walk around little and often

Step 7 (second week)
- Walk approximately 100 yards on flat ground, increasing by approximately 10 yards daily, e.g. walk to the corner shop
- Use the stairs four to five times daily

Step 8 (third week)
- Walk 250–300 yards, two or three times a day
- Use stairs as normal
- Begin to do light shopping, gardening or housework
- Take a bus

Step 9 (fourth week onwards)
- Begin to resume a normal way of life; participate in most normal daily activities, avoiding heavy gardening, moving heavy furniture, etc.
- Begin to take regular exercise, e.g. swimming and walking, progressing gradually
- Start driving again

option for some. Occupational health and community nurses can support the patient and family throughout convalescence.

The aim for all patients is that they will be able to resume their daily lifestyle without physical symptoms, but this depends on their residual left ventricular function. An important part of the rehabilitation process is teaching the person and family how to live with these new limitations. If there is residual ischaemic tissue and angina, medication will help to control this (see p. 18).

Breathing

Oxygen therapy should be given alongside analgesics, to ensure maximal relief of pain. A semi-upright position also eases breathing. Anxious people often hyperventilate and deep breathing exercises may help.

Smoking is not permitted if oxygen therapy is being given and the patient should be encouraged to give up this habit. Stopping smoking is not easy and the best results come with encouragement and support (Van Berkel et al 1999).

Sleeping

The importance of punctuating exercise with rest periods is vital and people should be encouraged to have catnaps at home. In hospital, night sedation may help the patient to settle in a strange environment where noise levels are often high. Interventions need to be coordinated to allow the patient undisturbed periods of rest. A patient who is unable to sleep at night often becomes worried and anxious. An observant nurse can talk to the patient and help to put these fears into perspective.

Fear of dying

This is a very real fear for someone who has had a myocardial infarction (Thompson et al 1995). Once the initial fear has subsided, the patient has to come to terms with the cause of the cardiac event and the consequences of atherosclerosis. Complications with a high mortality rate occur at two stages after myocardial infarction:

- in the first 48 h, when cardiogenic shock and arrhythmias cause death
- 7–10 days later, due to myocardial rupture and ventricular septal defect.

Family fears of death must also be discussed. If not put into perspective, relatives can become overprotective once the person returns home.

Nutrition

In the early stages of myocardial infarction, the patient may have little appetite and opiates may induce nausea. Antiemetics should always be given in conjunction with opiates. Dietary advice should be tailored to the individual and will be similar for all patients with CHD.

Diabetic patients are likely to have raised blood glucose levels following a myocardial infarction. There is evidence that rigorous control of plasma glucose by insulin infusion, followed by subcutaneous insulin, can have a positive effect on long-term prognosis, and therefore patients' blood glucose levels need to be monitored closely and insulin therapy altered accordingly (Yudkin 1998).

Eliminating and fluid and electrolyte balance

Fluid balance is a vital means of assessing renal function, as 25% of cardiac output goes to the kidneys. If left ventricular function is compromised, fluid intake may be restricted to prevent the onset of cardiac failure and pulmonary oedema (p. 43). Electrolyte balance must also be maintained within normal limits and any deviations from normal acted upon.

Potassium regulation is important in the cardiac patient, as both low and high levels of serum potassium lead to life-threatening arrhythmias. Hypokalaemia causes ECG changes and increases the susceptibility to digoxin therapy and therefore toxicity. It can result from acidosis and diuretic therapy with insufficient potassium replacement. Hyperkalaemia in the cardiac patient also results in bradycardia and heart block, and leads to other ventricular arrhythmias. Causes include renal failure and tissue breakdown, which leads to large amounts of intracellular potassium being released into the circulation.

Sodium levels also require to be kept within normal limits. Assessment for obvious signs of fluid overload, such as oedema in the ankles and other dependent parts, and a daily weight check are also part of fluid-balance monitoring.

An increased workload is placed on the heart if there is straining at stool to aid defaecation. Aperients may be used to soften stools and there should be sufficient fibre in the diet. A commode is usually easier to use than a bedpan and even someone confined to bed is likely to expend less energy using a commode than balancing on a bedpan.

Personal hygiene

Initially the patient will be dependent on nursing staff, but this is one of the first areas where independence can quickly be regained. It is possible even in bed to wash the face and upper body and by discharge to be fully independent. It is safer not to lock the bathroom door, in case of emergency, and the family should discuss how to maintain the person's privacy while using the bathroom.

Sexuality

Although discussion of this intimate aspect of life is often difficult, sexual counselling should be an integral part of cardiac rehabilitation. The severity of the infarction and resulting cardiac decompensation are much less important causes of sexual debility than the person's psychological state (Freidman 2000). Reasons for not resuming previous levels of activity include:

- fear of chest pain or another heart attack
- feelings of depression
- partner concern about symptoms
- lack of, or poor, sexual advice from health professionals.

The energy levels and demands placed on the heart during sexual intercourse are comparable to walking briskly or climbing two flights of stairs. It is very rare for sexual intercourse to trigger another heart attack and, as a general guide, intercourse can usually be resumed approximately 2 weeks after discharge, although touching and caressing may be comfortable for some earlier than this.

The subject of sexual activity is best approached as a routine part of the rehabilitation of all coronary patients. The patient needs to feel at ease and the nurse needs to be well informed and prepared for questions. Written information may be useful as a starting point for discussion (Albarran & Bridger 1997). The aim of sexual advice is to restore, as nearly as possible, pre-infarction levels of sexual activity.

Complications of acute coronary syndromes

There are a considerable number of complications of acute coronary syndromes which tend to be related to the site and size of damaged myocardium. The most common are listed in Box 2.7. It is not possible to look at each one in detail, but the nurse should be able to recognise and report the following major problems and carry out the appropriate nursing intervention.

Cardiac arrest

Cardiac arrest may be defined as failure of the heart to pump sufficient blood to maintain cerebral function. It is a term often used synonymously with sudden death, although death is not always the outcome of a cardiac arrest. The three main mechanisms of cardiac arrest are:

- ventricular fibrillation (VF)
- ventricular asystole
- pulseless electrical activity (PEA).

Brain death usually occurs because of the failure of oxygenation of brain cells associated with either failure in ventilation or failure of the heart to pump oxygenated blood to the brain. The brain can tolerate only 4–6 min of anoxia. The signs of cardiac arrest are:

- abrupt loss of consciousness
- absent carotid and femoral pulses
- absent respirations.

A rapidly developing pallor often associated with cyanosis follows. Apnoea, gasping and gagging may occur.

The risk of sudden death in myocardial infarction patients is great. In 25% of cases, this occurs within minutes of the onset of pain, before the patient has reached hospital. The nurse must be familiar with resuscitation procedures within the hospital but should also know how to perform basic cardiopulmonary resuscitation (CPR) without hospital technology. Training programmes in basic CPR for lay people are aimed at reducing this very high early mortality rate, as are the development of trained paramedical staff in ambulances, mobile coronary care units and defibrillators in public places.

To be effective in resuscitation, regular education and training update is necessary, ideally 6-monthly, particularly for those who do not use these skills frequently (Broomfield 1996b, Wynne et al 1999).

The risk of sudden death remains high for the first 24 h after infarction, following which it rapidly diminishes. In the CCU, cardiac arrest may be anticipated; in the ward it is often diagnosed by the nurse, who finds the patient unconscious and pulseless. This is an emergency and every nurse is responsible for:

- recognising that cardiac arrest has occurred
- knowing the procedure for summoning help within the hospital
- commencing effective resuscitation.

The priorities of CPR are:

- airway
- breathing
- circulation.

The nurse is also responsible for maintaining the person's comfort and dignity, anticipating events and procedures, and giving care and support to the patient and relatives after the event.

Restoration of an oxygenated blood supply to the brain involves artificial ventilation and external cardiac massage.

Medical help should be summoned once it has been established that the patient is not breathing. Presence of breathing is assessed by looking for a rise and fall in the chest wall, listening for any breath sounds and feeling for any expelled air.

Artificial ventilation

involves:

- maintaining a clear airway through the removal of loose-fitting dentures, food, sputum, vomit or other obvious debris
- performing the head tilt/chin lift method, or the head tilt/jaw thrust if suspected spinal injury, to allow maximum air entry with the patient in a supine position
- inserting an oesophageal airway, laryngeal mask or endotracheal tube if available
- ventilating the patient mouth to mouth, mouth to mask or with a self-expanding bag and valve mask and pure oxygen if available
- observing for a rise and fall in the patient's chest wall.

The patient should be given two effective rescue breaths, determined by a rise and fall in the patient's chest wall, before assessing for signs of circulation. Each rescue breath should last about 2 s, with a pause of 2–4 s before the next breath.

Box 2.7

Complications of acute coronary syndromes

- Sudden death
- Arrhythmias
- Cardiac failure
- Hypoxia
- Hypotension
- Cardiogenic shock
- Papillary muscle insufficiency
- Ventricular septal defect
- Ventricular aneurysm
- Myocardial rupture
- Pulmonary embolus
- Pericarditis
- Deep vein thrombosis
- Post-MI syndrome
- Emotional difficulty

Circulation
is assessed by feeling for a carotid pulse for up to 10 s. If there is no pulse then external cardiac massage needs to be commenced.

External cardiac massage
can provide only limited cardiac output. If the arrest is witnessed, an initial blow to the chest, precordial thump, may be attempted by professional health care providers, as this may restore the heart rhythm and takes only seconds to perform. Blood flow during cardiac massage is thought to occur due to increased intrathoracic pressure rather than direct heart compression. External cardiac massage involves:

- placing the patient supine on a firm surface
- placing the heel of one hand on the lower half of the patient's sternum, and the other hand on top of the first
- keeping the rescuer's arms straight and elbows locked
- kneeling level with the patient and applying firm downward pressure, depressing the sternum approximately 4–5 cm
- compressing the sternum at a rate of about 100/min.

The internationally recognised guidelines developed by the American Heart Association (2000) and the European Resuscitation Council recommend a cycle of two inflations followed by 15 compressions for both one and two rescuers (see Fig. 2.12).

Medication
Ideally, all medications used during CPR are best administered through a central line to ensure swift distribution, as circulation time is greatly reduced. CPR should continue for 3 min to allow circulation of the drug. Adrenaline (1 mg i.v.) is given every 3 min during cardiac arrest.

Defibrillation
involves the delivery of a direct current (DC) shock to the heart through the chest wall. This causes depolarisation of all the myocardial cells that are able to respond to a stimulus, thereby terminating the fibrillation and allowing the normal conducting pathways to regain control of the heart. Monophasic defibrillation, with the current going one way through the heart muscle, is increasingly being replaced with equipment that delivers a shock in two directions, biphasic defibrillation. This means that lower energy levels are required and damage to myocardial muscle is reduced. The current can be delivered through hand-held paddles placed over gel pads or via pads stuck to the patient's chest. One pad should be placed below the right clavicle and the other over the apex of the heart in the fifth intercostal space. Ideally, the first shock should be administered within 90 s of the cardiac arrest. Precautions should be taken to ensure that floor surfaces are dry and all personnel warned that the shock is about to be delivered. Defibrillators that interpret the patient's heart rhythm and advise about defibrillation are increasingly available in areas where health professionals are less experienced in advanced life support and also in public places such as shopping centres and airports.

After-care
After successful resuscitation, the patient will require skilled nursing care. Full recovery can only be said to have occurred when the patient is fully conscious, with full cardiac, cerebral and renal function. The chances of achieving this are greatly enhanced if the patient is in a CCU where the arrest is witnessed and treatment initiated promptly. Success is less likely in the street where resources are limited.

Several body systems need assessment post-arrest, including the cardiovascular, renal, respiratory and central nervous systems. The patient may have been incontinent, have a sore chest and feel exhausted and somewhat embarrassed by their current state. An assessment of their level of orientation, recall, anxiety and general feelings should be made. The psychological support needed will vary. Relatives and witnesses to the arrest and the resuscitation attempt will also need support.

Ethical considerations
Unsuccessful resuscitation attempts do not enhance the dignity that is hoped for when we die. The appropriateness of merely prolonging the process of dying is often the subject of heated debate (Cotler 2000). The decision not to attempt resuscitation should involve the patient and the family and be documented to avoid confusion. The decision needs to be reviewed on at least a 24-h basis.

The Resuscitation Council (UK) (2000) points out that 'do not attempt resuscitation' (DNAR) orders may be a potent source of misunderstanding and dissent amongst doctors, nurses and others involved in the care of patients. Issues surrounding this dilemma include whether resuscitation is appropriate, involvement of the patient and family in the decision-making process and communication difficulties between doctors and nurses once the decision is made (Mason 1996). Increasingly, living wills are being made by patients, and nurses need to be aware of the significance of these when making decisions about resuscitation. It is important that it is understood by all that DNAR orders apply only to the decision whether or not to initiate resuscitation in the event of cardiac or respiratory arrest and should not in any way limit other medical or nursing care (Shepardson et al 1999, Jackson et al 2004).

STOP THINK **2.5** Should relatives be permitted to witness resuscitation attempts? See Connors (1996).

Cardiogenic shock
This is a serious degree of heart failure, precipitated by extensive (>40%) left ventricular damage in which the cardiac output is not sufficient to give an adequate blood pressure to maintain perfusion. The patient develops clinical shock with low urine output, cold clammy skin and hypoxia. Lactic acid is produced in the skeletal muscle beds as the metabolism changes, giving rise to a metabolic acidosis. This process is cyclical, with the heart continually trying to pump harder for an ever falling stroke volume (see Ch. 18).

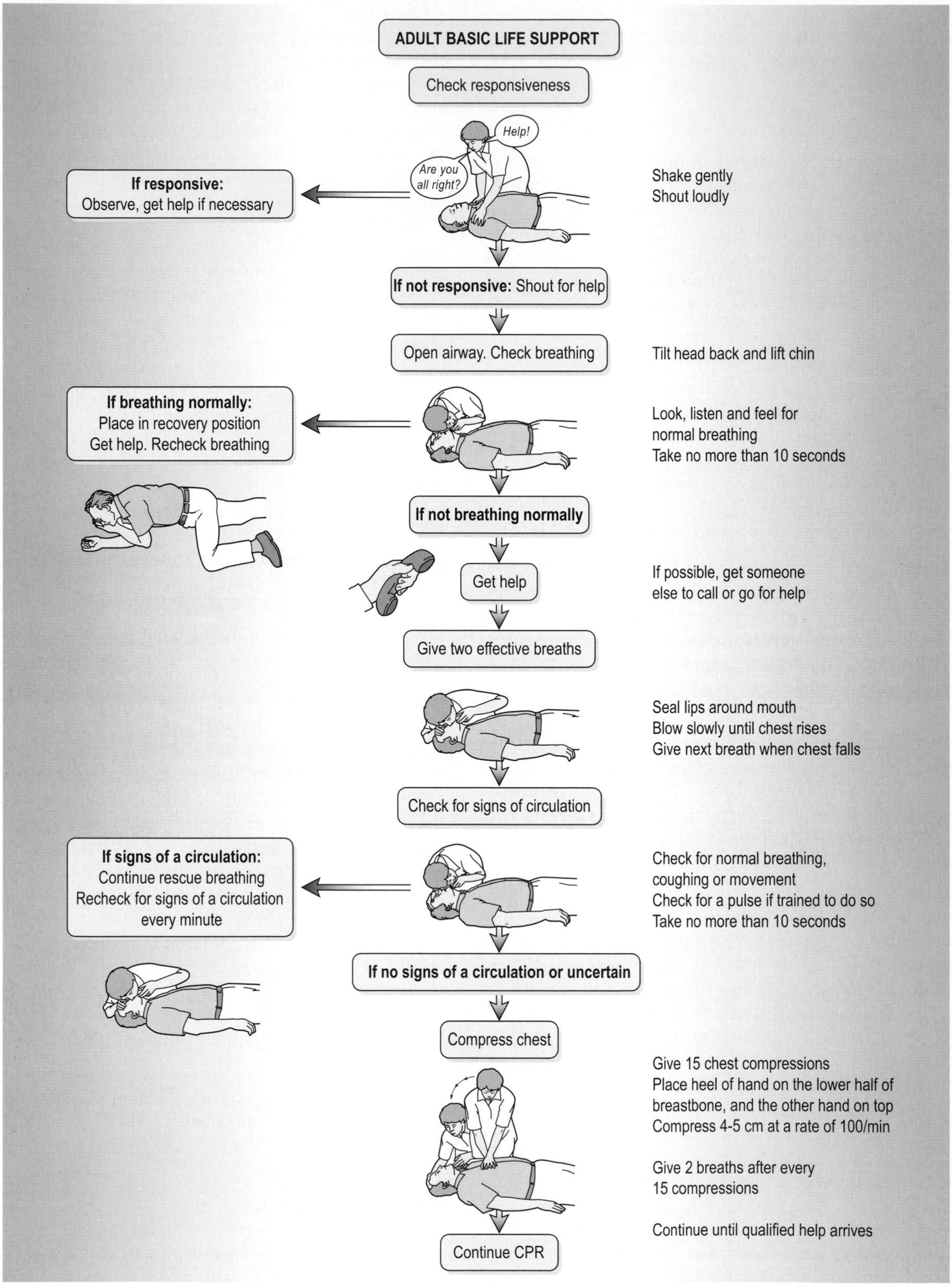
ADULT BASIC LIFE SUPPORT
Check responsiveness
Help!
Are you all right?
If responsive:
Observe, get help if necessary
Shake gently
Shout loudly
If not responsive: Shout for help
Open airway. Check breathing
Tilt head back and lift chin
If breathing normally:
Place in recovery position
Get help. Recheck breathing
Look, listen and feel for normal breathing
Take no more than 10 seconds
If not breathing normally
Get help
If possible, get someone else to call or go for help
Give two effective breaths
Seal lips around mouth
Blow slowly until chest rises
Give next breath when chest falls
Check for signs of circulation
If signs of a circulation:
Continue rescue breathing
Recheck for signs of a circulation every minute
Check for normal breathing, coughing or movement
Check for a pulse if trained to do so
Take no more than 10 seconds
If no signs of a circulation or uncertain
Compress chest
Give 15 chest compressions
Place heel of hand on the lower half of breastbone, and the other hand on top
Compress 4-5 cm at a rate of 100/min
Give 2 breaths after every 15 compressions
Continue until qualified help arrives
Continue CPR
A

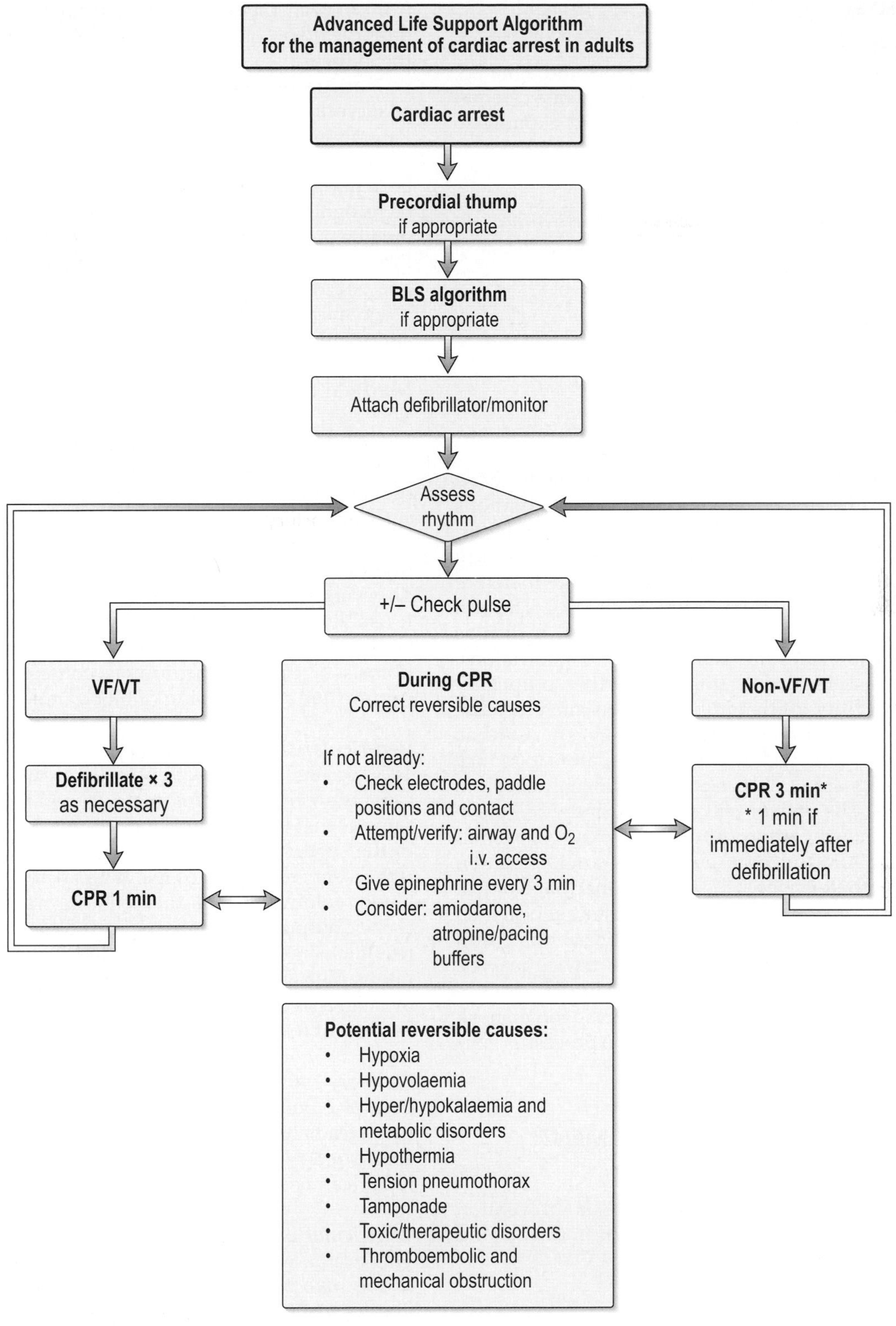

Fig. 2.12 A: An algorithm for basic life support. B: An algorithm for the management of cardiac arrest. (Reproduced with kind permission from the European Resuscitation Council.)

NB: Cardiopulmonary resuscitation – 2005 revised guidelines www.resus.org.uk

The Resuscitation Council (UK) recommends for adults:

- CPR with a chest compression to ventilation ratio of 30:2
- No initial ventilations before starting compressions
- When professional help is delayed for more than 4-5 minutes, one option is to give compressions for up to three minutes before attempting defibrillation
- Compressions for two minutes after defibrillation

If coordinated rhythm is not restored by defibrillation, second and further shocks should be given only after additional cycles of chest compressions.

PATHOPHYSIOLOGY

Clinical features
In the early stages, the patient may be restless and agitated, followed by mental confusion and lethargy as cerebral hypoxia increases. The skin becomes cold and clammy to touch.

Examination
There will be signs of central cyanosis. Vital recordings will reveal a rapid, thready pulse, hypotension, tachypnoea and hypothermia. Urinary output will be reduced.

MEDICAL MANAGEMENT
The priorities are to:

- enhance cardiac output
- restore tissue perfusion
- effect a diuresis through increased renal flow.

This often requires manipulation of several medications in order to obtain the best effect for the patient. Medications commonly used in myocardial infarction such as nitrates, beta-blockers, calcium antagonists and opiates may produce hypotension and worsen cardiogenic shock and therefore should be used with caution (Williams et al 2000). The aim is to improve cardiac output using inotropic drugs such as adrenaline, dopamine and dobutamine. These medications, often given via a central line, improve cardiac output by increasing contractility and often heart rate, which increase the demand on the myocardium for oxygen. Cardiac output can also be improved by using vasodilators to reduce afterload. Diuretics are widely used in cardiogenic shock to induce a diuresis. The patient will require urinary catheterisation to assess hourly urine output and may be haemodynamically monitored using a pulmonary artery flotation (Swan–Ganz) catheter (see Ch. 18). If pharmacological intervention is ineffective in treating cardiogenic shock, then more invasive therapy such as the intra-aortic balloon pump (IABP) (see p. 727) or left ventricular assist device may be required. Some patients may be appropriate for PTCA.

The outlook for patients developing cardiogenic shock is poor and mortality is high (45–80%), as the process is very difficult to reverse (Goldberg et al 1999).

NURSING PRIORITIES AND MANAGEMENT: Cardiogenic shock

The priority in caring for these patients is prevention or early recognition of the signs that shock is developing (O'Neal 1994, De Jong 1999).

Observation
Recording and assessment of all vital signs are important. The pulse will initially be rapid and thready as a compensatory response to the falling cardiac output; in the late stages, bradycardia develops.

Initially, systolic and later, diastolic pressure will fall. A fall in pulse pressure of more than 30 mmHg may be an indication that shock is developing in the hypertensive patient. The initial response to hypoxia is tachypnoea, which later becomes shallow and irregular. Most patients benefit from oxygen therapy. Urine output falls as a result of the falling cardiac output, leading to inadequate perfusion of the kidneys.

Nursing management of these patients requires careful observation and recording of response to medication. Patients are likely to become increasingly drowsy, confused, immobile and dependent on nursing care. They may also be lethargic or semi-conscious. Anxiety and fear need to be recognised and addressed (Williams 1993). Small doses of opiates may promote comfort and rest. The relatives need time spent with them to explain the condition of their loved one and how they can best help. The hospital chaplain or other spiritual advisor may provide comfort for the patient and family at this time.

Medical complications of myocardial infarction
The risk of complications following acute myocardial infarction is mostly dependent on the size of the infarcted area, the total loss of functional myocardium following previous ischaemic damage and the extent and severity of coronary artery disease.

Myocardial rupture
This very rare complication results in instantaneous death. It usually occurs 3–5 days after an extensive infarction in a heart with poor collateral blood flow. Necrosis occurs before fibrosis of the myocardium is complete, causing muscle rupture and the pumping of blood into the pericardium.

Ventricular septal defect
This occurs more frequently than rupture but in some cases is amenable to treatment. The pathophysiology is the same as that for myocardial rupture, with a hole developing in the septum separating the right and left ventricles. The right ventricle has to cope with increased pressures and blood volumes while the left ventricle suffers a fall in cardiac output. Rapid onset of cardiogenic shock may be the result. Operative repair can be undertaken but the mortality rate is high. If the patient can be supported for 2–4 weeks by aggressive medical management until the septum has become fibrosed, then the surgical results are slightly better.

Papillary muscle rupture
Loss of blood supply to the muscle supporting the mitral valve leads to prolapse and malfunctioning of the valve. If acute rupture occurs, then sudden death may result. Surgical repair can be attempted, but again survival rates are low.

Ventricular aneurysm
This occurs when the infarction involves the full thickness of the myocardium. As the necrotic tissue is replaced by fibrous tissue, it is subject to the high pressures in the left ventricle. This fibrous tissue balloons out to form a blood pouch, which does not contract. Blood stagnation in this pouch leads to the development of thrombi and systemic emboli complicate approximately half of cases of left ventricular embolism. If a large area of myocardium is affected then it can lead to cardiac failure; if the aneurysm is near the papillary muscle or mitral valve then incompetence will result. Surgical resection can be undertaken successfully with some of the smaller aneurysms.

Pericarditis

This is thought to be due to an autoimmune reaction in which antigens from the damaged myocardium cause inflammation of the pericardium. The patient presents with pain at any time from 24 h to 1 week after the myocardial infarction. On examination, a 'friction rub' caused by friction between the pericardium and myocardium is often heard, accompanied by an unresolving post-infarction pyrexia. Medical treatment and nursing care involve treating the pain with analgesics and non-steroidal anti-inflammatory agents. Reassurance that the pain is not an extension of the infarction is important.

Emboli

Embolism of a pulmonary or systemic vessel can occur after myocardial infarction. Emboli arise from clots forming in the healing myocardium or from circulatory stasis causing clot formation in the lower limbs. Nursing care involves maintaining passive exercises for the patient, whose mobility is restricted. The use of anti-embolism stockings should be considered. All post-myocardial infarction patients and those with known CHD should be given aspirin, which, taken daily, has been shown to be effective in reducing clot formation. In most patients this may be sufficient, but in people with pulmonary emboli or who are known to have mural thrombi, a more aggressive approach to anticoagulation is required.

ARRHYTHMIAS

The term arrhythmia is used to imply an abnormality in either electrical impulse formation or electrical impulse conduction within the heart. An arrhythmia may cause an effect by any one of the following changes:

- change in heart rate
- increase in myocardial oxygen requirement
- decrease in myocardial blood flow
- loss of synchronicity of ventricular contraction.

PATHOPHYSIOLOGY

Clinical features

The clinical manifestation of an arrhythmia depends on the ventricular rate, the conduction of the myocardium and the psychological response of the patient. Patient problems include:

- palpitations
- dizziness
- faintness
- shortness of breath
- chest pain
- headache
- reduced activity tolerance
- anxiety.

Nursing assessment includes the apparent effect of the arrhythmia on the patient, a history of any past experiences of the problem, a knowledge of any relevant medications or other treatments and identification of any possible precipitating factors.

In cardiac disease, the normal sinus mechanism can be altered if the disease affects the heart's specialised conduction tissue. Various conditions result in specific conduction disturbances, and while this chapter cannot deal with them all, it will concentrate on a few of the more common conditions with which the nurse should be familiar. In interpreting heart rhythms, the method used must be systematic and consider all components of the ECG complex.

Normal sinus rhythm should be recognisable to all nurses, as patients attached to cardiac monitors are increasingly nursed on general wards. The nurse's priorities are to:

- recognise and immediately report anything abnormal
- assess quickly the effect of the abnormality on the patient and take the appropriate action.

The normal electrocardiogram and the basic rules for observing cardiac monitors discussed earlier in the chapter apply here.

Sinus arrhythmias

The SA node is under autonomic control, primarily vagal, but is influenced by sympathetic stimulation, temperature, oxygen saturation and other metabolic changes. Sinus arrhythmias are often secondary to these influences.

Sinus arrhythmias are characterised by a constant PR interval but progressive beat-to-beat change in R–R intervals. During expiration, the reflex discharge of the vagal nerve slows the sinus mechanism; during inspiration this influence is diminished, allowing a speeding up of the sinus rhythm. Sinus arrhythmias are not life threatening and resolution of the primary cause resolves the arrhythmia.

Sinus bradycardia

This meets the criteria for sinus rhythm but the rate is less than 60 beats/min. It may result from increased vagal tone but also results from hypothermia, certain medications, e.g. beta-blockers, raised intracranial pressure and inferior myocardial infarction. Some individuals may experience sinus bradycardia when sleeping. It may be the norm in athletes. Intravenous atropine is given for symptomatic sinus bradycardia.

Sinus tachycardia

This also fits the criteria for sinus rhythm, but the rate is greater than 100 beats/min. It is a direct result of decreased vagal tone and often a response to sympathetic stimulation.

Narrow complex tachycardias

Atrial flutter

This is characterised by rapid and regular atrial excitation at a level above 200 beats/min. The AV node is not capable of conducting atrial rates above this level. The atrial waves form a sawtooth pattern. Ventricular deflections usually occur regularly within the atrial pattern and the block is described as a ratio, e.g. 4:1, which means four P waves per QRS complex.

Atrial flutter is not a stable rhythm and often progresses to atrial fibrillation.

Atrial fibrillation

When individual muscle fibres of the atria or ventricles contract independently, they are said to be 'fibrillating'. There is rapid disorganised atrial depolarisation because the atrial tissues have lost synchrony with each other. The atrial waves can occur up to 600 times per minute. Ventricular depolarisation is also irregular as a result of the variable response at the AV node, but the QRS complex is normal. It occurs in congestive cardiac failure and mitral valve disease, and commonly presents with ischaemic changes in old age.

MEDICAL MANAGEMENT

Atrial fibrillation can severely compromise cardiac output, as the loss of the effect of atrial systole can reduce stroke volume by up to 25%. With chronic atrial fibrillation, the danger of thrombi forming in the atria and then embolising is high.

Treatment

is aimed at reducing the rapid ventricular rate through chemical or DC cardioversion (see Box 2.8) to revert to sinus rhythm. Cardioversion after digoxin therapy may precipitate ventricular fibrillation if large doses of digoxin have been used. Anticoagulation in the form of heparin or warfarin may be prescribed to reduce the risk of thrombi.

Box 2.8

Cardioversion

Purpose

The term 'cardioversion' is used to mean the delivery of a specific and predetermined amount of energy to the heart, timed (synchronised) in such a way that the shock is delivered well away from the vulnerable period of the T wave on the ECG. It is usually performed electively, with the patient lightly anaesthetised. This differs from defibrillation, which usually involves the delivery of a larger amount of electricity to a patient in ventricular fibrillation without anaesthetic, as the patient is usually unconscious. Elective cardioversion is used to treat supraventricular and ventricular arrhythmias.

Electrical treatment has the advantage that it is free from pharmacological side-effects.

Procedure

Monophasic or biphasic electrical wave forms are used for cardioversion, the latter requiring lower energy settings. Energy levels are titrated upwards if an initial shock is unsuccessful. The patient is asked to remove any dentures or restrictive clothing. An ECG will be performed before and after the procedure, and the patient attached to a cardiac monitor throughout. Oxygen is given both before and after the procedure. A light anaesthetic is usually given and the patient asked to fast for 4–6 h prior to the procedure. Resuscitation equipment needs to be on hand. The defibrillator is set to the required output and the paddles or pads are placed in position, usually with one below the right clavicle and the other over the apex of the heart in order to depolarise an optimum mass of myocardial cells. The patient is usually awake and talking 5–10 min after the procedure; nausea and vomiting are not uncommon, as are a sore throat from the endotracheal tube and chest wall soreness due to the cardioversion. Cardioversion is often performed on a day-case basis and is frequently coordinated and led by nurses (Quinn 1998).

NURSING PRIORITIES AND MANAGEMENT: DC cardioversion

The procedure should be fully explained to the patient so that they are aware of what to expect. They will be prepared as for all patients prior to a general anaesthetic. The thought of an anaesthetic and an electric current being put across the heart may be frightening. Care should be taken to ensure that the area is dry and that all personnel are warned that the shock is about to be delivered. The patient is likely to want to know the outcome of the procedure and this should be explained. Topical creams may help to ease any chest soreness caused by the electric shock.

STOP THINK **2.6** Clarify the difference between emergency defibrillation and elective cardioversion.

Junctional tachycardias

The AV node, unlike the SA node, normally has no pacemaking role. Impulses must travel in both directions to stimulate atrial and ventricular contractions, so the position of the P wave varies. The QRS complex is of normal configuration and duration since the normal conduction pathway is followed below the AV node. Junctional tachycardia is characterised by the sudden onset of tachycardia greater than 150 beats per minute. There are three forms of junctional tachycardia: AV nodal re-entry tachycardia, AV re-entry tachycardia and paroxysmal atrial tachycardia. These are discussed in more detail in Jowett and Thompson (2003). The urgency of treatment depends on symptoms, which tend to be related to the ventricular rate. Carotid sinus massage may terminate junctional re-entry tachycardias and allows differentiation from atrial flutter.

Supraventricular tachycardia

This term is still often used but is anatomically incorrect because most narrow complex tachycardias incorporate both ventricular and atrial myocardium within the conduction circuit. Medical management of narrow complex tachycardia aims to reduce the rapid ventricular rate using carotid sinus pressure or antiarrhythmic drugs, e.g. amiodarone, adenosine or digoxin.

If these measures are unsuccessful then cardioversion may be indicated.

Ventricular arrhythmias

In these rhythms the ectopic focus arises below the AV node.

Ventricular tachycardia

This is a broad complex tachycardia with a QRS complex that looks wide and bizarre. The rate is regular at around 140–200 beats/min. It is generally caused by an irritable or ischaemic myocardium. Treatment, if the patient is symptomatic, is with immediate synchronised cardioversion and/or intravenous lidocaine. Other medication includes amiodarone, flecainide and mexiletine. Persistent episodes of ventricular tachycardia may be treated with override pacing or ablation therapy, where the ectopic focus or source of the arrhythmia is identified and removed.

Ventricular fibrillation
In this rhythm, there are no distinguishable complexes on the screen and only an erratic baseline trace is evident. Treatment is by immediate initiation of resuscitation procedures and defibrillation.

Cardiac electrophysiology studies and ablation processes

Electrophysiology studies involve the introduction of an intravenous or intra-arterial catheter with multiple electrodes positioned at various intracardiac sites for the purpose of recording or initiating electrical activity from specific areas of the atria or ventricles. These studies are performed on patients with arrhythmias which are resistant to medication, in order to identify the nature of the rhythm disturbance — also known as cardiac mapping.

Ablation therapy requires the delivery of a high-energy electric shock through a catheter in order to produce localised tissue damage in the unstable area identified as producing the arrhythmia, e.g. in Wolff–Parkinson–White syndrome.

Implantable cardioverter defibrillators

The implantable cardioverter defibrillator is an electronic device used to detect and terminate potentially lethal arrhythmias through the delivery of an electric shock. Current models weigh less than 200 g and are implanted without open chest procedures. They are particularly suitable for patients who have survived one episode of cardiac arrest not thought to be the result of myocardial infarction and for those with recurrent episodes of ventricular tachycardia unresponsive to optimal medication. Appropriate patients are likely to need individualised information and support to enable them to cope with the concept of being dependent on the device (James 2002).

Heart block

This arrhythmia results when there is a delay or interruption of impulse conduction from the atria to the ventricles at the AV node. It is described as:

- first-degree heart block
- second-degree heart block
- third-degree (complete) heart block.

Heart block is usually a complication of myocardial infarction.

First-degree block
appears as a prolonged PR interval with a mild bradycardia. It is asymptomatic and seldom requires treatment.

Second-degree block
appears as occasional blocking; for example, there may be alternate conducted and non-conducted atrial beats, giving twice as many P waves as QRS complexes. The patient may have no symptoms and require no treatment. If a fall in blood pressure or other signs of reduced cardiac output develop, the heart block is treated by the insertion of a pacemaker (see Box 2.9).

Complete heart block
exists when atrial and ventricular activity are uncoordinated. The atria and ventricles are electrically dissociated and desynchronised, with a subsidiary pacemaker developing in the ventricles. Cardiac output is reduced and the patient is haemodynamically compromised. The ventricles often contract at a rate of less than 40 beats/min and a pacemaker requires to be inserted immediately to restore cardiac output. The nurse's role is one of observation, reporting and patient support.

NURSING PRIORITIES AND MANAGEMENT: Arrhythmias

The clinical consequences of arrhythmias are extremely variable, but are likely to be more pronounced in those with chronic heart disease. Treatment usually aims to restore sinus rhythm and prevent recurrence of the arrhythmia. Nursing management involves anticipating and resolving patient problems, monitoring the patient, including their response to treatment, and providing information and support.

Pacemakers

Indications for pacing vary both nationally and internationally, although the American College of Cardiology, the American Heart Association and the North American Society for Pacing (ACC/AHA/NASPE 2002) have produced pacemaker guidelines. Nursing considerations include assessing pacemaker function, ensuring patient comfort and safety, preventing and dealing with complications, and teaching the patient about their condition and its management. The patient needs to be prepared for the procedure, even if it is done as an emergency (see Box 2.9).

Following pacemaker insertion, the patient should be attached to a cardiac monitor to assess whether the pacemaker is functioning properly. Cardiac output needs to be assessed frequently by recording the patient's blood pressure and asking them to report any symptoms of faintness, dizziness, chest pain or shortness of breath.

Limited mobility may make the patient more dependent on nursing care for a while. The patient with a temporary pacemaker should be aware of how long the temporary pacing is likely to continue and appreciate what is likely to happen next.

Removal of the temporary pacemaker is performed at the patient's bedside under aseptic conditions.

Permanent pacing

Initially, the nursing considerations are similar to those for temporary pacing. Some patients will be helped by a visit from a person who already has a permanent pacemaker, and also by being given an opportunity to handle a pacemaker. The patient needs to be reassured that the pacemaker will not be damaged by day-to-day activities. They should be taught to take their own pulse and be aware of the signs of

Box 2.9

Pacemaker insertion

Purpose
Pacemakers are used to gain control over the electrical activity of the heart. They have two basic components:

- a pulse generator containing a power source and electrical circuitry
- one or two pacing leads, each with an electrode on its tip.

Pacemakers may be either temporary or permanent, depending on whether the pulse generator is located externally or implanted. If pacing is planned for a short duration, an external source is used to deliver electricity to the heart via the skin. When long-term control of the heart is required, a permanent pacemaker is implanted. The two most common modes of pacing are:

- demand (ventricular inhibited) — senses intrinsic cardiac rhythm and stimulates myocardial depolarisation and contraction as necessary
- fixed rate — fires at a predetermined rate, irrespective of intrinsic cardiac activity.

Temporary pacing
This is used to maintain cardiac output during episodes of extreme bradycardia, heart block and asystole. It may also be used for the suppression of tachyarrhythmias, which are resistant to medication. It is usual for a special room to be set aside for temporary cardiac pacing, with ECG monitoring, fluoroscopy and resuscitation equipment being readily available.

Most commonly, a bipolar catheter is inserted into the subclavian vein, external jugular vein or antecubital fossa under local anaesthesia. The catheter is then passed into the right atrium and thence through the tricuspid valve and into the apex of the right ventricle, where the tip of the catheter is lodged against the ventricular wall. The external end of the catheter is stitched into place at the skin surface. The bipolar catheter is stimulated by the pacemaker's external pulse generator. Verification of pacing is judged from the appearance of a pacing spike preceding the QRS complex of the ECG. Pacing 'threshold' is obtained by determining the lowest voltage needed to elicit a paced beat, ideally less than 0.5 V. The threshold needs to be checked at least every 12 h, as it may increase over time.

Possible complications
These include arrhythmias, failure of the electrode to sense the heart's own electrical activity, failure of the electrode to generate a contraction, abdominal muscle twitching, pneumothorax and infection.

Permanent pacing
The decision to implant a permanent pacemaker is made after careful patient assessment. It is usually offered to patients with symptomatic bradycardias and heart block. The modern pacemaker is a small metal unit weighing between 25 and 30 g. It is powered by a lithium battery with a life of up to 15 years. Two types of pulse generator are currently available:

- single chamber with an electrode placed in either the atrium or the ventricle
- dual chamber with electrodes situated in both chambers.

The pacemaker is usually implanted under local anaesthesia in a cardiac catheterisation laboratory. The pulse generator is implanted in a subcutaneous pocket, usually under the clavicle, axilla or abdominal wall. The procedure is usually performed on a day-case basis.

reduced cardiac output. Signs of infection, such as redness or increased soreness at the implantation site, should also be reported. The importance of follow-up appointments should be explained. It is also useful to warn people that the pacemaker may trigger off alarms at airports. The patient should refrain from driving for 1 month (6 months for LGV and PCV, and re-licensing may be permitted thereafter providing there is no other disqualifying condition).

For further information see the Driver and Vehicle Licensing Agency (DVLA) website – www.dvla.gov.uk; for further information on the use of pacemakers and implantable internal defibrillators, see the ACC/AHA/NASPE (2002) guideline update for implantation of cardiac pacemakers and antiarrhythmia devices.

HEART FAILURE

The term 'heart failure' is used to describe a clinical syndrome that has a characteristic group of signs and symptoms. It results from an inability of the heart to provide an adequate cardiac output for the body's metabolic requirements. It is increasing in prevalence and the prevalence rises steeply with age. Statistical data suggest that after an initial diagnosis of heart failure, 16% of patients die within a year of diagnosis, 40% within the first 2 years and 61% within 5 years (British Heart Foundation 2004). Patients living with heart failure have been shown to visit their GP on average between 11 and 14 times per year (Gnani & Majeed 2001).

Heart failure is often referred to as either acute or chronic. Acute heart failure is a complex syndrome in which the patient's condition changes from moment to moment. It arises from the loss of functional myocardial tissue and the reduced contractility of the myocardium. It complicates between 25 and 50% of acute coronary syndrome patients. The clinical condition is often complicated by arrhythmias which reduce the cardiac output further. It may develop suddenly or during the first few hours or days after the infarction. Acute heart failure may resolve with medical therapy as the patient's condition stabilises. However, infarction may result in a long-term reduction of the functional capacity of the myocardium and chronic heart failure. Chronic heart failure can also occur as a result of hypertension, aneurysm, cardiomyopathy, arrhythmias and medication, such as beta-blockers and antiarrhythmics, often used in acute cardiac events.

The diagnosis of heart failure is not difficult to make, but identifying the underlying cause can be. Heart failure can result from primary heart disease or from non-cardiac causes (see Box 2.10). Many of these conditions are very

> **Box 2.10**
>
> **Primary cardiac conditions causing heart failure**
>
> **Right heart failure**
> - Pulmonary hypertension secondary to left heart failure
> - Congenital heart defect
> - Thromboembolism
> - Cor pulmonale
> - Atrial septal defect
> - Pulmonary venous stenosis
>
> **Left heart failure**
>
> **Ventricular origin**
> - Coronary artery disease
> - Aortic or mitral valve disease
> - Congenital heart defect
> - Hypertension
> - Ventricular septal defect
>
> **Atrial origin**
> - Atrial myxoma
> - Mitral stenosis

common, particularly in older people. They are often found in combination, making their individual contribution to the heart failure difficult to assess. Non-cardiac causes include chronic obstructive airways disease (COAD), hyperthyroidism and chronic anaemia (see Chs 3, 5 and 11).

PATHOPHYSIOLOGY

Heart failure can involve either ventricle independently or both together. Pure left or right ventricular failure may not exist for long because of their dependence on each other to maintain adequate blood flow. However, it is useful to look at the heart as two pumps. The left ventricle can cope better with alterations in pressure and the right with alterations in volume. Failure of the left side of the heart causes accumulation of blood in the left ventricle and left atrium with subsequent congestion of the lungs. Right-sided failure, where the right ventricle cannot effectively transfer deoxygenated blood to the pulmonary circulation, subsequently causes congestion of the circulation in the rest of the body (systemic circulation).

Cardiac reserve

The function of the heart is to pump blood to the body at sufficient volume and pressure to perfuse the tissues with oxygen. The requirements of many tissues are fairly constant, but the needs of the skeletal musculature vary with the level of physical activity. An increase in activity leads to an increase in cardiac output, this capacity to increase being the 'cardiac reserve'. The increase results mainly from increased heart rate and contractile force as a direct result of sympathetic nervous system (SNS) stimulation. In the patient with heart failure, the cardiac reserve is used to maintain baseline cardiac function and so the ability to respond to increased activity is limited. When the baroreceptors at various points in the body sense a fall in pressure and therefore a fall in cardiac output, the principal response is to increase stimulation of the SNS, followed up by a longer-term response.

Myocardial dilatation

Increased stretching of the myocardial cells, which occurs immediately after a sudden reduction in the ability to expel the stroke volume, increases their force of contraction and increases the cardiac output correspondingly. This compensatory mechanism becomes limited as myocardial oxygen demand increases.

Renal response

Reduced cardiac output has a depressant effect on the kidneys, which will not improve until the cardiac output returns to normal. The fall in blood pressure and sympathetic constriction of renal arterioles reduce the glomerular filtration rate (GFR). Reduced blood flow through the kidneys results in instigation of the renin–angiotensin–aldosterone mechanism and leads to increased angiotensin production, increased secretion of aldosterone and therefore increased sodium and water reabsorption. The fluid retention in itself does not interfere with the pumping ability of the heart, but it does increase venous return. The rise in extracellular fluid and blood volume increases systemic filling pressures, so more of the cardiac reserve has to be used to maintain perfusion, further reducing the heart's ability to respond to increased physical activity.

Congestive cardiac failure (CCF)

This term describes a state in which there is both right and left ventricular failure with a corresponding combination of systemic and pulmonary symptoms.

Myocardial hypertrophy

In response to the increased workload, the individual myocardial cells enlarge, thus increasing the total amount of contractile tissue. This compensation is usually of a temporary nature, and at this stage the prognosis is poor.

Oedema

Oedema may result when anything increases the movement of fluid from the bloodstream and impairs its return. One of the commonest causes is CCF, where the failure of the pump to move the blood volume forward results in back pressure, which raises the hydrostatic pressure such that it exceeds the colloidal pressure created by plasma proteins. As a result, the excess tissue fluid formed accumulates, exceeding the ability of the lymphatic system to drain the excess away.

In the early stages of heart failure, patients may complain of 'puffy ankles', being unable to fit comfortably into their shoes. There will also be sacral oedema.

Pulmonary oedema As systemic arterial pressure, and therefore afterload, increases, so does pressure in the left heart. Increased left ventricular end-diastolic pressure (LVEDP) results in increased pulmonary pressure and an accumulation of blood in the lungs. If the pulmonary pressure rises above 28 mmHg, there is movement of fluid from the capillaries into the alveoli and interstitial spaces. This causes pulmonary oedema. If this occurs as an acute event, it can lead to death in 30 min. In the congestive failure situation, it is a chronic progressive state where the reduced lung compliance and high pulmonary pressure lead to increased right heart pressures and blood congestion on this side. This further raises pressure in the systemic circulation,

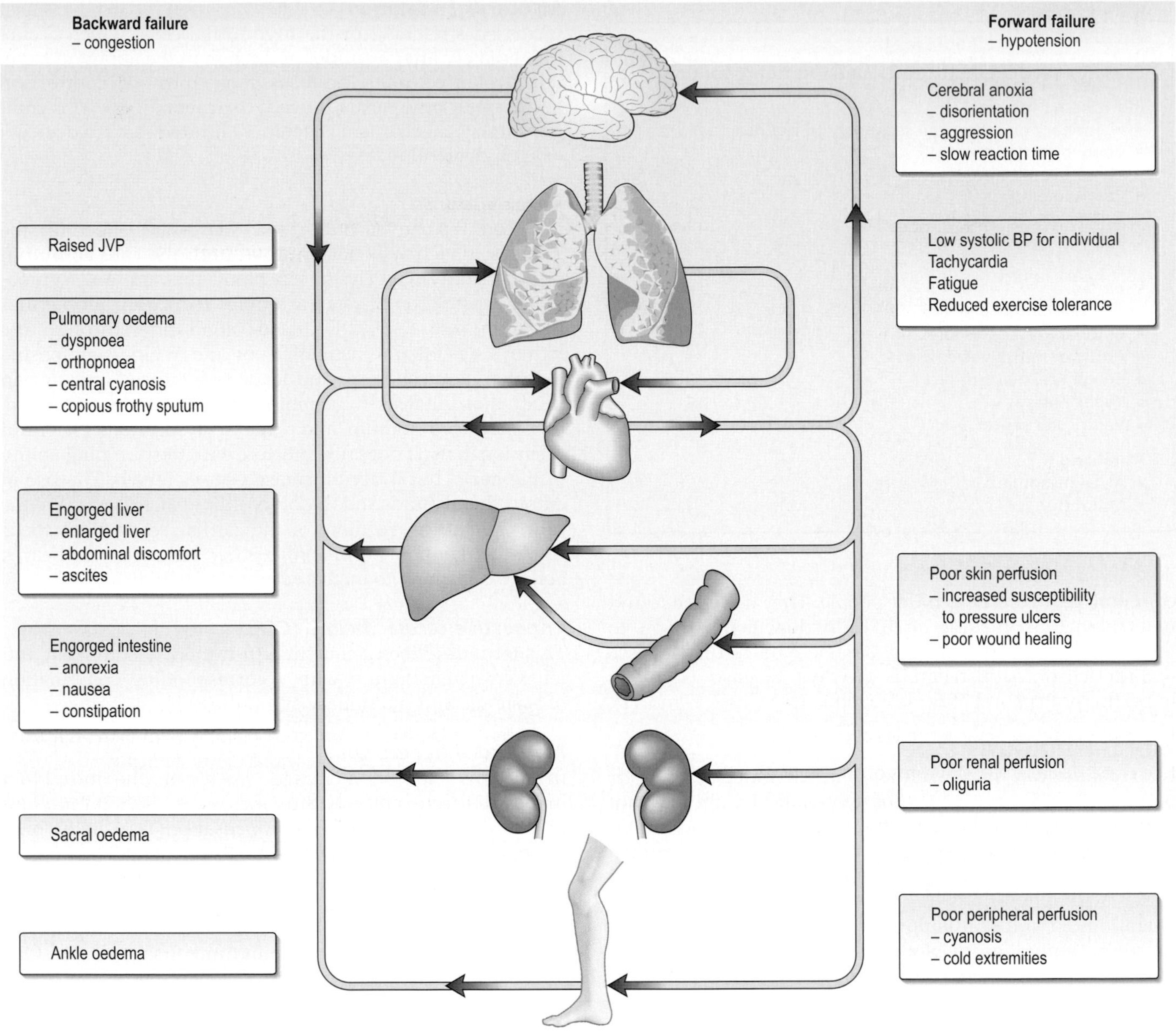

Fig. 2.13 Clinical effects of the decompensatory phase of ventricular failure.

making the whole process one of cyclical deterioration. As the systemic pressure rises, there is movement of fluid into the tissues giving rise to peripheral oedema. This is initially gravitational, but as the condition progresses the oedema becomes more widespread (see Fig. 2.13).

Common presenting symptoms

The presentation and history will depend on which side of the heart is failing. It may present gradually, as occurs in the ageing process, or suddenly, manifesting as acute pulmonary oedema with marked breathlessness, anxiety and tachycardia.

- Fatigue on exertion, dyspnoea with mild exercise and paroxysmal nocturnal dyspnoea are common early signs of failure of the left ventricle.
- Fatigue, awareness of fullness in the neck and abdomen, and ankle swelling are early signs of failure of the right ventricle.

Features appearing in systemic examination are listed in Table 2.6.

MEDICAL MANAGEMENT

Heart failure is suspected because of the patient's history, signs and symptoms. This diagnosis is then confirmed or excluded through a 12 lead ECG, which may show left ventricular hypertrophy, ischaemia or infarction; natriuretic peptides — B type natriuretic peptide (BNP) and its end terminal fragment N-BNP where available; a chest X-ray, blood tests, i.e. urea and electrolytes, creatinine, full blood count, thyroid function test, liver function test, glucose and lipids; echocardiography; urinalysis and peak flow.

Table 2.6 Systemic examination in heart failure

System	Points to note	Rationale
CVS	Chest X-ray	Evaluation of chamber enlargement Indication of primary cardiac abnormality
	Auscultation	Arrhythmia (especially AF) common A prominent third heart sound with a tachycardia (gallop rhythm)
	Vital signs	Venous hypertension common Observe jugular venous pressure
	Presence of oedema	Visible oedema in dependent parts, e.g. ankles, hands and sacrum, in bed-bound patients is a sign of inability to excrete sufficient water
Respiratory	Wheeze, bronchospasm	Possible increased pulmonary fluid
	Paroxysmal nocturnal dyspnoea	Evidence of poor left ventricle compensation
	Amount and consistency of sputum	Evidence of pulmonary oedema
	Pleural effusion on right side	Often found in patients with congestive cardiac failure
GIS	Chest X-ray	Recognition of oedema
	Diet	Sodium control is an important part of controlling fluid retention
	Palpation of abdomen	Signs of hepatic and splenic engorgement Presence of ascites
GUS	Micturition	Frequency and amount of urine passed; vital to assess effect of diuretic therapy
MS	Physical activity levels	Often severely limited by reduced cardiac reserve
CNS	Mental status	Signs of cerebral hypoxia
Skin	Skin integrity	Risk of pressure ulcers and delayed healing

Treatment

The main treatment approaches are:

1. oxygenation to improve myocardial contractility
2. rest to reduce cardiac workload
3. medication designed to improve cardiac function.

Diuretics, direct vasodilators and ACE inhibitors can be used to reduce symptoms, prolong life, or both, in heart failure patients.

- Diuretics, e.g. furosemide, induce sodium and water excretion, leading to decreased cardiac preload and wall tension, and an effective decrease of symptomatic pulmonary and systemic congestion. However, they have not yet been shown to prolong life in patients with congestive cardiac failure.
- Direct vasodilators, which induce venodilatation, arterial dilatation, or both, i.e. balanced vasodilators, may improve symptoms:
  - — venodilators, such as nitrates, exert a venous pooling effect, decreasing cardiac preload and symptoms of congestion
  - — arterial dilators, such as diltiazem hydrochloride and hydralazine, decrease afterload and improve cardiac output.
- The ACE inhibitors, e.g. enalapril and captopril, can cause haemodynamic and neurohormonal changes that lead to a reduction of preload and afterload, decreasing symptoms of heart failure. They might also deter the development of overt heart failure in some asymptomatic patients with left ventricular dysfunction.
- Beta-blockers are used to reduce the myocardial workload and myocardial contractility can be enhanced with, e.g. dopamine, but with caution, as inotropes increase myocardial oxygen demand and may produce arrhythmias. Arrhythmias associated with heart failure need to be treated to maximise cardiac output.

Patients with heart failure due to left ventricular dysfunction are usually prescribed a diuretic, an ACE inhibitor and a beta-blocker licensed for use in heart failure.

For further information on the pharmacological management of heart failure, see Gupta (2005).

Other treatment options for heart failure include intra-aortic balloon pump, revascularisation, biventricular pacing, valve replacement/repair, ventricular assist devices, cardiomyoplasty, ventricular volume reduction and heart transplant.

NURSING PRIORITIES AND MANAGEMENT: Heart failure

Patients with heart failure need a clinical assessment of cardiac output, cardiac rhythm, cognitive function, nutritional status and functional capacity. The patient's fluid balance status, blood urea, electrolytes and creatinine levels must be monitored to assess renal function and the effect of medication.

Acute heart failure may be a presenting problem in a CCU and heart failure following myocardial infarction is a poor prognostic sign. The manipulation of medication will form a major part of therapy for the patient admitted to hospital with an acute exacerbation of heart failure.

It is estimated that the average life expectancy of a patient with chronic heart failure is 4–5 years, and a reduced quality of life and concurrent depression are common (Mårtensson et al 2005). Patients and their families will need information and support to help them retain their independence for as long as possible. Nurse-led multidisciplinary intervention in chronic heart failure has the potential to yield substantial benefits for patients and family members, including reduced hospital admission rates and cost savings (McMurray & Stewart 1998). There is some evidence that nurse-led care of heart failure patients can increase quality of life for these patients (Mårtensson et al 2005).

The British Heart Foundation, the Department of Health and other national bodies (BHF et al 2003) have set out key aims for the local improvement of heart failure services and provide sources of information and examples of service models designed to help achieve the CHD National Service Framework (NSF) standards (DH 2000), the National Institute for Clinical Excellence (NICE) heart failure guidelines (NICE 2003) and the Scottish Intercollegiate Guidelines Network (SIGN) guidelines (1999).

For further reading about nurse-led care of the patient with heart failure, see Jaarsma & Stewart (2004).

Maintaining a safe environment

The prime concern for patients with heart failure is to restore haemodynamic stability, using a combination of medications to optimise cardiac function and control fluid loss through the kidneys. The effects of this therapy should be regularly assessed and practice nurses may be involved in monitoring the patient's weight, heart rate and rhythm. People living with heart failure should be taught how to monitor their pulse and to check their ankles for signs of oedema.

Breathing

The patient will often describe breathlessness, especially on exertion, as the main symptom. Difficulty in breathing can be a frightening and frustrating experience. Acute left ventricular failure leading to pulmonary oedema results in marked respiratory distress, agitation and production of copious frothy sputum. The priority is to reduce both the psychological and respiratory distress, using i.v. morphine, diuretics and oxygen therapy. Being with the patient and explaining what is being done in a reassuring way can allay anxiety and help the person through the alarming experience. The patient should be helped to sit upright and given high concentrations of oxygen to breathe. Reducing and spacing out energy demands may help to minimise difficulty in breathing. In hospital, the nurse is responsible for:

- ensuring that respiration is recorded regularly
- assessing the patient's subjective feelings about their breathing
- reporting acute episodes of dyspnoea
- administering oxygen therapy to help reduce anoxia, cautiously, in the patient with COAD (see Ch. 3)
- assessing the nature and amount of sputum
- working in partnership with the physiotherapist to apply chest physiotherapy and nasopharyngeal suctioning to help with sputum clearance.

At home the patient may need further advice around planning activities and symptom management. They should be supported to stop smoking.

Sleeping

Respiratory distress is often worse at night when the patient lies flat, and paroxysmal nocturnal dyspnoea is a very frightening experience. Sleeping supported with extra pillows helps. Patients with congestive failure may not sleep for long periods. Many doze for periods during the day. Some people stay in a chair at night, instead of going to bed, because of their respiratory distress. These factors should be remembered when patients are admitted to hospital. A restless patient awake in bed at 02.00 h may get more rest if they follow their normal pattern and are not constricted by hospital policy.

Elimination

Accurate estimation of fluid losses, in conjunction with daily weights, provides information on the effectiveness of diuretics; output should be in excess of 30 ml/h. Input of fluid and sodium should be restricted. Reducing sodium intake also often reduces the patient's thirst, which is very important if fluid intake is to be restricted to around 1 L/day. The use of loop diuretic therapy, such as furosemide, will cause loss of potassium. Potassium supplements are given and serum levels of potassium closely monitored to ensure they remain within normal limits, 3.5–5.5 mmol/L (see Ch. 20). To assist in the accurate assessment of haemodynamic status, a central venous catheter or pulmonary artery pressure catheter may be inserted.

Constipation should be avoided.

Oedema

Daily assessment of the extent of oedema will indicate the effectiveness of therapeutic intervention. All dependent areas should be assessed, including the spine and sacrum, if the patient is bed-bound. Patients at home should be taught how to monitor weight and the signs of oedema.

Nutrition

The patient should be encouraged to avoid salt at the table and to reduce the amount used in cooking. Herbs or salt substitutes can be used instead. In hospital, a low-salt diet may be rigidly enforced if the oedema is severe. Obese patients should also be on a reduced-calorie diet, to prevent further strain on the heart. Iron intake may need to be assessed if the person is anaemic.

Mobility

Rest is important for patients with congestive heart failure in order to reduce the cardiac workload and oxygen demand. In the acute phase, complete bed rest is advocated until pulmonary oedema is controlled. Activity is gradually increased until tolerated without signs of physical difficulty. A patient confined to bed or chair rest requires pillows for support to keep their breathing comfortable. With cardiac beds, both foot and head ends can be altered, helping to relieve respiratory distress, while aiding the peripheral drainage of fluid. Ankle swelling can be significantly reduced by walking and elevating the feet when sitting.

Work and leisure

People with heart failure may require help to live within their activity limits and to come to terms with the fact that they have a progressive disease for which there is no cure. Many people consider they are doomed to, and a few adopt, the role of invalid and dependant. The response to gradually increased activity is assessed to calculate the patient's functional capacity (see also the section on mobility for people with acute coronary syndrome, p. 31).

Personal hygiene

A patient with heart failure can usually retain independence in this area by taking certain precautions. Showers demand less energy expenditure than a bath, and a seat in the shower is helpful. A common difficulty is in drying the lower half of the body, because bending affects respiration, but by sitting, all parts of the body can be reached.

Someone with oedema will have very fragile, papery skin in the affected areas and great care must be taken not to break the skin by too much rubbing. Soap also has a drying effect on the skin; emulsifying oils may be better.

Communication

The importance of information being exchanged between the patient, family and health professionals cannot be overemphasised. It should be remembered that heart failure is a progressive disease which affects many people. The restrictions on mobility may confine these people to their home, further isolating them. Community cardiac specialist nurses, health visitors and practice nurses are increasingly involved in health assessment and screening. This assessment needs to take careful account of the social and psychological consequences, as well as the physical consequences, of disease processes and disability. It may be possible to arrange for attendance at a day hospital for those who wish it, or for a charity group such as Age Concern to provide transport to social events or day centres.

Sexuality

The patient's role within the family may have to alter as the disease increasingly restricts activities. Women may have to give up some household tasks to partners or to a home help. This can further demoralise them and requires tactful support from family and health professionals. Sexual activity may need to be modified if the individual's activity levels decrease or shortness of breath becomes a problem. The nurse needs to be equipped to offer realistic, non-judgemental advice (Westlake et al 1999).

VALVULAR DISORDERS

Adult valvular disease is either congenital or acquired. The effects of congenital problems largely manifest themselves in childhood and so are not discussed here.

The major causes of valve pathology are rheumatic heart disease (RHD), infective endocarditis and, to a lesser extent today, syphilis. Disease can cause narrowing (stenosis) of the valve, or regurgitation as a result of failure of the one-way valve, leading to blood back-flow through the valve. Major disruption can also result from papillary muscle dysfunction following myocardial infarction or penetrating chest wounds, when onset of symptoms can be sudden and severe.

Rheumatic heart disease

Rheumatic heart disease tends to be the result of rheumatic fever which is caused by group A streptococcal infection of the pharynx. It is usually a childhood ailment and shows seasonal variation, with a peak in colder months. Outbreaks of rheumatic fever are now more common in developing countries than they are in the West, especially within communities that are becoming progressively urbanised. In industrialised countries, the annual incidence is around 0.5 cases per 100 000 school-age children. However, in developing countries the annual incidence ranges from 100 to 200 children per 100 000 school-aged children (Olivier 2000). Poor housing and socioeconomic conditions exacerbate the problem. It may take up to 10 years before the signs of heart disease appear.

PATHOPHYSIOLOGY

The connective tissue of heart, joints and skin responds to infection by a proliferative and exudative inflammatory response with oedema and fragmentation of collagen fibres. The arthritic pain 'flits' from joint to joint and there is low-grade pyrexia. All layers of the heart can be affected. Endocarditis is most common, usually affecting the left side and involving the mitral valve, although any valve is at risk. The valve leaflets become inflamed and oedematous with small, firmly attached 'vegetations'. In the acute stages, this results in incompetence of the valve. Subsequent fibrosis deforms and thickens the leaflets and shortens the chordae tendineae, leading to stenosis with or without incompetence. Clinical outcome includes the need for surgical valve replacement, recurrence of rheumatic fever, endocarditis and thromboembolic events.

MEDICAL MANAGEMENT

Prophylactic antibiotic cover is instituted following the first occurrence of rheumatic fever and if this prevents recurrence then most of those who develop endocarditis will have a normal heart in the long term.

Infective endocarditis

The majority of cases are streptococcal or staphylococcal infections, although an increasing number of infective agents are being isolated, due to increasingly invasive medical techniques, such as in dental treatment or urinary investigation. Intravenous drug users also introduce bacteria into their body through use of contaminated needles.

PATHOPHYSIOLOGY

As well as being a cause of valvular disorder, those who have pre-existing valve disease or congenital lesions are at greater risk of developing bacterial endocarditis, as the underlying structures are already damaged and the blood flow is more turbulent. Certain sites are more favoured than others for bacterial proliferation. When blood flows from a high-pressure to a low-pressure system via a narrow orifice, the organisms tend to gather on the low-pressure side. If a high-pressure jet or regurgitant stream is created due to, for example, valve dysfunction, then satellite colonies will be seeded in the endothelial wall where the jet hits. In aortic regurgitation, for example, blood flows back from the high-pressure aorta via the supposedly closed aortic valve to the low-pressure left ventricle. Colonisation by bacteria would most likely occur on the ventricular surface of the aortic valve. Similar patterns can be elicited for other areas of dysfunction.

The vegetations of infective endocarditis, in contrast to those in rheumatic heart disease, are large and can aggregate to form up to 6 cm masses. This poses a double threat to the patient in that they:

- are more likely to embolise
- may cause ventricular insufficiency themselves by prolapsing into the valve orifice and obstructing flow.

Common presenting symptoms

Presentation may be slow and insidious, with general malaise, weight loss, lethargy, intermittent, often low-grade pyrexia, profuse sweating and joint pain. Microembolisation may manifest as splinter haemorrhages of the nail beds. If the infection has eroded tissue close to the valves where the conduction system lies, there may be evidence of rhythm and conduction disturbances. Evidence of embolisation may be seen in renal, cerebral, pulmonary and gastrointestinal systems. Myocardial infarction may also result from septic embolisation of the coronary arteries. Heart failure secondary to valve failure varies in its severity, depending on the valve affected and the acuteness of onset, and may give rise to shortness of breath and ankle oedema.

MEDICAL MANAGEMENT

Investigations should include ECG, chest X-ray and echocardiography. Cardiac catheterisation is also necessary for those referred for surgery to assess valve function, ventricular function and the patency of coronary arteries. Intravenous routes are normally used for long-term administration of antibiotic therapy. Patients should be advised about the importance of regular dental hygiene and prophylaxis when undergoing surgical procedures.

Valve stenosis and incompetence

Aortic stenosis

PATHOPHYSIOLOGY

The left ventricle becomes progressively hypertrophied, working at a higher pressure to eject blood past the stenosed valve. The chamber size of the ventricle is reduced by the increased muscle mass, which may itself contribute to outflow obstruction. This state is asymptomatic until the orifice is reduced to 0.5–0.7 cm^2 (normal 2.6–3.5 cm^2) when the patient may experience angina, as oxygen supply does not meet demand.

The other major effect is syncope, as cardiac output fails to rise in response to exercise. Hypertrophy may progress to decompensation and heart failure with rising LVEDP and pulmonary oedema. There is a link between aortic stenosis and gastrointestinal bleeding, known as Heyde's syndrome. However, the incidence of this is low (Pate & Mulligan 2005) and the problem usually subsides with valve replacement.

Mitral stenosis

PATHOPHYSIOLOGY

In this condition, the left atrium has to eject blood through a resistant valve. Left atrial pressure rises, and the atrium distends and eventually decompensates, with fibrous tissue interspersed between cardiac muscle. Conduction becomes aberrant and atrial fibrillation results, decreasing cardiac output as there is no atrial contribution to ventricular filling. If sinus rhythm persists, evidence of atrial hypertrophy can be seen on ECG. Since conduction takes longer to spread across the enlarged left atrium, the P wave becomes broadened and bifid. Left atrial pressure rises further with the stasis of blood within the chamber. This pressure increase is transmitted to the pulmonary vasculature, where vascular resistance rises with resultant greater right-sided afterload and possible failure. Acute elevations of pressure with exercise, for example, will precipitate pulmonary oedema. Stasis of blood allows the formation of mural thrombus within the atria. The obvious danger is that this may be dislodged and carried forward into the systemic circulation with profound ischaemic consequences for the area supplied by the embolised vessel (see Case History 2.2).

CASE HISTORY 2.2

K — living with mitral stenosis

K is an infant-school teacher in her early 30s. When she was 12 she developed rheumatic fever, thought to have resulted from a streptococcal throat infection, although it was not a common disorder and no-one else in her family had ever suffered from it. At that time she was in hospital for several weeks and left with inflammation of her mitral valve (valvulitis) which caused a progressive narrowing (stenosis) of her mitral valve over the years. On auscultation, K's mitral stenosis was identified by the characteristic diastolic murmur.

Until the age of 25, K felt quite healthy and often wondered just why she had to have regular medical checks and be prescribed antibiotics so quickly when some minor infection occurred. However, in her late 20s she began to experience breathlessness after various activities with the children at school. She often had to sit down, feeling light-headed, and developed a persistent, irritating cough. At first she dismissed it, but eventually she contacted her GP. Investigations showed that K's stenosis of the mitral valve was becoming worse and that she was developing the early signs of heart failure.

As a result of K's mitral stenosis, the pressure in the left atrium, pulmonary veins and capillaries increases. The left atrium dilates, fluid may accumulate in the alveoli, the pulmonary artery pressure rises, and the right ventricle hypertrophies. Systemic effects become apparent in the form of peripheral oedema, ascites and hepatic engorgement. Atrial fibrillation can occur which may potentiate pulmonary oedema and systemic emboli.

Managing such symptoms will include the use of anti-arrhythmic agents to control atrial fibrillation, diuretics, a low-sodium diet and anticoagulant therapy. K will have to adjust her lifestyle to accommodate her valvular disorder but she will be at home.

Aortic incompetence

PATHOPHYSIOLOGY

LVEDP is approximately one-eighth of the concomitant aortic pressure, and therefore any breach of the valve allows large amounts of blood to flow back into the ventricle. The ventricle dilates to accommodate this volume, LVEDP rises and stroke volume increases, as does systolic pressure. Diastolic pressure within the aorta is low because of regurgitation, and therefore there is a wide pulse pressure, often approximately 140 mmHg (190/50 mmHg). Chronic gradual aortic incompetence (AI) is well tolerated, but if there is an acute onset, left ventricular failure (LVF) quickly develops. AI also occurs when the valve annulus becomes dilated so that the cusps cannot coapt, e.g. in connective tissue disorders, syphilis and aortic dissection.

Mitral incompetence

PATHOPHYSIOLOGY

This allows back-flow of blood to the left atrium in systole, where regurgitated blood and the normal atrial volume mix and return to the ventricle during atrial systole. In order to cope with this increased load, the ventricle hypertrophies and then dilates. Forward flow diminishes, with progressive failure of the ventricle and with back-flow into the atria at systole. Weight loss and lethargy are marked as the heart can no longer provide the nutrition the blood usually carries. The left atrium dilates, and changes in conduction and rhythm occur.

Tricuspid stenosis and incompetence

PATHOPHYSIOLOGY

These result in increased right-sided pressure, with evidence of stasis and engorgement of the portal and peripheral circulations, e.g. ascites, liver dysfunction and peripheral oedema. If the right atrium becomes hypertrophied due to tricuspid stenosis, the P wave on the ECG will become peaked. The majority of right-sided failure is usually secondary to failure on the left; however, there is an increase in bacterial endocarditis of the right heart, with the increasing use, or abuse, of intravenous medication (see Ch. 36).

MEDICAL MANAGEMENT OF VALVULAR DISORDERS

The aim is to improve the haemodynamics by improving any aberrant rhythm, e.g. atrial fibrillation (AF), by digitalisation or cardioversion. This reduces the heart rate, allowing more time for filling the coronary arteries in the longer diastolic period. Atrial contribution to cardiac output is thereby regained. Congestive failure is relieved by diuretics and by reducing physical demands. Oxygen therapy may be of use for those with pulmonary congestion. Pyrexia should be investigated and treated appropriately. Anticoagulation may be commenced for those with evidence of previous embolisation, i.e. those in AF and those in low output states with left and right failure. The latter may require inotropic support to increase cardiac output and renal perfusion. Sudden onset with pulmonary oedema, e.g. with papillary muscle rupture post-AMI, requires artificial ventilation, full monitoring, afterload reduction and the possible aid of an intra-aortic balloon pump (IABP) as in cardiogenic shock (see Ch. 18) to gain time prior to urgent surgery.

Those with chronic disease processes may be maintained on long-term medication.

Valvuloplasty

This involves a catheter being introduced across the stenotic valve, the balloon is then inflated and the calcified stenosis cracked and opened up.

In the mitral position, the approach is across the septum, while with the aortic valve the catheter is introduced retrogradely. Problems include:

- bradycardias
- profound hypotension when the balloon is inflated
- embolisation
- tamponade
- possible myocardial rupture.

The aim of valvuloplasty is to increase the functional area of the valve and therefore cardiac output. It is particularly appropriate for older people with aortic stenosis, for whom a full operation would hold too many risks but whose life expectancy would be short without it. It has the advantage of a short hospital stay and the prompt resumption of normal life. An alternative would be prosthetic valve replacement. This surgery is used for patients where valvuloplasty is unsuitable or unsuccessful. Valve repair may be considered early on in the disease process before valve replacement is an option. Valve replacement with a mechanical or bioprosthetic valve, made from animal or human tissue, must be performed before the patient is too unwell to tolerate the operation. The choice of valve tends to be determined by the patient's age and the surgeon's preference. The patient undergoes a median sternotomy and valve replacement or repair using cardiopulmonary bypass. The patient who has had a mechanical device fitted needs to become accustomed to hearing it click during each cardiac cycle.

NURSING PRIORITIES AND MANAGEMENT: The patient with valvular disease

Breathing

Shortness of breath, often initially on exertion, is the hallmark of progressive heart failure and ongoing respiratory assessment is important. In some patients, sudden valvular failure may result in an alarming onset of breathlessness. In others, it is a slow progressive problem which starts with breathlessness on exertion and eventually also breathlessness at rest. Orthopnoea (breathlessness in the supine position) may also occur and the increasing number of pillows people require in order to breathe comfortably is an indicator of the progression of their disease. Diuretic therapy is used to reduce fluid in the pulmonary interstitium. Sudden valve failure can be very alarming and these patients may require an urgent operation. They should be within sight of the nursing staff and have means of summoning help. An upright position, well supported by pillows, helps chest expansion.

Nutrition

General fatigue may be the major limiting factor in maintaining adequate nutrition. Small, frequent meals may be more easily digested. They should be high in protein and carbohydrate, especially if the metabolism is raised by fever. Long-term mitral valve insufficiency does not allow sufficient forward flow of oxygenated blood to nourish the peripheries. The nutritional state of people with valvular disorders should be optimised prior to surgery, and liver failure may be a problem due to right-sided heart failure, secondary to the primary left-sided failure (see Ch. 4).

The advice of the dietitian will be valuable. High-protein, commercially available drinks can be given to supplement the diet; however, fluid restriction might also be necessary to prevent pulmonary oedema. Fluid restriction and oxygen therapy often leave the mouth dry, and sucking ice or frozen fruit juice helps to keep the mouth as fresh as possible, while minimising fluid intake.

Personal hygiene

The ability to look after personal hygiene may be limited by fatigue and breathlessness. The community nursing team can help at home with bathing and can arrange, through the occupational therapist, to provide aids that make getting in and out of the bath or shower easier. Helping patients in this way allows nurses to assess perfusion of the peripheries. Those who experience sweating associated with aortic insufficiency may need more frequent attention to personal freshness.

Sleeping

It can be difficult to sleep due to shortness of breath, even when sitting upright. Each person may have to amend daily activities to allow for periods of rest. Nursing care should be similarly planned.

Mobility

Movement may be limited by the symptoms of the individual. If restricted to bed rest, deep breathing and leg exercises should be encouraged. People whose activities are limited at home might benefit from a home help or may be eligible for mobility allowance. Advice can be sought from the social services department.

Local authorities issue car stickers for disabled people to allow greater access to public amenities and car parking.

Wheelchair use

Access to public buildings is slowly improving; public planning incorporates wheelchair access, and many older buildings have been adapted to cater for the less mobile. Lists of places that are suitable for access are available at tourist information centres, city council offices and certain website addresses. Wheelchairs can also be provided to enable people to tour exhibitions or to travel more easily between trains and aircraft, and most large travel organisations provide this service. Holiday brochures often specify which hotels are easily accessible. The Red Cross also hires out wheelchairs and aids for limited periods.

The government website www.direct.gov.uk has links to information on disabled access in the home, employment and for leisure pursuits.

For patients who have had surgery, mobility is regained gradually. Each person should set themselves the daily goal of walking a little further. Strenuous exercise should be avoided until the sternum heals; for example, any sport involving swinging movements of the arms, such as golf, could prevent the bone edges from knitting together. Some surgeons restrict strenuous exercise for longer, since they feel too great a pressure gradient can be developed across the prosthetic valve with the increased cardiac output brought about by exercise.

Work and recreation

Some lines of work may prove too strenuous, necessitating a change of job. After cardiac valve surgery, the patient will be unable to return to work for at least 3 months. Returning part-time is desirable, as people often tire easily at first. This can gradually be increased to full-time. Heavy physical work should be avoided for 6 months. The employer may be able to provide lighter work initially but still involve the person in the working environment. Some work is no longer possible after cardiac surgery, e.g. an HGV licence cannot be held. Advice from the social worker about claiming social security allowance and information about retraining schemes can be given, if appropriate. Worry about loss of income can add to the stress of undergoing major surgery.

Maintaining a safe environment

Once a prosthetic valve is in situ, the recipient should be aware of how to avoid putting the valve and themselves at risk. Anticoagulation with warfarin is required for life in those with metal valves, and for a shorter time for those with tissue valves. The person should understand the action of the drugs and their potential risks. They should also be aware of the risk of infection and should inform other health professionals, e.g. dentists, that they have a prosthetic valve and are taking warfarin. Antibiotic cover is given for dental treatment and any other invasive investigation.

Driving is to be avoided until the sternum heals, as sudden movement, e.g. to avoid an accident, could disrupt sternal wire sutures, as could sudden impact to the chest. A small pillow between the seat belt and the chest can reduce friction on the wound, but does not necessarily absorb impact. Eyesight, especially of those who wear glasses, and concentration span are both affected for some weeks after cardiopulmonary bypass.

Sexuality

In relation to sexual activity, avoiding strain on the sternal suture line is the most important limitation until the bone heals, but after that, resumption of relationships should not be excluded. Intimacy between couples can be maintained without full intercourse prior to this. Fear that the valve will fail under exertion should be allayed. Currently, there is no clear consensus on the optimal type of cardiac valve prosthesis that should be placed in women of childbearing age (Mihaljevic et al 2005). The risks of reoperative surgery for bioprosthetic valves must be weighed against those of anticoagulation therapy required for mechanical valves. Some surgeons recommend that young women with prosthetic valves do not become pregnant, because of the increase in circulating volume and cardiac workload. Although successful pregnancies have been completed, this should be as planned an event as possible. Women of childbearing age tend to be given tissue valves, as this allows the period of anticoagulation to be relatively short. Warfarin taken during pregnancy can cause birth defects, especially if taken during the first trimester of pregnancy. Oral contraceptives also inhibit the effects of warfarin. Some may find the prospect of sharing a bed with a partner who 'ticks' off-putting, especially as increases in heart rate can be clearly heard, which can increase fears that catastrophic events will take place during intercourse. These people can be reassured that the metallic noise becomes softened with time. For some patients, tissue valves might be considered, although they have a shorter life span and would require replacement within a few years.

For further information on valve disease, see Otto (2003).

STOP THINK

2.7 The continuing care of patients with valvular disorders is essentially carried out in the community. The desired outcome for someone like K in Case History 2.2 is that:

- she enjoys a full and happy life within the limitations imposed by her disorder
- she can cope with the medication and dietary restrictions
- she maintains nursing advice and support.

Which members of the primary health care team will support K? What will their priorities be in caring for K at home?

Grown up congenital heart (GUCH) disease

Whilst the demand for health care for children born with congenital heart disease is likely to remain relatively stable, the numbers of adults with complex congenital heart disease is predicted to increase significantly. The British Cardiac Society Working Party on grown up congenital heart disease estimated that by the year 2010 there will over 185 000 adults living with congenital heart disease in the UK (British Cardiac Society 2002). These patients may require admission to hospital for the control of arrhythmias, cardiac catheterisation and the treatment of heart failure. An accessible and dedicated ward area for these patients is recommended. Patients in the community may need support and advice on issues such as contraception and pregnancy, the risks of infective endocarditis and general lifestyle advice.

HYPERTENSION

Hypertension is difficult to define and there is controversy as to what level of pressure, systolic or diastolic, constitutes hypertension. In adults, the considered upper limit of normal is 130–139/85–89 mmHg and pressures consistently above this are defined as hypertension. The optimal blood pressure targets are a systolic blood pressure of less than 120 mmHg and a diastolic blood pressure of less than 80 mmHg (Williams et al 2004). The technique of measuring blood pressure can also vary, resulting in differences, principally in diastolic definition. The scope of the problem may well be underestimated since the majority of people are without symptoms until target organs are affected. They then present with major consequences such as renal failure, ischaemic heart disease, cerebral emboli or infarction.

Being aware of associated predisposing factors may enable health workers to target screening towards at-risk groups.

Associated factors

Several factors associated with hypertension have been identified:

- obesity
- sodium intake
- alcohol
- genetic factors
- smoking
- stress.

Obesity

The interaction between obesity and hypertension is not fully understood. Overweight adolescents are at significant risk of later hypertension. Those involved in health education and school nursing may play an important part in educating children about diet and exercise in general. An increased intake of sodium will result from general overeating and it is thought that the sodium pump may become impaired in this group. However, this is a reversible situation. Blood pressure has been shown to decrease with weight loss, particularly with a weight reduction programme that incorporates moderate sodium, high potassium and a low fat diet (Nowson et al 2005).

Sodium intake

The link between sodium and hypertension may result from increased sodium and water retention by the kidneys in response to an increased sodium load. Sodium accumulates within the arterial walls of hypertensive people. These vessels then become more responsive to substances that cause vasoconstriction. People who reduce their sodium intake also reduce their blood pressure. High sodium intake is a feature of Western lifestyle and more isolated peoples with a lower intake have a lower incidence of hypertension; once they adopt a Western diet the incidence rises. Adherence to low-sodium diets is poor, as they are so unpalatable. Emphasis is now laid on not adding salt after cooking and salt substitutes are widely available. There is a generally increased awareness of the contents of packaged foodstuffs; clear product labelling helps people at risk to identify substances that contain sodium.

An increase in potassium intake through consumption of fruits, vegetables and beans is reported to be beneficial in lowering blood pressure (Lydakis et al 1997).

Alcohol

The contribution of alcohol is difficult to assess, as there is a tendency to under-report alcohol consumption due to social pressures. However, blood pressure rises with increasing intake and a reduction in intake reverses this.

Genetic factors

A family history of hypertension predisposes individuals to the same condition. Certain ethnic groups are more susceptible to the condition: the black population in the USA has a 50% greater prevalence than their white counterparts. It appears that the mean resting renal blood flow of normotensive individuals with hypertensive parents is greater than in those with normotensive parents. The kidneys' ability to handle sodium is also thought to be genetically influenced.

Smoking

Nicotine promotes catecholamine release and so increases heart rate and blood pressure.

Stress

This is presumed to relate to increased sympathetic outflow (see Ch. 17). Certain occupations are associated with a higher risk of developing hypertension, e.g. crane drivers and air traffic controllers. People who work in noisy overstimulating environments also run a higher risk of occupational stress, especially if the tasks are repetitive and monotonous.

PATHOPHYSIOLOGY

Although difficult to define in terms of elevated blood pressure, hypertension is commonly classified according to cause:

- Primary or essential hypertension refers to a raised blood pressure where no cause can be found.
- Secondary hypertension is a result of the underlying conditions, most commonly:
  - — renal disease (see Ch. 8)
  - — an adrenaline-secreting tumour, e.g. phaeochromocytoma in the adrenal medulla
  - — diseases of the pituitary or adrenal cortex, where there is an elevation of glucocorticoids, e.g. Cushing's disease (see Ch. 5)
  - — coarctation (narrowing) of the aorta
  - — hyperthyroidism (see Ch. 5).

Hypertension can also be classified according to severity:

- mild — when elevation of blood pressure is only moderate and occurs over a long period of time
- malignant — when there is a sudden and severe blood pressure elevation.

The malignancy does not refer to cellular changes but to the fact that this is a life-threatening condition. Whatever form of hypertension is diagnosed, the concern is always the effect of this high blood pressure:

- on the heart, where the increased demand on its pumping capacity can lead to ventricular hypertrophy
- on the brain, where any elevation of blood pressure could precipitate a cerebral catastrophe (see Ch. 9).

Other organs that give rise to concern are the kidneys, where the delicate function of the nephrons can be impaired by constant high pressure, and the eyes, where fine retinal vessels may rupture and significantly impair vision.

Common presenting symptoms

People who are aware that they have a condition that predisposes them to hypertension will have been alerted to this potential problem and the symptoms may be more readily appreciated. However, many may be completely unaware of their hypertensive state, either having no symptoms at all or dismissing complaints such as headaches, vertigo, nosebleeds and fatigue.

MEDICAL MANAGEMENT

Examination

The elevated blood pressure may only be noticed at a routine examination for another reason, such as insurance cover. A single elevated reading does not justify a diagnosis of hypertension since anxiety about the examination itself may be the temporary cause; however, the person should be reassessed at a later date. Examiners should also be aware of the possible contribution their own technique and instrument calibration may make to errors in estimation, e.g. using inappropriately sized cuffs.

Generally, hypertension is defined by grading, with arbitrary cut-off points according to diastolic pressure.

Grade 1 hypertension is defined as a systolic blood pressure 140–159 mmHg or diastolic 90–99 mmHg or both. Grade 2 hypertension is a blood pressure greater than or equal to 160/100 mmHg (Williams et al 2004). The higher the diastolic pressure, the greater the risk of cerebrovascular accident (CVA), renal failure, coronary artery disease and heart failure.

Treatment of hypertension has been shown to reduce the relative risks of cardiovascular mortality and morbidity by 30% (Collins & Peto 1994). The management of the patient with hypertension is generally the responsibility of the primary health care team and hospitalisation is not usually required.

Investigations

include:

- blood pressure monitoring
- chest X-ray and ECG to determine the degree of left ventricular hypertrophy and heart failure
- full blood count, electrolytes, urea or nitrogen and creatinine, to exclude secondary causes and renal effects of the disease process
- urinalysis with microscopy, 24-h collections for creatinine clearance and vanillylmandelic acid (VMA)
- intravenous urogram (IVU) to assess renal perfusion.

Treatment

depends largely on how elevated the blood pressure is and the total risk of CVD. All adults should have their blood pressure measured routinely at least every 5 years. Those with 'high normal' systolic blood pressure (130–139 mmHg) or diastolic blood pressure 85–89 mmHg and those with previously elevated readings, should have their blood pressure measured annually (Williams et al 2004). All hypertensive patients should have a thorough history and physical examination. Medication is recommended in all patients with grade 2 hypertension. All patients with grade 1 hypertension should be offered treatment with antihypertensive medication if there is any complication of hypertension, target organ damage, diabetes mellitus or significant risk of CVD. Most people require more than one type of medication to control blood pressure. Care needs to be taken not to lower the blood pressure too far as this may cause feelings of light-headedness and fainting. Beta-blockers and ACE inhibitors are the first choice for younger patients. Calcium channel blockers and diuretics are more effective for older patients. The formulation used should ideally be effective for 24 h when taken as a single daily dose and titrated up to the manufacturer's recommendations.

STOP THINK **2.8** Using the *British National Formulary*, look at how the different antihypertensive medications exert their effect and why different agents might be used for different patients.

Certain lifestyle measures can reduce blood pressure (Williams et al 2004), including:

- maintaining a body mass index of 20–25 kg/m^2
- limiting alcohol consumption to three units a day or less for men and two units a day or less for women
- reducing intake of total and saturated fat
- eating at least five portions of fruit and vegetables a day.

Investigation for secondary causes of hypertension should ensue promptly. Tests should include assays for evidence of renal disease, primary aldosteronism, hypothyroidism and phaeochromocytoma, while urgent assessment and control of blood pressure take place. It may be that the hypertension is a side-effect of other treatment, e.g. oral contraception. Only 4–5% of women taking 'the pill' develop overt hypertension due to oestrogen ingestion, but it may take several months for it to settle. Other forms of contraception should be advised. Hypertension is also one of the signs of pre-eclampsia of pregnancy.

Overzealous treatment to achieve good blood pressure figures, rather than a good effect for the individual, should be avoided. Many people with hypertension have coexisting CHD, even if asymptomatic, and since the extraction of oxygen within the coronary circulation is close to maximum at rest, lowering the blood pressure may further compromise the coronary circulation, causing myocardial ischaemia.

Malignant elevation At any point in primary hypertension, sudden acute elevation of pressure can occur. This malignant hypertension can rapidly become life threatening. Death can ensue from CVA or from the cerebral oedema of hypertensive encephalopathy. Hypertension generally promotes the progression of atherosclerosis. Sudden increased pressure in vessels already compromised may lead to rupture or embolisation of existing thrombus. The importance of this depends on where the emboli occlude. Further occlusion of the afferent arterioles exacerbates the situation by stimulating increased renin release, which in turn contributes to the hypertensive state. Increased pressure may result in internal haemorrhage or infarction of the kidneys.

The progress of the increasing pressure is mirrored in changes to the vessels of the optic fundi, termed hypertensive retinopathy (see Ch. 12). Once papilloedema occurs, intracranial pressure has increased and the individual may complain of blurring of vision.

Management of hypertensive crisis

The aim of medical and nursing management of this life-threatening condition is a controlled reduction in blood pressure, with monitoring of other systems in order to minimise further damage or to prevent it from occurring (Shayne & Pitts 2003). Cerebral function should be assessed continuously. Blood pressure should be monitored, preferably by direct arterial cannulation, at least every 15 min to assess the efficacy of medication. Cardiac demand should be reduced as much as possible by bed rest and sedation. Straining at stool should be avoided. The patient should have urinary catheterisation and frequent observation of urine output. A 24-h urine collection should be commenced for excretory products of catecholamines, such as VMA, levels being twice that of normal in the presence of the adrenal tumour, phaeochromocytoma. The nurse should also be alert for haematuria or any other sign of blood loss. Complaints of ischaemic chest pain should be investigated and treated as already described.

Anxiolytic medication may benefit people whose condition is exacerbated by anxiety.

NURSING PRIORITIES AND MANAGEMENT: Hypertension

Where hypertension is secondary to an underlying condition, nursing priorities will reflect treatment of the primary problem. Hypertension will affect lifestyle and sense of well-being in many ways. However, since people with hypertension present in various ways, it is difficult to generalise about their management plans.

The experience of pain

Pain control is necessary for those experiencing headaches or anginal pain, with or without palpitations. Oral analgesics can be prescribed to combat headaches although the prescription may have to be tailored to the individual to find an effective agent. This symptom may only lessen once the level of hypertension is controlled and this may motivate the patient to comply with other treatments. Angina will be approached as previously discussed and will also be helped by other treatments aimed at lowering blood pressure, e.g. beta-blockade.

Nutrition

Dietary changes are aimed at the reduction of obesity, the control of any underlying problem such as diabetes mellitus, and the reduction of the salt content. A diet rich in fruits, vegetables and low-fat dairy food with reduced saturated total fat can substantially lower blood pressure (Cutler et al 1997). It is best to involve the whole family, as it is less socially disruptive if everyone can continue to sit down to the same meals together. Also, the hereditary aspect of hypertension would indicate that it is in the whole family's interest to prevent the problem developing. No salt added at table, or salt substitutes, are advised (see p. 51). The nurse may be able to assist patients in interpreting labels on food products.

Moderating alcohol intake is advised. This may be difficult for some, where entertaining forms a great part of their work; however, low-alcohol wines and beers are increasingly available.

Elimination

Diuretic medication can result in the need to pass urine at socially inconvenient times. This can often be avoided if the medications are taken first thing in the morning, so that their effect is largely over by the time the person leaves home. Discussing the person's daily routine and flexibility in the timing of treatment to adapt to the person's lifestyle can result in greater adherence to treatment. It is often difficult for an asymptomatic individual to realise the importance of continuing with medication, especially if there are undesirable side-effects. It is often best to broach the subject of side-effects before they occur and to point out that other medication can be tried if one medication does not suit.

Diuretics — apart from the aldosterone antagonist, potassium-sparing varieties — promote the excretion of potassium in the urine. Low levels of potassium can result in muscle weakness, fatigue and cardiac arrhythmias. It is therefore important that potassium supplementation is also adhered to by those taking diuretics. Many products combine both diuretic and potassium. A list of foods rich in potassium, e.g. bananas, can be supplied.

Sleeping

Relaxation and rest are important. Daily routines should be examined in order to find appropriate periods for rest. Night sedation may be necessary to ensure adequate sleep, although the patient should be encouraged to maintain their own relaxation habits, e.g. soaking in a warm bath. Referral to agencies that practise relaxation and stress management techniques may be of benefit to some (see Ch. 17).

Work and leisure

Some working environments may add to the stress experienced by individuals. Work routines should be re-examined to see if more opportunity exists for delegation of work and for rest. Smoking may be a habit engendered by stress and reinforced by working with a group of people in similar positions. Finding interests other than work may help the 'workaholic'. Sporting hobbies should be encouraged, as exercise will increase cardiac fitness as long as strenuous exercise is not embarked on without advice.

Breathing

Every effort should be made to stop smoking. Various approaches exist, from cigarette substitutes to hypnosis, acupuncture and sheer willpower. People should be encouraged to find their own way and, as in changing eating habits, the whole family can also be involved here.

Beta-blockade, using the non-cardioselective varieties, e.g. propranolol, may result in bronchospasm. This side-effect could be extremely alarming if the patient is not aware of the possibility.

Sexuality

Anxiety and tension between couples may lead to sexual dysfunction. Openness on the part of health professionals may help couples to feel they can discuss their fears with these professionals and with each other. Beta-blockade may also cause impotence.

For more information on hypertension, see Wilkinson et al (2002).

AORTIC ANEURYSMS

An aneurysm is a permanent dilatation of the aorta with a diameter at least 50% greater than would be expected. The aneurysm can be localised or extend along the length of the aorta.

The aorta is divided into three segments:

- the ascending aorta
- the arch
- the descending aorta, which consists of abdominal and thoracic portions.

Aneurysms are also classified by shape, as being:

- fusiform — involving a complete circumferential section
- saccular — an outpouching from one weakened area.

Saccular aneurysms can be tied off surgically at the neck of the sac, while fusiform types require excision and replacement with a tubular graft. If the graft is required close to the aortic valve, a composite prosthetic valve and tube graft may be employed, with reimplantation of the coronary arteries if necessary.

There are several causes of aneurysm formation:

- *Atherosclerotic disease*. This is the major cause of aneurysms, especially of the descending portion, 75% of the aorta being below the level of the diaphragm. Plaque formation reduces the nutritional supply to the aortic wall by hampering diffusion of nutrients from blood in the lumen.
- *Turbulence around bifurcations.*
- *Hypertension and medial degeneration*. The medial layer of the vessel wall undergoes degenerative changes associated with ageing. Since this is the layer that, due to its elasticity, withstands the most pressure, degeneration allows the wall to dilate. This often occurs without symptoms and may be found on routine examination. The patient is often hypertensive. Increased blood pressure, especially diastolic pressure, reduces the blood flow to the medial layer, which becomes ischaemic and weakened.
- *Cystic medial degeneration* also occurs as a consequence of connective tissue diseases, e.g. Marfan's and Ehlers–Danlos syndromes. These affect the ascending aorta and may cause the annulus of the aortic valve to dilate. This may result in an incompetent valve, as the cusps cannot completely cover the larger area. First presentation may be as a consequence of valvular failure.
- *Infection*. Aneurysms due to syphilis and other infectious causes are less prevalent today; they largely affect the ascending aorta.

Abdominal aortic aneurysms (AAAs)

The abdominal aorta is the most frequent site of aneurysm formation, affecting 2–5% of the male population over 60 years with a male:female ratio of 4:1 (Sternbergh et al 1998).

PATHOPHYSIOLOGY

Common presenting symptoms

The majority of AAAs are without symptoms, but a pulsating abdominal mass may be felt when lying in bed. Pain relates to compression of neighbouring organs. It is severe, unrelated to movement and radiates through to the low back, and possibly down into the thighs and buttocks. Presentation may be due to ischaemia of the end organs whose arterial supply originates within the aneurysmal section. Ischaemia may also be the result of embolisation of thrombus that gathers in the dilated portion due to sluggish blood flow and turbulence around atherosclerotic plaques. Diagnosis is made by ultrasonography, magnetic resonance imaging (MRI) and computed tomography (CT) scanning. Half of the dilatations greater than 6 cm will rupture within a year, so prompt surgical management is called for. Surgical repair involves either a midline incision for a retroperitoneal approach or a transverse approach above the umbilicus if the aneurysm is above the renal arteries and there is renal involvement. The aneurysm is clamped above and below the swelling and the thrombus removed. A synthetic graft is laid within the aneurysmal sac and sutured in place. The sac is trimmed and sewn over the graft. Older or cardiorespiratory-compromised patients may be unsuitable for surgical repair. Endovascular repair involving stent insertion into the affected lumen may be more appropriate for these patients (Ransome 1996). The risk of spontaneous dissection is that severe blood loss, hypotension and death will supervene. Emboli may enter the inferior vena cava and result in pulmonary infarction. Mortality in patients with a ruptured aneurysm is high. Emergency management aims to stabilise blood pressure by large volume infusion of colloid or other volume expanders and by pharmacological support with inotropic medication. Surgical repair should not be delayed.

For further information on the care of the patient undergoing surgical repair of an abdominal aortic aneurysm, see Collins (2003).

MEDICAL MANAGEMENT

Investigations
prior to planned surgery include abdominal X-ray, which will highlight any vessel calcification, echocardiography, ultrasound and CT scanning, all of which are non-invasive. Some centres also perform angiography; however, this may precipitate embolisation. Full cardiac investigation is required since atherosclerosis is a diffuse disease. Correction of any coronary insufficiency is recommended prior to surgical non-emergency aneurysm repair, since postoperative mortality is largely due to myocardial infarction.

Thoracic aneurysms

The aetiology is similar to aneurysms in the abdomen. False thoracic aneurysms can be secondary to blunt or penetrating injury to the chest in road traffic accidents, although they are more often associated with true rupture of the aorta, from which mortality is high. Some thoracic aneurysms are stabilised by surrounding tissue which can allow time for the patient to present at cardiothoracic services.

PATHOPHYSIOLOGY

Atherosclerosis affects the arch and descending thoracic aorta, while cystic medial degeneration and infections are found as causative agents in the ascending portion.

Common presenting symptoms
depend on the site of occurrence. Chest X-ray shows a widened mediastinum. Dilatation causes pressure on other structures: bronchospasm may result from deviation of the trachea, secretion retention and alveolar collapse from obstruction, shortness of breath and haemoptysis, if erosion occurs into the left main bronchus. Obstruction of the oesophagus may present as dysphagia, while fainting may be the result of reduced cardiac output due to obstruction of the superior vena cava.

Dissecting aortic aneurysms

PATHOPHYSIOLOGY

Tears in the intima due to the forces of hypertension, and the degenerative changes already discussed, allow a column of blood to enter and disrupt the media, creating a false lumen. Classification is by site of the tear. In addition to previously discussed predisposing diseases, there is a higher, but as yet unexplained, incidence of dissection among pregnant women.

Common presenting symptoms
depend upon the site and severity of the rupture. Severe anterior chest pain can be mistaken for acute myocardial infarction, but it is often described as tearing in nature. Pain may migrate as the dissection progresses. Alterations of neurological function may reflect involvement of the vessels originating from the arch of the aorta. As the dissection progresses, loss of peripheral pulses and palpable blood pressure will track its course. Renal artery dissection or occlusion will result in acute renal failure, exacerbated by the effects of profound hypotension. Alterations in rhythm or degrees of heart block may result from septal disruption as a consequence of aortic valve regurgitation. Leakage into the pericardium manifests as compression known as tamponade. The signs of cardiac tamponade are:

- hypotension
- tachycardia
- raised central venous pressure/jugular venous pressure
- oliguria
- peripheral vascular constriction
- fall in peripheral temperature.

If uncorrected, i.e. by pericardial aspiration of blood, this will lead to the state of pulseless electrical activity (PEA), cardiac arrest and death.

MEDICAL MANAGEMENT

Investigations
are identical to those used in AAAs.

Treatment
Operative correction is urgently required. If hypertension persists, this should be controlled by the use of arterial vasodilators, intensively and invasively monitored. If hypotension and collapse have supervened, then intervention is as for AAAs.

NURSING PRIORITIES AND MANAGEMENT: Aortic aneurysms

Pain control

The pain is often described as ripping or tearing in nature. Its location varies according to the section of artery affected and may progress as the dissection progresses. Intravenous opioids are the analgesia of choice because of their associated sedative effect and the slight vasodilatation achieved, both of which encourage a reduction in blood pressure.

Anxiety and fear of dying

The prospect of surgery is extremely frightening, whether emergency or elective, and this should be acknowledged by nurses. Operations carry high risks, but there is often no alternative intervention. Those going for elective procedures may wish access to legal advisors. The need for spiritual care should also be recognised. There may be times when a dignified, peaceful death is more appropriate than surgery.

Maintaining a safe environment

Rupture of an aneurysmal vessel is a potentially catastrophic and unpredictable event. Those with known aneurysms that do not yet merit surgery should be aware of signs that indicate a progression of their disease. Control of hypertension by medication is indicated (see p. 52).

Breathing

Shortness of breath may be experienced by those with aneurysms of the thoracic aorta as the vessel impinges on the trachea. This may also result in bronchospasm. Rupture of the vessel can create a fistula into the bronchus, with resulting haemoptysis. Changing the person's position to allow maximal lung expansion may help. Oxygen therapy will be required. Bronchodilators may be of limited use, as the problem is mechanical rather than irritant. Chest infection due to atelectasis, as the lung may collapse under the weight of the expanding aorta, is to be expected. Since maintaining the airway is a potential problem, an airway, suction equipment, an Ambu-bag and other resuscitation equipment should be available.

Mobility and rest

Anxiety may prevent the patient from sleeping, so sedation may be helpful if the blood pressure is not adversely affected. The patient's condition can be so unstable that even performing minimal care can be exhausting. Care should be planned so that people are left in peace for periods. Nurses sometimes have to accept that their patient's condition will not allow care that would otherwise be thought essential, e.g. pressure area care. Consider the use of aids to dissipate pressure on what is often already poorly perfused skin.

Elimination

Since approximately 25% of cardiac output perfuses the kidneys, urine output is an important indicator of cardiac function. Accurate observation and recording of fluid balance are essential.

Personal hygiene

Because of poor general status and poor tissue perfusion, this is an area where the patient becomes dependent on a nurse to maintain standards of personal hygiene.

Sexuality

People attending electively for resection of abdominal aneurysms may be offered counselling before surgery. There is a possibility of impotence and paraplegia postoperatively if the arterial supply to the spinal cord is interrupted. It is possible to arrange storage of sperm against this eventuality. These issues need to be handled with sensitivity by the nursing and medical staff.

Surgical intensive care

If the patient's condition has deteriorated and surgery is necessary, they are completely dependent on hospital staff for circulatory support. Accurate haemodynamic assessment is essential. Careful observation and documentation of the response to medication and large-volume colloid infusion are essential. This may require invasive monitoring and the specialist nursing skills of the intensive care unit, and the patient should be moved to such a unit as soon as is feasible. This may mean a journey of several hours by road or air, a daunting prospect for patient and escorting staff alike. It often necessitates the separation of the patient from their family at a time of great stress, so every effort should be made to ensure effective communication. The management of cardiogenic shock is described in Chapter 18. Postoperative care is similar to that following cardiac surgery (see Nursing Care Plan 2.1).

For further information on the care of the patient with an abdominal aortic aneurysm, see Collins (2003).

PERIPHERAL VASCULAR DISEASE

Peripheral vascular disease includes pathological processes affecting both the arterial and venous circulations. Arterial and venous peripheral disease can occur alone or together and it is important to be able to differentiate between the two.

Revise the vascular anatomy of the lower limbs (Waugh & Grant 2001). For information on the aetiology and pathology of vascular disease, see Ockenden (2003); for information on the assessment of patients with vascular disease, see Stubbling & Chesworth (2003).

ARTERIAL DISEASE

Arterial occlusions

Atherosclerosis is the commonest cause of arterial disease. It is characterised by the development of atherosclerotic plaques within the intima of the artery wall which inhibit arterial blood flow. Symptoms of impaired blood supply may be slow to appear if collateral circulation has had time to develop.

Arteriosclerosis obliterans

PATHOPHYSIOLOGY

This is the state of chronic occlusive atheroma of the arteries supplying the extremities. Turbulence at bifurcations, as occurs in larger vessels, predisposes to intimal changes. There is also a degenerative element in its development. The same process is found in the cerebral and visceral arteries. The factors influencing its development have been discussed in the section on CHD. It is typically a disease of middle-aged to older men, who may be hypertensive,

Nursing Care Plan 2.1

G is a 54-year-old unemployed welder who had an abdominal aortic aneurysm repair 36 h previously. This was an elective operation and involved the insertion of a synthetic graft. Since the operation G has been cared for in an intensive care unit. He had artificial respiratory support on a ventilator up until 12 h ago. A urinary catheter, nasogastric tube and central venous pressure line were inserted in theatre. G's wife and family are very concerned about his condition and his wife is spending most of the day at his bedside.

Nursing considerations	Action	Rationale	Expected outcome
1. Potential problem of hypovolaemic shock	• Continue to monitor vital signs, noting for: – fall in blood pressure – increase in heart rate • Observe for fall in hourly urine output • Observe for changes in mental state: restlessness, confusion • Note and report significant changes in temperature • Observe for signs of peripheral oedema and cold, pale peripheries • Observe wound site for excessive leakage • Give intravenous fluids as prescribed: colloids, crystalloids and inotropic support as necessary • Continue with central venous pressure recordings, noting and reporting trends	Hypovolaemic shock may arise due to excessive blood loss/inadequate fluid replacement or rapid warming	Stable vital signs Urine output >30 mL/h Stable neurological function
2. Possibility of developing hypertension	• Regular measurement of blood pressure • Monitor effects of any hypertensive medication • Ensure that G knows to report any pain/discomfort Assess and plan intervention, and evaluate pain relief measures • Observe wound site regularly for any sign of suture line being under stress due to increased blood pressure • Attempt to limit anxiety by providing information and support, and creating a calm, relaxed atmosphere for G and his family	May have been hypertensive prior to operation Systemic vascular response may increase as a result of: – decreased circulatory volume – increased sympathetic tone as a stress response High blood pressure may cause bleeding around the graft site and is controlled with i.v. GTN To control/relieve pain and anxiety	Vital signs within normal limits Is pain-free, comfortable and relaxed
3. Risk of infection	• Monitor temperature recordings at regular intervals • Give prophylactic antibiotics • Observe sites of intravenous and arterial access for redness/inflammation • Observe colour and consistency of urine	Risk of infection due to: – surgical procedure – immobility – urinary catheterisation – venous and arterial convolution	Remains apyrexial and free from infection

Continued

Nursing Care Plan 2.1 *(Continued)*

Nursing considerations	Action	Rationale	Expected outcome
4. **Possibility of gastrointestinal disturbance**	• Note nature of stools, especially diarrhoea and bloody stools • Observe for increase in abdominal girth • Maintain position and patency of nasogastric tube, gradually introducing fluids orally • Ensure that G knows to report abdominal pain • Ensure G is aware of the planned timescale for resuming eating and drinking • Mouth care	May develop as a result of handling the colon during surgery with resultant oedema May develop as a result of antibiotics Nasogastric tube to remain in place for 3–4 days, during which time oral fluids are gradually introduced	Remains free from gastrointestinal disturbance
5. **Possibility of cardiac arrhythmias**	• Monitor continuously heart rate and rhythm	Sinus tachycardia and atrial fibrillation are the most common arrhythmias	Heart rhythm stable
6. **Wound care**	• Check dressing with vital signs • Observe for signs of haemorrhage: may need to measure abdomen for increase in girth • Check drainage: vacuum drains may be used for 24–48 h		Wound healing problems identified promptly
7. **Possibility of difficulty in breathing**	• Administer 40–60% warm humidified oxygen • Ensure G knows to report any difficulty breathing • Observe respiratory rate and chest expansion • Offer oxygen therapy • Encourage turning 2-hourly to promote postural drainage • Encourage deep breathing and coughing • Liaise with physiotherapist regarding chest physiotherapy	Wound may limit deep breathing Abdominal distension may raise the diaphragm, reducing breathing capacity Signs of heart failure may suggest a rupture into the vena cava	Aim for oxygen saturation of 95% or above Is comfortable when breathing Displays no evidence of cyanosis or heart failure
8. **Potential problem of pain/discomfort**	• Ensure G knows to report any pain/discomfort • Give prescribed analgesics on a regular basis for abdominal pain at incision site • ECG if G experiences chest pain • Observe for signs associated with ischaemic pain: shortness of breath, nausea and vomiting	May experience abdominal pain at wound site May experience ischaemic chest pain as a result of decreased coronary artery blood flow Need to be aware of epidural anaesthesia masking haemorrhage or paralysis	Is pain-free and comfortable

Continued

Nursing Care Plan 2.1 *(Continued)*

Nursing considerations	Action	Rationale	Expected outcome
9. Potential problem of renal impairment	• Measure urine output hourly via urinary catheter • Maintain record of fluid input and output • Record weight at the same time daily • Give intravenous fluids at the rate prescribed • Note trends in urine output in relation to blood pressure and rates of medication infusion	May develop renal impairment as a result of embolisation; fall in blood pressure; trauma to the renal artery during surgery; or preoperative renal ischaemia due to renal artery involvement in development of aneurysm	Urine output >30 mL/h
10. Reduced mobility	• Record limb perfusion observations hourly • Complete pressure ulcer assessment tool preoperatively and immediately postoperatively • Use pressure-relieving mattress appropriately • Give subcutaneous heparin to prevent DVT	Epidural can lead to reduced sensation in lower limbs and prolonged pressure on vulnerable areas	
	• Assist to maintain desired activities of living: hygiene, personal grooming, mouth care, etc. • Place objects within reach Offer access to radio, papers, books as requested • Liaise with physiotherapist • Formulate plan for gradually increasing mobility, beginning with sitting out of bed for short periods on day 1 • Involve family members in care, if acceptable to them • Encourage frequent changes in position whilst in bed • Advise how to support wound when moving about	Mobility is reduced as a result of monitoring equipment, intravenous lines, urinary catheter, abdominal discomfort and uncertainty as to permitted safe level of movement	Effects of limited mobility will be minimised Mobility levels will be gradually increased
11. Anxiety and lack of information	• Explain all treatment and expected course of hospital stay to G and his family • Encourage B's family to visit when they can, promoting a welcoming and open atmosphere • Develop one-to-one relationship between nurse and G to foster open communication and individualised support and information giving • Provide realistic outlook for future and recovery • Avoid heavy lifting for 12 weeks • Return to work in 6–12 weeks	G and his family are likely to be anxious about the outcome of the operation and the future The ITU environment may exacerbate these feelings	G and his family will appear to be coping effectively with the operation and recovery G and his family will express that they feel able to cope and state that they understand the operation, treatment and plans for recovery

diabetic, have a diet high in lipids and who smoke, resulting in greater risk of atherosclerosis.

The result of increasing occlusion of the vessels, with medial calcification and loss of elastic fibres, is the slowing of blood flow. The blood becomes hypercoagulable. Thrombosis of the deep veins may occur, secondary to sudden arterial thrombosis. The ischaemia of surrounding tissue is evidenced by skin and muscle atrophy, loss of subcutaneous fat deposits and ischaemic neuropathy.

Severe occlusion can result in gangrene, usually first seen at the toes, then extending into the foot and leg. At the boundary between viable and necrotic tissue, an area of inflammation is often seen. The extent of the ischaemia will depend on how quickly occlusion developed and how extensive collateral circulation has become. Gangrene occurs when insufficient oxygen is conveyed to the tissue to sustain its life. This can be exacerbated by any other superimposed demand, e.g. infection, when oxygen demand rises but cannot be sustained by an impaired blood flow. Diabetic patients are more prone to infected ulceration in association with gangrene (see Ch. 5). Vasoconstriction should be avoided if at all possible.

Common presenting symptoms

may occur gradually or with sudden acute thrombosis, which may be the first indication of a process that has been silently progressing for some time (see Table 2.7).

Pain: intermittent claudication The term 'claudication' comes from the Latin 'claudicare' meaning to limp. Intermittent claudication is the commonest symptom of vascular disease and describes exercise-induced pain in muscle groups distal to the occluded vessel. Its nature varies from a numb cramp to severe pain. It is a manifestation of increased oxygen demand with exercise and the subsequent accumulation of metabolic wastes. It is relieved by rest. The calf muscles are the most commonly affected, but thigh and buttock muscles can also be involved, depending on the site of occlusion. The distance the individual can walk on the flat before onset of symptoms, the claudication distance, is an indication of the progress of the disease. Pain may eventually occur at rest, most often in the toes and foot and particularly at night, when limbs become warm and oxygen demand increases, thus interfering with sleep. Pain may become severe and difficult to contain if the patient develops gangrene. Neuropathy reduces sensation and may make the person unaware of the progressive gangrenous changes. Any exercise that can be tolerated should be encouraged.

MEDICAL MANAGEMENT

Investigations

Pulses should be assessed at rest in a warm room. They will remain intact until two-thirds of the lumen is occluded. Posterior tibial, popliteal and femoral pulses should be

Table 2.7 Presenting features of arterial and venous peripheral vascular disease

Assess	Arterial disease	Venous disease
Pain	Acute: sudden, severe pain, peaks rapidly Chronic: intermittent claudication; rest pain	Acute: little or no pain; tenderness along course of inflamed vein Chronic: heaviness, fullness
Impotence	May be present with aortoiliac femoral disease	Not associated
Hair	Hair loss distal to occlusion	No hair loss
Nails	Thick, brittle	Normal
Skeletal muscle	Atrophy may be present; may have restricted limb movement	Normal
Sensation	Possible paraesthesia	Normal
Skin colour	Pallor or reactive hyperaemia (pallor when limb elevated; rubor [red] when limb dependent)	Brawny (reddish-brown); cyanotic if dependent
Skin texture	Thin, shiny, dry	Stasis dermatitis; veins may be visible; skin mottling
Skin temperature	Cool	Warm
Skin breakdown (ulcers)	Severely painful; usually on or between toes or on upper surface of foot over metatarsal heads or other bony prominences	Mildly painful, with pain relieved by leg elevation; usually in ankle area
Oedema	None or mild; usually unilateral	Typically present, usually foot to calf; may be unilateral or bilateral
Pulses	Diminished, weak, absent	Normal
Blood flow	Bruit may be present; pressure readings lower below stenosis	Normal

Adapted from Bright & Georgi (1992).

included in the examination; dorsalis pedis pulses are not consistently present in all people. The volume of the pulses should be compared, as well as simple presence or absence. Many people find it difficult to differentiate between their own pulse and the patient's, and increasing the examiner's rate by exercising can help in this situation. The noise of turbulent blood flow (bruit) may also be heard as a murmur or abnormal sound when a stethoscope is placed over areas of turbulence in arteries that are still pulsating.

Colour and temperature As occlusion develops, the feet, and especially the toes, may be red in colour. This can later develop into bluish mottled areas or areas of pallor. With sudden occlusion, pallor may be marked. Elevation of legs with severe occlusion results in deathly pallor. Once legs return to the dependent position, colour normally returns. Superficial veins normally refill within 15 s, but in these cases it may take a minute or more. In severe cases, the limbs may become a cyanotic red colour (rubor). Temperature changes accompany reduced blood flow with cool pale extremities.

X-rays will show calcification of the vessel wall.

Doppler ultrasound When low-intensity sound is directed through the tissue towards a blood vessel, sound waves strike moving blood cells and are transmitted back. The frequency of these sound waves reflects changes in proportion to the velocity of the blood. Sound waves diminish in arterial occlusion and stenosis. Doppler ultrasound is used to assess the ankle brachial pressure index (ABPI) which decreases with arterial occlusion. Duplex scanners offer a sensitivity of 80% and are more reliable than angiography for detecting femoral and popliteal disease (see Fig. 2.14).

Helical or spiral computed tomography is a minimally invasive technique for vascular imaging which scans large areas in a short period of time, thereby reducing motion artefact.

Exercise testing will assess the functional limitations of arterial stenosis and differentiate occlusive arterial disease from other causes of exercise-induced lower limb symptoms.

Arteriograms are usually performed in order to assess occlusion prior to surgery.

Other examinations include ECG, a full blood count, urea, electrolytes and blood sugar estimation.

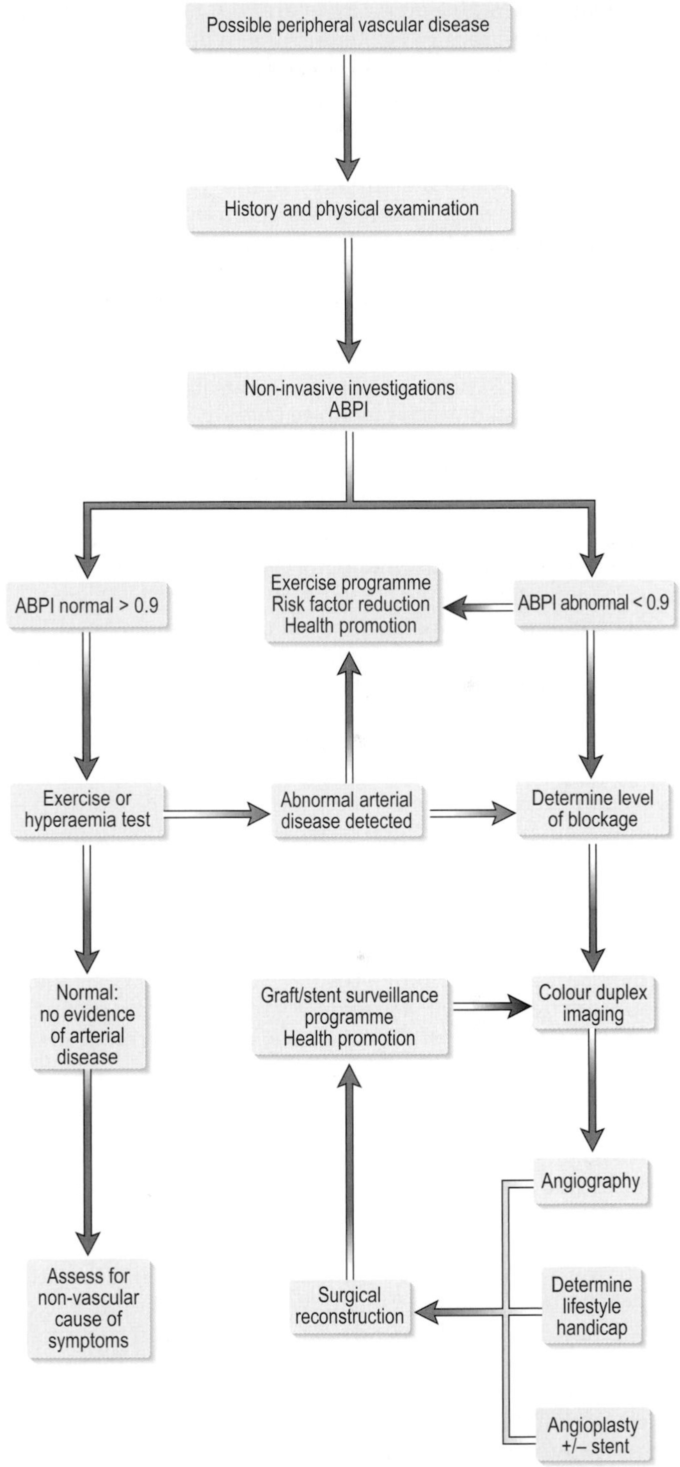

Fig. 2.14 The management of peripheral vascular disease. (Adapted from Murray 2003.)

Treatment

Underlying disease states, e.g. diabetes mellitus and infection, should be as well controlled as possible. Advice aimed at minimising symptoms and the risk of extending atherosclerosis should be given, as follows:

- Modify the diet to reduce lipid intake and reduce weight.
- Avoid the following which lead to vasoconstriction:
  — cigarette smoking
  — tight clothing
  — cold temperature.
- Avoid direct use of heat because of the risk of burns in a limb with decreased sensation.
- Avoid using hot water bottles, sitting too close to fires or radiators, taking hot baths and soaking the feet in hot water.
- Promote increased blood supply by a generally warm environment and elevation of the head of the bed.
- Avoid maintaining a completely dependent position since the resultant oedema will further reduce circulation.
- Encourage exercise up to the limit of pain, partly to maintain joint and muscle function and to promote

collateral circulation (Leng et al 2005). By walking three to four times a day, ischaemic time will decrease and pain control can also be improved by increasing blood flow; however, ischaemic pain is notoriously difficult to manage and may require opiate analgesics and night sedation.

- Avoid trauma to the impaired limb.
- Avoid wearing ill-fitting shoes; referral to a chiropodist may be required.

Patients will be prescribed regular aspirin or other antiplatelet medication to reduce the risk of coronary or cerebrovascular events.

For more information on the conservative management of intermittent claudication, see Murray (2003); on promoting health in vascular nursing, see Litchfield (2003); and on patients' experiences on living with peripheral vascular disease, see Gibson & Kenrick (1998).

Following assessment, sympathectomy may be considered to increase blood flow by obliterating neural control of vasoconstriction.

Percutaneous transluminal balloon angioplasty (PTBA) is a minimally invasive treatment for patients with atherosclerotic peripheral vascular disease. This surgical technique involves placing an intra-arterial balloon within an obstructing arterial lesion and forcibly dilating the balloon under fluoroscopy. In selected patients, the use of an intravascular stent may be an alternative to traditional bypass. Intravascular brachytherapy, whereby radiation is applied directly to the lesion, can inhibit re-stenosis (narrowing) of the vessels (Hansrani et al 2005).

If the occlusion is sudden and acute and the viability of the limb is in question, then surgical intervention, using either saphenous vein or prosthetic material, e.g. a femoropopliteal bypass, will be required to bypass the occlusion. Endarterectomy of the vessel may be performed first to core out the atheroma of the vessel.

Prior to surgery, the patient may undergo arteriography and should be rehydrated and have blood coagulation status assessed. There is a strong association with CHD, so full cardiac assessment is required prior to operation.

If the lesion is localised and accessible, embolectomy under local anaesthesia may be sufficient to reperfuse the limb. In this procedure, a catheter is inserted into the artery up to the level of the occlusion when the balloon at the end is inflated, aiming to fracture the plaque. Inflammation and re-endothelialisation occur secondary to this. Fibrinolytic drugs can be infused at the site of the occlusion. The advantage of embolectomy is that general anaesthesia can be avoided; however, reocclusion occurs more frequently than with bypass grafting.

For further information on peripheral artery bypass, see Galloway et al (2005).

Pain may become so severe and gangrene so advanced that the limb is no longer viable and amputation may become unavoidable. Bypass grafting may minimise the extent of amputation by restoring circulation, e.g. to a foot, but losing some of the toes. Amputation of a limb is traumatic for anyone but may be accepted as a means of relief from intolerable pain. It may, however, require skilled counselling before this fact can be faced by the patient and the full support of rehabilitation and limb-fitting services postoperatively is accepted (see Ch. 10).

STOP THINK **2.9** Find out about the rehabilitative care for any patient who has an amputation of a lower limb and is adapting to the use of a prosthesis.

For more information on the care of a patient faced with the prospect of an amputation, see Donohue (1997a–d).

Thromboangiitis obliterans or Buerger's disease

This chronic occlusive inflammatory disease has no known cause. It manifests in a younger population than atherosclerosis, is predominant in men and is strongly associated with smoking. It is postulated that carbon monoxide has a toxic effect on the arterial wall and nicotine has vasoconstrictive effects. In contrast to atherosclerosis, it affects small and medium vessels of the extremities. It is not a diffuse disease since only segments of arteries develop lesions. Thrombosis is a secondary feature. The lumen may become occluded and the intima thickened but the medial wall structure remains intact, in contrast to atherosclerotic disease. The diagnosis can often be made on the basis of a careful history and physical examination. A patient may present with cold hypersensitive fingers and toes on two or more limbs. Investigations aim to exclude other causes of ischaemia. Occasionally, arteriography is warranted to confirm the diagnosis. The patient is strongly advised to stop smoking. Besides the general treatment approaches used in ischaemic diseases of the limbs, including antibiotics, antirheumatics and corticosteroids, some specific surgical procedures may be considered.

Raynaud's disease

This is episodic vasospastic ischaemia of the small arteries and arterioles in the most distal part of the extremities in response to cold or, less commonly, emotional stress. It usually occurs in young women and is more prevalent in cool, damp climates. A distinction should be made between Raynaud's phenomenon, which results in no permanent damage, and Raynaud's disease, the more advanced condition associated with permanent damage. The fingers become pale and cold, but pulses are intact. Cyanosis may also be a feature. Pain is not always present, but function may be lost. Similar episodes of vasospasm can be found secondary to scleroderma, some neurological conditions and in some occupational groups, e.g. those that use pneumatic vibrating tools. Treatment includes avoiding situations that trigger the problem. This may mean a change in occupation, giving up smoking and keeping warm. Vasodilating medication, including calcium channel blockers, e.g. nifedipine, prostaglandin therapy and sympathectomy have been tried as means of improving the circulation. The nurse's primary role is patient education so that the onset of symptoms associated with this disease can be identified and minimised.

NURSING PRIORITIES AND MANAGEMENT: Arterial disease

Almost all the activities of life are affected by the distress of arterial disease.

Maintaining a safe environment

Possible loss of sensation increases the risk of trauma to tissue that has reduced ability to combat infection and to heal. The person's home and work circumstances can be considered, and hazards minimised. Useful advice includes the following points:

- Toenails may be best cut by the chiropodist in case soft tissue injury is inflicted, especially as some people with atherosclerotic disease, with or without diabetes, may also have poor sight.
- Caution should be exercised with electric blankets, hot water bottles, open fires and hot baths, as burns may not be felt.
- Cold can also be damaging.
- Constrictive clothing, e.g. tight underwear, is best avoided.
- Sitting cross-legged causes constriction of lower limb circulation.
- Remaining in one position for any length of time puts pressure on one area of tissue, allowing ischaemic changes to occur.

STOP THINK **2.10** Drawing on your experiences of visiting older people at home, identify the range of possible hazards for those susceptible to arterial disease. Think of your own home and work environment. How aware are you of actual and potential damage to your lower limbs from knocks, friction, pressure and cuts?

Pain control

The pain of claudication is relieved by rest; however, exercise to the limit of pain is to be encouraged in the hope of developing increased perfusion and collateral circulation. Controlling ischaemic pain is essential and will often require the use of opiate analgesics, which may cause drowsiness as a side-effect. Keeping warm, especially for people affected by vessel spasm, and positioning the affected limb in a dependent position from time to time are also advised. Anti-inflammatory medications are used in diseases with an inflammatory response. Distraction techniques can also be helpful (see Ch. 19).

Nutrition

Excessive weight increases circulatory demand, and people with diabetes need to be particularly careful about what they eat (see Ch. 5, Part 2). Dehydration contributes to the process of clot formation because of increased blood concentration, so taking plenty of liquids is recommended. A balanced diet, including the vitamins and trace elements that aid tissue healing and integrity, can help to prevent aggravation of symptoms (see Ch. 23). People with hyperlipidaemia could be encouraged to follow the diet suggested for those with CHD and may also be prescribed medication to reduce their lipid levels.

Sleep

This is often impaired by pain. Elevating the head of the bed is suggested to increase flow (see also Ch. 25).

Breathing

Smoking reduces the amount of oxygen the haemoglobin can carry and nicotine results in venous spasm. Encouraging the patient to give up smoking may therefore produce benefits.

Mobility

Maintaining as great a degree of mobility as possible can help to prevent general stiffness of all joints, which can develop if they are underused. Muscle wasting and weakness are associated problems; the patient can be encouraged to carry out a wide range of joint exercises.

Personal hygiene

Careful attention to hygiene helps to prevent infection, especially if the person is diabetic. After bathing, the skin should be thoroughly dried, especially between the toes. This gives the opportunity to assess the skin for any signs of ischaemia. Points to note are:

- bath water should be neither too hot nor too cold
- tight socks with elastic tops cause constriction
- clean clothing, daily, is preferred
- plastic shoes encourage sweating and maceration of the skin as water cannot evaporate.

Work

Consideration should be given as to the physical demands and environmental hazards at the person's work. The more potent analgesics may also impair work performance and safety.

Discharge planning

After successful surgery, it is important to consider how vascular improvement can be maintained to ensure a reasonable quality of life and prevent further hospital admissions.

STOP THINK **2.11** What type of discharge planning would be appropriate following femoropopliteal bypass grafting?

VENOUS DISEASE

Venous insufficiency

Venous disease results from:

- obstruction, by thrombus or thrombophlebitis
- incompetence of valves in the veins.

STOP THINK **2.12** Read Case History 2.3 and consider the following questions:

a) What is meant by the term gangrene?
b) Mr L was suffering from the pain of ischaemia prior to surgery. What is meant by the phantom limb pain that might occur after amputation and how do you think such pain could be alleviated?
c) Can you explain, in physiological terms, why his aching legs were relieved by rest?
d) Describe the tests Mr L might have undergone to assess his arterial insufficiency.
e) How does smoking affect the feet?
f) What vasodilatory medicine might have been prescribed?
g) What was the surgery that Mr L underwent?
h) It was clear that Mr L found it almost impossible to change his lifestyle. What role do you think

CASE HISTORY 2.3

Peripheral vascular disease: Mr L's memories

Mr L lay back on his hospital pillow, wishing he was at home. The powerful analgesic was at last easing the pain in his gangrenous foot. Tomorrow he would have surgery that would rid him of the limb, but losing a limb had been difficult to come to terms with — and what was this phantom pain he had heard so much about?

Thirty years ago Mr L had been strong and fit, fond of long country walks and watching football. His first complaint had been aching legs after his long walks, but it had not lasted long and was easily relieved by sitting down. However, the aching became a great deal worse and his walks became shorter and shorter. Fond of his food, he had gained weight and spent more of his leisure time smoking.

His GP had described his symptoms as intermittent claudication or limping. He had said it was due to impairment of the blood supply to his lower limbs and had organised several tests to confirm this. At first the treatment had seemed quite easy. Mr L had to cut down on his smoking, alter his diet to avoid rich and fatty food that could 'clog up' his arteries and avoid extremes of temperature, which would make the symptoms worse.

It had been hard to stick to his diet and give up smoking and, seeing no visible evidence of it working, he had soon abandoned this. The ache in his legs eventually became worse, developing into excruciating pain. At night he had to sit up in bed and hang his legs down to cool them and ease the pain. The GP had given him tablets to help dilate the blood vessels but they had not helped and not long afterwards he had found himself facing an operation to improve the blood supply.

Mr L had not minded the operation too much. One of his veins had been used to bypass the occlusion in the artery of his thigh. He had thought this rather clever at the time and he had quickly felt the benefits. After the operation he had felt much more enthusiastic about changing his lifestyle. The surgeon had stressed that the success of the operation in the long term would depend on his ability to stop smoking, and he had, for a while. Friends and family had said he looked so much better but somehow it did not last. He had lost weight but just could not stop smoking. He had known the pain was coming back. His toes were looking discoloured and often felt either very sensitive or numb. The skin on his right leg, particularly, was thin and dry and there had seemed to be less muscle. Once again, he had found himself in hospital, the circulation to his lower limbs being thoroughly assessed.

The night before his operation he was unable to sleep and feared both the immediate and long-term future.

hospital and community nurses can play in helping someone like Mr L?

i) Outline a plan of care for Mr L for the immediate postoperative period after his above-knee amputation of his right leg.

Some diseases, such as varicose veins, may seem trivial but can contribute to day-to-day discomfort and absence from work. Other venous diseases are associated with chronic health problems, such as venous ulcers, or a sudden medical emergency, such as pulmonary embolus following deep vein thrombosis.

Deep vein thrombosis (DVT)

Clot formation is more likely to occur when flow is reduced within the veins. This can occur due to obstruction and stasis but is also associated with increased blood viscosity, slower flow and damage to the endothelial wall of the vessel. Hypercoagulability may be a feature of dehydration or malignant disease. It seems that there is also an imbalance between fibrinolysis and coagulation in the postoperative patient, which predisposes them to DVT. Trauma may be mechanical or chemical. The increasing use of vascular cannulae predisposes the patient in hospital to the irritant effects of pharmacological preparations, the plastic of the cannula itself and the possibility of intimal trauma at insertion.

Stasis allows clotting factors that normally would be cleared from the circulation to remain active for longer. The effects of the muscle pumps of the leg and negative intrathoracic pressure during inspiration normally promote venous return. Any situation that obliterates their action predisposes to stasis of the venous circulation. Immobility and the recumbent position are frequently features of the postoperative patient and the older person. There has also been much debate about the risks of arising from sitting still for long periods during long-haul flights and passengers are now encouraged to exercise their limbs regularly. Muscle relaxant medications used during surgery abolish the muscle pump, and breathing is under positive pressure when ventilated mechanically. Stasis is more common in the dilated portions of varicosities. Mechanical obstruction to flow can be seen in pregnancy and abdominal tumours.

Prophylaxis is important and simple measures such as regular physical activity, avoidance of dehydration, elevation of the legs without calf compression, minimising periods of immobilisation and the use of graduated compression stockings are important (Kolbach et al 2005).

Other measures include intermittent pneumatic compression (IPC) devices and electrical muscle stimulation. Low dose subcutaneous unfractionated heparin is the most widely used form of prophylactic anticoagulation. Warfarin and dextran are also used.

For further information on assessing patients at risk of DVT, see Autar (1998).

MEDICAL MANAGEMENT

Clinical assessment includes the use of Homan's sign which involves sharply dorsiflexing the foot when the patient is lying flat with their legs straight. The test is positive if pain is felt in the calf. Alternatively, the knee can be slightly flexed and the gastrocnemius muscle compressed against the tibia. Again if pain is felt, the test is positive. More than 25% of DVTs produce no symptoms and are only detected on screening. In other cases, the affected area will be tender, swollen and hot. Compression ultrasonography has become a first line investigation with the measurement of circulating D-dimer concentrations. D-dimer, a by-product of fibrin production, is a useful adjunct to ultrasonography, with a 98% sensitivity for DVT and a high negative predictive value (Gorman et al 2000). Venography, plethysmography (use of infrared light to assess relative changes in blood volume) and isotope scanning may also be used. Once diagnosed, treatment includes pain relief and anticoagulation, first with heparin and later with warfarin. Prophylactic subcutaneous heparin is almost a routine postoperative prescription. Leg elevation, with some flexion at the knee, will be necessary until swelling and pain subside. Avoidance of dehydration, external pressure, immobility in those at risk and careful observation are all part of the preventive management. Home management is cost effective and likely to be preferred by patients (Schraibman et al 2001).

Chronic venous insufficiency

Of those suffering from chronic venous insufficiency, most will have had episodes of DVT previously. Pressure within the venous system remains high, resulting in increased capillary pressure and allowing chronic oedema to develop. The valves and elastic fibres of the vein wall are also destroyed by thrombophlebitis, aggravating the situation. Accumulation of interstitial fluid increases pressure locally. Eczema may occur secondary to this, possibly with pruritus. Owing to stasis, red blood cells may be trapped and haemolysed. This manifests as areas of brown pigmentation (haemosiderin). Melanin may also be deposited. Prolonged oedema reduces the nutrition available to subcutaneous tissue, which then fibroses. This induration further prevents drainage of any oedema.

Venous ulcers

Ulceration may follow trauma or dermatitis of such an area. Ulcers are commonly seen around the internal malleolus and tend to recur in the same place, as the scar tissue is atrophic.

Infection of ulcers is common. Venous ulceration is a major problem, particularly in older people, with district nurses spending a significant amount of time treating them. Compression therapy is considered to be the most appropriate non-invasive treatment of leg ulcers, although appropriate patients may benefit from surgery.

MEDICAL MANAGEMENT

Prompt and correct treatment of thrombophlebitis helps to prevent chronic venous insufficiency. Pain is worse in the dependent position, so elevation of the limb when seated and regular walking should be advised. Prolonged standing should be avoided.

Oedema is treated by elevation during bed rest. Once it is reduced, support stockings should be fitted. Any infection should be isolated and treated with appropriate medication. If varicose veins contribute to ulceration, they may be dealt with surgically. Chronic ulcers may have to be skin-grafted.

For information on the care and management of leg ulcers, see Chapter 23 (this volume) and Moffatt (2003).

Varicose veins

Varicosities are tortuous, dilated and incompetent veins, partly due to the effects of gravity. Dilatation causes the valves to become incompetent and retrograde flow is no longer prevented. It has a genetic component: about half the sufferers will have a family history of varicosities. The hormonal changes in pregnancy also reduce venous tone, while the obstruction to venous return by the gravid uterus combines to increase pregnant women's susceptibility. Simple obesity has a similar obstructive effect. Standing for prolonged periods maximises the force of gravity. Thrombophlebitis of the deep veins increases venous pressure, while inflammation destroys valve tissue. This increase in pressure is transmitted to the superficial veins which, being relatively less supported by surrounding structures, dilate. Most people complain of dull aching in their legs. Trauma may result in significant blood loss and should be guarded against. Ulcers are rare. Some individuals are concerned by appearance. Elevation and use of support stockings may reduce the aching and oedema.

MEDICAL MANAGEMENT

Diagnosis involves history taking, examination and investigation for reflux, including the Brodie–Trendelenburg test, i.e. selective clinical testing for reflux, which can identify sites of perforation or junctional incompetence in either the long or short saphenous system. Continuous wave Doppler or colour flow duplex ultrasonography is also used (see Fig. 2.15). Conservative treatment involves patient education, control of risk factors, advice on camouflage techniques and cosmetic treatments, e.g. laser therapy, microsclerotherapy. Support hosiery should be worn as routine. If symptoms persist, the most common management is the surgical stripping and ligation of the varicosed vein. For some, the injection of a sclerosing agent would be considered. Treatment is increasingly being carried out on a day surgery basis and this has an impact on nursing care priorities both in hospital and at home. There is potentially less time for providing accurate information to patients about the disease process, treatment options and interventions for its prevention. For further information on surgical intervention, see Chapter 26. Patients can usually return to driving in a week and to work between 1 and 3 weeks after the procedure. Some 20–30% of patients will develop recurrent varicose veins within 10 years (London & Nash 2000).

For a review of the treatment and prevention of varicose veins, see Vowden & Vowden (2003).

NURSING PRIORITIES AND MANAGEMENT: Venous insufficiency

Pain control

Bed rest or limb elevation reduces the throbbing pain of venous insufficiency. Walking rather than standing is advisable. Supportive anti-embolism stockings, by aiding venous return, reduce the feeling of pressure in the legs. However, they can be hot and uncomfortable. Once any oedema has reduced, the patient should be measured again, to ensure that the stockings fit properly and are still therapeutic. Similarly, swollen legs should not be squeezed into elastic stockings that have become too small. Anti-inflammatory medication may be prescribed to settle the inflammatory process of thromboembolism.

Mobility

Mobility should be maintained as much as possible. Patients should be advised to elevate the legs when sitting, in order to increase venous return and reduce oedema, and to avoid standing for long periods. After an operation for ligation of

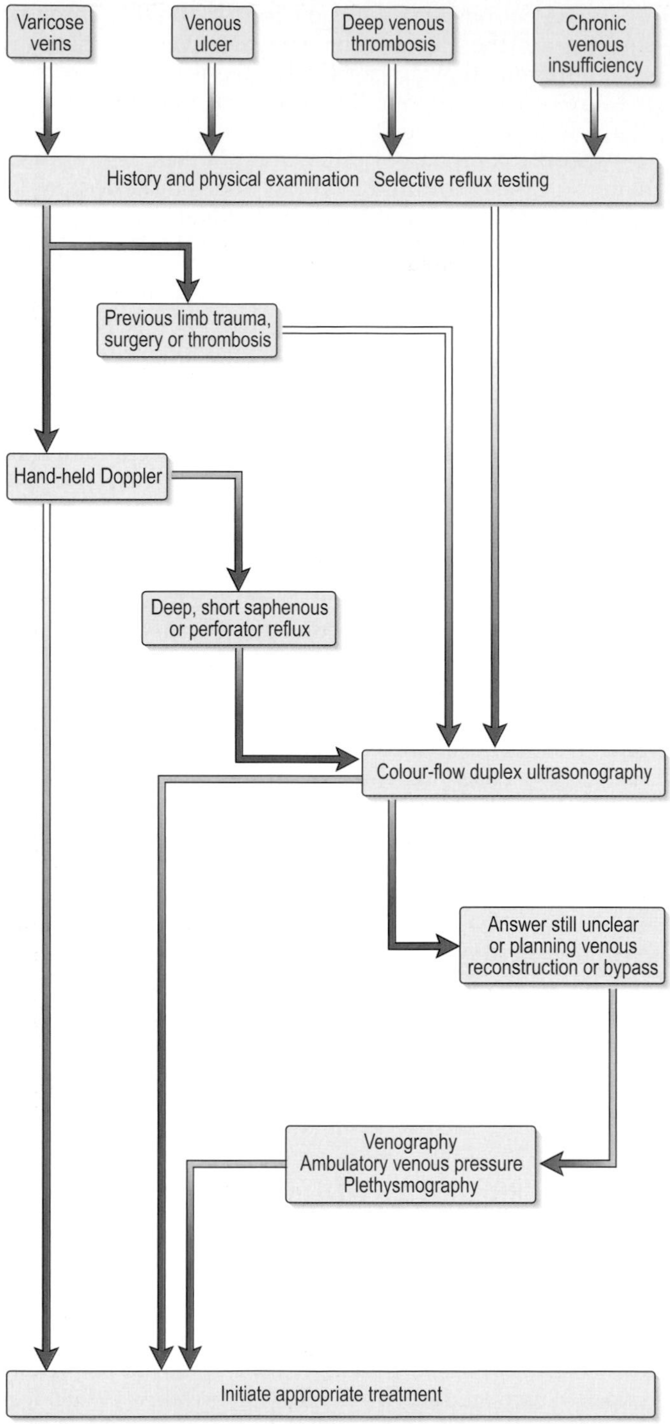

Fig. 2.15 Investigation pathway for patients presenting with venous disease. (Adapted from Murray 2003.)

varicosities, measures to prevent DVT should be considered. The patient will be advised to:

- walk a prescribed distance of perhaps 2 miles daily
- avoid standing for long periods
- always elevate the feet when sitting.

See Nursing Care Plan 2.2.

Nutrition

Adequate hydration and balanced nutrition assist flow and maintain vessel integrity. A diet deficient in fibre has been thought to predispose to varicose veins. Constipation and straining at stool can cause compression and dilatation of both the superficial and deep veins in the leg. Some supplementation of vitamins, trace elements and iron may have to be considered in the older person.

Maintaining a safe environment

Avoidance of trauma and infection is important, as in arterial disease. Blood loss can be severe, even from venous circulation.

Work

Occupations that involve standing for long periods, e.g. shop assistants, may present a problem. Prophylactic use of support hose by at-risk groups may be advised by the occupational health nurse.

Lifestyle issues

Women taking oral contraception run a slightly increased risk of DVT, especially if there is a family history of thrombosis. If a DVT was to develop, then oral contraception would be discontinued and another form adopted. Pregnant women are also more prone to DVT and varicose vein formation. The cosmetic effect of these problems can prove very upsetting, as wearing thick white stockings is far from attractive. Trousers and opaque-coloured tights may make them more acceptable. The perfect compression stocking, which would be easy to put on, comfortable to wear, give adequate graduated compression and look fashionably sheer, has not yet been invented!

STOP THINK **2.13** Health education leaflets related to cardiovascular disease are widely available. Where do these leaflets come from? Who uses them? Do health professionals and the public find them useful? Explore these questions during your placements in the community and in hospital.

Nursing Care Plan 2.2

J is a 68-year-old lady admitted to hospital 2 days previously for surgical stripping and ligation of varicose veins in her left leg. J lives alone and is concerned about how she will cope after discharge.

Nursing considerations	Action	Rationale	Expected outcome
1. Pain/discomfort	• Explain normal pains/ sensations likely to be felt over forthcoming days/weeks • Ensure support stockings are fitted correctly • Give analgesics to promote pain-free movement of affected extremities • Inspect bandages regularly for bleeding: a compression bandage is usually kept on the leg for 1–2 weeks	It is normal for the leg to feel painful and be very bruised. There may be a small amount of bleeding through the dressing. This may be a problem in the groin, particularly if the support bandage ends over a bruise Complaints of patchy numbness are to be expected, but these disappear over a year Sensation of pins and needles or hypersensitivity to touch in the involved extremity may indicate a temporary or permanent nerve injury as a result of surgery; the saphenous vein and saphenous nerve are in close proximity Local anaesthetic infiltration of groin and popliteal wounds can significantly reduce postoperative discomfort	Ultimately, is pain-free and comfortable Feels informed about the pains/sensations to expect Wears support stockings correctly
2. Leg needs to be supported	• Elevate leg 30° to provide adequate support for whole leg • Leg to be encased in pressure bandage from toe to groin for about a week, followed by knee-level stockings for 3–4 weeks after surgery • Ensure J has adequate supply of stockings	Long-term elastic support after discharge will promote circulation and limit likelihood of recurrence	Is aware of the importance of supporting the leg
3. Fear/difficulty in walking	• Encourage J to walk with normal gait, offering support if necessary • Encourage short frequent walks to regain confidence and promote circulation • Give analgesics to ease movement of affected extremity • Advise to continue leg exercises after discharge	Early ambulation needs to be encouraged to promote circulation	Feels confident about walking and is able to walk without discomfort

Continued ▶

Nursing Care Plan 2.2 *(Continued)*

Nursing considerations	Action	Rationale	Expected outcome
4. Potential for recurrence of varicosities	• Advise J to continue to avoid activities that cause venous stress by obstructing blood flow: – avoid wearing tight socks or tight girdle – avoid sitting or standing for long periods of time – avoid dangling legs (causes stasis of blood in lower leg) – avoid crossing legs at the knee for long periods whilst sitting (decreases circulation by 15%) • Elevate foot of bed 15–20° at night • Avoid excessive weight gain • Wear elastic support tights • Attend outpatient follow-up visits every 6 months • Avoid knocking/damaging leg	It is possible that varicosities may recur in approximately 20% of patients. Therefore conservative measures learned perioperatively need to be continued	Recurrence of varicosities will be avoided Will feel confident about practising preventive measures
5. Coping after discharge	• Ensure that she knows what to expect after discharge • Discuss availability of support from family and neighbours after discharge; assist in coordinating these resources • Discuss feelings about wearing support bandages; arrange to talk to someone who has previously had this operation to talk through feelings • Arrange for district nurse to visit to remove sutures • Advise about keeping bandage dry when washing • Ensure she is aware of outpatient follow-up	May feel isolated after support of hospital May have difficulty coping with activities of living at home May feel embarrassed about having to wear support stockings Sutures are removed after 2 weeks Phlebotomy stab incisions are usually closed with adhesive strips and larger wounds with subcuticular sutures	Feels more confident about coping after discharge home

REFERENCES

ACC/AHA/NASPE 2002 Guideline update for implantation of cardiac pacemakers and antiarrhythmia devices. Journal of Cardiovascular Electrophysiology 13: 1183–1199

Albarran J A W, Bridger S 1997 Problems with providing education on resuming sexual activity after myocardial infarction: developing written information for patients. Intensive and Critical Care Nursing 13: 2–11

American Heart Association in collaboration with the International Liaison Committee on Resuscitation 2000 Guidelines 2000 for cardiopulmonary resuscitation and emergency cardiovascular care. An international consensus on science. Resuscitation 46: 1–448

Ashworth P 1992 Cardiovascular problems and nursing. In: Ashworth P M, Clarke C (eds) Cardiovascular intensive care nursing. Churchill Livingstone, Edinburgh

Bright L D, Georgi S 1992 Peripheral vascular disease: is it arterial or venous? American Journal of Nursing 92(9): 34–47

British Cardiac Society 2001 Guidelines for the management of patients with acute coronary syndromes without ECG ST segment elevation. Heart 85: 133–142

British Cardiac Society 2002 Grown up congenital heart (GUCH) disease: current needs and provision of service for adolescents and adults with congenital heart disease in the UK. Heart 88: I1–I14

British Heart Foundation 2004 Coronary heart disease statistics. British Heart Foundation, London. Online. Available: www.heartstats.org/homepage.asp

British Heart Foundation, National Institute for Clinical Excellence, Department of Health, NHS Modernisation Agency, Coronary Heart Disease Collaborative 2003 Developing services for heart failure. DH, London

Broomfield R 1996a The named nurse in the coronary care setting. Professional Nurse 11(4): 256–258

Broomfield R 1996b A quasi-experimental research to investigate the retention of basic cardiopulmonary resuscitation skills and knowledge by qualified nurses following a course in professional development. Journal of Advanced Nursing 23: 1016–1023

Caunt J 1996 The advanced nurse practitioner in CCU. Care of the Critically Ill 12: 136–139

Collins R, Peto R 1994 Antihypertensive drug therapy: effects on stroke and coronary heart disease. In: Swales J D (ed) Textbook of hypertension. Blackwell Scientific, Oxford

Collinson J, Flather M, Fox K A et al 2000 Clinical outcomes, risk stratification and practice patterns of unstable angina and myocardial infarction without ST elevation. European Heart Journal 21: 1450–1457

Connors P 1996 Should relatives be allowed in the resuscitation room? Nursing Standard 10(44): 42–44

Cotler M 2000 The 'do not resuscitate' order: clinical and ethical rationale and implications. Medicine and Law 19: 623–633

Cutler T M, Windhausser M M, Lin P H, Jaranja N 1997 A clinical trial of the effects of dietary patterns on blood pressure. DASH Collaborative Research Group. New England Journal of Medicine 336: 1117–1124

De Belder A J, Thomas M R 1997 Primary angioplasty for the acute myocardial infarction. British Journal of Hospital Medicine 58: 35–38

De Bono D 1999 Investigation and management of stable angina: revised guidelines 1998. Joint Working Party of the British Cardiac Society and Royal College of Physicians of London. Heart 81(5): 546–555

De Jong 1999 Cardiogenic shock: changes in vital signs may signal impending circulatory collapse. American Journal of Nursing 97: 40–41

Department of Health 2000 National Service Framework for coronary heart disease. DH, London

Freidman S 2000 Cardiac disease, anxiety and sexual functioning. American Journal of Cardiology 86(Suppl F): 46F–50F

Fullard E M 1998 Organisation of secondary prevention of coronary heart disease in primary care. The nurses' perspective. Coronary Health Care 2(4): 177–236

Gershlick A H 2002 Intracoronary stenting: developments since the NICE report. Heart 87: 187–190

Gnani S, Majeed A 2001 Co-existing conditions of health services associated with heart failure: a general practice based study. Health Statistics Quarterly 12: 27–33

Goldberg R J, Samad N A, Yarzebski J et al 1999 Temporal trends in cardiogenic shock complicating myocardial infarction. New England Journal of Medicine 340: 1162–1168

Gorman W P, Davis K, Donnelly R 2000 Swollen lower limb-1: general assessment and deep vein thrombosis. In: Donnelly R, London N (eds) ABC of arterial and venous disease. BMJ Books, London

Hansrani M, Overbeck K, Smout J et al 2005 Intravascular brachytherapy for peripheral vascular disease (Cochrane Review). In: The Cochrane Library, Issue 2. Wiley, Chichester

Holland E, Foxcroft D 2000 Is nurse-led thrombolysis clinically safe, beneficial and acceptable? NT Research 5: 227–236

Howard C 1996 Fast-track care after cardiac surgery. British Journal of Nursing 4: 1112–1117

Jackson E A, Yarzebski J L, Goldberg R J et al 2004 Do not resuscitate orders in patients hospitalized with acute myocardial infarction: the Worcester heart attack study. Archives of Internal Medicine 164: 776–783

James J 2002 Management and support of patients with internal cardioverter defibrillators. In: Hatchett R, Thompson D (eds) Cardiac nursing: a comprehensive guide. Churchill Livingstone, Edinburgh

Joint Health Surveys Unit 2001 Health survey for England. The health of minority ethnic groups, 1999. TSO, London

Jowett N I, Thompson D R 2003 Comprehensive coronary care, 3rd edn. Baillière Tindall, London

Kamineni R, Alpert J 2004 Acute coronary syndromes: initial evaluation and risk stratification. Progress in Cardiovascular Diseases 46: 379–392

Kastrati A, Mehilli J, Nekolla S et al 2004 A randomized trial comparing myocardial salvage achieved by coronary stenting versus balloon angioplasty on patients with acute myocardial infarction considered ineligible for reperfusion. Journal of the American College of Cardiology 43: 734–741

Kegel L S 1996 Case management, critical pathways and myocardial infarction. Critical Care Nurse 16: 97–104

Khunti K, Samani N 2004 Coronary heart disease in people of south-Asian origin. Lancet 364: 2077–2078

Kolbach D N, Sandbrink M W C, Hamulyak K et al 2005 Non-pharmaceutical measures for prevention of post thrombotic syndrome (Cochrane Review). In: The Cochrane Library, Issue 2. Wiley, Chichester

Kucia A, Taylor K T N, Horowitz J D 2001 Can a nurse trained in coronary care expedite the emergency department management of patients with acute coronary syndromes? Heart and Lung 30: 186–190

Laitinen H 1996 Patients' experience of confusion in the intensive care unit following cardiac surgery. Intensive and Critical Care Nursing 12: 79–83

Leng G C, Fowler B, Ernst E 2005 Exercise for intermittent claudication (Cochrane Review). In: The Cochrane Library, Issue 1. Wiley, Chichester

Levine G N, Kern M J, Berger P B et al 2003 Management of patients undergoing percutaneous coronary revascularisation. Annals of Internal Medicine 139: 123–136

Linden B 1995 Evaluation of a home based rehabilitation programme for patients recovering from acute myocardial infarction. Intensive and Critical Care Nursing 11: 10–19

Lindsey G M, Smith L N, Hanlon P, Wheatley D J 2000 Coronary artery disease patients' perceptions of their health and expectations of benefit following coronary artery bypass grafting. Journal of Advanced Nursing 36: 1412–1421

Liu J L Y, Mandiadakas M, Gray A 2002 Cost of CHD to the National Health Service and social care system. Heart 88: 597–603

London N J M, Nash R 2000 Varicose veins. In: Donnelly R, London N (eds) ABC of arterial and venous disease. BMJ Books, London

Lydakis C, Lip G Y H, Beevers M, Beevers D G 1997 Diet, lifestyle and blood pressure. Coronary Health Care 1: 130–137

Lyons A, Fanshaw C, Lip G Y H 2002 Knowledge, communication and experiences of cardiac catheterization: the patient's perspective. Psychology, Health and Medicine 7: 461–467

Mårtensson J, Strömberg A, Dahlström U et al 2005 Patients with heart failure in primary health care: effects of a nurse-led intervention on health-related quality of life and depression. European Journal of Heart Failure 7: 393–403

Mason S 1996 The ethical dilemma of the do not resuscitate order. British Journal of Nursing 6: 646–649

Mayou R A, Gill D, Thompson D R et al 2000 Depression and anxiety as predictors of outcome after myocardial infarction. Psychosomatic Medicine 62: 212–219

McMurray J J V, Stewart S 1998 Nurse-led multidisciplinary intervention in chronic heart failure [editorial]. Heart 80: 430–431

Mihaljevic T, Paul S, Leacche M et al 2005 Valve replacement in women of childbearing age: influences on mother, fetus and neonate. Journal of Heart Valve Disease 14: 151–157

Moser D, Dracup K 2004 Role of spousal anxiety and depression in patients' psychosocial recovery after a cardiac event. Psychosomatic Medicine 66: 527–532

Murchie P, Campbell N C, Ritchie L D et al 2003 Secondary prevention clinics for coronary heart disease: four year follow up of a randomized controlled trial in primary care. British Medical Journal 326: 84–87

Murray S (ed) 2003 Chronic ischaemia. In: Vascular disease: nursing and management. Whurr, London

National Institute for Clinical Excellence (NICE) 1999 Coronary artery stents in the treatment of ischaemic heart disease. NHS HTA Programme, West Midlands Development and Evaluation Service, University of Birmingham

National Institute for Clinical Excellence (NICE) 2002 Guidance on the use of glycoprotein IIb/IIIa inhibitors in the

treatment of acute coronary syndromes. Technology Appraisal Guidance No 47. NICE, London
National Institute for Clinical Excellence (NICE) 2003 Chronic heart failure. National clinical guideline for diagnosis and management in primary and secondary care. Guideline No 5. Royal College of Physicians of London, London
NHS Centre for Reviews and Dissemination 1998 Cardiac rehabilitation. Effective Health Care 4: 1–12
Nicholson C 2004 A systematic review of the effectiveness of oxygen in reducing acute myocardial ischaemia. Journal of Clinical Nursing 13: 996–1007
Nowson C A, Worsley A, Margerison C et al 2005 Blood pressure change with weight loss is affected by diet type in men. American Journal of Clinical Nutrition 81: 983–989
O'Connor L 1995 Pain assessment by patients and nurses, and nurses' notes on it, in early acute myocardial infarction. Intensive and Critical Care Nursing 11: 183–191
Olivier C 2000 Rheumatic fever: is it still a problem? Journal of Antimicrobial Chemotherapy 45(Suppl): 13–21
O'Neal P V 1994 How to spot early signs of cardiogenic shock. American Journal of Nursing 94(5): 36–41
Pate G E, Mulligan A 2005 An epidemiological study of Heyde's syndrome: an association between aortic stenosis and gastrointestinal bleeding. Journal of Heart Valve Disease 13: 713–716
Quinn T 1998 Early experience with nurse led elective cardioversion. Nursing in Critical Care 3: 59–62
Quinn T, Morse T 2003 The interdisciplinary interface in managing patients with suspected cardiac pain. Emergency Nurse 11: 22–24
Radley A, Grove A, Wright S, Thurston H 1998 Problems of women compared to those of men following first myocardial infarction. Coronary Health Care 2(4): 202–209
Ransome P 1996 Transluminal aortic stenting. Nursing Standard 23(11): 52–53
Resuscitation Council (UK) 2000 Resuscitation Council guidelines. Resuscitation Council (UK), London
Rhodes M A 1998 What is the evidence to support nurse-led thrombolysis? Clinical Effectiveness in Nursing 2(2): 29–77
Roper N, Logan W W, Tierney A J 2000 The Roper–Logan–Tierney model of nursing: the activities of living model, 5th edn. Churchill Livingstone, Edinburgh
Scholte-op-Reimer W J M, Jansem C H, de-Swart E A M et al 2002 Contribution of nursing to risk factor assessment as perceived by patients with established coronary heart disease. European Journal of Cardiovascular Nursing 1: 87–94
Schraibman I G, Milne A A, Royle E M 2001 Home versus in-patient treatment for deep vein thrombosis (Cochrane Review). In: The Cochrane Library, Issue 2. Wiley, Chichester
Scott M 2002 Critical pathways: aiming for seamless care. In: Hatchett R, Thompson D (eds) Cardiac nursing: a comprehensive guide. Churchill Livingstone, Edinburgh
Scottish Intercollegiate Guidelines Network (SIGN) 1999 Diagnosis and treatment of heart failure due to left ventricular systolic dysfunction. SIGN, Edinburgh
Shayne P H, Pitts S R 2003 Severely increased blood pressure in the emergency department. Annals of Emergency Medicine 41: 513–529
Shepardson L B, Younger S J, Speroff T et al 1999 Increased risk of death in patients with do not resuscitate orders. Medical Care 37: 722–726
Sternbergh W C, Gonze M D, Garrad C L et al 1998 Abdominal and thoracicoabdominal aortic aneurysm. Surgical Clinics of North America 78: 827–834
Stewart S 2003 Refractory to medical treatment but not to nursing care: can we do more for patients with chronic angina pectoris? European Journal of Cardiovascular Nursing 2: 169–170
Taylor R S, Brown A, Ebrahim D M et al 2004 Exercise-based rehabilitation for patients with coronary heart disease: systematic review and meta-analysis of randomized controlled trials. American Heart Journal 116: 682–692
Thompson D R, Lewin R J P 2000 Management of the post myocardial infarction patient: rehabilitation and cardiac neurosis. Heart 84: 101–105
Thompson D R, Webster R A 2004 Caring for the coronary patient, 2nd edn. Butterworth-Heinemann, Oxford
Thompson D R, Webster R A, Sutton T W 1994 Coronary care unit patients' and nurses' ratings of intensity of ischaemic chest pain. Intensive and Critical Care Nursing 10: 81–88
Thompson D R, Ersser S J, Webster R A 1995 The experiences of patients and their partners one month after a heart attack. Journal of Advanced Nursing 22: 707–714
Thompson D R, Bowman G S, Kitson A L et al 1996 Cardiac rehabilitation in the United Kingdom: guidelines and audit standards. Heart 75: 89–93
Townsend P, Davidson N, Whitehead M 1992 Inequalities in health: the Black Report and the health divide. Penguin, Harmondsworth
Van Berkel T F, Boersma H, Roose-Hesselink J W et al 1999 Impact of smoking cessation and smoking interventions with coronary heart disease. European Heart Journal 20: 1773–1782
Westlake C, Dracup K, Walden J A et al 1999 Sexuality of patients with advanced heart failure and their spouses or partners. Journal of Heart and Lung Transplantation 18: 1133–1138
Williams A 1993 A case for emotional support and human contact. Management of cardiogenic shock. Professional Nurse 8: 520–523
Williams B, Poulter N R, Brown M J et al 2004 British Hypertension Society guidelines for hypertension management 2004: (BHS-IV) summary. British Medical Journal 328: 634–640
Williams G, Wright D J, Tan L B 2000 Management of cardiogenic shock complicating acute myocardial infarction: towards evidence-based medical practice. Heart 83: 621–626
World Health Organization (WHO) 2002 The World Health Report 2002. Reducing risks – promoting healthy life. WHO, Geneva
Wynne G A, Gwinnutt C, Bingham B et al 1999 Teaching resuscitation. In: Colquhoun M C, Handley A J, Evans T R (eds) ABC of resuscitation. BMJ Books, London
Yudkin J S 1998 Managing the diabetic patient with acute myocardial infarction. Diabetic Medicine 15: 276–281

FURTHER READING

ACC/AHA/NASPE 2002 Guideline update for implantation of cardiac pacemakers and antiarrhythmia devices. Journal of Cardiovascular Electrophysiology 13: 1183–1199
Autar R 1998 Calculating patients' risk of deep vein thrombosis. British Journal of Nursing 7: 7–12
Collins F 2003 Abdominal aortic aneurysm repair. In: Murray S (ed) Vascular disease: nursing and management. Whurr, London
Dinnes J, Kleijen J, Leitner M, Thompson D R 1999 Cardiac rehabilitation. Quality in Health Care 8: 65–71
Donohue S J 1997a Lower limb amputation 1. Indications and treatment. British Journal of Nursing 6: 970–972, 974–977
Donohue S J 1997b Lower limb amputation 2. Once the decision to amputate has been made. British Journal of Nursing 6: 1048–1052
Donohue S J 1997c Lower limb amputation 3. The role of the nurse. British Journal of Nursing 6: 1171–1174, 1187–1191
Donohue S J 1997d Lower limb amputation 4. Some ethical considerations. British Journal of Nursing 6: 1311–1314
Galloway S, Bubela N, McKibbon A et al 2005 Symptom distress, anxiety, depression and discharge information needs after peripheral artery bypass. Journal of Vascular Nursing 13(2): 35–40
Gibson J M E, Kenrick M 1998 Pain and powerlessness: the experience of living with peripheral vascular disease. Journal of Advanced Nursing 27(4): 737–745
Gupta S K 2005 The pharmacotherapy of heart failure. Anshan, Tunbridge Wells
Houghton A R, Gray D G 2003 Making sense of the ECG. Hodder Arnold, London
Jaarsma T, Stewart S 2004 Nurse-led management programmes in heart failure. In: Stewart D, Moser D K, Thompson D R (eds) Caring for the heart failure patient. Martin Dunitz, London
Jobin J, Maltais F, Poirier P, LeBlanc P, Simard C (eds) 2002 Advancing the frontiers of cardiopulmonary rehabilitation. Human Kinetics, Champaign, IL
Johnson M T 1997 Treatment and prevention

of varicose veins. Journal of Vascular Nursing 15: 97–103
Jolliffe J A, Rees K, Taylor R S et al 2005 Exercise-based rehabilitation for coronary heart disease. Cochrane Heart Group (Cochrane Review). In: The Cochrane Library, Issue 1. Wiley, Chichester
Jowett N I, Thompson D R 2003 Comprehensive coronary care, 3rd edn. Baillière Tindall, London
Levine G N, Kern M J, Berger P B et al 2003 Management of patients undergoing percutaneous coronary revascularisation. Annals of Internal Medicine 139: 123–136
Lindsay D, Gaw A 2003 Coronary heart disease prevention. Churchill Livingstone, Edinburgh
Litchfield B 2003 Promoting health in vascular nursing In: Murray S (ed) Vascular disease: nursing and management. Whurr, London
Moffatt C 2003 Leg ulcers. In: Murray S (ed) Vascular disease: nursing and management. Whurr, London
Murray S (ed) 2003 Chronic ischaemia. In: Vascular disease: nursing and management. Whurr, London
Nocton C 2003 Critical limb ischaemia. In: Murray S (ed) Vascular disease: nursing and management. Whurr, London
Ockenden L J 2003 Aetiology and pathology of vascular disease. In: Murray S (ed) Vascular disease: nursing and management. Whurr, London
Otto C M 2003 Valvular heart disease. Saunders, Philadelphia
Stubbling N, Chesworth J 2003 Assessment of patients with vascular disease. In: Murray S (ed) Vascular disease: nursing and management. Whurr, London
Vowden K, Vowden P 2003 Venous disorders. In: Murray S (ed) Vascular disease: nursing and management. Whurr, London
Waugh A, Grant A 2001 Ross and Wilson's anatomy and physiology, 9th edn. Churchill Livingstone, Edinburgh
Wilkinson I B, Cockcroft J, Waring S 2002 Hypertension: Your Questions Answered. Churchill Livingstone, Edinburgh

USEFUL WEBSITES

British Heart Foundation
www.bhf.org.uk

British Heart Foundation statistics
www.heartstats.org/homepage.asp

Driver and Vehicle Licensing agency (DVLA)
www.dvla.gov.uk

Society of Heart Valve Disease
www.shvd.org

Peripheral Vascular Diseases Group
www.link.med.ed.ac.uk/pvd

www.heartcentreonline.com
Useful pictures and animated clips

YourHeart
www.yourheart.org.uk
Information for cardiac patients and their families

DISORDERS OF THE RESPIRATORY SYSTEM

3

Cynthia B. Edmond
Jan McClean
Janice McGlone
Laura M. Wilson

INTRODUCTION

The respiratory system is one of the most vital systems in the human body. In health, it functions automatically and usually without our awareness. There are, however, few disease processes that do not have some disruptive effect on the respiratory system. There are also many respiratory disorders relating to environmental pollution, trauma, infection, genetic susceptibility and primary disease, as well as conditions secondary to other diseases. Although causative agents differ, the aetiology of each condition follows certain common patterns. To know the anatomy and physiology of the respiratory system is to understand how respiratory disorders inevitably relate to breakdown in ventilation, gaseous exchange or pulmonary perfusion. Symptoms differ only in degree and effect, and the treatment of symptoms will always have certain basic aims.

The effects of respiratory disorders range from the minor discomforts of the common cold to the distressing and life-threatening symptoms associated with respiratory failure. All are disabling to some extent to the individual and their family. As respiratory conditions and diseases cover such a broad spectrum and are common in both community and hospital settings, it is essential that nurses have a broad knowledge base relating to the basic concepts of normal respiration and an understanding of the factors that can lead to respiratory dysfunction.

Research indicates that some of the more serious respiratory disorders are related to lifestyle and are preventable. This chapter will therefore emphasise and outline various approaches to health promotion and disease prevention and the nurse's expanding role, opportunities and challenges in this field. It will also explore some of the more common disorders and, in discussing them, draw out the basic principles of management for all respiratory disorders. Although the emphasis is on nursing management, implicit in all discussions is the assumption that nurses work in close collaboration with other health care professionals and, in many instances, are responsible for coordinating the work of the whole team.

As you read this, you are probably unaware that you are breathing quietly and effortlessly; once you become attentive to the process of breathing, however, you can voluntarily vary the depth and pace of your respirations. You can sigh, cough or hold your breath for a time, and you can force air out through your vocal chords and sing or shout. When you go to sleep tonight, you can be reasonably confident that you will continue to breathe automatically and wake up in the morning feeling refreshed and well.

However, if for any reason your respiratory system were to break down, this whole picture would change. Case History 3.1(A) gives some insight into a patient's perspective on an acute episode of respiratory distress caused by a severe asthma attack (see p. 89).

STOP THINK

3.1 What is the critical response time in cardiopulmonary resuscitation (CPR) if you are to prevent irreparable brain damage? Refer to your first aid manual and, with appropriate guidance, be sure to practise CPR regularly throughout your nursing career: it is an essential procedure.

3.2 As well as following suggested reading and activities, you may find it useful to compile an information folder on essential procedures relating to respiratory care. It is also important when you are in the clinical area to observe the patients undergoing these procedures, to note their reactions and the effects of the procedures on them, and to talk to them about how they feel. Analyse the context. Reflect on your experiences. Make notes of critical incidents, and discuss them with your mentor or teacher.

The essential elements of life support are the essential elements of respiration. Airway, breathing (ventilation) and circulation are the ABC of life support. If any one of the three is cut off or becomes dysfunctional, the others are equally so, and an emergency situation exists which requires instant action if irreparable brain damage and death are to be prevented. An airway must be established and the individual's breathing and circulation restored in order to get oxygen to the vital organs and tissues.

ANATOMY AND PHYSIOLOGY

The reader is advised to review the anatomy and physiology of the respiratory system as a whole and to use a model of the thoracic cage to establish the relationship between all the structures illustrated in Figure 3.1. This section is intended as an overview of the most relevant points relating to normal respiratory function. Texts that can be consulted in conjunction with the present discussion are suggested below.

For further reading, see Waugh & Grant (2001) and Kindlen (2003).

Physiology of respiration

A continuous supply of O_2 and the elimination of CO_2 are necessary for the survival and functioning of body cells. The respiratory system in conjunction with the red blood cells (RBCs) of the circulatory system is responsible for this vital exchange. The process of respiration involves both external and internal respiration: external respiration involves oxygenation of the pulmonary capillary blood supply and elimination of CO_2 by diffusion across the alveolar and capil-lary membranes; internal respiration involves the exchange of O_2 and CO_2 at the cellular level and the use of O_2 and production of CO_2 in the tissues.

External respiration

External respiration involves ventilation, gaseous exchange and perfusion of the lungs with blood.

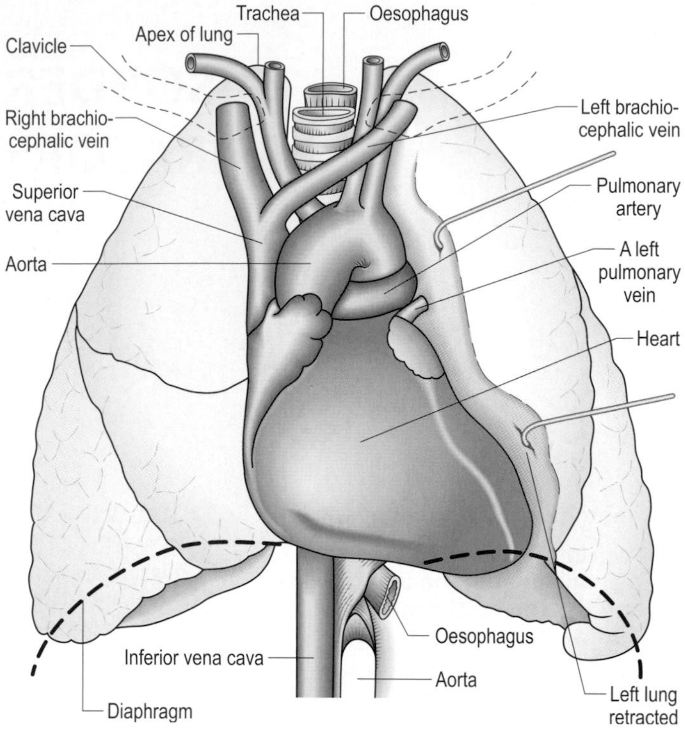

Fig. 3.1 Organs associated with the lungs.

Ventilation is the process by which air is moved in and out of the lungs via the airways. This process is powered by the respiratory muscles, mainly the diaphragm and the intercostal muscles, which work together to increase and decrease the size of the thoracic cavity. They are responsive to both voluntary and involuntary central nervous system (CNS) control. The thoracic cavity is lined with parietal pleura and the lung surfaces have a covering of visceral pleura. The negative pressure and serous lubricant between the parietal and visceral pleura have the effect of 'sticking' the lungs to the thoracic wall so that they expand and contract with these ventilatory movements. In health there is only a potential space between the pleural layers.

Central control Normally, the involuntary system maintains the regular automatic breathing cycle and is controlled by respiratory centres in the brain (see Fig. 3.2). These centres receive information from sensory receptors throughout the respiratory system and from chemoreceptors located in the carotid arteries, aorta and medulla.

The sensory receptors in the respiratory system itself monitor local irritants and lung expansion. A cough, for example, is a reflex response to airway irritants and a natural defence mechanism to clear the airways. The chemoreceptors monitor the levels of CO_2, O_2 and H^+ in the blood and of H^+ in the cerebrospinal fluid (CSF), and alter ventilation of the lungs to restore a normal balance of gases (see Table 3.1).

For a detailed explanation of gaseous exchange, see Chapter 7 in Kindlen (2003).

Pulmonary function — lung volume capacity and compliance It is important to bear in mind the basic principles relating to lung volume capacity and compliance and

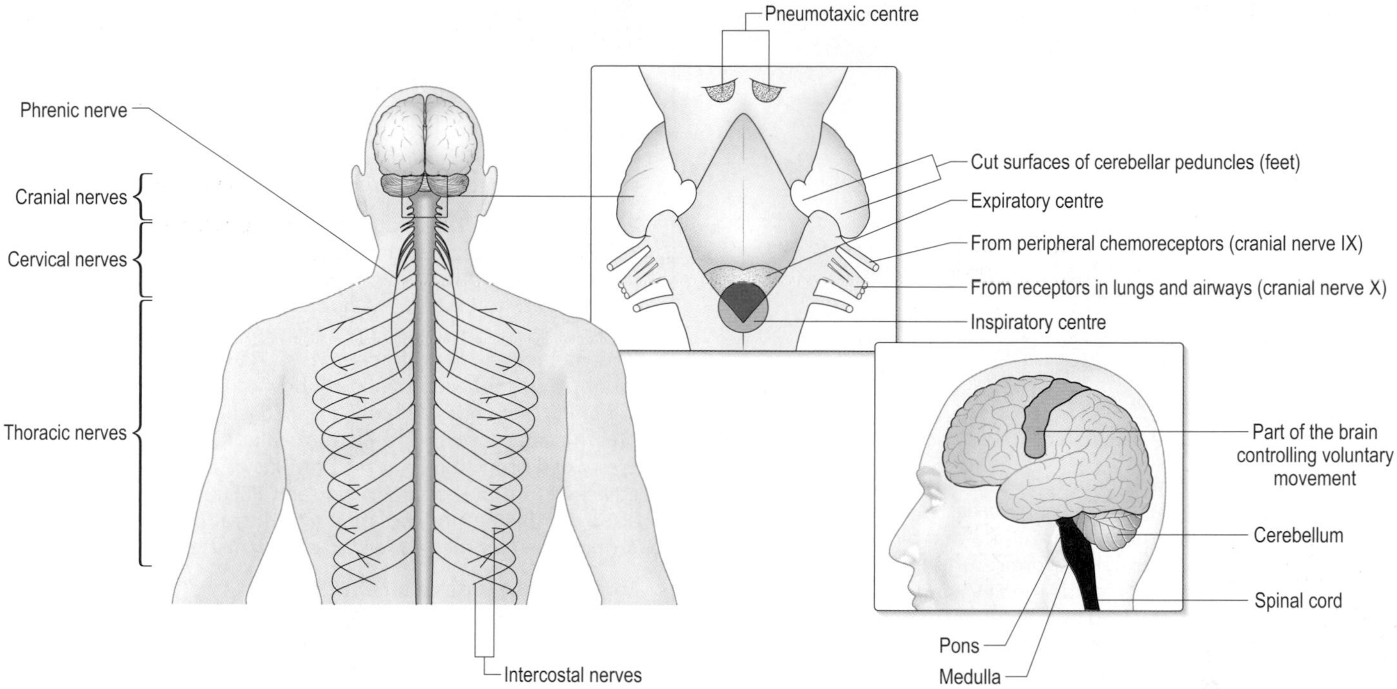

Fig. 3.2 Parts of the nervous system involved in controlling breathing: brain, brain stem, spinal cord and nerves. The enlarged inset shows the position of the respiratory centres in the medulla and pons of the brain stem as viewed from behind (the cerebellum, which sits on top of this, is not shown).

Table 3.1 Sensory receptors involved in the control of breathing

Type	Location	Stimulus	Effect on breathing
Within the respiratory system			
Irritant receptor	Airway epithelium: Nose, Trachea, Bronchioles	Inhaled particles and vapours	Sneeze Cough Increased rate and depth
Stretch receptors	Airway smooth muscle	Inflation	Slowed down
J receptors	Alveolar wall	Interstitial oedema Pulmonary emboli	Rapid and shallow
Muscle spindles	Respiratory muscles	Elongation of the muscles	Made smoother and more efficient
Elsewhere			
Chemoreceptors	Carotid artery Aorta	↑ CO_2, ↓ O_2, ↑ H^+ in blood	Increased rate and depth
	Brain (medulla)	↑ H^+ in CSF	Increased rate and depth

Reproduced with permission from Kindlen (2003).

to recognise the significance of their measurement. They are important factors in ventilation and are often affected by respiratory disorders. Lung volumes can be measured by spirometry (see Fig. 3.3).

The volume of air breathed in and out and the number of breaths per minute vary from one individual to another according to age, size and activity. Normal, quiet breathing gives about 15 complete cycles per minute in the adult. Lung volume can be assessed in the following terms:

- *Tidal volume (TV)* — this is the amount of air that passes in and out of the lungs during each cycle of quiet breathing (approximately 500 mL in the adult). Exchange of gases takes place only in the alveolar ducts

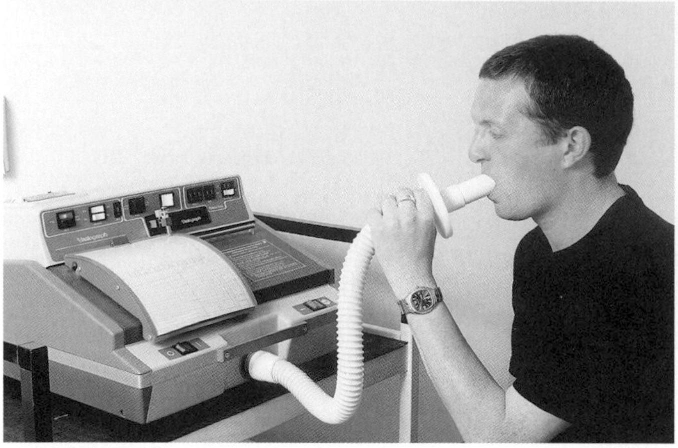

Fig. 3.3 Measurement of breathing flow and lung volumes by spirometry. The subject is instructed to breathe normally then fully inspire, put lips firmly around mouthpiece and blow out as hard, fast and completely as possible before returning to normal breathing. The spirometer records the FEV_1 and FVC. The standard test procedures are performed by trained technicians to ensure the quality of results. (Reproduced with kind permission of Medical Illustration Services, North Glasgow University NHS Hospitals Trust.)

and sacs. The rest of the air passages are known as 'dead space' and contain about 150 mL of air.

- *Inspiratory capacity* — this is the amount of air that can be inspired with maximum effort. This consists of tidal volume plus the inspiratory reserve volume (IRV).
- *Functional residual capacity (FRC)* — this is the amount of air remaining in the air passages and alveoli at the end of quiet respiration; it is composed of expiratory reserve volume (ERV) and residual volume (RV). The RV prevents collapse of the alveoli and makes continuous gaseous exchange possible as the alveolar gas mix remains constant.
- *Vital capacity (VC)* — this is the TV plus the IRV and ERV.
- *Total lung capacity (TLC)* — with maximum effort the adult lungs can hold 4–6 L of air. Most of this can be forcibly expelled, leaving a RV of about 1 L (see Box 3.1).

Lung expansion and recoil Elastic fibres in lung tissue and the surface tension of the fluid lining the alveoli give the lungs their natural recoil tendency. Ease of expansion and recoil depends on normal compliance and elasticity and on the presence of surfactant in the fluid lining the alveoli. Compliance can be reduced by the stiffening of normally soft alveolar tissue due to pulmonary oedema or to the ageing process. Conversely, compliance can be increased by extreme softening due to loss of lung tissue, as in emphysema.

Surfactant is a mixture of substances, mainly lipoproteins, secreted by cells of the alveolar epithelium, which lowers the surface tension of the alveolar fluid, making it easier for the alveoli to expand. Lack of surfactant in premature infants results in alveoli that remain collapsed (atelectasis) and leads to a ventilatory problem known as infant respiratory distress syndrome. A surfactant deficiency can also occur in adults as a response to severe shock, trauma or massive blood transfusion. This leads to increasing ventilatory difficulty, with rapid, shallow breathing and ineffectual respiration, a critical condition known as adult respiratory distress syndrome (ARDS) which may require artificial ventilatory support.

Ventilation, then, depends on CNS control, functioning respiratory muscles and adequate volume capacity of the lungs. Conditions which affect ventilation include some neurological diseases, diaphragmatic compression from constricting dressings or appliances, injuries to the chest wall, lungs or diaphragm, obstructive airways diseases such as asthma, space-occupying lesions, thoracic deformities and severe pain. In addition, certain opioid medications, such as morphine, are known to depress the central respiratory centre.

Gaseous exchange is the second vital component in the respiratory process. By a process of diffusion, O_2 passes from the alveoli into the bloodstream and CO_2 passes from the bloodstream into the alveoli. This exchange is dependent on adequate perfusion by the pulmonary blood supply.

Perfusion, i.e. the volume of blood passing through the lungs, determines the amount of O_2 taken into the body and the amount of CO_2 eliminated. In health, regulatory mechanisms ensure a balance between ventilation and perfusion such that well-ventilated parts of the lung receive an adequate blood supply and blood does not pass through the pulmonary circulation without being oxygenated (termed 'shunting'). Shunting occurs where there is an area of consolidation, as in pneumonia; although there is adequate perfusion, there is no ventilation.

STOP THINK **3.3** Revise the properties of gases.

Box 3.1

Assessment of air flow

Vital capacity
This is the sum of inspiratory reserve volume, tidal volume and expiratory reserve volume, approximately 4800 mL.

Peak expiratory flow rate (PEFR), or peak flow
This is an expression of the maximum rate of air flow when the individual is breathing out as hard and fast as possible, starting with full lungs. The normal range is 400–600 L/min. PEFR is measured with a simple instrument called a peak flow meter. Patients with diseases such as asthma are taught to record their own peak flow at regular intervals. A fall in PEFR provides a warning of bronchospasm before breathlessness occurs and therefore alerts patients to use prescribed bronchodilator medications or to seek medical advice before the condition worsens. PEFR measures are also recorded before and after administration of bronchodilatory medications to assess their effectiveness.

Forced expiratory volume (FEV)
FEV_1 (forced expiratory volume in 1 s) is the volume of air exhaled in the first second of a forced maximal expiratory manoeuvre. The FEV_1/VC ratio is the ratio between the volume exhaled in 1 s to the total volume of air exhaled. It will be reduced in an obstructive disorder, i.e. it will be less than 75%.

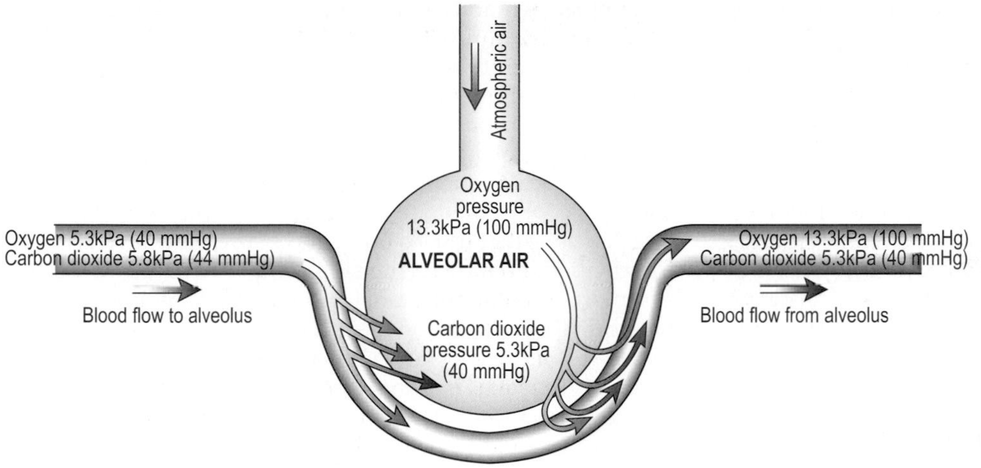

Fig. 3.4 The interchange of gases between air in the alveoli and the blood capillaries.

Gaseous exchange and lung perfusion Each microscopic, grape-like alveolus is surrounded by an intimate structural network of capillaries which together provide the lungs with an enormous capacity for gaseous exchange. This exchange is smooth and uninterrupted because the composition of the alveolar air remains constant due to the tidal ebb and flow of inspired air and the residual volume (RV) which is warmed and saturated with water vapour. As indicated in Figure 3.4, the gases in the blood leaving the lungs are in equilibrium with the air in the alveoli.

The total pressure exerted in the walls of the alveoli by the mixture of gases in air is the same as atmospheric pressure (100 kPa). Each gas in the mixture exerts a part of that total pressure proportional to its concentration; this is known as its partial pressure (P).

Arterial blood gas (ABG) levels Nurses may be involved in interpreting blood gas results, administering oxygen and monitoring respirators. A working knowledge of the properties of gases, of partial pressure and of gaseous exchange is therefore essential (see Table 3.2).

Table 3.2 Composition of air

	Dry atmosphere		Alveolar air (37°C)	
	%	kPa[a]	%	kPa[a]
Oxygen	21	21	13.2	13.2
Carbon dioxide	0.04	0.04	5.3	5.3
Nitrogen[b]	79	79	75.2	75.2
Water vapour	?[c]	?[c]	6.3	6.3

[a]Assuming barometric pressure is 100 kPa.
[b]Includes <1% rare gases (argon, helium, etc.).
[c]Amount of moisture in atmosphere depends on humidity and temperature. If moisture is present, percentage of other constituents will then be correspondingly decreased.
Reproduced with permission from Kindlen (2003).

Internal (cellular) respiration

Cellular respiration is an essential part of the whole process of respiration.

The haemoglobin of the red blood cells (RBCs) carries O_2 to the tissues where, by the process of diffusion, gaseous exchange takes place between the arterial end of the capillaries and the tissue fluid. CO_2, which is one of the waste products of carbohydrate and fat metabolism in the cells, transfers to the venous capillary blood, where it is carried to the lungs in three ways, i.e.:

- dissolved in the blood plasma
- combined with haemoglobin
- in combination with sodium as sodium bicarbonate.

These processes are described more fully in Kindlen (2003, pp. 136–138), where a clear description of both the oxygen–haemoglobin dissociation curve and the carbon dioxide dissociation curve is given.

PRINCIPLES OF NURSING MANAGEMENT IN THE PREVENTION AND TREATMENT OF RESPIRATORY DISORDERS

There are two main nursing priorities:

- health promotion and disease prevention
- developing clinical skills in order to ensure competent care.

The first priority will be addressed in relation to preventing serious respiratory diseases caused by environmental pollution and cigarette smoking; the second will be addressed in relation to specific respiratory disorders later in the chapter.

Conceptual framework

It is assumed in care planning for patients with respiratory disorders, whether in the hospital or in the community, that the care is underpinned by an appropriate driving philosophy and model of nursing care. It is suggested that a modified version of Orem's (2001) philosophy of promoting independence and balancing self-care deficit with nursing compensatory intervention could be appropriate in the care of an asthma patient. For example, on admission, during an acute attack of asthma (Case History 3.1(A), p. 89), C is unable to meet his self-care needs and requires major compensatory intervention by both medical and nursing staff. As he recovers, the deficit is reduced and nursing intervention, always in collaboration with other members of the health care team, moves through partly compensatory to supportive–educative as he is prepared for discharge home and is more able to control his asthma and maintain a higher degree of independence (see Case History 3.1(B), p. 94).

The nurse's role in health promotion and disease prevention

Promoting health and preventing disease are vital to the social and economic well-being of our society and their importance is reflected in government legislation and the development of large-scale screening and health education programmes (Donaldson 2004). With the cost of health care soaring, it makes good sense to prevent disease where possible rather than treating the consequences. This is particularly true of some respiratory diseases and nurses are well placed in their many roles in the hospital and community to plan an active and expanding role in the area of primary health care (Buck 1997).

Downie et al (1996) describe three basic orientations for health education: disease orientation, risk factor orientation and health orientation (see Box 3.2). The evidence suggests that while each of these models has a valid place, a comprehensive and collaborative approach is necessary to tackle the complexities of most health-related issues. Government initiatives are aimed at preventing specific diseases and eliminating risk factors while health-orientated programmes initiated by the health professionals reinforce government policies by offering a more positive focus and satisfying health outcome for the individual. Information should be presented in an innovative and effective way, which means that nurses must make sure they have accurate information, good teaching skills and adequate resources.

Environmental pollutants and cigarette smoking are two of the major risk factor areas which can affect the health of the respiratory system. When the lungs are continually exposed to such irritants there is, initially, an increase in mucus secretion. The cilia, which normally clear the air passages of mucus, become coated and dysfunctional and eventually die. The presence of irritants and excess mucus causes inflammation and narrowing of the airways, disrupting gas diffusion. Cigarette smoke also contains carbon monoxide (CO), which binds easily to haemoglobin and displaces oxygen. Other chemicals in tobacco smoke cause vasoconstriction and constriction of the airways (West et al 2000). Constant inflammation leads to the formation of fibrous tissue and permanent narrowing of the airways of chronic bronchitis. Alveolar tissue is destroyed, reducing lung area and resulting in emphysema (see p. 84). These destructive changes are irreversible, although further destruction can be avoided by eliminating the cause: a concept simple in theory but difficult to put into practice.

Box 3.2

Orientations for health education

Downie et al (1996) describe the following orientations for health education:

1. *Disease-orientated education*. This approach aims to prevent specific diseases. The emphasis is on measuring success in terms of progress towards target rates for morbidity and mortality.
2. *Risk factor-orientated education*. Efforts are aimed at eliminating particular risk factors to prevent associated diseases.
3. *Health-orientated education*. The aim is to enhance positive health as well as to prevent ill-health. This orientation recognises the physical, mental and social facets of both positive and negative health and acknowledges that:
   - Provision of information is not enough. The educational process needs to be participatory, to help people clarify their values, e.g. how they see themselves and their health, and acquire and develop life skills, e.g. decision making and assertiveness. The educator seeks to understand people's perspectives and opinions, to respect them rather than correct them or blame them for their behaviour
   - There are major constraints to freedom of choice in health-related behaviour, e.g. sociopolitical factors.

Environmental pollution and health

Exhaust fumes from motor vehicles are a major source of air pollution in cities in the UK and other heavily populated countries in the world. Government intervention is needed to control this and other environmental pollutants such as dust, smoke, chemical fumes, agricultural pollutants and cigarette smoke. Nurses can actively and usefully support such intervention through early detection of risk factors, innovative local intervention and health education in the hospital, the workplace, the school and the home.

Many industrial workplaces expose employees to pollutants such as dust, chemicals and toxic fumes. Miners of nickel, coal, cobalt and radium are exposed to fluorocarbons, which have been shown to be related to an increased incidence of serious lung disease, including carcinoma. Agricultural workers are exposed to biohazards such as grain dust, bacteria and their metabolites (endotoxins and exotoxins), fungi and their metabolites (glucans) and storage mites; they are also exposed to airborne insecticides, fungicides and pesticides and to animal parasites and debris. Epidemiological and clinical studies have identified strong associations between agricultural exposure and rhinitis and asthma. More serious diseases, although less common, are hypersensitivity, pneumonitis and respiratory infection (Linaker & Smedley 2002).

Occupational health and community nurses have a responsibility to educate employees and managers about environmental hazards and to press for the use of appropriate protective clothing and respiratory masks and for improved working conditions and leisure facilities.

The home can also be a source of respiratory risk factors. Use of aerosol hair and body sprays and household cleaning products, together with sidestream cigarette smoke, can be a constant source of respiratory irritation for the whole family. Again, it is the community nurse who can advise and educate families.

Cigarette smoking and health

The hazardous health effects of tobacco have been known for over 50 years (WHO 2002a). Although the prevalence of smoking has fallen in developed countries, it is increasing in many low and middle income countries, especially among young people and women. In 2000, an estimated 4.9 million deaths (8.8% of the global total) were attributable to use of tobacco, 45% higher than the number in 1990 (Shibuya et al 2003). Without additional interventions to reduce use of tobacco, the health burden will continue to increase. At current levels of consumption, the burden is estimated to double by 2020 (WHO 2002b).

The tobacco epidemic requires international action and, in 2003, the World Health Organization (WHO) for the first time used its constitutional authority to develop an evidence-based global public health treaty, the *WHO Framework Convention on Tobacco Control* (Shibuya et al 2003). This sets out a range of measures to reduce both the demand and the supply of tobacco. Governments have a key role in encouraging risk reduction strategies, for example, through taxation and restriction on tobacco advertising, promotion and sponsorship, but it is known that getting governments to agree on strategies for prevention or treatment is difficult. In the UK, legislation to ban advertising was only introduced in 2003 (Eaton 2003).

STOP THINK

3.4 Scan current journals and websites for articles relating to smoking and health. What is the current UK position regarding the following:

(a) tobacco advertising, promotion and sponsorship
(b) tobacco packaging and labelling
(c) protection from exposure to environmental tobacco smoke
(d) restriction of tobacco sales to and by minors?

Smoking tobacco is considered to be the most preventable cause of ill-health and early death in the UK. Reducing smoking and the harm it causes are major government health-related priorities (Scottish Executive 2004). It is estimated that every year in the UK, approximately 114 000 people die as a result of smoking which contributes significantly to disease of the heart, blood vessels, lungs, upper respiratory tract, oesophagus, stomach, bladder and other organs (Tobacco Advisory Group of the Royal College of Physicians 2000, British Heart Foundation 2004). In Scotland, adult smoking rates remain consistently higher than in the UK as whole for both genders, and there are marked differences by post-code sector; the highest smoking rates are found in areas of highest economic deprivation (Office for National Statistics 2002, NHS Health Scotland/ASH Scotland 2003).

The sidestream smoke inhaled in passive smoking has a higher concentration of some toxic and carcinogenic substances than has mainstream smoke, which is significant for families and workmates of smokers (Moher et al 2004). There is evidence that active or passive smoking during pregnancy is associated with increased health risks to the unborn child (Acharya et al 2002). Maternal smoking has been linked to sudden infant death syndrome (SIDS) and passive smoking to a high incidence of childhood asthma (Dezateux et al 1999). Passive smoking can also be linked to a high incidence of acute coronary syndromes (Pitsavos et al 2002) (see Research Abstract 3.1; see also Ch. 2).

RESEARCH ABSTRACT 3.1

Passive smoking increases the risk of developing acute coronary syndrome (ACS)

The purpose of this study by Pitsavos et al (2002) was to investigate the association between passive smoking and the risk of ACS. Patients with a first event of ACS (n = 848) and cardiovascular disease-free matched controls (n = 1078) completed a detailed questionnaire regarding their exposure to environmental smoke. From this, 297 (35%) of the patients and 259 (24%) of the controls were defined as non-smokers and passive smokers, respectively. The results showed that non-smokers exposed to cigarette smoke increased their risk of ACS by 51% when compared to non-smokers not exposed to smoke. It was estimated that 34 coronary events per 134 subjects would occur as a result of passive smoking during their lifetime.

Pitsavos C, Panagiotakos D B, Chrysohoou C et al 2002 Association between passive cigarette smoking and the risk of developing acute coronary syndrome: the CARDIO2000 study. Heart and Vessels 16(4): 127–130

Smoking cessation and nursing intervention

Although most adult smokers say they would like to give up smoking and are aware of its dangers, each year only 2% who try to give up will manage by will-power alone. There are a number of interventions that increase quit rates. These range from low intensity support, such as self-help materials and telephone helplines, to more intensive interventions including individual and group counselling. In general, the more intensive the intervention, the greater the increase in quit rate. When combined with pharmacological aids, i.e. nicotine replacement therapy (NRT) or bupropion (Zyban), quit rates double irrespective of the intervention (West et al 2000). However, even the most intensive interventions result in modest quit rates. Nevertheless, compared with other medical interventions, smoking cessation interventions are cost-effective and if widely available and properly applied, will contribute to a reduction in smoking prevalence. All NRT products are on the *Nurse Prescribers' Formulary* (British Medical Association 2002) and community nurses are now making an increasing contribution to smoking cessation (Percival 2003) (see Research Abstract 3.2).

STOP THINK

3.5 Design a smoking-related health education programme for early teenage children. What activities would you include? What teaching aids would you use? Access current websites that cover health promotion initiatives and look for local advertisements regarding one-to-one helplines.

RESEARCH ABSTRACT 3.2

Nursing interventions for smoking cessation

Health care professionals, including nurses, frequently advise patients to improve their health by stopping smoking. Such advice may be brief, or part of more intensive interventions. To determine the effectiveness of nurse-delivered smoking cessation interventions, the Cochrane Tobacco Addiction Group register was searched for studies of interventions using nurses or health visitors and an additional search made on CINAHL. Randomised trials with follow-up of at least 6 months were selected. Sixteen studies comparing nursing intervention to a control or usual care found intervention to significantly increase the odds of quitting. There was no evidence from indirect comparison that interventions classified as intensive had a larger effect than less intensive ones. There was limited evidence that interventions were more effective for hospital inpatients with cardiovascular disease than for inpatients with other conditions. Five studies of nurse counselling on smoking cessation during a screening health check found that under these conditions nursing intervention had less effect.

The results indicate the potential benefits of smoking cessation advice and counselling given by nurses to their patients, with reasonable evidence that interventions can be effective. The challenge will be to incorporate smoking cessation intervention as part of standard practice so that all patients are given an opportunity to be asked about their tobacco use and to be given advice to quit, along with reinforcement and follow-up.

Rice V H, Stead L F 2003 Nursing interventions for smoking cessation (Cochrane Review). In: The Cochrane Library, Issue 2. Wiley, Chichester

COMMON RESPIRATORY DISORDERS

Respiratory disorders reflect a breakdown in the integrity of the alveolar walls. They either cause, or are caused by, oedema, the presence of exudate or by inflammation, resulting in scarring and alteration in the process of gaseous exchange. Causes of respiratory inflammation are varied and range from common diseases such as influenza and colds, to bronchitis, pneumonia, tuberculosis, cystic fibrosis and the opportunistic infections of AIDS and other immunosuppressive conditions. While causative factors, organisms or irritants differ, the aetiologies of respiratory disorders are similar and they are, in varying degrees, similar in their clinical manifestations. Assessment of respiratory function is central to all clinical care (see Box 3.3).

For a detailed account of respiratory assessment, see Field (1997).

The incidence of COPD and malignancy due to environmental pollutants and cigarette smoking appears to have increased significantly in recent years (Office for National Statistics 2000). Additionally, the lungs are often involved in terminal or critical illness where pulmonary oedema, bronchitis, pneumonia or atelectasis, i.e. collapse of alveoli, may develop.

Box 3.3

Respiratory assessment: a clinical skill central to all patient care

- Visual observation — cyanosis, perfusion
- Respiratory rate, rhythm and depth
- Breath sounds
- Use of ancillary muscles
- Sputum and secretions
- Causes of variation from normal, e.g. pain, anxiety, disease
- Respiratory history
- Arterial blood gases
- Pulse oximetry
- Chest X-ray
- Pulmonary lung function tests
- Bronchoscopy
- Imaging, e.g. CT scan, MRI

Common clinical manifestations of all of these disorders include varying degrees of breathlessness, cough, sputum production and dyspnoea (difficulty in breathing), tachypnoea (increased respiratory rate), cyanosis (blue discoloration of the skin), hypoxia (low O_2 concentration in the tissues) and hypercapnia (high concentration of CO_2 in arterial blood).

Wherever there is disruption of the respiratory process, there is the probability that oxygen therapy will be necessary to relieve breathlessness and improve tissue perfusion (see Box 3.4).

Each of the processes involved in external respiration — ventilation, gaseous exchange and circulatory perfusion — is a critical component in maintaining the life and function of body cells. Disruption in any of these processes results in respiratory disorders of varying severity.

INFECTIONS OF THE RESPIRATORY SYSTEM

Infections of the upper respiratory tract are addressed in Chapter 14. This chapter will focus on bronchitis, pneumonia and tuberculosis.

Acute bronchitis and tracheobronchitis

Acute bronchitis is the inflammation of the mucous membranes of the bronchial tree. Tracheobronchitis, as the name implies, affects the trachea as well as the bronchi. Both conditions are associated with infections of the upper respiratory tract (see Ch. 14) but may also occur as a result of atmospheric pollutants, cigarette smoking or when some other chronic respiratory disorder already exists. They can affect people of all ages and are usually only of real concern in the very young, the very old and the debilitated. A normally healthy person will usually recover quite quickly. The concern in terms of health promotion is to ensure that acute bronchitis does not develop into bronchopneumonia and that acute attacks do not become so frequent that the condition becomes chronic (see p. 84).

For information on pulmonary pathophysiology, see West (2003).

Box 3.4

Oxygen (O_2) therapy

The need for O_2 therapy arises when oxygen transport to the tissues is insufficient due to breakdown in either the respiratory or the circulatory system. Clinical signs and blood gas levels are the main indicators of degree of hypoxia. Profound hypoxaemia will cause death in minutes, whereas death from carbon dioxide (CO_2) narcosis is a more lengthy process (see Box 3.6).

The aim of O_2 therapy is to administer sufficient oxygen to maintain tissue oxygenation at a functional level and eliminate detrimental compensatory responses to hypoxaemia, and to prevent serious or irreparable damage to vital organs and tissues.

The percentage of oxygen that is to be delivered is carefully determined, either by circumstances, as in life-threatening emergencies, where 100% pure oxygen may be given initially, or by carrying out arterial blood gas (ABG) measurement or pulse oximetry, and prescribing oxygen accordingly. A pulse oximeter is a small, non-invasive device which can register arterial oxygen saturation through the skin using a clip-on sensor (Cowan 1997).

For therapeutic purposes, the range of prescription is usually between 24 and 60% of O_2. Hyperbaric oxygen (oxygen given at greater than 1 atmosphere absolute) may be used to improve oxygen perfusion of the tissues by increasing the dissolved oxygen in the blood, as in treatment of CO poisoning or deep-sea divers' 'bends' (Bateman & Leach 1998).

In certain conditions, the amount of oxygen given is determined by prior knowledge of adverse effects. For example, in patients with known COPD (see p. 84) it is dangerous to give too much oxygen. In premature babies high oxygen tensions in the arterial blood may cause damage to immature retinal vessels and in severe cases may result in blindness. This condition is known as retrolental fibroplasia.

Oxygen is commonly administered via nasal cannulae or oxygen masks. Supplemental oxygen may also be delivered during mechanical ventilation or non-invasive ventilation (NIV). Hyperbaric oxygenation can be achieved in specialist centres using hyperbaric chambers.

Humidification chambers attached to the oxygen equipment ensure that the oxygen is moistened before being inhaled. In mechanical ventilators it is also warmed and therefore enters the respiratory tract as vapour, fully saturated and at body temperature.

Oxygen toxicity

Retrolental fibroplasia may develop in premature infants as described above. Mature lungs may be damaged if high concentrations of oxygen are given over several days. This is thought to increase alveolar permeability so that capillary walls break down and fluid and blood accumulate. Severe cases may progress to pneumonia, fibrosis, pulmonary hypertension and right-sided heart failure.

PATHOPHYSIOLOGY

Common presenting symptoms The individual feels generally unwell with, initially, a dry painful cough and a moderate pyrexia. The cough becomes increasingly productive as the inflamed mucosal cells pour out mucus and the sputum produced becomes increasingly mucopurulent. Bronchospasm can occur, causing wheezing and a degree of dyspnoea.

MEDICAL MANAGEMENT

Investigations For otherwise healthy individuals, investigations are usually unnecessary. However, if marked mucopurulent sputum is produced, a sputum culture will be taken to identify the causative organism and a chest X-ray will be required.

Treatment The treatment is aimed at relieving the symptoms. Bed rest is advocated until the pyrexia has resolved. Moist inhalations, as prescribed, can relieve the bronchial symptoms and a high fluid intake is encouraged. Expectorants will also help to relieve the congestion, and antibiotic therapy will be prescribed as appropriate.

NURSING PRIORITIES AND MANAGEMENT: Acute bronchitis and tracheobronchitis

The nurse's priority will be for those vulnerable individuals for whom acute bronchitis could prove serious. Overexertion must be avoided and such patients may need support with expectoration and sputum clearance and maintaining oral hygiene. Optimal nutritional and fluid intake will aid recovery and help to prevent further infection.

When the individual is well enough, advice should be given as to how further attacks can be prevented. Avoidance of cigarette smoke, dust and ill-ventilated, cold or crowded environments is encouraged but is not always easy to achieve. The advice given and the outcomes aimed for must be realistic and tailored to the lifestyle and socioeconomic circumstances of the individual. An influenza vaccination may prove an effective preventive measure in high-risk individuals. Currently it is recommended for people with underlying respiratory, heart and renal disease or impaired immune systems, for those over 65 years of age and for health care workers (Joint Committee on Vaccination and Immunisation 2003).

Pneumonia

Pneumonia is an infection of lung tissue and is most usefully classified according to the causative organism, which may be bacterial or viral.

Bronchopneumonia

PATHOPHYSIOLOGY

Bronchopneumonia is characterised mainly by patchy areas of consolidated lung tissue. Causative organisms are bacterial and fungal and include staphylococci, pneumococci, streptococci, *Haemophilus influenzae* and *Candida*. It usually occurs in individuals weakened by other conditions and often in the very old, the very young, the unconscious, and as a result of a pre-existing disease, such as chronic bronchitis, atelectasis or carcinoma in adults, or infectious diseases in infants.

Clinical features vary in severity depending on the overall condition of the patient but include varying degrees of pyrexia, cough with copious purulent sputum, exhalatory râles, dyspnoea and tachypnoea. On auscultation, consolidation of the lower lobes is found.

MEDICAL MANAGEMENT

The causative organism is isolated by sputum culture and sensitivity, and appropriate antibiotic therapies are commenced. The patient's general condition is improved by attention to nutrition, hydration and physiotherapy (Kleinpell & Elpern 2004).

NURSING PRIORITIES AND MANAGEMENT: Bronchopneumonia

The patient with bronchopneumonia will be very ill and both patient and family will need a great deal of comfort and reassurance. Attention to personal hygiene and physical comfort is important. The patient should be turned or encouraged to move regularly. An upright sitting position, where possible, will make breathing easier and, if oxygen is prescribed, this therapy should be monitored carefully. Aids to prevent pressure ulcers developing should be selected judiciously (see Ch. 23).

Bronchopneumonia can be prevented in many hospitalised high-risk patients by thorough nursing assessment and meticulous nursing care.

Lobar pneumonia

PATHOPHYSIOLOGY

This is an acute bacterial infection which sometimes involves a whole lobe. It occurs mainly in young adults, usually males, but its full-blown effects are uncommon now because of the early and effective use of antibiotics. However, if left untreated, lobar pneumonia can progress to further areas of consolidation as well as to pleurisy, pericarditis, bacteraemia and possibly death.

Viral pneumonia

PATHOPHYSIOLOGY

The main difference between viral pneumonia and other types of pneumonia is that the inflammatory reaction is localised within the septal walls of the alveoli and there is no exudate. Many cases are caused by agents such as *Mycoplasma pneumoniae*, *Legionella* and *Chlamydia*. This group was formerly known as primary atypical pneumonia (PAP). Although these diseases differ from pneumococcal pneumonia, there may be overlap in clinical presentation. Other highly contagious viruses which can begin as a 'common cold' and progress to more severe respiratory tract infections include influenza types A and B, respiratory syncytial virus (RSV), rubella and varicella, *Rickettsia* and echoviruses.

Clinical features Symptoms include pyrexia, muscular pains, headaches and a dry, hacking cough. Treatment is symptomatic, with attention given to general nutrition, hydration and antibiotic treatment of any intercurrent bacterial infections. The disease runs its course and, except in the more vulnerable individual, resolution is expected. However, the patient may be left feeling weak and exhausted for some time afterwards.

NURSING PRIORITIES AND MANAGEMENT: Viral pneumonia

Susceptible individuals — older people, the debilitated and health workers at high risk of infection — should be encouraged to attend the practice nurse clinic for influenza vaccinations in preparation for the winter months or where epidemics are forecast (Joint Committee on Vaccination and Immunisation 2003, Willcox 2003).

Most individuals can be treated at home. Some may need nursing advice or assistance to carry out the activities of daily living and to ensure they are properly nourished and hydrated. Individuals nursed at home will be referred back to their GP if medical treatment becomes necessary.

For further information, see British Thoracic Society (2001a). For information on severe acute respiratory syndrome, see Box 3.5.

Tuberculosis (pulmonary)

Tuberculosis (TB) is a chronic infectious disease mainly of the lungs (pulmonary tuberculosis) but, when infecting other parts of the body, it is known as miliary tuberculosis. In the early part of the 20th century, it was common in developed as well as developing countries. With the advent of compulsory chest X-ray, bacille Calmette–Guérin (BCG) vaccination and effective medication, the incidence in developed countries became almost negligible. However, the UK is now experiencing an increase in the incidence of TB due to increased immigration from Eastern bloc and developing countries and the rise of HIV (WHO 2004) (see also Ch. 37). The occurrence and rise in multidrug-resistant TB (MDR TB) has also been closely associated with HIV infection (Pozniak 2001).

For further information, see Joint Tuberculosis Committee of the British Thoracic Society (2000).

PATHOPHYSIOLOGY

Tuberculosis is a disease caused mainly by *Mycobacterium tuberculosis*, although *Mycobacteria avium* and *bovis* can also cause the respiratory form. The disease is characterised by two types of lesions: exudative and productive.

The exudative lesion arises from the inflammatory process in which the bacterial organism is surrounded by fluid containing polymorphonuclear leucocytes and monocytes. If the lesion fails to heal, it may become necrosed and develop into a productive lesion (tubercle).

A tubercle consists of a fibrous or a soft outer cover with a core of giant cells, lymphocytes, monocytes, fibroblasts and epithelioid cells. The mycobacterium can live in the centre of this tubercle for years. The soft tubercle can rupture and spread its contents into surrounding tissue. Spread of infection is by direct contact with the infected tissue, by the bloodstream or by the lymphatics. In pulmonary tuberculosis, spread to others is by droplet infection from coughing or saliva.

Clinical features vary in severity, depending on the virulence of the organism and the susceptibility of the

Box 3.5

Severe acute respiratory syndrome (SARS)

In 2003, the World Health Organization (WHO) reported the existence of a new atypical pneumonia called severe acute respiratory syndrome (SARS). SARS is defined as a serious respiratory illness, with patients exhibiting the following signs and symptoms:

- pyrexia (>38°C)
- cough, shortness of breath or difficulty in breathing
- changes on X-ray indicative of pneumonia.

The cause of SARS is the SARS coronavirus (SARS CoV). Corona viruses have a halo or crown-like (corona) appearance when viewed under the microscope. This group of viruses commonly cause mild to moderate upper respiratory illness in humans and are associated with respiratory, gastrointestinal, liver and neurological diseases in animals. Most SARS infections appear to be less infectious than influenza but the corona viruses can survive in the environment for as long as 3 h.

It is thought that the SARS CoV is closely related to the animal corona viruses and has jumped species. There is evidence that the SARS CoV may be able to survive longer than other forms of the virus. The incubation period is thought to be between 7 and 10 days.

The first outbreak of this life-threatening syndrome was in the province of Guangdong in China in mid-November 2002. From there it was spread to Hong Kong by an infected doctor. The exact means of transfer was unconfirmed. He seeded a cluster of cases among guests in the hotel where he stayed. The virus spread to other parts of China and to Canada, Singapore and Vietnam. It was then reported in Malaysia, the Philippines, Taiwan, Thailand and South Africa.

By 2003, the number of deaths reported as being due to SARS was: China, 348; Hong Kong, 298; Taiwan, 84; Canada, 38; Singapore, 32; Vietnam, 5; Malaysia, 2; the Philippines, 2; Thailand, 2; S Africa, 1 (BBC 2003).

Management of SARS CoV cases

Isolation is essential to limit the spread of the disease. It is recommended that patients are managed at home, if their condition permits, in order to limit cross-infection. Standard infection control precautions should be taken when examining or taking samples from a potential SARS case (see Ch. 16). Suspected SARS patients should be advised to cover their mouths with a tissue when coughing or sneezing. If respiratory status permits, the patient should wear a respirator or surgical mask when in close contact with a non-infected person. The health care worker or carer should wear a surgical mask.

At present there is no specific treatment for SARS, although antibiotics and antiviral drugs are being used to try to treat the symptoms.

For up-to-date information, see the WHO website: www.who.int/health.

individual. Manifestations include a productive cough, sometimes with bloodstained sputum, fatigue, weight loss, low-grade evening fever, night sweats and pleuritic pain. Advanced cases will manifest wheezing and râles, deviation of the trachea, pulmonary consolidation and haemoptysis, i.e. frank bleeding from the lungs.

MEDICAL MANAGEMENT

Investigations Mantoux/Heaf skin tests may be performed (see below). Specimens of sputum, bronchial washings or a lymph node biopsy may be sent for bacteriology. Chest X-ray will indicate the condition of the lungs. All forms of TB are compulsorily notifiable under the Public Health (Control of Disease) Act 1984. This allows contact tracing and provides surveillance data.

Treatment The patient is isolated until there is complete adherence to the medication regimen, usually 2–4 weeks. Medications include isoniazid, rifampicin, streptomycin, ethambutol and pyrazinamide. Until the specific sensitivity is determined, the patient is usually on a rotating regimen of several of these medications because of the high probability of bacterial resistance to some combinations. Therapy will then continue with long-term treatment with at least two of the medications. Regular clinic attendance and supervision of treatment are mandatory. Contacts are traced, tested and treated if necessary.

NURSING PRIORITIES AND MANAGEMENT: Pulmonary tuberculosis

Prevention

Prevention is based upon public health education and on screening and vaccination to protect those at risk. Specialist TB nurses, working closely with health visitors, public health nurses, school nurses, GPs, microbiologists and Consultants in Communicable Disease Control (CCDCs), are key in the prevention and control of TB.

Schoolchildren, health care workers and contacts of people identified as having TB are screened by the Mantoux/Heaf skin tests. These tests use a single intradermal injection of purified protein derivative (PPD). The result is read within 24–72 h.

Mantoux test With Mantoux testing, if the area of induration is >5 mm, the test is positive, which indicates either that a past subacute infection stimulated present immunity or that present infection exists which needs treatment. In the case of past infection, the result signifies that there is effective immunity and vaccination is not necessary. An area of 5 mm in a person recently exposed to tuberculosis indicates that a course of prophylactic treatment should be given. A negative Mantoux test, i.e. no reaction, indicates that there is no natural immunity and the BCG vaccination is necessary.

Heaf tests are similarly graded according to the reaction. Screening may prove difficult, especially in the homeless group. Education of carers working with homeless people is essential in detection of suspected cases. Currently, BCG is offered to children aged between 10 and 14 years and to certain groups at high risk of exposure to TB, including infants and children of certain immigrant populations known to be of high risk (Joint Tuberculosis Committee of the British Thoracic Society 2000).

Management of a newly diagnosed patient

The patient is isolated for 2–4 weeks and expanded infection control precautions are adopted (see Ch. 16). The patient will need reassurance that treatment will be effective, as well as rest, diversionary therapy, good nourishment and administration of prescribed medications. On discharge home, although treatment is standardised, the level of care required will vary from monthly review to directly observed therapy (DOT) three times per week. DOT is a treatment control strategy where health workers observe and record the patients swallowing the prescribed antituberculosis medication (WHO 2003). WHO (2004) recommends that in order to achieve global targets, government and national TB control programmes need to take a strategic approach to planning and match budgets more closely with plans.

OBSTRUCTIVE DISORDERS OF THE AIRWAYS

'Chronic obstructive pulmonary disease' (COPD), sometimes referred to as 'chronic obstructive airways disease' (COAD), is a term used to describe a group of disorders which cause obstruction to air flow. Included in this group are chronic bronchitis, emphysema, asthma and bronchiectasis:

- In chronic bronchitis, the inflammation and constant productive cough obstruct air flow
- In emphysema, the overdistended alveoli with reduced permeability result in impaired gaseous exchange
- In asthma, there is both inflammatory reaction and bronchospasm
- In bronchiectasis, there are chronic copious secretions filling the lungs.

Bronchiectasis is usually a separate condition, but the others often coexist and complicate each other in presenting as the set of symptoms commonly termed COPD (National Collaborating Centre for Chronic Conditions 2004).

Chronic bronchitis

The accepted definition of chronic bronchitis is the presence of a persistent productive cough for at least 2 months over 2 consecutive years. It can occur in any age group but is more common in middle-aged men, cigarette smokers and people exposed to high levels of environmental pollution.

PATHOPHYSIOLOGY

Chronic irritation causes hypertrophy and hyperplasia of the mucous glands of the tracheobronchial tree, which results in excessive mucus production and impaired ciliary action. The bronchi and bronchioles are usually the most severely affected and may become blocked with purulent mucus. This, together with the resultant oedema and congestion, can affect respiratory defence mechanisms and predispose to recurrent bacterial and viral infections.

Clinical features A chronic productive cough with mucopurulent sputum may persist for years, accompanied by gradual and increasing airway resistance and functional impairment. Untreated, this will lead to increasing dyspnoea, hypoxia and hypercapnia.

MEDICAL MANAGEMENT

Management is to advise the patient to avoid the causal irritant, if this is possible, and to treat the symptoms. This may involve prescribing physiotherapy, bronchodilatory medications, antibiotics and oxygen therapy.

NURSING PRIORITIES AND MANAGEMENT: Chronic bronchitis

Prevention of deterioration

The patient is advised and supported in avoiding causative agents.

When identifying patient problems and nursing priorities, it is useful to consider chronic bronchitis and emphysema together, as the two conditions often coexist (see p. 85).

Pulmonary emphysema

Pulmonary emphysema is a chronic destructive disease of the respiratory bronchioles, alveolar ducts and alveoli. It is most common in those aged over 40 and is often associated with other chronic lung disorders. There are two main types of pulmonary emphysema, which may coexist and which are exacerbated by persistent and severe coughing: alveolar emphysema and centrilobar emphysema.

Alveolar emphysema

PATHOPHYSIOLOGY

In this form of emphysema, the walls between adjacent alveoli break down, the alveolar ducts dilate and there is loss of interstitial elastic tissue. This results in distension of the lungs and loss of normal elastic recoil and therefore trapping and stagnation of alveolar air. As alveoli merge, there is loss of surface area for gaseous exchange, and this is further reduced by loss of permeability of the stretched and damaged alveolar walls. Predisposing factors include cigarette smoking, genetic deficiency of α_1-antitrypsin, which makes the individual more susceptible to environmental pollutants, acute lower respiratory inflammatory conditions and chronic coughing, which puts pressure on the already stretched tissues.

Centrilobar emphysema

PATHOPHYSIOLOGY

This type of emphysema involves irreversible dilatation of the bronchioles in the centre of the lobules, which affects airway pressure and ventilation efficiency. Predisposing conditions include recurrent bronchiolitis, pneumoconiosis and chronic bronchitis.

Clinical features Emphysema becomes symptomatic when approximately one-third of the lung parenchyma is affected. The patient is dyspnoeic, and in advanced cases the slightest physical activity can cause severe respiratory distress and cyanosis. Ventilation is forced and exhalation is particularly lengthy and difficult. The patient learns to push the air out through pursed lips, which automatically brings the upper abdominal muscles into play and helps maintain positive pressure in the airways. The hyperinflation of the lungs makes the chest barrel-shaped and rigid and exerts pressure on thoracic structures so that neck and facial veins are distended. There is a chronic, productive cough and wheezing.

Abnormal ventilation:perfusion ratios result in chronic hypoxia (low O_2 in tissues), hypercapnia (high CO_2) and polycythaemia. The clinical picture representing this is of peripheral cyanosis (due to low O_2) and facial flushing (because CO_2 is a vasodilator). Respiratory acidosis may occur in acute exacerbations of the disease, although the body may adapt its buffer system to some extent, given the chronic nature of the condition.

The patient is weakened by constant respiratory effort and becomes unable to tolerate normal basic activities of living.

MEDICAL MANAGEMENT

Investigations History, symptoms and clinical examination are diagnostic. Pulmonary function tests — spirometry (see p. 76) — indicate the type and extent of restricted function: reduction in all parameters indicates obstructive disease because of the prolonged exhalation time, and reduced FEV_1 (forced expiratory volume in 1 s) and FVC (forced vital capacity) indicate restrictive disease. Blood gas analysis and chest X-ray will confirm the stage and effect of the disease and influence treatment.

Treatment Oxygen is prescribed according to individual need and blood gas results (see Box 3.4). It is given in strictly controlled percentages because of the importance of the 'hypoxic drive' in COPD patients and the fact that too much oxygen can reduce this drive, resulting in CO_2 narcosis and respiratory arrest (see Box 3.6). Oxygen may be required constantly, both in hospital and at home.

Bronchodilator medication, corticosteroids and antibiotics are usually prescribed, and physiotherapy is essential.

STOP THINK

3.6 Maintaining a clear airway by regular aspiration of tracheal secretions is a common nursing procedure. As a rule of thumb, the procedure should not be carried out for more than 10–15 s at a time, with adequate periods of rest in between. What is the reason for this? Refer back to residual volume and the composition of alveolar air.

A full description of tracheal suctioning can be found in Jamieson et al (2003).

3.7 How would you explain the concept of hypoxic drive and its importance for self-treatment to a patient with COPD who is about to be sent home on O_2 therapy?

Box 3.6

Carbon dioxide narcosis

In healthy people, when CO_2 levels rise, the respiratory rate increases. This increase allows excess CO_2 to be blown off by the lungs. However, in chronic obstructive pulmonary disease (COPD), where chronic ventilatory problems result in constantly high levels of arterial CO_2, this mechanism becomes blunted and eventually PCO_2 has no effect on the respiratory centre in the brain.

With severe CO_2 retention, the respiratory drive is created by the low PO_2 stimulating the carotid and aortic bodies. This is known as the 'hypoxic drive'. A high concentration of O_2 will suppress this hypoxic drive, and if PO_2 is raised even to normal, breathing becomes shallow and more and more CO_2 is retained, further depressing the respiratory centre, and a condition known as carbon dioxide narcosis develops. This is characterised by increasing drowsiness and eventual death.

The hypoxic drive must always be considered when O_2 is prescribed for patients with COPD. Usually this is not more than 24% of O_2 — slightly more than the 21% in room air — which is enough to improve oxygenation without eliminating the hypoxic drive. Prior to and during O_2 therapy, it is essential to determine arterial blood gas levels and to prescribe O_2 accordingly. The correct percentage is ensured by using controlled-flow O_2 masks and other appliances.

Reproduced with permission from Rutishauser (1994).

NURSING PRIORITIES AND MANAGEMENT: Emphysema and chronic bronchitis

Major considerations

During acute exacerbation the patient may be very ill. The nurse will be involved in administering prescribed therapy, monitoring the patient's condition and detecting any deterioration.

In advanced cases of emphysema, even when stable, the patient will constantly strive for breath and will need maximum reassurance and calm support. Lifestyle will be drastically curtailed and every effort should be made to make a realistic assessment of the patient's capabilities and need for assistance in designing a care plan. Limitations may be extreme and affect even minor activities such as eating, drinking, combing hair, brushing teeth and moving about the room. Time should be spent helping, observing and listening.

Nursing Care Plan 3.1 describes the case of M, a 70-year-old lady admitted to hospital with exacerbation of COPD. She lives at home with her husband as sole carer. Over a period of 4 days she has developed increasing shortness of breath, chest pain on coughing and purulent sputum. She stopped smoking 5 years ago. She is very anxious regarding admission.

Oxygen therapy

Oxygen should always be administered strictly according to the prescribed amount, because of the danger of switching

Nursing Care Plan 3.1 M: exacerbation of COPD

Nursing considerations	Action	Rationale	Expected outcome
1. Potential problem of deterioration in M's condition following admission	• Monitor vital signs for: – increase in heart rate and respiratory rate – decrease in S_aO_2 • Observe for: – increasing oedema – changes in mental state: confusion, restlessness – increasing dyspnoea with use of accessory muscles	Despite optimal medical therapy patients with respiratory failure may develop respiratory acidosis or worsening hypercapnia, requiring consideration for invasive or non-invasive ventilation	Stable vital signs S_aO_2 remains above 90% (or at level stated by medical staff) No evidence of deterioration
2. Dyspnoea	• Administer oxygen therapy as prescribed and humidify where appropriate	Maintain adequate oxygenation	Minimise level of distress from dyspnoea
	• Administer prescribed medications (antibiotics, steroids, bronchodilators)	Maximise therapy	Gradual return to 'normal' level of dyspnoea
	• Refer to physiotherapist to assist with sputum clearance	Active cycle of breathing techniques can be taught to aid secretion clearance	
	• Position sitting upright in bed supported by pillows or leaning forward on the overbed table	To enable maximum expansion of the lungs and increase movement of the thoracic cage	
	• Provide nurse call bell near to hand and assist with personal hygiene	Minimise dyspnoea by minimising exertion/effort	
3. Pyrexia	• Administer antipyretic as prescribed • Nurse in cool room	Maintain temperature within normal range	Patient is apyrexial and comfortable
4. Anxiety	• Give support and reassurance • Explain care being administered and realistic expected progress • Avoid medical jargon	Information giving will improve patient knowledge and understanding	As a result of improved understanding patient will be less anxious
5. Maintaining adequate hydration and nutrition	• Commence fluid balance chart and carry out nutritional assessment • Refer to dietitian to set individual goals and provide high energy supplements • Provide nutritious and easily eaten diet • Change to nasal cannulae during meals	Monitoring and adjusting diet and fluid intake ensures optimal nutrition and avoids need for intravenous fluids	Patient will be well nourished and hydrated

Continued

Nursing Care Plan 3.1 M: exacerbation of COPD *(Continued)*

Nursing considerations	Action	Rationale	Expected outcome
6. Suitability for early discharge	• Refer to acute respiratory assessment team (or equivalent) for assessment for early supported discharge	M may be discharged home early under the care of Hospital at Home schemes, which provide continued monitoring and support for a limited period. Suitability depends on presence of other disease and level of physical functioning, social circumstances and M's preference	M is safely discharged home as early as possible
7. Potential problem of further hospital admissions with exacerbation of COPD	• Prior to discharge M and husband understand and are able to carry out medication and therapy regimens		
	• M has received advice on prompt response to symptoms of an exacerbation and on vaccines (flu/pneumococcal)	M is able to carry out treatment therapies and recognise when her respiratory function is compromised	Potential for admission with exacerbation of COPD will be reduced

off the patient's hypoxic drive. In hospital, a controlled ventimask is usually used. It is vital that the nurse understands this and can explain it in simple terms, especially if the patient is to use and control the oxygen supply at home. The patient and family will need both verbal and written information and plenty of opportunity for discussion (see Box 3.7). Nasal cannulae are often preferred when the patient is on long-term oxygen therapy (LTOT). At home, an oxygen concentrator machine is often used instead of oxygen cylinders with oxygen set at prescribed litres/min; use of nasal cannulae allows normal speaking, eating and drinking.

Non-invasive ventilation (NIV), delivered from a small ventilator via a mask, has been found to have significant beneficial effects for patients with acute exacerbations of COPD. In decompensated respiratory failure, the application of NIV can lead to improvement and prevent the need for intubation and mechanical ventilation. It is not suitable for individuals with impairment of swallow, cough or gag reflexes or excessive bronchial secretions (see Fig. 3.5 and Research Abstract 3.3).

Arterial blood gas (ABG) analysis

ABG analysis is the most reliable way to monitor blood gas levels and the nurse should be prepared to follow the required procedure for obtaining the blood sample (see Box 3.8). A basic understanding of normal levels is also assumed.

The nurse must be aware that cyanosis may be a late sign of hypoxia and should not be relied upon as an early indicator. As a rule of thumb, cyanosis is usually noticeable

Box 3.7

Patient teaching in O_2 therapy

Increasingly, patients go home on O_2 therapy and will need information on how to get a supply of medical O_2 and how to set it up at home. The following instructions, which should accompany the patient, should be discussed fully and reinforced on every contact.

Instructions for home use of oxygen

- Oxygen is highly combustible. Do not use it near a fire or open flame. Post a 'no smoking' sign on the cylinder and explain to relatives and friends the reason for so doing. Electrical appliances and kinetic toys that may produce a spark are also a source of danger.
- Adjust the flow meter to the flow rate the doctor prescribes and do not change it without the doctor's consent.
- Keep water in the humidifier to the correct level and change it daily.
- NOTIFY DOCTOR if any of the following occur:
  - — you have increased difficulty breathing
  - — you feel unusually restless or upset
  - — your breathing becomes irregular
  - — you feel abnormally drowsy
  - — your lips or fingernails look blue
  - — you have trouble concentrating or you become confused.

Do not assume that you will feel better if you take more oxygen. This may not be the case and you should consult your doctor or go to the nearest Emergency Department immediately if you experience any of these symptoms.

Reproduced with permission from Rutishauser (1994).

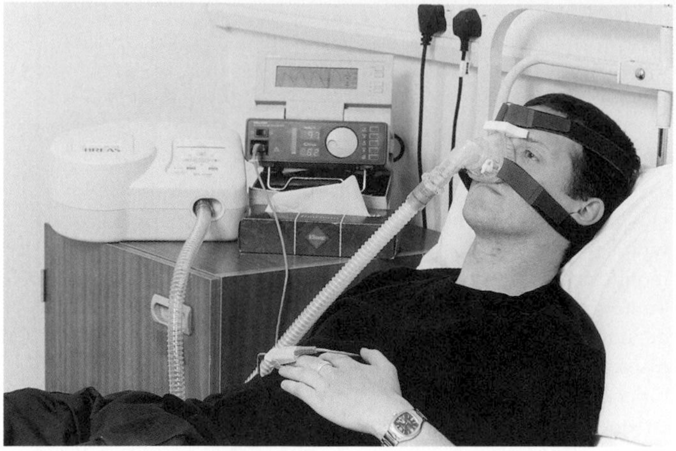

Fig. 3.5 Patient undergoing treatment with non-invasive ventilation. (Reproduced with kind permission of Medical Illustration Services, North Glasgow University NHS Hospitals Trust.)

RESEARCH ABSTRACT 3.3

Positive benefits of non-invasive ventilation (NIV)

NIV can improve gas exchange, optimise lung volumes and reduce the work of breathing. NIV is indicated in acute exacerbation of COPD when respiratory acidosis (H^+ >45 mmol/L) persists despite medical treatment on controlled oxygen therapy. NIV is also indicated in respiratory failure due to chest wall deformity or neuromuscular disease.

British Thoracic Society (BTS) 2002 Standards of Care Committee. BTS Guideline: Non-invasive ventilation in acute respiratory failure. Thorax 57(3): 192–211

Box 3.8

Monitoring arterial blood gas levels

In the clinical situation, arterial blood gas levels can be monitored by laboratory blood gas analysis. Blood is drawn from the radial or femoral artery, or from an established arterial line, using a heparinised syringe. Care is taken not to draw air into the syringe, which is capped and sent for immediate analysis.

Following the procedure, unless blood has been obtained from an arterial line (A-line), firm pressure must be applied to the puncture site for at least 5 min to ensure haemostasis under arterial pressure.

If on oxygen therapy, it is important to make sure that the patient has been receiving the prescribed amount for at least 15 min before and during the time when the sample is drawn. If the patient has been on a mechanical ventilator for a session of intermittent positive pressure breathing (IPPB), the nurse should wait at least 20 min before taking a sample and 20 min after commencing ventilation or post-tracheal suctioning. The prescribed amount of oxygen or the IPPB should be noted on the laboratory request form.

when the concentration of deoxygenated haemoglobin in blood exceeds 50 g/L. The distinction between central and peripheral cyanosis is an important one: central cyanosis is due to low oxygen content of the arterial blood (hypoxic hypoxia) and can be determined by inspecting the tongue and mucous membranes of the eye in addition to the skin; peripheral cyanosis is due to a sluggish circulation (stagnant hypoxia) where release of oxygen from the blood is slowed down even though the arterial oxygen content may be normal, as for example in cardiac failure and shock.

For further information, see Margereson & Esmond (1997a,b,c).

Positioning and breathing

The patient will be more comfortable sitting up and well supported by pillows. Breathing may be easier leaning forward on an overbed table with elbows extended to the side. Emphysematous patients tend to take short, shallow breaths and should be taught diaphragmatic breathing to improve and slow down ventilation. Pursed-lip exhalation is helpful because it improves positive airway pressure and brings the abdominal muscles into play.

Chest physiotherapy

The physiotherapist will teach the patient deep breathing and coughing exercises and postural drainage techniques and may perform frappage, patterns of clapping the chest wall, to loosen tenacious secretions. Deep breathing and coughing exercises should be reinforced by nursing staff and the patient should be taught to perform them independently and to continue them after discharge home.

Patient education

The patient should understand the disease process and the aims of treatment. If the disease is in the early stages, removal of predisposing factors such as cigarette smoking will help to prevent further deterioration. If the condition is advanced, the patient may need help to adapt to a severely compromised lifestyle and to preserve what pulmonary function remains.

Structured pulmonary rehabilitation programmes that include exercise, education, physiotherapy, nutritional support, smoking cessation and psychological support can be a way of ensuring that the patient achieves an optimal level of independence and functioning in the community. Structured programmes require an organised multidisciplinary approach, involving respiratory nurses and other members of the health care team. Trials have shown that such programmes have a positive effect on the person's quality of life (British Thoracic Society 2001a, Lacasse et al 2003).

Asthma

Asthma is a common chronic inflammatory condition of the airways, characterised by bronchospasm, severe dyspnoea, wheezing, chest tightness and expiratory exertion. As a result of inflammation, the airways are hyperresponsive and narrow easily in response to a wide range of provoking stimuli. Although much is known about asthma, it is a complex condition about which much remains to be understood.

CASE HISTORY 3.1(A)

C

C was brought into the Emergency Department one night by his wife, and this is the account of his first severe asthma attack:

'I just couldn't get my breath ... I was panicking and really scared. My chest felt it was in a steel vice ... I was wheezing and gasping for air and just couldn't get my breath. The nurse took one look and got into action straight away. The room was swirling ... I thought I was a gonner ... and I passed out.

When I came to, they'd put some powerful medication through a drip in my arm and an oxygen mask on my face.

I began to feel the panic again but then realised that the breathing was getting easier, and that calmed me down. That was my first bad attack of asthma and I never want to go through that again. I ended up in the Intensive Care and my family were worried sick.

Two years before this we'd been through a rough time ... I was made redundant from my regular job ... been unemployed then got this other job which I'm not happy with ... there's a lot of dust and fumes around. I'd started to wheeze and cough a fair bit and the GP said it was asthma ... which was a bit of a shock at my age — 40 years old! It must run in the family, though. Dad has asthma but I thought I'd got away with it. Anyway, the doctor had given me some pills and a puffer, which helped at times but I must admit I wasn't really good at taking them. This severe attack, though, made me want to know more about it so that it doesn't happen again.'

Broadly speaking, there are two types of bronchial asthma: extrinsic and intrinsic. The extrinsic form occurs in children and young adults who are hypersensitive to foreign proteins such as dust mites, pollens, animal dander and feathers. Familial allergic tendencies can often be traced. Intrinsic or chronic asthma occurs later in life and is often associated with chronic respiratory inflammatory disease. Although there may be no history of childhood asthma, there may be a family history of asthma and allergic tendencies (see Case History 3.1(A)). In many cases the role of allergens is still suspected.

A large group of asthma sufferers are found to be vulnerable to stimuli of both extrinsic and intrinsic origin. There is increasing evidence that the psychosomatic element is negligible and can no longer be regarded as a major causative factor in most cases (British Thoracic Society/Scottish Intercollegiate Guidelines Network 2003).

Research suggests that there is a critical trigger time early in the development of asthma when, if steroid therapy is introduced, the process can not only be controlled but also 'turned off' so that the condition does not progress or recur. However, there continues to be some resistance to steroid therapy from the general public, especially in relation to treating children. This is because of the misconceived fear of side-effects, which in fact are minimal with inhaled steroids (British Thoracic Society/Scottish Intercollegiate Guidelines Network 2003).

For current incidence of asthma in the UK, visit www.asthma.org.uk.

PATHOPHYSIOLOGY

Immunoglobulin E (IgE) is present in small amounts in normal sera but in increased amounts in asthma sufferers. In allergic extrinsic asthma, the disease process involves inhalation of antigens (allergens) which are absorbed by the bronchial mucosa and trigger production of IgE antibodies. These antibodies bind to mast cells and basophils around the bronchial blood vessels. When the allergen is encountered again, the antigen–antibody reaction releases histamines and bradykinin, resulting in bronchial muscle spasm, oedema and excessive secretion of thick mucus. In many cases, the severity of attacks lessens with age and good treatment, unless other factors are involved.

There are various theories of the pathogenesis of intrinsic asthma. Allergens may be implicated. Whatever the cause, the bronchi and bronchioles are chronically inflamed, oedematous, full of mucus and subject to bronchospasm. Air is trapped in the alveoli and expiration is difficult. The disease can be progressive and impaired ventilation can result in hypoxia, hypertension and right-sided heart failure.

Clinical features Asthma attacks can last for minutes, hours or days (status asthmaticus). They manifest as paroxysms of severe ventilatory difficulty with rapid, laboured breathing accompanied by wheezing. Expiration is forced and prolonged due to bronchospasm, hyperinflated lungs and trapped alveolar air. This may be accompanied by a dry or moist cough. There may be extreme anxiety, sweating, dyspnoea, orthopnoea and peripheral cyanosis with hypoxia and hypercapnia. Tachycardia is common because of anxiety and hypoxia and may be increased by bronchodilatory medication such as salbutamol (Hoskins et al 2000). If there is no response to treatment, exhaustion will occur rapidly and may be followed by respiratory failure.

MEDICAL MANAGEMENT

Investigations Diagnosis is by typical clinical presentation and past history. After an attack has subsided, lung function tests such as FEV_1 will be helpful in establishing the degree of impairment and in monitoring response to treatment. Prolonged FEV_1 indicates loss of elasticity of lung tissue. Chest X-rays will indicate clarity of lung fields and size of the heart. Skin sensitivity tests and a history of exposure to specific allergens may help in isolating and avoiding triggering factors.

Treatment Management of a patient with asthma is best coordinated by referring to the British Thoracic Society (BTS) guidelines (2003a,b,c) (see Figs 3.6–3.8). The guidelines are readily available to all GPs, Emergency Departments (EDs) and respiratory units and provide step-by-step guidance on treatment.

Depending on the severity of the asthma attack, the patient may be managed at home or be admitted to the local hospital Emergency Department. Respiratory status will be assessed by recording the peak expiratory flow (PEF), the type and rate of respirations and ability to complete a sentence without becoming breathless. The patient's general appearance and pulse rate will also indicate the level of respiratory distress.

Management of acute severe asthma in adults in general practice

Many deaths from asthma are preventable, but delay can be fatal.
Factors leading to poor outcome include:
- Doctors failing to assess severity by objective measurement
- Patients or relatives failing to appreciate severity
- Under use of corticosteroids

Regard each emergency asthma consultation as for acute severe asthma until it is shown to be otherwise.

Assess and record:
- Peak expiratory flow (PEF)
- Symptoms and response to self treatment
- Heart and respiratory rates
- Oxygen saturation (by pulse oximetry, if available)

Caution: *Patients with severe or life threatening attacks may not be distressed and may not have all the abnormalities listed below. The presence of any should alert the doctor.*

Moderate asthma	**Acute severe asthma**	**Life threatening asthma**
INITIAL ASSESSMENT		
PEF > 50% best or predicted	PEF 33–50% best or predicted	PEF < 33% best or predicted
FURTHER ASSESSMENT		
• Speech normal • Respiration < 25 breaths/min • Pulse < 110 beats/min	• Can't complete sentences • Respiration ≥ 25 breaths/min • Pulse ≥ 110 beats/min	• SpO_2 < 92% • Silent chest, cyanosis, or feeble respiratory effort • Bradycardia, dysrhythmia or hypotension • Exhaustion, confusion or coma
MANAGEMENT		
Treat at home or in surgery and ASSESS RESPONSE TO TREATMENT	**Consider admission**	**Arrange immediate ADMISSION**
TREATMENT		
High dose $ß_2$ bronchodilator: - Ideally via oxygen-driven nebuliser (salbutamol 5 mg or terbutaline 10 mg) - Or via spacer or air-driven nebuliser (1 puff 10–20 times) If PEF > 50–75% predicted/best: • Give prednisolone 40–50 mg • Continue or step up usual treatment If good response to first nebulised treatment (symptoms improved, respiration and pulse settling, and PEF > 50%) continue or step up usual treatment and continue prednisolone	• Oxygen 40–60% if available • High dose $ß_2$ bronchodilator: - Ideally via oxygen-driven nebuliser (salbutamol 5 mg or terbutaline 10 mg) - Or via spacer (1 puff $ß_2$ agonist via a large volume spacer and repeat 10–20 times) or air-driven nebuliser • Prednisolone 40–50 mg or IV hydrocortisone 100 mg • **If no response in acute severe asthma: ADMIT**	• Oxygen 40–60% • Prednisolone 40-50 mg or IV hydrocortisone 100 mg immediately • High dose $ß_2$ bronchodilator and ipratropium - Ideally via oxygen-driven nebuliser (salbutamol 5 mg or terbutaline 10 mg and ipratropium 0.5 mg) - Or via spacer (1 puff $ß_2$ agonist via a large volume spacer, repeated 10–20 times) or air-driven nebuliser
Admit to hospital if any: • life threatening features • features of acute severe asthma present after initial treatment • previous near fatal asthma **Lower threshold for admission if:** afternoon or evening attack, recent nocturnal symptoms or hospital admission, previous severe attacks, patient unable to assess own condition, or concern over social circumstances	**If admitting the patient to hospital:** • Stay with patient until ambulance arrives • Send written assessment and referral details to hospital • Give high dose $ß_2$ bronchodilator via oxygen-driven nebuliser in ambulance	**Follow up after treatment or discharge from hospital:** • **GP review within 48 hours** • Monitor symptoms and PEF • Check inhaler technique • Written asthma action plan • Modify treatment according to guidelines for chronic persistent asthma • Address potentially preventable contributors to admission

Fig. 3.6 Management of acute severe asthma in adults in general practice. (Reproduced from British Thoracic Society 2003a, with permission from the BMJ Publishing Group.)

Treatment in the Emergency Department will be in accordance with the BTS guidelines (2003b; see Fig. 3.7). Reference to the chart indicates that the treatment plan extends over a 2-h period, but the first 5 min are crucial. Response to treatment will determine whether the patient is admitted to hospital or discharged home. If discharged, the GP will follow the BTS guidelines for general practice (2003a; see Fig. 3.6). If admitted, the medical staff will follow the BTS guidelines for management of acute asthma in hospital (2003c; see Fig. 3.8).

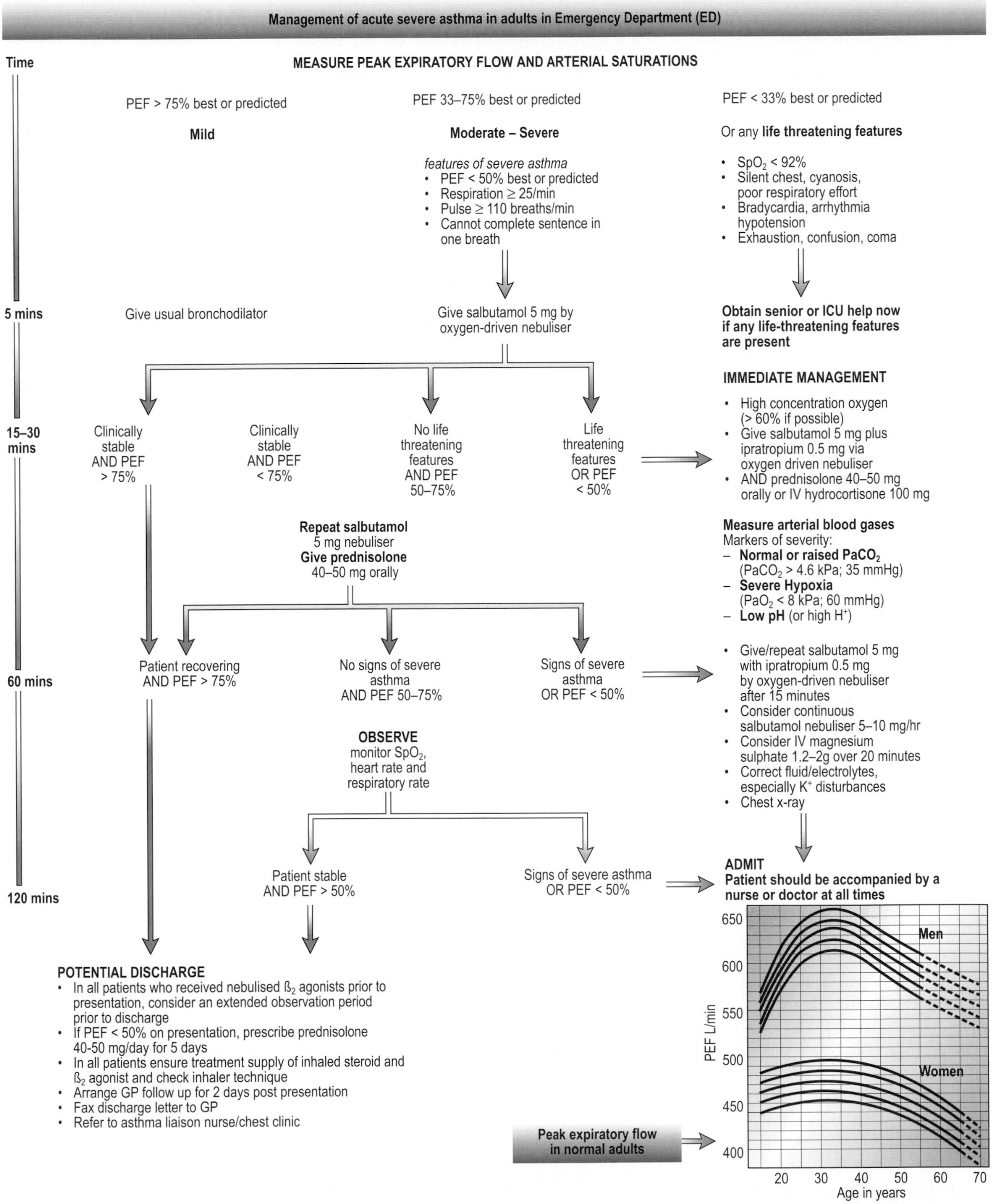
Management of acute severe asthma in adults in Emergency Department (ED)
Time
MEASURE PEAK EXPIRATORY FLOW AND ARTERIAL SATURATIONS
PEF > 75% best or predicted
Mild
PEF 33–75% best or predicted
Moderate – Severe
features of severe asthma
• PEF < 50% best or predicted
• Respiration ≥ 25/min
• Pulse ≥ 110 breaths/min
• Cannot complete sentence in one breath
PEF < 33% best or predicted
Or any life threatening features
• SpO2 < 92%
• Silent chest, cyanosis, poor respiratory effort
• Bradycardia, arrhythmia hypotension
• Exhaustion, confusion, coma
5 mins
Give usual bronchodilator
Give salbutamol 5 mg by oxygen-driven nebuliser
Obtain senior or ICU help now if any life-threatening features are present
IMMEDIATE MANAGEMENT
• High concentration oxygen (> 60% if possible)
• Give salbutamol 5 mg plus ipratropium 0.5 mg via oxygen driven nebuliser
• AND prednisolone 40–50 mg orally or IV hydrocortisone 100 mg
15–30 mins
Clinically stable AND PEF > 75%
Clinically stable AND PEF < 75%
No life threatening features AND PEF 50–75%
Life threatening features OR PEF < 50%
Repeat salbutamol 5 mg nebuliser
Give prednisolone 40–50 mg orally
Measure arterial blood gases
Markers of severity:
– Normal or raised PaCO2 (PaCO2 > 4.6 kPa; 35 mmHg)
– Severe Hypoxia (PaO2 < 8 kPa; 60 mmHg)
– Low pH (or high H+)
60 mins
Patient recovering AND PEF > 75%
No signs of severe asthma AND PEF 50–75%
Signs of severe asthma OR PEF < 50%
• Give/repeat salbutamol 5 mg with ipratropium 0.5 mg by oxygen-driven nebuliser after 15 minutes
• Consider continuous salbutamol nebuliser 5–10 mg/hr
• Consider IV magnesium sulphate 1.2–2g over 20 minutes
• Correct fluid/electrolytes, especially K+ disturbances
• Chest x-ray
OBSERVE
monitor SpO2, heart rate and respiratory rate
120 mins
Patient stable AND PEF > 50%
Signs of severe asthma OR PEF < 50%
ADMIT
Patient should be accompanied by a nurse or doctor at all times
POTENTIAL DISCHARGE
• In all patients who received nebulised ß2 agonists prior to presentation, consider an extended observation period prior to discharge
• If PEF < 50% on presentation, prescribe prednisolone 40-50 mg/day for 5 days
• In all patients ensure treatment supply of inhaled steroid and ß2 agonist and check inhaler technique
• Arrange GP follow up for 2 days post presentation
• Fax discharge letter to GP
• Refer to asthma liaison nurse/chest clinic
Peak expiratory flow in normal adults
PEF L/min
650
600
550
500
450
400
Men
Women
20
30
40
50
60
70
Age in years

Fig. 3.7 Management of acute severe asthma in adults in the Emergency Department. (Reproduced from British Thoracic Society 2003b, with permission from the BMJ Publishing Group.)

Management of acute severe asthma in adults in hospital

Features of acute severe asthma
- Peak expiratory flow (PEF) 33–50% of best *(use % predicted if recent best unknown)*
- Can't complete sentences in one breath
- Respirations ≥ 25 breaths/min
- Pulse ≥ 110 beats/min

Life threatening features
- PEF < 33% of best or predicted
- SpO_2 < 92%
- Silent chest, cyanosis, or feeble respiratory effort
- Bradycardia, dysrhythmia, or hypotension
- Exhaustion, confusion, or coma

If patient has any life threatening feature, measure arterial blood gases. No other investigations are needed for immediate management.

Blood gas markers of a life threatening attack:
- Normal $PaCO_2$ (4.6–6 kPa, 35–45 mmHg)
- Severe hypoxia: PaO_2 < 8 kPa (60 mmHg) irrespective of treatment with oxygen
- A low pH (or high H^+)

Caution: Patients with severe or life threatening attacks may not be distressed and may not have all these abnormalities. The presence of any should alert the doctor.

Near fatal asthma
- Raised $PaCO_2$
- Requiring IPPV with raised inflation pressures

Peak expiratory flow in normal adults

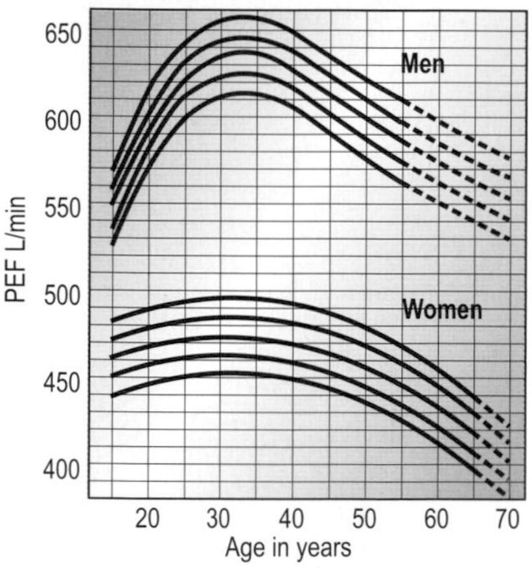

IMMEDIATE TREATMENT

- Oxygen 40–60% (CO_2 retention is not usually aggravated by oxygen therapy in asthma)
- Salbutamol 5 mg or terbutaline 10 mg via an oxygen-driven nebuliser
- Ipratropium bromide 0.5 mg via an oxygen-driven nebuliser
- Prednisolone tablets 40–50 mg or IV hydrocortisone 100 mg or both if very ill
- No sedatives of any kind
- Chest radiograph only if pneumothorax or consolidation are suspected or patient requires IPPV

IF LIFE THREATENING FEATURES ARE PRESENT:

- Discuss with senior clinician and ICU team
- Add IV magnesium sulphate 1.2–2 g infusion over 20 minutes *(unless already given)*
- Give nebulised β_2 agonist more frequently e.g. salbutamol 5 mg up to every 15–30 minutes or 10 mg continuously hourly

⇩

SUBSEQUENT MANAGEMENT

IF PATIENT IS IMPROVING continue:
- Oxygen 40–60%
- Prednisolone 40–50 mg daily or IV hydrocortisone 100 mg 6 hourly
- Nebulised β_2 agonist and ipratropium 4–6 hourly

IF PATIENT NOT IMPROVING AFTER 15–30 MINUTES:
- Continue oxygen and steroids
- Give nebulised β_2 agonist more frequently e.g. salbutamol 5 mg up to every 15–30 minutes or 10 mg continuously hourly
- Continue ipratropium 0.5 mg 4–6 hourly until patient is improving

IF PATIENT IS STILL NOT IMPROVING:
- Discuss patient with senior clinician and ICU team
- IV magnesium sulphate 1.2–2 g over 20 minutes *(unless already given)*
- Senior clinician may consider use of IV β_2 agonist or IV aminophylline or progression to IPPV

⇩

MONITORING

- Repeat measurement of PEF 15–30 minutes after starting treatment
- Oximetry: maintain SpO_2 > 92%
- Repeat blood gas measurements within 2 hours of starting treatment if:
  - initial PaO_2 < 8 kPa (60 mmHg) unless susequent SpO_2 >92%
  - $PaCo_2$ normal or raised
  - Patient deteriorates
- Chart PEF before and after giving β_2 agonist and at least 4 times daily throughout hospital stay

Transfer to ICU accompanied by a doctor prepared to intubate if:
- Deteriorating PEF, worsening or persisting hypoxia, or hypercapnoea
- Exhaustion, feeble respirations, confusion or drowsiness
- Coma or respiratory arrest

⇩

DISCHARGE

When discharged from hospital patients should have:
- Been on discharge medication for 24 hours and *have had inhaler technique checked and recorded*
- PEF >75% of best or predicted and PEF diurnal variability < 25% *unless discharge is agreed with respiratory physician*
- Treatments with **oral and inhaled steroids** in addition to bronchodilators
- Own PEF meter and **written asthma action plan**
- GP follow up arranged *within 2 working days*
- Follow up appointment in respiratory clinic *within 4 weeks*

Patients with severe asthma *(indicated by need for admission)* **and adverse behavioral or psychosocial features are at risk of further severe or fatal attacks**
- Determine reason(s) for exacerbation and admission
- Send details of admission, discharge and potential best PEF to GP

Fig. 3.8 Management of acute severe asthma in adults in hospital. (Reproduced from British Thoracic Society 2003c, with permission from the BMJ Publishing Group.)

The best treatment for asthma is avoidance of known causal factors and provision of patient education.

The majority of patients are treated by their GP and can administer their own treatment at home and avoid asthma attacks. Severe cases are referred to specialist respiratory units. Once diagnosed, if patients do not respond to the usual prescribed treatment and notice a significant drop in their peak flow readings or experience increasing difficulty, they may present and self-admit to the respiratory unit where they are known or to the nearest Emergency Department.

NURSING PRIORITIES AND MANAGEMENT: Asthma

Major considerations

The first priority is to ensure that the individual experiencing an asthma attack is seen by a doctor as quickly as possible. The condition can deteriorate rapidly.

Giving psychological support

An attack of asthma is extremely frightening. The patient will be fighting for breath and is often panic stricken. It is vital for the nurse to maintain a calm and reassuring manner and to stay with the patient throughout the attack. A sound knowledge base will enable the nurse to anticipate the course of the attack and the likely reactions to it and so help the patient to remain calm. Nebulised therapy is the method of choice in an acute episode of asthma (see Box 3.9 and Fig. 3.9).

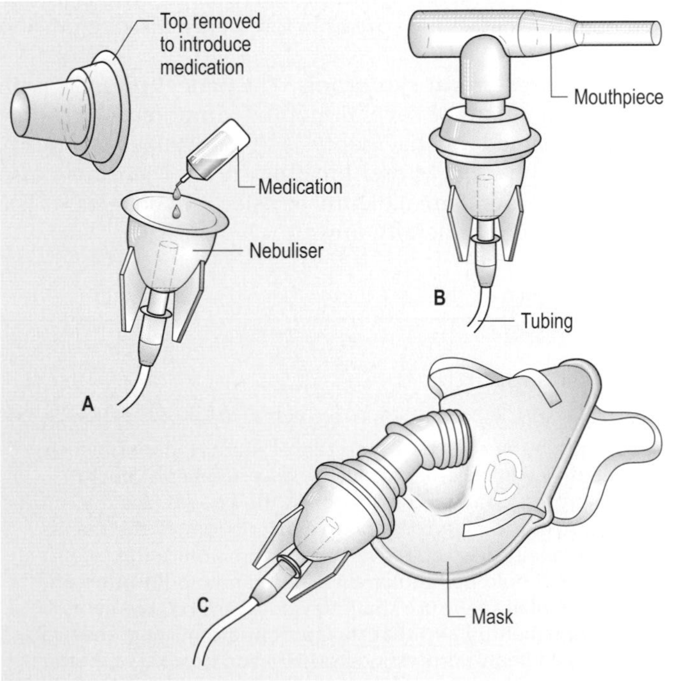

Fig. 3.9 Nebulisers. A: Nebuliser taken apart to introduce medication. B, C: Nebuliser attached to mouthpiece or face mask depending on drug to be used and/or patient preference. (Based on an original drawing by Nicole Rooth, Moreton Bay Design Co., Australia, with permission.)

Box 3.9

Assisting a patient to use a nebuliser

A nebuliser attached to a flow of oxygen or air converts a liquid into an aerosol mist. The medication is prescribed by the doctor. The procedure may be coordinated with chest physiotherapy, and peak flow of tidal volume may be measured and recorded before and after the treatment. The equipment is assembled according to the procedure illustrated in Figure 3.9.

The medication is checked and, if two medications are prescribed, they should not be mixed together. Separate nebulisers should be used and the bronchodilator medication given first.

- The equipment and purpose of the medication is explained to the patient. The medication is put into the nebuliser, which is assembled and attached to the air supply. If oxygen is ordered, a 'no smoking' sign is displayed and the reason explained. If the patient has chronic obstructive pulmonary disease (COPD), air is used instead of oxygen because of the danger of disrupting the patient's hypoxic drive (see Box 3.6).
- Peak flow is measured if required and the best of three attempts is charted.
- The patient sits up in a comfortable position.
- The air flow meter is adjusted to 5 L to ensure vaporisation of the medication.
- The nurse ensures that there is a fine vapour coming from the nebuliser and encourages the patient to breathe it in through the mouthpiece if possible. If this is too difficult, the patient may use an oxygen mask instead. The patient is instructed to breathe normally, taking an occasional deep breath. If the patient is on a respirator, a nebuliser can be introduced into the ventilator circuit.
- The nurse should stay with the patient until all the medication is nebulised and observe the respirations, checking how the patient feels and encouraging them to cough and expectorate if there is mucus in the lungs. A clean sputum container should be ready to hand.
- Half an hour after the treatment, peak flow readings are taken again and the best of three is charted.
- The procedure is documented and the equipment washed and dried and stored in the patient's locker until needed again.

Positioning and monitoring

The patient should sit up well supported by pillows or lean forward on an overbed table. Vital signs, oxygen therapy and ABGs should be monitored constantly and interpreted intelligently. The nurse should be alert for any sign of deterioration.

Prevention and treatment of non-acute asthma

Medication to prevent and treat asthma is also given via inhaler devices. The nurse, preferably with specialised education in asthma, should ensure that the patient is assessed for the correct inhaler device, understands the therapy and receives training in the correct use of the device. The choice may be influenced by the choice of medication or the patient's ability to use it. Figure 3.10 illustrates a selection of devices available.

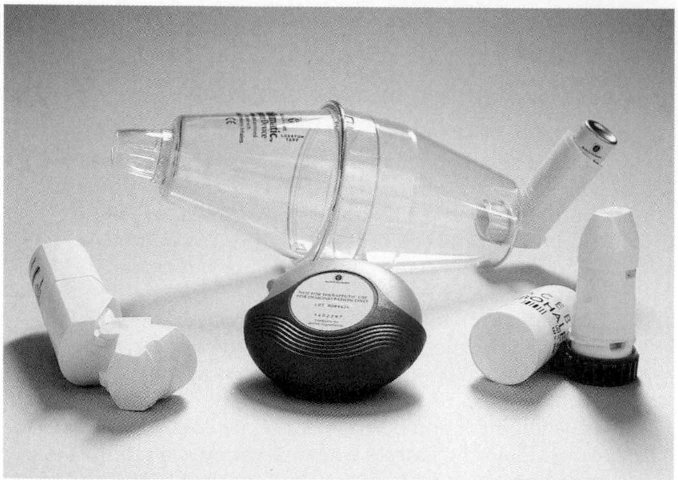

Fig. 3.10 Inhaler devices. Front row left to right: Easy Breathe Inhaler; Accuhaler; Turbohaler. Behind these is the Volumatic device with metered dose inhaler (MDI) attached. (Reproduced with kind permission of Medical Illustration Services, North Glasgow University NHS Hospitals Trust.)

Assisting with inhalation therapy

A common cause of failed home treatment is that the patient does not use the inhaler correctly and therefore does not get the full dose of the medication (Sayer 1999).

Adherence to prescribed treatment may be difficult to assess. Emphasis in therapy is on the concept of concordance which implies a negotiated agreement between nurse and patient. Non-adherence may be due to failure of the nurse to provide a treatment regimen which is acceptable and understood by the patient.

Health education

Practice nurses, community nurses and hospital nurses are in a good position to make a realistic assessment of patient capabilities and inhaler technique and to give advice accordingly. The effectiveness of received medication can be determined by measuring lung function (peak flow) before and after inhalation. Patients can be taught to do this themselves and to record the results.

For the hospitalised patient, a multidisciplinary care plan and critical pathway based on the latest British Thoracic Society's asthma guidelines (2003c) should be developed to ensure research-based practice, consistency of care and cost-effectiveness (see Case History 3.1(B) and Multidisciplinary Care Plan 3.2).

Specialist training

Audit has shown that specialist care of adult patients admitted with asthma is associated with improved outcome. The BTS recommends that health care personnel such as ambulance officers, ED staff, practice nurses and school nurses should have specific education in asthma care and be enabled to follow the guidelines that they recommend (see Figs 3.6–3.8).

LUNG CANCER

Lung cancer can be of primary origin or can occur as secondary metastatic spread from other primary sources.

CASE HISTORY 3.1(B)

C's story (cont'd)

At the team meeting just before C was discharged from hospital, he made the following comments:

'I just did not realise how important it was to know about asthma — and in particular to know about how it affects me and how the medications work. I hadn't given it much thought really before this severe attack and usually just had a few more puffs with the inhaler when I thought I needed them.

When I first came to this ward I remember how surprised I was that the other patients seemed to know so much and take such an active part in their own treatment. I thought you came into hospital to have things done to you, not to learn how to do it yourself, but I see now. They treated the unit a bit like a "club". Mostly they'd been in before and their good-natured "advice" was a great help, especially when I got depressed about being stuck with asthma. I realised it wasn't the end of the world.

Knowing about asthma makes me feel more in control; and now I've learnt how to use the inhaler properly and the peak flow meter, and you've explained what my safe limits are, I shall know what to do in future. Having it all written down, too, is somehow reassuring. I certainly don't want another episode like this last one, so it's worth taking a bit more time to understand things and look after myself. I don't intend to let asthma rule my life, though, but I will change my job and try to look after my general health more.'

PATHOPHYSIOLOGY

Lung cancer is classified according to basic cell type, i.e. squamous cell adenocarcinoma (the most common), undifferentiated carcinoma, and large- and small-cell carcinoma. The tumour may present as a cauliflower-shaped mass which slowly infiltrates the lung parenchyma. Because this form of cancer is difficult to detect in the early stages, it has a high potential for metastatic spread before being discovered.

Common presenting symptoms The patient presents with a persistent cough of several months' duration which may be accompanied by haemoptysis (bloodstained sputum), chest pain, hoarseness and breathlessness. There may also be weight loss, anaemia, pleural effusion and bone pain. The patient will look generally unwell.

Box 3.10

Cancer support

Patients with cancer move through a number of health care settings in the course of their cancer journey, during which time they will become involved with a number of health care professionals who will address their needs. For this, there needs to be a collaborative effort from all the teams involved and clear, effective lines of communication.

There should be regular evaluation and modification of the care plan to ensure that individual care requirements are implemented and that the appropriate nursing, medical and allied health professionals (AHP) and hospice support are being accessed to provide this package of care. Support will be available from oncology specialist nurses, the palliative care team, the pain control team, Macmillan nurses, district nurses, physiotherapists, dietitians, occupational therapists and social workers (see Chs 31 and 33).

Multidisciplinary Care Plan 3.2 C: acute asthma

Problem focus	Medical	Nursing	Patient	Physiotherapy	Social work
Transfer from ICU for stabilisation and establishment of self-care treatment regimen following an acute severe asthma attack	• Priority if called to review patient's condition	Coordinate team care • educative-supportive role • priority to any sign of deteriorating condition. Action STATIM • monitor vital signs and respiratory status		• Ensure clear airway – deep breathing, coughing exercises, use of ancillary muscles	• Problem with work environment
Patient involvement and understanding essential regarding: • disease process • symptoms • management • interpretation of symptoms and PEF • specific medication actions and side-effects • written self-care plan and action to be taken when pre-arranged signs of deterioration are evident	• Select and prescribe treatment and medications • Discuss with patient and care team: – asthma disease process – treatment and action of medications – taking and monitoring peak expiratory flow (PEF) – significance – nebuliser technique • Monitor ABGs • Establish individual acceptable range PEF • Establish written self-care plan for patient and action to be taken	• Reassurance • Reinforce and repeat doctor's explanations in lay terms • Teach use of peak flow meter. Repeat significance of PEF readings • Teach use of nebuliser and inhaler • Coordinate physio and medication times • Assist with ABGs • Medications as prescribed • Monitor effects • Assist C to work out role in care team and express questions and concerns • Contact Asthma Campaign • Assist with written self-care plan	• Cooperate with health care team to learn more about: – asthma – treatment – management – using nebuliser/inhaler – recording PEF and what readings signify Work out action to take at set points • Ask questions – discuss results • Practise use of equipment • Talk to social worker and get advice on work and family problems • Help to work out written self-care plan • Aim to control asthma and avoid further severe attacks	• Coordinate physiotherapy with inhalation regimen. Assist with nebuliser technique • Discuss general fitness • Teach C respiratory mechanics and exercises	• Advise on family benefits • Funding for peak flow meter • Advise on job change

MEDICAL MANAGEMENT

Investigations Diagnosis is confirmed by auscultation (listening to the chest with a stethoscope), chest X-ray or CT scan and sputum cytology. A bronchoscopy (direct visualisation of the trachea and bronchi using a bronchoscope, i.e. a flexible tube with a light source) may be performed. A small piece of lung tissue (biopsy) may be taken via the bronchoscope and sent for pathology.

Treatment A full explanation of the diagnosis and prognosis will be given to the patient and family so that an informed decision can be made regarding treatment.

Approximately 15% of primary lung tumours can be treated successfully by surgical removal. This will involve either lobectomy (removal of the affected lobe) or pneumonectomy (removal of the whole lung) followed by cytotoxic chemotherapy. Where there is invasive and metastatic spread, the treatment is usually conservative, involving chemotherapy, deep X-ray, intervention to alleviate symptoms and pain control (see Chs 19 and 31, and Box 3.10).

NURSING PRIORITIES AND MANAGEMENT: Care of the patient following lobectomy

General perioperative care is as described in Chapter 26. The reader should also review the position and function of the structures illustrated in Figure 3.1.

Specific considerations

The following points are of particular importance in postoperative management following lobectomy:

- The physiotherapist will manage the pre- and postoperative chest physiotherapy; however, the role of nursing staff in giving assistance and ensuring continuity is extremely important.
- Chest surgery can be very frightening and the patient and family will need careful explanations and constant reassurance.
- In order to allow full expansion of the operated lung, the patient must be nursed in a semi-upright position, well supported with pillows, following a lower lobectomy. Following an upper lobectomy, the patient must be nursed in the position requested by the surgeon; this will be detailed in the postoperative instructions.
- If oxygen therapy is required it will be prescribed by the doctor. The nurse will monitor the equipment, the amount given and the effect of the therapy on the patient.
- There are usually two chest drains in situ, one anterior to the apex and one posterior to the base. These are attached to underwater seal drainage and pleural suction (see Fig. 3.11). Their purpose is to allow air to escape from the lobectomy space and to allow drainage of haemoserous fluid caused by the surgical procedure. Management of underwater seal drainage is discussed in detail in Box 3.11.
- The patient can sit out of bed and walk short distances while the drains are in place, but care must be taken not to put traction on the tubes and to keep the drainage system below the level of the chest. Two pairs of chest drain clamps should accompany the patient at all times.

NURSING PRIORITIES AND MANAGEMENT: Care of the patient following pneumonectomy

Specific considerations

Postoperative positioning

It is vital to find out whether the pericardium has been opened during the operation or not. If it has been opened, the patient must not be allowed to lie on the operated side because of the danger of herniation of the heart through the pericardium and mediastinal shift, i.e. shifting of the heart

Box 3.11

Care of underwater seal drainage

Basic principles

The drainage system is sterile throughout. It is completely assembled prior to the chest drain being inserted. Connections are airtight and sealed with transparent tape to allow inspection. Water level in the drainage device is determined using the manufacturer's instructions. The water acts as a valve and prevents air re-entering the pleural space. The outlet tube allows expelled air to escape. Drainage may be by gravity and respiratory movements or may be assisted by attaching low grade suction to the outlet tube. Single-, two- and three-bottle systems are available.

The chest drain is sutured in place and has an additional purse-string suture around the skin entry site. A sterile dressing surrounds the entry site.

Nursing management

- Give a full explanation and reassurance to the patient to allay anxiety and gain cooperation.
- Assess for and provide appropriate pain relief.
- Keep the patient sitting up, well supported by pillows whilst in bed, and encourage deep breathing and coughing exercises as discussed with the physiotherapist.
- Ensure that two pairs of chest drain clamps accompany the patient at all times in case of accidental disconnection. If the system becomes disconnected, air will be drawn into the interpleural space, extending the pneumothorax.
- When clamping is necessary, it is critical that the clamps are not left on for more than the essential period as a tension pneumothorax may develop. The patient must never be left unattended while the tubing is clamped.
- Ensure that the drainage system is always kept below the level of the chest to prevent back-flow into the interpleural space.
- Check regularly to ensure that the system is airtight and the water level is correct.
- Note the presence of bubbling. If the tube is bubbling, air is being evacuated from the pleural space. If there are no bubbles, there should be a swinging movement of fluid in the down-tube which reflects the pressure changes in the pleural cavity with respiration. The amount of fluid swing should lessen as the lung re-expands. If there are no bubbles and there is no fluid swing, this may mean that either the drainage tube is blocked or that the lung is fully expanded. Chest X-ray will confirm.
- Prevent accidental disconnection by:
  - — supporting the chest drain on the chest wall with adhesive tape, taking care to loop the tube and not bend it
  - — securing the tubing to the bedclothes or the patient's clothes with tape and pins, taking care not to pierce the tubing
  - — stabilising the drainage device by housing it in a special cradle on the side of the bed or the floor.
- Maintain patency by gently lifting sections of the tubing at regular intervals to facilitate the gravitational drainage of blood and viscous fluid.
- Maintain sterility when changing the down-tube and drainage device.
- Measure and record the amount and consistency of drainage. There is a chart to record this on the side of the drainage device.

and greater vessels into the pleural space, causing kinking of the vessels and acute circulatory failure.

Unless otherwise indicated by the surgeon, the best practice is to nurse the patient upright, well supported by pillows.

Chest drains

Usually there are no drainage tubes in position, the main aim being for the space to fill with haemoserous fluid. This will slowly become organised into fibrous tissue and, together with contraction of the intercostal and diaphragmatic muscles and gradual slight shift of the mediastinum, will eventually fill the residual space.

However, if chest drains are in position, they will be attached to an underwater seal drainage system and double-clamped. There may be a request that the clamps be released for brief periods at given times to allow escape of excess fluid and air. If this is the case, the nurse must stay with the patient during the unclamped period and be prepared to clamp the tubings immediately if the patient is about to cough. Because a cough is a full inspiration followed by forced expiration, it will force air from the lung space out through the drainage tube, allowing a sudden mediastinal shift, which could be fatal (Allibone 2003).

Other considerations

The knowledge of loss of an entire lung, together with a degree of post-anaesthetic collapse of the alveoli, atelectasis, in the remaining lung, can cause a patient to panic and become extremely agitated. It is vital for the nurse to remain with the patient as much as possible and to maintain a calm and reassuring manner. Pain can be severe following pneumonectomy and prescribed pain relief should be given prophylactically. It should be borne in mind that effective pain control will help to promote calm, relaxed breathing and is therefore important to the patient's recovery. Oxygen will be given as prescribed. The nurse may need to explain that the lung space will be allowed to fill slowly with blood and serum which, over the following few weeks, will undergo fibrosis (see Ch. 19).

For further information on the management of pleural disease, see British Thoracic Society (2003).

RESPIRATORY EMERGENCIES

This section begins with a brief consideration of chest injuries, pulmonary oedema and respiratory failure. An introduction to endotracheal intubation and mechanical ventilation is also given. Pulmonary embolism, a fairly common and potentially lethal complication of surgery and trauma, is discussed in Chapter 26.

CHEST INJURIES

Fractured ribs and flail chest

PATHOPHYSIOLOGY

Any injury to the thoracic cavity has the potential to disrupt ventilatory mechanisms and compromise respiratory function. Penetrating injuries caused by sharp objects, bullets or fractured ribs may result in collapse of the lung or abnormal collections of blood or air in the pleural cavity. Non-penetrating injuries caused by blunt trauma or crushing can also disrupt ventilatory mechanisms, especially if the diaphragm or other structures are ruptured or contused. Both types of injury will involve disabling pain, and both will restrict surface area for gaseous exchange.

Clinical features Signs and symptoms common to all chest injuries include varying degrees of dyspnoea, chest pain, cyanosis, hypoxia, tachycardia and possibly haemoptysis.

MEDICAL MANAGEMENT

Investigations Diagnosis is confirmed by chest X-ray and the degree of hypoxia is determined by blood gas analysis.

Treatment Simple fractured ribs are usually stable and heal without intervention. Compound fractured ribs may cause a pneumothorax (see below).

When several successive ribs are fractured and become dissociated completely from the rest of the rib cage, the condition is known as flail chest and is characterised by paradoxical breathing. This is where the dissociated ribs rise and fall in opposition to the rest of the rib cage.

NURSING PRIORITIES AND MANAGEMENT: Fractured ribs and flail chest

Providing there are no complications or other serious injury, the patient with fractured ribs can be nursed at home. Flail chest, however, is often associated with more serious chest trauma requiring hospital care.

The main aim of nursing care is to promote rest and relieve pain until the intercostal muscles have had a chance to stabilise the fractured ribs. In the case of flail chest, the patient will need bed rest and probably opioid pain relief. In some cases, patient-controlled analgesia (PCA) may be appropriate.

On discharge, the patient should be advised to avoid heavy lifting or exertion until the fractures are healed.

Pneumothorax and haemopneumothorax

PATHOPHYSIOLOGY

The term 'pneumothorax' refers to the presence of air in the pleural space, and 'haemopneumothorax' to the presence of blood and air in the pleural space. Both conditions may cause partial or complete collapse of the lung on the affected side. However, tension pneumothorax is a more serious condition.

In 'tension pneumothorax', the opening into the pleural space from either the lung or the outside chest wall acts as a one-way valve and sucks air into that space during inhalation but does not allow it to escape during exhalation. Gradually there is a build-up of air in the affected side and a mediastinal shift occurs with resultant cardiopulmonary compromise.

Clinical features An open pneumothorax is characterised by the presence of an open wound and a sucking sound as air is drawn into the pleural cavity. In closed pneumothorax, air enters the space from torn lung tissue and there is little or no movement on the affected side.

MEDICAL MANAGEMENT

First aid The patient is kept in an upright position or lying on the affected side. Penetrating foreign bodies are not removed until intensive care facilities are available, in case their removal causes massive haemorrhage or mediastinal shift. Open wounds can be covered by a clean occlusive dressing; this must be released at intervals to avoid a tension pneumothorax developing.

On admission to the Emergency Department, the patient will have a chest X-ray. An apical intercostal chest drain will be inserted and connected to an underwater drainage system. If there is a haemopneumothorax, the patient will require a second chest drain in the basal chest wall. Opioid analgesics will usually be necessary to control the patient's pain and to relieve anxiety.

NURSING PRIORITIES AND MANAGEMENT: Pneumothorax and haemopneumothorax

Specific considerations

General principles of care for the initial period will be as described in Chapter 27. Specific considerations are as follows.

Observation and monitoring

Constant vigilance must be maintained in observing for any change in respiratory status. These injuries are potentially life threatening and the patient should never be left unattended. Changes in respiratory patterns, symptoms and vital signs should be monitored frequently and action taken accordingly.

Assisting with insertion of a chest drain

The patient will usually be given an opioid analgesic for sedation and pain relief. This will also result in slower, deeper and more effective breathing. The nurse assisting should offer simple explanations and reassurance. If possible, the patient should be assisted to sit up and lean forward with arms resting on an overbed table. This will help to expand the thoracic cavity and provide good support for the patient. The pressure needed to pierce the chest wall may be unpleasant but should not be painful. A complete, sterile chest drain set is kept pre-packaged in the Emergency Department. Before the chest drain is inserted, the drainage system should be opened, connected and the drainage chamber filled with sterile water to the requisite level. The whole system should be carefully checked to ensure that it is airtight. A local anaesthetic is then given at the chosen site. Once anaesthesia is achieved, a small incision is made and the chest drain is inserted into the pleural cavity. The chest drain is connected to the underwater drainage system and sutured in place (see Fig. 3.11). A chest X-ray is carried out to confirm the correct position. If low suction is required, a controlled underwater drainage system is connected between the suction source and the end drainage system.

Assisting with removal of a chest drain

This procedure must be carried out by two people, usually a doctor and an experienced nurse. A pre-procedural analgesic will be administered. A careful explanation of the procedure should be given to the patient, who should be shown how to practise the Valsalva manoeuvre which

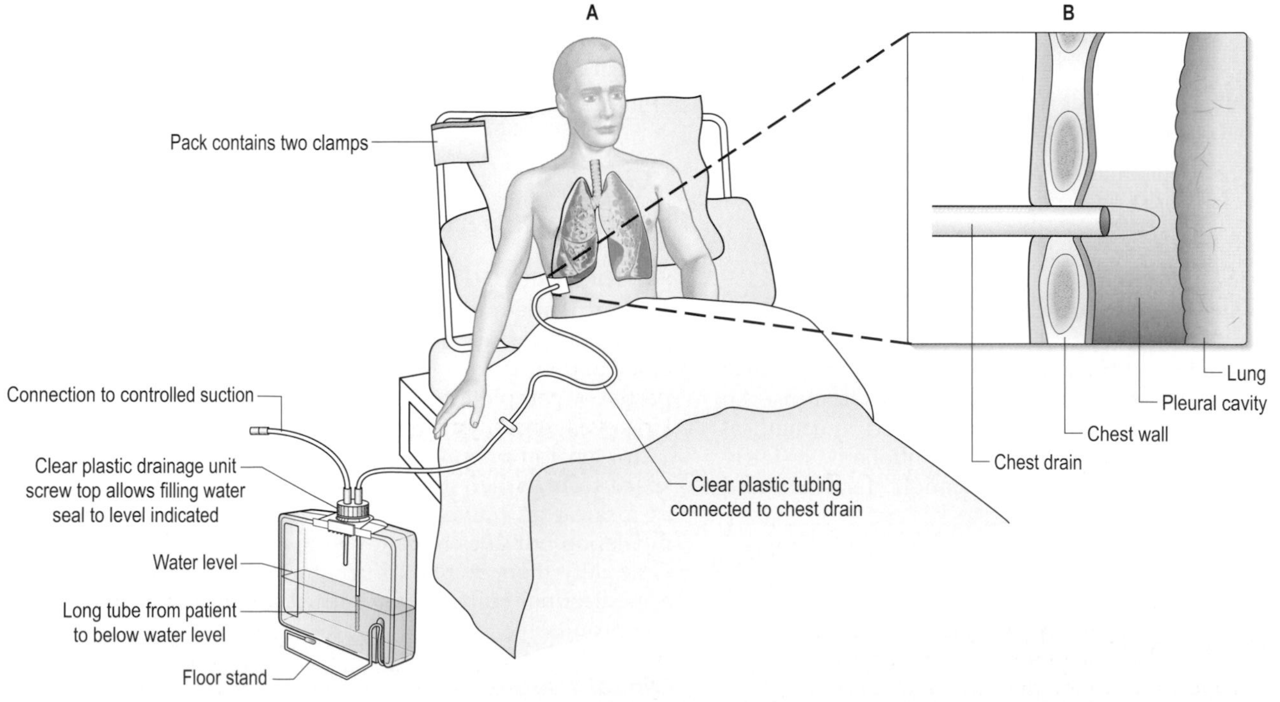

Fig. 3.11 Underwater seal chest drainage. A: Drainage system in position. B: Detail of the position of the chest drain in the pleural cavity. (Based on an original drawing by Nicole Rooth, Moreton Bay Design Co., Australia, with permission.)

involves forcible exhalation against a closed glottis. Alternatively, the patient can be asked to take a deep breath and hold it, as this prevents a rush of air into the puncture site and is more easily controlled than the Valsalva manoeuvre. An occlusive dressing and airtight tape must be ready to be applied to the insertion site. The purse-string suture holding the drain in position is located and the retaining suture removed. The drain is steadied and, as the patient performs the Valsalva manoeuvre, the drain is quickly removed and the purse-string suture tied to close the insertion hole. The dressing and airtight tape are then applied firmly and the patient observed carefully following the procedure. A check X-ray may be performed.

PULMONARY OEDEMA

Pulmonary oedema, excess fluid in lung tissue, is associated with many conditions, including inflammatory response to infections, shock, cardiac failure, nephrotic syndrome and severe allergic reactions.

PATHOPHYSIOLOGY

The lungs are susceptible to oedema because of the minimal tissue resistance offered by the thin alveolar and capillary cell walls. The condition is akin to drowning in that the lungs may be full of water, blood and mucus. Pulmonary oedema is usually acute and potentially life threatening, as it disrupts gaseous exchange.

Clinical features The patient presents with a moist cough that produces copious, frothy, pink sputum and is dyspnoeic, tachycardic and extremely distressed.

MEDICAL MANAGEMENT

Diagnosis is based on presenting signs and symptoms, auscultation, chest X-ray and medical history. The main principles of treatment are to remove the water from the alveolar sacs and to assist the respiratory process. Treatment consists of sitting the patient upright, giving oropharyngeal suction, diuretic therapy, opioid analgesics, bronchodilator medication and oxygen. In severe cases, it may be necessary to intubate and mechanically ventilate the patient.

NURSING PRIORITIES AND MANAGEMENT: Pulmonary oedema

As pulmonary oedema is usually associated with cardiovascular disease, specifically left ventricular failure, the principles of nursing management are discussed in Chapter 2.

RESPIRATORY FAILURE

If impending respiratory failure is recognised early, the actual state can be avoided; nurses should be alert for the following clinical signs:

- the patient appears restless and confused
- there is an increase in respiratory rate with laboured ventilatory effort and use of ancillary respiratory muscles (sternomastoid and abdominal muscles)
- forced and abnormal movement of the diaphragm
- pronounced flaring of the nostrils with each breath
- pale or deeply cyanosed and clammy skin.

Where impending respiratory failure is suspected, sedation must be withheld as it will further depress respiratory function. ABGs will confirm the diagnosis.

Respiratory failure is indicated when there is respiratory acidosis with a falling pH, PO_2 below normal and raised PCO_2 (see p. 91). Untreated, the condition will worsen steadily, and increasingly difficult ventilatory effort will leave the patient exhausted and hypoxic, and will eventually lead to a comatosed state and death. However, patients with impending respiratory failure are normally intubated and mechanically ventilated and are nursed in ITU. Only then can sedation be given with safety.

In order to cut down on dead space and improve respiratory efficiency, a tracheostomy, an opening directly into the trachea, is usually performed (see Ch. 14).

EMERGENCY AIRWAY MANAGEMENT, ENDOTRACHEAL INTUBATION AND MECHANICAL VENTILATION

Nursing priorities and management

The nurse must be prepared at all times to perform emergency airway procedures and to assist in endotracheal intubation and mechanical ventilation. These procedures are reviewed in Boxes 3.12 and 3.13 (see also Fig. 3.12).

For further information, see Armstrong & Salmon (1997).

STOP THINK **3.8** When a patient is mechanically ventilated, and in certain other instances, it is necessary to flood the lungs with pure oxygen both before and after carrying out aspiration. What is the reason for this? (See Ch. 29.)

GENETIC DISORDERS OF THE RESPIRATORY SYSTEM

There is considerable evidence of genetic predisposition and susceptibility to some of the more common respiratory diseases such as asthma. Of the classic genetic disorders, cystic fibrosis has the most dramatic and distressing impact on the respiratory system. This is a disease which disturbs the mucus-producing glands throughout the body, particularly those of the respiratory tract.

For a full description of the disease process and its nursing management, see Chapter 6.

CONTINUITY OF CARE: HOSPITAL AND COMMUNITY

Communication between hospital and community health care teams is vital for continuity and ultimate effectiveness of care, and issues relating to discharge planning, accountability and ethical implications are outlined in Box 3.14.

STOP THINK **3.9** During your community placement, ask your community nursing team leader to discuss the practice profile with you.

Select two respiratory care patients from the profile and collect as much relevant information about the

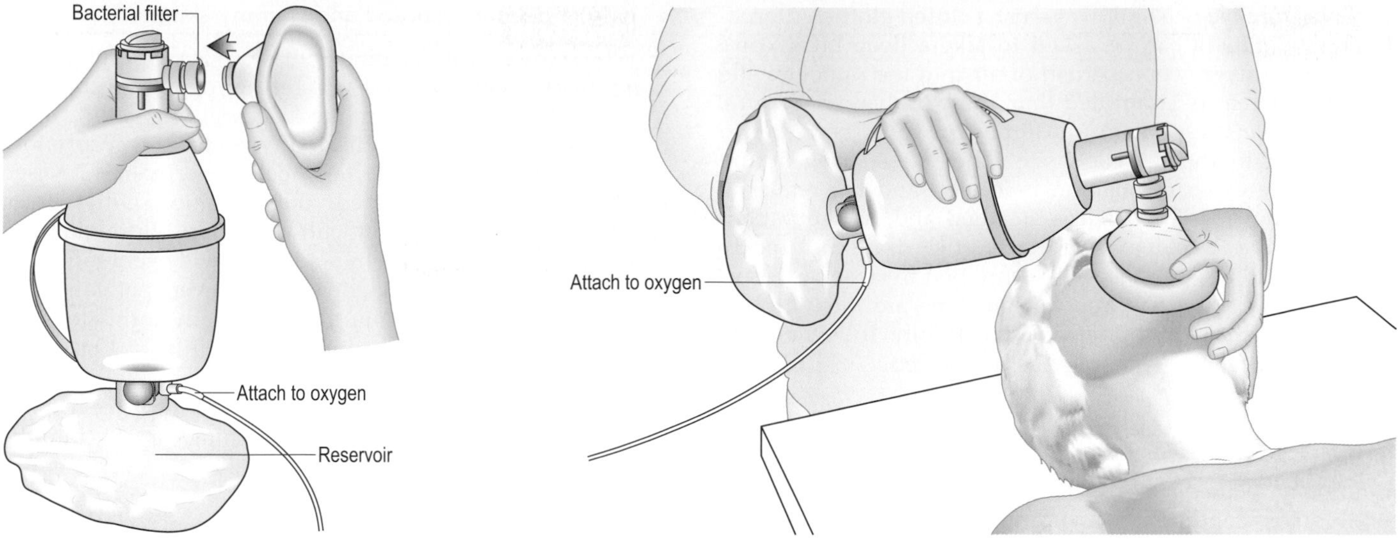

Fig. 3.12 Assembling and using the AMBU bag resuscitator. A: Attaching the face mask and bacterial filter. B: AMBU bag may be attached to oxygen supply if time permits. Patient's neck is hyperextended and mask placed firmly over mouth and nose. Jaw is supported forward. The bag is compressed every 5 s for an adult. (Based on an original drawing by Nicole Rooth, Moreton Bay Design Co., Australia, with permission.)

Box 3.12

Endotracheal intubation and mechanical ventilation

Endotracheal intubation and mechanical ventilation are both specialist procedures and will be performed and monitored by doctors and nurses specially educated in this area. However, it is necessary for the generalist nurse to be familiar with the relevant procedures and equipment in order to be prepared to assist in emergency situations and to better understand the needs of the patient who has been intubated and ventilated during general anaesthesia.

Endotracheal intubation

Maintenance of equipment

Equipment on resuscitation trolleys and in the anaesthetic room must be checked regularly to ensure that it is complete and functional. Equipment must include an appropriate range of sizes of both nasal and oral endotracheal (ET) tubes, at least two laryngoscopes with a supply of new batteries, universal connectors, catheter mounts, 20 mL syringes, artery forceps, Magill intubating forceps, introducers, masks, oral airways, laryngeal spray, suction, lubricant and scissors.

Assisting the anaesthetist

During induction of general anaesthesia, the anaesthetist will select the appropriate tube for the patient and will test and lubricate it. The nurse will ensure that suction is available and have the prepared tube ready for the anaesthetist. The patient is given a full explanation and the nurse should continue to reassure the patient until the i.v. anaesthetic, muscle relaxant and anaesthetic gas have taken effect. The anaesthetist will visualise the vocal chords with the laryngoscope, introduce the ET tube, inflate the cuff and connect the ET tube to the anaesthetic machine. The nurse may be asked to apply cricoid pressure during induction of the anaesthetic in order to prevent regurgitation of stomach contents, especially in emergency cases. This procedure involves using the thumb and forefinger to apply pressure to the patient's cricoid cartilage until anaesthetised and the cuff of the ET tube has been inflated.

Extubation

Following extubation, removal of the ET tube, the nurse must be alert for complaints of sore throat due to damage to the tracheal mucosa, or problems related to oedema of the larynx leading to tracheal obstruction. The nurse should raise the head of the bed unless this is contraindicated and report the symptoms to the surgical team.

Mechanical ventilation

There are many reasons why a patient may need mechanical help with respiration. Extrapulmonary causes which affect the respiratory process include:

- those which affect the respiratory control centres in the brain, e.g. CNS disease, brain contusion or haemorrhage, drug overdose or anaesthesia
- those of neuromuscular origin which cause respiratory paralysis, e.g. Guillain–Barré syndrome, myasthenia gravis, poliomyelitis, organic phosphate poisoning and cervical spine injury
- those which restrict expansion of the thoracic cavity, e.g. musculoskeletal injuries such as extensive flail chest and ruptured diaphragm.

In addition, disorders which affect gaseous exchange can result in severe hypoxia. These include adult respiratory distress syndrome (ARDS), cardiac disease resulting in pulmonary oedema, smoke inhalation and respiratory infection in a patient with chronic obstructive pulmonary disease (COPD).

If help with breathing is needed, the patient may be intubated and attached to a mechanical ventilator. The ventilator will simulate the bellows action normally provided by the diaphragm and thoracic cage and will deliver oxygen-enriched air to the lungs. The type of ventilator used will depend on the specific needs of the individual and will be prescribed by the respiratory specialist. The patient will be nursed in the intensive therapy unit (ITU) and will need specialist nursing care, the principles of which are described in Chapter 29.

Box 3.13

Emergency airway management

Emergency airway management is an essential clinical procedure. The nurse must be familiar with the assembly and use of the hand-held resuscitator known as the AMBU bag and should always be aware of its location in the work area. In cases of respiratory arrest, the AMBU bag will ensure more effective ventilation. The procedure for its use is as follows:

- First, clear the airway of any obstruction, mucus or vomitus. Position the patient to open the airway and insert an oral pharyngeal airway, e.g. Guedel airway.
- Position the face mask to seal the mouth and nose and compress the AMBU bag with the other hand every 5 s. This will deliver approximately 1 L of air with each compression. A smaller bag is used for a child. Oxygen may be attached to the AMBU bag if available.
- If it is necessary to aspirate mucus from the patient's airway, do so via the oropharyngeal airway. Avoid nasotracheal suctioning where possible because this can stimulate the sensory receptors of the vagus nerve, causing disordered heart rate and rhythm — usually bradycardia (slowing).

type of statutory and voluntary services available for these particular patients and add this to your resource folder; use pseudonyms for the patients to ensure anonymity.

Compare your findings with those of your colleagues who may have had placements where the emphasis and case load were different.

Suggested resource people: Local Council of Social Services Directory of Statutory and Voluntary Services, GP surgeries, local libraries, health education libraries, day hospitals, community nursing services.

CONCLUSION

In health we are seldom aware of the functioning of the respiratory system, but disorders and diseases that affect respiration have the potential to affect every aspect of daily living. Airway, breathing and pulmonary circulation are the ABC — the essential elements — of survival.

This chapter has emphasised the importance of a thorough understanding of the anatomy and physiology of the respiratory system — particularly its physiology, because to understand the function of the system is to understand the profoundly disrupting effects that respiratory disorders can have for the individual's health and well-being. A sound knowledge base in respiratory care must inform nursing interventions in every field of practice. Whether working in community settings or a hospital ward, in educational programmes or in an industrial setting, the nurse must be prepared to recognise and act upon any compromise, whether chronic or acute, in respiratory function. Nursing intervention will range from resuscitative procedures in an emergency to giving day-to-day advice on the prevention or management of respiratory disease.

Nursing today encompasses both community-based primary health care and the specialised 'high-tech' skills

Box 3.14

Principles of nursing management: dimensions of community respiratory care

Recent trends have highlighted certain basic issues involved in management of respiratory disorders in the community. These trends include early discharge home from hospital, a higher incidence of severe and chronic respiratory disorders being cared for in the home, and respiratory consultants visiting patients in the community and working alongside GPs, practice nurses and clinical nurse specialists (British Thoracic Society/Scottish Intercollegiate Guidelines Network 2003).

The discharge process

Patient education
Teaching self-care and teaching relatives to assist with care should begin early during hospitalisation so that an acceptable level of proficiency is achieved before discharge and problems are identified and addressed.

Liaison between hospital and home
When a patient is discharged home following acute hospital care, it is vital that there is close liaison between the hospital and the community health care teams. Ideally, the community nurse or another member of the multidisciplinary community care team is allocated time to visit the patient while they are still in hospital and to participate in planning for discharge. At the very least, the community nurse should have direct patient and family contact before discharge and may already know them and be able to provide valuable input into discharge planning. The earlier this is done, the better, so that arrangements can be made to have the necessary equipment and services in place.

In addition to basic aids to daily living, special equipment such as that required for oxygen therapy, inhalation and nebulisation therapy, airway suctioning or mechanical ventilation can be installed before the patient is discharged, and the patient and carers taught to manage it efficiently.

Linking
Knowing and utilising all the statutory and voluntary support bodies that are available and appropriate to the patient and family are crucial in ensuring effective community care.

Practice profile
A descriptive and statistical record, the practice profile is compiled by each community nurse and is a vital tool in overviewing case type, frequency and workload, and in planning maximum and effective use of resources and skill mix.

Documentation
Respiratory disorders and their management in the home can carry a fair degree of risk and hazard.

Documentation is important in all areas of nursing as a basis for accountability and quality assurance; however, for community nurses, detailed and accurate records are even more essential as they often practise alone and are especially vulnerable to the complex legal and ethical dimensions involved in entering a person's home and administering treatment and advice. Great care must be taken to ensure that entry and treatment are achieved with that person's consent and cannot be construed as intrusion or assault or, conversely, that the care given cannot be described as negligent.

required in acute care. Nurses are developing new interdependent and independent roles to meet the demands of new approaches to health care delivery. Increasingly, they are being employed in community and specialist clinics to screen, advise, immunise and treat patients and to promote disease prevention and health education. At the same time, technological and medical advances are demanding a higher level of clinical nursing skills.

This chapter has illustrated two of the major principles in nursing management of respiratory disorders: disease prevention and health promotion, and the active, reflective acquisition of a sound knowledge base and clinical skills. Although the emphasis has been on nursing management, the implicit assumption is always that nurses work in close collaboration with other health care professionals and, in many instances, will be responsible for coordinating the work of the whole team.

REFERENCES

Acharya G, Jauniaux E, Sathia L et al 2002 Evaluation of the impact of current antismoking advice in the UK on women with planned pregnancies. Journal of Obstetrics and Gynaecology 22(5): 498–500

Allibone L 2003 Nursing management of chest drains. Nursing Standard 17(22): 45–56

Bateman N, Leach R 1998 ABC of oxygen: acute oxygen therapy. British Medical Journal 317(7161): 798–801

BBC (British Broadcasting Corporation) 2003 News/Health/SARS: Global hotspots. Online. Available: http://newsvote.bbc.co.uk

British Heart Foundation 2004 Smoking statistics. Online. Available: www.heartstats.org

British Medical Association 2002 Nurse prescribers' formulary, 2002–2003. BMJ Publications, London

British Thoracic Society (BTS) 2001a BTS guidelines for the management of community acquired pneumonia in adults. Thorax 56(Suppl 4): iv1–iv64

British Thoracic Society (BTS) 2001b Standards of Care Committee on pulmonary rehabilitation. Pulmonary rehabilitation. Thorax 56: 827–834

British Thoracic Society (BTS) 2002 Standards of Care Committee. BTS Guideline: Non-invasive ventilation in acute respiratory failure. Thorax 57(3): 192–211

British Thoracic Society (BTS) 2003a Standards of Care Committee. BTS Guideline: Management of severe acute asthma in adults in general practice. Thorax 58(Suppl 1): Annex 1

British Thoracic Society (BTS) 2003b Standards of Care Committee. BTS Guideline: Management of severe acute asthma in adults in A&E. Thorax 58(Suppl 1): Annex 2

British Thoracic Society (BTS) 2003c Standards of Care Committee. BTS Guideline: Management of severe acute asthma in adults in hospital. Thorax 58(Suppl 1): Annex 3

British Thoracic Society (BTS) and Scottish Intercollegiate Guidelines Network (SIGN) 2003 British guideline on the management of asthma. Thorax 58(Suppl 1): i1–i4

Buck D 1997 The cost-effectiveness of smoking cessation interventions: what do we know? International Journal of Health Education 35(2): 44–51

Cowan T 1997 Pulse oximeters. Professional Nurse 12(10): 744–750

Dezateux C, Stocks J, Dundas I, Fletcher M E 1999 Impaired airway function and wheezing in infancy: the influence of maternal smoking and a genetic predisposition to asthma. American Journal of Respiratory and Critical Care Medicine 159(2): 403–410

Donaldson L 2004 On the state of the public health: Annual Report of the Chief Medical Officer 2003. Department of Health, London. Online. Available: www.dh.gov.uk

Downie R S, Tannahill C, Tannahill A 1996 Health promotion, models and values, 2nd edn. Oxford University Press, Oxford

Eaton L 2003 United Kingdom finally bans tobacco advertising. British Medical Journal 326(7385): 351

Field D 1997 Every breath you take. Nursing Times 93(26): 28–30

Hoskins G, McCowan C, Neville R G et al 2000 Risk factors and costs associated with an asthma attack. Thorax 55: 19–24

Jamieson E M, McCall J M, Blythe R, Whyte L A 2003 Guidelines for clinical nursing practices related to a nursing model, 4th edn. Churchill Livingstone, Edinburgh

Joint Committee on Vaccination and Immunisation 2003 Flu immunisation policy. Department of Health, London. Online. Available: www.dh.gov.uk

Joint Tuberculosis Committee of the British Thoracic Society 2000 Control and prevention of tuberculosis in the United Kingdom: code of practice. Thorax 55: 887–901

Kindlen M 2003 Physiology for health care and nursing. Elsevier, Edinburgh

Kleinpell R M, Elpern E H 2004 Community acquired pneumonia: updates in assessment and management. Critical Care Nursing Quarterly 27(3): 231–240

Lacasse Y, Brosseau L, Milne S et al 2003 Pulmonary rehabilitation for chronic obstructive pulmonary disease (Cochrane Review). In: The Cochrane Library, Issue 3. Wiley, Chichester

Linaker C, Smedley J 2002 Respiratory illness in agricultural workers [review]. Occupational Medicine 52(8): 451–459

Moher M, Hey K, Lancaster T 2004 Workplace interventions for smoking cessation. Cochrane Database of Systematic Reviews 1: 2004

National Collaborating Centre for Chronic Conditions 2004 COPD – National clinical guidelines on management of chronic obstructive pulmonary disease in adults in primary and secondary care. Thorax 59(Suppl 1): 1–232

NHS Health Scotland/ASH Scotland 2003 Reducing smoking and tobacco-related harm: a key to transforming Scotland's health. NHS Health Scotland, Edinburgh

Office for National Statistics 2000 Health Statistics Quarterly 2000(8) ID: 19418. TSO, London

Office for National Statistics 2002 Living in Britain: results from the 2000–2001 General Household Survey. TSO, London

Orem D E 2001 Nursing: concepts of practice, 6th edn. Mosby, London

Percival J 2003 The place of pharmacotherapy products in smoking cessation. Professional Nurse 19(2): 113–117

Pitsavos C, Panagiotakos D B, Chrysohoou C et al 2002 Association between passive cigarette smoking and the risk of developing acute coronary syndrome: the CARDIO2000 study. Heart and Vessels 16(4): 127–130

Pozniak A 2001 Multidrug resistant TB and HIV infection. Annals of the New York Academy of Sciences 953: 192–198

Rice V H, Stead L F 2003 Nursing interventions for smoking cessation (Cochrane Review). In: The Cochrane Library, Issue 2. Wiley, Chichester

Rutishauser S 1994 Physiology and anatomy: a basis for nursing and health care. Churchill Livingstone, Edinburgh

Sayer Q M 1999 Achieving compliance in asthma management. Professional Nurse 15(2): 97–99

Scottish Executive 2004 A breath of fresh air for Scotland – tobacco control action plan. TSO, Edinburgh

Shibuya K, Ciecierski C, Guindon E et al 2003 WHO framework convention on tobacco control: development of an evidence-based global public health treaty. British Medical Journal 327(7407): 154–157

Tobacco Advisory Group of the Royal College of Physicians 2000 Nicotine addiction in Britain. Royal College of Physicians, London

West R, McNeill A, Raw M 2000 Smoking cessation guidelines for health professionals: an update. Thorax 55: 987–999

Willcox A 2003 Ready for vaccination. Nursing Standard 18(3): 1–7

World Health Organization (WHO) 2002a WHO framework convention on tobacco control. A56/8. WHO, Geneva

World Health Organization (WHO) 2002b Integrating prevention into health care. Fact sheet 172, October. WHO, Geneva
World Health Organization (WHO) 2003 Publication on DOT. Topics/TB. WHO, Geneva. Online. Available: www.who.int/ health
World Health Organization (WHO) 2004 Global TB control. Topics/TB. Fact sheet 104. WHO, Geneva. Online. Available: www.who.int/health

FURTHER READING

Armstrong R F, Salmon J B (eds) 1997 Critical care cases. Oxford University Press, Oxford
Bourke S J, Brewis R A L 1998 Respiratory medicine, 5th edn. Blackwell Science, Oxford
British Thoracic Society (BTS) 2001 Guidelines for the management of community acquired pneumonia in adults. Thorax 56(Suppl 4): iv1–iv64
British Thoracic Society (BTS) 2003 Guidelines on the management of pleural disease. Thorax 58(Suppl 2): ii1–ii7
Field D 1997 Every breath you take. Nursing Times 93(26): 28–30
Joint Tuberculosis Committee of the British Thoracic Society 2000 Control and prevention of tuberculosis in the United Kingdom: code of practice. Thorax 55: 887–901
Kindlen M 2003 Physiology for health care and nursing. Elsevier, Edinburgh
Kumar P, Clark M 2002 Clinical medicine, 5th edn. Elsevier, Edinburgh, Ch. 14
Margereson C, Esmond G 1997a Professional development 'learning curve' 1(3), Unit 43: 5–8. Chronic obstructive pulmonary disease: Part 1. Knowledge for practice. Nursing Times 93(19)(Suppl)
Margereson C, Esmond G 1997b Professional development 'learning curve', Unit 43. Chronic obstructive pulmonary disease: Part 2. The role of the nurse. Nursing Times 93(20): 67–70
Margereson C, Esmond G 1997c Professional development 'learning curve', Unit 43. Chronic obstructive pulmonary disease: Part 3. Professional issues. Nursing Times 93(21): 57–62
Molyneux A 2004 ABC of smoking cessation. Nicotine replacement therapy. British Medical Journal 328: 454–456
Porter-Jones G 2001 Developing TB guidelines. Nursing Times 97(26): 59
Rutishauser S 1994 Physiology and anatomy: a basis for nursing and health care. Churchill Livingstone, Edinburgh
Waugh A, Grant A (eds) 2001 Anatomy and physiology in health and illness, 8th edn. Churchill Livingstone, Edinburgh
West J B 2003 Pulmonary pathophysiology: the essentials, 6th edn. Lippincott, Williams and Wilkins, Philadelphia, p 124–127
Wiltshire S, Bancroft A, Parry O et al 2003 'I came back here and started smoking again': perceptions and experiences of quitting among disadvantaged smokers. Health Education 18(3): 292–303

USEFUL WEBSITES AND ADDRESSES

Asthma UK Adviceline
Tel: 08457 010203

British Lung Foundation
www.lunguk.org

British Thoracic Society
www.brit-thoracic.org.uk

Department of Health
www.dh.gov.uk

UK National Asthma Campaign
www.asthma.org.uk

World Health Organization
www.who.int/health

4

DISORDERS OF THE GASTROINTESTINAL SYSTEM, LIVER AND BILIARY TRACT

Margot Miller   Alison Crawshaw   Lesley Logan
Rosemary Paterson

INTRODUCTION

The study of the gastrointestinal (GI) system is essential to nursing practice, as the digestive processes are the means by which foods and liquids are digested and absorbed and then transported by the blood for cellular metabolism. Nutrition and dietary factors are integral to the care of individuals receiving treatment for diseases affecting either the digestive system itself or other systems of the body.

Because the GI system comprises a large number of organs with a range of interrelated functions, disorders can produce diverse and often distressing symptoms, some of which may cause people considerable embarrassment, leading them to restrict their social lives. Symptoms include pain, dysphagia, anorexia, loss of weight, heartburn, vomiting, constipation and diarrhoea.

Disorders of the GI system may be acute, presenting as life-threatening emergencies, or chronic, requiring long-term management and sometimes admission to hospital for more intensive treatment and/or surgical intervention. The specific needs of patients with GI disorders will vary, although in GI surgery there are general principles of perioperative care, which can be followed. Although many advances in pharmacological treatment have been made over the years, surgery is still the treatment of choice for some conditions, allowing many patients to make a complete and rapid recovery. For those patients whose condition is such that palliative surgery is the only option, skilled nursing care will be required both in the hospital and in the community.

Essential to human health and well-being is the ability to maintain a regular intake of a balanced diet, and the nurse working in a community or hospital setting is in a key position to advise individuals on the constituents of such a diet and how it may be achieved. The nurse is also in a good position to provide explanations of any investigations, treatments, diagnoses and prognoses, and to follow up any information given by medical colleagues. The principles of holistic care should be adhered to and a process of continuous assessment, planning, intervention and evaluation followed. This process should be flexible, allowing priorities to be changed as the patient's condition and circumstances evolve.

This chapter begins with a review of the basic anatomy and physiology of the GI tract and its related structures, describing the basic functions of that system and how the specialised organs and tissues which it comprises contribute to its effective functioning. The disorders of the GI system, liver and biliary tract that will most commonly be encountered by nurses in hospital or community settings are then described. A separate chapter has been devoted to disorders of the mouth and its related structures (Ch. 15) and it is vital that nurses caring for patients undergoing surgery, the terminally ill or those with GI and related disorders should appreciate the importance of giving careful attention to mouth care.

ANATOMY AND PHYSIOLOGY

The gastrointestinal or digestive tract runs from the mouth to the anal canal and includes the oesophagus, the stomach, the duodenum and the small and large intestines. The ancillary organs of digestion which are connected to, but do not form part of the digestive tract include the liver, the pancreas and the gall bladder. In this chapter, the spleen will also be considered alongside the GI system.

The digestive tract is responsible for taking in food and fluids at the mouth (ingestion), breaking up the food into pieces of a manageable size, extracting the nutritional content of the food and expelling residues and waste products from the rectum via the anus (defaecation). This section will briefly describe the structure and function of the different components of the digestive tract in order to help the reader understand the adverse effects of diseases of this organ system.

The mouth

The mouth carries out three functions in the process of digestion (see Ch. 15 and Fig. 15.1): mechanically breaking down food (chewing or mastication), initiating the chemical breakdown of food (salivation), and swallowing food (deglutition) to allow it to proceed on its journey through the digestive tract.

Movement of food within the mouth is achieved mainly by the tongue, which is largely composed of skeletal muscle. The tongue is also a sensory organ, allowing the taste, texture and temperature of food and fluids to be perceived. The sensation of taste is enabled by the fungiform papillae, or taste buds, which house the relevant sensory nerve endings. The filiform papillae give the tongue a roughness that allows it to be used for manipulating semi-solid food (see Ch. 15).

Saliva is released from three pairs of glands located around the lower jaw. These are, moving anteriorly, the parotid, the submandibular and the sublingual glands. A constant stream of saliva is released into the mouth, of which the submandibular glands contribute about 70% in the absence of a food stimulus. However, the sight, smell or presence of food in the mouth will stimulate the parotid glands to make the major contribution.

Saliva is a mildly alkaline and slightly viscous fluid that serves to keep the mouth moist and clean. It is mildly antibacterial. In digestion, it helps to lubricate food prior to swallowing and, since it contains the enzyme amylase, it also initiates the digestion of starch.

The final process in which the mouth participates is that of swallowing, whereby food is passed into the oesophagus. After food has been sufficiently chewed, which is partly a subjective decision and partly determined by the texture of the food ingested, it is formed into a ball (bolus) between the palate and the tongue and pushed to the back of the mouth by the tongue. The swallowing reflex is initiated by the bolus touching the oropharynx and involves the following steps:

- the temporary cessation of breathing
- the soft palate shuts off the nasal passage
- the raising of the larynx and the lowering of the epiglottis to protect the trachea
- the opening of the upper oesophageal sphincter to receive the bolus of food.

The oesophagus

The oesophagus is a hollow, muscular tube connecting the pharynx to the stomach. It exists solely to enable the passage of food between these two areas and performs no digestive or absorptive roles. The oesophagus is composed of three layers of tissue: an inner mucosal layer with an underlying submucosal layer, a middle muscular layer and an outer connective tissue layer. The mucosal layer contains glands that secrete mucus for the lubrication of food as it passes down the oesophagus. The submucosal layer provides a nerve and blood supply. The muscles of the middle layer are arranged both circularly and longitudinally. The composition of this layer changes throughout the length of the oesophagus in such a way that there is more striated, or voluntary, muscle at the pharyngeal end. Towards the stomach end, the muscle becomes predominantly and then entirely smooth, or involuntary.

The propulsion of food towards the stomach is achieved by peristalsis, which can be described as follows:

1. A descending wave of contraction of circular muscle narrows the lumen of the oesophagus, thereby compressing the bolus of food
2. This is preceded by contraction of the longitudinal muscles to widen the lumen in order to receive the bolus.

Peristalsis is entirely under involuntary control. Relaxation of the lower oesophageal sphincter allows food to enter the stomach (see Fig. 4.1).

The stomach

Digestion continues in the stomach when the bolus of food enters through the lower oesophageal sphincter. The basic structure of the stomach is illustrated in Waugh and Grant (2001). On the inner surface of the stomach, a mucosal, secretory, layer of tissue is supplied with blood vessels and lymph glands by an underlying submucosal layer. Between the mucosal layer and the outermost, peritoneal layer lies a

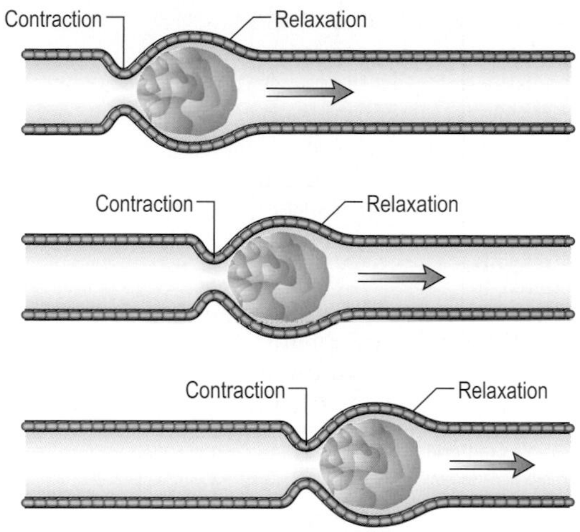

Fig. 4.1 Illustration of the movement of the bolus through the oesophagus by peristalsis.

muscular layer, which is itself composed of three layers: an inner layer of oblique fibres, a middle layer of circular fibres and an outer layer of longitudinal fibres. These layers of muscle allow increasingly stronger waves of contraction in three directions to mix the food in the stomach and allow maximum contact with gastric juice. Innervation of the stomach is from a branch of the Xth cranial (i.e. vagus) nerve, which provides parasympathetic nerve endings that stimulate the secretory cells of the stomach. The internal surface area of the stomach is increased by the arrangement of folds (rugae) in the lining.

Cells in the mucosa of the stomach produce mucus, hydrochloric acid and pepsinogen. This mixture is referred to as 'gastric juice' and, when combined with food in the stomach, as 'chyme'. Hydrochloric acid helps to maintain the acidity of the stomach at a pH of about 2. At this level of acidity, pepsinogen, an inactive precursor, is converted to pepsin, a protein-digesting enzyme that works optimally at this pH. The stomach, therefore, is mainly responsible for initiating protein digestion, although some carbohydrate digestion can continue inside a bolus of food by the action of any salivary amylase that has not yet become inactivated by the acidity of the stomach.

Release of gastric juice by the stomach mucosa is stimulated by the sight, smell and thought of food. This is known as the cephalic phase of digestion. The gastric phase of digestion begins when food reaches the stomach and continues until chyme enters the duodenum, where the intestinal phase of gastric digestion begins. The length of time taken to empty the stomach is variable and depends on the composition of the meal eaten. An average time for emptying of the stomach after a meal is about 4 h. Emptying takes place through the pylorus. The pyloric region holds about 30 mL of chyme; with each wave of contraction in the stomach about 3 mL of chyme is released into the duodenum. This process is regulated by the pyloric sphincter.

Digestion in the stomach is controlled by several factors. The presence of food in the stomach stretches the stomach wall, activating stretch receptors and stimulating the release of gastric juice. A hormone called gastrin is released by the stomach walls; this also stimulates the release of gastric juice. The presence of food substances such as protein and caffeine also stimulates gastrin release. Waves of contraction in the stomach are increased by stretching of the stomach wall and by the presence of protein. On the other hand, low pH inhibits gastrin release. Both the cephalic and gastric phases of digestion can be inhibited by emotional factors. The stomach is not involved in the main process of absorption, although some water, alcohol and certain medication, such as aspirin, are absorbed in the gastric phase.

The intestinal phase of digestion begins when chyme enters the duodenum. The main effect on gastric digestion of the entry of food into the duodenum is inhibitory. The enterogastric reflex, mediated via the medulla, leads to the inhibition of gastric secretion. In addition, the presence of food in the duodenum stimulates the release of three hormones — secretin, cholecystokinin and gastric inhibitory peptide — all of which inhibit gastric juice secretion and reduce gastric motility (see Fig. 4.2).

The small intestine

Extending from the pyloric sphincter to the ileocaecal valve, the small intestine is responsible for the completion of digestion, the absorption of nutrients and the reabsorption of most of the water that enters the digestive tract. The duodenum, which takes up the first 25 cm or so of the small intestine, plays a key role in the process of digestion. It collects chyme from the stomach and is the site where the secretions of the gall bladder and the pancreas are mixed with chyme. These secretions enter the duodenum through the ampulla of Vater, the joining of the common bile duct and the pancreatic duct, which meets the duodenum at the duodenal papilla. The emptying of the gall bladder is regulated by the sphincter of Oddi at the duodenal papilla.

In common with the remainder of the small intestine, the duodenum has a mucosal layer, a submucosal layer, a muscular layer and a peritoneal layer. Unlike the remainder of the small intestine, however, the duodenum is relatively immobile. Its regulatory role is fulfilled when the stimulus of chyme entering the duodenum triggers the enterogastric reflex as well as stimulating the release of gastrin, secretin, cholecystokinin and gastric inhibitory peptide. The effects of cholecystokinin and secretin on the functioning of the stomach have been mentioned above. Secretin also stimulates the cells of the liver to secrete bile, and cholecystokinin stimulates the release of digestive enzymes by the small intestine.

Chyme is very acidic because of its high concentration of hydrochloric acid. When it enters the duodenum, it is brought to a neutral pH by the effect of alkaline bicarbonate released by the pancreas. The effect of bile is to emulsify fats in the chyme, i.e. to break up fat globules into smaller particles more amenable to the effects of fat-digesting enzymes. The enzymes of pancreatic juice can then begin to digest their respective food substances in the duodenum; this action is continued as the chyme is passed down the small intestine.

The first two-fifths of the small intestine following the duodenum is called the jejunum and the remaining three-fifths the ileum. Two types of movement, segmentation and peristalsis, take place in the small intestine; these, respectively, mix and move the food along the tract.

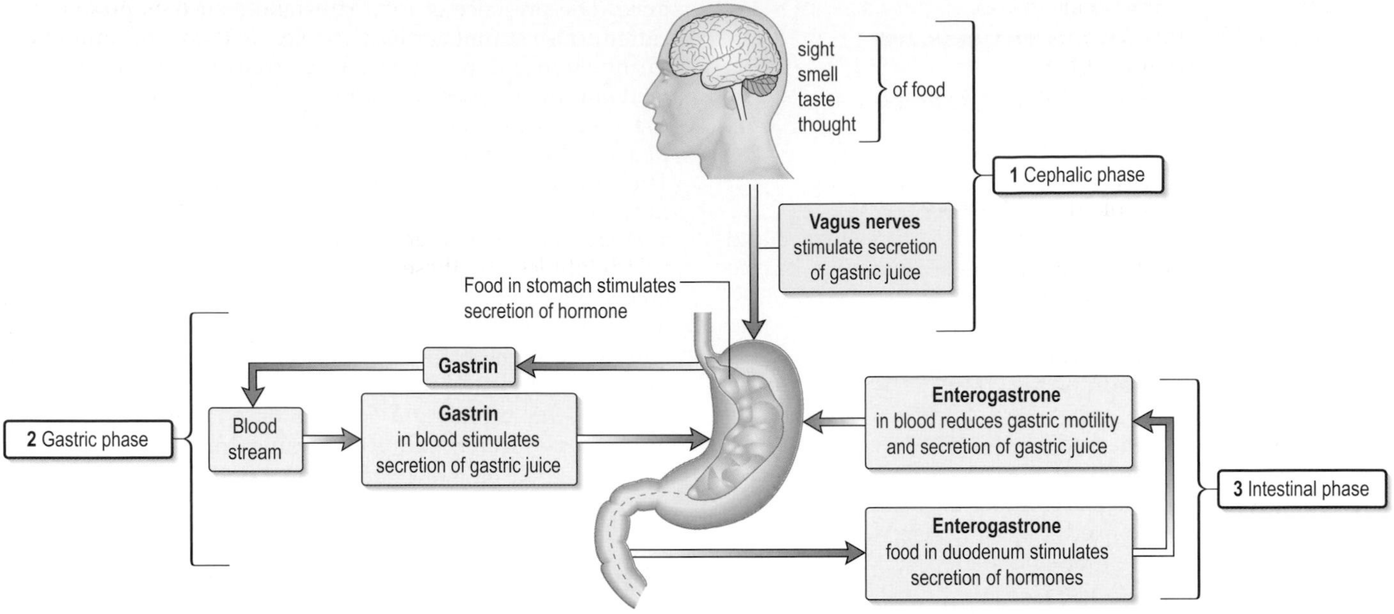

Fig. 4.2 The phases of secretion of gastric juices.

Secretory cells of the mucosa of the small intestine release a slightly alkaline juice containing mainly water and mucus. The remaining enzymes of digestion in the GI tract are located on the microvilli, which are microscopic finger-like projections of the cell membrane. The enzymes of the small intestine complete the digestion of all components of the diet, including protein, fat, carbohydrate and nucleic acids.

Absorption takes place along the full length of the small intestine, and 90% of all the products of digestion are absorbed here. The products of digestion are amino acids and peptides from protein, fatty acids and monoglycerides from fats, hexose sugars from carbohydrates, and pentose sugars and nitrogen-containing bases from nucleic acids. About 7.5 L of water are secreted into the small intestine daily and 1.5 L ingested. As only about 1 L enters the large intestine, the major portion of the water is reabsorbed in the small intestine. Absorption takes place at the villi, which greatly increase the digestive and absorptive area of the small intestine. Each villus contains an arteriole and a venule connected by a capillary network, and a central lacteal, which is a projection of the lymphatic system. Short-chain fatty acids, amino acids and carbohydrates are absorbed directly into the bloodstream. Triglycerides, which form structures called chylomicrons, are absorbed into the lacteals and then enter the bloodstream where the thoracic lymphatic duct empties into the left subclavian vein (see Fig. 4.3).

The large intestine

With most of the nutrients removed, the indigestible residue of food from the small intestine passes through the ileo-caecal valve and enters the large intestine. The mesentery attaches both the small and large intestines to the rear wall of the abdomen and provides both with their blood supply.

The large intestine can be divided into four portions: the ascending, the transverse, the descending and the sigmoid colon. The curves joining the ascending with the transverse colon and the transverse with the descending colon are

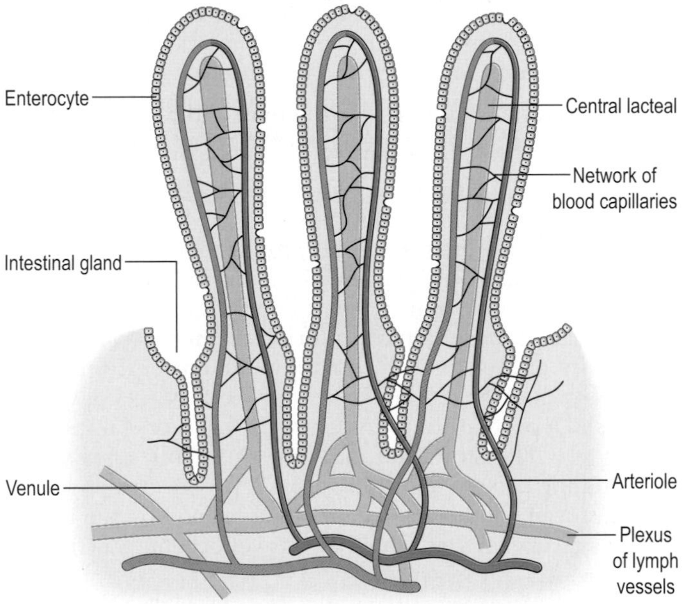

Fig. 4.3 Highly magnified view of the villi in the small intestine.

referred to as the hepatic and splenic flexures respectively. Near the ileocaecal valve, two features can be identified: the caecum, which is a pouch below the ileocaecal valve, and the appendix, which is a finger-like projection of the caecum. The descending colon leads to the sigmoid colon, which terminates in the rectum. Three muscular bands called the taeniae coli run the length of the large intestine. These maintain a slight longitudinal tension in the large intestine and give it its characteristic segmented appearance (haustration). The rectum stores food residue as faeces before expulsion via the anus. The anal canal, which opens externally at the anus, controls evacuation and has an internal anal sphincter of smooth muscle and an external anal sphincter of skeletal muscle.

In common with the small intestine, the large intestine has mucosal, submucosal, muscular and peritoneal layers, but it differs in appearance from the small intestine in that there are no villi. The large intestine is designed mainly for the absorption of water and the lubrication of food residue as it is passed, by the mass action of food entering at the ileocaecal valve, to the rectum. Any nutrients that do enter the large intestine are broken down by commensal bacteria, causing the gases methane, hydrogen, carbon dioxide and sulphur dioxide to be produced. Food can take up to 24 h to pass through the large intestine.

When faeces reach the rectum, a reflex is initiated whereby stretch receptors in the wall of the rectum send signals to the brain informing it of the presence of faeces. However, the desire to expel faeces (defaecation) can be suppressed until the time and place are appropriate. When it is appropriate to defaecate, the internal anal sphincter automatically relaxes and the external anal sphincter, under voluntary control, is relaxed. Intra-abdominal pressure is increased as the individual breathes in and holds the breath against a closed glottis (Valsalva's manoeuvre), and faeces are expelled from the rectum via the anal canal (see Fig. 4.4).

The hepatobiliary system, pancreas and spleen

The liver

With the exception of the skin, the liver is the largest single organ in the body. It is located mainly in the upper right quadrant of the abdomen, just below the diaphragm, and weighs about 1.5 kg. It is a compact lobular organ with large right and left lobes and two smaller caudate and quadrate lobes. Blood is supplied to the liver by the hepatic artery, as well as by the hepatic portal vein, which carries blood containing the products of digestion from the small intestine directly to the liver. The hepatic portal system also collects blood from the lower oesophagus, the stomach, the spleen and the large intestine.

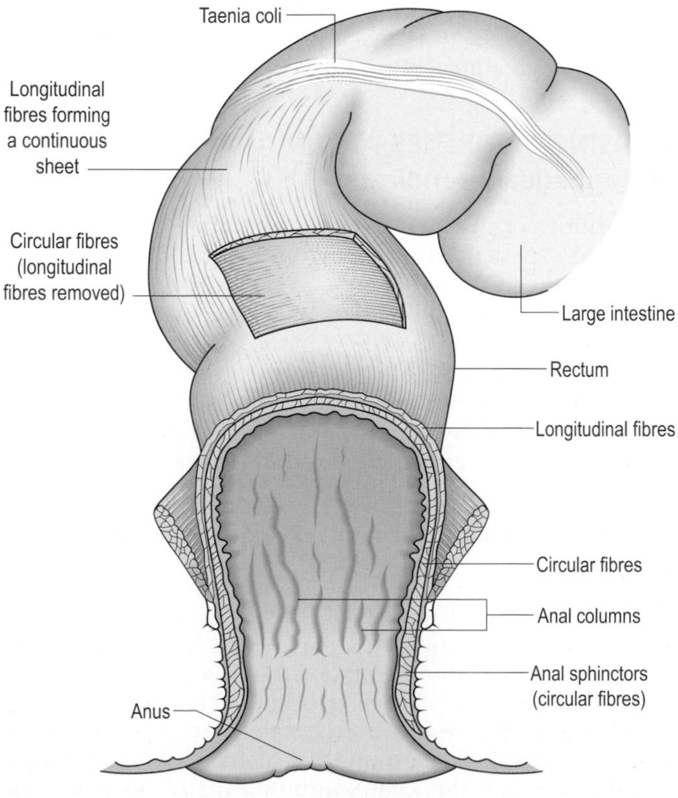

Fig. 4.4 The arrangement of muscle fibres in the colon, rectum and anus (sections have been removed to show layers).

Each lobe of the liver is subdivided into functional units called lobules. In these lobules, branches of the hepatic artery, the hepatic portal vein and a bile duct run concurrently in a structure known as the portal triad. All of the blood entering the liver mixes in spaces called sinusoids and is then drained into a central vein.

Due to its size and unique structure the liver has many diverse functions. These include the detoxification of blood by phagocytic, chemical and other processes, carbohydrate, protein and fat metabolism, protein synthesis and the manufacture and secretion of bile.

For further reading, see Waugh & Grant (2001).

The gall bladder

Lying beneath the liver, the gall bladder has the function of storing and concentrating bile, which is composed principally of bilirubin, derived from the breakdown of haemoglobin from erythrocytes, and bile salts, formed from excess steroid hormones. The gall bladder is a pear-shaped sac about 10 cm long. It lacks a submucosal layer but, in common with other parts of the digestive system, has a middle muscular layer comprising smooth muscle under vagal and hormonal control. Vagal stimulation causes the gall bladder to contract. The mucosal surface area of the gall bladder is increased by the presence of rugae; this promotes the reabsorption of water and a 10-fold concentration of the bile that enters from the cystic duct. The liver secretes bile at a rate of about 1 L per 24 h, but the capacity of the gall bladder is only 30 mL. Bile ducts in the right and left lobes of the liver empty their contents into the right and left hepatic ducts, respectively, which join to form the common hepatic duct. Bile is taken by the cystic duct from the common hepatic duct to the gall bladder, where it is stored and water is reabsorbed. When the gall bladder is stimulated, it contracts and the bile travels to the duodenum down the common bile duct. The release of bile is stimulated by cholecystokinin and secretin.

The pancreas

The pancreas, which lies below and behind the stomach, manufactures and releases pancreatic juice containing enzymes, including enzymes which digest protein, carbohydrate, fat and nucleic acids, and bicarbonate. These constituents of pancreatic juice are produced in the acinar cells of the pancreas.

The exocrine function of the pancreas is discrete from its endocrine function whereby insulin and glucagon are secreted into the bloodstream in response to fluctuating blood glucose levels. The exocrine secretory functions of the pancreas are under vagal and hormonal control. The initial stimulus for the release of pancreatic juice is food entering the duodenum and stimulating the release of cholecystokinin and secretin. Cholecystokinin is responsible for stimulating the release of the pancreatic enzyme portion of pancreatic juice and secretin is responsible for the release of bicarbonate. The pancreatic duct, which delivers pancreatic juice to the duodenum, and the common bile duct join at the ampulla of Vater. Release of bile and pancreatic juice into the duodenum is controlled by the sphincter of Oddi. This sphincter, a ring of smooth muscle, is relaxed by cholecystokinin.

The spleen

The spleen is composed of lymphatic tissue and lies in the upper left quadrant of the abdomen, between the stomach and the diaphragm. It is richly supplied with blood via the splenic artery. Blood flow through the spleen is slowed down by the fact that it must pass through sinuses in which the monophage/macrophage system scavenges old erythrocytes and pathogenic particles and passes the breakdown products on to the liver via the hepatic portal system.

DISORDERS OF THE GASTROINTESTINAL TRACT

DISORDERS OF THE MOUTH

The mouth and tongue are often examined by the physician during clinical examination, as local abnormalities or indications of disease elsewhere can often be detected in this manner. For example, a dry, furred tongue can indicate the presence of a digestive problem or dehydration.

Patients with gastrointestinal and liver disease require meticulous attention to oral hygiene as the mouth can be affected both directly, as in Crohn's disease, and indirectly, as in vitamin and iron deficiency in malabsorption and GI haemorrhage. Patients on steroid and immunosuppressive therapy are also prone to infections of the mouth and oesophagus.

The principles of mouth care and the treatment of a range of disorders affecting the mouth and related structures are described in detail in Chapter 15.

For further reading on oral care, see Evans (2001).

DISORDERS OF THE OESOPHAGUS

Because the oesophagus has a relatively narrow lumen, any obstruction rapidly affects the passage of food. The two most common symptoms that are experienced by patients with disease of the oesophagus are dysphagia and pain. The term dysphagia refers to difficulty in swallowing. This can present in varying degrees, ranging from slight and intermittent difficulty in swallowing solid food to total occlusion of the oesophagus, preventing the patient even from swallowing saliva. Oesophageal pain can be extremely severe and should not be underestimated. There are three main presentations:

- A burning pain (known as 'heartburn') felt high in the epigastrium and behind the sternum. This is usually due to the reflux of gastric contents and sometimes radiates to the neck and to one or both arms.
- A deep, boring, gripping pain across the front of the chest which may radiate to the back, neck or arms. This is usually due to spasm of the oesophageal muscle and is similar in nature to the pain of angina pectoris.
- Pain behind the sternum on swallowing, especially hot liquids. This is usually due to oesophagitis.

Oesophageal moniliasis

This condition is caused by the yeast-like fungus *Candida (Monilia) albicans*. Those who may be vulnerable to this condition are:

- patients with chronic oesophageal obstruction — oesophageal dysfunction causes stasis of saliva and food particles, which predisposes to infection
- patients with immunosuppressive disorders, e.g. diabetes mellitus, leukaemia, lymphoma, AIDS
- patients taking immunosuppressive therapy, e.g. chemotherapy or corticosteroids
- debilitated patients receiving long-term antibiotic therapy.

PATHOPHYSIOLOGY

Common presenting symptoms These will vary according to the severity of the infection, but may include dysphagia, heartburn and retrosternal pain. *Candida* affecting the mouth will show as white patches on the mucosa. A mild fever may be present.

MEDICAL MANAGEMENT

Diagnosis will be made using endoscopy, when biopsies and brushings will be taken. Treatment is with antifungal oral antibiotics such as nystatin suspension, amphotericin lozenges or parenteral fluconazole.

NURSING PRIORITIES AND MANAGEMENT: Oesophageal moniliasis

The priority of nursing care is to minimise the dysphagia and pain experienced on eating and drinking. The patient should be given a soft diet tailored to their likes and dislikes. Supplemental drinks should also be given to ensure weight loss does not occur. Oral hygiene is, of course, extremely important. Patients who prefer to wear their dentures at all times may have to be persuaded of the benefits of removing them at night, as the constant pressure and friction from the presence of dentures could exacerbate the problem.

Hiatus hernia and gastro-oesophageal reflux

A hernia is the protrusion of an organ through the wall of the cavity that contains it. It may apply to any part of the body but is most commonly thought of in terms of abdominal hernias, which are discussed later in this chapter (see p. 127).

A hiatus hernia results from herniation of a portion of the stomach through the oesophageal hiatus in the diaphragm. The opening of the diaphragm normally encircles the oesophagus tightly, and therefore the stomach lies within the abdominal cavity. When the opening through which the oesophagus passes becomes enlarged, part of the stomach protrudes into the thoracic cavity.

PATHOPHYSIOLOGY

Hiatus hernia disrupts the lower sphincter function and impairs oesophageal clearance (Quigley 2003). Hiatus hernias occur most frequently from middle age onwards. They are four times more common in women than in men and are often found in association with obesity. Such hernias can also result from a congenital abnormality presenting in early infancy. Hiatus hernias can be described as 'sliding' or 'rolling', the former being the more common. In sliding hernias, the oesophageal sphincter mechanism is defective, causing reflux of acid-peptic stomach contents.

Clinical features Although many individuals with a hiatus hernia are symptomless, the most common and significant symptom is heartburn as a result of the reflux oesophagitis. It occurs after eating and can be initiated by bending over and lying down. Waterbrash (pyrosis) and a feeling of fullness are common, but dysphagia is a relatively uncommon symptom. Bleeding may also be a feature, involving a chronic, small loss leading to anaemia. This may occur particularly in the older patient with reflux oesophagitis.

MEDICAL MANAGEMENT

Investigations Diagnosis is by medical history, barium swallow and meal or endoscopy.

Treatment In mild cases, it may be sufficient simply to advise the individual to make certain lifestyle adjustments, e.g. losing weight if appropriate, taking small meals at more frequent intervals, wearing loose clothing and avoiding bending over from the waist. Sleeping well supported by pillows is also helpful. It is essential for the individual not to smoke. Medication may include antacids and/or acid-inhibiting drugs.

Failure of medical treatment still remains a significant indication for surgery to reduce the hernia and re-form the angle between the oesophagus and stomach. The procedure is fundoplication (Griffin & Raimes 1997), commonly performed by laparoscopic technique. During the operation, a cuff of stomach is wrapped around the lower end of the oesophagus to tighten up the junction between the oesophagus and the stomach, thereby reducing the risk of reflux.

NURSING PRIORITIES AND MANAGEMENT: Gastro-oesophageal reflux

In many individuals, reflux occurs, without associated hiatus hernia, due to obesity, pregnancy or the use of drugs that may relax the gastro-oesophageal sphincter, e.g. anticholinergic drugs. Reflux can be most distressing and is often mistaken for angina. Most people are able to manage their symptoms by conservative means. For example, raising the head of the bed may be all that is needed to relieve symptoms at night. However, if reflux is chronic or severe, the inflammation of the oesophagus can lead to fibrosis and narrowing of the oesophagus, the development of dysphagia and a predisposition to malignant change (see p. 112).

Preoperative preparation

Preparation for surgery will be as for elective abdominal surgery on the GI tract (see p. 907 and Nursing Care Plan 26.1, p. 916).

Postoperative management

This is the same as that for patients undergoing laparoscopic surgery.

Adequate analgesia using opiate analgesics by patient-controlled analgesia (PCA) or i.m. administration must be given to ensure that the patient is pain-free and hence able to cooperate in deep breathing and coughing exercises. Causes of postoperative pain are described in Table 26.7 (p. 932). Analgesics commonly used in postoperative pain control are listed in Table 26.6 (p. 930).

The i.v. infusion must be monitored to ensure adequate hydration. Oral fluids may be withheld for 24 h. As bowel sounds return, sips of water can be given, increasing to 30 mL of water hourly and then greater amounts as they are tolerated. The nasogastric tube, if used, is removed at the discretion of medical staff, usually as the volume of gastric aspirate decreases.

Following this operation, patients will often have some difficulty in swallowing solid foods, but these symptoms usually settle within approximately 1 month of surgery. Approximately 5% of patients will have persistent problems with flatulence orally following surgery. This is termed 'gas bloat' and can be significantly reduced by encouraging the patient not to swallow air while eating or drinking and to reduce the intake of carbonated drinks. Prior to discharge the patient should be advised to take small, regular meals and to avoid heavy lifting. Return to normal activities will be possible as soon as the discomfort from the abdominal wound has settled, normally 5–10 days following laparoscopic surgery and 2–6 weeks following conventional surgery.

Achalasia

PATHOPHYSIOLOGY

This is a relatively rare motility disorder of the oesophagus (incidence = 1:100 000) (Heading & Tibaldi 1998). The cause is unknown but the pathophysiology is a loss of inhibitory innervation of the oesophageal body and the lower oesophageal sphincter (LOS). This impairment results in a loss of oesophageal peristalsis and failure of the LOS to relax. Unopposed cholinergic innervation can then compound the increased LOS pressure.

The condition can be complicated by respiratory pneumonitis and, very rarely, by oesophageal carcinoma.

Clinical features are as follows:

- dysphagia for solids and often liquids
- intermittent retrosternal chest pain
- regurgitation of oesophageal contents (especially at night)
- aspiration of oesophageal contents
- weight loss.

MEDICAL MANAGEMENT

Treatment There is no cure for achalasia and medical treatment is aimed at reinstating acceptable swallowing for the patient.

The principal treatment at present is pneumatic dilatation of the LOS and this seems to be effective in 60% of patients (Heading & Tibaldi 1998). Oesophageal perforation is a serious, but rare, complication of this procedure. Where dilatation is unsuccessful, a Heller's myotomy, i.e. laparoscopic division of the muscular fibres of the lower oesophagus to aid swallowing, may be performed.

Smooth muscle relaxants such as nitrates or nifedipine can be used in the short term to provide some relief from dysphagia whilst awaiting treatment.

Studies have shown that endoscopic injection of botulinum toxin is a safe and effective treatment for achalasia (Annesse et al 1996, Cuilliere et al 1997). This treatment inhibits the cholinergic effect on the LOS.

NURSING PRIORITIES AND MANAGEMENT: Achalasia

Nursing input is aimed at helping the patient come to terms with, and cope with, an imperfect swallow, although to many patients the fact that they can swallow at all is a significant improvement on their pretreatment condition.

The patient should be encouraged to eat slowly and drink fluids to ease the swallowing process. Dietetic referral may be necessary for patients with extreme weight loss prior to treatment and who require dietary supplementation.

For further reading on disorders of oesophageal motility, see Heading (1999).

Carcinoma of the oesophagus

The majority of carcinomas of the oesophagus occur in older people. Men are affected more frequently than women. This form of cancer is extremely unpleasant and distressing. The patient will rapidly become emaciated due to difficulty in eating and drinking, and skilled nursing care is essential to comfort and support the patient in coping with these and other effects of the illness. Several predisposing factors for oesophageal cancer have been identified:

- *Smoking* — this form of cancer is more prevalent among individuals who smoke (Kjaerheim et al 1998)
- *Alcohol consumption* — individuals who have had a high intake of alcohol are more likely to develop a malignant tumour; in England, a high incidence of oesophageal cancer among publicans and brewers has been noted
- *Achalasia* of the cardia, gastro-oesophageal reflux, Paterson–Kelly (Plummer–Vinson) syndrome and previous trauma are all associated with an increased risk of oesophageal cancer.

PATHOPHYSIOLOGY

Squamous cell carcinoma and adenocarcinoma form the majority of malignant oesophageal tumours. Globally, squamous cell carcinoma remains the most common, although the incidence of adenocarcinoma has been rising in the developed world since the 1970s. According to Pisani et al (2002) in squamous cell carcinoma, 10% occur in the upper oesophagus, 45% in the mid-oesophagus, and 45% in the lower oesophagus. Most adenocarcinomas occur in the lower third of the oesophagus and at the gastro-oesophageal junction, accounting for approximately 40–50% of all oesophageal cancers. The primary tumour can spread locally, up or down the oesophagus, and through its wall to the trachea, bronchi, pleura, aorta and lymph vessels. Distant metastases may occur in the liver and lungs.

Common presenting symptoms The most prominent presenting feature is dysphagia. In the initial stages, this symptom will occur only occasionally and the individual will probably not seek medical help. As the disease progresses and the tumour enlarges, dysphagia will increase and become a constant feature. There will be regurgitation of food, and vomiting and pain will become intense, indicating a spread of the cancer to surrounding tissues. Because of the dysphagia the patient will be anorexic and lose weight rapidly. Many patients develop a cough due to pressure on the bronchus, and a chest infection due to aspiration of oesophageal contents. Haematemesis and melaena occasionally occur as a result of bleeding from an ulcerated tumour.

MEDICAL MANAGEMENT

Investigations Diagnosis is confirmed by oesophagoscopy (see Box 4.1), during which biopsies will be taken. Computed tomography (CT) scan may be used to help identify local and metastatic spread to surrounding tissues. Bronchoscopy may be performed if the tumour is in the upper zone. This will identify whether the bronchus has been invaded and will have a bearing on treatment and care.

Endoscopic ultrasonography (EUS) is a recognised diagnostic tool for the staging of oesophageal and gastric carcinomas.

Treatment As the prognosis is poor, treatment is directed mainly towards the relief of symptoms. Each patient is carefully assessed as to the extent of the disease before a treatment plan is chosen and commenced. Time is also

Box 4.1

Endoscopy in GI medicine

Endoscopy refers to the visualisation of the interior of the body cavities and hollow organs by means of a flexible fibreoptic instrument (endoscope). The use of this technique has contributed greatly to diagnosis and therapy in many areas of medical practice. For use in the gastrointestinal tract, the endoscope is variously designed to view the oesophagus, the stomach, the duodenum, the colon and the rectum. It is also possible, by a modification of the gastroduodenoscope, to visualise the pancreatic and common bile duct; this is called endoscopic retrograde cholangiopancreatography (ERCP). Although most endoscopes are flexible, a rigid instrument may be used for a sigmoidoscopy. For further information, see Cotton and Ackerman (2003).

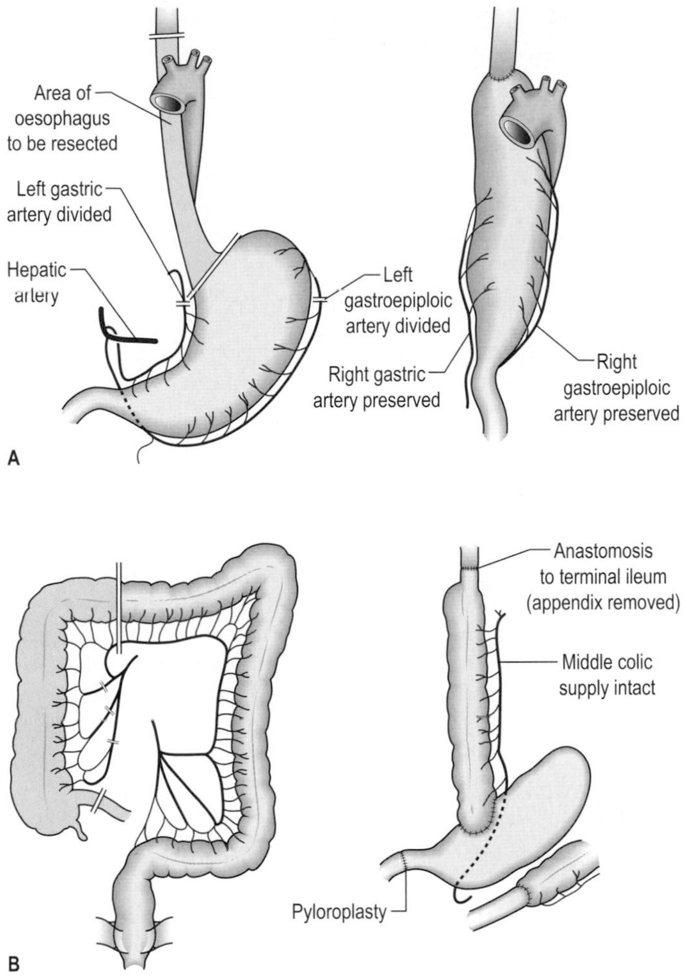

Fig. 4.5 Oesophagectomy and methods of reconstruction. A: Replacement by stomach. B: Replacement by colon.

spent on improving the general nutritional state of the patient by either nasogastric or parenteral feeds.

Surgical intervention will be attempted if the tumour is resectable and if there is no local spread or metastases (see Fig. 4.5).

Radiotherapy may be used if the tumour is radiosensitive, i.e. a squamous cell carcinoma. This treatment is usually used for tumours of the upper third of the oesophagus, but is also sometimes used for the relief of pain.

Malignant dysphagia may be relieved by oesophageal dilatation, endoscopic or open insertion of a stent, or tumour ablation with laser, heat, diathermy or injection of cytotoxic substances (Griffin & Raimes 1997).

NURSING PRIORITIES AND MANAGEMENT: Carcinoma of the oesophagus

Most patients with this form of cancer will be very distressed and emaciated, their life dominated by the symptoms of the disease and by the thought that there is no cure. However, by adopting a caring and sensitive approach, the nurse can do much to alleviate the patient's physical and emotional suffering (Lindars & Sergeant 1994).

STOP THINK **4.1** Mr J is a 65-year-old, newly retired accountant, with a wife and two married sons. He has recently been diagnosed as having oesophageal cancer with metastases in the bronchus and lungs. What would you consider to be the main priorities of his nursing care?

Major patient problems

Dysphagia

Some patients experience significant weight loss, for example, several kilograms over a period of months (Nicklin & Blazeby 2003). Weight should be recorded weekly and noted in relation to their pre-illness weight. An accurate account of daily dietary intake should be recorded with the dietitian's help. Consistency of food is important and the patient should avoid large pieces of meat, 'stringy' foods such as oranges, and 'stodgy' foods such as scones and pastries, as these food choices may lead to blocking of the oesophageal lumen.

The patient should be encouraged to take fluids with meals and to chew foods thoroughly, for example, twice as long as normal. In order to ensure adequate nutrition it may be necessary to provide a liquidised diet.

As the disease advances, the patient will be able to swallow liquids only and should be supplied with a variety of nutritionally supplemented liquids. Supplementary drinks are now available in a variety of sweet and savoury flavours.

Eventually, total dysphagia will occur. It cannot be overemphasised what a distressing condition this is for the patient and family. Nursing management is discussed on page 802.

In the case of a bolus obstruction, it may be necessary to perform an endoscopy to relieve the obstruction. The insertion of a stent is often used to relieve dysphagic symptoms. The oesophagus is dilated at endoscopy and the tube inserted. Following this procedure, the patient will lose the action of the gastro-oesophageal sphincter and will therefore suffer from reflux. The head of the bed should be elevated at all times. The patient will be prescribed an H_2 blocking agent, e.g. cimetidine, to help prevent reflux oesophagitis; this should be given in syrup form. Encouragement should be given to eat a semi-solid diet and to chew food well. The patient should take carbonated drinks, e.g., soda or tonic water, with every meal as this helps keep the stent clear.

Immediately after the insertion of a stent, the patient may suffer quite severe discomfort and it may be necessary to give an analgesic injection. A chest X-ray will be performed and the patient should not be allowed any food or fluid until this has been done in case of perforation of the oesophagus.

For further information, see Donahue (1990) and Owen (2001).

Pain

In the earlier stages of oesophageal cancer, if pain is present, mild analgesics such as paracetamol given in dispersible form may be all that is necessary. As the disease advances, opiates may be required. Initially, the patient may be able to swallow a morphine suspension, but if total occlusion of the oesophagus occurs, it may be necessary to give the morphine by injection. The most effective and convenient way of administering this is by the s.c. route via, for example, a Graseby syringe driver. This delivers a constant level of opioid and readily allows for a 'booster' dose to be given as necessary, to avoid the distress of breakthrough pain. The patient will be able to be at home, if circumstances allow, with a community nurse visiting daily to change the syringe. If necessary, an antiemetic can also be added to the syringe driver.

For further information, see Schofield & Dunham (2003).

Psychological distress

Time must be set aside to allow these patients to express their thoughts, fears and anger, which may be directed towards either the distressing nature of their symptoms or the poor prognosis of the disease, or perhaps both. In the final stages of the disease, every effort should be made to allow the patient to die in the environment of their own choosing. If the patient's choice is to remain at home, a Macmillan or Marie Curie nurse can provide the support and care required.

Oesophageal perforation

PATHOPHYSIOLOGY

Instrumental perforation may occur during endoscopy, especially if the oesophagus is friable due to disease. There is an increased risk of perforation with oesophageal dilatation and the insertion of an oesophageal tube in the palliative management of patients with oesophageal carcinoma.

Spontaneous perforation may occur following a sudden increase in oesophageal pressure caused by vomiting, straining, convulsions or blunt abdominal pressure, e.g. steering wheel pressure in a car accident.

Clinical features The individual will experience severe pain, which may be accompanied by dyspnoea, cyanosis, dysphagia and fever, due to leakage into the mediastinum.

MEDICAL MANAGEMENT

Treatment will be centred on managing potential shock, providing analgesics and prescribing antibiotic therapy. If perforation is severe, surgery may well be required. Such a patient may be acutely ill and require intensive nursing support (see Ch. 29).

Conservative management includes the administration of broad-spectrum antibiotics and ensuring the patient does not take food or fluid orally. These patients are fed either parenterally or via a feeding jejunostomy.

DISORDERS OF THE STOMACH AND DUODENUM

Disorders of the stomach and duodenum are the most common organic disorders of the GI tract. They are considered together here because disorders of one organ commonly affect the other. The overall incidence of acute upper GI haemorrhage in the UK is 103/100 000 adults per year. The incidence rises with age and the overall mortality is 14% (Rockall et al 1995).

Gastritis

PATHOPHYSIOLOGY

Gastritis is an inflammatory condition of the stomach that may be acute or chronic. Acute gastritis is commonly caused by the ingestion of an irritant substance such as aspirin or an anti-inflammatory drug, or by the excessive intake of alcohol. Chronic gastritis develops over many years and is found in patients with pernicious anaemia, autoimmune disorders, chronic alcohol abuse, peptic ulceration and gastric cancer, and following gastric surgery.

Clinical features The outstanding presenting symptom in gastritis is abdominal pain, accompanied by a feeling of distension, nausea, vomiting and anorexia. However, in chronic gastritis, the patient is often asymptomatic. Where symptoms are present, these are the same as those found with acute gastritis, pain being associated with eating and often being described as 'indigestion'.

MEDICAL MANAGEMENT

Investigations Diagnosis is made endoscopically by gastric biopsy. *Helicobacter pylori* is found in the biopsy of many patients with chronic gastritis and, if confirmed, antibiotic therapy will be prescribed.

Treatment An antacid may be prescribed to relieve discomfort and an H_2 blocker such as cimetidine prescribed to prevent histamine from stimulating the gastric parietal cells to secrete hydrochloric acid. Most important is dietary advice, as the patient should avoid causative agents such as alcohol and highly spiced foods.

NURSING PRIORITIES AND MANAGEMENT: Gastritis

In the very acute stage, when vomiting is present, an antiemetic will be given and i.v. fluid replacement therapy may be necessary for a short time. Frequent mouthwashes are given and an appropriate diet gradually reintroduced. The opportunity should be taken to explore the patient's dietary habits and to promote a healthy eating pattern. This is particularly important where the problem of alcohol abuse has been identified.

Peptic ulcer

A peptic ulcer occurs in those parts of the digestive tract that are exposed to gastric secretions, namely the stomach and duodenum.

In the past, peptic ulcer disease was thought to be a chronic relapsing condition that required long-term acid suppression therapy and often major surgical intervention. There was also an associated mortality due to major gastrointestinal haemorrhage and development of gastric cancer.

The identification of the *Helicobacter pylori* bacterium by Marshall and Warren in 1984, and its association with peptic ulcer disease, radically altered the management of this condition from the 1990s, especially with the shift in focus in the NHS from secondary to primary care.

PATHOPHYSIOLOGY

Peptic ulcer formation requires both the presence of gastric acid and damage to the mucosal defence barrier. *H. pylori* is known to be a major factor in causing this damage and is present in over 90% of all patients with duodenal ulcers and 75–80% of those with gastric ulcers (Chua et al 1997). Gastric irritant medication such as aspirin and non-steroidal anti-inflammatories (NSAIDs) are also known to cause mucosal damage. Cigarette smoking is considered to be a causative influence in the development of peptic ulcers and there is growing evidence that smoking prevents the healing of gastric and duodenal ulcers (Haslett et al 2002). The exact mechanisms by which this occurs are not clear, but it is known that long-term smoking increases gastric secretion and interferes with the actions of H_2-receptor antagonists.

The gastric mucosa is, in part, protected by being buffered by food, and erratic dietary habits may contribute to ulcer formation. There is also some conflicting evidence as to whether emotional factors such as stress and anxiety are also causative factors (see Box 4.2).

In *H. pylori* infection, the bacteria burrow beneath the mucosal layer and release a toxin that results in a local inflammatory and systemic immune response. Consequently there is inhibition of the release of somatostatin, a gastric hormone that inhibits gastric acid formation, and oversecretion results. *H. pylori* survive in this acid climate by enzymatically creating an alkaline microenvironment.

It was once believed that ulcers could not develop in the absence of gastric acid (achlorhydria) found in some conditions such as pernicious anaemia and gastric mucosal atrophy (Schwarz's dictum: 'no acid, no ulcer'). Research has shown that while this dictum holds for duodenal ulcers, gastric ulcers can be found in non-acid states (Bynum 1991).

Chronic peptic ulcers penetrate through the mucosa to the muscle layers and may damage blood vessels, causing bleeding. In the duodenum, they are found immediately beyond the pylorus and in 10–15% of cases are multiple. The resulting fibrosis can lead to pyloric stenosis, which in turn can lead to gastric outlet obstruction. Gastric ulcers are found on the lesser curvature of the stomach in 90% of cases.

Box 4.2

Stress ulceration

Unlike other forms of peptic ulceration, stress ulcers are superficial in nature and are often referred to as erosions, since they do not penetrate muscle layers. The pathogenesis is multifactorial and includes hypovolaemia, reduced cardiac output, increased vasoconstriction and splanchnic hypoperfusion. This contributes to acid back-diffusion and reduced bicarbonate secretion, mucosal blood flow and gastrointestinal motility. Within a clinical setting, these ulcers tend to occur after major surgery, trauma, burns or severe illness and commonly present with bleeding (which may be dramatic). The occurrence of stress ulcers will be less likely if prophylactic treatment is given. This is usually an i.v. H_2 antagonist, but proton pump inhibitors are being increasingly used (Daley et al 2004).

Common presenting symptoms The individual with a chronic peptic ulcer will describe a pattern of episodic pain and dyspepsia. Pain is a classic symptom and is described as a burning or boring pain in the epigastrium; often the patient points directly to where the pain is felt. The pain is sometimes more diffuse or radiates through to the back.

While studies show the relationship to food and mealtimes to be variable, the person with a duodenal ulcer is more likely to feel pain and 'hunger feelings' about 2–3 h after a meal, whereas with a gastric ulcer, pain is felt about 30–60 min after a meal and is not relieved by more food. Sometimes patients admit to inducing vomiting in an attempt to relieve the pain. Persistent non-induced vomiting of large amounts indicates an obstruction to the pylorus: pyloric stenosis. Other common features are belching and regurgitation which causes heartburn.

MEDICAL MANAGEMENT

Investigations A full medical history will be taken. An accurate diagnosis is made by endoscopy and/or barium meal. A full blood count is taken for haemoglobin estimation.

Diagnosis of *H. pylori* infection can be made by blood or serum tests for antibodies, and at endoscopy by taking a biopsy from the stomach lining and subjecting it to the rapid urease test, which detects the enzyme that *H. pylori* produces (also known as the 'campylobacter-like organism' (CLO) test). The CLO test, developed by Warren and Marshall in 1984, uses a well of urease indicator gel sealed inside a plastic slide. The gel is amber in colour and turns cherry red if *H. pylori* are identified in the tissue sample.

'Breath test' This is a non-invasive test that detects isotopic carbon dioxide after ingestion of radiocarbon-labelled urea. The *H. pylori* enzyme splits the carbon from the urea. It is then carried as carbon dioxide via the blood to the lungs, where it can be detected in exhaled breath. These tests are specific, as no other bacterium is known to produce the urease enzyme.

Treatment is dependent on the cause and severity of the ulcer. Removal of the causative factor followed by healing of the ulcer is the main aim of treatment, e.g. eradication therapy in *H. pylori* or discontinuation of NSAIDs or aspirin, followed by acid-suppressing medication.

Advice should also be given about avoiding known aggravating factors, such as smoking and erratic dietary patterns. Patient adherence to medication regimens is crucial to the success of *H. pylori* eradication and ulcer healing, and therefore patient education is essential. In some cases, surgical intervention may be necessary.

Medication may include:

- Antacids for the relief of dyspepsia. Many preparations are based on magnesium and may result in a degree of diarrhoea.
- H_2-receptor antagonists, e.g. cimetidine and ranitidine. These assist in ulcer healing by preventing histamine from stimulating the gastric parietal cells to secrete hydrochloric acid.
- A proton pump inhibitor, i.e. omeprazole, to inhibit the release of hydrochloric acid from the parietal cells.
- Eradication therapy which is now the standard treatment for *H. pylori*.

First-line treatment lasts for 1 week and consists of:

- proton pump inhibitor (lanzoprazole/omeprazole) twice daily
- amoxicillin 500 mg three times daily
- metronidazole 400 mg three times daily.

In patients with penicillin allergy, it is common practice to substitute clarithromycin 500 mg twice daily for amoxicillin. However, long-term acid-lowering therapy may be required if there are complicating factors, e.g. NSAID therapy.

Repeat endoscopy is essential to confirm that healing has occurred.

For further information, see University of York (1995), Cottrill (1996) and MacConnachie (1997).

Surgical intervention Indications for surgery for patients with peptic ulcer are as follows:

- failure of response to medical therapy
- recurrence
- development of complications, i.e. perforation, haemorrhage, pyloric stenosis.

The aim of surgical intervention is to reduce acid and pepsin secretion. This is achieved by interrupting the vagus nerve or by resection of the gastric acid-producing section of the stomach. The options for surgical intervention in peptic ulceration are summarised in Table 4.1.

NURSING PRIORITIES AND MANAGEMENT: Peptic ulcer

Preoperative preparation (see Case History 4.1)

The patient who is to undergo an elective procedure may be admitted 1 day prior to surgery or, if the patient is otherwise healthy, may be requested to attend a pre-admission clinic. This allows time for medical examination to be made regarding the individual's fitness for the operation and a general anaesthetic. A blood sample is required for grouping and cross-matching.

A full nursing assessment is made and a care plan formulated to meet the specific needs identified and to fulfil standard preoperative nursing requirements (see Ch. 26). Explanations are given of the timescale for the preparation that will take place. If the patient is a smoker, the importance of stopping smoking and support to do so is offered.

Preparation of the GI tract will include nil orally for 4–6 h preoperatively (see Ch. 26, p. 912). On the morning of the operation, the patient is prepared for theatre. A nasogastric tube is passed perioperatively.

Prior to emergency surgery, regular observations are made of blood pressure and pulse in order to detect any deterioration in the patient's condition. Analgesics are given for pain relief, and clear, concise explanations are given to the patient and the relatives regarding treatment.

STOP THINK **4.2** In the light of Mr R's identified needs in Case History 4.1, create a plan for this patient's preoperative care in hospital.

Postoperative management

On the patient's return to the ward, the nurse will monitor and/or observe the following:

- airway, respiratory rate, blood pressure and pulse and pulse oximetry
- nasogastric aspirate
- bleeding and drainage from the wound and the wound drain if present
- skin colour
- i.v. infusion and site
- urinary output.

These observations are maintained during the first 24–48 h, decreasing in frequency as haemodynamic stability is regained.

The nasogastric tube is usually left on free drainage between aspirations to allow air to escape. The aspirate should be observed for colour and amount. Normally the aspirate diminishes and bowel sounds are heard within 24–48 h. Should large amounts of aspirate continue, this would indicate that absorption from the stomach is not

Table 4.1 Surgical procedures used in the treatment of peptic ulceration

Site	Elective	Emergency
Gastric	Partial gastrectomy, or truncal vagotomy and pyloroplasty, or gastrojejunostomy	Partial gastrectomy Excision of gastric ulcer with truncal vagotomy and pyloroplasty or gastrojejunostomy Simple closure
Duodenal	Highly selective vagotomy Truncal vagotomy and pyloroplasty, or gastrojejunostomy Partial gastrectomy	Simple closure with truncal vagotomy and pyloroplasty, or gastrojejunostomy

After Whitehead (1988) and Forrest et al (1995).

CASE HISTORY 4.1
Mr R

Mr R has been diagnosed as having a duodenal ulcer with pyloric stenosis. He is 54 years old. He has lost a lot of weight over the last few months as a result of vomiting and does not eat much now. He is very thin and is also very anxious. He admits that he smokes 30–40 cigarettes a day and has difficulty sleeping. He has difficulty in hearing but does not use a hearing aid. His particular identified care needs are:

- relief of pain
- relief of anxiety caused by difficulty in hearing the doctor's explanations
- breathing exercises pre- and postoperatively, especially in view of his smoking
- pressure area care due to weight loss
- optimal maintenance of nutritional status
- getting adequate sleep.

occurring; it may also indicate the onset of paralytic ileus (see Ch. 26, p. 926).

Fluids are withheld for at least 24 h, after which period, if bowel sounds have returned, sips of water or ice chips may be given. Fluids may then be given at hourly intervals, beginning with 30 mL and gradually increasing until free amounts of fluid are well tolerated. Light, easily digested food is gradually introduced and the patient is encouraged to eat, but is asked to avoid drinking fluids for at least 30 min after meals (see 'dumping syndrome' below).

Care should be taken that the nasogastric tube is positioned comfortably and well supported. Nasal care is given as required. Oral hygiene is also important and the patient's mouth should be kept clean and moist using mouthwashes or by brushing the teeth if the patient can tolerate this.

The i.v. infusion must be maintained as prescribed, to preserve fluid and electrolyte balance and to prevent dehydration while oral fluids are not being taken.

STOP THINK **4.3** What observations could the nurse make of the patient that would indicate whether adequate fluid intake is being maintained? (See Ch. 20.)

Following surgery, patients should be encouraged to sit up, get out of bed and take a few steps as soon as possible. They should also be encouraged to breathe deeply and cough regularly to clear the lungs of anaesthetic gases and excess mucus. These measures will help to prevent chest infection. Regular gentle leg activity, even when in bed, can also help to prevent the development of deep vein thrombosis. Adequate analgesia and holding the wound firmly when moving or coughing will encourage the patient to cooperate actively with postoperative therapy.

Dumping syndrome

Dumping syndrome is a postoperative complication of gastric surgery that may occur following eating. Symptoms are varied and may consist of a feeling of epigastric fullness and discomfort, sweating, an increase in peristalsis, a feeling of faintness and sometimes diarrhoea.

These symptoms occur within 10–15 min of eating and usually settle within 30–60 min. Patients frequently have to lie down until symptoms subside. The symptoms are caused by the sudden emptying of hyperosmolar solutions into the small bowel, resulting in rapid distension of the jejunal loop anastomosed to the stomach and a withdrawal of water from the circulating blood volume into the jejunum to dilute the high concentration of electrolytes and sugars.

The symptoms of dumping may be alleviated by eating smaller portions of food more frequently, reducing carbohydrate intake and avoiding drinking fluids during meals. If symptoms persist, changes in dietary intake and further surgery may eventually be indicated.

Discharge planning

Patients who have undergone surgery for peptic ulceration are generally fit to be discharged within a week of the operation. However, older patients and those with intercurrent disease may need a longer period in hospital. Therefore, it is important for the nurse to be fully aware of the patient's social circumstances so that from the time of admission adequate preparation for discharge can be made and potential problems anticipated, e.g. Will the patient need transport home? Is a home help required? Does the patient have young children? Early communication with the patient's family or friends is essential in planning for discharge.

STOP THINK **4.4** In view of the patient profile given in Case History 4.1, what advice should be given to Mr R prior to his discharge?

An outpatient follow-up appointment may be arranged to ensure that a satisfactory recovery has been achieved, to discuss any ongoing management and to monitor the patient's rehabilitation. The GP is always given details of the patient's surgery and discharge and of any special aftercare that may be required. If continuing care of the wound is required, this will be arranged with the community nursing team or practice nurse prior to discharge.

Complications of peptic ulcer

The three major complications of peptic ulcer are:

- haemorrhage
- perforation
- pyloric stenosis.

Haemorrhage

Severe abdominal bleeding is a life-threatening emergency. Immediate measures must be taken to replace blood loss and arrest the bleeding (see Ch. 18, p. 725).

MEDICAL MANAGEMENT

Careful assessment of the extent of the bleeding is made, and fibreoptic endoscopy may be used to identify the exact site. In the first instance, an i.v. infusion is started and blood transfusion given if the patient is shocked. Intravenous ranitidine is given to reduce gastric secretion. Hourly oral fluids and a light diet are commenced when bleeding has stopped. Surgery is undertaken as an emergency if the bleeding does not cease. Elective surgery at a later date may be advised for patients who do not respond to conservative treatment.

NURSING PRIORITIES AND MANAGEMENT: Abdominal haemorrhage

Major nursing considerations

Nursing and medical staff must implement resuscitative techniques promptly as necessary. Oxygen therapy should be commenced and maintained at the prescribed rate. Blood pressure, pulse and respirations should be checked and recorded frequently to assess the patient's general condition and to observe for continuing haemorrhage. Central venous pressure monitoring may also be instituted.

Any vomit should be observed for amount and for the presence of fresh blood or a 'coffee ground' appearance. If the bleeding is severe and vomiting is continuous, a nasogastric tube will be passed to determine blood loss and to prevent further vomiting. Stools should be observed for melaena.

Pain is usually severe, requiring opiate analgesic relief. The patient should be monitored for response to analgesics (see Ch. 19, p. 742).

Urinary output must be monitored, as hypotension can affect renal function, diminishing filtration. A urinary catheter should be passed to assist in monitoring output.

Intravenous plasma protein substitutes or whole blood and plasma should be given promptly to restore circulating blood volume. Continuous monitoring must be maintained.

Efforts should be made to allay the patient's anxiety. Ongoing explanations will help to reassure both the patient and the relatives that appropriate treatment is available and that everything possible is being done to arrest the bleeding.

When the patient's condition has stabilised, preparation for surgery can be finalised. Alternatively, if conservative treatment has been successful, surgery may not be necessary.

Perforation

PATHOPHYSIOLOGY

Perforation of an ulcer allows the duodenal and gastric secretions to leak into the peritoneal cavity, resulting in peritonitis.

Perforation of a duodenal ulcer is two to three times more common than perforation of a gastric ulcer (Burkitt et al 2002).

Common presenting symptoms Haemorrhage is not a constant feature and the patient may have very few symptoms. The major presentation is the onset of severe epigastric pain, which becomes generalised abdominal pain and tenderness, made worse by any movement. Therefore, the patient typically stays remarkably still, as a result of which the abdomen develops a 'board-like' rigidity — a classic sign.

MEDICAL MANAGEMENT

Diagnosis is usually confirmed by plain erect X-ray of the upper abdomen. In a positive diagnosis, this will show air collected under the diaphragm. If the diagnosis is uncertain, barium examination may be undertaken. Gastroscopy, which requires inflation of the stomach, is contraindicated. Emergency surgery is the usual course of action, either to repair the perforation or to make a more extensive intervention.

NURSING PRIORITIES AND MANAGEMENT: Perforation

Nursing care will include the following:

- administering resuscitative therapy as necessary
- administering oxygen therapy
- monitoring blood pressure and pulse for shock
- administering i.v. fluids to correct electrolyte imbalance
- administering prescribed analgesics
- passing a nasogastric tube and performing regular aspiration to empty the stomach and prevent further peritoneal contamination
- commencing antibiotic therapy as prescribed
- preparing the patient for surgery
- giving careful explanations and calm reassurance.

Pyloric stenosis

PATHOPHYSIOLOGY

This complication of peptic ulceration is less common than haemorrhage or perforation, and most people associate the disorder with the congenital hypertrophy of the pylorus that sometimes occurs in babies. The stenosis occurs in the first part of the duodenum and in adults is due to repeated healing and breakdown of a chronic peptic ulcer. The build-up of fibrous tissues causes the stenosis, which results in partial or complete obstruction to the gastric outlet.

Common presenting symptoms include a feeling of fullness after meals, anorexia and occasional vomiting, which progresses to an overdistended stomach full of partly digested food, and projectile vomiting.

MEDICAL MANAGEMENT

Investigations Diagnosis is by clinical examination and a barium meal.

Treatment Dehydration and electrolyte imbalance, which may be severe due to the vomiting, are corrected by i.v. fluids. A nasogastric tube is inserted to alleviate vomiting. Once the patient is stable, surgical intervention may be necessary to prevent further ulceration and ensure gastric drainage. The most common procedures are vagotomy and pyloroplasty or vagotomy and gastrojejunostomy (Burkitt et al 2002, Garden et al 2002).

STOP THINK **4.5** What would you consider to be the nursing priorities for a patient with pyloric stenosis prior to surgical intervention?

Carcinoma of the stomach

Gastric carcinomas are more common in men than in women and are usually found in 55- to 70-year-olds. The highest incidence is in Japan. A diet high in carbohydrates and low in fat, fresh fruit and vegetables is thought to predispose to gastric cancer. An increased risk is associated with pernicious anaemia, chronic gastritis and following gastric surgery. The incidence is greater in individuals with blood group A (Garden et al 2002).

PATHOPHYSIOLOGY

Gastric carcinomas are almost always adenocarcinomas derived from the mucus-secreting cells of the gastric glands; 60% occur at the pylorus or in the antrum, 20–30% in the body and 5–20% in the cardia. The tumour spreads along the gastric wall to the duodenum and oesophagus and through the wall to the peritoneum. Adjacent organs become infiltrated. Metastatic spread may occur locally to neighbouring organs, within the peritoneal cavity, or via the lymphatic or blood vessels to the liver, lungs and bones. In most countries, the overall cure rate for gastric cancer remains around 10%. However, the results from Japan present a more encouraging picture, with an overall 5-year survival rate of over 50% (Griffin & Raimes 1997).

Common presenting symptoms The most common symptoms are anorexia, loss of weight and epigastric pain. Often such symptoms are either rationalised as trivial or tolerated despite the distress they cause; consequently, there may be considerable delay before the patient seeks medical help. By this time, the disease may be well advanced and may have spread to adjacent organs. Dysphagia indicates that the cardia of the stomach is involved. Vomiting suggests obstruction by a tumour at the gastric outlet.

MEDICAL MANAGEMENT

Investigations Diagnosis can be made by medical history, clinical examination and a barium meal, usually confirmed by CT scanning. Fibreoptic gastroscopy allows direct inspection and a biopsy to be taken.

Treatment The prognosis is poor. A partial or total gastrectomy — which is either palliative or so-called curative, depending on the extent of the tumour — may be undertaken. Details of surgery are given in Figure 4.6 (see also Griffin & Raimes 1997). Sadly, for some patients the carcinoma is so advanced that surgical intervention is inappropriate.

NURSING PRIORITIES AND MANAGEMENT: Carcinoma of the stomach

See Chapter 26 for details of perioperative nursing priorities in abdominal surgery.

Long-term care after palliative surgery

Major patient problems

After the patient has been discharged home, it is very likely that the symptoms of the cancer will gradually increase.

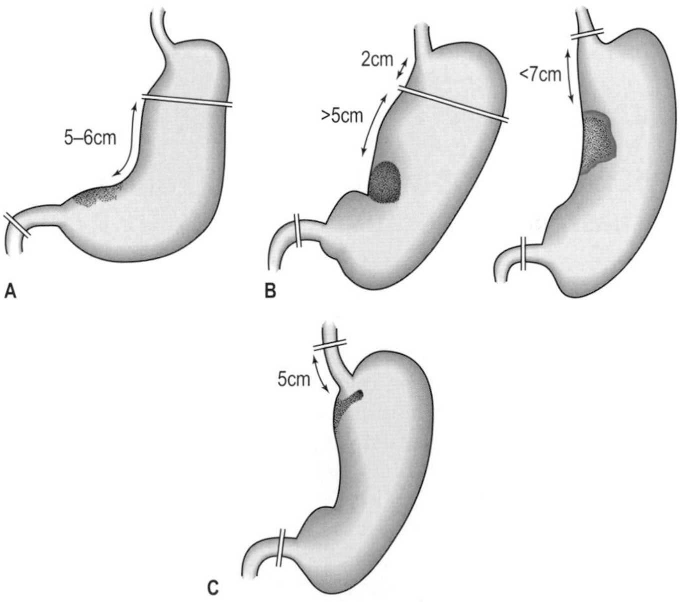

Fig. 4.6 Surgical resection for carcinoma of the stomach. A: Antral carcinoma — subtotal gastrectomy and resection of the first part of the duodenum. B: Carcinoma of the middle third — subtotal or total gastrectomy depending on the proximal margin of resection. C: Carcinoma of cardia — total gastrectomy and resection of lower oesophagus. (Reproduced with kind permission from Griffin & Raimes 1997.)

Skilful and sensitive nursing care will be required to help the patient to remain as comfortable and as free from anxiety as possible.

Pain from the tumour, metastases and ascites can be relieved initially by oral morphine sulphate (MST), progressing, as the need arises, to the judicious use of opioid analgesics, usually diamorphine, given subcutaneously via a syringe driver. Such delivery gives a consistent level of analgesia and is often the key factor in enabling the patient to be pain-free and to remain at home.

Dietary intake may prove a problem. Persistent nausea and vomiting may develop and be difficult to control. Regular and pre-emptive antiemetic medication can be most beneficial. Meals should be small and attractively served at times when the effect of antiemetics is at its optimal level. Nutritious drinks such as Ensure and Enlive can help to supplement nutrition without extra effort on the part of the patient.

Diarrhoea and constipation can both occur. A common side-effect of opiate analgesics is constipation, for which an oral laxative should be prescribed. Orally or rectally administered medications can help to control these symptoms, as can dietary advice.

Mouth infection As in all malignant disease, candidiasis is very common. Nystatin lozenges or suspensions may be given after meals and oral hygiene and dental/denture care must be meticulously maintained (see Ch. 15, p. 636).

Ascites For some patients, there may be the added distress of ascites, which is an accumulation of serous fluid within the peritoneal cavity that can cause pressure on other abdominal organs and the respiratory system. Abdominal paracentesis, whereby the ascitic fluid can be drained off, may be preferred to relieve the symptoms. Diuretics may also be used.

Psychological distress The support of the community nursing team and where possible the Macmillan or Marie Curie nursing services can prove indispensable in giving the patient the confidence to remain at home rather than in hospital. The daily visits of such a nurse, as well as ensuring that the practical aspects of care are achieved, gives the patient and the family the opportunity to talk about fears and worries. The visiting nurse is in an ideal position to monitor the well-being of both parties and to recognise when plans of care should be reviewed. Chapters 31 and 33 explore many ways in which a sensitive continuity of care can be achieved, whether in hospital, at home or in a hospice.

DISORDERS OF THE SMALL AND LARGE INTESTINES

Unlike disorders of the upper GI tract, in which the major problem is that of ingestion of nutrients, disorders of the small and large intestines result in problems of absorption of nutrients or the transit and elimination of bowel contents. People suffering from such problems complain of varying degrees of abdominal pain and discomfort, diarrhoea and/or constipation. Often the symptoms are insidious and/or embarrassing, such that they are ignored or tolerated and not mentioned even to close relatives.

Many health education strategies are now aimed at encouraging the early reporting of symptoms before serious changes have occurred. An American colon cancer screening initiative (Anderson et al 2003) successfully increased screening for, and raised awareness of, this condition. However, although mortality from colorectal cancer can be reduced by 90% using existing screening methods, these are utilised by less than 50% of the US population. In the UK, baseline findings from a multicentre study have shown that 71% of people aged 55–64, who showed an interest in screening in a questionnaire, actually attended for flexible sigmoidoscopy (Mayor 2002).

Malabsorption syndromes

PATHOPHYSIOLOGY

Malabsorption is a consequence of impaired digestion or absorption of nutrients from the intestinal lumen and is caused by a number of conditions. These include:

- lack of digestive enzyme activity, as in chronic pancreatitis and hypolactasia
- lack of bile salts, as in common bile duct obstruction and liver disease
- loss or damage to the absorptive area, as in coeliac disease, extensive bowel resection or Crohn's disease
- failure of adequate removal from the interstitial fluid of absorbed nutrients, as in obstruction of lymphatic drainage.

Common presenting symptoms Whatever the cause, the presenting signs and symptoms of malabsorption are essentially the same. Patients may complain of frothy, greasy and bulky stools that are difficult to flush away (steatorrhoea), diarrhoea, weight loss and abdominal distension.

Vitamin and mineral deficiencies due to malabsorption may result in anaemia, lack of iron, folate and vitamin B_{12}, bleeding disorders and purpura due to lack of vitamin K, and peripheral neuropathy due to lack of vitamins A and B.

Protein deficiency can result in oedema and the musculoskeletal system may also be affected by osteopenia due to lack of calcium, vitamin D and phosphate, and tetany due to lack of calcium.

MEDICAL MANAGEMENT

Investigations When a careful history and clinical examination suggest malabsorption, the following diagnostic tests will be carried out to determine the cause:

- faecal fat estimation
- glucose and lactose tolerance tests
- haematological studies
- radiological and barium studies
- endoscopic examination and biopsy.

Treatment The form of treatment offered will clearly depend upon the cause of the malabsorption. In coeliac disease, where there is sensitivity to gluten, or in lactose intolerance, the advice seems simple: avoid foods containing the offending element. However, for the individual, such advice is not always easy to follow and the condition can potentially cause disruption and stress in everyday life, undermining the sense of well-being.

Where malabsorption is part of, or has resulted from, some other disorder, nutritional supplementation may be required on a temporary or permanent basis.

NURSING PRIORITIES AND MANAGEMENT: Malabsorption syndrome

Major considerations

The assessment and planning of care will necessarily focus on the problems of nutritional impairment, diarrhoea and any associated feeling of embarrassment, anger or despair. For some, pain will be a distinctive feature, in which case providing analgesics must be a priority.

A full nutritional assessment should be made (see Ch. 21) with the assistance of the dietitian. While assessing eliminatory function, efforts should be made to minimise the physical misery and embarrassment caused by diarrhoea. Attention to hygiene and the provision of soothing creams for any excoriation can make all the difference. Ensuring rest and relaxation can help general malaise. This is not always easy, as the investigations may be many and frequent. Supporting the patient through such tests and ensuring full understanding will help in maintaining a positive attitude.

Counselling and teaching will be a priority once the diagnosis and management have been determined. This is especially important as discharge approaches and the patient begins to take responsibility for dietary modification. The community nurse, GP and self-help groups can give support in the community, but probably the best support can be gained from those closest to the patient. The involvement of family and significant friends in any teaching and health promotion programme should be encouraged.

Inflammatory bowel disease: Crohn's disease and ulcerative colitis

Inflammatory bowel disease is the term used to describe two chronic and debilitating conditions: Crohn's disease (CD) and ulcerative colitis (UC). Both disorders are relatively common in developed countries and usually affect people in young adulthood. The incidence of both conditions has risen in Western populations over the last century, associated with better diagnostic techniques (Logan 1998). As yet no definitive cause has been found but it is currently believed that a combination of genetic susceptibility and environmental factors such as bacteria, drugs, smoking and perhaps diet, are implicated (Jewell 2002). It would seem that UC and CD are different manifestations of the same disease; UC, however, affects the colon and rectum, whereas CD can affect any part of the GI tract from the mouth to the anus.

PATHOPHYSIOLOGY

In UC, inflammatory changes occur in the mucosa and submucosa. These changes are diffuse, with widespread superficial ulceration. In CD, the inflammatory changes affect isolated segments of all layers of the intestinal tract. The damaged mucosa develops granulomata, which give the bowel a cobblestoned appearance. Fibrosis and narrowing of the tract can occur and the transmural damage can lead to fistula formation whereby abnormal passageways develop between loops of the bowel.

In UC, the rectum is almost always involved (proctitis) and a variable amount of the rest of the colon. The entire colon can be affected. The inflammatory process affects primarily the mucosa and is continuous. Initially, there is reddening and oedema of the mucosa with bleeding points. This is followed by ulceration, which is usually superficial. In acute disease, especially of the transverse colon, there may be gross dilatation (toxic dilatation) causing the bowel wall to become thin and rupture. In chronic disease, the colon becomes shortened and narrowed. It should be noted that when Crohn's disease affects the colon or rectum, the presentation, treatment and prognosis are very similar to that of UC.

Common presenting symptoms Bloody diarrhoea with frequency, urgency and abdominal cramping are characteristic of UC. Pain may be relieved by defaecation. Pus and mucus may be present in the stool. Attacks vary in severity from being troublesome to life threatening.

The symptoms of CD depend on the site of inflammation, with large bowel CD presenting very similarly to UC. Small bowel CD may present with severe constant pain and weight loss. Oral and perianal lesions may also be present. As with UC, the severity of attacks varies. Both conditions may be associated with extra-intestinal symptoms that include arthritis, skin lesions and eye inflammation. Both UC and CD have minimal mortality rates but both have a substantial negative impact on quality of life (Love et al 1992).

Sometimes the disease is in quite an advanced state before help is sought. In such situations, the symptoms may reflect the more serious complications of rectal abscesses, fissures, fistulae or even obstruction and perforation, which will constitute an abdominal emergency.

MEDICAL MANAGEMENT

Investigations History and examination suggesting inflammatory bowel disease prompt hospital admission for diagnostic tests. Haematological studies will reveal a raised WBC, a raised ESR, a raised platelet count and lowered Hb, B_{12} and zinc. There is often hypoproteinaemia.

STOP THINK **4.6** Can you explain these abnormalities in the blood picture?

Other investigations will include:

- examination of the diarrhoea for blood, fat and infective agents
- radiological and barium examination to reveal characteristic features of inflammatory bowel disease
- endoscopic examination — proctoscopy, sigmoidoscopy and colonoscopy; great care must be taken with such examinations, which are in fact contraindicated in fulminating disease due to the risk of perforation of the bowel
- ultrasound and CT scanning to determine the presence of abscess formation.

Treatment As there is no real cure for inflammatory bowel disease, with the exception of total colectomy in UC, the aim of medical intervention is to bring about remission of active disease and maintain this for as long as possible. This may involve the initial correction of fluid and electrolyte imbalance (see Ch. 20), malnutrition and anaemia. Close observation will be made for signs of obstruction or perforation.

Treatment strategies will have the following aims:

- Relieving abdominal pain by the judicious use of analgesics.
- Controlling the inflammation by the use of steroid therapy and 5-amino-salicylic-acid (5ASA) medications such as mesalazine and sulfasalazine. Anti-inflammatory treatment can be given orally or rectally. The aim is to bring the inflammation under control with steroids and then to maintain remission with 5ASAs, thus avoiding long-term steroid usage. The immunosuppressant medications azathioprine and mercaptopurine are used in severe cases and when the patient cannot tolerate steroids. The monoclonal antibody to tumour necrosis factor alpha, infliximab, is being used increasingly in refractory CD (Carty & Rampton 2003).
- Preventing thrombosis in the acute stage, due to thrombocytosis by the administration of s.c. heparin 5000 units twice daily.
- Restoring nutritional and fluid and electrolyte status. In fulminating disease, enteral nutrition may not be possible and parenteral nutrition will be required (see Ch. 21, p. 806). If enteral nutrition is possible, an elemental diet free of residue may be necessary for a short while before a low-residue diet can be reintroduced. As the inflammation settles, dietary restrictions can be reduced. During any quiescent phase, a 'normal' healthy diet is recommended. Such a diet should have sufficient kilocalories to restore and maintain weight, as well as being high in protein and carbohydrate and low in fat. Supplements of vitamins, iron, folic acid, zinc and potassium may be required.

Surgical intervention Surgery is required in 20–30% of patients with inflammatory bowel disease, but it is always preferred that any surgery be postponed for as long as possible. As a result, living with this condition can mean living with the constant anxiety that symptoms will become severe and complications arise. Surgery becomes unavoidable when:

- acute episodes become more frequent or fail to respond to medical treatment and there is a deterioration, leading to generalised debility, malnutrition, fluid and electrolyte disturbance and anaemia
- obstruction is acute and/or fails to resolve by conservative means
- perforation occurs
- toxic megacolon occurs — the colon hypertrophies, dilates and could rupture
- fistulae develop — these may be internal or enterocutaneous

Box 4.3

Ileoanal pouch anastomosis

The surgical management of chronic ulcerative colitis and familial adenomatous polyposis was revolutionised in 1978 by the introduction of the ileoanal pouch anastomosis, following proctocolectomy and avoiding the necessity of a permanent stoma. Factors such as age, concurrent medical conditions and, most importantly, anal sphincter function are to be considered. Patient selection is of paramount importance to achieve good results. The use of a temporary ileostomy is recommended in most patients to prevent pelvic sepsis. Small bowel obstruction, pelvic sepsis, fistula formation and pouchitis are the most common complications. Sexual dysfunction represents a major concern for younger patients in need of this kind of surgical treatment. The primary advantages of this technique are that the disease is removed completely, adequate reservoir is restored and transanal defaecation and faecal continence are re-established, avoiding the necessity of a permanent stoma (Moreno et al 1996).

This procedure is not used in Crohn's disease because of the risk of disease recurrence in the pouch.

- abscesses fail to respond to intensive treatment
- malignant changes are considered to be a risk.

The choice of operation will depend on the extent and severity of the disease. It is generally accepted that the emergency operation of choice is colectomy with terminal ileostomy and preservation of the rectum. This leaves open for the future the option of proctectomy, ileorectal anastomosis or ileoanal anastomosis. Elective surgery may include total proctocolectomy with permanent ileostomy, colectomy with ileorectal anastomosis or restorative proctocolectomy with ileoanal reservoir.

Great strides have been made in recent years to develop sphincter-preserving operations which avoid creation of a stoma (Moreno et al 1996, Williams 2002) (see Box 4.3). Williams (2002) discusses the possible alternatives to conventional stoma formation, recognising the undoubted impact which stoma formation can have on the patient's self-concept and body image.

In CD, the patient may undergo more than one operation over many years, as surgery may initially be limited to resection of the affected segments of the bowel. However, because the disease affects the total GI tract, alternatives to stoma formation are less easily achieved.

NURSING PRIORITIES AND MANAGEMENT: Inflammatory bowel disease

General considerations

The nursing care of patients with inflammatory bowel disease is essentially symptomatic and must be individualised. Assessment will focus on nutritional status, pain and discomfort, eliminatory patterns, how much the patient knows about the condition and their ability to cope with it. It will also be important to get to know the patient's lifestyle, likes and dislikes, and to identify any sources of stress in their daily life. For some patients, developing a treatment plan will be much easier if a trusting relationship is developed with the nurse. Having a 'named nurse' can be a great comfort and support in coping with the stress of being hospitalised and undergoing a range of often exhausting investigations for which fasting and bowel preparation is required (see Case History 26.4, p. 906).

Confirmation of diagnosis can be a great source of relief in some patients, many of whom may have thought they had a much more serious illness. However, they will now have to accept the reality of a condition that is with them for life. Time must be spent on a regular basis helping the patient to adjust and to plan positively for the future. The National Association for Colitis and Crohn's Disease (NACC) can offer a great deal of support to both patients and their families (see Useful websites, p. 157).

In addition, nursing priorities must include assessing and relieving pain, providing comfort measures that will promote rest, ensuring a high standard of personal hygiene, and providing emotional support to the patient and the family.

It is essential that privacy and ease of access to a toilet or commode is ensured, as the patient will be embarrassed and sensitive about the frequent bowel movements. The patient should be encouraged to maintain an adequate nutritional intake. Small snacks between meals will help to increase calorie intake. The provision of regular oral hygiene and antiseptic mouthwashes is essential to prevent moniliasis. The use of an oil-based barrier cream will help to prevent excoriation around the anal area. Fatigue will be a constant feature. A tactful approach when disturbing an exhausted patient in order to carry out essential care is helpful in gaining cooperation, despite appearing unappreciative of the nursing care being carried out.

Nursing care in acute episodes

During fulminating episodes, the patient may be acutely ill. Abdominal pain can be severe and diarrhoea unremitting, and the presence of fissures, fistulae and rectal abscesses may make the symptoms worse. Dehydration and electrolyte imbalance must be corrected and nutritional status maintained by the parenteral route. The patient will be prone to infection, and the nurse should be alert for signs of pyrexia and tachycardia that may indicate the presence of infection. Toxic megacolon, when the colon becomes grossly dilated, is a life-threatening medical emergency that can result in perforation, haemorrhage and septicaemia. A sudden reduction in either bowel motions or bowel sounds in the acutely ill patient should alert the nurse to the possible onset of this grave complication. Pain and abdominal distension are not always present. This complication will require immediate surgical intervention.

Monitoring

Specific monitoring of the patient's physical condition should include:

- recording of vital signs, particularly any elevation in temperature or pulse rate or signs of impending shock
- recording fluid intake and output. This would include all fluid replacement, whether i.v. or oral, and all fluid

losses: urine, liquid diarrhoea and/or via any fistula. A drop in urine output may indicate fluid depletion. However, if parenteral nutrition is necessary, signs of fluid overload could occur (see Ch. 20, p. 769)
- recording frequency and nature of diarrhoea on a stool chart.

Perioperative care

The essential principles of perioperative care are discussed in Chapter 26. In inflammatory bowel disease there are additional concerns of which the nurse must be aware. Many patients are physically debilitated and, should they present as an abdominal emergency, it may not be possible to improve this state prior to surgery (see Case History 26.2, p. 903). The psychological preparation for surgery that may involve stoma formation is essential, even if time is limited. If optimal time is available, such preparation, in which the stoma nurse specialist plays a key role (see Box 4.4), has been shown to have a very beneficial effect in helping the patient come to terms with and manage the stoma.

> **Box 4.4**
>
> **The role of the stoma nurse specialist**
>
> Psychological preparation for ileostomy and colostomy is essential. The need for information, for emotional support and to develop new skills is vital for the total well-being of the patient (Porrett & Daniel 1999).
>
> The stoma nurse specialist specialises in the care of patients who undergo stoma surgery. In the case of elective surgery, the stoma nurse will visit the patient and the family prior to the operation to give information and support. It is essential that the patient is fully informed of the surgical options available in order to give informed consent to treatment. Clear explanations can help to ensure that the patient understands the changes in body function that will take place and help in adjusting to the accompanying alteration of body image and self-concept. An opportunity should be given to voice feelings and concerns. The spouse or partner should be included in these discussions if the patient wishes, and topics such as sexuality and fertility should be addressed. Referral for specialist counselling may be made as required. Part of the stoma nurse's function is to liaise with other members of the health care team in hospital and in the community, in order to ensure that optimal care and support are given during the patient's treatment and rehabilitation.
>
> The stoma nurse specialist is usually involved in helping to choose the stoma site; this decision should be made after observing the patient standing, walking and sitting, rather than just lying in bed (Black 2000). The chosen stoma site should be marked before the patient is transferred to theatre. The various appliances which are available should be demonstrated before the operation, and, if it seems appropriate, it may be helpful for an individual who has a stoma to visit the patient to talk about what it is like to cope with a stoma in day-to-day living and to reinforce the fact that general health will improve after the surgery.
>
> Research has shown that adequate counselling and education prior to surgery have a positive effect upon the individual's ability to cope following the procedure.

For further information, see Porrett & Daniel (1999) and Black (2000).

Stoma care

Postoperatively, the nurse must maintain close observation of the stoma to ensure that it is viable and has a good blood supply. The stoma should be pink; if it darkens in colour this indicates that the blood supply is threatened. Initially the stoma will be oedematous, but this should reduce over a few days. A clear drainage stoma bag will be in position to allow good observation of the stoma. If an ileostomy has been formed, digestive enzymes will be present and fluid faeces will become copious; care must be taken that the skin is protected by the correct application of the stoma bags. The stoma is formed so that it is approximately 3.5 cm long, thus protecting the surrounding skin. However, care is still necessary to protect the skin and position the appliance. No pressure should be put on the stoma during care.

The patient should be reassured that the output from the stoma will reduce and will become more 'paste-like' in consistency, as the small intestine recovers and adjusts. The stoma nurse specialist can demonstrate the various appliances available so that the patient has a supply of the most suitable ones prior to discharge. Initial care of the stoma is given by the nursing staff, with the patient gradually taking over under supervision and then performing care independently before going home. Continuity of care is given in the community by the primary health care team and the stoma nurse specialist. Advice is also available from the ward staff as required.

Dietary advice should be given by the dietitian and the stoma nurse specialist before discharge, and the patient and family should be advised of the likely protracted recovery and adjustment time that will be required before a return to good health and a full lifestyle can be achieved.

For further information, see Black (2000).

STOP THINK

4.7 Arrange to accompany a stoma nurse specialist on a follow-up visit if possible.

4.8 Ensure you are aware of the different stoma appliances that are available to ostomists. What are the arrangements for the supply and disposal of the appliances?

4.9 As part of your community studies, find out the allowances and benefits to which a person with Crohn's disease may be entitled.

Diverticular disease

Diverticular disease presents as small hernias or outpouchings of the mucosa through the muscular wall of the bowel. These occur predominantly in the sigmoid and descending colon. The presence of uncomplicated diverticulae with minimal or no symptoms is known as diverticulosis and is present in at least half the population aged 80 years and over (Tjandra et al 2001). If inflammation occurs, causing severe symptoms, the condition is referred to as diverticulitis and, if persistent, will be considered a chronic inflammatory disease. However, it is often impossible to distinguish one condition from the other on radiological examination, and hence it is useful to include both active and asymptomatic disease in the term 'diverticular disease'.

It is thought that a diet low in fibre is a major factor in the development of the disease. Research has shown that people with diverticular disease have diets low in fresh fruit and vegetables, brown bread and potatoes, and high in meat and milk products. It is also thought that chronic constipation and the excessive use of purgatives may cause diverticular disease by raising intraluminal pressure.

PATHOPHYSIOLOGY

It is thought that a low volume of colonic content leads to a reduction in the diameter of the colon. Increased luminal pressure during segmentation causes herniation of the mucosa through the muscle wall. Faeces may collect in the hernia(e), causing inflammation, perforation and abscess formation, the formation of fistulae into the small intestine, bladder or vagina, and peritonitis. Repeated attacks can eventually lead to obstruction.

Common presenting symptoms include the presence of intermittent grumbling, spasmodic pain in the left iliac fossa or suprapubic region, and a mass may be palpable on abdominal or rectal examination. Constipation, intermittent constipation or intermittent diarrhoea are usual. The majority of patients with diverticular disease are asymptomatic, but Figure 4.7 shows the range of clinical presentations that can occur.

MEDICAL MANAGEMENT

Investigations Diagnosis is made by barium enema. Flexible sigmoidoscopy is undertaken to exclude cancer. Colonoscopy is indicated when there is rectal bleeding or where a carcinoma is suspected. Most individuals are treated in the community by their GP.

Treatment The main treatment is dietary. The individual should be encouraged to increase fibre intake, including unprocessed bran, wholemeal bread, fruit and vegetables, and should drink plenty of water. Antispasmodics such as propantheline bromide can be used. It must be emphasised that stimulant laxatives should not be used, as they increase the pressure in the muscular wall of the colon and can cause more herniation of the mucosa.

In severe exacerbations, admission to hospital may be necessary if there is marked abdominal pain and pyrexia. Treatment will include broad-spectrum antibiotics, i.v. infusion and nasogastric aspiration until the inflammation subsides. Although many people who live with diverticular disease feel able to cope and have no difficulty in adhering to dietary advice, for about 25% of sufferers complications do occur and surgical intervention will be required. Those complications that may necessitate surgery are shown in Figure 4.7(C–H). Depending on the nature and severity of the problem, resection and temporary or permanent stoma formation may be necessary.

STOP THINK

4.10 Possible surgical procedures for diverticular disease might include:

(a) colectomy
(b) Hartmann's procedure (see Ch. 26)
(c) transverse loop colostomy.

An anxious older patient cannot remember what the surgeon actually said in describing these operations. How would you explain the nature and purpose of these procedures to the patient?

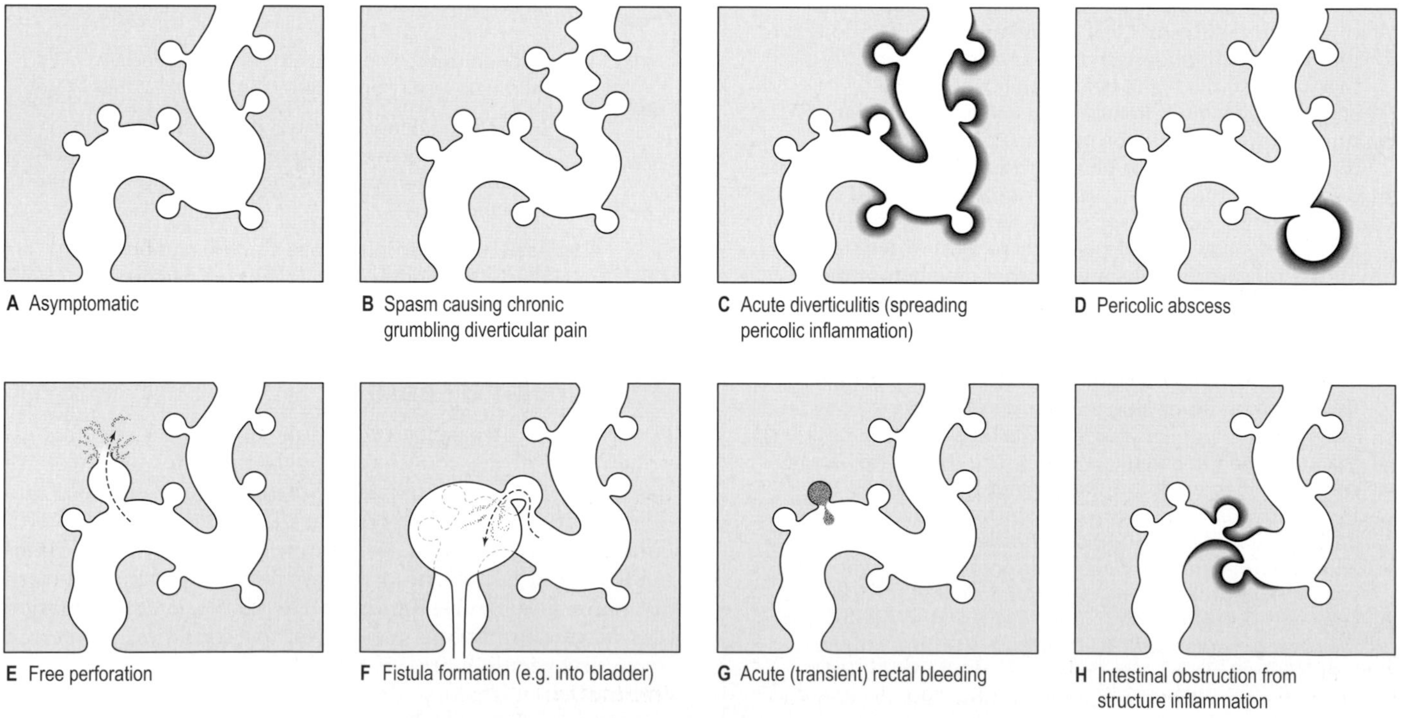

 Fig. 4.7 Clinical presentations in diverticular disease (Burkitt et al 2002).

Irritable bowel syndrome

PATHOPHYSIOLOGY

Irritable bowel syndrome (IBS) is an interaction of three major mechanisms: psychosocial factors, altered gut motility and altered sensory gut function (Camilleri & Choi 1997). Organic bowel disease must be excluded when making the diagnosis. IBS accounts for up to 50% of all referrals to gastroenterology clinics and has a prevalence of between 3 and 22% in European adults with women representing 80% of patients (Delvaux 2003). In IBS, the disorders of gut motility and sensation are mediated by psychological stress factors such as anxiety and depression, although other gut irritants, some food types and alcohol can exacerbate symptoms. In addition up to 40% of IBS patients report physical or sexual abuse (Delvaux 2003).

Common presenting symptoms are:

- diarrhoea and/or constipation
- abdominal pain (often relieved by defaecation)
- abdominal distension
- sensation of incomplete evacuation (tenesmus)
- urgency of defaecation.

MEDICAL AND NURSING MANAGEMENT

Investigations include a careful history, noting details of the paient's physical symptoms, life stressors and reactions to these, and general personality. The type of investigation will depend on presenting symptoms and the patient's age. For example a young person with no 'alarm' symptoms, e.g. weight loss, anaemia and/or rectal bleeding which would raise the suspicion of a pathological problem rather than a functional problem, would require only blood tests and no invasive procedures. However, patients over the age of 40 and anyone with the above 'alarm' symptoms would require flexible sigmoidoscopy to exclude any more serious pathology.

Once the diagnosis is confirmed, time is spent discussing the symptoms and findings and reassuring the patient that there is no underlying pathology.

Treatment is aimed at control of the predominant symptoms. If this can be achieved by avoiding known aggravating factors such as certain foodstuffs or psychological stressors, then the need for pharmacological intervention can be avoided. However, if no particular factor can be identified then antidiarrhoeal agents, bulking agents and antispasmodics should be prescribed.

Alternative therapies such as hypnotherapy have been shown to have significant and long-term value in symptom control in IBS (Gonsalkorale et al 2003). However, nurses must remember to be realistic when discussing coping strategies with patients, as alternative therapies are not readily available on the NHS and can be very expensive.

Appendicitis

The appendix develops from the dependent pole of the caecum as a blind-ended, worm-like sac. It has a large amount of lymphoid tissue in its walls and is covered by the peritoneum. The appendix is described as vestigial in that it constitutes the remnant of a structure whose function is no longer required. In adulthood it is about the size of an adult little finger (5–6 cm).

Inflammation of the appendix is the most common cause of abdominal sepsis in developed countries. The concern is always that the inflamed appendix might rupture, causing peritonitis. Appendicitis is a life-threatening condition and constitutes a surgical emergency.

Although in many people the appendix has virtually disappeared by their middle years, appendicitis can occur at any age. It is rare in infancy and less common in later life, but in the UK can affect 12–15% of those aged 8–15 years. Its prevalence is thought to be closely related to refined Western diets where faecolith residues may be retained in and obstruct the lumen of the blind-ended appendix. The incidence of appendicitis does appear to have fallen significantly over the past 10 years, perhaps reflecting the promotion of a healthier diet that is high in fibre. Less commonly, viral infections, contaminated food and intestinal (tape) worms can precipitate appendicitis.

PATHOPHYSIOLOGY

When the lumen of the appendix becomes obstructed, bacteria proliferate and cause an acute inflammatory response. The local end-arteries become thrombosed and gangrene sets in. This in turn leads to perforation and localised peritonitis. If left untreated, this becomes generalised peritonitis (see Box 4.5 and Fig. 4.8).

Common presenting symptoms Often appendicitis occurs 'out of the blue'. Many an anecdote tells of individuals who at 21.00 h were happily enjoying an evening at the theatre or a restaurant and at 03.00 h found themselves in a hospital bed minus their appendix.

For others, symptoms of colic and fever may 'grumble' on for some time before an acute episode occurs. In such cases, the obstruction has perhaps been partial and the inflammation transitory. These recurrent episodes can result in adhesions forming which can cause further problems (see Box 4.6).

The classic and cardinal features are usually seen in the young person and readily 'diagnosed' even by family and friends (see Case History 4.2).

STOP THINK **4.11** After reading Case History 4.2, try to answer the following questions:

(a) How do you account for the discomfort affecting P's right leg?
(b) Why would any delay in admitting P to hospital have been unwise?
(c) Why might P have experienced postoperative urinary retention? (See Ch. 26, p. 934.)

MEDICAL MANAGEMENT

Investigations Following a careful history and examination, only essential investigation will be carried out to confirm diagnosis. If this is in doubt, an ultrasound scan may be undertaken.

Treatment

Surgical intervention Appendicectomy is the treatment of choice. To remove the offending appendix, a small

Box 4.5

Peritonitis (inflammation of the peritoneum)

Acute peritonitis
Acute peritonitis is commonly caused by irritating substances, often bacterial in nature, entering the abdominal cavity due to:

- perforation of an organ by either trauma or disease, e.g. a penetrating injury, a perforated appendix, duodenal ulcer, or ruptured fallopian tube as a result of an ectopic pregnancy
- gangrene of an organ such as might occur in a strangulated hernia
- septicaemia, which may have originated in another part of the body.

The peritoneum becomes inflamed, inciting a dramatic increase in the production of serous fluid. This rapidly becomes infected and purulent in the presence of bacteria (typically *Escherichia coli* and *Bacteroides*). Toxins are absorbed from the inflamed and oedematous peritoneum and large amounts of fluid are lost into the peritoneal cavity, leading to paralytic ileus, abdominal distension, hypovolaemia, fluid and electrolyte imbalance and loss of protein.

Immediate and intense pain is felt at the site, followed by vomiting, pyrexia, extreme weakness and shock. Diagnosis is essentially clinical, supported by X-ray examination to detect the presence of free air, fluid levels, abdominal masses and perforations.

Treatment is by a combination of surgery, i.v. antibiotic therapy and specific intervention for the underlying cause. The peritoneal cavity may need to be opened to remove the toxic material and allow drainage of the peritoneal cavity. Supportive therapy includes i.v. fluids to maintain fluid and electrolyte balance, nasogastric aspiration to relieve distension, oxygen therapy and analgesics. If the patient continues to remain pyrexial, tachycardic and in pain, an abdominal abscess should be suspected as a complication.

Chronic peritonitis
This is far less common than acute peritonitis but may occur in association with tuberculosis (see Ch. 3) or as a complication of some long-standing irritant such as peritoneal dialysis or a foreign body. Symptoms are less severe and include low-grade fever, vague pain and malaise. Treatment will depend on the cause.

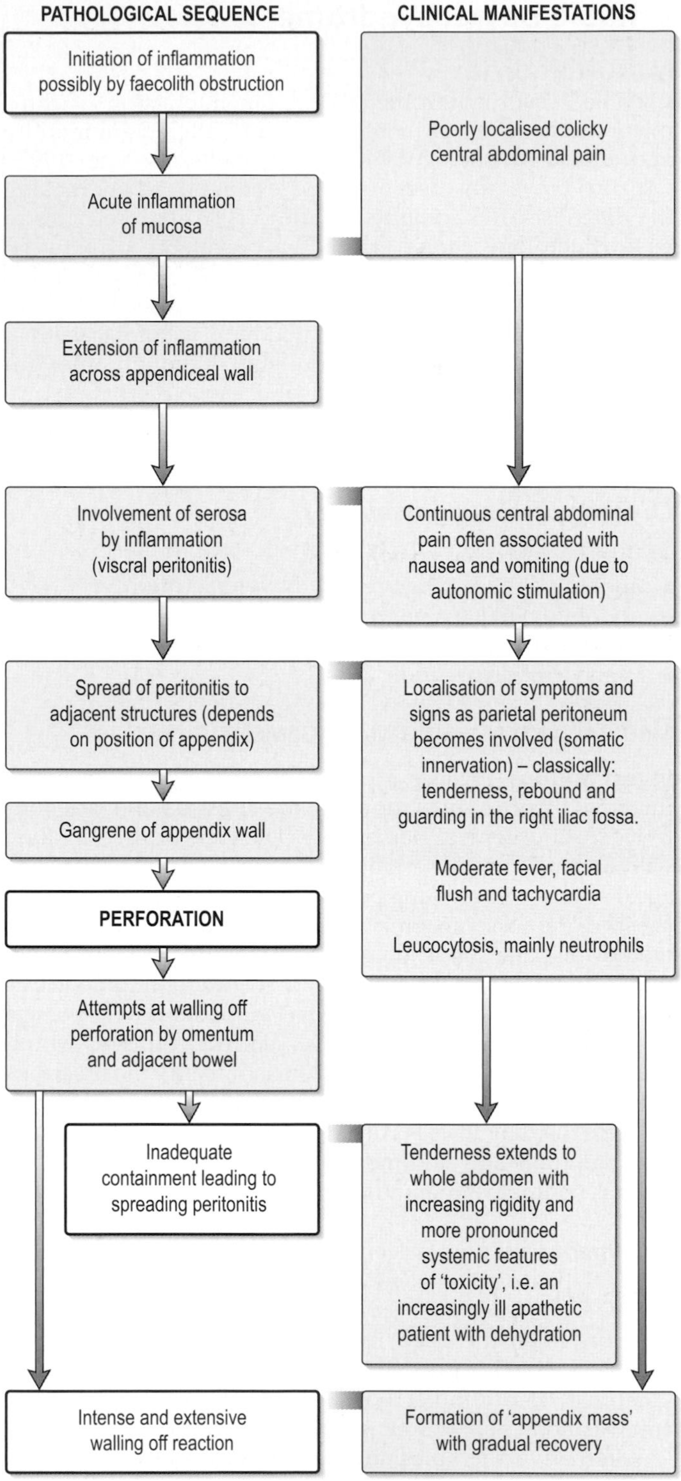

Fig. 4.8 The pathophysiology and clinical manifestations of acute appendicitis (Burkitt et al 2002).

incision is made, the appendix 'delivered' and the stump sutured. The cavity will be irrigated and a drainage tube inserted if any infected material is evident. Alternatively, the appendix may be removed using a less invasive laparoscopic technique.

NURSING PRIORITIES AND MANAGEMENT: Appendicitis

As appendicitis so often presents as an emergency, the patient may have to be prepared quickly. Every detail of safe physical preparation must be attended to, but psychological support must not be considered 'a luxury we can't afford'. The skilled nurse will blend clinical and interpersonal skills to support the patient and family during this crisis.

In the majority of cases, postoperative recovery will be uneventful and rapid. Pain relief should be ensured and vital signs monitored at regular intervals. Monitoring should be tailored to the patient's condition and continue until stability is restored (see Ch. 26, p. 921).

Box 4.6

Adhesions

An adhesion is the union of two surfaces that are normally separate. In the abdomen they are commonly the result of abdominal surgery, injury or inflammation. As healing occurs, fibrous scar tissue develops which may adhere to adjoining tissue, e.g. loops of bowel. These adhesions can distort tissue and, by so doing, impair function, e.g. the transit of intestinal contents. Adhesions may be asymptomatic, but they occasionally cause obstruction and require surgical division.

Such fibrous bands can also occur around pelvic organs, in the pleura, the pericardium and in damaged joints.

CASE HISTORY 4.2

P

P, an active 13-year-old boy, complained of having pains in his stomach and of feeling sick. He refused his breakfast and was reluctant to go to school. Kept at home 'just in case', he was listless and vomited the soup he tried at lunchtime. His friends came round after school; for a while he seemed to 'pick up' and laughter was heard from his room. However, by 20.00 h he could localise the pain to his right side. He curled up on the sofa and complained particularly when he tried to straighten out his right leg.

His mother, suspecting appendicitis, called the doctor. By the time the GP arrived, P was flushed, vomiting and in considerable pain, especially when the GP tried to examine his abdomen. He was immediately admitted to hospital, where a diagnosis of appendicitis was confirmed and he went directly to theatre for an appendicectomy. His designated nurse ensured that both he and his mother understood what was to happen. P's mother was relieved to know that an analgesic could now be given but understood that P's description of the pain had been important in aiding diagnosis. P was not given any bowel preparation, as it would only aggravate the condition. He had not eaten since lunchtime, but because he had vomited, and on examination appeared dehydrated, an i.v. infusion was started to correct any fluid and electrolyte imbalance (see Ch. 20). Intravenous antibiotics were administered in the perioperative period.

P appeared to cope well but was clearly comforted by his mother's presence; she helped him into his theatre gown and promised to safeguard his precious watch. Once prepared, P was taken to theatre, returning to the ward in the early hours of the next day. P's mother decided to go home, having reassured P that she would be back in the morning.

P recovered rapidly and there had been no evidence of perforation or peritonitis (see Box 4.5). He required little analgesic relief but the nurse remained alert to the possibility he was 'putting on a brave face'. The fluid balance record was maintained while the i.v. infusion continued, but this was discontinued after 24 h. By the next day, P was out of bed and taking a light diet and wanting to go home. His only problem had been an initial inability to pass urine that he found unpleasant and embarrassing. However, standing out of bed made things easier. The nurse running water from the tap, however, didn't impress him at all.

P was discharged on the third postoperative day. His sutures were dissolvable and would therefore not need to be removed. The discharge advice for this normally active boy was to ensure that he was not overly active too soon and his nurse took time to explain again that healing would not be fully complete for about 4–6 weeks.

Complications

Should perforation and peritonitis occur (see Box 4.5), the patient may become seriously ill. Intestinal peristalsis will be halted and the risks of dehydration, electrolyte imbalance and septic shock are very real. Treatment will involve the removal of the appendix and toxic material, drainage of any abscess and the administration of systemic antibiotics. Oxygen therapy may be necessary and vascular volume will be restored and maintained intravenously. Opiate analgesics will be given to ensure pain is not allowed to exacerbate an already serious situation. With effective and prompt intervention, the mortality rate of such complications is low.

Abdominal hernia

In the discussion on hiatus hernia (see p. 110), a hernia was defined as the protrusion of an organ through the structures that normally contain it. Abdominal hernias occur where there is an acquired or congenital weakness in the muscle wall of the abdomen, allowing an outpouching of peritoneum to form a sac (see Fig. 4.9). Acquired weakness can occur in any condition that may result in chronically

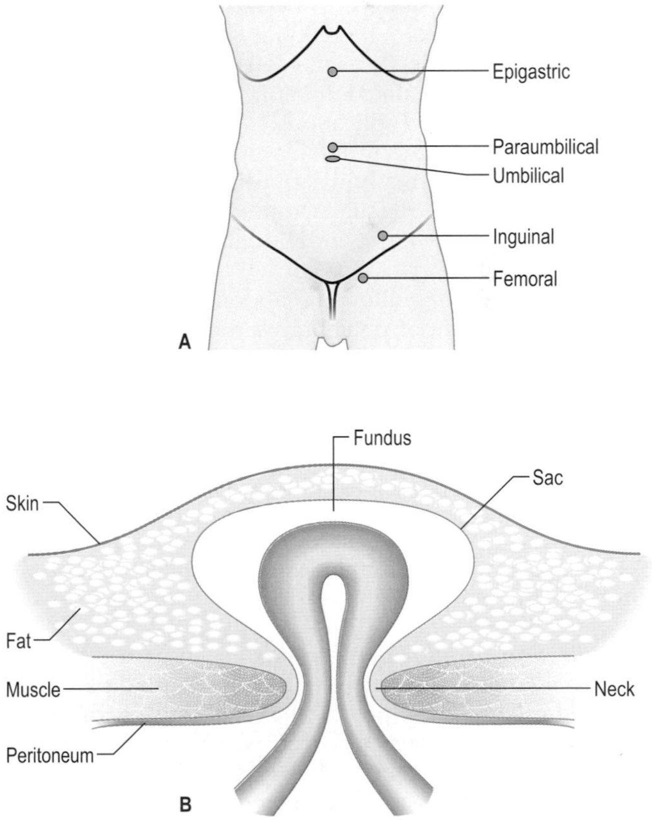

Fig. 4.9 A: Common abdominal wall hernias. B: The principles of the anatomy are the same in each case, although there are obviously individual differences. There is a protrusion of the peritoneum through a natural gap or weakness in the muscle wall of the abdomen. This gap narrows the sac of peritoneum into a neck before it opens out into the fundus. The sac may or may not contain some of the contents of the peritoneal cavity, e.g. omentum, small bowel. (Reproduced from Whitehead 1988, with permission from Edward Arnold.)

raised intra-abdominal pressure, e.g. chronic cough, constipation or heavy lifting, or where abdominal muscle weakness has developed, e.g. obesity, old age, illness or pregnancy.

An untreated hernia may progress to contain peritoneal contents, typically the small or large bowel. The major concern is that, due to twisting and/or constriction at the neck of the sac, the blood supply may become impaired at that site. Unless this is immediately resolved, all of the symptoms of intestinal obstruction will occur (see Box 4.7).

STOP THINK **4.12** How would paralytic ileus be managed?

PATHOPHYSIOLOGY

Abdominal hernias The most commonly occurring types of abdominal hernia may be described as follows.

Inguinal hernia This type of hernia may be indirect or direct, the former being the more common. In indirect inguinal hernia, congenital abdominal weakness causes the hernial sac to protrude through the inguinal ring and follow the round ligament or spermatic cord. A direct inguinal hernia protrudes directly through the posterior ring. Inguinal hernias are far more common in men than in women.

Femoral hernia This type of hernia is considered to be acquired, resulting from herniation through the femoral canal. This canal is wider in women, making such herniation more commonly a female complaint. Femoral hernias also have a greater risk of complications.

Umbilical hernia Many infants are born with an umbilical hernia. This normally disappears in the first year of life without surgical repair. Acquired umbilical hernias can develop in overweight individuals or in those with abdominal ascites (see p. 138).

Incisional hernia Following abdominal surgery, the incision site is a point of potential weakness. This becomes a problem if the patient experiences postoperative problems such as impaired healing, especially if drainage of the wound has been required, abdominal distension or generalised debility.

STOP THINK **4.13** It is often difficult to picture the anatomical features of inguinal or femoral hernias. Review again normal abdominal anatomy with the help of your physiology textbook and take time to understand for yourself how hernias develop.

Reducible and irreducible hernias In the early stages, a hernia may often be reducible, i.e. with manual palpation or a change to standing posture the sac will return to the abdominal cavity. However, as the hernia becomes larger and adhesions form, reduction becomes impossible and the hernia is described as irreducible or incarcerated. If the blood flow is then impaired and obstruction occurs, the hernia is described as strangulated.

Common presenting symptoms The term hernia is usually familiar to the public and the diagnosis, therefore, is often of no surprise. However, familiarity with the term must not be confused with full understanding of the condition. Many may live with the condition for some time, not appreciating the related problems that could occur. Often

Box 4.7

Intestinal obstruction

Intestinal obstruction occurs when the normal transit of intestinal contents is impeded due to mechanical obstruction, vascular occlusion or impaired innervation. Obstruction may be partial or complete.

Mechanical obstruction

Intraluminal causes
- Neoplasms
- Strictures
- Foreign bodies
- Faeces
- Intussusception: a telescoping of one part of the bowel into another part

Extramural causes
- Adhesions
- Strangulated hernia
- Volvulus: twisting of the bowel
- Neoplasms outwith the intestinal tract

When the obstruction occurs, the affected intestine becomes distended with GI secretions (as much as 8 L is formed each day). As the fluid accumulates, the pressure rises and the bowel responds by attempting to propel the contents forward. This serves only to increase secretions; eventually, the increase in pressure increases capillary permeability and fluid is forced out into the peritoneal cavity. The distension may cause respiratory embarrassment. Severe abdominal colic is experienced. If the obstruction is in the small bowel, vomiting occurs. Obstruction in the large bowel results in distension with air and faeces, and the eventual increase in pressure results in necrosis and the threat of perforation. The outcome of unresolved obstruction will be electrolyte imbalance, hypovolaemia and possibly peritonitis.

Vascular occlusion
Obstruction may occur if there is vascular occlusion of the major mesenteric blood supply by a thrombus or embolus. It is the resulting ischaemia that leads to obstruction. Although there is pain, there is no distension. As the condition deteriorates, the pain may actually decrease. If undiagnosed, gangrene and bacteraemia develop as toxins from the lumen invade the peritoneum and are absorbed into the bloodstream. If surgical intervention is not prompt, death may result. It should also be noted that any mechanical obstruction (e.g. strangulation) that impairs blood supply carries with it a significant mortality risk.

Impaired innervation: paralytic ileus
Paralytic ileus will occur when trauma, inflammation or pain in the thoracolumbar region interferes with the normal innervation of the bowel. It can therefore be a complication of such conditions as back and chest injury, renal pathology and peritonitis. Temporary (paralytic) ileus that follows the necessary handling of the bowel in certain abdominal surgical procedures usually resolves in 12–48 h (see Ch. 26, p. 926). Paralytic ileus will result in marked distension, causing discomfort and respiratory embarrassment.

Treatment
Treatment will involve the correction of fluid and electrolyte imbalance, the relief of the distension and pain, and surgical intervention to address the cause.

it is only when symptoms of local pain and tenderness arise that medical advice is sought. By that time the hernia will probably have become irreducible.

MEDICAL MANAGEMENT

The traditional treatment of choice is surgical repair, herniorrhaphy being the usual procedure. The abdominal contents are returned, the sac excised (herniotomy) and the abdominal wall repaired and strengthened with sutures. Laparoscopic techniques are now the more common approach to hernia repair. The minimally invasive nature of such surgery is proving increasingly beneficial to the patient. Follow-up in an outpatient clinic is not considered necessary unless there was an identified surgical problem.

On rare occasions, surgery is contraindicated due to pre-existing morbidity. In these situations a supporting truss may be worn to keep the hernia reduced and the patient free of symptoms. However, this option is not ideal. Surgery under epidural or local anaesthetic for those patients with chronic respiratory or cardiac problems has greatly improved patient outcome and obviated the need for many people to wear a truss.

Strangulation of a hernia This life-threatening complication presents with all of the symptoms of intestinal obstruction, i.e. vomiting, severe abdominal pain, distension and absolute constipation. The patient rapidly becomes shocked, dehydrated and pyrexial. Diagnosis is made by history and clinical examination. A plain X-ray may identify the location and the associated distended loops of bowel. Rapid preparation for surgery will be necessary and definitive therapy will include oxygen, opiate analgesics, i.v. correction of fluid and electrolyte balance, nasogastric aspiration and antibiotic administration. Surgery may well necessitate resection of the affected bowel and intensive nursing care will probably be required in the early postoperative period.

When such an occurrence is unexpected, relatives will find it especially hard to cope and will need regular contact with nursing staff for information, explanation and support. The patient is initially often too ill to appreciate more than clear and brief communications.

NURSING PRIORITIES AND MANAGEMENT: Abdominal hernia

Perioperative care

Ideally, the surgery will be elective and the patient fit. Care must be taken to ensure the patient is not suffering from a chest complaint, allergy or smoker's cough. In such situations, surgery should be postponed, as postoperative coughing could threaten the integrity of the hernia repair. Smoking is always discouraged, even if only for the perioperative period, and the physiotherapist and nurse should teach the patient how to support the wound and flex the hip on the affected side should coughing or sneezing occur. Postoperative recovery is usually uneventful and the patient is often discharged the next day. Potential problems that must be recognised are urinary retention, infection of the wound and pain, particularly scrotal discomfort when inguinal herniorrhaphy has been performed. A well-fitting scrotal support, used in conjunction with analgesics, usually eases any discomfort.

STOP THINK **4.14** What specific nursing care is required if the patient has had a hernia repair under epidural anaesthetic?

Hernia repair should never be considered lightly. Often surgery is more complicated than anticipated and the patient may experience considerable postoperative pain and temporary loss of peristalsis. If this is the case, postoperative recovery will necessarily take a little longer (see Ch. 26).

Discharge advice

Time must be taken to ensure that the patient and the family understand the precautions that are necessary to ensure optimal recovery and well-being. Although activity is encouraged, lifting or straining must be avoided. Older men may be troubled by an enlarged prostate gland and may strain to pass urine. Equally, coughs, colds, known allergens and constipation, i.e. anything that might raise intra-abdominal pressure during the weeks of healing, should be avoided if at all possible. The time allocated to give advice and support prior to discharge presents an ideal opportunity for general health promotion, e.g. on smoking, diet and alcohol, and, in the vulnerable patient, for a sensitive reappraisal of home circumstances and community support. Driving should be avoided until the patient is confident of being able to perform an 'emergency stop' if required.

Colorectal cancer

Neoplasms, both benign and malignant, can occur in the large bowel. The concern with benign neoplasms such as polyps is that, if they are extensive, large and of prolonged duration, there is a propensity for malignant change to occur. As a result, if polyps are diagnosed, they are usually removed surgically. Malignant tumour of the large bowel — colorectal cancer — is second only to cancer of the lung in causing death from malignant disease in Western society. It is the second most common cause of cancer-related deaths in Scotland (SIGN 2003). Although it affects all age groups, it is uncommon under the age of 40.

Cancer can affect any part of the large bowel but is most common in the rectum and sigmoid colon (Keighley & Williams 1999). It affects men and women equally, but rectal carcinoma is more common in men and colonic carcinoma is more common in women.

The exact cause of colorectal cancer is unclear. As it is virtually unknown in rural communities in the developing world, its association with the Western diet is increasingly accepted. The early work of Burkitt (1971), relating low-fibre diets to disease, has proved very influential. Certainly, a low-residue diet prolongs transit time in the intestine, thus allowing any potential carcinogen increased contact with the intestinal mucosa. Colorectal cancer is also associated with other disorders of the bowel, e.g. ulcerative colitis, adenomatous polyps and, significantly, the hereditary disorder known as familial adenomatous polyposis (FAP) (see Ch. 6).

PATHOPHYSIOLOGY

The tumours arise from the epithelial cells of glandular tissue — adenocarcinomas. As they grow, they progressively obstruct the bowel by extending into the lumen or spreading circumferentially to form a ring-like stricture (see Box 4.7). Metastatic spread is by direct infiltration of local tissues and organs via the lymphatic and portal circulation, or by implantation during surgery.

Common presenting symptoms Unfortunately, patients tend not to present until the disease is at an advanced stage. The symptoms are subtle, gradual and easily ignored or explained away. Symptoms will vary somewhat according to the site of the tumour but will essentially involve an alteration in bowel habit. Constipation alternating with diarrhoea is the presenting feature, combined with rectal bleeding and weight loss. Tenesmus and colic may well be present, as well as excess mucus in the stool. Pain is not a common feature and, perhaps due to this, medical advice is often not sought until either the patient is very anaemic and debilitated or the symptoms associated with obstruction are marked.

MEDICAL MANAGEMENT

Investigations Many patients will present with a palpable mass that can be detected on abdominal or rectal examination. Specific investigations to confirm diagnosis will include barium studies, sigmoidoscopy, colonoscopy and biopsies. CT scan, chest X-ray and ultrasound scan will be necessary to seek out metastases, particularly in the lung and liver. For the latter, liver function tests will also be carried out.

Staging The staging of the carcinoma is based on histological examination of a resected specimen (see Ch. 31). For colorectal cancer, Dukes' staging is the most widely used (Keighley & Williams 1999). At its simplest, it describes four stages:

- A — the tumour is confined to the bowel mucosa and submucosa
- B — the tumour has invaded the bowel wall to serosa but there is no lymph node involvement
- C — spread to involve lymph nodes
- C2 — distant metastases or severe local or nodal spread, making surgical 'cure' impossible.

Treatment Surgical removal of the tumour is the only effective management. The type and extent of surgery will depend on the site of the tumour. It may be possible for resection and end-to-end anastomosis to be performed (see Fig. 4.10), but often stoma formation is necessary on a temporary or permanent basis.

See also Young et al (1996) and Garden et al (2002) for further details.

STOP THINK **4.15** Turn to Chapter 26 and read Case History 26.2 (p. 903). Mrs B represents a common clinical reality. She had felt unwilling to talk about her symptoms, hoping they were just haemorrhoids. Ultimately she required emergency intervention and a stoma formation for which she was totally unprepared. Can you think (or discuss as a group) how such a situation might have been prevented?

NURSING PRIORITIES AND MANAGEMENT: Colorectal cancer

Major considerations

Psychological support

The realisation that seemingly minor ailments are actually symptoms of cancer is most stressful for any individual. From the moment a patient is referred, as an outpatient or inpatient, a sensitive and tactful approach is of paramount importance. This is not easy. Many registered nurses working in general hospital wards are worried about their lack of skills in communicating with cancer patients and, in particular, in giving psychological care (McCaughan & Parahoo 2000). Psychological care needs to include the family and significant others in order to develop a trusting relationship. The beneficial effect of spending time to allow

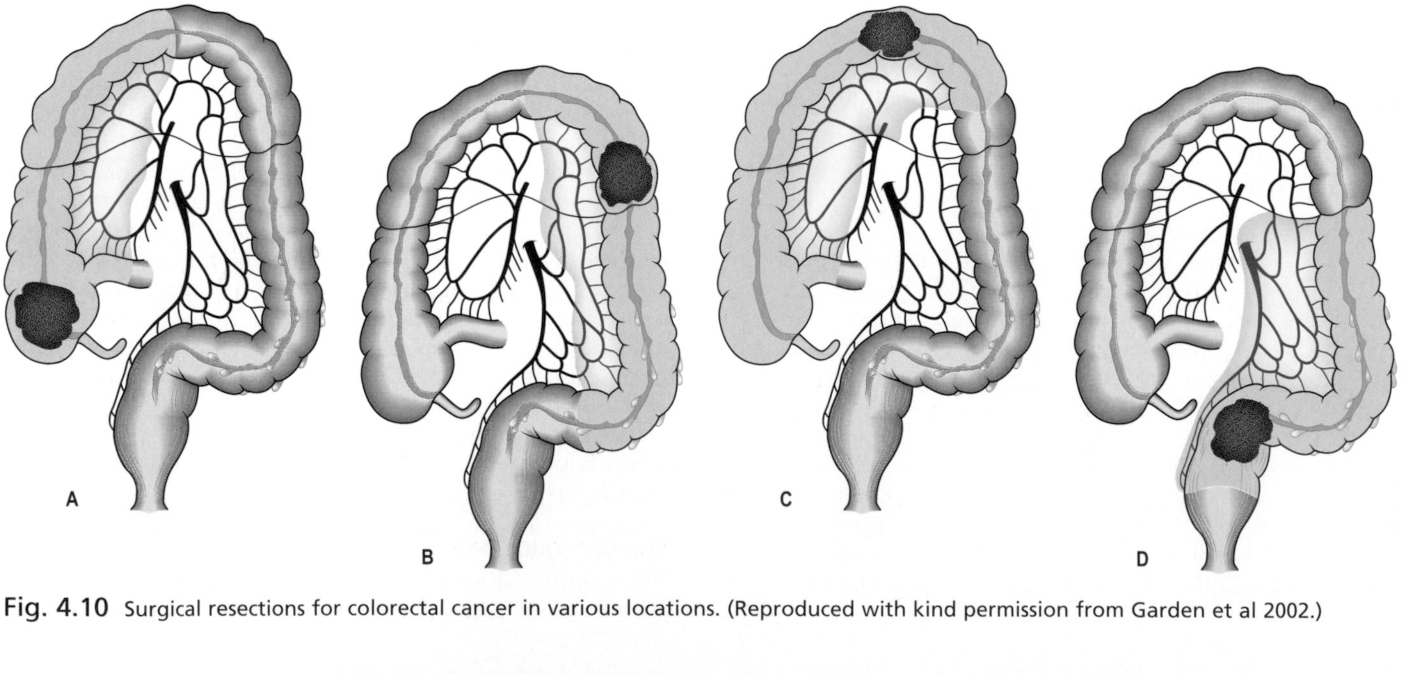

Fig. 4.10 Surgical resections for colorectal cancer in various locations. (Reproduced with kind permission from Garden et al 2002.)

fears to be expressed and explanations and support to be given cannot be overstated.

Perioperative care

The principles of perioperative nursing care are given in Chapter 26. If surgery is to include stoma formation, this will present a further source of stress. A cooperative team approach by the various health care professionals involved will greatly assist the patient's physical and psychological recovery and adjustment to what may prove to be major and perhaps only palliative surgery. For the specific input of the stoma nurse specialist, see Box 4.4.

Discharge planning

For those patients for whom cure is not a possibility, planning for discharge and home care should aim to maximise their independence and quality of life for as long as possible. This requires the coordination and integration of hospital and community services, and a respect for the wishes of both the patient and the family. The reader is referred to Case History 31.4 (p. 1060) for a more detailed examination of this issue.

Health promotion

Great efforts are being made to detect colorectal cancer early, when its prognosis is so much more favourable. The 5-year survival rate for localised lesions is 80–90%. This rate drops to 35–65% once the disease has spread to adjacent structures and lymph nodes (Porrett & Daniel 1999). Factors being addressed include fostering awareness of early warning signs and information for those especially at risk. Preventive measures also include providing advice concerning diet and health screening. See, for example, www.hebs.scot.nhs.uk.

ANORECTAL DISORDERS

Anorectal conditions such as haemorrhoids, abscesses, fissures, fistulae and sinuses are relatively common and always distressing, but are often tolerated for many months or even years before professional help and advice are sought.

Haemorrhoids

PATHOPHYSIOLOGY

Haemorrhoids, commonly called 'piles', are generally considered to be varices of the superior haemorrhoidal veins occurring as a result of congestion of the venous plexus. It would seem that a lack of dietary fibre is the most important predisposing factor (see Box 4.8). The resulting chronic constipation and straining during bowel movements raises intra-abdominal pressure, leading to venous plexus engorgement. The bulging mucosa is dragged down and, as the condition worsens, the haemorrhoids prolapse into the anal canal. Other conditions that can lead to or aggravate the congestion are pregnancy, where the development of haemorrhoids is often neglected, tumours and cardiac failure.

For further information, see Kamm & Lennard-Jones (1994).

Haemorrhoids may be internal or external. Internal haemorrhoids are classified according to the degree to which they prolapse into the anal canal. External haemorrhoids occur outside the anal canal and are less common.

Common presenting symptoms Commonly the patient complains of 'fresh' blood in bowel movements, which at first may be thought to be due simply to the passing of constipated motions. The experience of prolapse, at first transient, becomes increasingly frequent and is associated with pain, the discharge of mucus and pruritus. Often such symptoms have been managed by over-the-counter (OTC) remedies such as creams to reduce the itching and pain. Education of the patient in order to achieve the passing of soft bulky stools with minimal effort, often yields more relief in the long term than conventional treatments. The addition of supplementary dietary fibre and ensuring an adequate fluid intake are often seen as more acceptable (Porrett & Daniel 1999). However, many people find the adjustment of diet too much of a change in lifestyle. Should the haemorrhoidal vessels thrombose, pain is always severe and it may only be at this stage that the patient seeks help.

MEDICAL MANAGEMENT

Investigations

- History and examination to exclude other pathologies, particularly a carcinoma.
- Rectal examination, proctoscopy and/or sigmoidoscopy to confirm the diagnosis.

Treatment

If the haemorrhoids are identified in their early stages, management requires no more than attention to the patient's diet and perhaps a bulk laxative. If the constipation is corrected, the problem will usually resolve but the patient must understand this and feel confident in diet alteration. The practice nurse can play an important part in patient education and in arranging a follow-up appointment to monitor the patient's well-being.

Surgical intervention The following surgical treatments may be used to resolve haemorrhoids that do not respond to conservative management:

- *Injection*. For haemorrhoids in the early stages, injection of the haemorrhoidal veins with an irritant solution provokes fibrosis and atrophy with minimal discomfort.
- *Band ligation*. Bands are applied to the mucosa-covered haemorrhoidal pedicle, constricting the vessels, which then eventually shrink.
- *Infrared coagulation*. Infrared radiation is applied in pulses to the haemorrhoid by means of a fibreoptic probe, causing coagulation and shrinkage.
- *Haemorrhoidectomy*. The above interventions are the most commonly used and can be carried out on an outpatient basis. If, however, the haemorrhoids are not amenable to such therapies, haemorrhoidectomy to ligate and excise the haemorrhoids may be required. If thrombosis has occurred, this procedure will be required immediately.

Box 4.8

Constipation

Constipation may be defined as difficult and infrequent defaecation. The following factors can contribute to its development.

Diet
A diet that is low in fibre and bulk predisposes to small faecal bulk. A low fluid intake also contributes to small bulk. Small bulk predisposes the GI tract to reduced peristaltic action and slow passage of contents along the colon. Epidemiological studies indicate that low-fibre diets contribute to many of the GI diseases found in the Western world, such as diverticulosis, appendicitis and haemorrhoids.

Exercise
Lack of exercise contributes to reduced peristalsis, due to reduced muscle tone of the bowel and abdominal muscles. Individuals who take less exercise include the older person and those who are ill or have a physical disability. Hospital patients are, in general, restricted in their mobility, given their environment and their medical condition, and investigations and treatment often predispose patients to constipation.

Elimination habits
Neglecting to empty the rectum when the stimulation caused by faeces therein (the 'call to stool') is ignored results in constipation; if this occurs repeatedly, faecal impaction can result. Watery diarrhoea, caused by the breakdown of faecal material proximal to the hard impacted mass, can bypass the mass. Impacted faeces can press on the urethra and cause retention of urine (see also Ch. 24).

Socioeconomic factors
Nutritional and dietary intake is determined by eating patterns formed in childhood and influenced by familial and social norms and income levels. A low income can result in the exclusion from the diet of fresh fruit and vegetables, which can be relatively expensive. Low-income families and older people living alone may have to make difficult choices in spending their limited resources on food, heating and clothing. Lack of transport or reduced mobility can also limit shopping expeditions and therefore the choice of foods. The older person living alone may be less likely to cook nutritious meals for a number of reasons, e.g. lack of motivation, poor appetite and limited mobility.

Medication
Many medications have side-effects that cause constipation; these include ganglion-blocking drugs, psychotropic drugs, muscle relaxants, and morphine and its derivatives.

Dentition
Poor dentition makes chewing difficult, especially where there has been dental clearance and dentures do not fit well or comfortably. This can result in the avoidance of fresh fruit and vegetables, and an emphasis on soft, easily chewed foods that do not add fibre to the diet.

Motility of colon
Eating results in increased colonic motor activity that may be perceived by the individual as an urge to defaecate, but mobility or lack of regular exercise decreases gut motility and may contribute to constipation (Doughty 2000).

The bowel may become obstructed by a growth, a hernia or by adhesions following surgery. In addition, spasticity can occur in inflammatory conditions such as appendicitis or diverticulitis.

Rectal conditions
Local conditions such as haemorrhoids or anal fissure, which cause pain on defaecation, can result in avoidance of defaecation with eventual constipation.

Prevention and treatment
Dietary advice is important in the prevention of constipation. Wholemeal bread, fresh fruit and vegetables, and cereals such as porridge oats and All Bran are important. Unprocessed bran can also be added to soups or stews. The individual should be advised to drink plenty of fluid throughout the day. Older people who have urinary incontinence tend to take inadequate fluid in an attempt to avoid being incontinent of urine.

The importance of emptying the bowel regularly and of not ignoring the call to stool should be emphasised. The individual should be encouraged to take as much physical exercise as possible.

The initial treatment of constipation can include the use of laxatives. Bulk-forming preparations such as Fybogel and stimulant laxatives such as bisacodyl by mouth or by rectum may be used initially. Where there is a faecal mass, rectally administered faecal softeners such as arachis oil may be necessary.

Any condition, such as haemorrhoids, anal fissure or diverticulosis, which is predisposing the individual to constipation, should be treated.

NURSING PRIORITIES AND MANAGEMENT: Haemorrhoids

General considerations

Whether it is the cause or the effect, it is most important that difficulty with defaecation is effectively corrected. Measures to achieve this include:

- increasing dietary fibre
- maintaining a high fluid intake (2–3 L/day)
- prescribing a stool softener to facilitate water and fat absorption into the faeces
- ensuring sufficient exercise and activity.

In addition, nursing priorities must include measures to alleviate pain and itching, to ensure good personal hygiene, to provide appropriate privacy in a hospital setting and to prevent infection.

Preoperative preparation (see Box 4.9)

If surgery is required, the aim of nursing care in the preoperative period is to control the acute symptoms and to ensure that the patient feels comfortable and free from any distress when defaecating. One of the major postoperative fears in any form of anorectal surgery is the pain that might be experienced upon the first bowel movement. Time is

Box 4.9

Principles of nursing care for patients undergoing perianal surgery

Preoperative preparation

- Ensure the patient's privacy to reduce embarrassment
- Give analgesics for the acute pain that is often present
- Provide bowel preparation. This may include the administration of suppositories or an enema to clear the rectum. Some surgeons prefer not to give any bowel preparation prior to haemorrhoidectomy so that evacuation of the bowel after surgery can occur more quickly

Postoperative care

- Observe for haemorrhage during the first 24 h by monitoring vital signs and checking the anal area
- Give analgesics as this area can be very painful after surgery
- On the first postoperative day, encourage the patient to bathe
- Assess the patient for urinary retention
- Assess for return of bowel movement
- Administer a bulk-forming aperient to facilitate easier bowel evacuation. Analgesics may be required prior to the first bowel movement
- Give the patient a bath after the bowels have opened to keep the area clean and to relieve discomfort
- Advise the patient on avoiding constipation

well spent explaining postoperative care and how any pain and discomfort will be relieved or minimised. Patients are very often comforted merely by the fact that the nurse understands their fears and has the knowledge and skill to help them to manage the problem.

Postoperative care (see Box 4.9)

Care priorities in the postoperative period include:

- the relief of pain and promotion of comfort
- the prevention of postoperative haemorrhage
- the prevention of postoperative urinary retention
- the prevention of infection
- the promotion of optimal faecal elimination
- patient education prior to discharge regarding lifestyle and diet.

STOP THINK

4.16 Anaesthesia and pain may inhibit urination in the early postoperative period. What support and interventions might be considered?

4.17 What would be the key points in any pre-discharge advice and support given to a patient following anorectal surgery?

Other common anorectal disorders

Fissure in ano

PATHOPHYSIOLOGY

This is a tear in the lining of the lower anal canal. Pain is experienced only on defaecation. The cause of a primary fissure is uncertain, but it often follows an episode of constipation and the forceful passage of a hard stool. It is a common complication of Crohn's disease.

Common presenting symptoms The main symptom is extreme pain on defaecation that persists for some hours. Rectal bleeding may be seen on defaecation.

MEDICAL MANAGEMENT

Anal fissures can heal spontaneously with the local application of creams or suppositories. Constipation is treated and then avoided by a high-fibre diet. Surgical treatment is a lateral internal sphincterotomy.

Fistula-in-ano

PATHOPHYSIOLOGY

A fistula is an abnormal communication between two epithelial lined surfaces. A fistula-in-ano is a granulating track between the anorectum and the perineum. The cause is uncertain, but it may be associated with an anal gland infection that produces an abscess that then tracks. Fistulae are associated with Crohn's disease, ulcerative colitis, HIV infections, radiation damage and hidradenitis, i.e. a chronic suppurative condition that may affect the apocrine glands of the axillae, groin and perineum.

Common presenting symptoms Commonly an abscess is present, as well as pain, pruritus ani, rectal discharge and excoriation of skin.

SURGICAL MANAGEMENT

The fistula is laid open by fistulotomy and heals gradually by granulation over some weeks.

Pilonidal sinus

PATHOPHYSIOLOGY

This is a sinus that contains hair and occurs in the natal cleft. The hair curls and penetrates the skin, causing irritation. Secondary infection is common, which can lead to a pilonidal abscess.

Common presenting symptoms The individual will experience localised, throbbing pain. The site will be tender to the touch if an abscess is present. A discharge is often the first sign that a sinus is present.

MEDICAL MANAGEMENT

Antibiotic therapy is given prior to surgery if an infection is present, followed by excision of the sinus when the infection has cleared. The importance of good perianal hygiene and keeping the area free from future hair growth cannot be overemphasised (Porrett & Daniel 1999).

Anovaginal and rectovaginal fistulae

PATHOPHYSIOLOGY

Obstetric trauma is the most common cause for the development of these fistulae. Other causes include trauma, radiation damage, and inflammatory bowel disease, especially Crohn's disease.

Common presenting symptoms The patient complains of passing flatus and faeces per vagina. There may be vaginitis and recurrent urinary tract infections may also occur.

Diagnosis is readily made during examination under anaesthetic at which time multiple biopsies are taken.

SURGICAL MANAGEMENT

Direct repair of the defect or advancement of a mucosal–submucosal flap of rectum or vagina to cover the defect is often successful. Occasionally a bowel resection with or without a temporary defunctioning stoma is required.

NURSING PRIORITIES AND MANAGEMENT: Faecal incontinence

Faecal incontinence is a common and distressing symptom with many causes including:

- congenital malformation
- trauma
- obstetric injury
- rectovaginal fistula
- inflammatory bowel disease
- functional disorder
- postirradiation damage
- postoperative complications, e.g. following colorectal/perianal surgery
- neurological disease
- degenerative disorders.

Both a medical and a nursing history should be completed; in the latter the use of a checklist such as Norton (2001) may prove helpful. Investigations that may be indicated to confirm the diagnosis and determine treatment vary from digital examination to in-depth assessment of anorectal physiology and endo-anal ultrasound.

Treatment depends on the underlying cause but psychological support and education about methods of self-management must be given. Conservative treatment should be undertaken initially, including medication, biofeedback and sphincter exercises, control of bowel habit and advice about ensuring regular bowel motions. Surgical intervention may ultimately be necessary.

For a detailed description, see Keighley & Williams (1999).

DISORDERS OF THE HEPATOBILIARY SYSTEM

DISORDERS OF THE LIVER

The liver can be affected by a large number of diseases, some of which are more common than others. Because of the large number of functions that the liver performs, there are infinite combinations of manifestations, both specific and non-specific. The onset illness may be acute, as in an acute attack of viral hepatitis, or chronic, where disease processes have been progressing for many years before symptoms become evident. A patient with advanced chronic liver disease but who has little or no symptoms is said to be 'compensated'; when the liver begins to fail and symptoms appear, the patient is then said to be 'decompensating'.

Manifestations of liver disease

Non-specific symptoms such as anorexia, nausea, lethargy, malaise and vomiting are common. Weight loss also occurs in chronic liver disease, notably in malignant disease.

Specific features include enlargement of the liver, i.e. hepatomegaly, portal hypertension with associated ascites and splenomegaly, jaundice, oesophageal varices and hepatic encephalopathy.

ACUTE LIVER DISEASE

Acute hepatitis

PATHOPHYSIOLOGY

Hepatitis denotes inflammation of the liver that may be acute or chronic. Globally, viruses are the most common cause of acute hepatitis, but the disease may also be a response to certain medication (see Box 4.10) and alcohol. All types of hepatitis will cause similar symptoms, which can range from slight to severe and possibly life threatening, as in fulminant hepatic failure. This, fortunately, is very rare. Many patients with acute hepatitis will not require hospitalisation and some will not even contact a doctor. For patients who do have symptoms, these are considered in three phases as follows:

- *Prodromal or pre-icteric phase.* Flu-like symptoms which last from 2 to 7 days in hepatitis A virus (HAV), and slightly longer in hepatitis B virus (HBV). Symptoms include headache, low-grade fever (37.5–38.5°C), nasal congestion, sore throat, anorexia, lethargy, mild upper abdominal pain or discomfort in the right hypochondrium, arthralgia and arthritis. As the liver has no sensory innervation, pain is caused by stretching of the liver capsule. In inflammatory conditions such as hepatitis, pain is usually perceived as a dull ache in the right upper quadrant.
- *The icteric phase.* Prodromal symptoms usually disappear. Jaundice, of varying intensity, occurs but rarely causes plasma bilirubin to rise above 200 mmol/L. Jaundice is a yellowing of the skin and mucous membranes and occurs when the bilirubin level in the blood exceeds 50 mmol/L. There are three distinct types:
  — hepatocellular jaundice: hepatocyte destruction renders the liver unable to transport bilirubin; this is the type of jaundice seen in viral hepatitis

Box 4.10

Medication-induced hepatitis

Hepatitis may be caused by any drug, but the more common culprits include analgesics such as paracetamol taken in excess, psychotropic drugs such as the phenothiazines, antibiotics such as erythromycin, and anaesthetics such as halothane. Any patient with hepatitis should be questioned regarding medication taken recently, including those taken without medical advice, and including herbal remedies.

In most incidences of any medication-induced hepatitis, the biopsy shows changes as for viral hepatitis. However, some medications will also cause fatty changes in the liver cells.

— haemolytic jaundice: caused by excessive red cell destruction (see Ch. 11)
— cholestatic jaundice: caused by obstruction to the flow of bile through the liver ducts due to cirrhosis or malignancy. Obstruction of the larger extrahepatic ducts may be caused by gallstones or cancer of the head of pancreas (Fawcett & Smith 2004).

- *The convalescent phase.* Occurs approximately 2 weeks after the onset of jaundice. Jaundice lessens and eventually disappears. Other symptoms resolve.

Postviral syndrome It is recognised that hepatitis is a common cause of a postviral syndrome in which, despite liver function tests returning to normal, lethargy persists for some months. Patients need reassurance regarding recovery as many feel that they have developed chronic liver disease.

MEDICAL AND NURSING MANAGEMENT

There is no specific treatment for acute hepatitis, but advice can be given to help the patient cope with the illness. Any medication thought to have caused the hepatitis should be stopped, and no other medication should be taken without medical advice. Whilst strict bed rest is not necessary, it is advisable for the patient to rest as much as possible and to avoid strenuous exercise. The patient may have intolerance of fatty foods. A well-balanced, high-calorie diet should be encouraged. Alcohol should be totally avoided, as it can slow recovery and exacerbate symptoms. If required, referral can be made to an alcohol counsellor who can provide counselling and support for patients with alcohol dependency problems. The patient should be given education on the transmission routes of the hepatitis viruses in order that hygiene precautions may be taken (see p. 136).

Restrictions on certain professional activities may also be required if the hepatitis is viral in origin, e.g. to medical or dental personnel working in exposure-prone posts. Sexual intercourse during menstruation and sexual practices that may result in damage to the skin and mucous membranes should be avoided.

Fulminant hepatic failure

PATHOPHYSIOLOGY

This is a rare condition that results in sudden massive necrosis of liver cells and severe impairment of hepatic function. The most common causes are drug/medication-induced hepatitis and viral hepatitis; all other causes are extremely rare.

Clinical features The patient develops encephalopathy, in which confusion leads to stupor and progresses rapidly to coma. Jaundice and fetor hepaticus are present and ascites may develop later. Abnormal neurological signs, cerebral oedema, hypoglycaemia, circulatory and renal failure and coagulation defects develop.

MEDICAL MANAGEMENT

The medical management of fulminant hepatic failure is supportive care and management of complications such as infection. Liver transplant should be considered if early improvement does not occur, so that patients can be transferred to a transplant centre before severe coma occurs. Transplant for fulminant hepatic failure has a 71.7% 1-year survival rate and a 63.4% 5-year survival rate (UK Transplant Statistics Department 2004).

The prognosis without transplant is extremely poor, with the survival rate being approximately 10% once deep coma has occurred. However, there are patients who do survive and recover normal hepatic structure and function.

The nursing care of these patients is highly specialised and is of paramount importance to the patient's recovery. For this reason, patients with fulminant hepatic failure must be nursed in a specialist liver or intensive therapy unit.

Future management: the bioartificial liver As many patients die before a suitable liver transplant can be found, research is ongoing to find new treatment to support the patient until either a donor is found or the liver recovers sufficiently to support life.

For further information on research into the bioartificial liver, see Plevris et al (1988) and for information on an artificial recycling system such as the molecular adsorbent recirculating system (MARS), see Koivusalo et al (2003).

The bioartificial liver uses similar principles to renal dialysis. However, as there is no known artificial filter that can imitate the many functions of the hepatocyte, then human hepatocytes will be used. Originally it was thought that porcine hepatocytes would be used. However, in 1997 the United Kingdom Xenotransplantation Interim Authority was convened to advise on the ethical, safety and animal welfare issues that xenotransplantation raised, and to regulate its use. It is now very difficult to obtain permission to use animal cells and organs and most medical researchers prefer to use human cells.

The cells are loaded into a haemofiltration device known as a bioreactor and, using a delivery system similar to renal dialysis, blood is pumped through the bioreactor and back into the patient.

The MARS system is a novel dialysis system that removes albumin-bound substances from the blood.

These innovative treatment options remain in the early research stages, with many practical problems to be solved before they can be used routinely in the clinical setting.

VIRUSES THAT CAUSE HEPATITIS

All the hepatitic viruses can cause a similar initial illness. The differences between them would appear to be their modes of transmission and progression of disease:

- Common viruses
  — hepatitis A
  — hepatitis B
  — hepatitis C
  — hepatitis D (delta)
- Uncommon viruses
  — hepatitis E
  — hepatitis F (the status of hepatitis F as a true virus remains unconfirmed and its existence is now doubtful (Bowden 2001)
  — hepatitis G
  — Epstein–Barr (EB) virus
  — cytomegalovirus (CMV)
  — measles.

Hepatitis A

PATHOPHYSIOLOGY

Hepatitis A (HAV) is an acute condition. A chronic form does not occur. It is usually a mild illness, often occurring in epidemics in communities such as schools, prisons, army camps and psychiatric settings, or in areas where sanitation and hygiene are poor. It is transmitted by the faecal–oral route. The incubation period is 2–7 weeks, with faeces being the most important infective material. The person becomes infectious 2–3 weeks prior to the onset of the clinical illness and remains so for approximately 2 weeks thereafter. Blood and urine are rarely infectious. Male homosexuals are at risk of hepatitis A due to oral–anal contact. Patients with hepatitis A are usually only mildly unwell and are rarely admitted to hospital.

Improved standards of food and personal hygiene in the UK mean that most people have not been exposed to HAV and, as they will not have acquired natural antibodies, they are therefore susceptible to infection. Immunisation should be considered before travelling to regions where HAV is still prevalent (Crowcroft 2001).

HAV is not associated with a carrier state in that once the acute infective stage has ceased, transmission to another person is not possible.

MEDICAL MANAGEMENT

Investigations The diagnosis of HAV depends on the presence of antibodies to HAV in the patient's blood. The presence of anti-HAV IgM denotes recent or current infection. It is present from 1 week before onset of the clinical illness and disappears after approximately 3 months. The presence of anti-HAV IgG denotes previous infection and remains positive for life, conferring immunity.

Precautions If hospitalisation is required, the patient is usually independent and therefore the risk of infection is low. However, if a patient has diarrhoea and requires nursing assistance, the following precautions should be taken:

- plastic gloves and aprons must be used for all procedures
- linen and disposable wipes must be disposed of as per local policy
- thorough handwashing must be carried out after patient contact.

Immune serum globulin i.m. can prevent hepatitis A if given within a few days of exposure. A vaccine has now been developed which will give protection for 5–10 years and is recommended for food handlers, travellers in high-risk areas and homosexual men.

Hepatitis B

PATHOPHYSIOLOGY

Hepatitis B (HBV) can cause acute or chronic infection. Ten per cent of infected adults will become chronic carriers, of which there are an estimated 350 million worldwide and 1 in 1000 of the population of the UK. Of the 10% of chronic carriers, some will be asymptomatic and some will develop chronic hepatitis (Collier & Oxford 2000).

The virus is transmitted by the parenteral route. Patients receiving blood or blood products and i.v. drug abusers who share needles are greatly at risk. Tattooing can also spread the virus. The virus is present in body fluids such as saliva, urine and semen and therefore the disease can be spread by close personal contact, e.g. sexual intercourse, especially in male homosexuals, and particularly in areas of overcrowding, poverty and poor sanitation. The disease can also be transmitted from mother to baby either at birth or soon afterwards. Faeces will not transmit infection provided they are free of blood. The incubation period is approximately 2–6 months.

MEDICAL MANAGEMENT

Investigations The most important test in the diagnosis of HBV is for the hepatitis B surface antigen (HBsAg) in the blood. This appears from one to several weeks before the onset of the clinical illness and disappears 1–12 weeks later. However, this may not be present in patients who either clear the virus from the blood quickly or present late. It is therefore also necessary to look for antibodies to the hepatitis core antigen (anti-HBc). The presence of anti-HBc IgM denotes acute HBV; anti-HBc IgG denotes chronic HBV.

The presence of the hepatitis B 'E' antigen (HBeAg) in the carrier state reflects greater infectivity of blood and body fluids. It is also associated with a greater likelihood of progression to chronic liver disease.

Precautions There is great risk to medical and nursing staff when dealing with blood, blood products, body fluids and open wounds, e.g. venepuncture sites, skin lesions, and ulcers on injection sites of i.v. drug abusers. Care should also be taken in areas where the patient's identity is unknown, e.g. emergency departments. All precautions should be taken as per individual hospital policies, and hospital staff should be vaccinated against HBV infection.

Hepatitis B immune globulin i.m. can prevent hepatitis B if given within a few days of a high-risk exposure (e.g. a 'sharps' injury). Vaccination provides good long-term immunity but booster doses are needed every 3–5 years.

Treatment Current treatment for HBV is either interferon alpha, an immunomodulator, or lamivudine, a nucleoside analogue. Interferon has many side-effects and is poorly tolerated (see p. 677). Lamivudine is associated with increasing viral resistance the longer it is taken. Several new nucleoside analogues are currently being developed and it is hoped that these may increase the treatment options available for HBV (Younger et al 2004).

STOP THINK **4.18** A staff member sustains a 'sharps' injury. What procedure should be followed and how can the individual be prevented from developing hepatitis?

Hepatitis C

The hepatitis C virus (HCV) was identified in 1989 and is now known to be responsible for 90% of what was known as non-A, non-B hepatitis (Blair & Hayes 1997).

PATHOPHYSIOLOGY

Like HBV, HCV is transmitted parenterally and the highest incidences are in i.v. drug abusers and people who received blood products before 1991, when screening became available. Other risk factors include body piercing, tattooing and needlestick injuries. Unlike HBV, sexual transmission appears to be low in HCV.

Acute infection occurs in about 10% of patients, but about 80% will go on to develop chronic infection. Of these, approximately 20% will develop cirrhosis after 20 years of infection. There is also an increased risk of hepatocellular cancer associated with chronic HCV infection (Nissen & Martin 2002).

MEDICAL MANAGEMENT

Investigations Diagnosis is made serologically by the presence of antibodies to HCV. An active viraemic state will then be confirmed by a technique, which amplifies nucleic acids, known as the polymerase chain reaction (PCR) test. Blood will also be tested for HCV genotype. There are six known genotypes worldwide (1–6), of which types 1, 2 and 3 are common in Europe, the UK and North America. In the UK approximately 50% of known HCV positive patients have genotype 1. This genotype is known to be more resistant to treatment (Lee 2003).

Liver biopsy can be useful for staging the extent of any liver damage.

Treatment The British Society of Gastroenterologists now recommends the combination of pegylated interferon, a naturally occurring protein with complex effects on immunity and cell function, and ribavirin, an antiviral agent, for the treatment of HCV. Pegylated interferon is administered as a s.c. injection once per week; ribavirin is taken as an oral preparation on a twice-daily basis and the dose is weight dependent. Patients with genotype 1 are treated for 48 weeks and the success rate is approximately 50%. Types 2 and 3 are treated for 24 weeks and have a success rate of over 80%.

Nursing support is vital for patients undergoing interferon therapy and most patients are now treated in nurse-led clinics. There are many associated side-effects and the patient will require regular haematological monitoring, as well as help and advice on coping with physical side-effects, which include:

- flu-like symptoms that can be ameliorated by regular paracetamol
- poor appetite and weight loss
- fatigue
- anaemia
- reduction of the white cell and platelet count
- mood lowering and depression
- thyroid dysfunction
- allergic type skin problems.

All side-effects are reversible on stopping treatment, with the possible exception of some cases of thyroid dysfunction.

Therapy is self-administered and the patient will require education on self-injection techniques and the safe storage and disposal of equipment and medications. Advice on diet and lifestyle may be necessary and the patient should be encouraged to avoid alcohol and drugs.

Hepatitis D (delta) virus

The delta virus occurs either simultaneously with an acute hepatitis B infection or as an added infection in a chronic hepatitis B carrier. It never occurs when the B virus is not present. It is diagnosed by the presence of anti-delta (anti-HD) in the blood.

For further information, see Pratt (2003). Further information on the less common hepatitis viruses can be found in Shearman et al (1997).

CHRONIC LIVER DISEASE

Chronic hepatitis

Hepatitis is referred to as chronic when the patient continues to have clinical symptoms or abnormal liver function tests 6 months after the onset of the illness. The main causes of chronic hepatitis are:

- the B, C and D viruses as already described
- autoimmune hepatitis
- drug-related hepatitis
- cryptogenic hepatitis.

Autoimmune hepatitis

PATHOPHYSIOLOGY

The cause of this disease is unknown but it is thought to be immune mediated. It is a chronic condition but may present as an 'acute' illness similar to acute viral hepatitis. This 'acute' onset is probably an exacerbation of long-standing but asymptomatic disease. It is identified by detecting non-organ-specific antibodies to nuclei, smooth muscle and occasionally liver–kidney microsomes. About 80% of those affected are women and about 20% have other autoimmune disorders, e.g. rheumatoid arthritis and ulcerative colitis.

Prognosis is dependent on the severity of the inflammatory activity. Patients with severe multilobular necrosis on biopsy generally develop cirrhosis within 5 years.

Clinical features Patients who present with an 'acute' illness will show signs and symptoms similar to those of acute hepatitis (p. 134); however, other features such as ascites and hypoalbuminaemia may be present, indicating the chronic nature of the disease.

MEDICAL MANAGEMENT

Steroids and immunosuppressive medications, prednisolone and azathioprine, are used to achieve remission. The doses are gradually reduced until a maintenance dose is achieved. If cirrhosis is present, treatment will include symptomatic relief of the manifestations of chronic liver disease.

SURGICAL MANAGEMENT

Transplantation has been described by Sir Magdi Yacoub as one of the miraculous achievements of modern medicine (UK Transplant Statistics Department 2004).

Liver transplant for chronic liver disease has been available in the NHS since 1983 and improved patient management techniques have led to increased success rates. Each year in the UK around 650 people undergo liver transplant in one of nine specialist centres. There are approximately 160 people waiting for a liver transplant in the UK at any given time. Around 85% of the livers transplanted for chronic liver disease are functioning well a year after surgery (Neuberger & Lucey 1994).

NURSING PRIORITIES AND MANAGEMENT: Autoimmune hepatitis

Nursing intervention is dependent on the severity of the illness. Initially the patient may require full nursing care and nutritional support. Occasionally a high-dependency setting may be appropriate.

As the patient improves, education regarding the condition is important to aid understanding of the symptoms and the need for long-term immunosuppressive therapy. Alcohol should be avoided, especially if there is cirrhosis.

Alcoholic hepatitis

PATHOPHYSIOLOGY

Clinical features This condition usually follows years of alcohol abuse and often a recent prolonged bout of heavy drinking. The patient will complain of anorexia, vomiting, lethargy, diarrhoea and upper abdominal pain. A fever will be present and the patient will appear generally unwell and malnourished. There may be signs of chronic liver disease, i.e. ascites and oedema, encephalopathy, jaundice and the dilated capillaries of spider telangiectasis. GI bleeding may occur from erosions or peptic ulceration, and also as a result of bleeding tendencies, due to the liver's inability to synthesise adequate clotting factors.

The diagnosis is made from an accurate picture of the patient's alcohol intake (often obtained from relatives and friends), liver function tests and liver biopsy provided the patient's clotting time allows this.

Cirrhosis of the liver

Cirrhosis or scarring of the liver is an irreversible condition caused by many hepatic diseases. There are many clinical manifestations, which vary with the severity and duration of the disease. Alcohol is the commonest cause, with the other major players being viral hepatitis, primary biliary cirrhosis, autoimmune hepatitis and haemochromatosis.

PATHOPHYSIOLOGY

Prolonged low-grade inflammation causes progressive scarring and destruction of the liver cells. The remaining liver cells proliferate to form nodules; this results in the liver becoming irregular and distorted in shape. The blood vessels are also destroyed. The resistance to the flow of blood increases, which in turn leads to portal hypertension (see p. 141). The major complications of cirrhosis, resulting from hepatocellular failure, portal hypertension and portal systemic shunting, are ascites, GI bleeding, hepatic encephalopathy, renal dysfunction and hepatocellular carcinoma.

Common presenting features As the disease progresses, the patient feels increasingly fatigued and lethargic. Anorexia, nausea and weight loss are common. Jaundice, bruising, spider telangiectasis and finger clubbing are also seen. Pruritus is a common symptom of cirrhosis (see Nursing Care Plan 4.1) and is probably caused by bile salt deposition in the skin. It is a feature of cholestasis but is not always accompanied by jaundice. It is especially troublesome in primary biliary cirrhosis. Endocrine abnormalities such as gynaecomastia and impotence in males and amenorrhoea and infertility in females can also develop.

MEDICAL MANAGEMENT

The aim of treatment is the removal of any identifiable cause such as alcohol abuse and the management of the major symptoms and complications. Liver transplantation is considered when earlier treatment fails. Considerable counselling and support may be required to eliminate an alcohol problem and improve nutrition. The medical and nursing management of the major complications of cirrhosis of the liver are considered in more detail below.

Ascites

Ascites is the abnormal accumulation of serous fluid within the peritoneal cavity and is a serious prognostic development (Jalan & Hayes 1997). It results from a combination of the following factors:

- raised portal pressure
- increased lymphatic pressure in the liver
- low plasma protein — albumin
- sodium retention.

Box 4.11 gives further details on pathophysiology.

MEDICAL MANAGEMENT

The main components of treatment are restriction of sodium and fluid intake, administration of diuretics and abdominal paracentesis in refractory ascites (see Box 4.12).

NURSING PRIORITIES AND MANAGEMENT: Ascites

Major considerations

The main aims of nursing care are as follows:

- To promote bed rest in the position most comfortable for the patient. The legs should be elevated to help reduce peripheral oedema. The semi-prone position improves kidney perfusion and also the venous return to the heart, which in turn promotes a diuresis.
- To provide pressure area care. This is vital because oedema may compromise skin quality and the patient is likely to experience reluctance and difficulty in moving.
- To obtain baseline observations before commencing treatment. This should include the patient's weight and a record of the extent of ascites and oedema.
- To encourage the patient to eat a diet very low in salt. Daily sodium intake must be restricted to 60 mmol, and to 40 mmol in severe ascites.
- To ensure that the patient manages the restriction in fluid intake and understands why it is necessary. It is

Nursing Care Plan 4.1 Care plan for an older man with liver failure due to alcoholic cirrhosis

Problem (actual/potential)	Reason	Nursing action
1. Anxiety, anger and fear	Due to: lack of knowledge; fear of the unknown and perhaps denial of the reality of his condition	• Encourage fears to be expressed and questions to be asked. Explain all procedures and maintain a non-judgemental approach. Confidence will be restored and he will feel better able to cope
2. Loss of self-concept: **• body image** **• role performance** **• self-identity** **• self-esteem**	Due to: – physical alteration resulting from jaundice, ascites and weight loss – loss of libido, impotence and gynaecomastia due to retention of oestrogens normally broken down in the liver	• Restore optimal liver function • Provide a trusting relationship • Refer to a specialist counsellor as appropriate
3. Pain and discomfort	Due to: – the enlarged liver that stretches the liver capsule (the liver itself has no sensory nerve innervation) – biliary obstruction secondary to the cirrhosis – gastritis due to alcohol abuse – oedema, ascites, bowel disturbance, dyspepsia and itching	• Relieve pain and discomfort via: – comfort measures such as positioning, gentle movement and distraction techniques – medication for pruritus: • sodium bicarbonate baths • calamine lotion • colestyramine which binds the bile salts in the intestines • antihistamine – analgesics, used with caution to avoid hepatotoxic effects
4. Insomnia	Due to: pain, anxiety, dyspnoea induced by ascites, itching and the strange environment	• Relieve pain, anxiety, dyspnoea and itching (see above) • Provide optimal peace and quiet when appropriate
5. Nutritional impairment: anorexia, anaemia and weight loss	Due to: – the inability of the liver to perform its metabolic functions and the reduction in production of bile – reduction in iron, vitamin B_{12} and red blood cells – fetor hepaticus (a bad taste in the mouth and bad breath) – previous dietary neglect due to alcohol excess	• A diet high in calories: – protein to restore plasma proteins – glucose, thought to aid liver cell recovery • Supplements, e.g. vitamins and iron • Low salt to reduce oedema • Controlled fat intake according to degree of jaundice • Small tempting meals • Oral hygiene • Monitoring of weight If anaemia becomes severe a blood transfusion and oxygen therapy may be required
6. Fluid and electrolyte imbalance and impaired tissue perfusion	Due to: – reduced arterial flow, portal hypertension, ascites – salt retention due to loss of detoxification of aldosterone and the triggering of the renin–angiotensin mechanism	• Reduce salt intake to no added salt (NAS) or less as necessary • Fluid restriction (1–1.5 L/day) if hyponatraemia develops • Gentle use of diuretics • Paracentesis if necessary

Continued

Nursing Care Plan 4.1 Care plan for an older man with liver failure due to alcoholic cirrhosis *(Continued)*

Problem (actual/potential)	Reason	Nursing action
7. Infection	Due to: loss of Kupffer cell function and lymphocyte production and exacerbated by nutritional, circulatory and respiratory impairment	• Hygiene maintained at a high standard. Strict asepsis with any invasive techniques. Regular monitoring of vital signs • Chest physiotherapy as appropriate • Infection screening as appropriate • Antibiotics if necessary but used with caution
8. Impaired skin integrity	Due to: oedema, loss of protein, jaundice, weight loss and bleeding tendency (see problem 11)	• Regular relief of pressure • Sensitive care of the skin, nails and when shaving • Use of emollients • Optimal positioning and repositioning
9. Immobility	Due to: malaise, weakness, ascites, dyspnoea and perhaps confusion	• Ensure optimal activity and rest. Provide companionship • Relieve symptoms as described
10. Impaired detoxification of natural and medicinal substances	Due to: liver cell damage	• Careful and tactful enforcement of abstinence from alcohol • Vigilance with all medications
11. Tendency to bleed that might be insidious or dramatic leading to hypovolaemic shock	Due to: – portal hypertension and development of oesophageal varices – gastritis – loss of clotting factors – inadequate absorption of vitamin K – reduced reserves of blood in the liver	• Regular monitoring of vital signs • Monitoring of any vomit for blood, fresh or digested • Skin and mucous membranes observed for bruises or bleeding • Give vitamin K as necessary • Manage hypovolaemic shock (see p. 725) should severe bleeding occur
12. Encephalopathy: **• lethargy** **• flapping tremor (asterixis)** **• irrational behaviour** **• aggression** **• loss of ability to perform daily duties**	Due to: inability of the liver to convert ammonia to urea. Ammonia levels rise to such a level that cerebral cell damage occurs due to nitrogenous neurotoxins Note: 1 A GI bleed constitutes a 'high protein meal' and will exacerbate encephalopathy 2 Infection will exacerbate encephalopathy by inducing a catabolic state 3 Hypoxia will exacerbate encephalopathy	• Careful monitoring of behaviour and ability to communicate effectively • Observe for precipitating factors, e.g. 1, 2 or 3 • Manage encephalopathy: – reduce protein intake – give rectal and colonic washouts, if necessary, to remove blood from bowel – give oral lactulose, an osmotic laxative, to reduce ammonia by acidification of bowel environment and to help evacuate bowel contents, *and/or ...* – give oral neomycin (poorly absorbed from the gut) to reduce intestinal flora – monitor level of consciousness (LOC) – ensure safety and comfort

important to help the patient to 'pace' the fluid intake throughout the day. It is also important that the patient's family and friends are made aware of diet and fluid restrictions.

- To administer diuretics as prescribed. Spironolactone is the medication of choice because of its potassium-sparing properties. Fluid loss is measured by weighing the patient at the same time each day in similar clothes, with an empty bladder.
- To control pain. Pain may be mild and responsive to non-opioid analgesics. However, in malignant disease it can be severe and difficult to control. Strong analgesics and small doses of prednisolone are used to control this severe pain.

Box 4.11

Ascites

The term ascites refers to a marked increase in the volume of fluid in the peritoneal cavity. This is usually due to an underlying disease in which the total body fluid is increased. Hepatic cirrhosis accounts for over 80% of cases but ascites can also be caused by cardiac failure, nephrotic syndrome, malignancy in the peritoneum or infection such as tuberculosis.

In health, serous fluid is continually produced in the peritoneal cavity and is sufficient to provide lubrication only, but ascites occurs when fluid enters the peritoneal cavity more quickly than it can be returned to the circulation by the capillaries and lymphatics. Fluid normally leaves a capillary at its arteriolar end and returns at its venous end but, in cirrhosis, portal hypertension causes more fluid to be produced in the hepatic sinusoids which are unable to drain via impaired hepatic lymphatics. The failing liver cannot synthesise enough of the plasma protein, albumin, and the resulting hypoalbuminaemia lowers the osmotic pressure of the blood, reducing the amount of peritoneal fluid reabsorbed at the venous end. This picture is further complicated by sodium and hence water retention. The presence of ascites in liver disease is a poor prognostic sign as it implies poor liver function. Severe ascites can cause great discomfort: dyspnoea, anorexia and the ability to eat only small meals; inhibited mobility and discomfort when lying in bed or sitting upright in a chair. If pain occurs, it is often felt in the back. Many of the symptoms correspond to the discomfort of full-term pregnancy! Increased intra-abdominal pressure also leads to hernias, especially at the umbilicus.

Ascitic fluid in cirrhosis is usually straw-coloured; bloodstained ascites indicates malignant disease; bile staining indicates a communication with the biliary system; and cloudy fluid denotes infection. Chylous ascites, which has a milky appearance, is caused by lymphatic obstruction.

Gastrointestinal bleeding

GI bleeding is a direct result of portal hypertension. It may be slow and insidious, as in portal hypertensive gastropathy, or sudden and catastrophic, as in major oesophageal or gastric variceal rupture.

PATHOPHYSIOLOGY

Portal hypertension occurs when there is an obstruction in the intra- or extrahepatic circulation. Hepatic cirrhosis accounts for over 90% of cases of intrahepatic hypertension in this country. Extrahepatic portal hypertension is less common: in adults it is usually due to thrombosis, as occurs in polycythaemia rubra vera, local inflammation or sepsis, as in pancreatitis, or invasion by malignant tumours.

Common clinical features The cardinal signs of portal hypertension are splenomegaly, enlargement of the spleen, hypersplenism, splenomegaly and a deficiency in one or more types of blood cells, and a portosystemic collateral circulation. The collateral vessels open up to decompress the portal system and are present throughout the abdomen. They are, however, most problematic at the gastro-oesophageal junction where they can rupture and cause massive haemorrhage.

Box 4.12

Abdominal paracentesis

In intractable ascites, i.e. when sodium restrictions and diuretic therapy have little effect, it is possible to drain the fluid from the peritoneal cavity by means of a catheter inserted through the abdominal wall. This procedure is known as abdominal paracentesis. Such patients are already hypoproteinaemic and the sudden loss of fluid and protein by paracentesis is likely to lead to a shift of both from the rest of the body into the abdominal cavity, sometimes with consequent hypovolaemia, shock and even death. The protein is therefore replaced at the time of paracentesis by an infusion of salt-poor albumin. The patient's blood pressure should be monitored closely and the fluid drained no more quickly than at a rate of approximately 2 L/h. Strict aseptic technique should be used when inserting the catheter to avoid introducing infection that can lead to bacterial peritonitis. This procedure requires cooperation from the patient to lie relatively still in bed while the catheter is in situ over several hours. Help will be required from the nursing staff to maintain comfort over this period. Any leakage on removal of the catheter can be collected in a drainable bag (e.g. a stoma bag) until the puncture site heals (usually within 48 h).

MEDICAL MANAGEMENT

Investigations Portal hypertension is diagnosed by medical history, palpation of the abdomen, and ultrasound when splenomegaly is demonstrated. Angiography of the portal venous system will determine the cause and site of the obstruction. Endoscopy will demonstrate gastro-oesophageal varices. Hypersplenism will cause thrombocytopenia and leucopenia. Anaemia may also be present.

Treatment The presenting symptoms are treated. Bleeding from oesophageal varices is treated by blood transfusion and by variceal eradication. This can be done endoscopically, either by injection sclerotherapy or band ligation. Balloon tamponade, compression of the varices using inflated balloons, and medication such as vasopressin are used only to stop active bleeding until variceal eradication treatment is commenced. Patients who do not respond to endoscopic management of their varices will be treated with a transjugular intrahepatic portosystemic stent (TIPSS).

Sclerotherapy is a treatment for oesophageal varices involving the injection of an irritant solution. This causes thrombosis and obliteration of the varicosed veins.

Banding is an alternative for the long-term treatment of varices as it has fewer complications than sclerotherapy.

Splenectomy is particularly valuable where there is portal hypertension due to obstruction in the splenic vein.

Transjugular intrahepatic portosystemic stent (TIPSS) is a radiological intervention whereby a metal stent is inserted in the liver to connect the portal and systemic veins. It is effective in lowering the portal pressure and thus controlling variceal bleeding and re-bleeding. It is associated with a low complication and mortality rate (Redhead et al 1993).

For further information, see Miller (1996).

NURSING PRIORITIES AND MANAGEMENT: Oesophageal varices

If the patient is vomiting profusely from bleeding oesophageal varices, a high-flow suction catheter should be available for intermittent suction and maintenance of a clear airway.

Blood pressure and pulse should be observed quarter-hourly and the nurse should be alert for signs of hypovolaemic shock (see Ch. 18). Intravenous fluids and a blood transfusion should be maintained and an accurate record of all fluid intake and output kept. A urinary catheter is passed and urine output measured hourly during the acute phase, as underperfusion of the kidneys due to shock can result in renal impairment.

Intravenous infusion of a vasoconstricting agent such as vasopressin may be used to constrict the splanchnic arterioles and so reduce the blood loss at source.

The patient is fasted prior to transfer to theatre for endoscopic eradication of varices. Standard preparation is followed and on return to the ward, a clear airway and no oral fluids must be maintained until sensation and the ability to swallow have returned. The nurse will observe closely for recurrence of bleeding.

Because of the experience of either vomiting blood or passing melaena, the patient may be extremely anxious. A calm approach and clear explanations of treatment and care are essential in order to help relieve the natural fears that extensive bleeding causes.

Should the bleeding not be arrested endoscopically, a gastric or oesophageal tamponade is used to stop the bleeding by balloon tamponade, i.e. compression. A Sengstaken or Minnesota tube is passed well into the stomach and the gastric balloon inflated to approximately 300 mL of air. Gentle but firm traction is applied to maintain the balloon at the oesophagogastric junction. The oesophageal balloon is inflated only if bleeding persists, as it carries a risk of oesophageal perforation. Great care is required when inflating the oesophageal balloon (no more than 30 mL of air) and it must be deflated for 30 min every 4 h. The nurse will monitor the inflation pressures and times and move the tube from side to side in the mouth every hour to prevent pressure ulcers from forming there.

The tube should be in situ no more than 12 h and immediate therapy is required on removal, i.e. endoscopic eradication or TIPSS.

Anxiety and agitation can be relieved by small i.v. doses of a benzodiazepine sedative such as midazolam. As patients with liver disease are very sensitive to sedatives, the benzodiazepine antagonist flumazenil should be immediately available. Antiemetics such as metoclopramide should be given if the patient is nauseated and retching, as this increases the pressure in the varices and could cause further haemorrhage.

For further information, see Stanley & Hayes (1997) and Starr & Hand (2002).

Hepatic encephalopathy

PATHOPHYSIOLOGY

Hepatic encephalopathy (HE) is a neuropsychiatric syndrome that occurs only in significant liver disease. It may be overt or subclinical and is potentially fully reversible (Jalan & Hayes 1997). The subclinical form can be difficult to diagnose but the overt form can lead to bizarre and even violent behaviour. The exact cause is unclear, but one popular theory is that gut-derived neurotoxins which the failing liver has been unable to neutralise somehow cross the blood–brain barrier and cause changes in cerebral neurotransmission (Jalan & Hayes 1997). This gives rise to a range of behaviour patterns that are graded 1–4 in order of severity, as follows:

1. Lack of awareness, euphoria, short attention span and impaired ability for simple arithmetical calculations
2. Lethargy, apathy, disorientation in time and place, personality change and inappropriate behaviour
3. Semi-stupor, somnolence, confusion and gross disorientation
4. Coma.

MEDICAL MANAGEMENT

Medical treatment is aimed at reversing the commonly known precipitating factors of HE, which are:

- protein loading
- GI bleeding
- sepsis
- dehydration
- blood chemistry imbalances
- use of sedatives
- constipation.

For further information on the medical management of HE, see Riordan & Williams (1997).

NURSING PRIORITIES AND MANAGEMENT: Hepatic encephalopathy (HE)

Detection, avoidance and management of the above factors can be largely nurse-led. The better the nurse knows the patient, the easier it will be to detect subtle changes in the patient's personality and to reverse the encephalopathic process before coma develops. It is useful to involve family and friends in the monitoring process.

Good dietary advice is essential, not only to avoid protein excess but also to maintain a high calorie intake to avoid tissue catabolism. Dietary protein restriction is very rarely recommended nowadays as many patients with liver failure are malnourished due to ill health or alcohol excess. Constipation should be avoided and lactulose can be used to promote one to two bowel movements per day. Lactulose is especially beneficial following GI bleeding, as it alters bowel pH which then modifies colonic bacterial metabolism so that less ammonia is produced. A major GI bleed represents a large protein load in the bowel.

Close monitoring of fluid balance and daily weight is important to avoid dehydration, especially in patients on diuretic therapy or undergoing abdominal paracentesis.

Strict aseptic technique should be used for all invasive procedures and any focus of infection promptly reported and treated.

A safe environment must be maintained at all times for the patient who may be at risk of confusion and unsteadiness.

For further information on HE, see Shearman et al (1997).

Cancer of the liver

Tumours of the liver can be either primary or secondary growths. The liver is the most common site for metastatic spread and patients often present with symptoms from the secondary rather than the primary lesion.

Primary tumours

Hepatocellular carcinoma is the principal primary tumour. It is one of the major cancers of the world but the incidence varies greatly between countries. The highest risk populations are in sub-Saharan Africa and eastern Asia and males are more commonly affected than females (Chen et al 1997). Chronic hepatitis B and C virus infections are the main causes of the cancers in high-incidence areas. Hepatocellular carcinomas also occur in haemochromatosis and alcoholic cirrhosis of the liver.

PATHOPHYSIOLOGY

The tumour is highly vascular and occurs most frequently in the right lobe. It may invade the hepatic and portal veins, the obstruction to these vessels resulting in portal hypertension. There may be local spread to the peritoneum or metastatic spread to the lungs or lymphatic system.

MEDICAL MANAGEMENT

Investigations A very high serum alpha-fetoprotein (AFP >200 ku; normal: 2–6 ku) is diagnostic. Ultrasound with fine-needle aspiration or biopsy at laparoscopy is performed to obtain cells for histological examination. Ultrasound, CT scan and angiography are needed to define the extent of liver involvement and venous invasion prior to a decision being taken on treatment.

Treatment The first objective is to see whether the tumour is localised sufficiently in the liver to be resected surgically (see Box 4.13). Unfortunately, surgery is usually impossible, either because liver involvement is too extensive or because metastasis to other organs has occurred. Some patients may benefit from chemoembolisation of the vessels supplying the tumour, but as this treatment can have unpleasant side-effects, it is often reserved for patients with hepatic symptoms (see Box 4.14). Medical therapy also aims to relieve symptoms such as pain or ascites.

Secondary tumours

These are the most common malignant liver tumours and can originate from a primary growth in any part of the body.

PATHOPHYSIOLOGY

Multiple deposits are usually found and may be sited anywhere in the liver. The histology of the cells may indicate the primary site; however, the cancer cells may be anaplastic, giving no indication of their origin.

Clinical features are as for primary malignant tumours, with signs of associated cirrhosis. Pain is often the most common symptom for which the patient seeks medical help. The abdomen will become distended due to the enlarged liver, peritoneal invasion and ascites. The patient will have difficulty in bending and is usually anorexic. Jaundice may be present. Weight loss is usually marked.

MEDICAL MANAGEMENT

Diagnosis is by fine-needle aspiration under ultrasound imaging to obtain cells for histology. If the primary site is unknown and causing no symptoms, but there are metastatic deposits in the liver, the patient is not subjected to investigations to locate the primary tumour, as outcome is determined by the spread to the liver.

Treatment must generally be restricted to symptom control, although occasionally a localised metastasis from the colon can be resected.

Box 4.13

Surgical resection of liver tumours

Resection of liver tumours constitutes major surgery. In some cases, complete removal of the tumour may be possible, depending on the site and size of the tumour and on liver function. Resection is contraindicated in patients with extensive liver cirrhosis.

Because the liver has a good capacity to regenerate, following small hepatic lobectomy the prognosis is relatively good if the entire tumour has been resected. More extensive resections carry a higher mortality rate.

The nursing management of a patient following major liver surgery is intensive and should be carried out in a specialist unit.

Box 4.14

Hepatic artery ligation and tumour embolisation

Hepatic artery ligation may give worthwhile palliation in patients with hepatocellular carcinoma. Following ligation, tumour necrosis occurs. This treatment is contraindicated in patients with portal vein obstruction and cirrhosis because of the ensuing massive hepatic necrosis.

Tumour embolisation may also provide worthwhile palliation. During hepatic angiography, a gelatin sponge is injected into the branches of the hepatic artery, causing tumour infarction.

Chemotherapy may also be used; if so, the drug is delivered directly into the tumour to avoid systemic side-effects.

NURSING PRIORITIES AND MANAGEMENT: Cancer of the liver

Major patient problems

Nursing management is aimed at symptom control as well as providing the emotional support patients require when facing a terminal illness (see Chs 31 and 33). Time should be spent with the patient so that there is the opportunity to express thoughts, fears and anger. As the prognosis of this form of cancer is so poor, this patient may be left with a very short time to put their affairs in order and to prepare for impending death. Family and friends will also need support from nursing and medical staff.

Initially, the patient may be able to attend personal needs, and may also be able to return home. However, repeated admission may be necessary for abdominal paracentesis (see Box 4.12). As the disease advances, there will be progressive dependence on nurses and/or relatives for care. Due to extreme weight loss, much attention is required in maintaining intact pressure areas, and oral hygiene should be given regularly in the hope of preventing moniliasis. At this point, the patient and family may appreciate the privacy of a single room, but this should not be undertaken without prior discussion with them.

DISORDERS OF THE BILIARY SYSTEM

STOP THINK **4.19** With the help of your physiology textbook, review the structure and function of the biliary system.

Cholelithiasis

Cholelithiasis, the presence of gallstones, is the commonest disorder of the biliary tree. It is more prevalent among women than men and its incidence appears to be increasing. In developed countries, at least 20% of women over 40 will develop gallstones. Until about 20 years ago, the most likely person to develop gallstones was said to be an obese woman in her 40s with fair skin ('fair, fat, fertile, female and 40'). This categorisation is now considered outdated as, for unknown reasons, gallstones are affecting people at a much younger age. Other factors related to the development of gallstones include the use of oral contraceptives, diabetes mellitus and genetic history.

For further information, see Garden (2002).

PATHOPHYSIOLOGY

Gallstones are formed from the constituents of bile salts. Stones vary in size and shape, and may be solitary or multiple. Their colour can vary from yellow to dark brown. There are three main types:

- pure cholesterol stones (a 'solitaire' that fills the gall bladder): 10%
- pigmented stones ('jack stones', black and shiny): 2–3%
- mixed stones (mainly cholesterol often with some calcium): 80%.

Biliary colic

Gallstones can be asymptomatic. It is believed that only 10–30% of gallstones become symptomatic. At postmortem 12% of men and 24% of women will have gallstones present (Garden 2002). More often they cause biliary colic or an acute or chronic cholecystitis. Cholecystitis can also, less commonly, be caused by trauma and, even more rarely, by tumours.

PATHOPHYSIOLOGY

Biliary colic is caused by a transient obstruction of the gall bladder from an impacted stone.

Common presenting symptoms The patient complains of a sudden onset of severe gripping pain in the right hypochondrium that often radiates to the back. It can be associated with nausea and vomiting. The pain may vary in intensity and can last for several hours. The pain will ease when the stone either passes into the common bile duct or falls back into the gall bladder.

MEDICAL MANAGEMENT

The patient will recover quickly, but repeated bouts of colic are common. Following investigations a cholecystectomy may be performed.

Acute cholecystitis

PATHOPHYSIOLOGY

It is thought that, in this condition, gallstones irritate the mucous membrane lining of the gall bladder, which then becomes inflamed.

Common presenting symptoms The patient presents with an acute illness that is severe in nature, and may be in shock due to pain and vomiting.

A mass may be felt and Murphy's sign, a catching of the breath at the height of inspiration when the gall bladder is palpated, is usually positive. The pain will be severe in the right hypochondrium and may radiate to the right shoulder tip.

There may be tenderness and guarding of the whole abdomen and the patient may not tolerate examination. Sweating and pallor may be present.

There will be pyrexia and tachycardia due to infection. Jaundice may be present if there is obstruction of the common bile duct; in this case the patient will have a history of pale stools and dark urine. A history of fatty intolerance may also be described, and the pain often starts following a fatty meal.

MEDICAL MANAGEMENT

Investigations Tests that may be used to establish a diagnosis are as follows:

- blood tests — liver function tests, serum amylase and white blood count
- ultrasound
- CT scanning
- endoscopic retrograde cholangiopancreatography (ERCP)
- intravenous cholangiogram (used occasionally)
- oral cholecystogram (less common).

Ultrasound is now the main investigative procedure for patients with suspected gallstones. It is non-invasive and causes minimal discomfort to the patient. The scanning machine can be brought to the patient in the admissions ward, thus avoiding an uncomfortable journey to the radiology department. Ultrasound can identify stones in the gall bladder, thickening of the gall bladder wall and both intra- and extrahepatic duct dilatation. It can be done quickly and is relatively inexpensive.

Treatment Cholecystectomy is indicated in patients with biliary colic or acute cholecystitis and may be undertaken early in the acute admission. It may also be undertaken as an elective procedure around 6 weeks after an acute episode and following a full recovery. Antibiotic cover is always given. Moreover, with an 'early' cholecystectomy, the patient is not at risk of further attacks of acute cholecystitis while waiting for elective surgery. Removal of gallstones can also be performed by ERCP and sphincterotomy. In more specialised centres, surgeons are now performing laparoscopic cholecystectomy.

Laparoscopic cholecystectomy The advantages to the patient of this procedure are:

- reduced stay in hospital
- early mobilisation with lower risk of complications
- minor nature of surgical wounds
- reduced need for opioid analgesics
- speedy return to normal life.

The procedure is performed under general anaesthetic. The surgeon passes a laparoscope into the abdomen at the umbilicus. The abdomen is then insufflated with CO_2 to allow clear visualisation of the gall bladder.

Three more incisions are made in the region of the right hypochondrium to allow instruments to be manipulated. The cystic artery is identified and ligated. The cystic duct is identified, at which stage an intraoperative cholangiogram can be done to check for stones in the common bile duct. If stones are present, these can be removed.

By careful dissection, the gall bladder is then removed from the liver bed. It is brought to the undersurface of the umbilicus, where the stones are extracted and the gall bladder removed.

All stab wounds are then closed with a subcutaneous suture. On return from theatre, immediate nursing care is as for any routine general anaesthetic (see Ch. 26).

Free fluids can be given when the patient has fully recovered from the general anaesthetic. Normal diet is generally started the following day. Most patients are discharged on the first or second postoperative day.

STOP THINK **4.20** Complications, such as damage to the common bile duct, are rare and often insidious in their development.

(a) In the relatively short postoperative period in hospital, what observations or clinical signs might indicate a significant complication?
(b) What specific advice might be given to the patient and family members?

NURSING PRIORITIES AND MANAGEMENT: Acute cholecystitis

Immediate concerns

Patients experiencing an acute episode of cholecystitis will be severely ill and will be referred to hospital as quickly as possible after being seen by their GP or by contacting NHS Direct/24. The priorities of care while the attack is being managed prior to surgical intervention include the following:

- administration of an i.m. opiate analgesic at frequent intervals
- hourly recording of vital signs until the patient's condition stabilises
- fasting the patient and commencing i.v. fluids
- careful monitoring of fluid and electrolyte balance
- i.v. administration of a broad-spectrum antibiotic
- if vomiting is persistent, a nasogastric tube may be passed and an antiemetic given.

Major patient problems

The patient will be restless and uncomfortable due to the pain. The most comfortable position for the patient should be sought and analgesics given regularly. Fear of pain and of the unknown increases pain (see Ch. 19). It is therefore vital to explain what is happening and to assure the patient that the condition can be treated. When the condition is stable, the patient should be introduced to the surroundings and information about the ward can be provided.

Once the acute phase has passed, fluids can be given and foods gradually reintroduced. The i.v. infusion may be discontinued when the patient can tolerate an adequate oral intake. Intravenous antibiotics are usually given for 5 days and then discontinued.

Sweating can be a problem and frequent washes and changes of bedclothes may be necessary to keep the patient comfortable. Oral hygiene should be maintained as necessary.

While the patient is in bed, gentle exercises to prevent deep vein thrombosis should be taught and frequent changes of position should be encouraged to alleviate pressure. Taking deep breaths to avoid pulmonary complications should be encouraged and smoking should be discouraged.

Perioperative care

Cholecystectomy is carried out on patients with acute cholecystitis to relieve symptoms and prevent complications. Exploration of the common bile duct may be undertaken if there is evidence of stones. Open cholecystectomy used to be one of the most common surgical operations; however, since the advent of laparoscopic cholecystectomy in 1978, the use of this operation has fallen sharply (Garden et al 2002).

Nursing care following an open cholecystectomy

In this procedure, the surgeon approaches the gall bladder through a subcostal paramedian or midline incision. An intraoperative cholangiogram is performed to identify any stones in the common bile duct. If stones are present, the surgeon will explore the duct, remove the stones, and may occasionally insert a T-tube to maintain patency and prevent stricture of the duct. The long leg of the T-tube is brought out through a stab wound in the abdominal wall and then connected to a drainage bag. It is vital that this

Box 4.15

Management of a T-tube

A T-tube is inserted into the common bile duct following exploration. This tube is necessary as a 'safety valve' because following surgery the duct will become inflamed and oedematous, blocking the flow of bile into the duodenum. Approximately 300–500 mL of bile should drain in the first 24 h. This amount will gradually decrease over the next 8–10 days as the patency of the duct returns. An accurate recording of the amount of bile drainage must be made. The presence of insufficient or excessive bile must be reported. When there is a sudden cessation of bile drainage, a kinked or compressed tube must be suspected.

It is also important to support the bile drainage bag at all times to prevent traction on the tube and accidental removal. An aseptic technique must be used when emptying or changing the bag. Daily cleaning of the skin at the drain site is necessary and the nurse should check for bile leakage from around the tube, inflammation or excoriation of the skin. Any excess tubing should be coiled and taped to the abdomen. Prior to removal, a T-tube cholangiogram will be done to check the patency of the bile duct and the flow of bile into the duodenum. If the duct is patent, the tube is removed. If there are residual stones in the duct, the T-tube is left in situ. These residual stones may pass spontaneously into the duodenum; otherwise it will be necessary to remove them under X-ray vision.

Prior to performing a T-tube cholangiogram some surgeons ask for the T-tube to be clamped for 24 h. This procedure is, however, becoming less common. If there is any complaint of abdominal pain whilst the tube is clamped, it must be respected and the clamp removed immediately.

The patient will require an analgesic 30 min before the tube is removed. The skin suture is removed and a firm steady pressure applied to the tube. The nurse should observe the amount of bile leakage following removal and apply a sterile dressing. Observation of the patient for any signs of biliary peritonitis should be made for 24 h.

tube is not removed accidentally (see Box 4.15). A T-tube cholangiogram is done 8–10 days postoperatively to ensure patency of the duct prior to its removal. If the ducts are stone-free, the tube will be removed following instructions from the surgeon (see Fig. 4.11).

There is usually a wound drain inserted into the gall bladder bed. Regular observation of the colour and amount of blood draining postoperatively is vital. Excessive drainage of bright red blood must be reported immediately to the surgeon. This drain is usually removed 24–48 h postoperatively.

Immediate postoperative care is as for any major abdominal surgery requiring general anaesthesia. Adequate analgesia is vital so that the patient can perform deep breathing and coughing exercises to prevent atelectasis and pneumonia. In most cases, the anaesthetist will perform an intercostal nerve block and top it up at regular intervals so that the patient is pain-free. This can be supplemented with i.m. or i.v. analgesics given regularly over the first 24–48 h. The nurse should check at regular intervals that

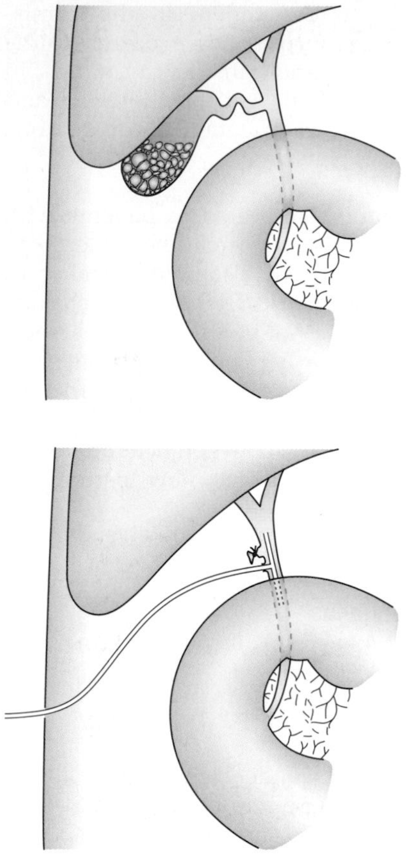

Fig. 4.11 The T-tube in the common bile duct (Forrest et al 1995).

the incision site and surrounding area are numb, to ensure the intercostal nerve block is working effectively. The patient should be raised to an upright position and encouraged to do breathing exercises to prevent pulmonary complications.

Other considerations

The patient may begin to take oral fluids gradually after the first 24 h (30–60 mL/h). If these are tolerated, free fluids may be given. Diet is gradually increased over the next 3 days. A nasogastric tube is not used unless the patient shows signs of paralytic ileus. In this case the patient should be fasted, a nasogastric tube passed and the stomach kept empty.

Sutures are removed 7–10 days postoperatively unless, as has become more common, an absorbable subcutaneous suture is used. If the wound is dry and clean, the dressing can be removed 24–48 h postoperatively and the wound left exposed.

Depending on the patient's fitness and age, discharge home normally occurs within 6–10 days. Discharge plans will need to be discussed with relatives or carers. The patient must be instructed to do no heavy lifting for 4–6 weeks to avoid wound herniation. Normal diet is allowed. In an uncomplicated recovery, the patient should be fit to return to work 4–6 weeks later. A detailed discharge summary will be sent to the GP, who will then certify when the patient is fit for work. A follow-up appointment will be given for 4 weeks after discharge so that the surgeon can make sure that the outcome is satisfactory (see Case History 4.3).

CASE HISTORY 4.3
Mrs G

Mrs G had suffered from episodes of cholecystitis and biliary colic for many months before she finally went to her GP. She was a busy mother of three and, as she recounted at a later date, 'There really was no time to be going to the doctor. Besides, the pain always went eventually, especially if my husband rubbed my back up between the shoulder blades'.

Eventually, when she felt so ill that she was forced to stay in bed, she 'gave in'.

The investigations and surgery passed uneventfully in surgical terms, as she had been quite well and free from symptoms at the time of admission. Unlike her sister in London, she had had an open cholecystectomy. It was the first time she had had an operation and, although she thought the nurses were wonderful and had explained everything, she later remarked: 'No one ever tells you just how awful the first day after the operation really is'.

Within 10 days, Mrs G was at home once more, delighted that at least her sutures were dissolvable ones. She knew that she must not do too much lifting and that although she should have a normal diet, she should avoid fatty foods as they might make her feel 'squeamish'. 'It's like only having weak washing-up liquid to deal with greasy dishes instead of good concentrated liquid,' she explained to a friend.

Three weeks after discharge, she visited the doctor. She was quite distressed and reported the following problems: 'I keep having episodes of diarrhoea and I'm so tired. No one said who was going to do the hoovering or put the shopping away in those high cupboards. The family thinks I'm back to normal because the wound is healed but I am so tired still. Everything is an effort'.

Chronic cholecystitis

PATHOPHYSIOLOGY

Chronic cholecystitis is caused by the presence of stones in the gall bladder. In this condition the gall bladder wall becomes thickened and fibrosed.

Common presenting symptoms The patient may present with biliary colic but more often complains of pain in the right upper quadrant of the abdomen, often following a big meal. There will be a history of fat intolerance, flatulence and heartburn. Abdominal distension may also be a problem following meals.

The pain is less severe than in acute cholecystitis and patients often put up with their symptoms for years before seeking medical advice. In chronic cholecystitis, the patient's general condition must be taken into account, particularly if elderly or suffering from other medical conditions that may increase the risks of surgery.

MEDICAL MANAGEMENT

Investigations are as for acute cholecystitis.

Treatment Usually the diseased gall bladder is removed, either by an open cholecystectomy or, more commonly now, by a laparoscopic cholecystectomy.

Choledocholithiasis

Stones in the bile duct occur in about 10–15% of patients with gallstones.

PATHOPHYSIOLOGY

Common presenting symptoms Colicky pain occurs if the stones impede the flow of bile through the sphincter of Oddi. Impaction of a stone at the sphincter will cause jaundice. The patient will have pale, fatty stools, dark urine and possibly complain of generalised itching. Some stones will clear spontaneously following passage into the small intestine.

If the stone becomes impacted, the bile duct will become dilated. Infection can cause cholangitis with rigors, severe pain and jaundice. Acute pancreatitis may develop due to obstruction of the sphincter of Oddi and reflux of bile salts into the pancreatic ducts (see p. 148).

MEDICAL MANAGEMENT

Investigations are as for acute and chronic cholecystitis.

Treatment Removal of the stones via ERCP and sphincterotomy to allow the stones to pass freely into the small intestine will be carried out either prior to surgery or in cases where surgery is contraindicated.

For further information, see Garden (2002).

Tumours of the biliary tract

Cancer of the gall bladder

PATHOPHYSIOLOGY

This is a rare cancer and is nearly always related to gallstones. It is more common in females than in males. Signs and symptoms are consistent with those for gallstones and a history of persistent obstructive jaundice may be present. A mass may be palpable. In most cases, surgery is not a chosen treatment and survival rates are poor. Eighty per cent of gall bladder tumours are adenocarcinomas. As with other tumours, the involvement of lymph nodes and the presence of metastases will determine the patient's prognosis.

Cancer of the bile duct (cholangiocarcinoma)

PATHOPHYSIOLOGY

The cause of bile duct cancer is unknown although there are strong associations with inflammatory bowel disease and primary sclerosing cholangitis (Garden 2002). It is more common in older people, and men are affected more than women. It is a rare cancer but its incidence appears to be increasing. Tumours can arise from the intra- or extrahepatic biliary tree. Direct spread and metastases are present in at least 50% of the patients who go for surgery.

MEDICAL MANAGEMENT

Treatment As cancer of the bile ducts carries a very poor prognosis, treatment is usually in the form of palliative therapy. Jaundice is a very distressing symptom and if this is not treated the patient may die from liver failure.

For some patients, palliation can be achieved by the insertion of a stent, either by ERCP or by percutaneous transhepatic techniques, e.g. percutaneous transhepatic cholangiography (PTC). In a few cases, where the tumour is at the lower end of the common bile duct, a radical resection

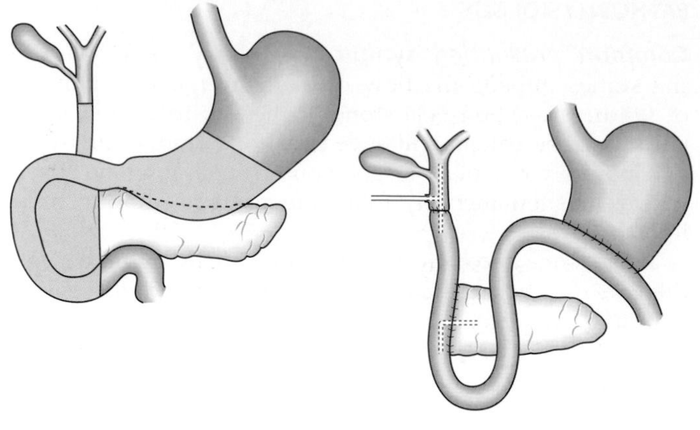

Fig. 4.12 Whipple's procedure. This extensive procedure involves resection of the head of the pancreas, the duodenum and the antrum of the stomach, as well as removal of the gall bladder. Reconstruction is carried out with choledochojejunostomy, pancreatojejunostomy and gastrojejunostomy. This is a major operation that carries a relatively high mortality rate. Leakage from the anastomosis, abscess formation and fistula are the main complications (Forrest et al 1995).

in the form of a Whipple resection may be possible (see Fig. 4.12). This is major surgery and should be considered only if the tumour is localised and if the patient is fit for surgery.

Tumours of the upper biliary tract are resectable in only 10% of cases. Following resection of the tumour, a Roux loop of jejunum is anastomosed to the biliary tract or, in some cases, the left hepatic duct. A hepaticojejunostomy then restores the continuity of the small intestine. A hepaticojejunostomy can also be performed to bypass the tumour and achieve palliation. Radiotherapy and chemotherapy have not been shown to improve survival.

NURSING PRIORITIES AND MANAGEMENT: Cholangiocarcinoma

The patient with a diagnosis of cholangiocarcinoma will require specialised nursing care. Only a few of these patients will be considered for major resection, following which they are cared for in a high-dependency ward for approximately 48 h. In some cases the patient is prepared for major resection but at the time of surgery it is discovered that only a bypass of the tumour may be carried out safely. These patients are usually devastated by this turn of events and require a great deal of support. Following palliation, jaundice will subside and the patient's appetite will improve. For a few months the patient may feel so well that they become unrealistic about the prognosis. Few patients survive more than a year following palliation. Following resection, the outlook is better. Good family support is necessary. It is important to take an honest approach and to give explanations to the patient and family as they request it. It will be necessary to spend time with the patient and the relatives to answer their questions and offer support. Close communication with the GP is also important so that community care can be provided when necessary.

DISORDERS OF THE PANCREAS

Pancreatitis

Inflammation of the pancreatic gland may be acute or chronic. Acute pancreatitis can range from mild oedema to severe necrosis and haemorrhage. Following an attack, the gland returns to normal. Chronic pancreatitis is associated with permanent anatomical and functional abnormality. The patient usually suffers from relapsing attacks with relative good health between episodes.

Acute pancreatitis

Acute pancreatitis can be life threatening, with approximately one in four patients presenting with severe disease; of these, one in four will die (Garden et al 2002). It can affect all adult groups. In the UK its two main causes are gallstones and excessive alcohol consumption. Other identified causes include smoking, infection, trauma, medication, e.g. corticosteroids, hypercalcaemia, hyperlipidaemia, pancreatic cancer and hereditary factors. In modern practice, intervention with ERCP can also cause pancreatitis.

PATHOPHYSIOLOGY

The pancreatic enzymes, trypsin and lipase, which are normally activated in the duodenum, are prematurely activated within the pancreas, causing autodigestion of the gland. This autodigestion leads to varying degrees of oedema, haemorrhage, necrosis, abscess and cyst formation in and around the pancreas. Spasm of the sphincter of Oddi with reflux of duodenal contents into the pancreatic duct is thought to be an important factor in this enzyme activation. Gallstones and alcohol are two contributing factors to spasm. Passage of stones down the common bile duct may also promote reflux of infected bile along the pancreatic duct when these ducts form a common channel to the ampulla of Vater.

Activated enzymes such as trypsinogen and chymotrypsinogen, phospholipase, elastase and catalase are responsible for increased capillary permeability. This permits large volumes of fluid to escape into the peritoneal and retroperitoneal cavity, causing damage to the surrounding tissue. This severe loss of circulating fluid leads to hypovolaemic shock and predisposes the individual to acute renal failure, which may result from local intravascular coagulation in the renal vascular bed. Development of pulmonary oedema with left-sided pleural effusion may result from release of toxins. The release of lipase causes fat necrosis in the omentum and areas adjacent to the pancreas. Calcium soaps become sequestered in areas of fatty necrosis, which may result in the development of hypocalcaemia.

MEDICAL MANAGEMENT

History and examination The patient usually presents with epigastric pain of acute onset radiating to the back, associated with nausea and vomiting. There may be a history of biliary tract disease or alcohol abuse.

Acute pancreatitis is often associated with severe shock. There may be signs of dehydration with rapid pulse and respiration, hypotension and pyrexia. Marked abdominal tenderness is usually present in the upper abdomen, which may appear distended. Bruising around the umbilicus

(Cullen's sign) and in the loin region (Grey Turner's sign) are rare late manifestations of acute pancreatitis due to petechial bleeding into the retroperitoneal space.

Investigations include blood analysis, urinalysis, X-ray ultrasound and CT scan, as follows:

- Serum lipase is one of the most reliable markers of acute pancreatitis.
- A serum amylase of above 1000 IU/L in the past 48 h is strongly suggestive of acute pancreatitis. Normal levels are 100–300 IU/L. Urinary amylase can remain elevated for 10–14 days.
- Plain X-ray films of the abdomen can reveal distended loops of small bowel with paralytic ileus; chest X-ray may reveal left-sided pleural effusion.
- Urea and electrolyte levels are important indicators of the state of hydration and are necessary for the correct management of the patient.
- A raised white blood cell count ($9–20 \times 10^9$) reveals an active inflammatory process.
- Hyperglycaemia and glycosuria are often present but are transient.
- Arterial blood gases may reveal severe hypoxia.
- Abdominal ultrasound and CT scan are used to detect the presence of peripancreatic collections and pancreatic necrosis.

Treatment

Conservative management Acute pancreatitis is usually managed conservatively; for mild attacks, treatment is generally symptomatic. The principles of management are as follows:

- *Pain relief.* This is usually provided in the form of opiate analgesics. Morphine can cause some spasm at the sphincter of Oddi, but is frequently prescribed as it is effective (Garden et al 2002).
- *Correction of shock.* If haemorrhagic pancreatitis is diagnosed, shock is treated by i.v. administration of large volumes of crystalloids, plasma, dextran or blood in order to maintain circulatory blood volume and adequate urine output. Oxygen therapy is essential to correct the associated hypoxia. PO_2 saturation levels should be monitored. Hypoxaemia may develop insidiously such that respiratory failure (ARDS) can develop. Arterial blood gases are closely monitored in case ventilatory support is required (see Chs 2, 18 and 29).
- *Suppression of pancreatic function.* The patient is fasted to decrease stimulation of pancreatic enzymes and a nasogastric tube is passed if the patient is vomiting persistently.
- *Controlling infection.* When there is evidence of infection, a broad-spectrum antibiotic is prescribed. For the majority of patients this supportive treatment will settle the acute attack and surgical treatment will not be necessary. If there is any doubt about the diagnosis, a laparotomy will exclude other causes of peritonitis, such as perforated peptic ulcer and mesenteric ischaemia.
- *Monitoring blood glucose levels.* This must be done as secondary diabetes mellitus can sometimes develop, requiring insulin therapy.
- *Monitoring cardiac status.* This will be required if electrolyte derangement is such as to cause potentially lethal dysrhythmias.

Surgical intervention At an early stage in management, gallstones as a cause of the acute attack are excluded by ultrasound scanning. Cholecystectomy during the course of the patient's admission is now advocated to avoid recurrent problems following discharge. Patients with gallstone pancreatitis can usually be identified by their slow clinical progress and by the use of various clinical and biochemical prognosis factors.

Early ERCP may demonstrate the presence of stones in the common bile duct, which can be extracted by a small balloon catheter or basket following sphincterotomy. The complication of peripancreatic necrosis or abscess can be detected by radiological imaging (see Appendix 1). Most patients will require necrosectomy, i.e. the removal of necrotic tissues, and drainage at laparotomy. It may be wise to put in place a gastrostomy and jejunostomy tube at this time, as recovery is slow and the patient may require prolonged nutritional support (see Ch. 21).

NURSING PRIORITIES AND MANAGEMENT: Acute pancreatitis

Major considerations (see Case History 4.4)

The care of patients with acute pancreatitis will vary according to the severity of the attack. Some individuals present with vague abdominal pain that resolves quickly. More often, patients present with severe epigastric pain, often radiating to the back, and with vomiting and shock. It should be borne in mind that the severity of the attack is not always easily judged by an initial assessment and that these patients therefore require close observation.

Priorities of nursing care are:

- to relieve pain and promote comfort (see Nursing Care Plan 4.2)
- to monitor vital functions
- to restore and maintain haemodynamic status, i.e. to restore volume deficit, correct electrolyte imbalance and correct impaired gaseous exchange
- to restore and maintain adequate nutrition
- to prevent or minimise potential complications (see Box 4.16)
- to prevent the development of pressure ulcers
- to maintain the nasogastric tube (if present) and provide frequent mouthwashes and oral hygiene

CASE HISTORY 4.4

Mr N (see also Nursing Care Plan 4.2)

Mr N, aged 36, is admitted with a history of sudden, central abdominal pain that is only partially relieved by sitting forward and hugging his knees. He describes the pain as 'boring through his back'. His skin is pale and clammy and his respirations rapid and shallow, his pulse is rapid and there is marked hypotension. Mr N is clearly in an advancing state of shock. In addition, he is nauseated and repeated vomiting has led to increasing dehydration, exacerbating his shocked state.

Nursing Care Plan 4.2 Care of a patient with acute pancreatitis: the management of pain (see Case History 4.4)

Nursing consideration	Action	Rationale	Desired outcome
1. ***Pain*** **Mr N has severe and potentially excruciating pain due to autodigestion of the pancreas, the 'chemical burn' of pancreatic exudate, inflammation, and distension caused by an adynamic bowel**	• Rapidly assess and then monitor verbal and non-verbal evidence of pain, noting factors that either aggravate or ease the pain	To assist in achieving effective pain relief	Mr N's pain is relieved, as evidenced by the verbal communication, body relaxation and corresponding changes in vital signs
	• Give the prescribed analgesic	All opiates may cause some spasm of the sphincter of Oddi, but they are very effective (Garden et al 2002). As analgesia is achieved, smaller and less frequent doses may be given	
	• Give other adjuvant medication, e.g. antibiotic therapy, sedative agents, H_2 antagonists, antiemetics	Such agents may be used to help control the acute attack and associated symptoms, particularly pain	
	• Pass an NG tube and aspirate stomach contents	This will relieve the pain associated with distension and minimise pancreatic stimulation	
	• Position Mr N as comfortably as possible, minimising any unnecessary activity	Pain will be minimised, as will Mr N's metabolic rate and pancreatic activity	

- to monitor blood sugar level in order to detect secondary diabetes
- to support the patient in maintaining personal hygiene
- to help the patient to be up and about as early as possible.

As the patient's general condition improves, clear oral fluids can be introduced, gradually progressing to a light diet.

An episode of pancreatitis can be a very traumatic time for both the patient and the family, who may have been unaware of the important functions that the pancreas performs. It is important to explain the rationale of all procedures and investigations carefully to alleviate anxiety. Showing the patient diagrams can be very helpful. The patient may be very worried about work, family and financial situation, and a visit from the social worker may be of value. Patients with alcohol-associated acute pancreatitis may, with their consent, be referred for counselling to address their dependency problem (see Ch. 36).

It is important to reduce the noise level on the hospital ward to a minimum to allow patients to have adequate sleep (see Ch. 25). It may be advisable to give some form of night sedation. Restricting visits from wider family and friends may reduce the strain on the patient during visiting hours. Communication with the family is of course vital. On the patient's admission to the ward, nurses should introduce themselves to the relatives and give a full explanation of what has occurred. Medical staff should be available to give regular updates on the patient's condition.

Further considerations

When the acute episode has resolved, and if gallstones are present, an early elective cholecystectomy with possible exploration of the common bile duct will be undertaken. If the attack has been due to alcohol, the patient must be advised prior to discharge to abstain totally or risk a life-threatening recurrence.

Advice regarding return to work is important. The patient often feels tired and it is often advisable not to return to work for perhaps 4–6 weeks. The patient will be reviewed in the outpatient clinic initially at 3–4 weeks. A detailed account of management will be sent to the GP so that continuity of care can be maintained.

For further information, see Garden (2002) and Fawcett & Smith (2005).

Box 4.16

Complications of acute pancreatitis

Pancreatic pseudocyst
This condition develops in about 10% of patients following acute pancreatitis or an exacerbation of chronic pancreatitis. A pseudocyst is a sac containing pancreatic juice, debris and blood within a lining of inflammatory tissue, directly connecting with a pancreatic duct. Small pseudocysts are often asymptomatic, but large cysts can compress surrounding structures, often causing pain, nausea, vomiting and, occasionally, obstructive jaundice. A raised serum amylase will be present. Ultrasound scan can be used in diagnosis and monitoring. Surgery is necessary if the cyst is symptomatic, since there is a danger that it may rupture or precipitate haemorrhage. Surgery consists of drainage of the pseudocyst into the stomach (cyst gastrostomy) or duodenum (cyst duodenostomy).

Pancreatic abscess
This is a more serious complication of acute pancreatitis. The patient is usually very ill, with pyrexia, a raised white blood cell count and tachycardia. Early diagnosis by CT scanning and the use of aggressive surgical intervention have improved mortality rates. Surgery consists of extensive drainage and debridement of infected tissues. Multiple large drains are used to drain the abscess cavity. Peritoneal lavage with normal saline 0.9% warmed to body temperature can be used to irrigate the cavity. Adequate nutrition following surgery is vital. Most surgeons establish a feeding jejunostomy and gastrostomy tube during surgery.

Pancreatic necrosis
This complication is a major cause of death in acute pancreatitis. Early diagnosis is essential. The patient often fails to improve with conservative management. A persistent pyrexia, raised white blood cell count, tachycardia, hypotension and poor respiratory function are ominous signs. At laparotomy, necrotic tissue is removed, peritoneal lavage is carried out and the pancreatic bed adequately drained. A feeding jejunostomy and gastrostomy tube are inserted.

In some cases, the surgeon may opt to leave the wound open to allow for packing of the wound and to minimise the need for repeated laparotomies to deal with recurrent intra-abdominal sepsis.

Duodenal ileus
Due to persistent pancreatic inflammation, duodenal ileus may persist. Nutritional status will need to be maintained either by parenteral means or by jejunostomy feeding. A gastroenterostomy may need to be performed.

Haemorrhage
Severe bleeding may occur from gastric or duodenal ulceration. Prophylactic i.v. cimetidine is given to patients with acute pancreatitis. On rare occasions, haemorrhage may occur into a pseudocyst or by erosion of a blood vessel by the inflammatory process.

Chronic pancreatitis

Chronic pancreatitis is a relatively rare condition in the UK but its incidence is increasing, due to the increase in alcohol consumption. However, the mechanism by which alcohol damages the pancreas is poorly understood.

PATHOPHYSIOLOGY

Chronic pancreatitis leads to permanent damage of the gland, with replacement by fibrotic tissue and calcification. The ducts become narrowed and the flow of pancreatic juice is obstructed. The cells slowly stop secreting pancreatic juice. The obstructed ducts can give rise to recurrent attacks of pancreatitis lasting a few days.

Common presenting symptoms The patient usually presents with a history of severe epigastric pain, often radiating to the back. The pain is often eased by bending forward. Nausea and vomiting may also be present. A history of recent alcohol abuse may be given.

Weight loss is common and may be due to the pain or to malnutrition associated with prolonged alcohol abuse. Malabsorption is also present as a result of pancreatic insufficiency. The stool may be pale, offensive and difficult to flush away. This type of bowel movement is known as steatorrhoea and is due to a high undigested fat content. It is often a distressing feature for the patient.

Diabetes mellitus develops in approximately one-third of these patients and may require treatment. Transient jaundice may be present due to inflammation of the head of the pancreas, which obstructs the common bile duct. The presence of jaundice may be upsetting for some people, who feel 'dirty' or 'old' due to the discoloration of the skin and the marked yellowness of the sclera.

STOP THINK **4.21** Why might bending forward ease the pain in chronic pancreatitis?

MEDICAL MANAGEMENT

Investigations Clinical assessment is as follows:

- Plain abdominal X-ray may show speckled calcification of the pancreas
- Ultrasound scan and CT scan may show an enlarged, swollen gland
- ERCP is performed to outline the pancreatic duct if surgery is contemplated
- Faecal fat estimation, although used less often now, may reveal malabsorption

- Fasting blood sugars are assessed and a glucose tolerance test may be necessary.

Treatment Management of chronic pancreatitis is mainly symptomatic. The patient should be advised to stop drinking alcohol and may need professional counselling to this end. Replacement of pancreatic enzymes with a commercial preparation may help to alleviate the steatorrhoea and reduce pain. Good control of diabetes will be necessary.

Pain control can be difficult, since some of these patients become addicted to opiates (Haslett et al 2002). Management advice from a pain control specialist is invaluable. In a small number of patients in whom severe pain persists, surgery will be indicated. It may be necessary to resect the head of the gland (Whipple's procedure; see Fig. 4.12) or the body and tail (distal pancreatectomy). Adequate drainage of the duct (pancreatojejunostomy) may be undertaken where ERCP shows the pancreatic duct to be dilated. A total pancreatectomy is rarely undertaken due to the resulting permanent diabetes mellitus and exocrine insufficiency.

NURSING PRIORITIES AND MANAGEMENT: Chronic pancreatitis

Nursing management of an acute attack in relapsing pancreatitis is similar to that for acute pancreatitis.

Major patient problems

Pain

Pain is often constant in nature, radiating through to the back. It is often described as being like a sharp knife twisting in the gut and presents a major challenge to pain control. Assisting the patient into a comfortable position often helps. The patient may find that bending forward while leaning on a bed table helps. The use of a heat pad to the back may give some relief, and NSAIDs such as diclofenac sodium (Voltarol) in suppository form can be of value. It is often necessary to use opioid analgesics to alleviate pain or it may be necessary to seek advice from a pain specialist (see Ch. 19). Many hospitals now have pain teams that can advise on all aspects of pain management.

Alcohol dependency

Alcohol abuse is the most common cause of chronic pancreatitis. Total abstinence will help to resolve the pain. If the patient has had a recent 'binge', sudden withdrawal may precipitate delirium tremens. Mild sedation is frequently used to prevent this. Expert help may be necessary to assist the patient to overcome an alcohol problem.

Patient education is vital in view of the progressive destruction of the gland by this disease. Family life is usually already disrupted by the patient's alcohol abuse, and help from a social worker will be useful in assisting the patient and family to cope with the situation. Good liaison with the GP and primary health care team is important so that support can be continued in the community. Caring for these patients can present a professional and personal challenge to members of the multidisciplinary team, who may feel inclined to blame the patient for the illness (see Ch. 36).

The patient's nutritional intake must be assessed. The patient is weighed and a well-balanced diet low in fat is given once the acute attack has resolved. Pancreatic enzyme supplements can be prescribed and taken prior to meals to aid absorption of nutrients. This should also alleviate the steatorrhoea. Concurrent administration of an H_2-receptor antagonist may improve the efficacy of these supplements.

Cancer of the pancreas

Tumours of the pancreas can arise from exocrine or endocrine tissue. Benign tumours are very rare. Insulinoma arises from the islet of Langerhans cells and results in oversecretion of insulin, causing hypoglycaemia. Gastrinomas also arise from the non-beta islet cells, secreting gastrin and giving rise to the overproduction of acid of Zollinger–Ellison syndrome leading to peptic ulceration. Adenocarcinoma is by far the most common malignant tumour of the exocrine pancreas.

The cause of pancreatic cancer is unknown, but smoking and a high-fat, high-protein diet are thought to increase the risk. It is twice as common in men as in women and its incidence is increasing; over 6000 people die from pancreatic cancer in the UK each year (Garden 2002). It is the fourth most common cause of cancer deaths in men in the UK and the sixth most common in women. It mainly affects individuals aged 50–70 years.

PATHOPHYSIOLOGY

Adenocarcinoma of the pancreas arises from the ductal tissue and is more commonly located in the head of the gland. Lesions frequently obstruct the pancreatic duct, causing chronic pancreatitis. The carcinoma can also obstruct the bile duct, giving rise to obstructive jaundice. Cancer of the pancreas carries a very poor prognosis because the disease has often spread to nearby organs by the time a diagnosis is made. Surgical resection has not been shown to improve the rate of survival. However, cancer of the duodenum, lower bile duct and periampullary regions often presents earlier with obstructive jaundice, and surgical resection offers a much better prognosis.

Common presenting symptoms Jaundice is often the symptom with which the patient first presents to the GP. The urine is dark in colour, the stool pale and fatty, and the skin and sclera have a yellowish tinge. Severe itch can be a very distressing symptom.

Severe weight loss and anorexia are associated with vague epigastric pain, often radiating to the back. Initially pain is intermittent, but gradually it becomes constant and severe.

MEDICAL MANAGEMENT

Investigations are as follows:

- Blood is taken for liver function tests and to check for the presence of a coagulation defect
- An ultrasound scan will detect a dilated biliary tree and exclude the presence of gallstones

- A CT scan may demonstrate a pancreatic mass, local invasion by tumour, or metastases
- Pancreatic tissue may be obtained for cytology by using CT scan or ultrasound-guided fine-needle aspiration
- ERCP can be used to define the site of obstruction and obtain biopsies.

Treatment Relief of obstructive jaundice and pain control are all that can be offered to the majority of patients with pancreatic cancer. ERCP with stenting of the biliary tree can relieve obstructive jaundice and may reduce the necessity for surgical intervention. Chemotherapy has been used but appears to have little effect. Surgery is usually palliative but jaundice may be relieved by cholecystojejunostomy or choledochojejunostomy.

In a minority of cases, pancreatoduodenal resection (Whipple's procedure) may be worthwhile, if the tumour is less than 2 cm in diameter and confined to the head of the pancreas (see Fig. 4.12).

NURSING PRIORITIES AND MANAGEMENT: Cancer of the pancreas

Investigative procedures are extensive and surgery in the majority of cases only offers palliation. The nurse has a very important role in helping both the patient and the family to cope during this very difficult time.

Major patient problems

Anxiety

Patients with pancreatic cancer are usually very anxious. They may have no previous history of illness and often deny the diagnosis. They are often the breadwinner in the family and may even be approaching retirement. They may have difficulty coming to terms with the diagnosis and are often angry and withdrawn, especially with close family members. Relatives often feel shut out and helpless. The nurse can help by offering support and advice to the patient and family members, who should be given opportunities to discuss the illness and its implications.

Extensive discussion with the patient and relatives prior to surgery is necessary. Some patients are prepared for a Whipple's procedure but then at surgery it is found that the disease is more extensive than expected and a bypass is all that can be safely attempted. This is devastating for the patient and family, who will have built up hopes for recovery.

Pain

Pain is often persistent, particularly when the disease is at an advanced stage. Oral opioids may be given and titrated to the patient's specific needs. Progression to s.c. diamorphine may be necessary as the disease advances and an oral laxative will also be given to prevent the side-effect of constipation.

As the disease advances, pain may become more difficult to control. A coeliac plexus nerve block may also be of benefit.

Close monitoring of the effectiveness of pain control is essential to ensure that the best possible quality of life can be maintained for the patient (see Ch. 19). If the patient is discharged home, liaison with the primary health care team is essential to ensure that full continuity of care is achieved. As the condition deteriorates, discussion with the patient and family is essential to ensure the best option for care at home, in hospital or in a hospice (see Ch. 33).

Jaundice

Jaundice is usually persistent and accompanied by severe itching (pruritus). The itching is usually all over the body and the patient often scratches until the skin bleeds. Patients may be so distressed by itch that they feel they are being driven mad. Every effort should be made to relieve itching that is believed to be caused by a deposition of bile salts in the skin. Antihistamines are used but they can cause sedation. A twice-daily bath with added sodium bicarbonate is very effective. Calamine lotion or Eurax cream applied locally may help. Night sedation is important, as itching is often worse at night.

For further reading on pruritus, see Bosonnet (2003).

Following ERCP and stenting, the jaundice and itch will subside over 7–10 days. The patient will feel much better as soon as the itch disappears and as the jaundice fades. Patients should be actively encouraged to drink extra fluids at this time. This helps the jaundice to abate by flushing bilirubin and bile salts out of the blood and tissues.

Anorexia and weight loss

Poor appetite and subsequent weight loss are further distressing aspects of the disease. Meals should be small and attractively presented. Liaison with the dietitian is necessary. High-protein drinks between meals may be tolerated well. If weight loss is severe, special care should be taken to prevent the development of pressure ulcers. Malaise associated with anorexia and weight loss will increase the patient's dependency; nurses and other carers will need to offer more and more assistance with many aspects of daily life (see Box 4.17).

For further reading on cancer care, see Corner & Bailey (2001).

Box 4.17

Reversal of cancer cachexia in pancreatic cancer

Cancer cachexia is characterised by numerous metabolic abnormalities which would appear to be driven by cytokines such as interleukin-6 and also, perhaps, specific tumour-derived factors (McNamara et al 1992). The resulting alterations in energy balance and loss of lean tissue very much impair the individual's quality of life and shorten survival.

Conventional nutritional supplements for cachexia have failed to demonstrate any significant benefit in terms of nutritional status. While previous studies have shown that the administration of oral eicosapentaenoic acid (EPA) will stabilise weight in patients with advanced cancer, a recent pilot study undertaken by Barber et al (1999) combining EPA with a conventional nutritional supplement has demonstrated that this combination may indeed reverse cachexia in advanced pancreatic cancer.

DISORDERS OF THE SPLEEN

Trauma

The spleen is highly vascular and is one of the organs most frequently damaged by abdominal trauma. In 20% of patients who present with splenic injury, associated rib fractures are found on X-ray examination. The spleen is particularly susceptible to injury when pathologically enlarged.

PATHOPHYSIOLOGY

Injury to the spleen can result in rupture, evulsion from its pedicle or tearing beneath the capsule, with possible formation of a subcapsular haematoma. Delayed rupture of the spleen occurs in about 5% of patients and is thought to be caused by haematoma bursting through the capsule wall. This usually occurs within 2 weeks of injury, but in a few cases can be delayed for months or even years.

Common presenting symptoms Rupture and evulsion of the spleen cause immediate intraperitoneal bleeding. As blood spreads throughout the peritoneal cavity, signs of haemorrhage and hypovolaemic shock may develop. Patients generally present as an acute abdominal emergency.

The patient experiences abdominal pain with particular tenderness in the left upper quadrant. Referred pain is often felt in the left shoulder tip. Bruising to the abdomen may or may not be evident.

Non-acute presentation Not all patients present with splenic injury in such a dramatic way. If a diagnosis is difficult to establish and splenic injury is suspected, vigilant and careful observation of the patient is vital. The patient will be admitted to hospital for close observation, which includes frequent monitoring of blood pressure, pulse, respiration and PO_2 saturations. Any pain experienced by the patient should be monitored, noting its site, type and duration. Whether the pain is increasing or decreasing may be relevant. Analgesics may initially be withheld, as they may mask the true situation. The patient will be fasted during this period of observation and should be given frequent oral hygiene.

Any change in the patient's condition should be reported immediately as, following rupture, temporary improvement in the patient's condition may precede sudden deterioration.

MEDICAL MANAGEMENT

Treatment Injury to the spleen is an indication for splenectomy, provided the organ cannot be conserved. Preference is given to conserving splenic tissue if at all possible by suturing capsular tears or by performing a partial splenectomy because of the risk of systemic infection following splenectomy (Forrest et al 1995). Another method used following injury is to wrap the spleen in an absorbable haemostatic mesh.

NURSING PRIORITIES AND MANAGEMENT: Splenectomy

General considerations

The patient may be in a distressed and anxious state and the nurse should give reassurance whilst measures are being taken to establish and administer i.v. fluids along with blood and blood products as required. Oxygen therapy may be commenced to raise the circulating levels and a urinary catheter is inserted to assess renal function. Blood pressure, pulse, respirations and PO_2 saturations should be closely monitored and any changes reported quickly. A nasogastric tube may be passed to empty the stomach contents and prevent aspiration. Analgesics to relieve pain should be given and their effect monitored.

Relatives should be kept informed of what is happening and comfort and support given during this stressful and worrying time.

Perioperative care

In preparation for splenectomy, a full assessment of the patient's blood count and coagulation status must be made. In the presence of any bleeding tendency, a transfusion of blood or platelets may be administered. In patients with thrombocytopenia, platelets should be made available for use to cover the intra- and postoperative phase.

An antipneumococcal vaccine is given to prevent or minimise chest infection postoperatively; *Haemophilus influenzae* type B vaccine is also given prophylactically.

Preparation for surgery is as for abdominal surgery requiring general anaesthesia. A nasogastric tube is passed because handling of the stomach during surgery results in a temporary ileus.

In the postoperative period, the physiotherapist plays an important role in the care of these patients because of the increased risk of collapse of the left lower lobe of the lung. The nurse must encourage the patient to perform deep breathing exercises and aid expectoration between physiotherapy sessions. Some doctors advise the administration of low-dose heparin in all patients undergoing splenectomy as there will be a transient increase in platelet and leucocyte levels. The nurse must therefore be aware of the importance of passive exercises whilst the patient is on bed rest and encourage movement and early ambulation.

A complication that may follow splenectomy is pancreatitis caused by the handling and bruising of the tail of the pancreas during surgery. The nurse must therefore be alert to any change in the patient's condition, especially any increase or change in the nature of the pain experienced.

Due to the loss of lymphoid tissue, there is an increased risk of infection. As most infections occur within 3 years of splenectomy, some surgeons advise the use of prophylactic penicillin for this period, or even longer. This cover is mandatory when the patient is a child (Garden et al 2002).

Postoperative care is as for abdominal surgery requiring general anaesthesia and the patient will usually be nursed in a high-dependency area (see Nursing Care Plans 26.2, p. 922, and 26.4, p. 927).

Hypersplenism

Hypersplenism is a syndrome consisting of splenomegaly and pancytopenia and is common in patients with cirrhosis and associated portal hypertension. The bone marrow is normal and no autoimmune disease is present.

PATHOPHYSIOLOGY

Primary hypersplenism is due to hypertrophy of the spleen as a response to the need to destroy abnormal blood cells.

Secondary hypersplenism occurs when inappropriate cell destruction is secondary to splenic enlargement. It is unclear why some patients with cirrhosis develop hypersplenism but it is thought that, in portal hypertension, splenic congestion may lead to splenomegaly and hypersplenism. Other conditions causing splenic enlargement are haemolytic anaemia, idiopathic thrombocytopenic purpura, myelofibrosis and lymphoma. As ethanol has a direct toxic effect on the bone marrow and consequently blood cell production, a history of alcohol consumption may potentiate the manifestations of hypersplenism in cirrhotic patients (Peck-Radosavljevic 2001).

Clinical features The effects of hypersplenism include expansion of the blood volume to fill the increased vascular spaces. There is increased pooling of blood in the cells with excessive destruction, possibly induced by metabolic damage as the cells are packed tightly together in the enlarged spleen. Increased amounts of urobilinogen are present in the urine. Blood analysis will show anaemia, leucopenia and thrombocytopenia, and marrow turnover will be increased.

Evidence has also shown that severe hypersplenism is an independent predictor of variceal bleeding and spontaneous bacterial peritonitis (Liangpunsakal et al 2003).

MEDICAL MANAGEMENT

Management of hypersplenism in the cirrhotic patient is aimed at coping with effects such as variceal bleeding, infection and anaemia. Very rarely is splenectomy an option but it would be considered in cases of severe life-threatening anaemia as this may reduce the rate of red cell destruction.

NURSING PRIORITIES AND MANAGEMENT: Hypersplenism

In the context of gastrointestinal nursing, the nursing care of the patient with hypersplenism will be as for a patient with cirrhosis (see p. 138).

CONCLUSION

The many medical conditions included in this chapter highlight the wide variety of skills, and the depth of knowledge required, to nurse in the field of gastroenterology. Nurses specialising in gastrointestinal nursing, in addition to the essential and established skills of care, are now performing diagnostic and therapeutic endoscopy, measuring GI tract manometry and siting gastrostomy tubes. These advances are in line with evolving technology and the increased patient demand for rapid access to health care services and it is likely that the role will continue to evolve and grow to meet the needs of a modern health service. It is hoped that this chapter will provide the building blocks of knowledge required for gastrointestinal nursing now and in the future.

REFERENCES

Anderson M, Mutlu E, Siempliski M, Dimou C, Aronis C 2003 Web based intervention to increase colorectal cancer screening in primary care practices. Journal of General Internal Medicine 18(1): 128

Annesse V, Basciani M, Perri F et al 1996 Controlled trial of botulinum toxin versus placebo and pneumatic dilatation in achalasia. Gastroenterology 111: 1418–1424

Barber M D, Ross J A, Voss A C, Tisdale M J, Fearon K C H 1999 The effect of an oral nutritional supplement enriched with fish oil on weight loss in patients with pancreatic cancer. British Journal of Cancer 81(1): 80–86

Black P K 2000 Holistic stoma care. Harcourt, London

Blair C, Hayes P 1997 Hepatitis C. Current concepts. Proceedings of the Royal College of Physicians of Edinburgh 27: 300–310

Bowden S 2001 New hepatitis viruses: contenders and pretenders. Gastroenterology and Hepatology 16(2): 124–131

Burkitt D 1971 Epidemiology of cancer of the colon and rectum. Cancer 28: 3–13

Burkitt H G, Quick C R G, Gatt D 2002 Essential surgery: problems, diagnosis and management, 3rd edn. Churchill Livingstone, Edinburgh

Bynum T E 1991 Non acid mechanisms of gastric and duodenal ulcer formation [review]. Journal of Clinical Gastroenterology 13(Suppl 2): S56–64

Camilleri M, Choi M 1997 Irritable bowel syndrome [review]. Alimentary Pharmacology and Therapeutics 11: 3–15

Carty E, Rampton D 2003 Evaluation of new therapies for inflammatory bowel disease. British Journal of Pharmacology 56(4): 351–361

Chen C, Yu M, Liaw Y 1997 Epidemiological characteristics and risk factors of hepatocellular carcinoma. Journal of Gastroenterology and Hepatology 12(9–10): S294–308

Chua E, Garvey C, Kingsnorth A N, Rhodes J M 1997 A 49-year-old with a duodenal ulcer and a mass in the head of her pancreas. Lancet 349(9046): 174

Collier L, Oxford J 2000 Human virology, 2nd edn. Oxford University Press, Oxford

Crowcroft N 2001 Guidelines for the control of hepatitis A virus infection. Communicable Disease and Public Health 4(3): 213–227

Cuilliere C, Ducrotte F, Metman E et al 1997 Achalasia: outcome of patients treated with intersphincteric injection of botulinum toxin. Gut 41: 87–92

Daley R, Rebuck J, Wellage L, Rogers F 2004 Prevention of stress ulceration: current trends in critical care. Critical Care Medicine 32(10): 2008–2013

Delvaux M 2003 Functional bowel disorders and irritable bowel syndrome in Europe. Alimentary Pharmacology and Therapeutics 18(3): 75–79

Doughty B 2000 Urinary and faecal incontinence. Nursing management. Mosby, St Louis

Fawcett T M, Smith G D 2004 Jaundice: its causes and care. Gastrointestinal Nursing 2(1): 23–27

Fawcett T M, Smith G D 2005 Acute pancreatitis: pathophysiology and patient care. Gastrointestinal Nursing 3(8): 31–39

Forrest A P M, Carter D C, McLeod I B 1995 Principles and practice of surgery, 3rd edn. Churchill Livingstone, Edinburgh

Garden O J 2002 Hepatobiliary and pancreatic surgery, 2nd edn. WB Saunders, London

Garden O J, Bradbury A W, Forsyth J 2002 Principles and practice of surgery, 4th edn. Churchill Livingstone, Edinburgh

Gonsalkorale W, Miller V, Afzal A, Whorwell P 2003 Long term benefits of hypnotherapy for irritable bowel syndrome. Gut 52(11): 1623–1629

Griffin S M, Raimes S A 1997 Upper gastrointestinal surgery. WB Saunders, London

Haslett C, Chilvers E R, Boon N A, College N A 2002 Davidson's principles and practice of medicine, 19th edn. Churchill Livingstone, Edinburgh

Heading R, Tibaldi M 1998 Oesophageal symptoms and motility disorders. Medicine 26(7): 1–6

Jalan R, Hayes P 1997 Hepatic encephalopathy and ascites. Lancet 350(1): 1309–1315

Jewell D P 2002 Pathogenesis of inflammatory bowel disease – an update. Immunology Supplement 107 Supplement 1 61

Keighley M R B, Williams N S 1999 Surgery of

the anus, rectum and colon, 2nd edn. WB Saunders, London
Kjaerheim K, Gaard M, Andersen A 1998 The role of alcohol, tobacco and dietary factors in upper aerogastric tract cancers: a prospective study of 10,900 Norwegian men. Cancer Causes and Control 9(1): 99–108
Lee S 2003 Indicators and predictors of response to antiviral therapy in chronic hepatitis C. Alimentary Pharmacology and Therapeutics 17(5): 611–621
Liangpunsakal S, Ulmer B, Chalasani N 2003 Predictors and implications of severe hypersplenism in patients with cirrhosis. American Journal of Medical Science 326(3): 111–116
Lindars J, Sergeant T 1994 Quality of life in patients with oesophageal carcinoma. Nursing Times 90(43): 31–32
Logan R F 1998 Inflammatory bowel disease incidence: up, down or unchanged? Gut 42(3): 309–311
Love J, Irvine E, Fedorak R 1992 Quality of life in inflammatory bowel disease. Journal of Clinical Gastroenterology 14: 15–19
Marshall B J, Warren J R 1984 Unidentified curved bacilli in the stomachs of patients with gastritis and peptic ulceration. Lancet 1: 1311–1315
Mayor S 2002 Single flexible sigmoidoscopy screening could help prevent colorectal cancer. British Medical Journal 324(7343): 934
McCaughan E, Parahoo K 2000 Medical and surgical nurses' perceptions of their level of competence and educational needs in caring for patients with cancer. Journal of Clinical Nursing 9: 420–428
McNamara M J, Alexander H R, Norton J A 1992 Cytokines and their role in the pathophysiology of cancer cachexia. Journal of Parenteral and Enteral Nutrition 16: 505–555
Moreno E F, Dominguez J M, Sagar P M, Pemberton J H 1996 Update on ileal pouch–anal anastomosis. Revista de Gastroenterologia de Mexico 61(4): 387–393
Neuberger J, Lucey M R 1994 Liver transplantation: practice and management. BMJ Publishing Group, London
Nicklin J, Blazeby J 2003 Anorexia in patients dying from oesophageal and gastric cancers. Gastrointestinal Nursing 1(7): 35–39
Nissen N, Martin P 2002 Hepatocellular carcinoma: the high risk patient. Journal of Clinical Gastroenterology 35(5)(Suppl 2): S79–S85
Norton C 2001 Nursing for continence, 2nd edn. Beaconsfield Publishers, Beaconsfield
Peck-Radosavljevic M 2001 Hypersplenism. European Journal of Gastroenterology and Hepatology 13: 317–323
Pisani P, Bray F, Parkin D M 2002 Estimates of the world-wide prevalence of cancer for 25 sites in the adult population. International Journal of Cancer 97(1): 72–81
Porrett T, Daniel N 1999 Essential coloproctology for nurses. Whurr, London
Quigley E M M 2003 New developments in the pathophysiology of gastro-oesophageal reflux disease (GERD): implications for patient management. Alimentary Pharmacology and Therapeutics 17(Suppl 2): 43–51
Redhead D N, Chalmers N, Simpson K, Hayes P 1993 Transjugular portasystemic stent shunting (TIPSS). A review. Journal of Interventional Radiology 8: 37–41
Rockall T, Logan R, Devlin H, Northfield T 1995 Incidence and mortality from acute upper gastrointestinal haemorrhage in the United Kingdom. British Medical Journal 311(6999): 222–226
Scottish Intercollegiate Guidelines Network (SIGN) 2003 Guideline 67: Management of colorectal cancer. SIGN, Edinburgh
Tjandra J J, Clunie G J A, Thomas R J S 2001 Textbook of surgery, 2nd edn. Blackwell Science, Oxford
UK Transplant Statistics Department 2004 Online. Available: www.uktransplant.org.uk
Waugh A, Grant A 2001 Ross and Wilson's anatomy and physiology, 9th edn. Churchill Livingstone, Edinburgh
Whitehead S 1988 Illustrated operation notes. Edward Arnold, London
Williams J 2002 The essentials of pouch care nursing. Whurr, London
Younger H M, Bathgate A J, Hayes C 2004 Nucleoside analogues for the treatment of chronic hepatitis B [review]. Alimentary Pharmacology and Therapeutics 20: 1211–1230

FURTHER READING

Black P K 2000 Holistic stoma care. Harcourt, London
Bosonnet L 2003 Pruritus: scratching the surface. European Journal of Cancer Care 12(2): 162–166
Corner J, Bailey C 2001 Cancer nursing: care in context. Blackwell Science, Oxford
Cotton P, Ackerman U 2003 Practical gastrointestinal endoscopy: the fundamentals, 5th edn. Blackwell Science, Oxford
Cottrill M R B 1996 Helicobacter pylori. Professional Nurse 12(1): 46–48
Donahue P A 1990 When it's hard to swallow: feeding techniques for dysphagia management. Journal of Gerontological Nursing 16(4): 6–9, 41–42
Evans G 2001 A rationale for oral care. Nursing Standard 15(43): 33–36
Garden O J 2002 Hepatobiliary and pancreatic surgery, 2nd edn. WB Saunders, London
Garden O J, Bradbury A W, Forsyth J 2002 Principles and practice of surgery, 4th edn. Churchill Livingstone, Edinburgh
Heading R C 1999 Disorders of oesophageal motility. In: Bianchi Porro G, Isselbacher K J (eds) Gastroenterology and hepatology. Clinical medicine series. McGraw-Hill, Milan
Kamm M A, Lennard-Jones J E 1994 Constipation. Wrightson, Petersfield
Keighley M R B, Williams N S 1999 Surgery of the anus, rectum and colon, 2nd edn. WB Saunders, London
Koivusalo A, Yildrim Y, Vakkur A, Lindgren L, Hockerstedt K, Isoniemi H 2003 Experience with albumin dialysis in five patients with severe overdoses of paracetamol. Acta Anaesthesiologica Scandinavica 47(9): 1145–1150
MacConnachie A M 1997 Eradication therapy in peptic ulcer disease. Intensive and Critical Care Nursing 13: 121–122
Miller F 1996 Using a stent to treat patients with portal hypertension. Nursing Standard 10(26): 42–45
Norton C 2001 Nursing for continence, 2nd edn. Beaconsfield Publishers, Beaconsfield
Owen W 2001 Dysphagia. British Medical Journal 323(7317): 850–853
Plevris J, Schina M, Hayes P 1998 The management of acute liver failure [review]. Alimentary Pharmacology and Therapeutics 12: 405–418
Porrett T, Daniel N 1999 Essential coloproctology for nurses. Whurr, London
Pratt R 2003 Prevention and control of viral hepatitis. Nursing Standard 17(33): 43–52, 54–55
Riordan S, Williams R 1997 Current concepts: treatment of hepatic encephalopathy. New England Journal of Medicine 337(7): 473–479
Schofield P, Dunham M 2003 Pain assessment: how far have we come in listening to our patients? Professional Nurse 18(5): 276–279
Shearman D J C, Finlayson N, Camilleri M 1997 Diseases of the gastrointestinal tract and liver, 3rd edn. Churchill Livingstone, Edinburgh
Stanley A, Hayes P 1997 Portal hypertension and variceal haemorrhage. Lancet 350: 1235–1239
Starr S, Hand H 2002 Nursing care of chronic and acute liver failure. Nursing Standard 16(40): 47–56
Tjandra J J, Clunie G J, Thomas R J 2001 Textbook of surgery, 2nd edn. Blackwell Science, Oxford
University of York, NHS Centre for Reviews and Dissemination 1995 Helicobacter pylori and peptic ulcer. Effectiveness Matters 1(2)
Waugh A, Grant A 2001 Ross and Wilson's anatomy and physiology, 9th edn. Churchill Livingstone, Edinburgh
Young G P, Rozen P, Levin B 1996 Prevention and early detection of colorectal cancer. WB Saunders, London

USEFUL WEBSITES

British Colostomy Association
www.bcass.org.uk

British Liver Trust
www.britishlivertrust.org.uk

Coeliac UK
www.coeliac.org.uk

IBS Network
www.ibsnetwork.org.uk

Ileostomy Association (ia – the Ileostomy and Internal Pouch Support Group)
www.the-ia.org.uk

National Association for Colitis and Crohn's Disease (NACC)
www.nacc.org.uk

Scottish Intercollegiate Guidelines Network
www.sign.ac.uk

UK Transplant
www.uktransplant.org.uk

ENDOCRINE AND METABOLIC DISORDERS

5

Maggie N. Carson

PART 1 **ENDOCRINE AND METABOLIC DISORDERS**

Kay Malloch, Joan Allwinkle

PART 2 **DIABETES MELLITUS**

PART 1 ENDOCRINE AND METABOLIC DISORDERS

INTRODUCTION

Endocrinology is the study of hormones — chemical messengers secreted by endocrine cells and neurones. Hormones, usually travelling in the bloodstream, maintain homeostasis by acting on and coordinating activity within target organs or tissues.

Endocrinology is a rapidly growing field (Wilson 2005). The word hormone was first used by Ernest Starling in 1905 and the study of endocrinology developed from that date. Considerable progress is being made, with important implications for other areas of medicine, e.g. neuroendocrinology, which in turn has important applications within psychiatry. Advances are constantly being made in this field and current research is adding to knowledge of genetic causes of many endocrine conditions. For example, the site of the mutation in the genes that causes both syndromes of multiple endocrine neoplasia (MEN I and MEN II) has been discovered (Thakker 1998, 2004). Identifying carriers of the mutation will allow biochemical screening of individuals before they are symptomatic, therefore providing an opportunity for earlier treatment (Bassett et al 1998). Genetic research is an area from which future treatments of endocrine disease will come. There are other areas of endocrinology that are not covered in this chapter, mostly rare conditions. A list of further reading at the end of the chapter will give the reader plenty of scope for further study.

Apart from diabetes mellitus and thyroid disorders, endocrine problems are not common. Many endocrine disorders are rarely seen and may be difficult to diagnose without complicated and exhaustive testing. As a result, patients may be referred by their general practitioner or local hospital to specialist centres for diagnosis. For the patient, this has the advantage of offering highly specialised care. It also means that relatively few nurses have the opportunity to treat and care for people with these disorders. However, given the wide-ranging effects of endocrine dysfunction, it is important that all nurses have a general understanding of endocrinology. Endocrine diseases can affect every system of the body, sometimes causing disfigurement and a change in body image or even posing a threat to life. These disorders can seriously affect the patient's psychological outlook, either as a direct result of the illness or by virtue of the individual's reaction to it.

It is well documented that individuals react differently to being ill. Some view their situation as a challenge, while others see it as a punishment, react with anger or try to apportion blame. Anger may be directed at family members or at nursing and medical staff (Sinclair & Fawcett 1991). This situation may be exacerbated by an unstable mental state, mood swings, depression or frank psychosis, which may, in fact, be sequelae of the disorder, e.g. Cushing's syndrome. The nurse must be aware of this possibility and react accordingly, offering support and understanding to the patient and their relatives. Identifying the patient's worries and concerns, providing factual information and educating the patient about their condition and its management will all help to minimise psychological distress. Explanations that the underlying illness may be influencing the patient's mood may help them and their relatives to cope (Ramirez & House 1997).

As the tests and investigations required to diagnose some of the rarer endocrine conditions are often long and exhausting, clear explanations are essential so that the patient understands the need for them and the procedures that will be followed. This will help to reduce anxiety and increase the patient's confidence in the health care team. The psychological support that the nurse can offer this group of patients cannot be overemphasised. Many benefit from referral to a patient support group (see 'Useful Websites', p. 189) and the contact this brings with other patients, who have the same condition. Often these patients are young and probably otherwise in good health, and therefore the impact of endocrine disease on their body image and/or self-esteem should not be underestimated. For example, patients experiencing sexual dysfunction may feel embarrassed to talk to and seek support from family members and friends — in such cases, support from the health care professional is crucial.

For further information on the psychological care of medical patients and recognition of need and service provision, see RCP/RCPsych (1995).

ANATOMY AND PHYSIOLOGY

The nature of the endocrine system, being one of control, means that it has far-reaching effects throughout the body on various target organs. In order to make this chapter as clear as possible, each endocrine gland will be considered separately. In cases where a disease is caused by the abnormal secretion of a trophic or control hormone, the disease will be discussed under the heading of the end organ. For example, in Cushing's disease, adrenocorticotrophic hormone (ACTH) is secreted in excess by the pituitary gland. This acts on the adrenal gland, causing it to produce excess amounts of cortisol. Therefore, as the adrenal gland is the end organ, and it is the secretion from this gland that causes unwanted effects on the body, Cushing's disease is discussed under the heading of the adrenal gland.

Hormones

The endocrine system is one of the two major control systems of the body, the other being the nervous system. The nervous system mediates its activity by means of nerves directly supplying the organs and structures to which it relates. The endocrine system operates by a system of hormones, which are secreted into the bloodstream for transport to their respective target organs.

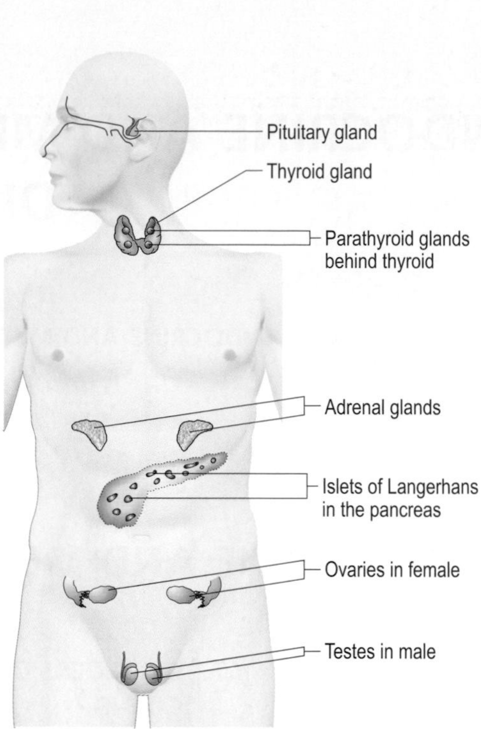

Fig. 5.1 The endocrine glands and their location in the body.

The endocrine glands and their anatomical position are shown in Figure 5.1.

Action

Although the hormones are carried to every cell in the body, they affect only those cells or organs upon which they have an excitatory or inhibitory action. This system allows individuals to respond to changes in their environment and is important in controlling growth and development, sexual maturation and homeostasis.

Many hormones are bound to proteins within the circulation. It is now known that only unbound or free hormones are biologically active, and that binding serves as a buffer against very rapid changes in plasma levels of a hormone. This principle is important in the interpretation of many tests of endocrine function.

Control

Most hormone systems are controlled by a feedback system which ensures that hormone levels, whilst fluctuating, remain within a preset range (see Table 5.1). Figure 5.2 illustrates how negative feedback operates in the hypothalamic–pituitary–thyroid axis.

Pattern of secretion

Hormone secretion is either continuous or intermittent. An example of the former is the secretion of thyroxine by the thyroid gland, in which hormone levels over a day, month or year show very little variation. Intermittent secretion is seen in three forms: circadian, menstrual and pulsatile.

Table 5.1 List of normal ranges (these may vary for different laboratories)

Hormone			SI units
Aldosterone (normal diet)	Pose	Upright (4 h) Supine (30 min)	330–830 pmol/L 135–400 pmol/L
Cortisol	Time	09.00 h 18.00 h 00.00 h (asleep)	200–700 nmol/L 100–300 nmol/L <50 nmol/L
11-deoxycortisol	Time	09.00 h	7–18 nmol/L
Dehydroepiandosterone (DHEA) sulphate	Time	09.00 h	7–31 nmol/L
DHEA sulphate	Population	Women Men Prepubertal	3–12 μmol/L* 2–10 μmol/L* <0.5 μmol/L*
Androstenedione	Population	Adults Prepubertal	3–8 nmol/L <1 nmol/L
Oestradiol	Population	Prepubertal Women Postmenopausal Follicular Mid-cycle Luteal Men	<20 pmol/L <100 pmol/L 200–400 pmol/L 400–1200 pmol/L 400–1000 pmol/L <180 pmol/L
Progesterone	Population	Women Follicular Luteal Men	 <10 nmol/L >30 nmol/L <6 nmol/L
Testosterone	Population	Prepubertal Men Women	<0.8 nmol/L 9–35 nmol/L 0.5–3.0 nmol/L
ACTH	Time	09.00 h	7–51 ng/L
FSH	Population	Prepubertal Women Postmenopausal Follicular Mid-cycle Luteal Men	<5 U/L >30 U/L 3.0–15 U/L up to 20 U/L 3.0–15 U/L 1–7 U/L
GH	Fasting between pulses		<1 mU/L
LH	Population	Prepubertal Women Postmenopausal Follicular Mid-cycle Luteal Men	<5 U/L >30 U/L 2.5–10 U/L 25–70 U/L <1–13 U/L 1–10 U/L
Prolactin			<360 mU/L
TSH			0.4–5 mU/L
Thyroxine (free)			10–20 pmol/L
Tri-iodothyronine (free)			5–10 pmol/L
Catecholamines	Taken with patient cannulated and lying for 30 min prior	Adrenaline Noradrenaline	0.03–1.31 nmol/L 0.47–4.14 nmol/L

Adapted from Besser & Trainer (1995).

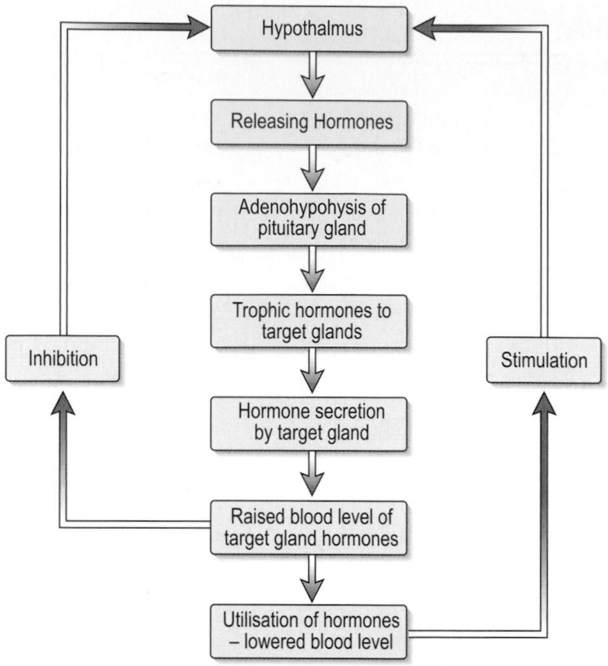

Fig. 5.2 Negative feedback regulation of the secretion of anterior pituitary hormones.

Other factors which affect hormone secretion include stress, disease, trauma, surgery or emotional upset. As in any complex regulatory system, it is likely that disequilibrium in endocrine function will have important consequences. Disorders of the endocrine system may be categorised most simply as those involving overproduction (hypersecretion) and those involving underproduction (hyposecretion).

For further information, see Montague et al (2005).

DISORDERS OF THE PITUITARY GLAND AND HYPOTHALAMUS

As stated above, disorders of the endocrine system result in either an oversecretion or an undersecretion of a hormone. Therefore, in principle, treatment should be straightforward, either replacing the missing hormone or removing, or suppressing the source of, the oversecretion. Advances have made the treatment of the wide range of endocrine disorders more successful, and the outlook for those suffering from them is becoming ever more hopeful.

Hypersecretion of a hormone usually arises from a so-called 'functioning' pituitary adenoma. As this adenoma grows, it is likely to 'crowd out' the normal function of other areas of the pituitary, and as a result progressive hypopituitarism occurs. This failure of the pituitary hormones occurs in a characteristic sequence (Besser & Thorner 2002). Secretion of growth hormone (GH) is lost first, followed by the gonadotrophins luteinising hormone (LH) and follicle-stimulating hormone (FSH), thyroid-stimulating hormone (TSH) and then adrenocorticotrophic hormone (ACTH). Prolactin (PRL) deficiency is rare except as seen postpartum in Sheehan's syndrome.

ANATOMY AND PHYSIOLOGY

The existence of the pituitary gland has been known for at least 2000 years. It lies immediately below the hypothalamus in the pituitary fossa. It is connected to the hypothalamus by the pituitary stalk and consists of two lobes — anterior and posterior — which function independently of each other (see Fig. 5.3). In the developing fetus the anterior lobe is formed from Rathke's pouch, which grows upwards and becomes separated from the oropharynx to become the adenohypophysis. The posterior lobe is a down-growth from the forebrain, which becomes the neurohypophysis. The posterior pituitary contains nerve fibres which grow into it from the hypothalamus via the pituitary stalk. The hormones secreted by the pituitary gland, together with their action, are listed in Table 5.2.

The hypothalamus is part of the floor of the third ventricle of the brain. It is an area of specialised cells or nuclei which produce hormones. These hormones regulate pituitary function and act as releasing factors for the anterior pituitary hormones (see Fig. 5.4). The hypothalamus also controls many centres for functions such as appetite, thirst, temperature regulation, sexual activity, sleeping and waking.

The pituitary stalk carries blood to both lobes of the pituitary in a portal system by which the hypothalamic releasing or inhibitory hormones are carried to the anterior pituitary. The trophic hormones produced in the anterior pituitary stimulate the peripheral endocrine glands. The posterior pituitary acts as a reservoir for antidiuretic hormone (ADH)/vasopressin and oxytocin.

The optic chiasm sits just above the pituitary fossa. Therefore, an expanding lesion from the pituitary or the hypothalamus may result in a defect in the visual fields because of pressure on the optic nerve or optic chiasm.

Hyper- or hyposecretion of hormones or local effects of a tumour will all disturb the balance of the system.

HYPERSECRETION OF THE ANTERIOR PITUITARY HORMONES

Hypersecretion of adrenocorticotrophic hormone: Cushing's disease

Cushing's disease is found when an excess of glucocorticoid secretions is stimulated by an ACTH-producing adenoma of the pituitary. As noted above, this disease will be discussed under 'Disorders of the adrenal cortex' (p. 178).

Hypersecretion of growth hormone: acromegaly and gigantism

Aetiology

Acromegaly is a rare condition caused by prolonged, excessive secretion of growth hormone (GH) from a benign tumour of the pituitary gland occurring after fusion of the epiphyses of the long bones. The word acromegaly comes from the Greek 'akron' meaning extremities and 'megas' meaning great. It has a prevalence of 40–60 cases/million in the UK and an incidence of four new cases a year

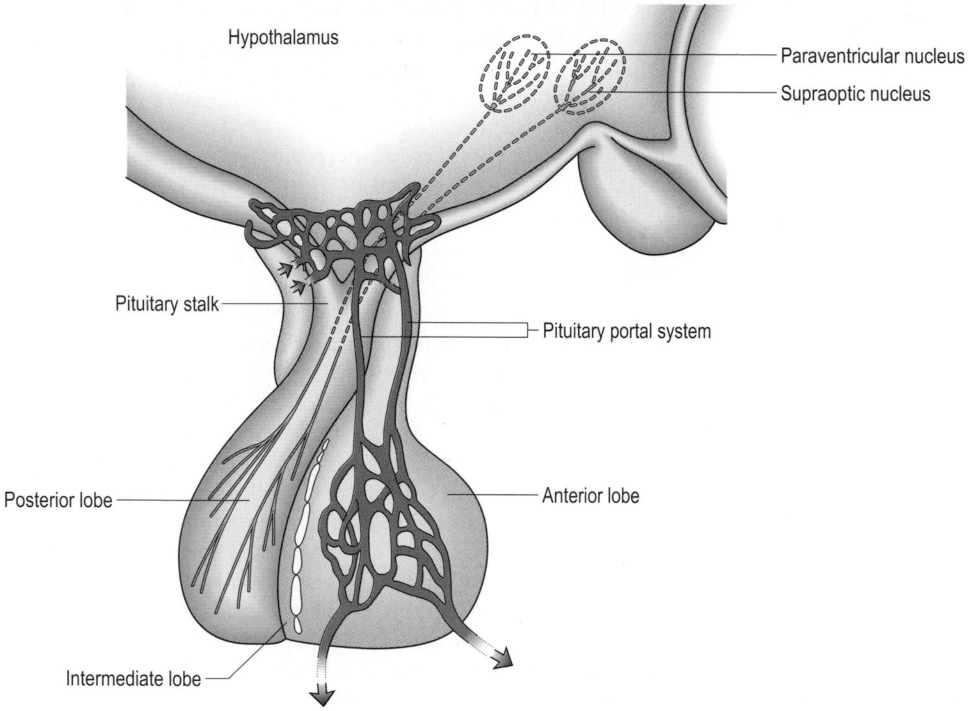

Fig. 5.3 Position of the pituitary and its associated structures.

Table 5.2 Hormones of the pituitary gland and their action

Hormone	Action
Anterior lobe Growth hormone (GH)	Pulsatile release. Does not have a single target gland but acts on a variety of tissues, e.g. bone, viscera and soft tissues. It is particularly important in children to stimulate growth. Action in adults recently thought to involve maintenance of cardiovascular activity, fat deposition and muscle development
Prolactin (PRL)	Main action is to stimulate lactation in females; also stimulates corpus luteum to secrete progesterone
Adrenocorticotrophic hormone (ACTH)	Secreted under circadian rhythm. Stimulates the adrenal cortex to secrete corticosteroids
Luteinising hormone (LH)	Promotes ovulation; stimulates formation of the corpus luteum
Follicle-stimulating hormone (FSH)	Stimulates the production of sex hormones and contributes to regulation of the menstrual cycle in women. In women, stimulates the production of ovarian follicles and secretion of oestrogen; in men, promotes the production of spermatozoa
Thyroid-stimulating hormone (TSH)	Stimulates the thyroid to release thyroxine
Posterior lobe Vasopressin — also called antidiuretic hormone (ADH)	Controls water homeostasis in the body by regulating water reabsorption from the renal tissues
Oxytocin	Induces uterine contraction during labour and ejection of milk from breasts postpartum

(Wass 2001). The incidence in men and women is equal. The mean age at diagnosis is between 40 and 50 years, although excessive secretion of growth hormone can occur at any age and, in children in whom fusion of the epiphyses has not yet occurred, leads to gigantism. Acromegaly leads to a reduction in life expectancy with a two- to four-fold increase in mortality rate (Colao et al 2004).

PATHOPHYSIOLOGY

Clinical features The onset of the disease is insidious, leading on average to a delay in diagnosis of around 8 years from the onset of symptoms, which include:

- excessive sweating, seen in >80% of patients
- headaches

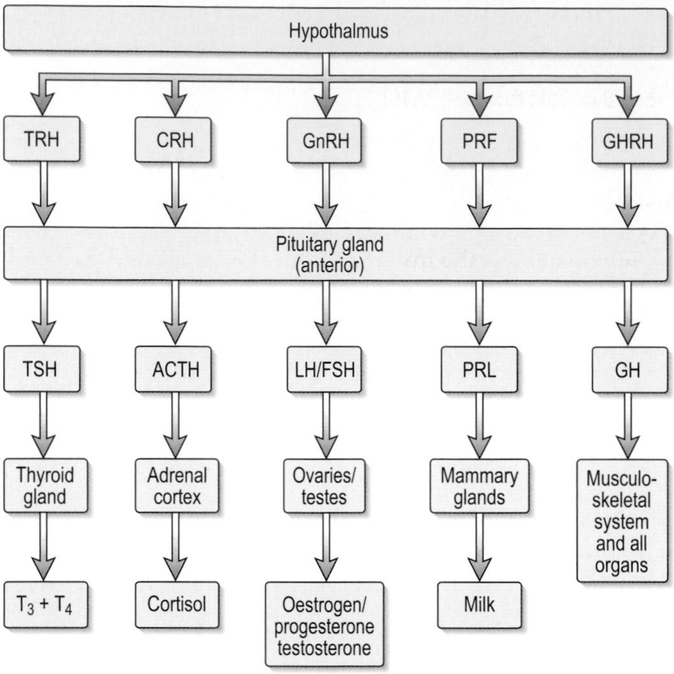

Fig. 5.4 Schematic diagram showing the relationship between the hypothalamus, the pituitary gland and their target organs. TRH, thyrotrophin-releasing hormone; CRH, corticotrophin-releasing hormone; GnRH, gonadotrophin-releasing hormone; PRF, prolactin-releasing factor; GHRH, growth hormone releasing hormone; TSH, thyroid-stimulating hormone; ACTH, adrenocorticotrophic hormone; LH/FSH, luteinising hormone/follicle-stimulating hormone; PRL, prolactin; GH, growth hormone.

- enlargement of the hands and feet, often resulting in the need for ring size and shoe size to be increased
- tiredness and lethargy
- joint pain and osteoarthritis
- coarse facial features, frontal bossing, enlarged nose, protruding jaw and increased interdental separation
- oily skin
- deep voice
- tongue enlargement
- soft tissue swelling
- goitre and other organomegaly
- features of hyperprolactinaemia
- visual field defects.

Complications include:

- hypertension in approximately 40% of patients
- insulin resistance, impaired glucose tolerance and diabetes mellitus in approximately 20% of patients
- obstructive sleep apnoea
- increased risk of colonic polyps and colonic carcinoma
- ischaemic heart disease
- cerebrovascular disease
- congestive cardiac failure (Colao et al 2004).

Common presenting symptoms The patient may notice an increase in their shoe size or the fact that they have had to have their wedding ring enlarged. Along with their family and friends they may notice a change in their facial appearance. Women often feel very self-conscious about this, and also about their deepening voice, as they may be mistaken for men on the telephone. The major symptoms, which prompt a consultation with their GP, are usually headache and sweating. Visual symptoms may be identified by their ophthalmologist, or their dentist may notice their enlarging jaw and/or increasing spacing between their teeth. Patients can therefore find themselves referred to an endocrinologist by a number of routes.

MEDICAL MANAGEMENT

Investigations Diagnosis can be confirmed following clinical examination and pituitary function testing. On clinical examination, some or all of the symptoms listed above may be present. Magnetic resonance imaging (MRI) usually shows the pituitary tumour and whether there is enlargement of the pituitary fossa. If acromegaly is suspected, a blood sample should be obtained and an insulin-like growth factor 1 (IGF-1) and random GH level measured. If the IGF-1 level is 'normal', when compared to the age-adjusted range, and GH <0.5 mU/L, the diagnosis of acromegaly can be excluded (Trainer 2002). Otherwise, the patient should proceed to have an oral glucose tolerance test (OGTT). The OGTT has been the gold standard for the diagnosis of acromegaly for many years. False positives may occur if the patient has diabetes mellitus, renal or liver disease, or anorexia nervosa. In acromegaly, measurement of GH levels during the OGTT are consistently elevated and fail to suppress to <2 mU/L in response to a 75 g oral glucose load. Normally, the level of GH would be undetectable. Acromegaly is therefore diagnosed on the basis of an elevated IGF-1 and failure to suppress GH during the OGTT (Giustina et al 2000). Further pituitary function tests may be performed to assess whether the remainder of the pituitary gland has been compromised. Prolactin is co-secreted in 30% of tumours.

For further information, see Bouloux & Rees (1994).

Treatment In untreated acromegaly, the mortality is nearly twice that of the normal population; early treatment is therefore essential. The aim of treatment is to relieve and, if possible, resolve symptoms associated with elevated GH and IGF-1 levels and the local effects caused by the tumour mass itself, and to prevent co-morbidity by lowering mean GH and IGF-1 levels to accepted 'safe' levels with minimal disruption to the patient's lifestyle. Treatment may take the form of surgery, radiotherapy or medication (Wass 2001).

Surgery This is currently regarded as the first-line therapy for acromegaly and, when performed by a pituitary surgeon, remains the treatment of choice. Hypophysectomy via the trans-sphenoidal route, which has a low morbidity and mortality, is the surgical procedure most commonly used. It results in a rapid fall in GH levels, often with no loss of any other pituitary hormones. As a mode of treatment it is both rapid and inexpensive when compared to medical therapies. In patients with microadenomas (tumours <1 cm diameter) it is curative in ~80% of cases. In macroadenomas (tumours >1 cm diameter) this figure is nearer 40% (Kaltsas et al 2001).

Radiotherapy Conventional external beam radiotherapy (4500 cGy over 25 fractions) results in a delayed fall in

GH and IGF-1 levels over the following decade which is paralleled by the development of hypopituitarism (Wass 1997). Sixty per cent of patients have a normal IGF-1 after 5 years, rising to 84% of patients after 15 years (Biermasz et al 2000). Although used less often nowadays, it is safe and radiation-induced visual damage is extremely rare. Patients must be advised that they may feel tired during the period of treatment and may experience some temporary alopecia at the site of entry of the beams. Anecdotally, many patients later complain that their short-term memory has been affected, but evidence to support this is scanty. It is a useful treatment for patients in whom surgery is contra-indicated or if GH/IGF-1 levels are not too high and/or there is a large tumour or residual tumour postoperatively, or where medical therapy fails to control GH/IGF-1 levels. Other forms of radiotherapy include stereotactic or gamma knife radiotherapy (radiosurgery) which takes the form of a single dose (upper limit 8–9 cGy) administered as many beams. This is more expensive than conventional radiotherapy but is a 'one-off' cost. Long-term data are required, but early results suggest that GH and IGF-1 levels fall more rapidly for radiosurgery than with conventional radiotherapy and there is less damage to surrounding tissues which may reduce the incidence of radiotherapy-induced hypopituitarism (Swords et al 2003). These two forms of radiotherapy can be given following conventional radiotherapy but cannot be used if the tumour is in close proximity to the optic chiasm.

Medication This has changed radically in recent years. It is now possible to control GH and IGF-1 levels in more than half of patients with a somatostatin analogue, a synthetic compound which acts on the somatostatin receptors of the tumour and suppresses the secretion of GH, e.g. lanreotide (Somatuline Autogel) or octreotide (Sandostatin Lar). These are given by deep intramuscular or subcutaneous injection by a nurse every 28 days and are the most widely used form of medical therapy. There is evidence of tumour shrinkage in a large minority of cases, probably due to cell shrinkage rather than cell death (Bevan et al 2002). If the patient is resistant to this class of medication, pegvisomant (Somavert), a GH receptor antagonist, i.e. it binds to GH receptors, blocking the impact of excessive circulating GH which in turn causes IGF-1 levels to fall, can be used. This medication is capable of achieving normal IGF-1 levels in >90% of patients (van der Lely et al 2001). It is given by a once daily subcutaneous injection; however, it is very expensive and is currently used only for patients with active disease who have failed to respond to other medical therapies. Previously, patients were treated using dopamine agonists, the first effective medical treatment for acromegaly, e.g. bromocriptine or cabergoline, both tablets, taken orally. However, 'safe' levels of GH were achieved in only approximately 10% of patients on bromocriptine and 39% of patients on cabergoline (Abs et al 1998).

Long-term treatment strategies for acromegaly have changed. Until recently, surgery and radiotherapy were used in conjunction, with medical therapy then used to control residual excess GH secretion, as radiotherapy only lowers GH levels gradually. Medical therapy may also be used preoperatively to control symptoms or to attempt to shrink a large tumour prior to surgery. In patients unfit for surgery, medical therapy alone may be used.

NURSING PRIORITIES AND MANAGEMENT: Acromegaly

Major considerations

Giving psychological support

Change in body image is an important feature of this disorder. The patient may have considerable difficulty in coming to terms with their changed appearance and may be anxious about the investigations they must undergo and the treatment that may be required.

It is important to create as relaxed an environment as possible and to reduce anxiety by spending time with the patient and their family, explaining the reasons for their changed appearance, the effect of therapy and the expected treatment outcome. They will be reassured to hear that biochemical cure may result in a return to a more normal appearance, although the degree will depend on the stage of the disease at the beginning of treatment. Some symptoms, such as sweating, may be cured almost immediately, while others, e.g. soft tissue swelling, may take longer to resolve. Bony changes are usually not reversible.

Some patients benefit from meeting other patients who have been treated successfully and, if the patient wishes, nursing staff should try to arrange this either directly or through a local patient support group.

Perioperative care

The reader is referred to Chapter 26 for principles of preoperative preparation and postoperative care, and to Chapter 23 for information on wound healing. Specific postoperative observations include neurological monitoring, with special care being taken to observe for leakage of cerebrospinal fluid from the nose which is a recognised complication (Baxter 1994). The patient is nursed well supported on pillows to ensure that an upright position is maintained. Recovery is usually rapid and the patient discharged home on the fourth or fifth postoperative day.

STOP THINK **5.1** Miss W, aged 45 years, has been diagnosed as having acromegaly. She has undergone trans-sphenoidal hypophysectomy for the removal of a GH-producing adenoma. Identify the specific or potential problems and devise a plan to meet her care needs. What long-term treatment and care will she require?

Prolactin hypersecretion

Aetiology

It is now known that prolactin is the most common hormone to be secreted by pituitary tumours and that small microadenomas (<1 cm in diameter) occur frequently (Haslett et al 2002). However, a wide variety of medications and diseases can cause high prolactin levels. Before carrying out extensive investigations for pituitary disease, it is important to exclude other pathological causes such as hypothyroidism and to take a detailed medication history. Medications that block the dopamine receptor and so elevate prolactin levels include tranquillisers, e.g. chlorpromazine (Largactil); antiemetics, e.g. metoclopramide (Maxolon); and some antidepressants, e.g. amitriptyline and fluoxetine (Prozac). The other key differential diagnosis is a hypothalamic or suprasellar space-occupying lesion which interferes with dopamine production. Dopamine is the natural prolactin inhibitory factor and therefore, in its absence, hyperprolactinaemia ensues; due to the mechanism this is known as disconnection hyperprolactinaemia.

PATHOPHYSIOLOGY

Hyperprolactinaemia causes galactorrhoea and amenorrhoea in women; the raised prolactin level suppresses gonadotrophin-releasing hormone (GnRH) secretion within the hypothalamus, leading to gonadotrophin deficiency (LH and FSH) and then oestrogen deficiency, resulting in infertility (Haslett et al 2002). In men, the galactorrhoea is much less frequent, but the elevated prolactin lowers LH and FSH levels which in turn lower testosterone levels, resulting in a reduced libido, impotence and infertility.

Common presenting symptoms in premenopausal women include menstrual disturbances, e.g. amenorrhoea, oligomenorrhoea (infrequent menstrual flow) and infertility. Galactorrhoea occurs in about 80% of these women (Schlechte 2003). The majority of prolactinomas in women are small (<1 cm diameter and referred to as a microprolactinoma) at the time of diagnosis, so headaches and neurological deficits are rare. Men, on the other hand, may present with headache, visual loss, cranial nerve defects and/or hypopituitarism due to the mass effect of the tumour which tends to be larger at the time of diagnosis (>1 cm in diameter and referred to as a macroprolactinoma). In both men and women elevated levels of prolactin over a long period can lead to low bone density which increases when prolactin levels are normalised but does not return to normal (Di Somma et al 1998).

MEDICAL MANAGEMENT

Investigations When other causes of the presenting symptoms have been excluded, prolactin levels should be measured in the unstressed patient. Because venepuncture is stressful, an intravenous cannula is placed in the patient's arm and the patient allowed to rest for 30 min prior to the blood sample being taken. The patient should not smoke or drink tea or coffee in this period. If the prolactin levels are raised, an MRI should be performed. If this shows a large pituitary tumour, tests of other pituitary functions should be carried out to see if there are any other pituitary hormone deficits. Visual field tests may also be carried out to assess if the tumour mass is causing pressure on the optic chiasm. Pituitary MRI will usually show even a small tumour of only a few millimetres in size. Prolactinomas are almost always benign.

Treatment The aim in the treatment of microprolactinomas is to lower the excessive levels of prolactin, thereby restoring gonadal function. In macroprolactinomas, the aim is to reduce tumour size, prevent tumour expansion and to restore gonadal function. Reduction of tumour size and lowering of hormone levels may be achieved by medication alone. Consequently, this is the treatment of choice (Molitch 2002). Prolactinomas respond well to dopamine agonists, e.g. bromocriptine (Parlodel), cabergoline or quinagolide. These result in a lowering of prolactin levels, restoration of gonadal function and termination of galactorrhoea, usually within a few weeks of starting treatment (de Rosa at el 1998). In most patients menstrual cycles resume and fertility is restored. Patients must therefore be given appropriate contraceptive advice. Trans-sphenoidal surgery is usually performed only in patients who are resistant to or cannot tolerate dopamine agonists. Irradiation of the pituitary gland results in a reduction in prolactin secretion, but this takes many years to achieve. Dopamine agonists are therefore continued while waiting for the effects of radiotherapy to occur, but the need for this treatment should be reassessed regularly.

NURSING PRIORITIES AND MANAGEMENT: Prolactin hypersecretion

Specific nursing care is aimed at ensuring that the medication regimen is followed correctly in order to avoid side-effects. Dopamine agonists, especially bromocriptine, often cause nausea, vomiting, constipation and postural hypotension mediated by dopamine release. Consequently, there should be a slow increase in dosage, the first doses being given whilst eating and on retiring to prevent the common symptoms of postural hypotension and gastric irritation. The dosage can then be built up gradually to 2.5 mg three times a day. Cabergoline, a longer acting dopamine agonist, need only be taken once or twice a week. It is more potent than bromocriptine and has a lower profile of side-effects (Webster 2000).

For further information, see Besser & Thorner (2002) and Liu & Couldwell (2004).

HYPOSECRETION OF THE ANTERIOR PITUITARY HORMONES

Hypopituitarism

The term hypopituitarism refers to partial or total deficiency of anterior pituitary hormone secretion. It may be associated with pathological processes that destroy the pituitary itself or with disturbance of the hypothalamic control of the pituitary. Total failure of all hormone production is termed panhypopituitarism.

Aetiology

As already stated, hypopituitarism is most commonly caused by the presence of a pituitary tumour. These are frequently benign. Pituitary carcinoma is very rare. Benign microadenomas having no clinical effects are surprisingly common and are found in up to 23% of people at postmortem (Bouloux & Rees 1994).

PATHOPHYSIOLOGY

Pituitary tumours can vary greatly in size and may extend outside the pituitary fossa to compress surrounding structures. They are generally classified as functioning or non-functioning, depending on whether they produce a hormone, e.g. GH or prolactin.

Common presenting symptoms Symptoms caused by local compression may arise (see Ch. 9, p. 408), but the individual usually presents with signs associated with pituitary hormone deficiency. The precise symptoms will vary in accordance with the particular hormone that is deficient (see Table 5.3).

MEDICAL MANAGEMENT

Investigations Diagnostic investigations include visual field testing and biochemical investigation to determine the severity and degree of pituitary failure and to distinguish between isolated hormone failure and complete anterior pituitary failure. MRI is also performed.

Treatment The choice of treatment will depend on the diagnosis of the cause of the pituitary failure and will aim to relieve the clinical effects and symptoms experienced by the patient. Treatment may involve surgery, radiotherapy to reduce the tumour and medication to replace the deficient hormones (see Table 5.4).

NURSING PRIORITIES AND MANAGEMENT: Hypopituitarism

Major considerations

Giving information

Effective nursing intervention depends upon the establishment of a good nurse–patient relationship in a friendly environment. As the effects of hypopituitarism can be widespread, causing diverse physical and psychological changes which can be difficult to comprehend, it is important to ensure that all of the patient's questions are answered in a way that is understood. Open and frank discussion about changes in body image and sexuality is essential to the individual concerned. Clear, ongoing explanations of the extensive and possibly uncomfortable investigations will help to relieve the patient's anxiety. The presence of a nurse known to the patient during these investigations can be reassuring.

Table 5.3 **Symptoms associated with anterior pituitary hormone hyposecretion**

Deficiency	Symptoms
LH/FSH	*Men* Poor libido and impotence Infertility Small soft testicles Loss of secondary sexual hair *Women* Amenorrhoea Infertility Dyspareunia Breast atrophy Loss of secondary sexual hair
TSH	*Children* Growth retardation *Adults* Decreased energy Constipation Sensitivity to cold Dry skin Weight gain
ACTH	*All* Weakness Tiredness Dizziness on standing Pallor Hypoglycaemia
GH	*Children* Growth retardation Short stature *Adults* Cardiovascular activity Muscle development Fat distribution General sense of well-being

Table 5.4 **Hormone replacement therapy**

Deficient hormone	Replacement	Check
Anterior pituitary		
Women		
LH	Ethinylestradiol	*Libido and symptoms of deficiency
FSH	Medroxyprogesterone	
Men		
LH	Testosterone	*Libido and potency
FSH		
Children	GH	Growth chart
ACTH	Hydrocortisone	Cortisol levels throughout the day
TSH	Thyroxine	T_3 and T_4 levels
Posterior pituitary		
ADH	Desmopressin	Plasma and urine osmolality

Reproduced with permission from Besser & Thorner (2002).

*For men and women, the only treatment of associated infertility entails regular injections of the deficient pituitary hormones (mainly FSH in the form of Pergonal or Metrodin) or, if the defect is hypothalamic, hourly parenteral injection of a gonadotrophin-releasing hormone via an implanted pump.

Neurosurgery or radiotherapy is a frightening prospect for most people. Preoperative preparation must include an explanation of procedures, the nature of immediate post-operative care and the expected long-term outcome. Reminding the patient that many of their symptoms will be relieved by surgery, radiotherapy and/or hormone replacement therapy will be of considerable psychological benefit.

Supporting the patient taking ongoing replacement therapy

Anterior pituitary hormone replacement

Cortisol Hydrocortisone, or sometimes prednisolone, is given to those who have ACTH deficiency. It is rapidly absorbed with a short half-life. The usual dose is 10 mg on waking, 5 mg at midday and 5 mg in the early evening. It can also be given as a twice-daily regimen with a total daily dose of 15–30 mg. It is important to monitor cortisol levels regularly, as over-replacement can be associated with hypertension, hyperglycaemia and hyperinsulinaemia, as well as reduced bone mineral density. The omission of even one dose may have serious consequences. Such patients should be advised to carry a steroid card and to wear a MedicAlert bracelet at all times, indicating they are cortisol deficient. Patients should also be given an emergency hydrocortisone pack to keep at home containing a vial of hydrocortisone for i.m. injection which they have been shown how to use. The nurse should demonstrate how to use this and ensure that the patient has practised and mastered the technique.

Thyroxine Thyroid replacement is given as an oral medication. The usual dose is 100–150 mcg/day, taken as one dose in the morning. As it has a very long half-life, the occasional missed dose is not critical. Thyroxine levels can be monitored by the patient's GP.

Growth hormone Until 1988 it was claimed that low levels of GH had little or no effect in adults, but studies have shown that replacement GH therapy in patients with adult onset GH deficiency has profound effects on patients' quality of life, vascular morbidity and cardiovascular mortality (Brooke & Monson 2003). It is now apparent that GH deficiency is associated with changes in body composition, bone density, lipid metabolism, physical performance and cardiovascular function (Mukherjee & Shalet 2004). GH replacement has been shown to improve symptoms and to reverse a number of the surrogate markers of metabolic and cardiovascular dysfunction. In 2003, the National Institute of Clinical Excellence (NICE) produced guidance for the prescription of GH in England and Wales which was subsequently ratified by the Health Technology Board for Scotland (HTBS). In order to be eligible to commence GH replacement, patients must fulfil several criteria, which include biochemical evidence of GH deficiency, and must demonstrate a reduced quality of life, as evidenced by their responses to a disease-specific questionnaire, the Adult Growth Hormone Deficiency Assessment – Quality of Life, or AGHDA-QoL (see www.nice.org.uk/pdf/AGHDA_questionnaire.pdf). Continuation of therapy is dependent on demonstrating that symptomatic benefit, based on improvement in questionnaire score, has been achieved (NICE 2003). GH is replaced by a daily subcutaneous injection which patients are taught to self-administer using a special pen device. Some of these pen devices offer needle-free delivery. GH is available in vials which contain either liquid GH or a powder and diluent which need to be mixed. The normal starting dose is 0.3–0.5 mg daily titrated over a 3-month period. During this time IGF-1 levels are checked every 6 weeks with the aim of keeping the levels within the age-matched reference range. The dosing schedule is adjusted to maximise benefits and minimise side-effects which can include transient oedema, arthralgia and headaches (Drake et al 1998). Older patients, women and those with a large body mass index (BMI) can be more prone to side-effects (Holmes & Shalet 1995). The usual maintenance dose is 0.2–0.6 mg/day. Women often require higher doses than men of the same age (Gaillard & Giusti 2004). Patients on GH replacement should be reassessed annually for evaluation of biochemical parameters (lipids and glucose), body composition (waist circumference, lean body mass and bone mineral density), exercise endurance and well-being using the AGHDA questionnaire.

For further information, see Piersanti (2004).

Gonadotrophins Testosterone replacement therapy has been available for over 50 years. Subcutaneous implants were developed in the 1940s, i.m. injections in the 1950s, oral tablets in the 1970s and transdermal patches and gels in the 1990s (Schubert et al 2004). Replacement can result in an improvement in sexual function, an increase in bone mineral density and improvements in body composition, e.g. increased lean body mass/decreased fat mass in hypogonadal men (Wang & Swerdloff 1997). In addition, positive changes are seen in erythropoiesis, prostate size and lipid profiles (Wang & Swerdloff 1999). Testosterone replacement is usually commenced when the diagnosis of hypogonadism is established and serum testosterone levels fall below a normal age-matched reference range.

There are now many testosterone preparations with differing routes of administration. Replacement depends on the formulation and there are advantages and disadvantages to each (Gooren & Bunck 2004). Most preparations have unfavourable pharmacokinetics which result either in sub- or supra-physiological and/or fluctuating levels of testosterone. Testosterone replacement can be by i.m. injection (250 mg every 3–4 weeks or 1000 mg every 3 months), implants (200–600 mg every 3–6 months), transdermal patches (2.5–7.5 mg/day or 4–EMG/day if scrotal patches are used), transdermal gel (1–2 sachets/day), oral tablets (25–40 mg t.d.s.) or buccal tablets (30 mg b.d.). Testosterone levels are monitored either immediately prior to an injection/implant or 8 h after the application of a patch.

Intramuscular injections have, for many years, been the most widely used and accepted form of testosterone replacement in the UK but these can be uncomfortable, are disruptive as the patient must make an appointment to see their GP or practice nurse every 3–4 weeks and can cause mood swings due to the fluctuating levels of testosterone, which are high immediately post-injection but then fall off over the next 2–3 weeks (Nieschlag 1998). Transdermal patches mimic the normal physiological and diurnal variations of testosterone but frequently cause skin irritation and are often discontinued for this reason. Transdermal gels result in more stable levels of testosterone (Swerdloff et al 2000). Both the patch and the gel are self-applied, making them a popular choice. Ultimately, the choice of testosterone replacement therapy should be made by the patient once they have been provided with the information they require to make an informed decision. Younger patients are more likely to choose a long-acting preparation whereas men over the age of 50 should be advised to opt for a short-acting one. This is to ensure that if the preparation has to be stopped due to a contraindication to testosterone replacement therapy, e.g. the development of prostate cancer, levels of serum testosterone will immediately fall (Nieschlag 1998).

For further information, see Nieschlag & Behre (2004).

Posterior pituitary hormone replacement Replacement of deficient hormones should alleviate many symptoms, allowing the patient to lead a near normal life. It is essential that the individual feels free to contact the appropriate doctor or specialist nurse at any time to discuss their condition or any related anxieties. As pituitary disease is a lifelong condition that will require ongoing monitoring, hospital attendance will continue on at least an annual basis for many years, giving the doctor or nurse the opportunity to build therapeutic relationships with their patients.

DISORDERS OF THE POSTERIOR PITUITARY: ANTIDIURETIC HORMONE (ADH)/VASOPRESSIN SECRETION

Diabetes insipidus

Diabetes insipidus (DI) is defined as the passing of large amounts (>3 L/24 h) of dilute urine (osmolality <300 mOsmol/kg) and exists in two main forms:

- cranial DI, due to a deficiency of hypothalamic secretion of ADH
- nephrogenic DI, a condition in which the renal tubules are resistant to the action of ADH.

Causes of both cranial and nephrogenic DI may be familial or acquired and include pituitary tumours, infection (meningitis, encephalitis), inflammatory conditions (tuberculosis, sarcoidosis), trauma (head injury, neurosurgery), vascular (Sheehan's syndrome, sickle cell disease), chronic renal disease, metabolic (hyper/hypocalcaemia, hyperglycaemia) and some medications (lithium). Primary polydipsia may be psychological (Lindholm 2004).

PATHOPHYSIOLOGY

Clinical features Deficiency of antidiuretic hormone (ADH)/vasopressin leads to polyuria, nocturia and a compensatory polydipsia. Urine output may reach 10–15 L or more per day, leading to severe dehydration if the individual's fluid intake is restricted in any way.

MEDICAL MANAGEMENT

Investigations Diagnosis is often made by single paired urine and plasma osmolality, obviating the need for the more stressful and prolonged water deprivation test. Plasma osmolality will show high concentration and urine will be dilute. However, sometimes the results are equivocal and a water deprivation test is required to make the diagnosis.

Treatment is by the administration of synthetic vasopressin (desmopressin or DDAVP). This may be given orally, intranasally or by i.m. injection.

Syndrome of inappropriate antidiuretic hormone (SIADH)

The causes of SIADH are many, but include oat cell carcinoma of the lung, pneumonia, tuberculosis (TB), meningitis, head injury, acute intermittent porphyria and medication, e.g. tricyclic antidepressants, some anticoagulants and some chemotherapeutic agents such as vincristine.

PATHOPHYSIOLOGY

Clinical features SIADH may present with vagueness, confusion, nausea and irritability which, if not corrected, may lead to epileptiform attacks and coma. It is caused by an excess of ADH, leading to a dilutional hyponatraemia. Biochemical investigation will reveal low plasma sodium, low plasma osmolality and an inappropriately high urine osmolality. Blood pressure, thyroid function, kidney function and adrenal function will be normal.

MEDICAL MANAGEMENT

Medical intervention may include:

- fluid restriction to 500–1000 mL/day
- treatment of the underlying cause
- administration of demeclocycline to inhibit the action of ADH on the renal tubules
- administration of hypertonic saline infusions (in severe cases in ITU).

NURSING PRIORITIES AND MANAGEMENT: Diabetes insipidus

Major considerations

The nurse's interventions will include accurate recording of fluid balance with the full cooperation and participation of the patient. It is essential for the patient to have easy access to toilet facilities. Samples of urine will be required for osmolality assessment.

The nurse will also be involved in medication administration and education of the patient with regard to self-administration of medicines, continued measurement of fluid balance and regular weight recording. Most patients rapidly become aware if the therapy is no longer effective and will contact their GP or the specialist physician or nurse supervising their care.

DISORDERS OF THE THYROID GLAND

ANATOMY AND PHYSIOLOGY

The thyroid is a small gland in the neck that sits anteriorly to the larynx and is attached to the thyroid cartilages and

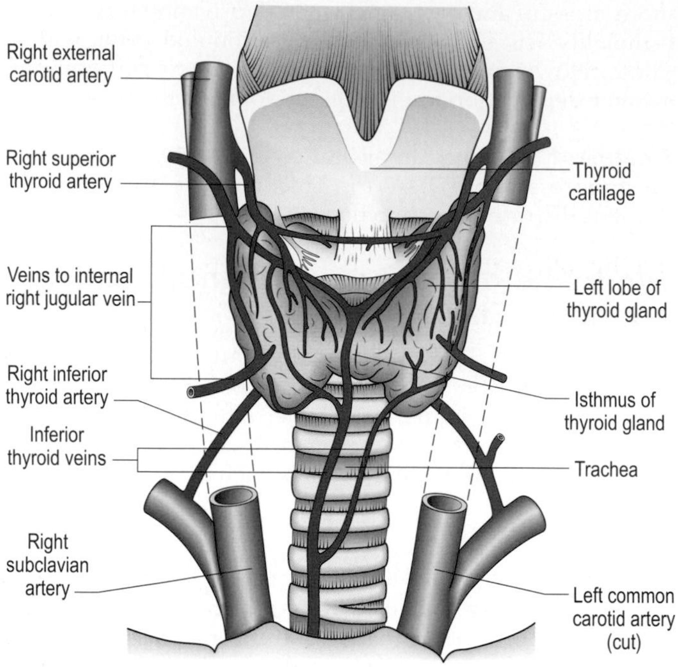

Fig. 5.5 The thyroid gland and associated structures.

the trachea. It consists of two lobes connected by an isthmus (see Fig. 5.5). Structures that lie in close proximity include the oesophagus, the parathyroid glands, the recurrent laryngeal nerves and the carotid arteries. These may all be affected by enlargement of the gland.

The thyroid receives a rich blood supply from the superior thyroid arteries, which branch from the external carotid arteries, and from the inferior thyroid arteries, which branch from the subclavian arteries. Each lobe is filled with hollow vesicles called follicles, which produce and store the thyroid hormones. Between the follicles are parafollicular cells ('C' cells), which secrete the hormone calcitonin; this, together with parathormone from the parathyroid glands, is involved in the metabolism of calcium.

The hormones, thyroxine (T_4) and 25% of circulating tri-iodothyroxine (T_3) are synthesised and secreted by the thyroid gland. This synthesis of thyroid hormones is dependent on the availability of iodine in the diet, e.g. from table salt, fish and milk. Dietary iodine is absorbed from the small intestine, changed to iodide and transported in the blood to the thyroid gland, where it is taken up by the thyroid cells. More T_4 than T_3 is produced, but T_4 is converted in some tissues to the more biologically active T_3. Over 99% of all thyroid hormone is bound to plasma thyroid-binding proteins. Only the free hormone is available for use by the tissues. If the levels of T_4 and T_3 in the blood fall, the hypothalamus releases thyroid-releasing hormone (TRH). As the levels of TRH rise, the pituitary gland secretes thyroid-stimulating hormone (TSH) which stimulates the thyroid gland to produce more T_4 and T_3. The principal effect of thyroid hormones is to influence the metabolism of cells and, therefore, the metabolic rate. Low levels of hormone are associated with a low temperature, i.e. patients will complain of feeling cold, slow heart rate and weight gain, whereas patients with high concentrations of thyroid hormones experience a rapid heart rate, heat intolerance and weight loss despite an increased appetite and high calorie intake.

STOP THINK **5.2** Describe how the thyroid hormones T_3 and T_4 are controlled.

Simple goitre

A goitre is an enlargement of the thyroid gland. It can occur without over- or underactivity of the gland. The term 'simple goitre' is a paradox as its cause is poorly understood. In young adults the gland is soft and diffuse, enlarged two to three times its normal size. Thyroid hormone and TSH levels are normal and there is no evidence of autoimmunity. If the stimulus to goitre formation remains, whatever it is, the gland becomes further enlarged and nodular over the ensuing 20 years or so (euthyroid multinodular goitre) and when patients are 60 years of age or beyond they may develop hyperthyroidism (toxic multinodular goitre).

HYPERSECRETION OF THE THYROID HORMONES

Hyperthyroidism, thyrotoxicosis, is a condition in which there are high levels of circulating thyroid hormones. Hyperthyroidism and diabetes mellitus are amongst the most prevalent of the endocrine diseases. (Diabetes mellitus is discussed in detail in Part 2 of this chapter.) The most common cause of hyperthyroidism is intrinsic thyroid disease; pituitary-driven hyperthyroidism is extremely rare. Hyperthyroidism mainly affects women aged between 30 and 50 years, but can occur at any age in either gender.

Graves' disease

Graves' disease is the most common form of hyperthyroidism. It is an autoimmune disorder in which antibodies (anti-TSH receptor) behave like TSH, stimulating thyroid hormone production and in some cases thyroid enlargement or goitre. Graves' disease tends to run in families and may be associated with ophthalmic features. The ophthalmopathy of Graves' disease, which affects the majority of patients to some extent, is also autoimmune in aetiology. The result of the immune process is fibroblast proliferation in the retro-orbital space, with water accumulation and enlargement of the extraocular muscles and increased fat. The increased pressure behind the eye pushes the eye forward (exophthalmos) and the swollen muscles work inefficiently, causing double vision (diplopia). Vision may be threatened. The swelling of the eyelids is due to prolapse of retrobulbar fat and poor lymphatic and venous drainage.

Toxic multinodular goitre

As mentioned above, this is often the outcome of the simple diffuse goitre in the young adult. It is the second most common cause of hyperthyroidism after Graves' disease. As it presents in older people, the clinical aspects of hyperthyroidism may be different, with cardiovascular features, e.g. atrial fibrillation, predominating.

Toxic adenoma (solitary nodule)

This type of tumour constitutes about 5% of hyperthyroidism. In these patients, the thyroid nodule acts autonomously and produces excess levels of thyroid hormone, leading to suppression of the normal thyroid.

PATHOPHYSIOLOGY

In hyperthyroidism, high levels of circulating thyroid hormones stimulate cell metabolism, resulting in a high metabolic rate. TSH secretion is suppressed. The cardiovascular system is affected with tachycardia and, in older patients, atrial fibrillation and cardiac failure. Patients complain of general fatigue, although for short spells they may become more active, and find that they are restless.

Common presenting symptoms There is increased irritability, inability to relax and sleep, heat intolerance with excessive sweating, palpitations, perhaps a feeling of shakiness and a fine tremor of the hands. By far the most common symptom, however, is weight loss, despite an increased appetite. Patients often complain of excessive watering and grittiness of the eyes. An enlargement of the gland (goitre) may have been noticed.

MEDICAL MANAGEMENT

Investigations Clinical examination will confirm the tachycardia and atrial fibrillation, goitre and ophthalmopathy. The skin will be hot and moist and a fine tremor of the outstretched hands may be discernible. Diagnosis is usually confirmed by elevated serum T_4 and a suppressed TSH.

Treatment The three approaches to treatment in hyperthyroidism (thyrotoxicosis) are:

- antithyroid medication
- surgery
- radioactive iodine therapy.

Medication Antithyroid medication (carbimazole 30–40 mg/day or propylthiouracil 300–400 mg/day) is prescribed to inhibit the synthesis of thyroid hormones. The patient will continue to take the medication until a euthyroid state (i.e. normal thyroid function) is achieved, after which serum T_4, TSH and the medication dose are monitored to ensure that the patient remains euthyroid and to avoid over- or undermedication. Treatment usually continues for some 18 months, with regular outpatient visits. The patient is asked to report unexplained fever or sore throat, as the major side-effect of antithyroid medication is agranulocytosis, which occurs in approximately 1 in 300–500 patients (see Ch. 11, p. 480). The most common adverse reaction is an urticarial rash which occurs in about 2% of patients. Other side-effects include fever and arthralgia which can occur in 1–5% of patients, usually within the first few months of starting therapy, and are more common in patients treated with higher doses (Cooper 1999). Symptomatic control of tachycardia is obtained by administration of beta-blockers such as propranolol until thyroid hormone levels are normal.

Surgical intervention Partial thyroidectomy is performed only after medication has produced a euthyroid state. In some centres, the patient is given potassium iodide for 1–2 weeks before surgery, which will inhibit thyroid hormone release, reduce the size and vascularity of the gland and reduce the risk of peri- and postoperative haemorrhage. Approximately 80% of patients are cured by surgery (Parwardhan et al 1993). Partial thyroidectomy is also a useful treatment for patients with large or unsightly goitres — complications of this procedure include postoperative haemorrhage, recurrent laryngeal nerve palsy, hypocalcaemia and hypothyroidism. Features of postoperative nursing care specific to patients who have undergone partial thyroidectomy are described in Nursing Care Plan 5.1.

For further information, see Braverman & Utiger (2004).

Radioactive iodine therapy Iodine-131 (^{131}I) acts by destroying functioning cells or by inhibiting their ability to replicate. It is usually administered as a single capsule on an outpatient basis. Patients are advised to avoid eating for 3–4 h after administration to allow adequate absorption of the iodine; they are also advised to drink at least 2 L of fluid over the next 24 h and to pass urine frequently in order to excrete free circulating radioactive iodine as rapidly as possible.

Patients present a radiation hazard for approximately 1 week following this treatment. This type of therapy is used when surgery is not appropriate, but is not usually offered to women of child-bearing age.

CARCINOMA OF THE THYROID GLAND

Carcinoma of the thyroid gland is rare, comprising around 1% of all cancers (Haslett et al 2002). It is three times more common in women than men and can occur at any age (Schneider & Ron 2005).

The five main types of thyroid carcinoma are:

- papillary (this is the most common type and accounts for ~80% of all thyroid carcinomas)
- follicular (less common, usually found in older people)
- anaplastic (rare, more common in older people)
- lymphoma (usually of the type known as non-Hodgkin's lymphoma; see p. 515)
- medullary cell (rare, may run in families).

Papillary and follicular thyroid cancers are sometimes also called differentiated thyroid cancer because they still retain histological features typical of the thyroid gland.

PATHOPHYSIOLOGY

Papillary or follicular carcinomas usually present with a lump which can cause hoarseness or difficulty in swallowing. Metastases from follicular carcinoma commonly involve the brain, liver, lungs and bones.

Common presenting symptoms Often the patient will have noticed a painless small nodule or swelling in the neck. They may be euthyroid or may have symptoms associated with either hyper- or hypothyroidism.

MEDICAL MANAGEMENT

Investigations Tests of thyroid function (T_3, T_4 and TSH levels) are carried out and are followed by radiological

Nursing Care Plan 5.1 Postoperative care for a patient who has undergone partial thyroidectomy

Nursing considerations	Action	Rationale	Outcome/further action
1. Compromise of airway as a result of anaesthesia and surgery to the neck area	• Sit the patient in an upright position with plenty of support for the neck. Oxygen may be ordered for 1–2 h after surgery	Support of the head will reduce strain on the suture line and improve the comfort of the patient, who may be very anxious about moving the neck	The airway will remain clear and strain on the suture line will be minimal
2. Risk of haemorrhage following surgery	• Record blood pressure and pulse half-hourly, watching for signs of irregular or laboured breathing or stridor. Clip removers should be kept by the bed for up to 24 h after surgery	A rise in pulse and a fall in blood pressure can indicate haemorrhage, which should be reported. If respiratory embarrassment occurs due to haemorrhage, the clips must be removed to allow the blood compressing the trachea to escape. The wound should be covered with saline-soaked gauze and the patient returned to theatre immediately	Early detection of possible haemorrhage should prevent a crisis from developing and allow bleeding to be stopped sooner rather than later
3. Risk of tetany due to accidental removal of the parathyroid glands	• Observe closely for tetany, including tingling of fingers and toes, a positive Chvostek's sign (facial asymmetry on tapping of the cheek) or Trousseau's sign (inflation of blood pressure cuff causes spasm of hand) (see Box 5.3)	Sudden drop in calcium levels can lead to tetany, resulting in airway obstruction and, if left untreated, fitting and death	Early indications of lowered calcium levels should be reported, allowing treatment in the form of i.v. calcium gluconate to be given
4. Risk of thyroid crisis (This is now rare due to improved postoperative preparation of the patient about to undergo thyroid surgery. It is a life-threatening situation)	• Measure pulse, blood pressure, temperature and respiratory rate half-hourly, reducing as recovery allows	As a result of trauma to the thyroid, enormous amounts of thyroid hormones are released into the bloodstream, causing tachycardia, a rise in blood pressure and hyperpyrexia (up to 41°C). The patient appears very restless and irritable. Death may result from heart failure	Once thyroid crisis has been diagnosed, treatment must be commenced immediately with i.v. beta-blockers (propranolol in high doses), carbimazole, steroid therapy (i.m. hydrocortisone 100 mg)
5. Risk of damage to laryngeal nerve	• Observe for breathing difficulties, noisy breathing, stridor, swallowing difficulties and hoarseness, and report problems	Damage to the recurrent laryngeal nerve can result in vocal cord spasm and paralysis of larynx leading to respiratory obstruction	If damage occurs, tracheostomy is usually necessary initially. The damaged nerve should recover in a few weeks. Inhalation of nitrous oxide may help in the acute period to relieve the spasm

examination (ultrasound) of the neck. Fine needle biopsy or aspiration is necessary to distinguish cancer from benign pathologies, to give a firm diagnosis and to differentiate between the types of thyroid cancer. Radioactive isotope scanning, using technetium or iodine, is a painless procedure which involves injecting the radioactive isotopes into a vein in the patient's arm and then, after 20 min rest, scanning the thyroid gland with a gamma camera. As cancer cells do not absorb the radioactive liquid as well as normal thyroid cells, any cancer cells will generally appear as 'cold areas' or 'cold nodules' on scanning. However, only 10% of such cold nodules are malignant. Many turn out to be cysts, and operative exploration may be avoided if aspiration cytology is normal.

Staging The stage of a cancer is a term used to describe the size of the tumour and whether or not it has metastasised. This information helps the clinician decide on the most appropriate treatment (see also Ch. 31, pp. 1041–1043).

Stages of thyroid cancers

- Stage 1. The tumour is <1 cm, is contained within the thyroid gland and has not metastasised.
- Stage 2. The tumour is between 1 and 4 cm, and is contained within the thyroid gland, i.e. has not metastasised.
- Stage 3. The tumour is >4 cm but is still contained within the thyroid gland *or* the tumour is of any size and has spread just outside the gland or to the lymph nodes in the neck.
- Stage 4. The tumour has spread into other structures in the neck *or* the tumour has spread to involve more lymph nodes in the neck or upper chest *or* the tumour has metastasised to other parts of the body. All patients with anaplastic thyroid cancer are considered to have Stage 4 disease.

When patients under the age of 45 are diagnosed with papillary or follicular thyroid cancer, different staging categories are used and there is no Stage 3 or 4 for these patients:

- Stage 1. The tumour can be of any size and the lymph nodes may also be affected but there is no spread to other sites.
- Stage 2. Any tumour that has metastasised, e.g. to the lungs or bones.

Treatment Surgery, radioactive iodine (^{131}I) or radiotherapy may be given alone or in combination. The treatment chosen will depend on several factors including the patient's age, general health, and the type and stage of the tumour. The treatment of choice is near-total thyroidectomy. This is usually followed by a large dose of ^{131}I to ablate any thyroid remnant. Any tissue showing radioiodine uptake subsequently must be assumed to be recurrent disease, and further ^{131}I may be taken up therapeutically by the tumour tissue. Follow-up is important and will usually be carried out at 6-monthly intervals initially. At follow-up, the tumour marker, serum thyroglobulin (Tg) is measured. It should not be detectable in a patient who has had a total thyroidectomy, ^{131}I ablation of remnant and is taking thyroxine in a dose sufficient to suppress serum TSH. If detectable, further surgery or ^{131}I therapy may be required.

NURSING PRIORITIES AND MANAGEMENT: Carcinoma of the thyroid gland

Major considerations

Caring for the patient receiving ^{131}I therapy

Before ^{131}I ablative therapy the patient will have discontinued thyroid hormones for 4–6 weeks to allow TSH to rise, which ensures better uptake of ^{131}I. In those in whom a period of hypothyroidism is best avoided, e.g. an older patient with ischaemic heart disease, high TSH levels in the blood can be achieved by giving Thyrogen (human recombinant TSH). Thyrogen is given as two i.m. injections 24 h apart, prior to commencement of ^{131}I, and negates the need to discontinue thyroid hormone replacement (Haugen et al 1999).

The patient and family should be given clear explanations regarding the effect of ^{131}I, the reasons for the patient being nursed alone with restricted access for staff and visitors, and procedures to be followed in the handling of body fluids. It should be explained to the patient that they cannot be discharged until their radiation level is safe.

Measures should be taken to prevent constipation, as this inhibits the subsequent excretion of radioactive material. A high fluid intake should be encouraged to promote a good urinary output. Commodes and bedpans should be designated for the patient's exclusive use. All body fluids will be highly radioactive following ^{131}I administration and the patient should be encouraged to bathe or shower regularly to remove contaminated perspiration.

The patient should be nursed in a single room containing a minimum of equipment. Film badges should be worn at all times by staff members to indicate radiation exposure. Duties should be coordinated so that each staff member spends a minimum amount of time with the patient.

As with all endocrine disease, prompt treatment should result in complete alleviation of all signs and symptoms; the patient should be reassured of this whilst undergoing treatment. Follow-up after treatment is essential. Nursing staff should encourage the patient to attend outpatient or GP clinics as advised. The patient should be reassured that, particularly with localised disease from a papillary carcinoma, the probability of 'cure' is extremely high (Dougherty & Lister 2004).

For further information, see Schafer (2005).

HYPOSECRETION OF THE THYROID HORMONES

Underactivity of the thyroid gland may be primary, resulting from disease of the thyroid, or secondary, due to pituitary failure.

Aetiology

Primary hypothyroidism as a result of autoimmune disease is the commonest cause of thyroid underactivity. It may be associated with other autoimmune disease. It is six times more common in women than in men.

Hypothyroidism (myxoedema) may also be iatrogenic, i.e. caused by previous treatment for thyrotoxicosis by means of surgery or radioactive iodine.

Iodine deficiency is another cause of hypothyroidism and is due to insufficient dietary intake of iodine. This leads to reduced thyroid hormone production. Goitre is a common feature of this condition. Endemic hypothyroidism is occasionally seen in areas where iodine levels in the water supply are low, usually inland areas far from the sea or mountainous regions. This was once a problem in Derbyshire in the UK. It is still seen in some areas of the world, such as parts of central Africa, central Asia and central and eastern

Europe as well as in the Andes and the Himalayas (Delange & Dunn 2005).

Congenital hypothyroidism occurs in approximately 1 in 4000 live births and usually results from congenital absence of the thyroid gland; it can also be caused by certain genetic enzyme defects. Some medications may also induce hypothyroidism; for example, lithium carbonate (used in bipolar disorders) can result in goitrous hypothyroidism (Haslett et al 2002).

PATHOPHYSIOLOGY

If congenital hypothyroidism is not detected and treated early, the child will not develop fully, either mentally or physically. Neonatal screening for congenital hypothyroidism is performed in most developed countries at 5–7 days. In primary hypothyroidism (myxoedema), serum T_4 is low and levels of TSH are high. The onset of myxoedema is slow and insidious. Because the affected individual is often an older person, it may be accepted as a normal part of ageing and it may be some time before a medical opinion is sought. The patient may report sensitivity to cold, weight gain, a general slowing down of body functions, lethargy, depression and an inability to 'think quickly'. The face will be puffy in appearance and hair sparse, coarse and brittle. In severe hypothyroidism, the patient may be admitted in a coma and perhaps be thought to be suffering from hypothermia. This represents a medical emergency in which intensive treatment and care are essential. Diagnosis of hypothyroidism is confirmed by low plasma levels of T_4 and raised TSH levels.

MEDICAL MANAGEMENT

Treatment Hypothyroidism is treated with replacement doses of thyroid hormone (thyroxine) commencing with a low dose of 25–50 mcg and increasing by increments of 25–50 mcg every 3–4 weeks until serum TSH is normal.

NURSING PRIORITIES AND MANAGEMENT: Hypothyroidism

It is usual to treat patients on an ongoing basis in the community. The community nursing team should follow up medical treatment and explanations and ensure that patients understand the reasons for the thyroxine replacement therapy and the importance of attending for regular checks to ensure that a euthyroid state is achieved and maintained. Patients are often seen in hospital for annual review at nurse-led clinics which are becoming more common.

DISORDERS OF THE PARATHYROID GLANDS

ANATOMY AND PHYSIOLOGY

The parathyroid glands are situated on the posterior lobes of the thyroid gland. They are usually four in number; however, more than four glands occur in up to 6% of individuals. This has been attributed to division of the glands during development. The blood supply is from the inferior and superior thyroid arteries.

The glands secrete parathormone (PTH), which is the most important hormone involved in calcium metabolism. Parathormone maintains plasma calcium levels within normal limits. It acts predominantly on the kidney tubules to increase reabsorption of calcium but also increases gut absorption of calcium and mobilises it from bone. Plasma calcium will therefore rise, and in turn suppress PTH secretion; conversely, a fall in plasma calcium will stimulate the secretion of PTH. In most instances, raised levels of calcium in the plasma are due either to hyperparathyroidism or malignancy.

Vitamin D and calcitonin are also involved in calcium metabolism (see Box 5.1).

Box 5.1

Vitamin D and calcitonin in calcium metabolism

Vitamin D is found in two forms: cholecalciferol (vitamin D_3), which is formed predominantly in the skin by the action of sunlight, and ergocalciferol (vitamin D_2), which is synthetic and added to food. It is the skin-synthesised form which is of greater importance and is perhaps best considered as a hormone.

Vitamin D is biologically inactive; only when it is metabolised by the liver (to form mildly active 25-hydroxycholecalciferol) and the kidney (to form very active 1,25-dihydroxycholecalciferol) does it have any action on calcium metabolism. The active metabolite increases calcium absorption from the gut and is essential for bone formation.

If 1,25-dihydroxycholecalciferol is present in excess, it causes increased resorption of calcium from bone, leading to hypercalcaemia. The kidney is able to detect rising levels and ceases production of the active form, producing an inactive form until the levels drop.

Bone is constantly being re-formed by deposition and reabsorption of calcium. Calcitonin reduces the reabsorption of calcium from bone. Local stress, such as weight bearing, is important in this process. Prolonged inactivity or immobility can result in calcium being lost from bone, while exercise increases bone formation and remodelling.

HYPERSECRETION OF THE PARATHYROID GLANDS

Hypercalcaemia

PATHOPHYSIOLOGY

In most instances, raised plasma levels are caused by hyperparathyroidism or are secondary to malignancy (see Box 5.2). Mild hypercalcaemia, which is often asymptomatic, occurs in about 1 in 1000 of the population (Kumar & Clark 2002).

Even mild symptoms can lead to an early diagnosis, due to advanced chemical analysis techniques; this means that it is now extremely rare to see the severe renal and bone problems associated with hypercalcaemia that occurred in the past.

Box 5.2

Causes of hypercalcaemia

Common

- Malignancy
- Myeloma
- Primary hyperparathyroidism

Rare

- Addison's disease
- Milk alkali syndrome
- Sarcoidosis
- Thyrotoxicosis
- Vitamin D poisoning
- Immobility
- Phaeochromocytoma
- Thiazide diuretics
- Tuberculosis

Common presenting symptoms Patients may present with symptoms of malignancy or of hypercalcaemia, including:

- constipation
- depression
- drowsiness, coma
- malaise
- nausea, vomiting
- nocturia
- polydipsia, polyuria
- psychosis
- weakness.

MEDICAL MANAGEMENT

Investigations Diagnosis is based on medical history, clinical examination and tests to ascertain the cause.

Treatment Hypercalcaemia caused by malignancy is usually seen only in patients with advanced carcinoma when bony metastases have occurred and signifies a poor prognosis (Ralston et al 1997). If possible, it should be treated, as this may improve the quality of the patient's life. Adequate hydration is of great importance and, in itself, is often enough to relieve the symptoms of the hypercalcaemia. However, it is now established that bisphosphonate medications (e.g. disodium pamidronate) are highly effective in lowering malignant hypercalcaemia (Fleisch 1998). These are administered by an intravenous infusion, but oral preparations, e.g. sodium clodronate or ibandronic acid, can be used in the long term to prevent a recurrence of hypercalcaemia (Ralston et al 1997). Other treatments include oral phosphate and steroid therapy.

Primary hyperparathyroidism

This condition is caused by the overproduction of PTH by the parathyroid glands. It affects three times more women than men and its incidence increases with age. It is usually idiopathic (Haslett et al 2002).

MEDICAL MANAGEMENT

Treatment Surgery is indicated for the management of hypercalcaemia due to excessive PTH secretion, as no long-term medication is available. However, asymptomatic hypercalcaemia requires no surgical intervention and can be treated conservatively with simple monitoring of calcium levels on an intermittent basis by the patient's GP or the hospital outpatient department.

Following parathyroidectomy, hypocalcaemia of either a transient or permanent nature may ensue. This should be treated promptly to prevent tetany. If severe hypocalcaemia occurs, i.v. calcium gluconate (10 mL of 10%) should be given immediately. Vitamin D and oral calcium supplements will be required. Calcium levels should be monitored closely until they have stabilised.

NURSING PRIORITIES AND MANAGEMENT: Primary hyperparathyroidism

Major considerations

The investigations for diagnosis of hypercalcaemia may require hospital admission, particularly if the hypercalcaemia is severe and/or is thought to be secondary to malignancy. The patient will probably have been unwell for some time and will be feeling very tired and weak on admission.

Careful explanations of the investigations and treatment are required. These will include a 24-h urine collection for calcium. As it is particularly important for the accuracy of this test that the urine collection is completed properly, it is essential that this is explained clearly, and is fully understood by the patient. If surgery is undertaken, the perioperative care is the same as for thyroidectomy (see p. 172). In addition, regular assessment for impending hypocalcaemia is undertaken (see Box 5.3).

Box 5.3

Detecting increased neuromuscular irritability (tetany) due to hypocalcaemia

Positive Chvostek's sign
The nurse can test for this sign by tapping the person's facial nerve about 2 cm anterior to the ear lobe. If hypocalcaemia (or hypomagnesaemia) is present, unilateral twitching of facial muscles, especially around the mouth, may be observed.

Positive Trousseau's sign
This may be observed when taking the blood pressure of a person with a low calcium level which, as yet, is not producing observable effects. The sphygmomanometer cuff is inflated around the person's arm and pressure is increased to above systolic pressure for 2–3 min. The constrictive effect of the inflated blood pressure cuff exacerbates the hypocalcaemia in the limb distal to the cuff. During blood pressure recording or shortly afterwards, muscular contraction or twitching will be noticed in the limb concerned.

Secondary and tertiary hyperparathyroidism

Secondary hyperparathyroidism occurs due to disease processes that cause hypocalcaemia, e.g. in vitamin D deficiency or in renal disease. The parathyroid glands strive to keep the calcium levels up, while calcium remains normal or is low. Rarely, this can lead to autonomous secretion of parathyroid hormone, leading to permanent hypercalcaemia, termed tertiary hyperparathyroidism. This is often seen in patients with renal failure.

HYPOSECRETION OF THE PARATHYROID GLANDS

Hypocalcaemia

The most common cause of hypocalcaemia is artifactual due to low albumin levels, i.e. the calcium is actually normal when the low albumin is corrected for by the biochemistry laboratory (Stewart 2005). Other relatively common causes include a low magnesium, renal failure and vitamin D deficiency (see Box 5.1). Autoimmune hypoparathyroidism is rare, but iatrogenic hypoparathyroidism following surgery to the neck is more common.

Rickets and osteomalacia

These are diseases of calcium and phosphorus metabolism resulting from a deficiency in vitamin D intake and synthesis. It may be questionable to discuss these under the heading of endocrinology, but as they are usually seen and treated by endocrinologists, as opposed to other physicians, they are considered in this chapter.

Vitamin D deficiency during growth produces abnormalities in the growing skeleton known as rickets. In childhood, rickets produces soft, painful bones in which the weight-bearing bones bend and may give rise to gross deformities. In the adult, where bone growth is completed, osteomalacia is the result; symptoms are generally diffuse bone pain and myopathy.

Rickets does not now occur commonly in the population of the UK, due to better nutrition and, possibly, to a reduction in industrial pollution which allows more sunlight through. It is, however, sometimes seen in the Asian community in the UK as they tend to cover up and avoid exposing themselves to sunlight, particularly those individuals with an increased vitamin D requirement, e.g. babies, children and pregnant women. The exact explanation for its prevalence is not clear, but it may be associated with an inability to synthesise vitamin D, as it occurs predominantly in people who eat a strict vegetarian or vegan diet.

Treatment is by vitamin D replacement, and prevention is the aim, particularly targeted to known vulnerable groups.

DISORDERS OF THE ADRENAL GLANDS

ANATOMY AND PHYSIOLOGY

The adrenal glands are situated on the upper part of the kidneys. They are highly vascular and derive their blood

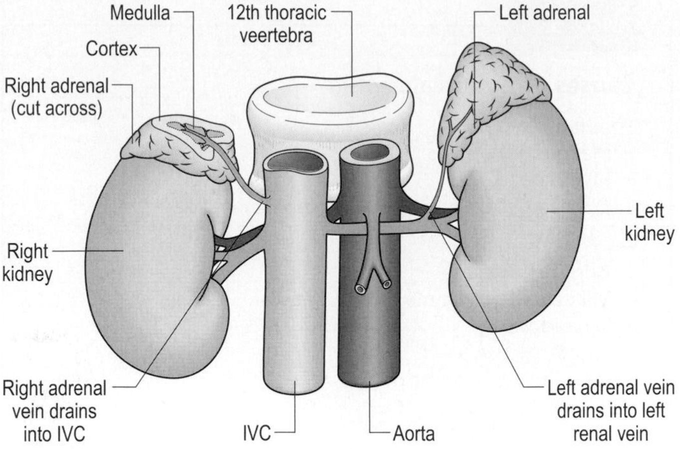

Fig. 5.6 The adrenal gland and associated structures. IVC, inferior vena cava. (Reproduced with permission from Jeffcoate 1993.)

supply from the renal arteries, the inferior phrenic arteries and directly from the aorta; they are drained by the suprarenal veins (see Fig. 5.6). The adrenal glands have a composite origin. The cortex, the outer part, has the same embryonic site of origin as the gonads. The medulla, the inner part, is derived from neural crest cells which have migrated from the developing neural tube and have become enclosed within the cortex. The latter can arguably be considered part of the nervous system. The secretions, and therefore the actions of the two separate parts of the glands, are quite different and will be discussed separately.

The adrenal cortex

The adrenal cortex produces three types of hormone, collectively termed corticosteroids:

- mineralocorticoids
- glucocorticoids
- adrenal androgens.

Mineralocorticoids The most important of the mineralocorticoids is aldosterone, which is the most potent regulator of sodium and potassium and hence of the acid–base balance of the body. Aldosterone acts on the distal convoluted tubules of the kidney and stimulates the cells to reabsorb and thus conserve sodium.

Glucocorticoids such as cortisol, the principal glucocorticoid, have varied and wide-ranging actions, many of which are not fully understood (see Fig. 5.7). They are essential to life and, in their absence, blood sugar, blood pressure and blood volume fall, sodium excretion increases and muscle contractility decreases. Death ensues due to low blood volume, myocardial weakness and shock. If present in excessive amounts, an opposite set of changes occurs: blood volume expands, blood pressure rises, potassium falls, glycogen storage is increased, blood sugar levels rise, connective tissue is reduced in quality and strength, and immunity is impaired. Wound healing and the process of inflammation are also inhibited.

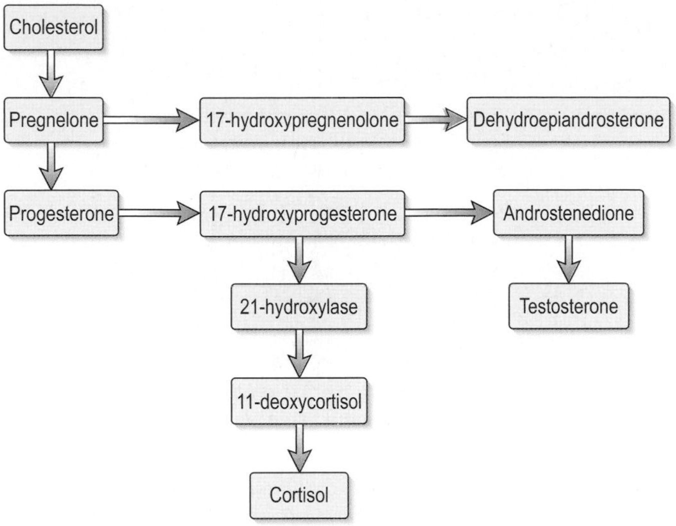

Fig. 5.7 Simplified schematisation of cortisol synthesis.

Adrenal androgens The adrenal cortex, in addition to the gonads, produces male sex hormones. The effects are appropriate in the male, but in the female excessive production may have a virilising effect.

The adrenal medulla

Adrenaline, noradrenaline and dopamine, i.e. the catecholamines, are secreted by the adrenal medulla. Eighty per cent of adrenomedullary secretion is adrenaline, most noradrenaline and dopamine being secreted by neurones and functioning as neurotransmitters.

In normal secretion, adrenaline probably has some effect on mean blood pressure; although it increases systolic pressure, it decreases diastolic pressure. When secreted under the control of the sympathetic nervous system (see Ch. 9, p. 407) it causes tachycardia, decreased gut motility and the closure of sphincters in the gut, pupil dilatation, bronchodilatation and piloerection.

Noradrenaline raises both systolic and diastolic blood pressure but has less effect on gut motility and does not produce bronchodilatation.

The difference between the effects of adrenaline and noradrenaline is partly explained by the presence of receptors on the surface of effector cells, i.e. those cells on which adrenaline and noradrenaline have their effect. These are termed α- and β-adrenoreceptors. Noradrenaline is most active at α-adrenergic receptors and adrenaline at β-adrenergic receptors. In addition, most cardiac receptors are termed B_1, to distinguish them from bronchodilator B_2 adrenoreceptors.

HYPERSECRETION OF THE ADRENAL GLANDS

The adrenal medulla

The main effect of the catecholamines (adrenaline, noradrenaline and dopamine) secreted by the adrenal medulla is on the cardiovascular system and the central nervous system, and on carbohydrate and lipid metabolism. Together, adrenaline and noradrenaline prepare the body for the 'fight or flight' response.

Phaeochromocytoma

Phaeochromocytoma is a very rare condition which causes about 1 in 1000 cases of hypertension (Kumar & Clark 2002). In this condition, a tumour of the adrenal medulla produces excessive adrenaline and noradrenaline. The tumour is small, with about 10% being multiple tumours and 10% being malignant.

PATHOPHYSIOLOGY

Clinical features The tumour produces the clinical effects of excessive catecholamine secretion which include hypertension and palpitations.

Common presenting symptoms Patients may present with anxiety, tachycardia, palpitations and panic attacks. Headaches, sweating and pallor may also occur. There may be a history of high blood pressure, which may be labile. Patients may present as an acute emergency with a hypertensive crisis (Spencer et al 1993) or may be asymptomatic (Bravo & Tagle 2003).

MEDICAL MANAGEMENT

Investigations A careful history and clinical examination may lead the physician to suspect a phaeochromocytoma. Investigations include 24-h urine collections for urinary free norepinephrine (NE) and epinephrine (E) and catecholamines or their two major metabolites, metanephrine and vanillylmandelic acid (VMA). Normal levels of NE/E and catecholamine secretion usually exclude a diagnosis of phaeochromocytoma. Abdominal X-rays and a CT scan may show a tumour of the medulla.

Treatment includes surgical removal of the tumour and administration of α- and β-adrenoreceptor blocking medications, e.g. phenoxybenzamine and propranolol.

NURSING PRIORITIES AND MANAGEMENT: Phaeochromocytoma

Major considerations

The first priority of care is to limit anxiety as much as possible and to nurse the patient in a quiet, non-stressful environment. Clear, concise explanations of the reasons for the symptoms will help to relieve the anxiety.

Blood pressure and pulse should be recorded 4-hourly, and any sweating or flushing noted. Antihypertensive medication must be maintained as the risk of postoperative hypotensive collapse is reduced by adequate preparation with adrenoreceptor blocking medication.

A care plan should be devised such that the patient can be as independent as possible in self-care tasks. Preoperative preparation is as for general abdominal surgery (see Ch. 26). Specific postoperative care includes $\frac{1}{2}$-hourly recording of blood pressure to observe for immediate postoperative hypotensive collapse brought on by the reduced blood volume characteristic of chronic vasoconstriction. Specialist medication such as sodium nitroprusside, a potent

Table 5.5 Unwanted effects of steroids on the systems of the body*

System	Pathological effect	Comments
Endocrine	Suppression of endogenous steroid production Diabetes Weight gain Amenorrhoea	Therapy should always be withdrawn gradually to enable the hypothalamic–pituitary–adrenal axis to recover
Cardiovascular	Elevation of blood pressure	Due to sodium retention
Gastrointestinal	Peptic ulceration/GI bleeding	
Renal	Polyuria Glycosuria	
Central nervous	Mood change Change in sleep pattern Appetite stimulation	May manifest itself as euphoria, depression and even so-called steroid psychosis
Musculoskeletal	Muscle wasting Osteoporosis Pathological fracture	Muscle wasting can be seen in proximal muscle; often severely affected patients cannot rise from a squatting position
Skin	Bruising Striae Thinning Poor wound healing 'Moonface' and acne	Skin becomes friable and may tear easily
Immune	Suppression	May mask signs of infection

*The use of steroids in medicine has proved to be beneficial in a wide variety of diseases, from asthma to bowel disease, and as an adjunct to other treatment in cancer therapy. They can provide effective pain relief in chronic musculoskeletal conditions. However, their use should be judicious and all patients having steroid therapy in the long term should be monitored and supervised. Short-term treatment, such as therapy used in the relief of an acute asthma attack, does not require such long-term follow-up. In the long term, use of steroid therapy, natural or synthetic, will mimic Cushing's syndrome, so-called iatrogenic disease.

All patients on steroid therapy should wear a 'MedicAlert' bracelet, and should inform doctors, dentists or nurses that they are on steroid therapy. Surgery or intercurrent illness will require dose increases to mimic the body's normal response to stress.

vasoconstrictor, should be available to control blood pressure in a hypotensive crisis.

The adrenal cortex

Cushing's syndrome

Cushing's syndrome is caused by the excessive and inappropriate circulation of glucocorticoids. It is most commonly seen in the therapeutic administration of synthetic steroids (see Table 5.5). Spontaneous causes of Cushing's syndrome are extremely rare. The major causes, excluding iatrogenic causes, are (Kumar & Clark 2002):

- pituitary-dependent disease (Cushing's disease)
- ectopic ACTH production
- adrenal adenoma
- adrenal carcinoma
- alcohol-induced.

PATHOPHYSIOLOGY

Clinical features Increased plasma cortisol levels have wide-ranging clinical effects on most systems of the body, i.e. altered fat and carbohydrate metabolism, diabetes mellitus and obesity, wasting of muscles, retention of sodium leading to hypertension, oedema, compromise of the immune system and osteoporosis. Other effects include thinning of the skin with bruising or purpura, hirsutism and oligomenorrhoea in women and impotence in men (see also Table 5.6).

Common presenting symptoms Because of the wide-ranging clinical effects of Cushing's syndrome, the patient can present with varying symptoms. Frequently, the patient will complain of infections which will not resolve, weight gain, bruising and discoloration of the skin.

MEDICAL MANAGEMENT

Investigations Diagnosis is confirmed by radiological and biochemical investigations (see Table 5.7). The differential diagnosis between pituitary disease, ectopic ACTH production and primary adrenal hypersecretion is important as the treatment and management of these three causes will vary considerably.

Treatment Surgery and medical therapy are the main forms of treatment. Metyrapone is commonly used to lower cortisol levels. An alternative approach is to remove completely endogenous cortisol by adrenalectomy and to supplement levels with an oral steroid.

Trans-sphenoidal surgery is the treatment of choice for removal of an ACTH-producing tumour of the pituitary. The antifungal medication ketoconazole may be used, due

Table 5.6 Signs and symptoms of Cushing's syndrome

Symptoms or sign	Aetiology
Muscle wasting which can be demonstrated by the patient being unable to stand from a squatting position	Catabolic effect of the steroids
Osteoporosis which can be so severe as to result in spontaneous fracture of vertebrae or ribs	Protein loss from the skeletal matrix
Skin thinning and purple striae, plethora, easy bruising and purpura	Atrophy of the elastic lamina allows disruption of the dermis so capillaries can be seen below the surface. Weakening of the capillaries leads to easy bruising (often without trauma)
Oedema	Weakening of the capillaries
Poor wound healing, immunocompromisation	The lymphocytes are destroyed, lowering the ability to fight infection. Signs of infection, e.g. swelling and redness, are masked
Obesity and 'buffalo hump' (pad of fat across shoulders)	Altered metabolism of fat. Fat is laid down over the trunk. Lipid levels may be raised
Hypertension	Sodium-retaining properties of glucocorticoids
Diabetes mellitus	Alteration in the normal metabolism of carbohydrate and the increased conversion of protein to carbohydrate
Depression, euphoria and frank psychosis	Unknown
Change in libido, impotence, oligomenorrhoea and infertility	Due to the general hormone imbalance that is occurring
Excess hair growth, hair loss (particularly of the male pattern type in women)	This is seen in Cushing's disease/syndrome but is not solely due to cortisol overproduction

Table 5.7 Radiological and biochemical tests for differential diagnosis of Cushing's syndrome

Test	Findings indicative of Cushing's syndrome
Radiological	
Adrenal CT scan	Adrenal adenomas and carcinomas are usually large and detectable on a CT scan
Skull X-ray	It is difficult to detect these often small pituitary tumours; 90% of X-rays are normal
CT scan of head and pituitary fossa, MRI scan	High-resolution scanning and increasingly sophisticated techniques often allow an enlarged pituitary to be detected
Chest X-ray	May show a bronchial carcinoma which may be a source of ectopic ACTH production
Venous catheterisation	This technique may be of value in confirming by blood sampling a pituitary origin of ACTH production as well as locating an ectopic source
Biochemical	
Dexamethasone suppression test	Under the principle that, as a result of the feedback system, high levels of steroids will switch off ACTH production and therefore steroid production, failure of suppression indicates Cushing's syndrome and at a higher dose may indicate pituitary disease. Ectopic ACTH production is not suppressed with a low or a high dose
Circadian rhythms	Patients with Cushing's syndrome may lose the normal variation in levels of cortisol. These should be measured at 09.00 h and at 24.00 h when the patient is sleeping and not warned. The patient should have been in hospital for at least 48 h before commencement of this test
Insulin tolerance test	This test, in which a dose of i.v. insulin is given, demonstrates that the normal rise in cortisol levels to hypoglycaemia is absent and will differentiate between true Cushing's, depression and alcohol-induced pseudo-Cushing's. It is performed mainly in specialist centres as a high level of supervision is required, and certain baseline measurements of pituitary function and confirmation of a normal ECG are recommended to ensure the patient's safety
Glucose tolerance test	This test will indicate that glucose metabolism is impaired; indeed, most people with Cushing's syndrome show a diabetic tendency
Urine collection	24-h urinary collections are performed and should show an elevation in excreted steroids. Accuracy in this test is difficult to achieve as it relies on the patient managing a complete, uncontaminated 24-h collection

to its activity in inhibiting steroidogenesis in the steroid synthesis pathway (see Fig. 5.7). Surgery for removal of a benign adrenal adenoma offers a good chance of cure, but adrenal carcinoma carries a poor prognosis. The medication mitotane (o,p′-DDD) is adrenolytic and may be used in the treatment of adrenal carcinoma (Allolio et al 2004).

Following adrenalectomy, patients will require lifelong hydrocortisone and mineralocorticoid replacement therapy. They must always wear a MedicAlert bracelet and carry a steroid card, and be informed of the dangers of hypocortisolaemia, a life-threatening condition.

Management of ectopic ACTH syndrome This condition most often occurs in patients with an oat cell carcinoma of the lung (see Ch. 3). The neoplastic cells themselves produce ACTH and give rise to Cushing's syndrome. Care is as for malignant disease (see Ch. 31), taking into account the additional complications of Cushing's syndrome.

There is another subgroup of patients with ectopic ACTH production from less malignant tumours, the so-called carcinoid tumours, who present with a picture of more classical Cushing's syndrome and who may survive for many years with appropriate treatment.

NURSING PRIORITIES AND MANAGEMENT: Cushing's syndrome

Major considerations

The main aim of nursing care is to relieve the symptoms of the disease. On admission, a full nursing history is taken and the patient's needs thoroughly assessed to provide a basis for a care plan.

A major consideration will be the psychological impact of the illness, e.g. related to a change in body image. Providing clear ongoing explanations of the hormonal changes that the patient is experiencing, the investigations and the subsequent treatment that they will undergo help provide optimal psychological support.

Ongoing follow-up after discharge from hospital is essential. Initially, 3-monthly tests will be carried out, gradually reducing to an annual check. If adrenalectomy or pituitary surgery has been performed, precautions will need to be taken regarding hydrocortisone replacement; this must be explained in detail. An information leaflet can be useful as a reference for the patient when at home. This should tell the patient when to increase the therapy, e.g. during illness, and when to seek medical advice.

STOP THINK **5.3** Recall the physical symptoms that commonly occur in Cushing's syndrome. Identify the potential care needs that the patient will have and formulate a care plan responsive to those needs (see Case History 5.1 and Nursing Care Plan 5.2).

HYPOSECRETION OF THE ADRENAL HORMONES

Addison's disease

Addison's disease is a rare condition in which there is total destruction of the adrenal cortex resulting in failure of cortisol secretion. It may occur at any age and is more common in females. Autoimmune adrenalitis is the most common cause in the developed world and is responsible for 80–90% of cases. Adrenal destruction by adrenalytic medication such as mitotane (o,p′-DDD), TB, HIV or malignancy are rare causes.

PATHOPHYSIOLOGY

Clinical features High levels of ACTH result in pigmentation of the skin and mucous membranes. Glucocorticoid, sex steroid and mineralocorticoid production are reduced. Plasma levels of proteins are low and potassium are high, with serum urea being elevated due to volume depletion.

Common presenting symptoms The onset of the disease is usually insidious, often starting with a feeling of general malaise and weakness. Skin discoloration may have been noticed, especially in the palmar creases and on the inside of the lips and cheeks. Some patients present as medical emergencies with an Addisonian crisis (see below). Untreated, this can be fatal.

MEDICAL MANAGEMENT

Investigations Diagnosis is by clinical examination and blood tests to confirm high levels of ACTH and low levels of cortisol. In the short Synacthen test (SST), a dose of 250 mg tetracosactide (synthetic ACTH) is given i.v. or i.m. and blood samples for plasma cortisol taken at 0, 30 and 60 min after its administration will show a failure of the adrenal glands to respond to the stimulus of the parenteral ACTH. Once this has been demonstrated, the cause of the adrenal failure needs to be identified. The most common cause, i.e. autoimmune, can be tested for with an assay to detect the presence of 21-hydroxylase antibodies. If there are no antibodies present, infectious or genetic causes should be investigated. Tests will include an MRI of the adrenal glands and screening for TB, HIV and cancer.

Treatment is by long-term replacement doses of mineralocorticoid and glucocorticoid. This should lead to an improvement in the patient's well-being. Levels of hydrocortisone should be checked regularly to ensure the dose is correct. Mineralocorticoid replacement with fludrocortisone should be checked by regular blood pressure readings, which should show no postural hypotension, and by measurement of plasma renin.

Addisonian crisis Adrenal crisis is a life-threatening event. It occurs in such situations as injury, infections, anaesthesia and surgical procedures where, unlike in the healthy individual, the stress response does not occur. The absence of the cortisol surge to a major stressor results in a severely shocked patient. Addisonian crisis requires immediate intervention. Symptoms may include:

- sudden penetrating pain in the abdomen, legs or lower back
- fever
- severe vomiting and diarrhoea leading to dehydration
- hypotension
- hypoglycaemia
- loss of consciousness (O'Donnell 1997).

CASE HISTORY 5.1

J

J was a 20-year-old woman admitted to the unit following transfer from her local hospital with a history of weight gain, hirsutism, acne on her back and face, pain and increasing weakness in her limbs, amenorrhoea and depression.

She was transferred in a wheelchair, being unable to walk at this point. Her parents and her fiancé accompanied her.

Once J was settled into the unit, clinical examination showed her to have centrally located obesity, severe acne, marked facial hair and some loss of occipital hair. She had severe pitting oedema of her ankles and had been amenorrhoeal for 6 months. Purple striae were present on her abdomen and thighs, and bruising was noticeable on her shins. She was unable to stand from the squatting position, indicating marked proximal myopathy. She was tearful and anxious and complained of a poor sleep pattern and waking at about 04.00 h. Observations showed her to be hypertensive at 170/110 mmHg; pulse and temperature were normal. J had some photographs of herself taken at her engagement party some 4 months before, showing a pretty, very slim, smiling young woman.

She was helped to settle into the unit and her nurse sat with her and explained the investigations that were to be performed. As many of these involved multiple venepunctures, she was reassured that a local anaesthetic cream would be applied. (It is inadvisable to leave cannulae in situ as the risk of infection in someone who is immunocompromised is high.)

On the first day, blood tests showed that J's baseline cortisol levels were well above the normal range. Her haemoglobin, liver function, urea and electrolytes were measured, as well as her sex hormone levels and thyroid function. A measurement of ACTH was made and found to be extremely high. Skull and chest X-rays were performed.

An insulin tolerance test showed elevated cortisol levels throughout, with no response to hypoglycaemia. A glucose tolerance test showed elevated glucose levels throughout; glycosuria was present 1 h post-glucose load. This had not resolved at 2 h, indicating a diabetic tendency.

On the third and fourth days, blood was taken at 09.00, 18.00 and 24.00 h and repeated the next night, the midnight samples being taken when J was asleep. This was to establish her circadian rhythm; the results showed that the levels of ACTH and cortisol did not fall at night and remained high throughout the day.

The finding that both the ACTH levels and the cortisol levels were high indicated that the high cortisol levels were being driven by ACTH. The source of the ACTH had to be established.

During this time J was seen by a psychiatrist, who established that she was depressed but not suicidal. Medical staff kept her informed about the results of her tests and their implications; further explanations were given by her nurse. A CT scan the following day showed an enlarged pituitary gland.

Based on this it was decided that petrosal sinus sampling (www.cushings-help.com/petrosal.htm) would be performed and samples taken for ACTH and cortisol after a catheter had been inserted into the right groin. The procedure was explained to J and her consent obtained. Her right groin was shaved and she was fasted overnight. Samples were taken at various points, including the petrosal sinuses (the point nearest the pituitary gland on both the left and right sides). No sedation is permitted prior to this test as it interferes with the results, and so extremely detailed explanation of the procedure was required to gain J's confidence and understanding. She was accompanied by her nurse, who remained with her throughout the procedure. When assayed, the results showed a higher level of ACTH on the left side of the pituitary.

Once a source had been found for the excess ACTH, J could be started on medication to control her symptoms. She was started on metyrapone 500 mg t.d.s. and her cortisol levels were checked daily to ensure she did not become hypocortisolaemic.

After review of her results and X-rays, it was suggested that to try to remove the pituitary tumour would be the best treatment option. After discussion with J, her consent for the operation was obtained. It was explained to her and her fiancé that there was a possibility that she may become deficient in all pituitary hormones following the surgery, including those which would affect her fertility. In this eventuality, hormone replacement could be given.

A small adenoma was removed from the left side of her pituitary gland. On return from theatre J was nursed on the neurosurgical ward initially. Hydrocortisone injections were given (100 mg every 6 h for 48 h) to ensure that if the tumour had been removed, J's cortisol levels would not fall too rapidly and predispose her to an Addisonian crisis. J returned to the endocrine unit looking rather bruised around the eyes and wearing a nasal bolster but otherwise well. Nursing staff continued to monitor her lying and standing blood pressures. Temperature and pulse were checked 4-hourly and nasal discharge was observed and tested for signs of CSF leak.

Three days postoperatively J's hydrocortisone was withdrawn. A measurement of her 09.00 h cortisol and ACTH was taken the next day. Her cortisol level was very low and correspondingly J felt weak and light-headed. Her blood pressure showed a postural drop. The next morning the exercise was repeated and the results were the same. J was losing weight around her face and her ankle oedema was reduced. She said she felt very positive for the first time in many weeks and was sleeping well. On the afternoon of the fourth postoperative day, she became weak and dizzy and felt nauseated. Her blood pressure was measured and found to be low. She was helped to lie down and the doctor informed. It was felt that an Addisonian crisis was impending and so a blood sample was taken for cortisol measurement and J was commenced on oral prednisolone. Some days later all of J's hormone levels were checked and, as she felt well on her replacement therapy, she was discharged home to the care of her family. It was arranged for her to return to the ward in 12 weeks' time.

By the time J returned for this visit, she had lost a considerable amount of weight, was walking unaided, had lost most of her facial hair and had started menstruating. Her steroid therapy was stopped and close observation maintained to observe for impending adrenal crisis. A blood test 48 h later indicated that her cortisol levels were in the normal range. It was decided to repeat all the pituitary function tests done prior to the surgery. These showed all hormones to be in the normal range and responses to hypoglycaemia, as demonstrated by the insulin tolerance test, to be intact. This showed that the pituitary had recovered its normal function. J was discharged home with a regular follow-up inpatient appointment every 12 weeks to ensure that all was well.

Some months after, the nurses received an invitation to J's wedding and 1 year later J was the very proud mother of a baby daughter.

Nursing Care Plan 5.2 Care of a patient with Cushing's syndrome

Nursing considerations	Action	Rationale	Expected outcome
1. Pain from fractured vertebrae or ribs as a result of osteoporosis	• Provide immediate pain relief. Administer as prescribed, noting the efficacy • Handle and position the patient carefully	Pain will cause the patient discomfort and will increase anxiety. Pain relief will reduce this. Fractured ribs will cause shallow breathing and will increase chances of chest infection. Gentle handling will reduce distress and prevent further fractures	The patient should be pain-free and comfortable and anxiety reduced
2. Infection as a result of immuno-compromisation	• Make 4-hourly recordings of temperature, pulse and blood pressure. Report any variation from the normal range immediately	Death from overwhelming infection can occur. Signs of infection will be masked, so infection may be advanced before signs are seen	Any infection will be identified early and correct treatment commenced
3. Damage to skin as a result of skin thinning and oedema or poor wound healing	• If the patient is immobile, care of pressure areas will be required to prevent tissue damage. Legs will need to be elevated to relieve the oedema and any wounds will require scrupulous aseptic technique when dressed	Tissue will be rapidly broken down and slow to heal, so preventive measures are essential. Susceptibility to infection requires precautions to prevent introduction of infection	Further tissue damage will be prevented and any present source of infection healed as rapidly as possible
4. Hypertension	• Record blood pressure 4-hourly after 10 min lying flat and 1 min standing. Report levels beyond the normal range or postural deficit	Increasing blood pressure may lead to stroke or heart failure and if persistently high will need to be treated with drugs. Postural deficit will indicate a problem with sodium excretion or retention	Blood pressure levels will remain within acceptable limits
5. Diabetes mellitus as a result of abnormal carbohydrate metabolism	• Record pre- and postprandial blood sugar levels and perform daily urinalysis	Persistently high blood sugars will lead to the complications of diabetes mellitus and may need to be treated with insulin	Blood sugar levels will remain within the normal range
6. Psychosis and mental disorder	• Ascertain the patient's psychological status early on. A psychiatric opinion should be obtained. Mood swings and bizarre behaviour should be reported. The patient may be so disturbed as to require 24 h psychiatric nurse observation	The patient's psychological state may change rapidly and close observation for this is necessary. Some patients can become suicidal	The patient will not be a danger to themselves or others and patient safety is maintained at all times

Treatment aims to restore steroid, sodium and glucose levels to within normal range by i.v. administration of 100 mg hydrocortisone, and i.v. infusion of normal saline given quickly with dextrose if glucose levels are low. Hydrocortisone is then given i.v. or i.m. 6-hourly until the patient is stable, following which steroid replacement can be given orally and mineralocorticoids introduced.

NURSING PRIORITIES AND MANAGEMENT: Addison's disease

Major considerations

Careful observation of temperature, pulse, and standing and lying blood pressure should be made. A raised temperature will indicate signs of infection which the patient may not be able to fight effectively. Any postural drop in blood pressure should be reported immediately.

The steroid replacement therapy should be administered with the patient's full involvement so that they have a full knowledge of dosage and timing and techniques for self-administration before discharge. The patient should be issued with a steroid card and advised to carry this and to wear a MedicAlert bracelet on their wrist or ankle at all times.

An ampoule of hydrocortisone 100 mg should be kept at home in case of serious illness or trauma, and the GP or community nurse called to administer it. It may be of value also to teach a member of the family how to do this.

It is vital that the patient and their relatives have a thorough understanding of their condition and the signs associated with complications. This will help to restore confidence and enable the patient to return to a full and active life.

STOP THINK

5.4 With a colleague, undertake a role-play exercise by acting out the education of the patient regarding steroid therapy. Formulate an information sheet which could be given to patients prior to discharge.

5.5 Check within the local hospital context what advice is available for patients with Addison's disease. Where do patients obtain the MedicAlert bracelet? Are these patients exempt from prescription charges?

CONGENITAL ADRENAL HYPERPLASIA (CAH)

This is a group of inherited disorders caused by a deficiency of one of the five enzymes involved in cortisol synthesis (Charmandar et al 2004). It is one of the most common autosomal recessive disorders with a prevalence in the USA and Europe of approximately 1:15 000–16 000 (van der Kamp & Wit 2004).

PATHOPHYSIOLOGY

To understand CAH it is necessary to understand the biosynthesis of steroids. To take the most common deficiency, which accounts for 95% of cases of CAH (Labarata et al 2004) as an example, if the enzyme 21-hydroxylase (CYP21) is absent because of a gene defect located on the short arm of chromosome 6, cortisol will not be produced in sufficient quantity. By means of the negative feedback system, ACTH production will be increased to stimulate the production of cortisol. This in turn will lead to hypertrophy of the adrenal cortex and elevated levels of 17-hydroxyprogesterone, androstenedione and testosterone — the hormones occurring before the enzyme block (see Fig. 5.7). This will result ultimately in virilisation.

Definitions of CAH CAH disorders can be divided into three main groups:

- severe or classic – with or without salt wasting (SW)
- moderate/less severe – simple virilising (SV)
- mild – non-classic (NC).

Common presenting symptoms If severe or classic, CAH presents at birth or in early infancy with sexual ambiguity and salt-wasting due to mineralocorticoid deficiency. It has an incidence of 1 in 15 000 (Labarata et al 2004). Life-threatening vomiting and dehydration can occur in the first weeks of life. In the female, the high level of androgens present cause clitoral hypertrophy and fusion of the labial folds resulting in ambiguous genitalia. The syndrome may not be recognised in the male. Internal genitalia may develop normally. If a diagnosis is not made at birth, a genotypical female (XX) may be labelled male. Furthermore, if not treated with corticosteroids, the individual may go into adrenal crisis and die.

Moderate CAH is sometimes referred to as simple virilising CAH and is typically recognised by signs of virilisation in prepubertal children. Effects can include premature development of pubic hair (precocious puberty), advanced bone age, accelerated growth velocity and diminished final height in both men and women as a result of premature fusion of the bony epiphyses (New 2004).

Mild or non-classic CAH has an incidence of 1 in 1000 and because prenatal virilisation does not occur, presents in late childhood/early adulthood (Labarata et al 2004). Symptoms of androgen excess include hirsutism, severe acne, temporal baldness and infertility in adolescents and adult women. Menarche may be normal or delayed and secondary amenorrhoea is common (Otten et al 2005). Polycystic ovarian syndrome (PCOS) may also be present. In young men, early beard growth, acne and a growth spurt may prompt the diagnosis. Men may also present with oligozoospermia or diminished fertility despite appearing asymptomatic and are only diagnosed when efforts to conceive fail.

MEDICAL MANAGEMENT

Investigations include blood tests to confirm high levels of ACTH and 17-hydroxyprogesterone (Azziz & Zacur 1989). Replacement of the glucocorticoid is usually given in the form of prednisolone to suppress the ACTH production and thereby reduce the overstimulation of the adrenals. Other requirements frequently include mineralocorticoids such as fludrocortisone.

NURSING PRIORITIES AND MANAGEMENT: Congenital adrenal hyperplasia (CAH)

General considerations

Information should be given to the individual regarding steroid replacement therapy (see p. 178). Nursing care should concentrate on the psychological support which will be required, especially if the diagnosis is made in adulthood.

The psychosocial and psychosexual implications of CAH are considerable, and formal counselling and psychotherapy should be made available. In female patients, hirsutism and acne can be especially distressing. Antiandrogens, e.g. cyproterone acetate, are now the treatment of choice (Spritzer et al 1990). Other important issues for women, which need discussion, include menstruation, sexuality, fertility and the possible need for plastic surgery, as some effects of virilisation are not reversible by medication (Hagenfeldt 2004). This is particularly important as the patient approaches adulthood, as sexual intercourse may be rendered difficult, painful or impossible. Prevention of subfertility should be implemented as a treatment goal from the start of puberty. The transition of care for the patient from the paediatric to adult endocrinologist is of utmost importance.

DISORDERS OF THE GONADS

ANATOMY AND PHYSIOLOGY

The gonads — ovaries in the female and testes in the male — are described in Chapters 7 and 8.

DISORDERS OF SEXUAL DIFFERENTIATION

In normal development, gonadal and phenotypic sex follow an orderly process of development determined by chromosomal sex at the moment of conception (see Ch. 6).

During the early stages of fetal life the gonad has the potential to develop female or male characteristics. In the presence of another X chromosome (i.e. 46, XX) or the absence of another chromosome (i.e. 45, XO), development will follow the female pattern. The presence of two X chromosomes is, however, necessary for normal ovarian function.

By the second month of fetal development the genital organs are undifferentiated duct systems, termed the Müllerian and Wolffian ducts. In the normal female, as development progresses, the Wolffian system regresses and the Müllerian system develops to form the fallopian tubes, the uterus and the upper vagina. The external genitalia undergo little change.

In the male, the Müllerian system regresses and the Wolffian system develops to form the testes, vas deferens, prostate and seminiferous tubules. The genital tubercle present in both systems forms the clitoris in the female and the penis in the male.

There is evidence to suggest that the normal development of a male child is hormone-dependent. It appears that testosterone inhibits the regression of the Wolffian duct and stimulates its development into the male sexual structures. In contrast to this, the ovary is not affected by hormones in utero.

Abnormalities of sexual differentiation may present with abnormal genitalia at birth, growth disturbance in childhood or abnormal secondary sexual development.

Abnormalities of gonadal development

True hermaphroditism, i.e. the presence of both male and female sexual characteristics in the same individual, is extremely rare (Karam & Baker 2004). It occurs when both the Müllerian and Wolffian systems continue to develop. Diagnosis requires a high index of suspicion for subtle abnormalities of the genitalia (Wiersma 2004). Ovotestes may exist or an ovary on one side and a testis on the other.

Chromosomal abnormalities

Chromosomal abnormalities affecting sexual differentiation may be described briefly as follows:

Klinefelter's syndrome is a condition in which phenotypical males have two X chromosomes and one Y chromosome. It is the most prevalent sex chromosome disorder in men with an incidence of 1 in 600 male newborns (Kamischke et al 2003). Men with Klinefelter's syndrome are typically tall, infertile and may exhibit a varying degree of Leydig cell failure resulting in testosterone deficiency. (Bojesen et al 2004).

Turner's syndrome is a condition in which the individual is phenotypically female, but has the genotype XO, i.e. complete or partial absence of one X chromosome. It is the most commonly occurring chromosomal abnormality in females, with an incidence of approximately 50 in 100 000 women and girls (Gravholt 2004). Affected individuals are of short stature with a 'web neck' and may have widely spaced nipples and peripheral oedema. The ovaries are atrophic and serum LH and FSH levels are elevated. They are prone to a variety of serious cardiac problems including coarctation of the aorta and aortic dissection. Women with Turner's syndrome are thought to have a reduced life expectancy, mainly due to these serious cardiac problems, but they may also have multiple co-morbidities, which can include hypothyroidism, deafness, osteoporosis, oestrogen deficiency and infertility (Ostberg & Conway 2003).

Kallman's syndrome In this condition there is a normal karyotype but a genetic defect in the pathway leading to gonadotrophin secretion; thus there is a deficiency of gonadotrophins and therefore sex steroid secretion is reduced. This condition is sometimes termed congenital hypogonadotrophic hypogonadism. Typically, the individual has a defect in their sense of smell (anosmia). Normal gonadal function can be restored with replacement of LH and FSH, meaning that fertility is possible. Otherwise, when fertility is not an issue, androgen replacement therapy is mandatory (John & Schmid 2000).

Testicular feminisation This is a syndrome of androgen resistance or complete androgen insensitivity (CAI syndrome) caused by mutations in the androgen receptor gene. While the karyotype is male (46, XY), the phenotype is female. Testes are present, but because of tissue resistance to circulating androgens but not oestrogen at puberty, breast tissue develops although pubic hair does not (Skordis et al 2005). Regression of the Müllerian system occurs due to tissue insensitivity but the Wolffian system does not develop and a blind-ended vagina results (Hannema et al 2004). The gonads may become malignant and are usually removed at the onset of adult life.

NURSING PRIORITIES AND MANAGEMENT: Disorders of sexual differentiation

Whilst disorders of the gonads are rarely life threatening or require admission to hospital, the psychological implications for the individual and their family cannot be overemphasised.

The role of the nurse in the investigation and treatment of these conditions is to offer psychological support to the individual, and, if they agree, their family, in an environment which is both relaxed and supportive.

Counselling on an informal and formal basis is essential during investigations, when complete privacy must be ensured. Feelings of inadequacy regarding sexuality and low self-esteem are common. An approach which demonstrates empathy with the individual helps to create a positive image during the initial examinations and investigations and during subsequent treatment.

EATING DISORDERS

Eating disorders can be divided into two main diagnostic categories: anorexia nervosa and bulimia nervosa (Garfinkel 2002). Patients who do not fit either of these categories but who have a clinically significant problem are diagnosed as having an atypical eating disorder. The discussion of eating disorders in this chapter may seem controversial, as many would classify these as psychological illnesses and among the most common of all psychiatric disorders in women (Morgan et al 1999). However, as endocrine disorder is often a manifestation of an eating disorder, e.g. amenorrhoea in the patient with anorexia, such patients may be seen in endocrine clinics. For this reason eating disorders are considered here.

Studies into the role of the hypothalamus have highlighted the influence it has on appetite control and it is considered almost certain that the hypothalamus has a function in some eating disorders (Costin 1999). Hypotheses include the identification of a negative feedback system involving a specific protein produced by the fat cell, known as leptin, which may be malfunctioning in the obese patient (Farooqi et al 1998).

ANOREXIA NERVOSA

Anorexia nervosa is an eating disorder characterised by self-inflicted starvation and a relentless pursuit of thinness (Bruch 1999).

Epidemiology

Anorexia nervosa is seen in all social classes and in both sexes. However, only 5–10% of cases occur in males and there is a higher prevalence in social classes 1 and 2 (Hoek 2002). Bruch (1999) indicated that anorexic individuals tend to be young girls who come from highly successful families in which the parents have high expectations of their children.

Aetiology

Contributory factors in the development of anorexia nervosa include:

- Family background, parental pressure, sibling disability, parental overprotection and negative changes within family relationships (Horesh et al 1996)
- The onset of puberty and psychosexual development in which there is denial and avoidance of sexuality marked by the development of the breasts and change of shape of hips and thighs
- Sociocultural expectations — there is an enormous emphasis on thinness in society's image of female beauty.

Studies also suggest that there is a genetic risk factor for anorexia. Studies of twins in the USA suggest that approximately half the risk of developing this eating disorder is inherited (Grice et al 2002).

PATHOPHYSIOLOGY

There is a complex relationship between nutritional, endocrine and psychological factors in this condition. Disorders in nutritional status result from prolonged insufficient intake of carbohydrates, fats and other nutrients. Metabolic disturbances, e.g. hypokalaemia, can occur following self-induced vomiting or the continual use of laxatives.

Clinical features Endocrine dysfunction appears to relate to weight loss and affects the hypothalamic–pituitary–gonadal axis. Blood tests reveal low circulating levels of LH, FSH and oestradiol. Injections of GnRH stimulate a rise in these, indicating that hypothalamic function is affected and the pituitary response is intact. Amenorrhoea occurs in girls as a result of this disturbance, secondary to the loss of body fat. The individual's metabolic rate slows down, resulting in hypotension, bradycardia, reduced core body temperature and cold extremities.

Individuals with anorexia nervosa often have underlying depression. It would seem that their psychological symptoms are aggravated by the undernutrition, and some professionals argue that patients are more receptive to psychological help when they are better nourished. The characteristic psychological state involves a denial of the illness, a failure to recognise the need for treatment and a need to exercise control over eating behaviour. The individual will have a distorted body image and insist that their abnormally thin, wasted, cachectic body appears obese.

Common presenting symptoms Most frequently, the anorexia will have been present for some months before individuals can be persuaded to see their GP. A determination to lose weight, coupled with the desire to change the shape of the body is typical, as is the denial of any problem or illness. In women, amenorrhoea, typically beginning 3–6 months from the start of weight loss, is often found.

MEDICAL MANAGEMENT

History and investigation Diagnosis is reached after investigations have proved that there is no underlying cause for the weight loss. Objective criteria have been developed to aid diagnosis. These include:

- a determination to diet and lose weight and maintain the weight loss
- a change of body shape to one of extreme thinness
- distorted body image
- avoidance of sexuality
- amenorrhoea in female patients.

Treatment Depending on the severity of the weight loss and its effect on general health, most patients can be managed in an outpatient setting, with psychological treatment regimens for a minimum of 6 months. If the patient's condition deteriorates or there is no improvement during this time, more intensive forms of treatment may need to be considered. These may require day care or inpatient care in a specialist mental health unit.

It is commonly accepted that an eclectic approach to treatment is appropriate. Psychological treatment should focus on the patient's eating behaviour, their attitude to their weight and body shape and any wider psychosocial issues that may be affecting them. Psychological therapy may include cognitive–behavioural therapy (CBT) to improve attitudes towards body image and individual and/or family interventions focused explicitly on eating disorders. Restoring body weight and nutritional status will be at the centre of whatever approach is used. If the weight loss has led to physiologically life-threatening conditions such as hypokalaemia or renal failure, it may be necessary to correct fluid and electrolyte imbalance by i.v. fluids and to improve nutritional status by parenteral or nasogastric feeding for as short a time as possible. Given the invasive nature of these procedures, they can be psychologically damaging for the individual. Force feeding of the patient must be done in strict accordance with the Mental Health Act of 1983. Rigid inpatient behaviour modification programmes should not be used. Following any inpatient episode, patients should be offered ongoing outpatient treatment for at least 12 months. They should be regularly reviewed for any signs of physical and psychological risk, e.g. suicidal thoughts or self-harm (NICE 2004).

A multidisciplinary team approach in which dietitians, occupational therapists, medical staff, psychologists and nurses work together with the anorexic individual in an agreed and consistent framework is essential. Current therapy combines the use of psychotherapy and antidepressants (Bardin 1997). Other studies have looked at the maintenance of weight using drugs that act on serotonin uptake (O'Dwyer et al 1996). However, there is limited evidence for the benefits of medical therapy in the treatment of anorexia nervosa and this should never be regarded as the primary treatment (NICE 2004). Side-effects, especially cardiovascular, must be carefully monitored.

NURSING PRIORITIES AND MANAGEMENT: Anorexia nervosa

Major considerations

The main aims of nursing care for patients with anorexia nervosa are to facilitate physical and psychological recovery by seeking to:

- establish a good relationship with the patient
- restore body weight and nutritional status by aiming for 0.5–1 kg/week average weight gain as an inpatient and 0.5 kg/week as an outpatient, achieved by increasing calories by ~3500–7000/week
- establish a good eating pattern and the enjoyment of mealtimes
- eliminate self-induced vomiting and the use of laxatives
- help the individual to acquire a positive self-image.

Because of their condition, patients will often present strong arguments as to why they cannot eat and will resort to devious methods to avoid taking in calories. Visits to the toilet after eating, to vomit or to dispose of food not eaten, should be monitored and, where possible, prevented. Dental treatment and advice is important to minimise effects of vomiting, e.g. patients should be told not to brush their teeth after vomiting and to avoid the use of acidic mouthwashes. It is important that mealtimes are handled in a relaxed manner. Realistic goals should be set and agreed to by each patient, with regard to foods eaten and weight gain. A written contract can help to create a climate of trust and help to prevent manipulation of staff and parents.

As an inpatient, if goals are met and maintained, short stays with the family can be arranged. If these visits are successful, plans can be made for discharge home. Continued support and monitoring of nutritional and weight status is essential, as relapse is common among anorexic individuals.

BULIMIA NERVOSA

Bulimia nervosa is an eating disorder characterised by episodes of binge eating, followed by episodes of fasting, self-induced vomiting and the misuse of laxatives and sometimes diuretics to prevent weight gain, coupled with an exaggerated preoccupation with the individual's weight and body shape (Lilly 2003). It occurs in about 1% of young women in the developed world, with women being ten times more likely to be affected than men (Hay 2003). These women are usually of normal weight but some may be obese. As with anorexia nervosa, bulimia nervosa often begins during adolescence. It is a chronic condition which affects a patient's quality of life; however, very few actively seek help because of feelings of shame associated with the binge eating and purging, which have often gone on in secret for many years, becoming deeply ingrained patterns of behaviour which can be hard to change. Once identified, however, patients should be encouraged to follow an evidence-based self-help programme. Specially adapted forms of CBT are available and 16–20 sessions over a 4–5 month period are recommended (NICE 2004). If there is no response, or the patient is not willing to undergo CBT, other forms of psychological therapy should be considered, e.g. interpersonal psychotherapy. This should be continued for 8–12 months (NICE 2004). As an alternative to psychological therapy, or as an additional first step, a trial of antidepressants may be instigated. These can decrease the frequency of episodes of binge eating and purging. As a first choice, selective serotonin reuptake inhibitors (SSRIs) are prescribed. The SSRIs are well accepted and tolerated, and have fewer side-effects than the tricyclic antidepressants.

For further information on both anorexia nervosa and bulimia nervosa, see Murphy & Manning (2003) and Nicholls & Viner (2005).

REFERENCES

Abs R, Verhelst J, Maiter D et al 1998 Cabergoline in the treatment of acromegaly: a study in 64 patients. Journal of Clinical Endocrinology and Metabolism 83: 374–378

Allolio B, Hahner S, Weisman D, Fussnacht N 2004 Management of adrenocortical carcinoma. Clinical Endocrinology 60(3): 273–287

Azziz R, Zacur H A 1989 21-Hydroxylase deficiency in female hyperandrogenism: screening and diagnosis. Journal of Clinical Endocrinology 69(3): 577–584

Bardin C W 1997 Current therapy in endocrinology and metabolism, 6th edn. Mosby, St Louis

Bassett J H D, Forbes S A, Pannett A A J et al 1998 Characterization of mutations in patients with multiple endocrine neoplasia type I. American Journal of Human Genetics 62: 232–244

Baxter M A 1994 Acromegaly and hypophysectomy: a case report. Association of American Nurse Anaesthetists 62(2): 182–185

Besser G M, Thorner M O 2002 Comprehensive clinical endocrinology. Mosby, Edinburgh

Besser G M, Trainer P J 1995 The Barts endocrine protocols. Churchill Livingstone, Edinburgh

Bevan J S, Atkin S L, Atkinson A B et al 2002 Primary medical therapy for acromegaly: an open prospective multicentre study of the effects of subcutaneous and intra-muscular slow release octreotide on growth hormone, insulin-like growth factor-1 and tumour size. Journal of Clinical Endocrinology and Metabolism 87: 4554–4563

Biermasz N R, Dulken H, Roelfsema F 2000 Long-term follow-up results of postoperative radiotherapy in 36 patients with acromegaly. Journal of Clinical Endocrinology and Metabolism 85: 2476–2482

Bojesen A, Jun S, Birkbaek N, Gravholt C H 2004 Increased mortality in Klinefelter's syndrome. Journal of Clinical Endocrinology and Metabolism 89(8): 3830–3834

Bouloux P M G, Rees L M 1994 Diagnostic tests in endocrinology and metabolism. Chapman and Hall, London

Bravo E L, Tagle R 2003 Pheocromocytoma: state of the art and future prospects. Endocrine Reviews 24(4): 539–553

Brooke A M, Monson J P 2003 Adult growth hormone deficiency. Clinical Medicine 3: 15–19

Bruch H 1999 Eating disorders. Basic Books, New York

Charmandar E, Brook C G, Hindmarsh P C 2004 Classic congenital adrenal hyperplasia and puberty. European Journal of Endocrinology 151(Suppl 3): U77–82

Colao A, Ferone D, Marzullo P, Lombardini G 2004 Systemic complications of acromegaly: epidemiology, pathogenesis and management. Endocrine Reviews 25(1): 102–152

Cooper D S 1999 The side effects of antithyroid drugs. The Endocrinologist 9: 457

Costin C 1999 The eating disorder sourcebook: a comprehensive guide to the causes, treatments and prevention of eating disorders, 2nd edn. Lowell House, Los Angeles

De Rosa M, Colao A, Di Sarno A et al 1998 Cabergoline treatment rapidly improves gonadal function in hyperprolactinomic males: a comparison with bromocriptine. European Journal of Endocrinology 138: 286–293

Delange F M, Dunn J T 2005 Iodine deficiency. In: Braverman L E, Utiger (eds) Werner and Ingbar's the thyroid: a fundamental and clinical text, 9th edn. Lippincott, Williams and Wilkins, Baltimore

Di Somma C, Colao A, Di Sarno A et al 1998 Bone marker and bone density responses to dopamine agonist therapy in hyperprolactinaemic males. Journal of Clinical Endocrinology and Metabolism 83: 807–813

Dougherty L, Lister S (eds) 2004 The Royal Marsden Hospital manual of clinical nursing procedures, 6th edn. Blackwell Publishing, Edinburgh

Drake W M, Coyte D, Carnacho-Hubner C et al 1998 Optimising growth hormone replacement therapy by dose titration in hypopituitary adults. Journal of Clinical Endocrinology and Metabolism 83: 3913–3919

Farooqi S, Rau H, Whitehead J, O'Rahilly S 1998 Ob gene mutations and human obesity. Proceedings of the Nutrition Society 57(3): 471–475

Fleisch H 1998 Bisphosphonates: mechanisms of action. Endocrine Review 19: 80–100

Gaillard R C, Giusti V 2004 Dosing and individual responsiveness to growth hormone replacement therapy. In: Abs R, Feldt-Rasmussen U (eds) Growth hormone deficiency in adults; 10 years of KIMS. Oxford Pharmagenesis, Oxford, Ch 10, p 103–116

Garfinkel P E 2002 Classification and diagnosis of eating disorders. In: Fairburn C G, Brownell K D (eds) Eating disorders and obesity: a comprehensive handbook. Guilford Press, New York

Giustina A, Barkan A, Casanueva F F et al 2000 Criteria for cure of acromegaly: a consensus statement. Journal of Clinical Endocrinology and Metabolism 85: 526–529

Gooren L J G, Bunck M C M 2004 Androgen replacement therapy, present and future. Drugs 64(17): 1861–1891

Gravholt C H 2004 Long-term follow-up of Turner's syndrome. International Growth Monitor 14(4): 2–6

Grice D E, Halmi K, Fichter M M et al 2002 Evidence for a susceptibility gene for anorexia nervosa on chromosome 1. American Journal of Human Genetics 70(3): 787–792

Hagenfeldt K B 2004 Congenital adrenal hyperplasia due to 21-hydroxylase deficiency – the adult woman. Growth Hormone IGF Research Suppl A: S67–71

Hannema S E, Scott I S, Hodapp J et al 2004 Residual activity of mutant androgen receptors explains wolffian duct development in the complete androgen insensitivity syndrome. Journal of Clinical Endocrinology and Metabolism 89(11): 5815–5822

Haslett C, Chilvers E R, Boon N A, Colledge N R 2002 Davidson's principles and practice of medicine, 19th edn. Churchill Livingstone, Edinburgh

Haugen B R, Pacini F, Reiners C et al 1999 A comparison of recombinant human thyrotropin and thyroid hormone withdrawal for the detection of thyroid remnant or cancer. Journal of Clinical Endocrinology and Metabolism 84: 3877–3885

Hay P J 2003 Quality of life and bulimic eating disorder behaviours: findings from a community based sample. International Journal of Eating Disorders 33: 434–442

Hoek H W 2002 Distribution of eating disorders. In: Fairburn C G, Brownwell K D (eds) Eating disorders and obesity: a comprehensive handbook. Guilford Press, New York

Holmes S J, Shalet S M 1995 Which adults develop side-effects of growth hormone replacement? Clinical Endocrinology 43: 143–149

Horesh N, Apter A, Ishai J et al 1996 Abnormal psychosocial situations and eating disorders in adolescence. Journal of the American Academy of Child and Adolescent Psychiatry 35(7): 921–927

Jeffcoate W 1993 Lecture notes on endocrinology, 5th edn. Blackwell Scientific, Oxford

John H, Schmid C 2000 Kallman's syndrome: clues to clinical diagnosis. International Journal of Impotence Research 12(2): 121–123

Kaltsas G A, Isidoi A M, Florakis D et al 2001 Predictors of the outcome of surgical treatment in acromegaly and the value of the mean growth hormone day curve in assessing post-operative disease activity. Journal of Clinical Endocrinology and Metabolism 86: 1645–1652

Kamischke A, Baumgardt A, Horst J, Nieschlag E 2003 Clinical and diagnostic features of patients with suspected Klinefelter's syndrome. Journal of Andrology 24(1): 41–48

Karam J A, Baker L AL 2004 Images in clinical medicine. True hermaphroditism. New England Journal of Medicine 350(4): 393

Kumar P, Clark M 2002 Clinical medicine: a textbook for medical students and doctors, 5th edn. WB Saunders, London

Labarata J I, Bello E, Ruiz-Echarri M et al 2004 Childhood onset of congenital adrenal hyperplasia: long-term outcome and optimization of therapy. Journal of Paediatric Endocrinology and Metabolism 17(Suppl 3): 411–422

Lilly R Z 2003 Bulimia nervosa. British Medical Journal 327(74): 380–381

Lindholm J 2004 Diabetes insipidus: historical aspects. Pituitary 7(1): 33–38

Molitch M E 2002 Medical management of prolactin secreting pituitary adenomas. Pituitary 5: 55–65

Morgan J F, Reid F, Lacey J H 1999 The SCOFF questionnaire: assessment of a new screening tool for eating disorders. British Medical Journal 319(7223): 1467–1468

Mukherjee A, Shalet S M 2004 Overview of growth hormone deficiency in adults. In: Abs R, Feldt-Rasmussen U (eds) Growth hormone deficiency in adults; 10 years of KIMS. Oxford Pharmagenesis, Oxford

National Institute for Clinical Excellence (NICE) 2003 Human growth hormone (somatropin) in adults with growth hormone deficiency. Technology Appraisal 64. NICE, London

National Institute of Clinical Excellence (NICE) 2004 Eating disorders: core interventions in the treatment and management of anorexia nervosa, bulimia nervosa and related eating disorders. Clinical Guidelines 9. NICE, London

New M I 2004 An update of congenital adrenal hyperplasia. Annals of the New York Academy of Sciences 1038: 14–43

Nieschlag E 1998 Therapeutic controversy VII: if testosterone, which testosterone? Which

androgen regimen should be used for supplementation in older men? Formulation, dosing and monitoring issues. Clinical Endocrinology 51: 757–763
O'Donnell M 1997 Emergency! Addisonian crisis. American Journal of Nursing 97(3): 41
O'Dwyer A M, Lucie J V, Russell G F 1996 Serotonin activity in anorexia nervosa after long term weight restoration: response to D-fenfluramine challenge. Psychological Medicine 26(2): 353–359
O'Riordan J H H, Malan P G, Gould R P 1982 Essentials of endocrinology. Blackwell Scientific, Oxford
Ostberg J E, Conway G S 2003 Adulthood in women with Turner's syndrome. Hormone Research 59(5): 211–221
Otten B J, Stikkelbroeck M M, Claahsen-van der Grinten H L, Hermus A R M M 2005 Puberty and fertility in congenital adrenal hyperplasia. Endocrine Development 8: 54–66
Parwardhan N A, Monront M, Rao S et al 1993 Surgery still has a role in Graves' hyperthyroidism. Surgery 114: 1108
Ralston S H, Thiebaud D, Herrmann Z et al 1997 Dose–response study of ibandronate in the treatment of cancer-associated hypercalcaemia. British Journal of Cancer 75: 295–300
Ramirez A, House A 1997 ABC of mental health: common mental health problems in hospital. British Medical Journal 314(7095): 1679–1681
Schlechte J A 2003 Prolactinoma. New England Journal of Medicine 349: 2035–2041
Schneider A B, Ron E 2005 Carcinoma of follicular epithelium: epidemiology and pathogenesis. In: Braverman L E, Utiger R D (eds) Werner and Ingbar's the thyroid: a fundamental and clinical text, 9th edn. Lippincott, Williams and Wilkins, Philadelphia
Schubert M, Minnemann D, Hubler D et al 2004 Intramuscular testosterone undecanoate: pharmacokinetic aspects of a novel testosterone formulation during long-term treatment of men with hypogonadism. Journal of Clinical Endocrinology and Metabolism 89: 5429–5434
Sinclair H C, Fawcett J N 1991 Altschul's psychology for nurses, 7th edn. Baillière Tindall, London
Skordis N, Lumbroso S, Penkleous M et al 2005 Complete androgen insensitivity syndrome caused by the R855H mutation in the androgen receptor gene. Journal of Paediatric Endocrinology and Metabolism 18(3): 309–313
Spencer E, Pycock C, Lyttle J 1993 Pheochromocytoma presenting as acute circulatory collapse and abdominal pain. Intensive Care Medicine 19(6): 356–357
Spritzer P, Billard L, Thalabard J C et al 1990 Cyproterone acetate versus hydrocortisone treatment in late-onset adrenal hyperplasia. Journal of Clinical Endocrinology and Metabolism 70(3): 642–646
Stewart A F 2005 Hypercalcaemia associated with cancer. New England Journal of Medicine 352: 373–379
Swerdloff R S, Wang C, Cunningham G et al 2000 Long-term pharmacokinetics of transdermal testosterone gel in hypogonadal men. Journal of Clinical Endocrinology and Metabolism 85: 4500–4510
Swords F M, Allan C A, Sibtain A et al 2003 Stereotactic radiosurgery XVI: a treatment for previously irradiated pituitary adenomas. Journal of Clinical Endocrinology and Metabolism 88: 5334–5340
Thakker R V 1998 Multiple endocrine neoplasia – syndromes of the twentieth century. Journal of Endocrinology and Metabolism 83: 2617–2620
Thakker R V 2004 Genetics of endocrine and metabolic disorders: parathyroid. Reviews in Endocrine and Metabolic Disorders 5(1): 37–51
Trainer P J 2002 Acromegaly—consensus. What consensus? Journal of Clinical Endocrinology and Metabolism 87: 3534–3536
Van der Kamp H J, Wit J M 2004 Neonatal screening for congenital adrenal hyperplasia. European Journal of Endocrinology 151(Suppl 3): U71–75
van der Lely A J, Hutson R K, Trainer P J et al 2001 Long term treatment of acromegaly with pegvisomant, a growth hormone antagonist. Lancet 358: 1754–1759
Wang C, Swerdloff R S 1997 Androgen replacement therapy. Annals of Medicine 29: 365–370
Wang C, Swerdloff R S 1999 Androgen replacement therapy, risks and benefits. In: Wang C (ed) Male reproductive function. Kluwer, Boston
Wass J A H 1997 Evidence of the effectiveness of radiotherapy in the treatment of acromegaly. Journal of Endocrinology 155(Suppl 1): S57–S58
Wass J A H (ed) 2001 Handbook of acromegaly. Bioscientifica, Bristol
Waugh A, Grant A (eds) 2001 Ross and Wilson's anatomy and physiology in health and illness, 9th edn. Churchill Livingstone, Edinburgh
Webster J 2000 Cabergoline and quinagolide therapy for prolactinomas. Clinical Endocrinology 53: 549–550
Wiersma R 2004 True hermaphroditism in South Africa – the clinical picture. Paediatric Surgery International 20(5): 563–568
Wilson J D 2005 The evolution of endocrinology. Clinical Endocrinology 62(4): 389–396

FURTHER READING

Agana-Defensor R, Proch M 1992 Pheochromocytoma: a clinical review. Clinical Issues in Critical Care Nursing 3(2): 309–318
Azziz R 2005 Diagnostic criteria for polycystic ovary syndrome: a reappraisal. Fertility and Sterility 83(5): 1343–1346
Besser G M, Thorner M O 2002 Comprehensive clinical endocrinology. Mosby, Edinburgh
Bouloux P M G, Rees L M 1994 Diagnostic tests in endocrinology and diabetes. Chapman and Hall, London
Braverman L E, Utiger R D (eds) 2004 Werner and Ingbar's the thyroid: a fundamental and clinical text, 9th edn. Lippincott, Williams and Wilkins, Philadelphia
Counsell C M, Gilbert M, Snively C 1996 Management of a patient with a pituitary tumour resection. Dimensions of Critical Care Nursing 15(2): 75–81
Hall R, Besser M (eds) 1989 Fundamentals of clinical endocrinology, 4th edn. Churchill Livingstone, Edinburgh
Kaltsas G A, Besser G M, Grossman A B 2004 The diagnosis and medical management of advanced neuroendocrine tumours. Endocrine Reviews 25(3): 458–511
Liu J K, Couldwell W T 2004 Contemporary management of prolactinomas. Neurosurgical Focus 16(4): E2
Montague S E, Watson R, Herbert R 2005 Physiology for nursing practice, 3rd edn. Baillière Tindall, London
Murphy B, Manning Y 2003 An introduction to anorexia nervosa and bulimia nervosa. Nursing Standard 18(14–16): 45–55
Nicholls D, Viner R 2005 Eating disorders and weight problems. British Medical Journal 330: 950–953
Nieschlag E, Behre H M (eds) 2004 Testosterone: action, deficiency, substitution, 3rd edn. Cambridge University Press, Cambridge
Piersanti M 2004 Growth hormone replacement for patients with adult onset growth hormone deficiency – what have we learned? Neurosurgical Focus 16(4): E12
Royal College of Physicians/Royal College of Psychiatry 1995 Psychological care of medical patients: recognition of need and service provision. RCP/RCPsych, London
Schafer J 2005 My story, thyroid papillary carcinoma. Online. Available: http://oncolink.upenn.edu/types/article.cfm

USEFUL WEBSITES

ACTH
www.cushingsacth.co.uk

Addison's Disease Self Help Group (ADSHG)
www.adshg.org.uk

AMEND (Association for Multiple Endocrine Neoplasia Disorders)
www.amend.org.uk

Anorexia Nervosa and Related Eating Disorders (ANRED)
www.anred.com

British Thyroid Foundation
www.btf-thyroid.org

Climb: Congenital Adrenal Hyperplasia UK Support Group
www.cah.org.uk

eXtra (Klinefelter's Syndrome Association UK)
www.ksa-uk.co.uk

MedicAlert Foundation
www.medicalert.org

The Pituitary Foundation
www.pituitary.org.uk

Thyroid Eye Disease (TED) Charitable Trust
www.patient.co.uk/showdoc/26739046

PART 2 DIABETES MELLITUS

INTRODUCTION

Diabetes mellitus is defined as a metabolic disorder of multiple aetiology. It is characterised by chronic hyperglycaemia with disturbances of carbohydrate, protein and fat metabolism which results from defects in insulin secretion, insulin action or both (World Health Organization 1999). In the UK, 1 in 20 people over the age of 65 has diabetes and in people over the age of 85 this rises to 1 in 5 (DH 2001). Diabetes UK (2003a) estimates that there are around 1.4 million adults with known diabetes and there could be as many as a further million who may have type 2 diabetes without yet knowing it.

Diabetes classification

In the past, diagnostic and treatment characteristics were the main classification criteria. Accordingly, diabetes was described as being insulin-dependent diabetes or non-insulin-dependent diabetes. This classification has been replaced by the World Health Organization (WHO) classification (WHO 1999) which recognises the main types of diabetes as follows:

- Type 1 diabetes (formerly insulin-dependent diabetes)
- Type 2 diabetes (formerly non-insulin-dependent diabetes)
- Gestational diabetes
- Impaired glucose regulation
- Other specific types.

For a detailed study of normal anatomy and physiology, see Tortora & Grabowski (2002); for information on gestational diabetes, see Diabetes UK (2004).

ANATOMY AND PHYSIOLOGY

The pancreas

The pancreas has both exocrine and endocrine functions. Exocrine tissue is responsible for the secretion of enzymes which are transported in ducts to the duodenum where they play a vital role in the digestion of food. The endocrine function of the pancreas is concerned with the secretion of hormones. Clusters of endocrine tissue, the islets of Langerhans, are found scattered throughout the pancreas. There are two principal types of cell contained within the islets: beta cells (β cells), which secrete insulin, and alpha cells (α cells), which secrete glucagon. Each has a role in the regulation of blood glucose.

Delta cells (δ cells), also within the islets, secrete somatostatin which contributes to the regulation of a variety of hormones throughout the body, including insulin and glucagon.

Blood glucose regulation

Within a 24-h period, the healthy human will alternate between the 'fed state' and the 'fasting state' several times. In the 2 h following a meal the blood glucose will tend to rise as absorption of nutrients takes place. This is termed

Table 5.8 The physiological effects of insulin

Process	Action	Tissue
Effects on carbohydrate metabolism		
Glucose transport	↑	Adipose, muscle
Glycolysis	↑	Adipose, muscle
Glycogen synthesis	↑	Adipose, muscle, liver
Glucose oxidation via pentose phosphate pathway	↑	Liver, adipose
Glycogen breakdown	↓	Muscle, liver
Glycogenolysis, gluconeogenesis	↓	Liver
Effects on lipid metabolism		
Lipolysis	↓	Adipose
Fatty acid synthesis	↑	Adipose, liver
Low-density lipoprotein synthesis	↑	Liver
Lipoprotein lipase	↑	Adipose
Cholesterol synthesis	↑	Liver
Effects on protein metabolism		
Amino acid transport	↑	Muscle, adipose, liver, others
Protein synthesis	↑	Muscle, adipose, liver, others
Protein degradation	↓	Muscle
Urea formation	↓	

↑, increase; ↓, decrease.
Reproduced with permission from Watkins et al (2003).

the postprandial or fed state. Once glucose has been taken up into the cells, blood glucose levels will tend to fall and will not rise again until the next meal is taken. This is termed the preprandial or fasting state. In health these fluctuations are very slight, as insulin is secreted at a low or basal level throughout the whole day, only rising to an increased stimulated level at mealtimes.

Insulin and glucagon are principally (but not exclusively) responsible for blood glucose regulation.

Insulin

Insulin, an anabolic hormone, is secreted in response to a rising blood glucose level. Its functions are (Table 5.8):

- to facilitate glucose uptake by the cells
- to promote glycogenesis, i.e. the conversion of glucose to glycogen for storage in the liver and skeletal muscle
- to promote protein synthesis
- to promote conversion of glucose to triglycerides for ultimate storage as body fat.

All of these functions have the effect of preventing an abnormal rise in blood glucose (hyperglycaemia) during the postprandial period (see Fig. 5.8). Insulin secretion is highest in the fed state and lowest in the fasting state.

Glucagon

Glucagon, a catabolic hormone, is secreted in response to a falling blood glucose level and has the following functions:

- to promote the conversion of stored glycogen to glucose (glycogenolysis) and its release from the liver
- to promote fat and protein breakdown in order to provide an alternative source of glucose via lipolysis and gluconeogenesis
- to influence the production of ketone bodies (ketogenesis). In total or near-total insulin lack, these weak acids are produced as a result of the chemical processes involved in fat breakdown.

The actions of glucagon and the other counter-regulatory hormones are all geared towards preventing an abnormal fall in blood glucose (hypoglycaemia). Glucagon secretion is highest in the 'fasting state' and lowest in the 'fed state'.

STOP THINK **5.6** Imagine that 1 h ago you finished a three-course meal. What hormonal response would you expect from the islet cells in the pancreas right now?

Other influences on blood glucose regulation

The anterior pituitary secretes two hormones of significance to blood glucose regulation:

- *Somatotrophin (growth hormone)* — this hormone tends to raise blood glucose and is therefore described as diabetogenic in action and anti-insulin in effect. It influences blood glucose in two main ways:
  - — by promoting glycogen-to-glucose conversion (glycogenolysis)
  - — by inhibiting muscle glycogen storage.
- *Adrenocorticotrophic hormone (ACTH)* — this hormone stimulates the adrenal cortex to release cortisol (see below). A negative feedback mechanism operates in response to the circulating levels of cortisol in the blood.

The adrenal cortex secretes a group of hormones known as glucocorticoids, the most significant of which is cortisol. Cortisol is released in a diurnal rhythm such that secretion is higher in the mornings and lower in the evenings.

Like glucagon, cortisol is a catabolic hormone. Secretion is increased during periods of physical or psychological stress, when its effect is to raise the blood glucose level in an effort to meet the additional metabolic demands posed

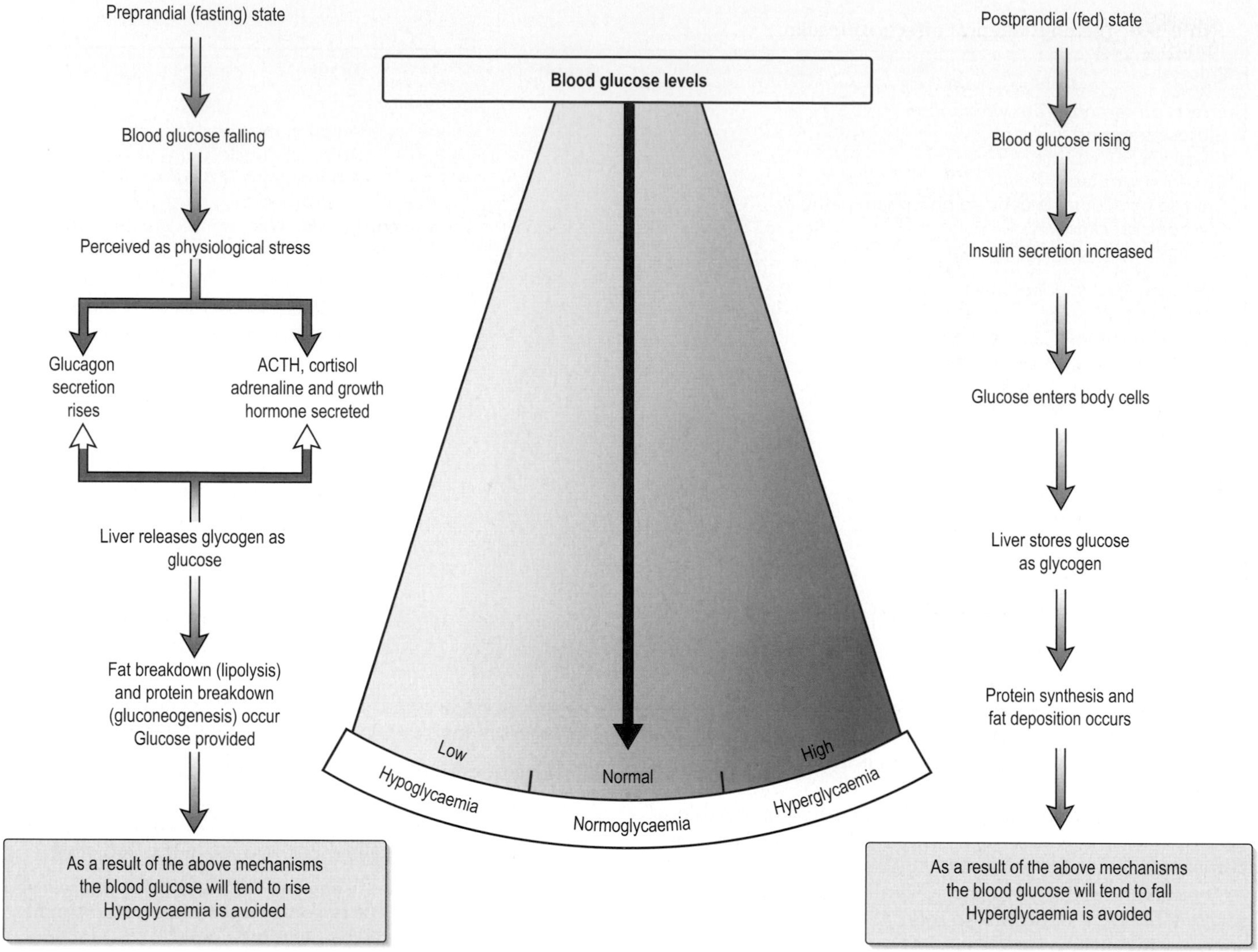

Fig. 5.8 The regulation of blood glucose in health.

by the stressed state. Cortisol causes stored glycogen to be converted to glucose and promotes the breakdown of fat (lipolysis) and protein (gluconeogenesis), thus providing an alternative source of glucose to meet the energy needs of the cells.

The adrenal medulla secretes adrenaline and noradrenaline, which together are known as catecholamines. These 'fight or flight' hormones are catabolic in their action. In response to stress, they place the body and brain in a state of 'high alert', causing blood glucose to rise as glycogen stores are released and fat/protein breakdown occurs. This increases the amount of available glucose and helps to prepare the body to meet increased energy demands.

The liver and skeletal muscle About 60% of absorbed nutrients are laid down as reserves in order to meet energy demands during fasting. Under the influence of insulin, the liver and, to a lesser extent, skeletal muscle can store glucose in the form of glycogen. The liver is also involved in protein and fat synthesis for subsequent storage.

During fasting, or in response to stress, glucagon (and other stress hormones) will promote the release of liver and muscle glycogen in the form of glucose. The liver also contributes to the chemical processes of gluconeogenesis by which body stores of fat and protein are converted to glucose (see Fig. 5.8).

TYPE 1 DIABETES

Aetiology

The pathogenesis of type 1 diabetes is complex and has been the subject of extensive research. It is currently thought that a genetic predisposition to the disease, possibly combined with environmental triggers, activates an autoimmune attack on the pancreatic β cells (see Box 5.4). In type 1 diabetes, insulin secretion is virtually totally absent, resulting in lifelong treatment with insulin.

PATHOPHYSIOLOGY

The process of islet destruction probably begins very early in life and is known to start several years before the clinical onset of diabetes (Watkins 2003). However, individuals often present with initial symptoms when the demand for insulin has been increased, e.g. in response to a physical or psychological stress such as illness, trauma, surgery, pregnancy

Box 5.4

Type 1 diabetes: the genetic link

A child with a mother with type 1 diabetes has a 1–2% increased risk of developing the same type of diabetes by 25 years; the risk is about three times greater if the father has this disease. If both parents have the disease the risk is further increased and genetic counselling should be sought in these rare circumstances (Watkins 2003).

Inherited susceptibility to type 1 diabetes depends on several genes. The strongest link has been traced to the DR3 and DR4 genes in the human leucocyte antigen (HLA) located on chromosome 6 (now called 'type 1 diabetes 1' locus) (Williams & Pickup 1999). Studies have revealed that in identical twins identified as HLA-DR3 'types', and in whom one suffers from type 1 diabetes, there is a high incidence of diabetes mellitus affecting the second twin. The HLA-DR3 group also shows persistent islet cell antibodies, indicating that genetic and immunological (possibly autoimmune) susceptibilities probably coexist. Within the general population it has been found that autoimmune disorders occur more frequently in people identified as HLA-DR3 types.

or bereavement. In such cases, the additional metabolic demands posed by the stressed state can no longer be met by the failing pancreas and symptoms of diabetes become evident for the first time.

Once insulin therapy has been started and good control achieved, the remaining β cell mass can temporarily provide sufficient insulin to meet the body's demands. In this case the external insulin can be reduced or stopped on occasions. Unfortunately, this 'honeymoon period' is short lived and, as the β cell mass reduces further, the symptoms will reappear, necessitating lifelong treatment with insulin.

The effects of lack of insulin The signs, symptoms and clinical features of type 1 diabetes can best be explained in terms of the effects of insulin lack, as follows:

- In the face of insulin lack, body cells are unable to obtain glucose for metabolism.
- Glucose which is unable to enter cells accumulates in the blood, causing an abnormally high blood glucose level — hyperglycaemia.
- Increased amounts of glucose are filtered at the glomeruli. The capacity of the kidneys to reabsorb glucose (the renal threshold for glucose) is exceeded and glucose appears in the urine — glycosuria.
- Glucose is highly osmotic, i.e. it attracts and holds water to itself. As glucose is lost in the urine, large volumes of water are lost with it — polyuria.
- As fluid loss continues, the patient will begin to experience symptoms of dehydration, the most common of which is copious drinking in response to severe thirst — polydipsia.
- The cells' requirements for glucose are not being met. The counter-regulatory response is an increased secretion of glucagon and other stress hormones in an attempt to increase cell glucose.
- Under the influence of these hormones specific mechanisms come into play:
  — glycogen is converted to glucose and is released by the liver (glycogenolysis)
  — glucose is produced from the breakdown of body fat and protein (gluconeogenesis)
  — the patient's appetite may increase (polyphagia).
- These efforts to meet the demands of the cells for glucose have the combined effect of raising the blood glucose even higher.
- Weight loss occurs due to the depletion of body fat and protein stores. This, together with cell deprivation of glucose and fluid–electrolyte imbalance, causes muscle weakness and exhaustion.
- In the absence of insulin, fat breakdown results in the production and accumulation of ketone bodies (β-hydroxybutyric acid, acetoacetic acid and acetone). This leads to ketonaemia and ketonuria. Additionally, acetone excreted by the lungs gives a characteristic sweet, 'pear drop' odour to the breath.
- Ketone bodies are weak acids which release free hydrogen ions to cause the serious condition of metabolic acidosis to develop.
- Excess acidity of the blood leads to corrective respiratory buffering. The patient hyperventilates, i.e. respirations become faster and deeper (Kussmaul's respirations), which is a very useful way of removing H^+ from the blood, i.e. blow off carbon dioxide.
- Uncontrolled lipolysis in the absence of insulin, gluconeogenesis, ketogenesis and glycogenolysis combine to raise the blood glucose level still further, increase osmotic diuresis, and exacerbate dehydration and metabolic acidosis. This is a life-threatening situation known as diabetic ketoacidosis (DKA).
- As a result of these profound biochemical disturbances, the patient may experience nausea and vomiting and, although unexplained, colicky abdominal pain.
- Unless a diagnosis is reached and urgent medical treatment is established, the patient will progress to coma and ultimately to death.

Onset and progress of the disease Although the onset of type 1 diabetes may appear abrupt, the patient may have had undetected clinical signs, such as glycosuria, in the absence of actual symptoms over a period of months. Once symptoms do appear, the disease will usually have a rapid progression. However, there will be variations in severity, some patients being much more acutely ill than others at the time of diagnosis.

The patient with type 1 diabetes may visit their general practitioner (GP) complaining of thirst, an increase in the amount of urine passed and weight loss. They may also complain of feeling exhausted. The GP is likely to have the patient's urine tested for glucose and ketones. Blood glucose will also be measured. The presence of ketonuria and hyperglycaemia combined with symptoms of polyuria and thirst will usually be sufficient evidence upon which to refer the patient to a diabetes consultant. In hospital, following a full assessment, treatment can be commenced and the patient's response to therapy closely monitored. Although most patients are referred to hospital, admission is not automatic. The majority of newly diagnosed patients with type 1 diabetes should be managed as outpatients under the care of a multidisciplinary diabetes care team giving a collaborative approach to care (Carson 2000).

Recently, care of people with type 1 diabetes has focused on diabetes centres and patients require admission to hospital less often, unless particularly unwell. The members of the diabetes care team in the hospital and community will have specialist knowledge about diabetes management. The central objective of care will be to help the patient acquire the knowledge and skills needed to resume an independent lifestyle. The patient will usually be asked to attend the diabetic outpatient clinic at specified intervals or, if unable to do so, may be visited at home by the diabetes specialist nurse. A shared care approach between community and diabetes specialist centre is essential for the ongoing care, treatment supervision and evaluation of progress of these patients.

TYPE 2 DIABETES

Aetiology

Type 2 diabetes seems likely to be multifactorial. Although these factors are not fully understood, they differ from those thought to cause type 1 diabetes.

Genetic factors leading to susceptibility Type 2 diabetes has a strong genetic component, manifest in the high concordance of diabetes in monozygotic twins, familial clustering and differences in prevalence between ethnic groups (Watkins 2003). One unusual form of type 2 diabetes has a clearly established autosomal dominant form of inheritance. It is non-insulin-dependent, commonly develops in those under 25, and is given the rather anomalous title of 'maturity onset diabetes of the young' (MODY; see British Diabetic Association 1997, Watkins et al 2003).

Age The prevalence of type 2 diabetes rises significantly with increasing age and can be as high as 1 in 10 in the over-70s (British Diabetic Association 1996). Glucose metabolism is known to become less efficient from the third or fourth decade of life onwards and this deterioration accelerates in people over 60 years of age. Whilst this alteration in glucose tolerance may not in itself be pathological, when compounded by other factors (see below) it can contribute to the onset of symptoms of diabetes.

Insulin resistance In type 2 diabetes, tissue sensitivity to insulin may decline. The result is that hyperglycaemia can occur even when the circulating levels of insulin are normal or raised. Several reasons have been suggested for the development of insulin resistance: these include resistance in peripheral tissues in obesity, the effects of ageing and the presence of anti-insulin antibodies in the blood. Whatever the cause, the result is the inefficient use of available insulin.

β cell deficiency There is a markedly reduced first phase insulin secretion in response to glucose and, in established diabetes, an attenuated second phase. Insulin pulsatility is also abnormal, thereby reducing tissue insulin sensitivity. In healthy individuals, insulin is secreted in a pulsatile manner during both the postprandial (after meal) and basal (between meals) periods. These pulses are separated from the insulin peaks induced by food (Williams & Pickup 1999).

Obesity Obesity is known to induce insulin resistance in body cells. However, only a minority of obese people develop type 2 diabetes and only around 60% of people with the disorder are obese. Glucose tolerance decreases as weight increases and can be reversed as weight loss occurs. Fat distribution would appear to be significant in that there is a relationship between central obesity and diabetes. Research data from Wei at al (1997) indicate that waist circumference is the best obesity-related predictor of type 2 diabetes, suggesting that distribution of body fat, especially abdominal localisation, is a more important determinant than the total amount of body fat.

Ethnic and environmental factors There are wide geographical variations in the incidence of type 2 diabetes. In western Europe, around 3% of the population develop type 2 diabetes, but in certain circumscribed societies incidences of up to 40% have been reported, e.g. among the Pima Indians of North America and the Nauru Islanders of the Pacific, where gross obesity is also very common. These remarkably high prevalences are probably due to the exposure of genetically isolated, diabetes-predisposed populations to influences such as a 'Westernised' diet and reduced physical activity. In many developing and newly industrialised nations, type 2 diabetes is thought to be epidemic (Griggs 1998). In the UK, the prevalence of type 2 diabetes is particularly high in Asian and Afro-Caribbean people, with 20% of Asians and 17% of Afro-Caribbeans over the age of 40 known to have type 2 diabetes (Watkins 2003). This presents a considerable health burden in some inner urban areas.

PATHOPHYSIOLOGY

Type 2 diabetes usually presents in those over the age of 40 and most commonly in people over 60. Typically the patient is overweight. The signs, symptoms and clinical features of type 2 diabetes, although still marked, are less severe than those of type 1 diabetes and are due to the more gradual onset and the effects of hyperglycaemia arising from a relative deficiency of insulin. In type 2 diabetes, there is still some insulin being secreted; as a result, ketogenesis is inhibited and, as the hyperglycaemia is less severe, dehydration is also much less common.

The effects of a relative lack of insulin are as follows:

1. *Hyperglycaemia-related symptoms* — nocturia, polyuria and thirst may develop gradually. The patient, who is often obese, may initially be gratified to note that weight loss is occurring.
2. *Genital or oral fungal infections* — candidal infections are common and result in the distressing symptoms of pruritus vulvae in the female and balanitis in the male. The sugar-rich urine around the genitalia appears to provide the yeast organism with favourable conditions in which to multiply.
3. *Staphylococcal skin infections* — these commonly result in boils and abscesses, and may provide the initial stimulus for the patient to visit their GP.

Table 5.9 Diagnostic glucose concentrations

Diagnosis	Venous whole blood (mmol/L)	Capillary whole blood (mmol/L)	Venous plasma blood (mmol/L)
Diabetes mellitus			
Fasting	≥6.1	≥6.1	≥7.0
2 h postprandial	≥10.0	≥11.1	≥11.1
Impaired glucose tolerance (IGT)			
Fasting and	<6.1 and	<6.1 and	<7.0 and
2 h postprandial	≥6.7	≥7.8	≥7.8
Impaired fasting glycaemia (IFG)			
Fasting and	≥5.6 and <6.1	≥5.6 and <6.1	≥6.1 and <7.0
2 h postprandial	<6.7	<7.8	<7.8

In the absence of diabetic symptoms, abnormality in both 2 h postprandial and fasting blood sugar is required to establish the diagnosis of diabetes mellitus. The 2 h postprandial test should be performed following the oral glucose tolerance test using 75 g glucose load (WHO 1999).

4. *Non-specific symptoms* — such as tiredness and lethargy — are also frequently reported. The cause is uncertain, but altered fluid and electrolyte balance may be responsible. Visual disturbance may occasionally be reported, as hyperglycaemia may cause opacity of the optic lens and accommodation may be affected by dehydration of the lens fluid.

Symptom-related complications At the time the patient first seeks medical attention, evidence of vascular and neurological complications such as proteinuria, sexual dysfunction, retinopathy and peripheral neuropathy may already have developed. Such patients have probably had asymptomatic diabetes with persistent hyperglycaemia for several years prior to diagnosis.

Onset and progress of the disease Type 2 diabetes may present in several ways. A diagnosis will usually be made on the evidence of glycosuria and a fasting or random venous plasma blood glucose concentration of more than 7.0 mmol/L and 11.1 mmol/L, respectively, in laboratory tests. The presence of symptoms and an elevated venous plasma blood glucose concentration of >11.1 mmol/L together are diagnostic of diabetes (WHO 1999) (see Table 5.9).

Ketonuria is not a feature of type 2 diabetes, as ketogenesis is inhibited by the presence of even small amounts of insulin.

Asymptomatic glycosuria may be discovered as an incidental finding, e.g. during a routine medical examination. Such a finding would normally prompt capillary and then venous blood glucose analysis. In the absence of symptoms, these results should be confirmed by repeat testing on a different day. If the fasting or random values are not diagnostic, a 2 h oral glucose tolerance test should be carried out (WHO 1999).

IMPAIRED GLUCOSE TOLERANCE (IGT) AND IMPAIRED FASTING GLYCAEMIA (IFG)

IGT and IFG are recognised as stages in the natural history of diabetes rather than as a class of diabetes (WHO 1999). It is not clear why some people may have blood glucose results at or just above the upper limit of 'normal'. Inconclusive results in the absence of symptoms may not necessarily be judged abnormal. For example, since glucose tolerance is known to decline with age and obesity, such factors would be considered in the overall assessment. To help determine to which category the patient should be assigned, an oral glucose tolerance test may be carried out.

It is known that some people with IGT or IFG will go on to develop diabetes mellitus and that they may have a greater risk of developing atherosclerosis.

Onset and progress of the disease Although it is clearly desirable that people should be spared the negative consequences of being inappropriately labelled as 'diabetic', they should nonetheless have access to regular medical screening and should be offered information about the prevention of atherosclerosis and its consequences (see Ch. 2). These health promotion functions will normally be carried out by the practice nurse or the GP and community nursing staff, although in some areas the patient may also be asked to attend a diabetic clinic for an annual review.

IGT has implications for women who are planning to conceive. Current evidence suggests that it is important to correct hyperglycaemia and ensure tight control of blood glucose prior to conception to reduce the risk of fetal abnormality (Williams 2003). Pre-conception advice should be made available and the patient's blood glucose brought within normal limits before conception and closely monitored throughout her pregnancy. Care of this kind may be provided at a combined 'diabetic–obstetric' clinic.

DIABETES MELLITUS SECONDARY TO OTHER DISEASES AND CONDITIONS

PATHOPHYSIOLOGY

In type 1 diabetes the fault is to be found in the islets of Langerhans where β cell output of insulin is either absent or insufficient to meet the needs of the cells. In type 2 diabetes, the islet cells may still produce insulin, but in insufficient amounts, or insulin function may be hindered in some way. In contrast, hyperglycaemia in type 2 diabetes may be iatrogenic, i.e. occurring as a side-effect of certain medications, or be secondary to other disease.

Some medicines, notably steroids, have a diabetogenic effect. The thiazide group of diuretics have been known to worsen established diabetes and in some older patients may actually hasten the onset of the disease. Excess secretion or administration of glucocorticoids, aldosterone, catecholamines or growth hormone will have a diabetogenic effect and can result in hyperglycaemia. Diabetes may therefore be a feature of Cushing's syndrome, Cushing's disease, phaeochromocytoma, primary aldosteronism and acromegaly (see Ch. 5, Part 1).

Pancreatitis and carcinoma of the pancreas may greatly reduce the number of functioning β cells and result in impaired insulin secretion. Chronic hepatic disease will have considerable consequences for carbohydrate, protein and fat metabolism. Glycogenesis and glycogenolysis may both be impaired and consequently hyper- and hypoglycaemia frequently feature in chronic disorders of the liver. Chronic renal failure can cause impaired glucose tolerance and insulin resistance, although the underlying mechanism by which this occurs remains unclear.

There are other rare genetic disorders which give rise to secondary diabetes (Williams & Pickup 1999). Friedreich's ataxia, an inherited disorder of balance and movement, is one example. Another is a condition with an autosomal character which is referred to by the acronym DIDMOAD (Wolfram's syndrome) as it incorporates **d**iabetes **i**nsipidus, **d**iabetes **m**ellitus, **o**ptic **a**trophy and **d**eafness.

Onset and progress of diabetes mellitus are characterised by hyperglycaemia with glycosuria. Associated features such as thirst and polyuria may be experienced, and in hepatic disease the patient may also experience hypoglycaemic episodes, with symptoms such as trembling, sweating and clouding of consciousness. The underlying disease process will influence the nature and severity of the symptoms. Urinalysis and blood glucose will be monitored and dietary adjustment may be prescribed; this may be combined with oral hypoglycaemic medication or insulin therapy.

MANAGEMENT STRATEGIES IN DIABETES MELLITUS

Diabetes care in the UK and Europe has been strongly influenced by the St Vincent declaration (Krans et al 1992). Such was the concern over the duration and quality of life of people with diabetes, that the countries concerned pledged to deploy resources for its resolution and to intensify research into prevention and cure of diabetes and its complications.

Diabetes management requires a multidisciplinary approach. For those patients who are not acutely ill at the time of diagnosis, management may be provided entirely within the community setting. However, many patients are more acutely ill at the time of onset and require hospital care to allow close monitoring of the effects of early treatment.

The professionals in the diabetes care team will share common goals for care, each contributing expertise in accordance with the patient's individual needs. It is worth remembering, however, that the patient is the most important member of the diabetes care team, and full participation by the patient is necessary to achieve the following aims:

- Attainment and maintenance of normoglycaemia
- Monitoring of response to therapy
- Prevention and detection of diabetes-associated complications
- Facilitation of self-care through education
- Promotion of social and psychological adjustment.

ATTAINING AND MAINTAINING NORMOGLYCAEMIA

There are three main therapeutic approaches to this management:

- dietary therapy
- oral hypoglycaemic therapy
- insulin therapy.

NUTRITIONAL ADVICE FOR PEOPLE WITH DIABETES

Appropriate dietary advice is essential in the effective management of diabetes. The aim is to give people with diabetes information to enable them to make informed choices about the type and quantity of food they eat. The Clinical Standards Advisory Group recommend that all newly diagnosed patients should be offered a consultation with a registered dietitian within 4 weeks of diagnosis (Clinical Standards Advisory Group 1994). Dietitians are skilled in translating nutritional guidelines into practice. Dietary recommendations are the same as those given to the general population (see Ch. 22).

Current nutritional standards are summarised in Table 5.10.

Carbohydrate

All food that contains carbohydrate (CHO) will cause blood glucose levels to rise. The extent of the glycaemic response (the rise in blood glucose after eating) caused by food varies. This is affected by the amount of food consumed, the source of the carbohydrate such as glucose or starch, the cooking method and other components of the meal.

The glycaemic index was devised to help explain some of the differences caused by different carbohydrates on blood glucose levels. It allows the glycaemic effect of foods to be ranked against a standard such as glucose. Foods with a high glycaemic index cause a rapid rise in blood glucose levels and should be used sparingly. Lower glycaemic index foods cause a more gradual glycaemic response and if taken as part of a meal can lower the glycaemic effect of the whole meal (Dyson 2004).

Table 5.11 shows examples of the glycaemic index of certain foods.

Sucrose is no longer considered to be any more harmful to blood glucose levels than other CHO. However, it is still

Table 5.10 Current nutritional standards

Component	Comment
Protein	Not more than 1 g/kg body weight
Total fat	Less than 35% of energy intake
Saturated and transaturated fat	Less than 10% of energy intake
n-6 polyunsaturated fat	Less than 10% of energy intake
n-3 polyunsaturated fat	Eat fish, especially oily, once or twice weekly. Fish oil supplements not recommended
Monounsaturated fat	10–20% of energy intake
Total carbohydrate	45–60% of energy intake
Sucrose	Up to 10% of daily energy
Fibre	No quantitative recommendation
Vitamins and antioxidants	Encourage food rich in these
Salt	6 g or less of sodium chloride per day

Data from Diabetes UK (2003b).

an empty calorie source and harmful for teeth and should be taken sparingly as part of a meal.

Fructose Fruit consumption should be encouraged as fructose has a low glycaemic effect. People with diabetes should be encouraged to eat five servings of fruit and vegetables per day. These foods are a good source of soluble fibre, which is also found in oats, pulses, nuts and grains. Excessive fruit intake can significantly increase blood glucose levels and therefore a sensible intake level should be encouraged.

Carbohydrate restriction is not recommended but some measure of control may be discussed, particularly in those with type 1 diabetes. Carbohydrate can be measured in 10 or 15 g portions or exchanges. Historically, dietitians advised people to measure their intake in 10 g exchanges to rigidly control their intake. This approach became less common in the 1980s when advice focused more on healthy eating guidelines. Quantifying CHO is now being used more frequently in view of the Dose Adjustment for Normal Eating (DAFNE) project findings (DAFNE Study Group 2002). The DAFNE education programme teaches people to adjust their insulin injections to fit their lifestyle, instead of adjusting their lifestyle to a particular insulin regimen, thus improving glycaemic control and quality of life in people with type 1 diabetes. However, the emphasis is markedly different, with the educated patient adjusting the amount of insulin given for the amount of carbohydrate consumed, irrespective of the source of CHO.

Table 5.11 Glycaemic index examples

Low GI	Intermediate GI	High GI
Porridge	Croissants	Cornflakes
Most fruit	Cheeries	White/wholemeal bread
Granary bread	Potatoes	Chips
Pasta	Pineapple	Jelly babies
Beans	Couscous	Cornchips
Pulses	Sucrose	Honey
Yoghurt	Full fat ice cream	Glucose

Fat

Fat should not be overlooked when providing dietary advice to people with diabetes. It is the major energy source of the diet. A reduction in intake is generally necessary for weight control. All sources of fat contain the same number of calories per gram. It is a common misconception that fat from vegetable sources contains fewer calories than that from animal sources but this is not the case. It does, however, have less atherogenic potential than animal fats and a high intake of saturated fat, which is mainly found in animal products, is linked to elevated cholesterol levels (Segal-Isaacson et al 2001). People with diabetes should generally be encouraged to eat less fat and, where possible, to choose fat from monounsaturated sources (see Table 5.12).

Weight control

Weight control is particularly important in people with type 2 diabetes, where obesity is a well-recognised problem. Losing weight is notoriously difficult. A loss of 1–2 kg/month by means of a 500–600 kcal reduction in intake per day is considered to be successful progress (Scottish Intercollegiate Guidelines Network (SIGN) 1996). Advice on increasing physical activity should also be included.

Table 5.12 Sources of fat

Type of fat	Food source
Saturated fat	Fatty meat Butter Cheese Cream Pastry Baked products, e.g. cakes and biscuits
Polyunsaturated fat	Sunflower seeds and oils Corn oil Oily fish Some soft margarine
Monounsaturated fat	Olive oil Most nuts Avocado Grapeseed oil Peanut oil (ground nut) Some soft margarine

Alcohol

It is not necessary for people with diabetes to avoid alcohol completely. As with the adult population in general, a maximum of 14 units of alcohol per week for women and 21 units for men should not be exceeded. Care should be taken by those treated with insulin to avoid hypoglycaemia when drinking by ensuring adequate CHO intake. Those who are overweight should be advised as to the high calorie content of alcohol.

For a more in-depth review of nutritional advice for people with diabetes, see Diabetes UK (2003b).

ORAL HYPOGLYCAEMIC THERAPY

Oral hypoglycaemic medication can be effective only if β cells are capable of secreting some insulin. This form of therapy is therefore used exclusively for patients with type 2 diabetes.

In the absence of persistent symptoms, dietary treatment should continue for at least 3 months before drug therapy is commenced. Oral hypoglycaemic therapy would then be reserved for patients with type 2 diabetes who have persistent hyperglycaemia despite a period of dietary adjustment (United Kingdom Prospective Diabetes Study Group (UKPDS) 1998a, DH 2001, SIGN 2001). Five main groups of oral agents are available for use in the UK (see Table 5.13).

The sulphonylureas

Mode of action These drugs stimulate the β cells of the pancreas to secrete more insulin in response to blood glucose levels, increase insulin sensitivity and reduce the hepatic metabolism of insulin.

Side-effects The most common side-effect is hypoglycaemia. This can be minimised by starting the patient on the lowest dose possible and gradually increasing the amount over a period of weeks. As sulphonylureas lower blood glucose, it is important that both the patient and carers are aware of the risks of hypoglycaemia. The medication should be taken 20–30 min before food. The relationship between exercise, medication and diet will form an important part of the patient education programme.

Other side-effects include weight gain, gastrointestinal disturbance and skin rash. Facial flushing following alcohol ingestion can occur with chlorpropamide. It should be noted that the effect of sulphonylureas is potentiated by other protein-bound medication, e.g. warfarin. This interaction increases the amount of available sulphonylurea and may therefore cause hypoglycaemia.

The biguanides

Metformin

Mode of action Metformin reduces glucose absorption in the gut, reduces peripheral insulin resistance and inhibits liver glucogenesis. Guidelines recommend first-line use of metformin following UKPDS findings of a survival benefit in this group (UKPDS 1998a, SIGN 2001).

Side-effects Gastrointestinal upset is the most common. Medication-induced hypoglycaemia is very uncommon

Table 5.13 Oral hypoglycaemic agents

Drug	Dose range (mg/day)	Points to note
Sulphonylureas		
Gliclazide	40–320	
Glipizide	2.5–20	
Glimepiride	1–6	Stimulation of β cells to secrete insulin and increases insulin sensitivity
Gliquidone	15–180	
Tolbutamide	500–2000	
Chlorpropamide	100–500	Avoid use in older people: risk of hypoglycaemia
Glibenclamide	2.5–15	
Biguanides		
Metformin	500–3000	Inhibition of liver glucogenesis. Increases peripheral uptake of insulin. Treatment of choice for overweight patients with type 2 diabetes. Contraindicated in renal, liver and cardiac disease
Prandial glucose regulators		
Repaglinide	0.5–16	Beta cell stimulation. Shorter acting than sulphonylureas — fewer hypos. Take only at meals
Nateglinide	60–540	
Thiazolidinediones		
Rosiglitazone	4–8	Combats insulin resistance. Increases insulin sensitivity. Increases peripheral uptake of glucose. Reduces hepatic liver production. Contraindicated in heart failure and poor liver function. Used in conjunction with other agents
Pioglitazone	15–30	
Alpha glucosidase inhibitor		
Acarbose	50–600	Delays carbohydrate absorption. Poorly tolerated due to gastrointestinal side-effects

with biguanide therapy as is vitamin B_{12} malabsorption. Lactic acidosis is a rare occurrence but should be noted and metformin is contraindicated in patients with renal, liver and severe cardiovascular disease or serious systemic illness.

Prandial glucose regulators

Mode of action These drugs are designed to stimulate extra insulin release to coincide with meal digestion. They should be taken up to 15 min before each meal and are rapidly absorbed. As they are also quickly eliminated from the body, the insulin effect is short lived, thus reducing the risk of hypoglycaemia.

Side-effects Side-effects are uncommon, but can include gastrointestinal upset, nausea and skin rash.

Thiazolidinediones

Mode of action The thiazolidinediones (glitazones) tackle insulin resistance and act by increasing insulin sensitivity within the peripheral tissue, increasing peripheral glucose uptake and reducing hepatic glucose production. They are used in conjunction with other oral agents.

Side-effects can include weight gain, headache and fluid retention. Use of thiazolidinediones is therefore not advised in patients with cardiac failure or poor liver function.

Alpha-glucosidase inhibitor

Acarbose is poorly tolerated due to prominent side-effects and is now less commonly used. However, it can be used alone or in combination with other oral agents.

Mode of action Acarbose acts by delaying the breakdown of starch and sucrose into monosaccharides which can be absorbed in the small intestine. In the patient with diabetes, the effect is to reduce the postprandial peak in blood glucose.

Side-effects The most common side-effects are flatulence and diarrhoea.

INSULIN THERAPY

For all patients with type 1 diabetes, insulin therapy is essential to maintain life, and will be required throughout life. Insulin cannot be given orally as its protein structure would be inactivated by digestive enzymes. Parenteral administration is therefore necessary and normally takes the form of subcutaneous (s.c.) injection.

In patients with type 2 diabetes, glycaemic control deteriorates as the condition progresses and 30% of patients will eventually require insulin therapy (UKPDS 1998a). Others may require insulin therapy during periods of stress or illness but this does not change the classification of their disorder.

The objectives of insulin therapy are:

- to maintain blood glucose within normal limits
- to relieve hyperglycaemia-associated symptoms
- to correct metabolic/biochemical disturbances
- to prevent diabetes-associated complications.

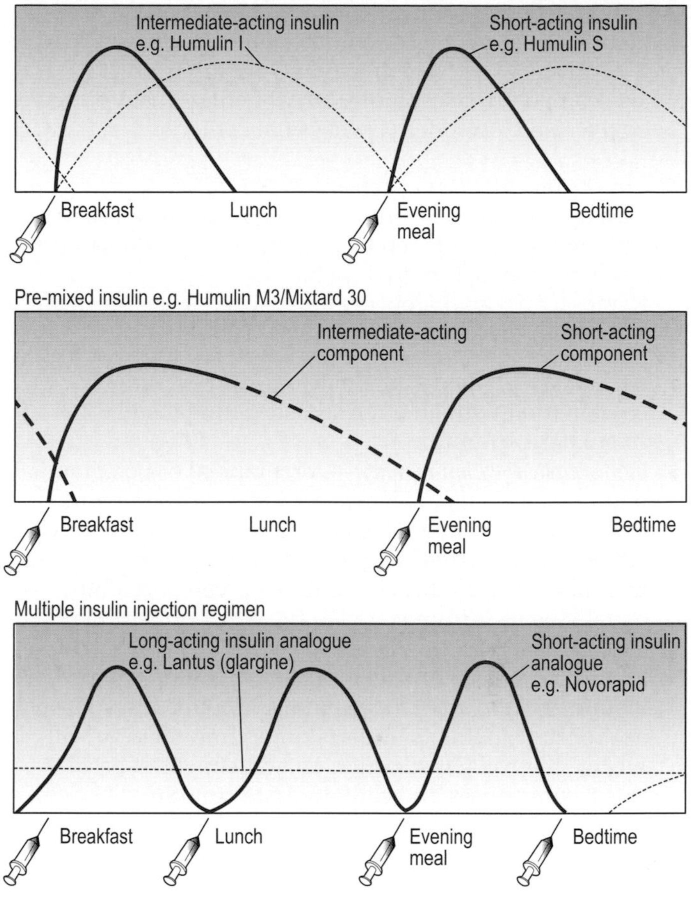

Fig. 5.9 Duration of action for short-, intermediate- and long-acting insulins and rapid- and long-acting analogue insulins.

Types of insulin

In the past, all insulin preparations were derived from animal sources, mainly beef and pork. Genetic engineering and other advanced techniques have resulted in the production of biosynthetic human insulin and purified or highly purified pork and beef insulin.

Throughout western Europe, biosynthetic human insulin is now the main source. Insulins are manufactured in various forms: soluble, isophane, insulin zinc suspension, analogue and ready-mixed in combination.

Duration of action

There are many insulin preparations on the market. These may be categorised as rapid-acting analogue, short-acting, intermediate-acting, long-acting (including long-acting analogue) and biphasic (see Fig. 5.9).

Rapid-acting analogue insulin (Humalog, NovoRapid) These are clear solutions. They have a rapid onset of action and therefore should be injected 0–15 min before meals. They are also licensed to be given up to 15 min after a meal. This may be a useful point if the patient is unsure of how much they will eat, perhaps as a result of illness or if the patient is a young child. The length of action is 4–5 h, and therefore this type of insulin is most commonly used within a basal bolus, multiple injection regimen. Its use is associated with lower postprandial hyperglycaemia, reductions in HbA1c (see monitoring methods for explanation of glycosylated haemoglobin — HbA1c, p. 202) and, when compared to soluble, short-acting insulin, fewer hypoglycaemic episodes (Owens et al 2001).

Short-acting insulins (Actrapid, Humulin S) These are also clear solutions. The onset of action is delayed for 30 min when injected subcutaneously; their maximal effect occurs in 3–4 h but can last up to 8–10 h.

Rapid-acting analogue insulin and short-acting insulin may be prescribed in the following ways:

- *twice daily* — given in the morning and evening in combination with an intermediate-acting insulin (Insulatard, Humulin I)
- *by multiple injection regimen* — preprandial or postprandial injections with the dose adjusted to correspond with carbohydrate intake. This is usually combined with either intermediate-acting insulin or long-acting analogue insulin (glargine), which would be given once daily, usually being administered at breakfast or bedtime
- *by continuous s.c. infusion using an insulin pump* — this allows for a basal or background, continuous release of insulin and the ability to administer bolus doses when appropriate; patients undertaking pump therapy will receive intensive instruction on adjustment of basal rates, bolus doses and carbohydrate counting
- *intravenously* — during acute metabolic emergencies when immediate insulin effect is required, e.g. in diabetic ketoacidosis (DKA).

Intermediate- and long-acting insulins are cloudy in appearance. Their onset of effect is delayed for 1–2 h. The intermediate-acting insulins achieve maximum effect in 4–6 h and have a duration of action of 12–20 h. Long-acting insulins have their maximum effect in 8–12 h and a duration of action of up to 36 h.

Intermediate-acting insulins come in two main forms:

- Isophane insulin comes as a suspension of insulin with protamine (Insulatard, Humulin I). This type of insulin may be used in combination with short-acting insulin. It provides a stable solution in which each insulin retains its own pharmacological properties even when mixed and stored in the same syringe.
- Lente insulins are combined with zinc in two forms: amorphous 30% and crystalline 70%. The zinc binds the insulin, and as a result onset of action is delayed and the duration extended. Lente insulins are now rarely used due to the introduction of new insulins with more suitable action profiles.

Intermediate-acting insulins can also be used in conjunction with oral hypoglycaemic agents, and given at bedtime to control fasting hyperglycaemia in patients with type 2 diabetes. This regimen can help to prevent weight gain but may require large doses to achieve effective control, especially at the post evening meal glucose test (Yki-Jarvinen et al 2000).

Long-acting insulin suspensions, e.g. Ultratard, have a greatly extended period of action of up to 36 h. They have been used in the past in multiple injection regimens and also as once daily injections. With advances in insulin production, the use of these insulins is rare as more people are prescribed long-acting analogue insulin.

Long-acting analogue insulin (glargine) is more slowly absorbed, providing a continuous level of insulin over a 24-h period. It is a true basal insulin with a peakless action profile, which therefore reduces the risk of hypoglycaemia. It is a once-daily insulin which is used in conjunction with a rapid-acting analogue insulin in a multiple injection regimen. It may also be used in conjunction with oral hypoglycaemic agents in the treatment of people with type 2 diabetes.

Biphasic insulin These ready-mixed insulins include a combination of short-acting, e.g. Humulin M3 or Mixtard 30, or rapid-acting analogue, e.g. Humalog Mix 25 or Novomix 30, and intermediate-acting insulin in set ratios. Most are now available in pen form, making the administration of insulin more user friendly.

STOP THINK **5.7** Using the *British National Formulary* or a current pharmacology text, e.g. Greenstein & Gould (2004), draw up a table which illustrates examples from rapid, short-, intermediate- and long-acting and biphasic insulins and indicate the species (source), onset and duration of action.

Administering insulin

The overall aim in administering insulin therapy is to achieve the best possible control of blood glucose throughout the 24-h period. The treatment should mimic the physiological response to normal variations in blood glucose. During the fasting state, there is a continual but low secretion of insulin. Following meals, a surge in blood glucose results in increased insulin secretion.

Frequency

To mimic normal blood glucose fluctuations, a single injection of insulin with a 24-h period of action, such as glargine, could be given once daily in combination with rapid-acting insulin with a short (4–5 h) duration of action, such as NovoRapid, before each meal. This multiple injection system has considerable advantages, not least of which are patient autonomy and flexibility of mealtimes and meal size. Patients using this system will carry an insulin injecting device in the form of a pen. This allows administration of insulin to be quick and discreet, enabling adaptability for the day-to-day changes in the patient's activity levels, eating pattern and lifestyle. This system is most effective if blood glucose levels are regularly monitored and patients are taught to adjust diet and insulin accordingly: the system does not, therefore, suit everyone. For many patients, twice-daily injections remain the preferred regimen, whereas some, especially older patients, who have perhaps been required to progress to insulin from diet and/or oral therapy, will be more willing to accept once-daily injections.

Mixing insulin

It is not advisable to mix zinc-based insulins and soluble insulins in a syringe for later use, as free zinc in the suspension can bind to the soluble insulin, extending the onset and duration of action. The injection should be given just

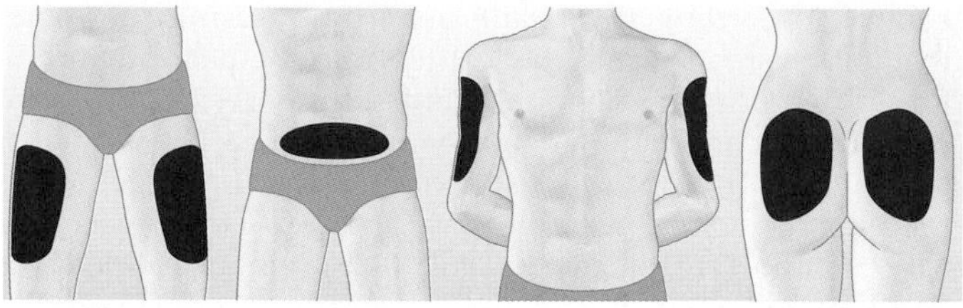

Thighs Abdomen Arms Buttocks

Fig. 5.10 Suitable injection sites for insulin. Repeated injections in the same area may cause pitting or lumpiness of the skin.

after preparation. This problem does not arise with isophane insulins as they do not contain zinc. Free mixing of two insulin types in this way is rare now with the availability of such a wide range of premixed biphasic insulins.

The insulin dose will vary from patient to patient according to carbohydrate intake and insulin sensitivity or resistance, and will take account of the patient's blood glucose levels, lifestyle, and growth and development needs. The patient and carers should receive information regarding the timing of injections in relation to food intake, as this differs depending on insulin type and is important in relation to avoiding hypoglycaemia. Information should also be provided about how to achieve a balance of food, exercise and insulin to avoid detrimental swings in blood glucose.

Injection sites

Insulin is given by s.c. injection. The most common sites for injection are the upper thighs and the abdominal wall. Patients can also use the outer aspect of the upper arms and buttocks but this may prove difficult when attempting to pinch up the skin. Overuse of one site can lead to lipohypertrophy, loss of sensitivity and impaired or erratic absorption of insulin. For this reason 'site rotation' is advised (see Fig. 5.10). Insulin is more rapidly absorbed from the abdomen and therefore the thighs are more useful for evening injections.

Injection technique

In the home environment there is no need to cleanse the skin with alcohol prior to injection. However, the site should be visibly clean. A mound of skin should be gently pinched up before injection to avoid intramuscular injection. The skin should not be pinched if 5 mm or 6 mm needle is used. The syringe or pen device should be held as illustrated in the appropriate device leaflets and the needle inserted straight into the subcutaneous tissue at a 90° angle. Insulin syringes and pen needles currently in use in the UK have a variety of needle lengths and gauges, and it is important to select the appropriate needle for the body weight of the patient to ensure a subcutaneous injection.

For further information on injection technique and pen use, see MacKinnon (2002).

The insulin should be injected steadily and the needle held in position for a further count of at least 6 s before withdrawing smoothly.

For a guide to insulin pens and needles, see Diabetes UK (2003b).

The care setting

The patient with type 1 diabetes may be managed in the primary care setting provided adequate supervision and support can be given to both patient and family during the early stages of treatment. It is still common for initial stabilisation on insulin to take place within the hospital diabetes unit and for outpatient attendance to be advised to allow for regular screening for diabetes-related complications. If ketoacidosis or dehydration is present, management in hospital will be essential.

MONITORING RESPONSE TO THERAPY

METHODS

The methods used for monitoring glycaemic control include:

- urinalysis
- blood glucose monitoring
- glycosylated haemoglobin
- body weight monitoring.

Urinalysis

Urine tests are performed to detect the presence of glucose and ketones. In order to screen for possible renal complications of diabetes mellitus, urine may also be tested for protein. Testing the urine for glucose is not completely accurate as it does not reflect the current blood glucose level. The urine may have remained in the bladder for some time before micturition and may therefore test high for glucose while the blood glucose may well be normal or low. In addition, the absence of glycosuria merely indicates a blood glucose level below the renal threshold for glucose, which in most people is around 10 mmol/L. Urinalysis cannot therefore detect hypoglycaemia. If there is any reason to suspect that the patient is suffering from, or is at risk of, episodes of hypoglycaemia, then instruction in blood glucose monitoring should be considered. Fewer people with diabetes are now being taught urine testing in the hospital setting.

Equipment

Chemically impregnated dipsticks (Multistix) are the usual means of urine testing on admission to hospital. Ketostix should also be used for the measurement of ketones. The manufacturer's instructions for use and storage of urine testing materials must be followed precisely.

Recording

Urinalysis results should be accurately recorded on the appropriate chart.

Blood glucose monitoring

Blood glucose monitoring is the most widely used method of testing glucose levels. Routine glucose measurement should be by near-patient blood testing, i.e. a blood glucose test performed at the patient's bedside on a suitable meter.

Advantages

Blood glucose monitoring offers increased patient involvement in diabetes management and helps to improve day-today glycaemic control. It is used by patients to adjust their insulin levels, assess if blood sugar levels are low for driving or exercise and monitor the effect of certain amounts and types of food eaten (DAFNE 2002). It can also give warning of impending metabolic crisis and guide subsequent intervention.

Blood glucose monitors are inexpensive and often provided free from diabetic clinics. Each model has different functions to suit the individual patient's capabilities. Some have integrated test strips with capillary-fill dosing, most have a large memory store for downloading results and all come with quality control solution to check the accuracy of the test.

Disadvantages
Blood glucose monitoring requires a fair degree of manual dexterity, visual acuity, cognitive ability and motivation. For severely visually impaired individuals, there are talking meters which can be purchased; patients require intensive training from a diabetes specialist nurse in the use of these devices. Although expensive, this is justified because of the independence gained by the patient. Near-patient testing in a hospital setting requires a standardised system throughout, with a quality assurance programme in place involving internal and external quality control. This is often more successful if there is a diabetes link nurse system in place within the hospital (DH 1996).

Blood glucose measurement

Equipment
This includes:

- a spring-loaded finger-pricking device
- a blood glucose meter and test strips — for some patients, a blood ketone meter combined with a blood glucose meter and test strips.

Some patients with erratic blood glucose levels may require continuous monitoring, measuring interstitial glucose levels every 10 s, using a sensor inserted under the skin of the abdomen. One example of these devices is the MiniMed Continuous Glucose Monitoring System which can be used to detect hypoglycaemia and provide a profile of glucose levels over a 24-h period. It is used to help improve glycaemic control.

Frequency
For patients with type 1 diabetes, preprandial and pre-bed tests, with the occasional postprandial test, can provide important feedback and aid learning for all seriously motivated people with diabetes and can be an essential tool in achieving tight diabetic control (Watkins 2003).

Method
The hands should be washed to avoid any contamination of the test strip. Blood of sufficient quantity should be obtained and the procedure detailed in the manufacturer's directions should be followed precisely (Craddock 1996). If the test is conducted by a health care professional, gloves should be worn.

Blood glucose measurement provides a simple and, if performed correctly, reliable method of monitoring glycaemic control. Recording the results may be by using the meter memory system or may be written into the patient's monitoring diary. In the hospital ward setting, results recorded on a chart should be regularly monitored. The nurse or patient carrying out the test should know the target levels for which to aim, usually 4.5–7.7 mmol/L before meals, 6.0–9.0 mmol/L after meals and 7.0–9.0 mmol/L at bedtime (Watkins 2003).

For further information on blood glucose measuring systems, see Batki et al (1998).

Glycosylated haemoglobin estimation (HbA1c)

Glucose in solution binds to haemoglobin by a process of glycosylation. The rate at which proteins bind to glucose is directly related to the current glucose concentration in the blood. The blood proteins in which glycosylation is most readily measured are haemoglobin, albumin and fructosamine. The normal ranges vary according to the laboratory technique and reference ranges should therefore be provided by the laboratory undertaking the test.

Advantages
Measurement of glycosylated haemoglobin provides an independent check of other measures of glycaemic control. It gives an indication of control over a period of time, normally 2–3 months, and not merely a one-off recording as in plasma glucose estimation. Additionally, it provides a tool with which to assess the effects of interventions such as diet, medication or education.

Disadvantages
Anything which interferes with normal haemoglobin levels, such as haemorrhage or anaemia, could potentially distort glycosylated haemoglobin results. Similarly, conditions which influence serum albumin levels, such as renal or hepatic disease, may result in problems in interpreting glycosylated albumin results.

Body weight monitoring

Weight is not a sensitive indicator of glycaemic control. However, the negative significance of rapid weight loss accompanied by thirst, glycosuria and ketonuria should be recognised. Similarly, it can be a positive sign if the patient's weight is stable and within an acceptable range. Body weight therefore forms part of the overall monitoring picture. However, body mass index calculation can provide a more accurate picture of the patient's weight in relation to their height and thereby an indication of whether they are overweight or obese. A patient is considered to be overweight if BMI is >25 (see Ch. 21 for calculation of BMI).

In type 2 diabetes, it is often seen as a priority to help the patient lose weight. Obesity increases insulin resistance and therefore correction of obesity can increase the sensitivity of cells to insulin. Weight reduction alone may bring the blood glucose down within normal limits.

Associated problems
Social attitudes can lead to overweight people feeling stigmatised. As a result, guilt or low self-esteem may affect

the patient's response to dietary advice. It is important that nurses involved in monitoring the patient's weight in the home, clinic or hospital adopt a sensitive approach.

Equipment and procedure

Scales should be checked regularly for accuracy. If possible, the patient should be weighed at the same time of day, ideally having just emptied their bladder. As far as possible, the patient should wear clothing of comparable weight each time.

Frequency

For hospital inpatients, weekly weighing should be adequate. Routine weighing at each outpatient clinic appointment is advisable. Frequency of self-weighing by a patient at home will be at the patient's discretion and in relation to the advice offered and the goals which have been set. On the whole, weighing more frequently than once a week is neither psychologically desirable nor valuable as a monitoring tool.

PREVENTING AND DETECTING DIABETES-ASSOCIATED COMPLICATIONS

ACUTE METABOLIC COMPLICATIONS OF DIABETES

The acute complications arising from diabetes are:

- diabetic ketoacidosis (DKA)
- hyperglycaemic hyperosmolar non-ketotic coma (HHNK)
- hypoglycaemia.

Diabetic ketoacidosis (DKA)

This condition can be defined as uncontrolled hyperglycaemia caused by an insulin insufficiency, accompanied by dehydration and acidosis.

Epidemiology

In the UK, DKA is the most common cause of death for people with diabetes below the age of 20 years. There is very little recent research showing incident rates of DKA, although it is thought that this has not declined significantly through the decades despite increasing knowledge and more sophisticated management in specialist units (Dave at al 2004).

Aetiology

Newly presenting diabetes may lead to DKA in patients where there has been a delay in diagnosis. In patients with established diabetes, DKA can be precipitated by infection, myocardial infarction, stroke or physical or emotional trauma, as these increase stress hormone secretion. Stress hormones raise the blood glucose and increase insulin requirements. DKA may therefore be caused by an inadequate dosage of insulin being taken during intercurrent illness or other major stress, or by insulin being omitted altogether. Persistently poor diabetic control related to poor concordance with treatment regimens can be a particular contributing factor, often associated with repeated hospital admissions.

Fluctuations in diabetes control are common during adolescence and this is reflected in the number of young people admitted to hospital with DKA. It is the major cause of diabetes-related deaths in young people with diabetes mellitus (Lebovitz 1995).

STOP THINK **5.8** Consider why diabetes may be unstable during adolescence.

PATHOPHYSIOLOGY

The symptoms of DKA are a consequence of the combined effect of insulin lack and increased secretion of catabolic, counter-regulatory stress hormones. As a result, two major biochemical disturbances occur simultaneously:

- Accelerated gluconeogenesis and glycogenolysis cause hyperglycaemia, which in turn results in osmotic diuresis, dehydration and electrolyte disruption with a loss of sodium (hyponatraemia) and potassium (hypokalaemia)
- Increased fat breakdown (lipolysis) results in the formation of ketone bodies which are weak acids and cause metabolic acidosis (see Box 5.5).

MEDICAL MANAGEMENT

Reversing the hyperglycaemia Short-acting, soluble insulin (Humulin S or Actrapid) is administered to lower blood glucose. Initially, 50 mL of sodium chloride 0.9% (1 unit/mL) is administered via syringe driver infusion at 6 units/h. The insulin dose will later be varied in accordance with the blood glucose level and can be reduced to 3–4 units/h when the blood glucose level is <16 mmol/L and then to 2–4 units/h when it is 10–15 mmol/L. The aim should be a gradual reduction in blood glucose over a period of 12 h. If blood glucose does not fall within the first hour, the insulin dose may be increased to 12 units/h. However, before doing this, it is important to ensure that the insulin delivery mechanism is intact, i.e. the venflon is patent and the infusion pump is working. Capillary blood glucose should be checked hourly. Venous blood glucose and plasma potassium (K^+) are measured 2-hourly.

Rehydrating Rapid restoration of circulating volume is necessary, followed by gradual correction of the interstitial and intracellular deficit. Sodium chloride (NaCl) 0.9% is given by rapid i.v. infusion: 1–2 L may be given over the first hour, and then 500 mL hourly for 2–5 h. The rate is then adjusted according to the patient's state of hydration; caution should be taken with older patients who may be at risk of cardiac failure. When blood glucose falls below 15 mmol/L, the sodium chloride is replaced by i.v. dextrose 5% to allow maintenance of blood glucose levels in the range of 10–15 mmol/L.

Replacing potassium Derangements in plasma potassium can vary. Hyperkalaemia may be evident in the very early stages due to severe metabolic acidosis, but once rehydration is underway, hypokalaemia is usual and may be severe. Intravenous potassium chloride (KCl) is prescribed in accordance with the blood biochemistry. Initially 10–30 mmol/h may be administered within the i.v. fluids. This must be administered by a regulated infusion delivery system.

Box 5.5

The development of diabetic ketoacidosis (DKA)

The key precipitating factors for DKA are inadequate supply of insulin and increased demand for insulin, often in combination. These are often triggered by:

- newly presenting type 1 diabetes
- infection, especially respiratory, urinary or abscesses
- trauma or surgery
- severe illness, e.g. myocardial infarction or cerebrovascular accident
- failure to take sufficient insulin — this may be accidental or deliberate; many young women in particular discover that ketosis will cause rapid weight loss.

As a result of reduced insulin and increased stress hormone levels, cells will be unable to utilise glucose, glycogen will be converted to glucose, protein will be broken down to provide glucose (gluconeogenesis) and fat will be broken down (lipolysis), releasing ketone bodies. The combined effects of these events are:

- hyperglycaemia and hyperketonaemia
- osmotic diuresis
- fluid and electrolyte disruption
- catabolism/wasting
- acidosis.

As a result the patient will exhibit the following symptoms, signs and clinical features:

Symptoms
- Polyuria
- Intense thirst
- Polydipsia
- Lethargy/weakness
- Nausea/vomiting
- Abdominal colic
- Muscle cramps
- Blurred vision

Complications
- Cerebral oedema
- Adult respiratory distress syndrome
- Thromboembolism

Signs and clinical features
- Hyperglycaemia and glycosuria
- Polyuria progressing to oliguria
- Ketonuria
- Ketone breath (sweet fruity odour)
- Weight loss
- Hypokalaemia
- Hypotension and tachycardia
- Acidaemia
- Rapid, deep (Kussmaul's) respirations
- Evidence of intercurrent infection/illness
- Skin flushed and warm
- Hypothermia may develop
- Confusion and drowsiness progressing to coma

Monitoring The patient will be closely monitored for the following:

Potentially mortal dysrhythmias Continuous cardiac monitoring commenced and a 12-lead ECG is performed to detect cardiac arrhythmias associated with serum potassium lack or excess.

Hyperglycaemia Capillary blood glucose is measured hourly and venous blood glucose 2-hourly until <20 mmol/L, then 4-hourly.

Dehydration Blood urea, electrolytes and plasma osmolality are checked 2-hourly.

Response to fluid and K^+ replacement Blood pressure and pulse are measured hourly as a guide to blood volume. Central venous pressure (CVP) or pulmonary capillary wedge pressure (PCWP) may be initiated and measured in the older patient or those with renal or heart failure.

Oxygen therapy This will be administered in accordance with blood gas results.

Nasogastric aspiration will be performed to protect the airway if the patient is vomiting, drowsy or unconscious.

Acidosis Arterial blood gases are checked initially, but venous bicarbonate levels are adequate for monitoring of acidosis 1- to 2-hourly thereafter.

Underlying infection A chest X-ray is performed. Blood cultures, full blood count, urine and sputum specimens are sent to microbiology. Temperature, pulse, pulse oximetry and respiration are recorded hourly.

Ketosis and renal function Urine is tested for glucose, ketones, protein, urea and electrolytes.

Additional therapy which can be used in the treatment of DKA includes:

The use of an alkaline — sodium bicarbonate This is not routinely used as it may exacerbate tissue hypoxia and hypokalaemia. As overcorrection may result in alkalosis, sodium bicarbonate is usually reserved for the treatment of very severe acidosis where the pH is below 7.0 and hydrogen ion concentration exceeds 100 mmol/L, and then only if the patient does not respond to adequate treatment with fluids and insulin.

Broad-spectrum antibiotics These may be given only if infection is suspected.

Anticoagulants Low-dose heparin 5000 IU s.c. twice daily may be given as standard venous thromboembolism prophylaxis.

Urinary catheterisation Urine volume is measured hourly as severe dehydration carries a risk of acute renal failure.

Space blanket This may be used if the patient is hypothermic due to the vasodilatory response to metabolic acidosis.

Subsequent medical management of DKA will address the following concerns:

Insulin When blood glucose is below 15 mmol/L, the i.v. prescription may be changed to an infusion of 50 units of soluble insulin in 50 mL of sodium chloride 0.9% (1 unit/mL) and infused using a syringe driver. The rate should be adjusted to allow a gradual reduction in blood glucose over 12 h, initially starting at 6 units/h and reducing to 2–4 units/h when glucose is 16 mmol/L.

Fluid and electrolytes If the patient is still dehydrated, or severely hyponatraemic, following the osmotic consequences of glycosuria and dehydration, further i.v. sodium chloride 0.9% can be given. Plasma electrolytes, osmolality and glucose levels will be checked 2- to 4-hourly. Capillary blood glucose is monitored hourly. The infusion rate will be adjusted in accordance with blood glucose and other biochemical results. When the patient is deemed to be clinically and biochemically stable, s.c. insulin and an oral diet are resumed. The i.v. insulin therapy is discontinued 1 h after the first s.c. injection of insulin and when the patient has eaten the subsequent meal.

Prevention Once the patient is stable, every effort should be made to establish the cause of DKA and, where appropriate, the patient should be referred to the diabetes specialist nurse to discuss any changes to their diabetic medication and issues of self-management in an effort to prevent recurrence. For many patients, however, the experience of DKA is what first makes them aware that they have diabetes mellitus.

NURSING PRIORITIES AND MANAGEMENT: DKA

Each patient admitted with DKA will have unique problems and needs. The biochemical disruption of DKA is profound and life threatening. Priorities for nursing care will be strongly influenced by the prescribed medical therapy and the need for complex monitoring. Whilst the nurse must draw upon technical skills in such a situation, it is vitally important to remember to care for the patient as a whole person.

Immediate priorities

The newly admitted patient with DKA is vulnerable in a variety of ways. The nurse should be sensitive to this vulnerability and try to accommodate individual needs when planning and implementing care.

Case History 5.2 and Nursing Care Plan 5.3 provide an example of how a patient may present with DKA and how nursing priorities may be met following admission and until consciousness is regained. It should be pointed out, however, that the vast majority of patients presenting with DKA will not be unconscious. Individuals with long-standing diabetes mellitus can usually recognise the signs and symptoms of impending ketoacidosis and will seek medical help at a much earlier stage in its development. Those newly diagnosed with type 1 diabetes are taught how to recognise and respond to indications of hyperglycaemia and ketoacidosis.

CASE HISTORY 5.2

R (see also Nursing Care Plan 5.3)

R is a lively 18-year-old and the eldest of three children. At present she lives with her family but is soon to leave home to undertake a secretarial course at a college some 30 miles away.

R and her two brothers have recently suffered a bad bout of flu. The boys are now fully fit but R is far from well. She has been passing an excessive amount of urine and is constantly thirsty. She has lost weight and has recently been complaining of feeling tired all the time.

This morning she is very drowsy. Her skin feels hot and dry and she looks flushed. She has vomited several times and has complained of abdominal pain and cramps in her limbs. Her breath has a peculiar sweet smell and her mouth is very dry. She has also been complaining of blurred vision.

Her parents are alarmed and have called the GP to request an urgent visit. Alerted by the 'acetone breath', her symptoms and the history of recent illness, the GP checks R's capillary blood glucose and finds it to be greater than the upper limit on his blood glucose meter (33.3 mmol/L). R is too drowsy to produce a urine specimen to check for ketones but the GP is in little doubt about the diagnosis. An ambulance is summoned and R and her parents are taken to hospital. The ward is alerted to expect an unconscious patient with diabetic ketoacidosis (DKA).

On admission, R is acutely ill and has complex care requirements. A nurse who has the appropriate levels of knowledge and skill is assigned to care for her. She has prepared for R's admission and will subsequently assess her nursing needs and plan and evaluate her care (see Nursing Care Plan 5.3).

Further considerations

When the patient is alert and able to respond, the focus of care will change. The nurse will work with the patient, the dietitian and the medical staff to stabilise blood glucose and to monitor the effects of therapy.

The subsequent care of the patient in hyperglycaemic crisis, whether due to DKA or hyperglycaemic hyperosmolar non-ketotic coma (HHNK), will be similar in many respects.

Hyperglycaemic hyperosmolar non-ketotic coma (HHNK)

This term refers to uncontrolled hyperglycaemia and dehydration in the absence of ketonaemia.

Epidemiology

HHNK is less common than DKA. It is most often seen in people with undiagnosed type 2 diabetes and tends to affect an older age group. Mortality rates can be as high as 30%.

Aetiology

As in DKA, severe physical or psychological stress such as cerebrovascular accident (CVA), myocardial infarction, trauma or bereavement can precipitate HHNK.

Dietary indiscretion such as a marked increase in refined carbohydrate intake, perhaps over Christmas or a holiday period, may account for the onset of HHNK. Some patients give a history of drinking large volumes of sugar-containing drinks in an effort to quench an ever-increasing thirst. In 50% of patients, however, the cause of this metabolic disturbance will remain unknown.

PATHOPHYSIOLOGY

HHNK may develop gradually over a period of days or weeks. This is different from DKA, in which the symptoms of uncontrolled diabetes appear rapidly over a period of hours or days. However, the course of HHNK can occasionally, and especially in the young, develop over a few hours (Watkins et al 2003).

Due to the absence of ketones, the patient does not initially appear acutely ill and therefore the onset of the condition is often very gradual. The signs and symptoms are similar to those found in DKA, with the following notable exceptions:

- ketonuria is absent or slight
- severe weight loss is unusual
- in the absence of the serious symptoms of ketosis, the blood glucose may be even higher than in DKA before the patient feels ill (usually >50 mmol/L) and seeks medical attention

- physiological response to dehydration can be more marked due to the degree of hyperglycaemia and to age-associated intolerance to fluid and electrolyte disruption
- symptoms associated with ketonaemia/acidosis will not be in evidence.

STOP THINK **5.9** Given the above differences, draw up a list of signs, symptoms and clinical features of HHNK. Compare this with the list given for DKA and discuss the reasons for the differences.

The features of HHNK may be further described as follows:

Hyperglycaemia can be severe but develops gradually. Although some insulin is still being secreted, there is a relative insulin deficiency and the blood glucose continues to rise. The severe hyperglycaemia in HHNK is due to the combined effects of cellular resistance to insulin and the generation of glucose by stress hormone-driven glycogenolysis and gluconeogenesis.

Hyperosmolality Normal plasma osmolality is around 280–300 mmol/kg. This is calculated using a formula which takes account of the sodium, potassium, urea and glucose levels in the blood. Hyperglycaemia accounts for much of the hyperosmolar state in HHNK. The high blood glucose will exert an osmotic pull and as a result fluid is drawn out of the cells into the circulation. Initially this will cause an increase in the glomerular filtration rate and large volumes of fluid will be lost by osmotic diuresis. As a result, the patient will develop polyuria, thirst, dehydration and hypovolaemia.

Hypernatraemia The normal range for plasma sodium (Na^+) is 135–145 mmol/L. In HHNK, Na^+ may be raised above this level. Hypernatraemia can develop in response to a reduction in circulatory volume. In order to conserve a falling blood volume, aldosterone is secreted by the adrenal cortex, causing the kidney to retain sodium and excrete potassium.

By the time the patient presents, the period of osmotic diuresis has usually passed and dehydration has developed. As a result, the glomerular filtration rate falls, oliguria develops and blood urea rises. The combined effect of fluid loss, raised sodium levels, high blood glucose and raised plasma urea is that the blood becomes highly 'concentrated', i.e. hyperosmolar (hyperosmotic).

Non-ketosis The production of ketones (ketogenesis) will be inhibited by the presence of insulin. Insulin also enables the small amount of ketones which result from lipolysis to be metabolised, thus preventing their accumulation in the blood.

Impaired level of consciousness This occurs due to the effects of dehydration (hyperosmolality) on brain cells, impairing cerebral function and leading ultimately to coma.

MEDICAL MANAGEMENT OF HHNK

This follows a similar approach to that of DKA, with some important differences, and centres on the following concerns.

Rehydration The fluid deficit is considerable and can be as much as 8–12 L. Replacement rate should be slower than in DKA and must be approached with a degree of caution, given the risks associated with over-vigorous fluid replacement to which older patients are especially vulnerable:

- Sodium chloride 0.9% (normal saline) is given if plasma Na^+ levels are either not yet known or lower than 145 mmol/L.
- If plasma sodium is higher than 145 mmol/L, then half-strength normal saline (0.45% NaCl) may be given.

The infusion is changed to 5% dextrose once blood glucose measures 10–15 mmol/L to allow maintenance of blood glucose levels in the range of 10–15 mmol/L.

Replacement of potassium As potassium levels are so variable and unpredictable in HHNK, extreme care is required during replacement to monitor cardiac effects. Continuous cardiac monitoring is strongly recommended.

Insulin therapy An infusion of 50 units of soluble insulin in 50 mL sodium chloride 0.9% is commenced. In HHNK, the patient is less insulin resistant than in DKA, so the insulin infusion is commenced at a lower rate, usually 3 units/h. Insulin resistance is a syndrome associated with type 2 diabetes, whereby there is reduced tissue sensitivity to the action of insulin, leading to a compensatory increase in insulin secretion.

Anticoagulant therapy A major cause of death in HHNK is thrombosis, often pulmonary or cerebral, which is presumed to result from dehydration and hyperosmolality. Patients who are comatose or who have severe serum osmolality should receive intravenous heparin. Patients with lesser degrees of hyperosmolality may be given heparin 5000 IU s.c. 8-hourly. Other therapy and monitoring is as for ketoacidosis.

NURSING PRIORITIES AND MANAGEMENT: Hyperglycaemic hyperosmolar non-ketotic coma (HHNK)

Aspects of medical management which have implications for the planning of nursing care (McHoy 2003) include:

- i.v. infusion (fluid replacement)
- i.v. insulin (by syringe driver)
- heparin (s.c. or by i.v. infusion pump)
- central venous pressure (CVP) monitoring
- neurological observations
- cardiac monitoring
- urinary catheterisation
- oxygen therapy
- nasogastric aspiration (if patient is unconscious).

Immediate priorities

These interventions will need appropriate attention to ensure the safety and comfort of the patient. In addition, the patient is likely to be vulnerable due to an impaired level of consciousness, dehydration, electrolyte imbalance, the hazards of immobility and diabetes-associated risk factors. Nursing interventions will therefore include the following.

Monitoring consciousness

In patients with HHNK the level of consciousness is of particular importance as there is a risk of cerebral thrombosis due to the combined effects of immobility, dehydration and diabetes-associated atherosclerosis.

Another reason for vigilance is that the patient may be prescribed an i.v. infusion of half-strength normal saline aimed at reducing hyperosmolality. If the fall in plasma osmolality is too rapid, cerebral oedema can develop, raising intracranial pressure. The nurse should therefore promptly report any evidence of deterioration in the patient's neurological function (see p. 412).

Monitoring dehydration and electrolyte balance

The nurse should observe for the following warning signs:

Evidence of persistent hypovolaemia Hourly monitoring is required. The nurse should report hypotension, a rapid thready pulse, a CVP reading lower than 5 cm H_2O and a urine volume of less than 30 mL/h. Measures to raise blood volume and blood pressure will probably be prescribed. This can include rapid infusion of i.v. fluids or plasma. Such treatment will require close monitoring in order to detect circulatory overload (see below).

Evidence of fluid overload The nurse should promptly report a rising CVP, especially if this is accompanied by breathlessness, moist breath sounds, distended neck veins and a full pulse. These may indicate that fluid replacement has been too vigorous, causing over-expansion of the circulatory volume and placing strain on the left ventricle.

Evidence of electrolyte disruption Changes in pulse rate and rhythm should be reported promptly, along with ECG changes associated with hypo- and hyperkalaemia (see Nursing Care Plan 5.3), in order to allow adjustment to therapy and to prevent development of life-threatening cardiac dysrhythmias.

Monitoring response to insulin

Capillary blood glucose should be measured hourly to assess the response to i.v. insulin and to prevent overcorrection leading to hypoglycaemia. Accurate measurement and recording of blood glucose will provide the basis for adjusting insulin dosage.

Preventing complications

Many patients with HHNK are older people (DH 2001) who are especially vulnerable to the effects of hospitalisation and the complications of immobility. Maintenance of comfort and hygiene, including oral care, is of great importance.

Diabetes can cause neurovascular and ischaemic skin changes leading to impairment in circulation and sensation. There may also be disordered sweating due to autonomic neuropathy and increased susceptibility to infections, which places the skin at particular risk. Avoidance of skin damage is therefore a priority. The patient's position should be frequently altered, suitable pressure-relieving devices should be used and the skin, clothing and bedding should be kept cool, clean and dry.

Care is required when lifting, moving or positioning the patient to avoid damage to skin, muscles or joints. Particular attention should be paid to avoiding damage to the heels. Due to vascular and neurological changes, the feet of people with diabetes require particular attention to avoid serious complications (DH 2001) (see also p. 212).

Atherosclerosis is common in patients with diabetes, thus placing them at particular risk of vascular complications. Passive limb exercises whilst the patient is unconscious, and active limb movements when they are able to cooperate, will help to prevent venous stasis, which may result in deep vein thrombosis and pulmonary embolism. The nurse and the physiotherapist should encourage limb exercises.

Breathing exercises are also important as older, bedfast patients are at considerable risk of developing chest infections. Moreover, older people, and in particular those with diabetes, are less able to resist infection and tend to recover less quickly than younger non-diabetic people.

Monitoring the patient for pyrexia or other evidence of infection will allow prompt intervention. It is also important to ensure that the care environment and the standards of nursing care provided are such that infection risks are minimised (see Ch. 16).

Providing psychological support

The experience of a hyperglycaemic crisis can cause great distress, not only to the patient but also to family and close friends. Adopting a warm, empathic approach and accepting the fears of the patient and family is important if trust and rapport are to be established. The nurse should provide essential information using brief, clear explanations and should check to ensure these are understood. Access to medical staff and information about the ward or hospital should be provided.

Further considerations in DKA and HHNK

When the patient is deemed to be clinically and biochemically stable, on the basis of observation, bedside monitoring and laboratory tests, ongoing care is planned to address changing needs. If urine volumes are satisfactory, the urinary catheter is removed. The nasogastric tube is removed and oral fluids are offered. Diet is introduced under the guidance of the dietitian. When oral intake is adequate and blood urea and electrolyte levels are within normal limits, the i.v. fluids will usually be discontinued.

Subcutaneous insulin

This will replace the i.v. insulin when the patient is well enough to eat. Prescribing insulin is the responsibility of the physician but the nurse will be closely involved in monitoring patient response by frequent estimation of blood glucose. The nurse may also be required to adjust the insulin dosage within guidelines laid down in the written prescription.

Oral hypoglycaemic therapy

If possible, the patient is re-established on oral hypoglycaemic therapy. However, some patients may need to continue insulin therapy for some time before changing back to oral medication. Others may need to make a

Nursing Care Plan 5.3 Nursing care for R, a patient with DKA, during the first 24 h after admission (see Case History 5.2)

Nursing considerations	Action	Rationale	Evaluation
Impaired consciousness	• Position and support R in semi-prone or lateral position • Keep artificial airway in position until voluntarily expelled	To prevent asphyxia and prevent aspiration of secretion/vomitus	Skin colour and respirations are normal
	• Perform oropharyngeal suction if secretions are audible		
	• Provide nasogastric (NG) aspiration	Due to unconscious state and recent vomiting	
	• Continuously monitor colour and breathing		Risk factors eliminated
	• Administer oxygen as prescribed, ensuring that fire safety rules are observed	To correct hypoxia and prevent O_2 combustion	Blood gases improving
	• Monitor neurological status hourly. Record/report findings	To detect improvement/deterioration in conscious level	R is progressively more responsive
Hyperglycaemia and ketonaemia	• Administer prescribed short-acting insulin i.v. by infusion pump	To correct hyperglycaemia and ketonaemia	Trends indicate blood glucose returning to within the normal range
	• Monitor capillary blood glucose hourly: record/report findings	To evaluate response to insulin therapy and prevent hypoglycaemia	
Fluid deficit/replacement	• Administer i.v. fluids as prescribed. Observe venepuncture site for redness, swelling or extravasation. Record all fluids in fluid balance chart	To correct hypovolaemia	No discomfort or swelling of venepuncture site
	• Monitor CVP, BP, breathing, temperature: observe neck veins, skin colour and urine volumes	To monitor effects of fluid replacement	Vital signs are returning to within their normal ranges
	• Catheterisation usually prescribed if unconsciousness persists and if patient is oliguric	To monitor renal function and detect renal insufficiency (urine <30 mL/h)	Urine volume >30 mL/h
	• Test urine hourly for ketones: record results		Ketonuria diminishing
Electrolyte imbalance/replacement	• Observe effects of potassium replacement; provide continuous cardiac monitoring	Overzealous K^+ replacement can cause ventricular fibrillation, leading to cardiac arrest	
	• Report tall peaked T wave (indicates hyperkalaemia)		K^+ should be 3.5–5 mmol/L

Continued ▶

Nursing Care Plan 5.3 Nursing care for R, a patient with DKA, during the first 24 h after admission (see Case History 5.2) *(Continued)*

Nursing considerations	Action	Rationale	Evaluation
Electrolyte imbalance/ replacement *(Continued)*	• Report flattened or inverted T wave (indicates hypokalaemia)		
	• REPORT ECG CHANGES PROMPTLY	Persistent hypokalaemia due to inadequate K^+ replacement can result in heart block, which may lead to cardiac arrest	Cardiac monitor should display normal tracing
Probable current infection/ potential risk of infection	• Collect throat swab, catheter specimen of urine and, when consciousness returns, a specimen of sputum. Monitor TPR. Take venous blood specimen for culture and full blood count	To detect/monitor current infection	Specimen analysis Blood culture results and TPR normal
	• Administer prescribed antibiotics and note/report side-effects	To safely administer therapy	
	• Reduce risks of infection by high standards of nursing care (e.g. personal and catheter hygiene)	To prevent hospital-acquired infection	Patient infection-free
Inability to meet or communicate comfort needs	• Ensure bed is smooth, cool and crease-free. Provide regular position change and use of pressure-relieving aids to protect skin. Ensure careful positioning of limbs	To promote general comfort	Skin unblemished and free from discomfort
	• Wash, rinse and dry skin: observe for signs of pressure	To protect skin from damage	
	• Clean oral cavity 2-hourly. Lubricate lips. Clean nostrils and apply lubricant	To prevent oral and nasal discomfort and drying due to O_2 and the effects of dehydration and nasogastric tube	Oral/nasal mucosa intact
	• Keep hair groomed in preferred style. Use R's own nightwear. Maintain privacy throughout	To maintain R's individuality/ dignity	Patient feels/looks comfortable
Fear and shock as consciousness returns and diagnosis becomes apparent	• Display calm, empathic manner. Provide brief, clear explanations of reason for hospital admission and current care and treatment		
	• Provide access to parents and family	To convey positive attitudes To provide relevant information	R appears less acutely distressed
	• Encourage patient to verbalise concerns and express emotions		

Continued

Nursing Care Plan 5.3 Nursing care for R, a patient with DKA, during the first 24 h after admission (see Case History 5.2) *(Continued)*

Nursing considerations	Action	Rationale	Evaluation
Fear and shock as consciousness returns and diagnosis becomes apparent *(Continued)*	• Avoid bombarding R with information at this stage • Show sensitivity to the emotional needs of this vulnerable young patient	To recognise R's rights as an individual	R is able to express her needs
R's parents are anxious and shocked due to their daughter's hospitalisation and diagnosis	• Provide a comfortable, private waiting area for parents • Explain (briefly at this stage) what has happened to their daughter		
	• Encourage/accept verbalisation of fears and expression of emotions	To provide essential information to answer immediate concerns	Parents are reassured and able to meet with and support their daughter
	• Provide access to R and to medical staff		
	• Supply information about the ward/hospital (booklets etc.)		
	• When parents feel able to cooperate, complete admission documentation and patient profile		
	• Assure parents of access to nursing staff to answer their questions as they occur		
	• Arrange a visit from the diabetes specialist nurse and dietitian at a mutually suitable time	To establish a trusting relationship, facilitate early educational interventions and offer support to the family	Parents' immediate needs have been met; they appear to feel supported

permanent change to insulin therapy in order to achieve better control of blood glucose levels.

Restoration of self-care

The physician, diabetes specialist nurse, dietitian and ward nurses will initiate the process of preparing the patient to assume responsibility for self-care, but a contribution will also be made by the GP and the community nursing staff once the patient returns home.

Patient education

The newly diagnosed patient will require information about how a balance between activity, food and medication can be achieved with the help of frequent blood glucose monitoring. This is especially important for patients with type 1 diabetes.

Once the crisis has passed, perhaps the most important aspect of care is to prevent further episodes of DKA or HHNK. This involves identifying the events which led up to the crisis and discussing with the patient where action might have been taken to avert the crisis or obtain help at an earlier stage. Glycosylated haemoglobin estimation can provide useful information about glycaemic control over the preceding weeks, as can the patient's record book containing blood glucose and urinalysis results.

It is all too easy to be wise in retrospect. It is therefore not helpful to blame the patient for any episode of DKA or HHNK. The main aims should be to help the patient understand their diabetes and have confidence in its management; therefore time should be spent re-assessing their knowledge and addressing any issues which may help to prevent further episodes of illness.

Emotional support

If severe underlying emotional distress or disturbance has precipitated the metabolic crisis, then the patient's difficulties may need to be sensitively explored. In accordance with the patient's wishes, appropriate counselling facilities may be provided. The newly diagnosed patient will require emotional support in meeting the immediate practical demands imposed by the condition.

Hypoglycaemia (insulin reaction/coma)

In people with diabetes, hypoglycaemia is a common side-effect of treatment and occurs when blood glucose falls below 4 mmol/L.

Epidemiology

Hypoglycaemia is the most common complication of insulin therapy. It occurs less frequently with oral sulphonylurea therapy. It can also feature in diabetes which is secondary to other disorders, e.g. in patients with certain liver diseases. Of those people with insulin-treated diabetes, 25–30% suffer one or more severe hypoglycaemic episodes every year (Williams & Pickup 1999).

Aetiology

There are several causes of hypoglycaemia. The three main causes are:

- excess insulin
- insufficient food
- increased exercise/activity.

For other causes, see Box 5.6.

Box 5.6

Hypoglycaemia: classification, causes and risk factors

Classification

- *Asymptomatic* — biochemical hypoglycaemia without symptoms
- *Mild* — easily recognised and corrected by the patient
- *Moderate* — patient conscious but requiring help from others
- *Severe/unconscious* — cerebral function severely affected by glucose lack

Causes

- Too much insulin
- Wrong type of insulin
- Inappropriate combination of insulins
- Excess dosage of oral sulphonylureas
- Delayed or missed meal
- More than usual amount of exercise
- Alcohol ingestion, especially when hungry
- Stress, such as hypothermia

Risk factors

- Impaired awareness of hypoglycaemia
- Strict glycaemic control
- Excess alcohol consumption
- Drug abuse

PATHOPHYSIOLOGY

Symptoms are idiosyncratic, often developing over a very short period of time of 5–15 min.

Endocrine/autonomic response Glucagon and counter-regulatory hormones are secreted in response to falling blood glucose and act to restore blood glucose to normal. The activation of the autonomic nervous system in response to the stress of hypoglycaemia provokes autonomic symptoms of hypoglycaemia (MacAuley et al 2001). These hormones potentiate the effects of the sympathetic nervous system to cause the following symptoms:

- pounding heart
- palpitations
- sweating
- trembling
- sensation of hunger
- sensation of anxiety.

Central nervous system response As brain cells are unable to metabolise alternatives to glucose for energy, a fall below the normal blood glucose will cause neuroglycopenic symptoms, such as:

- lack of concentration
- dizziness
- unsteady gait
- slurred speech
- tingling around the lips.

Other non-specific symptoms, including headache and nausea, can occur.

In addition, observers may notice abnormalities such as:

- pallor
- irrational behaviour
- muscle twitching/seizures
- extreme drowsiness or coma.

Some of these symptoms and signs could, with disastrous consequences, be mistakenly attributed to excess intake of alcohol.

Loss of sensitivity to symptoms Recently diagnosed patients tend to rely on autonomic symptoms such as sweating, tremor and pounding heart to alert them to a fall in blood glucose. However, after some years, patients may become less sensitive to these responses and come to rely on neuroglycopenic features such as visual disturbances and dizziness to alert them to impending hypoglycaemia.

In long-standing insulin-treated diabetes, the perception of the onset of symptoms of hypoglycaemia may become blunted, due to autonomic neuropathy or the effect of intensified insulin treatment (Williams & Pickup 1999). The patient may remain asymptomatic even when the blood glucose falls below 2 mmol/L, although at this level some signs may be obvious to others. This is known as impaired awareness of hypoglycaemia. Symptoms can also be masked by the following:

- *Alcohol* — if the patient is known to have consumed alcohol or smells of alcohol, this can lead others to mistake hypoglycaemia for intoxication, particularly as many symptoms and clinical features are similar.

- *Ageing* — in older people hypoglycaemia may cause neurological disturbances and the presenting symptoms can be mistaken for failing mental function or transient ischaemic attacks (cerebrovascular disease).
- *Time of day* — hypoglycaemia during sleep is asymptomatic. It is often not detected although features such as night sweats, restlessness, nightmares, stertorous breathing and headaches on waking may give the patient an indication of its occurrence. This causes rebound hyperglycaemia and is attributed to an increase in the release of counter-regulatory hormones during the night to correct the hypoglycaemia. This is known as the Somogyi phenomenon (Frier & Fisher 1999).
- *Sulphonylurea-induced hypoglycaemia* — long-acting preparations such as chlorpropamide and glibenclamide, even at normal therapeutic doses, have been implicated in severe, prolonged hypoglycaemic coma. This risk is increased in older people, particularly when they may be unwell and not eating, and in those with poor renal function (Burge et al 1999). This can lead to prolonged hypoglycaemia and may be fatal.

MEDICAL MANAGEMENT

Treatment of hypoglycaemia is simple and the effects are usually dramatic and gratifying. Nevertheless, the risks posed by hypoglycaemic coma and the importance of early detection and intervention must be stressed.

Hypoglycaemia can be treated with oral carbohydrate, s.c. or i.m. glucagon, or i.v. glucose — depending on the stage and severity.

The conscious patient should be given rapidly absorbed glucose as a glucose drink or as sweets, followed by a more gradually absorbed form of carbohydrate, e.g. glucose tablets or a glass of fruit juice, followed by biscuits or a sandwich. Hypoglycaemia can recur if food is not consumed after the initial treatment with glucose.

The confused or drowsy patient If the patient is too drowsy to eat or drink safely, glucagon 1 mg by i.m injection can be given. This will have the effect of raising the blood glucose. Where possible, relatives should be taught how to administer glucagon.

The unconscious patient Medical help should always be sought for the unconscious patient, although if hypoglycaemia is known to be the problem, glucagon i.m should be given while the doctor is awaited and the patient should be placed in the recovery position until consciousness returns. Nothing should be given orally whilst the patient is unconscious (MacKinnon 2002).

If glucagon is unavailable, or fails to bring a response within 10–15 min, i.v. dextrose in a dose of 30–50 mL of glucose 50% is required, which will usually raise the blood glucose sufficiently for consciousness to be regained. When coma persists, hospital admission will be necessary. Unconscious hypoglycaemia in the hospitalised patient may be treated by i.v. dextrose as first-line treatment.

The hospitalised patient with hypoglycaemic coma A specimen of venous blood will be taken for laboratory estimation of blood glucose. Continuous i.v. infusion of dextrose 10–20% will be commenced and the patient's clinical response monitored by regular measurement of blood glucose. Approximately 1–2% of patients with hypoglycaemic coma fail to respond promptly to parenteral therapy. For these patients, other causes of coma such as alcohol or drug overdose, hypothermia or cerebral haemorrhage should be excluded. As cerebral oedema can accompany prolonged hypoglycaemia, an i.v. infusion of mannitol (a hyperosmotic fluid) may have to be given and oxygen administered (Richmond 1996).

NURSING PRIORITIES AND MANAGEMENT: Hypoglycaemia

In hypoglycaemic coma the period of extreme vulnerability tends to be short. Nevertheless, the nurse must take the patient's vulnerabilities into account in nursing interventions by:

- ensuring the patient's airway is clear
- monitoring the patient's conscious level
- administering prescribed therapy
- monitoring capillary blood glucose
- exploring the possible cause of the hypoglycaemic coma
- providing information and encouragement for the patient to help improve diabetes control.

Metabolic complications of diabetes vary in cause, severity and outcome. All indicate a lack of stability of diabetes control which requires further assessment and investigation and possibly subsequent modification of treatment or lifestyle.

For a detailed account of the causes, symptoms, treatment and management of hypoglycaemia, see Frier & Fisher (1999).

CHRONIC COMPLICATIONS OF DIABETES MELLITUS

This section will consider chronic complications of diabetes mellitus which result in pathological changes in large blood vessels (macroangiopathies), small blood vessels (microangiopathies) and nerves (neuropathies). The Diabetes Control and Complications Trial conducted in the early 1990s (Diabetes Control and Complications Research Group 1993) is considered to be one of the most important pieces of diabetes research in the last 20 years. It demonstrated that tight control of blood glucose prevented or delayed the onset of complications in type 1 diabetes, particularly retinopathy, neuropathy and nephropathy. However, the risk of severe hypoglycaemic attacks increased three-fold.

In 1998, the United Kingdom Prospective Diabetes Study Group (UKPDS) reported their findings in relation to the reduction of long-term complications in patients with type 2 diabetes. It was found that, through tight control of blood glucose and maintenance of blood pressure within normal limits, the risk of deaths related to diabetes could be reduced. Additionally, the long-term complications of diabetes such as heart disease and stroke and the loss of sight and kidney damage could also be reduced (UKPDS 1998a,b).

STOP THINK **5.10** Consider the potential risks of poor diabetes control.

Detailed management of specific diabetes-related complications is provided in Chapters 2 and 11.

Atherosclerosis

Epidemiology

Although atherosclerosis is not peculiar to diabetes, it is known that myocardial infarction, cerebrovascular accident (CVA) and gangrene are relatively frequent complications and are major causes of death in people with diabetes. Atherosclerosis develops at a much younger age in people with diabetes than in non-diabetic individuals: this is most noticeable in females.

Both types of diabetes carry increased risk, but those with type 2 diabetes show the strongest tendency to develop atheroma. This is probably due to age-related factors and perhaps also to the effects of long-standing asymptomatic hyperglycaemia prior to diagnosis. In type 1 diabetes, microvascular disease such as retinopathy usually precedes evidence of atherosclerosis.

Aetiology

Up to 70% of adults with type 2 diabetes have raised blood pressure and more than 70% have abnormal cholesterol levels (DH 2001). There are several risk factors for coronary artery disease (Kirby 2003):

- Increased concentrations of low density lipoprotein (LDL) cholesterol
- Decreased concentrations of high density lipoprotein (HDL) cholesterol
- Raised blood pressure
- Hyperglycaemia
- Smoking.

It is therefore essential that management of people with diabetes should focus on managing these risk factors.

Onset and progress of the disease

The development and vascular distribution of atherosclerosis in diabetes are similar to that found in the non-diabetic population, the exception being the more severe peripheral arterial involvement which may affect the lower limbs of some people with diabetes.

Cardiovascular disease

When compared with the general population, diabetes in men is associated with a two- to three-fold risk of developing coronary heart disease. In premenopausal women this is increased to four to five times the risk if the woman has diabetes (British Diabetic Association 1995). In a study coordinated by the World Health Organization, it was found that, of a group of 497 people aged 35–54 years with diabetes at 8-year follow-up, the prevalence of cardiovascular disease was 45%: 43% had coronary heart disease, 4.5% cerebrovascular disease and 4.2% had peripheral vascular disease (British Diabetic Association 1995).

Atherosclerosis of the coronary vessels can impair oxygen delivery to the myocardium, resulting in angina pectoris or myocardial infarction (MI). Due to the effects of autonomic neuropathy the patient may develop a cardiac arrhythmia and may have a 'silent' (painless) MI. Indeed, MI is more often fatal in people with diabetes compared with MI in those without diabetes (Stevens et al 2004).

Myocardial infarction (MI)

Approximately 10% of all MIs occur in patients with diabetes mellitus and mortality rates are also approximately two-fold higher than in the non-diabetic population (Watkins 2003).

A study of post-MI diabetic patients started on insulin therapy showed a reduction in mortality rate (Malmberg 1997). Further confirmation of these results is required, but at present this study provides the best evidence available in support of insulin treatment for all such patients — for some indefinitely (Watkins 2003).

For further details of heart disease in diabetes, see Fisher (2003).

Cerebrovascular disease

The incidence of stroke in patients with diabetes is also high and mortality following stroke is increased compared to the non-diabetic population. The clinical presentation is similar to that in the non-diabetic subject (Bell & Ovalle 1999). Hypertension is probably the most important of those factors which contribute to the development of atherosclerosis. Lowering the diastolic blood pressure to <80 mmHg in those at risk is of benefit (Hanson et al 1998).

Retinopathy

Diabetes is the leading cause of blindness in people under the age of 60 in industrialised countries. It is also a major cause of blindness in older people (National Institute for Clinical Excellence (NICE) 2002). By 20 years after the onset of diabetes, almost all patients with type 1 diabetes and over 60% of patients with type 2 diabetes will have some degree of retinopathy. Even at diagnosis, it is estimated that approximately one-quarter of patients will already have established background retinopathy (Watkins 2003).

Retinopathy results from changes in the basement membrane of small blood vessels of the retina (retinal microangiopathy) and can be classified as:

- background (non-proliferative) retinopathy
- maculopathy
- proliferative retinopathy.

Background retinopathy

Background retinopathy rarely causes a major threat to vision unless the macula is affected. In the early stages of retinopathy, the capillaries of the retina become more permeable. This can cause fluid exudation (hard exudates) into the retina. Retinal veins may swell at localised spots, giving the appearance of 'beading'. Microaneurysms can develop; these can rupture, causing small bleeds. Arteriolar occlusions cause retinal infarcts or 'cotton wool spots' on the retina. More spots occur in rapidly developing retinopathy or where there is coexisting hypertension. Evidence of venous bleeding and 'cotton wool' spots suggests progression to pre-proliferative retinopathy.

Maculopathy

Maculopathy can cause severe loss of central vision and is most common in type 2 diabetes. In this condition, oedema, haemorrhages and exudates are concentrated on the macular area of the retina.

Proliferative retinopathy

Microvascular disease of the retina can result in areas of hypoxia. This will give rise to the compensatory development of new blood vessels (neovascularisation) which grow forward from the retina to invade the vitreous body. These new vessels are fragile and poorly supported; consequently, haemorrhages into the vitreous body are common. Progressive traction on the retina can result in retinal detachment. Proliferative retinopathy and retinal detachment will seriously threaten vision.

MEDICAL MANAGEMENT

The main priorities in the treatment of diabetic retinopathy are to reduce the risk of haemorrhage and to limit new vessel growth into the vitreous body. Photocoagulation by means of laser technology can be used to treat proliferative and pre-proliferative retinopathy. Treatment should be considered in all patients with visual potential (NICE 2002).

Screening Annual ophthalmoscopic examination for those with no identified retinopathy and 6-monthly for those with background retinopathy is strongly advised. This will enable swift and appropriate treatment to help prevent blindness. Where glycaemic control is poor, or where hypertension or renal involvement is more frequent, eye examinations may be recommended. Referral to an ophthalmologist should be made for maculopathy, proliferative and pre-proliferative retinopathy, a fall in visual acuity, retinal detachment or rubeosis iridis (NICE 2002).

Retinal photography should be carried out annually and it is now possible to do this using non-mydriatic retinal cameras which allow the retina to be photographed without prior dilatation of the pupil. Many health authorities are using mobile units to carry out retinal screening in the community.

Prevention The patient should be aware of the established link between poor blood glucose control and retinopathy and of the importance of promptly reporting changes in vision. As eye tests for patients with diabetes are free of charge, the optician should be made aware that the patient has diabetes. The risks of retinopathy increase if the patient is hypertensive.

Other eye disorders

Although retinopathy poses the main threat to vision in diabetes, there is also an increased risk of cataract and glaucoma. The reasons why this should be so are not entirely clear. It is possible that glycosylation of protein in the optic lens can cause the opacities of cataract (Hamilton & Ubig 1991). The management of cataract and glaucoma are described in full in Chapter 13.

Sadly, many patients with diabetes do ultimately suffer partial or total blindness. Maintaining independence in relation to diabetes management and general self-care will present quite a challenge but patients may be referred to local visual impairment services and the Royal National Institute for the Blind (RNIB). Allwinkle (2002) describes various devices which can enable the blind or partially sighted patient to administer insulin and monitor blood glucose. These include pre-filled disposable insulin pens with an audible dialling mechanism and information on how to obtain a talking meter which can be purchased from the USA. This meter uses capillary-fill test strips which make the task of blood sampling easy for the patient. The nurse and the visually impaired patient with diabetes should work together to seek out ways of reducing the patient's dependence on others. Diabetes UK (the national charity for diabetes) and the RNIB can provide invaluable up-to-date information about the help currently available for these patients (see 'Useful websites', p. 227).

Diabetic nephropathy

Approximately 20% of patients with type 1 diabetes develop proteinuria after a disease duration of 25 years (EURODIAB IDDM 1994) and up to 40% of patients with type 2 diabetes will eventually develop diabetic nephropathy, the incidence of which is related to the duration of their diabetes (Molitch 1997). Between 10 and 20% of patients with type 2 diabetes who have diabetic nephropathy will eventually progress to end-stage renal failure (Cooper 1998).

AETIOLOGY AND PATHOPHYSIOLOGY

The kidneys of people with diabetes are vulnerable with respect to the following:

- *Microvascular changes* — damage to the capillaries in the glomeruli can occur. The basement membrane initially thickens and, in the later stages, nodules of glycoprotein are deposited in the glomerular capsule. As a result, the filtering capacity of the glomeruli is reduced.
- *Macrovascular changes* — atheromatous changes in renal vessels can lead to poor renal perfusion which will ultimately impair renal function.
- *Hypertension* — a common feature in diabetes, hypertension can contribute to kidney damage and, conversely, can also result from kidney damage.
- *Urinary tract infection* — this can occur for several reasons:
  - — diabetes-associated predisposition to infection
  - — damaged renal tissue vulnerable to infection
  - — the need for catheterisation during metabolic crisis
  - — atonic bladder associated with autonomic neuropathy, causing urinary stasis and ascending urinary tract infection.

Screening

All patients with diabetes should have their urinary albumin concentration and serum creatinine measured at regular intervals, usually annually, and this should be measured using an early morning urine sample. Urinary albumin:creatinine ratio should be measured by a laboratory method or a 'near-patient' test specific for albumin at low concentration. Any abnormal result should be confirmed by a further sample (SIGN 2001).

Microalbuminuria is defined by a rise in urinary albumin loss of between 30 and 300 mg/day. This is the earliest sign of diabetic nephropathy and predicts increased total mortality, cardiovascular mortality and morbidity, and end-stage renal failure (SIGN 2001).

Blood pressure All patients with proteinuria should have their blood pressure measured at every clinic or surgery visit. The UKPDS demonstrated that reducing blood pressure from 154/87 mmHg to 144/82 mmHg in type 2 diabetes led to a risk reduction of 8% in developing microalbuminuria over 6 years (UKPDS 1998b). In the HOPE study, angiotensin-converting enzyme (ACE) inhibitor therapy for 4.5 years in type 2 diabetes was associated with an absolute risk reduction of developing proteinuria of 2% (HOPE 2000). Therefore, tight blood pressure control (<140/80 mmHg) in patients with type 2 diabetes should be maintained (SIGN 2001).Good glycaemic control should be maintained in all patients with diabetes. Both the Diabetes Control and Complications Trial (DCCT) (Diabetes Control and Complications Research Group 1993) and UKPDS (1998b) have shown that a reduction in mean HbA1c (glycosylated haemoglobin) was associated with a reduction in the occurrence of microalbuminuria and proteinuria.

MEDICAL MANAGEMENT

Diabetic renal disease is treated in the same way as renal disease in the non-diabetic population. The reader is referred to Chapter 8 for detailed coverage of early, advanced and end-stage renal failure. Only diabetes-related points will be mentioned in the short sections which follow.

Treatment choices for the patient in end-stage renal failure include haemodialysis, continuous ambulatory peritoneal dialysis (CAPD) or renal transplant using live or cadaver donors.

Renal transplantation using a live donor offers the best treatment for suitable patients. Careful selection of patients is important, given that other major diabetes-related complications usually coexist with the renal disease. Virtually all diabetic patients with end-stage renal failure have retinopathy, and 20–30% are blind. Retinopathy alone would not militate against active treatment by dialysis or renal transplantation but the presence of carcinomatosis, advanced dementia or severe cerebrovascular disease may do so. The prognosis in, for example, severe cardiovascular disease is also poor (Watkins et al 2003).

Oral hypoglycaemics Due to the danger of lactic acidosis, metformin (a biguanide) should not be used for patients with renal impairment. Chlorpropamide (a sulphonylurea) should also be avoided as it is mainly excreted by the kidneys and in renal failure can accumulate in the blood, causing serious hypoglycaemia. It may be necessary for some patients in renal failure, whose diabetes was previously controlled by oral medication, to be changed to insulin therapy.

NURSING PRIORITIES AND MANAGEMENT: Diabetic nephropathy

When renal function is impaired, diabetes control should be closely monitored by regular blood glucose measurement. Measurement and recording of fluid intake and output and body weight may be required to monitor renal function. Dietary and fluid restrictions may be imposed due to renal impairment. Patients and their families should be made aware of the vital importance of these measures.

Prevention of renal failure

By identifying early renal impairment by screening for microalbuminuria, making efforts to improve diabetes control and detecting and treating hypertension, it is possible to prevent or delay the progression of renal disease (Diabetes Control and Complications Research Group 1993).

Medical and nursing staff should exercise extreme caution in the introduction and subsequent care of urinary catheters in order to prevent infection. Prompt treatment of any established urinary tract infection will normally be required to minimise damage.

STOP THINK **5.11** Identify three treatment approaches which may be used in end-stage renal failure in a diabetic person and discuss the potential lifestyle implications of each form of treatment.

For further information on diabetic nephropathy, see Hasslacher (2001).

Diabetic neuropathy

Aetiology

Although the cause of diabetic neuropathy is uncertain, it is known that neural function in the diabetic patient deteriorates in response to pressure, metabolic changes and ischaemia (Watkins et al 2003). The incidence of diabetic neuropathy is known to rise in line with the duration of diabetes and with increasing age. A popular theory is that nerve damage occurs as a result of the accumulation of metabolites of glucose (such as sorbitol), causing osmotic swelling and subsequent damage to the nerve cell. Ischaemia as a cause of diabetic neuropathy, however, remains controversial but must be considered a contributory factor (Watkins et al 2003).

PATHOPHYSIOLOGY

Structural damage affecting the Schwann cells causes segmental areas of demyelination to appear, thus impairing conduction of the nerve impulses. There is no widely accepted classification of diabetic neuropathy, but a number of clinical syndromes are recognisable (see Table 5.14).

Peripheral neuropathy This is a distal symmetrical neuropathy, principally affecting the lower extremities and playing a major part in the aetiology of diabetic foot problems. It can affect either sensory or motor nerves and the patient's symptoms will reflect this.

Polyneuropathy This term refers to widespread neuropathic changes affecting many nerves. Again, the lower extremities are often affected (peripheral polyneuropathy).

Mononeuropathies Single nerves or their roots are affected. The condition is often of rapid onset and reversible, suggesting an acute vascular origin rather than chronic

Table 5.14 Diabetic neuropathy

Type of neuropathy	Body system/part affected	Symptoms/signs	Special points
Peripheral neuropathies Polyneuropathies: • Sensory	The lower extremities are the most frequently affected area	Reduced sensation: numbness, heaviness, insensitivity to heat, cold, and pressure Increased sensation: tingling, burning, pain (worse at night)	Serious risk of tissue damage as a result of heat, cold or pressure
• Motor — Amyotrophy — Muscle wasting	 Muscles of the pelvic girdle Muscles of the hands and feet	Severe muscle wasting and pain Loss of strength in hand grip Changes in walking pattern Pressure points altered Painless foot ulcers can develop	Physiotherapy Aids to assist hand grip Chiropody Adapted footwear Care of the feet
Neuropathic arthropathy	Joints in the feet: 'Charcot's joints'	See 'The diabetic foot'	
Mononeuropathies: • Sensory	Femoral, sciatic, radial or ulnar nerve 3rd cranial nerve	Acute pain with sudden onset Weakness and paralysis Ptosis: drooping of the upper eyelid	Provide pain relief Improve diabetes control Refer to an ophthalmologist
• Motor	3rd, 4th and 6th cranial nerves	Squint: diplopia	
Autonomic neuropathies	*Cardiovascular system* • Heart and blood vessels • Vasomotor centre	Postural hypotension Tachycardia at rest Painless myocardial infarction Reduced perspiration in lower extremities Increased perspiration in upper extremities	Symptoms such as syncope, dizziness and sweating; can be confused with hypoglycaemia
	Gastrointestinal system • Stomach	Diabetic gastroparesis (delayed emptying) Nausea, anorexia Feeling of fullness	Altered absorption rate of nutrients can affect diabetes control
	• Bowel	Constipation Diarrhoea	Adjust diet
	Urinary system • Bladder	Loss of sensation Incomplete emptying Retention of urine Atonic bladder Sphincter incompetence	Urinary stasis creates risk of infection which may lead to renal damage
	Reproductive system • Male genitalia	Erectile dysfunction Retrograde ejaculation Infertility	Neuropathic, vascular and psychological factors usually coexist

metabolic disturbance (Williams & Pickup 1999). Examples of mononeuropathy include ptosis (drooping eyelid) and diplopia which can occur as a result of damage to cranial nerve III.

Autonomic neuropathies Damage can occur within the autonomic nervous system, causing numerous abnormalities in many areas of the body. Common manifestations are abnormal sweating, postural hypotension, diarrhoea and erectile dysfunction. Less common are gastroparesis and bladder dysfunction (Williams & Pickup 1999).

Prevention

Major benchmark studies such as the DCCT and UKPDS have shown that strict glycaemic control can decrease the risk of complications, including neuropathy. Other sensible measures such as avoiding smoking and tight control of blood pressure, blood cholesterol and triglycerides are advised (see Ch. 2).

MEDICAL MANAGEMENT

Diabetic neuropathy affects many systems of the body. Management, which is essentially symptomatic, may involve the multidisciplinary efforts of the diabetes care team. A variety of treatment approaches may be adopted, including medication, surgery and physiotherapy.

NURSING PRIORITIES AND MANAGEMENT: Diabetic neuropathy

Devising ways to meet the particular comfort needs of the patient will be a central focus for nursing care. Reducing the risk of accidental tissue damage arising from severe sensory impairment will also be a priority.

Neuropathies can seriously interfere with lifestyle and emotional well-being. An example of this is erectile dysfunction which affects up to 35% of all men with diabetes (Williams & Pickup 1999). Erectile dysfunction can be devastating for both the patient and his partner. Many men with diabetes and erectile dysfunction would like help for this problem but are reluctant to seek advice. Once the diagnosis has been made, there are several treatment options available, including professional sexual counselling, vacuum devices, penile injections and oral agents such as sildenafil. The choice of treatment will depend on local circumstances, personal experience and, most importantly, the patient's own preference (Mills 2003).

For further reading on diabetic neuropathy, see Gries et al (2003); for more information on erectile dysfunction, see Alexander (2003).

The diabetic foot (see Table 5.15)

Successful management of the diabetic foot requires input from the multidisciplinary team including nurse, podiatrist, orthotist, physician and surgeon (Edmonds et al 1999).

Education of the patient is vital in the prevention of problems (see Box 5.7) and it is essential that the patient with diabetes is screened, at least annually, for foot disease (SIGN 2001).

Table 5.15 Clinical signs of the diabetic foot

Sign	Neuropathic foot	Ischaemic foot
Temperature	Warm	Cool
Pulses	Present	Absent
Pain	Loss of sensation	Intermittent claudication and rest pain
Skin	Dry cracking skin	Blanches on elevation
Deformity	Present	Absent
Position of ulcer	Plantar surface, toes or high pressure areas	Margins of foot and toes

Box 5.7

Measures to protect the feet in diabetes

General measures

- Do not smoke
- Take a healthy balanced diet
- Try to maintain body weight within normal limits
- Exercise — try to keep active; this will help improve the circulation
- Get blood pressure and blood fats checked regularly

Footwear

- Ensure correctly fitting shoes — ask for feet to be measured when buying shoes. Break in new shoes very gradually
- Ensure that socks or stockings fit comfortably — avoid constricting around ankles and avoid socks with thick seams
- Change footwear as soon as possible if wet
- Avoid walking barefoot — wear slippers and beach shoes to prevent injury
- Do not wear sandals if there is any loss of sensation in the feet

Foot care

- Bathe feet daily using lukewarm (not hot) water and soap
- Pat feet dry gently; pay special attention to the area between the toes
- Apply a moisturising cream daily to avoid dryness and keep the skin supple
- Avoid exposing feet to excess heat or cold
- Avoid sunburn to the feet and legs
- Cut nails according to the shape of the toes while they are still soft from bathing but do not dig down the side of the toenails
- Inspect feet daily for blisters, corns, calluses, cracks or redness (a mirror can help in seeing the underside of the foot)
- Do not burst blisters
- If a minor cut or abrasion does occur, wash thoroughly and cover with a clean dressing. See your doctor if the cut has not healed in 48 h
- Your chiropodist should be consulted for treatment of ingrown toenails, corns or calluses. Do not use home remedies or over-the-counter (OTC) products such as corn plasters
- Your general practitioner should be consulted for the treatment of verrucae
- A doctor or nurse should be consulted if foot problems such as tingling, numbness, swelling, pain or loss of feeling develop
- Ensure you have your feet inspected annually by a trained professional

Screening Foot examination by trained professionals should consist of:

- testing of foot sensation using a 10 g monofilament or vibration
- palpation of foot pulses and use of a Doppler if possible (see Box 5.8)
- inspection of foot appearance and footwear.

Box 5.8

Doppler ultrasound

A hand-held Doppler probe is a portable ultrasound designed to detect blood flow. It works by transmitting high frequency sound waves through the tissue and collecting the reflected signal (Grasty 1999). The movement of blood flow causes the reflected wave to undergo a frequency shift, the extent of this depending on the speed and direction of the flow. Systolic pressure can be measured by combining the use of the Doppler and a blood pressure cuff. The Doppler is now widely used by trained practitioners as a screening test to assess the peripheral arterial circulation (Vowden 1999).

Disorders of the foot in diabetes can occur as a result of two syndromes: the neuropathic foot and/or the ischaemic foot (Edmonds et al 1999).

Based on UK population surveys, diabetic foot problems are a common complication of diabetes, with prevalences of 23–42% for neuropathy, 9–23% for vascular disease and 5–7% for foot ulceration (SIGN 2001).

Painful peripheral neuropathy can be a major problem for many people, particularly at night. It can be treated with some success by tricyclic antidepressants such as amitriptyline. Gabapentin has also been shown to be effective, with fewer side-effects. Topical capsaicin should also be considered for localised neuropathic pain.

Deformity of the foot can lead to ulceration, particularly in the absence of protective pain sensation and with the contribution of unsuitable footwear. Early detection can initiate properly fitting shoes before ulceration occurs.

Charcot foot/Charcot joint is a neuroarthropathic syndrome with osteoporosis, fracture, acute inflammation and disorganisation of foot architecture (SIGN 2001). The patient may complain of a hot, red and swollen foot with or often without pain. Diagnosis should be made by clinical examination supported, where available, by the use of thermography (SIGN 2001). Immobilisation of the limb, usually by casting of the foot, and reduction of stress by decreasing the amount of weight-bearing on the affected limb through use of crutches are the current mainstays of treatment. However, other treatment options are being considered. One option is the use of i.v. pamidronate, a bisphosphonate which is a potent inhibitor of bone reabsorption with minimal effect on bone formation. This action stops the osteoclastic activity of bone breakdown, promotes healing and decreases local inflammation (Mrugeshkumar 2004).

For further information on pamidronate use, see Selby et al (1994).

Management of ulcers

Neuropathic ulcers are most frequently caused from callus build-up but can also be due to thermal injury, e.g. stepping into hot water, and to chemical injury, e.g. from use of corn plasters. Whatever the initial cause, the injury is usually not perceived by the patient, due to loss of pain sensation. In the neuropathic foot, the aim is to redistribute plantar pressures by some form of cast or cradled insole. However, in the neuroischaemic foot, the aim is to protect the vulnerable margins of the foot by using a wide fitting shoe (Armstrong & Lavery 1998).

The ulcer should be subjected to initial debridement and drainage of exudate. The larvae of the green bottle fly (maggots) can be a very effective method of debridement (Yates et al 2003). Stimulation of subsequent wound healing can be improved by a number of preparations such as becaplermin (Regranex) as well as the use of absorbent, non-adhesive dressings. Living human tissue replacement therapy can also be used for persistent wounds (SIGN 2001) (see Ch. 23).

Infection Initial prescription of broad-spectrum antibiotics is vital to help improve healing. A wound swab for culture should be taken before antibiotics are commenced. Progression to cellulitis and osteomyelitis will require hospital admission for administration of i.v. antibiotics, immobilisation and appropriate wound treatment. Stress hormones will be released in response to severe infection, which in turn cause hyperglycaemia. The resulting increase in insulin demand will present an increased challenge to the pancreas, and as a result metabolic crisis may ensue. Intravenous fluids and insulin may be required to stabilise the patient's condition.

Necrosis The ischaemic foot results from atherosclerotic changes in the distal vessels of the legs. It is important to explore the possibility of revascularisation in the infected neuroischaemic foot. Angioplasty is indicated in the treatment of single or multiple stenosis or short segment occlusions of blood vessels. If angioplasty is not possible because of long arterial occlusions, bypass should be considered (Edmonds et al 1999). In the neuropathic foot in which there is necrosis, surgical debridement will probably be required. However, severely affected patients may eventually require digital amputation or, in even more serious cases, a below knee amputation.

Nurses involved in the care of people with diabetes should undertake regular monitoring of the patient's feet and commence appropriate and timely treatment whenever necessary (Edmonds et al 1999).

Chronic complications of diabetes mellitus can have important implications for the planning of nursing care. Whether the patient is at home or in hospital, the nurse should carefully assess the individual's nursing needs, giving special consideration to risks associated with impaired circulation and sensation, increased risk of infection and delayed healing. Recognition of these risk factors will enable care to accommodate the patient's particular vulnerabilities and will help to ensure that suitable educational support is provided.

STOP THINK **5.12** Explain the way in which infection can have an impact on diabetic control and consider the role of the nurse in minimising the effect of intercurrent infections.

FACILITATING SELF-CARE THROUGH EDUCATION

In most hospital and community settings the overall coordination of patient teaching is undertaken by the diabetes specialist nurse working closely with the specialist dietitian and the patient's physician. The National Institute of Clinical Excellence (NICE) has published guidance on patient education, recommending that 'structured patient education is made available to all people with diabetes at the time of initial diagnosis and then as required on an ongoing basis, based on a formal regular assessment of need' (NICE 2003). In many cases, however, the care of patients with diabetes will be undertaken by community and hospital nurses who are not specialists in diabetes care. All such nurses may be required to undertake a teaching role and must therefore ensure that their own knowledge base is adequate.

Assessment

Before embarking on a teaching programme, the nurse must determine the needs of the patient and family for information, and plan teaching strategies that will make the learning experience pleasant and effective (Ley 1997). By establishing a rapport with the patient and family, the nurse will be better able to assess the patient's needs in relation to:

- current level of knowledge about diabetes
- understanding about the reasons for prescribed treatment
- knowledge and skills required for self-care
- emotional response to the diagnosis
- social support from family and friends
- barriers to learning, e.g. sensory loss, mobility and manipulation problems, language difficulties, reading and writing difficulties and intellectual impairment.

Planning a teaching programme

Personnel

Any member of the diabetes care team may be involved in teaching the patient and family about diabetes. However, it is likely that the main responsibility for patient teaching will rest with the nursing staff, and in particular with the diabetes specialist nurse who will work in partnership with the patient and family (Brown 2003).

Materials and methods

An impressive array of informative and attractive booklets is available, many of which are sponsored by manufacturers and written by diabetes health care professionals. These provide visual back-up for teaching and discussion sessions. Video and computer programs can be provided for patients to view individually or in groups. Diabetes UK is an excellent source of educational materials (see 'Useful websites', p. 227).

Teaching sessions

The NICE guidance suggests principles of good practice rather than recommendations on the type, setting and frequency of education (Avery 2003).

NICE guidance (2003) suggests education interventions should:

- reflect the principles of adult learning
- be provided by an appropriately trained multidisciplinary team
- be delivered to groups of patients unless considered unsuitable or inappropriate
- be accessible to all local people, taking into account cultural needs and disabilities
- use a variety of techniques to promote active learning.

Sessions should be short and information presented in small, easily assimilated and integrated sections with teaching points categorised into lists. Ordering presentation so that the most important point is always raised first can help the patient to prioritise information. Being direct and specific will aid retention, as will using simple words and brief sentences. Before going on to a new topic, the instructor should use sensitive questioning to check the patient's recall and understanding of the material already covered (Ley 1997). Patients should be encouraged to ask questions and discuss the topics within the group.

Staff members should be consistent in the information they provide. Adopting a friendly manner and taking time to talk about non-medical matters can relax the patient and set the scene for a more productive teaching session. It is important to consider the age group for which teaching materials have been designed in order to avoid giving inappropriate information.

The programme

The teaching programme should be tailored to suit the patient's individual needs but is likely to include some of the following topics:

- What is diabetes mellitus? — type 1 and type 2
- Treatment of diabetes
  - — oral hypoglycaemics
  - — insulin therapy
    - why insulin and how does it work?
    - types of insulin
    - storage and administration of insulin
- the diet–insulin–exercise balance — insulin dose adjustment (see Box 5.9)
- monitoring blood glucose
- recognising and treating hypo- and hyperglycaemia
- what to do during illness
- testing for ketones
- avoiding complications
- health screening
- lifestyle factors — alcohol, smoking, recreational drugs, driving, travel, pregnancy and sexual health.

STOP THINK **5.13** J is 15 years old and has insulin-dependent diabetes. He plays football for the school team, enjoys partying and goes swimming once a week. Consider how a short teaching session might be prepared to help J understand the significance of exercise to overall diabetes control, personal well-being and the prevention of chronic complications.

Box 5.9

Exercise in diabetes

Exercise and increased activity can provide many health benefits for the person with diabetes, such as improving insulin sensitivity, weight control and reduction, heart and circulatory protection, strengthening of joints and bones and many other benefits. Exercise will reduce blood glucose levels and a clear understanding of the role of exercise in blood glucose control is essential for every patient with diabetes. The nurse must find a way of explaining this role that is appropriate to the learning needs of individual patients. The analogy of 'fuel intake' (food) and 'energy output' (activity/exercise) is often useful for the purposes of illustration.

What happens during exercise?
When energy output is low, the demand for fuel in the form of glucose is also low. However, during bursts of activity the demand for glucose will rise and it is then drawn from reserves in the muscles and liver. The rate at which glucose is taken up by the cells is influenced by medication (insulin or tablets). If available supplies of glucose are depleted and are not replaced, the patient's blood glucose will fall and may continue to fall for several hours after prolonged or intense exercise, thus increasing the risk of hypoglycaemia.

Avoiding exercise-induced hypoglycaemia
Insulin-treated patients should be advised to monitor blood glucose before and after exercise and when to take extra carbohydrate to avoid hypoglycaemia. A quickly absorbable form of glucose such as glucose tablets or a glucose drink may be used to augment diet and help prevent an abrupt fall in blood glucose. Another strategy to avoid exercise-induced hypoglycaemia is for the insulin dose to be reduced prior to planned and prolonged strenuous activity. Insulin dose adjustment in relation to exercise is an important aspect of the patient's education programme when commencing insulin therapy. Blood glucose should then be monitored to gauge the effects of any reduction. Patients on oral antidiabetic therapy may, less frequently, also experience exercise-induced hypoglycaemia and consequently may need to adjust their carbohydrate intake to meet the additional energy demands imposed by the exercise.

Patients with type 1 diabetes should also be made aware that hyperglycaemia (blood glucose >14.0 mmol/L) with ketonuria is an absolute contraindication to exercise as this can indicate that there is a lack of circulating insulin and that the patient is metabolically unstable. Exercise in this situation could cause higher blood glucose levels and a risk of diabetic ketoacidosis (Burr & Dinesh 1999).

PROMOTING PSYCHOLOGICAL AND SOCIAL ADJUSTMENT

The emotional impact of diabetes mellitus

There is extensive literature that acknowledges the 'grief' that people experience in the face of any kind of loss of health or lifestyle and people diagnosed with diabetes may experience such grief and sense of loss. The diagnosis of diabetes has been likened to the experience of bereavement (Everett & Kerr 1998). In the context of diabetes, Jacobson (1996) describes that for some there is 'a clearly demarcated period of bereavement' and it has been suggested that the degree of early adjustment to their disorder can predict the subsequent development of anxiety and depression in youths with type 1 diabetes (Kovacs et al 1995).

The experience of loss in an individual, especially with type 1 diabetes, may be masked by the apparent acceptance of diabetes by virtue of the necessity to engage in specific self-care activities such as insulin injections and blood glucose monitoring. This can be described as at an intellectual level of acceptance. However, the degree of emotional acceptance may be hidden as the patient engages in an intensive programme of education designed to provide the knowledge and skills leading to self-management. Such intellectual acceptance and emotional acceptance are described as two stages in psychosocial adjustment to physical disability (Livneh & Antonak 1994). Examples of emotional non-acceptance include denial or part-denial, feeling stigmatised, alienated, angry, rebellious, self-blaming, guilt, isolated and unable to disclose their diagnosis (Brown 2001). The difference between intellectual and emotional acceptance can be understood from comments made by people with diabetes:

- *'You ask me anything about diabetes I could tell you … I'm right up to date with everything … I know everything about diabetes ... I'm one of those people who strives to know what I've got … to watch for the pitfalls …'*
- *'Probably the main reason I know I'm not in charge of my diabetes is because I've not accepted it yet … It's all to do with my brain … once I've accepted it, I know for a fact I will be more in control …'*

Psychosocial factors influencing self-management of diabetes

Diabetes self-management has been estimated to be seen as over 98% the patient's responsibility (Anderson & Funnell 2002). This is an enormous demand, not only on the person with diabetes, but also on the individual's family. One of the purposes of diabetes education is to impart knowledge and skills that enable the person with diabetes to make informed decisions about how they are going to lead their life with diabetes. However, there are other determinants of behaviour which can influence behavioural choices. These include health beliefs, locus of control, self-efficacy, behavioural intentions, quality of life and emotional adjustment.

Health beliefs

The health belief model (see Fig. 5.11) points to the significance to the person with diabetes of the perceived benefits, costs, severity and susceptibility within the diabetes experience that the person subjectively perceives in relation to themselves and their diabetes (Becker & Janz 1985):

- *A benefit might be perceived as: 'If I follow my regimen then I will avoid ill-health in the future'.*
- A cost might be perceived as: *'If I follow my prescribed regimen then my life will revolve around diabetes and there will be no time for anything else'.*

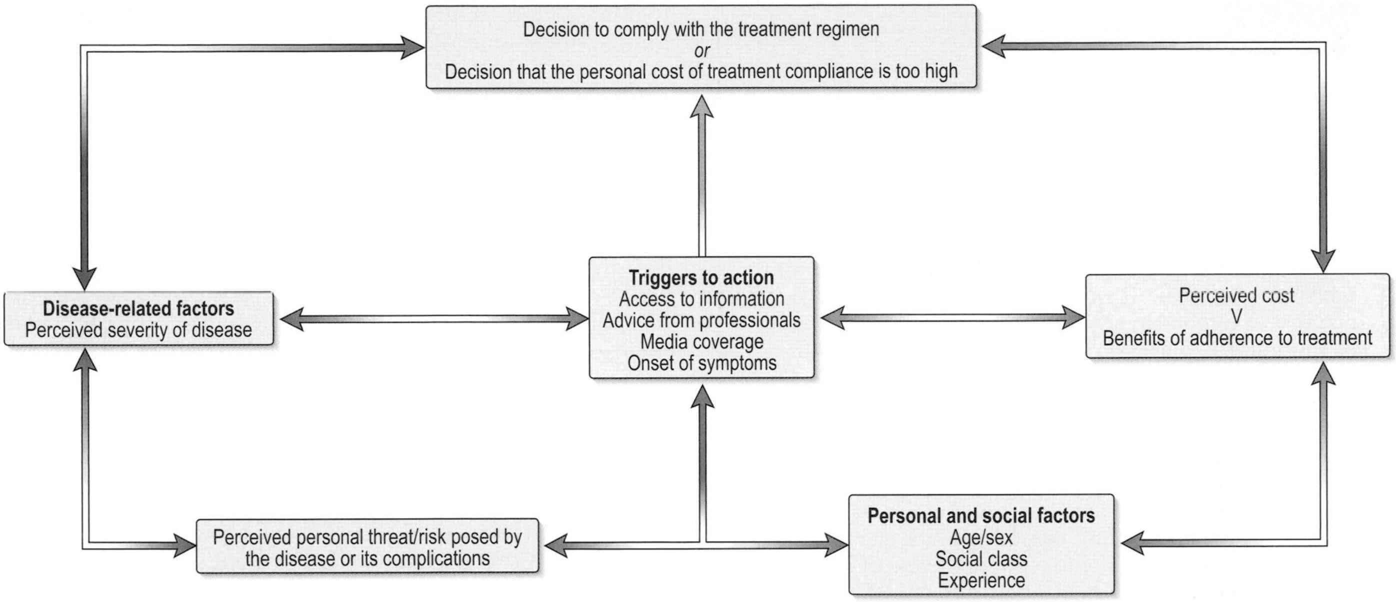

Fig. 5.11 The health belief model, summarised.

- Severity can be expressed as: *'Diabetes is serious and leads to complications'.*
- Susceptibility includes: *'If I have poor control then I will develop eye and kidney problems'.*

In order to live positively with their diabetes, people need to believe that benefits of self-care outweigh the costs.

People with type 2 diabetes may believe they are less susceptible to complications, particularly if they have been incorrectly told they have 'mild' diabetes.

Locus of control

Rotter's social learning theory of locus of control (1966) originally described the 'locus' as being either internal or external. It was suggested that a person operated somewhere along a continuum ranging from an internal locus, whereby the person felt personal responsibility for their health and subsequent outcomes, to an external locus, where the individual had no sense of influence over what happened to their health, perceiving it to be influenced by outside factors. The construct was further developed to recognise that some may see events as being in the hands of powerful others, such as health care professionals, or that events could be due to chance or fate (Wallston et al 1976). Bradley et al (1984), using a diabetes-specific multidimensional locus of control scale, found that when events were seen fatalistically, this was associated with poor glycaemic control.

Peyrot and Rubin (1994) designed a diabetes-specific locus of control instrument that helped them identify two components in internal locus of control that predict opposing outcomes in terms of self-management: the first component, autonomy, is linked with successful self-care; the second component, self-blame, may lead to negative outcomes because such self-blame results in an inability to access resources such as health care professional support. In addition, how the locus of control was perceived would influence how the individual would anticipate events happening in the future.

Self-efficacy

Self-efficacy theory describes the confidence, or otherwise, that an individual might have in expecting that a behaviour will result in a given outcome (Bandura 1977). Knowledge and understanding of the implications of health actions must be accompanied by a positive attitude and self-belief in individual capability to carry out those actions (Scriven & Orme 2001). Strengthening of self-efficacy is particularly important in older people to allow them to develop confidence and belief that they can reach desired outcomes (Heath & Schofield 1999).

Behavioural intentions

Peyrot and Rubin (1997) suggest that a person's intention to change their diabetes self-care practices leads to actual behaviour change but such change may not occur for several months. This is more likely to be the case for self-regulation behaviours such as blood glucose monitoring or taking medication on time, than for lifestyle change relating to diet or exercise.

Quality of life (see Box 5.10)

There are many definitions of quality of life (QoL) but, in general, QoL includes several domains such as psychological state, physical well-being, role functioning and social support (Everett & Kerr 2001). People with diabetes often have to make decisions about the balance between quantity of life versus quality of life; these issues are crucially important, because they may powerfully predict an individual's capacity to manage their diabetes and maintain long-term health and well-being (Rubin 2000). The most common decision may be about achieving a level of glycaemic control that prevents long-term complications against risking hypoglycaemia.

Box 5.10

Quality of life with diabetes mellitus: Mr P's experience

I have been an insulin-dependent diabetic for about 35 years, on two injections a day.

Over these years I have had a number of really bad 'hypos'. Some of them, my wife was able to bring me out of with the help of glucose drinks, chocolate or Dextrosol tablets. Other times, when I was saturated in sweat, and not able to respond in any way, and therefore appeared to be unconscious, only then would a doctor be called. This was usually in the night, and then 8 out of 10, an ambulance would be called, which was very alarming, for myself and also for my wife who felt unable to help me in those situations.

I had always regularly attended the hospital diabetic clinic, where the normal required checks would be carried out. However, a few months ago through the clinic I was offered the chance to go onto a different type of insulin given by using the pen system. I now give myself an injection of two different kinds before breakfast, then another before lunch, and another before tea.

The purpose of the changeover from pork insulin to synthetic human insulin, i.e. NovoRapid and glargine, was to try and eliminate high and low sugar readings in my numerous daily tests that I do, and to get them on a much more balanced level.

I have still had a number of episodes where my sugar level has become very low, when I have had to eat something sweet to push my blood sugar level up again. On the whole, the changeover is working out a lot better than before, and it just means minor adjustments to the amounts I give myself each day until I get it right. Since the changeover, I have been in contact with a specialist diabetic nurse and have spoken to her quite a number of times when I have had any queries. She also contacts me regularly just to see how things are, which I find very reassuring. I have always tried to lead a normal life, and to keep my diabetes under tight control, and to keep myself as fit as possible and my weight steady, as I know how important these factors are in keeping me as healthy as possible.

Some people will risk long-term complications in order to avoid hypoglycaemia. An example might be:

> *I'd rather not live so long, rather than live the way you have to live in order to keep the blood sugars low …*

Emotional well-being and depression

Emotional well-being correlates positively with optimal self-care practices (Rose et al 2002). In particular, high self-esteem relates positively to self-care; depression and/or anxiety relate negatively to self-management. The incidence of depression and anxiety, affecting one in five people with diabetes, is much higher than in the general population. Although the aetiology is unclear, it is probably related to the daily demands of self-care practices, the physiological effects of blood glucose changes, including hyper- and hypoglycaemia, and to the disease process with its long-term complications (Lloyd & Brown 2002). Depression is considered to have such a significant impact on the person with diabetes and their self-management abilities that regular annual screening for depression is recommended for all people with diabetes (SIGN 2001).

Education and behaviour change

The compliance model of diabetes education

Traditionally, diabetes education was delivered using what is described as the 'compliance model'. In this approach, health care professionals (HCPs) teach patients knowledge and skills, and set targets for them to achieve, based on the evidence available, in order to prolong a physically healthy life. When glycaemic control is not achieved, the HCP uses their expertise to diagnose the problem and to instruct the patient on the best course of action. People with diabetes are expected to follow the HCP's advice.

The empowerment model

Since the early 1990s, an alternative model of educational care has been advocated. The empowerment model (Funnell et al 1991) acknowledges the patient's expertise, their personal responsibility in self-management and their right to informed choice in treatment. It acknowledges the importance of both quality and quantity of life, taking into account the many determinants of behaviour that exist.

The concept of empowerment in diabetes 'emerged out of the realisation that patients cannot be forced to follow a lifestyle dictated by health care professionals' (Feste 1992).

More recently, the idea of the empowered patient has been supported in the National Service Framework for England and Wales (DH 2001) and in health policy for Scotland (Scottish Executive Health Department 2002).

The key to facilitating self-empowerment is in the nature of communication between the nurse and the person with diabetes (Brown 1997).

- An open questioning style will help the person with diabetes to decide what they want to change (*'What do you find most difficult about your diabetes?'*).
- Exploring thoughts and feelings around the chosen issue (*'What is that like for you? … How do you feel about that? … What are your thoughts about the situation? … How would this have to change for you to feel better about it?'*).
- Inviting commitment to that behavioural change. Working together to develop a plan to implement the change, taking into account the costs and benefits and the obstacles and support that might be experienced (*'Are you willing to take action to improve the situation for yourself? ... What steps could you take to bring you closer to where you want to be?'*) (Anderson & Funnell 2002).

The planned behaviour change should be evaluated so that options can be considered if the initial plan is unsuccessful.

For further reading on psychology in diabetes care, see Snoek & Skinner (2000).

Relationships

Family relationships

If the family unit was previously stable, diabetes is unlikely to have an adverse effect on family relationships. Indeed, patients who enjoy good support from their families show enhanced stability and are more likely to adopt recommended health maintenance behaviours (Maclean & Lo 1998).

However, the very nature of diabetes, with its attendant rules and restrictions, may allow the disorder to be used by family members or the patient as a means of manipulation or self-assertion. This is more likely to occur where family relationships were difficult prior to the diagnosis of diabetes (Laffel et al 2003).

Sexual relationships

Although embarking on a sexual relationship is anxiety-provoking for many people, it raises particular concerns for people with diabetes. Uncertainty may be felt about when, and if, to tell the other person about the diabetes. Practical issues such as what to do if a 'hypo' develops when out on a date or, even worse, during lovemaking, may cause real worry. Having to explain such things as set eating and injection times or dietary restrictions may cause embarrassment and may be seen as interfering with the spontaneity of a budding relationship. The mere presence of diabetes can affect the quality and quantity of a patient's relationships (Polonsky 2000).

Family planning

Information on pregnancy and contraception should be made available to all women with diabetes who are of child-bearing age. There are no contraceptive methods specifically contraindicated in women with diabetes. However, methods with a proven high degree of effectiveness are preferred, as unplanned pregnancy can lead to serious risks for the mother and baby. Low dose oestrogen preparations of the combined oral contraceptive group are safe for the majority of women. The presence of diabetes complications and other risk factors should be considered when deciding on the type of oral contraceptive pill, and progesterone only preparations may be more appropriate in women with these factors. It is important, with oral contraceptives, to monitor blood glucose levels regularly as some of these drugs can cause fluctuations in glycaemic control (Williams & Pickup 1999).

A healthy pregnancy and happy outcome is possible if excellent glycaemic control is achieved before and during pregnancy. Prospective parents may worry about passing on their diabetes to the baby and genetic counselling may be offered to enable the couple to make an informed decision (see Ch. 6). If the woman has severe complications of diabetes, the couple may be advised against pregnancy as it could lead to a worsening of her condition and put her at greater risk of illness during her pregnancy.

For a discussion of genetic and other pregnancy-associated risks, see Parker (1996).

Pre-conception Ideally the couple should attend for pre-conception counselling to help reduce the risks to mother and baby. Strict control of blood glucose before conception greatly helps towards improving the outcome of the pregnancy. Once pregnant, the woman's progress should be monitored on a regular basis by a specialist team, consisting of diabetes specialist nurses and midwives, diabetologists, obstetricians and dietitians.

For further information on diabetes and pregnancy, see Moshe (2003).

Gestational diabetes Gestational diabetes (GDM) is glucose intolerance, which presents or is first recognised during pregnancy and a diagnosis of GDM identifies the woman as at risk of developing type 2 diabetes in the future (SIGN 2001).

The Scottish Intercollegiate Network (SIGN 2001) details the management of both existing and gestational diabetes.

Social relationships

Patients with diabetes quite naturally resist being singled out and labelled. This can create real difficulties. On the one hand, coping with diabetes means that the individual may have to rely on others should a crisis occur. On the other hand, the person with diabetes may resent being treated differently from others. The patient's adjustment within their social milieu will involve a complex interplay of personal and social factors; the degree of success will vary considerably from person to person.

Access to counselling should be provided for those people who are experiencing relationship difficulties arising from their diabetes.

STOP THINK **5.14** What do you understand by the term 'labelling'? Why do you think people with diabetes may be concerned about being labelled?

Lifestyle implications

Employment

In view of the risk of hypoglycaemia, people with diabetes who are treated with insulin are excluded from some areas of employment, e.g. those which involve certain categories of vocational driving (see below for driving regulations), airline piloting and air traffic control, deep sea diving, working on offshore oil rigs, working at the coal face, at heights or near dangerous moving machinery. Diabetes would also exclude an applicant from joining the UK armed forces or the police. However, in many cases, if diabetes develops while in the job, it is sometimes possible to continue employment.

For further information, contact Diabetes UK (see 'Useful websites', p. 227).

Driving

The UK Driver Vehicle Licensing Authority (DVLA) must, by law, be informed when a driver is diagnosed as having diabetes mellitus and is receiving treatment with insulin or oral antidiabetic medication. Those who are treated with insulin will be issued with a licence for a period of 1–3 years to allow periodic review by the DVLA. A medical practitioner may be required to advise on the stability of the driver's diabetes control prior to re-licensing. The DVLA must be informed if any problems or diabetic complications develop which may affect safety.

A person holding a Large Goods Vehicle (LGV) and/or a Passenger Carrying Vehicle (PCV) licence will have their licence removed when they commence insulin therapy. There are also restrictions on lighter goods and smaller passenger vehicle licences.

For further information, contact the DVLA at www.dvla.gov.uk.

Box 5.11

Diabetes UK

Diabetes UK (formerly the British Diabetic Association) is a charitable organisation which raises money for diabetes research and provides information and advice for people with diabetes and professionals involved in their care. As well as being a national organisation, it has local branches throughout the UK. Different sections cater for particular groups, e.g. teenagers. Diabetes UK offers help and advice on a wide variety of topics such as monitoring and treatment approaches, insurance, holidays and travelling abroad.

Full members of Diabetes UK receive the bi-monthly journal *Balance* free of charge. This is an excellent publication which provides a forum for people with diabetes and their families to exchange ideas and keep up to date with current progress in diabetes management. *Balance* is also produced on audiotape for visually impaired subscribers.

Hypoglycaemia is the main danger when driving. People with diabetes should receive education regarding how to avoid and effectively manage hypoglycaemia when driving.

Car insurance

Patients whose diabetes is treated with medication must inform their insurer. Failure to notify the insurer can invalidate any claim. Diabetes UK have their own insurance broker who can advise on any insurance-related matter (see Box 5.11).

Travel

Altered mealtimes, travelling across different time zones, and dietary and climatic changes may all have an effect on diabetes stability. It is therefore essential for the person with diabetes to monitor their diabetes closely whilst travelling. Travellers with diabetes should seek specific advice from their GP or the diabetes team regarding insulin adjustment. All medication and monitoring equipment should be carried in hand luggage to allow for ready access and to reduce risk of loss. Also, the extremely low temperature of the hold can adversely effect the action of insulin.

Most airlines now require the traveller to carry a letter from a medical practitioner detailing the need to carry syringes, pen needles and blood glucose monitoring equipment in their hand luggage.

For further information on travel, see www.diabetes-travel.uk or contact Diabetes UK (see 'Useful websites', p. 227).

Eating out

Flexible insulin regimens, insulin pen devices and home blood glucose monitoring (HBGM) have simplified eating out for people with diabetes. People on insulin therapy are advised as to appropriate insulin adjustment to allow more freedom of choice when dining out.

Smoking

People with diabetes are at greater risk than others of developing vascular and neuropathic disorders. Smoking compounds these risks. The health care team should encourage smoking cessation and should discuss the availability of resources to provide support whilst the patient is trying to give up smoking (Haire-Joshu et al 2003). However, it must be accepted that the patient has freedom of choice and may decide to continue to smoke against advice.

Identification

Patients should be strongly advised to carry a card or wear a MedicAlert pendant or bracelet to identify themselves and to give details of the type of diabetes they have and its management.

FUTURE DEVELOPMENTS

Research in diabetes care is at an exciting stage. Combined kidney and pancreas transplants are now undertaken in a number of centres in the UK for those in renal failure as a complication of type 1 diabetes. Successful transplantation allows the patient to be free of the restrictions of renal dialysis as well as daily injections of insulin. Five years after transplantation, 60% of patients remain well without needing insulin injections (Watkins 2003).

Islet cell transplantation offers people with type 1 diabetes hope for a cure. This process is the subject of intensive research trials (Swift & White 2003). Islet cells are isolated from the donor pancreas and injected into the liver of the recipient. In the liver, the cells develop a blood supply and begin to produce insulin, a process called the Edmonton protocol. At Diabetes UK's Spring 2003 National Conference, James Shapiro, the surgeon taking the procedure forward, reported that 50 patients in the UK had received islet cell transplants and, of these, 85% were insulin independent within a year. This figure fell to 70% in 2 years. New combinations of immunosuppressive agents prevent the body rejecting the transplanted islet cells, thus eliminating the need for steroid therapy which could damage the newly transplanted cells. The major drawback to the increasing availability of this advance is that the equivalent of two donated pancreas is required to provide sufficient islet cells for transplantation.

For further information, see Diabetes UK (see 'Useful websites', p. 227).

Over the years, feasibility studies into the effectiveness of non-enteral routes of delivering insulin have been attempted. These have included ocular, buccal, rectal, vaginal, oral, nasal and uterine delivery systems. However, a growing body of evidence suggests that inhaled insulin is an effective, well-tolerated, non-invasive alternative to s.c. soluble insulin for patients with type 2 diabetes (Cefalu 2003).

It is increasingly recognised that diabetes is not merely a disease of a single hormone (insulin) but that the absence of multiple pancreatic hormones is implicated. C-peptide, traditionally thought to be biologically inert, has been shown to have an effect on appetite and reducing hypoglycaemia. Various other pancreatic hormones including GLIP-1 and Exendin-4 have been synthesised and shown to be effective in treating type 2 diabetes soon after failure of oral therapy (Edwards et al 2001). These hormones have some benefit in type 1 diabetes and the value outweighs the cost of added injections (Idris & Donnelly 2003).

The ultimate hope is that diabetes will at some future date be preventable. Researchers continue to seek definitive answers to the questions surrounding aetiological factors, with a view to finding ways of manipulating these factors to prevent the disease developing.

Trends in health care provision

The political and economic climate in the UK over the past two decades has given rise to significant changes in the structure and function of the primary care team and has shifted the focus of health care toward the community setting. Emphasis has been on developing further the role of the diabetes specialist nurse who 'can transform the standard of diabetic care, achieving liaison between hospital, general practitioner and patients at home and offering a wide range of clinical and educational expertise' (Watkins et al 2003).

The growth in the number of practice nurses has made it possible for many GPs to run their own clinics for diabetic patients. In some areas, community dietitians and podiatrists are available for consultation in the health centres where clinics are run.

Community nurses and health visitors may find themselves, to an increasing extent, taking high-quality diabetes care directly into the patient's home. Effective hospital–community liaison will become especially important to ensure continuity for the patient in 'shared care'.

Whatever the care setting, it is important that the patient has access to facilities for estimation of glycated haemoglobin and microalbuminuria and for screening for retinopathy and foot-threatening neuropathic or vascular disease. It seems likely that integrated hospital and community care will offer the best use of resources for diabetes screening. However, dealing with a severe metabolic crisis such as DKA will remain the province of the hospital.

Continuing education for all members of the diabetes care team must be a priority. National standards and guidelines such as the National Service Framework (DH 2001) and Scottish Intercollegiate Guidelines Network (SIGN 2001) are necessary to create best practice through a firm research base and to support provision of the highest possible quality of care for people with diabetes. Diabetes specialist nurses and community diabetes facilitators can make a significant contribution in the education of their colleagues. Providing the education and support which will enable the patient to move away from the despondency and fear which frequently accompany diagnosis, towards independence and autonomy, is surely both the science and the art of nursing care in diabetes mellitus.

REFERENCES

Allwinkle J 2002 Blood glucose monitoring for visually impaired people with diabetes. The Journal of Diabetes Nursing 6(5): 157–159

Anderson R M, Funnell M M 2002 Using the empowerment approach to help patients change behaviour. In: Anderson B J, Rubin R R (eds) Practical psychology for diabetes clinicians. American Diabetes Association, Alexandria, VA

Armstrong D G, Lavery L A 1998 Evidence based options for off-loading diabetic wounds. Clinics in Podiatric Medicine and Surgery 15: 95–100

Avery J 2003 NICE guidelines on the use of patient education models [editorial]. Journal of Diabetes Nursing 7(7): 258

Bandura A 1977 Self-efficacy: towards a unifying theory of behaviour change. Psychological Review 84: 191–215

Becker M H, Janz N K 1985 The health belief model applied to understanding diabetes regimen compliance. The Diabetes Educator 11(1): 41–47

Bell D S H, Ovalle F 1999 Stroke management in the diabetic patient. Journal of Critical Illness 14: 309–318

Bradley C, Brewin C R, Gamsu D S et al 1984 Development of scales to measure perceived control of diabetes mellitus and diabetes-related health beliefs. Diabetic Medicine 1: 213–218

British Diabetic Association 1995 Diabetes in the United Kingdom 1995. BDA, London

British Diabetic Association 1996 Counting the cost: the real impact of non insulin dependent diabetes. BDA/King's Fund, London

British Diabetic Association 1997 Two more diabetes genes identified. Diabetes Update Spring: 1–3

Brown F 1997 Patient empowerment through education. Professional Nurse Study Supplement 13(3): S4–S6

Brown F J 2001 Personal empowerment in adults with type 1 diabetes: a phenomenological study. MPhil Thesis (unpublished). University of Strathclyde, Glasgow

Brown F 2003 Progressing the relationship with patients: an overview. Journal of Diabetes Nursing 7(2)

Burge M R, Sood V, Sobhy T A et al 1999 Sulphonylurea induced hypoglycaemia in type 2 diabetes mellitus: a review. Diabetes, Obesity and Metabolism 1(4): 199

Burr B, Dinesh N 1999 Exercise and sport in diabetes. Wiley, Chichester

Carson C 2000 Working collaboratively to provide diabetes care for adolescents. Diabetes and Primary Care 2(2)

Cefalu W T 2003 Novel routes of delivery for patients with type 1 or type 2 diabetes. Annals of Medicine 33(9): 579–586

Clinical Standards Advisory Group 1994 Standards of clinical care for people with diabetes. HMSO, London

Cooper M E 1998 Pathogenesis, prevention and treatment of diabetic nephropathy. Lancet 352: 213–219

Craddock S 1996 Diabetes mellitus at diagnosis. Nursing Standard 10(30): 41–48

DAFNE Study Group 2002 Training in flexible, intensive insulin management to enable dietary freedom in people with type 1 diabetes: dose adjustment for normal eating (DAFNE) randomised controlled trial. British Medical Journal 325: 746–749

Dave J, Chatterjee S, Davies M et al 2004 Evaluation of admissions and management of diabetic ketoacidosis in a large teaching hospital. Practical Diabetes International 21(4): 149–153

Department of Health 1996 Hazard warning, June 1996. Safety Notice MDA SN 9616. Extra-laboratory use of blood glucose meters and test strips: contra-indications, training and advice to users. DH, London

Department of Health 2001 National Service Framework for diabetes: standards. DH, London

Department of Health/British Diabetic Association 1995 St Vincent Joint Task Force for Diabetes: the Report. DH/BDA, London

Diabetes Control and Complications Research Group 1993 The effect of diabetes on the development and progression of long term complications in insulin dependent diabetes. New England Journal of Medicine 329: 977–986

Diabetes UK 2003a News. Diabetes Update Autumn: 7

Diabetes UK 2003b Current nutritional standards. Diabetic Medicine 20: 886–887

Dyson P 2004 Diet and diabetes – the new recommendations. Journal of Diabetes Nursing 8(4): 127–131

Edmonds M, Wilson S, Foster A 1999 Diabetic foot ulcers. Nursing Standard 14(12): 39–45

Edwards C M, Stanley S A, Davis R et al 2001 Exendin-4 reduces fasting and postprandial glucose and decreases energy intake in healthy volunteers. American Journal of Physiology, Endocrinology and Metabolism 281(1): 155–161

EURODIAB IDDM 1994 Complications study: microvascular and acute complications in IDDM patients. Diabetologia 37: 278–285

Everett J, Kerr D 1998 A picture of the impact of newly diagnosed type 2 diabetes. Journal of Diabetes Nursing 2(6): 170–175

Everett J, Kerr D 2001 Measuring quality of life in diabetes. Journal of Diabetes Nursing 5(2): 53–55
Feste C 1992 A practical look at patient empowerment. Diabetes Care 15(7): 922–925
Frier B M, Fisher M 1999 Hypoglycaemia in clinical diabetes. Wiley, Chichester
Funnell M M, Anderson R M, Arnold M S et al 1991 Empowerment: an idea whose time has come to diabetes education. The Diabetes Educator 17: 37–41
Grasty M S 1999 Use of the hand-held Doppler to detect peripheral vascular disease. The Diabetic Foot 2(1)(Suppl)
Griggs K 1998 Global contender. Nursing Times 94(22): 65–66
Haire-Joshu D, Glasgow R E, Tubbs T L 2003 Smoking and diabetes. Diabetes Care 26: s89–90
Hamilton H, Ubig M 1991 The eye in diabetes. The Practitioner (symposium) 235: 780–782
Hanson L, Zanchetti A, Carruthers S G et al 1998 Effects of intensive blood pressure lowering and low-dose aspirin in patients with hypertension: principal results of the Hypertension Optimal Treatment (HOT) randomized trial. HOT Study Group. Lancet 351: 1755–1762
Heath H, Schofield I 1999 Healthy ageing: nursing older people. Mosby, London
HOPE (Heart Outcomes Prevention study) 2000 Effects of ramipril on cardiovascular and microvascular outcomes in people with diabetes mellitus. Results of the HOPE study and MICRO-HOPE sub-study. Lancet 355: 253–259
Idris I, Donnelly R 2003 Analogues of GLP-1 and exendin. New therapeutics developments in type 2 diabetes. Modern Diabetes Management 4: 13–16
Jacobson A 1996 The psychological care of patients with insulin-dependent diabetes mellitus. New England Journal of Medicine 33(19): 1249–1254
Kirby M 2003 Lipid management in people with diabetes. Diabetes and Primary Care 5(4): 152–157
Kovacs M, Goldston D, Obrosky S D et al 1995 Psychiatric disorders in youths with IDDM: rates and risk factors. Diabetes Care 20(1): 36–44
Krans H M J, Porta N, Keen H (eds) 1992 Diabetes care and research in Europe. The St Vincent Declaration action programme. World Health Organization Regional Office for Europe, Copenhagen
Laffel L M B, Connell A, Vangsness L et al 2003 General quality of life in youth with type 1 diabetes. Diabetes Care 26: 3067–3073
Lebovitz H E 1995 Diabetic ketoacidosis. Lancet 345(8952): 767–772
Ley P 1997 Communication with patients: improving communication, satisfaction and compliance. Croom Helm, London, Ch. 2
Livneh H, Antonak R F 1994 Psychosocial reactions to disability: a review and critique of the literature. Critical Reviews in Physical and Rehabilitation Medicine 6(1): 1–100
Lloyd C, Brown F 2002 Depression and diabetes. Current Women's Health Reports 2: 188–193
MacAuley V, Deary I J, Frier B M 2001 Symptoms of hypoglycaemia in people with diabetes. Diabetic Medicine 18(9): 690–705
MacKinnon M 2002 Providing diabetes care in general practice, 4th edn. Class Publishing, London
Maclean D, Lo R 1998 The non-insulin-dependent diabetic: success and failure in compliance. Australian Journal of Advanced Nursing 15(4): 33–42
Malmberg K 1997 Prospective randomised study of intensive insulin treatment and long term survival after an acute myocardial infarction of patients with diabetes mellitus. DIGAMI (Diabetes Mellitus, Insulin Glucose Infusion and Acute Myocardial Infarction) Study Group. British Medical Journal 314: 1512–1515
McHoy A 2003 The clinical management of diabetic ketoacidosis in adults. Journal of Diabetes Nursing 7(9): 332–336
Mills L S 2003 Erectile dysfunction: assessment and treatment in diabetes. Journal of Diabetes Nursing 7(4): 146–149
Molitch M E 1997 Management of early diabetic nephropathy. American Journal of Medicine 102: 392–398
Mrugeshkumar S 2004 Charcot arthropathy. Online. Available: www.eMedicine.com
National Institute for Clinical Excellence (NICE) 2002 Management of type 2 diabetes retinopathy – early management and screening (Guideline E). NICE, London
National Institute for Clinical Excellence (NICE) 2003 Guidance on the use of patient education models for diabetes. Technology appraisal 60. NICE, London
Owens D R, Zinman B, Bolli G B 2001 Insulins today and beyond. Lancet 358: 34
Peyrot M, Rubin R R 1994 Structures and correlates of diabetes-specific locus of control. Diabetes Care 17(9): 994–1001
Polonsky W H 2000 Understanding and assessing diabetes – specific quality of life. Diabetes Spectrum 13(1): 36
Richmond J 1996 Effects of hypoglycaemia: patients' perceptions and experiences. British Journal of Nursing 5(17): 1054–1059
Rose M, Fliege H, Hildebrandt M et al 2002 The network of psychological variables in patients with diabetes and their importance for quality of life and metabolic control. Diabetes Care 25(1): 35–42
Rotter B 1966 Generalised expectancies for internal versus external control of reinforcement. Psychological Monographs 80: 1–28
Rubin R R 2000 Diabetes and quality of life. Diabetes Spectrum 13(1): 21
Scottish Executive Health Department 2002 Scottish diabetes framework. Scottish Executive, Edinburgh
Scottish Intercollegiate Guidelines Network (SIGN) 1996 Management of obesity. A national clinical guideline. SIGN, Edinburgh
Scottish Intercollegiate Guidelines Network (SIGN) 2001 Management of diabetes. A national clinical guideline. SIGN, Edinburgh
Scriven A, Orme J 2001 Health promotion: the empowerment imperative. In: Health promotion: professional perspectives, 2nd edn. Open University, Milton Keynes, p 10–11
Segal-Isaacson C J, Carello E, Wylie-Rosett J 2001 Dietary fats and diabetes mellitus: is there a good fat? Current Diabetes Reports 1(2)
Stevens R J, Coleman R L, Adler A I et al 2004 Risk factors for myocardial infarction: case fatality and stroke case fatality in type 2 diabetes. Diabetes Care 27(1): 210–206
Swift S, White S 2003 Could islet transplantation be a potential cure for diabetes? Nursing Times 99(15) (Diabetes Supplement)
United Kingdom Prospective Diabetes Study Group 1998a Intensive blood glucose control with sulphonylureas or insulin compared with conventional treatment and risk of complications in patients with type 2 diabetes (UKPDS 33). Lancet 352(9131): 837–853
United Kingdom Prospective Diabetes Study Group 1998b Tight blood pressure control and risk of macrovascular and microvascular complications in type 2 diabetes (UKPDS 38). British Medical Journal 317: 703–713
Vowden P 1999 Doppler ultrasound in the management of the diabetic foot. The Diabetic Foot 2(1)(Suppl)
Wallston B S, Wallston K A, Kaplan G D et al 1976 Development and validation of the health locus of control (HLC) scale. Journal of Consulting and Clinical Psychology 44: 580–585
Watkins P J 2003 ABC of diabetes, 5th edn. BMJ Publishing, London
Watkins P J, Amiel S A, Howell S L 2003 Diabetes and its management, 6th edn. Blackwell Publishing, Oxford
Wei M, Gaskill S P, Haffner S M, Stern M P 1997 Waist circumference as the best predictor of non-insulin dependent diabetes mellitus (NIDDM) compared to body mass index, waist/hip ratio and other anthropometric measurements in Mexican Americans: a 7 year prospective study. Obesity Research 5(1): 16–23
Williams G, Pickup J C 1999 Handbook of diabetes, 2nd edn. Blackwell Science, Oxford
Williams J 2003 Overview of the care of pregnant women with pre-existing diabetes. Journal of Diabetes Nursing 7(1): 12–15
World Health Organization 1999 Definition, diagnosis and classification of diabetes mellitus and its complications. Report of a WHO Consultation. WHO, Geneva
Yates I, Fox M, Crewdson M, Woodyer A B 2003 Larvae – a key member of the multidisciplinary foot team? – Larval therapy. The Diabetic Foot 6(4): 166, 168, 170–171
Yki-Jarvinen H, Dressler A, Ziemen M 2000 Less nocturnal hypoglycaemia and better post-dinner glucose control with bedtime insulin glargine compared with bedtime NPH insulin during insulin combination therapy in type 2 diabetes. HOE 901/3002 Study Group. Diabetes Care 23: 1130–1136

FURTHER READING

Alexander W D 2003 Treatment of erectile dysfunction in men with diabetes. Diabetes and Primary Care 5(2): 64–69

Angel A, Dahalla N, Peirce G et al 2001 Diabetes and cardiovascular disease. Kluwer, Amsterdam

Batki A, Garvey K, Thomason H et al 1998 Blood glucose measuring systems. Professional Nurse 13(12): 865–873

Bilous R 2002 HOPE and other recent trials of antihypertensive therapy in type 2 diabetes. In: Amiel S (ed) Horizons in medicine. Royal College of Physicians, London

British National Formulary. Online. Available: www.bnf.org

Diabetes UK 2003a The implementation of nutritional advice for people with diabetes. Diabetic Medicine 20: 786–807

Diabetes UK 2003b Insulin pens available in the UK. Balance July–August: 39–41

Diabetes UK 2004 Recommendations for the management of pregnant women including gestational diabetes. Diabetes UK, London

Edmonds M E, Foster A V M 2000 Managing the diabetic foot. Blackwell Science, Oxford

Fisher M 2003 Heart disease and diabetes. Martin Dunitz, London

Frier B M, Fisher M 1999 Hypoglycaemia in clinical diabetes. Wiley, Chichester

Greenstein B, Gould D 2004 Trounce's clinical pharmacology for nurses, 17th edn. Churchill Livingstone, Edinburgh

Gries F A, Cameron N E, Low P A et al 2003 Textbook of diabetic neuropathy. Thieme, Stuttgart

Hasslacher C 2001 Diabetic nephropathy. Wiley, Chichester

MacKinnon M 2002 Providing diabetes care in general practice, 4th edn. Class Publishing, London

McConville D, Buchanan J, Lee B 2003 Infection control in diabetic foot disease. The Diabetic Foot

Moshe H 2003 Textbook of diabetes and pregnancy. Taylor and Francis, London

Parker C 1996 Pre-pregnancy monitoring for women with diabetes. Professional Care of Mother and Child 6(5): 135–138

Royal College of General Practitioners (RCGP) 2000 Clinical guidelines for type 2 diabetes. Prevention and management of foot problems. RCGP, London

Selby P L, Young M J, Boulton A J 1994 Bisphosphonates: a new treatment for diabetic Charcot neuroarthropathy? Diabetic Medicine 38(1): 34–40

Snoek F J, Skinner T C 2000 Psychology in diabetes care. Wiley, Chichester

Tortora G J, Derrickson B 2006 Principles of anatomy and physiology, 11th edn. John Wiley & Sons Inc., New York

United Kingdom Prospective Diabetes Study (UKPDS) 1998 (Original publications in British Medical Journal and Lancet)

Williams G, Pickup J C 1997 Textbook of diabetes, 2nd edn. Blackwell Science, Oxford

Williams R, Wareham N, Kinmonth A M et al 2001 Evidence base for diabetes care. Wiley, Chichester

ADDITIONAL RESOURCES AND USEFUL ADDRESSES

Sources of information

General Practitioner Information Pack
Directory of Diabetes Specialist Nurses

Both available free of charge to health care professionals from:

Diabetes UK
www.diabetes.org.uk

Diabetes in General Practice — clinical series

Royal College of General Practitioners
www.rcgp.org.uk

The Diabetes Handbook: Non-insulin Dependent Diabetes, and Insulin Dependent Diabetes

Both by Dr John L Day, available from Diabetes UK (www.diabetes.org.uk)

USEFUL WEBSITES

Sources of educational material

Abbott Diabetes Care (Abbott Laboratories)
www.diabetesnow.co.uk

Diabetes UK
www.diabetes.org.uk

Diabetes journals
www.diabetesjournals.com

Royal National Institute of the Blind (RNIB)
www.rnib.org.uk

Measurement of insulin and injection technique
Becton Dickinson (UK) Ltd
bdukcustomerservice@europe.db.com

Insulin and mode of action
Aventis Pharma UK
www.aventis.co.uk

Eli Lilly & Co Ltd
www.lilly.co.uk

Novo Nordisk Pharmaceuticals Ltd
www.novonordisk.co.uk

Blood and urine glucose monitoring

Bayer plc
www.bayerdiag.com

Lifescan UK
www.lifescan.co.uk

Roche Diagnostics Ltd
www.roche.com

Clinical Standards Board for Scotland
www.show.scot.nhs.uk/crag/topics/csbs/csbsmain.htm

National Service Framework for Diabetes
www.dh.gov.uk/PolicyAndGuidance/HealthAndSocialCareTopics/Diabetes/fs/en

Scottish Intercollegiate Guidelines Network (SIGN)
www.sign.ac.uk

GENETIC DISORDERS

Kathleen MacDonald
Susan Hook
Yvonne Robb
South East Scotland Genetic Counsellors
Scottish Huntington's Advisory Team

6

INTRODUCTION

Genetics is the study of genes and their relationship to hereditary characteristics. Genes are units of deoxyribonucleic acid (DNA) found in the chromosomes within the nuclei of living cells. They carry coded information that influences physical and psychological characteristics and susceptibility to many major life-threatening diseases.

This chapter provides a basic outline of the mechanics of genetic inheritance, raises awareness of the genetic aspects of common diseases and outlines nursing roles in genetic counselling. A small number of classic but rare genetic conditions are described and the principles of cancer genetics are introduced.

Our genes play a fundamental role in determining our health. Greater knowledge of genetics has had, and will continue to have, a major impact on the understanding of human illness, disease prevention, diagnosis and treatment. It is estimated that 6 out of 10 people by the age of 60 will develop a disease which is at least partially genetically determined (DH 2003). The wide range of genetic influences in health and disease will mean that nurses in most areas of practice will require an understanding of genetics and the ability to apply this to practice. As our understanding of the genetic predisposition to common diseases, such as cancer, heart disease, diabetes mellitus and asthma increases, genetics becomes an integral part of many nursing roles. The combination of environmental and genetic factors will determine whether a predisposition manifests in actual disease. Increasing public awareness of the environmental factors may help people avoid some of the consequences of their genetic makeup.

Within the specialised field of genetics, there is the more focused role of the specialist nurse, who is involved in non-directive counselling, diagnosis, testing and support of individuals and families with genetic conditions (Skirton et al 1997).

THE MECHANICS OF GENETIC INHERITANCE

Chromosomes

Each human cell contains 46 chromosomes within the nucleus, with the exception of the gametes (ova and spermatozoa), which contain 23 chromosomes. Of the 46 chromosomes, 23 come from one parent and 23 from the other. These chromosomes are paired, giving 22 pairs called autosomes 1–22 and one pair of sex chromosomes, either XX for females or XY for males.

By staining, photographing and arranging according to size, the chromosomes extracted from a cell can be organised into a karyotype. A normal female karyotype would be reported as 46, XX and a normal male karyotype as 46, XY (see Fig. 6.1). Chromosomal abnormalities can be identified by this method.

Cell division

To understand the mechanisms of genetic inheritance, it is necessary to be familiar with the basic processes of cell division, i.e. mitosis and meiosis.

Mitosis

is the normal process of cell division for growth and replacement of cells. The genetic information in one parent

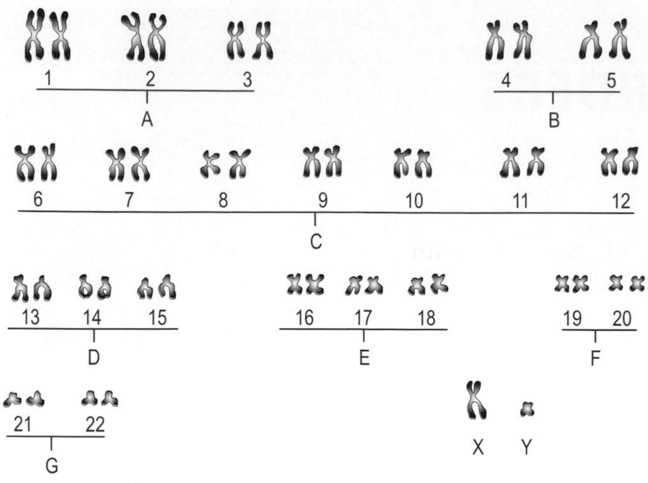

Fig. 6.1 Karyotype of a normal male.

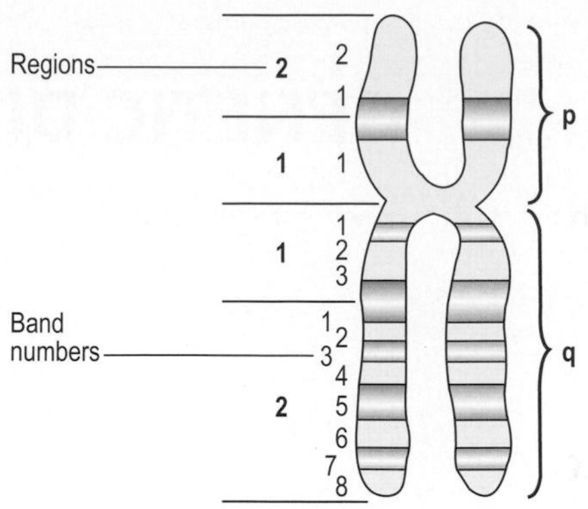

Fig. 6.2 The X chromosome: regions and bands. Each chromosome has a narrow waist called the centromere and a long and a short arm. The short arm is labelled p (from the French petit) and the long arm is labelled q. The tip of each arm is called a telomere. Chromosomes can be divided for reporting purposes into numbered chromosome regions, with region 1 closest to the centromere. Each region is further divided into bands.

cell replicates and divides to produce two daughter cells, each with 46 chromosomes carrying the identical genetic information.

Meiosis

is the process of cell division, which results in the production of gametes, ova or spermatozoa. Unlike mitosis, the four resulting cells have only one copy of each chromosome pair (23 chromosomes). New pairings are established when the ova and spermatozoa come together at fertilisation, re-establishing the full chromosome complement of 23 pairs (46 chromosomes). Within this process, rearrangement of chromosomal material results in the individual differences seen in offspring, whilst familial genetic patterns are still maintained. If meiosis is not successful, one gamete may end up with abnormal chromosomes or an incorrect number of chromosomes. The results of this are seen in the classic chromosome conditions. An example is Down's syndrome (trisomy 21) where the individual has 47 chromosomes, with three copies of chromosome 21. Chromosomal abnormalities often lead to miscarriage, usually early in pregnancy. However, some pregnancies may result in the birth of an affected child.

DNA and RNA

In 1944, chromosomal nucleic acid was shown to be the carrier of genetic information. Two types are recognised: DNA (deoxyribonucleic acid) and RNA (ribonucleic acid).

A molecule of DNA is composed of two nucleotide chains spiralled round one another to form a double helix. Genes are carried in this DNA.

Genes

Genes are units of DNA, consisting of coded hereditary information and are carried on the chromosomes. As chromosomes are paired, each pair carries two copies of each gene (with the exception of the genes on sex chromosomes in males). Each gene is located at a specific point on a chromosome known as its locus. Chromosomes can, for identification purposes, be divided into numbered chromosome regions and bands so that, if known, their position can be charted (see Fig. 6.2). Genes at the same locus on chromosomes are called alleles. If the two alleles at a locus are identical, the individual is said to be homozygous at that locus and if they are non-identical, the individual is said to be heterozygous.

With the exception of identical twins, each individual carries unique sequences or patterns of DNA. These genetic patterns can be recorded by a technique known as DNA fingerprinting and can identify individuals, as for example in forensic medicine or paternity testing (see Box 6.1).

There are at least two kinds of genes: structural genes, which specify protein synthesis, and genes that act as 'switches' to activate or deactivate structural genes and maintain homeostasis.

The coded information contained in the structural genes is translated with the help of RNA into specific proteins. The RNA becomes a mobile copy of the corresponding encoded blueprint in the DNA (messenger RNA, or mRNA).

Box 6.1

DNA fingerprinting

Paternity testing has been revolutionised by the technique known as DNA fingerprinting. Throughout the human genome, there are repeats of short sequences (tandem repeats) called minisatellite DNA. They have no known function but are valuable tools for genetic analysis. After DNA digestion with a restriction enzyme and electrophoresis, a DNA minisatellite probe will identify multiple DNA fragments from many chromosomal regions. The number and size of these fragments are unique to each individual, except for identical twins. In other words, one can generate a unique genetic fingerprint specific only to that individual. Each band is inherited from one parent and therefore a putative father can be either excluded or positively identified. DNA can be extracted from dried bloodstains or semen; for this reason this technique has had important implications for forensic medicine.

Some of these proteins are enzymes that catalyse specific chemical reactions. Others form part of the structure of body cells and tissues. Molecular biology has been able to describe the process of enzyme movement and matching of chemical bases along the coding strand of the DNA double helix, which is involved in translating genetic codes into mRNA for protein synthesis.

For information on genes and genetic inheritance, see Skirton & Patch (2002).

THE HUMAN GENOME PROJECT

The Human Genome Project (HGP) originally arose because of the need to develop new mutation detection methods and was a unique collaboration to determine the entire nucleotide sequence of the human genome.

The aims of this project were to:

- identify all of the genes in human DNA. There are approximately 30 000 genes in human DNA, fewer than were anticipated
- determine the sequences of the 3 million chemical base pairs that make up human DNA
- store the information on a database
- improve the tools for data analysis
- transfer related technologies to the private sector
- address the related ethical, legal and social issues.

Identification and understanding of the genes responsible for disease may help towards the future treatment of genetic conditions. Currently, however, there is very little available in the form of curative treatment.

For information on the Human Genome Project, see Venter et al (2001), Francis et al (2003) and www.genome.gov.

CATEGORIES OF GENETIC CONDITIONS

The three main categories of genetic conditions are:

- chromosomal anomalies
- single-gene or Mendelian conditions
- multifactorial or polygenic conditions.

Chromosomal anomalies

Autosomal variations

Numerical autosomal chromosome variations

Abnormalities can arise if, during meiosis, non-disjunction takes place and both of one pair of chromosomes passes to one gamete and the other gamete does not get a copy of that chromosome. If fertilisation takes place, the zygote will then have either three copies of the chromosome (trisomy) or only one copy (monosomy). One example of a trisomy is Down's syndrome (an extra copy of chromosome 21) with its characteristic appearance, a degree of learning disability, and sometimes cardiac and intestinal abnormalities.

Autosomal chromosomal deletions and translocations

Structural variations arise if a part of a chromosome breaks off and attaches itself to another chromosome. This will result in the gamete either having part of a chromosome missing (a deletion) or having a rearrangement (a translocation).

A balanced translocation does not cause any abnormality because chromosomal material is not gained or lost. However, there will be a higher risk of an unbalanced chromosome complement occurring when that individual has a child. This may result in a spontaneous abortion or an affected child with possibly physical and/or learning difficulties.

Chromosomal abnormalities are often found in spontaneously aborted fetuses. The risk of a couple having another affected child with a chromosomal abnormality is usually low. The risk to other family members is even lower. However, if one of the parents is found to carry a balanced translocation, the risk of another affected child is greatly increased. Balanced translocations account for approximately 5% of chromosomal abnormalities. In this situation, all relatives can have their chromosomes checked for the translocation (Bonthron et al 1997).

Sex chromosome variations

Although the psychological implications of the diagnosis of a sex chromosome anomaly may be profound, the problems caused by these abnormalities tend to be less severe than those resulting from autosomal abnormalities. Consequently, a significant number of people may have a sex chromosome variation without being aware of it. It is now known that numerical abnormalities of the sex chromosomes are not as rare as was once believed (Harper 2004).

Sex chromosome variations often result in infertility; therefore, the diagnosis may only be made for the first time following fertility investigations. Occasionally an affected fetus may be diagnosed during antenatal screening. Diagnosis in children may be made at a paediatric growth or endocrine clinic following investigation of abnormal growth patterns.

An example of a sex chromosome variation is Klinefelter's syndrome (an extra copy of the X chromosome in a male). The boys have a normal physical appearance and usually a normal level of intelligence. The personality may be more reticent. After puberty the testes are small, facial hair is scant and sometimes there can be a degree of breast enlargement. Most of those with Klinefelter's syndrome are infertile, but it is important to note that sexual performance is not impaired.

It is rare for sex chromosome abnormalities to recur in a family, even in the offspring of affected fertile individuals.

Single-gene or Mendelian conditions

These conditions are caused by a mutation in one of our genes. An individual who carries a genetic mutation is at risk of passing the mutation to the next generation. The risk of having an affected child can be calculated if the mode of inheritance and details of the family history are known.

The inheritance of single-gene conditions can be:

- autosomal dominant
- autosomal recessive
- X-linked.

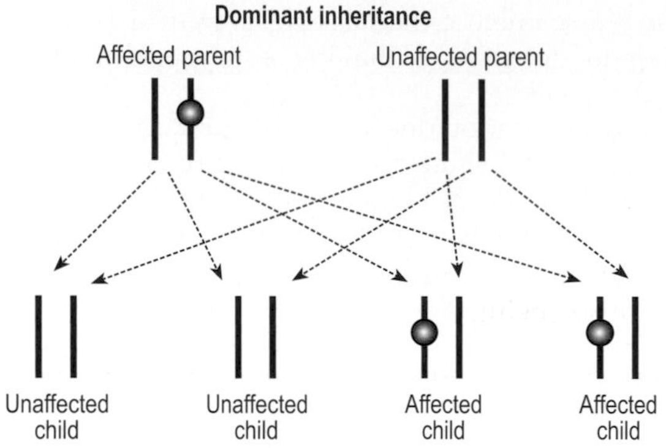

Fig. 6.3 Autosomal dominant inheritance.

Autosomal dominant inheritance

Autosomal dominant conditions are caused by a mutation in a dominant gene on one of the 44 autosomes. One gene on a pair of autosomes will be normal, while the corresponding gene on the other autosome will have a mutation. If the mutated gene is dominant, it will overrule the normal gene. As a result, the individual who carries the mutation will ultimately be affected by the condition. Those who carry a dominant gene mutation will have a 1 in 2 (50%) chance of passing it on to each of their children (see Fig. 6.3). This is because during meiosis only one of each pair of chromosomes will pass to each ovum or sperm. Whether the disease is or is not transmitted from the parent will depend on whether the ovum or sperm contains the chromosome with the normal gene or the chromosome with the gene mutation.

It is important to note that there is a 50% chance, in each pregnancy, of the fetus inheriting the gene mutation. Therefore, if there are two children, it is not inevitable that one will inherit the mutation and the other will not. It could be that both inherit the mutation, neither inherits it, or one will and one will not.

As the mutation is on an autosome rather than a sex chromosome, the sex of the individual is of no consequence to inheritance. If an individual tests negative for a known gene mutation in their family, they cannot pass on the mutation to their children.

Four distinct features can complicate genetic counselling in dominant conditions:

- non-penetrance or reduced penetrance
- variable expression
- anticipation
- new mutations.

Non-penetrance or reduced penetrance

In autosomal dominant disorders it is possible for an individual to have inherited a mutation from their affected parent, to show no detectable signs of the disease themselves and yet the disease manifests itself in their children. Although the disease may appear to have skipped a generation, the gene mutation must have been present in all three generations. This is known as 'reduced penetrance' or 'non-penetrance'. Hereditary breast cancer is a good example of this. Individuals who carry a BRCA1 mutation (one of the genes known to predispose to breast cancer) will not inevitably develop breast cancer. Their lifetime risk of breast cancer is high but approximately 15% will not develop the disease (Thompson et al 2002). This feature of autosomal dominant inheritance complicates the genetic counselling process as an extra element of uncertainty is introduced. However, it is possible, in a general way, to relate the degree of penetrance to the risk of developing the condition. Where penetrance of a condition is high, it is unlikely that an unaffected individual will carry the genetic mutation and where penetrance is low, even individuals who carry the gene mutation have only a small risk of developing the disorder.

Variable expression

is where a genetic disorder presents itself with varying severity or in different ways in individuals who carry the causative mutation. Individuals may be mildly or severely affected or may present with a variable clinical picture (phenotype). One example of this is tuberous sclerosis. Tuberous sclerosis is a multisystem genetic condition, the most commonly involved systems being the skin, central nervous system and the renal system. Apparently unaffected parents can have a child who is severely affected with uncontrollable epilepsy, severe learning difficulties and behavioural problems. During the process of genetic counselling, thorough investigation of the parents may reveal mild features of the condition (such as the skin features). Although in this case scenario the couple will have a 50% risk of having a second affected child, it is not possible to predict how severely affected the child may be. The child may be mildly affected like the parent, or severely affected like the sibling.

The age of onset of dominantly inherited conditions can also be variable. With some conditions, symptoms may not appear until young adulthood or middle age. Examples of these are myotonic dystrophy (see p. 243) and Huntington's disease (see p. 244).

Anticipation

In some conditions, the nature of the gene mutation allows it to increase in size as it passes down to the next generation. This is known as 'anticipation' and tends to result in a more severe form of the resulting disease. One example of this is myotonic dystrophy (see p. 243).

New mutations

A genetic disorder may be caused by a new mutation in that individual rather than the individual having inherited the mutation from the previous generation. This is a very important factor in the genetic counselling process as the risk of the couple having a second affected child will be very different. In tuberous sclerosis, two-thirds of newly diagnosed cases will be the result of a new mutation. If the disorder is the result of a new mutation, the risk of a second child being affected will be very low (1–2%), compared with the 50% risk if the mutation was inherited from either one of the parents.

The rate of identification of genes responsible for classic genetic conditions is small but is steadily increasing. Consequently, the availability of genetic testing for autosomal dominant conditions is also increasing. If the gene mutation responsible for causing a condition is identified in an affected individual (proband), other family members can be offered a test to identify whether or not they have inherited the mutation. Knowing that they do not carry the mutation offers certainty that they will not develop the condition and cannot pass the condition on to their children. Knowing that they do carry the mutation means that they have a 50% risk of passing the mutation on to their children. However, in conditions where non-penetrance, variable expression or anticipation may be a factor, uncertainty remains regarding if, when and how the condition will manifest itself.

Autosomal recessive inheritance

Autosomal recessive conditions are caused by mutations in both copies of the same autosomal gene. An example of an autosomal recessive condition is cystic fibrosis (see p. 236). Parents have two copies of each gene and both pass on one copy to each child. If they have a gene mutation in one of their autosomes then there is a 50% (1 in 2) chance that they will pass that mutation on to each of their children. As the parents have one normal and one mutated copy of the gene, they are carriers and are not affected by the condition. The risk of having a son or daughter affected by the condition is 25% (1 in 4) (see Fig. 6.4). The risk that the child will inherit only one copy of the gene mutation from either parent is 50% (1 in 2), making them a carrier of the condition like their parents. There is a 25% (1 in 4) risk that the child does not inherit a mutation from either of the parents and this means that they will not be a carrier or be affected. Parents who are closely related (consanguineous) are more likely to have a child with a recessive condition, as they will share a greater percentage of the same genes and possibly the same genetic mutations. Population screening in subgroups of the population at high risk can detect carriers of certain conditions so that detection and early treatment can be offered if appropriate (Kingston 2002). In autosomal recessive conditions, the precise risk depends on the frequency of heterozygotes in the population. Screening can also be offered to relatives, usually following a diagnosis of a condition in the family. Many autosomal recessive conditions are severe and include complex malformation syndromes and recognised inborn errors of metabolism, e.g. phenylketonuria. It is not unusual to have an affected child born where there is no known family history of the condition (Harper 2004).

X-linked inheritance

X-linked conditions are caused by a mutation in a gene on the X chromosome. Males are affected by the condition as they only have one copy of the gene, whereas females are less likely to be affected as they have two copies. Females inherit one X chromosome from their father and one from their mother. If a female carries a mutation on one copy of her X chromosomes she will have a second normal copy. This results in her being a 'carrier' but she is unlikely to develop the condition. Occasionally a female can show signs of an X-linked condition; this is known as a 'manifesting carrier'.

A male inherits a Y chromosome from his father and an X chromosome from his mother. If he inherits a mutated X chromosome from his mother, he has no second copy and will therefore have the condition associated with the gene mutation.

If a carrier female passes on her mutated X chromosome to a daughter, the daughter will be a carrier like her mother. In the case of an affected male with an X-linked condition, all of his daughters will be carriers but none of his sons will either be affected by or carry the condition (see Figs 6.5 and 6.6).

Genetic testing can only be offered to family members if the causative mutation is identified in the affected child. Complicating features of X-linked conditions include new mutations (see autosomal dominant) and gonadal mosaicism. Gonadal mosaicism is when the mutation arises in the

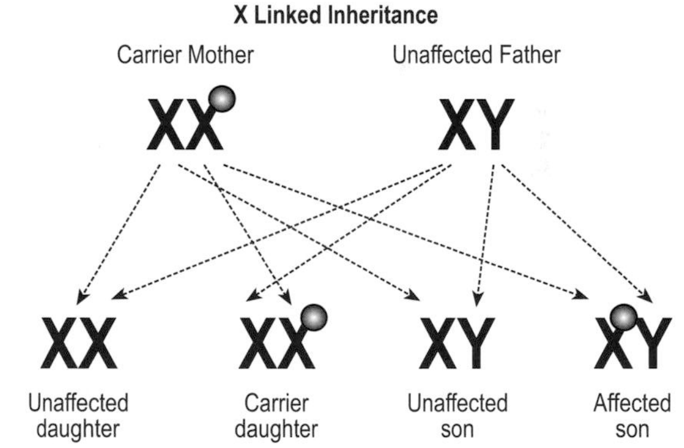

Fig. 6.5 X-linked inheritance — carrier mother.

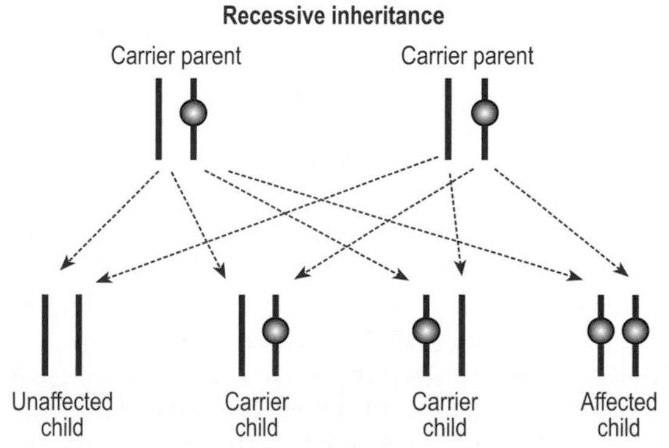

Fig. 6.4 Autosomal recessive inheritance.

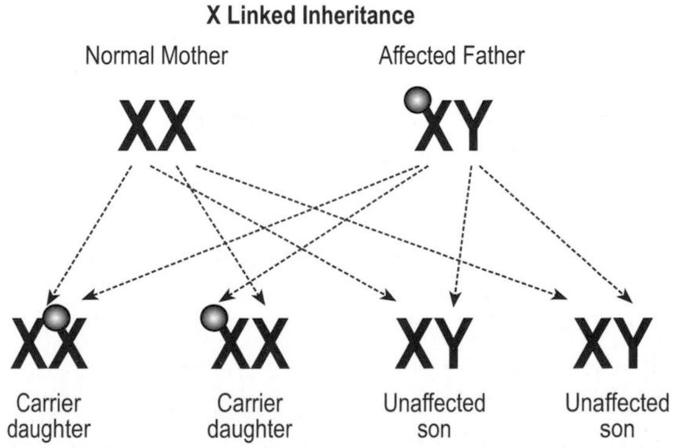

Fig. 6.6 X-linked inheritance — affected father.

cells of the mother's ovaries. This means that the risk of the mother having another affected son or carrier daughter can rarely be ruled out. However, in both new mutations and gonadal mosaicism there will be no risk to the wider family.

Multifactorial or polygenic conditions

In many conditions, genetic and environmental factors combine to give rise to disease. Risks of recurrence of these conditions within a family are generally regarded as low, the greatest risk being to first- and second-degree relatives (approximately 1%). When environmental factors are known, e.g. diet, smoking and exercise in coronary heart disease, these can be modified with beneficial effect. However, this approach is not possible for the majority of multifactorial conditions.

Factors that increase the risk of multifactorial conditions are (Harper 2004):

- the genetic component of the disease
- the closeness of the relationship to the affected person
- the presence of the condition in more than one family member
- the severity of the condition in the affected person
- the presence of the condition in a person not of the sex usually affected.

Common conditions which are considered to be multifactorial in origin include:

- asthma
- coronary artery disease
- congenital heart disease
- diabetes mellitus
- essential hypertension
- schizophrenia
- cleft lip and palate
- neural tube defects.

TESTING FOR GENETIC CONDITIONS

Testing for genetic conditions can be divided into four main categories:

- Antenatal
- Diagnostic
- Presymptomatic
- Carrier.

Antenatal testing, also referred to as prenatal testing, is used to predict whether a fetus is affected by a genetic condition or has inherited a gene mutation.

Techniques for antenatal diagnosis

Diagnostic ultrasound

Various abnormalities can be detected using high-resolution ultrasound imaging. Congenital abnormalities can, in some instances only, be detected by ultrasound scans from around 14 weeks' gestation.

Conditions detectable by ultrasound scanning include:

- skeletal abnormalities, e.g. severe short-limbed dwarfism, osteogenesis imperfecta
- neural tube defects, e.g. spina bifida
- major organ malformations, e.g. severe congenital heart disease, renal agenesis
- polyhydramnios, i.e. excess amniotic fluid
- oligohydramnios, i.e. decreased amniotic fluid
- hydrops, i.e. abnormal accumulation of serous fluid in a body cavity or tissues.

Amniocentesis

During pregnancy, fetal cells slough off into the amniotic fluid. It is possible to withdraw a sample of amniotic fluid between 16 and 20 weeks' gestation and to culture and test the fetal cells for chromosomal abnormalities. Alphafetoprotein (AFP) levels can be measured to detect neural tube defects such as spina bifida. Amniocentesis has the potential to diagnose around 200 genetic disorders. The risk of spontaneous abortion after the procedure is estimated to be less than 1%.

Conditions detectable by amniocentesis include:

- chromosomal disorders, using karyotyping
- inherited diseases, using biochemical and DNA studies
- open neural tube defects, indicated by amniotic fluid AFP.

Chorionic villus sampling (CVS)

This is carried out between 10 and 12 weeks of pregnancy and is thus termed first-trimester prenatal diagnosis. Essentially, this test provides the same diagnostic information as amniocentesis but gives a result more quickly as the cells grow faster; however, it is not suitable for diagnosing all genetic disorders.

Under ultrasound guidance, a catheter is inserted through the abdomen or the cervical os to the placental insertion site. Villi are aspirated and the cells are analysed. Conditions detectable by CVS are chromosomal disorders (using karyotyping) and inherited diseases (using DNA studies).

Transabdominal CVS can be done at any stage of pregnancy, providing the placenta is in an accessible position. Depending upon the type of analysis, results may be available within days. The risk of spontaneous abortion after CVS is estimated to be 2–4%.

Fetal blood sampling

This is occasionally used for diagnosis of disorders when DNA diagnosis is not possible. Under ultrasound guidance, a special sampling needle is passed transabdominally. A fetal vessel near the umbilical cord insertion is punctured and fetal blood withdrawn. This is carried out at 18 weeks' gestation (Proud 1995).

Diagnostic testing

Diagnostic testing, in the form of direct gene testing, is now available for a small number of conditions. However, the diagnosis of genetic conditions often relies on the presence or absence of signs and symptoms and the results of other investigations. Molecular confirmation of the underlying genetic mutation in the affected individual is required before presymptomatic testing can be offered to at-risk relatives. The main techniques used in the diagnosis of genetic conditions are:

- chromosomal analysis or karyotyping (see Fig. 6.1)
- mutation analysis
- direct gene testing
- clinical examination
- biochemical tests
- radiography
- ultrasonography.

Presymptomatic testing

This is used to predict whether or not an individual 'at risk' of inheriting a genetic condition has inherited the gene mutation before there are any signs or symptoms. The benefits of presymptomatic testing are clear where treatment is available to prevent the occurrence of the disease. However, when no treatment is available to prevent, cure or alleviate the disease, the 'at risk' individual must examine the advantages and disadvantages of knowing their status. Presymptomatic protocols have been developed to enable individuals to make informed decisions (Bates et al 2002).

For further reading on presymptomatic testing, see Skirton & Patch (2002).

Carrier testing

Carrier testing is used to find out whether an individual carries a particular autosomal recessive or X-linked gene mutation. It has mainly been offered in families with a known genetic condition or to individuals in an at-risk group.

GENETIC COUNSELLING

> *Genetic counselling is the process by which patients or relatives at risk of a disorder that may be hereditary are advised of the consequences of the disorder, the probability of developing or transmitting it and the ways in which this may be prevented, avoided or ameliorated.*
>
> (Harper 2004)

A genetic team normally consists of consultant medical geneticists, genetic counsellors who may either be genetic nurses or non-medical health professionals, a data manager, scientists/laboratory staff and an administrative team. Referral to most genetic departments can be from any health professional involved in the care of the individual or family requiring referral. Indications for referral include:

- several family members with a classic genetic condition
- women, or couples, seeking advice on increased pregnancy risk of fetal abnormality
- individuals seeking advice on interfamily relationships
- the presence of dysmorphic features
- unexplained stillbirth
- unexplained developmental delay
- recurrent miscarriages
- family history of chromosomal abnormality
- family history of breast, ovarian or colorectal cancer.

Referral for genetic counselling should only be made with the consent of the individual or family.

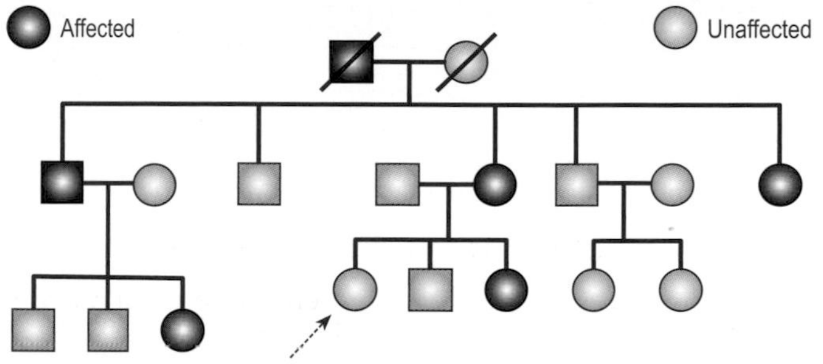

Fig. 6.7 Three-generation pedigree.

Family history is the first and very important part of genetic counselling. A three-generation family history is taken and a pedigree constructed (see Fig. 6.7). This pedigree gives a visual representation of the family and their relatives as to illnesses, miscarriages, deaths and consanguinity. The pedigree can demonstrate the inheritance pattern and may provide indicators for the diagnosis of a genetic condition. In some genetic conditions, the family history is also used to assess whether family members are at risk and/or are eligible for screening programmes.

Box 6.2 lists the information that should be included in a pedigree. The universal symbols used to construct a pedigree are illustrated in Figure 6.8.

The family pedigree is referred to throughout the genetic counselling process. There may be additions to the pedigree as more individuals from the extended family are seen. In many cases the original information is incomplete and requires confirmation by death certificate, medical notes or postmortem reports. However, it is not uncommon for the diagnosis to remain unclear and as a result families may be left with uncertainty. If a diagnosis can be made, the person receiving counselling will be encouraged to share the information with family members, enabling them to seek further advice. Genetic counselling aims to be non-directive (Harper 2004), i.e. it presents individuals with information in a way they understand and encourages them to explore in detail all the options available in order to make decisions without influence from the genetic counsellor.

Box 6.2

Drawing up a pedigree

Details are required from both sides of the family over three generations:

- Record dates of birth
- Record those who have died, plus cause and age of death
- Ask specifically about infant deaths, stillbirths and miscarriages
- Ask about consanguinity (marriage between relatives, e.g. cousins)
- Record maiden name of married women
- Record specific information related to the specific condition if known.

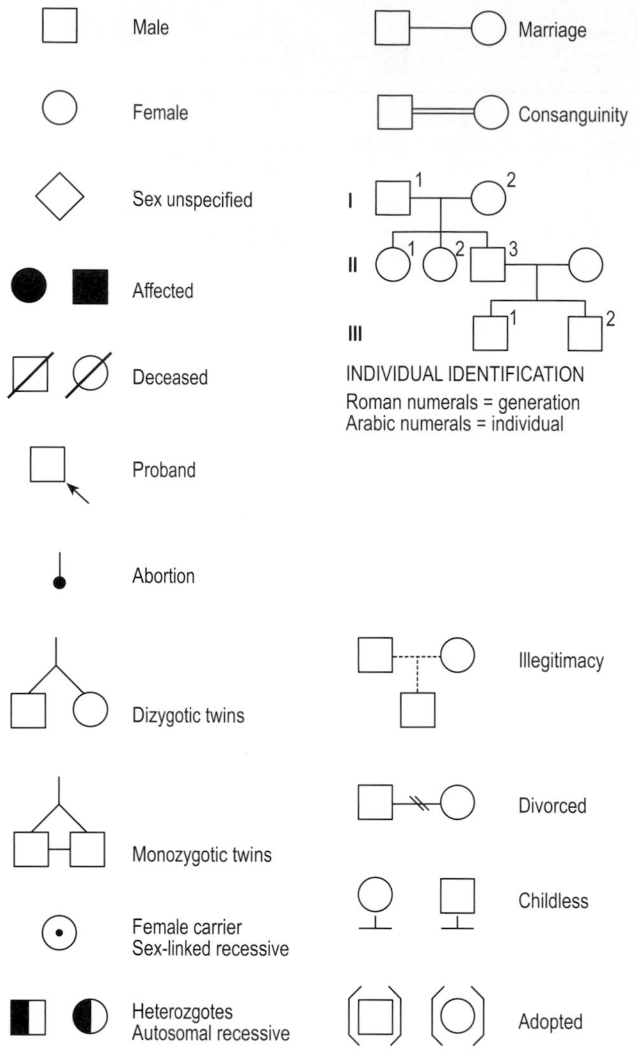

Fig. 6.8 Standard symbols used in constructing a pedigree.

Genetic counsellors

Genetic counsellors are an emerging professional group, related to, but separate from, existing health professions (Skirton & Patch 2002). There are two career pathways to becoming a genetic counsellor: the nursing pathway and the scientist pathway. The Association of Genetic Nurses and Counsellors (AGNC) developed and introduced a registration system ensuring that each professional practises at a competent level. This aims not only to ensure standards and safety but also to provide a framework for education in the clinical setting. It is envisaged that registration will be a statutory requirement for practice in genetic counselling.

CLASSIC GENETIC CONDITIONS AND THEIR MANAGEMENT

CYSTIC FIBROSIS

Cystic fibrosis (CF) is a single-gene, autosomal recessive disorder which disturbs the mucus-producing glands throughout the body, leading to respiratory problems, incomplete digestion and abnormal sweating. In the UK, it affects 1 in 2500 newborns and approximately 1 in 25 individuals carries a CF gene. There are 7500 affected individuals in the UK (Cystic Fibrosis Trust 2001).

There is no complete cure for CF. However, advances in treatment have resulted in a steady rise in survival rates over the past several decades and median life expectancy in the UK is currently 31 years (Hodson et al 2002). Despite this, affected individuals continue to have numerous medical problems requiring exhaustive and expensive therapy.

PATHOPHYSIOLOGY

In CF there is a defect in the passage of sodium and chloride ions in and out of the epithelial cells of a number of organs which affects fluid secretion in various glands.

Common presenting symptoms

Presentation usually occurs in early life with recurring respiratory problems, frequent bulky offensive-smelling stools and failure to gain weight satisfactorily. A proportion present neonatally with meconium ileus. A small number are not diagnosed until adulthood: 1 in 12 patients in the UK are diagnosed after 18 years of age (Cystic Fibrosis Trust 2001).

Clinical features

The air passages of people with CF secrete large amounts of thick, sticky mucus which plugs up the small airways and creates an ideal environment for bacterial infection in the respiratory tract. In the intestine, thick, abnormal mucus is also produced which clogs the ducts leading from the pancreas to the intestine. Food is incompletely digested; weight loss occurs despite a good appetite; and fatty, bulky, foul-smelling stools are passed. The pancreas regresses and may be completely destroyed; however, 10–20% of patients retain at least partial pancreatic function. The prevalence of CF-related diabetes mellitus (CFRDM) rises with life expectancy, with up to 30% of those surviving into their third decade displaying abnormal glucose tolerance (Liddle et al 1998). Five per cent of patients develop hepatic cirrhosis; some of these go on to develop portal hypertension and splenomegaly. Oesophageal varices may develop in these patients which, whilst treatable, can be fatal. The sweat glands also malfunction, secreting too much chloride and sodium in the sweat.

Most males with CF are infertile, as a result of an abnormality of the epididymis and vas deferens which end in blind channels instead of leading through to the urethra. In the female, fertility may be impaired because thick cervical mucus impedes the passage of spermatozoa. Delayed secondary sexual development is an almost universal finding in adolescents.

The gene responsible for cystic fibrosis is on chromosome 7 and has been labelled the 'cystic fibrosis transmembrane regulator' (CFTR) gene.

The clinical consequences of CF are outlined in Figure 6.9.

Prognosis

Elborn et al (1991) predicted that individuals with CF born in the 1990s would survive into their 30s and 40s. This is indeed the case, but some still die as young adults (Nir et al

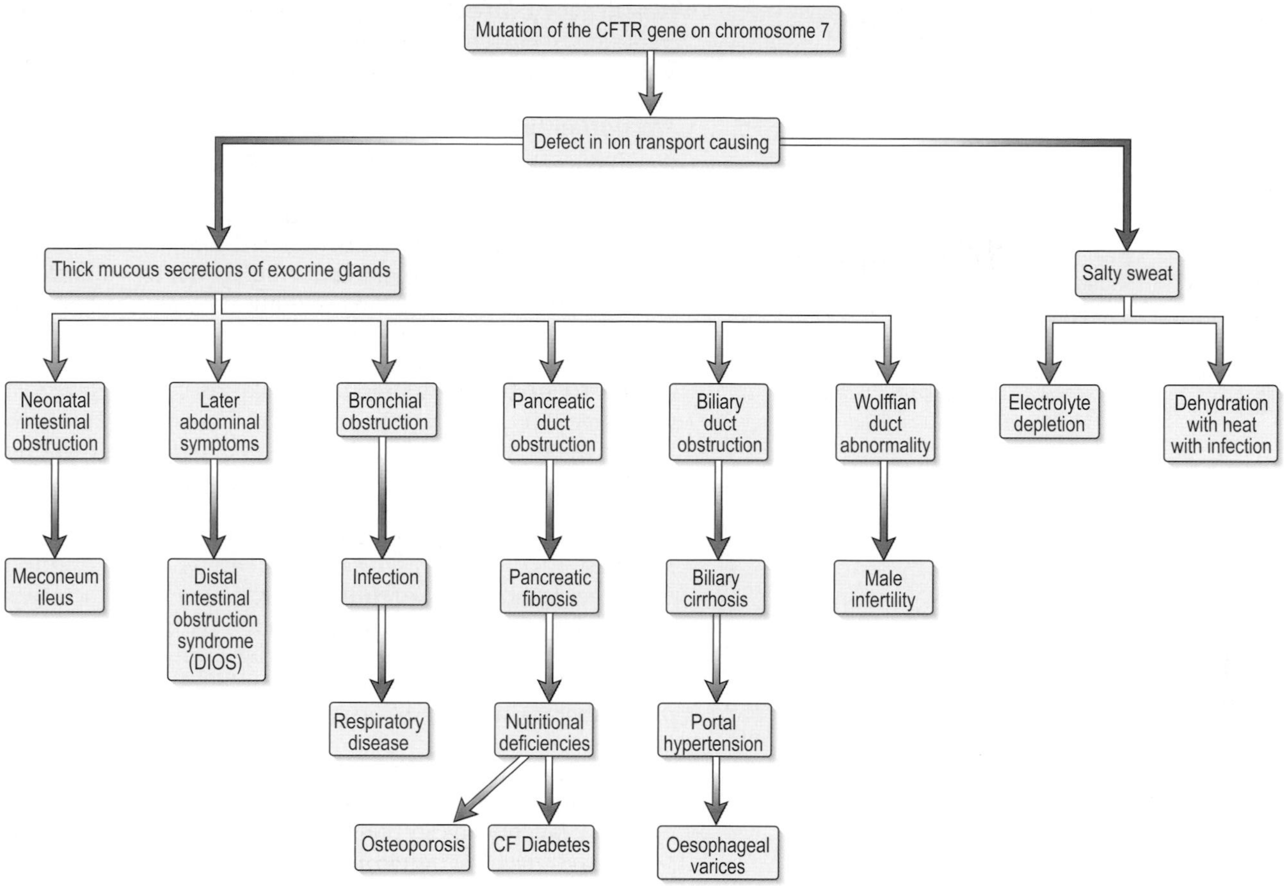

Fig. 6.9 Clinical consequences of cystic fibrosis.

1996, Cystic Fibrosis Trust 2001). Advances in treatment are largely due to improved nutrition and aggressive antibiotic therapy.

The psychological burden of living with a debilitating disease which needs constant drug therapy and physiotherapy is great for both those affected and their families, particularly during adolescence; however, this does not deter many sufferers from living full and productive lives (Walters et al 1993, Lowton & Gabe 2003).

MEDICAL MANAGEMENT

Investigations

Until the CFTR gene was identified, testing to determine high levels of sodium and chloride in the sweat was the single most important method for diagnosing CF.

In CF the potential difference between interstitial fluid and the respiratory surface epithelium is abnormally large. This can be measured in the nasal epithelium and may aid diagnosis.

Other supporting evidence is based on X-ray examination, CT scanning and sputum cultures. There may also be pancreatic insufficiency or a history of recurrent respiratory infection. In some cases there may be a family history of CF.

Genetic diagnosis

At least 900 different mutations within the CFTR gene have been found. One common mutation, called Delta F508, is found in 60–70% of the affected UK population. This mutation, along with a number of others, allows detection of most affected individuals by analysing their DNA. At present, most suspected CF cases are diagnosed by a combination of a sweat test and genetic testing.

Genetic screening

To have cystic fibrosis, an individual must inherit one copy of the mutated gene from each parent (see Fig. 6.10). It is a recessive disease, where both parents are carriers or heterozygotes and have a CF gene on one chromosome 7 and a normal gene on the other chromosome 7. Carriers have no symptoms of the disease, as the normal gene compensates fully for the CF gene (see p. 233). Using DNA from a mouthwash sample, it is possible to detect 85% of those who carry a CF gene by testing for the most common CF mutations. It is not practicable to test routinely for all 900 mutations. If both partners are found to be carriers, they are given the option of prenatal diagnosis.

Newborn screening, by a heel prick test, at around 6 days has been introduced in Scotland, Wales and Northern Ireland and will be made available throughout the UK (NHS Scotland 2003).

Aims of treatment

The overall aim of management is to help affected individuals reach adulthood, leading as normal a life as possible

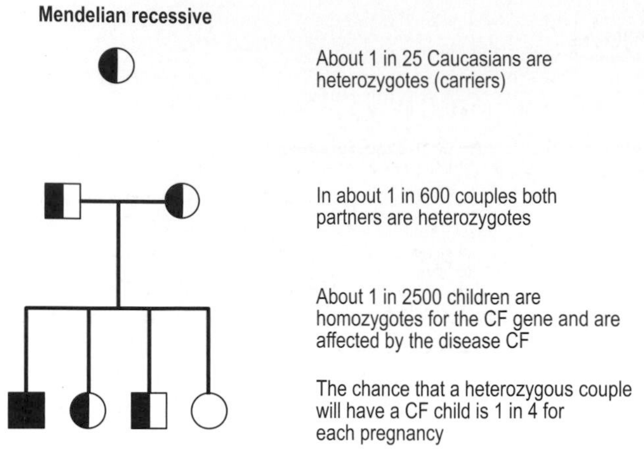
Mendelian recessive
About 1 in 25 Caucasians are heterozygotes (carriers)
In about 1 in 600 couples both partners are heterozygotes
About 1 in 2500 children are homozygotes for the CF gene and are affected by the disease CF
The chance that a heterozygous couple will have a CF child is 1 in 4 for each pregnancy

Fig. 6.10 Genetic inheritance of cystic fibrosis.

with minimal dependency. The ultimate aim is a self-determining life, and from the time of diagnosis this concept should be fostered in the parents and, in turn, in the affected individual. This aim is promoted by a multidisciplinary team whose skills, along with close cooperation between the parents, patient and family, are put into action from the time of diagnosis. Regional cystic fibrosis treatment centres lead the way in management.

The treatment programme

At a regular clinic visit 6–12 weekly, the patient is weighed, lung function tests are carried out and sputum is sent for culture and sensitivity. At regular intervals, exercise testing and chest X-rays are carried out and blood is taken for biochemistry and haematology. Aspects of dietary regimens and physiotherapy techniques are checked and specific problems requiring detailed involvement of particular team members identified. A standard form is used to record findings, including details of physical examination.

Improved survival is largely due to improved nutritional status and earlier antibiotic treatment against staphylococcal and pseudomonal infections. If *Pseudomonas* colonises the lungs, it is almost impossible to eradicate and causes deterioration of lung function. Many CF centres practise segregation of patients in hospital and at clinics to reduce the incidence of cross-infection. However, this segregation has potentially detrimental psychosocial implications for peer and family support.

Pancreatic enzyme supplements are taken at each meal or snack. The amount of capsules required varies greatly between individuals and is also dependent on the size and fat content of the meals or snacks. Small snacks between meals require a lower dose of capsules.

NURSING PRIORITIES AND MANAGEMENT: Cystic fibrosis

Cystic fibrosis is a long-term, life-threatening multisystem disorder and there are a number of essential areas of management.

Respiratory infection

Persistent recurrent lower respiratory tract infections result in lung damage and impaired function.

Physiotherapy

is accepted as an essential part of respiratory tract management and daily performance of airway clearance techniques (ACT) is generally recommended. There is a variety of ACTs and treatment should be tailored to individual needs and preferences of the patient (Fig. 6.11). These include postural drainage and percussion, the active cycle of breathing technique, autogenic drainage and oscillatory positive expiratory pressure devices, such as flutter, cornet and positive expiratory pressure mask (PEP) (Association of Chartered Physiotherapists in Cystic Fibrosis 2002). Much time is spent with adults, children and parents educating them in physiotherapy techniques, as this is a key element of the treatment programme.

Exercise

It has been shown that regular exercise not only increases the efficiency of the lungs, heart and circulation but also improves the general physique and self-esteem (Webb & Dodd 2000). Activities must complement, not replace, physiotherapy and can be adapted to all stages of the illness trajectory.

To reduce the length of stay in hospital, parents and older children are taught to administer their own antibiotic drugs intravenously so that treatment initiated in hospital can be completed at home. This allows patients to feel more in control of the situation and less dependent on hospital staff. An implantable venous reservoir has greatly improved acceptance of home intravenous treatment.

The increased use of intravenous antibiotics has resulted in a rise in anaphylactic and anaphylactoid reactions in CF patients and must be taken into account when prescribing home intravenous treatment.

Nebulised antibiotics have been shown to be effective (Hodson et al 2002), and require a special compressor and nebuliser system. Other nebulised drugs such as bronchodilators and antimucolytic agents may be an integral part of the treatment regimen.

Nutrition

It has been shown that CF patients require 20–50% more than the normal daily food intake. Individuals with CF have a higher basal metabolic rate and resting energy requirement; extra energy is also needed to combat chest infections. Due to a loss of bile and pancreatic enzymes, a significant amount of nutritional intake is lost in frequent, bulky, greasy stools. However, pancreatic enzyme preparations are now so effective that fat absorption can reach 80–90% of normal. Three daily meals and supplemental snacks are usually required to bring the energy level up to that desired.

Distal intestinal obstructive syndrome (DIOS) can occur in adults with CF. Symptoms include colicky abdominal pain, bloating and constipation. Treatment includes oral aperients and occasionally the use of gastrograffin enemas to detect potential for perforation. Following an attack of DIOS, enzyme dosage should be reviewed to ensure its appropriateness. Fat-soluble vitamin supplements are given to compensate for loss in the stools. Osteoporosis is

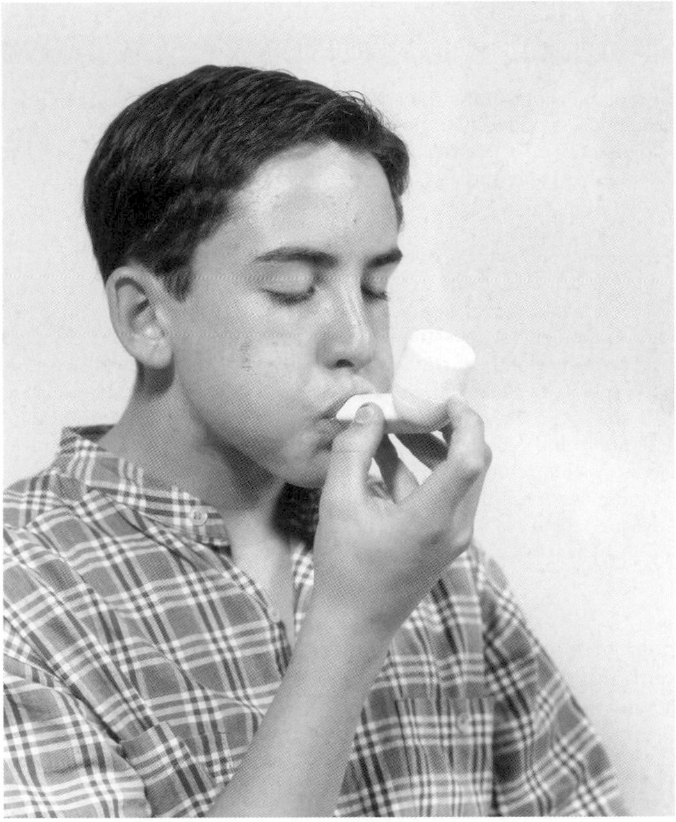

A

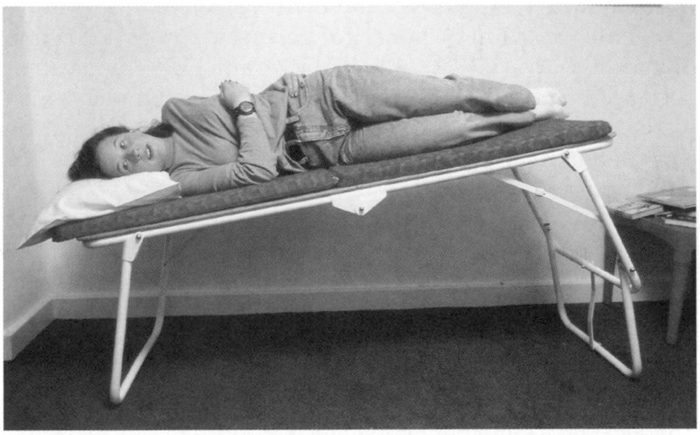

B

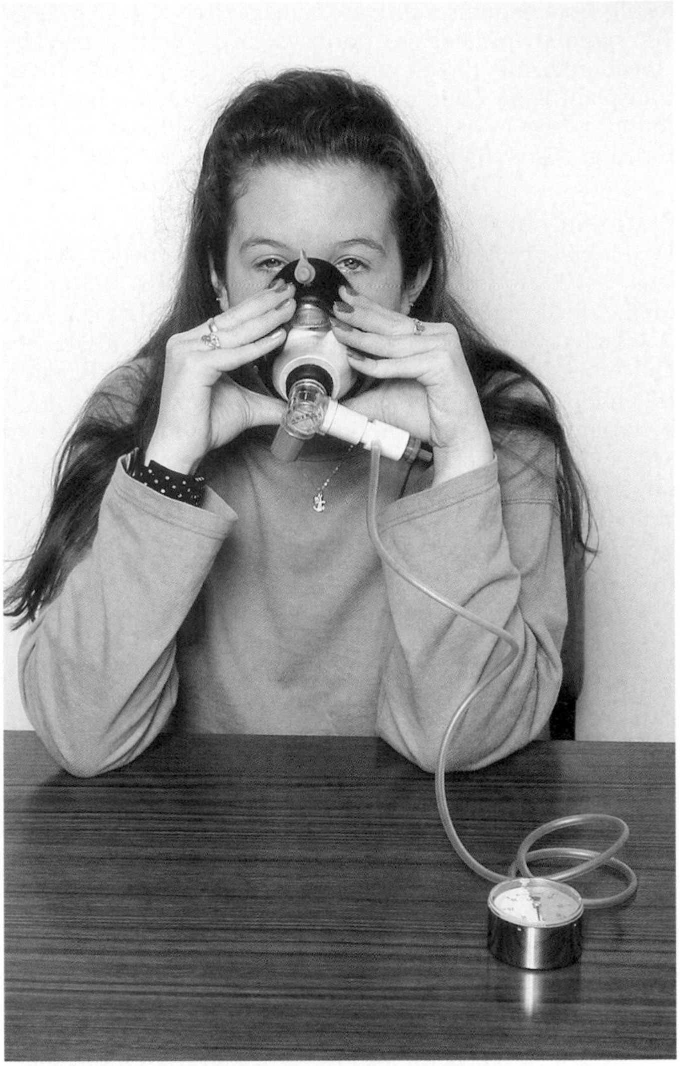

C

Fig. 6.11 Physiotherapy techniques for cystic fibrosis. A: Using the 'flutter' device which produces a vibrator effect during expiration. B: Teenager doing her own treatment using the active cycle of breathing, with self chest clapping. C: Using the positive expiratory pressure (PEP) mask. (Photographs published with permission from the Cystic Fibrosis Trust from *TREATMENT: Physiotherapy for Cystic Fibrosis,* September 2001. Photographer (A, B), Camilla Jessel; (C) photograph courtesy of Clement Clarke International.)

increasingly recognised as a complication of poor nutrition due to the loss of absorption of fat-soluble vitamins in CF (Haworth et al 1999) and the use of bisphosphonates and calcium supplements is increasingly recognised as beneficial.

Salt depletion can occur in hot weather or as a result of strenuous exercise, and salt supplements are recommended where appropriate.

Enteral feeding is encouraged in children who fail to gain weight over a 6-month period and in adults who are chronically underweight (body mass index <19, see Ch. 21, p. 797), either by the nasogastric route or via a gastrostomy tube. Good nutrition, by whatever means, correlates positively with increased survival (Corey et al 1988, Hallyar et al 1997).

Control of diabetes mellitus

An annual oral glucose tolerance test is recommended for patients over 10 years of age. If a modest glucose intolerance is demonstrated, no action is taken. If patients progress to develop diabetes mellitus, insulin is the treatment of choice and blood glucose is regulated by insulin dose adjustment. Diabetic complications are rare (Koch & Lang 1995).

Liver disease

Significant disease may already have occurred by the time the liver function tests (LFTs) become abnormal. Ursodeoxycholic acid may improve the LFTs but long-term effects are unclear (Nousia-Arvanitakis et al 2001). Banding can be performed to halt variceal bleeding that can result from significant liver damage (see Ch. 4, p. 142). Transjugular intrahepatic portosystemic shunting may be considered for those with portal hypertension. Liver transplant is an option in end-stage disease and has been found to be associated with an improvement in lung function post-surgery (Westaby 1995, Genyk et al 2001).

Pregnancy and infertility

Development of secondary sexual characteristics occurs later in CF. However, women with CF can still reproduce, unlike their male counterparts. However, pregnancy in a woman with CF may cause deterioration in health. Outcomes are closely linked to pre-pregnancy lung function (Edenborough et al 2000) and it is a time of close cooperation between the CF multidisciplinary team and the obstetrician. Moreover, the woman with CF must also consider the impact of a potential shortened life expectancy upon her children. Progression of the disease may prevent her from carrying out day-to-day care of her child. Those who become pregnant require increased supervision, more physiotherapy and carefully managed antibiotic therapy. Adult males with CF are now in a position to seek help at assisted reproduction clinics, where techniques such as artificial insemination by donor (AID) and microscopic epididymal sperm aspiration (MESA) with intracytoplasmic sperm injection (ICSI) are allowing fatherhood to become a reality. These techniques are expensive, not always easily available and may also raise further ethical dilemmas.

Transplantation

Lung transplant has brought renewed hope for those with CF, but may also cause new problems as a direct result of the surgery, or from tissue rejection. Moreover, there are psychosocial problems which can be difficult to foresee. The idea of a lung transplant should be introduced very sensitively, as consenting to this procedure is a grave decision. Patients, relatives and professionals may have differing viewpoints and conflicting emotions (see Case History 6.1). The overwhelming shortage of cadaveric donor organs has resulted in the use of living donor transplants, which creates further ethical dilemmas. Survival from lung transplant is approximately 60% at 5 years (Egan et al 2002). However, approximately a third of those on a transplant list will die whilst awaiting transplant.

CASE HISTORY 6.1

Individuals with cystic fibrosis — J, A and S

J thought about a lung transplant for over a year but elected not to attend for assessment at the transplant centre. She eventually chose to discontinue active treatment because she wished to avoid coping with a protracted terminal illness. J died in relative peace and dignity in her local hospital within a short time.

A was keen to find out if he was a suitable candidate for transplant and was pleased to be accepted and placed on the waiting list. Everything in the family centred on the time when the bleeper would go off calling him for transplant. Alas, A ran out of time and died before a suitable donor was found.

S was one of the lucky few. He finally underwent lung transplant after three false alarms; on each previous occasion when he was called, the donor lungs were found to be unsuitable. S leads a full life and is back working full time. He has had two rejection episodes requiring hospitalisation and suffers from immunosuppressant-induced peripheral neuropathy. His wife worries about the future in terms of further rejection.

Psychosocial considerations

Patients, parents and siblings are profoundly affected by the psychosocial and emotional stresses of living with CF. The CF nurse is in an ideal position to recognise that problems exist, and to plan and implement measures to help deal with issues such as the transition from paediatric to adult care, education, careers, relationships, body image and coping with the terminal stages of illness (UK Cystic Fibrosis Nurse Specialist Group 2001). Case History 6.2 describes some of the difficulties that might be faced by a teenage boy with CF, and how the sensitive intervention of a specialist nurse might help. The advent of segregation policies in and out of hospitals has seen the demise of the social networks once so strong in the CF community. Other innovative ways to help support and bring together patients and their families without direct contact are being utilised, such as the use of advocates, CF magazines, websites and teleconferencing.

Outlook for the future

Since the discovery of the CF gene, advances in the understanding of the role of CFTR and ion transport have been made. Future therapies will involve correction of the faulty gene either by viral or non-viral gene therapy or correction of the defective CFTR protein by 'trafficking' medication such as the prodrug thapsigargin, a tumour promoter which increases intracellular calcium stores. Studies to optimise current therapies include the long-term use of the macrolide antibiotic azithromycin (Equi et al 2002); its mode of action may include anti-inflammatory as well as antimicrobial activity.

Whilst some of these therapies give hope for an eventual cure for CF, the focus continues to be on supportive treatment such as physiotherapy, antibiotics and intensive nutritional support. The prospect of CF sufferers surviving into their fourth, fifth and sixth decades reflects real progress but also creates further challenges for those individuals and for the health professionals involved in their care.

HAEMOPHILIA

Haemophilia is an inherited disorder in which there is a defect in the clotting mechanism of the blood. It is present from birth, is lifelong and is characterised by recurrent and persistent bleeding episodes involving mainly the deep tissues of muscles and joints (Rizza 1997).

PATHOPHYSIOLOGY

There are two types of haemophilia: haemophilia A, where bleeding is due to the deficiency of the clotting factor VIII (FVIII) and haemophilia B, also known as Christmas disease, where bleeding is due to the deficiency of clotting factor IX (FIX).

CASE HISTORY 6.2

G

G is a small, thin, red-haired 16-year-old in his fourth year at high school. He is judged to be academically average by his headmaster. G is a particularly keen cyclist and is a member of the school cycling team. He was diagnosed with cystic fibrosis (CF) at the age of 3. Since that time, his care has been shared by his GP, the local hospital and the regional CF centre. G attends the centre every 3 months. At these visits he has spirometry, a sputum sample is taken and he sees the physiotherapist, dietitian, CF nurse and the doctor to review all aspects of his care. Once a year he has a full review, which includes an X-ray, blood tests, a glucose tolerance test to screen for diabetes and a meeting with the psychologist to assess his psychological well-being.

G has been admitted twice in the last year for intensive intravenous therapy for Pseudomonas respiratory infections. He has recently had a Portacath device inserted for ease of administration.

Today G is going to talk to the specialist nurse, who will suggest that he sees a careers guidance officer. She knows G well and has already submitted a report to the careers office. G has had periods of absence from school when his condition necessitated admission to hospital. Some teaching was given while in hospital and he had extra tuition at home. His father helps with physiotherapy and they have a close relationship.

The specialist nurse knows from discussions with G that he is quite sensitive about his illness. He is smaller and thinner than his classmates; he weighs 50 kg and is currently 1.62 metres tall. His friends have entered puberty at the normal time but he is lagging behind and there is no sign of secondary sexual characteristics. He is self-conscious about this and gets embarrassed when using the shower and communal changing rooms at school. Reassurance from the CF consultant that he will catch up is little consolation.

For a time G had shown signs of depression and stopped adhering to his treatment regimen. He questioned what the point of it all was if he was going to die anyway.

His parents were concerned and asked the CF nurse to chat to him. Because of the problems of cross-infection between patients, the nurse was unable to arrange for G to meet with other patients to share experiences and thus support each other. However, she was able to give G some details of websites and chat rooms used by other sufferers and to get him subscribed to the CF magazine. Through these forums he learnt he was not alone and shared many of the same thoughts and feelings as his peers. He learnt that he was not the only one who had to cope with an average twice daily routine consisting of physiotherapy, nebulisers and enzymes before and after school. He found out that his peers wore jogging bottoms under their trousers to make them look more bulky and tried this out. Knowing that he was not alone and being able to express this made him feel better. In addition, he realised through the chat lines that there were people out there with CF who were in their thirties and forties with careers and wives and families, and this gave him hope for the future.

Within the UK, the incidence of haemophilia is approximately 1 in 10 000 live male births, haemophilia A being five times more common than haemophilia B (World Federation of Haemophilia 2004). Both share the same symptoms and inheritance patterns and no differentiation is made between them with regard to bleeding tendency.

The severity of the condition depends upon the level of circulating factor VIII or IX. The unit of activity of factor VIIIc/IXc is the amount of factor VIII/IX coagulant activity in 1 mL of fresh normal plasma (Colman et al 1994). Normal values are expressed in reference to average normal plasma, and range from 50 to 150 IU/dL. Levels less than 50 IU/dL are regarded as abnormal. A frequent classification of haemophilia is to define the severity of the condition as severe, with FVIII/FIX level of 0–2 IU/dL; moderate, with FVIII/FIX level 2–10 IU/dL; and mild, levels >10 IU/dL. Although the severity of the disease is variable, it is constant within a family.

Mode of inheritance

Haemophilia is sex linked and recessive in nature. The abnormal gene responsible for the disorder is carried on the X chromosome. As males only have one X chromosome, affected males will pass the faulty gene to each of their daughters. All daughters will be carriers and are termed obligate carriers. These daughters have a 1 in 4 chance of producing a son with haemophilia and a 1 in 4 risk of having a carrier daughter. All sons of a man with haemophilia will be unaffected, as they inherit his Y chromosome which does not carry an affected gene (see Fig. 6.12). Prenatal diagnosis is possible for carrier women by chorionic villus sampling at 10 weeks' gestation, or amniocentesis at approximately 14 weeks' gestation, to obtain material for genetic analysis by looking for a particular gene mutation in the DNA of the fetus. In families where the genetic mutation has not been identified, linked markers can be used in DNA-based family linkage analysis if there is a suitable family structure. Carrier testing is also available for other family relatives. These tests are offered by specialised genetic units (Bonthron et al 1997).

Two-thirds of children diagnosed with haemophilia have a family history of the disorder which can be traced through the maternal family tree. The remaining third has no family history, suggesting that the child or his mother may represent a spontaneous new genetic mutation, or it may have been transmitted undetected through generations with no affected boys being born.

Common presenting symptoms

In haemophilia, although the factor VIII/IX levels are reduced at birth, babies rarely present with bleeding from the umbilical cord. Children with severe haemophilia are usually diagnosed within the first year of life when they start to crawl. Often the first symptom is that they start to bruise easily. Unfortunately, if there is no known family

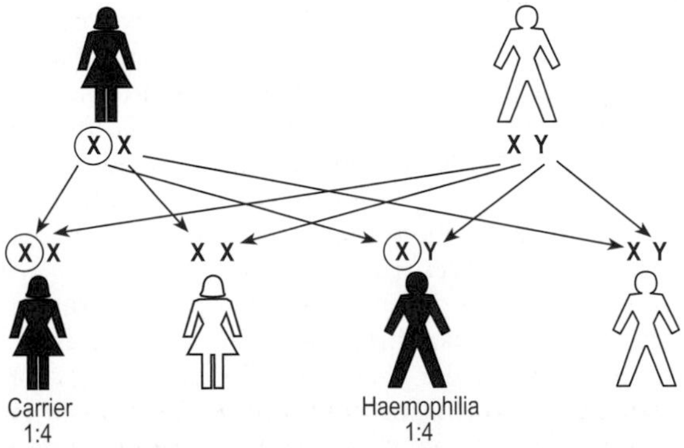

Fig. 6.12 Genetic inheritance of haemophilia.

history, the early signs of haemophilia can sometimes be wrongly interpreted as non-accidental injury (Haemophilia Society 1997a). The individual who has severe haemophilia can present with spontaneous internal bleeding, most commonly into joints and muscles. This type of bleeding may result from normal daily living but can present with life-threatening bleeds such as intracranial haemorrhage or gastric bleeding. Frequent and severe bleeding, particularly into the joints, can result in arthropathy and disability. The main joints affected are the hinge joints, namely the knee, elbow and ankle.

Mild and moderate haemophilia may not be diagnosed until later in childhood, or even adulthood. As some clotting factor activity is present in the blood, minor injuries heal normally. It may not be until surgery, dental extraction or if an injury occurs that the deficiency is revealed.

Individuals with haemophilia can experience a tingling sensation at the onset of a spontaneous bleed which then results in pain. As the bleeding progresses, the pain increases, the joint/muscle may feel warm to touch and may begin to swell, thus restricting movement.

Prognosis

The life expectancy of those with haemophilia should not differ from that of the average person and most individuals reach adult life with only a moderate degree of disability. This contrasts greatly with the past when it was a debilitating condition which resulted in a shortened lifespan (Harper 2004).

Great advances in treatment products and regimens have helped to change the outlook for young haemophilic children. Historically, patients with haemophilia have suffered from repeated bleeds into joints, causing damage and leading to disablement. New treatment regimens have dramatically lessened the likelihood of this.

MEDICAL MANAGEMENT

Diagnosis

Any individual with prolonged or unexplained bleeding should be tested for haemophilia. Diagnosis is made, within specialised haematology laboratories, via a blood sample which can differentiate which clotting factor is deficient.

Treatment of a bleeding episode

The goals of haemophilia treatment are to minimise permanent damage, minimise suffering and pain, permit tissue healing and restore function. By giving intravenous factor replacement therapy, raising the circulating factor level to within the normal range, joint damage and subsequent arthropathy can be prevented. There are two different modes of delivery of replacement therapy: on-demand therapy, where treatment is given on the first evidence of a bleed, and prophylaxis, where treatment is given in order to prevent bleeding from occurring.

Intravenous treatment with the appropriate factor concentrate is given for bleeding into a joint or muscle, or injury, for example, to the head, eye, mouth, tongue or neck. It is imperative that pain is controlled and activity reduced by resting the affected joint/limb, supporting it with pillows and applying cold packs to the affected area. The use of aspirin must be avoided due to its antiplatelet activity and intramuscular injections should never be given as they may cause a haematoma. Any weight or pressure on a joint must be avoided and, after the acute phase has passed, referral made to the physiotherapist.

Some patients develop inhibitors to FVIII and FIX. This is because, lacking factor VIII or IX, the body considers replacement coagulation factor concentrates to be a foreign protein, and produces antibodies which combine with the clotting factor and inhibit its action (Haemophilia Society 1997b).

Prophylaxis involves administering replacement factor concentrate, in advance, to prevent bleeding. It can be given as a single dose, for example, prior to an event that may result in bleeding, as a short-term procedure to counter a temporary increase in the frequency of bleeding or as a long-term procedure in order to prevent haemarthrosis and the development of arthropathy.

Within the UK, practice is guided by the United Kingdom Haemophilia Centre Doctors' Organisation (UKHCDO 1994). Guidelines recommend prophylactic treatment for all severe haemophilic boys to protect them from long-term joint damage and arthropathy. It is generally started in children when they are 1–2 years old. An infusion of the replacement factor concentrate is given three times a week in haemophilia A and twice a week in haemophilia B.

Complications

When a bleed occurs within a joint, the patient will stop using the joint because of severe pain and the muscles can become slack and wasted. The joint, no longer supported adequately, becomes susceptible to injuries which cause further bleeding. Blood enters the joint space causing damage to the articular cartilage, the synovium and the joint surface. The joint space becomes smaller, leading to permanently restricted movement and cysts can develop. Repetitive bleeding episodes result in arthritis, particularly if not adequately treated (Rodriguez-Merchan 2000).

Muscle bleeding, if untreated, can cause contractures and compression, leading to nerve damage, permanent palsy and loss of the use of the affected limb, e.g. ' foot drop' from a bleed into the calf muscle or 'claw hand' from a bleed into the forearm. Bleeding into muscles can weaken them, rendering them unable to support joints and causing risk of joint damage. If blood is lost into a large muscle it can cause a drop in the haemoglobin level; if blood loss is rapid, hypovolaemic shock can occur (see Ch. 18).

NURSING PRIORITIES AND MANAGEMENT: Haemophilia

The Haemophilia Centre

There is a network of haemophilia centres throughout the UK that aim to provide the best care and management for haemophilia patients. These may be comprehensive care centres or local haemophilia centres. At a comprehensive care centre, potential patients are tested for haemophilia by using the specific factor assays; new patients are registered and special medical cards issued. Some of the initial investigations include specialised laboratory testing which cannot be carried out in smaller centres. Twenty-four hour emergency cover is supplied by a multidisciplinary team of consultant haematologists, specialist nurses, physiotherapists, social workers, orthopaedic surgeons, liver specialists and dentists. Patients are reviewed on a regular basis.

Home treatment

In the past two decades there has been a move to deliver care in the home and community setting rather than in hospital. Specialised nursing posts have been developed to help to deliver and facilitate care that can meet the needs of the patient and their family (Haemophilia Alliance 2001). This is particularly visible in haemophilia care.

Many patients, both adults and children, are selected for home treatment after being taught and carefully supervised to proficiency in all aspects of care. This includes the recognition of bleeds and the administration of factor concentrate either through direct venepuncture or using an intravascular access device such as a Portacath. This allows immediate treatment of bleeding episodes and consequently the need for less factor concentrate. Pain is minimised and hospitalisation often avoided, allowing the patient to maintain as normal a life as possible. Self-management of treatment allows a degree of control over the disorder, raises confidence and increases independence. Initially it is the parents who are involved with the home treatment of their child and when the child gets older they too become increasingly involved in their own treatment.

The haemophilia nurse plays the key part in the education and care of the patient and their family. 'It is the role of the haemophilia nurse to provide flexibility, experience and knowledge, to give support, regular home assessment and act as a bridge between the family and the multidisciplinary hospital-based team' (Vidler 1999). Lasting relationships are formed with the nursing staff as this service is likely to be continued throughout the patients' entire lives.

Outlook for the future

The development of effective therapy for haemophilia has been a story of success combined with tragedy. Haemophilia treatment has been hampered by the human immunodeficiency virus (HIV) and hepatitis C transmitted via the early factor concentrates. However, the development of factor VIII/IX concentrates during the last three decades has revolutionised haemophilia care.

The introduction of plasma donor screening, viral inactivation methods and DNA technology into concentrate manufacturing has minimised the problem of new viral transmissions by clotting factor concentrate (Lusher 1995). The range of products available today for the treatment of haemophilia reflects the advances made in biotechnology and includes products produced in animal cell culture by recombinant gene therapy (Watson & Ludlam 1997).

Advances are also being made in gene therapy and trials have already started in some centres in the USA. It is hoped that gene therapy will result in the release of FVIII/FIX which may effectively convert someone with severe haemophilia into someone more mildly affected, thus reducing the number of episodes of spontaneous bleeding. With safer products and the possibility of 'cures', the future outlook looks positive for patients with haemophilia.

MYOTONIC DYSTROPHY

Myotonic dystrophy is a multisystem autosomal dominant condition (see p. 232) that presents with myotonia, slow relaxation of voluntary muscle after contraction, and progressive weakness and wasting of the facial, sternomastoid and distal muscles. The disorder is due to an expansion of the myotonic dystrophy gene located on the long arm of chromosome 19. The size of the expansion correlates broadly with the severity of the disease in the individual. The age of onset is variable but the majority of those who have the expanded myotonic dystrophy gene show some symptoms by the time they reach adult life. There is great variation in severity: some people with the expanded myotonic dystrophy gene can be so mildly affected that they are unaware of it, while others can have major problems. As inheritance is autosomal dominant, an affected individual of either sex has a 50% risk of passing the gene on to a child of either sex (see p. 232). The genetic abnormality is unstable and tends to increase in size as it is passed from one generation to the next. This explains the progressively earlier age of onset and greater severity of the disease as it is passed from generation to generation. Affected females are at risk of having a child with the severe congenital form of the disorder, as the expanded gene is thought to be more unstable when maternally inherited. Babies affected by congenital myotonic dystrophy present with respiratory failure, feeding difficulties and ongoing developmental problems requiring specialist multidisciplinary support. New mutations are thought to be rare and it should be assumed that all cases have been inherited unless there is positive evidence to the contrary. Myotonic dystrophy is no longer thought to be a rare disorder and is regarded as the most frequently occurring muscular dystrophy of adult life, affecting approximately 1 in 8000 of the population (Harper et al 2004).

Common presenting symptoms

The main muscle groups involved are facial, sternomastoid and the distal limb muscles. Other systems and associated problems may include:

- eyes — cataracts, ptosis (see Ch. 13)
- endocrine — diabetes mellitus (see Ch. 5)
- cardiac — mainly conduction defects (see Ch. 2)
- gastrointestinal tract — swallowing difficulties, constipation, diarrhoea and abdominal cramps (see Ch. 4)
- central nervous — variable cognitive impairment, specific personality changes in adults, somnolence (see Ch. 9)
- respiratory — muscle weakness, hypoventilation, anaesthesia risks (see Ch. 3).

NURSING PRIORITIES AND MANAGEMENT: Myotonic dystrophy

Major considerations

The prevention and management of complications

It is important that medical problems are diagnosed early and treated appropriately to prevent exacerbation and avoid complications. This should be stressed, both to those at risk and to those already affected. The severe degree of apathy characteristic of myotonic dystrophy can be a major obstacle to overcome and can be responsible for low attendance rates at clinics and lack of motivation in treatment regimens.

Myotonic dystrophy affects a number of body systems and thus requires careful management both in daily living and when particular medical problems arise. The multi-disciplinary team should be aware of the following points:

- Problems with anaesthesia may arise because the surgeons and anaesthetists are unaware that the patient has such a neuromuscular disorder. Individuals should be encouraged to wear a MedicAlert bracelet or to carry an alert card in case of accidents requiring surgery.
- Breathing exercises may help to reduce the tendency to hypoventilate. If there are signs of nocturnal hypoventilation, such as recurrent chest infections, morning headaches and increased daytime sleepiness, referral to the respiratory team will be required.
- When there is evidence of oesophageal/pharyngeal muscle weakness causing swallowing difficulty, it may be necessary to adjust the diet and to refer to the speech and language therapist (SALT), who may also help with speech difficulties due to weak facial muscles.
- Regular electrocardiograms (ECGs) should be carried out with appropriate medication as required. If there is evidence of conduction defects, a cardiac pacemaker may be considered.
- Cataract surgery is often required.
- Special obstetric care is necessary during pregnancy and delivery due to uterine muscle involvement, the increased risk of miscarriage and the risk of a congenitally affected baby.
- A high-fibre diet will help to alleviate constipation. Laxatives may be necessary.
- Sternomastoid weakness makes the use of headrests in cars imperative.
- Below-knee calipers or plastic moulded splints may help to control foot drop should it occur.

Psychological support

The diagnosis of a hereditary, slowly progressive muscle disorder of varying severity with associated multisystem involvement can have a profound psychological effect upon the individual and the family.

Living with myotonic dystrophy is not easy either for those affected, who have little energy or motivation, or for their partners or offspring. To live with someone who has an expressionless face, a monotonous voice, a marked lack of enthusiasm and may keep falling asleep, can put a great strain on a relationship. Sympathy and understanding are necessary for all family members.

Other forms of progressive muscular dystrophy include:

- Duchenne muscular dystrophy — inherited in an X-linked recessive form which usually affects boys and is severe
- Becker muscular dystrophy — also inherited in an X-linked recessive form which also affects boys but is less severe
- Facioscapulohumeral dystrophy — inherited in an autosomal dominant form with variable expression.

The Muscular Dystrophy Campaign (see 'Useful websites') is a charitable organisation which funds advisors who offer support and information to individuals affected by muscular dystrophy and their families.

HUNTINGTON'S DISEASE

Huntington's disease (HD), previously known as Huntington's chorea, is a progressive inherent neurodegenerative disorder, mainly of adult onset. Symptoms become apparent at any age but the average age of onset is normally between 40 and 50 years (Kremer 2002). There are, however, rare exceptions, with reports of symptoms starting as early as 2 years of age or as late as 80 years (Huntington's Disease Collaborative Research Group 1993). Approximately 7% of individuals with HD show symptoms before age 20 and are classed as having juvenile HD (Wells & Warren 1998).

The disease has a particularly rich historical literature which can be traced back to well over a century. The remarkable description of HD by George Huntington, an American physician, in 1872 has subsequently borne his name. The disease is characterised by an insidious onset which progresses over 15–20 years to a prominent and complex movement disorder, with changes in behaviour, mood and cognition. The incidence in the UK tends to vary between 5 and 10 per 100 000 (Bates et al 2002).

NEUROPATHOLOGY

The manifestation of symptoms and progression in HD is related to its neuropathology, characterised by loss of specific neuronal populations in many areas of the brain. The most striking neuropathological feature at autopsy of advanced HD patients is the gross atrophy of the caudate nucleus and putamen (see Ch. 9).

Genetics and testing

Huntington's disease is an autosomal dominant condition and therefore affects both sexes equally. Any offspring has a 50% chance of inheriting the faulty gene which will almost always mean that they will develop HD in their lifetime.

The gene mutation is confined to a small section on the short arm of chromosome 4 and has been named IT15. The gene codes for a protein called huntingtin whose function is not clearly understood. The gene is composed of three chemical bases — cytosine, adenine and guanine (CAG) — and is often referred to as a trinucleotide repeat. In the mutated HD gene, the first section is longer than normal and is associated with a CAG repeat size of 36 or more (Quarrell 1999). Individuals with a repeat size greater than 36 will eventually develop HD in almost every case.

In 1993 the Huntington's disease gene was identified. Following this, direct genetic testing became available and testing is now available at genetic centres throughout the UK.

Three categories of testing are discussed: predictive testing, diagnostic testing and prenatal testing.

Predictive testing

This test is carried out by DNA analysis of a blood sample and is available to asymptomatic individuals who should normally be 18 years or older and who have a family history

CASE HISTORY 6.3

E

E is 33 years old. Her father suffers from Huntington's disease (HD) and is cared for in a hospital for the chronically ill. Her younger sister, P, has early signs of the disease and the diagnosis has been confirmed by direct gene testing which shows that she is carrying the HD gene.

E has asked her general practitioner if she can be referred for genetic counselling. E is seen at the genetic department and is given information on the HD presymptomatic test protocol. She decides to go ahead with the test programme and understands that it involves four counselling sessions with staff in the genetic unit, including one with a specialist psychiatrist who will assess her coping mechanisms. Three months later, at the end of the programme, she is still sure that she wants a test because, for her, the uncertainty of being at risk of HD is even worse than knowing for certain that she has inherited the altered gene.

of HD. Genetic centres follow a strict testing protocol developed from guidelines set up by the Committee of the International Huntington's Association (IHA) and the working group on HD of the World Federation of Neurology (WFN) in 1994. The guidelines recommend that individuals at risk and considering testing should be seen for genetic counselling on two to four occasions over at least a 3-month period to allow them to consider fully the implications of testing prior to a blood sample being taken (see Case History 6.3). Post-test counselling should also be available and most centres will offer ongoing support whilst the individual remains asymptomatic, as well as monitoring of the disease as symptoms develop.

Diagnostic testing

This would also be undertaken by means of a blood test, but unlike predictive testing, it is carried out in someone thought to be symptomatic of HD, thus helping to confirm the diagnosis.

While the development of direct genetic testing has made the diagnosis of HD easier, it is still very much a clinical diagnosis matched by the demonstration of an expanded CAG repeat in the HD gene. A firm diagnosis will only be given with certainty when someone presents with specific extrapyramidal motor abnormalities, as opposed to minor motor abnormalities, subtle cognitive changes or psychiatric problems (Kremer 2002).

Prenatal testing

The isolation of the HD gene has given reproductive choices to couples who have an increased risk of passing on the genetic mutation associated with HD, although it has not proven to be a widely chosen option (Simpson et al 2002).

A parent who has tested positive for the faulty HD gene can have direct genetic testing carried out on the fetus during early pregnancy by means of chorionic villus sampling or amniocentesis. The decision to have this test is a considerable one with many complex questions to discuss including the ethics of such a procedure.

For further information about genetic testing, contact your nearest genetics department.

It is also possible for prenatal exclusion testing to be carried out when a parent is at 50% risk of having the faulty HD gene and does not want to risk passing it on, but does not want to have direct genetic testing themselves. This test is also carried out in early pregnancy using chorionic villus sampling or amniocentesis. Blood samples are required, however, from both parents and if possible, both grandparents on the affected side of the family or from several other family members. Family linkage analysis is used in this technique. If the fetus has inherited the gene from the grandparent who is from the unaffected side of the family, then the child has virtually no risk. If the gene is inherited from the grandparent who is affected, the risk to the fetus is 50%, which is the same as that of the at-risk parent, as it is not identified whether it is the affected grandparent's 'normal' or faulty gene that is passed on.

Ethically, this also leaves difficult decisions to be made, as the parents may decide to terminate a pregnancy where there is only a 50% risk.

It is also important to consider that invasive tests in early pregnancy do carry an increased risk of miscarriage.

Preimplantation genetic diagnosis (PGD) is a relatively new technique combining in vitro fertilisation (IVF) with genetic testing. Using PGD in Huntington's disease offers an opportunity to couples where one partner has the faulty HD gene, to avoid passing the faulty gene on to their children. This specialist technique is only offered at a limited number of centres in the UK.

Common presenting symptoms

The early symptoms of adult onset Huntington's disease can be very subtle. Throughout the illness, individuals usually demonstrate a combination of complex motor, cognitive and emotional or psychiatric symptoms, but there is wide individual variation in how these symptoms present.

Motor symptoms There are two parts to the movement disorder of HD: the presence of involuntary movements and the impairment of voluntary movements. Some people with the illness initially have problems with motor control. This can lead to choreic movements, which may be noticed as jerks, twitches or exaggerated gestures. Changes in balance and coordination can also occur at this stage, leading to clumsiness and difficulty carrying out tasks that require fine motor control.

As the disease progresses, chorea tends to become more obvious and incapacitating. In many patients, however, chorea eventually peaks and then begins to decline, with rigidity and bradykinesia (slowness of movements) becoming more significant.

Over a number of years, motor symptoms worsen, such that walking difficulties become more pronounced. As a result, the individual is at high risk of falls with significant associated morbidity and, ultimately, confinement to a wheelchair (Kremer 2002). Speech is often affected early in the illness, often as a mild disturbance of clarity which deteriorates as the disease progresses, causing significant communication difficulties. Dysphagia generally occurs late in the illness, resulting in an increased risk of aspiration. In the advanced stages of the disease, there is a significant loss of independence and functioning with patients being highly dependent on others for most, if not all, aspects of their care.

Although the motor symptoms of Huntington's disease are often the most visible, it is often the non-motor symptoms that have the greatest impact on patients' and families' daily lives. For some people, changes in mood or personality may be the first symptoms of the disease, for example having sudden changes in mood, being irritable or making irrational judgements. Depression and anxiety can also occur at this stage, as well as difficulty concentrating and forgetfulness. As a result, it is often only in retrospect, once a diagnosis has been made, that families recall these changes as being the onset of the disease.

Cognitive symptoms The cognitive disorder in HD is characterised by impaired memory and executive function, and slowed thinking.

Executive functions which are affected include organising, prioritising and regulating information, as well as impulse control and flexible thinking. Impairments in executive functioning can lead to difficulties in judgement, problem solving, divided attention, irritability and disinhibition. Processing of information is also slower so that more time is required to answer questions and complete routine tasks. Cognitive changes vary in severity between individuals but in most cases become more severe as the disease progresses (Craufurd & Snowden 2002).

Psychiatric symptoms can occur at any stage of the disease and vary amongst individuals.

The most common psychiatric disorder in patients with Huntington's disease is depression, which is thought to occur in up to 40% of individuals at some stage of the disease (Quarrell 1999). Anxiety, changes in personality and apathy are also common symptoms (Caine & Shoulson 1983).

Other less common psychiatric disorders that can occur include bipolar disorder, obsessive–compulsive symptoms and psychosis.

Management

Huntington's disease is a very complex condition and the issues that confront patients and their families span the expertise of many professionals and are best met by a coordinated multidisciplinary approach. As there is currently no preventive or curative treatment for HD, the goals of management are to reduce symptoms, maintain independence and improve quality of life.

Most people with Huntington's disease will live at home with support until the more advanced stages of the disease, when some will need long-term care. Nursing staff may, however, come into contact with patients with HD at any stage of their illness in a variety of settings.

In the early stages of the disease, management is mainly concerned with ensuring that individuals have accurate information and access to support services. The main issues with which patients may need support at this stage include employment, driving and finance as well as emotional support for themselves and their families. Cognitive changes may be apparent and the patient will benefit from assistance in looking at strategies to aid daily living such as using reminders, calendars and lists and establishing routines.

Baseline assessments of cognitive functioning, nutritional state and dysphagia may also be carried out.

As the disease progresses, management of symptoms should be regularly reviewed.

MEDICAL MANAGEMENT

It is important that the clinical features of HD are assessed and disease progression monitored. Patients may be seen by a variety of medical specialists at different stages of their illness, depending on the most significant clinical problems, or be monitored solely by their GP. Pharmacological treatments of the psychiatric features of the disease are available and can be successful in treating these symptoms. Such treatments are also available to manage the involuntary movements present in HD.

Chorea, whilst being a highly visible symptom, may not be distressing to the patient, however, and it is important to remember that medications used to suppress chorea can have side-effects, including worsening of voluntary motor control. It is advisable, therefore, to consider non-pharmacological interventions in the management of chorea, which can include exercise, massage, stress reduction and relaxation.

As the symptoms of HD change over time, any medication used should be reviewed regularly.

NURSING PRIORITIES AND MANAGEMENT: Huntington's disease

Mobility

The movement disorder present in HD affects an individual's mobility, which will deteriorate over time, with falls becoming common. The main management of falls involves risk assessment of the patient and modification of the environment. It is important to involve occupational therapists and physiotherapists to assess functioning and mobility, advise on strategies and provide aids and adaptations to assist daily living. For example, furniture with sharp corners should be avoided and obstacles minimised. Specialist seating, padded bed sides and adapted wheelchairs can assist with the patient's comfort and minimise the risks or injury.

Swallowing

Dysphagia is common in HD and is, directly or indirectly, a common cause of death in people with advanced stage HD. This is often due to choking, aspiration or malnutrition. Dysphagia results from impaired voluntary control of the muscles involved in swallowing, impaired respiratory control and impaired judgement, which can result in eating too quickly or taking too large mouthfuls. A referral to a speech and language therapist will allow for an assessment of the patient's swallowing and provide advice on the most appropriate consistency of food and fluids.

Devices such as large-grip cutlery, non-slip mats, plate guards and spout-lid cups can help maintain independent eating. Patients should be encouraged to eat slowly and deliberately, to take small bites and to clear their mouth of food between bites. Sitting upright with the chin tucked down is the optimal position for swallowing as this reduces the risk of aspiration. Distractions should be kept to a minimum whilst eating, as patients may be distracted by noise such as from the television. Patients may need observation and supervision at mealtimes and will eventually require assistance with eating. Dysphagia may result in weight loss.

Diet

Weight loss is common in HD and patients will generally require a higher calorific intake to maintain their body weight. This is partly to do with increased energy requirements due to choreic movements and partly (though not yet fully understood) to increased resting basal expenditure. Referral to a dietitian will be made for nutritional assessment and nutritional supplements may be recommended. Patients should be weighed and reviewed regularly.

For patients who have severe dysphagia and/or significant weight loss, alternative feeding methods may be considered, the most common of these being percutaneous endoscopic gastrostomy (PEG) tube feeding. This is, however, a very individual decision and ideally an individual should be given an opportunity to discuss this early in their illness, as their capacity to make decisions may be affected as the disease progresses.

Communication

Communication is greatly compromised in HD and deteriorates over time due to impairment of the muscles involved in speech production as well as cognitive changes, such as lack of initiation and word retrieval. It is extremely important that communication is maintained for as long as possible and general strategies include allowing more time for conversation, minimising distractions, using prompts, simple closed questions and communication boards. Assessment by a speech and language therapist is recommended. For individuals whose ability to communicate is impaired it is often helpful to make up a life story book with photos and information about their life, friends and family and likes and dislikes. This allows for a means of communication as well as ensuring that any new staff are able to learn about the patient. It is important to remember that it is very likely that a high degree of awareness and comprehension will still be present even when the patient is unable to communicate verbally.

Behavioural changes

Due to the cognitive changes that occur in HD, a patient may be distracted, irritable, confused, uncooperative or withdrawn. They may demand that you respond immediately, become aggressive if their needs are not met, and may not be able to consider the consequences of their actions. This can be very challenging, but it is vital not to take the patient's behaviour personally and remember that the behaviour is a direct result of the changes taking place in the brain. Patients with HD can have little control over their impulses and emotions, become very inflexible and appear to make irrational judgements.

It is important to look carefully at any difficult situations to try to establish the exact cause and any precipitating factors that might be avoided in future. It is also important, when managing behavioural changes, to be willing to try several strategies and develop a team approach. Ensuring that the patient has a very structured routine and that distractions are minimised can also help manage behavioural changes. Any sudden changes in behaviour may have been caused by head injury following a fall, infection, side-effects of medication or other illnesses that may need further investigation.

Personal care

As the disease advances, patients will have more difficulty managing their personal care and will require assistance in areas such as bathing and dressing. Patients sometimes find it difficult to make judgements about their personal appearance and may resist taking a shower or brushing their teeth, or may have difficulties with initiation and simply require prompting. In order to help a patient maintain some independence as well as being more practical, it is often easier if clothing is loose and comfortable with limited buttons and zips. Many patients with HD have problems with temperature control and may complain of being too hot or too cold. It is necessary therefore to attempt to ensure that the environment is comfortable for the patient's individual needs.

Incontinence can be a problem for some patients in the later stages of the illness and should be investigated to rule out causes such as urine infection. Patients may benefit from protective underwear and regular toileting (see Ch. 24). Using the toilet can also cause difficulties for patients who are still mobile and, due to a decreasing ability to regulate movement and possible problems with visual and spatial impairment, patients often 'flop' down onto the toilet seat, potentially loosening fixtures or causing injury.

Many patients with HD smoke and it is important to ensure that this is done safely to reduce the risk of fire and burns.

It is important to ensure that patients who are losing their independence are treated as valued individuals and are cared for with dignity and respect. Seeing a loved one becoming more debilitated by HD can be devastating for families and their grief is compounded by the fact that other family members may also be affected or at risk of HD. It is therefore vital that a support network is put in place, not only for the patient with HD but also for their family. Caring for a patient with HD is undoubtedly challenging, but can also be greatly rewarding and optimal care can result in a major improvement in the patient's quality of life.

The Scottish Huntington's Association and the Huntington's Disease Association of England and Wales have professional advisors who can offer emotional support to individuals and families as well as offering specialist assessment, advice and information on HD and its management (see 'Useful Websites').

CANCER GENETICS

Cancer genetics is a relatively new subject and is becoming an increasingly demanding aspect of the work of all genetics departments. As knowledge advances and more is understood about cancer genetics, the possibilities for testing will increase.

At a cellular level, all cancers, both sporadic and inherited, are genetic (Kingston 2002). The latter may be due to inherited changes in the genes directly involved in normal cellular growth and proliferation or to genetic changes resulting in the increased possibility of a mutation in the genes related to cell growth. The formation of a human cancer is a multistep process and is the result of a series of mutations in a single cell. Genes with a positive effect on growth and proliferation of cells are known as oncogenes, and those with a negative effect as tumour suppressor genes or anti-oncogenes (Hodgson & Maher 1999). Oncogenes and tumour suppressor genes are often referred to as the 'gatekeeper' genes (Kinzler & Vogelstein 1997). Activation of oncogenes and inactivation of tumour suppressor genes are both important in the formation of the malignant cell (Hodgson & Maher 1999).

A third class of genes has been identified which is also known to predispose to malignancy. These genes are involved in DNA mismatch repair. Their role is to maintain the integrity of the genome (Hodgson & Maher 1999) and they are referred to as the 'caretaker' genes (Kinzler & Vogelstein 1997).

The aims of cancer genetics include:

- the identification of a subgroup of the population who are at significantly increased risk of developing cancer
- reduction of mortality from 'common' cancers, e.g. breast, ovarian and colorectal, by offering appropriate screening or surgery for those at increased risk
- reassurance and discharge from screening for those not at increased risk compared with the general population risk.

Cancer is a common disease, said to affect 1 in 3 people in their lifetime (see Chs 31 and 35). Therefore, chance may account for the apparently high incidence of 'common' cancers in some families (Eeles et al 2004). However, factors which may imply a genetic predisposition to cancer are:

- a family history of cancer on one side of the family with an autosomal dominant pattern of inheritance. The cancers may be the same or with a known association, e.g. breast and ovarian
- onset of cancer at a young age (under 50 years)
- the presence of multiple primary tumours or bilateral tumours in an individual
- the presence of rare cancers.

The detection of an identifiable germline mutation in a relevant gene, in an affected family member, would be regarded as confirmation of an inherited predisposition to cancer within a family (Hodgson & Maher 1999).

Familial breast cancer

Two genes (BRCA1 and BRCA2) have been found to influence the occurrence of familial breast cancer and may be responsible for approximately 5–10% of breast cancers (Mitchell & Eeles 1999). The BRCA1 gene was cloned in 1994 (Futreal et al 1994) and over 100 different mutations have been identified so far. The overall lifetime risk of breast cancer for those with a BRCA1 mutation is up to 87% (Thompson et al 2002). The BRCA2 gene was cloned in 1995 (Wooster et al 1995). The overall lifetime risk of breast cancer for those with a BRCA2 mutation is up to 84% (Ford et al 1998). There is an increased risk of ovarian cancer in those with a BRCA1 or BRCA2 mutation. Mutations in BRCA2 are more likely to be implicated in families with cases of male breast cancer. It is apparent that BRCA1/BRCA2 do not account for all familial breast/ovarian cancer families. Research is ongoing for new gene mutations.

Unless the history is from the paternal side of the family, women at increased risk of breast cancer are recorded as those with a first-degree relative (mother, father, sister, brother, daughter or son) affected by cancer within a family that meets one of the following criteria:

- one first-degree relative who developed breast cancer under the age of 40 years or a male with breast cancer at any age
- two first- or first- and second-degree relatives on the same side of the family who developed breast cancer under the age of 60 years or with ovarian cancer
- three first- or first- and second-degree relatives on the same side of the family with breast or ovarian cancer at any age. One first-degree relative unless history is from the paternal side
- one first-degree relative with breast cancer in both breasts (separate primary cancers)
- one first-degree relative with breast and ovarian cancer.

Screening

The options available for women at an increased risk of developing breast cancer include screening by mammography and breast examination. Screening protocols vary nationally. The following approach is adopted in Scotland (Scottish Cancer Group 2001):

- From age 35 or 5 years younger than the earliest onset of breast cancer in the family (rarely under the age of 30) mammography is offered every 2 years and clinical breast examination every year.
- From age 40–50 years a mammography and clinical breast examination is offered every year.

The National Breast Screening Programme offers 3-yearly screening with mammography for women from age 50 to 70 years (see Ch. 7).

High-risk women over age 50, e.g. BRCA1 or BRCA2 gene carriers, may be offered 18-monthly breast examination and mammography; however, this depends on local amendments to guidelines.

The sensitivity of mammography improves with age as the glandular tissue is replaced by fat (involution) so the breast becomes less radiodense, softer and droopy. This process of involution begins after the age of 30.

The UK National Study of Magnetic Resonance Imaging (MRI), called the MARIBS research, has assessed the value of MRI as a method of screening for young women at an increased risk of developing breast cancer (Leach 2002).

Clinical trials assessing the value of tamoxifen in the prevention of breast cancer in women with a family history have reported mixed results. The overall risks with tamoxifen use and benefits in prevention remain unclear (IBIS 2002) (see Chs 7, Part 2, and 31).

Prophylactic surgery — risk-reducing mastectomies

Women who have, or are likely to have, a gene mutation may elect for prophylactic surgery. This may seem a drastic course of action (Hatcher et al 2001), but is acceptable to some women who have seen a number of their relatives suffer from breast cancer.

Aspects for discussion regarding this include (Eeles 1996):

- the surgical technique to be used — subcutaneous or total mastectomy

- surgery to remove enough breast tissue to prevent the development of invasive breast cancer, i.e. wide local incision (WLE)
- minimisation of psychological complications.

Women with a high risk of developing breast cancer due to a family history or to being a carrier of a BRCA1/BRCA2 mutation, also have the option of prophylactic salpingo-oophorectomy. This has been shown not only to reduce their risk of ovarian cancer, but also to significantly reduce their risk of breast cancer by up to 50% (see Ch. 7, Part 2).

Familial ovarian cancer

Two types of ovarian cancer susceptibility genes have been identified: the breast and ovarian cancer tumour suppressor genes (BRCA1 and BRCA2) and the mismatch repair genes associated with hereditary non-polyposis colon cancer (HNPCC) families (see p. 249). Mutations in the BRCA1 gene are estimated to confer an increased ovarian cancer risk of up to 66% (Thompson et al 2002) and mutations in the BRCA2 gene an increased risk of up to 27% (Ford et al 1998). The mismatch repair genes confer an increased lifetime risk of ovarian cancer of approximately 12% in addition to an increased risk of endometrial cancer (Aarnio et al 1999).

At present, relatively few patients are classed as high risk because a mutation in a cancer predisposing gene has been detected in their family. In most cases, risk estimates are based on family history. The following list defines women who are at greater than five times the population risk of ovarian cancer based upon family history (Thompson et al 2002). Screening protocols vary nationally.

Women at increased risk of ovarian cancer are those with a first-degree relative (mother, father, sister, brother, daughter or son) affected by cancer within a family that meets one of the following criteria:

- two or more individuals with ovarian cancer, who are first-degree relatives of each other
- one individual with ovarian cancer at any age, and one with breast cancer diagnosed under age 50 years, who are first-degree relatives of each other
- one relative with ovarian cancer at any age, and two with breast cancer diagnosed under 60 years, who are connected by first-degree relationships
- known BRCA1 or BRCA2 (or other relevant cancer gene mutation) carrier
- untested first-degree relative of a predisposing gene carrier
- three or more family members with colon cancer, or two with colon cancer and one with stomach, ovary, endometrial, urinary tract or small colorectal cancer in two generations, one with cancer under age 50 years
- an individual with both breast and ovarian cancer.

The options available to these women to manage their increased risk of ovarian cancer include screening or prophylactic salpingo-oophorectomy.

Screening

Survival in ovarian cancer is dependent on stage at presentation. The 5-year survival rate for Stage I disease is over 85%, whereas Stage IV is approximately 10%. Therefore, detecting ovarian cancer early through screening has the potential to have a major impact on prognosis. Unfortunately, the effectiveness of screening for ovarian cancer has yet to be demonstrated (Scottish Cancer Group 2001). Studies are investigating the use of the CA125 tumour marker and transvaginal ultrasound at variable frequencies.

Prophylactic surgery

The alternative to screening for women at an increased risk is prophylactic salpingo-oophorectomy. Recent studies have confirmed that the risk of both ovarian and primary peritoneal carcinoma (a cancer indistinguishable from ovarian cancer) is reduced by 90% following prophylactic surgery in BRCA1/BRCA2 mutation carriers (Kauff et al 2002, Rebbeck 2002). There is also a reduction in breast cancer risk, which is very significant given that most women at increased risk of ovarian cancer are also at increased risk of breast cancer.

Hereditary non-polyposis cancer of the colon (HNPCC)

Almost all cases of HNPCC are due to a germline mutation in one of the known DNA mismatch repair (MMR) genes (Vasen et al 1991). HNPCC is defined by the number of individuals in a family diagnosed with an HNPCC-related cancer (see below), their age at diagnosis and their relationship to each other.

There are internationally agreed diagnostic criteria, known as Amsterdam criteria, for identifying HNPCC families. Initially, only colorectal cancers were considered in these criteria. Further research has identified a spectrum of cancers in HNPCC families and the modified Amsterdam criteria have been established (Vasen et al 1999). Families meeting the criteria below are given a high genetic risk.

At least three relatives must have a cancer associated with hereditary non-polyposis colorectal cancer (colorectal, endometrial, stomach, ovary, ureter or renal pelvis, brain, small colorectal, hepato-biliary tract or skin (sebaceous) tumours):

- one must be a first-degree relative of the other two
- at least two successive generations must be affected
- at least one of the relatives with cancer associated with hereditary non-polyposis colorectal cancer should have received the diagnosis before the age of 50 years
- familial adenomatous polyposis must have been excluded in any relative with colorectal cancer
- tumours should be verified whenever possible.

Several HNPCC genes have been identified. The three genes most commonly associated with HNPCC are MLH1, MSH2 and MSH6. HNPCC gene carriers have an increased risk of developing the cancers shown in Table 6.1.

The options available to these individuals to manage their increased risk of cancer include screening and/or prophylactic surgery. Screening recommendations for those at high risk differ throughout the country but all include colonoscopy at varying intervals. Screening recommendations in Scotland (Scottish Cancer Group 2001) are:

- 2-yearly colonoscopy, from age 30 or 5 years younger than the youngest affected until age 70

Table 6.1 Gene carrier risk of developing cancer

Cancer type	Gene carrier risk (%)
Colorectal, male	74
Colorectal, female	30
Endometrial	42
Ovarian	12
Gastric	7
Biliary tract	9
Uroepithelial	8
Kidney	5
Brain	4.5

Adapted from Aarnio et al (1999).

- gynaecological screening for ovarian and endometrial cancer, from age 35 years
- 2-yearly upper gastrointestinal endoscopy, from age 50 or 5 years younger than youngest onset of stomach cancer.

In addition, consideration needs to be given to screening for other cancers which may occur in specific families that are part of the HNPCC spectrum.

Prophylactic colorectal surgery may be considered, particularly if numerous polyps are identified through screening. Women may wish to consider prophylactic gynaecological surgery.

Only a small proportion of families will meet the modified Amsterdam criteria. However, a greater proportion of families will be identified at a moderately increased risk above the population risk; for these moderate risk families, colonoscopy screening is offered less frequently.

Familial adenomatous polyposis coli (FAP)

FAP affects 1 in 8000 of the population (Burn & Chapman 1994). It is inherited in an autosomal dominant fashion with almost complete penetrance, although 25% of cases seem to arise from a new (sporadic) mutation (Dunlop 2002). FAP is characterised by hundreds to thousands of adenomatous polyps, which are present mainly in the large intestine and rectum but can occur in the upper digestive tract. The vast number of polyps makes it highly likely that a cancer will occur (Scott et al 2001, Dunlop 2002). As these polyps are usually present by the teenage years, at-risk individuals are screened by flexible sigmoidoscopy from the age of 13. Annual screening is recommended until the age of 30 years and thereafter screening can be offered on a 3- to 5-yearly basis until age 60 years (Dunlop 2002). If no polyps are identified by the age of 60 years, the individual is deemed not to be at risk and screening is usually discontinued. Cancer commonly occurs at the mean age of 40 years (Jarvinen 2003) and prophylactic colectomy is indicated in the early 20s in individuals with recurrent polyps at screening. The operation of choice is a proctocolectomy and ileoanal pouch (Dunlop 2002).

Extracolonic tumours can be found in FAP. These can be bone and soft tissue abnormalities such as papillary thyroid tumours, abdominal desmoid tumours, osteomas, epidermoid cysts and hepatoblastomas. Tumours can also occur in the upper gastrointestinal tract (Chung et al 2003). Screening of the upper gastrointestinal tract is offered at 3-yearly intervals from the age of 25 years.

FAP is caused by a single gene fault on chromosome 5 (APC gene) and mutations can be unique to individual families (Jarvinen 2003). The disease and severity within the family can be variable (Crabtree et al 2001). There are some families where the gene fault cannot be identified and direct gene testing will not be available to other family members at risk. There is a milder form of this condition called attenuated FAP, where the onset is in the later years and there is a reduced number of polyps present. The mutations in these cases are generally located in the extreme end of the APC gene. Early identification of cases and prophylactic surgery have improved the survival rate in FAP (Dunlop 2002).

Genetic testing for cancer predisposition

The availability of gene testing is currently limited to families with a strong history of breast, ovarian or colorectal cancers. However, as more cancer susceptibility genes are identified and more is understood about their role in the aetiology of cancer, an increasing number of tests may become available. Cancer genetics is a rapidly developing field and guidelines for risk assessment, screening and genetic testing are continuously being reviewed and developed.

Genetic modification and gene therapy

There are a number of ways in which human gene therapy could potentially be used (Resnick & Langer 2001): genes could be deleted from somatic cells, genetic mutations corrected or missing genes introduced. This would affect only the individual being treated and has been judged by controlling committees as acceptable practice in most cases. Currently gene therapy is not part of clinical practice but this may change with future advances. Debate continues over ethical issues related to the potential practice of gene modification or therapy.

CONCLUSION

In the field of human genetics the use of scientific knowledge raises ethical and moral problems, particularly where every advance has an enormous potential for good and evil. Recognition of the destructive potential of genetic engineering has prompted the imposition of strict controls on biotechnology and genetic research. This chapter has presented an outline of current developments in genetics and molecular biology. It has outlined nursing involvement in genetic counselling and care of patients with genetic disorders. The information gained from the Human Genome

Project and related genetic research will undoubtedly create significant changes in health care practice. As public awareness continues to grow, individuals and families are increasingly requesting genetic counselling. All health care providers, in particular nurses, will therefore require a fundamental understanding of basic genetic concepts and genetic influences on health and disease. Consequently, it is imperative for nurses to be well informed.

REFERENCES

Aarnio M, Sankila R, Pukkala E et al 1999 Cancer risk in mutation carriers of DNA mismatch repair genes. International Journal of Cancer 81: 214–218

Association of Chartered Physiotherapists in Cystic Fibrosis 2002 Clinical guidelines for the physiotherapy management of cystic fibrosis. CF Trust, Kent

Bates G, Harper P, Jones L 2002 Huntington's disease, 3rd edn. Oxford University Press, Oxford

Bonthron D, Fitzpatrick D, Porteous M et al 1997 Clinical genetics – a case-based approach. Saunders, Philadelphia

Burn J, Chapman P 1994 Familial adenomatous polyposis. Archives of Disease in Childhood 71: 103–107

Caine E D, Shoulson I 1983 Psychiatric syndromes in Huntington's disease. American Journal of Psychiatry 140: 728–733

Chung D C, Mino M, Shannon K M 2003 Case 34-2003. A 45 year old woman with a family history of colonic polyps and cancer. New England Journal of Medicine 349: 1750–1760

Colman R W, Hirsh J, Marder V J et al 1994 Haemostasis and thrombosis: basic principles and clinical practice, 3rd edn. Lippincott, Philadelphia

Corey M, McLaughlin F J, Williams M et al 1988 A comparison of survival, growth and pulmonary function in patients with cystic fibrosis in Boston and Toronto. Journal of Clinical Epidemiology 41: 583–591

Crabtree M D, Tomlinson I P M, Talbot I C et al 2001 Variability in the severity of colonic disease in familial adenomatous polyposis results from differences in tumour initiation rather than progression and depends relatively little on patient age. Gut 49: 540–543

Craufurd D, Snowden J 2002 Neuropsychological and neuropsychiatric aspects of Huntington's disease. In: Bates G, Harper P, Jones L (eds) Huntington's disease. Oxford University Press, New York

Cystic Fibrosis Trust 2001 Growing older with CF. A handbook for adults. CF Trust, Kent

Department of Health 2003 Our inheritance, our future – realizing the potential of genetics in the NHS. TSO, London

Dunlop M G 2002 Guidance on gastrointestinal surveillance for hereditary non-polyposis colorectal cancer, familial adenomatous polyposis coli, juvenile polyposis and Peutz–Jeghers syndrome. Gut 51: 21–27

Edenborough F P, Mackenzie W E, Stableforth D E 2000 The outcome of 72 pregnancies in 55 women with cystic fibrosis in the United Kingdom 1977–1996. British Journal of Obstetrics and Gynaecology 107: 254–261

Eeles R 1996 Testing for the breast cancer predisposition gene BRCA1. British Medical Journal 313: 572–573

Eeles R, Easton D F, Ponder B et al (eds) 2004 Genetic predisposition to cancer, 2nd edn. Hodder Arnold, London

Egan T M, Detterbeck F C, Mill M R et al 2002 Long term results of lung transplantation for cystic fibrosis. European Journal of Thoracic Surgery 22(4): 602–609

Elborn J S, Shale D J, Britton J R 1991 Cystic fibrosis: current survival and population estimates to the year 2000. Thorax 46: 881–885

Equi A, Balfour-Lynn I M, Bush A et al 2002 Long term azithromycin in children with cystic fibrosis: a randomized placebo-controlled crossover trial. Lancet 360(9338): 978–984

Ford D, Easton D F, Stratton M 1998 Genetic heterogeneity and penetrance analysis of the BRCA1 and BRCA2 genes in breast cancer families. American Journal of Human Genetics 62: 676–689

Futreal P A, Lui Q, Shattuck-Eidens D et al 1994 BRCA1 mutations in primary breast and ovarian carcinomas. Science 266(5183): 120–122

Genyk Y S, Quiros J A, Jabbour N et al 2001 Liver transplantation in cystic fibrosis. Current Opinions in Pulmonary Medicine 7(6): 441–447

Haemophilia Alliance 2001 A national service specification for haemophilia and related conditions. Haemophilia Alliance, London

Haemophilia Society 1997a Haemophilia and school – guidelines for teachers of children with haemophilia and von Willebrand's disease, 3rd edn. The Haemophilia Society, London

Haemophilia Society 1997b Haemophilia and inhibitors. The Haemophilia Society, London

Hallyar K M, Williams S G, Wise A E et al 1997 A prognostic model for the prediction of survival in cystic fibrosis. Thorax 52: 313–317

Harper P 2004 Practical genetic counselling, 6th edn. Hodder Arnold, London

Harper P, von Engelen B, Eymard B et al 2004 Myotonic dystrophy: present management, future therapy. Oxford University Press, Oxford

Hatcher M, Hern R, Fallowfield L 2001 The psychological impact of bilateral prophylactic mastectomy: prospective study using questionnaires and semistructured interviews. British Medical Journal 322: 76

Haworth C S, Selby P L, Webb A K 1999 Low bone mineral density in adults with cystic fibrosis. Thorax 54: 961–967

Hodgson S, Maher E 1999 A practical guide to human cancer genetics. Cambridge University Press, Cambridge

Hodson M E, Gallagher C G, Govan J 2002 A randomized clinical trial of nebulised tobramycin or colistin in cystic fibrosis. European Respiratory Journal 20(3): 658–664

Huntington's Disease Collaborative Research Group 1993 A novel gene containing a trinucleotide repeat that is expanded and unstable on Huntington's disease chromosomes. Cell 72: 971–983

IBIS 2002 First results from the International Breast Cancer Intervention Study (IBIS-1): a randomised prevention trial. Lancet 360(9336): 817–824

Jarvinen H J 2003 Genetic testing for polyposis: practical and ethical aspects. Gut 52(Suppl 1): ii19–ii22

Kauff N D, Satagopan J M, Robson M E 2002 Risk-reducing salpingo-oophorectomy in women with BRCA1 or BRCA2 mutation. New England Journal of Medicine 346(21): 1609–1615

Kingston H M 2002 ABC of clinical genetics, 3rd edn. BMJ Books, London

Kinzler K W, Vogelstein B 1997 Cancer susceptibility genes: gatekeepers and caretakers. Nature 386(6627): 761–763

Koch C, Lang S 1995 Other organ systems. In: Hodson M, Geddes D (eds) Cystic fibrosis. Chapman and Hall, London

Kremer B 2002 Clinical neurology in Huntington's disease. In: Bates G, Harper P, Jones L (eds) Huntington's disease. Oxford University Press, New York

Leach M O 2002 The UK study of magnetic resonance imaging as a method of screening for breast cancer (MARIBS). Journal of Experimental Clinical Cancer Research 21(Suppl): 3

Liddle K, Charlton J, Innes J A et al 1998 Collaborative care in cystic fibrosis related diabetes mellitus. Paediatric Pulmonology 17(Suppl): 350

Lowton K, Gabe J 2003 Life on a slippery slope: perceptions of health in adults with cystic fibrosis. Sociology of Health and Illness 25(4): 289–319

Lusher J M 1995 Considerations for recurrent and future management of haemophilia versus its complications. Haemophilia 1: 2–10

Mitchell G, Eeles R 1999 The breast cancer predisposition genes, BRCA1 and BRCA2: cancer risks and predictive genetic testing. Cancer Topics 11: 1

NHS Scotland 2003 Information for health professionals in pregnancy and newborn screening. Scottish Executive, Edinburgh

Nir M, Laang S, Johansen H K et al 1996 Long term survival and nutritional data in patients with cystic fibrosis treated in a Danish center. Thorax 51: 1023–1027

Nousia-Arvanitakis S M D, Fotoulaki M M D, Economou H et al 2001 Long-term prospective study of the effect of ursodeoxycholic acid on cystic fibrosis-related liver disease. Journal of Clinical Gastroenterology 32(4): 324–328

Proud J 1995 Ethics and obstetric ultrasound. British Journal of Midwifery 3(2): 79–82
Quarrell O 1999 Huntington's disease: the facts. Oxford University Press, New York
Rebbeck T R 2002 Prophylactic oophorectomy in BRCA1 and BRCA2 mutation carriers. European Journal of Cancer 38(Suppl 6): S15–17
Resnik D B, Langer P J 2001 Human germline gene therapy reconsidered. Human Gene Therapy 12(11): 1449–1458
Rizza C 1997 Clinical features and diagnosis of haemophilia, Christmas disease and von Willebrand's disease. Haemophilia and other inherited bleeding disorders. Saunders, London
Rodriguez-Merchan E C, Goddard N J, Lee C A 2000 Musculoskeletal aspects of haemophilia. Blackwell Science, Oxford
Scott R J, Meldrum C, Crooks R et al 2001 Familial adenomatous polyposis: more evidence for disease diversity and genetic heterogeneity. Gut 48: 508–514
Scottish Cancer Group 2001 Cancer genetic services in Scotland. Guidance to support the implementation of genetic services for breast, ovarian and colorectal cancer predisposition. Scottish Executive, Edinburgh
Simpson S, Zoeteweij M, Nys K et al 2002 Prenatal testing for Huntington's disease: a European collaborative study. European Journal of Human Genetics 10(11): 689–693
Skirton H, Patch C 2002 Genetics for health care professionals. BIOS Scientific, Oxford
Skirton H, Barnes C, Curtis G et al 1997 The role and practice of the genetic nurse: report of the AGNC Working Party. Journal of Medical Genetics 34(12): 141–147
Thompson D, Easton D F, Breast Cancer Linkage Consortium 2002 Cancer incidence in BRCA1 mutation carriers. Journal of the National Cancer Institute 94(18): 1358–1365
UK Cystic Fibrosis Nurse Specialist Group 2001 National consensus standards for the nursing management of cystic fibrosis. CF Trust, Kent
UKHCDO 1994 United Kingdom Haemophilia Centre Doctors' Organisation guidelines. UKHCDO, Oxford
Vasen H F A, Mecklin J P, Khan P M et al 1991 The international collaborative group on hereditary non-polyposis colorectal cancer (ICG-HNPCC). Diseases of the Colon and Rectum 34: 424–425
Vasen H F A, Mecklin J P, Khan P M 1999 New clinic criteria for hereditary non-polyposis colorectal cancer (HNPCC Lynch syndrome) proposed by the International Collaborative Group on HNPCC. Gastroenterology 116: 1453
Vidler V 1999 Teaching parents advanced clinical skills. Haemophilia 5: 349–353
Walters S, Britton J, Hodson M E 1993 Demographic and social characteristics of adults with cystic fibrosis in the United Kingdom. British Medical Journal 306(6877): 549–552
Watson H G, Ludlam C A 1997 Replacement therapy and other therapeutic products. Haemophilia and other inherited bleeding disorders. Saunders, London
Webb A K, Dodd M E 2000 Exercise and training for adults with cystic fibrosis. In: Hodson M E, Geddes D M (eds) Cystic fibrosis, 2nd edn. Arnold, London
Wells R, Warren S 1998 Genetic instabilities and hereditary neurological diseases. Academic Press, New York
Westaby D 1995 Liver and biliary disease. In: Hodson M, Geddes D (eds) Cystic fibrosis. Chapman and Hall, London
Wooster R, Bignell G, Lancaster J et al 1995 Identification of the breast susceptibility gene BRCA2. Nature 378: 789–791
World Federation of Haemophilia 2004 What is haemophilia? WFH, Quebec

FURTHER READING

Calzone K A, Biesecker B B 2002 Genetic testing for cancer predisposition. Cancer Nursing 25: 15–25
Emery J, Lucassen A, Murphy M 2001 Common hereditary cancers and implications for primary care. Lancet 358: 56–63
Francis S, Collins M M, Aristides P 2003 The Human Genome Project: lessons from large-scale biology. Science 300: 286–290
Haemophilia Alliance 2001 A national service specification for haemophilia and related conditions. Haemophilia Alliance, London
Harper P S, van Engelen B, Eymard B et al 2004 Myotonic dystrophy: present management, future therapy. Oxford University Press, Oxford
Hately P 2001 Respiratory infections. In: Esmond G (ed) Respiratory nursing. Baillière Tindall, London
Jones P 2002 Living with haemophilia, 5th edn. Oxford University Press, Oxford
Kirkwood S C, Su J L, Conneally M, Foroud T 2001 Progression of symptoms in the early and middle stages of Huntington's disease. Archives of Neurology 58(2): 273–278
Lowton K 2002 Parents and partners: lay carers' perceptions of their role in the treatment and care of adults with cystic fibrosis. Journal of Advanced Nursing 39(2): 174–181
Lowton K 2003 Double or quits: perception and management of organ transplantation by adults with cystic fibrosis. Social Science and Medicine 56: 1355–1367
Lui T, Wahlberg S, Burek E et al 2000 Microsatellite instability as a predictor of a mutation in a DNA mismatch repair gene in familial colorectal cancer genes and chromosomes. Cancer 27: 17–25
Lynch H T, de la Chapelle A 1999 Genetic susceptibility to non-polyposis colorectal cancer. Journal of Medical Genetics 36: 801–818
National Human Genome Research Institute. The Human Genome Project. Online. Available: www.genome.gov
Rodriguez-Merchan E C, Goddard N J, Lee C A 2000 Musculoskeletal aspects of haemophilia. Blackwell Science, Oxford
Scottish Intercollegiate Guidelines Network (SIGN) 2000 Epithelial ovarian cancer: a national clinical guideline. SIGN, Edinburgh
Skirton H, Patch C 2002 Genetics for health care professionals. BIOS Scientific, Oxford
Venter J C, Adams M C, Myers E W et al 2001 The sequence of the human genome. Science 291(5507): 1304–1351

USEFUL WEBSITES

Association of Genetic Nurses and Counsellors
www.agnc.co.uk

Contact a Family
www.cafamily.org.uk
The CaF Directory of specific conditions and rare syndromes in children with their family support networks

Department of Clinical Genetics, Molecular Medicine Centre, Western General Hospital, Edinburgh
www.genisys.hw.ac.uk

Human Genome Project
www.genome.gov

Muscular Dystrophy Campaign
www.muscular-dystrophy.org

Muscular Dystrophy Support Group
www.mdsguk.org

Scottish Huntington's Association (SHA)
www.hdscotland.org

The Haemophilia Society
www.haemophilia.org.uk

The Huntington's Disease Association (HAD)
www.hda.org.uk

World Federation of Hemophilia
www.wfh.org

DISORDERS OF THE REPRODUCTIVE SYSTEM AND THE BREAST

7

Anne C. H. McQueen
PART 1 THE REPRODUCTIVE SYSTEMS
Karen L. Burnet
PART 2 THE BREAST

PART 1 THE REPRODUCTIVE SYSTEMS

INTRODUCTION

Any threat to an individual's reproductive capacity affects that person's body image, self-esteem and gender identity. Since these are influenced by personal attitudes, social customs and cultural background, people respond differently to such a threat. Reproduction of the human species involves a complex series of events affected by physical and psychological capacities and the state of health. Attitudes towards sexual reproduction, underlying beliefs held and feelings experienced are influenced by cultural norms, current social values, religious background, lifestyle and parental and peer pressure.

Human reproduction and the ability to procreate are important issues, evidenced by the incidence of subfertility in the United Kingdom (UK) and the growing development of reproductive technologies. While the physiological aspects of reproduction are concerned with continuance of the species, the psychosocial aspects of reproduction are of significance to the feelings of health and well-being for both men and women.

Human beings are individuals with their particular aspirations and values. Thus, for some people, having their own children and raising a family are perceived as important parts of their role in life. For others, these are inconsequential. For yet others, they may be desirable but unobtainable, giving rise to sadness and regret. Whether or not individuals wish to use their reproductive capacity to have children, sexuality is an important concept of self-expression and interaction with others.

The ethos of disease prevention is paramount in health care. Practice nurses, in particular, have an important role in advising and encouraging good health awareness and in facilitating and conducting screening and health monitoring. However, screening is not always possible and some diseases can be far advanced before diagnosis.

Although scientific advances and more sophisticated technology may become available, there are economic constraints on practical therapeutics, and choices must be made when resources are limited. In addition, the rapid progress of science and technology creates ethical issues that society has yet to debate and fully explore as a basis for action and future directions in health care. The Joint Report of the Council on Scientific Affairs and the Council on Medical Science (1992) recognised that the proliferation of health care technology requires thorough evaluation of new technologies in terms of safety and effectiveness.

Advanced minimal invasive techniques also have the advantage of a shorter anaesthetic, allowing patients a shorter stay in hospital. This has implications for nursing and patient care following hospital treatment to adapt to the dynamic nature of nursing in a changing society.

The anatomy and physiology of the male reproductive system appear in Chapter 8.

ANATOMY AND PHYSIOLOGY OF THE FEMALE REPRODUCTIVE SYSTEM

The primary function of the reproductive system is the propagation of the human species. Sexual drive and anticipated pleasure help to meet the reproductive need. The female reproductive system is structured to produce gametes (ova or eggs), to receive the male penis during sexual intercourse and to facilitate the passage of sperm. It accommodates and promotes the growth of the embryo before birth and feeds the newborn infant.

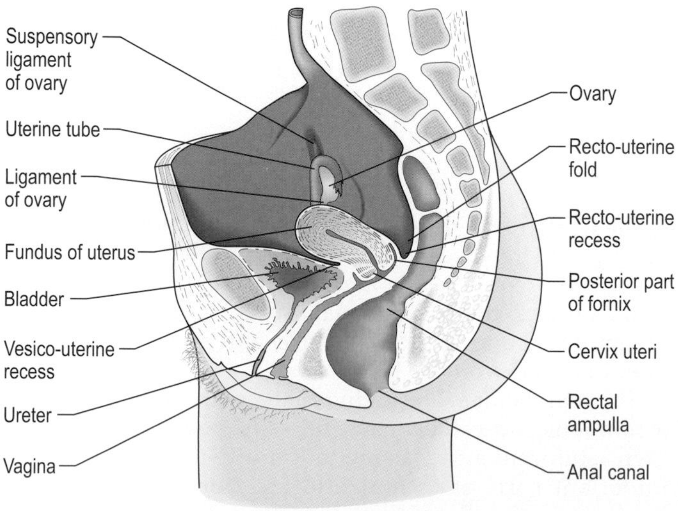

Fig. 7.1 The relationship of the female reproductive organs: sagittal section.

These complex functions are maintained by the following structures (see Figs 7.1 and 7.2):

- the internal organs
  - — the ovaries
  - — the uterus
  - — the uterine (fallopian) tubes (or oviducts)
  - — the vagina
- the external organs
  - — the vulva
  - — the mammary glands or breasts.

The ovaries

Women have two ovaries, the size and shape of large almonds, one on either side of the uterus. The surface of the ovary consists of a single layer of germinal epithelium surrounding connective tissue that forms the stroma of the ovarian cortex and medulla. The ovarian follicles develop in the cortex. A woman is born with approximately 100 000 follicles, although this may fall to approximately 30 000 by adolescence. Each follicle contains an immature ovum known as an oocyte. The medulla, in the centre of the ovary, consists of fibrous connective tissue, blood vessels and nerves.

The production of ova and hormones

The ovary has two functions:

- ovum production
- internal secretion of hormones.

Ovum production

The ovarian cycle begins at around 12–13 years of age. Follicles begin to mature under the influence of the follicle-stimulating hormone (FSH) and luteinising hormone (LH), released by the anterior pituitary gland. During the cycle, follicles can pass through five stages (see Fig. 7.3):

- *primary follicle* — each oocyte is surrounded by a thin layer of epithelial cells
- *developing follicle* — the follicular epithelium proliferates, the oocyte moves to a side position, and a fluid-filled cavity develops within the epithelium

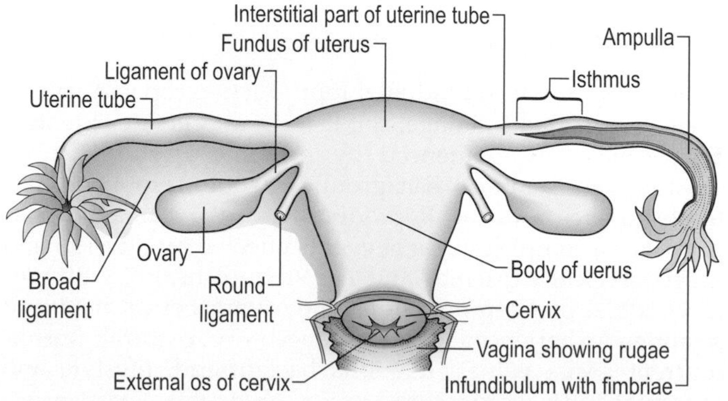

Fig. 7.2 The organs of the female reproductive system and attachments.

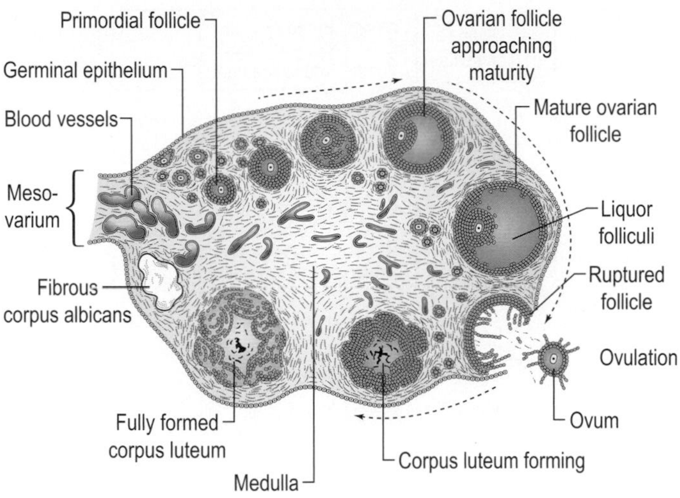

Fig. 7.3 Sequence of development of the ovarian cycle.

- *mature (Graafian) follicle* — the follicle reaches its maximum size
- *corpus luteum* — a yellow mass which forms in the ovarian follicle after ovulation
- *corpus albicans* — scar tissue on the surface of the ovary when the degenerated corpus luteum atrophies.

The maturing follicle is surrounded by a layer of ovarian tissue, known as the theca. Several follicles may develop together but only one will mature fully, as others regress. The mature (Graafian) follicle ruptures at the surface of the ovary and discharges the ovum and fluid into the peritoneal cavity, a process called 'ovulation'. Wafting movements of the finger-like ends of the uterine tubes assist the transfer of the ovum into the tube (oviduct). It is thought that fertilisation of the ovum usually occurs in the ampulla of the uterine tube.

The ruptured follicle contracts around leaked blood after discharging the ovum. The epithelial cells (granulosa) multiply and the corpus luteum is formed under the influence of LH, secreted by the anterior pituitary gland. The corpus luteum synthesises steroid sex hormones for at least 8–10 days. If the ovum is not fertilised, the corpus luteum degenerates, stops its hormone production and forms scar tissue called the 'corpus albicans' near the surface of the ovary. If the ovum is fertilised, the corpus luteum continues to develop, increasing its size and hormone production for about 2 months.

Secretion of hormones

The production of sex hormones is influenced by the hypothalamus of the brain. The hypothalamus produces gonadotrophin-releasing hormone, which stimulates the anterior pituitary gland to release FSH and LH: FSH stimulates the initial development of ovarian follicles and their secretion of oestrogen; LH stimulates further development of the ovarian follicles, initiates ovulation and incites production of ovarian hormones. FSH and LH control the secretion of two types of ovarian steroid hormones: oestrogens and progestogens.

The oestrogens Oestrogens have three main functions:

- development and maintenance of female reproductive structures
- control of fluid and electrolyte balance
- increase of protein anabolism.

The compound secreted by the theca interna cells of the developing follicle is oestradiol, and its metabolite (waste product) is oestriol. Many other oestrogens may be identified in the urine. Oestradiol is also produced by theca interna cells that invade the corpus luteum.

The progestogens The main compound of this group is progesterone, produced by the luteinised granulosa cells of the corpus luteum. The metabolite of progesterone is pregnanediol, which is also excreted in the urine.

The uterus (see Figs 7.1 and 7.2)

The uterus is a pear-shaped organ approximately 7.5 cm long. It has three main parts:

- the fundus
- the body
- the cervix.

The uterine tubes enter the uterus at its upper outer angles or cornua. The body of the uterus narrows towards the cervix, an area known as the isthmus. The cavity of the uterus connects with the cervical canal at the internal os. The cervical canal opens into the vagina via the external os. The cervix occupies the lower third of the uterus and half of the cervix projects into the vagina. The uterus normally lies in an anteverted position, almost at right angles to the vagina (see Figs 7.1 and 7.4).

Structure

The uterus has three coats:

- endometrium — mucous lining
- myometrium — smooth muscle
- parietal peritoneum — serous coat.

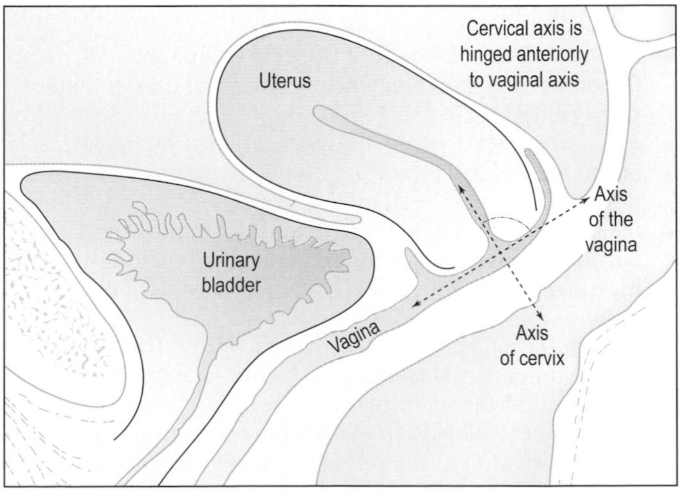

Fig. 7.4 The anteverted position of the uterus.

Endometrium

This is the tissue lining the uterus. This mucosa is continuous with the vagina and the uterine tubes. There are three layers of endometrial tissue:

- *the compact surface layer* — partially ciliated, simple columnar epithelium (stratum compactum)
- *the spongy middle layer* — composed of loose connective tissue and glands (stratum spongiosum)
- *the dense, inner layer* — responsible for the regeneration of the endometrium after menstruation (stratum basale).

During menstruation the compact and spongy layers slough away from the inner layer. The thickness of the endometrium varies from 0.5 mm just after menstrual flow to about 5 mm near the end of the endometrial cycle.

Myometrium

The myometrium is formed from three layers of muscle fibres that extend in all directions:

- the outer layer of longitudinal fibres
- the intermediate layer, in which fibres run irregularly, transversely and obliquely
- the inner layer of circular fibres.

Parietal peritoneum

Peritoneum forms the external coat of the uterus but does not cover the lower anterior quarter of the uterus and the cervix.

Blood supply

The blood supply to the uterus is from the uterine artery, a branch of the internal iliac artery. Veins accompany the arteries and drain into the internal iliac veins. Tortuous arterial vessels enter the layers of the uterine wall and divide into capillaries between endometrial glands.

Nerve supply

The nerves supplying the uterus and the uterine tubes are formed from parasympathetic fibres from the sacral outflow and sympathetic fibres from the lumbar outflow.

Supporting structures

The uterus is maintained in position in the pelvis by fascia and muscle structures (see Fig. 7.5). The uterine ligaments are:

- *the broad ligament* — a fold of peritoneum and fibromuscular tissue extending from the uterus to the pelvic side wall
- *the cardinal ligaments* — these are formed by dense fascia at the base of the broad ligaments, from the cervix to the pelvic side wall
- *the round ligaments* — these extend from the anterior cornua of the uterus forwards and down through the inguinal canal to the subcutaneous fat of the labia majora
- *the uterosacral ligament* — this passes from the cervix and cardinal ligaments backwards to the sacrum, dividing to pass around the rectum
- *the pubocervical ligament* — this passes from the anterior cervix forwards to the pubic bone, dividing to pass around the urethra.

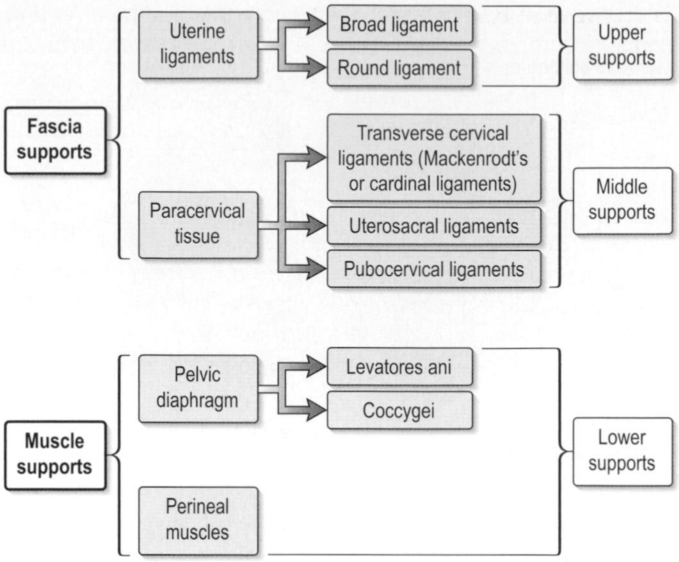

Fig. 7.5 The supports of the uterus.

These ligaments support the position of the uterus within the pelvis. Paracervical tissue, fatty and connective tissue form a supportive sling, allowing the uterus to pivot either backwards or forwards. This gives the uterus mobility anteriorly and posteriorly. Lateral and downward movements are limited by the muscles of the pelvic floor.

The axis of the vagina is considered to be a straight line that is related to the axis of the cervix. When the cervical axis is hinged anterior to the vaginal axis, the uterus is 'anteverted' (see Fig. 7.4), which is its normal position. When the cervical axis is hinged backwards to lie posterior to the vaginal axis, the uterus is 'retroverted'. This can be a normal position for the uterus to occupy provided that the retroversion is mobile and not fixed.

Functions

The functions of the uterus are:

- *menstruation* — sloughing off of compact and spongy layers of endometrium attended by bleeding from torn vessels
- *maintenance of pregnancy* — an embryo implants itself in the endometrium and takes all its nourishment throughout fetal life
- *initiation of labour* — it develops powerful, rhythmic contractions of the muscular wall for the birth of the infant.

The uterine tubes (fallopian tubes or oviducts) (see Fig. 7.2)

The uterine tubes (10–14 cm long) turn posteriorly as they extend laterally from the cornua (or horns) of the uterus towards the lateral pelvic wall. The ends open as funnel-shaped structures with finger-like projections (fimbriae). The broad ligament of peritoneum forms the outer serous layer of the tubes. The middle coat, of muscular tissue, is arranged in two layers: an outer longitudinal layer and an inner circular layer. The lining of mucous membrane, comprised mainly of ciliated columnar epithelium and secretory cells, lies in folds. The lumen of the tube is narrow. The ends of the tubes are mobile and at ovulation the fimbriae enfold the adjacent ovary to take up the released ova.

Functions

The functions of the uterine tubes are to convey ova from the ovary to the uterus and to allow the sperm and ova to meet for fertilisation within the tube. Passage of the ova along the tube is facilitated by the action of cilia and peristalsis.

The vagina

The vagina is a fibromuscular channel extending downwards and forwards from the cervix to the labia, thereby connecting the internal and external reproductive organs. The cervix of the uterus is inserted into the upper end of the vagina, known as the vault. This creates anterior, posterior and lateral fornices (see Fig. 7.1). The anterior wall of the vagina is approximately 7.5 cm and the posterior wall about 9 cm in length. The vagina is composed mainly of smooth muscle with a lining of mucous membrane arranged in folds or rugae. In the virginal state, a fold of mucous membrane, the hymen, forms a border around the external opening of the vagina, partially closing the outlet. Normally the anterior and posterior walls lie in apposition but the vagina is capable of considerable distension during childbirth.

The vagina is kept moist during the reproductive years by mucus from the cervix and transudation of fluid through the vaginal wall. Glycogen produced in the vagina is fermented by the Doderlein bacilli (normally inhabiting the vagina) to produce lactic acid. This maintains a slightly acid environment in the vagina, inhibiting the growth of other microorganisms.

Functions

The vagina:

- receives semen from the male, deposited in the posterior fornix during sexual intercourse
- provides an outlet for the fetus and other products of conception
- provides an outlet for menstrual flow
- provides a barrier to infection.

The vulva

The vulva comprises the female external genital organs, consisting of:

- the mons pubis
- the labia majora
- the labia minora
- the clitoris
- the fourchette
- the urinary orifice
- the vaginal orifice
- Bartholin's glands.

The pelvic floor

The pelvic floor is formed by tissues that fill the pelvic outlet and support the pelvic organs.

- The *levator ani muscles* form a broad muscular sheet extending from the pubic bone to the sacrum and coccyx and laterally to the pelvic walls. The urethra, vagina and rectum perforate this muscular sheet.
- The *superficial perineal muscles* lie under the levator ani muscles. They pass from the pelvic side walls, the pubis and the sacrum to unite centrally between the vagina and the rectum, where they form the superficial part of the perineal body.
- The *perineal body* consists of wedge-shaped muscle and fibrous tissue lying between the lower vagina and lower rectum.

The endometrial cycle

The ovarian cycle (see 'Ovarian functions', p. 254) and the endometrial cycle together constitute the menstrual cycle. The endometrial cycle is driven by the hormonal events of the ovarian cycle and can be divided into four phases:

- the menstrual phase
- the proliferative phase (follicular or pre-ovulatory)
- the secretory phase (luteal or post-ovulatory)
- the ischaemic phase.

The menstrual phase

Menstruation is believed to be caused by low levels of progesterone and oestrogens causing vasospasm of arteries to the endometrium. The menstrual phase lasts for 3–6 days and is characterised by bleeding from the uterus, with 50–60 ml of blood being lost at each menstrual period when necrotic parts of the compact and spongy layers of endometrium slough away, leaving a thin, bleeding area of tissue. By the third day of menstruation new epithelial cell growth has begun to cover the disorganised basal layer of endometrium; by the fifth day, epithelium covers the whole surface.

The proliferative phase

The proliferative phase begins while bleeding is still continuing. It is a time of regrowth of endometrium, under the control of oestradiol from the maturing follicle. The growth of epithelium, glands, blood vessels and connective tissue produces thickening of the endometrium. This phase extends to the 14th or 15th day of the cycle, when the peak of proliferation is reached.

The secretory phase

Soon after ovulation, glycoprotein secretory granules appear in the endometrium and can be seen with an electron microscope as large, clear vacuoles developing under the nuclei. Progesterone produced by the corpus luteum promotes the secretory phase. The endometrial glands become enlarged, the arteries coil, connective tissue hypertrophies and tissues rich in glycogen become oedematous. At 7–8 days following ovulation, the endometrium is 5–6 mm in depth and is in a state of readiness to implant a fertilised ovum.

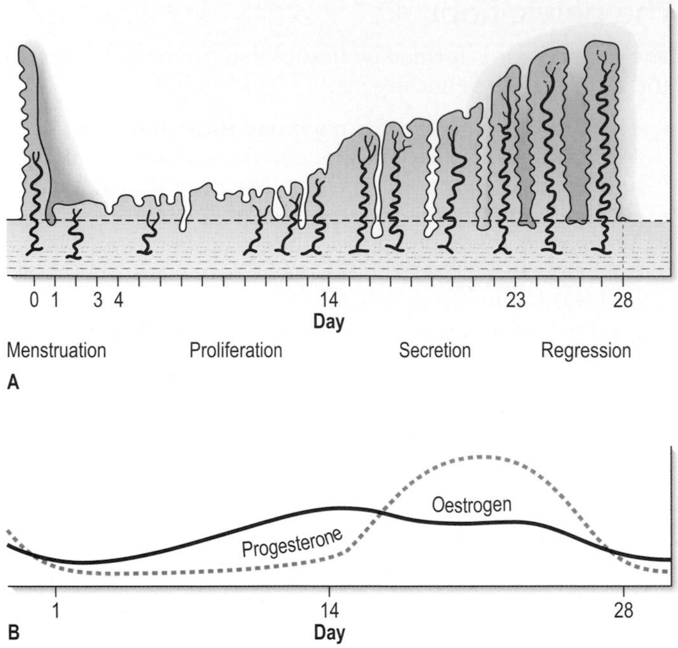

Fig. 7.6 The hormonal control of the menstrual cycle.

If implantation occurs, the corpus luteum continues to produce progesterone and maintains the pregnancy (see Fig. 7.6).

The ischaemic phase

In the absence of implantation, the corpus luteum degenerates and the production of oestrogen and progesterone declines. A leucocytic infiltration of the endometrium takes place, the stroma starts to disintegrate, oedema disappears and the endometrium shrinks. Vasoconstriction occurs. There is lack of nourishment to the endometrium and it begins to slough and separate; menstruation begins again 14 (±1) days after ovulation. This time relationship is constant.

Fluctuations in the length of the cycle occur in the preovulatory phase, as follicles may not mature at the same rate each month. Thus there may be variation in the time of onset of menstruation. Most women establish an average pattern that is normal for each, although many young women have irregular patterns.

The menarche

In Western cultures, girls first menstruate (reach the menarche) within the age range of 9–16 years. Nutrition and body weight influence menstruation and sexual development. This has cultural ramifications in that amenorrhoea and infrequent menstruation are more common in developing countries, especially in the rural areas (Helman 1997). The onset of menstruation may be delayed by intensive physical activity.

Some oestrogen synthesis stimulates early physical sexual changes to occur some time before the first menstruation. There may be follicular growth and some oestrogen withdrawal bleeding to give the early periods of the first few months. These periods are anovular, ovulation having not yet occurred. Such periods are painless. More discomfort may be experienced with the menstruation that follows ovulation. A rise in basal temperature may be a guide to whether ovulation has occurred.

Variation in menstrual cycle length occurs in response to significant life events. Excitement, stress, anxiety or change of environment can delay the maturing of a follicle, ovulation and menstruation. Excessive exercise, as in athletes, can result in irregular periods, anovulatory cycles and amenorrhoea.

The climacteric and menopause

The word climacteric comes from the Greek word klimacter, meaning a step or rung of a ladder. This signifies a step or phase in life from the child-bearing years to a period of infertility associated with age-related changes. The process of the climacteric is usually gradual and may extend over several years. Most women experience the climacteric or perimenopause over a period of 2–3 years, but it may extend over 10 years. During this time the body adjusts to lower levels of oestrogen.

The ageing process of the ovaries results in ripening of fewer follicles and a decreased stimulation by the pituitary hormones. The ovaries atrophy and less oestrogen is released into the circulation. Initially this reduced oestrogen level in the blood results in excessive production of FSH from the anterior pituitary gland, and this feedback mechanism can continue for several years. The withdrawal of oestrogen and the increase in pituitary hormone contribute to the changes associated with the climacteric.

The menopause is sometimes confused with the climacteric. However, the menopause is defined as the cessation of menstruation and is marked specifically by the date of the last menstrual period. It follows, then, that the time of the menopause (last menstrual period) can only be identified in retrospect some months after the event. The menopause is only one effect of the climacteric. 'Postmenopausal' is a term applied to events occurring after menstruation has stopped for at least a year.

The menopause signifies the end of a woman's reproductive capacity. This normally occurs between 45 and 55 years of age, with the mean age for cessation of periods being 51 years. This has remained constant for many years (Abernethy 1997).

A premature menopause is one which occurs before the age of 40 years. This can occur naturally or may be induced iatrogenically. The age of menarche, socioeconomic factors, race, use of oral contraceptives and number of pregnancies appear to have no effect on whether a woman has an early or a late menopause (Abernethy 1997).

Endocrine changes influencing the climacteric

Endocrine changes occur prior to changes in a woman's menstrual pattern when there is an alteration in the ratio of the pituitary gonadotrophins (FSH and LH). FSH levels begin to rise between the ages of 35 and 40 years, affecting the oestrogen feedback mechanisms and resulting in altered ovarian function. As a consequence, some anovular menstruation occurs and there is a reduction in progesterone produced by the theca-lutein cells. During this period the amount of oestrogen produced shows considerable fluctuation.

Although ovarian cycles may become anovular many years before the menopause occurs, women between the ages of 40 and 45 can still become pregnant as regular ovulation may continue.

Eventually there is further deterioration in ovarian response to the pituitary gonadotrophins and disturbance to the feedback between the hypothalamus–pituitary and the ovaries. There is then a further alteration to the FSH:LH ratio, with an elevation in LH and a steep rise in FSH. However, fewer follicles are stimulated so oestrogen secretion is reduced. The fluctuations in oestrogen production, while following a gradual decline, alter the menstrual pattern in many women, showing considerable variation amongst women until the menopause.

After the menopause there is continued secretion of oestradiol and oestrone, although in varying and declining amounts. Oestrone becomes the predominant oestrogen. Small amounts of oestrogen can be found in the blood and urine of postmenopausal women. Some of this oestrogen may be derived from adrenal activity and the conversion of some androgens into oestrogen. Some oestrogen may be produced by residual ovarian stroma.

Uterine bleeding patterns

The climacteric is characterised by irregular menstruation. Periods may become scanty, or bleeding may be heavy. The menstrual cycle shortens, associated with a decrease in oestradiol secretion. As this continues, LH levels rise and then menstrual cycles lengthen. Anovulatory cycles result in oestrogen-withdrawal bleeding patterns, irregular cycles with intermittent and prolonged spotting (low oestrogen profile) or prolonged amenorrhoea followed by sudden, profuse bleeding (high oestrogen profile).

Somatic changes associated with the climacteric

The somatic changes associated with the climacteric occur as a consequence of a decrease in circulating oestrogen and an increase in gonadotrophins. Since the diurnal secretion of oestrogen varies from woman to woman, the changes experienced vary in severity but are progressive.

The ovaries atrophy and follicles disappear or fail to respond to gonadotrophins. Uterine atrophy is accompanied by a transformation of the muscle fibres to fibrous tissue. The endometrium becomes thinner. The cervix tends to remain dilated and the external os more lax. The fallopian tubes become smaller and the fimbriated ends retract from the ovaries. Atrophy of the vaginal epithelium results in thinning of the vaginal wall, a loss of folds, elasticity and lubrication, and an increase in pH. Vaginal dryness can result in pruritus and dyspareunia. Loss of acidity within the vagina allows organisms to multiply more easily. There is an increase in connective tissue beneath the mucosa, causing narrowing and shortening of the vagina. The vagina is more prone to ulceration and bleeds easily to touch. Senile vaginitis may occur in older women. The labia become thin and lose their sexual responsiveness. Skin over the vulva loses support due to a decrease in subcutaneous tissue and lack of tone of the underlying tissues. Hair growth in this area decreases with advancing years. The muscles and connective tissue of the pelvic floor lose tone and elasticity, and consequently become less effective in supporting the pelvic contents. The urethral mucosa may also show atrophic changes, resulting in symptoms of urethritis and cystitis, although no bacteria are isolated in the urine. In the breasts, subcutaneous fat is reabsorbed and glandular tissue atrophies.

Some of these physiological changes, resulting in lack of lubrication, loss of libido and dyspareunia, can contribute to sexual problems for the woman. Hormone replacement therapy (HRT) may be a possible treatment option or psychosexual counselling may be of benefit. Many factors contribute to a satisfying sex life — satisfaction in a relationship, psychological well-being and emotional security can all make a significant contribution, illustrating the need for a holistic approach.

Vasomotor disturbances

Vasomotor disturbances commonly accompany the climacteric changes (see Box 7.1). Hot flushes (or hot flashes) are the most common but perspiration, headache, fainting and palpitations may also be experienced. Hot flushes can start with a sensation of extreme warmth in the chest, quickly followed by flushing of the face and neck. The feeling of heat may become generalised. This is caused by dilatation of the blood vessels to the skin and an increased blood flow. The flush may be accompanied by sweating and palpitations. Dizziness and nausea may also be experienced. Shivering is often reported after the flush, probably due to compensatory constriction of the blood vessels. While vasomotor symptoms will eventually subside with no long-term effects, hot flushes and sweats are embarrassing,

Box 7.1

Hot flush

It has long been postulated that dysfunction of central thermoregulatory centres in the hypothalamus, caused by changes in oestrogen levels at the time of menopause, result in hot flushes. Oestrogen withdrawal, rather than low circulating oestrogen levels, seems to be the main factor that leads to hot flushes. Weir (2004) describes a model of the pathogenesis of hot flushes whereby oestrogen withdrawal leads to decreased levels of endorphin and catecholestrogen (a metabolic by-product of oestrogen). This results in increased hypothalamic release of norepinephrine and serotonin. Norepinephrine and serotonin lower the set point in the thermoregulatory nucleus, allowing mechanisms of heat loss to be triggered by subtle changes in core body temperature. Thus, it is suggested that endorphins play a key role in the regulation of norepinephrine release, and that agents that increase oestrogen and endorphin levels, or that decrease central norepinephrine release, would be expected to reduce hot flushes.

While oestrogen therapy effectively relieves hot flushes, for women who do not wish hormonal therapy, some antidepressants that affect the release and uptake of serotonin and norepinephrine provide a promising alternative. Venlafaxine, fluoxetine and paroxetine have been found to reduce hot flushes significantly (by 50–60%) when compared with placebo (Shanafelt et al 2002).

RESEARCH ABSTRACT 7.1

Efficacy and safety of estradiol transdermal system compared with placebo on vasomotor symptoms in menopausal women.

A double-blind, placebo-controlled, parallel-group, multicentre trial involving 196 menopausal women complaining of symptoms was conducted to evaluate the efficacy and safety of three doses of Esclim (0.025, 0.050 or 0.100 mg) 17beta-estradiol/24 h as a therapy for moderate to severe vasomotor symptoms. The women received continuous, unopposed treatment with one of three doses of Esclim or a matching placebo transdermal patch for 12 weeks. Findings indicated that the frequency of moderate to severe vasomotor symptoms was reduced significantly compared with the effect of the placebo ($P<0.05$). The severity of the symptoms was also reduced. The adverse effects of oestrogen, notably endometrial hyperplasia and metrorrhagia, were less frequent in the smallest dose.

Utian W H, Bury K A, Archer D F et al 1999 Efficacy and safety of low, standard and high dosages of an estradiol transdermal system (Esclim) compared with placebo on vasomotor symptoms in highly symptomatic menopausal patients. The Esclim Study Group. American Journal of Obstetrics and Gynecology 181(1): 71–79

uncontrollable and can be distressing for many women. Porter et al (1996) report on a Scottish survey of 6096 women aged 45–54 years and note that 84% experienced at least one of the classic symptoms associated with the menopause and 45% of the women reported one or more symptoms as a problem. Randomised controlled trials (RCTs) have indicated the value of oestrogen in reducing the severity of vasomotor symptoms when compared with placebo (see Box 7.1 and Research Abstract 7.1).

In addition to oestrogen therapy, other treatments, such as vitamin E and/or B_6, clonidine, plant oestrogens, propranolol and oil of evening primrose, have been used. Progestogens have been shown to alleviate hot flushes (Loprinzi et al 1994). Phytoestrogens, found in soya, can be taken as a supplement and have been suggested as a remedy for menopausal symptoms. While some women do find them valuable, there is controversy about advocating them as a therapy for menopausal symptoms (Davis 2001, Naftolin & Stanbury 2002).

Emotional changes

Some women complain of irritability, anxiety, difficulty in concentration, dizziness, a bloated feeling and depressive feelings after the menopause. In addition to hormonal changes occurring at the perimenopause, women may also be facing other psychological or social changes which can affect their emotional state. While HRT is commonly accepted as a method of treating a negative mood and is promoted by pharmacological companies, it is difficult to establish a causal relationship between oestrogen deficiency and the emotional behaviour of women (Stephens & Ross 2002).

CONDITIONS AFFECTING MENSTRUATION

Amenorrhoea

Amenorrhoea means the absence of menstruation and is a symptom, not a disease. It is described as primary or secondary.

Primary amenorrhoea is defined as non-appearance of menstruation in a female by the age of 16 years. A delay in the onset of menstruation may be a cause of concern. There may be an anatomical fault or some disturbance in hormonal secretions. Delayed puberty may be familial or constitutional. Secondary amenorrhoea is the absence of menstruation for a period of time which is twice the length of the normal menstrual cycle for a woman who has previously menstruated. Thus, if two or more menstrual periods are missed then secondary amenorrhoea may be said to exist. This often means that the woman may wait until menstruation has been absent for a year before seeking investigation.

Physiological amenorrhoea

Amenorrhoea is physiological before puberty, during pregnancy and lactation, and after the menopause. Inheritance, race, climate and general nutrition influence when menstruation begins. The potential for maturation of ovarian tissue is in place before birth. After puberty, full regulation of ovarian activities by the hypothalamus and pituitary gland is achieved and menstrual cycles are established, but the exact time for this is unpredictable.

Before puberty

A teenage girl may be seen by her GP because of delay in the onset of menstruation. The doctor may undertake a general physical examination to determine if other secondary sex characteristics are present; if so, menstruation will follow in due course. If secondary sex characteristics or menstruation fail to develop, the doctor will refer the patient to a consultant gynaecologist and endocrinologist for investigation.

During pregnancy

After ovulation has occurred, the lining cells of the ovarian follicle are stimulated by LH to develop the corpus luteum which produces progesterone. This hormone in turn stimulates the endometrium and its secretory glands into a state of readiness to receive the fertilised ovum from the uterine tube. When the fertilised ovum becomes embedded in the wall of the uterus, it produces the hormone human chorionic gonadotrophin (hCG). This hormone enables the corpus luteum to continue its production of progesterone for 3–4 months until the placenta grows and produces its own progesterone and oestrogen. The presence of the growing fetus and the continued production of progesterone prevent the loss of endometrium and the menstrual flow.

Amenorrhoea is frequently one of the first symptoms that lead a woman to suspect that she is pregnant. Levels of hCG in the urine provide a positive diagnosis when a test for pregnancy is completed in the clinic or laboratory. The doctor usually confirms the pregnancy by abdominal palpation and a vaginal examination, when the uterus is found to be increased in size.

During lactation

Mothers who totally breast feed their baby may not ovulate or menstruate during the first 6 months after the birth or until they start to wean the baby. Breast feeding therefore exerts a measure of birth control, but it cannot be recommended as 100% effective as a contraceptive. Sutherland (2001) claims that the contraceptive effectiveness of lactational amenorrhoea has been reported as 98% effective provided the woman is fully breast feeding, is within 6 months of the birth and menstruation has not returned. However, Hartmann (1991) states that fertility may return as early as 2 weeks after birth in some women who are fully breast feeding and Farrer (1990) indicates that most women will ovulate before their first menstruation following childbirth.

Total nipple stimulation is important for suppression of ovarian function. The suckling stimulus to the nipple leads to a neurohormonal reflex production of prolactin by the anterior pituitary gland and the consequent maintenance of high circulating levels of prolactin inhibits gonadotrophin hormone release, preventing ovulation and menstruation.

Suppression of the ovaries declines where supplements comprise more than 50% of the diet of the baby who is breast feeding. The incidence of ovulation and the risk of pregnancy then rise rapidly.

A poor state of nutrition in the mother is also known to inhibit ovulation, particularly in developing countries (Lunn 1992). To ensure contraception during the period of lactation, the mother may be advised to use a barrier method. The progestogen-only pill is considered safe during lactation since it does not affect the milk supply and only insignificant quantities enter the milk. The combined oral contraceptive pill, however, inhibits lactation and small quantities enter the milk (Everett 1997).

After the menopause

The menopause, or date of the final menstrual period, may not be fully acknowledged until a year without periods has passed. Many women pass this milestone without regrets and without unpleasant physical symptoms. Medical intervention may be sought if physical discomfort such as hot flushes, headaches or sweating is experienced.

Information and support from the nurse, outlined later in this chapter (p. 273), can be helpful.

Pathological amenorrhoea

Uterine lesions, congenital abnormalities

PATHOPHYSIOLOGY

- *Congenital absence of uterus and vagina* may occur, although ovaries and secondary sex characteristics have developed.
- In *primary deficiency of endometrium* a diagnostic test can be performed by giving ethinyl oestradiol 0.05 mg by mouth, twice a day for 21 days. If withdrawal bleeding occurs within 7–10 days then there is not a failure of endometrium but probably failure of stimulation by the ovaries. If there is no bleeding, an endometrial problem exists. The endometrium may be absent, deficient or unable to be stimulated by oestrogen. In this case, the amenorrhoea is entirely of uterine origin.

Ovarian lesions

Failure of normal development is a rare condition of the ovary. Chromosomal abnormalities such as Turner's syndrome may occur.

PATHOPHYSIOLOGY

Turner's syndrome is a condition that results from the absence of one female chromosome. The chromosome complement is written as 45XO. The woman is reported to be 'chromatin negative'. The condition shows infantile development of the genitalia, absence of breasts, short stature and a webbed neck. There may be associated congenital cardiac lesions (see Ch. 5).

MEDICAL MANAGEMENT

Chromosomal studies confirm the diagnosis. Early diagnosis is important and investigations can usually be initiated before puberty, suspicion being aroused by the short stature of the child.

Treatment, such as ethinyl oestradiol 0.01 mg twice daily, in 3-week cycles, given for several months, then norethisterone added for the last 10 days of each cycle, can be used to stimulate development of the breasts and uterus. Menstruation may occur with this treatment.

Pituitary disorders (see also Ch. 5)

- *Deficiency of gonadotrophin secretion* may occur without deficiencies of other trophic hormones. No cause may be found but it is often associated with emotional responses.
- *Infantilism* may result from congenital failure of the pituitary gland, causing dwarfism, lack of sexual development and amenorrhoea. FSH is absent or low. Oestrogens may be undetectable in the urine.
- *Fröhlich's syndrome* is a disturbance of the hypothalamus, resulting in underdevelopment of genital tissues, amenorrhoea, obesity, hirsutism and retardation of mental responses.
- *Ischaemic necrosis* of pituitary tissue may result from thrombosis of pituitary vessels following profound shock and anaemia, often due to severe postpartum haemorrhage. The production of trophic hormones ceases or is reduced. The condition is characterised by lethargy, weight gain, reduced metabolic rate, hypotension and amenorrhoea. HRT gives some psychological benefit only, by withdrawal bleeding effects.
- *New growths* of the pituitary cause acromegaly and amenorrhoea, with signs of Cushing's syndrome due to effects on the suprarenal glands.

Other endocrine disorders

- *Adrenogenital syndrome* results from overactivity of the adrenal cortex due to the presence of a tumour or hyperplasia. Excessive production of androgens occurs, giving signs of virilism — a deepening voice, hirsuteness, an enlarged clitoris and the development of acne and amenorrhoea.
- *Cushing's disease* is caused by hyperplasia of the adrenal cortex, which leads to an excess of glucocorticoids, stimulating the conversion of protein into carbohydrate. Obesity, glycosuria, hypertension, increased androgen

activity and amenorrhoea from regressive changes in the genital organs are the main features of the condition.

The following endocrine disorders may also be accompanied by amenorrhoea:

- Addison's disease
- myxoedema
- thyrotoxicosis
- diabetes mellitus.

Emotional stress

PATHOPHYSIOLOGY

Emotional disturbance is likely to affect menstrual function through the hypothalamic–pituitary axis since the hypothalamus controls the output of gonadotrophins from the pituitary gland. Emotional distress caused by some traumatic event, such as receiving bad news or being involved in a major disaster, may contribute to amenorrhoea. If a woman has sexual intercourse without contraception, the fear of becoming pregnant may itself cause temporary amenorrhoea.

MEDICAL MANAGEMENT

Following discussion with the doctor, it is expected that the patient will understand and be reassured about the effects of stress on menstruation. When she makes a positive adjustment to the critical event that has preceded the problem, physical and mental relaxation will promote a spontaneous return of menstruation.

Anorexia nervosa (see also Ch. 5)

PATHOPHYSIOLOGY

Anorexia nervosa is a psychological illness, the distress being manifest as disordered eating behaviour. It is associated with dieting routines and distortion of body image and is characterised by extreme weight loss and dislike for foods, particularly carbohydrates. It occurs most commonly in adolescent girls with a peak age of 17–18 years and an incidence of 1–2 per 1000 (Fombonne 1995). There is failure in hypothalamic stimulation of LH release and amenorrhoea occurs.

MEDICAL MANAGEMENT

Women with anorexia nervosa are usually reluctant to accept they have a problem or to seek help. Their weight loss may be being investigated or they may present to their GP with another problem but when a diagnosis is made, care is usually maintained by a psychiatrist. A behavioural therapy programme is negotiated with the patient to ensure an improvement in food intake, while a cognitive therapist may assist her to think more rationally and improve her feelings of self-esteem and her body image. Positive physical and psychological changes can promote a return to menstruation.

Psychotic illness

PATHOPHYSIOLOGY

Psychotic illness may be a cause of amenorrhoea. The person with a schizophrenic reaction may not menstruate for many months or years. A life crisis can contribute to disturbances in the activity of neurotransmitter catecholamines in the brain. The chemistry of the hypothalamic– pituitary axis may be disrupted, resulting in amenorrhoea.

MEDICAL MANAGEMENT

The psychiatrist would check that a pregnancy has not developed in the patient with a psychotic reaction. A reliable source of information will be needed, whether the patient herself or her partner. A laboratory pregnancy test may be necessary. The acute symptoms of the patient's illness may be treated by neuroleptic medication or psychotherapeutic intervention. A return of the normal menstruation pattern would be expected when the body chemistry becomes more stable.

Severe general illness

PATHOPHYSIOLOGY

The stress of severe illness may induce ineffective functioning in multiple body organs and may temporarily suppress menstrual function. Stress, as experienced by prisoners of war or refugees, associated with malnutrition, minimal protein and vitamin intake, leads to amenorrhoea.

MEDICAL MANAGEMENT

The amenorrhoea is secondary to the general illness. Thus the particular illness condition must be treated before the amenorrhoea can be relieved. The influences of emotional and physical stress are complex, and sometimes assisting the patient to relax and lower anxiety levels may promote menstruation before the general illness is fully relieved.

NURSING PRIORITIES AND MANAGEMENT: Amenorrhoea

The nurse caring for a patient with amenorrhoea may do so in any of the hospital specialties or in the community — the nursing management will be similar in all of these locations.

Assessment

As part of the routine assessment of the patient, the nurse should enquire about the date of the last menstrual period and whether there are any problems with menstruation. The nurse should ascertain whether the patient has any knowledge of the reason for the absence of menstruation. As the patient shares information, the nurse should be able to establish how the patient feels about the amenorrhoea that is described. The patient may not regard amenorrhoea as a problem or, conversely, it may be a source of some distress. Assessment should take account of her lifestyle, including nutrition, eating pattern, body weight, level of exercise and any stressful life events.

Care planning

In negotiation with the patient, the nurse should plan time to give her information about the absence of menstruation. This can perhaps be associated with potential worries about the condition. The patient's level of anxiety should be documented in the plan. The nurse may wish to emphasise the need for self-relaxation and may teach a simple relaxation exercise. Relaxation audiotapes may be available from the physiotherapy department, occupational therapy or the department of clinical psychology.

If, following a medical assessment, puberty is deemed to be delayed, reassurance and counselling are part of nursing care. Nurses can encourage optimism, provide general information about diet, exercise and lifestyle, and offer support, but in some cases skilled counselling may also be of value.

Evaluation of care

The patient's long-term goal of 'a return of the menstrual period' may not be achievable within the early weeks of care and should be modified to include a short-term realistic target. This may include an evaluation of the level of anxiety experienced by the patient. Nurse and patient should negotiate and evaluate it, to check on the response to self-relaxation activity during the first 2 days of care. The patient may need more help from the nurse and new target times for evaluation of goal achievement will then need to be set.

The patient should be asked to report menstruation. Achievement of such a long-term goal may occur as a result of medical treatment, particularly if hormonal or anxiolytic sedative drugs have been prescribed.

Cryptomenorrhoea

This is a condition of concealed menstruation and it is important to differentiate it from amenorrhoea. Menstrual blood is unable to pass through the vagina due to an obstruction. This may be due to an imperforate hymen, a transverse vaginal membrane, or complete or partial vaginal atresia. Incomplete canalisation of the lower end of the Müllerian cords will result in atresia of the upper vagina. There may be a complete absence of the vagina or cervical stenosis after cautery to the cervix or amputation of the cervix.

PATHOPHYSIOLOGY

In this condition, the uterus, ovaries and the pituitary gland are functioning normally, but the menstrual outflow is obstructed. Conditions such as an imperforate hymen or a transverse vaginal septum will result in an accumulation of blood in the vagina (haematocolpos). In addition to vaginal distension, retrograde flow to the fallopian tubes (haemosalpinx) and accumulation of blood may cause pelvic congestion and displacement of structures. Symptoms are cyclical pain and lower abdominal swelling.

MEDICAL MANAGEMENT

The condition is relieved by surgical drainage. There is a risk that the fallopian tubes may be damaged due to retrograde flow and consequent distension.

NURSING PRIORITIES AND MANAGEMENT: Cryptomenorrhoea

Assessment

The patient will be admitted as an emergency for early transfer to the operating theatre. The nurse assessing the patient on admission will uncover the following symptoms:

- pelvic pain
- potential retention of urine from pressure on the urethra
- anxiety about the condition, the strange environment and unknown procedures.

Care planning

If time allows before transfer to the operating theatre, the relief of the patient's pain will be a priority, according to medical prescription. A comforting, positive attitude of open regard shown by the nurse may help to reduce the patient's anxiety. Giving information will prepare the patient for the procedures to be expected before surgery and in the first 24 h after the operation (see Ch. 26).

A urethral catheter may be introduced unless there is an obstruction of the urethra. This may be undertaken once the patient is anaesthetised. An empty bladder facilitates the work of the surgeon and reduces risk of injury to the bladder.

Postoperative care

This will ensure the patient's safe recovery from anaesthesia and that pain is fully relieved. The patient's vaginal blood loss will be observed and documented. The patient should quickly recover, without any complications of anaesthesia or surgery. Full information should be given about what the surgery entailed and expected future progress.

Evaluation of care

The patient should quickly achieve the following outcomes:

- freedom from pain
- minimal blood loss, reducing daily
- no nausea or vomiting
- return to self-care activities within 24 h
- no hospital-acquired infection
- able to explain, before discharge, the action to be taken if the condition recurs
- discharge within a day or two, with an outpatient clinic appointment for 1 month's time.

If these outcomes are not achieved then discharge will be delayed while care is modified, until the patient's condition improves. Surgical treatment should result in subsequent menstrual blood flow per vagina.

Dysmenorrhoea

Dysmenorrhoea is pain associated with menstruation. Many women experience minor discomfort associated with menstruation, but dysmenorrhoea is more disabling. Before the start of the period, the breasts may feel larger and ache; there may also be feelings of abdominal distension, constipation may be a problem, and the woman may feel unwell. The symptoms may persist for 1–2 days and are relieved or replaced by the symptoms of backache, frequency of passing urine and loose bowel action with the onset of menstruation.

For some women, the first hours or the first day are the most painful. Dragging sensations from the umbilical area down to the groins and thighs may be experienced, or the pain may be severe, colicky or spasmodic in nature across the abdomen and back. The pain may be so distracting as to interfere with the woman's usual daily activities. Dysmenorrhoea affects 40–95% of menstruating women, and has been reported as the most common cause of regular absenteeism among young women (Jones 2004).

Two types of dysmenorrhoea are described:

- primary dysmenorrhoea (spasmodic) is due to physiological activities of the menstruation, with muscle contraction
- secondary dysmenorrhoea (congestive) is associated with organic pelvic disease.

Primary dysmenorrhoea is seen in young women in their late teens and early 20s. At first they may have anovulatory, pain-free menstruation. Later, when ovulation becomes established, they experience pain 24 h before the flow begins. The pain is of the severe colic type over the lower abdomen, often radiating to the thighs and back, and lasts for at least 12 h. Nausea, fainting and diarrhoea may accompany the acute phase and the girl looks pale and drawn with a tense facial expression.

PATHOPHYSIOLOGY

Dysmenorrhoea is associated with an increased production of prostaglandin from the endometrium, resulting in intense uterine contractions. Arterioles in the uterus can go into spasm and the resulting muscle ischaemia can produce uterine pain similar to that of angina.

Misunderstandings about the physical changes of menstruation and the nature of dysmenorrhoea may underlie ineffective management (see Research Abstract 7.2). Education about the nature of dysmenorrhoea and its effective management should therefore be addressed with young girls and their parents as appropriate.

The excess prostaglandin (F2) circulating in the blood may cause nausea, vomiting, diarrhoea or faintness. Muscular incoordination may be the result of improper functioning of the autonomic nervous system. This may cause spasm of muscles of the uterine isthmus and of the internal os.

Rarely, dysmenorrhoea may be due to an obstruction to the flow of blood as a result of a clot being lodged in the cervix. Other possible causes include pelvic inflammatory disease, endometriosis and congenital abnormalities.

MEDICAL MANAGEMENT

Detailed interviews may be carried out with the girl and her mother, separately and together. In this way, shared and different attitudes to the subject can be identified and problems defined. Vaginal or possibly a rectal examination may be carried out.

Efforts are made to educate the girl and her mother, as necessary, about normal menstrual function. It is important to test their understanding by giving them opportunities for feedback about attitudes and old wives' tales. A period of rest and the application of warmth to the abdomen or back may be helpful. The need to rest should not be used as an excuse for avoiding school or work. Regular exercise, the avoidance of constipation and the prevention of anxiety and tension are emphasised. Exercise encourages the release of endogenous endorphins which have natural analgesic properties. A series of exercises to stretch the ligaments that support the uterus in the pelvis may relieve menstrual pain. Attention should be paid to maintaining good posture.

Treatment Non-habit-forming analgesics can be of value, particularly aspirin, which reduces prostaglandin synthesis.

RESEARCH ABSTRACT 7.2

How adolescents manage menstrual discomfort

Campbell and McGrath (1997) surveyed 386 adolescent girls, at public high school, aged between 14 and 21 years. Eighty-five per cent of the subjects were English Canadian. Two hundred and ninety-one cases were used for analyses. The Menstrual Distress Management Questionnaire (designed for their study to measure disability and medication use) and the Symptom Severity Scale were the measurement tools used. Ninety-three per cent of the subjects reported menstrual discomfort during the last three menstruations but there was great variability in the reported degree of menstrual discomfort and the treatments employed by the subjects.

Seventy per cent of those who reported dysmenorrhoea had used over-the-counter (OTC) medications to manage their discomfort. Users of OTC medications reported greater symptom severity and disability than non-OTC users. Seventy-five per cent of the OTC medication users took within the recommended dose of 1–2 pills, but 57% took medication less often than the maximum daily frequency. Seventeen per cent used prescription medication and reported significantly greater symptom severity and disability than non-prescription medication users. Of the prescription drug users, 71% took the prescribed amount, 13% took less and 16% took more.

The authors concluded that adolescent girls frequently suffer from menstrual discomfort and self-medicate with OTC medications. However, they may not be using these medications effectively or using prescribed medications appropriately.

Campbell M A, McGrath P J 1997 Use of medication by adolescents for the management of menstrual discomfort. Archives of Pediatrics and Adolescent Medicine 151(9): 905–913

An antiprostaglandin synthetase inhibitor such as mefenamic acid or naproxen may be prescribed to reduce the pain. Mefenamic acid can be taken three times per day, the analgesic effect persisting for longer than that of aspirin (Trounce 1997). Antispasmodic drugs such as hyoscine butylbromide may help with colicky pain. In cases of severe pain, the combined oral contraceptive pill may be taken for 6 months to suppress ovulation and reduce blood loss. This relieves pain for that period, and when normal cycles return, the pain should be less severe. Progesterone alone may be given to the young girl whose skeletal growth is incomplete. Progesterone from day 5 to day 25 will relax the arteriole spasm in the myometrium without inhibiting ovulation. It is thus also useful for those with pain who wish to become pregnant.

Dilatation and curettage may be performed to relieve cervical spasm or obstruction but is not advised as a routine intervention in dysmenorrhoea due to the risk of incompetence of the cervix. In severe cases, hysteroscopy may be necessary to exclude uterine pathology. A laparoscopy may be required to exclude endometriosis which can occur 3–4 years after the onset of menstruation (Hoshiai et al 1993). A pregnancy and vaginal delivery may improve or cure primary dysmenorrhoea.

NURSING PRIORITIES AND MANAGEMENT: Primary dysmenorrhoea

Assessment

An assessment should be made of the general health of the patient. The patient's own description of the nature of her painful periods should be recorded along with any observations she makes about her physical and emotional symptoms on particular days of the cycle. Any medication used for pain relief or contraception, and its effectiveness, should be noted. Dietary habits and exercise activities are also relevant. By sensitively questioning the patient as to whether she has any special worries or has recently experienced stressful events, useful information may be obtained for inclusion in the care plan.

Care planning

The care plan should be designed in collaboration with the patient. It may be necessary to help the woman recognise signs of impending menstruation so that analgesics can be taken in time to prevent pain. The nurse and patient should discuss strategies other than pharmacological interventions to relieve pain.

The stress of hospital admission or the illness condition may induce menstruation at an earlier date than expected. The nurse may then have to write up appropriate interventions to ensure the patient is 'pain-free' or 'pain is reduced to a tolerable level'. Where possible the patient's preferred methods of pain relief should guide the nursing actions planned.

A teaching plan should be completed in preparation for the patient's discharge as follows:

- Give a simple explanation of the functioning of hormones in the menstrual cycle and the effects of excessive prostaglandins; perhaps use diagrams.
- Discuss the beneficial effects of a diet adequate in fibre, vitamins and polyunsaturated fats, and low in sodium chloride.
- Compare the patient's present level of physical exercise with that of a more beneficial programme. Explain the effects of exercise and good posture in stimulating the function of all organs and the release of pain-relieving endorphins (see Ch. 19).
- Teach a simple relaxation exercise. Ask the patient to practise the exercise regularly. Explain the effects of muscular relaxation in counteracting anxiety or tension and muscle spasm. Refer to massage and local heat application.
- Discuss the use of drugs that reduce the development of prostaglandins, particularly any drug prescribed for the patient.
- Ask the patient to explain, in her own words, some of the changes she would like to make in future. Reinforce her understanding and resolve, and check whether she needs further explanation.

Evaluation of care

A pain verbal rating scale, such as the visual analogue scale, could be used by the patient (see Ch. 19). If the goal of optimal pain relief is not achieved it may be necessary to change the analgesic. Relaxation exercises should be used while the effects of analgesics are awaited. The achievement of the patient's goals will be her first step in a change of lifestyle. Further support and encouragement may be given by her mother, friend, partner, a school or practice nurse or the GP.

Secondary dysmenorrhoea

PATHOPHYSIOLOGY

Secondary dysmenorrhoea is experienced in later menstrual life by women in their mid-20s after previous years of painless menstruation. Women usually complain of a dragging pain in the lower abdomen, pelvic area and breasts, accompanied by headache. The pain occurs some days before the menstrual flow and may continue throughout the period.

The condition is usually associated with some pelvic pathology, although anxiety or depression can be an aggravating factor:

- *Adenomyosis* is a state of increased tension in the uterine muscles, due to accumulating blood in the cystic spaces.
- *Fixed retroversion of the uterus* can cause severe pain, especially if associated with a low-grade pelvic infection.
- *Partial stenosis of the cervix*, following cautery or cone biopsy.
- *Endometriosis* interferes with normal rhythmic contractions of the uterus.
- *Pelvic congestion*, due to increased blood supply to the uterus, and menorrhagia.
- *Pelvic inflammation*, particularly salpingitis, might contribute to pain.
- *Fibromyomata and polyps* interfere with normal rhythmic contractions of the uterus and cause muscular spasms as the uterus attempts to empty itself of the abnormal tissue.

MEDICAL MANAGEMENT

History and examination A detailed history of the problem is recorded and a full physical examination is completed. An accurate history of the pain is important, noting the age of onset, and the site, radiation, duration, character and time of onset in the menstrual cycle. The doctor seeks information about any related symptoms, possible abnormal uterine bleeding, pain on sexual intercourse (dyspareunia), pruritus and premenstrual tension.

Treatment Medical treatment may involve examination under anaesthetic (EUA), dilatation of the cervix and curettage of endometrium. A laparoscopy may be performed when endometriosis is suspected. The presence of fibroids or polyps will be treated appropriately (see p. 274). Pelvic inflammation can be treated by antibiotics. An analgesic drug can be prescribed that is suitable for inhibiting prostaglandin synthesis, e.g. mefenamic acid.

NURSING PRIORITIES AND MANAGEMENT: Secondary dysmenorrhoea

On assessment, actual or potential pain episodes will be identified as a problem. Goals and interventions will be similar to those described for primary dysmenorrhoea, particularly education for the maintenance of personal health. Additional problems will be identified and appropriate nursing interventions planned depending on the specific underlying pathology and the treatment interventions recommended.

Social and psychological issues vary with women's individual circumstances and needs. Pre- and postoperative care planning will be needed if surgical procedures are planned. The nurse needs to be able to promote trust and develop a warm relationship with the patient in order to counteract the patient's fears and communicate effectively. At the time of discharge the patient's future prospects for an improved pattern of menstrual cycles should be much better.

ABNORMAL UTERINE BLEEDING

Abnormal uterine bleeding is described according to the rhythm or pattern of the blood loss episodes:

- *Menorrhagia* refers to heavy or profuse menstrual bleeding. The flow of blood occurs at normal intervals but is increased in amount or duration.
- *Polymenorrhoea* describes menstrual periods that occur with a frequency of less than 21 days.
- *Polymenorrhagia* refers to periods that are both heavy and frequent.
- *Metrorrhagia* describes irregular or unusual bleeding from the uterus between periods.
- *Dysfunctional uterine bleeding* is the descriptive diagnosis used when no organic cause for the abnormal bleeding can be identified.

When abnormal uterine bleeding occurs, the passing of blood clots from the uterus is significant. The menstrual flow is greater than normal if the usual anticlotting agents released by the endometrium are not able to control the volume or rate of flow of the blood.

Menorrhagia

PATHOPHYSIOLOGY

There is hormonal imbalance from any variation in the pattern of oestrogen and progesterone secretion; it is usually of endocrine origin with oversecretion of gonadotrophins. Emotional stress may result in excesses of these hormones being produced.

Ovarian lesions are of two types:

- *Polycystic growths* — may disturb the normal production of ovarian hormones and excessive endometrial growth occurs.
- *Immature follicles* — may fail to result in ovulation. The corpus luteum fails to form, so progesterone cannot be produced. Oestrogen levels continue to rise and there is a proliferation of the endometrium.

Uterine lesions consist of the following types:

- *Fibroids* — increase the surface area of the endometrium that bleeds with greater flow. They may prolong the flow by restricting or disturbing contractions.
- *Polyps* — increase the surface area of endometrium.
- *Adenomyosis* — interferes with contractions by infiltrating the myometrium with endometrial cells.
- *Multiparity* — may result in loss of tone in the uterine muscle fibres. These may be replaced by fibrous tissue which will interfere in the normal contractions.
- *Developmental disorders*, e.g. a bicornuate, septate or duplicated uterus — may impede contractions.
- *Endometriosis* — this is a condition in which ectopic endometrium deposits may be found in the muscle wall or in scattered areas of the pelvic cavity; it is accompanied by increased blood supply to the uterus.
- *Tumour formation* — increases blood supply and bleeding.
- *Intrauterine contraceptive devices* — cause some irritation of the endometrium. Excessive bleeding may be problematic during the first 3 months after insertion.
- *Fallopian tubal ligation* — involves some alteration in the course of blood vessels that increases uterine blood supply. Following the operation, menstruation is usually heavier and may lead to the need for hysterectomy in some women.

MEDICAL MANAGEMENT

Medical examination seeks evidence of stress, worry or tension in the patient and will try to establish whether bleeding is a problem of quantity or rhythm, or both. Pelvic examination may reveal tenderness, masses or irregularities. If no pelvic abnormality is found, then a provisional diagnosis of dysfunctional uterine bleeding is made.

Investigations Special investigation is made of haemoglobin level and full blood count to assess any anaemia present. An EUA and a diagnostic curettage can be performed to show the endometrial response to hormones, to identify any uterine polyps and to exclude carcinoma. Hope (2000), however, asserts that endometrial assessment is not required at an early stage. An estimation of urinary gonadotrophins, oestrogens and progestogens as indicators of hormonal activity may be completed.

Treatment This will depend on the amount of blood lost. Hope (2000) suggests either mefenamic acid 500 mg or tranexamic acid 1 g, three times daily on the first day of the period and on other days with a heavy flow, for a period of 3 months, followed by a review. A dilatation and curettage investigation may in itself relieve the problem, especially in cases of an endometrial polyp. In some instances it may be necessary to nurse the patient in bed and to administer an anxiolytic sedative medication as prescribed to encourage relaxation and reduce stress responses. Any anaemia identified should be corrected as appropriate.

Hormone therapy may be given. Progesterone may be prescribed to provide a balance with oestrogens and reduce excessive endometrial growth. One of the combined contraceptive pills may be given to suppress hormone production, e.g. norethisterone 10–20 mg daily for 10 days, from the 15th day of the cycle. Progestogen administration will modify flow in heavy, but regular, cycles in dysfunctional uterine haemorrhage.

Endometrial ablation is another treatment option for menorrhagia. The aim of this procedure is to remove the endometrium and up to 3 mm of the myometrium. There are several methods of achieving this: transcervical resection of the endometrium (TCRE), laser ablation of the endometrium, rollerball endometrial ablation or thermal uterine balloon therapy (Rosevear 2002). If suitable for this treatment, the woman may be prescribed danazol 4–6 weeks in advance of the procedure to reduce endometrial thickening. The surgery can be performed as a day case. The procedure involves the use of a hysteroscope, inserted vaginally, and through which other instruments are passed to remove the endometrial lining. Following the procedure slight vaginal bleeding can be expected for a few days. Menstrual periods will become lighter or may cease, but dysmenorrhoea and premenstrual symptoms may continue. This procedure may require to be repeated at a later stage or a hysterectomy may eventually be necessary. Disadvantages of this procedure include the possibility of severe haemorrhage or uterine perforation which would necessitate hysterectomy at the time of TCRE. Women should therefore be aware of this before consenting to the procedure.

When a hysterectomy is deemed necessary it may be possible to undertake this without major surgery by means of laparoscopic surgery. This requires insertion of a number of small trocars through the abdominal wall, providing entry sites for instruments. The viewing laparoscope is inserted below the umbilicus, two other insertion sites will be positioned just above the pubic hair line and accessory insertion sites will be used for electrosurgical techniques, a stapling device or to insert sutures via the abdominal cavity. The procedure is performed using video monitoring. The woman can be discharged from hospital within 2 days.

If large fibroids or endometriosis exist, an abdominal hysterectomy is required. Alternatively, in the case of fibroids, a myomectomy may be appropriate. Here the fibroids are shelled out of the myometrium. This conserves the uterus for child bearing.

Metrorrhagia

PATHOPHYSIOLOGY

- *Lowered oestrogen level* may occur just prior to the formation of the corpus luteum, resulting in vaginal blood spotting at the time of ovulation.
- *Changes in the cervix*, e.g. inflammation, erosion, polyps or carcinoma, may cause slight bleeding, especially after intercourse or vaginal examination.
- *Changes in the vagina*, e.g. inflammation, ulceration and atrophy, may cause bleeding.
- *New growth*. Endometrial carcinoma is a major cause of irregular bleeding.
- *Complications of an early pregnancy*. As a fertilised ovum settles into the endometrium, slight bleeding may occur. This loss may be repeated during several months of the pregnancy. Haemorrhage might also occur in a pregnant woman due to 'placenta praevia', when the placenta has implanted abnormally low in the uterus.

MEDICAL MANAGEMENT

Investigations A visual examination with a vaginal speculum is an early investigation. A more detailed examination using the colposcope apparatus completes the colposcopy examination, where magnification of the cervix allows for diagnosis of cervical neoplasia through observation of the epithelial vascular pattern, surface contour and colour. In 95% of patients, premalignant intraepithelial neoplasia is visible through the colposcope.

Punch biopsies are taken for histological examination and examination of tissue complements the colposcopy observations. The Papanicolaou (Pap) smear test is a routine investigation to evaluate changes in cells shed or scraped from the cervix. A high vaginal swab of secretions will allow the identification of bacterial infection, or fungal or parasitic infestations.

The dilatation and curettage operation will provide evidence to support any further investigations.

Treatment Infections of the reproductive tract will be treated with the appropriate broad-spectrum antibiotic. Vaginal thrush (candidiasis) is relieved by nystatin pessaries. *Trichomonas vaginalis* is treated with metronidazole (Flagyl).

In ovulation spotting, small quantities of oestrogen may be given for 6–7 days, 3 days before ovulation.

Any malignant changes that are identified are usually treated by surgical excision, radiotherapy or cytotoxic medication as advised.

PREMENSTRUAL SYNDROME

Premenstrual syndrome (PMS) refers to physical and psychological symptoms occurring in the latter half of the cycle, 2–12 days prior to menstruation, and subsiding after the menstrual flow begins. As luteal phase symptoms, they are present for no longer than 16 days. There is a symptom-free week following menstruation. The symptoms vary from one woman to another, but also show variability from cycle to cycle in individual women with respect to severity, timing and duration.

In establishing a diagnosis, Reid (1991) stresses the importance of the severity of symptoms experienced by women. While mild physiological symptoms are experienced by approximately 95% of women in their reproductive years (Wyatt et al 1999), around 5% of women have symptoms severe enough to disrupt their lives (O'Brien 1993). Hylan et al (1999) estimate that 1.5 million women in the UK experience such symptoms, 35% of them seeking medical help. Symptoms of PMS frequently start after discontinuing the oral contraceptive pill or after a pregnancy, and become progressively worse with age.

Abraham (1987) subdivides symptoms as follows:

- nervous tension, mood swings, irritability and anxiety
- weight gain, swelling of extremities, breast tenderness, abdominal bloating and pelvic pain
- headache, craving for sweets, increased appetite, heart pounding, fatigue and dizziness or fainting
- depression, forgetfulness, confusion, crying and insomnia.

Leather et al (1993) found that symptoms of PMS had greatest effect in the home, with 82% of women reporting relationships with their partners to be seriously affected and 61% reporting relationships with their children to be severely affected, associated with disturbed body image and low self-esteem.

PATHOPHYSIOLOGY

Numerous theories have been suggested to explain PMS, but the precise cause remains unknown. PMS is concluded to be a multifactorial psychoneuroendocrine disorder (see Box 7.2).

Prostaglandins Prostaglandins are produced in response to changing levels of oestrogen and progesterone. They exert sedative effects on the central nervous system and affect both aldosterone and antidiuretic hormone (ADH) activity. If premenstrual changes are influenced by prostaglandins, it may be the balance between the prostaglandins that is of greatest importance.

Fluid retention or redistribution Since the 1930s it has been suggested that PMS might be related to hormones responsible for fluid retention, but research studies can only suggest that there may be a redistribution of body fluids in intracellular and extracellular compartments. They have failed to demonstrate a pattern of fluid retention in most women that suffer from PMS.

Hypoglycaemia Abnormalities of glucose metabolism in the luteal phase of the menstrual cycle that exaggerate glucose swings during the luteal phase might account for premenstrual hypoglycaemic symptoms. However, a causal relationship with PMS is inconclusive (Reid et al 1986).

Vitamin B_6 (pyridoxine) deficiency Vitamin B_6 increases inhibitory amines such as dopamine and serotonin, and also acts as a coenzyme in converting excitatory amino acids to corresponding inhibitory amino acids, with sedative effects. Vitamin B_6 can reduce the excitatory biogenic amines.

Research suggests a central neurotransmitter abnormality, causing a reduced platelet uptake of serotonin and reduced peripheral blood serotonin levels found in the luteal phase of the cycle in women with PMS (Menkes et al 1992, Sundblad et al 1992).

Progesterone withdrawal Although many researchers have suggested that PMS is the result of unopposed oestrogen effects, due to deficiency of progesterone production, many PMS patients have been shown to have adequate corpus luteum functioning. This suggests that it may be the rate of fall of progesterone level during the late luteal phase that is causative in PMS rather than a deficiency state.

Endorphin withdrawal Endorphins are a group of substances which are endogenous opioid peptides. They appear to be important in the physiology of pain and mood change. Studies have shown that there is a change in endorphin levels in women who experience PMS, endorphins declining as the cycle progresses or in the week preceding menstruation (Facchinetti et al 1987).

O'Brien (1993) suggested that PMS is probably related to ovarian function, which in turn is linked to gonadotrophins, which may well be dependent on endorphin function. The current state of knowledge suggests that the primary causal factor lies somewhere in the hypothalamus–pituitary–ovarian mechanism or in the higher centres which influence it.

Serotonin Serotonin is a neurotransmitter that influences mood, appetite and behaviour. In women with PMS it can be significantly lower in the luteal phase of the menstrual cycle than in control subjects, hence the serotonergic system has become a focus of study in PMS (see Research Abstract 7.3).

Box 7.2

Theories related to premenstrual syndrome

Imbalance
- Oestrogen/progesterone
- Prostaglandins

Excess
- Aldosterone
- Angiotensin II
- Oestrogen
- Androgen
- Antidiuretic hormone
- Endorphin
- Prolactin

Deficiency
- Progesterone
- Androgen
- Essential fatty acid
- Blood glucose
- Magnesium
- Endorphin
- Zinc
- Vitamin B_6

Physical changes
- Sodium and water retention
- Abnormal water distribution
- Leakage of albumin/tissue fluid
- Allergy related to progesterone
- Dietary abnormality
- Serotonin or aspartine neurotransmitter disturbance

RESEARCH ABSTRACT 7.3

Selective serotonin reuptake inhibitors in the treatment of premenstrual syndrome

Wyatt et al (2002) carried out a systematic review on the effectiveness of selective serotonin reuptake inhibitors (SSRIs) in the treatment of women with severe premenstrual syndrome (PMS). An electronic search of the Cochrane Menstrual Disorders and Subfertility Group specialised register of controlled trials, Cochrane Controlled Trials Register, MEDLINE, EMBASE and PsychLit was conducted. All trials in which women were randomised to receive SSRIs or placebo in a double-blind trial for the treatment of premenstrual syndrome were considered. Fifteen trials were included in the systematic review and 10 trials in the main analyses.

The findings indicated that SSRIs were very effective in treating premenstrual syndrome, both physical and behavioural symptoms. Side-effects resulted in some withdrawals (2.5 times more likely in the treatment group, particularly with high doses). The reviewers concluded that there is good evidence for the use of SSRIs in the treatment of severe premenstrual syndrome.

Wyatt K M, Dimmock P W, O'Brien P M S 2002 Selective serotonin reuptake inhibitors for premenstrual syndrome. Cochrane Database Systematic Review (4): CD001396.www.update-software.com/Abstracts/AB001396.htm

While researchers have been keen to find one reason for PMS, it is more likely that it is a combination of physical, psychological and social factors.

MEDICAL MANAGEMENT

Recommended treatment focuses on identifying and controlling individual symptom clusters. Drug treatments are used cautiously. Many research studies have shown marked placebo effects of 40–60% in PMS sufferers. The patient–doctor relationship is thought to be an important influence on some women, relieved that their condition is being taken seriously.

Investigations A thorough examination is required to diagnose PMS accurately and exclude or identify any underlying pathology. Other medical, psychiatric and gynaecological conditions must be excluded or be identified as coexisting with PMS.

Breast cancer must be excluded, as hormone-dependent cancers may be stimulated by hormone therapy. A patient with pelvic pain may have an inflammatory condition, or endometriosis, that needs further investigation. Some patients may have a depressive illness, as well as PMS. This may be referred to as secondary PMS, the depressive symptoms persisting through what is expected to be a symptom-free week in the cycle.

Estimations of oestrogen, progesterone, prolactin, gonadotrophin or electrolytes are not usually helpful in making a diagnosis of PMS.

Treatment An integrated treatment programme can be adopted whereby patients are asked to record in a diary, on a daily basis, personal experiences in mood, behaviour, thinking patterns and physical discomforts, for at least 3 months. Symptom clusters and symptom-free times can be thus easily identified.

In addition, women should be advised to:

- take regular exercise
- avoid coffee, tea and chocolate
- take a diet that is low in sugars and high in lean proteins
- take vitamin supplements B_6 and E_1 and the mineral magnesium
- restrict salt intake
- limit fluid intake
- chart their weight daily
- avoid alcohol and smoking
- avoid stress.

These general measures contribute to good health and can maximise physical and psychological well-being.

While some women have found evening primrose oil can relieve symptoms of PMS (Campbell et al 1997), the beneficial effects have not been substantiated in research (Khoo et al 1990, Robinson & Garfinkel 1990, Budeiri et al 1996). Robinson and Garfinkel (1990) included factors such as diet, exercise and stress control in their recommendations for effective management of PMS.

Some women find aromatherapy helpful for specific PMS symptoms, such as headache or fluid retention. A few drops can be added to bathwater or mixed in a massage oil. Rosemary or peppermint can be used to relieve headache; fennel, juniper or geranium to reduce fluid retention; bergamot and jasmine to elevate mood; and lavender and rose to help balance hormone production (Rich 1996).

Drug treatments used in PMS depend partly on the preference of the doctor providing care and the particular cluster of symptoms experienced by the patient. Many women who have already tried over-the-counter remedies expect or request hormonal treatment.

Hormonal treatment Hormonal treatment of PMS is as follows:

- Some doctors continue to use progesterone or progestogen for all PMS symptoms. The drug may be given orally, by injection, by suppository, in the combined contraceptive pill or by means of an implant. However, Wyatt et al (2001) present evidence from a meta-analysis that does not support the use of progesterone or progestogens in the treatment of PMS.
- The drug danazol, which inhibits pituitary gonadotrophin secretion, is prescribed selectively for some patients, particularly those with severe mastalgia and other PMS symptoms (Halbreich et al 1991). Danazol completely suppresses the menstrual cycle and reduces breast tenderness, but varying degrees of improvement in other symptoms have been documented. Patients are advised to use alternative, non-hormonal contraceptive methods. The major disadvantage of danazol is that high doses cause masculinisation (Deeny et al 1991). Other minor side-effects such as nausea, dizziness and rashes are troublesome to certain patients.
- Analogues of gonadotrophin-releasing hormone (GnRH), such as buserelin, will inhibit the release of gonadotrophins and so suppress follicular development, ovulation and the endocrine changes of the cycle. A 'medical oophorectomy' is thus created. Suffling (2001) claims that GnRH analogues are most effective if administered by depot injection and their use limited to 6 months, minimising the side-effects associated with sudden oestrogen withdrawal. The treatment is expensive and is generally reserved for women with severe symptoms, when other treatment options have failed.
- Oestrogen therapy, in the form of transdermal patches or subcutaneous implants, can be used to suppress menstruation. Natural oestrogen administered by this route avoids the liver and so prevents problems with clotting factors and lipid metabolism. For women with a uterus, the use of this percutaneous oestrogen therapy requires to be complemented by the use of cyclical progestogen, to prevent endometrial hyperplasia. Unfortunately some women experience mild PMS-like symptoms during this phase of the treatment.
- Bromocriptine is a stimulant of dopamine receptors in the brain and also inhibits the release of prolactin by the pituitary. The role of prolactin in PMS is poorly understood, but bromocriptine has been shown to be effective in the treatment of breast symptoms.
- Schellenberg (2001) suggests that one tablet daily of *Agnus castus* (dry extract) is well tolerated and can be effective in women's self-assessment of their symptoms, e.g. mood, headache, breast fullness and bloating.

Diuretic treatment In women who have a measured weight increase, the diuretic spironolactone may be prescribed. This medication blocks the body's use of the hormone aldosterone. Some investigators have found it to be useful for symptoms of depressed mood.

Analgesic treatment Where pain is a primary symptom, the anti-inflammatory analgesic and prostaglandin inhibitor mefenamic acid may be helpful, but research as to how many PMS symptoms this medication will relieve is contradictory. There is agreement that the medication is of benefit for some PMS symptoms.

Psychological support Supportive psychotherapy and techniques that improve coping skills and stress management should be part of the care programme. Women who experience secondary PMS, whereby their unhappy mood and agitated behaviours persist throughout their cycles, may need the clinical help of a psychiatrist. Wyatt et al (1999) suggest that vitamin B_6, up to a dose of 100 mg/day, can be helpful for premenstrual depression and other premenstrual symptoms.

Surgery In cases of severe PMS or those compounded by other gynaecological problems, hysterectomy with bilateral salpingo-oophorectomy followed by HRT may be considered. Oophorectomy must be included to prevent the ovarian cycle, otherwise the cyclical problems will persist.

NURSING PRIORITIES AND MANAGEMENT: PMS

Assessment

The nurse may encounter women who experience PMS symptoms not discussed with their doctors. Nurses have opportunities to provide such women with information suggesting daily recording of physical changes, discomforts, emotional feelings and behaviour.

Care planning

A supportive–educative approach combines the giving of information and advice, and also allows the woman to suggest how best the aims can be achieved in her particular circumstances. The nurse should discuss options with particular care to avoid causing any financial embarrassment to the woman who may have little money to spare from her family budget for vitamin supplements or evening primrose oil, which may be costly.

Useful advice includes the following:

- Undertake physical exercise as a stimulant to the circulatory system, improving functioning of all bodily organs and relieving congestion. As a result concentration and sleep should improve, and feelings of well-being may increase.
- Reduce fat, sugar, salt, coffee and tea consumption.
- Aim to eat five servings of fresh fruit and vegetables per day (Williams 1995).
- Reduce smoking and alcohol intake.
- Avoid stressful situations to reduce tension and feelings of frustration, particularly at trigger times in the cycle.
- Incorporate relaxation exercises.
- Obtain massage, carried out by a partner, nurse or therapist.

A counselling approach by the nurse can encourage the woman to verbalise her preferred choices. Information should be given to the patient about the nature of any drugs prescribed. Referral to a health visitor may be necessary if the patient requires continuing support at home. The possible value of self-help groups can also be discussed with the woman, but the value of family support, emphasised in some cultures, should not be undermined.

Evaluation of care

Some symptoms may have greatly improved, but there may be no feeling of improvement in other areas. Where unresolved problems remain, each planned action should be reviewed. Evidence of a sustained unhappy mood or other severe symptoms should be referred to the GP or PMS clinic doctor or the added interventions of a psychiatrist or psychotherapist.

DISORDERS OF THE MENOPAUSE

Physiological, psychological and social changes associated with the menopause have been described earlier. The long-term effects of oestrogen withdrawal on women's health will now be addressed.

Decreased oestrogen formation is associated with the development of osteoporosis and cardiovascular disease, resulting in an increased risk of bone fractures, myocardial infarction, angina and stroke. The literature suggests that there is some cultural variation in the experience of post-menopausal symptoms and in the incidence of disorders related to the withdrawal of oestrogen (Lock 1994, Robinson 1996, Chow et al 1997). Gasperino (1996) proposes that there is ethnic variation as well, suggesting, for example, that the greater bone and muscle mass and lower fat, as a percentage of body weight, in black women is relevant to the lower incidence of osteoporosis and cardiovascular disease in this ethnic group.

Factors contributing to an increased risk of osteoporosis and cardiovascular disease include:

- inherited factors
- sedentary lifestyle
- low calcium intake
- low body weight
- early menopause
- cigarette smoking
- excessive salt intake
- excessive stress
- high protein intake
- moderate to excessive alcohol intake
- caffeine
- pre-existing disorders of the kidney or thyroid, rheumatoid arthritis and diabetes.

Osteoporosis

Osteoporosis is a disease characterised by a decrease in bone density per unit volume, predisposing to fracture with even minimal trauma. The demineralisation and consequent weakening of bone are more marked in trabecular bone. The World Health Organisation (WHO) defines osteoporosis as bone mineral density of more than 2.5 standard deviations below the mean value for young adults (WHO 1994). This definition has been used to diagnose osteoporosis based on bone mineral density assessed at the hip and spine using dual energy X-ray absorptiometry (DEXA). Peripheral densitometry devices have been introduced with the advantage of low cost and portability, allowing assessment at the heel or forearm. However, since bone mineral density is not consistent throughout the skeleton there is the potential for misdiagnosis if the WHO's definition is applied at all sites. Such discordance between sites is more common in younger women, and Miller et al (1998) recommend that more than one site is used in women younger than 65 years. Quantitative ultrasound at the heel can be used to assess bone strength (rather than bone density) and can provide a useful measure from which predictions can be made about the risk of future fractures in older women (Hans et al 1996, Hodson & Marsh 2003). The most common sites for fractures are the wrist, spine and hip, causing pain, deformity and possible hospitalisation.

Oestrogens play an important part in achieving a strong bone structure. They determine the sensitivity of bone to parathyroid hormone, limit resorption of bone and increase calcium absorption from the gut. In early adult life, the rate of bone formation exceeds that of resorption, thus building strong bone. When oestrogen levels decline prior to the menopause, bone resorption increases and bone loss accelerates after the menopause. This is most marked in the first years after the menopause when there is a significant decline in oestrogen. During the first 5–10 years after the menopause, bone density decreases significantly. Thereafter the rate of bone loss gradually decreases. Failure to achieve maximum skeletal mass in early adulthood will be aggravated by oestrogen deprivation after the menopause. HRT after the menopause, however, is not recommended as the first choice for preventing osteoporosis (Singh 2003).

Cardiovascular disease

Before the age of 50, deaths from breast cancer outnumber deaths from ischaemic heart disease and stroke in women, but in postmenopausal women the mortality rate for arterial disease greatly exceeds that of breast cancer. Payne (1997) suggests that cardiovascular disease is the most common cause of death among women in the UK. Withdrawal of oestrogen at the menopause causes changes in lipid and lipoprotein metabolism, resulting in a low high-density lipoprotein:low-density lipoprotein ratio. Such metabolic disturbances can contribute to the incidence of cardiovascular disease in this group (Stevenson 1996). Recent research suggests that HRT offers women no protection against ischaemic heart disease (Løkkegaard et al 2003). A consensus statement on HRT by the Royal College of Physicians (2003) indicates that its value remains controversial and that although effective in relief of vasomotor symptoms, mood changes and insomnia associated with the menopause, evidence is lacking to support the use of HRT in treating osteoporosis, heart disease or Alzheimer's disease. Grant (2003) suggests that this underestimates the dangers of HRT, indicating an increased risk of breast cancer (Rossouw et al 2002, Beral et al 2003), ischaemic heart disease (Rossouw et al 2002) and ovarian cancer (Gottlieb 2003).

MEDICAL MANAGEMENT: LONG-TERM EFFECTS OF THE MENOPAUSE

Hormone replacement therapy (HRT) Once bone loss has occurred it cannot effectively be replaced. There is evidence that oestrogen prevents bone loss in early menopausal women (Stevenson et al 1990) by decreasing the rate of bone resorption. Bone loss occurs most rapidly at the time of the menopause or shortly after. Prophylactic HRT has been recommended in the past for osteoporosis, but there is now the suggestion that side-effects outweigh the benefits (Singh 2003).

Other therapies which reduce the rate of bone resorption are calcitonin and bisphosphonates. Calcitonin can prevent postmenopausal trabecular bone loss (MacIntyre et al 1988, Overgaard et al 1989) by decreasing osteoclast activity, as do bisphosphonates (Reginster et al 1989). Gottlieb (2001) suggests that parathyroid hormone may offer short-term treatment in cases of established fractures (see Research Abstract 7.4).

Research in the 1990s suggested that oestrogen replacement after the menopause decreased the risk of cardiovascular disease (Hunt et al 1990, Stampfer & Colditz 1991) and stroke (Finucane et al 1993). The main beneficial effects on the cardiovascular system appeared to be on vessel walls, blood flow and lipid metabolism (Whitehead & Godfree 1992). Nabulsi et al (1993) suggested that taking oestrogen postmenopausally can reduce the risk of coronary artery disease by 42%, and if progestogen is included the benefits may be even greater. However, this remains controversial and further research is ongoing.

In hormone replacement therapy oestrogen is administered continuously. Progestogens are given for 12–14 days per month on a cyclical basis to women with a uterus, for endometrial protection, reducing the risk of erratic bleeding, endometrial hyperplasia and endometrial cancer (Whitehead et al 1990). This results in a withdrawal bleed. Tibolone (Livial) is a synthetic steroid with properties of

RESEARCH ABSTRACT 7.4

Parathyroid hormone in the treatment of established fractures

In a randomised controlled study of 1637 postmenopausal women with previous vertebral fractures (Gottlieb 2001) the women were given either 20–40 mcg parathyroid hormone or a placebo subcutaneously daily. In addition all patients took calcium and vitamin D supplements daily. The women receiving parathyroid hormone showed a significant reduction in the risk of new fractures when compared with those taking the placebo. Women in the treatment group also showed significant increases in vertebral, femoral and total-body mineral density. While there is some concern about the possible side-effect of bone tumours (identified in rats having high doses in earlier trials) this may prove to be a possible option for short-term treatment in cases of established fractures.

Gottlieb S 2001 Human parathyroid hormone may prevent osteoporosis. British Medical Journal 322(7296): 1200–1201

RESEARCH ABSTRACT 7.5

The effect of hormone replacement therapy on women's menopausal symptoms

Gelfand et al (2003) evaluated the effects of a regimen of constant-oestrogen, intermittent-progestogen hormone replacement on women's menopausal symptoms in a randomised, double-blind, placebo-controlled multicentre study conducted over 90 days. One hundred and nineteen postmenopausal women with vasomotor symptoms participated in the study. All the women still had their uterus and had reported amenorrhoea for at least 6 months. The active treatment group showed a marked reduction in menopausal symptoms as measured by the Kupperman Index when compared with the placebo group after 45 days of treatment and this was maintained until the end of the study (90 days). The active treatment group also showed greater improvement in quality of life as measured by the Menopause Quality of Life summary score. The authors concluded that the regimen of constant-oestrogen, intermittent-progestogen was effective in relieving menopausal symptoms and improving quality of life. The treatment was well received by the sample of women.

Gelfand M M, Moreau M, Ayotte N J, Hilditch J R, Wong B A, Lau C Y 2003 Clinical assessment and quality of life of postmenopausal women treated with a new intermittent progestogen combination hormone replacement therapy: a placebo-controlled study. Menopause 10(1): 29–36

oestrogen, progestogen and androgen; if taken continuously, it should not cause a withdrawal bleed.

Short-term HRT may be prescribed for specific menopausal symptoms such as hot flushes and atrophic vaginitis, for as long as treatment is required. Long-term HRT may be prescribed for women under 40 years who have had a premature menopause, occurring naturally, as a result of surgery or iatrogenically.

While HRT can confer benefits for women experiencing adverse effects of the menopause (see Research Abstracts 7.1 and 7.5), it can also have side-effects, and risks are associated particularly with long-term use. In addition, there are some contraindications to be considered regarding the use of HRT.

Although many preparations of HRT are available, the reported adherence rate is poor, with a significant number of women discontinuing therapy. Treatment is abandoned because of the side-effects experienced or because of fear of risks associated with the treatment. Possible side-effects include:

- breast pain/tenderness
- leg cramps
- vaginal discharge
- vaginal bleeding
- fluid retention/bloating
- mood changes
- increased appetite.

Such side-effects might be reduced or eliminated by changing to a different preparation. However, women are encouraged to persist with one form of therapy for at least 3 months as some of the early side-effects can be temporary.

While it is acknowledged that unopposed oestrogen increases the risk of endometrial cancer, Whitehead et al (1990) suggested that this risk can be eliminated if progestogens are administered for 12–14 days of the cycle. Wells et al (2002) demonstrated a degree of hyperplasia with sequential oestrogen/progestogen but, in most cases, this can be prevented with a regimen of continuous progestogen with oestrogen.

The link between HRT and breast cancer has been the subject of research for some time. Schairer et al (2000) indicated that an oestrogen–progestogen regimen increases breast cancer risk beyond that associated with oestrogen alone. Beral (2003) confirmed earlier findings that the present use of HRT is associated with an increase in breast cancer, the effect being substantially greater when oestrogen–progestogen combinations are used. There is a need for further research.

Contraindications to HRT are usually described as absolute or relative. Absolute contraindications generally include:

- pregnancy
- undiagnosed endometrial bleeding
- endometrial cancer
- breast cancer
- severe active liver disease
- porphyria.

While HRT is not recommended for women with these problems, individual women may still wish to take HRT for severe acute symptoms or for protective effects. Such women are referred to a specialist centre to be fully informed and closely monitored if they decide to embark on the therapy. Possible contraindications are identified to highlight the likelihood of complications, to ensure that underlying disorders are treated or monitored, and to monitor the appropriate therapy, which may differ from uncomplicated cases, if the woman and her doctor decide on HRT. Caution is therefore required in prescribing HRT in association with the following:

- endometrial hyperplasia, endometriosis or fibroids
- hypertension — treat prior to HRT
- clotting problems — refer to a haematologist (Whitehead & Godfree 1992)
- diabetes — monitor glucose levels to identify any change required in insulin
- gallstones — may be aggravated, rather than develop as a new disease (Whitehead & Godfree 1992); if treated, they are not of concern
- otosclerosis — Whitehead and Godfree (1992) recommend referral to an ENT specialist since they have anecdotal experience of increasing deafness in such patients.

Menopause clinics Some GPs prescribe HRT directly, whereas others refer women to menopause clinics which have become established in many hospitals throughout the

UK, staffed by a gynaecologist with a special interest in the management of problems associated with the menopause. Specially trained nurses and paramedic personnel contribute to the overall assessment and care of those attending the clinics. Treatments can be more easily controlled and supervised within such a clinic, protocols are established, dietetic and diagnostic facilities are more readily available, and screening, general health and patient education programmes can be introduced.

NURSING PRIORITIES AND MANAGEMENT: The postmenopausal woman

Women should be encouraged to make an informed choice about HRT. The role of the nurse involves the development of trust within the nurse–patient relationship and the giving of information to enable women to come to an informed decision. The educative and supportive aspects of the self-care nursing model (Orem 1991) are useful. Whilst not recommending HRT for all postmenopausal women, it is not justifiable to withhold treatment from a fully informed patient who requests it.

Since women worry about the risks of HRT, the nurse should raise these, both to allow a discussion of personal feelings and to clarify any misunderstandings. It is important to warn about the early side-effects of the sudden rise in oestrogen levels at the start of HRT. Women should understand that there are a range of medications, doses and types of HRT, so that if one is found to be unacceptable, another regimen may be tried.

The following is a guide for nurses interviewing women facing the menopause:

- Provide information and advice according to the problems and concerns of individual women and any ongoing postmenopausal symptoms.
- Encourage a healthy lifestyle and continuing health awareness.
- Give dietary information to encourage selecting low-fat, calcium-rich foods; explain physiological links to vascular conditions and the maintenance of bone mineral content.
- Check the patient's usual physical exercise pattern; reinforce the need for regular exercise, stressing the importance of the pull of muscle on bone for bone formation and health; discuss a weight-bearing exercise programme.
- Discuss the benefits and possible side-effects of HRT.
- Explain the need for self-examination of breasts and teach the technique.
- Provide opportunities for questions.
- Check the patient's understanding of the information given by encouraging feedback.
- Give the patient a copy of free booklets prepared by the health authorities relating to the menopause and a healthy lifestyle, for example the Health Education Board for Scotland booklets *The Time of Your Life, Well Woman, Eat to your Heart's Content, Look after Yourself*.
- Give the name and telephone number of a person to contact in the event of any problem occurring.

DISORDERS OF THE FEMALE REPRODUCTIVE SYSTEM

BENIGN TUMOUR OF THE OVARY

Benign cystic teratoma or dermoid cyst

Dermoid cysts may develop in women of all ages and comprise 25% of all ovarian tumours. There is a 3% possibility of such cysts becoming malignant.

PATHOPHYSIOLOGY

The dermoid cyst is believed to develop from the aberrant division of an unfertilised oocyte, but the cause remains uncertain (Lewis & Chamberlain 1995). It is formed from accumulated sebaceous material from the glands of the neoplasm. It is a thick-walled cyst, whitish-yellow in colour, lined with skin, hair follicles, hair and sweat glands. Teeth may be found emerging from primitive sockets, and bone cartilage, lung and intestinal epithelium can be identified within the cyst.

MEDICAL MANAGEMENT

The patient may present with abdominal pain. Following an abdominal and vaginal examination, she is referred to a gynaecologist for assessment. Pain may be caused by peritoneal irritation from the cyst. Peritonitis may result from rupture of the cyst contents into the abdomen. The cyst may become infected if salpingitis, appendicitis or diverticulitis is present. Dense adhesions may occur between an infected cyst and the peritoneum or bowel. Torsion or twisting of the pedicle or stalk of the cyst may develop and this may reduce the blood supply, particularly the venous return, to the cyst and cause pain. Malignant change may occur in any of the primitive tissues of the cyst.

Investigations A Pap cervical smear test may be completed at the time of vaginal examination by the GP. Any malignant cells present might be associated with an ovarian cancer. An ultrasound scan can identify the ovarian cyst.

Treatment Surgery will be undertaken by laparoscopy or laparotomy. The extent of surgery will vary according to the age of the woman. In younger women, with child-bearing years ahead of them, the benign cyst alone may be shelled out of the ovary, leaving the normal ovarian tissue to continue functioning. Both ovaries will be assessed, as the cysts are often bilateral.

Women who already have a family or are over 50 years of age would be advised to have the ovary removed. In the event of malignancy of the dermoid cyst, both ovaries and the uterus would be removed. Involvement of the peritoneum in the spread of malignancy would necessitate the instillation of a cytotoxic agent, such as thiotepa (see p. 1053), into the abdominal cavity at the time of surgery.

NURSING PRIORITIES AND MANAGEMENT: Dermoid cyst

Nursing care will depend upon the extent of the surgery undertaken and will be described in the section on ovarian cancer (p. 286).

BENIGN TUMOURS OF THE UTERUS

Endometrial polyps

Polyps are benign neoplasms of the endometrium of the uterus. They may develop from an overgrowth of endometrial glands and stroma. The polyp may produce a stalk and may descend towards the vulva. Single or multiple polyps may occur commonly in women of any age group. Vaginal bleeding may be slight but occurs between menstrual periods or following coitus. Under anaesthetic the polyp can be removed from the uterus by twisting it off at its stalk or by curettage of the endometrium. Histological examination of all polyps is routine as recurrent multiple polyps may undergo malignant change.

Fibromyomata

Myomata or fibroid tumours of the muscle of the uterus can occur in women between 35 years of age and the onset of the menopause. The growth of fibroids is stimulated by ovarian hormones, particularly oestrogens. Women who have not had children are more liable to develop such tumours.

PATHOPHYSIOLOGY

The fibroid is spherical in shape and firm in consistency. Some fibroids are small, while others may grow large enough to fill the abdominal cavity. The tumour is encapsulated and the capsule contains the blood vessels supplying the tumour. As it grows, the centre of the tumour becomes less vascular and liable to degenerative change.

Multiple fibroids may be present, giving the uterus an irregular shape (see Fig. 7.7) or causing displacement of the uterus and uterine vessels.

Common presenting symptoms Menstruation becomes heavier and is prolonged when there are fibroids in the uterus. If the tumours are submucous then menstruation may become irregular and there may be bleeding between periods, but this is not common. Uterine pain may result as the uterus strongly contracts to attempt expulsion of the fibroid. Pressure upon pelvic nerves may cause back or leg pain; pressure on pelvic organs may lead to:

- frequency of micturition
- retention of urine
- obstruction of the gastrointestinal system
- oedema of a leg.

A fibroid may become infected and necrotic, causing a purulent vaginal discharge.

The most noticeable change is that of increasing girth of the abdomen; rapid increase may indicate that malignant change has taken place in the fibroid. Polycythaemia is associated with uterine fibroids but is a rare condition.

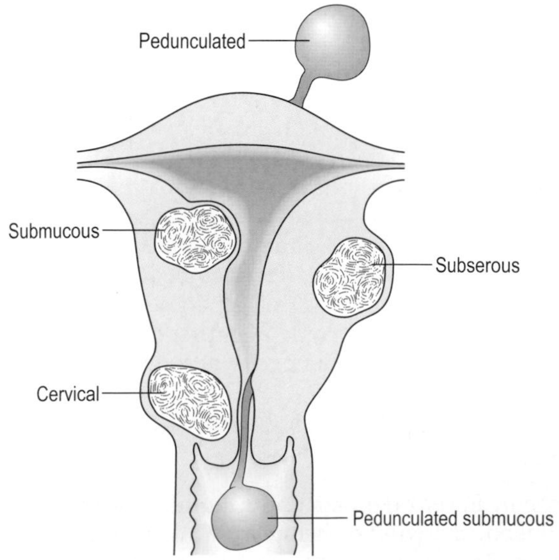

Fig. 7.7 Common sites of fibromyomata in the uterus.

MEDICAL MANAGEMENT

On abdominal and vaginal examination, the uterus is usually found to be symmetrically enlarged. It feels harder than it does in pregnancy, unless there is some degeneration of the fibroid(s) as occurs after the menopause. The uterus may feel nodular due to the presence of multiple tumours. The lower part of a tumour may be felt through the cervix and the difference between fibroid and carcinoma of cervix may be difficult to ascertain.

Investigations Pelvic X-ray and ultrasound scan may assist with diagnosis of fibroids. Diagnostic curettage may be performed to exclude endometrial carcinoma. An EUA is helpful in diagnosis. A sigmoidoscopy or barium enema may be performed to exclude carcinoma of the bowel.

Treatment Small fibroids may not be treated and any symptoms should disappear with the menopause. Medical treatment may be prescribed in the interim to relieve symptoms. Goserelin, a gonadotrophin-releasing hormone analogue, may be prescribed. In a woman who desires a future pregnancy it may be appropriate to shell out the fibroids from the myometrium (myomectomy); an older woman may be treated by hysterectomy. If the fibroids are small, a vaginal hysterectomy may be possible. Any anaemia experienced by the patient is rectified by blood transfusion before surgery.

Embolisation of uterine arteries has been introduced as an alternative treatment to hysterectomy (Thomas 1997). This involves cannulating the right femoral artery after administration of a local anaesthetic to the inguinal region. Under screening control, a catheter is passed through the arterial system and eventually to the right and then left uterine arteries which are individually embolised with polyvinyl alcohol solution. Contrast medium is injected to ensure effective arterial occlusion. Thomas (1997) stresses that patients require good opiate pain control following this procedure, but once pain is controlled patients can be discharged.

NURSING PRIORITIES AND MANAGEMENT: Fibromyomata

Nursing care will be prioritised depending upon the type of surgery completed. Observations of pulse, blood pressure and vaginal blood loss are recorded to monitor internal bleeding from the operation site.

Care following hysterectomy will be similar to that described on page 280, but the patient will not have the worry of having a malignant disease that may continue to cause problems. Fibromyomata may recur in some women (Fedele et al 1995).

TROPHOBLASTIC TUMOURS

Trophoblastic tumours arise from the primitive tissues destined to develop into the placenta. They may be benign or malignant.

Hydatidiform mole (vesicular mole)

The hydatidiform mole results from hydropic degeneration and vesicle formation of the chorionic villi. These project from the outer mass of cells forming the trophoblast and are destined to become the placenta when the fertilised ovum settles into the endometrium. The uterus fills with grape-like vesicles which produce large quantities of chorionic gonadotrophin. The chromosomal pattern is 46XX, but all the chromosomal material is derived from the sperm, which doubles its chromosomes and takes over the ovum. No fetus develops.

PATHOPHYSIOLOGY

A hydatidiform mole is a benign tumour mass of chorionic cells in the uterus, which exists as though it were a developing pregnancy. Ovarian follicles are enlarged and there is an increase in blood and urine levels of human chorionic gonadotrophin (hCG). The uterus increases in size, sometimes faster than in a pregnancy. The villi of the trophoblast become swollen and the villi or vesicles cluster together like grapes.

Common presenting symptoms A woman may visit her doctor complaining of a vaginal discharge of fresh or altered blood which does not seem like normal menstruation. She may have noticed that some jelly-like mole vesicles have been expelled. She may be feeling unwell with some nausea and vomiting that resembles early pregnancy. Pelvic pain is not usually a problem.

MEDICAL MANAGEMENT

A general physical and vaginal examination will be performed. The uterus may be increased in size. A 'blighted ovum' might be suspected but the watery vesicles of the mole, if identified or reported, will alert the doctor to the condition.

Investigations A series of pregnancy tests will be completed. Pregnancy tests are positive, although there is no fetus present. The urine is diluted 1:10, 1:100 and 1:1000 — a positive pregnancy test in the 1:100 dilution is strongly suggestive of the mole. The diagnosis is confirmed by ultrasound investigation and by the finding of high levels of hCG in urine or serum. Choriocarcinoma is a serious complication following hydatidiform mole in 1 in 30 cases.

Treatment The uterus may be stimulated to contract by administration of oxytocin, in order to expel the mole, or it may be evacuated vaginally by suction apparatus. The uterus is in a soft, delicate state and is gently curetted to prevent perforation. A hysterectomy may be advised for a woman who has a family or is past child-bearing age. Thorough follow-up of the patient is necessary if hysterectomy has not been performed. At weekly or 2-weekly intervals for 2 years there must be measurement of urinary output of hCG by radioimmunoassay.

Complications A rising level of hCG with negative curettings of the uterine cavity suggests that the mole has become invasive of the muscle of the uterus and may even erode through the uterine wall. Deposits of molar tissue may be found in other parts of the body, in the peritoneum or in the lungs, and may cause death.

Choriocarcinoma

In 50% of cases choriocarcinoma of the uterine wall occurs after hydatidiform mole. The malignant condition may appear to arise spontaneously from the ovary but it is more likely to be associated with other neoplastic tissues, such as a teratoma. It may follow a normal pregnancy, an abortion or an ectopic pregnancy.

PATHOPHYSIOLOGY

The uterus becomes ulcerated, causing an offensive, blood-stained vaginal discharge. Metastatic spread of the cancer is speedy and extensive; the brain, lung, liver and other organs may be involved. Early deterioration is expected if the condition is not treated early.

Diagnosis is difficult but confirmed by hCG estimations in urine and plasma. The tissues contain malignant syncytioblast and cytotrophoblast cells.

MEDICAL MANAGEMENT

Follow-up arrangements after mole removal are usually stringent and early signs of development of the malignant tumour should become obvious, but there are greater risks if a woman delays consultation.

Investigations The tumour produces large amounts of hCG, used as a tumour marker. Uterine curettings provide histological evidence that confirms diagnosis and excludes a rare ovarian teratoma. hCG levels are also used to monitor the response to therapy.

Treatment Choriocarcinoma is highly sensitive to single-agent chemotherapy. If the tumour is confined to the uterus then intensive cytotoxic drug treatment is given using the drug methotrexate, toxic to the decidua, with almost 100% successful results. Folinic acid is given to protect the bone marrow. Special facilities are needed to protect patients who have a lowered resistance to infection because of diminished white blood cells.

If there is metastatic disease, methotrexate may be combined with other cytotoxic agents. The drugs induce marked side-effects during the treatment period and cardiac toxicity may occur. Early detection and treatment of the condition are advised, the disease being known to be curable even after systemic spread. Eighty per cent of patients may make a complete recovery if the disease is identified within

6 months of onset. Good prognosis from metastatic disease is associated with hCG titre levels of less than 40 000 mIU/mL before chemotherapy. hCG levels above 40 000 mIU/mL give a poor prognosis.

Some women may need a hysterectomy before treatment is completed but, as the condition occurs in child-bearing years, women may wish to become pregnant after a period of 2 years from recovery.

NURSING PRIORITIES AND MANAGEMENT: Hydatidiform mole/choriocarcinoma

Hydatidiform mole

Nursing care following evacuation of hydatidiform mole will be similar to that following curettage of the uterus. Recovery from anaesthetic should be speedy and the patient will become self-caring soon after returning to the ward. Following an anaesthetic, the nurse should check on the level of vaginal blood loss, which should be minimal within 24 h, diminishing quickly. Persistent bleeding should be reported to the doctor.

Minimal abdominal discomfort should be experienced by the patient. A mild analgesic will be prescribed, if necessary. If a patient experiences more severe pain, she should be closely observed. Intensive curetting of the uterus might, in rare cases, result in perforation of the uterus and even damage to the bowel. Any cause for concern should be reported to the doctor.

A series of postoperative urine and blood specimens will be required to estimate hCG levels. Specimens may need to be sent to one of the specialised centres in the UK where there is greater experience in assessing the significance of hCG levels and reporting results.

Choriocarcinoma

In the event of persistently high levels of hCG, a diagnosis of choriocarcinoma would require transfer of the patient to a specialised centre for chemotherapy. The patient may be very anxious, having to face up to the seriousness of her illness and the urgency of treatment. The nurse will reinforce the information already given to the patient by the doctor, emphasising the positive aspects of the care and the expertise of the staff at the specialised centre. The nurse must be prepared to cope with any outpouring of emotion and facilitate special wishes the patient may have. The partner can be fully involved in the events and can accompany the woman to the treatment centre.

Special facilities are available for reverse barrier nursing of the patient to protect her from infection as chemotherapy progresses and her immune system is compromised (see Ch. 16). Physical, psychological and social aspects of nursing care will be of primary concern. Many weeks of treatment may be involved before recovery is achieved and the patient returned to normal family life. Follow-up and further hCG monitoring are essential.

GYNAECOLOGICAL CANCER

The organs of the female reproductive system are susceptible to benign or malignant overgrowth of tissues. Cancerous or malignant tumours are generally differentiated from benign tumours by the following properties:

- they are not encapsulated and invade tissues in which they arise
- they show disorderly reproduction
- they tend to show loss of structural differentiation
- they can produce metastases.

The cervix, body of the uterus, ovary and vulva are potential sites for primary cancerous growth.

Carcinoma of the cervix

The cervical tissue is at particular risk of carcinomatous change. Hughes (2001) suggests cervical cancer affects 4200 women in the UK annually. Department of Health (1999) records indicate that 4000 new cases of invasive cancer of the cervix were registered in 1998–1999. In Scotland in 2002 there were 100 deaths from cervical cancer but over the most recent 10-year period there has been a fall in incidence and mortality (Scottish Health Statistics 2003).

Cancer of the cervix occurs most often in women between 30 and 50 years of age. It is preceded by a pre-invasive condition that can be simply and effectively treated if identified by cervical cytological screening. The peak age for pre-invasive lesions is 25–35 years and for invasive cancer 40–50 years. Although there is difficulty in providing a high-quality smear, and programmes can still be improved in terms of accessibility and education for all women, cervical cytology remains the most effective screening test in medical oncology, contributing to a reduction in the morbidity and mortality rates of cervical cancer (Masood 1997).

Pre-invasive cancer of the cervix

PATHOPHYSIOLOGY

The endocervical canal is lined with columnar epithelium one cell thick. Deep branching compound racemose glands exist within these cells and secrete alkaline mucus. Adenocarcinoma, which is relatively rare, arises within these cells (5–12% of cervical cancers). This type of cancer is not normally diagnosed from a cervical smear.

The area where the columnar cells of the endocervix join with the squamous cells of the ectocervix is called the squamocolumnar junction (SCJ). A natural physiological process exists whereby the columnar cells migrate down to the ectocervix, moving the SCJ to a new position and causing a red area of columnar epithelium around the cervical os (Hopwood 1990). The migrated columnar cells then start to break down in the acid environment of the vagina and the squamous cells beneath grow to replace them. The area where the normal replacement of the columnar cells with squamous cells takes place is called the transformation or transitional zone and is most commonly where precancerous changes occur. Cervical smears must therefore be taken from this area using specially shaped instruments.

A specific 'oncogene' has been identified as giving a cell its cancer potential (see Ch. 31). Adolescence, the time of menstruation, the first pregnancy and the prenatal period are times of maximum cellular activity in the cervix, when the tissues are more sensitive to a carcinogen that has been sexually transmitted and more prone to genetic mutation.

The relationship between cervical squamous pre-cancer and sexual intercourse appears to be conclusive since the condition is virtually unknown in celibate women. Epidemiological observations indicate that the age of onset of intercourse and the number of sexual partners influence the development of cervical pre-cancer and cancer (Lewis & Chamberlain 1995). The condition is also more common in lower socioeconomic groups. The more sexual partners the woman has had, the more likely she is to be exposed to the unknown carcinogen(s). Two viruses have been proposed as possible carcinogens:

- the human papilloma virus (HPV) (Eluf-Neto et al 1994)
- the herpes simplex virus type 2 (Hildesheim et al 1991, Jones 1995).

The specific high-risk viruses thought to be linked with cervical cancer (HPV16, 18, 31 and 33) cannot be identified from a cervical smear test alone — the DNA needs to be examined.

Studies of the role of the male sexual partner suggest the possible transmission of viruses but also refer to the possible carcinogenic effect of human sperm. It is suggested that the basic proteins of histone and protamine fraction of the sperm heads may act as carcinogens. Barrier methods of contraception can offer protection.

There is a possible increased risk of cervical cancer associated with cigarette smoking although there may be several coexisting factors contributing to the risk (Phillips & Smith 1994, Szarewski et al 1996). Factors currently considered to be important are listed in Box 7.3. These factors may change as research continues.

Box 7.3

Risk factors and possible causes of carcinoma of the cervix

Risk factors

- Early intercourse (before 17 years of age)
- Multiple sexual partners
- Early pregnancy
- Living in an urban environment
- Low socioeconomic status
- Smoking
- Immunosuppression
- Use of oral contraception
- Previous abnormal smear
- Failure to participate in screening
- Nutritional deficits — vitamins A, C, folic acid
- High-risk male partner
- In utero exposure to diethylstilbestrol

Possible causes

- Human papilloma virus
- Herpes simplex virus
- Sperm from high-risk tissue-type male
- Smoking
- In utero exposure to diethylstilbestrol
- Immune deficiency

Reproduced with permission from Shingleton & Orr (1987).

Carcinoma of the cervix is now classified as a preventable disease if certain examinations are undertaken regularly by women. Cervical cancer that is identified in the pre-invasive stage is curable.

Common presenting symptoms The earliest knowledge of a malignant change in the cervix may be from a report on a cervical smear test. A clear vaginal discharge may occur in the early stages, whereas later the discharge may be bloodstained or have a bad odour. Irregular vaginal bleeding may be associated with prolonged menstruation, occur between periods, follow sexual intercourse, or be postmenopausal. Pain may be experienced when metastases are present or if there is nerve involvement.

Where there is advanced disease, venous or lymphatic obstruction may lead to extensive oedema within the pelvis. Blocked ureters may result in renal failure, and the spread of growth may lead to fistula formation between the vagina and rectum, or the vagina and the urinary bladder, in which case incontinence will be unavoidable. Massive haemorrhage may occur and death may be related to kidney failure or intestinal complications.

MEDICAL MANAGEMENT

Investigations The following procedures may be completed:

- traditional Papanicolaou smear test or a smear test using liquid based cytology
- Schiller test
- colposcopy and biopsy
- histological examination of smears and tissue specimens.

Papanicolaou (Pap) smear test Papanicolaou and Traut showed the value of smears in detecting cervical cancer as early as 1941, but it was not until 1964 that cervical screening was introduced in the UK. From the 1980s a number of initiatives were introduced in the UK to improve the organisation of cervical screening services and reduce mortality from cervical cancer. Women are generally recalled on a 3- or 5-yearly basis. On the basis of research, the Cancer Research Campaign (1994) and Ibbotson and Wyke (1995) recommended that women aged between 20 and 64 years should have a smear test every 3 years. However, for maximum personal benefit women may wish to have a Pap test every 1–2 years from the time they are sexually active until the age of 70. Cervical cancer remains a significant health risk for older women and it is suggested that a revision of the guidelines for cessation of screening may be appropriate (Colgan et al 2002). Women who are not or have never been sexually active are excluded. A woman who has had a total hysterectomy for benign reasons will not require subsequent smear tests, but if a hysterectomy has been performed for pre-cancer or cancer, subsequent vault smears should be taken. Women who have had a subtotal hysterectomy will still require to have cervical smear tests.

The cells identified from the cervical smears are classified as shown in Box 7.4. This information is supplemented as appropriate with the histological grade of pre-invasive disease, i.e. CIN1, CIN2 or CIN3 (see Box 7.5).

Women may be asked to have a smear test repeated where there is an inconclusive diagnosis or if minor cytological abnormalities are detected.

Box 7.4

Papanicolaou smear test results in graded classes

Class 1	Cells are normal in appearance
Class 2	Abnormal cells are present but are not malignant; the patient may have suffered from vaginal inflammation
Class 3	Abnormal cells are present and are suggestive of malignancy
Class 4	Abnormal cells are present and appear to be malignant
Class 5	Abnormal cells are present and definitely malignant

Box 7.5

Histology of cervical intraepithelial neoplasia (CIN)

Current terminology for cervical intraepithelial neoplasia describes three grades of change as part of a continuum of pre-invasive disease:

- CIN1 corresponds to mild dysplasia
- CIN2 corresponds to moderate dysplasia
- CIN3 corresponds to severe dysplasia and carcinoma in situ.

Liquid based cytology Liquid based cytology (LBC) is a new method of preparing a cervical cell sample. Samples are collected from the woman as for a Pap test but a brush-like device is used instead of a spatula. The head of the collecting device is rinsed or broken off into a small container of preservative fluid, most or all of the cells being retained. In the laboratory the sample is mixed to disperse the cells. Cellular debris is removed. A thin layer of the cervical cells is placed on a microscope slide and is stained for examination by a cytologist (NICE 2003). Following a pilot programme this method of obtaining cervical cells is now in operation across the UK. Advantages of this technique over the Pap smear are:

- improved slide preparation, allowing a more homogeneous sample for examination
- increased sensitivity and specificity
- improved handling procedures for laboratory samples.

Colposcopy and biopsy Colposcopy is recommended immediately for all women with a smear that suggests CIN2 or CIN3 and involves examination of the vagina and cervix using magnification and illumination to identify and assess pre-invasive changes. Saline may be applied to the cervix to identify blood vessel patterns. Acetic acid is applied to the transformation zone, mucus is removed with a cotton wool ball or a swab and the area is carefully examined for abnormal epithelium. Iodine can be used (the Schiller test; see Appendix 1) to outline abnormalities. Several biopsies are taken from abnormal areas. Histological examination of the biopsies will confirm the diagnosis of pre-invasive disease. If the transformation zone cannot be completely visualised because it extends too high in the cervical canal, a cone biopsy is performed for diagnosis.

A diagnostic biopsy method may be that of punch biopsy or low-voltage diathermy loop excision biopsy. The punch biopsy tends to crush the sampled tissue and may not include stroma which can lead to missing invasive disease. The diathermy loop excision method can provide tissue samples of better size and allows better control of bleeding.

Treatment options

Conservative treatment Pre-invasive cancer of the cervix that can be fully visualised within the transformation zone can be treated by destruction of the entire transformation zone down to a depth of 6 mm. This depth will ensure the destruction of diseased crypts and glands without destroying normal tissue. Accurate assessment of depth is difficult. Conservative treatment is important to the woman who has not yet started a family and who needs to avoid developing an incompetent cervix to prevent loss of a future pregnancy.

Destructive treatment The following destructive treatment methods may be used:

- *Cryotherapy*. Cryonecrosis is produced by crystallisation of intracellular water using nitrous oxide or carbon dioxide. Freeze–thaw–freeze techniques produce the best results. Little or no analgesia is required. Patients can expect a copious watery vaginal discharge after this procedure.
- *Electrocoagulation diathermy*. Temperatures of over 700°C are used to induce tissue destruction to a depth of at least 7 mm. Traditionally carried out under general anaesthesia, Chanen (1989) demonstrated that the procedure can be carried out successfully with intracervical infiltration with a local anaesthetic. Bleeding and discharge can be expected in the postoperative period.
- *Cold coagulation*. A thermasound heated to 120°C is applied for 20 s to five areas of the surface of the cervix. The procedure is completed under local anaesthetic and has a reported cure rate of 94% (Gordon & Duncan 1991).
- *Laser vaporisation*. The carbon dioxide laser (pulsed or continuous) may be applied to the cervix to ablate the pre-invasive cancer. The procedure can be performed under local anaesthetic. Postoperatively, primary or secondary haemorrhage may occur. A 94% success rate has been reported (Baggish et al 1989); however, Dey et al (2002) suggest that loop diathermy excision is a more effective treatment of CIN than laser vaporisation.
- *Excision of the transformational zone*. This procedure can be performed using laser or a diathermy loop. The latter method is easier to perform and more economical in terms of time. Large loop excision of the transformation zone (LLETZ) may be achieved under colposcopic guidance by low-voltage diathermy — an alternative to cone biopsy. The procedure is performed under local anaesthetic. A bloodstained vaginal discharge usually follows for 1–2 weeks. Severe secondary haemorrhage may occasionally occur.
- *Cone biopsy*. When a transformation zone is not fully visible for colposcopy then an excisional method of treating the pre-invasive cancer has to be used. The

entire transformation zone is excised, which provides a large specimen for histological examination and allows confirmation that all diseased tissue has been removed or that the disease was more extensive than originally diagnosed. The procedure, performed under a general anaesthetic, may be complicated by secondary haemorrhage, infection, cervical stenosis or incompetence. Care is required to prevent uterine perforation and pelvic abscess.

NURSING PRIORITIES AND MANAGEMENT: Pre-invasive carcinoma of the cervix

The person with pre-invasive cancer is treated as an outpatient or as a day patient. Diagnosis, treatment and follow-up are completed in separate visits to a colposcopy clinic. An appointment for colposcopy is given to correspond with the middle of the menstrual cycle, which is a favourable time for the procedure. The nurse will need to ensure at all stages that the patient understands the procedures planned and the expected outcome.

Anxiety levels amongst women presenting for colposcopy have been found to be higher than those of women going for surgery, concerns about the procedure being as great as those about the illness condition (Marteau et al 1990). Sensitive approaches are required to help the patient to express her feelings and think rationally about the future after treatment.

When the patient feels calmer, other information can be given, as it is more likely to be retained. The nurse should tell the person to expect vaginal discharge and some bleeding after the treatment, and explain what to do if bleeding becomes suddenly very heavy or if she suspects she has an infection. The opportunity for health promotion regarding avoiding smoking can be taken.

Arrangements for a follow-up cervical smear test are discussed as part of the pre-discharge routine, as well as the need for future annual check-ups.

Invasive carcinoma of the cervix

PATHOPHYSIOLOGY

Commonly, carcinoma develops from the vaginal surface of the cervix, and less often from the cervical canal. It may form an ulcer on the cervix or become a fungating cauliflower-type growth and is of the squamous cell type. Tissues become eroded and infected, forming an unpleasant vaginal discharge.

The carcinoma spreads by direct infiltration of surrounding tissues and via lymphatic vessels. Blood-borne metastases in more distant organs occur less often. The prognosis for cervical cancer relates to the extent of the growth at the time of diagnosis rather than to the histological type of the cancer. The international classification of carcinoma of the cervix is shown in Box 7.6 (see also Ch. 31).

Common presenting symptoms A woman may have no particular symptoms at the time a cervical smear result confirms that cancer of the cervix exists. On the other hand, she may visit the doctor because of irregular vaginal bleeding, perhaps associated with sexual intercourse,

Box 7.6

International classification of carcinoma of the cervix

Stage 0	Pre-invasive carcinoma, also known as carcinoma in situ (CIN3)
Stage IA	Microinvasive carcinoma; less than 5 mm in depth
Stage IB	Neoplasm confined to the cervix
Stage IIA	Neoplasm has infiltrated adjacent parametrial tissue or upper vagina; if the carcinoma is endocervical then it has extended up into the uterus in this stage
Stage IIB	Tumour extending to the parametrium but not to the pelvic wall
Stage IIIA	Lower third of the vagina is involved or the parametrium
Stage IIIB	Involves lymph nodes as far as the pelvic wall or there are isolated metastases in the pelvis, often obstructing a ureter
Stage IVA	Spread of growth to adjacent organs
Stage IVB	Spread of growth to distant organs

micturition or defaecation. An ulcerated area or an overgrowth of tissue on the cervix may be directly visible to the doctor on examination using a vaginal speculum.

A vaginal discharge becomes more continuous; a thin bloodstained loss may change to a thicker, brown, offensive discharge or heavier bleeding episodes. Lower abdominal pain develops as the growth increases in size, spreads and exerts pressure on surrounding structures. Very severe lower back and sciatic pain may occur and lymphatic nodes adhere to the sacral plexus. Pressure on the pudendal nerve and blood vessels causes obstruction to the venous return and oedema of the legs.

Incontinence of urine and faeces may occur as the bladder and rectum are inflated with growth or react to radiation side-effects. Ureters may become blocked and renal failure may ensue.

MEDICAL MANAGEMENT

Investigations A number of investigations are required before any treatment is planned to establish the spread or otherwise of the disease. A chest X-ray and intravenous pyelogram are completed to gain information on obstruction of the flow of urine from the kidneys, which indicates involvement of the parametrium. A cystoscopy may be performed. A lymphangiogram and a CT scan will assist with identification of disease spread to lymph nodes.

The patient with carcinoma of the cervix requires a general physical examination and a thorough pelvic examination. Haematological and blood chemistry and nutritional studies will be completed. An EUA is carried out at the time of cone biopsy or the insertion of radioisotopes. The EUA increases the accuracy of identifying the stage of development of the growth. It allows better examination of the upper vagina and improved palpation of the abdomen, pelvis and enlarged pelvic, inguinal and para-aortic lymph nodes. Fine-needle aspiration of nodes under sonar or CT guidance may be performed to delineate the spread of the cancer. The information gained is used to confirm, modify or extend treatment plans.

Serum markers Tumour-derived and tumour-associated markers in the plasma of patients with carcinoma of the cervix continue to be researched (Ngan et al 1996, Sliutz et al 1997). Individual marker levels may be used at the assessment stage, in the planning of treatment, when monitoring the response to treatment and in the follow-up years of care. Marker measurement values tend to increase with the stage of disease and decrease with effective treatment. Initial levels before treatment may be an aid to prognosis. The following are examples of serum markers that may be studied:

- *Carcinoembryonic antigen (CEA)* — squamous cell carcinoma and adenocarcinoma have significantly different capacities for CEA release.
- *Plasma histaminase* falls during radiotherapy with a value that is inversely proportional to the radiation response.
- *Tumour-associated antigen (TA-4)* provides a means for monitoring squamous cell tumours.
- *Immunosuppressive acid protein (IPA)* — patients with recurrent cervical cancer have shown elevated IPA, whilst 83% of patients previously treated but without evidence of recurrence did not have elevated levels.

Treatment

Surgery When the carcinoma is confined to the cervix, resection of the malignant tissue is necessary. This may be achieved by laser beam therapy, cone biopsy of the endocervical tissue or amputation of the cervix. Where there is extension of the growth up into the uterus, hysterectomy and removal of pelvic lymph nodes will be necessary.

Radical surgery may be planned for some patients who are at earlier stages of the disease and are more generally fit. This surgery may be combined with radiotherapy as tumours of the cervix are particularly radiosensitive. Care is jointly planned by the surgeon and radiotherapist. The Wertheim–Bonney–Meigs operation involves removal of the uterus, cervix, the upper third of the vagina, pelvic cellular tissue lateral to the uterus and vagina, and the uterosacral and cardinal ligaments. The lymphatic glands in the obturator fossae and along the external and internal iliac vessels are removed. The ovaries are preserved in premenopausal women.

To facilitate the excision of the cervix, vagina and supporting ligaments, the ureters are dissected free during the operation. Postoperatively there may be a breakdown of the ureteric anastomosis, leading to a urinary fistula. The autonomic nerve supply to the bladder may be disturbed, resulting in incomplete bladder emptying as a complication.

Pelvic exenteration Where there is extensive recurrent disease, an anterior pelvic exenteration may be performed, involving removal of all the reproductive organs and the urinary bladder. The ureters are implanted into an artificial bladder fashioned from a loop of ileum — a urinary diversion (see Ch. 8). If the rectum is also removed, a terminal colostomy is formed. This extremely radical surgery may be combined with cytotoxic drug therapy using cisplatin and other chemotherapeutic agents.

Radiotherapy Radiotherapy is initially to reduce the size of tumour, inhibit its growth and reduce its blood supply before surgical removal by hysterectomy. Caesium-137 rods may be inserted under general anaesthetic into the uterine cavity and vaginal vault to provide a radiation dose to the whole pelvis. The treatment will reduce the blood supply to the growth and exert a lethal effect on the cancer cells. Hysterectomy may be performed after local irradiation by caesium or standard supervoltage techniques. Stages III and IV of carcinoma of the cervix are usually inoperable. Palliative irradiation therapy is then indicated. Radiation may be administered via sophisticated machinery such as the Cathetron, which can pass high-intensity radiocobalt radiation from a protected store along ducts to applicators already positioned in the uterus and vagina. The patient is treated in a protected room, reducing radiation risks to others.

The dose of radiation necessary to kill the tumour cells may leave a very low level of protection for healthy tissue cells. Short- or long-term radiation reactions may be induced by therapy. The bladder and rectal tissue may become swollen, inflamed, friable or fibrosed and there is a risk of the development of a fistula. The patient may become distressed by urinary problems or diarrhoea. Symptoms are relieved as they occur. Minor surgical repair operations may be necessary. The patient's general comfort is of prime importance.

NURSING PRIORITIES AND MANAGEMENT: Hysterectomy

Preoperative care

Assessment

The assessment process will identify the patient's gynaecological details, individual problems and needs for nursing assistance and support. The patient who has previously been prescribed an oral contraceptive drug will have been advised to discontinue the contraceptive pill and use an alternative barrier method for 6 weeks prior to the operation to reduce the risk of thrombus formation during surgery or in the postoperative period. The nurse should check that this advice has been followed.

Identification of actual and potential problems

Anxiety

The woman may experience considerable anxiety related to surviving the operation and the illness condition. A change in body image may occur, a sense of loss and some alteration in sexuality and sexual identity may be feared. The woman's loving relationship with her partner may appear to be threatened by the surgery, particularly if her child-bearing potential is lost. Anxiety may also be focused on the family members who remain at home: how will the children and her partner cope whilst she is in hospital? She may be worried that her illness will affect her ability to work and support the family in future. A gentle approach by the nurse may help the patient to speak about her main concerns. Being able to do this at the time of assessment may be the first step towards making a positive adjustment and thereby reducing anxiety. The nurse will be able to plan to utilise opportunities to help the patient manage her anxiety during the hospital period.

The need for information

In preparation for surgery, the patient will need information about the events to be expected during both the lead-up to the operation and the recovery period. The benefits of planned information-giving preoperatively, based on nursing research findings, are described in Chapter 26. An information booklet explaining the operation and its resultant internal changes and answering many questions about the future should be provided for the patient to read at her leisure. This provides a permanent reminder of what she may have been told and reinforces her understanding.

The surgeon will advise when sexual intercourse may be resumed. Normally this will be several weeks after the operation, to allow internal healing and to reduce the incidence of infection. The patient will benefit from knowing that a sexual climax will again be achievable even though the uterus has been removed. The nurse can explain that the pleasurable sexual experience is achieved from the stimulation of the external clitoris within the vulva and the psychological experience associated with stimulation of the penis in the vagina. The patient may already be aware of this, but will be pleased to know that the experience should not change. It is helpful if the patient's partner can be included in the information-giving session. The patient may then approach surgery more calmly and confidently, and recover with minimal physical or emotional problems (see also Research Abstract 7.6).

Exercise

Patients will have limited mobility in the first 48 h after a hysterectomy. There will be a risk of venous stasis and pressure ulcer development. Patients should be encouraged to practise foot and leg exercises before the operation, so that they understand how to carry out the exercises while resting in bed after surgery. A short course of subcutaneous heparin may be prescribed prophylactically. Patients will also benefit from experiencing how it feels to be moved by nurses using a mechanical hoist, and from knowing what they can do to assist the process. This should help to reduce apprehension about being moved at a time when dependent. A visit by the physiotherapist will prepare the patient for moving, and for deep-breathing and coughing exercises to be used after the operation.

Protection from hazards (see Ch. 26)

The doctor is responsible for fully informing the patient about the planned operation and is required to obtain the patient's informed consent in writing. The nurse preparing the patient checks that the consent form has been signed before completing the other major surgery preoperative procedures. The patient will wear anti-embolism stockings to counteract venous stasis during the operation period. A premedication is given as prescribed. The patient leaves the ward escorted by her nurse who completes a safe transfer to the operating theatre staff.

Postoperative care

The patient's individual needs and actual problems will transfer from a preoperative care plan to a postoperative care plan, but a major new focus will be that of maintaining a safe internal and external environment for the patient. There are a number of potential problems that will feature in the care plan and will have been explained to the patient preoperatively. The general care of a patient following major abdominal surgery is described in Chapter 26, and in Nursing Care Plan 7.1.

RESEARCH ABSTRACT 7.6

A study of self-concept and social support after hysterectomy

Webb and Wilson-Barnett (1983) studied depression, self-concept and sexual life in 128 women during recovery from hysterectomy as part of a nursing study. At the time of operation, 103 were premenopausal and 102 were sexually active. The women were interviewed 1 week and 4 months after the hysterectomy. The results showed that women felt physically and emotionally much better, were less tired and irritable, had gone back to work and had resumed leisure and social activities. Responses showed that:

- 94% were happy to have no more periods
- 84% were glad they could no longer become pregnant
- 90% of those who were sexually active said their sex life was now as good as, or even better than, previously
- 92% were glad they had the operation.

The small numbers who gave 'negative' replies to these questions were still not completely recovered and gave this as the reason for their answers. They referred to physical complications of wound, urinary or vaginal infections which delayed recuperation rather than the psychological problems suggested in medical studies.

In studying the social support of these women results showed:

- 70% had been told 'old wives' tales' of pessimistic outcomes; 11% felt there was some truth in them after their own experiences
- 23% of partners (n = 103) had been given no extra help in the home.

The greatest area of dissatisfaction was in the lack of information from medical and nursing staff. Women would have liked guidance on what they could do, how they might feel as they progressed and what symptoms or complications could occur.

Webb C, Wilson-Barnett J 1983 Self concept, social support and hysterectomy. International Journal of Nursing Studies 20(2): 97–107

Carcinoma of the body of the uterus

Carcinoma of the body of the uterus is more common with advancing age, most cases occurring in the sixth and seventh decades (Blake et al 1998). The condition is associated with infertility, diabetes mellitus, oestrogen replacement therapy, obesity and hypertension. An excess of oestrogen is common to all the risk factors. As women are living longer, the present rate is expected to increase.

PATHOPHYSIOLOGY

The columnar epithelium that covers the surface of the endometrium and forms the lining of the glands gives

Nursing Care Plan 7.1 Care of a patient following a hysterectomy

Potential problems	Expected patient outcomes	Nursing care	Rationale
1. Irregularity in vital signs	• Pulse and BP measurements are within acceptable limits for the patient • Blood loss through wound or drainage tubes is minimal in any 24 h	Record BP and pulse: ______ Inspect wound/drains Observe for any pv loss Record temperature: ______	Haemorrhage due to loss of haemostasis at operation site would result in hypovolaemia, requiring blood transfusion. Fine drainage tube is in position in wound. Pyrexia may occur due to infection in chest, urinary tract, wound or veins
2. Body fluid imbalance	• No sign of dehydration or fluid overload • Patient is adequately hydrated • Signs of fluid overload are detected from fluid balance record	Maintain intravenous therapy as prescribed Observe i.v. puncture site for signs of infection or fluid being given extravenously Record fluid intake and output Dress cannula site with: ______ Change giving set: ______	Major surgery depletes body potassium, sodium and water levels Fluid and electrolyte replacement is needed by the intravenous route
3. Patient to have nil by mouth	• Peristalsis returns within 48 h	Patient to be given no fluid or food by the oral route until prescribed by doctor Record any bowel activity	Peristaltic movement of the intestines stops when the abdomen is opened and the gut is handled. Food and fluid, if taken, could not be digested. Bowel sounds are heard when peristalsis returns. Patient passes gas
4. Urinary bladder is drained by a self-retaining catheter (suprapubic or transurethral) Risk of bladder dysfunction after catheter removal Risk of urinary tract infection	• Urine drains freely to minimise pressure on operation sites Urine is clear and has low bacterial count	Observe and record urinary output Obtain catheter specimen of urine: ________ for laboratory culture and sensitivity Complete catheter toilet: ____ Remove catheter on: ______	During the radical hysterectomy the ureter is either partially dissected to allow resection of the medial portion of the cardinal ligament, or more extensively dissected to sever the cardinal ligament at the pelvic side wall. There may be oedema and bruising of posterior urethral wall. Diminished bladder sensation, reduced bladder compliance and stress incontinence may occur. Urinary tract infection is a risk with a catheter in the urinary bladder

Continued

Nursing Care Plan 7.1 Care of a patient following a hysterectomy *(Continued)*

Potential problems	Expected patient outcomes	Nursing care	Rationale
5. Possibility of patient becoming distressed or uncomfortable due to postoperative pain	• Patient expresses verbally or by body language that pain has decreased to an acceptable level on a pain scale of 1 = 'low' to 5 = 'high'	Remind the patient of the availability of analgesia Reposition the patient as necessary for comfort Give analgesia as prescribed or supervise the patient-controlled analgesia system (PCA) Ask patient if analgesia is adequate using pain scale 1 = 'low' to 5 = 'high'	Patients have different pain tolerance levels. It may not be possible to keep the patient pain-free at all times. A degree of pain control that is acceptable to the patient should be planned
6. Limited mobility with risk of: **• venous stasis** **• pressure ulcers**	• No limb tenderness, pain, swelling or redness during hospital stay • Moves safely within limits allowed • Pressure areas remain intact	Supervise limb exercises whilst patient in bed, to be performed ______ -hourly Move patient to relieve pressure over bony prominences: 2-hourly Anti-embolism stockings to be worn until ______ Mobilisation programme: ______________________ ______________________	The patient who is immobilised by major surgery and confined to bed may experience reduced muscular stimulation to the venous system. The blood flow in the veins of the limbs is slowed down, increasing the potential for blood clot formation, inflammation of the vein and surrounding tissues (phlebitis and cellulitis) with accompanying swelling and pain and possible embolism. Body pressure exerted over pressure areas for more than 2 h will result in compromise of the blood supply to the tissues and the development of pressure ulcers. Exercising of limb muscles and the wearing of anti-embolism stockings are preventive measures that reduce risk. Measures to relieve pressure over pressure areas are effective in preserving skin and other tissue integrity

Continued ▶

Nursing Care Plan 7.1 Care of a patient following a hysterectomy *(Continued)*

Potential problems	Expected patient outcomes	Nursing care	Rationale
7. **Needs information or new skills in readiness for discharge**	• With information/instruction/ practice will be able to function independently in: ______ ______ ______ by discharge on: ______	Patient preparation: ______ ______ ______	Depending upon progress during the hospital stay, the patient will need an individualised pre-discharge programme. Advice and counselling in areas of the activities of living may be needed. Personal care, including wound management, the importance of exercise and restricting of lifting activity, should be related to the surgical removal of ligaments and supporting structures in the pelvis and the slow healing of abdominal muscle and other tissues The patient may be discharged with a suprapubic catheter in situ. Practice will be needed in the management of the closed drainage system. The patient may have the support of a community nurse when at home to complement self-care. The patient will need to know what to do if problems occur, and who to contact: GP or hospital. The patient should be encouraged to ask questions and talk about any concerns. Information about a local group of the Hysterectomy Association should be provided should the patient feel in need of support and social contact. Medical staff will need to give specific instructions about when sexual intercourse may be resumed and what follow-up surveillance will be maintained in the observation for recurrence of disease; 20-year follow-up may be achieved

origin to carcinoma of the body of the uterus. The growth is usually an adenocarcinoma. In a small number of cases of adenocarcinoma, there may be a squamous metaplasia. This squamous element may be benign or malignant.

Endometrial carcinoma develops in an atrophic senile uterus. The lesion penetrates the endometrium, spreads laterally and grows slowly. With time it penetrates the myometrium deeply, reaching the peritoneal covering, and the lymphatic glands become involved. Secondary deposits may affect pelvic and aortic lymph nodes and the ovary. Metastases to the lung, bone, liver or brain may be late, blood-borne complications. There are different grading systems that can be applied to endometrial cancer. Staging relates to the tumour size, location and spread beyond the uterus. Walczak (2000) describes a system that coincides with recommendations of the International Society of Gynaecological Pathologists (see Box 7.7). Scholten et al (2004) claim that the most widely used grading system for endometrial cancer is the International Federation of Gynaecology and Obstetrics (FIGO) system. However, this three-tiered system is now being challenged by a binary grading system, based on the amount of solid growth, the pattern of invasion of the myometrium and the presence of tumour cell necrosis (Lax et al 2000, Scholten et al 2004). While both the FIGO and binary systems show good prognostic power, the binary grading system is said to have better prognostic power and greater interobserver and intraobserver reproducibility.

Common presenting symptoms From the age of 45 years, a woman expects changes in the menstrual cycle related to the menopause. The early signs of carcinoma of the uterus may be difficult to distinguish from the changes of the climacteric. Unexpected or irregular vaginal bleeding is a significant sign. Bleeding that is too heavy, occurs too often or happens after cessation of periods at the menopause needs to be investigated. Low abdominal pain may be a late experience for the woman with uterine carcinoma. The vaginal discharge may be clear or brown with an offensive odour.

Box 7.7

Staging of endometrial cancer

Stage IA	Tumour is limited to the endometrium
Stage IB	Tumour invasion to less than one-half of the myometrium
Stage IC	Tumour invasion to more than one-half of the myometrium
Stage IIA	Involvement of endocervical glandular tissue
Stage IIB	Invasion of cervical stroma
Stage IIIA	Invasion of serosa and/or peritoneum
Stage IIIB	Metastatic spread to pelvic and/or para-aortic lymph nodes
Stage IVA	Invasion of the mucosa of bladder and/or bowel
Stage IVB	Distant metastases — intra-abdominal and/or inguinal lymph nodes

Reproduced with permission from Walczak (2000).

MEDICAL MANAGEMENT

Investigations In some cases a routine cervical smear test may yield the first evidence of malignant endometrial cells. Initial investigations include a transvaginal scan (TVS) and endometrial biopsy. If the endometrial biopsy is insufficient for histological identification of malignant cells or if there is thickening of the endometrium shown on the TVS (indicative of pathology), the diagnosis can be concluded by a hysteroscopy followed by dilatation and curettage of the endometrium.

Treatment

Total hysterectomy Cancer of the uterus is usually treated by total hysterectomy and bilateral salpingo-oophorectomy, i.e. surgical removal of the uterus, cervix, fallopian tubes and ovaries. The abdominal or vaginal surgical approach may be used. A vaginal hysterectomy is suitable if the uterus is small and not distended with bulky tumour.

Extended hysterectomy An extended hysterectomy also includes removal of pelvic lymph nodes. Surgical treatment may be combined with radiotherapy to the pelvic wall. Alternatively, the uterine tumour may be irradiated to shrink it and deplete its blood supply before surgery. Postoperative radiotherapy may be given either as external beam only or in combination with vault caesium.

Cytotoxic and hormonal treatments Cytotoxic medication may be used as early as possible following surgery to counteract metastatic seeding. Carcinoma of the endometrium is often sensitive to hormone therapy. High doses of medroxyprogesterone acetate (Depo-Provera) or hydroxy-progesterone caproate (Delalutin) may suppress the progress of the disease in advanced cases and limit metastatic activity. The 5-year survival rates in women treated for early cancer of the uterus are 60–70%.

NURSING PRIORITIES AND MANAGEMENT: Carcinoma of the uterus

The nursing care of the patient with cancer of the uterus involves pre- and postoperative care for hysterectomy. Care will be individualised but will be similar to that for the patient with carcinoma of the cervix (see p. 276).

Total or extended hysterectomy does not involve dissection of the ureters, as in radical hysterectomy. The patient should therefore have less difficulty with recovery of bladder function postoperatively, as there will be no disturbance of the nerve supply or any bladder wound. A self-retaining urethral catheter may be used in the first few days, to avoid distending the urinary bladder and exerting pressure on the posterior urethral wall, which may be swollen and bruised.

A haematoma in the vault of the vagina is a potential complication of vaginal hysterectomy. This will result in prolonged abdominal discomfort, raised body temperature and a sustained feeling of being unwell, until the haematoma is diagnosed and drained.

The patient will need information about her progress at regular intervals in the postoperative period. Of particular concern may be the need to have cytotoxic drug therapy at an early, vulnerable stage after major surgery. The patient may feel greatly debilitated by the side-effects of nausea and vomiting. Psychological support from the nurse should help the patient to view the chemotherapy as the final safety net in the treatment process. Positive improvements should be seen within 3 months of treatment being completed. Medical follow-up is essential to monitor progress and identify early signs of recurrent disease.

Malignant disease of the ovary

Ovarian cancer is the sixth most common cancer in women and the leading cause of death from a gynaecological malignancy. The incidence and mortality of ovarian cancer has shown little change in the past two decades, despite an increase in the proportion of women receiving surgical treatment to manage the disease (Laurvick & Semmens 2002).

Ovarian cancer is more common in developed countries (Lambert et al 1992). A relationship is said to exist between multiple ovulation in women in well-nourished communities and the incidence of ovarian cancer, the disease being more common in the better-nourished and upper social groups. Pregnancy and the oral contraceptive pill have a protective effect. The condition is more common in infertile and nulliparous women and in women who have not taken a sexual partner. A previous problem of endometriosis is linked to malignant change. The peak incidence is between 50 and 70 years of age (Blake et al 1998).

To date there is no effective screening procedure for early detection of this disease in the population. The tumour is often widespread before symptoms appear. As a result, late detection of the condition prohibits effective treatment and the mortality rate is higher than for other genital malignancies.

PATHOPHYSIOLOGY

Ovarian tumours comprise tissues of the normal ovary, most commonly arising from the epithelial lining. The tumour may occur unilaterally or bilaterally. Carcinoma developing in other organs can metastasise to the ovary. Carcinoma of the body of the uterus may spread directly to the ovary, although this is less common with carcinoma of the cervix or vagina. The pylorus, sigmoid colon, rectum, gall bladder, breast and kidney are possible sites of primary growth. The lymphatic channels and blood vessels facilitate the spread of ovarian cancer. Box 7.8 outlines the international classification of ovarian cancer.

Ovarian cancer is histologically classified according to the type of cell from which it originates, the most common source being surface epithelium, formed from embryonic mesothelium. Three types of tumour may develop:

- serous (tubal)
- endometrioid (endometrial)
- mucinous (endocervical).

Serous papilliferous carcinoma The malignant serous tumour is the commonest type of primary ovarian cancer and often affects both ovaries. The growth penetrates the capsule of the ovary and projects on the outside surface. Tumour cells are disseminated into the peritoneal cavity to form multiple seedling metastases. In most cases there is rapid spread in the peritoneal cavity secreting excessive amounts of fluid into the abdominal cavity.

Serous papilliferous cystadenoma The cysts of this serous new growth contain many papillary processes and are lined with a single layer of cubical epithelium on a vascular connective tissue base. The epithelium resembles that of the fallopian tube, the cells being ciliated.

Mucinous cystadenoma Mucinous tumours are formed from columnar epithelium, similar to the tissue of the endocervix. The tumours are described as multilocular, consisting of several cysts clustered together and separated from each other by a septum. The cysts have mainly fibrous tissue walls and contain viscid mucin, a glycoprotein. This tumour can grow to a very large size.

Mucinous cystadenomas may rupture spontaneously or be damaged during surgery, spilling epithelial cells into the peritoneum where seeding and further growth occur, with secretion of mucin forming a jelly-like mass in the abdominal cavity.

Mucinous carcinoma Approximately 10% of ovarian cancer is classified as mucinous and 5% of mucinous cysts are found to be malignant (Lewis & Chamberlain 1995). Many of these tumours are identified at an early stage of growth, which gives a better prognosis for the patient.

Endometrioid carcinoma In the ovary, this type of cancer resembles adenocarcinoma of the endometrium of the uterus. The tumour consists of tubular gland cells as found in the endometrium. It may be secondary to uterine disease or a primary ovarian growth that coexists with cancer in the body of the uterus.

Germ cell tumours Similar tumours may arise in the germ cells of either gender and may be benign or malignant. Benign conditions are very common; malignancy is rare. The commonest type of germ cell tumour is the dermoid cyst or cystic teratoma. Dermoid cysts usually occur in the ovary but are very rare in the testes; malignant teratoma is more common in the testes.

Amongst the malignant germ cell tumours, the highest incidence is of the dysgerminoma histologically resembling a seminoma of the testis. It shows large round cells separated by fibrous septa and is highly malignant, perforating its capsule and spreading cells into the blood and lymphatics.

MEDICAL MANAGEMENT

Ovarian cancer is insidious in its growth and the woman may be quite free from discomfort or suspicion of disease until an advanced stage. Approximately 70% of women have the disease diagnosed when it has spread beyond the ovaries (Blake et al 1998). Late symptoms are related to increased pressure in the abdominal–venous channels,

Box 7.8

International classification of ovarian cancer

Stage I	Disease limited to one or both ovaries
Stage II	Growth extending beyond the ovaries but confined within the pelvis
Stage III	Growth with widespread intraperitoneal metastases
Stage IV	Cases with other distant metastases and/or parenchymal liver involvement

causing oedema in the legs and pain from pressure on nerves to the legs. Metastatic growth in the peritoneum will contribute to extensive ascites, abdominal pain, frequency of micturition, nausea, vomiting, emaciation and breathlessness. A thrombosis may form in an iliac vein or in the inferior vena cava. If growth has spread to other organs then other symptoms may occur, such as obstruction of the small bowel or the colon.

Investigations A full pelvic examination is necessary, with palpation of the ovaries. Ultrasonic scanning and laparoscopy are useful diagnostic procedures. A Pap smear may show ovarian malignant cells in a specimen taken from the posterior fornix of the vagina. X-rays of the pelvis and vertebrae may show bony metastases. An intravenous pyelogram may be performed to assess the degree of involvement of the urinary system. A ureter may become obstructed, hydronephrosis occurring. A full blood count and serum biochemistry are included in investigations and tumour markers have a place in diagnosis. Ovarian tumours are always surgically removed. It is important that the ovary and peritoneal cavity should be fully assessed to define the spread of the disease.

Treatment When malignant disease of the ovary is diagnosed, both ovaries need to be removed and total hysterectomy completed. The tumour may involve the peritoneum and other organs. As much malignant tissue as possible will be removed. The infracolic omentum is removed since it is a common site for microscopic disease (Blake et al 1998). Adjuvant chemotherapy is normally given except in early stages of the disease. Radiation is generally confined to palliation. In advanced states, palliative treatment only may be possible. Abdominal paracentesis may be performed to relieve the pain and respiratory distress caused by ascites. Hospital admission is arranged as needed to make patients more comfortable. They may be cared for in a hospice or live their last months with their families at home.

NURSING PRIORITIES AND MANAGEMENT: Ovarian cancer

In addition to physical care, the patient with ovarian cancer will need much psychological support from the nurse. Anxieties associated with investigations, diagnosis and the effects of hysterectomy and cytotoxic drug therapy will need to be anticipated and managed in all aspects, as described earlier in the chapter. The patient may make a full recovery quite quickly or, if secondary disease remains, may be debilitated for longer. She may or may not be aware of the seriousness of the cancer condition, as full details of the illness may have been withheld in her best interests. However, openness is generally found to be more helpful for both the patient and her carers (Glaser & Strauss 1965, Hinton 1980, Knight & Field 1981, McQueen 1997).

The nurse will work towards helping the patient make physical and emotional adjustments. Attention will be given to the relief of pain, nausea and vomiting after surgery and chemotherapy. As physical problems are relieved, the patient may cope better emotionally, but in terminal cases, time is needed to adjust to the sad news. If a warm, trusting relationship has been developed with the nurse at the acute stage of treatment, it will sustain the patient who needs to return to the ward to continue with cytotoxic drug therapy or for palliative paracentesis. This can be emotionally demanding for the nurse but can also provide immense satisfaction, and patients appreciate the time and individualised attention given to their emotional needs (McQueen 1995). In caring for terminally ill patients, the nurse's empathetic feelings extend to the patient's family, and part of holistic patient care incorporates the giving of information and support to the relatives (McQueen 1997).

OTHER GYNAECOLOGICAL DISORDERS

Displacements of the uterus

The basic criterion of uterine normality is mobility rather than position. The cervix is laterally anchored but the fundus is free to move widely in an anteroposterior position. If the long axis of the endometrial cavity is hinged forwards in relation to the cervical canal, the body of the uterus is anteflexed in relation to the cervix. Similarly, if the long axis of the endometrial cavity is hinged backwards in relation to the axis of the cervical canal, then the body of the uterus is retroflexed in relation to the cervix (see Fig. 7.8).

Careful assessment of the position of the uterus is necessary to prevent perforation of the uterus during diagnostic or therapeutic curettage.

Cervicovaginal prolapse

The cervix can become prolapsed and elongated by the opposing forces of pull of the transverse and uterosacral ligaments against prolapsed vaginal walls. The cervix prolapses but the uterus stays in the pelvis.

Anterior vaginal wall prolapse

- *Cystocele* — the upper part of the vaginal wall prolapses due to underlying failure of the fascia and the bladder base descends.
- *Urethrocele* — the lower part of the vaginal wall prolapses and the urethra descends. This is caused by stretching of the urogenital diaphragm, which holds the urethra to the pubic bone.

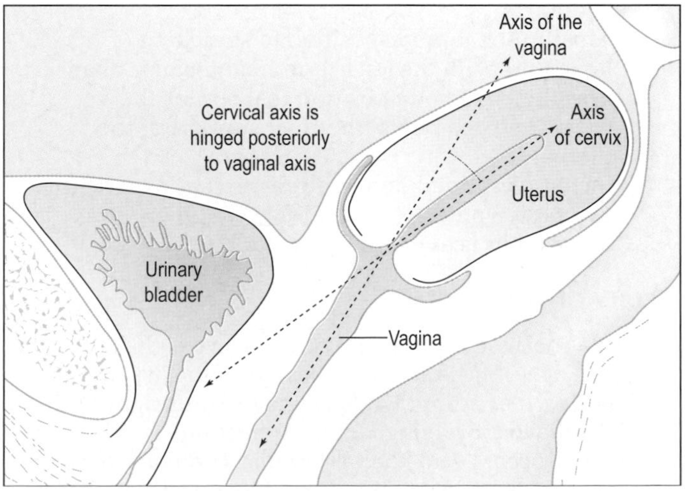

Fig. 7.8 The retroverted uterus.

Posterior vaginal wall prolapse

- *Rectocele* — if the prolapse is at the level of the middle third of the vagina, the retrovaginal septum is involved and the rectum prolapses with the vaginal wall. If the lowest part of the vaginal wall prolapses, the perineal body is involved rather than the rectum.
- *Enterocele* — if the upper part of the posterior vaginal wall prolapses, the pouch of Douglas is elongated and the small bowel or omentum may descend.

Both anterior and posterior vaginal walls may be involved in the prolapse. When a cystocele is present, bladder emptying tends to be incomplete, causing hypertrophy of the bladder. The uterus may become distorted, leading to reflux of urine and, ultimately, hydronephrosis. Urinary tract infection is inevitable and this contributes to hypertension and raised blood urea levels in women with prolapse.

Uterovaginal prolapse

When the ligaments and muscles supporting the uterus and vagina become ineffective, the genital tract descends, prolapses or herniates through the gap between the muscles of the pelvic floor.

The uterus descends in the axis of the vagina taking the vaginal wall with it. This prolapse is essentially but not exclusively a postmenopausal condition.

Three degrees of uterine prolapse are described:

- *first degree* — the cervix is still within the vagina
- *second degree* — the cervix appears at the introitus
- *third degree* — the uterus and vagina are completely prolapsed and lie outside the vulva. Rectal prolapse may also occur. This is sometimes called complete 'procidentia' or 'vault prolapse'. The vaginal rugae are smoothed out, and the epithelium becomes thickened and keratinised. The uterus becomes dry, sore, swollen, inflamed, congested and ulcerated from contact with clothing. Contributing factors are:
  - — stretching of muscle and fibrous tissue from repeated child-bearing. It is suggested that it is due to the action of progesterone relaxing muscles during pregnancy
  - — injury to the muscles of the pelvic floor during childbirth
  - — constitutional predisposition to stretching of ligaments with the long-term maintenance of an upright, erect body position that strains the transverse ligaments (the chief support of the uterus)
  - — increased intra-abdominal pressure, as experienced by obese women with a chronic cough or those engaged in heavy industrial work.

MEDICAL MANAGEMENT

History The woman is likely to be overweight and suffer from backache. She is aware of feelings of the internal organs coming down at a time when she is in an upright position. This is relieved by lying down or resting. Pelvic venous congestion occurs and the abdominal contents exert pressure on the inadequate, weakened pelvic floor. There is frequency of micturition, incomplete bladder emptying and the residual urine is a focus for infection. Stress incontinence may be a major problem for some women (see Ch. 24). There may be difficulty in voiding urine and in defaecation. The cystocele or rectocele may have to be supported or pushed upwards vaginally before urine can be passed or the bowel evacuated. Physical movements become difficult and uncomfortable.

Examination Severe prolapse may be diagnosed by inspecting the vulva with the patient lying on her back and straining downwards. A vaginal speculum is used to allow direct vision of a prolapsed anterior vaginal wall and any rectocele or enterocele formed by a prolapsed posterior vaginal wall. A rectal examination is needed to confirm the latter type of displacement. The degree of uterine prolapse is usually assessed before surgery when the patient is anaesthetised.

Investigations Apart from an EUA, no routine procedures are necessary to assist with diagnosis of uterine displacement. Preoperative assessment will usually involve a full blood count, urinalysis, and a midstream specimen of urine for culture and sensitivity. Other procedures, such as a chest X-ray, ECG or blood chemistry estimation, may be necessary to assess the patient's general medical fitness for surgery.

Treatment Surgical treatment is curative for prolapse but a small number of women may be unfit for surgery due to advanced age or poor physical condition. The uterus may be supported by the use of a ring pessary made from polyethylene or flexible vinyl. Such pessaries may have the disadvantage of acting as a foreign body in the vagina, causing some local inflammation. Pessaries are changed every 4–6 months when the vaginal walls can be examined for inflammation or ulceration. A course of vaginal oestrogen may be prescribed to diminish atrophic changes, inflammation, infection and discharge.

Surgery to conserve the uterus If there is only a first-degree descent of the uterus or if the woman prefers to retain her uterus, although prolapsed, then the Manchester (Fothergill) operation is performed. This involves partial amputation of the elongated cervix and the joining of the cut transverse cervical ligaments to the stump of the cervix. The shortened ligaments antevert and elevate the uterus. The vaginal walls are repaired as necessary.

Repair of uterovaginal prolapse Reconstruction of the pelvic floor involves restoring the pelvic aperture to its previous competent state. This is achieved by bringing together skeletal muscle between the anus, vagina and bladder, and approximating the medial borders of the pubococcygeus muscles. Childbirth can result in supporting structures being torn, separated and overstretched. These structures are identified at operation and reconstructed. An elongated cervix may be amputated. The fascia supporting the bladder and bladder neck is tightened across the midline. The parametrial tissues supporting the uterus are shortened to raise the uterus to its normal position.

Repair of cystocele is known as anterior colporrhaphy, supporting the urethra and urethrovesical junction. A rectocele is repaired by a posterior colpoperineorrhaphy, the repair of the perineal body. Bladder, perineum and vulva have an excellent capacity for repair, related to a rich blood supply and good venous drainage. Surgery is usually very successful.

A complete uterine prolapse will usually be treated by hysterectomy.

NURSING PRIORITIES AND MANAGEMENT: Displacements of the uterus

Preoperative care

Preoperative assessment and care of patients for gynaecological operations has been fully described earlier in the chapter. Care is always individualised according to needs, but some problems and interventions are similar.

- *Information.* Information about procedures before and after the operation, in order to increase patient understanding and cooperation and to reduce anxiety and risk of venous stasis are required.
- *Potential embarrassment.* A woman admitted for repair of prolapse may experience embarrassment in having to identify that she has a problem of stress incontinence requiring her to wear some form of protection. The nurse will ensure that her special requirements are met discreetly.
- *Evacuating the lower bowel before surgery.* According to the surgeon's requirements, the patient will be given two rectal suppositories or an evacuant enema on the evening before the operation day.
- *Preparing the operation site.* An antiseptic vaginal douche can reduce the numbers of bacteria inhabiting the area and inhibit their multiplication, allowing healing of the vaginal wounds without infection.

Postoperative care

- *Risk of strain on internal suture lines from a full bladder.* An indwelling catheter is required and a continuous urinary drainage system is maintained. Precautions are taken to prevent the introduction of infection when collecting specimens or changing drainage bags.
- *Loss of bladder tone.* This is possible after catheter removal. Catheterisation is completed after the patient has passed urine once daily to assess the level of urine retained in the bladder. A residual urine of less than 60 mL is satisfactory.
- *Risk of wound infection.* The use of a bidet for perineal toilet twice daily can minimise the risk of infection.
- *Constipation.* This will potentially cause strain on the repaired posterior vaginal wall. A stool-softening agent can be prescribed to promote easy bowel evacuation.
- *Strain on healing ligaments and muscles.* The patient is advised to avoid jarring or lifting activities for 2 months.
- *Pre-discharge counselling.* An opportunity is created for the patient to discuss her feelings and worries about the level of recovery from surgery, bladder functioning, future return to sexual activity and work. An appointment is given for a medical follow-up in the outpatient department. The patient is given the name of the nurse to contact in the ward if further advice is needed.

Salpingitis

Infection of the fallopian tubes, salpingitis, usually affects both tubes simultaneously. It may result from an ascending infection from the vagina, cervix or uterus or it can occur directly from appendicitis, a pelvic abscess or bowel inflammatory disease such as diverticulitis. The ovaries may also be involved in the inflammatory process. Salpingitis may therefore be part of generalised pelvic inflammatory disease (PID).

Acute salpingitis may follow childbirth, abortion, diagnostic or operative procedures involving the uterus, or the insertion of intrauterine devices.

PATHOPHYSIOLOGY

Ascending infection of the fallopian tubes through the vagina, cervix and uterus is most commonly caused by the organism *Chlamydia trachomatis.* Gonococcal infection, which is sexually transmitted, may also be the cause. Streptococcal and staphylococcal organisms are associated with salpingitis following abortion, childbirth or the insertion of an intrauterine device. These causes may reflect reactivation of pre-existing disease. Intestinal tract commensals, *Escherichia coli* or *Streptococcus faecalis,* may be involved if the infection is linked to appendicitis or bowel infection. The blood-borne tubercle bacillus may unobtrusively inflame the reproductive organs.

The fallopian tubes become engorged and swollen, possibly filled with a seropurulent exudate. Epithelium cells are shed, damaging the delicate ciliated, transporting function of the tubes.

Common presenting symptoms The patient experiences a generalised feeling of being unwell, with:

- raised body temperature and associated sweating
- nausea
- vomiting
- aching joints
- severe pelvic and abdominal pain
- dyspareunia.

MEDICAL MANAGEMENT

Salpingitis may be identified for the first time at laparoscopic surgery, the tubes observed as red, oedematous, distended and blocked. Adhesions may form between the fallopian tubes and other pelvic structures and peritonitis may be evident.

Abdominal and vaginal examinations identify tenderness over the cornua of the uterus. Vaginal discharge may not be observable if the salpingitis has been from lymphatic spread and the muscle of the fallopian tube is mainly involved in the inflammatory process. Infection spread via the mucous membrane of the genital tract will affect the lumen of the fallopian tube, creating a purulent, foul discharge that is drained through the vagina. Scar tissue may form, causing narrowing or closure of the fallopian tube and the severe complication of sterility may result. Adhesions may form between the inflamed tubes and the peritoneum. Peritonitis may occur if pus leaks out of the tubes into the peritoneal cavity. Rarely, a pelvic abscess may form in the rectovaginal pouch or abscesses may form on the ovaries.

Investigations High vaginal or cervical swabs of discharge are pathologically investigated. Throat, urethral and rectal swabs may be taken. During surgery, exudates from the fallopian tubes or the pouch of Douglas may be obtained. Causative organisms are identified by cell culture or antigen detection, using immunofluorescence or enzyme immunoassay. Examination for specific antibody may assist in diagnosis. The antibiotic sensitivities of organisms are established.

Diagnosis may be confirmed by laparoscopy.

Treatment Antibiotic therapy is administered at the earliest opportunity. Analgesic medication will be necessary. Paracetamol, pentazocine or pethidine may be used at different levels of assessed pain severity.

Patients appreciate rest in bed in the acute phase of the illness. An upright position is considered helpful to promote simple downward drainage within the abdominal cavity, towards the uterocolonic pouch of Douglas, reducing the possible spread of infection to structures nearer to the diaphragm. Salpingitis may follow a chronic course and surgical removal of fallopian tubes, ovaries and uterus may be necessary.

NURSING PRIORITIES AND MANAGEMENT: Salpingitis

Nursing care will be organised to relieve the patient's pain, pyrexia and associated sweating, nausea, vomiting and potential dehydration. Analgesics and antibiotic drugs are administered as prescribed. Increased amounts of fluid, 3–4 L in 24 h, will require to be taken orally, or intravenously if vomiting is a problem. When the patient's pain is more tolerable, she may appreciate tepid sponging and a change of linen as a general comfort measure and to reduce body temperature. The doctor will usually explain to the patient the extent of her problem and the treatment given. In addition to giving information, a counselling approach may be helpful in giving support while encouraging the woman to look to the future. Information will need to be shared with her about the prevention of infection, the risk of infertility and the possibility of an ectopic pregnancy following salpingitis.

PATHOPHYSIOLOGY

A fallopian tube may fail in its usual function of transporting a fertilised ovum to the uterus, and the ovum will then implant in the tube. This delayed passage of the ovum, or obstruction, may be due to a deficiency in peristaltic movement, damage to the ciliated epithelium, a developmental abnormality or adhesions from an earlier inflammation. The trophoblast erodes through the epithelium and connective tissue, embedding itself in the muscle wall of the tube, where the pregnancy develops and erodes into blood vessels, causing bleeding around the embryo and into the muscle wall. Increased tension in the tube may lead to rupture.

Common presenting symptoms The woman experiences the early indications of pregnancy: amenorrhoea, breast changes, early-morning sickness and frequency of micturition. Amenorrhoea may not occur in one-third of women with a tubal pregnancy and this may result in delayed diagnosis.

The trophoblast slowly erodes the tubal wall, which results in gradual or sudden rupture of the tube before the 10th week of gestation. The woman complains of spasms of abdominal pain that are not too severe at first. Shoulder pain may be experienced. This is referred pain from the diaphragm, which is irritated by blood in the abdominal cavity.

Tubal rupture causes severe localised pain, which is followed by intense, more generalised abdominal pain. The products of conception are expelled into the peritoneal cavity and there is haemorrhage from the tubal placental site. Uterine bleeding may occur at this time. The patient is in a state of shock, with rapid, feeble pulse rate, lowered blood pressure, sighing respirations and pallor — an acute abdominal emergency exists. Diagnosis of the condition is difficult because similar symptoms and signs may occur in other abdominal emergencies such as perforation of a peptic ulcer or torsion of an ovarian tumour.

MEDICAL MANAGEMENT

Investigations

Pregnancy tests Standard immunological pregnancy tests are not helpful as a tubal pregnancy may not produce enough hCG to give a positive result. Estimation of the b subunit of hCG in the serum is of greater value. Absence of b-hCG excludes pregnancy. A level of 6000 mIU/L suggests a normal pregnancy in the uterus, whereas a level below 6000 mIU/L suggests a tubal pregnancy or a missed abortion.

Ultrasound scanning By the sixth or seventh week of pregnancy, a gestational sac can be identified within the uterus on ultrasound scanning. From the sixth week onwards, it may be possible to show a gestational sac and fetal cardiac echoes outside the normal uterus, directly confirming an ectopic pregnancy.

Laparoscopy Direct vision of the fallopian tubes using a laparoscope allows diagnosis of an ectopic pregnancy when there is uncertainty in clinical diagnosis. Laparoscopy involves giving the patient a general anaesthetic, which should be avoided if there is the possibility that a pregnancy exists in the uterus. The use of hCG estimations and ultrasound scanning may reduce the need for patients to undergo laparoscopy.

Treatment An ectopic pregnancy always requires urgent surgical intervention. The damaged tube is usually removed. An unruptured ectopic pregnancy may be removed from a linear incision in the tube, ensuring conservation.

A ruptured ectopic pregnancy quickly produces a state of hypovolaemia in the patient and a blood transfusion is necessary. This will sustain the patient through surgery and partially relieve the hypotensive symptoms. Immediate surgery is essential even though the patient is in a poor physical condition. Improvement is speedy once the intraperitoneal bleeding is controlled.

The ruptured fallopian tube is removed but the ovary is conserved if possible. Recovery after salpingectomy is usually rapid and uncomplicated. Prompt surgery ensures a low mortality rate from a ruptured ectopic pregnancy. A woman who has suffered one ectopic pregnancy is at risk of developing a similar pregnancy in the second fallopian tube. It is usual for the patient to be encouraged to be optimistic about the future and having a normal pregnancy by means of the remaining fallopian tube.

NURSING PRIORITIES AND MANAGEMENT: Ectopic pregnancy

Preoperative care

Risk of hypovolaemia

The nurse assesses and monitors the patient's physical state intensively from the time of admission to the ward. There are life-threatening concerns as the patient is at risk of hypovolaemic shock and cardiac arrest if the tubal pregnancy ruptures. Vital signs are recorded every 15 min. Problems of increased pulse rate, lowered blood pressure and the patient's pain experience are communicated to the doctor. A state of readiness is maintained to resuscitate the patient if necessary.

Pain

Pain is a major problem for the patient. It may be moderate, but may become intense and intolerable if the pregnancy ruptures through the tube, with bleeding and spillage of gestational sac fluid into the peritoneal cavity. Analgesia is given as prescribed.

Preparation for general anaesthesia

Emergency surgery will be planned. Fasting from food and fluid by mouth prior to laparotomy will be as described in Chapter 26. In the case of emergency surgery it is important for the anaesthetist to know the last time the patient ate or drank and of any vomiting. It may be necessary to introduce a nasogastric tube prior to surgery to reduce the risk of regurgitation and inhalation of gastric contents when the patient is anaesthetised.

Anxiety and the need for information

The patient may be fearful about the operation to come and distressed about losing a pregnancy. She will need information about the surgery and postoperative care, and needs to be encouraged to talk about any worries she may have. It is possible that she may be too weak to talk and the nurse must show empathy and understanding of the patient's feelings and concerns. The nurse may indicate that she will talk with the patient some time after the operation and that she will accompany her to the operating theatre and be responsible for her care when she returns to the ward.

Postoperative care

Postoperative care will be individualised according to patient need, but will follow the general principles of postoperative care described in Chapter 26. Her condition will begin to stabilise as soon as the ectopic pregnancy is removed and bleeding is controlled. Her main problems will be similar to those of other patients who have had abdominal surgery, when organs and the peritoneum have been handled by the surgeon and tissues have been cut through, as follows:

- *Change in vital signs.* The nurse monitors pulse rate, blood pressure and body temperature. Wound, drainage tube and blood loss from the vagina are observed for more than minimal drainage. Primary and secondary haemorrhages are risks. Wound dehiscence may occur. Any causes for concern will be shared with the doctor.
- *Postoperative pain.* The level of pain can be assessed using a verbal rating scale (VRS 1–10). Analgesics are prescribed and administered to control pain.
- *Post-anaesthetic nausea.* This problem may be prevented or treated by giving an antiemetic medication with analgesics as prescribed.
- *Fluid and electrolyte imbalance.* Intravenous fluid and electrolyte replacement therapy is administered as prescribed, until oral intake is resumed. Fluid intake and output are recorded.
- *Venous stasis and pressure-area damage.* The patient is actively encouraged to exercise her legs hourly whilst confined to bed. Assistance is given to change the patient's position every 2 h to protect pressure areas. A programme of early mobilisation will be introduced.
- *Personal care.* Whilst intravenous therapy is in situ, assistance will be given to maintain the patient's preferred standard of personal care until fully mobile.
- *Loss and grieving.* Time is planned for counselling the patient. She needs to know that she can talk about her feelings and express emotion freely. Information should be shared about the possibility of future pregnancies. Details of local support groups for those who suffer loss should be given.

Further considerations

Psychological support

A woman who is suffering a second ectopic pregnancy will become infertile. She may become emotionally distressed at any time during her hospital stay and may show behaviour associated with a crisis of loss and a grief reaction. She will need support whilst expressing her feelings of regret and possibly guilt. Both the nurse and the patient's partner may be helpful in assisting the woman to be realistic about future options and limitations. Some reorganisation of the woman's life will emerge as she accepts her inevitable situation.

Special services

As a result of media coverage, the public are now aware of techniques such as in vitro fertilisation (IVF) and embryo transfer into the uterus (ET) and the possibility of surrogacy for infertile couples. Nurses need to know about such special services and policies within their own units, so that they are informed and can respond to the patient with appropriate caution and discretion and refer enquiries to the patient's doctor.

FAMILY PLANNING SERVICES

Birth control was considered 'social' medicine prior to 1950 and responsibility for family planning advice was established within the Family Planning Association (FPA) and its clinics. The National Health Service Reorganisation Act of 1973 made provision for free family planning advice within the NHS. The FPA clinics and domiciliary services were merged into the NHS in 1974, when a completely free contraceptive service became available at clinics and hospitals and was extended into primary care in July 1975 (Loudon 1985).

Free contraceptive services are now available from general practitioners, family planning clinics in hospitals and the community, and voluntary organisations such as the FPA and Brook Advisory Centres. The voluntary groups receive grants from central government or from purchasing health authorities.

All contraceptive supplies are available free of charge from family planning clinics, and GPs provide prescriptions, except for condoms. Male and female sterilisations are available free in NHS hospitals. Vasectomies may be performed in some large family planning clinics and by some GPs in the surgery. Item-of-service payments are made to GPs and hospital staff.

Postnatally, community midwives, health visitors and GPs routinely discuss birth control methods with the new mother. This is invaluable in reminding women of their fertility and the possibility of another early pregnancy if precautions are not taken when resuming sexual activities.

Women who discontinue attending the GP or family planning clinic may do so because they have changed their birth control method. Women who have completed their family may have chosen sterilisation or their partners may have chosen vasectomy for a permanent form of birth control. Others may be abandoning contraception because the time is favourable for them to begin a family.

The contraceptive needs of young people

Provision of extra contraceptive services for young people after puberty, under 16 years and up to 20 years of age, is controversial and, in the past, was given a low priority. With more recent concern about AIDS and HIV transmission, young people have been specially targeted for health education and advice about their sexual behaviour. Grimley and Lee (1997), in a study of 15- to 19-year-old American females, found that subjects perceived the male condom to be acceptable for both prevention of pregnancy and sexually transmitted diseases. The Contraceptive Choices Survey (Family Planning Today 1996) commissioned by the Contraceptive Education Service showed condoms to be the second most popular method of birth control. The most popular method of contraception, especially for younger women, is still the contraceptive pill, used by 43% of those aged 16–24 years. The combined pill of progestogen and low oestrogen is favoured for high contraceptive protection and ease of use.

ABORTION

The term 'abortion' refers to the premature delivery of a non-viable fetus, spontaneously or by induction. The term 'miscarriage' is sometimes used when the pregnancy loss is spontaneous and is a term generally considered to be more acceptable to women who lose a wanted pregnancy. Debate surrounds the issue of 'non-viability' and the accepted stage at which a fetus is considered viable or capable of independent existence varies between countries. In the UK, a fetus is considered viable from the 24th week of pregnancy. This viability is recognised and safeguarded in the Infant Life (Preservation) Act 1929 and its amendment under the Human Fertilisation and Embryology Act 1990. It has been proposed that the fetus should be deemed viable as early as 18–20 weeks because of the possibility that life-support equipment can maintain the vital functions of such a small fetus and it has been argued that technological advances in medicine have the potential for saving the life of an infant weighing as little as 500 g. Such debates continue, reflecting different social attitudes and scientific developments.

Abortion may be discussed in terms of:

- the level of certainty of the abortion occurring
  — threatened
  — inevitable
  — missed
  — induced
- the cause or relative incidence of the abortion
  — spontaneous
  — habitual (recurrent)
- the degree of success in expulsion of the products of the pregnancy
  — incomplete
  — complete.

Threatened abortion

PATHOPHYSIOLOGY

An abortion is presumed to threaten when a woman known to be pregnant develops vaginal bleeding during the first 24 weeks of pregnancy. Some lower abdominal pain related to uterine muscle contractions may be experienced at the time of bleeding, but there may be no uterine contractions and no pain. The blood loss may be brown or red.

It is not unusual for a show of blood to coincide with the woman's regular date of menstruation. This type of bleeding is due to the fertilised ovum becoming more deeply implanted in the uterine wall. There is little risk of loss of the pregnancy if the bleeding settles quickly (see Fig. 7.9A).

MEDICAL MANAGEMENT

The presence of bleeding, slight uterine contractions and a closed cervical os established by medical examination assist in identifying threatened abortion; 70–80% of women can be expected to continue to full-term pregnancies and give birth to a healthy infant.

Treatment While the woman is continuing to lose blood vaginally, rest in bed is prescribed to ensure that the best possible adjustments can be made within the uterus and to allow a better blood flow to the uterus. Bed rest is usually maintained as long as the blood loss is bright red. One week of bed rest may result in considerable improvement for the patient.

NURSING PRIORITIES AND MANAGEMENT: Threatened abortion

The patient will be very concerned about the possible loss of the pregnancy. This may result in tearfulness, anxiety,

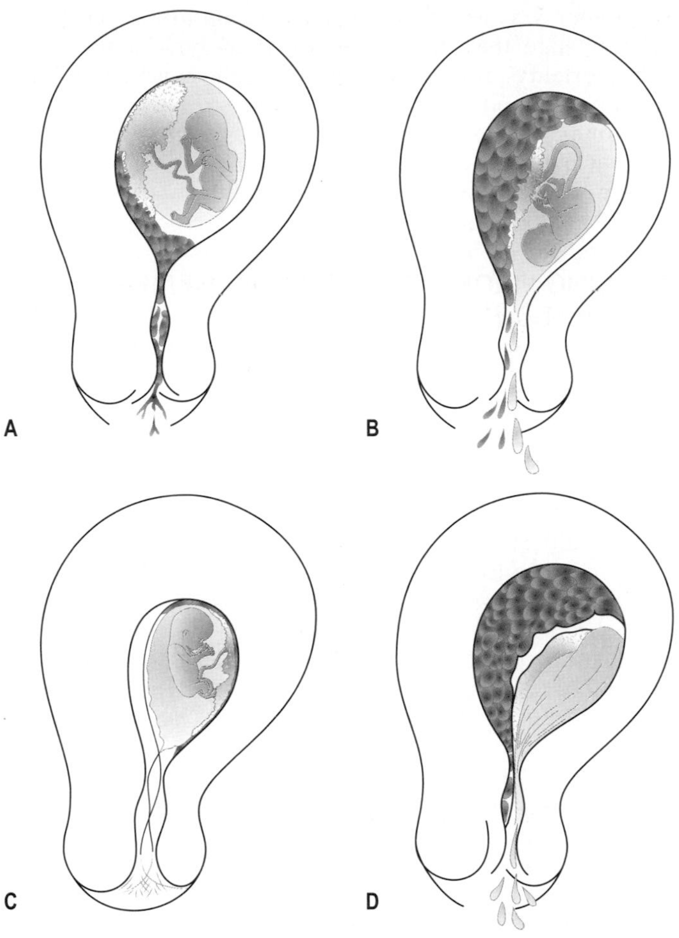

Fig. 7.9 The types of abortion that may be seen. A: Threatened abortion. B: Inevitable abortion. C: Missed abortion. D: Incomplete abortion.

irritability and feelings of frustration. The immediate and long-term future may be feared. The patient may be apprehensive of pain and uncertain of what to expect. Small doses of anxiolytic–sedative drugs and progesterone may be prescribed to encourage rest and to help sustain the pregnancy.

Nursing care will be planned with the goal of reducing anxiety and inducing relaxation in the patient. Vaginal bleeding will be observed and quantified. The patient's experience of abdominal discomfort or pain will be assessed and recorded. The supportive, counselling contact time with the nurse will be appreciated by the patient and her partner. When talking with the patient and partner, both doctor and nurse will usually refer to a threatened miscarriage of the pregnancy rather than using the term abortion.

Inevitable abortion

PATHOPHYSIOLOGY

A threatened abortion can progress to an inevitable abortion if bleeding continues. Inevitable abortions occur in 20% of all pregnancies. An abortion becomes inevitable, with no possibility of saving the pregnancy, when the following are present:

- vaginal blood loss
- strong uterine contractions
- pain
- dilatation of the cervix.

Contractions will increase, the fetal sac membranes will rupture and the uterine contents move through the cervical os. Part or all of the products of conception will be voided from the uterus (see Fig. 7.9B). An inevitable abortion may be complete if all products of conception are voided, or incomplete if some products are retained.

MEDICAL MANAGEMENT

The aborting process will involve blood loss. Estimation of blood loss, and assessment of pulse, blood pressure and appearance of the patient will indicate whether shock is developing. Blood transfusion may become essential and analgesic medication will be prescribed as necessary.

The fetus that has been expelled is retained and examined to assess whether the fetal sac and contents are intact or whether remnants have been retained. Ergometrine maleate 125–500 mg will be given intramuscularly or intravenously according to blood loss which will induce strong contraction of the myometrium, to exert and sustain pressure on the multiple open-ended blood vessels of the placental bed. Thus, bleeding will be controlled until the uterus itself reduces size gradually.

Ultrasonography can be useful to classify the type of abortion (complete, incomplete, missed, etc.) and, based on this, appropriate information can be given to the woman about the likely outcome and therapeutic options. If any of the products of conception are thought to have been retained, several treatment options may be available and it is recommended that women are involved in the choice of approach. The options are:

- surgical evacuation of the retained products from the uterus, an invasive procedure involving a general anaesthetic (GA)
- medical management that avoids a GA and invasive surgery
- expectant management ('wait and see'), whereby four out of five women with an incomplete abortion will complete their abortion within 14 days (Nielsen et al 1995).

NURSING PRIORITIES AND MANAGEMENT: Inevitable abortion

Assessments of vaginal blood loss may need to be maintained for a further period of 12 h. When the effects of ergometrine diminish and the uterine muscle relaxes, blood vessels open up and bleeding and blood clots continue as problems. Further doses of ergometrine, in tablet form, may then be prescribed to control the bleeding and expel blood clots. The blood clots will cause further pain for the patient until they are finally voided from the vagina.

The patient may be distressed by the blood loss, pain, sight of the fetus and the anguish of losing a pregnancy to which she had become emotionally attached. She is likely to experience considerable physical and emotional distress and will need the nurse to be readily available to support, reassure, comfort and assist her through the procedures and experience of pregnancy loss. The patient will need to have the opportunity to talk about her feelings of loss. In this respect, time and empathy from the nurse will be appreciated (Leask 1991, Nazarko 1992). It may be that she has already had a previous miscarriage and will also be recalling that experience as part of her grieving process. The patient's sadness may be sustained for many months after the abortion occurs. To plan some continued support, the nurse in hospital can refer the patient to the community midwife, who is able to provide bereavement counselling until resolution of the grief reaction takes place.

Missed abortion

PATHOPHYSIOLOGY

The term 'missed abortion' describes the intrauterine death of a fetus that has not been expelled. The size of the uterus fails to increase over a 2-month period and the expected signs of a normally developing pregnancy will be missing. The death of the fetus may occur at any week of gestation. Some placental tissue survives to produce progesterone and prevent expulsion (see Fig. 7.9C).

MEDICAL MANAGEMENT

The woman may have experienced movements of the fetus in the uterus, but later reports that recently she has not felt the baby kicking. The doctor will no longer be able to hear the fetal heart beat on auscultation of the abdomen. The uterus may seem to have increased in size due to increased fluid level in the uterus, known as 'hydramnios'. The patient may state that she feels empty and has lost feelings of being pregnant. She is asked to record on a chart any sensation of the baby moving or kicking.

Investigations An ultrasound scan of the uterus and a cardiotocograph reading will assess the status of the fetus and the position of the placenta.

Treatment The diagnosis of a missed abortion will require the doctor to decide whether to allow some time for the fetus to be aborted spontaneously as a natural labour response or whether to evacuate the uterus immediately after diagnosis. The decision may be to let nature take its course and wait for labour to begin. However, the doctor is also likely to take account of the preference of the woman, who has already had to adjust to the loss of the pregnancy and may be further distressed by the dead baby within her.

A risk exists, with missed abortion, that hypofibrinogenaemia will occur. One-third of patients may develop defective blood coagulation due to lowering of fibrinogen levels. Death of the fetus leads to major utilisation of clotting factors at the placental site, and this reduces clotting factors in the woman's blood. Disseminated intravascular coagulation (DIC) is the mechanism that is said to bring about the change in the woman's systemic circulation from the release of thromboplastins at the site of the damaged placental tissue.

The missed abortion may be evacuated from the uterus by vacuum extraction under general anaesthetic if the pregnancy was less than 12 weeks. Chia and Ogbo (2002) acknowledge that this procedure does have a morbidity and mortality and suggest that medical evacuation using mifepristone and misoprostol is a safe and effective alternative for patients who do not require a hospital admission, general anaesthetic and surgery. Gronlund et al (2002) found that misoprostol, alone, effectively induced labour in most patients with missed abortion.

NURSING PRIORITIES AND MANAGEMENT: Missed abortion

A counselling approach will be necessary to provide the patient with opportunities to express her needs and feelings freely.

If evacuation of the uterus under general anaesthetic is planned, the patient will need the usual pre-anaesthetic care in terms of fasting, a shower, and precautions against mis-identification and maintenance of personal safety (see Ch. 26). Following treatment, observations of vital signs and vaginal blood loss will be required to assess recovery.

If the products of conception are to be evacuated, the products of pregnancy should be expelled 4 h later. The nurse must be available to observe the patient's vital signs and need for pain relief. The patient may experience side-effects of nausea, vomiting or diarrhoea, but these are usually transitory. The presence of the nurse can be comforting to the patient, reducing feelings of isolation while treatment progresses.

The way in which individual patients cope emotionally is unpredictable, but the nurse can anticipate that any patient may feel sad and angry about the lost pregnancy. Follow-up counselling can be arranged by the nurse with the community midwife or health visitor, when the woman's level of adjustment can be assessed.

Spontaneous abortion

PATHOPHYSIOLOGY

A spontaneous abortion is a response to a naturally occurring phenomenon such as hormonal problems, uterine abnormality, cervical incompetence, a genetic malformation in the fetus or psychological factors. Pearce (1991) estimated that 25% of all pregnancies terminate in miscarriage in the first trimester; reasons include both fetal and maternal factors. Some women may not be aware that they have aborted a blighted ovum. Congenital abnormalities of the reproductive tract or long-standing medical problems may have an unfavourable influence on the pregnancy. Abortions in the early weeks of the second trimester of pregnancy are often found to be due to an incompetent cervix that responds to the increasing weight of the fetus. The cervical os dilates, the membranes rupture and the pregnancy is lost.

MEDICAL MANAGEMENT

To counteract recurrence of abortion, it is necessary to identify the pregnancy and any incompetence of the cervix at an early stage. In the case of cervical incompetence, a Shirodker's suture can be inserted surgically, closing the internal os, to increase the resistance of the cervix until the pregnancy reaches full term. When the patient goes into labour, the suture is removed to enable delivery to occur.

NURSING PRIORITIES AND MANAGEMENT: Spontaneous abortion

The physical care of the patient with a spontaneous abortion is similar to that of the patient with an inevitable abortion. The patient will normally be distressed by the loss of the pregnancy and will need psychological support from the nurse. A counselling approach to communication will encourage the expression of feelings. Continued support should be arranged by referral to the community midwife.

Habitual (recurrent) abortion

Recurrent abortion refers to a spontaneous abortion that occurs in three or more successive pregnancies. Many factors may contribute to recurrent abortion.

PATHOPHYSIOLOGY

Genetic, hormonal, anatomical, infectious and immunological factors have been implicated in the causation of recurrent abortion.

Tumbo-Oeri et al (2001), in a literature review on the state of thinking among researchers and clinicians on recurrent spontaneous abortion, suggest that there is evidence of involvement of immunological factors in successful pregnancies. However, the underlying mechanisms are poorly explained and largely speculative. They conclude that more focused investigation is required to provide a complete understanding of the mechanisms involved in recurrent pregnancy loss.

MEDICAL MANAGEMENT

Treatment Patients with immunological problems have been treated with leucocyte transfusions with successful results. Identified hormonal deficiencies are treated by replacement hormones, thyroid preparations and progesterone. Vaginal suppositories of progesterone 25 mg, twice daily, beginning 3 days after ovulation, are given and continued throughout the luteal phase, until the 10th week of gestation. At this time the placenta should be sufficient to maintain the pregnancy.

The administration of antibiotic medication is routine, where culture and sensitivity of organisms are known. Otherwise, the tetracycline group is given to offset an infective focus that might disrupt the pregnancy. Reconstruction surgery has achieved considerable success in treating structural abnormalities of the uterus and eventual successful pregnancies.

NURSING PRIORITIES AND MANAGEMENT: Recurrent abortion

Physical and psychological care are paramount at the time that the abortion occurs. Sensitivity in responding to the woman's needs is central. Potential for future assisted maintenance of a pregnancy will be fully discussed by the doctor and reinforced by the nurse. The patient who is anxious can be helped to learn relaxation techniques that may be used for self-induction of relaxation as an everyday activity, and one that can be practised in future pregnancies.

Incomplete abortion

An incomplete abortion is one in which only part of the products of conception are expelled from the uterus (see Fig. 7.9D).

PATHOPHYSIOLOGY

Portions of placenta and membranes are retained, some bleeding continues and could possibly be heavy.

MEDICAL MANAGEMENT

The residual products may be voided spontaneously by the patient but usually a dilatation and curettage is required to clear away the retained remnants of the pregnancy. Ergometrine 500 mg is administered intravenously to control uterine bleeding. Heavy blood loss will necessitate blood transfusion.

NURSING PRIORITIES AND MANAGEMENT: Incomplete abortions

The patient may experience continuous abdominal pain while the uterus retains products of conception. Nursing care involves the administration of analgesics as prescribed to reduce the discomfort, which may continue until the curettage is complete. Vaginal blood loss will need to be observed. Heavy, continuous blood loss may reduce the patient's circulating blood volume, resulting in signs of shock. Observations of vital signs will facilitate early recognition of shock and prompt correction of the condition by transfusion.

The patient will normally be worried about her condition and the operation planned and upset about the miscarriage. Adjustment to the loss will be gradual over time. Counselling time spent with the nurse may help to begin the adjustment process, and continuity may be gained by follow-up support from the community midwife or health visitor.

Induced abortion: termination (voluntary) of pregnancy

An unwanted pregnancy creates potential anguish and difficulties for a woman. She may experience feelings of conflict about both wanting and rejecting the pregnancy. She may fear having to explain it to her family and admit to sexual activities and her incompetence with contraception. Family standards of behaviour, cultural norms and religious beliefs may appear to be violated both by the pregnancy and by the possibility of an abortion. The woman may feel very alone, may be indecisive and under pressure from a partner who may reject the pregnancy. The conditions of the Abortion Act require decision-making to be completed early in the pregnancy.

The Abortion Act 1967 and 1990 amendments

In the UK, the Abortion Act 1967 became operative in 1968 and applies to England, Wales and Scotland but not to Northern Ireland. The Act states that the termination of pregnancy by a registered practitioner is not illegal under certain conditions. Notification of a termination must be given on a prescribed form to the Chief Medical Officer of the Department of Health within 7 days of the termination.

The Human Fertilisation and Embryology Act 1990 has amended the Abortion Act 1967, recognising viability of the fetus at 24 weeks.

Conditions of the Act and statutory grounds

A legally induced abortion must be:

- performed by a registered medical practitioner
- performed, except in an emergency, in a National Health Service hospital or in a place for the time being approved for the purpose of the Act
- certified by two registered medical practitioners as necessary on any of the following grounds:
  - — the continuance of the pregnancy would involve risk to the life of the pregnant woman greater than if the pregnancy were terminated
  - — the continuance of the pregnancy would involve risk of injury to the physical or mental health of the pregnant woman greater than if the pregnancy were terminated
  - — the continuance of the pregnancy would involve risk of injury to the physical or mental health of any existing child(ren) in the family of the pregnant woman greater than if the pregnancy were terminated
  - — there is a substantial risk that if the child were born it would suffer from such physical or mental abnormalities as to be seriously handicapped
- in emergency, certified by the operating practitioner as immediately necessary:
  - — to save the life of the pregnant woman
  - — to prevent grave permanent injury to the physical or mental health of the pregnant woman.

The conscience clause of the Abortion Act 1967

The Act states that no-one shall be under any legal obligation to participate in any treatment authorised by the Act to which he or she has a conscientious objection unless the treatment is necessary to save the life or prevent grave permanent injury to the physical or mental health of a pregnant woman.

The conscience clause does not only apply to members of a particular religion or faith. In England and Wales, a person must prove conscientious objection in the event of any legal proceedings. The clause also makes it explicit that the conscientious objector is not exempt from participation in the emergency care of the patient should such a situation arise. This is affirmed in the *Code of Professional Conduct* (NMC 2002).

Counselling of the pregnant woman requesting termination

In many hospitals the woman who requests a termination of pregnancy is referred to the Assessment and Counselling Service. The social worker seeks to understand what the pregnancy and termination mean to the woman, identifies any contraindications to termination and provides evidence for the final decision-making and the best solution.

It is valuable to interview couples together for counselling. Adolescent girls are often accompanied by parents who may be angry and rejecting of their daughter's pregnancy. The risk is then that the girl passively acts in accordance with her parents' wishes. The counsellor would usually speak with them together and then separately.

Counselling clarifies the woman's conflicting feelings about the pregnancy and strengthens her capacity to face up to her responsibilities. She may be more confident in making a decision in an unpressured atmosphere. The counsellor may have established that contraindications to the termination exist or that the request for termination be supported. In either case the information is made available to the gynaecologist. The counselling service ensures that adequate assessment and advice are provided for the woman who seeks a termination. It is suggested that in this way she will experience less regret, guilt or long-term psychological problems.

MEDICAL MANAGEMENT

Vacuum aspiration (suction curettage) This is the most commonly used abortion method for early termination of pregnancy. It may be performed with a general anaesthetic or a paracervical nerve block with lidocaine 0.5%. The cervix is dilated, a flexible cannula is inserted and the contents of the uterus are aspirated by suction. The uterus is then curetted to ensure total removal of the products of conception, and to reduce haemorrhage and the possibility of infection. Ergometrine 0.5 mg is administered intravenously to promote contraction and involution of the uterus.

Medical termination The main treatment schedule consists of oral mifepristone 200–600 mg followed by oral misoprostol 0.4–0.6 mg, 36–48 h later for pregnancies up to 49 days' gestation and vaginal gemeprost 1 mg or misoprostol 0.8 mg for periods of up to 63 days amenorrhoea (Bygdeman & Danielsson 2002).

Following administration of misoprostol the patient remains under observation for a further 6 h. The nurse monitors pulse, blood pressure, blood loss and other signs and symptoms experienced by the patient. The medical abortion is usually complete within 4–6 h. Anti-D Rhesus immunisation is given before discharge and an appointment is made for the patient to return in 5–9 days to assess the outcome.

While this method of terminating a pregnancy has its advantages — the woman can carry on her daily activities following administration of the tablets and there is no anaesthetic or surgical intervention — there are also potential problems of which the woman should be made aware. These include:

- a 5% chance that the termination will be unsuccessful/incomplete, resulting in the need for surgical abortion
- the possibility of pain following administration of gemeprost, necessitating powerful analgesics
- possible psychological distress for the woman seeing the expelled fetus.

Dilatation and evacuation of contents Abortion that is induced in the second trimester of pregnancy may be completed by dilatation of the cervix with graduated dilators. Preoperatively the patient may have a prostaglandin pessary to soften the cervix and facilitate easier dilatation. A curette is introduced into the uterus and the products of conception and the superficial layer of endometrium are curetted or scraped from the walls of the uterus. Care is taken to avoid damage to the pregnant uterus. Ergometrine 0.5 mg is administered and few side-effects to the procedure are expected. Patients are followed up at the clinic.

Prostaglandin abortion Prostaglandin may be used in young women in the second trimester of pregnancy (13–18 weeks), when the cervix is soft and more easily damaged, or in older women when the pregnancy is beyond 18 weeks. Prostaglandin can be administered intravenously, extra-amniotically, intra-amniotically or in the form of pessaries. If pessaries are used these can be administered 4-hourly (maximum five doses). Abortion can take place within 12–20 h but this varies. Observations of pulse, blood pressure, blood loss, uterine contractions, cervical dilatation and any side-effects of the medication are noted and treated as appropriate. This more prolonged procedure causes more side-effects and can be more traumatic for patients. Psychological care and emotional support constitute an important part of their care.

Intra-amniotic injection The instillation of prostaglandins or other substances into the amniotic sac to induce labour and expulsion of the fetus may be used between the 14th and 20th week of pregnancy but this method carries a higher risk of complications.

Since there appears to be no consensus as to the most efficient method of procuring late abortions, Paz et al (2002) compared the efficacy of intra-amniotic injection of prostaglandin F2 alpha (PGF2alpha) and intravaginal application of misoprostol in terminating second trimester pregnancies after pretreatment with intracervical laminaria in a randomised trial. Laminaria primes the cervix, reducing resistance and minimising trauma. Following intracervical laminaria, vaginal misoprostol was more effective and less painful, compared with intra-amniotic PGF2alpha, for the termination of second trimester pregnancies with live fetuses.

NURSING PRIORITIES AND MANAGEMENT: Termination of pregnancy

Preoperative care

The procedure is generally completed on an outpatient basis or as a day patient in hospital. There is only a short time available for the nurse to build a relationship with the patient whilst documentation is completed. Every effort must be made to show acceptance of the woman and understanding of the difficulties she has been experiencing. Opportunities must be created for her to express her feelings as she wishes and the nurse should be available to listen. A consent form is signed for the termination and consent for anaesthetic is given. Blood tests such as haemoglobin and haematocrit, ABO grouping and the Rhesus factor are necessary precautions prior to the procedure.

Postoperative care

Vital signs related to bleeding and abdominal cramping pain must be observed by the nurse. Inspection of vulval pads will indicate the degree of blood loss. Heavy bleeding will usually require further administration of ergometrine to sustain contraction of the uterus and to evacuate blood clots. Pyrexia may indicate the onset of infection. Mild analgesics may be ordered to relieve cramping pain and also for their antipyretic properties. Women with Rhesus-negative blood require an injection of anti-D immunoglobulin.

The patient is advised to avoid the use of tampons, douching, strenuous activities or sexual intercourse for 2 weeks to reduce the risk of infection and aid healing. The patient's contraception methods are reviewed with her so that any changes needed are understood and appropriate decisions made. A follow-up outpatient examination is completed 2–3 weeks after the abortion to exclude the possibility of a failed abortion, an ectopic pregnancy or other complications. It also allows for an assessment of the patient's acceptance of and comfort with her decision to terminate. Relief is often expressed. Sadness, regret and depression are sometimes short lasting but at other times prolonged. The patient's relationship with her sexual partner may also be discussed; it may have been strengthened or weakened by the abortion experience. Referral to a postabortion support group may be helpful, if there is one active in the area.

Complications of abortion/pregnancy termination

- Pelvic infection — inflammation of the endometrium (endometritis) and fallopian tubes (salpingitis) may occur
- Perforation of the uterus — may occur accidentally during insertion of cannula or use of the curette
- Haemorrhage — bleeding should not be more than a normal menstrual period
- Laceration of cervix, cervical incompetence and recurrent abortion
- Ectopic pregnancy — related to previous salpingitis
- Incomplete removal of uterine contents
- Hydatidiform mole
- Delayed menstruation
- A live fetus at the time of delivery
- Possible susceptibility to subsequent pregnancy loss and premature births
- Infertility.

With improved services, the numbers of complications to abortion can be greatly reduced. Effective networks of outpatient facilities with good access, to avoid delays in uptake of services and reduced travel for women in need, should be the aim of authorities responsible for service provision.

CHILDLESSNESS

While some couples living together choose not to have children, the majority clearly do raise a family. For many people this is an important role, and when childlessness is a reality it brings disappointment. In addition, many other feelings, associated with social and cultural expectations and religious beliefs, may be experienced.

Barbour (1997) suggested that, until recently, much attention relating to treatment and counselling in this area has been directed towards women. Her experience with infertile couples, however, suggests that the feelings and reactions of men also require to be addressed. Mason (1994) also recognised the significance of fatherhood in the context of male infertility. Hjelmstedt et al (1999) found that women reacted more strongly to their infertility than men but distress experienced by men concerned their male role and the social pressure to become a parent.

Some couples choose not to have children in the early years of their relationship but later may experience difficulty in conceiving. It is well documented that one in six couples will seek specialist help for a fertility problem (Winston 1991, Templeton 1992). In one-third of couples experiencing subfertility, the problem lies with the woman, in one-third with the man and in the remaining third both the man and the woman contribute some causative factor (see Tables 7.1 and 7.2).

The provision of general facilities to investigate and treat subfertility and to assist in conception are well established at the endocrinology and gynaecological surgery level in the NHS, but the specialist in vitro fertilisation services have been slow to develop, hampered by lack of finance. This has led to an increase in the fertility business in private health care. The need for subfertility services is expected to grow due to the trend towards later first pregnancies and an increasing number of remarriages. Demand is increased due to raised public awareness of treatment possibilities (Effective Health Care Consortium 1992).

Childlessness is deliberately maintained in women who use birth control methods. This is regarded as voluntary childlessness. Sterility refers to an absolute factor preventing procreation in either the man or the woman. The condition may be induced by ligation and separation of the fallopian tubes or by vasectomy.

Subfertility

A couple is said to be subfertile if there is a lack of conception after a 12-month period of unprotected sexual intercourse (Thonneau et al 1991). Primary subfertility refers to those cases where a pregnancy has never occurred, and secondary subfertility to those cases where there has been a previous pregnancy, irrespective of the outcome. The literature suggests that 10–15% of couples have difficulty conceiving or having the number of children they want and seek fertility services (Evers 2002, Kolettis 2003).

The principal causes of subfertility are shown in Tables 7.1 and 7.2. In some couples there will be more than one cause of subfertility. In 5–10% of cases after thorough investigation the cause of the infertility is unexplained (Adamson & Baker 2003). As diagnostic testing becomes more accurate, the proportion of unexplained cases of subfertility may decrease. The contribution of psychological factors to prolonged subfertility is not yet clearly established by research. A small proportion of cases of subfertility may be preventable, particularly tubal damage associated with sexually transmitted diseases.

MEDICAL MANAGEMENT

The diagnosis and management of subfertility is complex. The couple may require to undergo a variety of tests and investigations which can cause embarrassment and stress (see Tables 7.1 and 7.2).

Female subfertility

Female subfertility may be due to failure to ovulate, irregular egg release from the ovary, obstructed fallopian tubes, hostile cervical mucus, endometriosis or uterine conditions which inhibit implantation.

Ovulation disorders

These are among the commonest causes of subfertility (Power 2001). Failure to ovulate is linked with the functioning of hormones from the hypothalamus, pituitary and ovary (HPO axis). Anovulation is categorised into five groups:

- Hypergonadotrophic hypogonadism — elevated FSH and LH to within the accepted menopausal range; no response to ovulation induction.
- Hypogonadotrophic hypogonadism — hypothalamic suppression of gonadotrophin-releasing hormone (GnRH) release causes very low levels of pituitary gonadotrophin and results in suppression of ovulation.
- Eugonadotrophic hypogonadism — functional disturbance of the HPO axis, generally with oligomenorrhoea.
- Polycystic ovarian disease — small cysts on the ovarian surface coupled with hormonal imbalance. Multiple small follicles partly develop but none reaches maturity.
- Hyperprolactinaemia — high levels of prolactin suppress pulsatile secretion of GnRH and oestradiol production mediated by LH.

Treatment seeks to remedy problems arising from imbalances in the HPO axis. Ovulation induction is aimed at encouraging development of one follicle, leading to a single pregnancy. Clomiphene citrate can be used in women with eugonadotrophic hypogonadism or polycystic ovaries. This anti-oestrogen stimulates gonadotrophin release by inhibiting the negative feedback of gonadal steroids on the hypothalamus.

Treatment should commence in the early follicular phase. In amenorrhoeic women or those with severe oligomenorrhoea, treatment begins after an induced withdrawal bleed. Generally 50 mg clomiphene is administered daily for 5 days. Ovulation is expected 5–10 days after the last clomiphene tablet and intercourse is best timed between days 10 and 16. In successive anovulary cycles, clomiphene can be increased by 50 mg/day to a maximum of 200 mg/day.

For women who do not respond to clomiphene therapy, human menopausal gonadotrophin (hMG) may be used for direct ovarian stimulation. Careful monitoring of the dose is required to reduce the risk of multiple pregnancy.

Pulsatile GnRH is a suitable therapy for women with hypogonadotrophic hypogonadism. This is administered as a pulse dose via an infusion device and stimulates pituitary gonadotrophin release, resulting in the menstrual cycle with positive and negative feedback loops.

Elevated prolactin levels can result in chronic anovulation by inhibiting GnRH release and LH-mediated oestradiol production. Bromocriptine, a powerful dopamine agonist, inhibits prolactin release and may therefore be a therapy considered for such patients.

Table 7.1 Subfertility: summary of causes, investigations and treatment in women

Causes	Investigations	Treatment
Disorders of ovulation		
Stein–Leventhal syndrome Failure of one or both pituitary gonadotrophins (trauma or vascular disorder) Failure of hypothalamic releasing factor (stress, anorexia nervosa) Primary ovarian failure Tumours of ovary Cysts of ovary Endometrial hyperplasia (causing upset ovarian function) XO karyotype Drugs — post-pill amenorrhoea, phenothiazines, tricyclic antidepressants Adrenal dysfunction Thyroid, hyper- and hypothyroidism	• History • Examination (bimanual) • Skull X-ray • Endometrial biopsy, histology and culture • Plasma progesterone level • Urinary oestrogens level • Ovarian biopsy • Cervical mucus specimen (can be used as a parameter of ovulation) • Full blood count and ESR • Thyroid function tests • Chromosome studies	• Clomiphene • Bromocriptine — for raised prolactin only • LH releasing hormone (LHRH) by pump injection • Pergonal and human chorionic gonadotrophin (hCG) • Buserelin with human menopausal gonadotrophin (hMG) is useful for those with polycystic ovaries • Surgical wedge resection of ovary under laparoscopy. May be effective when drug treatment failed • Gamete intrafallopian transfer (GIFT)
Disorders of fallopian tubes		
Congenital absence Blocked due to infection: — tuberculosis — recurrent appendicitis — gonococcal infection — septic abortion Hydrosalpinx Disturbance of tubal secretions	• History • Examination • Hysterosalpingogram • Laparoscopy • Biopsy of fallopian tube • Hormone studies (no oestrogen surge)	• Salpingolysis • Salpingostomy • Tubal reconstruction — by microscopy • Tubal excision and transplantation • Oral oestrogens • In vitro fertilisation (IVF) and embryo transfer (ET)
Endometrium lining of the uterus		
Not prepared due to disorder of ovulation Endometriosis Endometritis Fibroids Endometrial hyperplasia Endocervicitis	• History • Examination (bimanual) • Hysterosalpingogram • Endometrial biopsy • Evidence of discharge	• Treatment of disorders of ovulation • Dilatation and curettage • Myomectomy • Endometriosis IVF-ET/GIFT
Factors in the cervical mucus		
Hostile mucus Cervical mucus not prepared due to deficiency of oestrogen as a result of disorders of ovulation Sperm antibodies in cervical mucus	• Postcoital test • Mucus/sperm match test • Spinnbarkheit test • Fern test • Sperm invasion test	• Deficient oestrogen — clomiphene • Ethinyl oestradiol (0.01 u daily for a 3-day period before ovulation) • Refrain from intercourse for a set period or use condom during intercourse. At the end of this time, there may be a decrease in antibodies
Psychosexual problems		
Frigidity Vaginismus Stress-affecting hypothalamic function Decreased sexual libido	• History and interview	• Psychological referral • Use of vaginal dilators
Others		
Congenital abnormalities (e.g. bicornuate uterus) Obesity Retroverted uterus Hirsutism and virilism (disorders of ovarian or adrenal function, also by certain drugs)	• Examination • Hysterosalpingogram	• Lose weight • Ventro-suspension surgery • Surgical restructuring of genital organs as possible

Table 7.2 Subfertility: summary of causes, investigations and treatment in men

Causes	Investigations	Treatment
Testes Congenital absence of both Klinefelter's syndrome Cryptorchidism Trauma Testicular failure: — torsion — infections — unrestricted pituitary output	• History • Examination • Testicular biopsy • Urinary gonadotrophins • Chromosome investigations	• Cryptorchidism should be detected early in school career and requires surgical intervention • Hormone therapy
Vas deferens and epididymis Congenital absence of both Blockage due to infections: — partial — complete Venereal disease Vasitis Epididymitis	• History • Vasogram • Semen analysis • Postcoital test	• No treatment for congenital absence • Vaso-epididymostomy • Microsurgery — removal of blocked section of vas
Spermatozoa Oligospermia (less than 20 million in 1 mL) Varicocele Hernia Physical exhaustion and overwork Aspermia Factors in the testes, vas deferens and epididymis (see above) Endocrine abnormalities, failure of pituitary, adrenal and thyroid glands	• History • Examination — consistency of testicles, presence/absence of varicocele • Semen analysis • Postcoital test • Seminal plasma analysis for fructose content and its glycerol phospherol choline • Interstitial cell-stimulating hormone, follicle-stimulating hormone and testosterone levels • Testicular biopsy • Thyroid tests • Urine analysis — gonadotrophins, ketosteroids • Vasogram	• Surgical treatment of varicocele or hernia • Moderation with alcohol, tobacco and work • Wearing loose underpants • Intrauterine insemination by donor • Vaso-epididymostomy • Assisted conception techniques using partner sperm
Semen volume Too low — sperms fail to contact cervical os Too high — overdilution Quality	• Semen analysis • Postcoital test	• Pooling of two or more semen samples and intrauterine insemination by partner • High doses of gonadotrophins • Split ejaculate and intrauterine insemination by partner
Agglutination of spermatozoa Sperm autoantibodies Hostile mucus Sperm antibodies in cervical mucus (penetrate the mucus but become agglutinated and immobilised and die)	• Seminal fluid analysis • Rosette formation of head-to-head clumping, or a wheatsheaf formation of tail-to-tail clumping in seminal fluid • No sperm invasion is seen	• It may be possible to wash the antibodies off these sperm and then, after centrifuging, produce a concentrated specimen; they can be inseminated directly into the cervix • Corticosteroid therapy
Ejaculatory disorders Hypospadias Epispadias Retrograde ejaculation	• History • Examination	• Collection of semen and artificial insemination by partner • Surgical treatment

Table 7.2 Subfertility: summary of causes, investigations and treatment in men *(Continued)*

Causes	Investigations	Treatment
Sexual problems Impotence Premature ejaculation Stress Decreased sexual libido	• History • Interview	• Psychological referral • Help regain self-confidence • Apply local anaesthetic to penis before coitus. Treatment for premature ejaculation • Monoamine oxidase inhibitor drugs
Others Poor general health Febrile illness Emotional shock Acute allergic response	• History • Examination • ESR	• Full recovery ensues naturally

Tubal disorders

Where tubal factors are the cause of the subfertility, tubal surgery may be advised but this depends upon the nature, site and severity of the condition of the tube, the presence and extent of adhesions, and the skill of the surgeon. Diagnostic procedures will include laparoscopy and hysterosalpingography for full assessment of the condition.

Treatment Surgical procedures used to treat tubal infertility include fimbrioplasty, salpingostomy, salpingo-ovariolysis, tubotubal anastomosis, uterotubal anastomosis and tubal cannulation. Results of such reconstructive surgery show great variation depending on the degree of tubal damage and the adequacy of the surgery performed. Audebert et al (1998) suggested that results from a laparoscopic fimbrioplasty are as good as results from microsurgery.

The World Health Organization (WHO) (1997) cautions against quoting statistics to patients since the 'success' rates reported in studies are often not defined in terms of achieving an intrauterine pregnancy and delivery of a live baby. Reversal of sterilisation, however, is more likely to be successful if the occlusive technique used for sterilisation caused minimal damage to the tubes. Clips, for example, generally have minimal traumatic effect and are associated with the highest proportion of intrauterine pregnancies following reversal. Successful reversal can also depend on the site of occlusion (WHO 1997).

Endometriosis

The association between endometriosis and infertility is complex (Mahutte & Arici 2002). Many women with the condition conceive successfully without intervention.

Treatment There is controversy over the treatment of infertile women with endometriosis without distortion of the pelvic viscera. Martin (1995) suggests that surgery should only be performed where symptoms such as pain and deep dyspareunia are attributable to endometriosis.

The use of laparoscopic surgery in the treatment of minimal and mild endometriosis may improve success rates but further research in this area is needed (Jacobson et al 2002). Surgery, however, is recommended in cases of distortion of pelvic tissues. Surgery to remove endometrial tissue, correct anatomical relationships and enhance the possibility of fertility can be successful by laparotomy or laparoscopic techniques (Candiani et al 1991, Redwine 1991). Other options for women with endometriosis include in vitro fertilisation (IVF), embryo transfer (ET) and gamete intrafallopian transfer (GIFT) (Effective Health Care Consortium 1992).

Male subfertility

Iammarrone et al (2003) suggest there is an increasing incidence of male reproductive problems. Male fertility problems can be categorised into three therapeutic groups: untreatable sterility, treatable conditions and subfertility. Subfertility is the most common (Baker 1995). Impaired semen quality and sperm dysfunction can occur as a result of many factors. The cause may be unknown, but it may be associated with a previous infection or factors such as stress, excessive smoking or alcohol intake. Obstruction of the vas deferens will result in ejaculate without sperm. Antisperm antibodies which attack sperm or inhibit their motility may be present in semen. Iammarrone et al (2003) claim recent studies suggest an increased incidence of genetic disorder relating to male infertility.

Common presentations are:

- oligozoospermia — reduced number of sperm
- asthenozoospermia — reduced motility
- tetratozoospermia — abnormal morphology
- oligoaesthenotetratozoospermia — a combination of the above three
- azoospermia — absence of sperm.

Semen analysis includes an assessment of volume; sperm concentration, motility and morphology; and the number of white cells present. Sperm mucus interaction can be examined in a postcoital test.

Men presenting with subfertility should be fully investigated to ascertain the type of subfertility and identify any related health issues requiring independent treatment.

Treatment should be aimed at achieving natural conception. If male antibodies to spermatozoa are produced, prednisolone has been shown to be effective as an immunosuppressant (Hendry et al 1990). When natural conception is not possible, assisted reproductive techniques (ARTs) offer another possibility. ARTs involve the collection of sperm and eggs and either the immediate placement of the gametes into the fallopian tubes (GIFT) where fertilisation takes place or in vitro fertilisation (IVF) and subsequent transfer of the embryos (ET). Microinsemination techniques such as partial zona dissection (PZD) or subzonal insemination (SUZI) may be appropriate in, for example, oligozoospermia or tetratozoospermia (Fishel et al 1993). Green et al (1997) suggest that almost all cases of male infertility can be treated by intracytoplasmic injection (ICSI) if viable sperm can be obtained; however, there is some concern that ICSI may result in transmission of defects to the offspring since the natural selection of the spermatozoa is bypassed (Iammarrone et al 2003). Recognising this potential problem, Tournaye (2003) recommends that all men for ICSI should be rigorously screened and fully informed about the limitations of current knowledge and screening methods available.

While ARTs allow many subfertile men to father children, these techniques do not meet the needs of men who do not produce sperm. Donor insemination (DI) may be an option in such cases. DI may also be considered by couples where the man is known to be a carrier of a genetic disease or where couples do not wish to take the risk of having a child born with a genetic disorder transmitted by recessive genes. Kovacs (1997) suggests that a reasonable conception rate from DI in most units is about 10% per cycle. The cumulative conception rate increases to approximately 40% over five treatment cycles.

Provision of information and counselling

The stressful nature of investigations and treatment of subfertility and the psychological impact of the condition on couples require information about the nature of investigations, the implications of and alternatives to treatment. Emotional support and therapeutic counselling should be easily available to the couple. The Committee of Inquiry into Human Fertilisation and Embryology (1984) recommended that 'counselling should be available to all infertile couples and third parties at any stage of the treatment'. Infertility counselling is recognised by counsellors as a specialised area (Jennings 1995) and Monarch (2003) emphasises the continuing role of counsellors in helping patients, and the conception team, deal with the difficult psychosocial and ethical issues they face in practice. Boivin (2003) also draws attention to the added value of group interactions that focus on education and skills training, e.g. relaxation, claiming that these approaches are significantly more effective in producing positive outcomes across a range of issues.

In vitro fertilisation and embryo transfer (IVF-ET)

The work of Edwards and Steptoe in 1978 (summarised in Edwards & Steptoe 1983) led to the birth of the first human infant after conception in vitro (IVF). In the intervening decades the success rate of IVF has improved as a result of advances in ovulation induction regimens, oocyte retrieval, embryo culture, embryo transfer and improved facilities of cryopreservation (Fauser & Devroey 2003). IVF is now widely accepted as a form of treatment for unexplained subfertility. However, the success rate, measured by the end result of live healthy babies, depends on many factors, including the age of the woman, duration of infertility, existing fertility problem(s) of the couple and previous pregnancy history (see Box 7.9). The estimated live birth rates per cycle are reported to be between 13 and 28% but effectiveness of IVF has not been properly evaluated against other treatments (Pandian et al 2002). Some pregnancies terminate with spontaneous abortion or ectopic pregnancy (Talbot & Lawrence 1997).

Box 7.9

Indications for selection into IVF programmes

- Husband and wife are generally healthy
- Ovaries are accessible
- The uterus is functioning normally
- Menstrual function is normal or correctable
- Age preferred below 40 years but a flexible individual approach is taken
- The couple have an uncorrected problem, e.g.:
  — tubal
  — inadequate sperm for normal reproduction
  — endometriosis
  — cervical hostility
  — immunological
  — anovulation
  — undiagnosed by available methods.

Ovarian stimulation Various protocols are in use to achieve controlled hyperstimulation of the ovaries. Agents used include clomiphene citrate, purified FSH, exogenous gonadotrophin and gonadotrophin-releasing hormone agonists (GnRHAs). Modifications to protocols depend on the patient's response.

Clomiphene citrate acts in a negative feedback system to increase endogenous gonadotrophin. A hypothalamic site of action has been reported with increased pulsatile release of GnRH. Clomiphene results in synchronous development of multiple follicles, allowing many oocytes to be retrieved. A disadvantage can be a premature rise in LH, resulting in premature ovulation. To avoid the patient's spontaneous ovulation, hCG is used to induce timed ovulation for ovum retrieval. Medication used to stimulate ovarian function have improved and the three gonadotrophins are now available as recombinant products. In some situations the near-100% pure FSH preparations can cause abnormally low LH levels. The addition of LH may be necessary in these cases and Ludwig et al (2003) believe that r-LH may become available in sufficient dosages to replace hCG for ovulation induction, reducing the incidence of ovarian hyperstimulation syndrome due to its shorter half-life.

The dose of exogenous gonadotrophin is determined on the basis of the patient's age and history.

GnRHAs have increased pregnancy rates per cycle (Hughes et al 1992) and can be used in combination with hMG for improved folliculogenesis. Fauser and Devroey

(2003) advocate a more patient-tailored approach to ovarian stimulation.

Harvesting of eggs Eggs (oocytes) for fertilisation can be recovered from mature ovarian follicles by:

- ultrasound scanner-guided follicle needle puncture and aspiration
- laparoscopy and needle aspiration.

The laparoscopy method requires a general anaesthetic. The ultrasound method can be completed with either a light general anaesthetic or with the patient sedated. The ultrasound probe is introduced into the vagina and the pelvis is inspected, noting the position of viscera and blood vessels. An appropriate pathway for the aspirating needle through the pelvis is selected. The laparoscopic method may be used when it is difficult to access the ovaries vaginally. Aspirated oocytes are transferred to the embryologist.

Laboratory procedures For maximum efficiency and effectiveness there must be close proximity between the operating theatre and the embryology laboratory. There must also be ease of communication between the surgeon and the embryologist; direct verbal and visual contact between the two is needed. Theatre time is usually booked in advance, with 24 h notice, but sometimes egg recovery may need to be done at short notice because of the patient's endogenous LH surge.

The embryologist examines the follicular aspirate for oocytes. The eggs are examined for the level of maturity, washed in clean culture medium and transferred to the culture container. On completion of the oocyte collection, they are placed in an incubator until insemination. This may be 3–6 h later for IVF. In GIFT the oocytes and prepared sperm are placed into a catheter to be inserted into the fimbrial end of the fallopian tube, where the gametes are deposited for fertilisation.

Collection of semen can be a stressful experience for the man, who needs to be assured of a secure private environment to produce a specimen of semen by masturbation (Jackson & Burden 1997). A toilet and hand basin should be available. Erotic video and literature may be helpful. However, some couples may wish to be together for this procedure, so a bed with washable covers should be in the room. Men may produce a semen sample in their own home if they are able to deliver it to the laboratory within 1 h.

Insemination involves mixing of sperm, prepared by the embryologist, and eggs in the appropriate concentration. Between 16 and 20 h later the oocytes are examined for fertilisation and once normal fertilisation has been established the embryos are returned to culture in fresh medium for another 24 h.

Embryo replacement This is usually performed 2–3 days after oocyte retrieval or about 48 h after insemination when the embryos are at the two- or four-cell stage. Placement of the embryos in the uterus is a delicate procedure that does not necessarily result in successful implantation and pregnancy. In some centres nurses are taught to perform this procedure, following a specified protocol, as part of their extended role (Peddie 1998). The incidence of pregnancy increases with the number of embryos replaced, but an attempt is made to reduce the risk of multiple pregnancy with the possibility of premature births. Usually two or three embryos are transferred, a painless procedure for the patient.

On discharge from hospital the patient is given instructions to send samples of urine to the unit on the 8th and 11th days after replacement so that pregnancy tests can be completed and to notify the unit if menstruation occurs so that she can be advised about future treatment. If her pregnancy is confirmed and develops, the unit will maintain an interest in the pregnancy and celebrate the success of childbirth.

Transport IVF

While there is an increasing demand for IVF treatment in the UK, a lack of funding limits the number of clinics able to offer IVF treatment. Transport IVF, however, makes this treatment more widely available to infertile couples. Here gynaecologists in local communities make arrangements with regional specialist IVF units to share the care of the patients (Kingsland et al 1992). The ways in which the services required at different stages of IVF are organised between the two centres vary. One possibility is for ovulation stimulation and oocyte retrieval to be undertaken at the satellite centre, with subsequent transfer of the oocytes to the central unit for insemination, fertilisation and embryo transfer.

Treatment of low-powered sperm in IVF-ET

Such treatments involve manipulating ovum and sperm together to improve penetration of the ovum by sperm in cases of sperm dysfunction such as poor motility. A deliberate injection of a single sperm into an ovum can be achieved using a sophisticated microscope and special instruments. The human embryos so formed have led to successful pregnancies for a few women.

See Green et al (1997) for further information regarding intracytoplasmic sperm injection.

Prenatal analysis of DNA for genetic abnormality

Prenatal diagnosis of genetic abnormalities is now possible by analysing DNA for a known gene defect (see Ch. 6). A single cell is removed from a 4–16 cell embryo. Information regarding a genetic defect can become available within a few hours, soon enough to allow the embryo to be implanted when it is known to be healthy. Diseases such as cystic fibrosis and Duchenne muscular dystrophy can thus be avoided. Some women have already been treated in this way, but long-term information is needed on whether the loss of a single cell from an embryo is likely to have any adverse effect.

Gamete intrafallopian transfer (GIFT)

GIFT offers an alternative treatment to IVF when women have at least one patent fallopian tube. It is primarily used in patients who have unexplained subfertility and cervical hostility. It is contraindicated in women with stage III and IV endometriosis, active infection and intrauterine abnormalities. GIFT can be performed in hospitals that do not have IVF facilities. However, where such facilities exist, surplus oocytes can be fertilised in vitro and cryopreserved. Thus IVF and later ET may be an option if GIFT is unsuccessful. Wood (1997) demonstrated that between 1990 and 1993 the live birth rate from GIFT was double that from IVF.

The technique involves giving follicle-stimulating drugs to stimulate the ovaries. Retrieval of eggs follows, as in IVF. The eggs are then mixed with the freshly donated sperm and transferred into the fimbriated ends of the fallopian tube(s) (see Fig. 7.10). GIFT is normally performed laparoscopically but it can be achieved vaginally or by means of a colposcope. The eggs, being placed directly in the fallopian tube, have the opportunity to become fertilised more naturally and continue along the tube to implant in the uterus.

Zygote intrafallopian transfer (ZIFT)

Here the gametes are fertilised before transfer to the fallopian tube. In this treatment, therefore, fertilisation is known to have occurred and embryos have the opportunity to benefit from the tubal environment and to enter the uterine cavity naturally.

NURSING PRIORITIES AND MANAGEMENT: IVF

The couple may have experienced many tests, investigations and surgical interventions before being offered the opportunity to seek pregnancy by the IVF method, and, though always hopeful for success, must recognise that this is not guaranteed.

Pre-laparoscopy care

Reducing anxiety

Pretreatment counselling looks to give a realistic picture of the chances of cumulative success rather than encouraging the couple to focus on success of the first cycle (Anderson & Alesi 1997).

The nurse will need to prepare a plan of care that will minimise the stress level and help the patient to relax. High stress levels are well known to disturb hormone levels and activity. Planned counselling sessions may be needed. Similarly, information-giving sessions will need to be planned. Slides and videotapes can be invaluable supplements for group work when the special needs of individuals can be identified and met within a supportive group. A system of open communication is important, whether the information is favourable or disappointing.

Self-care in the follicular stage

The patient is not ill and her role in maintaining self-care can be explained. She will need to learn how to collect her urine, required for laboratory testing, and record the time and amount passed. Verbal instructions can be complemented by a written explanation available in the toilet area. A patient whose first language is not English will need written instructions in her own language.

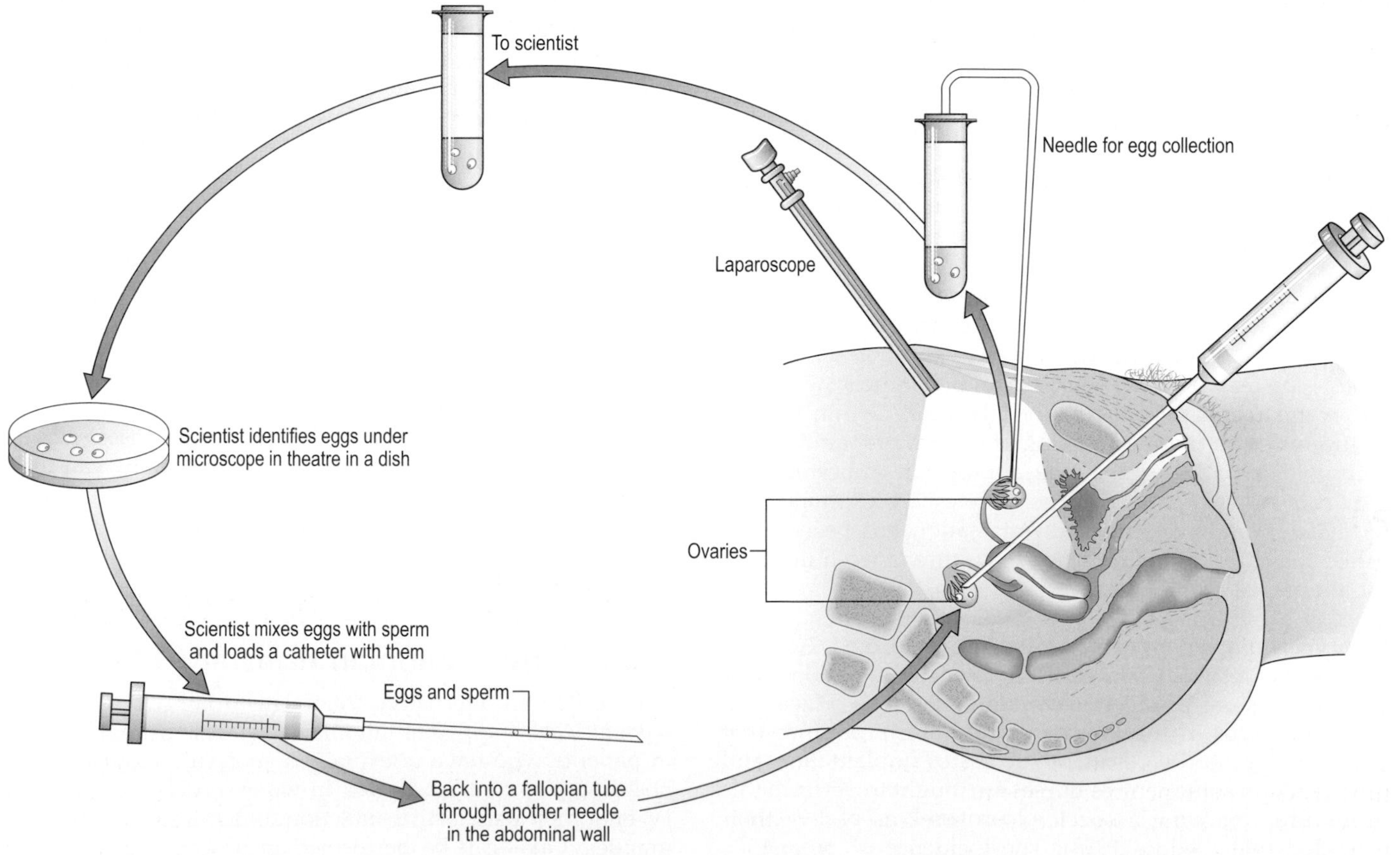

 Fig. 7.10 The GIFT treatment.

Blood and urine samples will be required for laboratory testing. Ovarian stimulants are given according to the individual patient's needs. Patients should understand that there are differences in need between individual women and the nurse's explanations can alleviate concerns.

Preparation for egg cell recovery

The procedure of ultrasound scanning should be explained in terms of checking the number of follicles maturing and their stage of development. Once the estimated time of ovulation is known, preparation for theatre begins. Blood is taken for haemoglobin estimation. Skin is prepared according to the policy of the unit; some surgeons still prefer the pubic area to be shaved prior to laparoscopy and oocyte recovery. Fasting arrangements are maintained according to protocol, in preparation for a general anaesthetic. No premedication drugs are prescribed, to avoid compromise of the patient's physiological balance and that of the ripened follicles.

The nurse should encourage the patient to relax and be calm for transfer to theatre. The eggs are generally recovered vaginally with ultrasound guidance but can also be retrieved via a laparoscope. Each mature follicle is carefully aspirated and the eggs are collected in the culture tube. The aspirate is immediately passed to the laboratory for examination and identification of oocytes.

Post-laparoscopy care

Recovery from the laparoscopy is rapid. Rest in bed for a maximum of 8 h is usually necessary to avoid referred pain in the shoulder from retention of residual gas in the abdomen. Mild analgesics such as paracetamol may be prescribed for relief of pain. The patient will be keen to know whether the laparoscopy was successful and how many eggs were recovered.

Sometimes the time of ovulation has been misjudged and the follicles have already ruptured prior to laparoscopy or the recovered eggs are too immature to be viable. During laparoscopy, adhesions may obscure the ovarian tissue, thus negating the procedure.

The nurse should adopt a sensitive approach when giving news of the failure of the procedure. The surgeon concerned may prefer to explain the difficulties to the patient and her partner. The nurse may have to repeat the information for the patient together with possible details of re-entry into the programme at a later date.

Preparation for embryo transfer

After a woman's eggs have been successfully recovered, it may be necessary to wait 2–3 days while the eggs are matured in vitro. 100 000 specially prepared motile sperm from her partner are added for each egg and fertilisation should occur within 18–24 h if there is no male problem. The embryos are observed in the laboratory as they develop to a two- or four-cell stage prior to transfer. Failures may also occur at this delicate laboratory stage and this is a further worrying time for the patient.

As soon as a positive decision is made for embryo transfer, the patient takes a shower and dresses in a clean gown. A bath is avoided to ensure there is no water in the vagina. The bed is prepared with clean linen and taken to the theatre. Once there, the patient is positioned in the modified lithotomy in the Trendelenburg position for the procedure of embryo transfer.

Following transfer the woman can resume her normal activities. Although resting does not increase the chance of pregnancy (Power 2001), the woman may prefer to have a quiet day.

STOP THINK

7.1 Think about how the patient will feel if failure occurs at any of the stages of the IVF treatment programme.

7.2 Write down the patient's possible thoughts about failure:
- during the follicular stage
- at the oocyte recovery stage
- at the embryo development stage in the laboratory
- after embryo transfer into the uterus.

7.3 Write down a few sentences of what you might say to the patient at each of the above stages.

7.4 Discuss with your mentor whether what you have written down could be used as a guide to communication with the patient, with allowances made for differences between patients and their partners.

Continuing need for support and counselling

Nurses working in hospital or in the community must be prepared to use their counselling skills with clients who wish to enter, are involved in, or have terminated a programme of subfertility treatment. Community midwives may participate in the care of women who are pregnant following subfertility treatment and others who have experienced a miscarriage. Health visitors also have a role in counselling following the loss of a pregnancy or an infant after subfertility treatment. Couples may continue to need to talk about their feelings of inadequacy or failure and to be allowed to grieve for their losses (see Case History 7.1).

For some couples, treatment options for subfertility will not prove successful and it may be necessary for them to accept that they will not have children of their own. Other possibilities can be sensitively discussed.

EMBRYO RESEARCH

The main aim of human embryo research has been the prevention of genetically transferred diseases. Embryo research

CASE HISTORY 7.1

K

K achieved a pregnancy during her programme of subfertility treatments. Unfortunately, she aborted a twin-boy pregnancy and was devastated by the loss. She returned to the programme and became a mother with the birth of quadruplets: three girls and a boy. Unfortunately the boy subsequently died. K visits the unit with her lovely girls in a triple buggy but still grieves over the boys. She has asked to re-enter the programme because she still wants a boy. K has been referred to an independent counsellor.

improves the understanding and management of genetic diseases.

Pre-implantation diagnosis in embryos is possible by removing and examining a single cell, although it is not known whether this cell removal might cause a defect in the child. The treatment offers hope to those who carry genetic defects that can affect the well-being of the child. Further embryo research may help with the understanding of miscarriage of pregnancies, which involve 100 000 women per year, with consequent effects on health and future fertility. Further understanding of the way embryos implant might shed more light on contraception, miscarriages and ectopic pregnancies. It is also expected that embryo research will improve the understanding and treatment of cancer by the study of 'oncogenes' which control cell division and growth.

The Human Fertilisation and Embryology Act 1990

A consequence of reproductive technology and in vitro fertilisation is the production of surplus embryos. This has created public concern about the potential for undesirable experimental work on embryos.

The Human Fertilisation and Embryology Act 1990 prohibits certain practices and has established the Human Fertilisation and Embryology Authority (HFEA) to license and regulate the activities of IVF centres. The Act applies only to the creation of embryos outside the human body. The embryo is not to be kept or used after the appearance of the primitive streak, at the end of 14 days. The primitive streak, or groove, is formed by invagination from the ectoderm, in the formation of the mesoderm between the ectoderm and the endoderm of the embryo. Identification of this structure is used to denote the beginning of human life (Morgan & Lee 1991). Frozen embryos can generally be stored for 5 years and gametes may be stored for 10 years. There are, however, exceptional conditions when storage periods can be extended. All centres involved in IVF must prepare a code of practice, which is subject to inspection, and are required to send 12-monthly reports to the HFEA. The Act has a conscientious objection clause. Consequently anyone who can show a conscious objection to any of the activities governed by the Act is not obliged to participate in them (HFEA 2003). Nurses must make known any conscientious objection to the appropriate person as soon as possible (NMC 2002).

Surrogate motherhood

The Human Fertilisation and Embryology Act defines the woman who carries the embryo as the mother of the child. If the woman then gives the baby to a married couple in a surrogacy agreement, a parental order can be made by a competent court (in private) to make the couple the child's legal parents, providing specified criteria are met (Human Fertilisation and Embryology Act 1990). Regardless of any prior agreement regarding the surrogacy, the Human Fertilisation and Embryology Act renders surrogacy contracts unenforceable.

The right of any childless couple to have a child is generally accepted, but after infertility treatments fail to help the woman to conceive, there may be less support for her seeking another fertile woman to assist in developing a pregnancy. Financial inducement and contractual arrangements cannot guarantee that the surrogate mother will be prepared to hand over the newborn baby to the infertile couple. If the intended parents do not wish to accept the child the surrogate (legal) mother is responsible for its welfare. In the event of the child being rejected by the birth mother and the intended parents the child can be placed for adoption or fostering.

DISORDERS OF THE MALE REPRODUCTIVE ORGANS

The anatomy and physiology of the male reproductive system is described in Chapter 8.

MALDESCENT OF THE TESTES (CRYPTORCHIDISM)

PATHOPHYSIOLOGY

Cryptorchidism is a condition in which one or both testes have not descended into the scrotum before birth. It is a common condition seen in approximately 1% of boys after their first year and may be self-correcting or require surgery in the form of orchidopexy. Normal descent keeps the testes cooler in the scrotum and avoids the germ cell degeneration that is possible in the higher temperature of the abdomen, which carries a risk of malignancy. Three different grades of maldescent are described:

- a retractile testicle is normally found in the scrotum but on stimulation is pulled up into the superficial inguinal pouch by an active cremaster muscle
- an ectopic testicle is prevented, by tissue structures, from descending from the inguinal canal into the scrotum
- an undescended testicle is possibly abnormal: it remains in the abdomen and fails to enter the inguinal canal and pass into the scrotum.

MEDICAL MANAGEMENT

The aim of treatment is to promote normal function of the testicle. Treatment should be completed by the boy's eighth year, before the testicle starts functioning. Untreated cryptorchidism results in sterility, since the cells involved in the initial development of sperm cells are destroyed by the higher body temperature within the body. The testicle may migrate spontaneously, or hormone treatment may be prescribed to stimulate migration. Otherwise, an orchidopexy is performed to bring the testicle into the scrotum. It is held there by means of a suture passing through the wall of the scrotum and into the thigh. The suture is removed 7–10 days postoperatively.

More extensive surgery may be needed with actual removal of the abnormal testicle and repair of an inguinal hernia if this has occurred. In addition to the risk of infertility, there is also a high risk of malignancy if the testes are left in the abdomen.

NURSING PRIORITIES AND MANAGEMENT: Maldescent of the testes

The nurse should identify any deficit in the patient's understanding of his condition and the operation to be performed. The patient who is still a child may feel embarrassed about asking questions and the nurse must judge where to begin and end when giving information and a health education programme. The facts of sexual life may need to be explained to the child with a parent present, or the parent may prefer to be the one to give the child the information. In some cases, the nurse may find it more relevant to focus on the parents' need for education, information and advice. While care should be taken not to cause undue anxiety, the suggested link with an increased risk of testicular cancer, at a later age, should be broached to encourage vigilance in adult life (see p. 308).

TORSION OF THE TESTES

Testicular torsion is an acutely painful condition caused by the twisting of the testicle on its spermatic cord. It may occur spontaneously or as the result of strenuous exertion. It commonly occurs in adolescents aged 12–18 years, but can also occur in adults. This condition is classified as a surgical emergency requiring immediate treatment.

PATHOPHYSIOLOGY

Testicular torsion results when an abnormality of the tunica vaginalis allows increased mobility of the testis and axial rotation of the spermatic cord above. The resulting ischaemia can lead to cell damage and infection within approximately 6 h.

Extravaginal torsion, a rare form, can occur in utero or in the newborn. In this case the testis is not painful but on examination is found to be a firm, large mass in the scrotum.

Common presenting symptoms The patient will present with sudden onset of acute pain in the groin, often radiating to the scrotum and abdomen. Exercise may be the precipitating factor, but the onset of pain can also occur at rest. Nausea and vomiting are common.

MEDICAL MANAGEMENT

The patient may give a history of previous, less severe episodes which resolved spontaneously. Examination of the testis may be hampered by the severity of the pain. The affected testis will be elevated, but abnormality of mobility ('bellclapper' deformity) may be present in the other testis.

Treatment Treatment is by immediate surgery to relieve the torsion and secure testicular fixation. However, if the torsion is detected at an earlier stage, it may be possible by gentle external manipulation to rotate the twisted testis in the appropriate direction. This may immediately resolve the emergency, but the testis should later be surgically secured to prevent recurrence.

NURSING PRIORITIES AND MANAGEMENT: Torsion of the testes

The patient will normally be young and fit and his stay in hospital brief. Although the surgery is not considered major, the acute onset of pain and the nature of the problem may give rise to considerable anxiety and embarrassment. Giving the patient adequate information will help to relieve anxiety and promote recovery. He should be informed that analgesics can be given immediately and that the acute pain will go away once the operation has been performed.

Postoperatively, the patient will have a small inguinal wound and perhaps some scrotal swelling. He will normally be able to return to school or to work in about 2 weeks, at which point he should feel comfortable walking and sitting. Lifting, heavy work and sports involving running, jumping or stretching should be avoided for about 6 weeks. An athletic support should always be worn when sports activities are resumed.

The patient who has received treatment in good time should also be reassured that no impairment to sexual function or fertility will result.

STOP THINK **7.5** Write a care plan for a patient following surgery for fixation of the testes. Consider what problems the patient might have. The care plan should include:

- checking the wound for oozing, swelling and infection
- ensuring the wearing of a scrotal support to prevent swelling
- relieving pain by bed rest and analgesics
- ensuring that the patient passes urine within a specific time postoperatively (it may take him up to 24 h)
- checking temperature, pulse and blood pressure
- informing the patient when he may eat and drink again
- giving discharge advice.

HYDROCELE

PATHOPHYSIOLOGY

A hydrocele is a collection of serous fluid in the membranous sac (the tunica vaginalis) that surrounds the testes. It may occur spontaneously without any cause or it may be secondary to an acute or chronic inflammatory condition of the testis or epididymis. The hydrocele usually occurs on one side only, is painless, and can swell to a considerable size. It may accompany a condition that causes oedema of tissues, such as congestive heart failure or nephrotic syndrome.

Common presenting symptoms Hydrocele is usually asymptomatic, but an increase in scrotal size and associated discomfort will often prompt the patient to seek advice. The embarrassment caused by the swelling may be such that the individual curtails social activities, swimming, sunshine holidays and sexual relations.

MEDICAL MANAGEMENT

The presence of fluid within the scrotal sac is dull to percussion and provides a red glow on transillumination. A tense hydrocele can be differentiated from a tumour in that the latter does not illuminate (Gillespie et al 1992). As a hydrocele can form around a testicular tumour, the possibility of cancer should be excluded.

Treatment The condition may be reducible by the wearing of a scrotal support, but it is often necessary to introduce a fine trocar and cannula to drain off the fluid. Bleeding and infection are common complications, and recurrence at 6–15 weeks is common.

VARICOCELE

A varicocele occurs when the veins draining the testes become distended and tortuous. This may cause enlargement of the spermatic cord. Palpation of the scrotum will reveal a mass of enlarged varicose veins. The condition most commonly occurs in men aged 15–30 years and sometimes resolves without intervention when there is regular sexual intercourse. A persistent varicocele may induce a raised temperature within the scrotum due to the increased blood supply and contribute to a subfertile state.

MEDICAL MANAGEMENT

The patient who complains of a dragging discomfort in the scrotum may find that this is relieved by the wearing of a scrotal support. If the condition is more severe, ligation of the veins may be needed. A small length of vein may be removed.

TESTICULAR CANCER

Testicular cancer is an uncommon condition, accounting for 1–2% of all cancers in men. It is, however, the commonest malignancy in men aged 20–34 years (Huyghe et al 2003). In the last 50 years, the condition has become more common among white racial groups but has remained only one-third as common among black racial groups. Its incidence is highest in Scandinavian countries and lowest in Asian and African countries. In Denmark, testicular cancer accounts for 6.7% of all cancers. In Japan, it accounts for 0.8%. There is a genetic component to testicular cancer; offspring of men with testicular cancer are 6–10 times more likely to develop the disease (Dearnaley et al 2001). Cryptorchidism (undescended testicle) and exogenous oestrogens have been linked with an increased incidence of testicular cancer. While exposure to exogenous oestrogens, in utero, can increase the risk of testicular cancer, Vessey (1989) indicated that such findings are not conclusive. Garner et al (2003) suggest the possibility of a link between testicular cancer and a high intake of dairy produce and Huyghe et al (2003) report an association with environmental factors and hormonal changes. More research is required to assess future trends and incidence rates and to identify risk factors.

As survival depends on early detection and treatment, Peate (1997) recommended that men should be encouraged to practise testicular self-examination at least every 6 months. The value of screening programmes for testicular cancer remains a matter for debate (see Research Abstract 7.7).

PATHOPHYSIOLOGY

The cell types of testicular cancer are classified in terms of embryonal tissue rather than adult testes tissue. Almost all the cancers arise from the primordial germ cell, the multipotent cell found in the yolk sac of the embryo. This multipotent cell will have many varieties of cell types as offspring, and a primary testicular tumour may have a wide variety of cell types. The normal cells of the testis have high proliferative potential and can become malignant under the influence of an abnormal environment.

Testicular cancers are grouped as:

- Originating from germinal tissue (97%)
  - — seminoma (typical, anaplastic or spermocytic)
  - — non-seminomatous
    - i. embryonal
    - ii. teratocarcinoma
    - iii. teratoma
    - iv. choriocarcinoma
- Arising from stromal tissue (3%)
  - — interstitial cell tumour
  - — gonadal stromal tumour.

RESEARCH ABSTRACT 7.7

Testicular cancer screening

A report of a working party of the Royal College of Physicians (1991) concluded that as testicular self-examination has never been evaluated and because chemotherapy now achieves cure rates of 90% or more, even in advanced cases of testicular cancer, screening is probably unnecessary. Moreover, because there is no identifiable pre-invasive stage, screening cannot reduce the incidence but might even increase it by overdiagnosis of borderline tumours. Thus screening for testicular cancer is not indicated.

Royal College of Physicians 1991 Report on preventive medicine. RCP, London

Germinal testicular cancer

PATHOPHYSIOLOGY

The germinal cancer types may develop from a single cell or a multifocus. The malignant growth is fairly rapid in one testis. Metastases may occur by extension locally or via the lymphatics to the retroperitoneal lymph nodes. Lymph node invasion may cause displacement of the ureters or kidneys. The ureters may become obstructed. By direct extension the tumour may invade the epididymis, extend up the spermatic cord or extend through the tunica vaginalis to the scrotum. Late metastases may be found in the lung, liver, adrenal gland or bone.

Common presenting symptoms The first sign of testicular tumour is painless enlargement of the testicle. This may be discovered by accident or by self-examination (see Box 7.10). A dragging sensation may be felt in the scrotum from the weight of the tumour.

MEDICAL MANAGEMENT

There is usually a lack of pain on palpation of the testis. Any painless lump in the testis that does not respond

Box 7.10

Teaching testicular self-examination

The nurse can make a valuable contribution to health promotion by teaching testicular self-examination. An effective teaching plan will explain the reasons for self-examination of the testes, the best time to perform self-examination, the steps to follow in self-examination and the types of abnormality that should be reported to a doctor.

Teaching plan

- Enquire about any previous information the patient may have gained about examination of the testes
- Respond to what the patient says about the topic and build on that knowledge. Give the patient the opportunity to ask questions and seek clarification regularly
- Use a simple diagram of the scrotum and testes to describe the structures involved
- Explain that it is necessary to be aware of the normal condition of the testes so that any later change can be recognised at an early stage
- Advise that the best time to perform self-examination is immediately after taking a shower or bath, when the body tissues are warm, the scrotum is relaxed and the testes easy to feel
- Emphasise the need to look at the scrotum for its colour, texture, any change in shape or any swelling that may be noticeable
- Instruct the patient that it is necessary to hold the scrotum in the palm of the hand and to examine each testicle by rolling the testis between his thumb and fingers:
  - — each testicle should feel smooth and be about the size of a small hen's egg
  - — the epididymis, which lies behind each testicle, should also be felt and should feel soft and slightly spongy to the touch.
  - — the spermatic cords, which extend upwards from the epididymis, should feel like round, firm tubes
- Explain that any abnormality in the shape of the testicle and any lump or swelling should be investigated by a doctor irrespective of how trivial it may seem
- Check that the patient knows why he is completing the self-examination. Help him to understand that a cancerous lump can now be successfully treated

promptly to antibiotics should be thought of as cancer until proven otherwise. Metastases may cause lumbar pain and abdominal or supraclavicular lymph node masses.

Investigations Laboratory studies of serum alpha-fetoprotein (AFP) and serum beta-human chorionic gonadotrophin (hCG) help in the diagnosis of germ cell cancer as tumour markers. AFP is high in aggressive non-seminomatous tumours; hCG is elevated in 30% of seminomas. These markers corroborate diagnosis but are also useful in monitoring treatment. Chest X-ray, chest CT scan, tomography, lymphangiography, abdominal CT scan, abdominal ultrasonography and intravenous pyelography may all be used diagnostically.

Treatment is by surgery with adjuvant radiotherapy and chemotherapy. The specific therapy will depend on the type of cancer and the stage of the disease.

Surgical intervention This involves a high radical inguinal orchidectomy. The testis, epididymis, a portion of the vas and parts of the gonadal lymphatics and blood vessels are removed. The remaining testis will undergo hyperplasia and produce enough testosterone to maintain sexual capacity, male characteristics and libido. The semen, however, may be of poor quality. Ejaculatory ability may be reduced.

Radiotherapy Following surgery, radiotherapy is recommended for seminomas. Standard treatment in the UK for stage 1 seminomas is adjuvant radiotherapy to the para-aortic area, over a period of 3 weeks, for lymph node treatment. In more advanced disease, radiotherapy is extended to the ipsilateral pelvic area and chemotherapy can also be administered (Dearnaley et al 2001). Fatigue, bone marrow depression and diarrhoea may be experienced as side-effects.

Chemotherapy In stage 1 non-seminomatous germ cell tumours there are two main approaches to therapy. When there is no vascular invasion a strict surveillance protocol can be followed; in cases of vascular invasion the patient can either have a surveillance protocol or immediate treatment with two courses of adjuvant chemotherapy. In more advanced disease additional courses of chemotherapy are employed (Dearnaley et al 2001). A number of cytotoxic agents are used as an adjunct to surgery and radiotherapy (e.g. bleomycin, cisplatin and etoposide). Cisplatin-based combined therapy has been a major advance in treating disseminated disease with a cure rate of 80% (Chaudhary & Haldas 2003). However, serious long-term complications from chemotherapy are now recognised and close follow-up of patients after completion of treatment is advocated. Significant side-effects include secondary leukaemia, azoospermia, nephrotoxicity, bone marrow suppression, neurotoxicity and vascular toxicities (Hawkins & Miaskowski 1996, Hilkens et al 1997, Chaudhary & Haldas 2003). Reduced sexual function and infertility are possible persisting side-effects following treatment for testicular cancer (Arai et al 1997, Jonker-Pool et al 1997). However, Taksey et al (2003) point out that a low sperm count does not necessarily prevent fatherhood.

NURSING PRIORITIES AND MANAGEMENT: Testicular cancer

The pre- and postoperative needs of a patient having orchidectomy are as for major surgery (see Ch. 26). The need for information, relief of anxiety, pain relief and protection from wound infection are primary. The young adult patient with insight into his cancer condition will undoubtedly be worried about the future, the course of the illness, his family responsibilities and his career.

Postoperatively the patient will require a short period of fully compensatory care whilst recovering from the anaesthetic. A short period of partially assisted care will follow. In the long term the patient will need planned educative and supportive care (see Case History 7.2).

CASE HISTORY 7.2

Mr W

Mr W is 32 years of age. He is married and has two young daughters aged 2 and 4. His wife looks after the children well but has always been very dependent on him for organising the family and helping with domestic chores and the shopping. They have usually enjoyed an average social life, babysitters permitting. Mr W works as a computer engineer. He likes to leave work promptly so that his wife isn't left too long on her own at home. She has had episodes when she has become reliant on alcohol, particularly when she is worried about the children.

STOP THINK

7.6 Mr W had his left testis removed 48 h ago. He has extensive lymphatic gland metastases. The medical plan includes radiotherapy and chemotherapy over the coming months.

Consider the circumstances of the family described in Case History 7.2 and:

(a) identify Mr W's needs for education and support
(b) prepare a teaching plan
(c) list the ways in which you as the nurse can provide support for Mr W during the postoperative period
(d) explain the ways that Mr W can continue to be supported after discharge from hospital
(e) identify the needs of the family in the short and long term.

For further information, see Moynihan (1996).

VASECTOMY

Couples who have used a range of birth control methods over the years may decide that permanent sterilisation by surgical means would now be preferable. According to Amundsen and Ramakrishnan (2004) vasectomy is one of the most reliable and cost-effective permanent methods of contraception. When compared with other Western European countries, the UK has a high rate of sterilisation: 23% of couples of reproductive age use this method (Roberts 2000).

Preoperative counselling

Before such a decision is taken the couple should meet with their GP or family planning counsellor to discuss their needs and circumstances and their reasons for considering sterilisation as a birth control method. The counsellor should provide information about both female and male sterilisation and the risks, side-effects and failure rates of the procedures available. The long-term effects and prospects for reversal of the sterilisation should be explained. The couple should also be encouraged to consider the implications of a breakdown of their marriage or partnership, or the loss by death of one of the couple or of their children.

A man contemplating vasectomy may have particular anxieties about the effect of the procedure on his masculinity and sex drive. He must be assured that, as the testes will not be removed, his hormone production, virility and sex drive will be unaffected. The nature of the operation should be described with the aid of a simple diagram. It should be explained that the ejaculation fluid will be free from sperm and that unused sperm will be broken down and reabsorbed. Further information that the patient will require is summarised in Box 7.11.

Box 7.11

Information for the patient undergoing vasectomy

Every patient undergoing vasectomy should be given an information leaflet containing the following information:

- The type of anaesthesia that will be given (i.e. general or local)
- The operation will be completed via the scrotal sac
- A portion of vas may be removed on each side
- A dressing will be applied to the wound and a scrotal support will be applied and should be worn for 2 weeks
- Some swelling and bruising will occur around the operation site. This may extend down over the thighs or up towards the umbilicus
- Some pain will be experienced, but this can be relieved by paracetamol or codeine tablets
- Skin sutures will dissolve spontaneously within approximately 1 week of the operation
- Strenuous exercise should be avoided for 2 days
- The patient will not become infertile immediately after the operation due to sperm being stored upstream of the operative site. Therefore, he must continue to take contraceptive precautions until two successive sperm samples are proved to be free of sperm
- Normal sexual intercourse can take place from the third postoperative day. As the operation site may be tender, the individual may prefer to wait longer than this
- At least 12 ejaculations should have occurred before the first semen test to clear sperm. A second semen test will be completed 2 weeks later. In a small proportion of cases, sperm persists in the seminal fluid for many months
- There is a 0.5–1.0% failure rate associated with the operation:
  - — the ends of a vas may join up again early or late after operation
  - — the surgeon may remove some structure other than the vas
  - — some men have anatomical abnormalities, such as a double vas that is not fully removed
- Reappearance of fertility after two negative semen tests may mean that the tests were not accurately completed or the ends of a vas have reunited
- Severe, prolonged pain may indicate some slow seepage of blood into tissues from a small blood vessel. A haematoma may have formed, causing the scrotum to swell. Rest in bed should ease the condition. Otherwise the site may need to be drained at the clinic
- The wound may become infected, in which case the GP will prescribe antibiotics
- There is a reasonable chance that the operation can be reversed should this be desired. Reversibility cannot be guaranteed, however, and a return to the previous level of fertility may not be achieved.

MEDICAL MANAGEMENT

The surgical procedure Vasectomy is the ligation or division of the vasa deferens, the genital ducts that store and

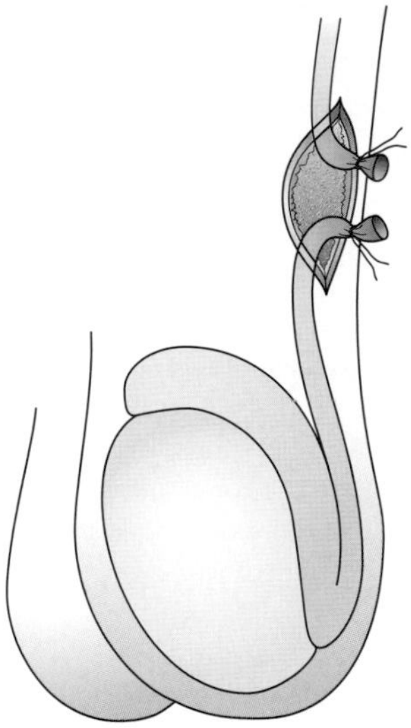

Fig. 7.11 The vas divided.

transport sperm to the urethra in the process of ejaculation (see Ch. 8), and is performed under either general or local anaesthetic. In the traditional method of vasectomy, the vas is palpated in the upper scrotum and an incision of 1 cm is made over the vas. The fascia around the vas is incised and the vas drawn out and ligated in two places.

The vas is then simply divided or a small segment is excised (see Fig. 7.11). One end of the vas is enclosed again in the fascia envelope. The other end of the vas is repositioned outside the fascia. Alternatively, the cut ends of the vas may first be cauterised or the cut ends looped back on themselves. The skin is closed with absorbable sutures and the procedure is repeated on the opposite side. The possibility for reversal of the operation is retained. Using this method there is some controversy over whether a section of vas should be removed. Roberts (2000) reports on observational studies that suggest an increased incidence of recanalisation after removal of segments less than 14 mm long. Hence, removal of 15 mm is recommended.

In 1974 a no-scalpel method of vasectomy was introduced by a Chinese surgeon. This procedure is carried out using a local anaesthetic. A vas-fixing forceps encircles the vas through the skin. A specially designed curved haemostat with sharp points is used to puncture the skin and vas sheath. The puncture hole is stretched to form a small opening in the scrotum through which the vas can be lifted out. It is then cut, tied or cauterised as in other vasectomy techniques. The midline puncture site can be used to isolate and interrupt the second vas. No skin sutures are required (Huber 1988). This procedure has been positively evaluated (Burket-Piccolino & Costa 1992, Holt & Higgins 1996, Black & Francome 2003), showing comparable intra-operative pain levels, less pain and bleeding postoperatively and fewer infections. These advantages are attributable to the minimal dissection and handling required for the procedure.

Outcome Following vasectomy the man should have two consecutive sperm analyses 2–4 weeks apart showing azoospermia to confirm effective contraception. The majority of men are pleased with the vasectomy operation. They usually consider it to have been minor surgery and to have caused no ill effects. They can approach sexual intercourse with greater relaxation and increased enjoyment. A minority experience regret after the operation, feeling that their sexual drive and performance have been reduced. Others who have taken new partners or remarried may regret being unable to have another child within the new relationship. A new wife who has no child may feel deprived and frustrated.

Reversal An increasing number of men are requesting reversal of their vasectomy. Surgeons are now attaining 70–90% success rates with such reversals, which are technically feasible, but the pregnancy rate achieved is disappointingly low: only one-third of the reversed vasectomies lead to pregnancy. This low rate may be due to the formation of sperm antibodies.

NURSING PRIORITIES AND MANAGEMENT: Vasectomy

Preparation for the procedure

The nurse may be responsible, jointly with the surgeon, for ensuring that the individual undergoing vasectomy and his partner understand what the procedure entails and its anticipated results.

Postoperative care

Postoperatively, the nurse on the ward will be involved in pain management and wound care and will have an important contribution to make in instructing the patient in postoperative self-care and in informing him about procedures for follow-up and assessment. The nurse should also alert him to the possible complications or problems that should be reported (see Box 7.12).

Many men are concerned about the development of scrotal swelling and haematoma in the postoperative period. Scrotal support, rest and analgesics are necessary for general comfort and to improve the condition over time. Any bleeding from the wounds may be relieved by the use of butterfly sutures to pull the wound edges together. Psychological after-effects of vasectomy should be few if preoperative counselling and information-giving have been adequate. Some men complain of an adverse effect on sexual performance after vasectomy, but they are usually those who have had similar difficulties before surgery.

The possibility of an association between vasectomy and prostate cancer has attracted some attention; however, studies suggest no increase in prostatic cancer in men who have had a vasectomy (Chacko et al 2002, Cox et al 2002) (see Research Abstract 7.8). There has also been some debate about a possible link between vasectomy and testicular cancer but Jorgensen et al (1993) and Moller et al (1994) have found no causal relationship. Jorgensen et al (1993) suggest that vasectomy might precipitate the development of testicular cancer from a pre-invasive carcinoma in situ lesion but Moller et al (1994) claim that vasectomy does not accelerate the growth or diagnosis of pre-existing testicular neoplasms.

Box 7.12

Inflammatory conditions of the male reproductive organs

Balanitis and balanoposthitis
The term balanitis refers to inflammation of the glans penis. The term balanoposthitis refers to inflammation of the prepuce or foreskin as well as the glans penis. Both conditions are the result of bacterial infection. They are painful, irritating and produce a discharge. They may be associated with inadequate hygiene and phimosis. A swab from the inflamed area is sent for pathological culture and sensitivity tests. Specific antibiotic therapy can be prescribed. Local treatment will involve bathing the affected areas with normal saline to relieve discomfort.

Epididymo-orchitis
In this condition, infection and inflammation of the testis and epididymis occur together. It may be caused by prostatitis, a urinary tract infection or a sexually transmitted disease. The testes are swollen, tender and painful. The patient is pyrexial and suffers from aches and pains. He may experience nausea and vomiting. Bed rest, extra fluids, analgesics and antibiotics are necessary. Cold packs applied locally to the scrotum and the wearing of a scrotal support will help to relieve discomfort and swelling.

Orchitis
This condition is most often caused by mumps occurring after puberty. It may result in atrophy of the testes and sterility. Males who have not had mumps in childhood should try to avoid contact with the disease. Early administration of gammaglobulin may reduce the severity of mumps in those who have been exposed.

Prostatitis
This is an acute or chronic inflammation of the prostate gland and is usually bacterial in origin. Urgency, frequency and pain with micturition are experienced. Acute retention of urine, cystitis, low back pain, chills and haematuria may occur. The prostate gland is enlarged and tender when examined. Midstream urine specimens are sent to the laboratory for culture and sensitivity. Antibiotics, analgesics and a high fluid intake are prescribed. The condition is liable to recur.

RESEARCH ABSTRACT 7.8

Vasectomy and risk of prostate cancer

Vasectomy has become a popular method of contraception but concern has been raised regarding a possible association with prostate cancer. Cox et al (2002) investigated this with a national population-based case-control study in New Zealand, involving 923 new cases of prostate cancer among men aged 40–74 years. Controls were randomly selected from the electoral register with frequency matching to cases in 5-year age groups. Cases and controls were interviewed by telephone. Their findings suggest no association between prostate cancer and vasectomy, and no association with time since. The authors therefore concluded that vasectomy does not increase the risk of prostate cancer, even after 25 years.

Cox B, Sneyd M J, Paul C, Delahunt B, Skegg D C 2002 Vasectomy and risk of prostate cancer. Journal of the American Medical Association 287(23): 3110–3115

The nurse should take the opportunity to check whether the patient understands how to self-examine the testes for the development of a lump (see Box 7.10). The patient should accept the need to complete a self-examination at appropriate intervals. However, it would be inappropriate to associate the risk of tumour with vasectomy until more research data are available.

Occupational health nurses can take a significant role in promoting testicular self-examination in the working male population, the majority of whom seldom need to visit their general practitioner.

ERECTILE DYSFUNCTION

Erectile dysfunction (or impotence) is the persistent inability, due to organic causes, to obtain an erection sufficient for sexual intercourse. The word impotence has wide social and psychological connotations and it is recommended that the use of this term with patients is discouraged and the disorder referred to as erectile dysfunction or another appropriate descriptive expression (Bancroft 1993). It is difficult to show the true prevalence of erectile dysfunction because of the nature of this disorder and the shame, guilt or embarrassment associated with it, but Bancroft (1993) suggests 7–8% of men may be affected, the incidence increasing with age.

PATHOPHYSIOLOGY

Erectile dysfunction may be a primary or secondary condition. The former implies that the patient has never had an erection. This is rare and is usually associated with gross abnormality of the penis or with hormone deficiency from childhood. Secondary erectile dysfunction is much more common and may be due to psychological or organic factors, or to a combination of both.

Most men will occasionally fail to gain or maintain an erection attributed to stress, overwork or some other reason.

Causes Psychological causal factors have been categorised by Kolodny et al (1979) as follows:

- Developmental
  - maternal or paternal factors
  - conflict in parent–child relationship
  - severe negative family attitude to sex
  - traumatic childhood sexual experience
  - gender identity conflict
  - traumatic first coital experience
  - homosexuality
- Affective
  - anxiety about performance
  - guilt
  - depression
  - poor self-esteem
  - hypochondria
  - mania

— fear of causing pregnancy
— fear of sexually transmitted diseases (STDs)

- Interpersonal
  — poor communication
  — hostility towards partner
  — distrust of partner
  — lack of physical attraction to partner
  — sex role conflict
  — divergent sexual preference, or sex value systems, e.g. time, place, type
- Cognitive
  — sexual ignorance
  — acceptance of cultural myths
  — performance demands
- Miscellaneous
  — premature ejaculation
  — isolated episode of erectile failure
  — iatrogenic influences.

Organic causes of secondary erectile dysfunction include:

- poor arterial inflow caused by atherosclerosis and aneurysm
- venous leaks between the corpora and venous system
- neurological diseases
- endocrine dysfunction
- drugs, including antihypertensives, narcotics and alcohol
- major surgery — cystectomy, radical prostatectomy (see Ch. 8).

For further information, see Bennett (1994).

MEDICAL MANAGEMENT

Investigations are carried out to provide an understanding of the problem (Gregoire & Pryor 1993):

- clinical interview to explore the nature of the problem, sexual behaviours and attitudes, relationship with a partner, personal and family history, medical history, psychiatric history and current therapy or medications
- physical assessment, including examination of penis, testes, prostate and seminal vesicles; neurological examination; vascular examination
- blood screen for evidence of endocrine imbalance, diabetes mellitus, renal failure
- assessment of penile blood flow by Doppler studies and angiography
- assessment of neurogenic factors by monitoring nocturnal penile tumescence (NPT), response to visual erotic stimuli, assessment of autonomic nerve function and neurophysiological studies
- psychological testing.

Treatment options:

Local injection A local injection at the base of the penis using the α-adrenergic receptor blocking agents, papaverine or a combination of papaverine and phentolamine can cause an erection. The action is by vasodilatation and vasocongestion within the spongy tissue of the penis. An erection can be maintained for a period of about 30 min. Patients can be taught to self-inject at home. Complications include fibrosis at the base of the penis and priapism requiring emergency hospital treatment. Priapism is persistent, painful erection of the penis, unrelieved by sexual intercourse or masturbation. Priapism lasting more than 4–6 h can result in necrosis and fibrosis of the cavernosal tissue as a consequence of ischaemia (King et al 1994).

Penile prosthesis There are various types of penile prosthesis available, ranging from semi-rigid, non-inflatable devices to multicomponent, inflatable implants. A full discussion with the patient (and his partner as appropriate) prior to surgery should include an explanation of the various types, the patient's expectations and possible complications.

The semi-rigid prosthesis consists of two semi-rigid silicone-covered or malleable rods inserted into the shaft of the penis, in the corpora cavernosum. It is important that the correct size is used by the surgeon if the prosthesis is to be effective. They give a permanent erection which is firm enough to allow the patient to have intercourse. A hinged prosthesis allows movement into the upward or downward position. Flaccidity and erection are possible with mechanical and inflatable prostheses.

Individual factors such as motivation, intelligence, dexterity and strength require to be considered in choosing an appropriate prosthesis, to avoid implanting a device that the patient cannot operate (Montague & Lakin 1994).

Infection and erosion are possible complications and usually require removal of the device. The probability of mechanical failure usually relates to the complexity of the device and failure generally requires re-operation.

Revascularisation of the penis This advance in surgery can help patients who have arterial problems. It involves anastomosing an abdominal artery to the penile vein to improve the blood supply. Although not considered major surgery, it does leave the patient with a fairly large abdominal scar. Infection may be a postoperative problem. This procedure has the advantage of restoring normality. Success rate is reported to vary from 50 to 81% (Sharlip 1994), depending on the selection of patients and the surgical procedure adopted.

Vacuum suction machine The machine produces a partial vacuum around the penis, causing it to engorge. An elastic band is then placed around the base of the penis to maintain the erection for a maximum of 15 min. The advantage of this treatment is that the patient can control the erection, but the duration of the erection is limited by the ischaemic effect of the tourniquet.

Psychotherapy Impotence judged to be psychological in origin may be helped by psychotherapy for the patient and his partner.

NURSING PRIORITIES AND MANAGEMENT: Erectile dysfunction

Psychological considerations

A man who develops erectile dysfunction is likely to be shocked and dismayed and reluctant to talk about the problem. This can become a complex matter, not only for the individual but also for his partner and family. Failure to accept or understand the problem can lead to the break-up of relationships. Moreover, organic causes of impotence, such as multiple sclerosis, diabetes and circulatory problems, may have already caused the patient to change his lifestyle and placed the family under stress. The patient may be very reluctant to discuss the problem openly with a doctor or nurse. He may present to his GP ostensibly with another problem, only managing with difficulty to mention his real concern. Occasionally it is at an outpatient appointment such as a diabetic clinic that the subject is brought up. Medical and nursing staff must treat the patient with empathy and sensitivity. While the condition is not life-threatening, once the patient presents he will want something done quickly.

Practical considerations for the patient receiving a penile implant

The nurse should ensure that the patient is given sufficient information about the procedure and recovery. He should be told that his hospital stay will be 4–7 days, and that regular analgesics will be given to control any pain. Catheterisation will be required for at least 24 h. Bed rest will not be required, but the patient should not spend too much time walking around or sitting in a chair for the first few days, to encourage healing and reduce discomfort. A scrotal support for a few weeks will help prevent swelling and minimise discomfort.

The consultant will discuss how soon the prosthesis may be used, usually recommending that it is not used until after the first outpatient appointment in 6 weeks. Sutures are normally dissolvable. It is helpful to assure the patient that visitors or other patients on the ward will not know what procedure he is undergoing unless he tells them himself. Nor will other people know that he has a prosthesis, although it may be necessary to avoid wearing tight trousers or swimming trunks.

OTHER DISORDERS OF THE MALE REPRODUCTIVE ORGANS

Inflammatory disorders of the male reproductive organs are briefly described in Box 7.12, page 312. Disorders affecting the prostate, urethra and urinary function are described in Chapter 8.

CULTURAL AWARENESS IN REPRODUCTIVE HEALTH

Sociological change and economic progress have contributed to the integration of immigrants into the UK and some have been in this country for generations. Inevitably, when people move from their particular culture to another, they bring with them their own beliefs and values. Some of these will remain with them, giving direction to their life and practices. Older members of a family tend to rely on tradition and may be reluctant to adopt new ideas, whereas younger generations growing up in a new environment are more influenced by different cultural perspectives and more likely to adapt to or adopt some of the dominant views of the indigenous population around them. This can cause tension within families as views associated with sex, marriage and family affairs come into conflict.

If health care workers are to provide sensitive care to individuals from different cultural backgrounds, they need to be aware that the beliefs and values associated with a particular culture. While the views of some will conflict with those held by the nurse, a non-judgemental approach is required. In this respect, Item 2 in the nurses' *Code of Professional Conduct* (NMC 2002, p. 4) states that nurses, midwives and health visitors must respect the individuality of patients 'irrespective of gender, age, race, ability, sexuality, economic status, lifestyle, culture and religious or political beliefs'.

Nurses are not expected to have a wide knowledge of all cultural and religious beliefs but should find out about the customs relevant to the cultural groups presenting in clinical practice. In some cases, problems with communication can be exacerbated in cross-cultural interactions, not only because English may not be the first language of patients, but also because they may feel embarrassed to ask for clarification or further explanation. Obtaining leaflets with information in different languages is required when this is a potential problem. Younger members of a family may be more fluent in English than their older relatives and effective communication may be achieved by sensitively incorporating them for translation and clarification. The services of an interpreter may need to be employed.

While reproductive functioning, sexuality and health disorders affecting the reproductive systems are felt to be very personal and intimate issues in British culture, this attitude may in fact be much more exaggerated in other cultures. Open communication, required for the sharing of information and the giving of health care advice, may therefore be made more difficult. The performance of a necessary vaginal examination, for example, may be seen as a major procedure with significant emotional implications.

While it has been suggested that treatment of fertility problems should incorporate the couple, Muslim or Sikh men may be extremely reluctant to attend a fertility clinic with their wife and can feel humiliated or angry at the suggestion that they might be responsible for the fertility problem. The beliefs held about fertility and the sanctity of semen in its life-giving potential can have important implications for the way men and women view contraception and the options available to them for regulating their family. While the nurse may not be conversant with specific options acceptable in different cultures, an awareness of the existence of such restrictions on individual choice allows a more sensitive, exploratory approach with clients.

Different cultural and religious perspectives view marriage and the production of offspring in different ways. Similarly, family networks vary and the extended family may have a significant influence on younger members, showing a sense of responsibility with regard to provision of information and support.

Thus, both culture and religion can have a powerful influence on sexual practices, family support networks and how individuals feel about their own sexuality and self-concept. In introductory interactions with patients — taking a history and building up a rapport — the nurse can learn much from them by showing an interest in their beliefs and their perspective on life and encouraging them to discuss these. This knowledge can then help nurses to be more aware and sensitive to cultural influences in health care and facilitate more individualised nursing.

Male circumcision — excision of the foreskin — is a procedure with religious connotations for those of Jewish or Muslim faith. This can be performed by a Jewish rabbi or by a family doctor. Harbinson (1997) indicates that circumcision is carried out in the USA for hygienic and social reasons, but in the UK the operation is only performed within the NHS for medical reasons.

Female circumcision is widely practised in some African and Egyptian ethnic groups, in parts of the Middle East and in South East Asia. In the UK, female circumcision is considered to be female genital mutilation. Female genital mutilation is a term used to refer to procedures resulting in different degrees of mutilation of the external genitalia of females (Royal College of Nursing 1996) and has been illegal in the UK since 1985. However, immigrant families can return to their home country to have this procedure carried out on the daughter (usually from the early days of birth to 16 years of age). The effects of the procedure are also seen in the UK amongst women who have been mutilated prior to arrival. Within the culture valuing this procedure, there may be difficulty in securing a husband for a female who has not been so treated.

Female mutilation can take various forms:

- Female circumcision involves excision of the hood of the clitoris.
- Clitoral excision may be performed with or without removal of the labia minora.
- Infibulation is a more extensive procedure involving removal of the clitoris, labia minora and some of the labia majora. The vulva is sutured together leaving only a small orifice for passage of urine and menstrual blood.

Although the risk of infection after these procedures is high, women may not present with problems until later in life. Problems may include recurrent urinary tract infections, vaginal infections, non-consummation, infertility and psycho-sexual problems. During pregnancy the women require sensitive care. Special antenatal care may be available to allow women to express their fears about labour and childbirth and for the provision of information and counselling. For some women a vaginal delivery will be feasible and de-infibulation may be possible to avoid a caesarean section (Toubin 1994). De-infibulation can be performed during a pregnancy or during labour but Omer-Hashi (1994) suggests that the earlier this is performed the better the outcome in terms of decreased pain during labour and a shorter recovery time after delivery.

Educating, advising and counselling people who have quite different beliefs, values and attitudes concerning health issues from those of the health professionals providing help and support requires tact and sensitivity. Understanding and empathy can help nurses to appreciate what others consider to be important. A balance is required between giving sound advice and respecting the social, cultural and religious views of others.

REFERENCES

Abernethy K 1997 The menopause. In: Andrews G (ed) Women's sexual health. Baillière Tindall, London, p 336–364

Abraham G E 1987 Premenstrual tension: current problems in obstetrics and gynaecology. In: O'Brien P M S (ed) Premenstrual syndrome. Blackwell Scientific Publications, London, p 1–39

Adamson G D, Baker V L 2003 Subfertility: causes, treatment and outcome. Best Practice Research in Clinical Obstetrics and Gynaecology 17(2): 169–185

Amundsen G, Ramakrishnan K 2004 Vasectomy: a 'seminal' analysis. South Medical Journal 97(1): 54–60

Anderson J, Alesi R 1997 Infertility counseling. In: Kovacs G (ed) The Subfertility Handbook. Cambridge University Press, Cambridge

Arai Y, Kawakita M, Okada Y, Yoshida O 1997 Sexuality and fertility in long-term survivors of testicular cancer. Journal of Clinical Oncology 15(4): 1444–1448

Audebert A J, Pouly J L, Von Theobald P 1998 Laparoscopic fimbriotoplasty: an evaluation of 35 cases. Human Reproduction 13(6): 1496–1499

Baggish M S, Dorsey J H, Adelson M 1989 A ten year experience treating cervical intraepithelial neoplasia with the CO2 laser. American Journal of Obstetrics and Gynecology 161: 60–68

Baker H W G 1995 Male infertility. In: de Grost L J (ed) Endocrinology, 2nd edn. Saunders, Philadelphia

Bancroft J 1993 Impotence in perspective. In: Gregoire A, Pryor J P (eds) Impotence: an integrated approach to clinical practice. Churchill Livingstone, Edinburgh, p 3–13

Barbour D 1997 How does infertility affect men? Fertility Nurses' Newsletter 20: 2–5

Beral V 2003 Breast cancer and hormone-replacement therapy in the million women study. Lancet 362(9382): 419–427

Black T, Francome C 2003 Comparison of Marie Stopes scalpel and electrocautery no-scalpel vasectomy techniques. Journal of Family Planning and Reproductive Health Care 29(2): 32–34

Blake P, Lambert H, Crawford R (eds) 1998 Gynaecological oncology: a guide to clinical management. Oxford University Press, Oxford

Boivin J 2003 A review of psychosocial interventions in infertility. Social Science Medicine 57(12): 2325–2341

Budeiri D, Li Wan Po A, Doran J C 1996 Is evening primrose oil of value in the treatment of premenstrual syndrome? Controlled Clinical Trials 17(1): 60–68

Burket-Piccolino A, Costa F J 1992 No-scalpel vasectomy (NSV) procedure and nursing care. Journal of Urological Nursing 11(2): 83–92

Bygdeman M, Danielsson K G 2002 Options for early therapeutic abortion: a comparative review. Drugs 62(17): 2459–2470

Campbell E M, Peterkin D, O'Grady K, Sanson-Fisher R 1997 Premenstrual symptoms in general practice patients. Prevalence and treatment. Journal of Reproductive Medicine 42(10): 637–646

Campbell M A, McGrath P J 1997 Use of medication by adolescents for the management of menstrual discomfort. Archives of Pediatrics and Adolescent Medicine 151(9): 905–913

Cancer Research Campaign 1994 Cervical cancer (factsheet 12); cervical screening (factsheet 13). CRC, London

Candiani G B, Vercellini P, Fedele L, Bianchi S, Vendola N, Candiani N 1991 Conservative surgical treatment for severe endometriosis in infertile women: are we making progress? Obstetrical and Gynaecological Survey 46: 490–498

Chacko J A, Zafar M B, McCallum S W, Terris M K 2002 Vasectomy and prostate cancer: characteristics of patients referred for prostate biopsy. Journal of Urology 168(4 Pt 1): 1011–1048

Chanen W 1989 The efficacy of electrocoagulation diathermy performed under local anaesthesia for the eradication of pre-cancerous lesions of cervix. Australian and New Zealand Journal of Obstetrics and Gynaecology 29(3 Pt 1): 189–192

Chaudhary U B, Haldas J R 2003 Long-term complications of chemotherapy for germ cell tumours. Drugs 63(15): 1565–1577
Chia K V, Ogbo W I 2002 Medical termination of missed abortion. Journal of Obstetrics and Gynaecology 22(2): 184–186
Chow S N, Huang C C, Lee Y T 1997 Demographic characteristics and medical aspects of menopausal women in Taiwan. Journal of Formosan Medical Association 96(10): 806–811
Colgan T J, Clark A, Hakh N, Seidenfeld A 2002 Screening for cervical disease in mature women: strategies for improvement. Cancer 96(4): 195–203
Committee of Inquiry into Human Fertilisation and Embryology (Chairman, Dame Mary Warnock) 1984 Report. HMSO, London
Cox B, Sneyd M J, Paul C, Delahunt B, Skegg D C 2002 Vasectomy and risk of prostate cancer. Journal of the American Medical Association 287(23): 3110–3115
Davis S R 2001 Phytoestrogen therapy for menopausal symptoms? British Medical Journal 323: 354–355
Dearnaley D P, Huddart R A, Horwich A 2001 Managing testicular cancer. British Medical Journal 332(7302): 1583–1588
Deeney M, Hawthorn R, McKay Hart D 1991 Low dose danazol treatment of the premenstrual syndrome. Postgraduate Medical Journal 67: 450–454
Department of Health 1999 Cervical screening programme 1998–99, Bulletin 1999/32. DH, London
Dey P, Gibbs A, Arnold D F, Saleh N, Hirsch P J, Woodman C B 2002 Loop diathermy excision compared with cervical laser vaporisation for the treatment of intraepithelial neoplasia: a randomised controlled trial. British Journal of Obstetrics and Gynaecology 109(4): 381–385
Edwards R G, Steptoe P C 1983 Current status of in vitro fertilisation and implantation of human embryos. Lancet ii: 1265–1269
Effective Health Care Consortium 1992 The management of subfertility. Effective Health Care 3. University of Leeds
Eluf-Neto J, Booth M, Munoz N et al 1994 Human papilloma virus and invasive cervical cancer in Brazil. British Journal of Cancer 69: 114
Everett S 1997 Contraception. In: Andrews G (ed) Women's sexual health. Baillière Tindall, London, p 173–217
Evers J L 2002 Female subfertility. Lancet 360(9327): 151–159
Facchinetti F, Martignoni E, Petraglia F, Sances M G, Nappi G, Genazzani A R 1987 Premenstrual fall of plasma beta-endorphin in patients with premenstrual syndrome. Fertility and Sterility 47(4): 570–573
Family Planning Today 1996 Contraceptive choices survey: how women decide [editorial]. Family Planning Today, First Quarter, UNIPATH, London
Farrer H 1990 Maternity care. Churchill Livingstone, Edinburgh
Fauser B C, Devroey P 2003 Reproductive biology and IVF: ovarian stimulation and luteal phase consequences. Trends in Endocrinology and Metabolism 14(5): 236–242
Fedele L, Parazzini F, Luchini L, Mezzopane R, Tozzi L, Villa L 1995 Recurrence of fibroids after myomectomy: a transvaginal ultrasonographic study. Human Reproduction 10(7): 1795–1796
Finucane F F, Madans J, Bush T, Wolfe P H, Kleinman J C 1993 Decreased risk of stroke among postmenopausal hormone users. Results from a national cohort. Archives of International Medicine 153(1): 73–79
Fishel S, Dowell K, Timson J, Green S, Hall J, Klentzerio L 1993 Micro assisted fertilisation with human gametes. Human Reproduction 8: 1780–1784
Fombonne E 1995 Anorexia nervosa: no evidence of an increase. British Journal of Psychiatry 166: 462–471
Garner M J, Birkett N J, Johnson K C, Shatenstein B, Ghadirian P, Krewski D 2003 Dietary risk factors for testicular carcinoma. International Journal of Cancer 106(6): 934–941
Gasperino J 1996 Ethnic differences in body composition and their relation to health and disease in women. Ethnicity and Health 1(4): 337–347
Gelfand M M, Moreau M, Ayotte N J, Hilditch J R, Wong B A, Lau C Y 2003 Clinical assessment and quality of life of postmenopausal women treated with a new intermittent progestogen combination hormone replacement therapy: a placebo-controlled study. Menopause 10(1): 29–36
Gillespie I E, Nasim A, Zawawi A R 1992 A guide to surgical principles and practice. Churchill Livingstone, Edinburgh
Glaser B, Strauss A L 1965 Awareness of dying. Aldine, Chicago
Gordon H K, Duncan I D 1991 Effective destruction of cervical intra-epithelial neoplasia (CIN) 3 at 100°C using the Semur cold coagulator: 14 years' experience. British Journal of Obstetrics and Gynaecology 98: 14–20
Gottlieb S 2001 Human parathyroid hormone may prevent osteoporosis. British Medical Journal 322(7296): 1200–1201
Gottlieb S 2003 HRT may increase risk of ovarian cancer. British Medical Journal 327(7418): 767
Grant C G 2003 Flawed advice from HRT specialists. British Medical Journal 327: 359
Green S, Fishel S, Stoddart N, Garrett L 1997 Microinsemination for the treatment of male factor infertility. In: O'Brien P M S (ed) The yearbook of obstetrics and gynaecology, Vol 5. RCOG Press, London
Gregoire A, Pryor J P (eds) 1993 Impotence: an integrated approach to clinical practice. Churchill Livingstone, Edinburgh
Grimley D M, Lee P A 1997 Condom and other contraceptive use among a random sample of adolescents: a snapshot in time. Adolescence 32(128): 771–779
Gronlund A, Grolund L, Clevin L, Anderson B, Palmgren N, Lidegaard O 2002 Management of missed abortion: comparison of medical treatment with either mifepristone + misoprostol or misoprostol alone with surgical evacuation. A multi-center trial in Copenhagen County, Denmark. Acta Obstetrica et Gynecologica Scandinavica 81(11): 1060–1065
Halbreich U, Rojansky N, Palter S 1991 Elimination of ovulation and menstrual acyclicity (with danazol) improves dysphoric premenstrual syndrome. Fertility and Sterility 56: 1066
Hans D, Dargent-Molina P, Schott A M, Sebert J L, Cormier C, Kotzki P O 1996 Ultrasonographic heel measurements to predict hip fracture in elderly women: the EPIDOS study. Lancet 348: 511–514
Harbinson M 1997 The arguments for and against circumcision. Nursing Standard 11(32): 42–47
Hartmann P E 1991 The breast and breastfeeding. In: Philipp E, Setchell M (eds) Scientific foundations of obstetrics and gynaecology, 4th edn. Butterworth-Heinemann, London
Hawkins C, Miaskowski C 1996 Testicular cancer: a review. Oncology Nursing Forum 23(8): 1203–1213
Health Education Board for Scotland (HEBS) booklets: The time of your life; A fresh look at the menopause; Eat to your heart's content; Look after yourself; Well woman. HEBS, Edinburgh
Helman C G 1997 Culture, health and illness, 3rd edn. Butterworth-Heinemann, Oxford
Hendry W F, Hughes L, Scammell G 1990 Comparison of prednisolone and placebo in subfertile men with antibodies to spermatozoa. Lancet 335: 85–88
Hildesheim A, Mann V, Brinton L A, Szklo M, Reeves W C, Rawls W E 1991 Herpes simplex virus type 2: a possible interaction with human papilloma virus types 16/18 in the development of invasive cervical cancer. International Journal of Cancer 49(3): 335–340
Hilkens P H, Pronk L C, Verweij J, Vecht C J, Van Putten W L, Van Den Bent M J 1997 Peripheral neuropathy induced by combination chemotherapy of docetaxel and cisplatin. British Journal of Cancer 75(3): 417–422
Hinton J 1980 Whom do dying patients tell? British Medical Journal 218: 1328–1330
Hjelmstedt A, Andersson L, Skoog-Svanberg A, Bergh T, Boivin J, Collins A 1999 Gender differences in psychological reactions to infertility among couples seeking IVF- and ICSI-treatment. Acta Obstetrica et Gynecologica Scandinavica 78(1): 42–48
Hodson J, Marsh J 2003 Quantitative ultrasound and risk factor enquiry as predictors of menopausal osteoporosis: comparative study in primary care. British Medical Journal 326: 1250–1251
Holt B A, Higgins A F 1996 Minimally invasive vasectomy. British Journal of Urology 77(4): 585–586
Hope S 2000 10-minute consultation: menorrhagia. British Medical Journal 321(7266): 935–938
Hopwood J 1990 Background to colposcopy and the treatment of the cervix. Schering Health Care, Burgess Hill
Hoshiai H, Ishikawa M, Sawatari Y 1993 Laparoscopic evaluation of the onset and progression of endometriosis. American Journal of Obstetrics and Gynecology 169: 714
Huber D H 1988 The no-scalpel vasectomy: a new technique. Association for Voluntary Surgical Contraception News 26(1): 1–2
Hughes C 2001 Cancer of the uterine cervix. In: Ganger E A (ed) Gynaecological nursing:

a practical guide. Churchill Livingstone, Edinburgh, p 215–230
Hughes E G, Federkow D M, Daya S, Sagle M, Dekoppel P, Collins J 1992 The routine use of gonadotrophin-releasing hormone agonists prior to in vitro fertilisation and gamete intrafallopian transfer: a meta-analysis of randomised controlled trials. Fertility and Sterility 58: 888–896
Human Fertilisation and Embryology Act 1990 HMSO, London
Human Fertilisation and Embryology Authority 2003 Code of practice, 6th edn. www.hfea.gov.uk/HFEAPublications/CodeofPractice/Code%20of%20Practice%20Sixth%20Edition%20-%20final.pdf
Hunt K, Vassey M, McPherson K 1990 Morbidity in a cohort of long-term users of hormone replacement: an update analysis. British Journal of Obstetrics and Gynaecology 97: 1080–1086
Huyghe E, Matsuda T, Thonneau P 2003 Increasing incidence of testicular cancer worldwide: a review. Journal of Urology 170(1): 5–11
Hylan T R, Sundell K, Judge R 1999 The impact of premenstrual symptomatology on functioning and treatment-seeking behavior: experience from the United States, United Kingdom, and France. Journal of Women's Health Gender Based Medicine 8: 1043–1052
Iammarrone E, Balet R, Lower A M, Gillott C, Grudzinskas J G 2003 Male infertility. Best Practice and Research Clinical Obstetrics and Gynaecology 17(2): 211–229
Ibbotson T, Wyke S 1995 A review of cervical cancer and cervical screening: implications for nursing practice. Journal of Advanced Nursing 22(4): 745–752
Jackson P, Burden J 1997 Laboratory techniques. In: Kovacs G (ed) The subfertility handbook. Cambridge University Press, Cambridge, p 220–234
Jacobson T Z, Barlow D H, Koninckx P R, Olive D, Farquhar C 2002 Laparoscopic surgery for subfertility associated with endometriosis. Cochrane Database Systematic Review (4): CD001398
Jennings S E 1995 Infertility counselling. Blackwell Science, Oxford
Joint Report of the Council on Scientific Affairs and the Council on Medical Science 1992 Technology assessment in medicine. Archives of Internal Medicine 152(1): 46–50
Jones C 1995 Cervical cancer: is herpes simplex virus type III a cofactor? Clinical Microbiological Review 8(4): 549–556
Jones A E 2004 Managing the pain of primary and secondary dysmenorrhoea. Nursing Times 100(10): 40–43
Jonker-Pool G, Van Basten J P, Hoekstra H J et al 1997 Sexual functioning after treatment for testicular cancer: comparison of treatment modalities. Cancer 80(3): 454–464
Jorgensen N, Giwercman A, Hansen S W, Skakkebaek N E 1993 Testicular cancer after vasectomy: origin from carcinoma in situ of the testis. European Journal of Cancer 29A(7): 1062–1064
Khoo S K, Munro C, Battistutta D 1990 Evening primrose oil and treatment of premenstrual syndrome. Medical Journal of Australia 153(4): 189–192
King B F, Lewis R W, Mckusick M A 1994 Radiologic evaluation of impotence. In: Bennett A H (ed) Impotence diagnosis and management of erectile dysfunction. WB Saunders, Philadelphia
Kingsland C, Aziz N, Taylor C, Manasse P, Haddan N, Richmond D 1992 Transport in vitro fertilisation – a novel scheme for community based treatment. Fertility and Sterility 58: 153–158
Kiran U, Amin P, Penketh R J 2004 Self-administration of misoprostol for termination of pregnancy: safety and efficacy. Journal of Obstetrics and Gynaecology 24(2): 155–156
Knight M, Field D 1981 A silent conspiracy: coping with dying cancer patients on an acute surgical ward. Journal of Advanced Nursing 6: 221–229
Kolettis P N 2003 Evaluation of the subfertile man. American Family Physician 67(10): 2165–2172
Kolodny R G, Masters W H, Johnston V E 1979 Textbook of human sexuality for nurses. Little Brown, Boston
Kovacs G T (ed) 1997 The use of donor insemination. In: The subfertility handbook. Cambridge University Press, Cambridge
Lambert H E, Blake P R, Coulter C, Dawson T, Mason P, Soutter P (eds) 1992 Gynaecological oncology. Oxford University Press, Oxford
Laurvick C L, Semmens J B 2002 Trends and outcomes for women diagnosed with ovarian cancer in Australia. Australian Family Physician 31(11): 1005–1011
Lax S F, Kurman R J, Pizer E S, Wu L, Ronnett B M 2000 A binary architectural grading system for uterine endometrial endometrioid carcinoma has superior reproducibility compared with FIGO grading and identifies subsets of advance-stage tumors with favorable and unfavorable prognosis. American Journal of Surgical Pathology 24(9): 1201–1208
Leask R 1991 Too common a story? Nursing Times 87(2): 22–23
Leather A T, Holland E F N, Andrews G D et al 1993 A study of the referral patterns and therapeutic experiences of 100 women attending a specialist premenstrual syndrome clinic. Journal of the Royal Society of Medicine 86(4): 199–201
Lewis T L T, Chamberlain G V P (eds) 1995 Gynaecology by ten teachers, 16th edn. Edward Arnold, London
Lock M 1994 Menopause in culture context. Experimental Gerontology 29(4): 307–317
Løkkegaard E, Pedersen A T, Heitmann B L et al 2003 Relation between hormone replacement therapy and ischaemic heart disease in women: prospective observational study. British Medical Journal 326: 426
Loprinzi C L, Michalak J L, Quella S K et al 1994 Megestrol acetate for the prevention of hot flashes. New England Journal of Medicine 331: 347–352
Loudon J D O 1985 Family planning in the United Kingdom: services and training. In: Loudon N (ed) Handbook of family planning. Churchill Livingstone, Edinburgh
Ludwig M, Westergaard L G, Diedrich K, Andersen C Y 2003 Developments in drugs for ovarian stimulation. Best Practice and Research Clinical Obstetrics and Gynaecology 17(2): 231–247
Lunn P G 1992 Breast feeding patterns, maternal milk output and lactational infecundity. Journal of Biosocial Science 24(3): 317–324
MacIntyre I, Stevenson J C, Whitehead M I, Wimalawansa S J, Banks L M, Healy M J 1988 Calcitonin for prevention of postmenopausal bone loss. Lancet 1(8591): 900–902
Mahutte N G, Arici A 2002 New advances in the understanding of endometriosis related infertility. Journal of Reproductive Immunology 55(1–2): 73–83
Marteau T M, Walker P, Giles G, Smail M 1990 Anxieties in women undergoing colposcopy. British Journal of Obstetrics and Gynaecology 97: 859–861
Martin D C 1995 Pain and infertility – a rationale for different treatment approaches. British Journal of Obstetrics and Gynaecology 102 (Suppl 12): 2–3
Mason M C 1994 Male infertility – men talking. Routledge, London
Masood S 1997 Why women still die from cervical cancer. Journal of the Florida Medical Association 84(6): 379–383
McQueen A 1995 Gynaecological nursing: nurses' perceptions of their work. MPhil thesis, University of Edinburgh (unpublished)
McQueen A 1997 The emotional work of caring, with a focus on gynaecological nursing. Journal of Clinical Nursing 6: 233–240
Menkes D B, Taghavi E, Mason P A Spears G F S, Howard R C 1992 Fluoxetine treatment of severe menopausal syndrome. British Medical Journal 305: 346–347
Miller P D, Bonnick S L, Johnston C C et al 1998 The challenges of peripheral bone density testing. Which patients need additional central density skeletal measurements? Journal of Clinical Densitometry 1: 211–217
Moller H, Knudsen L B, Lynge E 1994 Risk of testicular cancer after vasectomy: cohort study of over 73,000 men. British Medical Journal 309(6950): 295–299
Monarch J 2003 Counselling – its role in the infertility team. Human Fertility 6(Suppl 2): S17–21
Montague D K, Lakin M M 1994 Penile prostheses. In: Bennett A H (ed) Impotence diagnosis and management of erectile dysfunction. WB Saunders, Philadelphia
Morgan D, Lee R G 1991 Blackstone's guide to the Human Fertilisation and Embryology Act 1990. Blackstone Press, London
Moynihan C 1996 Psychosocial assessments and counseling of the patient with testicular cancer. In: Horwich A (ed) Testicular cancer, 2nd edn. Chapman and Hall Medical, London
Nabulsi A A, Folsom A R, White A et al 1993 Association of hormone replacement therapy with various cardiovascular risk factors in postmenopausal women. New England Journal of Medicine 328: 1069–1075
Naftolin F, Stanbury M G 2002 Phytoestrogens: are they really oestrogen mimics? Fertility and Sterility 77(1): 15–17
National Institute for Clinical Excellence (NICE) 2003 Guidance on the use of liquid-based cytology for cervical screening. NICE, London

Nazarko L 1992 Miscarriage and injustice. Nursing Standard 7(12): 44–45
Ngan H Y, Cheung A N, Lauder I J, Wong L C, Ma H K 1996 Prognostic significance of serum tumour markers in carcinoma of the cervix. European Journal of Gynaecological Oncology 17(6): 512–517
Nielsen S, Hahlin M, Oden A 1995 Using a logistic model to identify women with first trimester spontaneous abortion suitable for expectant management. British Journal of Obstetrics and Gynaecology 104(6): 755–756
Nursing and Midwifery Council (NMC) 2002 Code of professional conduct. NMC, London
O'Brien P M 1993 Helping women with premenstrual syndrome. British Medical Journal 307(9617): 1471–1475
Omer-Hashi K H 1994 Commentary – female genital mutilation: perspectives of a Somalian midwife. Birth 21(4): 224
Orem D 1991 Nursing: concepts of practice, 4th edn. McGraw-Hill, New York
Overgaard K, Riis B J, Christiansen C, Popenphant J, Johansen J S 1989 Nasal calcitonin in treatment of established osteoporosis. Clinical Endocrinology 30: 435–442
Pandian Z, Bhattacharya S, Nikolaou D, Vale L, Templeton A 2002 In vitro fertilisation for unexplained subfertility. Cochrane Database Systematic Review (2): CD003357
Payne E 1997 Menopausal problems. In: Luesley D (ed) Common conditions in gynaecology. Chapman and Hall, London
Paz B, Ohel G, Tal T, Degani S, Sabo E, Levitan Z 2002 Second trimester abortion by laminaria followed by vaginal misoprostol or intrauterine prostaglandin F2alpha: a randomized trial. Contraception 65(6): 411–413
Pearce J M 1991 Spontaneous abortion. In: Varma T R (ed) Clinical gynaecology. Edward Arnold, London
Peate I 1997 Testicular cancer: the importance of effective health education. British Journal of Nursing 6(6): 311–316
Peddie V L 1998 A prospective analysis of embryo transfer, performed by nurses in training. Report of a paper (presented by Barbour D) at the British Andrology Society, British Fertility Society and The Society for the Study of Fertility Annual Conference, July 1997. Fertility Nurses' Newsletter 21: 9
Phillips A N, Smith G D 1994 Cigarette smoking as a potential cause of cervical cancer: has confounding been controlled? International Journal of Epidemiology 23(1): 42–49
Porter M, Penney G, Russell D, Russell E, Templeton A 1996 A population based survey of women's experience of menopause. British Journal of Obstetrics and Gynaecology 103: 1025–1028
Power M 2001 The management of subfertility. In: Andrews G (ed) Women's sexual health, 2nd edn. Baillière Tindall, London
Redwine D B 1991 Conservative laparoscopic excision of endometriosis by sharp dissection. Life table analysis of reoperation and persistent or recurrent disease. Fertility and Sterility 58: 628–634
Reginster J Y, Deroisy R, Denis R et al 1989 One year controlled randomised trial of prevention of early menopausal bone loss by tiludronate. Lancet 2: 1469–1471
Reid R L 1991 Premenstrual syndrome. Current Problems in Obstetrics and Gynaecology and Fertility 8: 1–57
Reid R L, Greenaway-Coate A, Hahn P M 1986 Oral glucose tolerance during the menstrual cycle in normal women and women with alleged premenstrual 'hypoglycaemic' attacks: effects of naloxone. Journal of Clinical Endocrinology and Metabolism 62: 1167
Rich P 1996 Practical aromatherapy. Paragon, Bristol
Roberts H 2000 Good practice in sterilization. British Medical Journal 320(7236): 662–663
Robinson G 1996 Cross-cultural perspectives in the menopause. Journal of Nervous and Mental Disease 184(8): 453–458
Robinson G E, Garfinkel P E 1990 Problems in the treatment of premenstrual syndrome. Canadian Journal of Psychiatry 35(3): 199–206
Rosevear S K 2002 Handbook of gynaecology management. Blackwell, Oxford
Rossouw J E, Anderson G L, Prentice R L et al 2002 Risks and benefits of estrogen plus progestin in healthy post-menopausal women. Journal of the American Medical Association 288(3): 321–333
Royal College of Nursing 1996 Female genital mutilation. The unspoken issue. RCN, London
Royal College of Physicians 1991 Report on preventive medicine. Royal College of Physicians, London
Royal College of Physicians 2003 Final consensus statement on hormone replacement therapy, www.rcpe.ac.uk/esd/consensus/hrt_03.html
Schairer C, Lubin J, Troisi R, Sturgeon S, Brinton L, Hoover R 2000 Menopausal estrogen and estrogen-progestin replacement therapy and breast cancer risk. Journal of the American Medical Association 283: 485–491
Schellenberg R 2001 Treatment for the premenstrual syndrome with agnus castus fruit extract: prospective randomised placebo controlled study. British Medical Journal 322: 134–137
Scholten A N, Smit V T, Beerman H, van Putten W L, Creutzberg C L 2004 Prognostic significance and interobserver variability of histologic grading systems for endometrial carcinoma. Cancer 100(4): 764–772
Sharlip I D 1994 Vasculogenic impotence secondary to atherosclerosis/dysplasia. In: Bennett A H (ed) Impotence diagnosis and management of erectile dysfunction. WB Saunders, Philadelphia
Scottish Health Statistics 2003 Scottish Health Statistics Website of ISD Scotland www.isdscotland.org/isd/info3.jsp?pContentID=1430&p_applic=CCC&p_service=Content.show&
Shanafelt T, Barton D, Adjei A, Loprinzi C 2002 Pathophysiology and treatment of hot flashes. Mayo Clinic Proceedings 77: 1207
Shingleton H M, Orr J W (eds) 1987 Cancer of the cervix: diagnosis and treatment. Churchill Livingstone, Edinburgh
Singh D 2003 HRT no longer first choice for preventing osteoporosis. British Medical Journal 327: 1364
Sliutz G, Tempfer C, Hanzal E et al 1997 Serum M3/M21 in cervical cancer patients. European Journal of Cancer 33(6): 973–975
Smithson A 1992 Girls will be women. Nursing Times 88(6): 46–48
Stampfer M J, Colditz G A 1991 Oestrogen replacement therapy and coronary heart disease: a qualitative assessment of the epidemiological evidence. Preventive Medicine 20: 47–63
Stephens C, Ross N 2002 The relationship between hormone replacement therapy use and psychological symptoms: no effects found in a New Zealand sample. Health Care Women International 23(4): 408–414
Stevenson J C 1996 Metabolic effects of the menopause and oestrogen replacment. Baillière's Clinical Obstetrics and Gynaecology 10(3): 449–467
Stevenson J C, Cust M P, Ganger K F et al 1990 Effects of transdermal versus oral hormone replacement therapy on bone density in spine and proximal femur in post menopausal women. Lancet 336: 265–269
Suffling K 2001 Premenstrual syndrome. In: Gangar E A (ed) Gynaecological nursing: a practical guide. Churchill Livingstone, Edinburgh
Sundblad C, Modigh K, Anderson B et al 1992 Clomipramine effectively reduces premenstrual irritability and dysphoria: a placebo controlled trial. Acta Psychiatrica Scandinavica 85(1): 39–47
Sutherland C 2001 Women's health: a handbook for nurses. Churchill Livingstone, Edinburgh
Szarewski A, Jarvis M J, Sasiem P et al 1996 Effects of smoking cessation on cervical lesion size. Lancet 347(9006): 941–943
Talbot J McK, Lawrence M 1997 In-vitro fertilisation: indications, stimulation and clinical techniques. In: Kovacs G T (ed) The subfertility handbook. Cambridge University Press, Cambridge, p 88–108
Taksey J, Bissada N K, Chaudhary U B 2003 Fertility after chemotherapy for testicular cancer. Archives of Andrology 49(5): 389–395
Templeton A A 1992 The epidemiology of infertility. In: Templeton A A, Drife J O (eds) Infertility. Springer, London
Thomas S 1997 Embolisation of uterine fibroids. Nursing Standard 11(44): 27
Thonneau P, Marchard S, Talle A et al 1991 Incidences and main courses of infertility in a resident population (1 850 000) of three French regions (1988–1989). Human Reproduction 6: 811–816
Toubin N 1994 Female circumcision as a public health issue. New England Journal of Medicine 331(11): 712
Tournaye H 2003 ICSI: a technique too far? International Journal of Andrology 26(2): 63–69
Trounce J 1997 Clinical pharmacology for nurses, 15th edn. Churchill Livingstone, Edinburgh
Tumbo-Oeri A G, Omwandho C A, Muchiri J M 2001 Possible immunological basis for recurrent spontaneous abortions: a review. East African Medical Journal 78(11): 586–589
Utian W H, Bury K A, Archer D F et al 1999

Efficacy and safety of low, standard and high dosages of an estradiol transdermal system (Esclim) compared with placebo on vasomotor symptoms in highly symptomatic menopausal patients. The Esclim Study Group. American Journal of Obstetrics and Gynecology 181(1): 71–79
Vessey M P 1989 Epidemiological studies of the effects of diethylstilboestrol. IARC Publication No. 96. IARC, Lyon
Walczak J R 2000 Endometrial cancer. In: Yarbro C H, Froffe M H, Goodman M, Groenwald S L (eds) Cancer nursing principles and practice, 5th edn. Jones and Bartlett, Sudbury, MA, p 1168–1178
Waugh A, Grant A (eds) 2001 Ross & Wilson anatomy and physiology in health and illness, 9th edn. Churchill Livingstone, Edinburgh
Webb C, Wilson-Barnett J 1983 Self concept, social support and hysterectomy. International Journal of Nursing Studies 20(2): 97–107
Weir E 2004 Hot flashes ... in January. Canadian Medical Association Journal 170(1): 39–40
Wells M, Sturdee D W, Barlow D H et al 2002 Effect on endometrium of long term treatment with continuous combined oestrogen-progestogen replacement therapy: follow up study. British Medical Journal 325: 239–242
Whitehead M I, Godfree V 1992 Replacement therapy – your questions answered. Churchill Livingstone, Edinburgh
Whitehead M I, Fraser D, Schenkel L, Crook D, Stevenson J C 1990 Transdermal administration of oestrogen/progestogen hormone replacement therapy. Lancet 335: 310–312
Williams C 1995 Healthy eating: clarifying the advice about fruit and vegetables. British Medical Journal 5992(310): 1453–1455
Winston R M C 1991 Resources for infertility treatment. Baillière's Clinical Obstetrics and Gynaecology 5(3): 551–573
Wood C 1997 The role of gamete intrafallopian transfer. In: Kovacs G (ed) The subfertility handbook. Cambridge University Press, Cambridge, p 109–123
World Health Organization 1994 Assessment of fracture risk and its application to screening for postmenopausal osteoporosis. WHO, Geneva
World Health Organization 1997 Female sterilisation. WHO, Geneva
Wyatt K M, Dimmock P W, Jones P W, O'Brien P M S 1999 Efficacy of vitamin B-6 in the treatment of premenstrual syndrome: systematic review. British Medical Journal 318: 1375–1381
Wyatt K, Dimmock P, Jones P, Obhrai M, O'Brien P M S 2001 Efficacy of progesterone and progestogens in management of premenstrual syndrome: systematic review. British Medical Journal 323(7316): 776–788
Wyatt K M, Dimmock P W, O'Brien P M S 2002 Selective serotonin reuptake inhibitors for premenstrual syndrome. Cochrane Database Systematic Review (4): CD001396 www.update-software.com/Abstracts/AB001396.htm

FURTHER READING

Bennett A H (ed) 1994 Impotence diagnosis and management of erectile dysfunction. WB Saunders, Philadelphia
Green S, Fishel S, Stoddart N, Garrett L 1997 Microinsemination for the treatment of male factor infertility. In: O'Brien P M S (ed) The yearbook of obstetrics and gynaecology, Vol 5. RCOG Press, London
Moynihan C 1996 Psychosocial assessments and counseling of the patient with testicular cancer. In: Horwich A (ed) Testicular cancer, 2nd edn. Chapman and Hall Medical, London

PART 2 THE BREAST

INTRODUCTION

The breast is the human organ of lactation which develops in puberty to enable a mother to feed her offspring. In Western society the breasts are strongly associated with femininity and sexuality as well as with motherhood. Images of femininity and sexuality presented in advertising and other media use breasts, often large and perfectly formed, as symbols of sexual desirability promoting an idealistic beauty which few women can attain. It is not surprising, therefore, that breast disease often has profound implications not only for a woman's physical health but also for her social and familial roles, body image and self-confidence. Women who suffer any alteration or disfigurement of the breast often experience anxiety, depression and loss of sexual satisfaction.

This chapter will begin by discussing the anatomy and physiology of the healthy breast before considering the benign disorders of the breast, mammary dysplasia, fibroadenomas, breast pain and breast infections. In addition, the rare condition of gynaecomastia will be described in view of its important psychological implications for the individual.

Breast cancer and its treatment will then be discussed in detail as breast cancer is one of the most common malignant conditions in the United Kingdom. Related health care issues such as breast reconstruction, care of the fungating breast lesion and the management of lymphoedema will be given particular attention. Consideration will also be given to measures for the early detection of breast cancer.

Finally, the significance of diseases of the breast for a woman's psychological well-being will be discussed. Patient education will be considered in relation to promoting breast health and the early detection of disease. The importance of involving the patient and her family in making informed treatment choices and in carrying out subsequent self-care will also be considered.

ANATOMY AND PHYSIOLOGY OF THE BREAST

Structure of the breast

The breast is made up of glandular, fatty and fibrous tissue which is covered by skin. Men and women both have breast tissue, but in the male it remains rudimentary and normally does not develop in puberty.

The glandular tissue of each breast is divided into 12–20 lobes or segments (see Fig. 7.12). Each is made up of hundreds of lobules which are activated during pregnancy to produce milk. They are connected by terminal ducts which join to form lactiferous ducts before ending in approximately 10 openings in the nipple. Breast tissue is supported by Cooper's ligaments, fibrous bands which connect the skin of the breast to the underlying fascia. These ligaments may contract when affected by tumour causing dimpling of the skin (peau d'orange). With increasing age and weight, these ligaments stretch, causing the breasts to droop, otherwise known as ptosis.

The nipple contains smooth muscle and becomes erect when stimulated, allowing a baby to suck more easily. It is surrounded by the areola, on the surface of which are Montgomery's tubercles, or glands which lubricate the nipple during breast feeding.

Blood and lymph vessels

The breast is highly vascularised. It is supplied by thoracic branches of the axillary arteries laterally, and medially by branches of the internal mammary artery. Venous drainage follows arterial supply, and the lymphatic channels follow the main blood vessels outwards, branching to the regional lymph nodes. Most lymph drainage of the breast is via the axillary lymph nodes, proceeding from there to the supraclavicular lymph nodes. Drainage from the medial part of the breast is via the internal mammary nodes which lie beneath the ribs and lateral to the sternum.

Nerve supply

Branches of the IV, V and VI thoracic nerves, containing sympathetic fibres, supply the breast. Many sensory nerve endings exist around the nipple. When touched, these cause reflex erection and, after childbirth, the release of milk.

Associated muscles (see Fig. 7.13)

Behind the breast and overlying the rib cage is the pectoralis major muscle. This large triangular muscle, which attaches to the clavicle, sternum and upper six costal cartilages, is

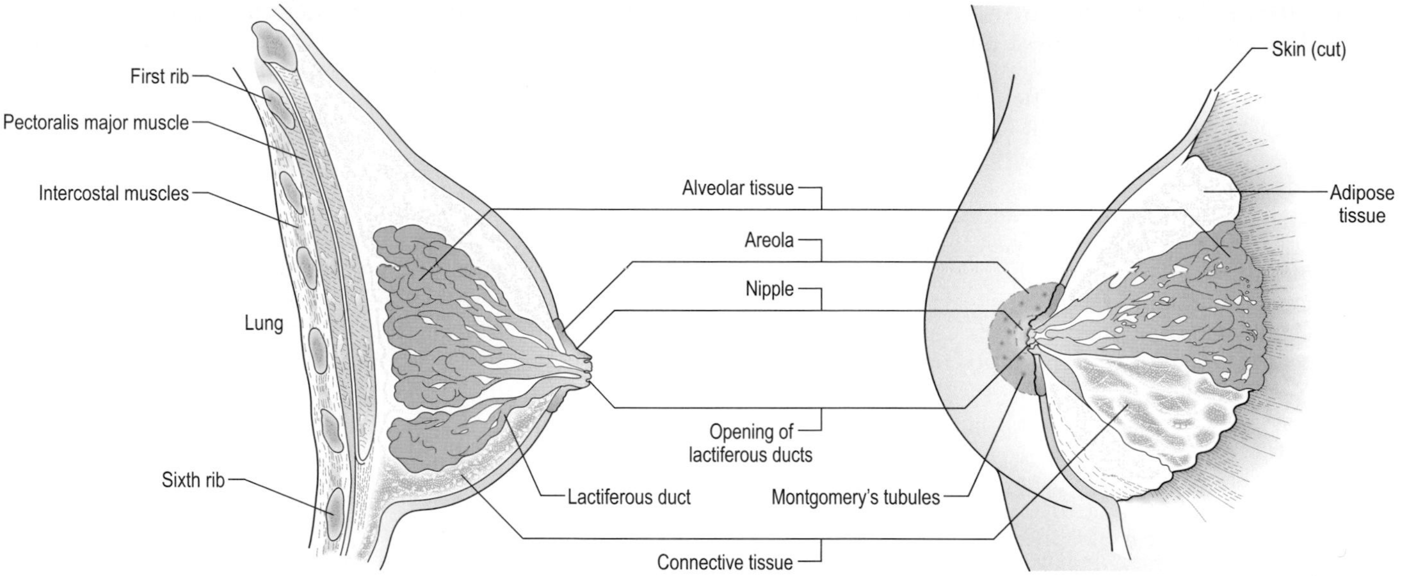

Fig. 7.12 Lateral cross-section of the breast.

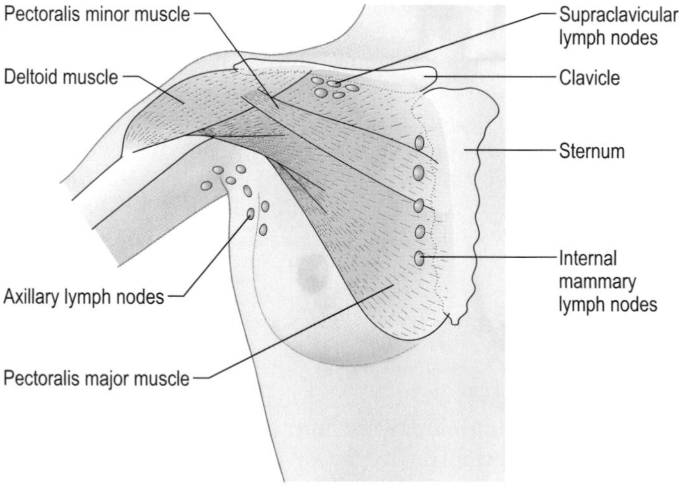

Fig. 7.13 The breast and associated structures.

used to adduct the arm. Behind the pectoralis major muscle lies the pectoralis minor. This muscle attaches to the third, fourth and fifth ribs and the front of the scapula. Its function is to stabilise the shoulder girdle, serratus anterior and the latissimus dorsi muscle from the base and back of the axilla, respectively. These structures and their nerve supply are important considerations when axillary surgery is performed.

Normal breast changes

The breasts constantly change as a normal consequence of ageing. Natural changes also occur with menstruation, pregnancy and lactation.

Puberty

A girl's breasts will begin to develop at puberty. The pituitary gland in the brain begins to produce the gonadotrophins, follicle-stimulating hormone (FSH) and luteinising hormone (LH). As the level of these hormones increases, egg follicles within the ovaries are stimulated to release oestrogens, which in turn stimulate an increase in the breast connective tissue, a lengthening of the ducts in the breast and the formation of the breast lobules.

Menstruation

At the start of each monthly cycle, blood oestrogen levels rise, causing the breast ducts and lobules to enlarge. After ovulation, the corpus luteum produces progesterone which causes further breast changes. At this time, tenderness and heaviness of the breasts may be noticed. If pregnancy does not occur, the hormone levels fall, the ducts and lobules regress, and the breasts lose their tenderness and swollen feeling. This usually precedes the onset of menstruation.

Pregnancy

If pregnancy does occur, the levels of oestrogen and progesterone continue to rise, causing the ducts and lobules to increase in size and number in order to prepare for lactation. The enzymes necessary for milk production are stimulated by prolactin (produced by the anterior pituitary gland) and by placental lactogen, but milk production is suppressed during pregnancy by high progesterone levels.

Milk production

After birth, progesterone levels drop and milk synthesis can begin. As the baby sucks, prolactin is released (from the anterior pituitary), initiating milk synthesis, and oxytocin is released (from the posterior pituitary), causing milk to be emptied from the ducts. The more the baby sucks, the more milk is produced. Sucking also inhibits the release of FSH and LH by the pituitary gland, so blocking ovulation. However, this effect is usually short lived and cannot be relied upon for contraception. When breast feeding stops, the ducts and lobules start to regress, and milk production slows and then ceases.

Once the baby is born, the breasts produce colostrum for 2 or 3 days before the true breast milk production begins. Colostrum is a yellowish fluid with a lower lactose content than milk and contains very little fat, but more vitamin A, protein and minerals. Like milk, colostrum is rich in IgA antibodies which protect the baby's gastrointestinal tract against bacteria and viruses (Newman 1995). Breast milk contains all that is necessary for an infant in the first few months of its life. Cells of the breast lobules extract amino acids, fatty acids, glycerol and glucose from the blood and build them into proteins, fats and lactose. Milk also contains calcium, phosphorus, vitamins A, B, C and D, and small amounts of iron, but the exact composition depends on the mother's dietary intake.

Menopause

As a woman approaches the menopause, changes in ovarian function and a subsequent drop in hormone levels cause glandular breast tissue to atrophy. This process of involution where breast tissue is replaced by fatty tissue causes the breasts to become softer and less lumpy. Consequently, the breasts are easier to examine and assess by mammography.

BENIGN BREAST DISORDERS

Benign breast disorders account for approximately 90% of all breast problems. The largest category of benign breast disorders occur as a result of 'anomalies of normal development and involution' (ANDI). The most common ANDI categories — structural disorders, benign mammary dysplasia, breast pain and breast infection — are considered here. Gynaecomastia is also mentioned because, although rare, it is the most common breast disorder in men.

ABNORMAL BREAST DEVELOPMENT

It is estimated that about 1% of men and 5% of women are born with one or more extra nipples. These extra nipples, or polythelia, usually develop whilst the foetus is in the womb, the most common site being along the milk line or the ectodermal ridge. Extra breasts can also develop and often occur in the lower axilla (Dixon & Mansel 2000).

Aberrations of normal breast development can cause the absence (amastia) or underdevelopment (hypoplasia) of one breast. This can occur in conjunction with a defect in the pectoral muscle and the upper limbs (Poland's syndrome). There is usually some difference in breast size for a woman, with the left breast being larger than the right, but the difference should not be extreme. If it is, then surgical intervention involving augmentation of one breast and reduction of the other breast is offered by many plastic surgeons (Reshef et al 1996).

Juvenile or virginal hypertrophy

Prepubertal breast enlargement is quite common and only requires investigation if it is associated with other signs of premature sexual development. The overgrowth of breast tissue can occur in adolescent girls whose breasts develop during puberty but then continue to grow. Usually no hormone abnormality can be detected. The treatment of choice for these women is a reduction mammoplasty, i.e. surgical removal of breast tissue from each breast (Dixon & Mansel 2000).

Epithelial hyperplasia

This is a common condition amongst women of all ages but particularly affects women between the ages of 30 and 55. This is often called fibrocystic disease but the term is misleading in that it is really not a disease but a natural occurrence in women as they approach the menopause. It is thought to be caused by the incomplete involution of breast tissue during each menstrual cycle, causing an increase in the number of cells lining the terminal duct lobular unit. This, in turn, leads to cystic changes, fibrosis and nodularity. If biopsied, the cells show hyperplasia, but with no alteration in individual cellular appearance. However, where atypical hyperplasia is present, the risk of breast cancer developing in the breast is raised, and regular screening may be advised.

Nodularity

This may present as diffuse lumpiness or thickening of the breast tissue which may contain single or multiple cysts. Commonly, it is bilateral, although it may occur in only one breast. Premenstrual tenderness is often experienced coinciding with an increase in nodularity. Cysts usually develop as a woman is nearing her menopause and they present as tender, fluctuant entities which, when examined under ultrasound, are shown to be fluid-filled. They may increase in size or stay the same and sometimes they just disperse.

MEDICAL MANAGEMENT

Investigations Assessment of a woman who complains of a lump or lumpiness within her breasts will involve clinical examination, mammography, ultrasound and sometimes fine-needle aspiration cytology or core biopsy. Cystic fluid is usually sent for examination if the fluid is bloodstained, as this may indicate cancer.

Whenever a cyst or area of nodularity is slightly suspicious in its presentation, excision biopsy will sometimes be recommended to exclude cancer (see p. 323). Follow-up examinations are not usually required unless histology reveals atypical hyperplasia in a younger woman or if there is a family history of breast cancer.

Nodularity is sometimes aggravated by oral contraceptive pills or the contraceptive coil. If this appears to be the case, a change in method of contraception may be recommended.

Fibroadenomas

Fibroadenomas are considered as aberrations of normal breast growth and are composed of both fibrous and glandular breast tissue. Under the same hormonal influences as the rest of the breast, a fibroadenoma grows as a centrifugal small nodule that is usually well circumscribed and freely movable within the surrounding breast tissue. They are very common, accounting for 13% of all palpable breast lesions, and in women aged 20 years or less, they account for 60% of breast masses (Dixon & Mansel 2000). Juvenile or giant fibroadenomas are rare and occur in adolescence. They are characterised by a fast-growing lesion that can grow up to 5 cm in size and will distort the breast. These lesions require surgical excision for cosmetic reasons.

NURSING PRIORITIES AND MANAGEMENT: Excision biopsy of lesions and fibroadenomas

Major considerations

Assessment

Surgery is not usually undertaken for benign lesions unless a diagnosis is not possible. Fibroadenomas are not usually removed unless they are large or of particular concern to the patient. Nursing assessment should include the presenting symptoms and, in particular, the presence of any discomfort and any aggravating or alleviating factors. The nurse should determine the patient's knowledge about her condition, her fears and concerns, and the ways in which the condition is affecting her normal life.

Perioperative care

General pre- and postoperative nursing practices are discussed in Chapter 26. Surgery is usually minor. Reassurance that this is not cancer may be needed but the nurse should not give false reassurance where doubt exists as to the nature of the lump. As postoperative recovery is usually rapid, surgery is frequently performed on a day-case basis or may require a 1-night stay in hospital. Postoperatively, the priority of nursing will be wound management and pain control. Because the breast is very vascular, there may be bruising even though the surgery is minor. A wound drain is sometimes needed, but, if present, is usually removed the following morning.

The breast is likely to be very painful for several days. Paracetamol is usually sufficient for pain relief, but if bruising and oedema are very extensive, a stronger analgesic may be required, e.g. an opiate-based drug. Wearing a supportive bra is usually advised for the first 2 weeks postoperatively to improve comfort and avoid strain being placed on the wound. The woman should be encouraged to bring a good fitting bra into hospital with her so that she may wear it very shortly after the surgery.

Patient education

The nurse should take the opportunity to promote breast health by discussing breast screening and breast awareness. It may be appropriate to discuss how breast comfort can be enhanced by a correctly fitting bra. Women who have premenstrual breast discomfort may find reducing salt or omitting caffeine from their diet helpful. Others find that a course of evening primrose oil brings relief.

BREAST PAIN

Breast pain (mastalgia) has been reported in over 50% of women who attend benign breast clinics (Mansel 2000). For most women, some breast discomfort is accepted as a part of the normal changes in their breasts each month. However, some women suffer more intense pain which affects their quality of life, usually from mid-cycle onwards, and is often relieved by menstruation. The pain can differ from cycle to cycle and can continue for many years. Evening primrose oil and reducing caffeine and fat intake have been found to be of benefit for some patients. Hormone manipulation using danazol, bromocriptine or a luteinising hormone releasing hormone agonist have all been used to some effect. Such drug interventions should be medically supervised at a benign breast disease clinic (Purushotham et al 2000).

Non-cyclical breast pain, usually experienced in women over 40, is the main type of mastalgia. Often localised within the breast, this type of pain can be relieved by infiltrating the area with a local anaesthetic and steroid. For both cyclical and non-cyclical mastalgia, wearing a firm and well-fitted bra can help (Mansel 2000).

BREAST INFECTIONS

PATHOPHYSIOLOGY

Breast infections, such as mastitis, are relatively common, causing swelling, tenderness and pain, which may be associated with a breast abscess or nipple discharge. Breast abscesses are most commonly seen during or following lactation. Infection may arise from a cracked nipple, but often there is no apparent cause. Staphylococcal organisms are the most common causes.

MEDICAL MANAGEMENT

Systemic broad-spectrum antibiotics are the usual treatment. However, a persistent abscess may require surgical drainage and excision of the surrounding capsule. A persistent nipple discharge may be treated by a microdochectomy, which involves removing one of the major ducts behind the nipple, or a duct clearance which involves removing the major duct system behind the nipple. Surgery is usually through a circumareolar incision, and this surgery often can be performed on a day patient basis.

Duct ectasia

Duct ectasia occurs during breast involution when the major subareolar ducts dilate and shorten. Normal breast secretions are retained behind these blocked ducts. Women with duct ectasia present with nipple discharge, nipple retraction, inflammation or a palpable mass. Surgery is indicated if the discharge is a problem (Curling & Tierney 1997).

NURSING PRIORITIES AND MANAGEMENT: Breast infections

Giving psychological support

Until the presence of infection has been established, fear of a more serious problem, particularly cancer, may remain. An explanation of the nature and possible cause of infection will help to reassure the patient, particularly as recurrent infections are quite common and may cause frustration and distress.

Reducing discomfort

The discomfort and pain accompanying a breast infection are usually the most distressing features of the condition. A supportive bra, applications of heat or cold 'packs' and padding to protect a sore nipple may all reduce discomfort, but mild to moderate analgesic medication is usually necessary to achieve a satisfactory level of comfort.

Surgical management

Where surgical excision of the abscess is required, nursing management will be similar to that for a woman undergoing an excision biopsy (see p. 328). The nurse must be particularly vigilant in observing for signs of wound infection.

OTHER DISORDERS OF BREAST STRUCTURE

Duct papillomas

Duct papillomas are benign wart-like lesions which form in the lactiferous duct wall. Most of these occur beneath the areola. Papillomas present with pain or bloody discharge and are usually soft and difficult to locate. Surgical resection is usually the treatment of choice (Blackwell & Grotting 1996).

Lipomas

When examined, these fatty lumps can be mistaken for cysts within the breast tissue. They do not cause major problems and diagnosis by ultrasound and cytology should be all that is needed.

Mondor's disease

Caused by a superficial thrombosis of a vein in the breast, this condition is usually very painful, requiring analgesics. Malignancy should always be excluded, but no other treatment should be necessary and the condition usually resolves in 6 months (Curling & Tierney 1997).

Galactocele

This is a cystic lesion which occurs in the breasts of pregnant or lactating women. Once diagnosed, treatment is by aspiration. This may have to be performed on several occasions to allow the walls of the cyst to adhere (Curling & Tierney 1997).

Fat necrosis

Presenting as a painful mass, fat necrosis can imitate breast cancer and should be diagnosed with care. About half of the cases of fat necrosis are caused by a blow to the breast, although the other cases have no history of trauma. The treatment is surgical excision to be absolutely sure that the area is not malignant (Blackwell & Grotting 1996).

GYNAECOMASTIA

This is a rare benign disorder which occurs in men and involves overdevelopment of male breast tissue as a result of oestrogen production either in puberty (30–60% of boys aged 10–16 years) or at a later age. This may be due to idiopathic excess oestrogen, e.g. in choriocarcinomatous teratoma or cirrhosis of the liver, to decreased testosterone, e.g. in Klinefelter's syndrome (see Ch. 6), or to drugs, e.g. amfetamines, antidepressants, certain antihypertensives, digoxin, spironolactone or oestrogen administration.

MEDICAL MANAGEMENT

Surgery is not usually recommended, as 80% of cases resolve within 2 years, unless the gynaecomastia is mistaken for a possible carcinoma; in such instances a biopsy may be advised. If the condition has arisen following the administration of a particular medication, modification of that medication can be considered. Hormone manipulation may be of benefit where gynaecomastia is due to the oversecretion of oestrogen (Dixon & Mansel 2000).

NURSING PRIORITIES AND MANAGEMENT: Gynaecomastia

Giving psychological support

Breasts are considered to be a female characteristic, and for this reason the overdevelopment of breast tissue in a man may cause an altered body image and emotional distress. Some men with gynaecomastia believe they have lost their masculinity and experience anxiety and depression as a result. When gynaecomastia occurs in adolescence, such feelings may be particularly acute.

The nurse must be sensitive to such feelings and show an understanding of them. It may be difficult for a man to express these feelings to a female nurse, especially if she is relatively young, but he is more likely to do so within a professional relationship where trust exists. A clear explanation of why the breast tissue has developed and of any treatment that may be given is essential.

For more information, see Dixon (2000) and Purushotham et al (2000).

MALIGNANT DISORDERS OF THE BREAST AND THEIR SEQUELAE

BREAST CANCER

Incidence and mortality

Breast cancer is the most common malignancy in women, accounting for 25% of all of female cancers (Breast Cancer Care 2003). Approximately one in nine women in the UK will develop breast cancer at some time in their lives. There are 40 000 new cases of breast cancer and 13 000 deaths due to breast cancer each year (Breast Cancer Care 2003). Less than 1% of all breast cancers occur in men. It is important for nurses to be aware of the special problems that men may experience when they are diagnosed with a disease that almost exclusively affects women (Perkins & Middleton 2003).

Risk factors

The main risk factors associated with breast cancer are listed in Box 7.13. Of these, only increasing age is known to be of any substantial significance.

Box 7.13

Factors increasing the risk of developing breast cancer

- Early menarche
- Increasing age
- Family history of breast cancer
- Age at birth of first child
- Geographical location
- Late menopause
- Nulliparity (no pregnancies)
- Social class (class I has highest risk)
- Other possible factors under evaluation
- High alcohol intake
- High-fat diet
- Stress

Increasing age Breast cancer in women is very rare below the age of 35 years, but incidence rates increase steadily from then, reaching over 300 per 100 000 of the population by the time women are 85 years old. The largest number of women are diagnosed between the ages of 45 and 75 years (see Fig. 7.14).

Geography England and Wales have the highest standardised mortality figures per 100 000 for breast cancer in the world, followed by Scotland and Denmark, Northern Ireland and the Netherlands, Canada and the United States of America (McPherson et al 2000). Generally, incidence in Western Europe, North America and Australia is approximately five times higher than in Asia and Africa. Japanese women have low rates of breast cancer, but incidence rates are seen to rise by the second generation among Japanese–Americans. This suggests that environmental and social risk factors may exist.

Diet Populations with a high rate of breast cancer generally have a diet high in fat. Obesity has also been found to be

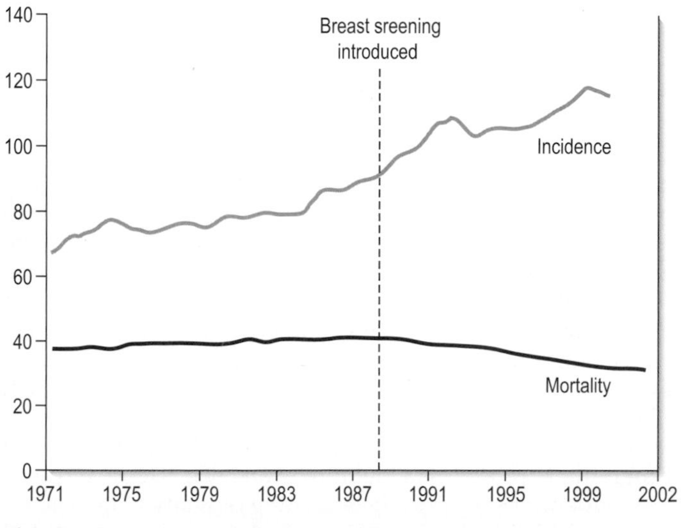

Fig. 7.14 Age-standardised incidence of and mortality from female breast cancer, England and Wales; rate per 100 000. From Office for National Statistics, www.statistics.gov.uk.

associated with a slightly increased risk of breast cancer. However, a clear link between diet and the risk of breast cancer has not been established.

Social class Breast cancer is slightly more common amongst women in social class 1, suggesting that breast cancer is a disease of affluent societies.

Hormone-related factors Women who have their first child after the age of 35, those who experience early menarche, and those who have a late menopause are all found to have a slightly increased rate of breast cancer. This has led to the belief that the hormone oestrogen may be implicated in the development of breast cancer (Wren 2004). In recent years, there has been much speculation as to the effects of the contraceptive pill and hormone replacement therapy on the incidence of breast cancer. Studies do not give a clear picture as yet, as oral contraceptive use was not common until the early 1970s and any effect is thought to be long term. There is no increased risk for women in their early 20s who have used oral contraceptives to space their pregnancies. However, use of oral contraceptives for 4 years or more by younger women before their first pregnancy may increase the risk of premenopausal breast cancer. More research is needed, particularly as today's contraceptive pills contain lower levels of oestrogen or none at all (Hemminki 1996).

Family history Between 5 and 10% of breast cancers are due to genetic predisposition (Arden-Jones 2003). The likelihood of a woman carrying a genetic abnormality is higher if:

- there are several cases of breast cancer in a single family
- those affected in that family have an early onset of cancer
- there is a diagnosis of a different epithelial cancer in one family, e.g. bilateral breast cancer, ovarian cancer, colon or prostate cancer. The combination of ovarian and breast cancer is particularly common in families who carry a cancer predisposing gene (Page et al 2000).

In families suspected of having a cancer predisposing gene, it is important to get a family history, or pedigree, going back several generations to assess who developed cancer and the type of cancer it was. This information is usually taken by a geneticist or a genetics nurse who is working in a specialised genetics clinic (see Ch. 6, p. 235). These details will usually allow the geneticist to confirm that a cancer gene is present and to estimate the likelihood or risk that any member of the family has the gene. Family histories are often difficult to recall and sometimes it is necessary to extend and verify details of family histories by using public records of births, deaths and marriages, pathology reports and hospital records. Patterns in the family pedigree can then be clarified and the breast cancer predisposing genes such as BRCA1 or BRCA2 can be identified by genetic linkage analysis. This involves taking tissue or blood samples from family members and using specialised genetic techniques to search for the problematic gene.

Women who are at an increased risk of developing cancer because of a genetic predisposition will be offered genetic counselling and psychological support by the geneticist and specialist nurses who work in the clinic. Counselling is a very important part of the process because of the implications for that individual and other members of the family who may not wish to know their risk of cancer. Family relationships can be seriously disrupted if risk assessment and genetic testing are not explored fully with all those involved (Arden-Jones 2003).

If the chance of the woman developing cancer is very high, this will be discussed with the woman and her future care will be considered. Interventions are regularly evaluated as this is a relatively new area of cancer care and there is uncertainty about the best way of screening or prevention for women (and men) at risk. Instituting regular clinical examination is debatable but contact with an established breast/genetics clinic is recommended for women at risk (Arden-Jones 2003). Regular mammographic screening commencing 5–10 years younger than the youngest relative already to have developed the disease is a current recommendation but this is not useful in women less than 35 years old. Both magnetic resonance imaging (MRI) and ultrasound are presently being evaluated as potential screening tools for women at high risk. Cuzick et al (2003), in an overview of the use of the oestrogen blocking tablet tamoxifen for women at risk, showed a reduction in breast cancer occurrence in high-risk women, so the use of this agent may be a future solution. Some women will have the BRCA1 or BRCA2 gene confirmed by DNA analysis and may then be offered bilateral subcutaneous mastectomy and bilateral oophorectomy as a preventive treatment, although this is clearly a serious undertaking (see p. 248). Research into this area of cancer care will continue far into this millennium. The implications for breast care are potentially very exciting, as women who are likely to develop breast cancer could be identified and treated prophylactically (McPherson et al 2000, Page et al 2000).

Prevention in the present

Over the last 30 years, advances in treatments, and more recently the multidisciplinary approach to breast cancer care, have made an impact on survival (Peto et al 2000). We also know that if women are diagnosed at an early stage in their disease, treatment is likely to be more effective (see Fig. 7.14). Therefore, taking measures to detect breast cancer earlier would appear to be one way of reducing breast cancer mortality.

Breast awareness

For many years there has been debate as to the value of monthly breast self-examination in the diagnosis of early breast cancer. Research has been unable to demonstrate that it alters survival from the disease. However, a woman who is aware of any changes that occur in her breast and, if she wishes, practises self-examination, is likely to notice any changes. This may aid diagnosis when a cancer is small, so enabling a wider choice of surgical treatment options to be offered. It also encourages an individual to participate in their own health care. Breast awareness helps a woman to know what is normal for her and to detect the following changes:

- A change in size of the breast, noticeably smaller or larger
- Newly inverted nipple or a nipple that has changed its shape
- Discharge from one or both nipples
- Change in colour
- A new lump or thickening in the breast that feels different from the rest of the breast tissue
- A rash or eczema-like changes around the nipple
- Pain in one part of the breast or in the armpit
- Puckering or dimpling of the skin of the breast (peau d'orange; see p. 328).

If a woman wishes to examine her breasts regularly she should do so when she feels comfortable although just after menstruation, e.g. day 8 of her cycle, can be convenient. Obviously, this does not apply to postmenopausal women. At this time, the breasts will be least lumpy and easiest to examine. Breast tissue can be lumpy and so each woman will need to become used to how her own breasts feel and learn to identify her ribs, which are often mistaken for lumps.

To carry out self-examination the woman should sit in front of a mirror and lift her arms above her head, noticing the shape and size of her breasts and any changes. She should examine her skin for dimpling and discoloration and the nipple for discharge, crusting and any new inversion.

Lying flat on a bed or when standing in the shower, with one arm behind her head, she should then examine her breasts using the flat of her fingers of the opposite hand. Breast tissue is very extensive, running vertically from the clavicle to the costal margin and the sternum to the axilla, and breast examination should cover all these areas systematically. Usually a hollow is noticed beneath each nipple. If any lumps, thickening or other changes are noticed, the woman should contact her GP immediately for an examination and advice.

Breast cancer screening

In 1986, the Forrest report (Department of Health and Social Security 1986) recommended the introduction of a national breast screening programme. Screening units are now in operation throughout the UK and women between 50 and 70 years are invited to attend for screening using mammography, i.e. X-ray examination of the breast.

The aim of breast cancer screening by means of mammography is to detect breast cancer at an earlier stage than is possible by clinical examination or breast self-examination, i.e. before a lump is palpable in the breast. In addition, it is hoped that more women with pre-invasive disease (in situ) cancer will be detected before the cancer cells have shown any evidence of spread. A research study by Sjönell and Ståhle (1999) questioned the mammography and screening programme in Sweden and this has raised fresh doubts about the effectiveness of the breast screening programme in the UK. Some clinicians involved in breast care would prefer to see the resources used for the screening programme invested in research into breast cancer treatment (Baum 1996). This debate is likely to continue until long-term evaluation of the effectiveness of the breast screening programme provides a definitive answer. There is much less evidence to support the screening of women aged 40–49 years, which is why, at present, the screening programme in the UK is offered only to women over the age of 50 (Kerlikowske et al 1995).

Mammography will detect 85–90% of all breast cancers in the women examined. It is most effective in postmenopausal women in whom breast tissue has been largely replaced by fat. For young women, in whom breast tissue is more dense, and detection of abnormalities therefore more difficult, mammography is frequently used in conjunction with breast ultrasound.

The success of the national screening programme will depend on a high uptake of the service. A Swedish study demonstrated an uptake rate of 70% (Tabar et al 1995) and this will have to be matched in the UK if the hoped-for 30% reduction in mortality is to be achieved. If fewer women participate in the programme, the cost per life saved increases and, although some women will clearly benefit, the cost-effectiveness of the programme will be called into question. Poor attendance at screening units may result from various factors, such as GP registers not being up to date, fears of discomfort or radiation, or a lack of understanding of the value of mammography. To further explain breast screening, all women invited into the programme are sent a leaflet entitled *Breast Screening – The Facts* (NHSBSP 2001).

Procedures Screening may take place in static or mobile units. The screening itself involves taking an oblique mediolateral and a cranial–caudal mammogram. Mammograms are repeated every 3 years and, although the screening starts from age 50 years, a woman may not be called until she is 53 years old. The woman is notified by letter of the result. If an abnormality is detected, the letter will ask her to attend for re-screening at an assessment centre (see Fig. 7.15). Here, a fresh two-view mammogram may show the detected lesion to be merely an overlapping of normal structures or a benign lesion requiring no intervention. In some instances, further assessment of the suspicious area using ultrasound and fine-needle aspiration cytology or a core biopsy may be required.

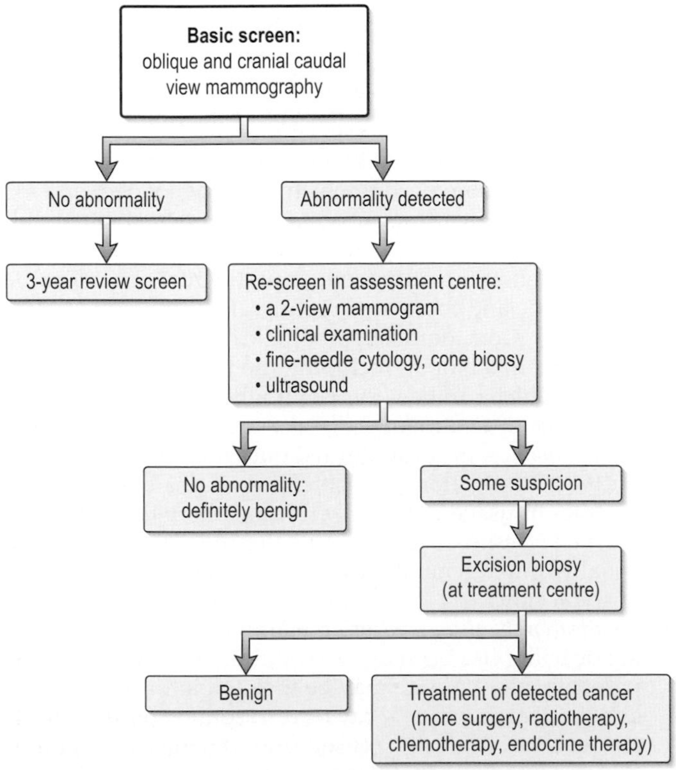

Fig. 7.15 Flow diagram of breast cancer screening procedure.

Psychological considerations Most women who present for breast screening are asymptomatic; apparently healthy people who, on the whole, come to be reassured that all is well. Inevitably, screening reminds the individual that breast cancer is a potential threat. It is therefore important that within the screening programme efforts are made to reduce anxiety where possible. It is particularly important that results are sent quickly. If the first screening is a positive experience, the woman will be more likely to attend 3 years later and may urge her friends to do likewise.

The nurse's role The Forrest report (Department of Health and Social Security 1986) recommended that qualified nurses should be available to support women who are undergoing screening. The report stressed the importance of having specialist nurses with an in-depth knowledge of breast disease and its treatment and with good communication skills to give support to women recalled to assessment centres following the detection of an apparent abnormality.

However, all nurses have a role in health education and should take every appropriate opportunity to raise women's awareness of the availability and benefits of screening programmes. Community nurses, in particular, can encourage women to attend for screening and can answer queries or discuss worries about breast screening as part of their general health promotion on an individual basis or through group discussion, e.g. in well woman clinics.

PATHOPHYSIOLOGY

Common presenting symptoms (see Table 7.3) Discovery of a non-tender, hard, usually irregular lump or thickening in the breast is the most common presentation of breast cancer. Increasingly, it is also diagnosed after a mass or microcalcifications are seen on a mammogram during routine breast screening.

Pain is not usually a presenting feature, but sometimes a sharp, pricking pain is the first symptom experienced. A change in breast size or shape may be noticed. Signs of inflammation and tissue oedema may also be present, and superficial veins may dilate and become more visible if partially obstructed by a tumour. If the tumour is advanced at the time of presentation, it may be fixed to the muscles beneath the breast. There may also be large palpable axillary lymph nodes or ulceration of the tumour through the skin, causing an infected, weeping, malodorous wound, although most women are sufficiently well informed to present to their GP before this advanced stage. Oedema of the arm may result if the cancer in the axilla is blocking the drainage of blood and lymph from the arm.

Histology Breast cancers may be classified according to the type of tissue from which they arise and their appearance under the microscope. The histological type of a cancer is often relevant to the choice of treatment.

Carcinomas arising from the epithelial cells of the ducts are known as ductal carcinomas and account for

Table 7.3 Signs and symptoms of breast cancer

Sign/symptom	Comment
Breast lump	Usually hard and irregular
Change in breast size or shape	
Impalpable mammographic abnormality	Mass/microcalcifications
Pain	Sometimes
Skin dimpling	Retraction of Cooper's ligaments
Peau d'orange	Thickening and oedema of skin
Nipple discharge	Usually bloodstained
Nipple retraction	Due to disease in main ducts
Nipple crusting	Usually Paget's disease of nipple
Dilatation of superficial veins	Result of partial obstruction of veins by tumour
Palpable axillary lymph nodes	Usually in advanced cancer
Ulceration of skin	Usually in advanced cancer

the majority of all breast cancers (Sainsbury et al 2000). Medullary, colloidal and tubular carcinomas are all types of breast cancer arising from ductal tissue. They usually arise in one area of the breast, but they can be multifocal; they are rarely bilateral. Cancers arising from cells of the breast lobules are known as lobular carcinomas. These account for approximately 15% of breast cancers and are more commonly multifocal and bilateral than ductal carcinomas (Crowe & Lampejo 1996).

In Paget's disease of the nipple, malignant cells are found in the epidermis of the nipple and are usually associated with small multifocal areas of ductal cancer behind the nipple and deep in the breast. Other breast cancer types, such as squamous cell or inflammatory carcinomas, are less common. Sarcomas and lymphomas may also arise in the breast, as may metastatic cancer tumours, although these are rare.

Breast cancers are classified as non-invasive or in situ (located only in the ducts or lobules) or invasive (having the ability to invade the basement membrane of the duct or lobule). This distinction has a bearing on prognosis and treatment. Ductal carcinoma in situ represents a very early stage of breast cancer which is often seen as microcalcifications on a mammogram. It cannot be predicted when, or if, a non-invasive breast cancer will become invasive.

Cellular differentiation, i.e. the degree to which cancer cells resemble their tissue of origin, is another important histological factor in determining prognosis: cells are described as well-differentiated, moderately differentiated or poorly differentiated, or grades I, II or III. Poorly differentiated cancers tend to be more aggressive, with the ability to metastasise at an earlier stage, and hence carry a poorer prognosis.

For more detailed information on the histology of breast cancers, see Dixon (2000).

MEDICAL MANAGEMENT

Investigations Once a breast abnormality has been detected, further diagnostic investigation will be carried out following referral to a specialist. This may involve:

- clinical examination of the breast
- mammography (see p. 326)
- ultrasound to distinguish solid from cystic lesions
- fine-needle aspiration to drain cysts and to obtain samples for cytological study
- biopsy.

Fine-needle aspiration cytology of the breast In this procedure, a syringe with a small-bore needle is inserted into the breast mass and suction is applied. The contents are withdrawn, placed on a slide and sent to the laboratory for cytological studies. Where a mass is found to be a cyst and a large amount of fluid is aspirated, it is usually discarded, unless it is found to be bloodstained, in which case a sample will be sent for examination. Cytological results are graded C0–C5:

- C0 represents an insufficient specimen
- C1 and C2 = benign cells
- C3 and C4 = cells suspicious of carcinoma
- C5 = carcinoma.

Fine-needle aspiration cytology is a useful diagnostic tool but is not conclusive on its own. A benign result may simply indicate that the needle missed the target; where other signs are suspicious, a biopsy will still be recommended. This method of gaining a provisional diagnosis can be very fast and is often used in clinics where the woman (or man) is given a diagnosis by the end of the clinic visit.

Biopsy On the basis of the investigations listed above, a decision is made as to whether a biopsy should be performed to confirm diagnosis. Biopsy may be of the following types:

- *A core biopsy* — removal of a core of tissue using a special large-bore needle which is spring loaded, and when guided by ultrasound, can accurately obtain good specimens of the suspicious lesion. This is often undertaken in the outpatient department using a local anaesthetic and the woman returns for her result several days later. Considerable pathological information can be gained from a biopsy, including the type of breast cancer, which can be very useful when planning the next stage of treatment.
- *Mammotome* – an X-ray-guided outpatient biopsy, useful for the investigation of calcifications in the breast. Many samples of tissue can be taken from a defined area.
- *Excision biopsy* — excision of the lump in its entirety, usually under general anaesthesia, requiring a 1-day hospital stay.
- *Localisation biopsy* — where a mammographic abnormality has been detected but there is no associated palpable mass. A wire may be inserted into the abnormal area under X-ray or ultrasound control. This tissue, once surgically excised from the breast, will be X-rayed to ensure that the surgeon has removed the area of abnormality.

Box 7.14

Staging of breast cancer tumours using the TNM and UICC classification system combined

Stage I	Tumour ≤2 cm, not fixed, no axillary node involvement
Stage II	Tumour ≤5 cm, with/without axillary node involvement. No detectable metastases
Stage IIIa	Tumour >5 cm, or chest wall involvement
Stage IIIb	Any tumour with supraclavicular node involvement, fixation to the chest wall, inflammation, ulceration
Stage IV	Any size tumour, positive lymph nodes and presence of distant metastatic disease

Treatment The choice of treatment in breast cancer will depend on several factors, including:

- the size, position and type of tumour (see Box 7.14)
- the spread of the disease
- the woman's general health
- the woman's priorities and wishes.

Surgical intervention Surgery is still considered to be the most effective treatment for early breast cancer. Formerly, radical mastectomy was the treatment of choice, but for many women, less extensive surgery followed by radiotherapy can be just as successful (Fisher et al 1990, Veronesi et al 1995).

Surgical procedures that may be used are as follows:

- *Lumpectomy* — removal of the breast lump with very little surrounding tissue. May be equivalent to an excision biopsy.
- *Wide local excision* — removal of the abnormal areas together with a 1–2 cm margin of normal tissue to reduce the possibility of incompletely excising the cancer. When the pathologist indicates that excision may be incomplete, re-excision is usually recommended. The amount of tissue removed in this operation can be considerable, depending on the size and location of the tumour in relation to the breast and may leave the breast smaller and somewhat altered in contour.
- *Partial mastectomy* — removal of a portion of the breast, usually the nipple and areolar complex. Invariably the breast is left smaller and its contour is changed.
- *Simple mastectomy* — removal of the breast tissue and overlying skin and nipple; all muscles are left intact and the scar is horizontal.
- *Mastectomy* — removal of all the breast tissue, overlying skin and the nipple. The pectoralis major and minor muscles remain and the axillary skin fold remains intact. The scar is oblique but less extensive than with a radical mastectomy.
- *Radical or Halsted's mastectomy* — this is rarely used nowadays unless there is extensive local spread of the breast cancer. This operation involves the removal of the pectoralis major and minor muscles, as well as the breast tissue and overlying skin, the nipple and the axillary lymph nodes. A long, oblique scar remains. The axillary skin fold is usually removed and the chest wall may appear concave and the ribs more prominent.
- *Axillary dissection* — this is usually performed if the patient has a confirmed *invasive* breast cancer to determine whether the cancer has spread to the lymph nodes or glands. When the tissue is examined pathologically the presence of cancer cells in these nodes indicates that micrometastatic spread is likely and hence adjuvant drug therapy is indicated. Where possible, axillary dissection, removing some or all of the lymph nodes, may be undertaken through the same incision as that made for the breast surgery. This would include some mastectomy and wide local excision procedures.
- *Sentinel lymph node biopsy* — axillary dissection can lead to chronic swelling, lymphoedema, of the affected arm in approximately 10–20% of individuals. Sentinel node biopsy is a new diagnostic procedure used to determine whether there is spread to the axillary lymph nodes. The procedure requires the removal of only one to three nodes for close review by the pathologist. If the sentinel nodes do not demonstrate cancer cells, this may eliminate the need to remove additional lymph nodes in the axillary area (see Appendix 1).

Primary or neoadjuvant chemotherapy For a woman who presents with a tumour greater than 3 cm in size many breast units across the UK are now offering primary chemotherapy, sometimes called neoadjuvant chemotherapy, to shrink the tumour prior to surgery (Mansi et al 1989, Richards & Smith 2000). In rare circumstances, often for the older patient, hormone therapy is used to achieve the same result. Any micrometastases that may have spread from the original tumour in the breast are also systemically treated by the chemotherapy or hormone therapy.

Throughout the chemotherapy (up to eight courses), the tumour will be assessed clinically by measurement, and radiologically by ultrasound and mammogram. When the maximum response to the medication has been achieved, surgery is considered and a mastectomy should be the surgery of choice. Sometimes, at the end of the chemotherapy, the tumour is no longer detectable radiologically, but limited surgery in the previous location of the tumour is recommended as small lesions are not always seen radiologically. Radiotherapy is then given to the breast or the chest wall to complete the local treatment.

Radiotherapy Otherwise known as teletherapy, this local treatment is usually advised following a wide local excision to reduce the risk of cancer recurrence in the remaining tissue and to protect the woman from the disease recurring systemically. Research has demonstrated that women with high-risk breast cancer survived significantly longer if they were treated with both chemotherapy and radiotherapy, supporting the use of radiotherapy as a local treatment (Overgaard et al 1997). If the axillary lymph nodes are not all removed and are found to contain cancer, they are also commonly irradiated. The supraclavicular region may also be irradiated. Radiotherapy is not always considered necessary following a mastectomy although it may be used if the tumour was large or multifocal.

Treatment is given at a measured dose of 2.0 gray/day to 25 doses, or fractions, or at 2.67 gray/day in 15 fractions (see Ch. 31). Radiotherapy is usually given to the breast over a period of 3–6 weeks, three to five times a week. Radiotherapy travels in straight lines only and is given at different angles to protect the delicate lung tissue and the heart from receiving high doses of radiation. The potential side-effects are erythema and soreness of the skin over the treated area, and a general feeling of tiredness towards the end of the treatment period. All patients should be given clear advice about skin care during their radiotherapy treatment. They should be encouraged to use aqueous cream or E45 to moisturise the area that is receiving the radiotherapy and should wash or shower the area during the treatment period using tepid water and a very mild soap. Patients should wear loose-fitting, cotton clothing next to their skin and avoid wearing underwired bras. Towards the end of treatment some women may need to wear a loose tee-shirt or an unstructured bra support. The College of Radiographers has produced helpful guidelines on the assessment and care of skin reactions and how to look after them (Glean et al 2001).

Psychologically it may be quite distressing for the woman to attend an oncology/radiotherapy department several times a week, as this is a continual reminder that she has had breast cancer. Tiredness seems to be a problematic issue for women who are undergoing breast radiotherapy and support for the woman during this time is important (Faithfull 1998).

Radiotherapy may be administered wholly or partly by iridium wire implants, otherwise known as brachytherapy. The patient may be nursed in an isolation room for around 5 days until the required dose of radiotherapy has been given. The radioactive wires are then removed. The main advantage of this method is its ability to deliver high doses of radiotherapy to the area from which the tumour was removed. Radiotherapy is discussed in more detail in Chapter 31.

Adjuvant chemotherapy Over 50% of women who present with an invasive breast cancer will already have micrometastatic spread, so adjuvant systemic medical therapy should be given with the aim of destroying the cancer cells that have escaped from the original tumour (Powles et al 1998). When breast cancer is present in the axillary lymph nodes, the chance of a woman developing distant metastases is high. Systemic medication circulating to all areas of the body have been shown to reduce the chance of metastases developing or to increase the length of time before metastases become apparent.

Premenopausal women who have positive axillary lymph nodes are likely to benefit from cytotoxic chemotherapy. A commonly used regimen was cyclophosphamide, methotrexate, 5-fluorouracil (CMF) although this has been superseded by the combination of CMF with epirubicin. Eight courses of this chemotherapy given over 7 months have been shown to be more effective in the adjuvant setting than the classic CMF regimen (Poole et al 2003).

Postmenopausal women are also being offered chemotherapy, particularly if they have positive axillary lymph nodes. Pre- and postmenopausal women whose axillary lymph nodes are free of cancer have traditionally not received adjuvant therapy. However, some doctors are now advising adjuvant chemotherapy or endocrine therapy, as studies have indicated improvements in survival and time to recurrence (EBCTCG 1998a). More detailed information on chemotherapy and its management is given in Chapter 31. The common side-effects of chemotherapy for breast cancer are listed in Table 7.4.

Table 7.4 Possible side-effects of chemotherapy regimens used in the treatment of breast cancer

Side-effect	Comment
Lethargy	All drugs to some degree, but especially doxorubicin, epirubicin, cyclophosphamide
Anorexia/altered taste	Usually only temporary with most regimens
Nausea and vomiting	More common with doxorubicin
Mouth ulceration	Particularly methotrexate, epirubicin and doxorubicin
Diarrhoea	Rarely, but more commonly with 5-fluorouracil (5FU)
Bone marrow depression, specifically neutropenia	Greater where doxorubicin and taxanes used
Alopecia	CMF: some; doxorubicin, epirubicin and taxanes: complete (but scalp cooling may reduce this if available)
Red urine	Doxorubicin
Reactivation of radiotherapy sites	Doxorubicin
Nail pigmentation	5FU
Hypersensitivity reaction	Taxanes

High-dose chemotherapy In some solid tumours there is a direct correlation between the dose of chemotherapy and the response of the tumour. Giving higher doses of chemotherapy can lead to greater cell kill, but it will also cause more side-effects and toxicities. High-dose chemotherapy was assessed as part of several randomised trials throughout the world for women with a high number of involved lymph nodes. As it was not demonstrated to be very effective, it is not used routinely at present (Lake & Hudis 2004).

Further research will be necessary to determine if this treatment provides a real survival advantage.

Endocrine therapies Many breast cancers are thought to be stimulated by female sex hormones, particularly oestrogen. Endocrine therapies act by interfering with the synthesis of oestrogen or preventing it from exerting an effect on cells.

The medication tamoxifen, which competes with oestrogen receptors in the cytoplasm of the cell and so blocks oestrogen from stimulating breast cancer cell growth, has been found to be effective in many women with breast cancer. Tamoxifen is generally more effective in women who are postmenopausal and who have high levels of oestrogen receptors. When the woman's tumour is biopsied or removed, it is stained immunocytochemically for oestrogen receptors. A percentage value is given for the number of receptors that stain positive, e.g. 75%, and this indicates whether the tumour is particularly sensitive to oestrogen. Because it is fairly well tolerated, tamoxifen is given to most post- and premenopausal women as an adjuvant therapy, regardless of whether there is spread to the lymph nodes.

A selection of aromatase inhibitors are now being offered to women as alternatives to tamoxifen. As selective inhibitors of the aromatase enzymes involved in the synthesis of oestrogen, anastrozole (Arimidex), exemestane (Aromasin), formestane (Lentaron) and letrozole (Femara) are all available for clinical use. By preventing oestrogen formation these drugs may cause oestrogen withdrawal symptoms such as hot flushes and night sweats. There is also the potential problem in the long term of musculoskeletal changes causing aching joints and possibly a loss of bone density (Fenlon 2003).

Ovarian suppression is particularly relevant for women who are still menstruating and have an oestrogen-positive tumour. Suppression may be achieved by surgical removal of the ovaries or radiotherapy to ablate the ovaries. For younger women who have not had a child, luteinising hormone releasing hormone (LHRH) analogues such as goserelin (Zoladex) can be used. Goserelin is given as a subcutaneous bolus injection and prevents the ovaries producing oestrogen. Once the injections are stopped, the effect is usually reversed.

Biological therapies New therapies for the treatment of cancer are regularly discovered. Trastuzumab (Herceptin), a monoclonal antibody that binds to the cell surface receptor human epidermal growth factor receptor 2 (HER_2) has recently been utilised for treating metastatic breast cancer. The cancer must be tested for the overexpression of HER_2 (Lewis et al 2004) and, if present, trastuzumab is administered as a weekly i.v. infusion. Trastuzumab targets the cancer cells and binds to the HER_2 cell surface receptors, preventing the cell from dividing. The medication also stimulates the immune system further to kill the breast cancer cells. Side-effects may include infusion-related chills and fever, usually following the first infusion, for which antihistamines usually prove effective treatment. Trastuzumab may cause cardiac dysfunction, particularly if given with anthracycline chemotherapy. Trastuzumab is now given as a single agent or with taxane chemotherapy.

STOP THINK **7.7** When is a woman likely to be advised that a mastectomy would be the best treatment for her?

NURSING PRIORITIES AND MANAGEMENT: Breast cancer

The pretreatment phase

The period prior to admission to hospital is usually characterised by anxiety and uncertainty. Diagnosis has often been confirmed by biopsy and so the patient's concerns are focused on her cancer, how far it has spread and the physical effects on her body of the impending surgery, chemotherapy, radiotherapy and hormone therapy. Nursing intervention at this time will include assessing the patient's situation, helping her to cope with anxiety, providing education and psychological support and assisting her in making informed choices with regard to treatment options.

Assessment

There may be limited time available for assessment at this stage, but where possible the nurse should try to identify the following:

- The woman's reaction, and that of her family, to the diagnosis or potential diagnosis of breast cancer
- The major fears and concerns of the woman and her family
- The woman's feelings about body image changes that may result from any proposed treatments
- The woman's knowledge of breast cancer and cancer generally, how much information she has been given by medical staff, how much she has understood and how much she wants to know
- Whether the woman has any previous experience of another member of her family having breast cancer or any other kind of cancer
- The kind and degree of support available to the woman through family and friends. Northouse et al (1995) found that patients and their partners who reported high levels of social support also reported fewer adjustment difficulties after surgery. Husbands consistently reported that they received less support than their wives from friends, nurses and doctors
- Concurrent stressors, e.g. recent bereavements, divorce, financial difficulties
- Previous anxiety/depression. Watson (1991) found that women who had experienced previous anxiety/depression were more likely to re-experience this following diagnosis and treatment.

The treatment phase

Assessment

On the patient's admission to hospital, the nurse should undertake a more comprehensive assessment, including medical history, family history and a full physical and psychological assessment. In particular, the factors relevant in the pretreatment phase should be reassessed to determine if the woman's needs and concerns have changed. Particular note should be made of preoperative shoulder function if axillary surgery is to be performed. Good communication between the patient, ward nurses and the specialist breast care nurse will help to identify any particular psychological or social issues important to the patient that may affect her coping abilities and recovery from the surgery.

Preoperative preparation

The reader is referred to Chapter 26 for a detailed discussion of clinical considerations in preoperative care.

Giving psychological support

The nurse should give each patient the opportunity to discuss her fears but must respect her wishes if she prefers not to disclose her feelings. Where possible, a quiet, private room should be set aside for patients to spend some time in solitude or to talk privately with a nurse, doctor or family members.

Relaxation tapes can be comforting at a time when the patient may feel isolated and insecure. A relaxed but professional atmosphere on the ward will also help, as will allowing women to remain in their day clothes, open visiting and permitting them to go out for meals or a walk.

Patient education

In addition to the issues discussed in the pretreatment phase (see above), the preoperative routine should be explained, including the approximate time of surgery and the timing and type of premedication to be administered.

The patient should be told that she may have drainage tubes in situ on return from theatre, sometimes in the breast wound and often in the axilla to prevent the collection of blood and serous fluid beneath the suture line. The patient should be advised that she can pick up the drains and walk around with them in place and reassured that it is difficult to dislodge the tubing as it is sutured in place. Sutures to the breast and axillary wound are usually subcutaneous and dissolvable, with paper stitches such as Steri-strips to the skin holding the wound edges together. A light dressing is all that is needed to cover the breast scar, although surgeons may have their own dressing preferences. It is worth telling the woman what sort of dressing to expect as she may think that the breast wound will be exposed on her return from theatre, which might be distressing.

A patient undergoing axillary dissection should be warned that she may experience discomfort on moving her arm for a few weeks postoperatively. The nurse should stress the importance of postoperative exercises and should refer the patient to a physiotherapist who can assess shoulder function preoperatively and teach exercises that can be used following surgery. Written information about the arm exercises is provided so that the woman can continue with them after she has been discharged. Because the axillary lymphatic system has been compromised by the surgery, nursing care should include informing the patient about their risk of lymphoedema and how to take preventive measures. Advice should address the following:

- Taking care not to develop infection in the affected arm by avoiding injections and vein puncture in that arm. An infection in the arm could further compromise the lymphatic system by causing localised swelling and inflammation.
- Avoiding the affected arm when blood pressure is manually recorded.
- Trying to avoid cuts and scratches in the arm and if damage to the arm does occur washing the area carefully with soap and applying an antiseptic cream to the wound.
- Reporting any signs of infection to the GP or the hospital.
- Wearing protective gloves when gardening.
- Avoiding insect bites by using insect repellent.
- Using a thimble for sewing.
- Avoiding the use of a wet-shave razor for removal of underarm hair by using depilatory cream or an electric razor instead.
- Taking care not to burn in the sun and using protective sun cream.
- Using the arm as normally as possible as regular movement will help lymph drainage.

The possibility of an intravenous fluid or blood transfusion in the immediate postoperative period should also be explained so that the patient does not become alarmed at finding one in place.

Patients often find it helpful to be told of the expected appearance of the surgical scar. Wound size and position, and the type of suturing to be used can be mentioned. Drawings and photographs may be helpful aids. It is important to warn the patient that, because the breast is so vascular, bruising and swelling are expected postoperatively. She should be reminded of this when she first looks at the scar.

Postoperative care

The nursing care of patients following surgical intervention is discussed in detail in Chapter 26. The following discussion will focus on considerations that are particularly relevant to breast surgery. The reader is also referred to Nursing Care Plan 7.2.

Wound management (see also Ch. 23) The size and position of the wound will depend on the operation performed. Generally, a low-suction drain is placed beneath the breast wound and another to the axillary region to reduce the likelihood of a seroma (see p. 343) forming. Initially, the drains and the wound dressing should be observed frequently for signs of excessive blood loss. Undue blood loss should be reported to medical staff immediately.

The wound drains will remain in situ for 2–5 days until the wound drainage is minimal, usually less than 50 mL/day. The nurse should ensure that the drains are patent and that, unless informed otherwise, suction is maintained; drainage volume should be recorded. Removal of the drains can be painful; this should be explained to the patient and removal should be preceded by the administration of oral analgesics or Entonox.

Some breast units permit patients to go home with the axillary drain still in situ. The woman, and a member of her family, are given instructions on management of the wound drain and wound care. The district nurses should be involved in the patient's early discharge, and will empty and finally remove the surgical drains at home (Chapman 2001). Close contact is usually maintained with the hospital and patients are asked to notify the hospital should the drain become loose or blocked or cause pain. Early discharge with the axillary drain still in situ is a new area of research. The work that has been done shows that, with good support, it is safe and does not cause any greater psychological distress for patients (Bundred et al 1998, Chapman 2001).

The wound should also be observed for signs of infection, i.e. redness, swelling, pain and discharge. Temperature and pulse should be monitored 4- to 6-hourly and a raised temperature brought to the attention of the medical staff.

Wound dressings should be changed only if they are being saturated by wound exudate. Unnecessary dressing changes reduce the rate of wound healing and increase the risk of infection. The wound dressing can be removed 48 h after the surgery if the wound is clean and dry (see Ch. 23). The patient can have a shower or bath at this point, providing that the wound is not soaked and the patient carefully pats the area dry with a clean towel.

The nurse must also consider other factors, such as nutritional intake, medication, stress and concurrent illness

Nursing Care Plan 7.2 Care for a woman who has undergone a mastectomy

Nursing considerations	Action	Rationale	Expected outcome
1. Potential problem of wound complications (infection, haematoma, seroma) and delayed wound healing	• Check drains half-hourly for blood loss. Change drainage if necessary and record volume of drainage. Check wound for swelling	Haemorrhage may occur, compromising patient's health, and may necessitate return to theatre	Prevention of infection where possible and early detection of problems and promotion of wound healing
January 10	• Observe wound for signs of infection (erythema, oedema, heat, pain, discharge)	Infection may delay wound healing and compromise general health. Medical treatment may be needed to control infection	There will be no signs of infection or bleeding
	• 4-hourly temperature and pulse	Increased temperature and pulse may indicate infection	
	• Aseptic dressing change only when absolutely necessary	Wound will heal more quickly if undisturbed, providing drainage is not excessive and there is no infection. Remove dressing 48 h after operation to allow air to get to the wound. Paper stitches to be removed at 10 days postop unless there is a wound infection or haematoma	
	• Assess nutritional intake and encourage balanced diet with plenty of vitamin C and protein	Vitamin C and protein are particularly important in wound healing	Patient will eat a balanced diet while in hospital
	• Assess amount of sleep and rest patient has had postoperatively. Where inadequate, consider anxiety reduction, pain control, night sedation to promote rest	Adequate sleep and rest are important in promoting wound healing	She will have at least 6 h sleep each night and report feeling stronger each day

Evaluation

January 11

Returned from theatre 12.30 h. All vital signs stable, now checked 4-hourly. Wound drainage 40 mL in last 4 h. Wound covered by light adhesive dressing.

January 12

Slight pyrexia of 37.4°C, but no other sign of infection. Wound discharge was 100 mL in 24 h (axilla 60 mL; breast 40 mL). Not sleeping well at night but managed to sleep a little today and does not wish for night sedation to be given.

January 13

Apyrexial and wound drainage reduced to 40 mL in 24 h. Slept better last night. Did not want early discharge with axilla drain in situ despite district nurse making contact prior to patient's admission.

January 14

Both wound drains removed today and wound dressing replaced. Wound is moist close to axilla and has oozed a little serous fluid but temperature remains normal.

January 15

Wound still a little moist close to axilla. Going home today so discussed signs of infection and advised visit to GP if they occur. Also advised that a seroma could form in axilla and to contact ward if this happens and arrange for an aspiration. Patient stated that she was worried about anything happening to her wound, particularly that it would open up, but said she was reassured following our discussion.

DISCHARGED

Continued ▶

Nursing Care Plan 7.2 Care for a woman who has undergone a mastectomy *(Continued)*

Nursing considerations	Action	Rationale	Expected outcome
2. Anxiety/distress due to altered body image as a result of mastectomy and diagnosis of cancer (Salter 1988)	• Give patient time and opportunity to express and explore feelings concerning cancer diagnosis and breast loss	Expression of feelings may help patient to clarify how she feels and relieve anxiety	Some anxiety will be alleviated
January 12	• Encourage patient to discuss feelings with partner where appropriate	Partner may then be more easily able to understand and support and give reassurance that she is still attractive	Patient will have more acceptance of changed body image
	• Give information about scarring, e.g. bruising, sutures, position (photos shown pre-op may help)	May help to have realistic expectations of wound and know that bruising etc. will fade	
	• Offer to remain with patient when she first looks at wound, assess reaction and give support in discussing feelings afterwards	Moral support may help patient to sum up courage to look at the wound	Patient will be able to look at scar before discharge
	• Fit temporary prosthesis after removal of the drains and show how to use. Show silicone prosthesis if desired and make fitting appointment	A prosthesis may increase a woman's confidence to face the outside world and regain a healthy body image	Patient will be able to fit temporary prosthesis into bra before discharge
	• Discuss possibility of breast reconstruction if not previously mentioned	Breast reconstruction is known to be helpful for some women in coping with breast loss. Woman herself is best one to judge value for her	Patient will understand types of reconstruction possible
	• Refer to specialist nurse if one exists	Specialist nurses have been shown to aid rehabilitation and may lower anxiety and depression postoperatively	
	• Offer written information on breast cancer, prostheses, clothing, etc.	Practical help may increase a woman's confidence to take up her usual social activities and feel she is still the same as ever	
	• Ask if she would like voluntary visitor to be put in touch and arrange if desired	Some women find others who have had similar operations a great help and encouragement	

Evaluation

January

Stated that she is very frightened that cancer may recur in the future. Her friend died 2 years ago from breast cancer metastases and this fills her with fear.

Temporary prosthesis fitted today and appointment made for 6 weeks after discharge. Mrs X also looked at her scar for the first time. She found it was better than she imagined. She has asked that the nurse stay with her tomorrow whilst she shows her husband before she goes home.

Mrs X showed her husband the scar today. He also told her it was much better than he had imagined and that having her was much more important than her having two breasts. Breast reconstruction was mentioned again but Mrs X is sure she will not want this. To be followed up by clinical nurse specialist who saw her again today and gave her a booklet from Breast Cancer Care.

Continued ▶

Nursing Care Plan 7.2 Care for a woman who has undergone a mastectomy *(Continued)*

Nursing considerations	Action	Rationale	Expected outcome
3. Difficulty moving arm due to discomfort following axillary dissection	• Refer to physiotherapist • Analgesics before physiotherapy • Encourage to practise arm exercises four times a day	Shoulder exercises are known to decrease the problems of reduced shoulder functioning that can result after an axillary dissection	To achieve and maintain full shoulder movement in 4 weeks and prevent 'frozen shoulder'
January 11	• Give written information sheets to reinforce what exercises to do and when	Written information will reinforce that given verbally and serve as a reminder after discharge home from hospital	Will be able to demonstrate physiotherapy exercises and perform four times each day
4. Pain January 10	• Regular analgesics initially postop. Assess effectiveness. Particularly important prior to physiotherapy	Regular analgesics more likely to be effective than PRN medication	Patient will report that pain is under control
	• Use pillow to support arm on affected side postop	Pillow provides a soft, comfortable support and encourages drainage of fluid back from arm	
	• Consider relaxation techniques and massage to relieve tension	Tension is known to increase experience of pain	

Evaluation

January 14

Seen by physiotherapist and commenced exercises. Patient says that she is able to move arm quite freely without much discomfort.

January 15

Has been practising arm exercises but a little more uncomfortable today and requested paracetamol prior to exercises this afternoon. She said this helped.

January 10

i.v. analgesic had been given in recovery but Mrs X has declined any further analgesics since returning to the ward.

January 11

Particularly uncomfortable when moving her arm. Had declined analgesics this morning but was persuaded that regular paracetamol for 2 or 3 days will not harm her and will help her move her arm, which is important.

January 14

Much more comfortable today and has again refused analgesics.

January 15

Requested analgesics prior to exercises today as arm feeling stiff and sore.

Continued ▶

Nursing Care Plan 7.2 Care for a woman who has undergone a mastectomy *(Continued)*

Nursing considerations	Action	Rationale	Expected outcome
5. Potential problem of lymphoedema of the arm, postoperatively or at some time in the future January 11	• Explain what lymphoedema is, how it is caused and when it may occur • Explain signs of lymphoedema and encourage to report to doctor as soon as it occurs	Information will help the patient to understand the pathological basis of lymphoedema and encourage early detection of lymphoedema should it occur	Risk of lymphoedema occurring will be reduced The patient will understand what lymphoedema is, and what to do if it occurs
	• Discuss hand and arm care: – Avoid lifting heavy objects with affected arm – Avoid injections, blood tests, blood pressure recordings in affected arm – Use gardening gloves when gardening, kitchen gloves with abrasive cleaners, thimbles when sewing – Clean any cut on hand or arm very thoroughly and apply antiseptic. If any signs of infection appear see GP for antibiotics – Use depilatory creams to remove hair under arm, rather than a razor – Elevate arm whenever possible, particularly initially after surgery – Use a gentle moisturising cream on arm to prevent cracking if skin is dry	Following removal of lymph nodes by surgery and radiotherapy, there is an increased risk of infection in the arm. These precautions reduce the risk of infection, and also the risk of infection precipitating lymphoedema	She will be able to recount how to look after her hand and arm
	• Encourage arm and shoulder exercises	Exercise is thought to reduce the possibility of lymphoedema occurring	

Evaluation

January 14

Long discussion in preparation for discharge. Her friend had lymphoedema so she is very concerned this shouldn't happen to her.

Very keen to have advice on hand and arm care and has been given a leaflet about this. Stressed that she can contact clinical nurse specialist at any time if she is concerned that her arm is swollen.

(e.g. diabetes mellitus), which may affect the rate of wound healing and resistance to infection (see Ch. 23).

Alleviating discomfort Pain from the wound will always be experienced to some degree, but pain on shoulder movement is often more of a problem. Pain is sometimes more intense a day or so after the operation when the initial numbness has faded. Patients should be encouraged to take analgesics regularly for the first 48 h, but many women find that the wound is less painful than they had expected and require oral analgesics infrequently beyond this period. It should be stressed, in any event, that it is preferable to take analgesics and continue arm exercises than to take no analgesics and avoid the exercises.

The experience of pain is influenced by many factors, such as anxiety and emotional distress (see Ch. 19). These must be considered by the nurse in her efforts to promote the patient's comfort after surgery.

Women who have had a mastectomy may experience phantom breast and nipple sensations at some point following surgery. This may be very distressing and requires the nurse to reassure her that these sensations will not continue for long. In rare cases damage to the intercostal brachial nerve may occur during surgery. If the nerve has only been bruised patients may complain of an uncomfortable tenderness (neuropraxia) but this sensation should fade over a period of weeks to months. Referral to a physiotherapist and a review of the patient's oral analgesics may help. As the bruising subsides so will the symptoms of pain and altered sensation although this may take several weeks to months.

Promotion of shoulder movement Patients who have undergone surgery involving dissection of the axillary lymph nodes are at risk of developing problems with shoulder movement. This risk is greater if radiotherapy to the axilla is given postoperatively (Lichter 1998). Postoperative exercises will help to ensure that a full range of shoulder movement is attained following surgery.

Ideally, exercises should be taught by a physiotherapist. The nurse must know what they involve, however, so that she can encourage the patient to practise them. Generally, gentle exercises are begun on the first or second postoperative day and gradually increased in extent and frequency as drainage from the wound diminishes and the axillary drain is removed.

Preparing the patient for discharge

Looking at a breast scar for the first time is often very difficult and may confirm a woman's fears about breast loss and intensify her grief. However, others find the scar neater and less distressing than they had imagined. Women who have wide local excisions may have a similar range of reactions.

The nurse should encourage a woman to look at her scar before she goes home, as this represents a significant step in rehabilitation (Denton & Baum 1983). The woman may wish to be accompanied by her partner or a nurse when first seeing her scar and this may also be the first time she talks about the loss or alteration of her breast. The woman must never be forced to look at her wound and it may not be until the first postoperative outpatient visit that she is able to take this step.

Rehabilitation proceeds at different rates, but the nurse should explain to each woman that it may take several months before she feels that her energy has returned to normal. Persistent fatigue may cause frustration and may give rise to anxiety that the cancer has returned. Fatigue is more likely if chemotherapy or radiotherapy is given postoperatively, but where it is profound, depression should also be considered as a possible contributing factor.

Most women can begin driving again in 2–3 weeks, providing they feel confident, their arm movement is not too uncomfortable and the seat belt is not pressing on the scar line. They must be confident enough to perform an emergency stop if necessary. Light household duties can be undertaken when the woman feels well enough, usually 2–3 weeks postoperatively, and she may return to work at around 6 weeks. This will, of course, depend on the extent of the surgery, the particular individual and the type of work she does.

Pain and discomfort from the wound will steadily reduce, but some discomfort often remains for 2–3 months. Paraesthesia around the scar and axilla may fade over several months, but some may always remain and can be made a little worse by local radiotherapy.

A collection of serous fluid in the breast wound or the axilla may occur postoperatively and is called a seroma. Some women believe that the large lump they can feel is cancer that has suddenly grown after surgery. Prior explanation of this and the possibility of seroma formation is likely to reduce any anxiety. The problem can be resolved by the aspiration of the fluid and may be performed as a simple outpatient procedure. Many specialist breast care nurses and nurse practitioners have been trained to carry out this intervention and patients should be informed who to contact should this problem arise.

Lymphoedema, or swelling of the arm with lymph fluid, is a possible long-term complication that can occur in anyone who has axillary surgery or radiotherapy. Women should be advised to contact their GP or hospital if they notice any swelling, and not to leave it until it becomes a problem. Lymphoedema following breast surgery is discussed on pages 344–346.

Prior to discharge, any woman who has had a mastectomy or a significantly wide local excision should be given a temporary prosthesis, shown how to position it in her bra and alter its shape, and advised how to wash it (see Box 7.15).

STOP THINK **7.8** Prepare a 10-min teaching session for your ward colleagues or fellow students on the subject of breast prostheses, including what types are available and why they are important for the patient.

Adjuvant therapy

Postoperatively, the woman will probably attend a surgical outpatient clinic where she will hear the results of her surgery, i.e. the number of lymph nodes involved with cancer, the size and grade of the tumour and the oestrogen status, all factors that will determine the need for adjuvant treatment. Following two meta-analyses published in *The Lancet*, many more women are now being offered adjuvant hormone and chemotherapy treatment. The first analysis showed that chemotherapy given to a woman with early breast cancer meant a statistically significant longer time to recurrence and a small but significant increase in survival (EBCTCG 1992). The second analysis showed that premenopausal women who are treated for an early breast cancer with adjuvant therapy have a 7–11% absolute improvement in 10-year survival (EBCTCG 1998a).

Information on radiotherapy and drug therapies should be given, as relevant, both verbally and in writing. The patient should understand why adjuvant treatment has been advised, for what period and at what intervals it will be administered, and what the side-effects may be. At this point the woman may be invited to join a research study, as several current national trials looking into effectiveness of different types of chemotherapy and hormone therapy are ongoing. The timing of this decision may put yet another strain on a woman who is already facing up to having cancer, so the support and information she receives from her oncologist, ward nurse and breast care nurse will be crucial at this time.

Box 7.15

Breast prostheses

The fitting of a breast prosthesis is an integral part of the rehabilitation of a woman who has had a mastectomy or partial mastectomy. The aim of the prosthesis is to match as closely as possible the woman's other breast in terms of size, shape, weight and feel, so that she may look natural and feel confident in clothing. This is important in helping her to resume her normal social activities and regain a healthy body image.

Temporary prostheses

A temporary prosthesis (sometimes known as a cumfie) is fitted as soon as the wound drains have been removed and is worn until a permanent prosthesis can be fitted. It is soft, light and washable, and can be pinned securely into the cup of a bra. If a bra cannot be worn because of discomfort, the prosthesis can be pinned into a camisole or slip. The woman may find that wearing loose clothing helps to achieve a balanced appearance. However, it is important that the nurse spends time fitting this prosthesis well, as it is with this that the woman will first face the outside world again.

Permanent prostheses

A permanent prosthesis is usually fitted 5–6 weeks after surgery or 2 weeks after the completion of radiotherapy, when the wound is well healed. The fitting may be undertaken by a specialist nurse, surgical appliance officer or visiting prosthesis company fitter. A private room with a full-length mirror is necessary and it is essential that each woman is treated with respect and sensitivity.

Today most permanent prostheses are made of silicone gel which feels soft and comfortable next to the skin and takes on the body's temperature. Many shapes and sizes are available; it should be possible for all women to be fitted with a prosthesis that gives a balanced appearance in a bra. Partial prostheses are available for women who have breast conservation. Silicone prostheses generally last for 2–3 years, but a woman is entitled to a replacement whenever the prosthesis begins to show signs of wear and tear or if she loses or gains weight or changes shape.

Special 'mastectomy bras' are not necessary, but the bra does need to be supportive and of the correct cup size, covering all of the tissue of the remaining breast. It is helpful if the nurse can give basic advice about bras and instruct a woman where she may be fitted for a bra locally, if her previous bras are now inappropriate. Volunteer organisations such as Breast Cancer Care give helpful advice about bras, swimwear and other clothing (see 'Useful addresses', p. 356).

Radiotherapy The possible side-effects of adjuvant radiotherapy in breast cancer are listed in Table 7.5. The nurse should also give advice on skin care for women undergoing radiotherapy.

Table 7.5 Possible side-effects of adjuvant radiotherapy used in the treatment of breast cancer

Side-effect	Comment
Erythema and soreness of the area treated	Not easily predictable
General tiredness	Especially toward the end of the treatment period
Photosensitivity	See Chapter 12; sun barrier creams should be worn for a year after therapy
Moist desquamation	Now rare because of the improved delivery of radiotherapy
Breast becomes firmer to the touch	Long-term effect due to fibrosis of tissue
Narrowing or blockage of lymph vessels	Increases risk of lymphoedema

Chemotherapy A variety of chemotherapy regimens are used and the woman may have already received chemotherapy treatment prior to her surgery. The nursing care for patients on chemotherapy regimens will be discussed separately.

Neoadjuvant (primary) chemotherapy These treatment regimens often contain an anthracycline-type drug and may need to be administered (see p. 337) via a pliable central venous catheter, sometimes known as a Hickman line. This central line is inserted through the chest wall and into the subclavian vein whilst the woman is under light sedation (see Fig. 7.16 and Box 7.16).

Peripherally inserted central catheters (PICC lines) are also a useful way of administering chemotherapy (see Ch. 31). Inserted through the antecubital fossa, the PICC line has the advantages of the Hickman line in that it can help prevent long-term damage to veins, relieves needle phobia and allows easy access for blood sampling. Central lines can represent a significant assault on the woman's body image as they protrude out of the chest wall or arm for the duration of the treatment (see Ch. 31 for the nursing care of patients receiving chemotherapy and p. 501 for disorders of white blood cells and lymphoid tissue).

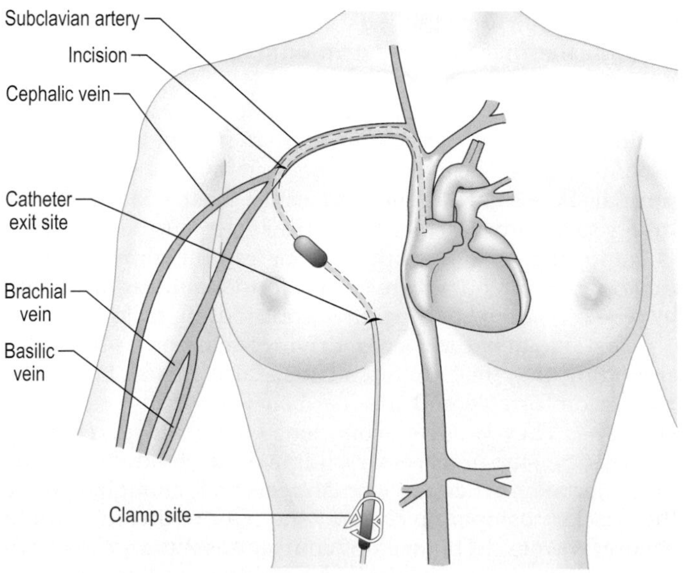

Fig. 7.16 Central line insertion.

Box 7.16

The central venous catheter for the administration of chemotherapy for breast cancer

Insertion of the central line may involve the woman having light sedation. The line is usually inserted by an anaesthetist but specialist nurses have extended their role to include this skill. The line is X-rayed after the operation to ensure that it is positioned correctly. The incision wounds will be covered with a light gauze dressing or an occlusive plastic dressing. The wound site must be cleaned and dressed regularly either by the woman herself or by the practice or community nurse; the frequency of the dressings is decided locally. The stitches should be removed from the incision site 7–10 days after the line has been inserted and from the exit site 6–8 weeks after insertion, but only if the central line was cuffed. This timing allows scar tissue to form around the line and to anchor it within the subclavian vein if it is a Hickman line. If the line is uncuffed, the exit site stitches remain in for the duration of treatment.

The woman (and often another member of her family or a close friend) will have been taught how to care for her central line. Community back-up is essential to continue the care that has been started in the hospital and to assist with the central line dressing. Infection of the exit site of the central line is common and this should be recognised quickly and treated with antibiotics, as septicaemia can develop. If this occurs, the line should be removed and the woman should be treated with i.v. antibiotics. Thromboses forming around the central line in the subclavian vein can be a problem and are indicated by blockage of the line, sometimes swelling of the arm on the side of the line and pain at the site of the thrombosis or referred into the side of the neck. An ultrasound scan or X-ray will be taken of the line for a definitive diagnosis and the woman will be started on anticoagulants. The line will be kept in situ unless the woman does not respond to the anticoagulants in which case it will have to be removed.

Provided that the site has completely healed, the woman can continue with some of her physical activities but should first check with her clinician. She can lightly shower over the central line site but, if receiving chemotherapy via a portable pump, should not get the pump wet. The line should be long enough with an extension to leave the pump outside the shower. Written instructions are often given by the hospital, including contact numbers should any problems occur.

Adjuvant therapy The patient should be reassured that the adjuvant chemotherapy regimens used in breast cancer tend to have milder side-effects than those used in the treatment of other cancers and can usually be managed by the outpatient department.

Nausea is commonly experienced but is normally mild and can be controlled by the range of antiemetics, including 5-HT_3 antagonists such as ondansetron or granisetron that are now available. Vomiting should be rare.

Thinning of the hair is to be expected in at least three-quarters of patients receiving CMF (Fisher et al 1990), though scalp cooling might help. Other breast cancer chemotherapy regimens containing an anthracycline such as adriamycin or epirubicin will cause total hair loss and the whole experience can be very stressful. Cooling the scalp with the use of ice caps can restrict the amount of chemotherapy reaching the hair follicles in the scalp and so may prevent complete hair loss, although the hair may thin and become drier and of poorer quality. Gentle shampoos should be used, and perms, colourants and the use of heated rollers and tongs should be avoided.

Bone marrow depression occurs with all cytotoxic drugs, but it is rare for neutropenia to be severe or for septicaemia to result. Nevertheless, every patient should be advised about good oral hygiene and the avoidance of obvious sources of infection. If the woman's temperature rises above normal she is usually advised to contact the hospital and to have a full blood count taken to ensure that her white cells are at an acceptable level. If the white cells are low and she is neutropenic, she may be prescribed oral antibiotics or, if necessary, admitted to hospital for intravenous antibiotics.

Fatigue is the most common problem and can be quite debilitating for the woman. Generally it is worst in the middle of a month's treatment cycle, when blood counts are at their lowest level.

A sore mouth and a susceptibility to mouth ulcers can be helped by using a soft toothbrush, salt water or medicated mouth washes.

Menstruation is usually affected, with periods becoming irregular or stopping, and this is yet another assault on the woman's body. Menopausal symptoms, e.g. hot flushes, may be experienced, but if the woman is in her early 30s, menstruation has a 90% chance of returning after chemotherapy finishes. Women in their early 40s are much more likely to go into early menopause.

Endocrine therapy Adjuvant tamoxifen is widely given in view of its relatively few side-effects and its proven efficacy (EBCTCG 1998b) although anastrozole is now being given in certain circumstances. Both pre- and postmenopausal women will usually experience menopausal symptoms, which can be very distressing. These may include fatigue, hot flushes, night sweats, joint pain, headaches and difficulty sleeping (Carpenter & Andrykowski 1999). There are vitamin and mineral preparations, often containing evening primrose oil (gamolenic acid), that can help with such symptoms; otherwise the woman's consultant or GP can prescribe medication to reduce the hot flushes. Unfortunately, these are not without side-effects and many women prefer to manage without such intervention.

Gastric upsets are uncommon but may occur, particularly if the tamoxifen tablets are not taken with food. Very occasionally, thrombocytopenia is a problem. The individual should be advised to report increased bruising or bleeding from her gums. A small increase in deep vein thrombosis and pulmonary embolus has also been noted with tamoxifen use (Fisher et al 2001) and women must inform their clinician of any new pain and swelling in their calves or sudden and unusual shortness of breath. Many women complain about an increase in weight, particularly around the abdomen, soon after starting the tablets. This may be due in part to fluid retention and in part to a reduction in physical activity following surgery. Other rare and more serious side-effects include endometrial cancer and cataract formation. Any abnormal vaginal bleeding should be investigated as well as any rapid deterioration in eyesight (Bruzzi 1998).

METASTATIC BREAST CANCER

Metastatic disease is sometimes obvious at the time of diagnosis but can occur months or many years later. Women in whom the cancer has spread to the axillary lymph nodes at the time of diagnosis are known to be at a greater risk of developing metastases at a later date. Often these metastases are too small to be detected by scans or other investigations. The rate at which breast cancer grows and metastases to other areas of the body varies and it is difficult to assess the long-term prognosis of an individual woman or to say that she is cured of the disease. It is estimated that over 50% of women who present with a breast lump already have metastatic spread (Richards & Smith 2000).

Once breast cancer has metastasised systemically, the oncologists will aim to put the disease into remission and to improve survival for the woman. The disease is no longer considered curable and the challenge for the oncologist is to give the woman prolonged life without distressing side-effects. The decision to treat should be considered carefully with the woman and her partner.

PATHOPHYSIOLOGY

The spread of breast cancer appears to be by direct invasion into the surrounding tissue and via the lymphatic and arteriovenous systems to distant areas, although this has not been proven absolutely. If untreated, local invasion of the breast cancer will cause ulceration, fixation to the chest wall and oedema of the arm. It may also, in extreme circumstances, erode blood vessels, causing haemorrhage, and invade the ribs or lungs and pleura, causing pleural effusion. Invasion of the brachial plexus can cause severe pain with functional and sensory loss in the arm. Invasion of the cutaneous nerves causes irritation and burning pain in the affected area. Because such aggressive local disease is not necessarily accompanied by metastatic spread, a woman may survive for many years with these problems.

Spread of breast cancer to distant sites is a common occurrence but may not become apparent for months or many years after the initial diagnosis and treatment. Metastases can occur anywhere and do not follow a systematic course. However, metastatic spread may be first discernible in the axillary and then supraclavicular lymph nodes, following the pattern of lymphatic drainage from the breast. The most common sites of metastases are bone, lungs, liver and brain. Less frequently, they occur in the ovaries and mediastinum and, rarely, in the stomach, oesophagus and intestine. The problems most commonly caused by metastasised breast cancer are listed in Table 7.6.

MEDICAL MANAGEMENT

Surgery rarely has a part to play in the management of metastatic breast cancer but can help with locally recurrent disease. Chemotherapy and endocrine therapy are the treatments of choice, given their systemic effectiveness. Radiotherapy plays an important role in the relief of bone pain and in the oncological emergencies of spinal cord compression, cerebral metastases and superior vena cava obstruction, where tumour pressure must be reduced quickly. In these contingencies, steroids are used in conjunction with radiotherapy to reduce the oedema in tissues surrounding the tumour and hence relieve pressure further.

The menopausal status of the patient, the site of the metastatic spread and the apparent aggressiveness of the tumour will determine which drug therapies are considered most appropriate.

Table 7.6 Common problems caused by metastatic disease in patients with breast cancer

Site of disease	Problem	Treatment
Bone	Bone pain Hypercalcaemia Spinal cord compression	Non-steroidal anti-inflammatory drugs, opiates, radiotherapy to site, chemotherapy Emergency: hydration, bisphosphonates, chemotherapy Emergency: radiotherapy and steroids
Bone marrow	Pancytopenia	Supportive blood + platelet transfusions. Chemotherapy (may cause further problems)
Lung/pleura	Pleural effusion Reduced expansion/shortness of breath with persistent cough	Pleural aspiration ± pleurodesis Low-dose morphine, codeine cough suppressant Chemotherapy/endocrine therapy
Liver	Liver pain	
Ascites	Opiates, steroids, chemotherapy Paracentesis, chemotherapy	
Skin	Ulceration/fungation Pain/irritation	Radiotherapy, chemotherapy, endocrine therapy, dressings, analgesia. For nerve pain, steroids and anti-inflammatory drugs
Brain/CNS	Confusion, headaches, nausea, vomiting, altered behaviour, convulsions	Emergency: radiotherapy and steroids Intrathecal methotrexate
Mediastinum	Superior vena cava obstruction	Emergency: radiotherapy and steroids
Axilla/supraclavicular fossa	Lymphoedema Brachial plexus pain and paraesthesia/paralysis of arm	Chemotherapy, endocrine therapy, radiotherapy Anticonvulsants, steroids and non-steroidal anti-inflammatories

Chemotherapy Disease that appears to be advancing rapidly or which involves the liver is most likely to be treated by chemotherapy. Regimens, including the taxanes paclitaxel (Taxol) and docetaxel (Taxotere), are given as outpatient infusions in conjunction with a premedication of steroids and chlorphenamine maleate (Piriton) to prevent hypersensitivity reactions. Currently, both paclitaxel and docetaxel are undergoing clinical trials as single agents or in combination with other chemotherapy agents and the short-term results are promising (Crown et al 2004).

The anthracyclines, alkylating agents, antimetabolites and vinca alkaloids are all effective at treating metastatic breast cancer and can all be given as single agents or in combination, depending on the previous treatment the woman has received.

The side-effects of chemotherapy regimens are described in Table 7.4 (p. 330).

Endocrine therapy Disease that is progressing more slowly may respond to endocrine therapies. These work more slowly but have fewer side-effects. Endocrine agents that may be used include the following:

Tamoxifen (see p. 331) This can be used in both pre- and postmenopausal women if it has not been used before as a neoadjuvant or adjuvant therapy.

Luteinising hormone releasing hormone (LHRH) analogues, e.g. Zoladex These interfere with the production of luteinising hormone and therefore oestrogen. Side-effects are the symptoms of menopause, e.g. amenorrhoea and hot flushes. These drugs are administered by subcutaneous injection every month and are only used for premenopausal women.

Anastrozole This medication inhibits aromatase enzymes that help to convert androgens to oestrogen and thus prevents the production of oestrogen. Other aromatase inhibitors can also be used (see p. 331).

Aminoglutethimide This medication inhibits the synthesis of aromatase, an enzyme needed to convert androgens produced by the adrenal glands to oestrogen. Allergic rashes are common but usually resolve if treatment continues. This is given only to postmenopausal women.

Progestogens, e.g. medroxyprogesterone acetate and megestrol acetate These are usually used as a third-line treatment when others have failed. Side-effects include an increase in appetite and euphoria. This can be helpful if a patient is depressed, nauseated and has lost her appetite; however, the steroid-type 'moon face' can develop (see Ch. 5). Weight gain is a problem, as is fluid retention, making progestogen a medication to be given with caution to any patient who has a history of cardiac disease. Glucose intolerance may be a problem so the patient should be monitored for the development of diabetes mellitus.

NURSING PRIORITIES AND MANAGEMENT: Metastatic breast cancer

Major nursing considerations

Assessment

Nursing assessment should address the physical, psychological and social impact of the disease, with particular consideration of the patient's own perception of these problems. The difficulties faced by the patient are likely to be determined in part by the site(s) of cancer spread. It should be remembered that medical priorities will not necessarily match the personal priorities of the patient and the decision to treat should be discussed carefully.

The reaction of the patient and her family to the news of progressive disease should be sensitively explored, and the nurse should assess how well they are coping. For many, the diagnosis of metastatic disease is more devastating than the original diagnosis of breast cancer, as the realisation dawns that treatment is now aimed at controlling rather than curing the illness. The patient and her family may once again experience shock, anger, denial, depression and despair as they try to come to terms with the implications of the diagnosis. They may feel that they had 'paid the price' at the time of the original diagnosis and that disease recurrence is very unfair (see Case History 7.3).

Even where cure is no longer possible, the philosophy of rehabilitation will remain at the centre of care, so that the highest quality of life can be maintained for as long as possible.

Palliative care

For a fuller discussion of the various aspects of long-term and palliative care that will be relevant to the patient with metastatic breast cancer, the reader is referred to Chapters 31 and 33. The important contribution of the nurse in controlling and managing symptoms such as pain, nausea and vomiting, fatigue, sexual problems, anxiety and shortness of breath is described in Chapters 3, 19 and 33.

STOP THINK **7.9** Consider the following questions with reference to Case History 7.3:

(a) Mrs J has extensive metastatic disease of her lumbar vertebrae. What implications does this have for nursing care?
(b) What side-effects is Mrs J likely to experience with chemotherapy?
(c) What information should the nurse give to Mrs J to prepare her for her first course of chemotherapy?

CASE HISTORY 7.3

Mrs J

Mrs J is a 54-year-old married woman with two adult children. She has a part-time job in a school, but spends a large part of each day looking after her elderly mother, who is disabled with rheumatoid arthritis and is unable to move around.

Mrs J was diagnosed as having cancer of the right breast 4 years ago. This was treated by a wide excision of the tumour with axillary clearance. Adjuvant radiotherapy was also given. At this time four axillary nodes were found to contain cancer, and Mrs J was prescribed four courses each of epirubicin and CMF chemotherapy and subsequently tamoxifen 20 mg, which she has been taking ever since. She was well until a month ago, when she began to experience pain in her back; this has since increased in intensity. On admission to hospital, a bone scan revealed extensive metastatic cancer in her lumbar spine, and a chest X-ray showed pulmonary metastases. Doctors have advised a course of taxane chemotherapy, to which she has agreed, but she is 'devastated' by the news of cancer recurrence and is extremely frightened by the thought of chemotherapy. Her other major concern is how she will manage to continue to look after her mother.

(d) Discuss other ways in which the nurse can help to allay Mrs J's anxiety about chemotherapy.

BREAST RECONSTRUCTION

Breast reconstruction may be achieved by several surgical methods but frequently includes the insertion of silicone breast implants or the transfer of a skin and tissue flap from another part of the woman's body (autologous). It may be undertaken for cosmetic reasons when women feel their breasts are too small, where one breast has failed to develop at puberty, or following breast cancer surgery which has removed part, or all, of a woman's breast. However, only the latter will be considered here.

Immediate breast reconstruction can be undertaken at the time of the mastectomy, or as a delayed reconstructive procedure. The aim of breast reconstruction following breast cancer surgery is to create a breast form which resembles the woman's other breast as closely as possible in size, shape and consistency. Complete symmetry when the woman is naked is not possible to achieve but the aim of the surgery should be that any differences are slight when she is wearing a bra.

As far back as 1986 the King's Fund Forum consensus committee statement on breast cancer treatments suggested that 'the possibility of reconstructive surgery should be discussed with all women in whom a significant loss of breast tissue will be necessary'. The recent National Institute for Clinical Excellence (NICE) guidelines on the treatment of breast cancer state that every woman should be offered the opportunity of breast reconstruction, delayed or immediate, if they need a mastectomy as part of their breast cancer treatment (NICE 2002). Breast reconstruction may help to reduce the psychological or emotional problems experienced by women after surgery or it may enable a woman to undergo a mastectomy which she would have otherwise found intolerable (Hart 1996).

The presence of bone metastases should not prohibit a woman from having reconstructive surgery if she perceives that this will improve her quality of life and she is generally well enough to undergo surgery. Only uncontrolled metastatic breast cancer is considered an absolute contraindication to breast reconstruction.

MEDICAL MANAGEMENT

Routine surgical preparation involving blood tests, chest X-ray and ECG will be undertaken prior to surgery. Photographs will be taken to aid the reconstructive surgeon during the surgery and afterwards when trying to match the shape and symmetry of the woman's reconstructed breast to her remaining one.

Several surgical techniques can be used to achieve breast reconstruction. The most common are described below.

Submuscular implant This involves inserting a silicone implant beneath the muscle overlying the chest wall. Generally this can be done only where the remaining breast is small and droops very little.

Tissue expansion An inflatable double-lumen silicone bag is inserted beneath the muscle overlying the chest wall and gradually inflated with sterile saline over a period of several weeks via a port valve and connecting tube which lie just beneath the skin. The aim of this is to slowly stretch the skin until the tissue expander is larger than the other breast. It is left overexpanded for several months and then some fluid is removed to create the natural ptosis of a breast. If the surgeon has used a 'Becker' type implant the port and the connecting tube are surgically removed, leaving a sealed prosthesis in the same 'pocket'.

Tissue expansion methods are useful when the breast reconstruction is delayed, i.e. the woman has chest wall skin that is good quality but inadequate quantity.

There has been much debate about the side-effects of using silicone because of recent claims that silicone prostheses can cause connective tissue disorders such as rheumatoid arthritis (Lipworth et al 2004). Because of the uncertainty surrounding its use many surgeons in the UK favour implants that contain sterile saline rather than silicone gel. Research into the use of silicone implants has been implemented and a study, conducted in Sweden, using a large nationwide cohort showed no association between breast implants and connective tissue disease (Nyren et al 1998).

Myocutaneous flap This involves transposing part of the latissimus dorsi muscle and overlying skin from the back, or the transrectus abdominus muscle (TRAM) and overlying skin from the abdomen, to the chest wall. If necessary, an implant can then be placed behind this. Oval scarring on the breast form results, as well as scarring on the abdomen or back and there is often a bulge where the attached muscle is folded over as it is moved to form the reconstructed breast (West 2003).

A newer surgical technique similar to the TRAM technique uses the abdominal fat and tissue only. The deep inferior epigastric artery and veins are identified and disconnected with the fat and tissue flap and then re-anastomosed with the internal mammary artery and vein. This means that the patient has less abdominal weakness than with a TRAM flap and, thus, very little risk of hernia.

These methods are generally used where a larger breast form is desired, following a radical mastectomy in which all chest wall muscle has been removed, or where radiotherapy has been given to the chest wall, causing the skin to lose its elasticity.

Reduction mammoplasty Surgery to the remaining breast may be advised if it is very large or pendulous in order to achieve as much symmetry as possible. Scarring following this procedure may be extensive and nipple sensation may be lost. These effects must be discussed with the woman beforehand.

Nipple areola reconstruction Sometimes the surgeon is able to do a subcutaneous mastectomy and leave the nipple intact. More often the nipple is not saved because of fear of cancer being present there. If this is so, a nipple areola reconstruction can be undertaken. Generally, this is done around 3 months after the initial reconstruction. The nipple may be created from the skin overlying the reconstruction, saved from the other nipple or a graft taken from the labia. The areola is usually created from an upper inner thigh skin graft. Some women do not want to undergo further surgery and opt for adhesive silicone nipples.

Breast augmentation following partial mastectomy This is usually carried out, if desired, at the time of the original surgery as it is more difficult after radiotherapy has been given. The implant is inserted into the area where tissue has been removed to reduce any alteration in breast size and shape and hence problems associated with altered body image.

Potential postoperative complications

Seroma/haematoma formation This is more likely to occur after an immediate reconstruction than if reconstruction is delayed. Serous fluid and blood may build up behind the implant in spite of the presence of wound drains, increasing discomfort and the risk of infection. Aspiration may be necessary and, occasionally, removal of the prosthesis.

Wound infection If wound infection occurs, antibiotics will be prescribed. If the infection fails to respond to these, it may be necessary to remove the prosthesis and re-attempt insertion after a 3-month recovery period. To try to avoid infection, prophylactic antibiotics will be prescribed at the time of surgery.

Necrosis This uncommon problem occurs where blood perfusion of the skin flap is inadequate and some of the tissue dies. It is more likely to occur when myocutaneous flaps are used.

Potential long-term complications

Capsular contracture A fibrous layer of tissue forms around the implant and, over time, will contract. If this contracture is severe, the implant will become hard to the touch, uncomfortable and cause the reconstructed breast to change in shape. Manual compression under local anaesthetic may break the capsule; the only alternative is to remove the implant and scar tissue and insert a replacement prosthesis. The incidence of capsular contracture requiring removal is difficult to ascertain but is likely to be around 15%; this figure increases significantly if radiotherapy is given to the breast after the reconstruction. There is some evidence that new textured implants result in a lower incidence of capsular contracture (Mulata et al 1997).

Abdominal herniation This infrequent problem may follow a TRAM flap reconstruction. The weakness in the abdominal wall resulting from this surgery is strengthened by the insertion of surgical mesh to reduce the possibility of herniation.

NURSING PRIORITIES AND MANAGEMENT: Breast reconstruction

Preoperative considerations

Assessment

Nursing assessment prior to breast reconstruction should address the following points:

- The woman's reasons for wanting a breast reconstruction. These may include wanting to eliminate the need for an external prosthesis, a desire to improve self-confidence and self-esteem or to 'feel more whole', and a desire to have greater freedom in choice of clothing (Goldberg et al 1984, Watson et al 2002, West 2003).
- The woman's expectations of breast reconstruction. A woman who has realistic expectations is more likely to be satisfied with the overall result of her reconstruction. Expectations for both physical appearance and quality of life should be assessed as, however good the reconstruction, it will not be an identical replacement for the breast that has been lost.
- The woman's knowledge of breast reconstruction and her understanding of what the surgeon has told her about the procedure and possible complications.

Giving information

The nurse has an important role in promoting realistic expectations of breast reconstruction. Showing photographs of breast reconstructions is one way of helping women to imagine what it will be like. Photographs that show the effect of the reconstruction unclothed, in a bra and under clothing are useful, but photographs should not show only the very best results.

It may also help to arrange for the patient to talk to another woman who has undergone a reconstruction, preferably by a similar method. Breast Cancer Care may be able to put the patient in touch with someone in her area if no-one is known to the nurse or consultant. Some women may also like to see an implant.

Giving psychological support

The woman who is undergoing breast reconstruction at the same time as her breast cancer surgery will be dealing with her recent diagnosis of cancer as well as with the idea of reconstruction. It may be particularly difficult for her to come to a decision about reconstruction at this time and so it should be made clear to her that refusing an immediate reconstruction does not prohibit surgery at a later date. The woman needs to have time to make her decision and should have access to a specialist nurse to go over what has been discussed (Reaby 1998).

Women considering a delayed reconstruction frequently have second thoughts about undergoing further surgery. The nurse can help by taking time to clarify with the patient her worries and concerns and her desire for reconstruction. Concurrent stresses and the woman's family situation should also be assessed and discussed, as these may influence how she feels about undergoing reconstruction and how she will cope postoperatively.

Postoperative considerations

Wound management

The aims and principles of wound management are described in detail in Chapter 23.

The following points are of particular relevance to wound healing following breast reconstruction.

The nurse should observe the wound for signs of necrosis, haematoma, seroma and infection. Wound drainage should be observed and the volume recorded every 30 min for the first 2 h after return from theatre and then at gradually increasing intervals. Circulatory perfusion of skin flaps should be checked with the same frequency. The skin flap should be gently pressed using a blunt tongue depressor; it should blanch and then quickly return to a pink colour once the pressure is released. This is particularly important where an autologous flap has been used in reconstruction and where tissue expansion is placing the wound under some tension. If the colour returns slowly, the flap looks blue or feels cold to the touch, the doctor should be informed in case it is necessary to take the patient back to theatre.

Temperature and pulse should be recorded 4-hourly. Dressings should be changed only if they become saturated with wound exudate or if it becomes essential to view the wound. Frequently, pressure dressings are applied in theatre and remain in place for 1–3 days. When these are removed, transparent dressings such as OpSite or Tegaderm are useful. Subcutaneous sutures are normally used and remain in situ for 10–14 days unless they are of the dissolvable variety. Discomfort from wounds will vary. Immediate reconstructions involving the removal of axillary lymph nodes and the more complicated surgical procedures involving raised tissue flaps will be the most uncomfortable. Opiate analgesics may be required by i.v. injection or continuous infusion pump for the first 2 days; after this time, oral analgesics are usually sufficient. Promoting comfort will increase rest and sleep and so encourage healing and general rehabilitation.

Patient education

Postoperative exercises should be taught, preferably by a physiotherapist, to all patients that have undergone breast reconstruction. Some surgeons prefer shoulder movement to be restricted to 90° flexion and abduction for 2–3 weeks, particularly if the scar is very tight or if they fear movement of the implant. Because the silicone implant is usually placed behind muscle, as the muscle contracts, tightening or discomfort may be experienced. This should disappear as the muscle accommodates the implant.

Advice about bras is commonly sought. Some support is likely to increase comfort and sports bras are usually the best option. Underwired bras should be avoided for the first few months. Surgical breast supports may be recommended for a few weeks. A partial prosthesis will need to be fitted to obtain a symmetrical appearance during tissue expansion and sometimes following reconstruction.

Giving psychological support

Although having a reconstruction after a mastectomy may help a woman to cope and foster rehabilitation, research indicates that many women mourn the loss of their breast and suffer from anxiety and depression following surgery (Dorval et al 1998). The nurse should not assume that a woman who has had an immediate reconstruction will have no problems related to a changed body image.

Women undergoing tissue expansion often experience frustration at the length of time the process takes to complete reconstruction. Some find it difficult to cope with an inequality in breast size and shape during this time (Goin & Goin 1988). Acknowledgement of these feelings, adequate opportunity to discuss them and access to counselling may help the woman to cope.

When complications do occur and an implant has to be removed, the individual may suffer further psychological distress. A wait of about 3 months is generally required before another implant can be inserted; during this time the woman will have to cope with another alteration in body image. Anxiety, depression and feelings of anger or despair may result. Some women may decide that they do not wish to undergo a further attempt at reconstruction. The nurse should support the patient whatever her decision and encourage her to express her feelings about the reconstruction and what it means to her.

LYMPHOEDEMA IN BREAST CANCER

Lymphoedema is the accumulation of a high-protein fluid in the interstitial spaces between cells in the tissue of a limb or other area. It is the result of a defective mechanism of lymph drainage due to tissue fibrosis, disease or a congenital disorder.

Approximately 28% of women with breast cancer will develop some degree of lymphoedema (Mortimer et al 1996), characterised by a swollen arm, often with some swelling of the adjacent chest and back. This condition can cause considerable physical and psychological distress (Woods 2003).

PATHOPHYSIOLOGY

All women with breast cancer who have axillary surgery to remove some or all of their axillary lymph nodes, or those who receive radiotherapy to the axillary region, are at risk of developing lymphoedema of the limb on the affected side. Scarring from these treatments will result in the closure or narrowing of many lymph vessels and so reduce the efficiency of lymphatic drainage from the arm. For most women, the drainage remains adequate and collateral vessels may develop to increase the pathways for drainage. However, lymphoedema may develop weeks, months or years after surgery or radiotherapy, sometimes following a wound complication, cording, infection or injury, but often without an obvious reason. It may remain mild or gradually progress until the arm is so heavy that it is difficult to lift and to use. Over time, fibrosis within the tissue of the arm may occur, causing hardness. There is also a higher risk of infection and cellulitis, as the high-protein fluid is an ideal breeding ground for bacteria.

Disease within the axillary area which causes an obstruction to lymph flow will also cause lymphoedema. This may be seen when cancer has recurred or when a woman presents with an advanced carcinoma of the breast. Signs of venous obstruction are sometimes seen. These are commonly a pink colouring of the arm and distended veins visible on the upper arm and chest wall.

Brachial plexus nerve damage is rarely seen, but may also result from radiation fibrosis or cancer infiltration of the nerve plexus, causing weakness, paraesthesia or nerve pain.

MEDICAL MANAGEMENT

Treatment Options for medical management are at present limited. The choice of treatment depends on whether the lymphoedema has been caused by fibrosis or by axillary disease. Assessment may include CT scanning and colour

Doppler ultrasound to determine the amount of scarring, venous obstruction or disease.

Previously, attempts to reduce the size and weight of the arm by surgically removing a large amount of tissue have had very little success and have frequently caused further problems with infection, swelling and pain as well as extensive scarring. Where venous obstruction is due to a thrombosis, anticoagulation therapy with warfarin may be used.

In the case of axillary disease, surgery to remove as much of the cancer as possible may be of use by reducing the obstruction of lymph and venous flow. However, chemotherapy or endocrine therapies, which have the advantage of not causing the same disruption to normal structures as surgery, are more likely to be used.

Pain relief Analgesics ranging from paracetamol to opiates will be used as required. If, however, the pain is due to brachial plexus damage by disease or radiotherapy, it is unlikely to respond adequately to opiates since nerve pain is only partly opiate responsive (Twycross 1996). Anticonvulsants, serotonin reuptake inhibitor antidepressants, steroidal and non-steroidal anti-inflammatory drugs (NSAIDs) and, in some cases, anti-arrhythmics may be effective. These should be used under the guidance of the palliative care team (Twycross 1996).

Cellulitis The risk of infection in a swollen limb is high. A small cut or insect bite may provide an entry point for infection and result in severe cellulitis requiring treatment by antibiotics. If cellulitis is recurrent, patients are often given a prescription to have on hand so they may obtain antibiotics as soon as infection occurs.

NURSING PRIORITIES AND MANAGEMENT: Lymphoedema

Major considerations

Treatment effectiveness is measured in terms of the reduction in size and weight of the arm, and for most people this is possible. However, sometimes all that can be done is to increase the softness and movement of the arm and to reduce the discomfort, but these improvements can represent a substantial increase in the quality of life for the patient.

Assessment

Nursing interventions must be preceded by an assessment to identify the physical and psychosocial needs of the individual patient.

Physical assessment should address the following areas:

- General information such as medical history, particularly of any surgery or radiotherapy, disease in the axilla and any information that the patient feels is relevant to their limb swelling
- Physical examination of the limb including the condition of the skin of the arm: colouring, presence of cuts/infection, previous cellulitis
- The size of the arm. Both arms should be measured at 4-cm intervals from a fixed point at the wrist to the root of the limb so that a comparison can be made and the severity of the oedema estimated to form a baseline for treatment. There are specialised calculators available that can take these circumferential measurements and convert them into a volume, providing a more accurate estimate of lymphoedema swelling
- The duration of the oedema and any precipitating or aggravating factors
- Presence of oedema in the adjacent tissue of the chest wall
- Any previous treatment for lymphoedema
- The type and severity of any discomfort experienced
- The individual's range of shoulder movement and ability to use the arm in activities of daily living.

Psychosocial assessment should include:

- how the lymphoedema has affected the woman's self-esteem and body image
- how the lymphoedema has altered the woman's lifestyle, work and social role and how she feels about this
- whether the swelling has affected the type of clothing she can wear.

Nursing interventions

The aim of nursing interventions in the management of lymphoedema are:

- to reduce arm size
- to improve the use of the arm
- to improve the comfort of the arm
- to improve the shape of the arm.

All treatments involve compression of the limb to try to push more fluid back into those lymph vessels that are patent.

There are now four recognised elements to the treatment of lymphoedema: (1) skin care, (2) exercise and movement, (3) lymph drainage and (4) external containment using compression sleeves or bandaging (Woods 2003).

Patient education is very important to explain clearly the aim of each treatment regimen and to promote a realistic expectation of outcome. Although therapy is aimed at control rather than cure, the patient who is given sufficient information and is encouraged to participate in treatment is likely to adopt a more positive attitude towards her situation.

The main treatment methods are related to the degree of severity of the lymphoedema:

1. *Skin care*. Treatment would begin with emphasis on the importance of skin hygiene and care. Advice given at the time of the axillary surgery should be re-emphasised. Any infection should be treated with antibiotics and the skin of the arm should be moisturised and kept as healthy as possible.
2. *Exercise and movement*. Lymph drainage can be promoted through movement and appropriate exercise of the arm as the muscle contraction and expansion stimulates the superficial lymphatics to drain (Woods 2003). Hughes (2000) identified swimming as an ideal as the water supports the body and provides some resistance to the muscles.
3. *Lymph drainage*. Manual lymph drainage (MLD) involves specialised movements of the thumbs, fingers and hand. This type of massage can only be carried out by trained

MLD therapists. Simple lymphatic drainage (SLD) has been developed from MLD for use by patients and their relatives. The aims of SLD as with MLD are:

- to stimulate normal lymphatic drainage
- to 'milk' fluid away from the congested areas
- to improve superficial lymphatic drainage (Woods 2003).

This type of massage is light, aiming to stimulate the lymphatic vessels in the skin. Deeper massage would cause increased blood flow to the muscles causing more fluid to accumulate in the tissues and would thus be counterproductive.

4. *External containment*. This would include the use of compression sleeves or enclosing the limb with pressure bandages.
   - For women with severe lymphoedema, lymphorrhoea (leakage of lymph fluid), skin problems or difficulty using a sleeve, *compression bandaging* is the treatment of choice. Low-stretch bandages are used to bandage the fingers and hand before the arm is encased. The pressure applied should be graduated, greater pressure being applied at the lower end of the limb. The bandages should be reapplied daily. Due to the large size of the arm and of the bandages required, this may need to be undertaken on an inpatient basis which also affords an opportunity for the provision of physiotherapy, occupational therapy and psychological support. However, community nurses experienced in this technique can undertake compression bandaging in the patient's home. This is particularly helpful for those who have advanced disease and feel unwell. Bandaging of a large arm may provide great comfort and relief from pain even if it offers little hope of reducing arm size.
   - *Compression sleeves* are often used for lymphoedema management. Several specialised ready-made varieties are available, e.g. Medi, Pan-Med and Sigva. Compression must be fairly strong (around 40 mmHg) if it is to be effective. Supports such as Tubigrip are not adequate. Sleeves may be difficult to put on but once fitted are supportive and comfortable. They should be worn during the day when the patient is most active. The sleeves should not be allowed to form creases, as this will cause ridging in the swollen tissue. The sleeve, easily laundered, may need to be worn for several weeks, during which time the patient must be monitored regularly to assess the effect. If the oedema is modest, it may be possible for the arm to return to its normal size.

Lymphoedema of the arm is a difficult condition for any patient to face, particularly if they have been treated for breast cancer. With the specialist care now available, patients should be quickly assisted to manage this chronic condition (Woods 2003).

MALIGNANT FUNGATING BREAST TUMOURS

Breast cancer is the most common cancer to cause ulceration. The result can be an unpleasant, weeping, malodorous, infected wound which is psychologically very difficult to cope with. Women often express feelings of disgust and revulsion and curtail social activities because of their embarrassment. An altered body image may lead to anxiety, depression and sexual problems.

Nurses have an important role to play in supporting women with fungating tumours. By rising to the challenge of wound management and controlling symptoms such as odour and excessive wound exudate, they can help to improve the quality of life for these women. Frequently it is the community nurse who has the greatest involvement with these women and their families (see Case History 7.4).

CASE HISTORY 7.4

Mrs S

Mrs S has been referred by her GP to the community nurse for management of a large ulcerating left breast carcinoma and for psychological support. She is 65 years old and a retired civil servant. She lives with her husband in a large house, which they own. She visited her GP ostensibly to have her blood pressure checked but broke down in tears and told him that she had had a breast lump for 3 years. She hadn't told anyone, including her husband, because she 'feared the worst'. Now the lump was smelly and oozing and she could no longer hide it from her husband, who had made her visit the GP.

On visiting Mrs S for the first time, the nurse finds a withdrawn and depressed lady who has stopped going out. She is embarrassed to show the nurse her breast, which is a large ulcerating mass with nodules extending to the surrounding tissue on the chest wall. The wound is malodorous, with a large amount of necrotic tissue and a profuse discharge. Mrs S has been covering it with gauze pads but has not cleaned it for some time, as she cannot bear to look at it.

Mrs S describes her husband as supportive and loving, but she will not allow him near her any more because she feels that she is 'disgusting'. She has taken to sleeping in a separate room and avoiding him when she can.

The nurse is able to speak very briefly to Mr S, who appears caring but very anxious about his wife's condition. He is not allowed by his wife to be present during her discussion with the nurse.

PATHOPHYSIOLOGY

Ulceration occurs when breast cancer infiltrates the epithelium and causes a breakdown of the skin. The resulting wound may be superficial or deep; it may affect a small area of the breast or may be very extensive, involving part, or all, of the chest wall. Frequently, as a tumour grows, its blood supply becomes inadequate, causing central tissue death and necrosis. When such a tumour ulcerates, a large necrotic mass is revealed, providing an ideal environment for infection to develop. This in turn will increase exudate and cause odour.

As the disease progresses, ulceration becomes more extensive and may erode blood vessels, causing haemorrhage but also occlusion of the blood vessels. A lack of oxygenation of the tissues leads to tissue breakdown and a build-up of bacteria at the tumour site causing the classic malodour associated with fungating lesions (King 2003). The severity of bleeding will depend on the size of the blood vessel. Capillary bleeding causing a slow loss of blood is commonly seen, but blood loss may be life threatening if a large vessel is eroded.

Tumour involvement of the cutaneous nerves can cause pain and irritation. There is often tenderness due to inflammation in the surrounding tissues. Whilst many women have remarkably little pain from these wounds, some have severe pain.

MEDICAL MANAGEMENT

Treatment will depend on the extent and position of the tumour and on what therapy for breast cancer, if any, the woman has previously received. Management may be considered in terms of treatments to try to control the disease and interventions aimed at symptom control.

Surgery For women who have an ulcerating tumour that appears confined to the breast region, it may be possible to remove the tumour surgically by performing a mastectomy (sometimes, unfortunately, called a toilet mastectomy). Where the tumour extends to the chest wall or a large area of skin, the surgery will be more extensive and surgical closure will require a skin graft or the use of a muscle and skin flap from the abdomen or back. These have been successfully used in some women to increase their quality of life, but careful discussion with the patient beforehand is important to ensure that she understands what the surgery entails, what benefits can be expected and what risks are involved. If the woman's general health is reasonable and she has a life expectancy of more than a few months, she may feel that this approach is the best for her even if recovery is protracted.

Radiotherapy can be used with great success in controlling some breast tumours. Complete remissions are occasionally seen, but more commonly radiotherapy achieves a reduction in tumour size and in the wound symptoms.

Chemotherapy and endocrine therapy may also be used, sometimes in combination with radiotherapy. Systemic drug therapies have the added advantage of treating disease elsewhere in the body as well as in the breast.

Symptom control measures are as follows:

- Analgesics may need to be provided frequently to alleviate constant pain or to make dressing changes more comfortable. The choice of analgesic will depend on the type and severity of the pain (see Ch. 19).
- Antibiotics may be required in the fight against infection.
- Supportive transfusion may be indicated where blood loss has caused anaemia.
- Surgical debridement may be very useful in removing necrotic tissue from the wound, but it is often not possible to carry out in view of the risk of haemorrhage. Streptokinase and streptodornase have also been used in combination for the debridement of necrotic tissue, although this treatment is time consuming and there is little evidence to support their use (King 2003).
- Diathermy can be helpful in controlling bleeding points but should be used with caution, given the necrosis it causes. In severe cases of bleeding, topical adrenaline may also be applied; this too should be used with caution.

NURSING PRIORITIES AND MANAGEMENT: Fungating breast tumours

Major considerations

Assessment

The nursing assessment of a woman with a fungating breast tumour must include far more than an assessment of the wound itself. It must consider psychosocial factors such as age, concurrent disease and disabilities, drug therapies and pain. All of these factors may influence the possibility of wound healing or infection.

The woman's psychological state, her reaction to the wound, her ability to cope with it and the way it has affected her life and her family are all equally important. The nurse should bear in mind that anxiety and depression can have a significant impact on treatment outcome. Frequently it is the community nurse that has the greatest involvement with these women and their families, as hospitalisation is rarely required. Women often live for many years with a slowly progressing fungating tumour, which makes it all the more important that every effort is made to improve their quality of life.

Wound management (see also Ch. 23)

Malignant breast lesions have a pathological cause, i.e. cancer. Unless this cause is being treated, wound healing is unlikely to occur. It is important that the nurse promotes realistic expectations in the patient, so that, if she is not receiving treatment for breast cancer, she is not hoping for complete healing of the wound.

The general aims of wound management are:

- to control the symptoms produced by the wound
- to minimise possible complications, e.g. infection
- to maximise comfort and minimise discomfort
- to promote healing where possible.

Many types of wound dressing are available. In order to choose products which are likely to be most effective for a given wound, the nurse must first identify the problems that are present. The most common problems associated with ulcerating lesions are discussed below (see also Nursing Care Plan 7.3).

Tissue necrosis Where tissue necrosis exists it is likely to increase the risk of infection. Debriding the wound of dead tissue will reduce this risk. Although it may be possible to remove the bulk of necrotic tissue by surgical debridement, the risk of haemorrhage sometimes prohibits this, making topical preparations, such as the hydrogels or the hydrocolloids, the preferred treatment, even though it is a slower process.

Infection is suspected where there is a purulent wound discharge, odour, inflammation and a raised body temperature. A wound swab should be taken by the nurse so that the appropriate systemic antibiotic can be prescribed. Preparations such as metronidazole gel may be applied topically to help fight infection (King 2003). The pharmacist and the infection control team will advise about the use of particular cleaning solutions when there is wound contamination by particular organisms such as *Pseudomonas*.

Nursing Care Plan 7.3 Caring for a woman with an ulcerating breast tumour (see Case History 7.4)

Nursing considerations	Action	Rationale	Expected outcome
April 6 1. **Ulcerating left breast cancer: the wound is malodorous, necrotic, and has a profuse discharge**	• Take wound swab for culture and sensitivity	Odour and discharge may be due to infection in wound	By April 13: A reduction in wound odour
	• Twice a day: – Cleanse wound with saline using syringe and quill – Remove any areas of *loose* necrotic tissue with forceps and sterile scissors – Apply thick layer of natural live yoghurt and leave for 15 min, covering patient with sterile towel – Remove yoghurt using saline in syringe again	Quill allows gentle but thorough cleansing (no cotton wool fibres may be left which act as focus for infection). This will increase speed of debridement but should only be done on loose dead tissue and should not be painful Natural *live* yoghurt very good at deodorising but need to leave 15 min to work	Reduction in necrotic tissue Amount of wound drainage will be reduced and controlled by wound dressings Mrs S will state that she finds her dressing comfortable and that the symptoms have improved
	• Apply Hydrogel wound dressing		
	• Cover with dressing, taking care to protect sore and friable areas with petroleum jelly	Dressing necessary to ensure Hydrogel is kept in place	
	• Apply absorbent secondary dressing containing charcoal, e.g. CliniSorb	Absorbent secondary dressing used because of profuse discharge. Charcoal helps to deodorise	
	• Keep in place with Netelast	Using Netelast reduces trauma to friable skin on chest wall	
	• Suggest change bedclothes frequently and open windows each day	These measures will help to prevent the odour lingering in the house	
April 10	• Apply Sorbsan instead of Hydrogel. Continue with rest of dressing	Sorbsan has a haemostatic action. Though more gentle than Varidase, it is also very absorbent	

Evaluation

April 10

Hydrogel debriding wound well but wound bleeding close to medial edge. Using Sorbsan to stop bleeding. Will continue with yoghurt.

April 13

Discharge reduced and now controlled by Sorbsan dressing. Odour much less obvious but still present, therefore will continue with yoghurt, Sorbsan and charcoal dressings.

Wound swab indicates *Staph. aureus* infection. GP will visit tomorrow and prescribe a course of antibiotics.

Continued ▶

Nursing Care Plan 7.3 Caring for a woman with an ulcerating breast tumour (see Case History 7.4) *(Continued)*

Nursing considerations	Action	Rationale	Expected outcome
April 6 **2. Embarrassment and disgust at wound causing:** (a) Difficulty in communicating with husband (b) Social isolation (c) Reduced self-esteem	• Dress wound to control symptoms of odour and discharge	If symptoms of odour and discharge are controlled Mrs S will be more likely to go out again and not feel so self-conscious	
	• Encourage Mrs S to express her feelings about her wound and the way it is affecting her life	This may help Mrs S to 'let go' of tension, to see her situation more clearly and to allow her to accept support from the nurse. It will also help the nurse to identify specific problems/concerns	Mrs S will verbalise her feelings about her wound
	• Encourage her to talk about her relationship with her husband and how it has altered	This will help the nurse to understand how they used to communicate and how close their relationship was. This will help her to plan intervention which may improve communication and mutual support	She will identify how her relationship with her husband has changed
	• Assess her social support and what sort of activities she used to do	This will indicate what the norm was for Mrs S and how things have changed. It will allow the nurse to know what activities and relationships she might encourage Mrs S to take up again	
April 10	• Suggest that Mr and Mrs S sit down together and discuss how they feel about the cancer, the wound and how it has altered their life	This would allow Mr and Mrs S to begin communicating again and to break down barriers so that they can support each other	Mr and Mrs S will discuss together how they both feel about Mrs S having breast cancer and an ulcerating lesion
April 13	• Suggest Mrs S should go out to her daughter's next week for tea	Mrs S is close to her daughter. As her wound is improving, this is an appropriate first step in taking up her social life again	She will arrange to go out to visit her daughter by April 20
	• Arrange for Mrs S to visit hospital for partial prosthesis to be fitted	Mrs S has voiced concern about her appearance in clothes. A partial prosthesis will enable her to regain a balanced appearance	
	• Discuss the choice of loose clothing to minimise the altered shape due to the dressings		

Continued

Nursing Care Plan 7.3 Caring for a woman with an ulcerating breast tumour (see Case History 7.4) *(Continued)*

Evaluation

April 10

Mrs S says she feels very down today. Expressed feelings of guilt that she hadn't sought help before and believes she has let her husband down. She knows that he loves her but believes he cannot possibly want to be near her because of her wound's odour. She describes her marriage as previously very strong. They used to talk about most things but both find it difficult to express their feelings to each other and have not spoken of the cancer diagnosis or what will happen now. She has spoken to her daughter, who has said they should all talk about it. She would like to, but doesn't feel she can. I reinforced that I felt it would be a good idea and offered to be present if that would help. She will think about it.

April 13

Mrs S is feeling better. She is very pleased that her wound is more manageable and particularly that it is less smelly. I suggested she might consider going out. She is hesitant about this but I suggested perhaps a couple of hours with her daughter. She is still conscious of the wound and feels everyone will know something is wrong because her appearance is not balanced due to the dressings and tumour itself distorting her breast shape. I suggested partial prostheses may help this and she is very keen on this idea.

Nursing considerations	Action	Rationale	Expected outcome
April 6 **3. Fear of breast cancer**	• Assess Mrs S's information needs by finding out what her knowledge of breast cancer is and identifying misconceptions she may have	Providing appropriate information may help to allay anxiety and remove misconceptions	Mrs S will specify the fears she has about breast cancer
	• Encourage Mrs S to express and explore her feelings concerning breast cancer	This is often therapeutic in itself but also allows the nurse to more accurately identify her fears	She will define her information needs concerning breast cancer and its treatment
	• Offer literature about breast cancer	Written information reinforces verbal information	
April 7 **4. Fear of dying in pain. Fear of nausea and vomiting**	• Reassure Mrs S that effective pain control is available. (Discuss worries about taking opiates if this is a problem for her.) Stress that nausea and vomiting can normally be controlled by medication		Mrs S will understand that pain from cancer can be effectively controlled and that nausea and vomiting, if they occur, can also be controlled by medication

Evaluation

April 7

Very upset today. Feels very guilty that she didn't go to the GP before. Feels she has let her husband down. Has always been frightened of having breast cancer, although she doesn't know anyone who has had breast cancer. She knows that it is likely that she will die from this, in spite of any treatment she may be given, and she is frightened about how this will happen. She equates cancer with a painful death and cannot bear the thought of pain or feeling nauseated.

April 10

Given booklet by Breast Cancer Care. Suggested that she should let her husband read it too. Also wanted to know about possible treatments for breast cancer of this stage. Discussed chemotherapy, radiotherapy and hormone therapy.

Continued

Nursing Care Plan 7.3 Caring for a woman with an ulcerating breast tumour (see Case History 7.4) *(Continued)*

Nursing considerations	Action	Rationale	Expected outcome
April 6	• Arrange a time to sit down and talk to Mr S	This will ensure the nurse has time specifically with Mr S	By April 13, Mr S will define areas of anxiety
5. Anxiety of Mr S due to Mrs S's condition and withdrawn behaviour	• Encourage him to express and explore his feelings and define the particular anxieties he has regarding his wife and any other areas of stress	Expression and exploration of feeling are therapeutic in reducing anxiety and will enable the nurse to assess the home situation more fully	Mr S will discuss his feelings concerning Mrs S's illness, behaviour and the ulcerating cancer
	• Assess the support systems that Mr S has and emphasise that the nurse is concerned for his welfare as well as his wife's	Many carers do not consider their own needs and consider the nurse only as a support for the patient	
	• Provide information about breast cancer and its treatment	Appropriate information may help to reduce anxiety by enabling Mr S to feel more involved and more in control of the situation	

Evaluation

April 6

Arranged to speak to Mr S tomorrow following visit to his wife.

April 7

Reluctant to discuss his feelings about his wife, preferring to dwell on his wife's problem and her feelings. Mr S fought back tears when discussing the future. However, he did say he feels angry with himself and his wife that the cancer got to this stage before medical help was sought. He feels guilty he didn't know about it and frustrated with his wife's withdrawn behaviour as he believes she will just give up and die. We discussed how control of the wound problems may give her the confidence to go out again, and how she will require his support, which he appears very willing to give.

Mr S appears to have very little support, only talking to his daughter on rare occasions about his wife. He used to talk over everything with his wife but now she won't allow this.

April 13

Seen briefly. Looks more relaxed. Has talked to GP about possible treatments and appointment to see consultant oncologist has been made for next week. Also believes that his wife is brighter because her wound has improved.

Excessive wound exudate is often due to a wound infection and hence the first action would be to treat the infection and to debride the wound as necessary. The aim of wound dressing is to absorb the maximum volume of exudate with the minimum bulk of dressing. This requires the use of a high-absorbency primary dressing, e.g. Kaltostat or Sorbsan, alginate hydrofibres, and a high-absorbency secondary dressing, e.g. CliniSorb, which has the added benefit of containing charcoal to reduce odour from the wound.

It is important to remember that once there is 'strike-through' of the secondary dressing (i.e. saturation of the dressing) a pathway exists for bacteria to move from the outside through the dressing into the wound. This should be prevented by frequent changes of the outer dressing. Waterproofing is also important. Dressings such as OpSite or Tegaderm may sometimes be used as a tertiary dressing as are disposable nappies where greater absorbency is needed.

Hydrocolloid or hydrogel dressings, available in sheet or gel format, may have an important role to play. Their high water content allows the rehydration of the wound and they have high absorption qualities for wound exudates. They do, however, promote a moist environment which can encourage the growth of bacteria, so constant evaluation of their use is necessary (King 2003).

Odour Despite the lack of research to legitimise the use of natural live yoghurt in reducing wound odour, it is in fact widely used and appears to be effective. It is thought that the application of yoghurt creates an acid medium which inhibits the growth of bacteria, and that the lactobacilli in the yoghurt also act directly on the bacteria within the wound.

Yoghurt is usually applied thickly for around 20 min before it is removed with saline or gently showered off in the bath. A further dressing such as Kaltostat or Sorbsan can then be used on the wound. Where odour is a severe problem, yoghurt can be applied three or four times a day to try to reduce the odour as quickly as possible. A secondary dressing containing charcoal can also be used.

Metronidazole gel is also effective, but the problem of bacterial resistance to antibiotics must be considered.

External deodorisers may be helpful, e.g. Ozium, Neutradol, Nilodor, but sometimes the smell of air fresheners or deodorisers is unacceptable to the patient or her family, and may even cause nausea. Fresh air is probably the most effective agent for removing odours from a room, and changing clothes daily will help to prevent odours from penetrating clothing.

Haemorrhage/capillary bleeding Capillary bleeding is commonly seen in malignant wounds and is often difficult to stop. Again dressings such as Kaltostat, an alginate hydrofibre, have a haemostatic property and are particularly useful where capillary bleeding exists.

It is extremely important that dry dressings are not applied to wounds that bleed, as removal is likely to cause further bleeding. To reduce trauma, adherent dressings should be removed only after soaking. Dressings such as Kaltostat and Sorbsan absorb exudate and turn to a gel which is then easily removed by syringing the wound with saline or when the patient showers. Where possible, wounds which are liable to bleed should be irrigated, for even the gentle use of cotton wool may be enough to cause bleeding.

The use of pressure may help to control bleeding, but if a major vessel is eroded, bleeding may be very difficult to control and alarming to the patient. Weak solutions of adrenaline may be advised by medical staff in such a situation, but these should be used with caution because of the possibility of systemic absorption.

Care must also be taken when using tape to hold dressings in place. The skin around an ulcerated wound is often inflamed, tender and delicate. As tape may cause trauma, it is a good idea to rotate the sites to which tape is applied. In fact, it is preferable for dressings to be held in place by net body bandages such as Netelast, which obviates the need for tape.

Pain Wound pain can range from very slight to severe. The nurse must assess the severity and type of pain being experienced and whether it is always present or affects the patient only during dressing changes. Pain assessment should be ongoing so that the effectiveness of pain control measures can be evaluated (see Ch. 19). Where dressing changes cause discomfort, analgesics should be offered to the woman at least 30 min before each change. The use of Entonox during the dressing procedure may also be helpful. The use of non-adherent dressings and, where possible, cleansing of the wound by irrigation will also reduce discomfort.

Patient education

Wound care As much information as the woman requires concerning her wound, dressings and general condition should be given. The degree to which the patient and her family are involved in wound management will depend largely on their own wishes and sensitivities. Some women prefer to be taught how to dress their own wounds completely at home, with only minimum supervisory involvement by the community or hospital nurse. This may originate in a desire to be independent or it may be prompted by embarrassment. Some patients feel unable to have anything to do with their wound and do not want family members to intervene either. No woman should be made to look at her wound if this is intolerable to her; to do so may destroy the only way in which she knows how to cope.

Diet Dietary advice may be appropriate if a woman is malnourished, has an infection, is anorexic or is considering starting a 'cancer diet'. The nurse should be able to give basic advice about a balanced diet (see Ch. 21) but may wish to refer the patient to a dietitian for further advice. The decision to go on to a cancer diet rests with the patient. There are many such diets: some are reasonably well balanced, but others are likely to cause extreme weight loss. Where this is likely to be detrimental to the individual, the nurse should discuss this with her. Ultimately, however, the nurse should support the patient in whatever decision she makes.

Prostheses and clothing Practical advice about clothing may be appreciated if the disease has radically altered the contour of the chest or where a large amount of absorbent dressing is necessary to control the wound exudate. The use of partial prostheses fitted over the dressings may restore a more normal breast contour. A larger soft bra may enable the dressing to be held in place comfortably but securely whilst maintaining a normal appearance in clothing. Where a bra cannot be worn due to discomfort, loose clothing will help to disguise any altered shape without causing any restrictions around the wound.

STOP THINK **7.10** Consider the following questions with reference to Case History 7.4:

(a) Identify the main problems that Mrs S has.
(b) Consider the effects a fungating lesion might have on a woman's body image.
(c) It is important that Mrs S does not feel that her nurse is disgusted by her wound. Consider how the nurse might demonstrate both verbally and non-verbally that this is not the case.
(d) How might the nurse endeavour to reduce Mr S's anxiety about his wife?
(e) What properties should the wound dressing have? Can you suggest any appropriate products for such a wound?

THE PSYCHOLOGICAL IMPACT OF BREAST DISEASE

Nurses have a particularly important role to play in supporting patients through the traumatic experience of breast disease. Although many women with breast cancer will face similar problems, no two individuals will respond to their diagnosis and treatment in exactly the same way. As this chapter stresses, ongoing assessment is the key to providing psychological and emotional support that is genuinely responsive to each woman's needs and priorities.

For most women, a diagnosis of breast cancer is devastating. They may have to cope with the prospect of mutilating surgery to a part of the body associated with femininity, sexuality and motherhood, the prospect of several months of intensive medical treatment and the possibility that they may eventually die of the disease. Some women with breast cancer discover their lump when washing or during self-examination whilst others are not aware that anything is wrong but find out when they attend for a screening mammogram. Symptoms of acute anxiety, panic, palpitations, tachycardia, loss of concentration and insomnia may be experienced in the period when a medical opinion is sought and a diagnosis awaited. Some women describe this time of flux as the most agonising period of their illness. For some women, the fear of cancer or its treatment is so great that they deny the presence of a lump or delay seeking medical help.

Some of this fear may be based on misconceptions about the nature of cancer treatments. It is important for nurses, especially those in community practice, to dispel myths about cancer therapy, to raise awareness of the success rate of breast cancer treatment, and to emphasise the importance of early detection.

Some women who undergo surgery for breast cancer initially experience euphoria that the cancer has been removed. Others deny the removal of their breast or find themselves unable to talk about it or to look at the scar. Much research has been carried out into the psychosocial sequelae of breast surgery. It has been reported that one-third of women develop severe anxiety or depression within a year of their diagnosis (Maguire 2000). It was thought that this was related mainly to the altered body image of mastectomy, but Fallowfield et al (2000) found that women who had a wide local excision had levels of anxiety and depression similar to those experienced by women who had chosen to undergo mastectomy. In their study, Dorval et al (1998) found that having a partial or total mastectomy did not significantly affect quality of life but that the individual's response to the surgery was affected by her age. Their study suggested that having a partial mastectomy may have lessened the negative effect of breast cancer for younger women.

Following diagnosis and surgery, a period of adjustment occurs which is characterised by fluctuating emotions. Northouse (1989) found that following mastectomy the major concern for most women and their partners surrounded issues of survival, in particular the extent of the cancer and the possibility of recurrence. Patients may also be worried about changes in lifestyle, treatment regimens and altered appearance.

For the majority of women who have undergone breast surgery, anxiety begins to reduce after about 3 months and the activities of normal life will be resumed. Some women, however, will continue to experience great anxiety, show signs of depression, withdraw from social contact or have sexual problems. These women are likely to benefit from more in-depth counselling and psychological support. Nurses, particularly those in the community and in outpatient departments, should be able to recognise emotional problems and, where necessary, suggest referral to a counsellor, psychiatrist or psychologist via the GP or hospital medical staff.

PATIENT EDUCATION

Being a recipient of the bewildering treatments for breast cancer can take self-determination away from the woman and this can lead to psychological morbidity. Research has shown that many patients find that information helps them to make sense of their situation, and hence to feel more in control, less vulnerable and less anxious (Fallowfield et al 2000). Most women have some general knowledge of breast cancer, but will not be familiar with the details of the tests or treatments they are to undergo. Many will, in fact, have misconceptions about breast cancer and its prognosis because of the misinformation that may be found in the popular media. Research by Macleod et al (2004) has demonstrated that different groups of women receive differing amounts of information from the available sources, the affluent group accessing more information than the deprived group. They state that health care professionals need to be aware that there may be greater psychological distress in the deprived group of women, perhaps not helped by the lack of informational support (see Research Abstract 7.9).

The nurse must bear in mind that the amount of information each woman wants about her disease or proposed treatment will vary. As too much information is likely to cause confusion and anxiety, it is important for the nurse to find out what each individual wants to know, and to

RESEARCH ABSTRACT 7.9

Psychosocial aspects of care in breast cancer: affluent vs deprived women

A postal questionnaire was sent out to affluent (n = 158) and deprived women (n = 263) with breast cancer to compare their psychosocial aspects of care with the purpose of understanding the balance of care and to explain why deprived women have poorer outcomes. Data were collected regarding reported sources of information, SF-36 scores and ongoing causes of anxiety. The results demonstrated that affluent women were more likely than deprived women to have received information from their hospital specialist (94.8 vs 76.0%) and from a breast care nurse (70.1 vs 40.0) than deprived women. They were also more likely to have received information from magazines (50.6 vs 33.0%), newspapers (45.5 vs 22.0%) and television news (45.5 vs 26.0%). Deprived women had poorer SF-36 scores than affluent women, and reported greater anxiety about money (12.2 vs 2.8%), other health problems (22.1 vs 8.2%) and family problems (17.5 vs 6.9%).

Personal and professional support is clearly important for patients with breast cancer. Health professionals need to be aware of the greater psychological distress demonstrated by deprived women, even some years after diagnosis with breast cancer, and seek to address it.

Macleod U, Ross S, Fallowfield L, Watt G C M 2004 Anxiety and support in breast cancer: is this different for affluent and deprived women? A questionnaire study. British Journal of Cancer 91: 879–883 clarify what has been understood. It is also important to remember that, in times of stress, information is more difficult to assimilate and remember. It is often necessary for the nurse to repeat information.

If the nurse feels unable to answer any questions, she should either find someone who can do so or arrange a further consultation with medical staff. The nurse may be able to facilitate communication by helping the patient to articulate her concerns and by clarifying concepts or terminology unfamiliar to the patient.

Areas of information that are likely to be relevant include:

- how breast cancer is and is not caused, e.g. it is not caused by a knock on the breast
- the aim of treatment and what outcome may realistically be expected
- the nature and likely cosmetic effect of any proposed surgery
- the possibility of breast reconstructive surgery if all, or a large part, of the breast is removed
- if axillary lymph node removal is advised, the effects of removal and the postoperative exercises necessary to ensure the return of full shoulder movement (see p. 332)
- staging tests that will need to be performed prior to or following surgery
- the availability of prostheses, when this is appropriate.

The nurse should ensure that the patient understands what the operation involves and the likely pre- and postoperative experiences, including the presence of wound drains, i.v. infusions, pain, scarring and any possible short- or long-term complications. Photographs or diagrams may be useful to demonstrate likely scarring or alteration in breast shape or size, and patient videos are becoming a popular way of reinforcing what has already been said.

Information given verbally may be reinforced in written form. Booklets on breast surgery and breast cancer can be obtained from Breast Cancer Care (BCC) and the British Association of Cancer United Patients (BACUP) if local literature is not available (see 'Useful websites', p. 354). These publications can also be useful for family and friends to read. Admission booklets providing information about the hospital, its facilities and visiting hours are also helpful.

Women who wish to have more in-depth knowledge about breast cancer may find Sampson & Fenlon (2000) useful. This book is written for the informed lay public.

THE ISSUE OF INFORMED CONSENT

The patient's rights

In order to give informed consent to an operation or treatment, a patient must be told what the procedure or therapy entails and its consequences, and must understand the information that she is given. Since the Alderhey tissue retention scandal (Hunter 2001), most centres now present women with individualised consent forms that clearly state in detail the type of surgery they will undergo and the expected effect of that surgery. The retention of tissue specimens for research is also made explicit and the woman has the right to refuse to donate her tumour tissue for research.

A woman who is diagnosed as having breast cancer has the right to be told of all the possible medical options and to decide which, if any, of these options she will take. She may wish to seek a second opinion from another specialist and to gather information to help her make a decision as to which is the best treatment for her. Research about particular aspects of treatment is becoming the norm in breast cancer care and most women being treated for cancer will be approached about entering one or more studies. In this event the study should be clearly explained and written information given as back-up. The woman must be assured that she has the absolute right to refuse entry without incurring any detrimental effect to her future care.

The nurse's role

The issue of informed consent is an important one for all nurses who aim to give truly patient-centred care. Doctors have the responsibility for obtaining informed consent, but nurses, including research nurses and specialist breast care nurses can help to ensure that this occurs by asking patients to explain what they understand is to happen to them and by providing any additional information that is desired. Often patients feel very vulnerable when consulting a doctor and a nurse may act as advocate by representing the patient or supporting her in meetings with the doctor.

For many women with breast cancer, the consultant will be able to give treatment options. In order for the woman to make an informed decision, she must understand what each operation or treatment involves, and any side-effects which may result. Most women find the thought of losing a breast very distressing and will prefer a wide excision of the cancer, while preserving the breast, if this is a safe option. However, mastectomy may be a better choice for tumours which are multifocal or involve a large portion of the breast. Mastectomy may also be preferred by women with small tumours to reduce the risks of local recurrence and the need for adjuvant radiotherapy.

A tumour that is multifocal (i.e. occurs in several areas of the breast) cannot safely be removed by conservative surgery as the risk of local recurrence would be unacceptably high. The cosmetic result of removing a large tumour from a small breast or removing a tumour that is centrally sited beneath the nipple could be so poor that a mastectomy would be more acceptable, although only the individual woman will know how she feels about this.

Some women facing breast surgery are not aware of the possibility of reconstructive surgery. In part, this reflects the lack of facilities and skills in many areas to undertake such surgery. The long waiting lists at centres where breast reconstructions are done may cause professionals to hesitate in disclosing the possibility of this surgery. Nonetheless, in fairness to the woman, all options should be explained so that she can decide whether breast reconstruction is right for her in light of the benefits and the possible complications.

THE ROLE OF THE CLINICAL NURSE SPECIALIST IN BREAST CARE

The role of the clinical nurse specialist in breast care has developed largely in response to the recognition that women with breast cancer benefit from the support and expertise of nurses specialising in this area (Watson et al 1988, McArdle et al 1996, Maguire 2000, NICE 2002). It must be stressed that the clinical nurse specialist provides an additional service to that provided by hospital and community nursing staff, and not an alternative to that service. The clinical nurse specialist functions as a resource for patients, their families and other nurses.

Ideally, the clinical involvement of the nurse specialist with the patient will begin at the time of diagnosis and prior to hospital admission. This may involve meeting patients in screening assessment units, and requires the cooperation of outpatient nurses and doctors in informing the nurse specialist of new patients. Many specialist nurses follow a limited intervention strategy of seeing patients in hospital before and after their surgery and then visiting them at home or making contact by telephone postoperatively to assess how they are coping. Where problems arise, referral for more in-depth psychological support can be made, but the nurse is likely to continue her involvement with the patient and her family. Because of the increasing complexity of the treatments available, the larger centres may employ more than one nurse specialist, and each is then able to focus her expertise on different aspects of the woman's care.

The nurse specialist also provides a contact point for patients and their family should they require advice or support at any time. She should facilitate communication between the community care team and the hospital but should also be able to use discretion on the patient's behalf if a large number of carers become involved. She will resume contact with patients should metastatic breast cancer develop. Many breast care nurse specialists also provide prosthetic and lymphoedema services.

REFERENCES

Arden-Jones A 2003 Breast cancer genetics. In: Harmer V (ed) Breast cancer, nursing care and management. Whurr, London, p 37–59

Baum M 1996 The breast screening controversy. European Journal of Cancer 32A(1): 9–11

Blackwell R E, Grotting J C 1996 Diagnosis and management of breast disease. Blackwell Science, Oxford

Breast Cancer Care 2003 www.breastcancercare.org.uk

Bruzzi P 1998 Tamoxifen for the prevention of breast cancer. British Medical Journal 316: 1181–1182

Bundred N, Maguire P, Reynolds J et al 1998 Randomised control effects of early discharge after surgery for breast cancer. British Medical Journal 317: 1275–1279

Cancer Research Campaign 1996a Factsheets 6.1 to 6.6. CRC, UK

Cancer Research Campaign 1996b Factsheet 6.2 Breast cancer. CRC, UK

Carpenter J S, Andrykowski M A 1999 Menopausal symptoms in breast cancer survivors. Oncology Nursing Forum 26(8): 1311–1317

Chapman D 2001 There's no place like home. Nursing Standard 16(11): 18–19

Crowe D R, Lampejo O T 1996 Malignant tumours of the breast. In: Blackwell R E, Grotting J C (eds) Diagnosis and management of breast disease. Blackwell Science, Oxford

Crown J, O'Leary M, Ooi S 2004 Docetaxel and paclitaxel in the treatment of breast cancer: a review of clinical experience. Oncologist 9(Suppl 2): 24–32

Curling G, Tierney K L 1997 Breast screening and breast disorders. In: Andrews G (ed) Women's sexual health. Baillière Tindall, London

Cuzick J, Powles T, Veronesi U et al 2003 Overview of the main outcomes in breast-cancer prevention trials. Lancet 361: 296–300

Denton S, Baum M 1983 Psychosocial aspects of breast cancer. In: Margolese R (ed) Breast cancer. Churchill Livingstone, Edinburgh

Department of Health and Social Security 1986 Breast cancer screening: the Forrest report. HMSO, London

Dixon J (ed) 2000 The ABC of breast diseases. BMJ Publishing Group, London

Dixon J, Mansel R 2000 Congenital problems and aberrations of normal breast development and involution. In: Dixon J (ed) The ABC of breast diseases. BMJ Publishing Group, London

Dorval M, Maunsell E, Deschenes L, Brisson J 1998 Type of mastectomy and quality of life for long term survivors. Cancer 15(10): 2130–2138

Early Breast Cancer Trialists' Collaborative Group (EBCTCG) 1992 Systemic treatment of early breast cancer by hormonal, cytotoxic, or immune therapy. Lancet 339: 1–15

Early Breast Cancer Trialists' Collaborative Group (EBCTCG) 1998a Polychemotherapy for early breast cancer: an overview of the randomised trials. Lancet 352: 930–942

Early Breast Cancer Trialists' Collaborative Group (EBCTCG) 1998b Tamoxifen for early breast cancer: an overview of the randomised trials. Lancet 351: 1451–1467

Faithfull S 1998 Fatigue in patients receiving radiotherapy. Professional Nurse 13(7): 459–461

Fallowfield L J, Hall A, Maguire G P, Baum M 2000 Psychological outcomes of different treatment policies in women with early breast cancer outside a clinical trial. British Medical Journal 301: 575–580

Fenlon D 2003 Hormones as a treatment for breast cancer: In: Harmer V (ed) Breast cancer, nursing care and management. Whurr, London, p 188–213

Fisher B, Brown A M, Dimitrov N V et al 1990 Two months of doxorubicin–cyclophosphamide with and without interval reinduction therapy compared with 6 months of cyclophosphamide, methotrexate, and fluorouracil in positive-node breast cancer patients with tamoxifen-non-responsive tumours: results from the National Surgical Adjuvant Breast and Bowel Project B15. Journal of Clinical Oncology 8(9): 1483–1496

Fisher B, Anderson S, Tan-Chiu E et al 2001 Tamoxifen and chemotherapy for axillary node-negative estrogen receptor negative breast cancer: findings from National Surgical Adjuvant Breast and Bowel Project B32. Journal of Clinical Oncology 19(4): 931–942

Glean E, Edwards S, Faithfull S et al 2001 Intervention for acute radiotherapy induced skin reactions in cancer patients: the development of a clinical guideline recommended for use by the College of Radiographers. Journal of Radiotherapy in Practice 2: 75–84

Goin M K, Goin J M 1988 Growing pains: the psychological experience of breast reconstruction with tissue expansion. Annals of Plastic Surgery 21(3): 217–222

Goldberg P, Stolzmann M, Goldberg H M 1984 Psychological considerations in breast reconstruction. Annals of Plastic Surgery 13(1): 38–43

Hart D 1996 The psychological outcome of breast reconstruction. Plastic Surgical Nursing 16(3): 167–171

Hemminki E 1996 Oral contraceptives and breast cancer. British Medical Journal 313: 63–64

Hughes K 2000 Exercise and lymphoedema. In: Twycross R, Jenns K, Todd J (eds) Lymphoedema. Radcliffe Medical Press, Oxford

Hunter M 2001 Medical research under threat after Alderhey scandal. British Medical Journal 322(7284): 448

Kerlikowske K, Grady D, Rubin S M, Sandrock C, Ernster V L 1995 Efficacy of screening mammography. A meta-analysis. Journal of the American Medical Association 273: 149–154

King R 2003 Fungating wounds. In: Harmer V (ed) Breast cancer, nursing care and management. Whurr, London, p 233–249

King's Fund Forum 1986 Consensus development conference: treatment of primary breast cancer. British Medical Journal 293: 946–947

Lake D E, Hudis C A 2004 High-dose chemotherapy in breast cancer. Drugs 64(17): 1851–1860

Lewis F, Jackson P, Lane S, Coast G, Hanby A M 2004 Testing for Her2 in breast cancer. Histopathology 45(3): 207–217

Lichter A S 1998 Breast cancer. In: Leibel S A, Phillips T L (eds) Textbook of radiation biology. WB Saunders, Philadelphia

Lipworth L, Tarone R E, McLaughlin J K 2004

Silicone implants and connective tissue disease: an updated review of the epidemiological evidence. Annals of Plastic Surgery 52(b): 598–607
Macleod H, Koelling P 2003 Physiotherapy for patients with breast cancer. In: Harmer V (ed) Breast cancer, nursing care and management. Whurr, London, p 102–121
Macleod U, Ross S, Fallowfield L, Watt G C M 2004 Anxiety and support in breast cancer: is this different for affluent and deprived women? A questionnaire study. British Journal of Cancer 91: 879–883
Maguire P 2000 Psychological aspects. In: Dixon J (ed) The ABC of breast diseases. BMJ Publishing Group, London, p 85–89
Mansel R E 2000 Breast pain. In: Dixon J (ed) The ABC of breast diseases. BMJ Publishing Group, London, p 16–20
Mansi J L, Smith I E, Walsh G E et al 1989 Primary medical therapy for operable breast cancer. European Journal of Cancer and Clinical Oncology 25(11): 1623–1627
McArdle J, George W D, McArdle C S et al 1996 Psychological support for patients undergoing breast cancer surgery: a randomised study. British Medical Journal 312: 813–816
McPherson K, Steel C M, Dixon J M 2000 Breast cancer – epidemiology, risk factors and genetics. In: Dixon J (ed) The ABC of breast diseases. BMJ Publishing Group, London, p 26–32
Mortimer P S, Bates D, Brassington H, Stanton A, Strachan D, Levick J 1996 The prevalence of arm oedema following treatment for breast cancer. Quarterly Journal of Medicine 89: 377–380
Mulata C M, Feldberg L, Coleman D J, Foo I T, Sharpe D T 1997 Textured or smooth implants for breast augmentation? 3 year follow up of a prospective randomized controlled trial. British Journal of Plastic Surgery 50(2): 99–105
National Health Service Breast Screening Programme (NHSBSP) 2001 Breast screening. The facts. Health Promotion England in conjunction with NHS Cancer Screening Programmes. DH, London
National Institute for Clinical Excellence (NICE) 2002 Guidance on cancer services, improving outcomes in breast cancer. Manual update. NICE, London
Newman J 1995 How breast milk protects newborns. Scientific American December: 58–61
Northouse L 1989 The impact of breast cancer on patients and husbands. Cancer Nursing 12(5): 276–284
Northouse L, Dorris G, Charron-Moore C 1995 Factors affecting couples' adjustment to recurrent breast cancer. Social Science Medicine 41(1): 69–76
Nyren O, Yin L, Josefsson S et al 1998 Risk of connective tissue disease and related disorders among women with implants: a nationwide retrospective cohort study in Sweden. British Medical Journal 316: 417–422
Overgaard M, Hansen P S, Overgaard J et al 1997 Post-operative radiotherapy in high risk premenopausal women with breast cancer who receive adjuvant chemotherapy. New England Journal of Medicine 337: 949–954
Page D L, Steel C M, Dixon J M 2000 Carcinoma in situ and patients at high risk of breast cancer. In: Dixon J (ed) The ABC of breast diseases. BMJ Publishing Group, London
Perkins G H, Middleton L P 2003 Breast cancer in men. British Medical Journal 327: 239–240
Peto R, Boreham J, Clarke M, Davies C, Beral V 2000 UK and USA breast cancer deaths down 25% in year 2000 at ages 20–69 years [research letter]. Lancet 355(9217): 1822
Poole C J, Earl H M, Dunn L 2003 NEAT (National Epirubicin Adjuvant Trial) and SCTBG BR 9601 (Scottish Cancer Trials Breast Group) Phase III adjuvant trials show a significant relapse-free and overall survival advantage for sequential ECMF. Proceedings of the American Society for Clinical Oncology 22: 4 [abstract 13]
Powles T J, Eeles R, Ashley S et al 1998 Interim analysis of breast cancer in the Royal Marsden Hospital tamoxifen chemoprevention trial. Lancet 352: 98–101
Purushotham A D, Britton P, Bobrow L 2000 Benign breast disease. In: Borgen P I, Hill A (eds) Breast diseases. Landes Bioscience, Georgetown, TX
Reaby L L 1998 Breast restoration decision making: enhancing the process. Cancer Nursing 21(3): 196–204
Reshef E, Sanfilippo J S, Levine N S 1996 Breast dysfunction: congenital abnormalities of the breast. In: Blackwell R E, Grotting J C (eds) Diagnosis and management of breast disease. Blackwell Science, Oxford
Richards M, Smith I E 2000 Role of systemic treatment for primary operable breast cancer. In: Dixon J (ed) The ABC of breast diseases. BMJ Publishing Group, London
Sainsbury J R C, Anderson T J, Morgan D A L 2000 Breast cancer. In: Dixon J (ed) The ABC of breast diseases. BMJ Publishing Group, London
Salter M 1988 Altered body image: the nurse's role. Wiley, Chichester
Sjönell G, Ståhle L 1999 Scientific foundation of mammographic screening is based on inconclusive research in Sweden. British Medical Journal 319: 55
Tabar L, Gad A, Holmberg L H et al 1995 Efficacy of breast cancer screening by age. New results of the Swedish two-counties trial. Cancer 75: 2507–2517
Twycross R 1996 Symptom management in advanced cancer. Radcliffe Medical Press, Oxford
Veronesi U, Salvadori B, Luini M et al 1995 Breast conservation is a safe method in patients with small cancer of the breast. Long term results of three randomised trials on 1,973 patients. European Journal of Cancer 31A: 1574–1579
Watson J D, Sainsbury J R C, Dixon J M 2000 Breast reconstruction. In: Dixon J (ed) The ABC of breast diseases. BMJ Publishing Group, London, p 97–104
Watson M (ed) 1991 Breast cancer. In: Cancer patient care: psychological treatment methods. Cambridge University Press, Cambridge
Watson M, Denton S, Baum M, Greer S 1988 Counselling breast cancer patients: a specialist nurse service. Counselling Psychology Quarterly 1(1): 25–34
West N 2003 Breast reconstruction. In: Harmer V (ed) Breast cancer, nursing care and management. Whurr, London, p 82–101
Woods M 2003 Lymphoedema and breast cancer. In: Harmer V (ed) Breast cancer, nursing care and management. Whurr, London, p 214–232
Wren B G 2004 Do female sex hormones initiate breast cancer? A review of the evidence. Climacteric 7(2): 120–128

FURTHER READING

Andrews G (ed) 2004 Women's sexual health. Baillière Tindall, London
Cancer Research Campaign 1997 Factsheets 7.1–7.5: Breast cancer screening. CRC, UK
Dixon J (ed) 2000 The ABC of breast diseases. BMJ Publishing Group, London
Harmer V 2003 Breast cancer, nursing care and management. Whurr, London
Macleod U, Ross S, Fallowfield L, Watt G C M 2004 Anxiety and support in breast cancer: is this different for affluent and deprived women? A questionnaire study. British Journal of Cancer 91: 879–883
Purushotham A D, Britton P, Bobrow L 2000 Benign breast disease. In: Borgen P I, Hill A (eds) Breast diseases. Landes Bioscience, Georgetown, TX
Sampson V, Fenlon D 2000 The breast cancer book. A personal guide to help you through it and beyond. Vermilion, London

USEFUL WEBSITES (see also Ch. 31)

Breast Cancer Care
www.breastcancercare.org.uk/home

British Association of Cancer United Patients (BACUP)
www.cancerbacup.org.uk

DISORDERS OF THE URINARY SYSTEM

8

Lesley Selfe

INTRODUCTION

The practice of urology as a specialty in its own right is commonplace in many general hospitals. Most patients who once would have been treated by a general surgeon are now referred to consultants in urology. This has come about partly in response to advances in technology, especially in the field of endoscopic and laser surgery. It is accepted that patients with urological disorders deserve the same level of understanding and sensitivity as those with gynaecological problems.

The movement within nursing towards patient-centred care in combination with the evolution of new, less traumatic and non-invasive treatments has allowed more individuals to be treated as outpatients or day cases. The appointment of clinical nurse specialists, including stoma care nurses and continence advisors, has also done much to improve standards of care.

It is important for nurses to bear in mind that patients with urological disorders often suffer from intense psychological distress. Nurses in this area of practice must develop good interpersonal skills so that they can discuss problems openly, sensitively and non-judgementally.

This chapter begins with a brief overview of the anatomy and physiology of the urinary system and of the male reproductive organs. With respect to the latter, this chapter complements the anatomy and physiology described in Chapter 7. Common disorders of the urinary tract and their treatment are then described, including infections, obstructive disorders, disorders of the bladder and some of the more significant renal disorders. With regard to the male urinary system and reproductive organs, only prostatic disorders and conditions primarily affecting the urethra are considered here. Conditions more directly affecting reproductive and sexual function, such as testicular cancer and impotence, are discussed in Chapter 7.

ANATOMY AND PHYSIOLOGY

The urinary system comprises the kidneys, the ureters, the urinary bladder and the urethra. Its function is to excrete the waste products of metabolism in the form of urine.

The kidneys

Structure

The kidneys are a pair of slightly lobulated organs which lie on the posterior abdominal wall, extending from the twelfth thoracic vertebra to the third lumbar vertebra. Because of the position of the liver, the right kidney is normally slightly lower than the left. Anteriorly, the kidneys are covered by the peritoneum and the contents of the abdominal cavity. Three layers of supportive tissue surround each kidney: an inner fibrous capsule, a middle fatty layer and an outer fascia. This fatty encasement is necessary for maintaining the kidneys in their normal position. Beneath this, a dark outer cortex surrounds a paler medulla, which consists of pale conical striations called the renal pyramids (see Fig. 8.1).

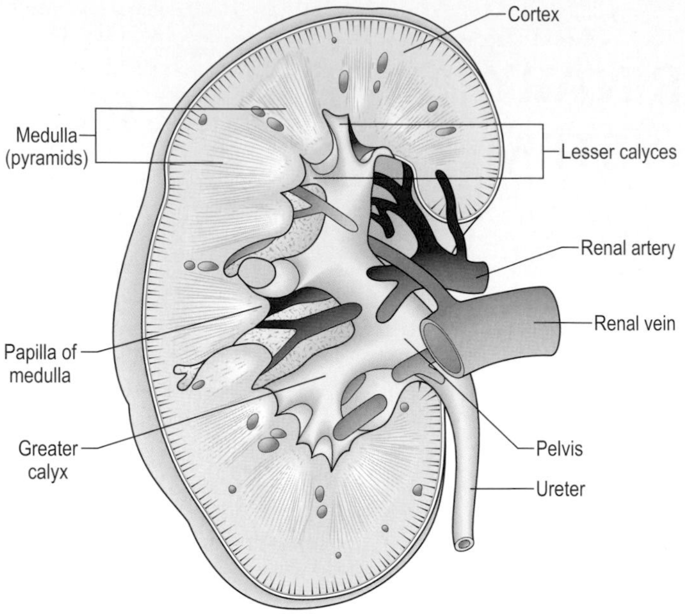

Fig. 8.1 Longitudinal section of the right kidney.

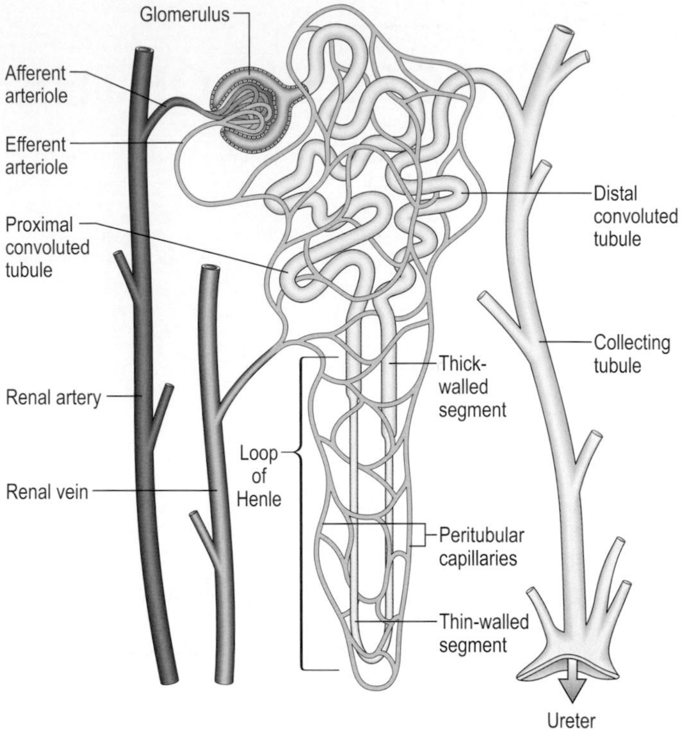

Fig. 8.2 Nephron with long loop of Henle (deep nephron).

At the hilus, i.e. the concave medial border of the kidney, blood vessels, lymph vessels and nerves enter and leave the organ. Medial to the hilus is the flat, funnel-shaped renal pelvis, which is continuous with the ureter leaving the hilus. Extending from the pelvis into the medulla are the cup-shaped calyces; these receive from the renal papillae the urine that has been formed in the nephrons and has passed through the collecting tubules. From the calyces the urine passes into the renal pelvis, which acts as a reservoir.

The nephron Each kidney is composed of approximately 1 million functional units called nephrons, which produce and channel urine into collecting tubules. A nephron consists of a convoluted tubular system and a tuft of capillaries known as the glomerulus. The glomerulus is enclosed in the cup-shaped upper end of the tubule (Bowman's capsule; see Fig. 8.2).

The tubule has three sections: the proximal convoluted tubule, which is the longest segment; the loop of Henle, which forms a hairpin-shaped curve; and the distal convoluted tubule. The distal convoluted tubules merge to form straight collecting tubules; these ultimately terminate at the renal papillae. Cortical nephrons are found in the cortex and have short loops of Henle. Juxtamedullary nephrons have long loops of Henle, allowing them to concentrate urine effectively.

Blood supply The kidney is supplied with blood by renal arteries arising directly from either side of the abdominal aorta immediately below the superior mesenteric artery. The renal arteries branch into smaller and smaller vessels, ultimately becoming afferent arterioles which lead into the nephrons. Each afferent arteriole subdivides further into a glomerulus. These capillaries then merge again to form an efferent arteriole which leaves the capsule and subdivides into a second network of peritubular capillaries which supplies the proximal and distal tubules, the loop of Henle and the collecting ducts. The capillaries merge into venules and then veins, eventually joining the renal vein, which in turn flows into the vena cava.

Function

The kidneys process about 180 L of blood-derived fluid daily. Of this, only about 1–2 L actually leave the body as urine, the remainder is returned to the blood. The kidney's basic function of producing urine takes place in the nephron. Here, the processes of glomerular filtration, selective reabsorption and tubular secretion result in the removal of wastes and toxins from the blood as it passes through the kidney and in the maintenance of fluid and electrolyte balance (Thomas 2002). The characteristics of normal urine are summarised in Box 8.1.

Glomerular filtration The initial filtration of blood takes place across a semi-permeable membrane in which fluid, electrolytes and certain non-electrolytes pass into the Bowman's capsule. Filtrate formation is a passive process and follows the same principles that account for all tissue fluid formation (see Ch. 20). However, the renal corpuscle is much more efficient because the filtration membrane is highly permeable and the glomerular pressure much higher than in other capillary beds. Hence the kidneys are able to filter the above mentioned 180 L of fluid daily, as compared with the 3 L/day produced by other capillary beds in the body.

The chemical composition of the glomerular filtrate is identical to that of plasma, i.e. plasma proteins are absent (the presence of protein in the urine can therefore be an indication of abnormality).

Box 8.1

Physical characteristics of urine

Volume (24 h)	1500 mL, but varies greatly according to fluid intake and insensible losses
Clarity	Transparent or clear; on standing, becomes cloudy
Colour	Amber or straw-coloured; varies according to amount voided; diet may change colour
Odour	'Characteristic'; on standing, develops pungent odour from formation of ammonium carbonate
PH (normal range 4.6–8.0)	Acidic when freshly voided, stale urine has an alkaline reaction from decomposition of urea forming ammonium carbonate. May become alkaline if diet consists largely of vegetables; a high-protein diet increases acidity
Specific gravity	1.015–1.020; highest in morning specimen

Chemical composition

Urine is approximately 95% water, in which is dissolved several kinds of substances. The most important of these are:

- Nitrogenous wastes from protein metabolism such as urea (most abundant solute in urine), uric acid, ammonia and creatinine
- Electrolytes, mainly the following ions: sodium, potassium, ammonium, chloride, bicarbonate, phosphate and sulphate — the amounts vary according to diet and other factors
- Toxins. During disease, bacterial poisons leave the body in the urine; this is an important reason for 'pushing' fluids on patients suffering from infectious diseases, as a high fluid intake dilutes the toxins that might damage the kidney cells if they were eliminated in a concentrated form
- Pigments
- Hormones
- Abnormal constituents such as glucose, albumin, blood, casts or calculi are sometimes found.

Adapted from Thibodeau & Patton (1999).

In order for glomerular filtration to take place, there must be adequate blood volume in the intravascular space and sufficient glomerular hydrostatic pressure. It is the glomerular hydrostatic pressure that essentially forces the water and solutes across the filtration membrane. This pressure (55 mmHg) is opposed by the colloid osmotic pressure exerted by the glomerular plasma proteins (30 mmHg) and the capsular hydrostatic pressure (15 mmHg). Thus the net filtration pressure responsible for filtrate formation is 10 mmHg. The rate at which fluid filters from the blood to the glomerular capsule is directly proportional to the net filtration pressure. The normal filtration rate is 120–125 mL/min.

Selective reabsorption The greater part of reabsorption takes place in the proximal convoluted tubule. Sodium, chloride, bicarbonate and potassium are returned to the blood by passive or active transport. Glucose is actively reabsorbed. Normally, all of the glucose is reabsorbed such that none appears in the urine. However, if blood levels of glucose are too high, some will be excreted in the urine.

About 99% of the water in the filtrate is reabsorbed. The continuous removal of sodium, chloride, bicarbonate, glucose and other materials from the tubule increases the osmotic forces such that water follows the dissolved materials. This is often referred to as obligatory water reabsorption.

One of the major functions of the kidney is to maintain a constant concentration of body fluids by regulating urine concentration. It is still uncertain exactly how this is achieved, but it would appear to be the result of the function of the loop of Henle, which may act as a 'counter-current multiplying system' in which the concentrations of sodium and negative ions move through a gradient, being greatest at the base of the loop. This allows the urine to be more dilute when leaving the loop of Henle than when it left the proximal tubule. This urine remains essentially unaltered unless the need to conserve fluid results in the release of antidiuretic hormone (vasopressin) by the posterior pituitary.

For further information, see Thomas (2002).

Tubular secretion In the distal convoluted tubule and in the collecting duct, sodium is reabsorbed from the tubular fluid while hydrogen and potassium ions are secreted into the fluid. This helps to regulate acid–base balance and rid the body of excessive potassium. In addition, tubular secretion can eliminate substances such as urea and uric acid, which may have been returned to the blood by passive processes, and can also dispose of substances not already in the filtrate, e.g. certain drugs.

Hormonal control of the kidney

Two hormones, antidiuretic hormone (vasopressin) and aldosterone, are important regulators of renal function.

Antidiuretic hormone (ADH) (vasopressin) is produced in the hypothalamus and stored and secreted by the posterior lobe of the pituitary gland. It affects water permeability in the distal convoluted tubule and the collecting ducts, allowing sodium, other ions and water to be reabsorbed, making the urine more concentrated. In the absence of ADH, sodium and other ions are reabsorbed, but not water. This makes the urine more dilute.

Pain, exercise, emotion and the use of narcotics or barbiturates can increase the secretion of ADH. Factors that decrease output are low plasma osmotic pressure, venous distension and alcohol consumption.

Aldosterone is produced in the outermost layer of the adrenal cortex. It acts on the distal tubule, where it increases the reabsorption of sodium (see Ch. 5, p. 176).

Other functions of the kidney

In addition to its role in removing waste products from the blood, the kidney has the following functions:

- Regulation of blood pressure through the maintenance of fluid volume.
- Production of the hormones renin, erythropoietin and 1,25-dihydroxycholecalciferol.

Renin is liberated through the juxtaglomerular cells and acts on angiotensinogen (a glycoprotein made in the liver and normally found in plasma), converting it into angiotensin I. Another enzyme in the pulmonary capillary bed acts on angiotensin I to convert it into angiotensin II. Angiotensin II has the following functions:

- Stimulation of the release of aldosterone, which helps to enable sodium reabsorption and therefore water reabsorption. This in turn helps to maintain plasma volume.
- A powerful vasoconstricting effect, acting on the arterioles and precapillary sphincters to shut down the capillaries, allowing blood volume to be maintained.

Erythropoietin is produced in response to lowered O_2 in the blood. It acts on the bone marrow, stimulating the production of red blood cells (erythropoiesis; see Ch. 11, p. 481).

1,25-dihydroxycholecalciferol is synthesised in the renal tubule cells and is the active form of vitamin D which enables calcium uptake from the small intestine (see Box 5.2, p. 175).

The ureters (see Fig. 8.3)

Urine is conveyed from the pelvis of each kidney to the bladder via the ureters. The ureters are tubular structures approximately 25–30 cm long, ranging in diameter from 2 to 8 mm at various points along their length.

Each ureter descends behind the peritoneum from the renal hilus to the level of the bladder and comes obliquely through the bladder wall before opening into the bladder cavity on its posterior inner surface. This arrangement is such that, when the bladder fills or empties, it is compressed, closing the distal ends of the ureters; in this way, there is no back-flow into the ureters.

Each ureter is composed of three layers of tissue:

- an outer fibrous layer which is continuous with the fibrous renal capsule
- a middle layer consisting of muscle fibres spiralling clockwise and anticlockwise; contraction of the muscle layer produces peristaltic movement of urine along the ureter into the bladder
- an inner mucosa of transitional epithelium.

The urinary bladder

The bladder is a muscular sac which acts as a reservoir for urine before it is expelled from the body. It lies behind the peritoneum in the pelvic cavity, with its anterior surface located just behind the symphysis pubis. In males, the bladder lies in front of the rectum, inferiorly to the urethra and the prostate gland. In females, it lies just anterior to the ureters and the superior section of the vagina.

Structure

The bladder is composed of four layers: an outer fibrous adventitia (except where the peritoneum covers the superior surface), a muscular layer, a submucosal layer of connective tissue and a mucosal layer of transitional epithelium. The muscle layer consists of intermingled smooth muscle arranged in inner and outer longitudinal layers and a middle circular layer and is called the detrusor muscle.

The interior of the bladder has three orifices, two for the ureters and one for the opening of the urethra. This forms a triangle called the trigone (see Fig. 8.4).

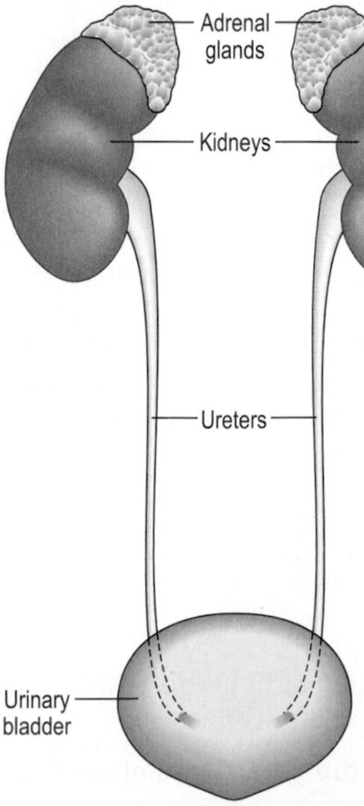

Fig. 8.3 The ureters and their relationship to the kidneys and the bladder.

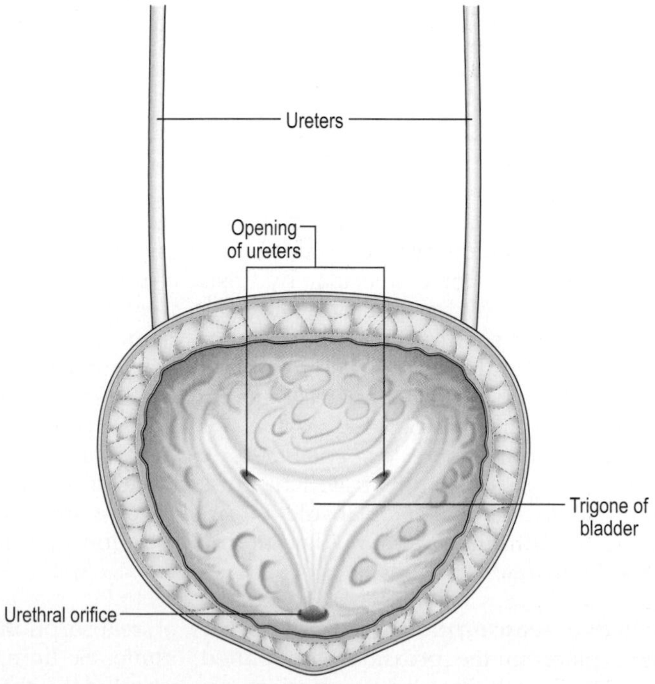

Fig. 8.4 The trigone.

Nerve supply to the bladder is both sensory and motor. Sympathetic nerves arise from T9 to L2 and parasympathetic and somatic nerves from S2 to S4. The motor innervation involves the parasympathetic supply to the detrusor muscle and the sympathetic supply to the trigone. Pudendal nerves under voluntary control supply the external sphincter and muscles of the perineum.

The urethra

The urethra is a tube 8–9 mm in diameter which extends from the neck of the bladder to the exterior. In males, it is about 21 cm long and in females about 4 cm long. It has an outer layer of smooth muscle continuous with that of the bladder. Beneath this lies a thin, spongy layer supplied with blood vessels, lymph vessels and nerves. The innermost layer is a lining of mucous membrane continuous with that of the bladder.

The male urethra is a shared pathway by which both urine and semen reach the exterior. Originating at the urethral orifice in the bladder neck, it is surrounded by the prostate gland and ends at the tip of the glans penis. It is lined with a large number of small mucus-producing glands (Littre's glands). It has an internal sphincter composed of smooth muscle which responds to parasympathetic and sympathetic stimulation. The external urethral sphincter lies at the point where the urethra leaves the prostate; this sphincter is composed of skeletal muscle and is hence under voluntary control.

The female urethra runs behind the symphysis pubis, opening at the external urethral orifice (the meatus) located between the clitoris and vagina. The passage of urine from the bladder through the urethra is governed by two sphincter muscles. At the opening from the bladder is an internal sphincter composed mainly of elastic tissue and smooth muscle and controlled by autonomic nerves. Near the external urethral orifice the smooth muscle is replaced by striated muscle to form an external sphincter under voluntary control.

Micturition

Micturition, the act of passing urine, is a complex physiological process governed by a number of neural controls. The bladder is very distensible, to allow for the storage of urine. An empty bladder is pear shaped and its walls are thick, falling into folds. As urine fills the bladder, it expands and becomes more oval to accommodate the increasing quantity of fluid. The muscle walls stretch and become thinner such that the bladder can comfortably hold 500 mL of urine. In extremis the bladder could hold more than 1 L. If this occurs it can be palpated above the symphysis pubis.

When the bladder contains 300–400 mL of urine, nerve fibres in the wall which are sensitive to stretch are stimulated (Downey 2000). In the infant or young child, this triggers a spinal reflex which results in contraction of the bladder muscle and relaxation of the internal urethral sphincter. When the nervous system is more mature, the individual is aware of a desire to pass urine and can inhibit the reflex action for a time.

Micturition is normally a painless function that occurs four to six times during the day. Decreased bladder capacity and weakened sphincter and detrusor muscles can, in older people and others, necessitate voiding once or twice during the night.

The composition of urine is given in Box 8.1.

STOP THINK **8.1** Keep a fluid balance chart for yourself over a 24-h period. Record all your fluid intake and the amount and frequency of all urine output. In addition, record your activities for this period. Then compare your results with those of your colleagues. If possible, also compare your results with a patient's fluid balance chart.

The male reproductive organs

The male reproductive organs are those structures responsible for the production, maturation, and delivery into the female reproductive tract of spermatozoa necessary for the fertilisation of ova. The essential organs of this system are the two testes, in which spermatogenesis occurs. The accessory organs which support the reproductive process include:

- the genital ducts — the epididymis (2), vas deferens (2), ejaculatory ducts (2) and urethra, which convey sperm to the exterior
- the glands — the seminal vesicles (2), the prostate gland and the bulbourethral (Cowper's) glands (2), which produce fluid as a vehicle for sperm
- the supporting structures — the scrotum, penis and spermatic cords.

The essential organs

The testes are paired oval organs 4–5 cm in length weighing 10–15 g each. They are suspended in the scrotum by the spermatic cords and are encased in three layers of tissue, as follows:

- the tunica vaginalis, or outer layer — a down-growth of the abdominal and pelvic peritoneum
- the tunica albuginea — a layer beneath the tunica vaginalis which consists of fibroelastic connective tissue containing some smooth muscle cells
- the tunica vasculosa — an inner layer made up of delicate connective tissue supplied by a network of capillaries.

Each testis contains 200–300 lobes, within which are tightly coiled seminiferous tubules. It is here that the primitive sex cells (spermatogonia) present in male babies at birth become transformed into spermatozoa (spermatogenesis). This process starts at puberty and continues throughout life.

A spermatozoon provides one-half of the genetic material required to create a new life. Each spermatozoon has a head, neck, body and tail, each with a specialised function. The head contains a highly compact package of genetic material encased in a specialised covering, called the acrosome, which contains digestive enzymes that can penetrate the ovum during fertilisation. The body contains mitochondria and the tail adenosine triphosphate (ATP); these provide energy for sperm locomotion.

The testes also produce androgens (masculinising hormones), the most important of which is testosterone, which is produced by interstitial cells (Leydig's cells). Testosterone promotes:

- maleness and male sexual behaviour
- the development and maintenance of male secondary sex characteristics and the functions of the accessory organs
- protein anabolism
- growth of bone and skeletal muscle and closure of the bony epiphyses
- a mild stimulant effect on the kidney tubule, with reabsorption of sodium and water and excretion of potassium
- inhibition of anterior pituitary secretion of the gonadotrophins follicle-stimulating hormone (FSH) and interstitial cell-stimulating hormone (ICSH). FSH stimulates the seminiferous tubules of the testes to produce spermatozoa. A negative feedback mechanism operates whereby, when testosterone levels are high, FSH and ICSH production is inhibited.

At the upper pole of the testis, the tubules combine to form the rete testis and then penetrate the tunica vaginalis to empty into the epididymis. The epididymis leaves the scrotum as the deferent duct (vas deferens) through the spermatic cords. The testes are well supplied with blood, lymph vessels and nerves from both divisions of the autonomic nervous system.

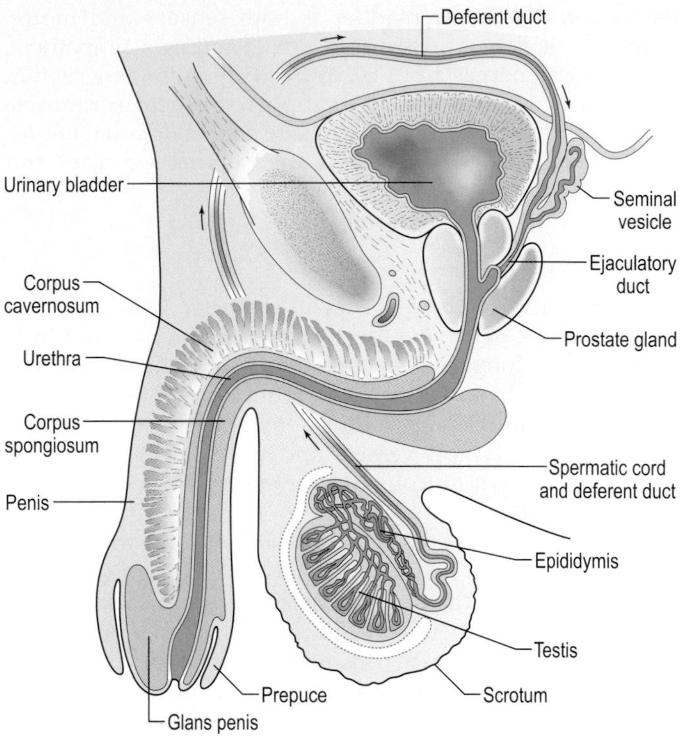

Fig. 8.5 Section of male reproductive organs. Arrows show the structures through which the spermatozoa pass.

The ductal system

The epididymis is the first part of the ductal system and forms a collection of tubules arising from the testis. The vas deferens, which is continuous with the epididymis, loops through the inguinal canal and joins the ejaculatory ducts, which pass through the prostate gland and lead into the urethra (see Fig. 8.5).

Sperm undergo a ripening process as they pass through the ductal system before ejaculation. They remain in the vas deferens for varying periods of time, depending upon the individual's degree of sexual activity. Sperm may remain in storage in the vas deferens for more than a month with no loss of fertility.

The accessory glands

The seminal vesicles are small, lobulated glands lined with secretory epithelium which lie to the posterior of the bladder at the base of the prostate. The lower end of each vesicle opens into a short duct, which joins with the deferent duct to form the ejaculatory duct.

The seminal vesicles secrete a thick, nutritive alkaline fluid that mixes with sperm on ejaculation. This fluid accounts for 30% of the volume of the seminal fluid and contains fructose and protein, which are essential to sperm motility and metabolism.

The prostate gland is a lobulated structure which lies in the pelvic cavity in front of the rectum and behind the symphysis pubis, surrounding the uppermost part of the urethra. It is palpable on rectal examination. The prostate gland secretes a thin, milky, alkaline fluid that makes up 60% of the seminal fluid; this fluid creates an environment more hospitable to sperm by giving protection from the normally acidic environment of the male urethra and female vagina. A neutral or slightly alkaline medium also increases sperm motility.

The prostate is susceptible to hyperplasia, which, because the urethra passes through it, can lead to urinary problems (see p. 375).

The bulbourethral glands are two pea-sized glands opening onto either side of the urethra. They produce a lubricating alkaline mucus that is expressed into the urethra during ejaculation, further reducing its typically acidic state, and contribute less than 5% to the volume of seminal fluid.

The supporting structures

The penis is a pendulous, soft tissue structure with a root and a body. The root lies in the perineum and is attached to the anterior and lateral walls of the pubic arch. The body, which surrounds the urethra, consists of three elongated masses of erectile tissue and involuntary muscle.

The erectile tissue is supported by fibrous tissue and covered with skin. The three elongated masses, which are longitudinal in shape, consist of an encompassing central column (the corpus spongiosum) containing the urethra, and two parallel columns (the corpora cavernosa) which provide the organ's main structural support. These structures are richly supplied with blood vessels.

At the distal end of the penis, the corpus spongiosum and the corpora cavernosa expand to become the glans penis, which surrounds the urethral meatus. The covering of skin folds upon itself at the glans penis to form a movable double layer called the prepuce.

Coitus and fertilisation The penis is supplied by autonomic and somatic nerves. Tactile, visual or mental stimulation causes a parasympathetic reflex leading to engorgement of the penis with blood and consequent erection. In the next phase, emission, sperm and secretions from the accessory glands are deposited in the posterior urethra. Finally, during ejaculation, the bladder neck closes and is followed by relaxation of the distal sphincter mechanism and spasmodic contraction of the bulbourethral muscles. This forces semen out through the urethra in spurts and is accompanied by the intensely pleasurable sensation of orgasm. Once ejaculation has taken place, the corpora cavernosa and the corpus spongiosum empty their excess of blood and the penis resumes its flaccid state.

The sperm, although anatomically complete and highly motile, undergo a further maturation process referred to as capacitation after introduction into the vagina. This enables the head of the sperm to use its hydrolytic (splitting) enzymes to penetrate the encasing membrane (the zona pellucida) of the ovum.

The millions of sperm ejaculated act collectively to produce hyaluronidase to liquefy the intracellular substance surrounding the ovum. This mass action is necessary for a single sperm to penetrate the ovum and bring about fertilisation.

The scrotum is a thin-walled pouch continuous with the abdominal wall. It is deeply pigmented and divided into two compartments, each of which contains one testis, one epididymis and the testicular end of the spermatic cord. The temperature of the testes is 2–3°C below body temperature, which helps to preserve sperm viability.

The spermatic cords Leading from each testis is a spermatic cord consisting of a testicular artery, a testicular venous plexus, lymph vessels, a deferent duct (vas deferens) and nerves; these are all surrounded by a fibrous connective sheath.

DISORDERS OF THE URINARY SYSTEM

URINARY TRACT INFECTIONS

Urinary tract infections are second only to respiratory infections in incidence. Infection can occur in both the upper and lower urinary tracts. The risk of developing a urinary tract infection varies throughout life. In childhood and adulthood, urinary infections are common in females; in women, infections are often precipitated by sexual intercourse (O'Callaghan & Brenner 2000). In healthy individuals, bacteriuria of the lower urinary tract increases transiently following sexual intercourse. In men, urinary infections are often associated with bladder outflow obstruction and/or in the presence of a urinary catheter.

PATHOPHYSIOLOGY

Normally, the anterior urethra and, in women, the entrance to the vagina contain microorganisms. The posterior urethra and the urinary tract are sterile. The urethral mucosa has antibacterial properties and is frequently washed by sterile urine, which discourages the passage of bacteria up the urethra to the bladder, ureters and kidneys. The female ureter is short, wide and straight, and allows the passage of organisms into the urinary tract more readily than does the longer male ureter.

The predisposing factors for urinary tract infections are as follows.

Vesico-ureteric reflux (the retrograde flow of urine) This can be:

- *Congenital primary reflux*. This occurs when there is a defect of the muscles around the vesico-ureteric junction (i.e. junction of the bladder and ureter). Abnormalities such as duplication and ectopic ureters can give rise to vesico-ureteric reflux which is often a cause of primary and recurrent infections in children (Downey 2000).
- *Acquired reflux*. This may be seen in patients with neuropathic dysfunction, urethral valves and (more rarely) in those with bladder outflow obstruction due to strictures. Injury to the ureteric orifice during surgery may also result in reflux. Tuberculosis and interstitial cystitis are other causes.

Obstruction Stones or strictures can prevent the free flow of urine and interfere with the ability of the kidneys to decontaminate themselves of organisms:

- *Tumours* of the prostate, bladder and kidney can give rise to urinary tract infections.
- *Pregnancy*. Hydroureter (distension of the ureter with urine) and hydronephrosis (distension of the kidney pelvis) can occur during pregnancy and persist for some months after childbirth. It is caused by relaxation of the muscles due to the high level of progesterone and by the obstruction of the ureters by the uterus.
- *Intubation*. Nephrostomy tubes inserted into the kidney pelvis, urethral or suprapubic catheters and other drainage tubes that communicate with the urinary tract predispose the individual to infection.

Fistulae Abnormal communication between the urinary tract and other structures (especially between the bladder and the colon) will allow organisms to enter the urinary tract.

Sexual trauma During sexual intercourse the female urethra can be traumatised. The movement of the penis in the vagina may also milk organisms along it into the bladder and cause infection. Varied sexual practices, inadequate personal hygiene and the use of foreign bodies can all play a part.

Iatrogenic factors Surgical and diagnostic procedures such as urethral and ureteric catheterisation, cystoscopy and other endoscopic instrumentations may exacerbate existing infections or send infection further up the urinary tract.

Pyelonephritis

Pyelonephritis, or inflammation of the renal pelvis, may occur in one or both kidneys. Bacteria may enter the urinary tract, especially the kidneys, via the bloodstream, or more commonly the bladder. Most organisms causing urinary tract infection — *Escherichia coli, Klebsiella, Proteus, Pseudomonas, Streptococcus faecalis* and *Staphylococcus albus* — are found in the bowel and the perineum.

Acute pyelonephritis

PATHOPHYSIOLOGY

In acute pyelonephritis, the kidney is usually swollen and soft and the pelvis and calyces may contain pus. The mucosal lining of the pelvis may be congested and oedematous.

Common presenting symptoms The patient typically experiences a sudden onset of severe pain in the loin (the area of the back immediately above the buttocks) radiating to the iliac fossa. Other common features are pyrexia, rigor, nausea and vomiting.

Where cystitis (inflammation of the bladder) coexists, dysuria, frequency of micturition and discoloured urine will be noted.

MEDICAL MANAGEMENT

Investigations Procedures will include the following:

- The collection of a midstream specimen of urine (MSU) to be cultured for evidence of a causative organism and antibiotic sensitivity. The specimen must be collected in clean conditions to prevent the introduction of contaminants (Inglis 2003).
- A full blood count and urea and electrolyte estimation. A raised white blood cell count and erythrocyte sedimentation rate (ESR) may be revealed in response to infection.
- An intravenous urogram (IVU) to locate any obstruction in the urinary tract (see Box 8.2). An ultrasound scan may also be performed for the same purpose.

STOP THINK **8.2** What might the nurse do or say to reduce anxiety and help the patient to understand the reasons for the investigations being performed?

Treatment The main aim of treatment is to eradicate the infection by means of antibiotic therapy. This may be commenced even before organism sensitivities are known. A more specific antibiotic can then be used following urine culture results. Analgesics, antiemetics and antipyretics may be prescribed. Oral fluids are recommended, up to 3 L/24 h.

In addition, the doctor will endeavour to determine and resolve any predisposing cause. Urine cultures will be repeated at 7 days to ensure that the infection has been eradicated.

NURSING PRIORITIES AND MANAGEMENT: Acute pyelonephritis

Major considerations

The patient with acute pyelonephritis of sudden onset will feel lethargic and is likely to require a period of bed rest.

In the acute phase, nursing priorities will include the administration of prescribed antibiotics and other medications. Attention should be given to the patient's personal hygiene and comfort, as well as to maintaining an accurate fluid balance record. Increasing fluid intake to as much as 3 L/24 h is to be encouraged (Thomas 2002) as this may reduce the osmotic pressure in the renal medulla and thereby decrease the proliferation of bacteria.

As the patient recovers, the nurse should focus on giving advice regarding hygiene. The importance of attendance at outpatient appointments for assessment of renal function and investigation of further urine infection should be stressed. Follow-up may be particularly problematic if the patient feels well and is symptom-free.

Box 8.2

Intravenous urogram or pyelogram (IVU or IVP)

This investigation, which involves the i.v. injection of an iodine-based contrast medium which is then excreted by the kidneys, allows a series of X-ray pictures of the kidneys, ureters and bladder to be taken.

Prior to the IVU, a control X-ray of the kidneys, ureters and bladder (KUB) is taken. The patient is requested to abstain from food for several hours and fluids for 1 h before the start of the X-rays. This helps the contrast medium to be excreted more quickly. The patient is also given an aperient to clear the bowel and thus ensure a clear image of the contrast medium on the X-ray. The patient should void beforehand to prevent the contrast medium becoming overdilute, resulting in a poor picture. Following the investigation, the patient is allowed to eat and drink again. The contrast medium will be passed when the patient voids urine, with no after-effects or change in the colour of the urine.

The IVU X-rays may show:

- absence of kidney
- obstruction of kidney
- obstruction of the ureter
- irregularities of the bladder wall — this finding may indicate the presence of a bladder tumour, diverticulum, calculi or foreign body.

STOP THINK **8.3** Mrs V is 6 months pregnant and has been admitted to the antenatal ward for investigation and monitoring of a raised blood pressure. Early one evening she complains of feeling very unwell and feverish and is visibly shivering. She is known to have a history of recurrent urinary tract infection. Refer now to Chapter 22. What would be your priorities for Mrs V's immediate care?

Chronic pyelonephritis

Chronic pyelonephritis results from recurrent urinary tract infection. In children, vesico-ureteric reflux is often present.

PATHOPHYSIOLOGY

Chronic pyelonephritis is focal and irregular and may affect both kidneys. Progressive infection causes fibrosis and scarring, which gradually destroys the parenchyma. Eventually, the kidney becomes small, granular and infected.

Common presenting symptoms This condition may be asymptomatic until the patient finally presents with features associated with renal failure. These include uraemia, lethargy, hypertension and proteinuria. Urinary frequency and dysuria may be reported.

MEDICAL MANAGEMENT

Investigations As with acute pyelonephritis, diagnosis can be made by IVU. Urine culture should be performed and urinary tract obstruction excluded.

Treatment Antibiotic treatment can be administered as either a short course in response to organism sensitivities or a long-term course where chronic infection proves difficult to eradicate. Where inflammation persists, renal impairment may progress to end-stage renal failure requiring treatment by dialysis (see p. 391).

NURSING PRIORITIES AND MANAGEMENT: Chronic pyelonephritis

Major considerations

Where the patient experiences acute episodes of inflammation, priorities may be the same as for patients with acute pyelonephritis. However, some individuals with chronic pyelonephritis only experience feelings of tiredness or of being 'under the weather'. Nevertheless, recurrence of infection is common and disturbances of renal function and end-stage renal failure are possibilities that must be taken seriously. The nurse should educate the patient regarding the condition, treatment and potential long-term complications and should emphasise the importance of attending outpatient clinics for assessment even when there are no symptoms. Where long-term antibiotic therapy is required, the patient may have concerns about the necessity for such treatment and the chronic nature of the condition. The nurse should provide opportunities for the patient to ask questions and voice concerns.

In the event that progressive renal failure occurs, the nurse should help to prepare the patient and family for the treatment options available and for the lifestyle adjustments that will need to be made.

For further information, see Wagenlehner & Naber (2000) and Nicolle (2002).

Cystitis

Cystitis may be chronic or acute and is characterised by severe inflammation of the bladder walls. More commonly affecting women, cystitis may result from predisposing factors such as the presence of foreign bodies or stones, obstruction, tuberculosis, carcinoma in situ, chronic urinary infection and schistosomiasis.

PATHOPHYSIOLOGY

Common presenting features are scalding pain on micturition, often followed by bladder spasm, resulting in an urge to pass urine a second time. Frequency, urgency, nocturia and incontinence may also be present. The patient may have a fever and complain of fatigue and abdominal discomfort.

MEDICAL MANAGEMENT

Investigations Urine culture will identify the causative organism, although antibiotic therapy may be commenced before sensitivities are known.

Treatment Repeat urinary cultures should be examined. Persistent infection may require long-term antibiotic treatment. The patient should be encouraged to increase their fluid intake during the day, thereby increasing the flushing effect of the urine flow. The measurement and recording of fluid balance, temperature and pulse are necessary until the patient's clinical symptoms are eradicated.

Many people, however, suffer from recurrent cystitis over several years and attempt to manage the associated problems, often depending on such things as lemon barley water, over-the-counter preparations and advice found in popular magazines. This is an example of a condition for which self-help often plays an important role.

For further information, see Wagenlehner & Naber (2000) and Nicolle (2002).

OBSTRUCTIVE DISORDERS OF THE URINARY TRACT

Disorders that cause obstruction to the flow of urine (see Fig. 8.6) are not uncommon. Although the early stages may cause only mild symptoms which are easily ignored, the progressive damage caused by abnormal pressure, infection and stone formation can lead to renal failure. The importance of early detection and intervention cannot be overemphasised.

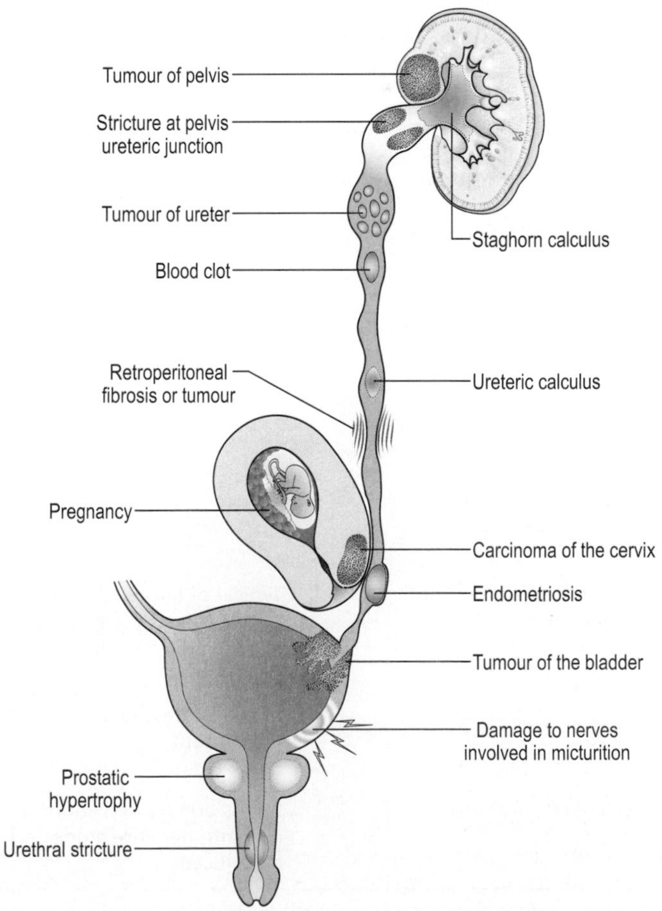

Fig. 8.6 Conditions causing obstruction to the urinary tract.

Urinary stones (renal calculi)

The formation of stones or calculi in the urinary tract is common in Europe, North America and Japan. According to Brewster et al (2001), in the developed world, 1–13% of the population is affected. The increasing incidence of calculi reflects affluence and a diet rich in refined sugar and proteins, but it is acknowledged that a wide variety of aetiological factors influence stone formation (Blandy 1998). Stone formation is more common in men than in women (M:F = 3:1). Interestingly, children and people of black African extraction are rarely affected.

PATHOPHYSIOLOGY

Table 8.1 summarises the features of the main types of stone that can form. In the majority of cases, however, unless there is an underlying disorder, no cause is evident. Box 8.3 identifies the predisposing factors.

Clinical features Stone formation may occur at any point in the urinary tract. Presenting symptoms and features will depend on the stone site:

- Stones that have formed in the renal calyces are often asymptomatic, but obstruction can occur at the calyx neck, resulting in infection and giving rise to pyrexia and pain. Scarring, renal atrophy and pyocalyx can occur.
- Stones found in the calyx can travel to the renal pelvis, causing pyrexia, nausea, vomiting and renal colic.
- The main presenting symptom of upper ureteric stones is colicky pain extending across the abdomen. Haematuria (gross and microscopic) may also be noted.
- The main presenting feature of mid-ureteric and lower ureteric stones is colicky pain radiating towards the scrotum in men and labia in women, together with urgency, frequency and abdominal distension.
- The main presenting symptoms of stone formation in the bladder are pain, dysuria, frequency and urgency.

Box 8.3

Predisposing factors in stone formation

- Idiopathic (most common)
- Stasis of urine, e.g. congenital abnormalities, chronic obstruction
- Chronic urinary infection (urea-splitting organisms, e.g. *Proteus*, cause alkaline urine and the development of magnesium-ammonium-phosphate stones, typically the 'staghorn' calculi of the renal pelvis)
- Excess urinary excretion of stone-forming substances, e.g. idiopathic hypercalciuria (calcium stones), hyperparathyroidism (calcium stones), hyperoxaluria (oxalate stones), gout (uric acid stones), cysteinuria (cysteine stones), xanthinuria (xanthine stones)
- Foreign bodies, e.g. fragments of catheter tubing, self-inserted artefacts, parasites (*Schistosoma* ova)
- Diseased tissue, e.g. renal papillary necrosis
- Multifactorial, e.g. prolonged immobility, children in developing countries

Reproduced with permission from Burkitt et al (1996).

Table 8.1 **Chemical composition, clinical features and aetiology of urinary tract stones**

Chemical composition	%	Clinical features	Aetiology
Calcium oxalate	40	Three types of stone are described: — small smooth 'hempseed' stones — small irregular 'mulberry' stones — small spiculate 'jack' stones	Most cases are idiopathic; predisposing factors include urinary stasis, infection and foreign bodies. Some are due to metabolic disorders: — hyperparathyroidism causing hypercalcaemia rather than hypercalciuria — hyperoxaluria (rare inherited disorder)
Mixed calcium oxalate and phosphate stones	15		Some are due to disorders associated with hypercalcaemia, e.g. sarcoidosis, multiple metastases, multiple myeloma, milk–alkali syndrome, overtreatment with vitamin D
Calcium and phosphate (hydroxyapatite)	15		Some patients excrete abnormally large amounts of calcium (idiopathic hypercalciuria, but without hypercalcaemia)
Magnesium ammonium phosphate	15	Typical of large 'staghorn' calculi of the pelvicalyceal system and some bladder stones	Caused by chronic infection by organisms capable of producing urease. This enzyme splits urea, forming ammonia if the urine is alkaline
Uric acid	8	Stones tend to absorb yellow and brown pigments. Pure stones are radiolucent	Occur in primary gout and also hyperuricaemia following chemotherapy for leukaemias and myeloproliferative disorders. Childhood urate bladder stones occur in some underdeveloped countries when urine pH is low
Cystine or xanthine	2	Excess urinary excretion of cystine or xanthine. Pure stones are radiolucent	Autosomal recessive inherited disorders

Reproduced with permission from Burkitt et al (1996).

MEDICAL MANAGEMENT

Treatment Small calculi (5 mm or less in diameter) may pass unobstructed through the urinary tract and be excreted in the urine. Intervention is indicated if there is evidence of anaemia, infection or hydronephrosis.

Conservative management The use of calcium-chelating agents and limiting calcium and sodium intake in the diet may be indicated where increased absorption of calcium is responsible for calculi formation. Acidification or alkalination of urine may prevent stones which form in these conditions. Fluid intake should be enough to ensure a urine output of 2 L/24 h. The drinking of large quantities of fluid serves no useful purpose. The rationale behind this practice is to produce sufficient urine flow to flush out the stone, but in practice the presence of a continued obstruction will simply result in further distension of the collecting system and make matters worse. Normal hydration is therefore recommended.

For further information, see Blandy (1998), Brewster et al (2001) and Tiselius (2003).

MANAGEMENT OF ACUTE RENAL COLIC

Investigations Procedures are listed in Table 8.2.

Treatment The patient with renal stones may be acutely ill, suffering from excruciating pain arising in the loin and radiating to the groin, which can last 5–6 h. Pain is caused by small calculi being moved along the ureter by peristaltic movements, by impaction and by obstruction of urine. Bed rest, warmth to the site of pain (Haslett et al 2002) and analgesics are the first line of treatment.

Medications include the opioid morphine (10–20 mg) intramuscularly. Pethidine should be avoided as it is associated with a higher incidence of vomiting (Holdgate & Pollock 2004). Diclofenac sodium (100 mg per rectum, usually at night) is a prostaglandin synthetase inhibitor which reduces renal blood flow and urination. It has an antispasmodic and anti-inflammatory effect and is long acting. Nausea may be relieved by an antiemetic such as i.m. prochlorperazine (12.5 mg) (Trounce & Gould 2000).

Flush-back of calculi and stenting This procedure affords temporary relief when a calculus causes obstruction and pain in the ureter. The stone is flushed back to the pelvis of the kidney. A small silicone tube, called a stent, is positioned in the ureter from the pelviureteric junction to the bladder. This stent is left in position to hold the stone in place. Further treatment to remove the stone can now be planned. The stent should not be left for more than 6 weeks. If the planned treatment cannot be carried out by the end of this period, the stent should be changed.

Insertion of a nephrostomy tube is indicated when obstruction in the kidney or the ureter cannot be relieved by flush-back and stenting (see Fig. 8.7 and Box 8.4). This is carried out under X-ray control, usually with a local anaesthetic. A small silicone tube is placed percutaneously into the collecting system of the kidney. The tube is held in place by a suture and connected to a closed-system drainage bag.

Ureteroscopic removal of calculi This procedure is suitable in the treatment of small calculi in the ureter. The ureteric orifice is dilated cystoscopically and a ureteroscope, to which a 'stone basket' is attached, is introduced into the ureter. The basket is opened out to ensnare the stone. The basket and stone are then withdrawn.

Rigid ureteroscopes are now available which can be inserted under direct vision. The surgeon is able to see the stone and can disintegrate it in situ before removing the smaller fragments in a 'basket' (Underwood et al 2003).

Extracorporeal shock wave lithotripsy (ESWL) This procedure is the treatment of choice for the majority of calculi, both renal and ureteric (Downey 2000). It effectively treats 70–80% of cases. Large calculi are broken up by means of this technique before percutaneous removal.

There are several lithotripsy centres in the UK, but some patients have to travel some distance for this treatment. Second-generation lithotripsers allow most patients to be

Table 8.2 Some investigations used for patients with renal calculi

Type of investigation	Test	Purpose
Investigation of urinary tract	Examination of urine for protein, RBC, WBC	Indicates abnormality of urinary tract
	MSU	Urinary infection
	Plain film abdomen	Shows opaque calculi, nephrocalcinosis
	IVU	Shows all calculi obstruction and abnormalities of urinary tract
Investigation of renal function	Blood urea, plasma creatinine	
	Creatinine clearance	
Investigation to determine underlying cause	Chemical analysis of calculus	Provides information as to what investigations to pursue
	Plasma calcium, phosphate	Hypercalcaemia
	Plasma parathyroid hormone	If hypercalcaemia is present to investigate possible hyperparathyroidism
	24-h urine calcium (2)	Hypercalciuria
	Plasma urate, 24-h urine urate (2)	In patients with urate stones or calcium stones
	24-h urine cystine (2)	In patients with cystine stones
	24-h urine oxalate (2)	Hyperoxaluria

Adapted from Haslett et al (2002), with permission.

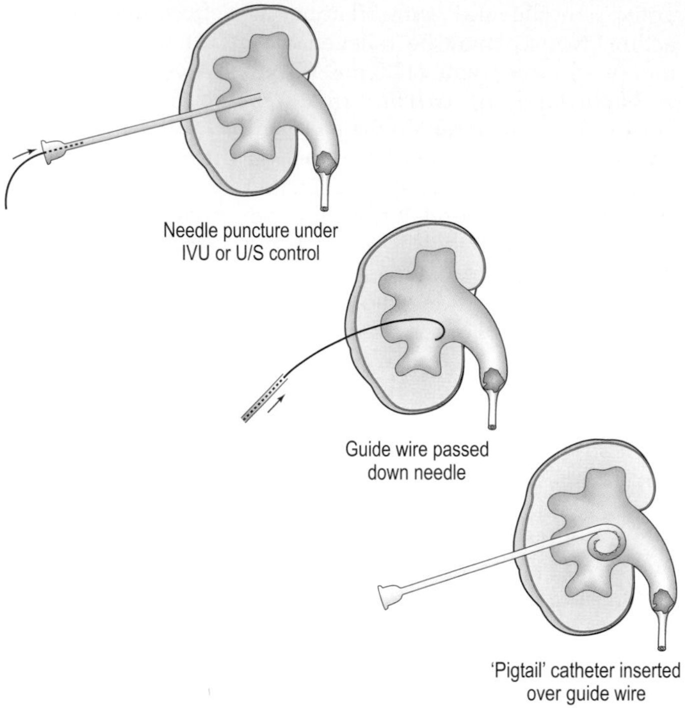

Fig. 8.7 Percutaneous nephrostomy.

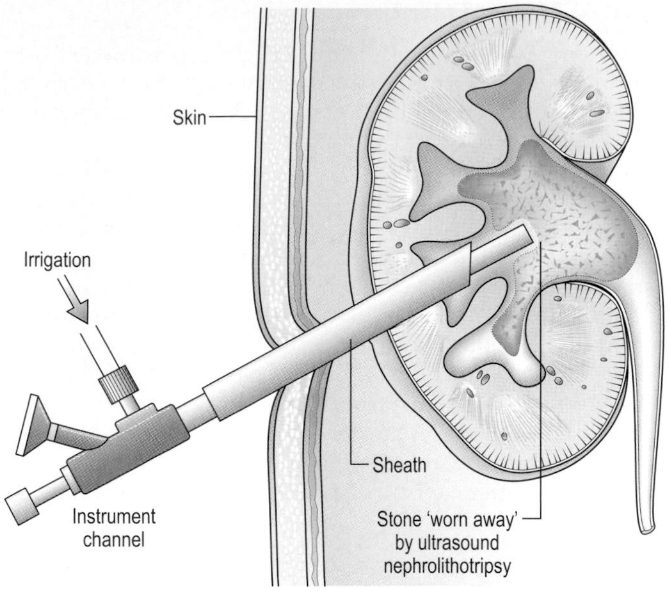

Fig. 8.8 Percutaneous stone removal.

Box 8.4

Stenting

The stents used by most surgeons are called 'double-J' or 'pigtail' stents and have small holes down most of the length of their tubing. These stents are self-retaining and must be removed endoscopically.

Some surgeons use an infant feeding tube as a stent following pyeloplasty, pyelolithotomy or ureterolithotomy. Infant feeding tubes are self-retaining to a degree, but the patient will need a urethral catheter in situ to keep the tube in place. When the catheter is removed the patient may pass the feeding tube without intervention. If this does not happen within 24 h, endoscopic removal will be required.

treated without anaesthetic. Depending on the density of the stone more than one treatment may be required. The patient lies on a special table, which allows shock waves produced by the lithotriptor machine to pass through it. The force of the shock waves causes the stone to disintegrate and fragment. The position of the patient on the table is dependent on the location of the stone. The whole procedure is performed under specialised X-ray and ultrasonic control. The disintegrated or powdered calculus is then allowed to pass down the ureter over the next few days.

Percutaneous nephrolithotomy (PCNL) This procedure is used to remove calculi lying within the kidney. Large staghorn calculi may need to be broken up first, using ESWL.

PCNL is performed under X-ray and ultrasound control. The patient will normally have a general anaesthetic. The kidney is punctured and the tract into the kidney is dilated to allow the nephroscope and a variety of grasping instruments to be inserted. The stone can then be removed or broken down into fine powder by ultrasonic probes (see Fig. 8.8). This powder can be aspirated through the centre of the probe.

Sometimes an electrohydraulic probe is used. This produces shock waves in the irrigating fluid to the kidney and results in the stone splitting into several fragments.

At the end of the procedure, a large nephrostomy tube with a smaller tube running down its centre is left in position to allow drainage and to prevent haematoma formation. This also allows access for a nephrogram 24–48 h postoperatively to assess the effectiveness of treatment.

Nephrogram No anaesthetic is required for this procedure. A contrast medium is injected down the smaller tube of a nephrostomy tube into the kidney. X-rays can then be taken and any fragments of calculi identified. Provided that there are no fragments left, the tubes can be removed.

Ureterolithotomy This open surgery is appropriate in the treatment of calculi occurring mid-ureter and causing obstruction that cannot be dealt with in any other way. An X-ray to identify the position of the stone will determine the incision to be made. The ureter is exposed and opened and the stone removed. The ureter is repaired either by removing a small section or by suturing the opening. A stent is usually left in place, positioned along the length of the ureter. This allows the ureter to heal and prevents leakage.

A wound drain will be left in position to prevent haematoma formation. The stent will normally be removed after 7 days.

Pyelolithotomy This open surgery can be used for the removal of calculi in the pelvis of the kidney which are causing an obstruction that cannot be removed by ESWL or PCNL. The procedure involves first exposing the affected kidney and then opening the pelvis of the kidney to remove the stone. Sometimes it is not possible to remove all of a staghorn calculus (see Table 8.1) in this way, in which case further incisions into the surrounding renal tissue (nephrolithotomy) are necessary. A stent will be left in place for 7 days.

NURSING PRIORITIES AND MANAGEMENT: Acute renal colic

Major considerations

A patient admitted with renal colic can often do little more than cope with the excruciating pain, and is often unable to answer questions or to follow advice and instructions until the pain is relieved. Once the acute attack has subsided, the patient should be allowed to rest since only then will it be possible to absorb all the necessary explanations relating to investigations and treatment. Nursing Care Plan 8.1 outlines the priorities of nursing care for a patient admitted with acute renal colic.

Following specific interventions

Flush-back and stenting

Medium-sized stones in the upper half of the ureter are associated with obstruction. Under direct vision the calculi are flushed back into the renal pelvis and a stent is inserted;

Nursing Care Plan 8.1 Nursing care for a patient admitted with acute renal colic

Potential problem	Action	Desired outcome
1. **Pain of a potentially excruciating nature**	• Administer prescribed analgesics • Evaluate effect of analgesics: return to patient in 30 min: – ask if she is pain-free and record a pain score using an appropriate pain assessment tool – observe for evidence of pain, e.g. raised pulse rate, sweating and evidence of neurogenic shock (see Ch. 18)	Pain is relieved
2. **Frequency and urgency of micturition**	• Locate urinal within reach of patient	Sensations decline as pain is relieved
3. **Nausea and vomiting**	• Administer prescribed antiemetics • Evaluate effect of treatment: return to patient in 30 min • Locate vomit bowl within patient's reach	Patient obtains relief from feelings of nausea and from vomiting
4. **Fluid and electrolyte imbalance**	• Institute i.v. fluids if patient is unable to take adequate fluid orally	Fluid and electrolytes are maintained at satisfactory levels
5. **Ureteric obstruction**	• Check and record blood pressure • Observe BP trends and report elevations • Measure urine output; report reduction in volume • Observe for haematuria and passage of stones	Any obstruction is recognised immediately
6. **Urinary tract infection**	• Check and record temperature; report pyrexia • Check and record pulse rate; observe trends and report elevations	Infection is prevented or immediately recognised
7. **Non-passage of small calculi**	• Encourage normal volumes of fluid intake • Alleviate nausea and vomiting • Check urine for presence of calculi (use plastic urinal to prevent sticking of calculi)	Passage and collection for analysis of small calculi
8. **Inability to perform personal hygiene**	• Offer wash and change of bed gown as required, particularly if sweating is profuse	Patient is clean and comfortable Self-esteem is maintained
9. **Difficulty in finding a comfortable position in bed**	• Assist patient to find a comfortable position • Evaluate position regularly; ask the patient if she is comfortable	Patient is relaxed and comfortable
10. **Anxiety**	• Give patient the opportunity to voice concerns • Provide information about the condition, investigations and treatment • Ensure the nurse call system is close at hand at all times	Patient has an understanding of the condition and has reduced anxiety about outcome

ESWL can then be performed. The patient should be prepared for a general anaesthetic as discussed in Chapter 26. Normally, only a short-acting anaesthetic is required. Priorities in postoperative nursing care are as follows:

- To record observations, temperature, pulse and blood pressure and to watch for signs of infection.
- To monitor urine output and record volume and colour of urine on the fluid chart. A decrease in volume may indicate obstruction. Haematuria may indicate trauma, but some haematuria is to be expected.
- To encourage a fluid intake of 3 L daily to prevent infection.
- To administer analgesics if the patient is in pain. Severe pain must be reported to medical staff, as this may indicate trauma, a misplaced stent or return of obstruction.

Discharge advice The patient should be advised:

- to continue to drink 3 L daily
- to take mild analgesics such as paracetamol or co-proxamol if in pain
- to seek help from the GP if urine output is bloodstained or 'burning'.

The patient should also be advised when follow-up treatment will take place and what this will entail. If treatment is not within 6 weeks, it must be impressed upon the patient that it is very important to have the stent changed. If it is not changed, sediment and crystals will build up around it and form more calculi.

Extracorporeal shock wave lithotripsy (ESWL)

The role of the nurse in the ESWL unit includes giving reassurance to both the patient and the family, explaining what to expect, administering any prescribed medication, encouraging the patient to drink following the procedure and giving discharge advice.

The patient may receive an oral premedication such as diazepam or temazepam prior to treatment. The treatment is not normally painful. Anxiety may be experienced due to the noise from the shock waves and the requirement to lie still for 1–1.5 h. Playing recorded music may help to alleviate anxiety and boredom.

The patient will normally stay in the ESWL unit until urine has been passed. Prophylactic antibiotics and analgesics may also be given.

Most patients will be able to return home and continue with their normal daily activities. However, a small percentage will need hospital admission during the first week post-treatment because of colicky pain, oedema and, occasionally, obstruction of the ureter. This will sometimes settle with no further treatment, but a stent may need to be inserted to allow the oedema to subside.

Discharge advice The patient should be advised:

- to drink 3 L of fluid a day, to help prevent infection and to help the gravel to pass down the urinary system
- to expect some haematuria and gravel when passing urine
- to take prescribed analgesics, but if pain increases to see the GP or report back to the hospital
- to attend a follow-up appointment about 6 weeks later to have further X-rays taken to assess the effect of the treatment.

Percutaneous nephrolithotomy (PCNL)

Preoperatively, the patient should be prepared for a general anaesthetic (see Ch. 26). Postoperatively, the patient is likely to return to the ward with:

- a urethral catheter in situ
- an i.v. infusion of clear fluids
- a nephrostomy tube in the affected kidney.

The nephrostomy tube is a large-bore tube with a narrower tube running down its centre. These tubes will normally be sutured into position and enclosed in a urostomy drainage bag attached to a large 2 L drainage bag.

Priorities in the management of the nephrostomy tube are to maintain a closed drainage system in order to prevent infection, and to monitor drainage. The nurse responsible must:

- check the position and the placement of the nephrostomy tube
- help the patient into a position that is comfortable and allows the tube to drain
- empty the drainage bag when necessary and record the volume and colour of output
- remember that the urine will take the path of least resistance, so most of the output from the affected kidney will discharge via the nephrostomy tube.

The urethral catheter is normally removed 24 h following surgery. The i.v. infusion is discontinued at the same time, if the patient is able to drink normally. A nephrogram is carried out 48 h following surgery, and the nephrostomy tube removed if treatment has been successful. Following removal of the nephrostomy tube, the patient may continue to pass urine via the puncture site. This will normally cease after 12–24 h.

The patient may have colicky pain following the removal of the tube, as the urine must now redirect itself via the correct route. Analgesics can be given, and the patient should be asked to lie on the affected side. This will take the pressure off the affected kidney, and the drainage will pass via the puncture site.

Once drainage from the puncture site has ceased, a small, dry dressing can be applied and the patient discharged home. Occasionally the nephrostomy tube may need to be left in situ for a prolonged period because further treatment may be necessary. In this case, the patient may be discharged home into the care of the GP and community nurse.

Ureterolithotomy or pyelolithotomy

Preoperative preparation is as normal, including skin preparation and any necessary shaving of the area to be operated upon (see Ch. 26).

If there has been an uneventful 2- or 3-day postoperative period, and a double-J stent or pigtail stent has been used, the patient may be discharged home into the care of the GP and community nurse, returning as a day case to the hospital for removal of the stent. The community nurse will check the wound and take note of the patient's temperature and urine output. Sutures are removed from the wound

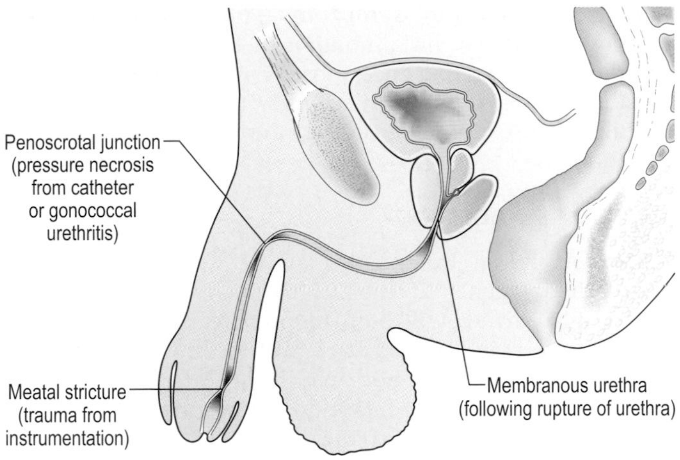

Fig. 8.9 Common sites and causes of urethral stricture.

at 7–10 days. If an infant feeding tube has been used as a stent (see Box 8.4), then the urethral catheter will remain in situ for 5–6 days. In this case, the patient may need to stay in hospital until the stent and sutures have been removed.

Urethral strictures

PATHOPHYSIOLOGY

A stricture is a narrowing within a structure which may arise from inflammation, muscular spasm or neoplastic occlusion. Urethral strictures can be congenital, caused by trauma, as in pelvic fracture, as a consequence of investigative instrumentation of the urethra (e.g. cystoscopy) or result from the presence of an indwelling urethral catheter (see Fig. 8.9). Infections such as non-specific urethritis and gonorrhoea may also result in stricture formation. It is a condition that more commonly affects men because of the length and structure of the male urethra.

Common presenting symptoms which can prove to be both distressing and frustrating are poor urinary flow, a feeling of incomplete bladder emptying, frequency, dysuria or haematuria, and dribbling incontinence, secondary to chronic urinary retention.

MEDICAL MANAGEMENT

Tests and investigations required are flow rate studies, retrograde urethrogram, urethroscopy, and full blood screening.

Treatment options include the following:

Urethrotomy The optical urethrotome allows the surgeon, under direct vision, to divide the urethral stricture. A silicone catheter would normally be left in place for a specified period to allow healing. However, the length of time it will be left in situ is variable.

Self-dilatation Often used in conjunction with urethrotomy, this technique involves the patient using a self-lubricating urethral catheter on a regular basis to increase the urethral diameter and keep the urethral passage open.

Urethroplasty Usually performed in two stages, this procedure involves excision of the stricture and anastomosis. In some cases a graft is required to replace the excised urethral tissue. This surgery requires a longer stay in hospital and is normally performed only after other treatments have failed.

NURSING PRIORITIES AND MANAGEMENT: Urethral strictures

STOP THINK **8.4** As a nurse looking after Mr E (see Case History 8.1), what could you do to help him come to terms with the idea of performing self-dilatation and to feel more positive about it?

Major patient problems

In many cases urethral strictures are difficult to correct and recurrence is likely, thus the person must learn to live with the condition.

Self-dilatation

The patient faced with the prospect of needing to perform self-dilatation on an ongoing basis will need moral support and encouragement from the health care team. A specialist nurse will explain and demonstrate the procedure initially and then guide the patient through it, ensuring that continuing support is provided as needed. It will also be helpful for the nurse to emphasise the following points:

- No-one need know that the individual is using this technique.
- Although the idea may be difficult to accept, this treatment will minimise the risk of further admission to hospital and time off work.
- There is always a risk of infection, but this can be minimised with good hygiene, washing of hands and meatus, and adequate intake of fluids.

CASE HISTORY 8.1

Mr E

Mr E, a 35-year-old fireman, was having difficulty in passing urine. Two years previously, he had been involved in an accident in which he suffered crush injuries to his pelvis and urethra. At that time he had had a suprapubic catheter (i.e. a catheter inserted into the bladder via the abdominal wall) for 6 weeks.

On the more recent occasion, he was referred to the urologist by his GP for two reasons: firstly, Mr E had had repeated urinary tract infections over the last year; secondly, he had noticed that for the last 6 months there was a difference in the time it took him to pass urine and that the stream was thinner than usual.

After a full investigation, the surgeon decided that the best course of action would be to perform an optical urethrotomy, followed by the patient being taught to perform self-dilatation. Mr E agreed to have the operation, although he did not like the idea of performing self-dilatation. When given the opportunity to discuss this, he expressed the following concerns:

- 'What if my friends and relatives find out?'
- 'I don't want to put a tube up there. How do I do it?'
- 'What about infection?'
- 'How often will I need to do this?'
- 'I work shifts. How can I do this?'

- Dilatation will be necessary once a day at first, but as time goes on it can normally be reduced to once a week depending on individual needs.
- Irregular working schedules should not pose a problem, and the patient can work out a routine that is convenient.

Fibrosis

PATHOPHYSIOLOGY

Fibrosis is the formation of excessive fibrous connective tissue within a structure. Fibrosis around the ureters predisposes them to obstruction. The cause of the fibrosis is often unknown. This condition, known as retroperitoneal fibrosis, is not neoplastic but can result in damage to renal function. Other external causes of fibrosis are post-radiotherapy treatment, scarring arising from other surgical procedures, and aortic aneurysm. Fibrosis within structures (e.g. ureters/urethra) is usually secondary to instrumentation.

DISORDERS OF THE PENIS AND MALE URETHRA

Phimosis

In this condition, the foreskin or prepuce of the penis is too tight to be retracted over the glans penis. It is most frequently due to balanitis xerotica obliterans, a fibrosing condition of unknown aetiology (Brewster et al 2001). Other causes include infection, trauma as a result of early attempts to draw back the foreskin before it has naturally separated or developed fully in size, or a poorly performed circumcision operation.

PATHOPHYSIOLOGY

The natural separation of the two layers of skin from the glans penis normally occurs by about the age of 2 years. Following separation, daily bathing is necessary to ensure hygiene is maintained. Poor personal hygiene can give rise to inflammation and infection and has been implicated as a cause of carcinoma of the penis (Downey 2000).

Box 8.5

Circumcision

Circumcision, the surgical removal of the prepuce (foreskin), may be indicated for penile carcinoma, balanitis, candidal infection, phimosis or adherent prepuce. These conditions generally affect adults. Circumcision may also be performed in accordance with religious beliefs, in which case the procedure is usually performed in childhood.

The main complications of circumcision are infection and bleeding. Painful erections in the immediate postoperative period can usually be relieved by the application of a local anaesthetic gel. Postoperative swelling or oedema may make micturition difficult. Dribbling or urinary leakage to the wound area can delay or prevent wound healing and cause secondary infection. The insertion of a urethral catheter may be necessary to relieve this problem in order that wound healing may take place.

Common presenting symptoms Phimosis often causes balanoposthitis, i.e. inflammation of both the glans penis (balanitis) and the prepuce (posthitis). Presenting features include itching, a white discharge, pain, discomfort and bleeding at sexual intercourse, and sometimes urinary retention.

MEDICAL MANAGEMENT

Treatment Initial treatment may be with antibiotics or anticandidal agents. If the individual is sexually active, he and his partner will both require treatment to prevent the infection being passed back and forth. Circumcision is the treatment of choice and may have to be performed as an emergency if urinary retention has occurred (see Box 8.5 and Case Histories 8.2 and 8.3).

CASE HISTORY 8.2

Mr A

Mr A, aged 20, presented to his GP with bleeding from the foreskin following sexual intercourse. He was concerned as this was the sixth occurrence.

On examination the foreskin was found to be very tight, and the GP advised circumcision. Referral was made to the local consultant urologist, and Mr A was put on the waiting list. After only a few weeks he was admitted as a day case for circumcision. Before discharge, he was given the following advice verbally and in written form by nursing staff:

- Take daily baths
- Do not go straight back to work. Avoid walking around for the next few days
- Change underwear daily. Do not wear anything tight until the wound has healed
- You must be able to pass urine before leaving hospital, and you should drink at least 3 L of fluids in 24 h to prevent urinary tract infection
- If you have pain, take a simple analgesic such as paracetamol every 4–6 h for the first 48 h
- At any sign of swelling, redness or fever, go and see your GP
- Sexual intercourse should be avoided until the skin is healed and feels normal
- Should any other problems arise, report to your GP or, if necessary, return to the hospital
- Change the dressing if it becomes wet with urine. Use a non-stick dressing.

CASE HISTORY 8.3

Mr C

Mr C, a 70-year-old widower, was referred by his GP to a urologist as an emergency, because he was in pain and having difficulty passing urine. On examination it was found that he had a tight foreskin and it was difficult to see the meatus. On abdominal examination he appeared to be retaining urine. Ultrasound confirmed that there was approximately 500 mL in his bladder.

Mr C was admitted to the ward with instructions that he would be operated on within the next 2 h for circumcision and urethral catheterisation. He was told that the catheter may need to stay in position for 24–48 h, depending on his general condition, and that his stay in hospital would be between 48 h and 1 week.

NURSING PRIORITIES AND MANAGEMENT: Phimosis

Prevention

Health education of the parents is important in the early years. It should be stressed that retraction of the foreskin for cleansing is unnecessary. Normal bathing or showering routines should suffice.

Promoting wound healing after circumcision

The nurse can promote wound healing by the following means:

- teaching good personal hygiene to the newly circumcised person
- washing the wound area daily with soap and water and applying a protective, non-adhesive dressing to prevent clothing disturbing wound healing
- providing more frequent washing and dressing changes should urine leakage occur onto the wound or dressing
- counselling the sexually active patient to refrain from sexual intercourse until the wound is well healed.

STOP THINK **8.5** How would your discharge advice to Mr A in Case History 8.2 compare with that given to Mr C in Case History 8.3? Would you make any changes, omissions or additions in your advice to the older man? What assumptions would prompt such changes? Are all of these assumptions fair?

Paraphimosis

Paraphimosis is a condition in which a foreskin that has been retracted over the glans penis cannot be returned to its usual position. The swollen band of foreskin obstructs the circulation to the glans, which in turn becomes swollen and painful. It is classed as a medical emergency as delayed action may lead to gangrene of the glans (Downey 2000).

Cold compresses applied to the penis may help to relieve the swelling and pain. The doctor or nurse may be able to manipulate the glans back under the foreskin with or without anaesthesia. Because of extreme pain, patients may require a penile nerve block, topical analgesic or oral opioids. If manipulation is unsuccessful, a dorsal slit may be made in the foreskin. There remains a risk of recurrence of the paraphimosis and a circumcision may be advisable at a later date.

Congenital disorders of the urethra and penis

At birth, an infant is examined to confirm its sex and to make sure that expected bodily structures are present. In boys, the urethral meatus is normally seen at the anterior tip of the glans penis. Occasionally a malformation of the urethra is identified as a congenital defect.

Hypospadias

Hypospadias is a condition where the meatus of the urethra is found in a position on the undersurface of the glans penis. It is the commonest congenital penile abnormality (Brewster et al 2001, Underwood et al 2003). The condition is usually treated quite effectively by enlargement of the meatus by plastic surgery. In some cases the urethral orifice is positioned further back on the lower surface of the penis, and this will complicate treatment. Surgical reconstruction should take place before the age of 2 years, as this avoids cosmetic and fertility problems in later life. The position of the meatus, distal urethra and presence or absence of chordee (downward curvature of the penis) will influence the surgical approach adopted.

Epispadias

The condition of epispadias is one in which the urethra opens onto the upper surface, or dorsum, of the penis. The meatus of the urethra may be positioned anywhere along the length of the penile surface. Epispadias may coexist with other serious congenital abnormalities involving a poorly developed anterior section of the urinary bladder and abdominal wall. Surgical reconstruction is likely to be complex and may involve transplantation of ureters.

DISORDERS OF THE PROSTATE

Benign prostatic hyperplasia

The prostate gland increases in size with age, reaching about 20–25 g by the time the individual is 20 years old. In individuals over the age of 45, the smooth muscle segments atrophy and are replaced by collagen fibres. As ageing progresses, connective tissue accumulates, resulting in benign prostatic hyperplasia (BPH), the most common neoplastic growth in men. Fifty per cent of men over the age of 60 will have BPH, but not all will have symptoms (Thorpe & Neal 2003). Demographic trends suggest that as people age, symptoms will become more prevalent (Wilt 2002). The cause of BPH is unknown, but it is thought that it may be associated with reduced androgen secretions.

Bladder outflow obstruction can occur for a number of reasons (see Box 8.6), but the most common cause is benign prostate hyperplasia.

PATHOPHYSIOLOGY

Stasis of urine in the bladder and a build-up of pressure in the bladder and ureters predispose the individual to infection, the formation of stones and possible renal failure. The bladder becomes enlarged, forming bundles called trabeculae. Diverticula may also be noted. If left untreated, obstructive effects will develop (see Fig. 8.10).

Common presenting symptoms The enlargement of the gland may be asymptomatic, perhaps noted only on a routine rectal examination. However, as the hyperplasia increasingly distorts and compresses the urethra and even the bladder, an inability to void normally will become obvious. Many men tolerate symptoms indefinitely, seeing them as just 'old men's problems' that have to be accepted. Presenting symptoms include:

- Irritative symptoms
  — frequency >7 times/day
  — urgency
  — nocturia

Box 8.6

Bladder outflow obstruction

Causes
- Benign prostatic hyperplasia
- Bladder calculi
- Bladder tumour
- Diuretics
- Neurological disturbances
- Phimosis
- Prostatic carcinoma
- Urethral strictures, stenosis, trauma

Common symptoms
- Double voiding
- Dribbling post-voiding
- Dysuria
- Diminished force of urine flow/stream
- Frequency
- Hesitancy
- Haematuria (occasional)
- Nocturia
- Incontinence
- Interrupted stream
- Urgency
- Urinary retention

Inadequate emptying of the bladder can result in a build-up of residual urine, increasing the risk of urinary tract infection and the incidence of bladder stone formation.

Diagnosis
Diagnosis of bladder flow obstruction may be assisted by:

- Blood screen of urea, electrolytes and creatinine
- Endoscopy — urethroscopy and cystoscopy
- History of symptoms
- Physical examination
- Ultrasound scan — residual urine volume and upper urinary tract
- Urinalysis
- Urine culture
- Urodynamic evaluation
- Voiding cystometrogram

- Voiding symptoms
  — hesitancy
  — poor stream
  — incomplete emptying
  — terminal dribbling
  — prolonged voiding times.

In addition, a history of recurrent urinary tract infections may be given. Increasing pressure due to obstruction, if untreated, can eventually result in renal impairment.

Acute urinary retention may be the single presenting feature, particularly if the prostate gland suddenly increases in size or if infection occurs. Some patients present with chronic urinary retention, sometimes associated with haematuria and urethral bleeding. Abnormal voiding patterns and disruption of daytime activities or sleep patterns can affect the individual's ability to work and interact normally with colleagues, partners and family. Bedwetting or urinary incontinence may cause embarrassment and distress. Embarrassment about such symptoms may also

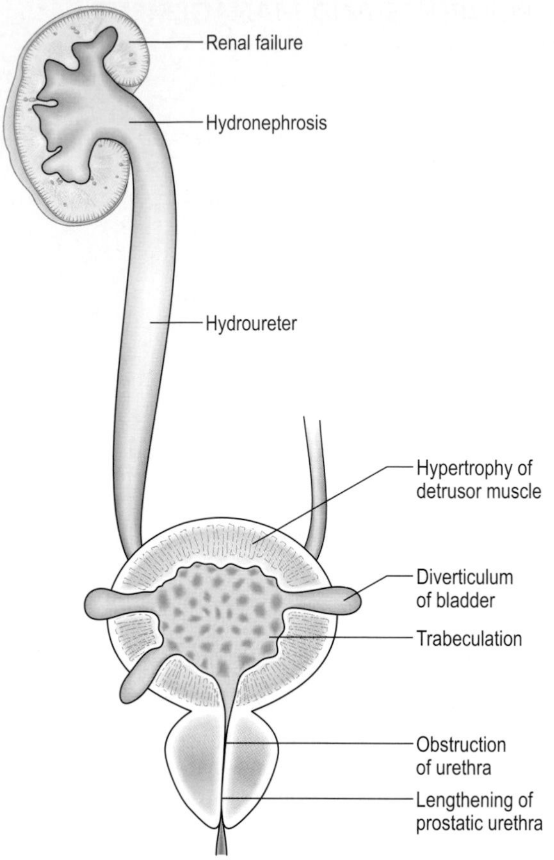

Fig. 8.10 Late sequelae of prostatic obstruction.

result in failure to seek professional help until the condition becomes unbearable.

MEDICAL MANAGEMENT

Investigations Diagnosis can be made by rectal examination; the prostate gland will feel large, elastic and uniform. Investigations will include:

- ultrasound scan
- urinary flow rates
- renal function tests
- full blood count
- symptom score to quantify symptoms and measure how 'bothersome' they are, for example, International Prostatic Symptom Score (IPSS) (Haslett et al 2002)
- serum acid phosphatase or serum prostate-specific antigen (PSA) to eliminate diagnosis of carcinoma in selected patients
- MSU.

Treatment is dependent on individual wishes, severity of symptoms and degree of obstruction (Underwood et al 2003).

Treatment options include:

- watchful waiting
- surgery
- laser therapy
- transurethral ablation
- transurethral microwave therapy (Thorpe & Neal 2003).

For further information, see Downey (2000), Garden et al (2002) and Thorpe & Neal (2003).

Transurethral resection of the prostate gland (TURP) is the surgical operation of choice. Where the gland is too large to resect transurethrally, an open procedure is used, most commonly taking the retropubic or transvesical approach. Prior to commencing the resection, a cystoscope is passed to view the bladder (see Box 8.7). A resectoscope is then passed and small sections are chipped away from the prostatic lobes, removing the material that had been intruding into the urethra and bladder neck. Irrigation fluid of a non-electrolyte solution, glycine, constantly flushes out the bladder during the procedure; an electrolyte solution is contraindicated in the presence of diathermy as this does not transmit electrical current effectively. Most commonly, irrigation continues postoperatively, as the operative bed can give rise to considerable bleeding and clots could lead to obstruction.

Potential postoperative complications of TURP are:

- haemorrhage — evident as haematuria
- clot retention
- infection — urinary tract, epididymis or testis
- extravasation — escape of urine into surrounding tissue due to bladder or urethral damage
- deep vein thrombosis and pulmonary embolism.

Possible late complications are:

- urethral stricture
- incontinence
- impotence
- retrograde ejaculation
- bladder neck stenosis.

For further information, see Reilly (1997).

Box 8.7

Cystoscopy

This procedure allows the surgeon to visualise the interior of the bladder and to take biopsies where suspicious lesions are evident. It may be carried out either under general anaesthetic with a rigid cystoscope or under local anaesthetic with a flexible cystoscope. The method selected will depend on the condition of the patient.

Cystoscopy under general anaesthetic

The standard procedures for preparing a patient for general anaesthesia will apply. The lower bowel should be free of faeces so that insertion of the cystoscope is not impeded or the view restricted.

Once recovered from the anaesthetic, the patient should be encouraged to drink and should be able to pass urine within 6 h of the procedure. The nurse should collect the first specimen passed and record its colour and amount.

Upon discharge, the patient should be advised that he may experience some frequency of desire to pass urine. He should watch for blood in the urine and, should this appear, increase his fluid intake. If the frequency does not settle, or if any bleeding continues, the patient should contact his GP or the hospital.

Cystoscopy under local anaesthetic

There is no restriction on the taking of food or fluids prior to this procedure, but the lower bowel should be free of faeces. The local anaesthetic is placed directly into the urethra in the form of lidocaine (lignocaine) gel. In a male patient, a penile clamp is applied to the penis to allow the gel to move along the urethra. A period of 10–20 min should normally be allowed for the local anaesthetic to take effect.

Following the procedure, the patient will normally pass urine sooner than under general anaesthetic, as there will have been no restriction applied to fluid intake prior to the operation.

NURSING PRIORITIES AND MANAGEMENT: Benign prostatic hyperplasia

General considerations

Patients with acute retention

Most patients presenting with acute retention as a result of BPH will be discharged home with a catheter in situ and will return for planned surgery at a later date; this reduces perioperative inpatient stay (Pickard et al 1998). Once the obstruction is relieved there is no urgency to perform surgery, which allows the treatment of any associated medical conditions and, when appropriate, the patient can be placed on the operating list.

Patients with chronic retention

Chronic urinary retention is usually the result of a crescendo of symptoms of prostatism. These men do not always complain of symptoms of bladder outflow obstruction, but mainly of urge incontinence, dribbling urine or wet beds at night. They usually have no pain and, although they have a large amount of residual urine, their bladder distension is not always obvious to the eye or palpable on physical examination.

Because of the large amount of residual urine, these patients are at risk of developing upper urinary tract dilatation and impaired renal function. However, if there is no renal impairment, it is not essential that these individuals are catheterised. It is urgent to make a diagnosis and proceed to prostatectomy once rehydration and renal function have returned to normal.

Catheterisation will permit bladder drainage and allow renal function recovery (see Boxes 8.8 and 8.9). Once catheterised, the patient may have a huge diuresis. His thirst mechanism will not allow adequate fluid replacement, making parenteral fluid replacement necessary. Large fluid replacement volumes put the patient at risk of heart failure and it should be borne in mind that impaired renal function may have precipitated anaemia.

Once the patient has been catheterised, his renal function restored and any anaemia corrected, there is no urgency to proceed to surgery. The individual may in fact benefit from a period of recuperation and bladder rest with the catheter in place. Depending upon the general well-being of the individual and upon community resources, care may be given in hospital or in the patient's home.

A trial without the catheter should not be made, as this would again lead to chronic retention followed by renal failure.

Box 8.8

The use of catheters

Indications for catheterisation

- Acute or chronic retention of urine
- Diagnostic investigations of the bladder function
- Pre- and postoperative needs
- Following trauma, burns, road traffic accidents or any trauma to the lower urinary tract
- Therapeutic instillations of specifically prescribed medication
- Intractable incontinence where all other methods have failed
- Protracted loss of consciousness

Choice of catheter

Points to consider when choosing a catheter are:

- The purpose of the catheterisation
- The length of time the catheter must remain in situ
- Whether a self-retaining catheter is necessary
- The gender of the patient.

Features of the catheter

- The smallest catheter that will adequately drain the bladder should be used: size 12–16 Fg for adults with clear urine; size 18–22 Fg for adults with haematuria
- The lumen of the catheter will vary depending on the material used. A latex catheter is made up of several layers of material, often coated inside with silicone, and its lumen will be smaller than that of a silicone catheter, which is extruded from one piece of material (Pomfret 1996)
- Balloon size: the larger the balloon, the higher the drainage eye lies in the bladder. This can impair drainage and cause more irritation to the sensitive trigone of the bladder. The balloon should be just large enough to stop the catheter falling out or being pushed out if the patient bears down. The recommended balloon size for routine use is 5–10 mL. A 30 mL balloon should be used only following surgery on the prostate gland

Note that underinflation of a large-capacity balloon causes distortion of the tip of the catheter and occlusion of the drainage eye. Therefore a large balloon should be filled with at least 20 mL of water. A smaller-ballooned catheter, because the water must reach the balloon, should be filled with at least 10 mL.

- Catheters for short-term use are made of a latex material that can cause irritation of the urethra and build-up of crystals in the bladder. Therefore it is not recommended to use this type of catheter for longer than 2 or 3 weeks
- Catheters for long-term use are made of 100% silicone material; they are less irritating, softer, and cause less build-up of crystals

For those with milder symptoms, it is a matter of discussion between the patient and his doctor as to whether symptoms are interfering with the individual's lifestyle sufficiently to warrant an operation and whether he stands a good chance of improvement from surgery. In rare cases where there is poor life expectancy or the patient is too unfit for surgery, prostatectomy may not be offered and a permanent indwelling catheter may be considered the best management.

Specific considerations for the patient undergoing TURP

Informed consent

The patient must be given a clear explanation of the after-effects of TURP, so that he can give his informed consent prior to the procedure. Since many men have retrograde ejaculation after prostatectomy, it is essential that they are counselled adequately beforehand. Retrograde ejaculation does not cause impotence, but a patient who has not been given adequate reassurance on this point could suffer psychological upset resulting in impotence. Retrograde ejaculation will not render the patient sterile, but neither will it necessarily permit him to father children easily. It should not be presumed that all older men are not sexually active, and all patients are entitled to preoperative information (see Case History 8.4 and Box 8.10).

STOP THINK **8.6** Identify and consider all the information that it will be necessary to give to Mr M in Case History 8.4. How could this information best be given to ensure he can really understand and remember the details?

Major patient problems

Patients who have undergone TURP may have the following problems and concerns postoperatively:

- Anxiety
  - — about the success of the surgery and the outlook for recovery
  - — about bleeding from the prostatic bed
  - — about the embarrassment of having a catheter in situ
- Pain
  - — from the raw area in the bladder
  - — from clots forming in the prostatic bed and blocking the catheter
  - — from the catheter itself
  - — from bladder extravasation
- Immobility
  - — due to inability to get out of bed because of the surgery
  - — because of irrigation
  - — due to fear of moving
  - — due to i.v. infusion

CASE HISTORY 8.4

Mr M

Mr M was admitted for a TURP. He was 73 years old and had been suffering from the miserable symptoms of an enlarged prostate gland for some time. He was glad to be in hospital but did not feel well. His joints and bones ached from long-standing osteoarthritis. His chest was not good and his feet and hands were always cold. He knew smoking did not help and he had been cutting down.

The surgeon and anaesthetist visited him and explained the surgery and that he would have an epidural anaesthetic. The physiotherapist visited him and discussed breathing techniques and encouraged him to stop smoking. Nursing staff were always at hand. They explained all the tests and procedures involved in preparation for surgery as well as how he could expect to feel after the procedure.

Box 8.9

Principles of catheter management

Performing catheterisation

The nurse performing catheterisation must introduce the catheter into the bladder using aseptic technique, without causing trauma and with minimum discomfort to the patient. The following considerations are essential:

- Adequate cleaning of the genital area
- Working under good light, especially when catheterising females
- Positioning the patient correctly
- Ensuring the patient's privacy
- Providing adequate anaesthetisation of the urethra for both male and female patients. An anaesthetic-containing antiseptic should be instilled and left to take effect for a minimum of 5 min.

Management of the indwelling catheter

The main priorities of catheter care are to prevent infection and to safeguard the dignity of the patient. To minimise the risk of infection the nurse should:

- Establish and maintain a closed system of drainage
- Promote good personal hygiene
- Carry out catheter hygiene once a day and after each bowel movement, using soap and water
- Encourage a fluid intake of 2–4 L daily, according to the individual's needs
- Encourage maximum mobility
- Change the catheter only when necessary, rather than routinely
- Avoid causing trauma to the urethra and bladder neck
- Give bladder washouts only when absolutely necessary, i.e. when the catheter is blocked or when washouts have been prescribed as a treatment (Getliffe & Dolman 2003). Bladder washouts should not be employed as a prophylactic treatment for urine infections.

Maintaining the dignity of the patient

The following measures will help to preserve the patient's dignity and self-esteem:

- Providing education and promoting self-care where possible in catheter toilet, the use of a bidet, emptying and changing bags
- Using a female length catheter for a female patient to allow her to wear skirts
- Encouraging the use of leg bags so the catheter is not in view
- Encouraging maximum mobility to promote confidence and give better drainage.

Problems and possible interventions

The nurse should be prepared for the following potential problems:

Bypassing

- Check to see if the catheter or drainage tube is blocked, kinked or looped
- Consider changing to a smaller catheter. It is a misconception that if the catheter bypasses, a larger catheter is required
- Check whether or not medication which can cause spasm has been prescribed
- Exclude constipation — relieve constipation immediately and emphasise the importance of a high-fibre diet
- Check with the doctor about the possibility of prescribing anticholinergic drugs if the bypassing still persists

Balloon not deflating

- Attach syringe to the valve in position without aspiration. It may self-deflate
- The balloon may be burst by injecting 2–5 mL of dilute ether via the balloon inflating channel
- A fine sterile wire may be passed up the inflating channel and the balloon burst
- Never cut off the end of the inflation channel of the catheter

Blockage

- This may be caused by medication, e.g. aperients causing phosphatic debris in the urine — change or stop the drug, encourage the patient to take a high-fibre diet and encourage more exercise
- Infection must be treated with the correct antibiotic. Check the amount of fluid intake and where possible try to increase this. Check the standard of personal hygiene
- If clots occur, carry out a bladder washout with normal saline

Urethral discharge

- Normal secretion of the urethral mucosa is increased with the presence of a foreign body, i.e. the catheter. To prevent this becoming troublesome to the patient, adequate meatal toilet should be instituted from the first day of catheterisation

---

- Difficulty eating and drinking
  - — due to nausea
  - — due to immobility
- Disturbed sleep
  - — due to irrigation changes, checks on temperature, pulse, blood pressure
  - — due to pain
  - — due to noise in the ward.

Major nursing considerations

Risk of haemorrhage Since haemorrhage is a major risk after prostatectomy, preoperative care should involve determining baseline haematological values. Careful consideration must be given to those individuals receiving oral anticoagulants for any other disease, since the risk of haemorrhage is considerable. It may be necessary to discontinue oral therapy preoperatively and to use i.v. heparin postoperatively until the oral regimen can be recommenced and stabilised. This may take some weeks to achieve and will require the patient to make additional visits to the hospital or GP surgery.

Anaemia Preoperative anaemia should be corrected and blood transfusion given postoperatively if required to replace blood loss. Blood is not routinely cross-matched due to the availability of protein and plasma products.

Fluid and electrolyte balance Preoperative determination of urea and electrolyte levels will provide baseline measurements and permit correction before surgery if required. This may involve urethral catheterisation to enable adequate

Box 8.10

Information for patients undergoing prostatectomy

Your doctor has already explained to you that you require an operation on your prostate gland. The prostate is situated at the base of the bladder and it is quite common in older men for the prostate to enlarge, causing the symptoms which you have been experiencing. In order to relieve these symptoms it is necessary to remove that part of the prostate gland which is causing a blockage to the flow of the urine from the bladder.

The anaesthetic

The operation may be performed under a general anaesthetic, when you will be completely asleep, or a spinal anaesthetic, which involves an injection in your back and makes the lower half of your body completely numb. This decision is usually made by the anaesthetist.

The operation

There are two ways of removing the prostate gland. Generally it is possible to do the operation through a telescopic instrument which is passed up through the penis. This operation is known as a transurethral resection of the prostate (TURP). The prostate tissue is cut away in small pieces which are washed out of the bladder and any bleeding is stopped using a special electrocautery probe.

Alternatively, it is sometimes necessary to remove the prostate by an open operation through an incision in the lower part of the abdomen. The same amount of tissue is removed by both operations and the end result is the same. Your surgeon will naturally try to remove your prostate with the tele-endoscopic instrument but it may be necessary to perform the 'cutting' operation, especially if the prostate is unusually large.

After the operation you will have a tube (catheter) draining the urine from your bladder into a bag which will be emptied regularly by the nursing staff. Immediately after the operation the catheter will contain blood, so the bladder, prostate and catheter are washed continuously with fluid that runs through an extra tube attached to the catheter. This is disconnected when the urine is clear, usually the morning after the operation. After the operation you will also have an infusion into a vein for about 24 h to provide extra fluid or blood if necessary.

After the operation

As soon as possible after the operation we like you to start drinking large quantities of tea, squash, fruit juice or water, but fizzy drinks are not recommended. An occasional can of beer is permissible. This will speed up your recovery by producing more urine to wash away the blood in the catheter and prevent infection. The catheter will be removed when the urine is clear, usually in the evening or the next morning after the operation. This is not painful. After it has been removed you should continue to drink as much as possible and pass urine every 2–3 h. This may be uncomfortable to start with and you may have to hurry or experience some dribbling but these minor symptoms improve rapidly. Once you are satisfied that you are passing urine well and your surgeon is satisfied with your progress, you may return home, usually 1–2 days after removal of the catheter.

At home

When you get home you should continue to drink well and avoid constipation, strenuous exercise and heavy lifting. You should not drive a car for 2 weeks, or play golf or go jogging for at least 3 weeks. Sometimes you may see some blood in your urine 7–10 days after the operation. This is rarely serious and if you drink plenty of fluids and rest it should disappear. If bleeding persists you should contact your family doctor. Infection and other problems are unusual. The bladder may be 'irritable' for several weeks after a prostate operation with frequency and urgency, but any remaining symptoms should disappear within 12 weeks.

You will be seen again in the urology outpatient clinic 2–3 months after your operation. You can return to work at that time or even sooner, if you feel able to do so.

Sexual activity after prostatectomy

This operation will alter your sex life but it is unlikely that there will be any change in the quality of the erections or climax. Sexual intercourse can take place 5–6 weeks after the operation. During sexual climax, however, you will not emit any semen from your penis. The ejaculation (semen) may flow into the bladder instead of down the penis and the first time you pass urine after intercourse it will be cloudy. This is not harmful. You are unlikely to produce any children following this operation but this should not be relied on as safe contraception.

Reproduced with permission from the Department of Urology, The Freeman Hospital, Newcastle upon Tyne.

bladder drainage and the use of i.v. fluids to achieve hydration.

During TURP, the bladder is irrigated with fluid to provide a clear view for the surgeon. Some of this fluid is usually absorbed, and if there is an interruption in the venous system during the resection, the fluid absorbed can be excessive. The fluid used in irrigation is usually isotonic glycine, excessive absorption of which can cause the patient to become hyponatraemic. This can cause confusion, a restless mental state and, in some cases, unconsciousness. This imbalance can be corrected by restricting fluid intake and encouraging the patient to increase the amount of salt in his diet.

Water is not used for irrigation because it can be readily absorbed and cause haemolysis. Saline interferes with the use of diathermy, and so is also unsuitable for irrigation during surgery. It is, however, the solution of choice for postoperative bladder washouts.

Urinary infection Men who have an indwelling urethral catheter preoperatively are at a high risk of developing infective complications. The effectiveness of prophylactic antibiotics is uncertain, but it would seem that those who do not receive systemic therapy at the time of operation, followed by a postoperative course, will be likely to develop bacteraemia and become unwell.

Urinary infection is common after prostatectomy, even in those who had sterile urine preoperatively. About one-third of men who have bacteria in their urine postoperatively are asymptomatic but should receive the appropriate oral therapy. This reduces the incidence of secondary haemorrhage caused by infection.

Management of irrigation

An irrigation set with a Y-connection will be used to allow two 3 L bags of normal saline to be erected at any one time, with one bag running at a time. The irrigation runs into the bladder via the irrigating channel of the catheter, diluting the urine, which then drains out through the outlet channel of the catheter into a drainage bag. Irrigation prevents blood clots forming and obstructing the catheter. The irrigation is regulated, via a clamp, to run at a speed sufficient to keep the bladder clear of blood clots. The bags are numbered and the amount of irrigation fluid recorded on a fluid chart. The patient's total output, i.e. urine and irrigation fluid, should be measured and recorded. The amount of irrigation fluid used should be subtracted from the measured output to give the urine output volume.

Specific assessment points are as follows:

- Observe and palpate the patient's lower abdomen. Abdominal distension may indicate clot retention or extravasation. Clot retention is a common complication in the first 12–24 h. Bladder washout or deflation and reinflation of the catheter balloon may be required.
- Note the colour of the irrigation fluid: a bright red colour may indicate fresh bleeding; a dark red colour would suggest old blood.
- In an uncircumcised male patient, check that the foreskin is over the glans penis to prevent paraphimosis.

The morning following surgery, the irrigation will be discontinued, provided the patient is able to drink large quantities of fluid to help flush the prostatic bed of any further bleeding or clots.

Pain relief should be adequate to allow the patient to rest and feel comfortable.

Catheter care (see also Boxes 8.8 and 8.9) A common problem while the catheter is in situ is the bypassing of urine around it. This is sometimes difficult to resolve, and the nurse should take the following preventive measures:

- Check that the catheter is not blocked by clots or debris and that it is in the bladder.
- Check the amount of water in the balloon. If it is 30 mL, then reduce it to approximately 20 mL or so, but not less than 15 mL.
- Give anticholinergic medication as prescribed, e.g. oxybutynin.
- Encourage the patient to continue to drink large quantities of fluid.

The catheter will stay in position for 2–3 days following surgery or until the urine output is clear. Before removing it, the nurse should ensure that the patient's bowels have moved, as straining following catheter removal can lead to further urethral bleeding. Following removal, the patient may experience urgency and frequency as before. He should be reassured that this is normal and that it may take up to 8 weeks for a normal voiding pattern to be established. The patient should be educated to tighten the sphincter muscle and to hold on as long as possible before passing urine.

Patients who had chronic retention before surgery often fail to void postoperatively. A long-term catheter will normally be inserted in such cases, and the patient allowed home for several weeks (usually 6). This time period allows the bladder to rest and regain its elasticity.

Patient involvement

The patient's dependence on nursing care will gradually decrease as blood loss and hence the need for irrigation lessens. Involvement of the patient in aspects of his own care is to be encouraged and may include:

- making entries in his own fluid chart; drinking at least 3 L in 24 h; emptying his own drainage bag; recording amount and colour (most patients will be happy to do this but may need guidance on colour and amount)
- attending to own personal hygiene; this would include cleaning the urethral catheter once or twice a day using soap and water (Pratt et al 2001)
- taking regular, if somewhat gentle, exercise (it should be remembered, however, that some patients feel embarrassed about carrying around a urinary drainage bag).

Discharge

Once the urine is clear, the catheter can normally be removed. This is usually done in the morning to allow the patient to establish a normal voiding pattern before retiring to bed. Provided the patient is able to pass urine without difficulty, he may be discharged from hospital the following day.

For further information, see Doherty & Winder (2000), Evans & Godfrey (2000), Pratt et al (2001), Pomfret (2001) and Robinson (2003).

Many patients feel, after the operation, that they have gained no relief from their problems. It must be understood that it will take about 6 weeks for the prostatic bed to heal, such that full urinary control is possible. During the early postoperative weeks, the patient should refrain from vigorous exercise. He should drink plenty of fluids and avoid becoming constipated. The community nurse will give advice and support should urinary problems occur.

It should be noted that at about 14 days postoperatively, when desiccated tissue has sloughed off the prostatic bed, haemorrhage can occur (secondary haemorrhage; see Ch. 26, p. 921).

Occasionally, urethral stricture occurs as the urethral mucosa in the prostatic region heals.

For further information, see Thorpe & Neal (2003).

Cancer of the prostate

Cancer of the prostate gland is the second most commonly diagnosed malignancy in men (Gray 2002). The incidence of prostatic cancer increases with age and postmortem studies have shown that approximately 30% of asymptomatic men over the age of 50, and 90% over the age of 90, have microscopic foci, evident only on histological examination. About 10% of men thought to have a benign prostate on examination are later found by histological examination to have prostatic cancer.

PATHOPHYSIOLOGY

The cause of prostatic cancer is not clear, but there is some evidence to show that hormonal activity plays a part in the transformation of certain normal cells into cancerous ones. Benign hyperplasia and carcinoma arise in different parts of the gland. Carcinoma occurs in the peripheral gland. Metastases often move to bone, where they are associated with severe pain. In cases of extreme bony destruction, pathological fractures may occur. It has been known for spinal destruction to cause paraplegia.

Common presenting symptoms Diagnosis of this disease is difficult because the patient is often asymptomatic. The GP is likely to see patients who present with advanced disease which is already beyond cure. Patients with locally advanced disease are likely to complain of bladder outflow obstruction, a sudden onset of urgency to void urine, and possibly haematuria.

Chronic urinary retention secondary to bladder outflow obstruction may cause renal damage by dilating the upper renal tracts. The patient may present with a palpable bladder or with renal failure; he is likely to be generally unwell and losing weight. Renal failure may also be caused by ureteric infiltration of tumour or by para-aortic lymph node obstruction causing ureteric obstruction. Those who feel unwell and are anaemic are likely to have suffered bone marrow infiltration and/or renal failure. A complaint of persistent backache may suggest bone metastases.

An irregular, enlarged, hard prostate gland does not prove diagnosis, although most advanced carcinomas will be felt as such on rectal examination. However, prostatitis or prostatic stone disease may feel similar on rectal examination. Moreover, if there is a tumour within the anterior part of the gland, rectal examination will reveal no abnormality.

MEDICAL MANAGEMENT

Investigations The only certain means of making a diagnosis is by histological examination. Fine-needle transrectal prostatic biopsy can be done without anaesthetic for this purpose. Specimens (prostatic chips) resected at the time of transurethral or open prostatectomy should be sent for histological examination. However, this may yield a false negative if the sample is not taken from the peripheral part of the gland. Prostatic cancer is graded histologically to assess malignant potential.

Additional investigations to provide evidence of local and metastatic spread include IVU, CT scanning, magnetic resonance imaging (MRI), ultrasound scanning, skeletal X-rays and lymphangiography.

Treatment The nature of the treatment offered and whether it is given on an outpatient or an inpatient basis will depend upon the extent of the disease and on how the patient presents symptomatically and clinically.

Surgery TURP is normally carried out to relieve urinary symptoms and retention. This does not, however, afford a cure.

Radical prostatectomy and clearance of any pelvic lymphatic involvement are performed in the hope of achieving a cure. This treatment is restricted to those with disease localised to the prostate, a life expectancy of greater than 10 years and no significant co-morbidity. The patient should be counselled preoperatively about his disease and the almost certain complication of urinary incontinence.

Radiotherapy This is given as either external beam or interstitial seed implantation (brachytherapy). For external beam radiotherapy, if the patient is generally fit, he will probably attend for daily treatment as an outpatient. Should the patient or medical team prefer, inpatient treatment may be given (see Ch. 31, p. 1044).

The side-effects of treatment vary from person to person. Liaison with the patient's relatives and with the community health care team will help to ensure that the patient is given optimum support in dealing with these (see Ch. 31, p. 1047). In some cases, the side-effects will necessitate hospitalisation, e.g. when nausea, vomiting and diarrhoea cause dehydration, or when urinary frequency or incontinence causes severe physical and psychological distress.

Treating advanced disease The aims of treatment in advanced disease are to provide symptomatic relief and to preserve an acceptable quality of life for the individual. The outlook for improvement will depend upon various factors; those with renal failure, anaemia or urinary retention and metastases have a poor prognosis.

Those who have metastatic disease and are symptomatic are normally offered hormonal treatment. Hormonal manipulation can be achieved by bilateral orchidectomy (excision of the testes) or by the administration of oestrogens or of luteinising hormone-releasing hormone agonists (LHRH), e.g. diethylstilbestrol, or non-steroidal anti-androgens. Of patients given hormonal treatment, 70% will experience symptomatic relief for a period, but will have recurrent symptoms in the long term.

The treatment of those with metastatic disease who are asymptomatic will usually be deferred until symptoms develop. Once hormonal treatment has been given and relapse occurs, the outlook is poor.

It would appear that chemotherapy is ineffective in treating advanced prostatic carcinoma. However, radiotherapy is sometimes beneficial in the relief of bony pain caused by metastases. Vertebral collapse caused by metastatic disease of the spinal column requires emergency radiotherapy or laminectomy and hormonal manipulation. If effective, these measures may prevent neurological symptoms and/or paraplegia from developing.

Pain control by means of opiate analgesics may cause constipation; this in turn can cause urinary retention. It may be more appropriate to administer non-steroidal anti-inflammatory medication to avoid this side-effect. Should analgesics be required, they should be given in doses which prevent pain occurring (see Ch. 19, p. 750). Sustained or slow-release medication is often very useful.

NURSING PRIORITIES AND MANAGEMENT: Carcinoma of the prostate

General considerations

The nursing management of the patient with prostatic cancer is very much influenced by the particular presentation of the disease in each individual. The nurse should take a problem-solving approach to care, and promote independence and self-care for as long as possible. The nurse should bear in mind that constipation and urinary retention or urinary incontinence are commonly encountered and can be very distressing both for the individual and for his family. Ongoing liaison between hospital and community teams will help to ensure that care is effective and genuinely responsive to the individual's unique situation (see Ch. 33).

A range of medical interventions may be necessary at different stages in the disease process. Nursing involvement will then include assisting with procedures such as:

- correction of anaemia by blood transfusion
- TURP to relieve retention
- bilateral subcapsular orchidectomy to reduce the hormone level, help prevent the spread of metastases and reduce pain.

In many cases, medical intervention can offer only temporary improvement, and the emphasis of care will turn to palliation. Treatment of advanced disease is usually shared between hospital and home, and the patient and his family will need a great deal of moral and practical support in both settings. It is important to convey a sense of optimism so that life can continue to be enjoyed to the fullest degree possible. In the last stages of the illness, however, it should not be seen as a defeat or failure to help the patient to let go of life and face death with dignity (see Ch. 33).

For further information, see Donovan et al (2001).

Table 8.3 Presenting features of bladder cancer

Sign/symptom	Reason
Haematuria, urine retention	Tumour growth Tumour spread
Dysuria, urgency, hesitancy, frequency	Stimulation of reflex micturition arc Secondary infection
Urinary incontinence	Irritability of bladder
Chills and cystitis	Obstruction/infection
Backache, pain	Ureteric obstruction Dependent upon the stage: infiltration Symptoms of cystitis or burning
Lower limb oedema	Venous obstruction Lymphatic obstruction
Infection	Obstruction Tumour necrosis
Malaise, anaemia	Frequency causing lack of rest or sleep Bleeding
Suprapubic mass, abnormal mass on rectal examination	Tumour size Tumour spread

DISORDERS OF THE BLADDER

Cancer of the bladder

Tumours of the bladder, usually transitional cell carcinoma, occur more commonly in men than in women (M:F = 4:1). The peak incidence of bladder cancer in the UK occurs at around 65 years of age. Bladder tumours are histologically similar to tumours of the renal pelvis and ureter. About 95% are malignant, and benign tumours often recur after apparently successful treatment.

There are geographical variations in incidence — tumours are more common in industrialised regions than in underdeveloped regions. Possible causative agents or factors include:

- occupational exposure (industrial dyes, solvents)
- cigarette smoking
- calculi
- diverticulae
- chronic inflammation due to indwelling catheterisation.

Screening of those in high-risk groups may help to reduce incidence and to monitor factors associated with bladder cancer, but as many years may elapse between exposure to a carcinogen and the development of cancer, direct connections are difficult to establish.

STOP THINK **8.7** What part can the occupational health nurse play in prevention?

Refer to Royal College of Nursing (2004).

PATHOPHYSIOLOGY

Tumour growth usually commences in the epithelial lining of the bladder, often as a papillary growth. (Papillae are minute nipple-shaped projections.) Benign growth will, without treatment, usually progress to malignancy and then, by stages, from superficial to deep muscle tissue involvement, eventually spreading locally into surrounding tissue and other parts of the urinary tract or organs.

Common presenting symptoms (see Table 8.3) Approximately 80% of people with bladder cancer will notice haematuria. This may be the only presenting feature of the disease. Dysuria, frequency, symptoms of obstruction and infection may also be noticed, but embarrassment may prevent the individual from visiting their GP. Symptoms may not persist following initial presentation, e.g. if associated infection is resolved by a course of antibiotics. Investigations should, however, be undertaken if the cause of haematuria is unclear.

STOP THINK **8.8** A 35-year-old man notices blood in his urine each morning. He has no discomfort and is otherwise well. Unless the haematuria persists this man may decide not to visit his GP. How might you encourage him to report the haematuria? What anxieties might he have about reporting to his GP?

MEDICAL MANAGEMENT

Investigations Diagnosis may be aided by physical examination, a full blood count, urea and electrolyte estimation and other biochemical assays. Examination of an MSU specimen will exclude evidence of infection. If the patient has microscopic or macroscopic haematuria and an infection has been excluded, the patient's upper urinary tract and bladder must be investigated. Table 8.4 lists the principal diagnostic investigations; in many respects these will be similar to those used in diagnosing prostatic disorders.

Table 8.4 Principal diagnostic investigations for tumours of the bladder

Investigation	Reason
Intravenous urogram (IVU)	If presenting feature is haematuria, IVU may exclude renal pelvic carcinoma
Cystoscopy and biopsy	Suspicious lesions can be examined for abnormal cells
CT scan	If local spread of tumour is suspected
Chest X-ray	If metastatic spread is suspected
Bone scan	
Liver function tests	

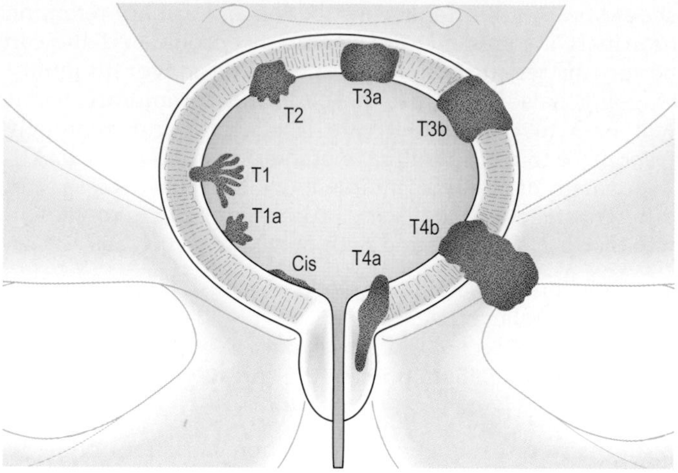

Fig. 8.11 Categories of bladder tumours. Cis, carcinoma in situ. (Garden et al 2002.)

Staging The staging of bladder tumours is illustrated in Figure 8.11 (see also Ch. 31). In addition to staging according to the actual tumour, the pathologist will grade transitional cell tumours according to the invasion differentiation of the lesion (National Institute of Clinical Excellence 2002).

Treatment The choice of treatment will depend on the type of tumour and the degree of invasion of local tissue, as determined by cystoscopy (see Table 8.5). Superficial lesions without muscle invasion can be treated by excision of the tumour through the urethra — transurethral resection of tumour (TURT) or cystodiathermy. Irrigation of the bladder may be used to keep the bladder clear of blood clots following transurethral resection (see p. 379).

For invasive bladder tumours, a combination of surgery (i.e. total cystectomy), radiotherapy and chemotherapy may be used.

Total cystectomy involves removing the lower ureters, bladder, prostate, urethra and lymphatics in men, and also, in women, the gynaecological organs. Urinary diversion is required and is most commonly ileal conduit and stoma formation (see Fig. 8.12). With this type of diversion, the ureters are anastomosed to an isolated section of the bowel (ileum with blood supply) and the loop brought to the abdominal surface as a stoma. This is a major procedure which will fundamentally affect the lifestyle of both the patient and family members.

Developments in reconstructive surgery have led to the use of bladder substitutes in place of urinary diversion, i.e. part of the intestine is anastomosed directly to the membranous urethra which provides a reservoir for urine; however, this technique is not appropriate for everyone as it requires major surgery.

For further information, see Downey (2000), Trotto (2000) and Pashos et al (2002).

Radiotherapy is normally given as an external treatment for bladder carcinoma over a 6-week period. It may be used as a palliative measure or in conjunction with surgery and/or chemotherapy, pre- or post-treatment. The age and general condition of the patient will determine whether treatment is given on an outpatient or inpatient basis. Sometimes the severity of the patient's symptoms leads to conversion from outpatient to inpatient care and a short period respite from the treatment plan to allow the patient to recuperate before progressing to the next treatment.

Chemotherapy Treatment of invasive bladder cancer with systemic chemotherapy is under investigation. Regimens of treatment vary. Some patients receive care on a

Table 8.5 Treatment choices in tumours of the bladder

Tumour	Treatment	Comment
Localised, well-differentiated tumour	Diathermy	Annual cystoscopy to check for recurrence
Histologically malignant tumours: — extensive superficial — locally invasive	Chemotherapy: intrarenal Radiotherapy Transurethral resection of tumour (TURT)	Annual cystoscopy to assess effect and check for recurrence
Failure to control tumour spread/severe symptoms	Cystectomy and ureter transplant to ileal conduit (urinary diversion)	Radiotherapy may be used to reduce size of tumour prior to surgery
Inoperable tumour	Analgesics Palliative radiotherapy	
Metastatic spread	Systemic chemotherapy	An option although success is limited

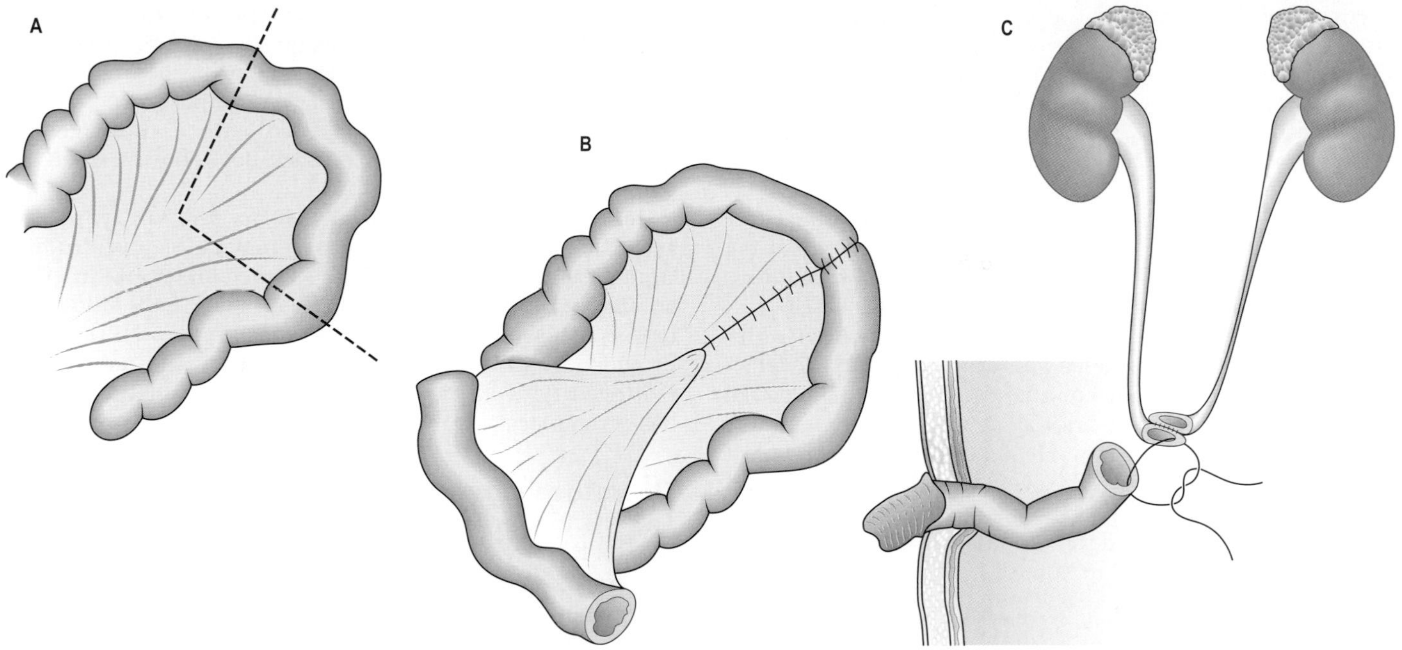

Fig. 8.12 Ileal conduit urinary diversion. A, B: Isolation of segment of terminal ileum. C: Fashioning of ureteroileal anastomosis. The stoma is made to protrude from the skin to minimise skin contact with urine and so reduce irritation.

day-care basis, receiving i.v. injections, while others attend for inpatient hospital care involving 2–3 days in hospital for each cycle of treatment. (For further details on systemic chemotherapy, refer to Ch. 31.)

Intravesical chemotherapy may be offered in some cases. The recurrence of superficial bladder tumours resected endoscopically is approximately 65%. Recurrent tumours are usually of the same type and stage as those previously resected. Further endoscopic resection may be the treatment of choice, but intravesical chemotherapy is also given. A urethral catheter is inserted and the chosen medication is instilled via the catheter. Treatment may be weekly, monthly or bimonthly, depending upon the type of tumour and the medication used.

Once the medication is instilled the catheter can be removed. The patient is asked to try to avoid passing urine for an hour and is asked to turn from back to front to sides every 15 min, in order to wash the medication around the bladder. The nurse administering the treatment should bear in mind that this patient may have difficulty in postponing the passing of urine for up to 1 h because of symptoms of frequency and bladder irritability. The patient should be reassured that an inability to comply with this request is not a sign of 'failure'.

The side-effects of the medications used in this treatment vary, but chemical cystitis leading to inflammation and bladder irritability, urgency and frequency is common. Sensitivity rashes are seen less commonly, as are more severe effects such as systemic toxicity and bone marrow suppression.

Since the medications used are toxic agents, precautions should be taken, such as wearing protective goggles, gloves and gowns when preparing and administering treatments and when discarding used equipment.

After the treatment has been completed, the patient should be advised that urine passed will contain chemical substances that will irritate the skin and that leakages or dribbles should be washed off immediately.

Effectiveness of treatment with intravesical chemotherapy varies considerably from individual to individual.

NURSING PRIORITIES AND MANAGEMENT: Total cystectomy and urinary diversion

Preoperative care

Psychological preparation (see Case History 8.5)

The patient admitted for cystectomy and urinary diversion may already know the nursing and medical staff on the ward from a previous admission. Staff should endeavour to build upon this rapport and provide information both verbally and in written form to prepare the patient for the physical effects of the operation, particularly the formation of a stoma. Considerable psychological adjustment may be required on the part of the patient to come to terms with the lifestyle changes that will be necessary and with the alteration in body image that may occur.

The patient is likely to have concerns relating to any pain that will be experienced, whether the operation will effect

CASE HISTORY 8.5

Mr L

Mr L, a 58-year-old married man employed as a bus driver, was diagnosed 5 years ago with cancer of the bladder. He was treated with regular cystoscopy and transurethral resection of tumour. Six months ago the tumour was found to be stage T2, and a course of chemotherapy was prescribed. Recent cystoscopy showed that this treatment had not been successful. Total cystectomy is now being considered for this patient.

a 'cure', how his family will cope in his absence and after his return home, and how he will appear to other people. The contribution of the named nurse and the stoma therapist in answering questions and allaying fears in the preoperative period is invaluable. It may be helpful to arrange for the patient and his family to meet with someone who has a stoma.

It should be noted that patients rarely ask about the effect surgery may have on sexual function. However, one of the side-effects for male patients of this life-saving procedure is impotence. This important matter must be discussed with male patients and their partners prior to the surgery in order to help them return to and lead a normal life (Black 2000).

The patient may gain confidence from the knowledge that his community nurse and GP as well as a stoma nurse are available to support him. He should be given a contact telephone number to use in the event of difficulty. He should be reassured that any problems and concerns, however small, can be discussed as he makes the challenging adjustment from hospital to home.

For further information, see Black (2000).

STOP THINK

8.9 How can the nurse help Mr L in Case History 8.5 to come to terms with his disappointing news and the prospect of total cystectomy?

8.10 Mr L is provided with an indwelling catheter which will remain in situ until he can be admitted to hospital. What advice and support could you offer to Mr L and his wife to ensure that no catheter-related problems develop? What part can the community nurse play? Review Boxes 8.8 and 8.9.

Physical preparation

The stoma will be sited on the abdomen below the waist, normally on the right-hand side. Considerations in choosing the exact site include:

- the patient's build
- access for the surgeon
- previous surgery
- access for the patient following surgery
- type of clothing to be worn after the surgery.

The following procedures are carried out in preparation for surgery:

1. The patient is kept on a fluid only or low-residue diet at commencement of bowel preparation.
2. The bowel is cleared of faeces. This may be by means of an enema or a high colonic washout and is carried out 2 days prior to the operation. Bowel sterilisation with systemic and local antibiotics may be prescribed.
3. Prophylactic antibiotic therapy is commenced preoperatively (and continued postoperatively).
4. The skin is shaved from nipple to knee, or according to the surgeon's wishes (see Ch. 26).
5. The chosen site for the stoma is marked.

Postoperative care

Return from theatre (see Nursing Care Plan 8.2)

Following surgery and recovery from anaesthetic, the patient will return to the ward. A nasogastric (NG) tube will be in place for aspiration of gastric contents. Examination will reveal a midline incision, covered by a surgical dressing, and a wound drain. The stoma, in the pre-marked position, should have a moist, red appearance and be covered by a collection bag fitted with a drainage tap and autoreflux valve to prevent back-flow of urine when the patient is lying flat.

Infant feeding tubes which form temporary splints across the ureteroileal anastomosis may be seen protruding from the stoma. The splints, one for each ureter and inserted at surgery, pass through the ileal loop and along the ureters across the junction of the anastomosis. The support provided by the splints maintains patency and reduces the risk of urine leakage from the anastomosis before healing has taken place.

The recovery period

The NG tube will be in place for 24–48 h, or until bowel sounds have returned. Drains may be removed when discharge is less than 50 mL/24 h; this is usually at 4–5 days postoperatively. Removal of splints from the stoma can usually be done at 10–14 days, and removal of sutures at 10 days. Assessment by the dietitian and provision of a diet plan may aid wound healing and recovery by ensuring an adequate nutritional intake.

During this time, the stoma nurse will visit. Working with the named nurse, they will teach the patient how to clean the stoma and change the bag and flange on a daily basis. The patient should be shown how to cut the flange to shape and fit it in position with the bag.

Patients differ in the time it takes them to come to terms with management of their stoma. Some show no interest at first in looking after the stoma and need a lot of encouragement to do so. Planning a programme with the patient, identifying goals to be attained and involving close relatives/carers will help to ensure successful self-care. A second visit from an individual who has already made the adjustment to life with a stoma may also help.

Discharge

Provided no complications have arisen, by 10–14 days after the operation the patient and nurse should be planning for discharge home. The first follow-up appointment will usually be scheduled for 6–8 weeks after the operation. Thereafter, outpatient appointments will be arranged at longer intervals, but will continue for life. To ensure optimal function and prevent long-term complications (see Box 8.11), periodic i.v. urograms or loopograms may be performed. A loopogram is the radiological examination of the bowel segment used to form the urinary diversion; this investigation may reveal any disorder of filling or capacity.

RENAL DISORDERS

Glomerulonephritis

The term 'glomerulonephritis' refers to a group of disorders characterised by inflammation of the glomeruli of the kidney. The disease may be primary to the glomeruli or secondary to a systemic disorder. Box 8.12 lists primary and secondary causes of glomerulonephritis.

Nursing Care Plan 8.2 Nursing care in the first 24 h following total cystectomy and urinary diversion

Potential problem	Action	Desired outcome
1. **Cardiovascular instability and hypovolaemic shock due to haemorrhage and pain**	• Record vital signs and report any deviations from normal range • Monitor and mark extent of blood loss evident on wound dressing • Record blood loss in drains and report if in excess of 100 mL/h	Cardiovascular stability Minimal blood loss Minimal pain
2. **Pain**	• Observe patient for distress. Assess pain using an appropriate pain assessment tool (NB: generalised abdominal pain may indicate peritonitis caused by leakage from anastomosis) • Administer prescribed analgesics • Evaluate effect after 30 min by asking patient if pain has been relieved	Patient is pain-free
3. **Fluid and electrolyte imbalance**	• Measure and record hourly urine output (NB: output <30 mL could indicate obstruction or possible leakage from ureteroileal anastomosis leading to peritonitis) • Balance all fluid output against all fluid input in 24 h • Observe for evidence of dyspnoea and dehydration, e.g. dry skin and mouth • Observe for vomiting	Fluid and electrolytes maintained at satisfactory levels
4. **Paralytic ileus**	• Remain nil by mouth • Perform NG aspirations hourly/free drainage • Administer antiemetics as necessary	Comfort is maintained until return of bowel sounds
5. **Deep vein thrombosis (DVT) and/or pulmonary embolism (PE)**	• Supply anti-embolic stockings preoperatively • Encourage movement of lower limbs • Observe for evidence of DVT or PE	Circulatory integrity is maintained
6. **Chest infection**	• Encourage deep breathing and coughing • Refer to physiotherapist • Position patient as upright as possible	Chest is clear with no evidence of infection
7. **Wound infection**	• Observe wound for leakage, check drains hourly • Record temperature and report pyrexia • Leave dressings undisturbed for 48 h if dry	Wound heals without infection
8. **Development of pressure ulcers**	• Change patient's position regularly and observe for reddening • Use a risk assessment scale to assess patient's needs • Ensure skin is clean and dry • Use Spenco mattress if necessary	Skin integrity is maintained
9. **Inability to perform personal hygiene tasks**	• Provide bed bath and mouth care	Patient is clean and comfortable
10. **Anxiety**	• Ensure the nurse call system is close at hand at all times • Discuss any concerns with patient. Provide information, but take post-anaesthetic drowsiness into account • Evaluate patient's understanding of information given. Return next day and ask if there are further questions or concerns	Patient understands what is happening and feels secure in the care provided

Box 8.11

Complications following total cystectomy

Specific complications post-cystectomy
- Breakdown of anastomosis
- Breakdown of blood supply to stoma (necrosis)
- Pelvic abscess
- Poor wound healing post-radiotherapy
- Prolapse of stoma
- Renal failure
- Retraction of stoma
- Urinary infection

Later complications
- Depression
- Prolapse of stoma
- Recurrence of tumour
- Retraction of stoma
- Stenosis of stoma
- Stone formation
- Urinary infection
- Urinary reflux

Box 8.12

Causes of glomerulonephritis

Primary causes
- Minimal change glomerular disease
- Proliferative glomerulonephritis
  - — mesangial (mesangium is a cellular network in the glomerulus that supports the capillary loops)
  - — diffuse capillary
  - — focal
  - — IgA nephropathy
  - — mesangiocapillary
  - — crescentic (Goodpasture's syndrome)
  - — membranous glomerulonephritis
  - — focal segmental glomerulonephritis

Common secondary causes
- Systemic lupus erythematosus
- Polyarteritis
- Diabetes mellitus
- Amyloidosis
- Henoch–Schönlein purpura
- Malarial nephropathy

Proteinuria, haematuria, hypertension, nephrotic syndrome and renal impairment characterise this disease but the severity of these effects will vary between individuals. Presentation is usually described in terms of a range of clinical syndromes, but accurate diagnosis requires histological investigation.

PATHOPHYSIOLOGY

Histological examination of renal tissue will demonstrate inflammation in the majority of cases, but it is also possible to find minimal change and no evidence of an inflammatory process. The disease process results from a defect in the immune response, such as a hypersensitivity to an exogenous antigen. The antigen–antibody reaction results in the formation of insoluble immune complexes that circulate in the blood and, instead of being ingested by macrophages, reach the kidney, where they become 'trapped' and set up a damaging inflammatory reaction in the delicate filtration structure. As a result of this:

- protein and red blood cells pass through the filtration fenestration
- the osmotic pressure of the blood plasma falls, leading to oedema
- sodium and water are retained, as are waste products and potentially toxic substances.

It would seem that many cases of acute glomerulonephritis occur 1–3 weeks after an 'innocent' streptococcal infection such as tonsillitis or otitis media, most commonly in children or adolescents; however, only 5% of these infections lead to glomerulonephritis. In recent years, there has been a significant reduction in the incidence of post-streptococcal glomerulonephritis as a result of better hygiene and the use of antibiotics. The disease can range from a mild, transitory, asymptomatic condition to a very severe form that precipitates acute renal failure, cardiac failure and convulsions.

Common presenting symptoms are exemplified in Case History 8.6.

For further information, see O'Callaghan & Brenner (2000) and Thomas (2002).

MEDICAL MANAGEMENT

Tests and investigations A patient such as T (see Case History 8.6) would probably be admitted to hospital, where investigations would confirm the diagnosis. This would be especially likely if there were symptoms of breathlessness or a risk of convulsions, which would indicate cardiac or cerebral complications. Investigations would include:

- urinalysis
- MSU
- full blood count and urea and electrolyte estimation
- throat swab

CASE HISTORY 8.6
T

T was an active 15-year-old schoolgirl. In September she developed a sore throat which completely robbed her of her voice for several days. It didn't last long and she was used to such minor ailments. In early October she began to notice a feeling of weariness that was quite uncharacteristic. She found herself longing for her bed as the day progressed and declined evening invitations for the usual lively events. On waking one morning, she noticed that her face appeared rather puffy and, on close inspection, found she had puffy ankles. Her parents became concerned and T made an appointment to see her doctor. She now began to consider other problems. She had lost her appetite, often felt rather sick and had noticed that her urine had been rather smoky and darker in hue.

T's GP identified significant proteinuria and haematuria, an elevated blood pressure and marked oedema. A diagnosis of acute glomerulonephritis was made.

Box 8.13

Life-threatening complications of glomerulonephritis

Acute hypertensive encephalitis leading to convulsions (see Ch. 9)

Management
- Maintain airway
- Monitor level of consciousness (e.g. with Glasgow Coma Scale)
- Give anticonvulsant therapy, e.g. i.v. diazepam
- Give hypotensive agents

Pulmonary oedema/cardiac failure (see Chs 2 and 3)

Management
- Give oxygen therapy
- Monitor cardiovascular status
- Give diuretic therapy, e.g. i.v. furosemide
- Give opiate analgesics, e.g. i.v. morphine combined with an antiemetic

Acute renal failure

Management
- Dialysis

- chest X-ray
- ECG
- ultrasound scan
- biopsy.

Treatment The aim of treatment is to reduce renal workload, restore and maintain fluid and electrolyte status and prevent uraemia. Thus management aims to prevent serious complications from occurring (see Box 8.13).

NURSING PRIORITIES AND MANAGEMENT: Glomerulonephritis

Major nursing considerations

Promoting rest

Bed rest is a necessity, especially in the early period, to reduce the workload of both the kidneys and the heart. This can pose quite a challenge in the care of younger patients. Time needs to be spent with the patient, explaining why rest is so important.

Maintaining fluid and electrolyte balance

While renal function is impaired and fluid overload poses a very real problem, fluid and sodium intake must be restricted. Potassium levels in the blood must be closely monitored and, if necessary, dietary modification made or ion exchange resins given. If hypertension is marked, antihypertensive medication may be required.

Preventing uraemia

While the kidney is impaired, the waste products of metabolism will build up in the blood. To prevent this, a protein-restricted diet will be necessary. Calorie intake can be maintained with carbohydrates, and vitamin supplements can be given. This diet must also be low in salt and many patients find meals unpalatable. The dietitian can contribute greatly to the patient's well-being by ensuring that the restricted diet includes at least some of the patient's favourite foods.

Preventing infection

If a streptococcal link is confirmed, penicillin may be prescribed. All patients with renal impairment are prone to infection. All procedures necessary for the prevention of cross-infection must be adhered to (see Ch. 16, p. 664).

Promoting convalescence and the maintenance of health

Most patients make a full recovery, but convalescence may take as long as 2 years. The acute condition can resolve fairly rapidly, and the majority of people recover normal renal function within a couple of months. Such patients often feel better quite quickly and it can be hard to persuade them that restrictions are still needed. Proteinuria can persist and regular monitoring will be necessary. After discharge, support for the patient and family will ensure that necessary lifestyle adjustments are made for the initial months. Exercise should be gentle and energetic sports activities avoided. Any infection should be treated seriously and medical advice sought.

Incomplete resolution and permanent glomerular damage can result in chronic glomerulonephritis and all the associated symptoms of renal impairment. Failure of function may be such that dialysis is required (see p. 391).

Nephrotic syndrome (see Case History 8.7)

Nephrotic syndrome encompasses a group of symptoms including proteinuria, oedema and lipidaemia. It can be a manifestation of certain forms of glomerulonephritis but may also occur as a complication of diabetes mellitus or amyloid disease, whereby insoluble starch-like deposits occur in kidney tissue. Often no cause can be found.

PATHOPHYSIOLOGY

In the normal kidney, protein molecules passing across the glomerular membrane are reabsorbed in the kidney tubules. However, where increased glomerular permeability occurs, increased numbers of protein molecules enter the tubules. When the capacity of the tubule to reabsorb protein is exceeded, protein is lost in the urine. Further protein is lost following catabolism of protein reabsorbed in the tubule, resulting in hypoproteinaemia. Muscle wasting can result from the catabolism of muscle protein as the body tries to maintain normal plasma protein levels. A low plasma protein reduces plasma osmotic pressure and fluid leaks into the extracellular areas. The resultant oedema occurs in dependent areas and may give rise to ascites in severe cases. Intravascular volume is maintained in many cases. How this occurs is not fully understood, but activation of the renin–angiotensin–aldosterone mechanism is thought likely.

Clinical features This syndrome is characterised by heavy proteinuria and hypoproteinaemia and by oedema. These patients generally have a low urine output and low urine

CASE HISTORY 8.7
Mrs Y

Mrs Y, aged 29, presented to her GP with a 3-week history of anorexia and tiredness. Examination revealed no muscle wasting but did show a moderate degree of ankle and sacral oedema. Mrs Y said that her complexion was naturally pale but that her face seemed to have become puffy in the last week or so. Urine testing showed heavy proteinuria. Blood samples were taken for biochemical analysis.

A clinical diagnosis of nephrotic syndrome was made and she was prescribed 80 mg of furosemide daily and a diet with no added salt. Mrs Y was advised that a renal biopsy might be necessary. She resisted immediate admission to hospital and the GP and district nurse arranged to attend Mrs Y's home on alternate days.

Mrs Y wished to stay at home as she had a 3-year-old son and a 6-month-old daughter to care for. On weekday mornings she took her son to a nursery half a mile away and collected him at midday. The family were dependent financially on Mr Y, who worked 200 miles away and was able to return home only at weekends.

One of the major difficulties Mrs Y will face is dealing with the increased diuresis that results from diuretic therapy. A heavy diuresis will occur for about 4 h following each dose. This may make it virtually impossible for Mrs Y to leave the house. Taking her son to the nursery and shopping for household necessities may become difficult. Confined to the house with two small children and a husband 200 miles away, Mrs Y may become socially isolated. The 'no-added-salt diet' may also pose a problem for Mrs Y, particularly if she enjoys salty foods.

The symptoms that Mrs Y has experienced are uncomfortable and frightening. It has been suggested to her that she might need a renal biopsy to determine the cause of her symptoms. It is likely that she will be worried and may need time to voice her concerns and perhaps obtain information and reassurance about her physical condition. It is possible that she may feel unable to carry out all the care for her children and require assistance at some times during the day.

sodium. Derangement of lipoproteins is evident and loss of fibrinogen in the urine can occur. Infection and thrombosis are common complications.

MEDICAL MANAGEMENT

Treatment The main aim of treatment is to reduce oedema. Diuretic therapy can be adjusted according to the severity of the oedema and small maintenance doses can be administered when the oedema is under control. Severe oedema may also be treated by the administration of salt-poor albumin to temporarily increase plasma osmotic pressure. Patients are advised to adhere to a diet free from added salt.

Identification of the underlying disease process, possibly by renal biopsy and histological examination, will dictate the nature of ongoing treatment. In many patients, chronic renal failure will eventually develop.

STOP THINK **8.11** Since Mrs Y in Case History 8.7 has young children, the health visitor will already know this family well. The effectiveness of intervention will depend on the quality of communication between members of the primary health care team. What are the essential features of teamwork that will contribute to the well-being of Mrs Y and her family? Draw from the following reference as you consider these issues in a discussion group.

For further information, see Thomas (2002).

Acute renal failure (ARF)

Acute renal failure, the sudden and severe reduction in previously normal renal function, may result from primary renal disease but is more frequently associated with other organ failure. Failure is often reversible, but should the kidneys fail to recover, permanent treatment will be required.

A mortality rate of up to 50% is associated with acute renal failure, the actual risk depending on the type of patient, the cause of failure and other organ involvement (Thomas 2002). Where death occurs, renal failure is often not the primary cause.

PATHOPHYSIOLOGY

Causes The causes of acute renal failure may be classified into three categories — pre-renal, renal and post-renal — each having a different physiological location.

Pre-renal causes are those in which a loss or decrease in renal perfusion results in renal ischaemia. They include:

- extracellular depletion, resulting from large GI loss such as vomiting, diarrhoea or NG aspiration; urinary loss due to polyuria or diuresis; loss from the skin, e.g. sweating or burns
- circulating volume loss, as in haemorrhage or hypoalbuminaemia
- reduced cardiac output, as in cardiac arrest, valvular disease, cardiac tamponade
- vascular disease, e.g. renal artery thrombosis or embolism.

Renal causes include conditions that impair renal function by damaging the structure of the kidney (tubules, interstitium, glomeruli or capillaries). If tubular damage occurs, this is termed acute tubular necrosis (ATN), although microscopically the tubules usually show dilatation rather than necrosis. ATN is often caused by prolonged pre- and post-renal events.

Nephrotoxic substances can also result in acute failure. These include:

- medications, e.g. cephalosporin antibiotics and non-steroidal anti-inflammatory drugs
- exogenous chemicals, e.g. heavy metals, phenols, carbon tetrachloride, chlorates, ethyl glycol
- bacterial toxins, particularly those released in Gram-negative septicaemia (see Ch. 18, p. 727).

Post-renal causes are mainly attributed to obstruction. The most common of these is bladder output obstruction which may be due to prostatic hypertrophy, tumours or calculi.

Clinical features Acute renal failure proceeds through four phases: onset, oliguric, diuretic and recovery. The onset phase is the time from the initial insult to the onset of oliguria. The oliguric phase is characterised by a urine output of less than 400 mL/24 h; however, some patients may be anuric. The oliguria is accompanied by abnormal plasma levels of creatinine, urea and electrolytes. The effects of acute fluid overload and hyperkalaemia (K^+ >6 mmol/L) can result in sudden death.

The patient may complain of anorexia, nausea and vomiting. Increased respiration due to pulmonary oedema and acidosis can occur. Drowsiness, confusion and coma may follow.

MEDICAL MANAGEMENT

Tests and investigations will depend on the suspected cause and on the immediacy of the presentation but may include:

- full blood count and urea and electrolyte estimation
- urinalysis, MSU, 24-h collections of urine for creatinine clearance
- X-ray of kidneys, ureters and bladder
- ultrasound
- renal biopsy.

Treatment The goal is to restore biochemical balance and prevent ARF progressing. The onset of renal failure must be identified early to minimise damage and, if possible, prevent the necessity for dialysis. The priorities of treatment are as follows.

Treating the cause, e.g. correcting hypovolaemia and increasing renal perfusion; managing sepsis; relieving any urinary obstruction.

Reversing, restoring and maintaining fluid and electrolyte status:

- *Hyperkalaemia.* Immediate measures may be required to correct hyperkalaemia, which could cause lethal dysrhythmias. Cardiac monitoring is essential, in particular observing for any changes in cardiac rhythm. Hyperkalaemia can be corrected in the short term by i.v. insulin–glucose infusion or sodium bicarbonate, either of which will shift potassium into the cells. Other measures include the administration of ion exchange resins, which when administered orally or rectally remove potassium ions.
- *Hyponatraemia and hypernatraemia.* In the oliguric state there is a danger of hyponatraemia, due to the risk of fluid overload and to the failure of the damaged tubules to reabsorb sodium. However, hypernatraemia can also be a problem in pre-renal ARF, as mechanisms instituted retain sodium in order to restore blood volume. Fluid intake must be restricted to the equivalent of insensible loss plus the previous day's urinary output. Sodium intake must be monitored closely.
- *Uraemia.* The inability to excrete the waste products of metabolism is managed by dietary restrictions, but ensuring adequate calorie intake to prevent the patient becoming catabolic. Parenteral nutrition may be necessary and potassium intake will be restricted (see Ch. 21, p. 806).
- *Metabolic acidosis.* The loss of the kidneys' buffering function, the electrolyte imbalance and the increased anaerobic respiration by damaged renal cells all result in acidosis. In the short term, this is managed by i.v. sodium bicarbonate.

If acute renal failure is very severe, persists or worsens, dialysis will be necessary.

NURSING PRIORITIES AND MANAGEMENT: Acute renal failure

Major nursing considerations

The care of patients with ARF will involve a large multidisciplinary team and may be carried out either in an intensive care setting or on a ward, depending on the condition of the patient. Priorities of nursing intervention will be as follows:

- to reduce the patient's anxieties and recognise the risk of altered consciousness due to uraemia and electrolyte imbalance
- to control fluid and electrolyte balance by:
  - — monitoring cardiac status for signs of dysrhythmias
  - — monitoring pulse, respiration and blood pressure for signs of overload and hypertension
  - — restricting fluid intake and measuring and recording urine output and other losses; daily weighing may be required
  - — administering prescribed medication and carrying out urinary assays as required
- to maintain nutritional status within the necessary limitations by the oral, enteral or parenteral route and to monitor the nutritional status of the patient
- to prevent infection due to uraemia by strict asepsis with regard to infusion sites and catheter management and by close monitoring of temperature and the patient's reported symptoms
- to manage anaemia by the safe administration of blood transfusions, if required
- to promote comfort at all times.

STOP THINK **8.12** Reconsider the care of T, who had acute glomerulonephritis (see Case History 8.6). Severe forms can result in acute tubular necrosis and acute renal failure. Draw up a care plan that would have met T's needs should ARF have developed.

The diuretic and recovery phases

The oliguric phase of renal failure may last 1–2 weeks and is followed by the diuretic phase, which indicates that renal function is returning. This is often a time of relief, but because the kidneys will not yet have regained their capacity for selective reabsorption, urine output can be as much as 4 L/day. This, in itself, could potentiate dehydration and electrolyte imbalances. Close monitoring must therefore continue. The recovery phase that follows can last several months and will require close medical follow-up of renal function. Convalescence in the form of rest, restricted activity, the avoidance of infections and alertness to any symptoms that might indicate renal problems may be a source of considerable stress to the patient, who may also be concerned about fulfilling family and work responsibilities.

For further information, see Albright (2001) and Thomas (2002).

STOP THINK **8.13** What community support services might help to alleviate such stress?

Chronic renal failure

Chronic renal failure is the gradual and progressive reduction in renal function. Failure may occur over weeks, months or even years. Each year, acceptance rates for renal replacement therapies are increasing, at a rate that exceeds death rates, and this is predicted to continue for the next 10 years (DH 2004). The available treatments are dialysis, haemodialysis, peritoneal dialysis or transplantation, which may be from cadaveric or living related donors (Thomas 2002).

PATHOPHYSIOLOGY

Any disorder which damages kidney function can result in renal failure (see Box 8.14).

Clinical features In the initial stages of failure the patient may be asymptomatic. Proteinuria, hypertension, anaemia or an elevated blood urea are, however, common presenting features.

As renal failure progresses, the patient may complain of fatigue, lethargy, pruritus, nausea, vomiting and indigestion. Breathlessness on exertion, headaches, visual disturbances, pallor and loss of libido may also be noted. A reduced immune response occurs, making the patient prone to infection, particularly of the urinary tract (see Ch. 16).

Metabolic bone disease, generalised myopathy, neuropathy and metabolic acidosis can be seen in advanced stages of renal impairment. Atherosclerosis due to altered lipid and carbohydrate metabolism and hypertension may also occur. Vascular calcification and pericarditis may also be identified.

Box 8.14

Aetiology of chronic renal failure

Congenital and inherited diseases
- Polycystic kidney disease (infantile or adult)
- Alport's syndrome
- Fabry's disease

Vascular disease
- Arteriosclerosis
- Vasculitis (polyarteritis nodosa [PAN], systemic lupus erythematosus [SLE], scleroderma)

Glomerular disease
- Proliferative GN
- Crescentic GN
- Membranous GN
- Mesangiocapillary GN
- Glomerulosclerosis
- Secondary GN (PAN, SLE, amyloidosis, diabetic glomerulosclerosis)

Interstitial disease
- Chronic infective interstitial nephritis (chronic pyelonephritis)
- Vesicoureteric reflux
- Tuberculosis
- Analgesic nephropathy
- Nephrocalcinosis
- Schistosomiasis
- Unknown origin

Obstructive uropathy
- Calculus
- Retroperitoneal fibrosis
- Prostatic hypertrophy
- Pelvic tumours
- Other causes

Reproduced with permission from Haslett et al (2002).

MEDICAL MANAGEMENT

Treatment aims to identify the cause, extent and complications of the renal failure and to preserve useful renal function for as long as possible.

Where hypertension is evident, antihypertensive drugs may be used to reduce and control blood pressure gradually. Lifestyle advice should also be given to assist with reducing blood pressure, e.g. stopping smoking and losing weight.

Fluid restriction may be required if the glomerular filtration rate is less than 5 mL/min as fluid overload can exacerbate problems with hypertension. Poor urine concentration can, however, result in a urine output of more than 2.5 L/24 h, in which case an intake of about 3 L/day is required.

Dietary measures are likely to include potassium and phosphate restrictions. Sodium restriction is not indicated unless there is evidence of oedema, hypertension or cardiac failure. In the case of salt-losing conditions, sodium supplements may be required. A diet with no added salt may be appropriate in some cases.

Regular monitoring of biochemistry and assessment of symptoms allow treatment to be readjusted and progression of the disease to be assessed.

Dialysis in the form of haemodialysis or peritoneal dialysis are the treatments available to replace the excretory functions of the kidneys (see Box 8.15). At present, transplantation is restricted by a lack of available cadaver donor kidneys. However, for some patients, it may be possible to consider a close family member as a live donor.

NURSING PRIORITIES AND MANAGEMENT: Chronic renal failure

General considerations

Nursing management requires a strategy to help the patient and family come to terms with an illness for which there is no cure and in which sudden death can occur. Nursing intervention should aim to help the patient maintain a good quality of life by developing ways to cope with the constraints of the treatments and the possibility of complications occurring.

Adherence with treatment

Patient beliefs about the value and benefit of a treatment may differ markedly when compared with the priority given to the same treatment by the nurse. Failure to adhere to diet and fluid restrictions may indicate that the patient has an underlying problem, or is not coping with some aspect of the treatment; alternatively, there may be a lack of understanding of the importance of the treatment regimen.

Box 8.15

Dialysis

Principles

Dialysis requires a semi-permeable membrane to combine three principles — diffusion, osmosis and filtration — in order to permit the removal of metabolic wastes, excess electrolytes and fluids from patients with renal failure.

Diffusion

Diffusion is the movement of molecules from an area of high concentration, across a semi-permeable membrane, to an area of low concentration. This process continues until the concentrations in each compartment are the same.

Osmosis

Osmosis is the movement of a fluid or solvent from a lower concentration to a higher one.

Filtration

Filtration is the movement of both solvent and solute across a semi-permeable membrane under pressure.

Types

Haemodialysis

Haemodialysis requires a means of vascular access, e.g.:

- *Percutaneous access*, including subclavian, femoral and jugular lines which are either temporary or permanent.
- *Arteriovenous fistula and arteriovenous grafts (synthetic).* A fistula involves the anastomosis of an artery and a vein. The increased blood flow causes increased pressure on the vein walls which leads to thickening and dilatation (arterialised); this allows the repeated insertion of needles for dialysis. This developmental stage takes about 12 weeks. The fistula can be seen as well as felt.

The blood is pumped from the patient to an artificial kidney (the dialyser) and back to the patient, having now been cleansed by the dialysate. The artificial kidney is normally a disposable hollow fibre or flat plate dialyser; different dialysers consist of different membranes. The type of membrane used is important as part of the patient's individualised dialysis prescription. Issues to consider are desired clearance, fluid removal and biocompatibility.

Peritoneal dialysis

The peritoneal membrane serves as the semi-permeable membrane for dialysis. A temporary or permanent Tenckhoff catheter is placed into the abdomen. The dialysate is instilled into the abdomen (usually 2 L at each session). A set time elapses and the dialysate is drained out.

Continuing ambulatory peritoneal dialysis (CAPD)

Two litres of dialysate are instilled into the peritoneal cavity and left in place, usually for 6 h, when it is exchanged. Once patients have been instructed in this method, they can be independent, visiting the hospital only for clinic appointments or when any problems arise; the main potential problems are peritonitis, dehydration and constipation.

Other methods

Other methods of renal replacement therapy are often used in intensive care, including:

- continuous arteriovenous haemofiltration (CAVH)
- continuous arteriovenous haemodiafiltration (CAVHD)
- continuous venovenous haemofiltration (CVVH)
- continuous venovenous haemodiafiltration (CVVHD).

Knowing the patient and having an understanding of the patient's social and cultural background can give insight into behaviour with regard to a particular treatment.

Major patient problems

Fatigue and lethargy characteristic of chronic renal failure can reduce both ability and performance at work. Absence from work due to sickness or attendance at hospital may result in unemployment or reduction of income. Feelings of helplessness, hopelessness and depression are often expressed by patients with a chronic illness (Thomas 2002). Loss of control over many aspects of life and low self-esteem are likely to influence family relationships. Transplantation is acknowledged as the treatment of choice for a person with end-stage renal disease. A successful transplant offers the patient freedom and independence as well as an enhanced quality of life (see Ch. 32).

For further information, see Thomas (2002).

Living with peritoneal dialysis

Peritoneal dialysis (PD) is performed either as continuous ambulatory peritoneal dialysis (CAPD) or automated peritoneal dialysis (APD). CAPD is a continuous treatment, generally performed four times a day; APD is achieved by machine, generally overnight in the patient's own home. PD offers patients a greater degree of control over their treatment and lifestyle. While the number of fluid exchanges per day will be prescribed by the doctor, the timing of each exchange can be decided by the patient, to fit in with family life or work commitments. In addition, freedom to be away from home for visits or holidays is possible. For holidays abroad, the dialysate manufacturer may be able to deliver fluid requirements to the holiday destination.

The need for regular fluid exchanges and aseptic technique can be limiting for some patients. Performing the exchange in a designated area at home can give confidence and reassure patients that they have done all they can to reduce the risk of peritonitis. There may be a reluctance to perform exchanges in the homes of friends and relatives, particularly if the patient's illness is poorly understood and a source of embarrassment.

STOP THINK **8.14** How might you help a patient to gain confidence in dealing with the treatment in order to take advantage of the relative freedom that PD offers?

The insertion of a tube and presence of fluid in the abdomen can alter body image and sexuality, thus discouraging those who are conscious of their appearance. A further disadvantage of CAPD is that it presents a constant reminder to the patient of their illness.

For further information, see Levy et al (2001) and Thomas (2002).

Living with intermittent haemodialysis

For some patients, haemodialysis may be the preferred option. This is generally hospital based, or in some areas satellite treatment centres are available. In some cases the patient may opt for home haemodialysis. A patient opting for home haemodialysis will undergo a training programme with their partner/carer before commencing the treatment.

Hospital or satellite haemodialysis is performed on an outpatient basis, two or three times a week.

Dialysis as a treatment does have a number of drawbacks, including the following:

- the need for transport to and from hospital
- the need to be away from home and dependants two or three times a week
- the difficulty of fitting in dialysis sessions with work and family commitments
- the increased fluid load prior to dialysis
- the need to restrict the diet
- the financial implications of lost work time
- the side-effects of dialysis and the continuing feeling of not being fully fit
- living with the uncertain hope of a kidney transplant
- the stress and strain on the family of dealing with the lifestyle constraints imposed by treatment.

STOP THINK **8.15** Consider the problems listed above and, for each, suggest ways in which the health care team can help.

Nursing support during dialysis

Assessments to be performed before haemodialysis are:

- Record patient's weight — compare with weight after last dialysis and the patient's recognised dry weight, i.e. the weight at which there is no clinical evidence of oedema, increased jugular venous pressure, shortness of breath or hyper/hypotension.
- Record temperature, pulse and blood pressure — compare these with values after the last dialysis. Any temperature increase could indicate an infected dialysis site. Raised blood pressure may indicate fluid overloading.
- Enquire how the patient has been feeling, i.e. well or unwell.
- Assess any known specific medical problem, e.g. blood sugar level in patients with diabetes mellitus.
- Once a month, take blood for urea and electrolyte levels pre- and post-dialysis; a full blood count should be checked every month.

During dialysis, the nurse should record the pulse and blood pressure. A drop in blood pressure may mean that the patient needs extra fluid. If necessary, the nurse should check the patient's weight halfway through the session.

At the end of dialysis, the patient's temperature, pulse, blood pressure and weight should be recorded in order to assess the effectiveness of the treatment. Any prescribed medications should be administered and the patient should be given the opportunity to raise any further concerns.

CONCLUSION

This is a challenging and rapidly developing area of practice in which to work, one in which the role of the nurse is constantly developing.

Caring for patients who have problems within the urinary system is complex and demanding. Conditions that affect the urinary tract can be either acute or chronic and it is important that the nurse recognises that the patient's needs are often multifactorial.

In order to provide high quality nursing care, when caring for these patients the nurse must demonstrate not only a good understanding of anatomy and physiology, the disease process and the potential complications but also good interpersonal skills and sensitivity in the experience of illness.

REFERENCES

Black P 2000 Holistic stoma care. Baillière Tindall, London

Blandy J 1998 Lecture notes on urology, 5th edn. Blackwell Science, Oxford

Brewster S, Canston D, Noble J, Reynard J 2001 Urology. A handbook for medical students. BIOS Scientific Publishers, Oxford

Bullock N, Sibley G, Whitaker R 1994 Essential urology, 2nd edn. Churchill Livingstone, Edinburgh

Burkitt H G, Quick C R G, Gatt D 1996 Essential surgery: problems, diagnosis and management, 2nd edn. Churchill Livingstone, Edinburgh

Department of Health 2004 The National Service Framework for Renal Services. Part One: Dialysis and Transplantation. DH, London

Downey P (ed) 2000 Introduction to urological nursing. Whurr, London

Garden J O, Bradbury A W Forsythe J 2002 Principles and practice of surgery, 4th edn. Churchill Livingstone, Edinburgh

Getliffe K, Dolman M 2003 Promoting continence. A clinical research resource, 2nd edn. Baillière Tindall, London

Gray M 2002 A prostate cancer primer. Urologic Nursing 22(3): 151–169

Haslett C, Chilvers E R, Boon N A, Colledge N R (eds) 2002 Davidson's principles and practice of medicine, 19th edn. Churchill Livingstone, Edinburgh

Holdgate A, Pollock T 2004 Systematic review of the relative efficacy of non steroidal anti-inflammatory drugs and opioids in the treatment of acute renal failure. British Medical Journal 328(7453): 1407

Inglis T J J 2003 Microbiology and infection. A clinical core text for integrated curricula with self assessment, 2nd edn. Churchill Livingstone, Edinburgh

National Institute for Clinical Excellence (NICE) 2002 Guidance on cancer services. Improving outcomes in urological cancers. The manual. NICE, London

O'Callaghan C, Brenner B M 2000 The kidney at a glance. Blackwell Science, London

Pickard R, Emberton M, Neal D E 1998 The management of men with acute urinary retention. British Journal of Urology 81: 712–720

Pomfret I 1996 Catheters: design, selection and management. British Journal of Nursing 5(4): 245–250

Pratt R J, Pellowe C, Loveday H P et al 2001 The EPIC Project: developing national evidence-based guidelines for preventing healthcare associated infections. Journal of Hospital Infection 47(Suppl): S3–46

Thibodeau G A, Patton K T 1999 Anatomy and physiology, 4th edn. Mosby, St Louis

Thomas N (ed) 2002 Renal nursing, 2nd edn. Baillière Tindall, London

Thorpe A, Neal D 2003 Benign prostatic hyperplasia. Lancet 361(9366): 1359–1367

Trounce J, Gould D 2000 Clinical pharmacology for nurses, 16th edn. Churchill Livingstone, Edinburgh

Underwood M, Alexander R, Gurun M, Jones G 2003 Key topics in urology. BIOS Scientific Publishers, Oxford

Waugh A, Grant A 2001 Ross and Wilson's anatomy and physiology in health and illness, 9th edn. Churchill Livingstone, Edinburgh

Wilt T J 2002 Treatment options for benign prostatic hyperplasia. British Medical Journal 324(7345): 1047–1048

FURTHER READING

Albright R C 2001 Acute renal failure: a practical update. Mayo Clinic Proceedings 76(1): 67–76
Black P 2000 Holistic stoma care. Baillière Tindall, London
Blandy J 1998 Lecture notes on urology, 5th edn. Blackwell Science, Oxford
Brewster S, Canston D, Noble J, Reynard J 2001 Urology. A handbook for medical students. BIOS Scientific Publishers, Oxford
Doherty W, Winder A 2000 Indwelling catheters: practical guidelines for catheter blockage. British Journal of Nursing 9(18): 2006–2014
Donovan J L, Frankel S J, Neal D E, Hamdy F C 2001 Screening for prostate cancer in the UK. British Medical Journal 323(7361): 763–764
Downey P (ed) 2000 Introduction to urological nursing. Whurr, London
Evans A, Godfrey H 2000 Bladder washouts in the management of long-term catheters. British Journal of Nursing 9(14): 900–906
Garden J O, Bradbury A W, Forsythe J 2002 Principles and practice of surgery, 4th edn. Churchill Livingstone, Edinburgh
Levy J, Morgan J, Brown E 2001 Oxford handbook of dialysis. Oxford University Press, Oxford
Nicolle L E 2002 Epidemiology of urinary tract infections. Clinical Microbiology Newsletter 24(18): 135–140
O'Callaghan C, Brenner B M 2000 The kidney at a glance. Blackwell Science, London
Pashos C L, Bottemann M F, Laskin B L, Redaelli A 2002 Bladder cancer, epidemiology, diagnosis and management. Cancer Practice 10(6): 311–322
Pratt R J, Pellowe C, Loveday H P et al 2001 The EPIC Project: developing national evidence based guidelines for preventing healthcare associated infections. Journal of Hospital Infection 47(Suppl): S3–46
Pomfret I 2001 Selecting the appropriate method of catheterisation. Journal of Community Nursing 15(4): 39–42
Reilly N J 1997 Benign prostatic hyperplasia in older men. Lippincott's Primary Care Practice 1(4): 421–430
Robinson J 2003 Choosing a catheter. Journal of Community Nursing 17(3): 37–42
Royal College of Nursing 2004 Competencies: an integrated career and competency framework for occupational health nursing RCN London
Thomas N (ed) 2002 Renal nursing, 2nd edn. Baillière Tindall, London
Thorpe A, Neal D 2003 Benign prostatic hyperplasia. Lancet 361(9366): 1359–1367
Tiselius H G 2003 Epidemiology and medical management of stone disease. BJU International 91: 758–767
Trotto N E 2000 Contemporary management of bladder cancer. Patient Care 34(7): 72–90
Underwood M, Alexander R, Gurun M, Jones G 2003 Key topics in urology. BIOS Scientific Publishers, Oxford
Wagenlehner F M E, Naber K G 2000 Hospital acquired urinary tract infections. Journal of Hospital Infections 46: 171–181

DISORDERS OF THE NERVOUS SYSTEM

9

Douglas Allan

INTRODUCTION

Many nurses may have only brief contact with patients suffering from neurological disorders, either while they are waiting to be transferred to a specialist neurological unit or following their return from such a unit. Community nursing staff, however, are increasingly involved with patients recovering at home, either from acute neurosurgical interventions or long-term neurological disorders, where the disorder cannot be cured. Recent years have also witnessed a growth in the number of specialised liaison or support nurses for patients with disorders such as epilepsy and multiple sclerosis.

This chapter considers the more common neurological and neurosurgical disorders and, where appropriate, makes reference to the less common disorders. The specialised neuroscience textbooks listed at the end of the chapter provide more detailed information. It is hoped that the information contained here will raise awareness of this specialised field of nursing, and stimulate further discussion on how best to meet the needs of the patient with a neurological condition and of their family and/or significant others.

ANATOMY AND PHYSIOLOGY

The nervous system is a complex, interrelated body system responsible for many functions including communication, coordination, behaviour and intelligence. It constantly receives data from the external and internal environments, interprets these, and then responds by adapting appropriately to demands.

The nervous system can be considered in two distinct parts, namely the central nervous system (CNS), comprising the brain and spinal cord, and the peripheral nervous system (PNS), consisting of the cranial and spinal nerves. The peripheral nervous system has two functional parts, the sensory division and the motor division (see p. 406).

Basic tissue structure

Nervous tissue consists of neuroglia (or 'glial cells') and neurones (or 'nerve cells'). The neuroglia markedly outnumber the neurones and form a supportive and protective network for the nervous system, e.g. by attaching neurones to their blood vessels and protecting the nervous system through phagocytic action, as the white cells do elsewhere in the body. In the peripheral nervous system, supporting cells, called 'Schwann cells', form the myelin sheath as well as having a phagocytic role.

Myelin protects and electrically insulates nerve fibres from one another, and potentiates, i.e. speeds up, nerve impulse transmission. Myelinated nerve impulses are transmitted by saltatory conduction, whereby the impulse jumps from one node of Ranvier to the next (see Fig. 9.1). Impulses in myelinated nerves are therefore transmitted very much faster than in unmyelinated nerves and require very much less energy. The importance of myelin in nerve impulse transmission is painfully clear to those suffering from demyelinating diseases such as multiple sclerosis. In this condition, the myelin sheath is destroyed, impulse conduction ceases and the affected individual loses the ability to control voluntary muscle movement (p. 430).

Neurones

Although fewer in number, neurones form the basis of the structural and functional unit of the nervous system. They are capable of conducting impulses throughout the nervous system and to other excitable tissues, including the muscles and glands. The structure of a typical multipolar neurone is shown in Figure 9.1.

The axons of sensory and motor neurones constitute the nerve fibres. They are bundled together in the peripheral nervous system by connective tissue to form the peripheral nerves (see Fig. 9.2). In the CNS, the axons of connector neurones are held in distinct tracts by the glial cells.

Classification of neurones Neurones are classified according to their structure and function. The functional classification is determined by the direction in which the impulse travels and the structural classification is based on the number of poles on the cell body.

Sensory or afferent neurones transmit impulses from receptors in the skin, sense organs and viscera to the brain and spinal cord. Structurally, these are unipolar, i.e. cells with processes projecting from one pole, or bipolar, where processes project from two poles at opposite ends of the cell. Bipolar neurones are found only in special sense organs, e.g. the retina of the eye.

Motor or efferent neurones transmit impulses in the opposite direction, from the brain and spinal cord to muscles and glands in the body (the effectors). Typically, these are multipolar, i.e. cells with processes projecting from many points all over the cell body (see Fig. 9.1).

Connector neurones or interneurones convey impulses within the CNS. Typically, these are also multipolar.

The nerve impulse

A nerve impulse can be initiated by a stimulus such as a change in temperature, pressure or the chemical environment, or impulses can be generated spontaneously by pacemaker cells. The impulse is described as a self-propagating wave of electrical charge along the membrane of the neurone, effecting changes crucial to the conduction of the impulse.

At rest, the nerve cell has an unequal distribution of ions on either side of the plasma membrane. These comprise potassium and sodium and are necessary to maintain the chemical difference which produces an electrical difference: the inside of the cell is negatively charged in relation to the outside. This has been measured at –70 mV and is termed the resting membrane potential. The cell is maintained in this condition by a system whereby ions are exchanged between the intracellular and extracellular fluids. A property of all nerve cells is their ability to respond to stimuli by producing an impulse when the stimulus is sufficient to initiate certain electrical and chemical changes within the cell membrane. These positive–negative changes occur in rapid succession, spreading to the end of the axon.

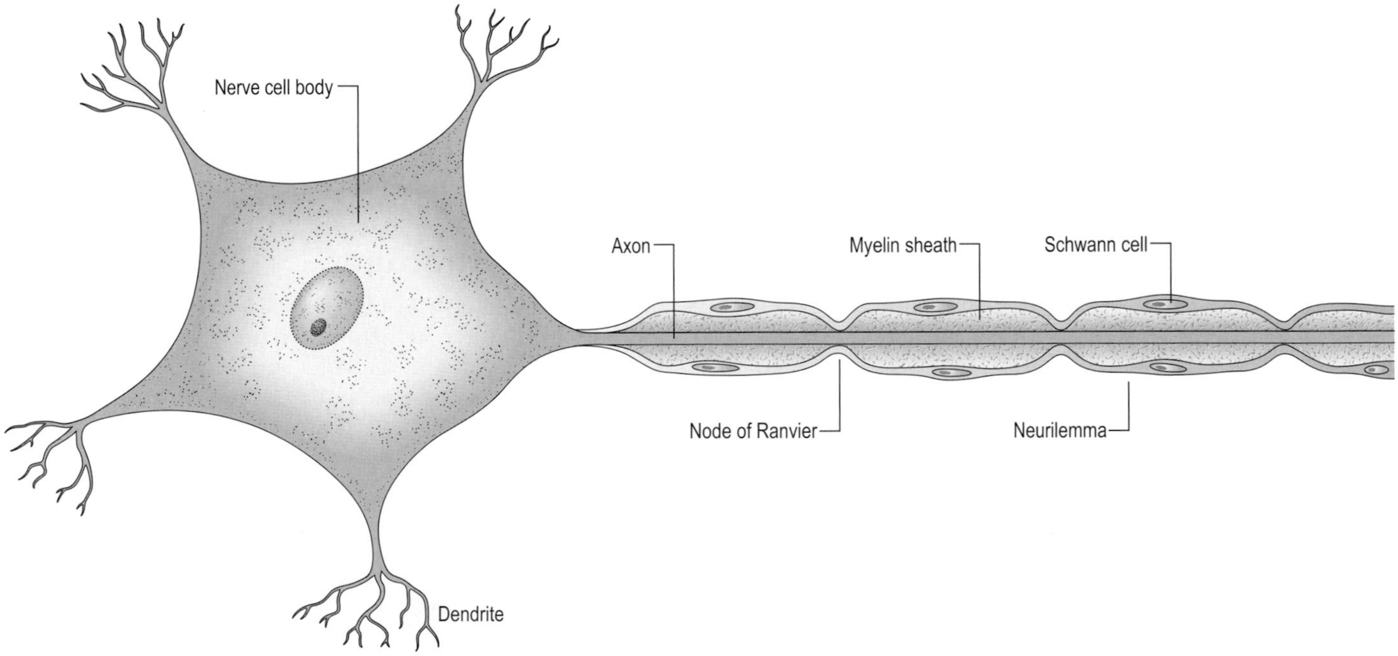

Fig. 9.1 Structure of a multipolar neurone. It consists of three parts: (1) The nerve cell body, which is grey in colour. Each cell body is enclosed in a selectively permeable membrane, which also extends along the cell processes. The cell body contains a nucleus surrounded by cytoplasm which also contains other structures called organelles. (2) The dendrites are thread-like extensions of the cell body which increase the surface area available to receive signals from other neurones. (3) The axon is a single long process that conducts impulses away from the cell body. In many large peripheral axons, the axolemma is surrounded by another covering called the myelin sheath. This is a multiple-layered covering of fatty material which is white in colour. Its function is to insulate the neurone electrically and thus speed up the conduction of the nerve impulse, by segmentation. Each interruption of the sheath is known as a node of Ranvier and the speed of the impulse is increased by its 'jumping' from node to node. The axon and its collaterals branch into axon terminals, the ends of which form a bulb-like structure. These help to transmit an impulse from one neurone to another across the gap (synapse) between them or at the junctions with effector cells.

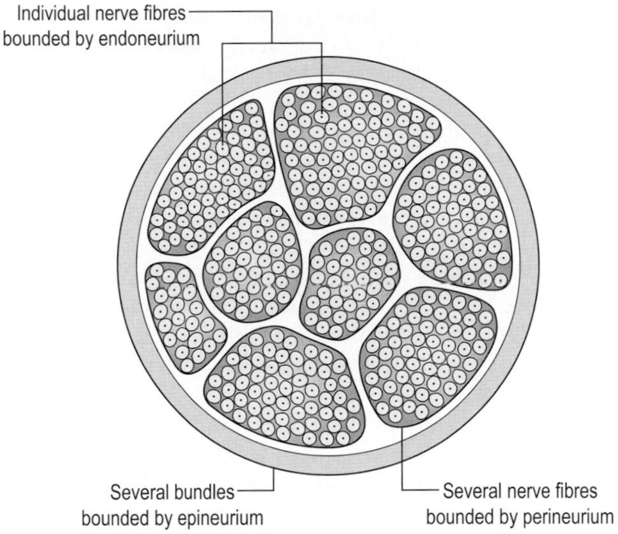

Fig. 9.2 Transverse section, peripheral nerve. The nerve fibres are surrounded by a fine connective tissue covering called the endoneurium. Several nerve fibres are bound together by another connective tissue covering called the perineurium and a number of these bundles may be surrounded by another covering called the epineurium.

Other more subtle and complex changes also occur.

For further information, see Marieb (2004) and Tortora & Derrickson (2006).

Generally, the larger the diameter of the axon, the quicker the nerve impulse travels, but the alternative device of saltatory conduction is found in myelinated neurones, as shown in Figure 9.3.

Neurotransmitters

The junctions between one neurone and another, and between neurones and muscles or glands, are known as synapses. Nerve impulses are transmitted across the gap at these synapses by chemical transmitters (neurotransmitters). The chemical is stored in vesicles in the expanded end of the axon and is released when the nerve impulse reaches this point. Several chemical transmitters have been identified, the most common ones being acetylcholine and noradrenaline. Many of these neurotransmitters are excitatory, resulting in the nerve impulse being transmitted to the receiving tissue and thus producing an effect such as contraction of muscle cells. Some, however, have an inhibiting effect and prevent the onward transmission of impulses, allowing, for example, muscle cells to relax. The effect of the neurotransmitter is terminated when it is destroyed by enzymes or reabsorbed into the neurone.

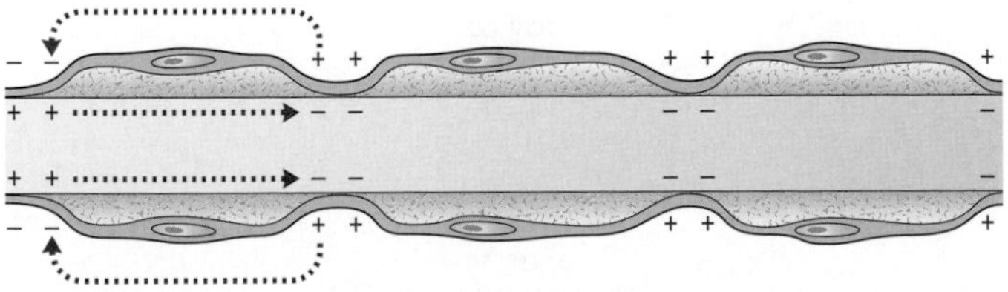

Fig. 9.3 Saltatory conduction in a myelinated nerve.

The central nervous system

The central nervous system consists of the brain and spinal cord.

The brain

The cerebrum, the largest constituent of the nervous system, forms the bulk of the brain. The outer surface, the cortex, is of grey matter and consists of nerve cell bodies. The surface area of the cerebral cortex is increased by a series of grooves (sulci) and ridges (gyri). The deeper grooves are termed fissures and some form landmarks, e.g. the longitudinal fissure which almost splits the brain into two hemispheres (see Fig. 9.4).

Each hemisphere is subdivided into four lobes, and each lobe is named according to the skull bones it underlies:

- frontal
- temporal
- parietal
- occipital.

The cerebral cortex is responsible for three main functions:

- receiving and interpreting a mass of sensory information from various sources in the internal and external environments
- initiating and controlling voluntary movement in response to the sensory information received
- integrating crucial functions such as memory and consciousness.

Certain areas of the cerebral cortex have been identified as being responsible for these functions, and these areas form a map, as illustrated in Figure 9.5.

Relative size The lips, thumbs and face use many more receptors than the trunk and legs: similarly, the thumbs, fingers, lips, tongue and vocal cords are more sensitive than the trunk, due to the greater number of receptors found in them. The homunculus (see Fig. 9.6) illustrates how the various parts of the body are represented in the corresponding motor and sensory areas of the cerebral hemispheres,

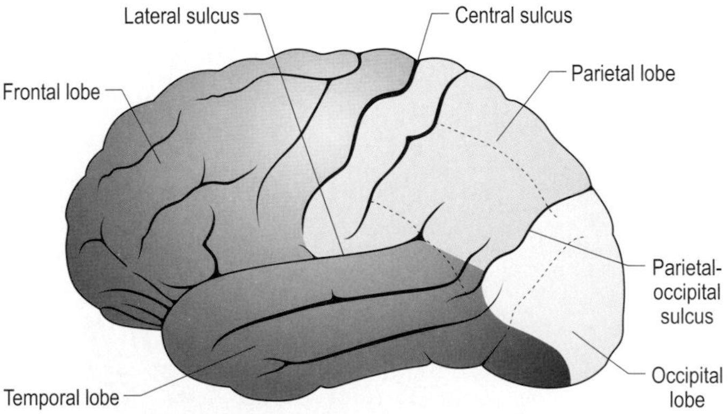

Fig. 9.4 The lobes and sulci of the cerebrum. Each of the lobes is bounded by 'landmark' fissures: the frontal lobe is separated from the parietal lobe by the central sulcus; the temporal lobe is separated from the frontal and parietal lobes by the lateral sulcus; and the occipital lobe is separated from the temporal and parietal lobes by the parietal–occipital sulcus.

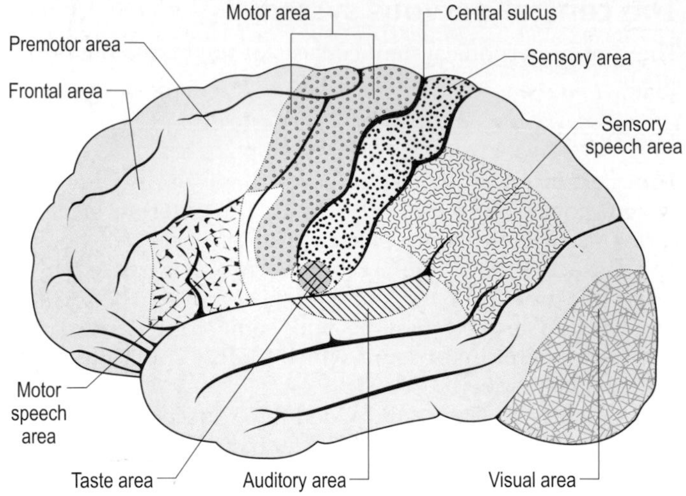

Fig. 9.5 The cerebrum showing the functional areas.

i.e. representation is proportional not to the relative size of the body parts, but to each part's complexity of movement or the extent of its sensory innervation.

For further information, see Waugh & Grant (2001).

STOP THINK **9.1** Discuss with your lecturer or mentor how this strange-looking representation might impact on the perceptions and experiences of a patient, for example, following limb amputation or where there has been stroke damage.

The concept of dominance The functions of speech and motor control are usually more highly developed in one cerebral hemisphere than in the other. This is referred to as dominance. Approximately 95% of the population are dominant in the left hemisphere and, as most of the spinal pathways cross over in the medulla (see p. 399), they are right-handed. However, if the dominant hemisphere is damaged, the opposite hemisphere is capable of taking over and assuming a dominant role.

Association areas Some areas of the brain remain unmapped (see Fig. 9.5). These are called 'association areas' and are thought to be responsible for complex functions such as integration of the senses, memory, learning, thought processes, behaviour and emotion.

Connecting pathways Below the outer cortical layer can be found areas of white matter (myelinated nerve fibres) that form connections between the cerebral cortex and other areas of grey matter in the CNS. Three types of connecting pathways (see Fig. 9.7) have been identified:

- association fibres — these connect between gyri in the same hemisphere
- commissural fibres — these connect between gyri in different hemispheres; one important group of commissural fibres is the corpus callosum
- projection fibres — these provide connections between the brain and spinal cord in ascending and descending pathways; one example is the internal capsule.

For further details on these interconnecting pathways, see Montague et al (2005).

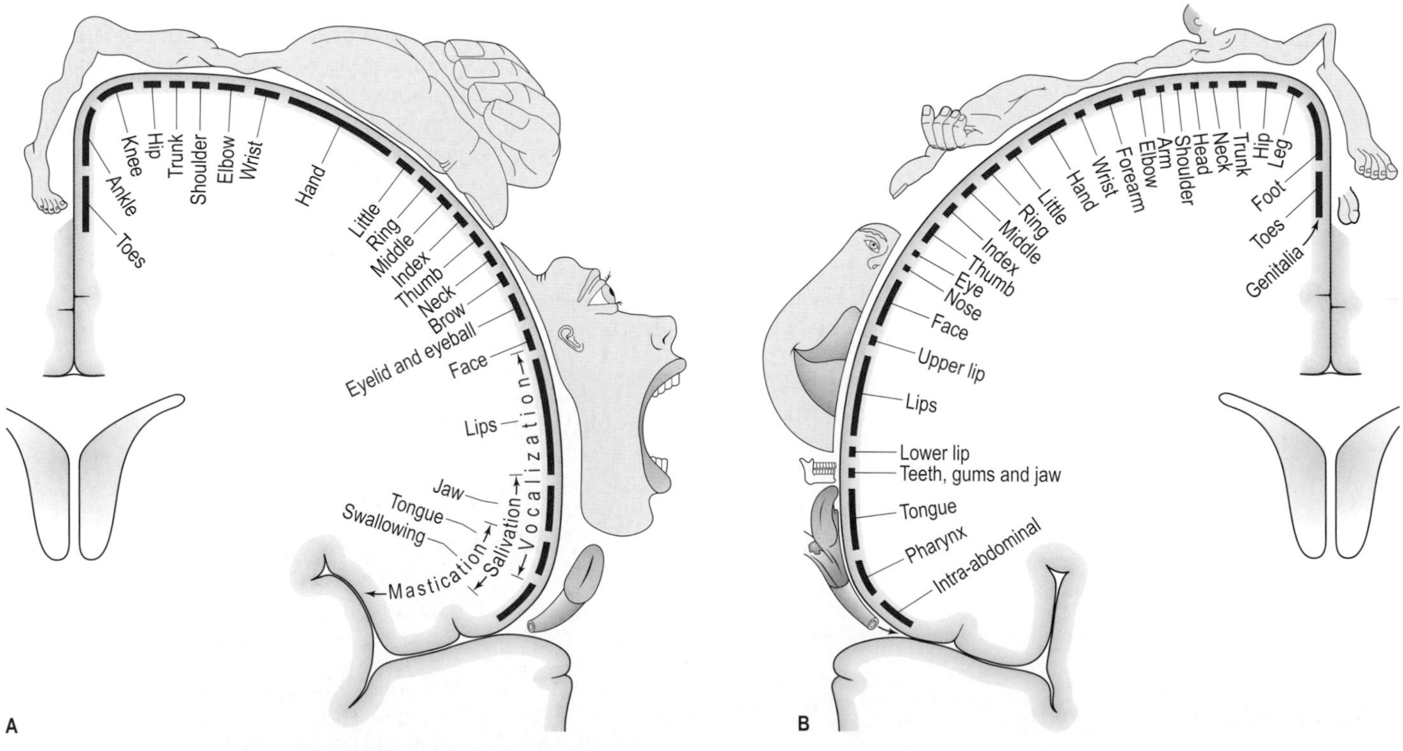

Fig. 9.6 A: The motor homunculus showing how the body is represented in the motor area of the cerebrum. B: The sensory homunculus showing how the body is represented in the sensory area of the cerebrum.

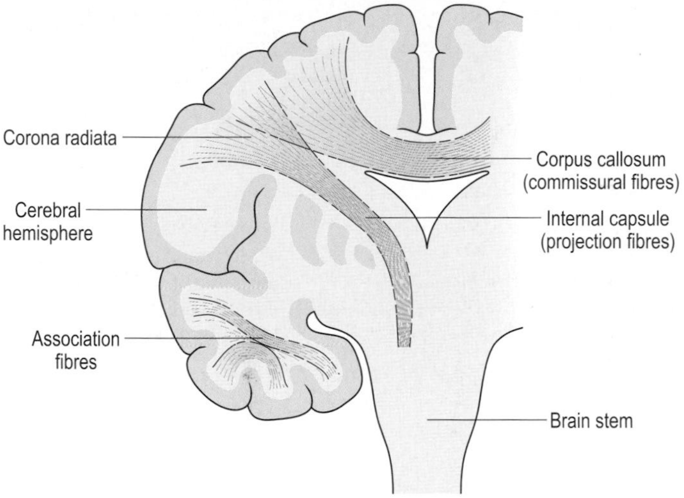

Fig. 9.7 White matter of the cerebrum.

Basal nuclei (ganglia) Within the white matter of the cerebrum are paired islands of grey matter called the 'basal nuclei'. They control large subconscious movements, such as swinging the arms while walking and regulating muscle tone for specific body movements, a function that is lost in Parkinson's disease.

Other structures closely associated with the cerebrum are the cerebellum and the pituitary gland.

The cerebellum is located below the posterior part of the cerebrum and is separated from it by a fold of dura mater. It consists of two hemispheres separated by a narrow strip called the 'vermis'. The cortex of the cerebellum consists of grey matter which has many folds to increase its surface area. The interior comprises white matter presented in a branching configuration termed the arbor vitae or 'tree of life'. There are three connections, called the 'cerebellar peduncles', which link the cerebellum to the rest of the brain and spinal cord. These allow the cerebellum to receive sensory information and thereby to maintain equilibrium and modify voluntary movement, making it smooth and coordinated.

The pituitary gland The pituitary gland is situated at the base of the brain in a depression in the sphenoid bone called the 'sella turcica' (Turkish saddle). It is attached to the brain via a stalk which is continuous with the hypothalamus, and communication is by means of nerve fibres and blood vessels. It has three lobes, an anterior, a middle and a posterior lobe, which secrete hormones that exert an influence on other parts of the body (see Ch. 5, Part 1, for details of the actions of pituitary hormones).

Diencephalon Three bilaterally symmetrical structures comprise the diencephalon:

- the thalamus
- the hypothalamus
- the epithalamus.

Collectively, these three structures enclose and form the boundaries of the third ventricle.

The thalamus consists of two oval-shaped masses (thalami), mainly consisting of grey matter with some white matter, and is situated within the cerebral hemispheres just below the corpus callosum. Sensory impulses associated with pain, temperature, pressure and touch are conveyed to the thalamus, which acts as a 'gateway'. Chaos would reign if all the sensory information flooding into the nervous system were allowed to reach the sensory cortex.

The hypothalamus is situated below the thalamus and forms the walls and floor of the third ventricle. It controls the output of the hormones from the pituitary gland and is located directly above it. Other functions include the regulation of hunger, thirst and body temperature (see Ch. 22). The last function is significant for patients with a hypothalamic disturbance following head injury.

The epithalamus is the most dorsal part of the diencephalon and forms the roof of the third ventricle. Extending from its posterior border is the pineal gland, thought to be concerned with growth and development (Hickey 2002).

The brain stem This is the collective name given to three structures: the medulla, the pons and the midbrain. Inferiorly, the medulla is continuous with the upper spinal cord and connects with the pons above. The pons is continuous with the midbrain, which connects with the lower portion of the diencephalon.

The medulla All the spinal pathways pass through the medulla, constituting its white matter. Some of these cross to the opposite side in triangular-shaped structures called the 'pyramids', a process known as 'decussation'. The purpose of this has never been established.

- It contains the reticular formation, a diffuse area of grey and white matter that has connections with the rest of the brain stem and cerebral cortex, within which is a structure known as the reticular activating system, responsible for consciousness and arousal.
- It accommodates three reflex centres, which control vital functions; these include:
  - — the cardiac centre, which regulates heartbeat and force of contraction
  - — the medullary rhythmicity area, which adjusts the basic rhythm of breathing
  - — the vasomotor centre, which regulates the diameter of blood vessels (important in control of blood pressure).

  Other non-vital centres include those responsible for coordinating swallowing, vomiting, coughing, sneezing and hiccupping.
- It also contains the nuclei of cranial nerves VIII to XII (see Table 9.1).

The pons The pons acts as a bridge between the medulla and the midbrain. It comprises fibres and nuclei. The fibres run in two directions: the transverse fibres connect with the cerebellum and the longitudinal fibres maintain the vital link between the spinal cord and the brain. The nuclei are the origins of cranial nerves V–VIII inclusive (see Table 9.1). Other important nuclei also exert an influence on respiration.

The midbrain The third component of the brain stem is the midbrain, which contains the central centres for visual, auditory and postural reflexes. It is located above the pons

Table 9.1 Cranial nerves

Number	Nerve	Origin	Termination	Functions
I	Olfactory	Olfactory mucosa	Olfactory cortex	Sensory: Smell
II	Optic	Retina	Visual cortex	Sensory: Vision
III	Oculomotor	Midbrain Proprioceptors in extrinsic eye muscles	Upper eyelid muscle Extrinsic eye muscles Ciliary muscles Sphincter muscle of the iris Midbrain	Motor: Eyelid movement Eyeball movement Accommodation of lens Pupillary constriction Sensory: Proprioception
IV	Trochlear	Midbrain Proprioceptors in extrinsic eye muscle (superior oblique)	Extrinsic eye muscle superior oblique Midbrain	Motor: Eyeball movement Sensory: Proprioception
V	Trigeminal	Pons Ophthalmic branch takes sensory fibres from skin of upper eyelid, eyeball, lacrimal glands, nasal cavity, side of nose, forehead and anterior half of scalp Maxillary branch takes sensory fibres from mucosa of nose, palate, parts of pharynx, upper teeth, upper lip, cheek and lower eyelid Mandibular branch takes sensory fibres from anterior two-thirds of tongue, lower teeth, skin over mandible and side of head in front of ear	Muscles of mastication Midbrain, pons and medulla	Motor: Chewing Sensory: Touch, pain, temperature, proprioception
VI	Abducens	Pons Proprioceptors in lateral rectus	Extrinsic eye muscle (lateral rectus) Pons	Motor: Eyeball movement Sensory: Proprioception
VII	Facial	Pons Taste buds on anterior two-thirds of tongue Proprioceptors in muscles of face and scalp	Facial, scalp and neck muscles Lacrimal and salivary glands Gustatory cortex	Motor: Facial expression Salivation Lacrimation Sensory: Taste Proprioception
VIII	Vestibulocochlear	Cochlear and vestibular portions of the ear	Cochlear nuclei in pons Vestibular nuclei in the medulla	Sensory: Hearing Equilibrium
IX	Glossopharyngeal	Medulla Taste buds on posterior one-third of tongue Carotid sinus Proprioceptors in muscles of face and scalp	Swallowing muscles in the pharynx Parotid gland Gustatory cortex	Motor: Swallowing Salivation Sensory: Taste Regulation of blood pressure Proprioception
X	Vagus	Medulla Receptors in the same structures that the motor portion innervates	Visceral muscles (muscles of pharynx, larynx, respiratory tract, oesophagus, heart, stomach, small intestine, proximal half of large intestine, gall bladder, liver, pancreas) Medulla and pons	Motor: Swallowing, digestive movements and secretions Sensory: Range of sensory inputs from organs supplied and proprioception from muscle

Table 9.1 Cranial nerves *(Continued)*

Number	Nerve	Origin	Termination	Functions
XI	Accessory	Bulbar portion: medulla	Muscles of pharynx, larynx, soft palate	Motor: Swallowing
		Spinal portion: cervical spinal cord	Sternocleidomastoid and trapezius muscles	Head movements
		Proprioceptors in muscles supplied by motor fibres	Medulla	Sensory: Proprioception
XII	Hypoglossal	Medulla	Muscles of tongue	Motor: Tongue movements
		Proprioceptors in tongue	Medulla	Sensory: Proprioception

For further information, see Tortora & Derrickson (2006).

and is the origin of the nuclei of cranial nerves III and IV (see Table 9.1). Cranial nerves I and II originate in the cerebrum.

The meninges

The brain and spinal cord are surrounded and protected by three meninges:

- the innermost layer, the pia mater
- the middle layer, the arachnoid mater
- the outer layer, the dura mater.

The pia mater is of the same structure as the arachnoid mater (see below), except that it has its own blood supply. The pia closely follows and adheres to the contours of the brain and spinal cord.

The arachnoid mater consists of collagenous and elastic fibres, covered by squamous epithelium. Fine strands of connective tissue connect the arachnoid with the pia below. The arachnoid mater projects into the sinuses as arachnoid villi, which are the structures responsible for the absorption of cerebrospinal fluid, and at certain points it joins the linings of the ventricles to form the choroid plexus, where cerebrospinal fluid is produced.

The dura mater is a double layer of dense fibrous tissue. The outer, periosteal layer adheres closely to the underside of the cranial bones, whilst the inner, meningeal layer is much thinner. The spinal dura mater has only one layer, which corresponds to the meningeal layer of the cranium. The two layers of the dura mater separate at several locations and these spaces contain the venous sinuses, e.g. the falx cerebri and the tentorium cerebelli. The former forms an incomplete division dipping down between the two cerebral hemispheres and is attached to the ethmoid bone at the front and the occipital protuberance at the back (see Fig. 9.8).

The tentorium cerebelli forms a division between the occipital lobes of the cerebrum and the cerebellum. It is attached along the midline to the falx cerebri, which draws it upwards to produce a tent-like appearance.

The ventricular system

The ventricular system consists of four fluid-filled irregular cavities (ventricles) interconnected by narrow pathways (see Fig. 9.9) and is connected with the central canal of the spinal cord and the cranial subarachnoid space. There are two lateral ventricles, one in each cerebral hemisphere, one

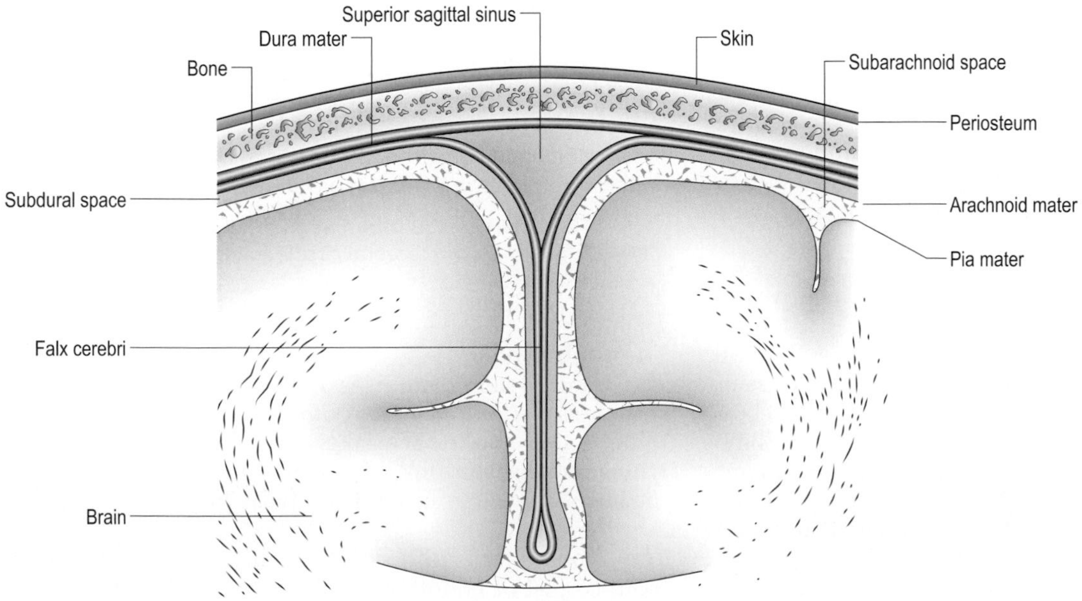

Fig. 9.8 Meninges of the brain.

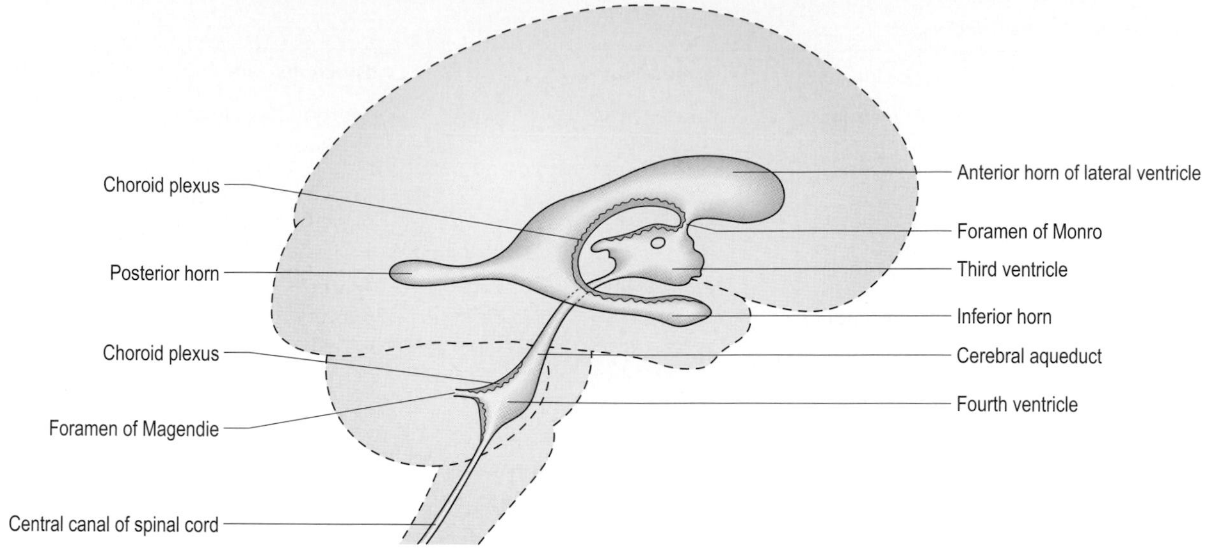

Fig. 9.9 Ventricular system.

Box 9.1

Normal features of cerebrospinal fluid

Colour: crystal clear
Pressure: 80–160 mmH_2O
Volume: 120–150 mL
Cells:
- red blood — none
- white blood
  - — polymorphonuclear leucocytes — none
  - — lymphocytes 0–5/mm^3

Protein: 0.2–0.4 g/L
Gamma globulin (IgG): less than 13% of total protein
Sugar: 3.6–5.0 mmol
Wassermann reaction: negative

ventricle (the third) located in the diencephalic region and another located in the medulla, called the fourth ventricle.

Cerebrospinal fluid (CSF) circulates within the closed ventricular system. Healthy cerebrospinal fluid is clear and colourless. Its normal features are as outlined in Box 9.1.

The CSF production–absorption cycle is continuous, and a fairly constant volume of 120–150 mL is maintained. When this process is interrupted and the volume is increased beyond normal limits, hydrocephalus occurs.

The main source of production of CSF is the choroid plexus, a collection of specialised capillaries located within the internal lining of the ventricles, the largest amount being produced in the lateral ventricles. From here, the CSF passes through two interventricular foramina (foramen of Monro) to the third ventricle, then via the single cerebral aqueduct (aqueduct of Sylvius) to the fourth ventricle. Some CSF passes down into the central canal of the spinal cord but most passes up through the two lateral and one medial foramina in the roof of the fourth ventricle, to circulate round the brain and spinal cord in the subarachnoid space before being reabsorbed into the blood via the arachnoid villi.

The functions of CSF are:

- protection and cushioning of the brain and spinal cord
- provision of nourishment
- maintenance of a uniform intracranial pressure
- removal of waste products.

Blood supply and drainage

The supply of blood to the head arises from the left and right common carotid arteries, which subdivide to form the internal and external carotid arteries. These supply blood to the anterior part of the brain, and the vertebral arteries supply the posterior part.

The greater part of the brain is supplied with blood by the circle of Willis, an unusual configuration of anastomosed blood vessels located in the base of the brain (see Fig. 9.10).

Venous drainage is by small veins in the brain stem and cerebellum, and external and internal veins draining the cerebrum. Some of the external and internal veins empty into one large vein called the vein of Galen (great cerebral vein). Unlike other parts of the body, these veins do not correspond with their arterial supply. All these veins empty directly into a system of venous sinuses, which is shown in Figure 9.11.

The principal sinuses are the superior and inferior sagittal, the straight, transverse, sigmoid and cavernous sinuses.

For more detailed information on the areas of the brain supplied by the cerebral circulation, see Montague et al (2005).

The limbic system

The limbic system comprises an interconnected complex of structures, including the hypothalamus. These are thought to be responsible for special types of behaviour associated with emotions, subconscious motor and sensory drives and the intrinsic feelings of pain and pleasure.

The blood–brain barrier The capillaries supplying the brain consist of endothelial cells with very tight junctions,

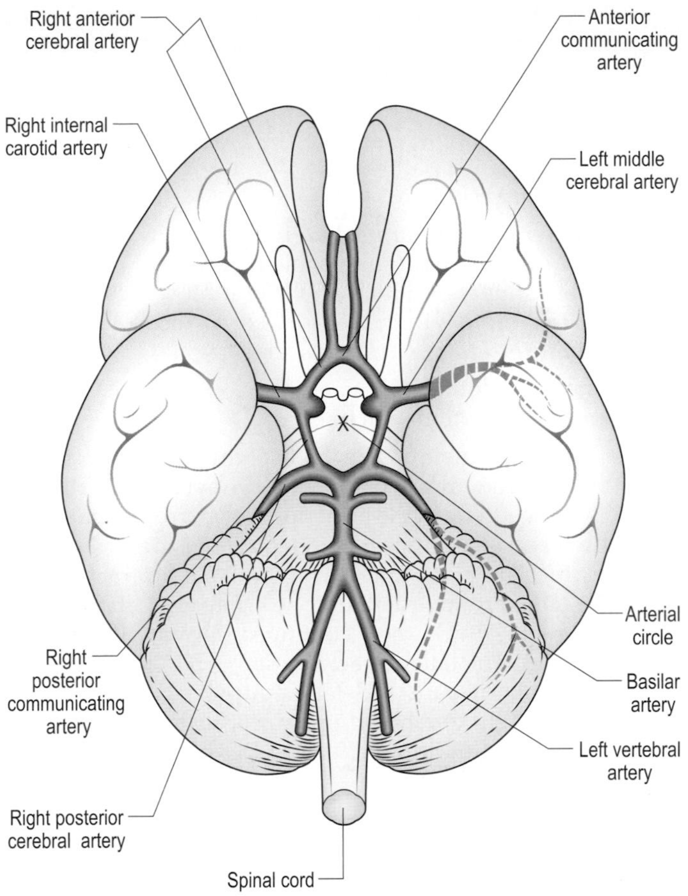

Fig. 9.10 Blood supply to the brain.

which make their permeability relatively low. This means that, as a protective mechanism, some substances are prevented or hindered from gaining access to the brain; this is termed the 'blood–brain barrier'.

For further information, seen Tortora & Derrickson (2006).

The spinal cord

The spinal cord is an oval cylinder that lies within the spinal cavity of the vertebral column. In adults, it is approximately 45 cm in length and extends from the medulla above to the first or second lumbar vertebrae at its lower end. Beyond this, the spinal nerves from the lumbar and sacral segments of the cord form the cauda equina, or 'horse's tail'. The cord is surrounded by the three meninges and CSF circulates in the subarachnoid space. The lower part of the cord is attached to the coccyx by the filum terminale and is tapered in shape (see Fig. 9.12).

The cord is segmented into five parts or regions, each corresponding to a specific number of vertebrae (in brackets):

- cervical (7)
- thoracic (12)
- lumbar (5)
- sacral (5)
- coccyx (1).

A shorthand labelling system has evolved to identify different levels within the spinal cord and vertebrae. For example, the third cervical vertebra becomes C3 and the fourth lumbar vertebra becomes L4 and so on.

Two enlargements of the spinal cord can be noted. The first is in the cervical region, extending between C4 and T1 and containing the nerve supply for the upper limbs. The second enlargement is lower in the lumbar region and is called the 'lumbosacral enlargement'. It extends from L2 to S3 and supplies innervation to the lower limbs. The spinal nerves, which are considered to be part of the peripheral nervous system, are attached by two short roots to the cord. There is a pair of spinal nerves equivalent to each of the vertebrae outlined above and these are labelled and numbered in a similar way. More detail on the spinal nerves can be found in the section on the peripheral nervous system (see p. 406).

The structure of the spinal cord is illustrated in cross-section in Figure 9.13.

The spinal pathways are described as:

- sensory — these ascend from the periphery of the body, e.g. cutaneous receptors in the hand, and are conveyed to the sensory cortex for interpretation

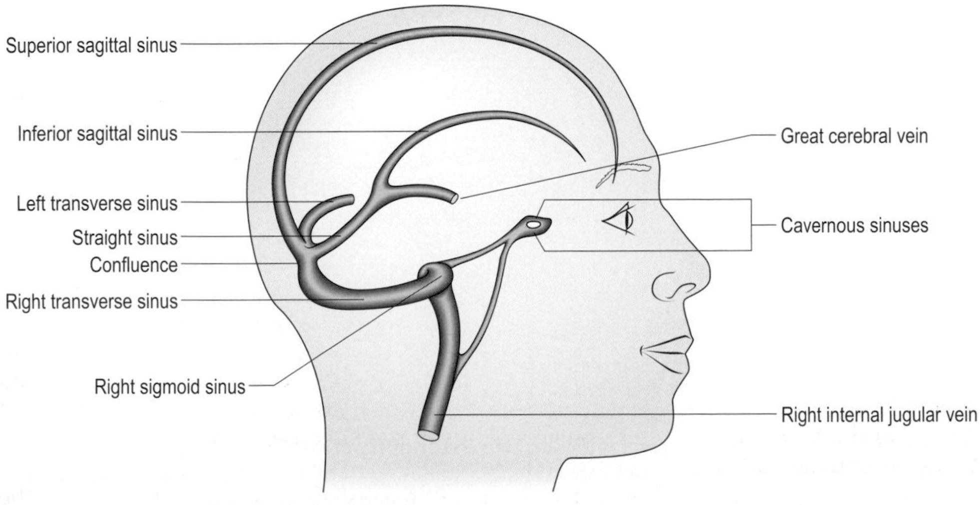

Fig. 9.11 Venous drainage of the brain.

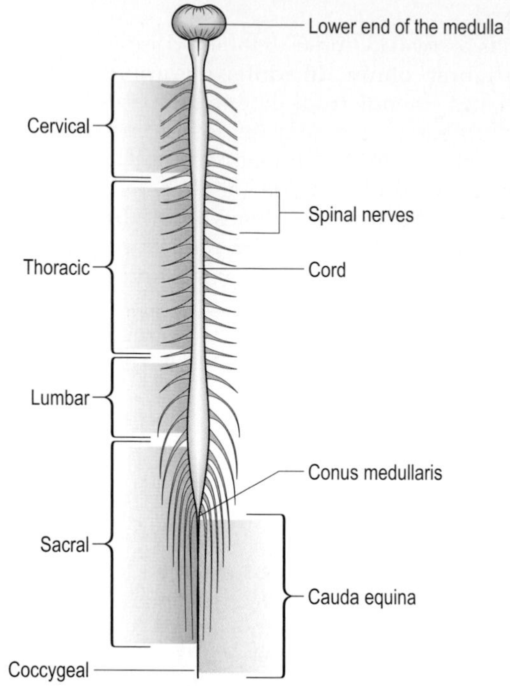

Fig. 9.12 Spinal cord.

- motor — these descend from the brain down to the periphery of the body, e.g. to skeletal muscles, where they initiate a motor response.

Each pathway has a name, derived from the white column in which it travels, the origin of the cell bodies and the termination of the axon. For example, the medial spinothalamic tract is located in the anterior white column, originates in the spinal cord and terminates in the thalamus.

The sensory pathways consist of:

- the posterior column pathway
- the spinothalamic pathway
- the cerebellar pathway.

The posterior column pathway Each pathway consists of a chain of three neurones, which transmit information such as discriminative touch and vibration sense from the appropriate receptors to the sensory cortex (see Fig. 9.14).

The spinothalamic pathways are:

- the lateral spinothalamic tract
- the medial spinothalamic tract.

The first order neurone in both pathways connects the receptor with the spinal cord where it synapses with the second order neurone in the posterior grey horn. The pathway crosses over to the opposite side of the cord and ascends in either the lateral or anterior spinothalamic tract to the thalamus. The second order neurone synapses with the third order neurone, which then continues, terminating in the sensory cortex. The lateral tract is responsible for conveying information about pain and temperature, and the medial tract conveys light touch and pressure (further information on pain can be found in Ch. 19).

The cerebellar tracts are:

- the posterior spinocerebellar tract
- the anterior spinocerebellar tract.

Both tracts are concerned with conveying impulses about subconscious muscle sense. Proprioceptors in the muscles and joints convey information via the spinal pathways, terminating in the cerebellum instead of the cerebral cortex.

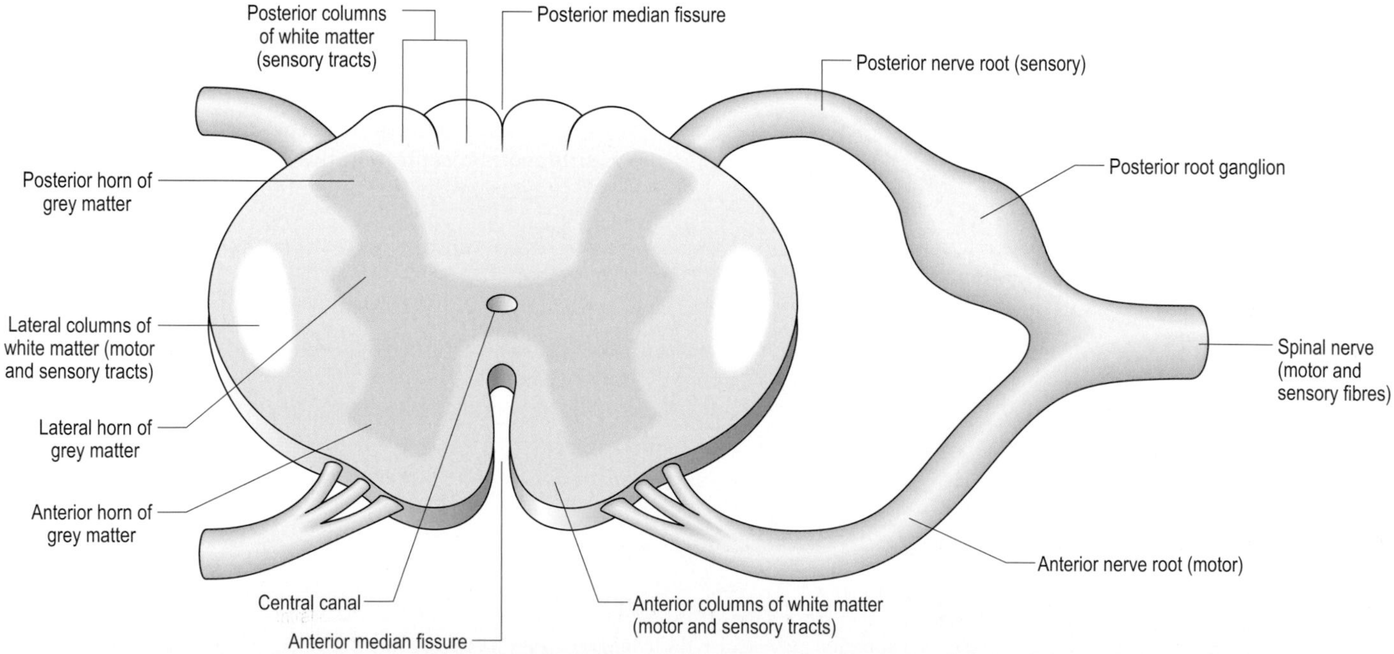

Fig. 9.13 Cross-section of spinal cord. It can be seen that the cord is incompletely divided into right and left halves by the posterior and anterior median fissures. In the centre is the central canal which contains cerebrospinal fluid originating from the fourth ventricle. Extending the entire length of the cord, this is located within an H-shaped area of grey matter with posterior and anterior and, at some levels, lateral horns. The remainder of the cord is made up of white matter organised in columns in the posterior, lateral and anterior segments.

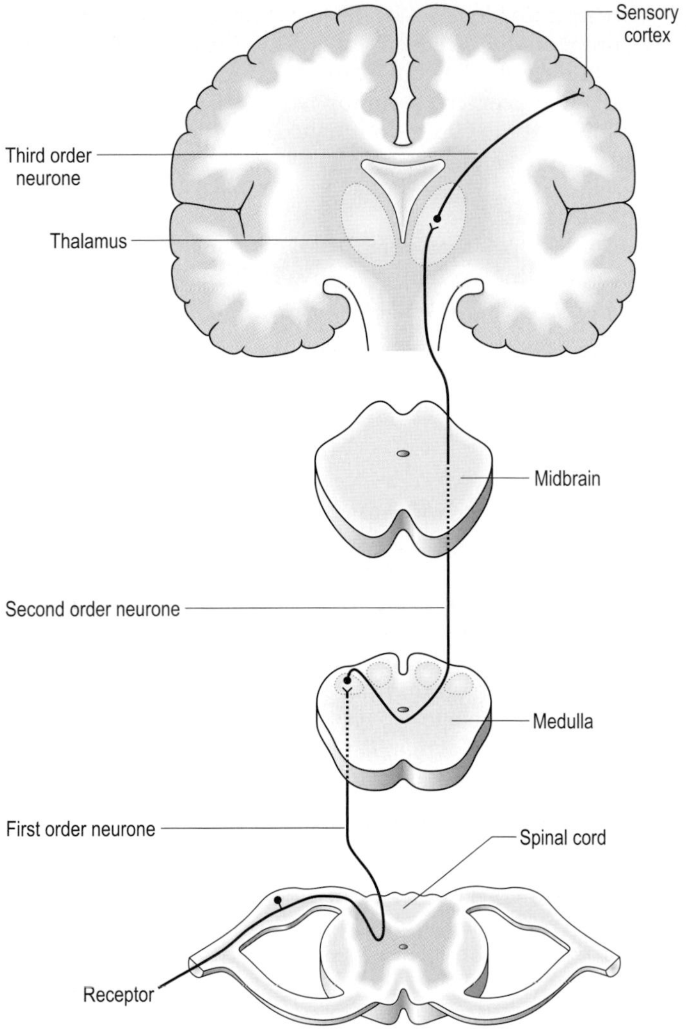

Fig. 9.14 The posterior column pathway. The first order neurone connects the receptor with the spinal cord and medulla on the same side of the body. In the medulla, the first order neurone synapses with the second order neurone, which decussates and then passes upwards to the thalamus where it synapses with a third order neurone which completes the sensory pathway, terminating in the sensory cortex.

This time there are only two neurones involved, synapsing in the posterior grey horn (see Fig. 9.15).

The sensory pathways are responsible for conveying a mass of information into the central nervous system. This information forms part of a large pool and decisions are made regarding the response to a given situation. The response is manifested by the motor system via its own set of pathways; this is described as 'integration' (Hickey 2002).

Motor pathways Once the motor process is initiated within the motor area of the cortex, the impulses descend via two main motor pathways, classified as the:

- pyramidal tracts — this indicates that the pathway passes through the internal capsule and forms the main pathway for impulses to the voluntary muscle
- extrapyramidal tracts — these are complex tracts which provide separate pathways between the cerebral hemispheres, the basal nuclei, the brain stem and the spinal cord. These tracts include all descending motor tracts, other than those corticospinal tracts which pass through the medulla (the pyramidal tracts). Extrapyramidal tracts collectively assist in maintaining muscle tone and gross automatic skeletal muscle movements.

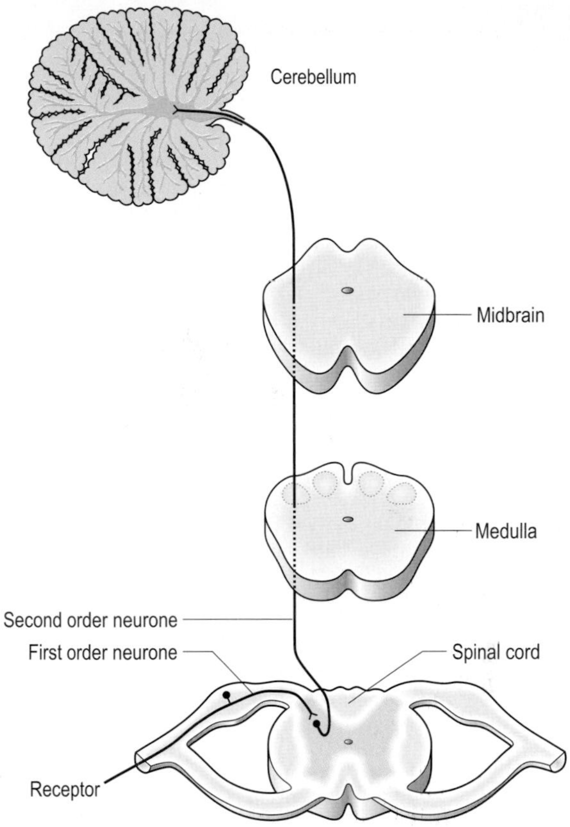

Fig. 9.15 The spinocerebellar tracts.

It is important to clarify the terms upper and lower motor neurones. These are the functional units of the motor system and they convey motor impulses. Damage to one or the other will result in very different functional impairment. An example of lower motor neurone disease is poliomyelitis.

The upper motor neurones extend from the motor cortex of the brain and pass down the pathways to end at the cranial nerve nuclei in the brain stem and the anterior horn of the spinal cord. This means that the upper motor neurone is contained entirely within the central nervous system (Tortora & Derrickson 2006). These are described in Box 9.2.

STOP THINK **9.2** Can you find some examples of upper motor neurone disease?

The lower motor neurones start at the anterior horn of the spinal cord and pass via the anterior nerve roots of the spinal nerves and the motor end-plate of muscles. Some start in the brain stem and are contained in the cranial nerves.

Box 9.2

The motor pathways

Pyramidal tracts

The pyramidal pathway comprises three main tracts:

- lateral corticospinal
- anterior corticospinal
- corticobulbar.

The lateral corticospinal tract

This is the actual pyramidal tract. It originates in the motor cortex and descends to the medulla where 85% of the fibres decussate. They continue downwards in the lateral white column of the corticospinal tract. Most synapse in the anterior grey horn with the lower motor neurone, which then exits the spinal cord via the spinal nerves to terminate on the appropriate skeletal muscle.

The anterior corticospinal pathway

These fibres follow a similar pathway to the lateral, except that they travel in the anterior white column and most of the fibres do not decussate.

The corticobulbar tracts

These are important in that they terminate in the nuclei of the cranial nerves in the medulla. They follow the same pathway as the corticospinal pathway.

Extrapyramidal tracts

These consist of all the descending motor pathways that do not pass through the pyramids. They are concerned with functions of tone and posture such as control of head movement and maintaining balance.

There are three of these pathways:

- *The rubrospinal tract*, which originates in the midbrain, decussates and descends in the lateral white column. It is concerned with tone and posture.
- *The tectospinal tract* also originates in the midbrain, decussates and descends in the anterior white column and enters the anterior grey horns of the cervical cord.
- *The vestibulospinal tract* originates in the vestibular nucleus of the medulla and descends on the same side in the anterior white column and terminates in the anterior grey horn at the cervical and lumbosacral levels of the cord. It is concerned with regulating muscle tone in response to movements of the head and therefore has an important part to play in maintaining equilibrium.

Peripheral nervous system

The peripheral nervous system has two functional parts:

- the motor division — this is further divided into:
  - — the somatic nervous system, which conducts impulses from the CNS to skeletal muscles
  - — the autonomic nervous system, which conducts impulses from the CNS to smooth muscle, cardiac muscle and glands
- the sensory division.

The cranial nerves

The cranial nerves pass from their origin, principally from the brain stem, out via small openings in the skull to innervate the appropriate structures. Each pair of nerves is named according to its distribution or function and is also numbered I–XII (see Table 9.1). Cranial nerves were formerly described as either motor or sensory, or a mixture of both; however, most motor nerves are now considered to be mixed, but with a dominance of motor fibres (Tortora & Derrickson 2006).

Spinal nerves

There are 31 pairs of spinal nerves, named and grouped according to the vertebrae with which they are associated (number of nerves in brackets):

- cervical (8)
- thoracic (12)
- lumbar (5)
- sacral (5)
- coccygeal (1).

It should be noted that there is one more cervical spinal nerve than there are vertebrae. This is because the first pair leave the vertebral canal between the occipital bone and the atlas, and the eighth pair leave below the last cervical vertebra. Thereafter, the spinal nerves are named and numbered according to the vertebra immediately above.

As can be seen from Figure 9.13, each spinal nerve has an anterior and a posterior root. The anterior root consists of motor nerve fibres, whereas the posterior roots are sensory. The posterior root can be distinguished by its root ganglion, a cluster of nerve cell bodies.

Shortly after leaving the intervertebral foramina, both roots join together to form a mixed nerve. From here the spinal nerves continue to form a complex network all over the body, carrying motor signals to effectors such as the skeletal muscles and conveying sensory information such as touch to the CNS for interpretation.

Further details of this complex network can be found in Tortora & Derrickson (2006).

The autonomic nervous system

The autonomic nervous system is outwith voluntary control and is the most complex and perhaps least understood part of the nervous system. Its involvement in, and effect upon, everyday activities is vague until its delicate mechanisms are upset. The effects are then readily felt by the individual.

The autonomic nervous system consists only of the nerves carrying motor impulses to the internal organs; thus it is exclusively peripheral and motor. Its activity is influenced by many factors, including sensory information from the internal organs, numerous peptides and hormones, and signals from higher control centres such as the hypothalamus. It is described as having two divisions, the sympathetic and parasympathetic, each imposing different effects (see Figs 9.16 and 9.17).

HEAD INJURY AND RAISED INTRACRANIAL PRESSURE

In 2000/2001, statistics demonstrated that almost 113 000 people were admitted to hospital in England as a result of head injury; 72% of these were males and 30% were under the age of 15 (DH 2000/2001). Of all people with a head injury, 90% will present with a mild injury, whilst the

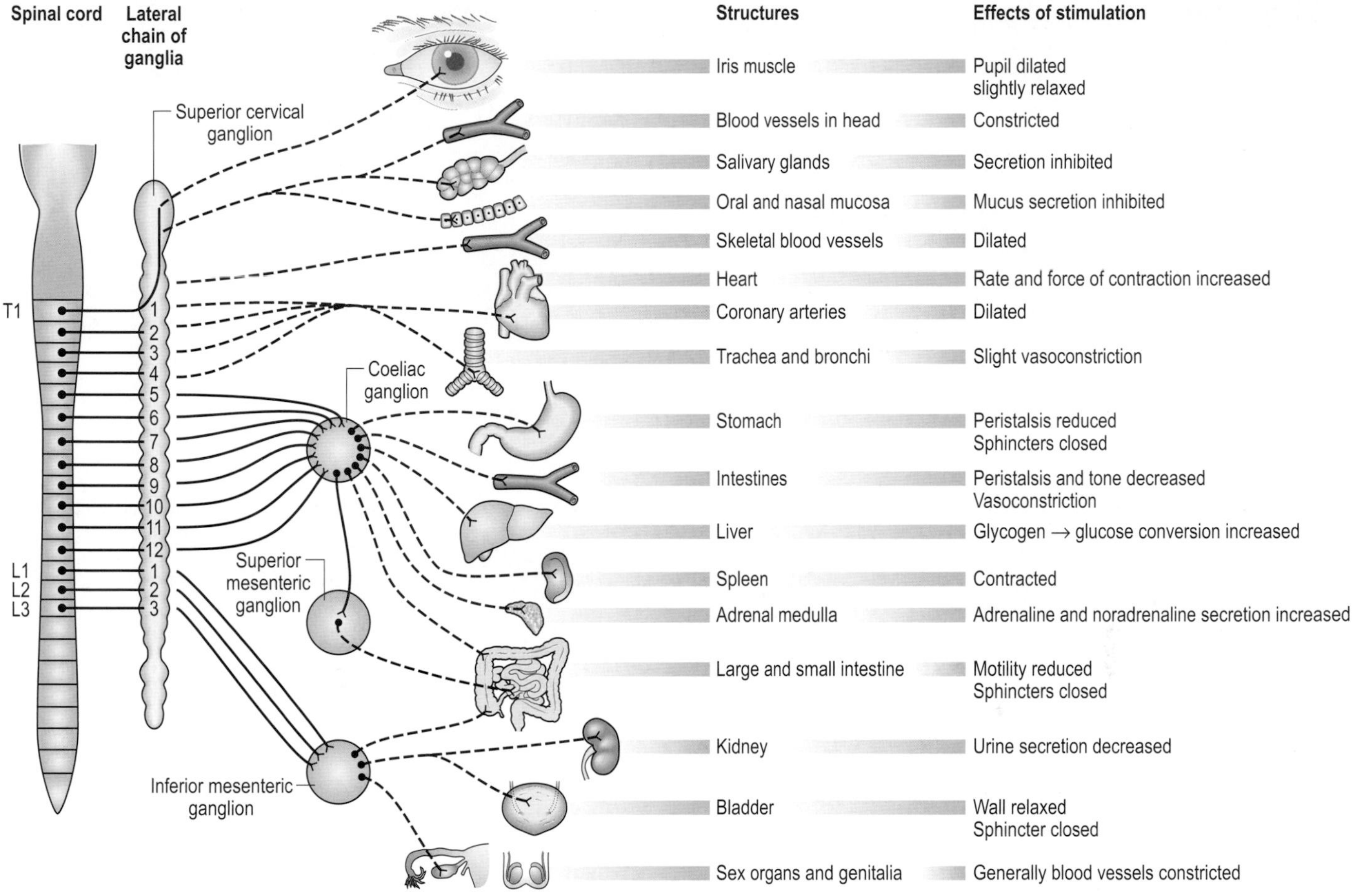

Fig. 9.16 The sympathetic outflow, the main structures supplied and the effects of stimulation. Solid lines, preganglionic fibres; broken lines, postganglionic fibres.

remaining 10% are classified as moderate or severe, but it is these 10% who are more likely to develop subsequent complications (Swann & Teasdale 1999).

Falls (24–43%) and assaults (30–50%) are the most common causes of mild head injury in the UK, followed by road accidents (25%), although these account for a far greater proportion of moderate to severe head injuries. Alcohol may be implicated in up to 65% of all adult head injuries (NICE 2003a).

Head injury is preventable. This is an area in which nurses should exercise their health education skills, e.g. by emphasising the dangers associated with head injury and its detrimental effects when communicating with patients who have experience of minor head injury with good recovery, and with their families. This may include consideration of driver behaviour or unsafe work practices. The use of seatbelts for the driver and all car passengers has led to a reduction in head injuries, as has the use of protective headgear for motorcyclists and horse riders (Headway 2004). Because a common contributing factor in head injury is overindulgence in alcohol, where appropriate, the patient can be encouraged to consider personal lifestyle and the consumption of alcohol.

PATHOPHYSIOLOGY

The adult skull can be considered as a rigid box divided into two major compartments, containing non-compressible components. A uniform pressure, called 'intracranial' pressure (ICP), is maintained. It is defined as the pressure exerted within the cerebral ventricular system. When an individual sustains a head injury or there is some abnormal pathology, e.g. a tumour, it can alter this delicate balance. When an increase in ICP occurs, the pressure in one compartment is higher than that in its counterpart, and abnormal movement of tissue from an area of high pressure to one of low pressure occurs, a process known as 'herniation' or 'coning'.

Three intracranial components are involved in the process of maintaining ICP:

- the brain
- the cerebrospinal fluid (CSF)
- blood.

The brain is the largest of these, occupying 80% of the content. The remaining 20% is taken up in equal proportion by the CSF and the blood. Under normal circumstances, ICP is maintained within normal limits, but when there is an alteration to the volume of one of these components within the confined space of the skull, the other two are compressed, resulting in a rise in ICP. The normal range of ICP is 0–15 mmHg and anything over 15 mmHg is considered abnormal. Transient rises in pressure occur with activities such as coughing or sneezing and this is a normal physiological response.

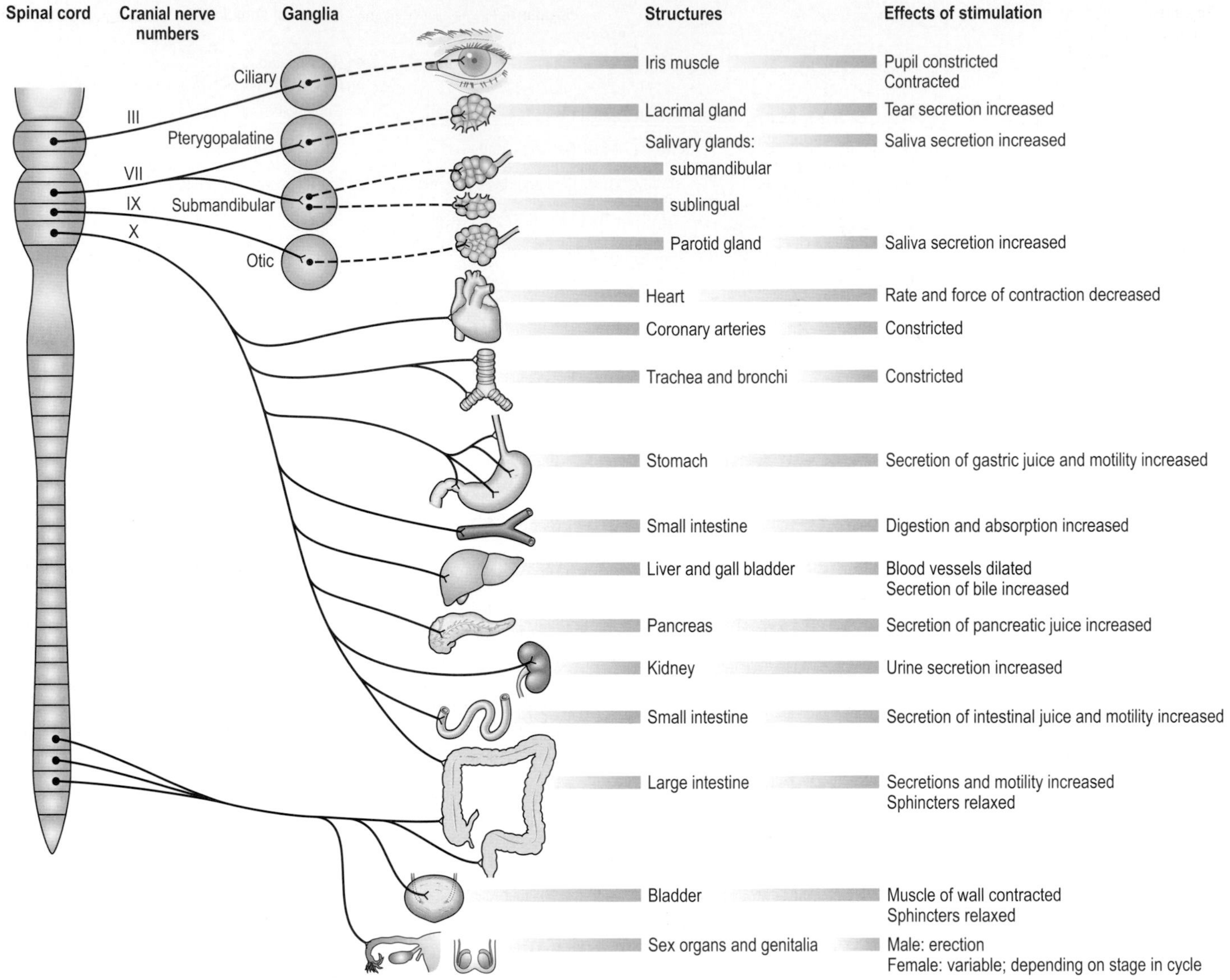

Fig. 9.17 The parasympathetic outflow, the main structures supplied and the effects of stimulation. Solid lines, preganglionic fibres; broken lines, postganglionic fibres. Where there are no broken lines, the second neurone is in the wall of the structure.

Changes to the brain and its associated structures following trauma may cause ICP to rise to a dangerous level, resulting in coma and leading to permanent brain damage.

The causes and presenting symptoms of raised ICP

Causes of raised ICP can be classified according to the intracranial components involved.

- *Brain* — brain tissue volume can be increased due to the presence of an expanding intracranial lesion, such as a brain tumour or a haematoma following head injury.
- *CSF* — increased production, decreased absorption or blockage of a CSF pathway will result in an abnormal accumulation of CSF within the cerebral ventricular system. This is a condition known as hydrocephalus.
- *Blood* — cerebral blood flow can be increased principally as a result of an abnormally high level of carbon dioxide in the blood (hypercapnia) and to a lesser extent due to a lack of oxygen in the tissues (hypoxia). These lead to congestion within the cerebral circulation, culminating in a raised ICP. Such a situation can be precipitated by neglect of the patient's airway during the postoperative period following neurosurgery or following head injury.

A rise in ICP can develop over a variable period of time. It can occur over a number of years in a slow-growing brain tumour, with the patient hardly noticing any symptoms, or it can occur in a matter of minutes following severe head injury, when the patient becomes profoundly unconscious. The underlying principle remains the same and is centred on the volume–pressure relationship curve (see Fig. 9.18).

A distinct correlation exists between ICP and conscious level. As ICP rises, conscious level deteriorates.

During the initial rise in ICP, compensatory mechanisms come into play, principally the ability of the cerebral ventricular system to reduce the volume of CSF by displacing it into a distensible spinal dural sac. A reduction in cerebral blood volume also occurs as a result of autoregulation, the ability of blood vessels to alter their diameter according

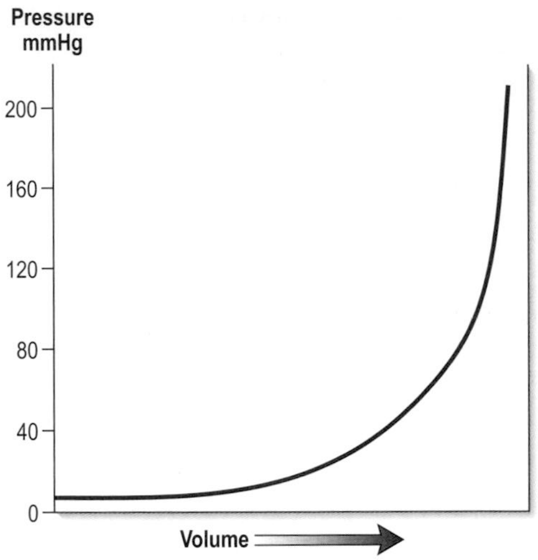

Fig. 9.18 Volume–pressure curve.

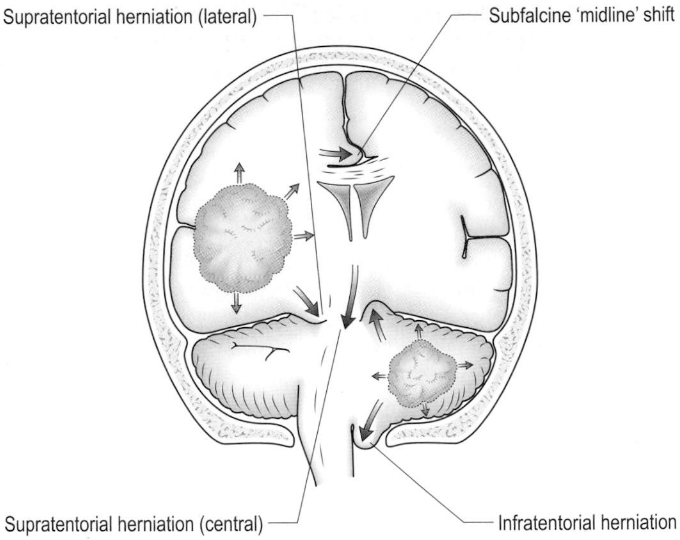

Fig. 9.19 Types of herniation.

to local conditions. This is represented by the flattened part of the curve. However, this is only a temporary measure and, as the volume of the expanding lesion increases, compensation is overcome and the steep part of the curve is entered. The addition of the same volume to that which was added previously and produced very little change in ICP now results in dramatic increases. This process has four identifiable stages, as described in Box 9.3.

Other factors which have an influence on this complex process include cerebral blood flow and cerebral oedema.

For further information on influencing factors, see Hickey (2002).

Herniation

Herniation is the process by which tissue in a high-pressure compartment is compressed and forced through an available opening into an adjoining low-pressure compartment.

Box 9.3

Stages of the volume–pressure relationship in raised intracranial pressure

Stage 1	The compensation phase: there is no rise in ICP, and conscious level remains unaltered.
Stage 2	The early phase of reversible decompensation: a slight increase in brain mass will produce an elevated ICP. Early signs of deterioration in conscious level are noted.
Stage 3	The late phase of reversible decompensation: ICP is now very high and conscious level is deteriorating rapidly. Detrimental changes occur in the respiratory rate and pattern. ICP will soon equal mean arterial pressure with, ultimately, cessation of cerebral blood flow.
Stage 4	The irreversible decompensation phase: further deterioration leading to death will occur if intervention is not initiated.

Such a situation can exist in the patient with raised ICP. The skull has two compartments:

- the supratentorial, the region above the tentorium
- the infratentorial, the region below the tentorium.

The opening that permits supratentorial herniation is the tentorial notch, and that which permits infratentorial herniation is the foramen magnum.

Supratentorial herniation is either central tentorial herniation or lateral transtentorial herniation.

Central tentorial herniation is when symmetrical herniation is produced by a midline expanding lesion or generalised swelling of brain tissue. It involves the downward displacement of the cerebral hemispheres, diencephalon and midbrain. The nerves and posterior cerebral arteries are stretched and compression of the oculomotor nerve (IIIrd cranial nerve) occurs, resulting in a non-reactive pupil that may also be dilated. These and other structures are displaced into the posterior fossa.

Lateral transtentorial herniation occurs in the presence of an expanding lesion located close to the temporal lobe. The medial part of the temporal lobe (the uncus) is forced downwards. This type of herniation can inflict pressure on the reticular activating system, resulting in a decrease in conscious level (see Ch. 28). Lateral transtentorial herniation can subsequently develop into a central herniation (see Fig. 9.19).

Infratentorial herniation is the downward displacement of the lower part of the cerebellum (the cerebellar tonsils) through the foramen magnum, where compression of the medulla results. The offending lesion is located in the posterior fossa. This type of herniation is less common.

MEDICAL MANAGEMENT

Common presenting symptoms The head-injured patient with raised ICP may be fully alert and orientated or may range from experiencing drowsiness to being deeply unconscious. Neurological deficits can be found, e.g. alteration of conscious level, onset of confusion or occurrence of a seizure. Answers to the questions listed below should be obtained as they have an influence on the management and outcome:

- *How long has the patient been unconscious?* The period of unconsciousness relates to the severity of brain damage, i.e. the longer the patient is unconscious, the more severe the damage.
- *Does post-traumatic amnesia (PTA) exist and for how long?* The patient's memory for events following injury is an indicator of the severity of brain damage, i.e. the longer the period of PTA, the worse the brain damage.
- *What were the cause and circumstances of the injury?* This may indicate if other extracranial injuries exist.
- *Does the patient have any headache or vomiting?* These would indicate the possibility of intracranial haemorrhage.

Table 9.2 lists the signs and symptoms of raised ICP.

Investigations In the head-injured patient, skull X-ray may reveal a fracture and computed tomography (CT) or magnetic resonance imaging (MRI) may demonstrate cerebral contusions or lacerations and/or an intracranial haematoma (Hickey 2002). Box 9.4 gives a description of the types of injury the brain may suffer.

ICP monitoring One of the most important diagnostic measures is the monitoring of ICP. This is an invasive technique involving direct measurement of ICP. A typical system comprises a fibreoptic transducer-tipped catheter, which can be placed in the lateral ventricle, subdural space or extradural space. The level of ICP is then transmitted to a digital data display or as a waveform. A pulsatile waveform will be demonstrated along with a pressure level indicating if the patient's ICP is within normal limits (≤15 mmHg) (see Fig. 9.20).

Treatment In the past, the treatment of head injury focused primarily on the interventions required to reduce ICP. However, greater emphasis is now placed on maintaining cerebral perfusion pressure (CPP) which is the blood pressure gradient across the brain, at more than 70 mmHg. This is because it has been shown that those patients with a high ICP, low blood pressure and low CPP make a poorer recovery. The means by which this is achieved are varied according to circumstances; however, the methods described here must not be used indiscriminately.

STOP THINK **9.3** How is CPP calculated? (see Haslett et al 2002).

Hyperosmolar agents An intravenous infusion of 100 mL of 20% mannitol over 15 min will reduce ICP by establishing an osmotic gradient between the plasma and brain tissue, thus removing water from the oedematous brain tissue to the blood. This will 'buy' time to allow the patient to be prepared for transfer to a specialist unit or for surgery. However, if repeated boluses are administered, its effect is neutralised, leading to a rebound increase in ICP.

Controlled hyperventilation In the past it was recommended that the reduction of P_aCO_2 would reduce ICP. However, it also causes vasoconstriction, thus reducing cerebral blood volume. It is suggested by Lindsay and Bone (2004) that the resultant reduction in cerebral blood flow may itself cause ischaemic brain damage. Maintaining the blood pressure and CPP appear to be as important, if not more important, than lowering ICP.

Fluid management Views on the management of fluids have been contentious for some time. Some advocate restricting fluid in order to induce slight dehydration. By controlling intake, the extracellular fluid, including that of the brain, is decreased, thus reducing ICP. The intake may be set at 1–2.5 L/24 h. However, some now advocate achieving normovolaemia or increasing fluids. Doing this increases cerebral blood flow and thus improves oxygen delivery to the brain.

Sedatives After years of advocating that patients with a head injury should never be sedated, as this would impede assessment of conscious level, there are now special circumstances under which sedation may be used. If ICP fails to respond to standard measures then sedation, under carefully controlled conditions, may help by reducing cerebral

Box 9.4

Description of injury to the brain

Contusions
Described as a bruising of the cerebral tissue. Most commonly affects the frontal, occipital and undersurface of the temporal lobes. There are two types:

- coup — indicates haemorrhage and oedema immediately under the injury site
- contrecoup — damage occurs directly opposite the injury site. This is caused by the rapid acceleration or deceleration movement of the brain within the skull following severe trauma. Contused brain tissue affects the blood supply to that area, resulting in swelling of the brain which will raise ICP.

Lacerations
Brain tissue is lacerated as a result of, for example, a skull fracture, resulting in disruption to cellular activity which will produce focal neurological deficits such as hemiparesis. Contusions and cerebral oedema may also occur.

Haematoma
A localised collection of blood. These are named according to their location:

- extradural — situated or occurring outside the dura mater
- subdural — between the dura mater and the arachnoid
- intracerebral — within the brain substance.

Diffuse brain injury
Here, there is no specific focal pathology. Shearing of the white matter occurs, causing disruption and tearing of the axons.

Table 9.2 Signs and symptoms of raised intracranial pressure (ICP)

<table>
<tr><th>Clinical parameter</th><th>Signs/symptoms</th><th>Reasons</th></tr>
<tr><td>Conscious level</td><td>Deterioration in conscious level</td><td>Raised ICP will reduce the amount of oxygen received by the oxygen-sensitive cells of the cerebral cortex.</td></tr>
<tr><td>Respiration</td><td>Deterioration in respiratory pattern</td><td>A particular respiratory pattern will be seen in relation to the non-functioning area in the medulla and pons.
<table>
<tr><td>Breathing pattern</td><td>Non-functioning area</td></tr>
<tr><td>Cheyne–Stokes</td><td>Affects various areas</td></tr>
<tr><td>Apneustic</td><td>Pons varolii</td></tr>
<tr><td>Ataxic</td><td>Medulla</td></tr>
<tr><td>Central neurogenic</td><td>Lower midbrain</td></tr>
<tr><td>Hyperventilation</td><td>Upper pons</td></tr>
<tr><td>Cluster breathing</td><td>Medulla</td></tr>
</table></td></tr>
<tr><td>Pupils</td><td>(a) Alteration in pupil size
(b) Reaction to light
(c) Blurring of vision/diplopia
(d) Ocular muscle paresis/paralysis</td><td>All the pupillary and eye movement responses to raised ICP are as a result of compression of the IIIrd cranial nerve (oculomotor). The ipsilateral pupil is usually affected first, followed by the other one.</td></tr>
<tr><td>Blood pressure</td><td>(a) An increase in systolic blood pressure followed by
(b) a fall</td><td>The increase in blood pressure occurs as result of ischaemia (due to raised ICP) of the vasomotor centre. Implicated in this is a widening pulse pressure. If this is not corrected, the ICP continues to rise and the blood pressure then begins to fall dramatically until it is unrecordable.</td></tr>
<tr><td>Pulse</td><td>Initially bradycardia (<60 beats/min) develops with a full and bounding pulse. In the later stages the pulse becomes weak and thready</td><td>This is brought about as a result of increased workload on the heart which is attempting to overcome cerebral blood vessel resistance by pushing more blood into the cerebral circulation.</td></tr>
<tr><td>Motor function</td><td>Contralateral hemiparesis/ hemiplegia</td><td>The raised ICP affects pyramidal tract function, and continued deterioration will ensue until the limbs are unresponsive to deep painful stimuli.</td></tr>
<tr><td></td><td>Headache usually in the early morning</td><td>Headache due to raised ICP is thought to be the result of displacement of the cerebrospinal fluid cushion producing dilatation of cerebral blood vessels, stretching of arteries at the base of the brain and traction of bridging veins. ICP will be adversely affected following REM sleep and by the retention of carbon dioxide during sleep, resulting in exacerbation of ICP in early morning.</td></tr>
<tr><td>'Cushing's triad'</td><td>Headache, becoming more severe or persistent</td><td>This indicates that the ICP is rising and the intracranial contents are being compressed; 'herniation' may occur.</td></tr>
<tr><td></td><td>Vomiting: may occur with early morning headache</td><td>The mechanism involved is not well understood.</td></tr>
<tr><td></td><td>Projectile vomiting and problems with swallowing</td><td>These indicate that there is increasing pressure on the brain stem, where the control centres for these functions are located.</td></tr>
<tr><td></td><td>Papilloedema</td><td>Occurs as a result of raised ICP being transmitted down the optic nerve to produce a swollen nerve head. This may be seen on direct fundoscopy. An unreliable sign, which is not constantly seen in all patients with raised ICP.</td></tr>
<tr><td></td><td>Problems with speech or comprehension</td><td>These may indicate that ICP is rising and that there is pressure on the cerebral cortex.</td></tr>
</table>

No order is implied within the above set of signs and symptoms. Any combination in varying degrees can occur in each patient. Individually, each of the signs and symptoms can be caused by other pathology, including extracranially.

metabolism and thus offering a degree of protection for the brain (Lindsay & Bone 2004). Drugs that may be used include propofol and etomidate. However, each has associated side-effects that require to be countered. Propofol causes vasodilatation that may require to be counteracted to prevent blood pressure from falling and causing a reduction in cerebral perfusion. Etomidate inhibits steroid synthesis, and thus steroid cover will be required.

Surgical intervention Surgery may be performed to remove a focal lesion such as an expanding haematoma and this may be combined with decompression. Withdrawal of small amounts of CSF via a ventricular catheter results in a reduction of ICP, but this provides only temporary relief. To be effective, drainage would require to be continuous, but this is often impractical. Examples of neurosurgical approaches are given in Box 9.5.

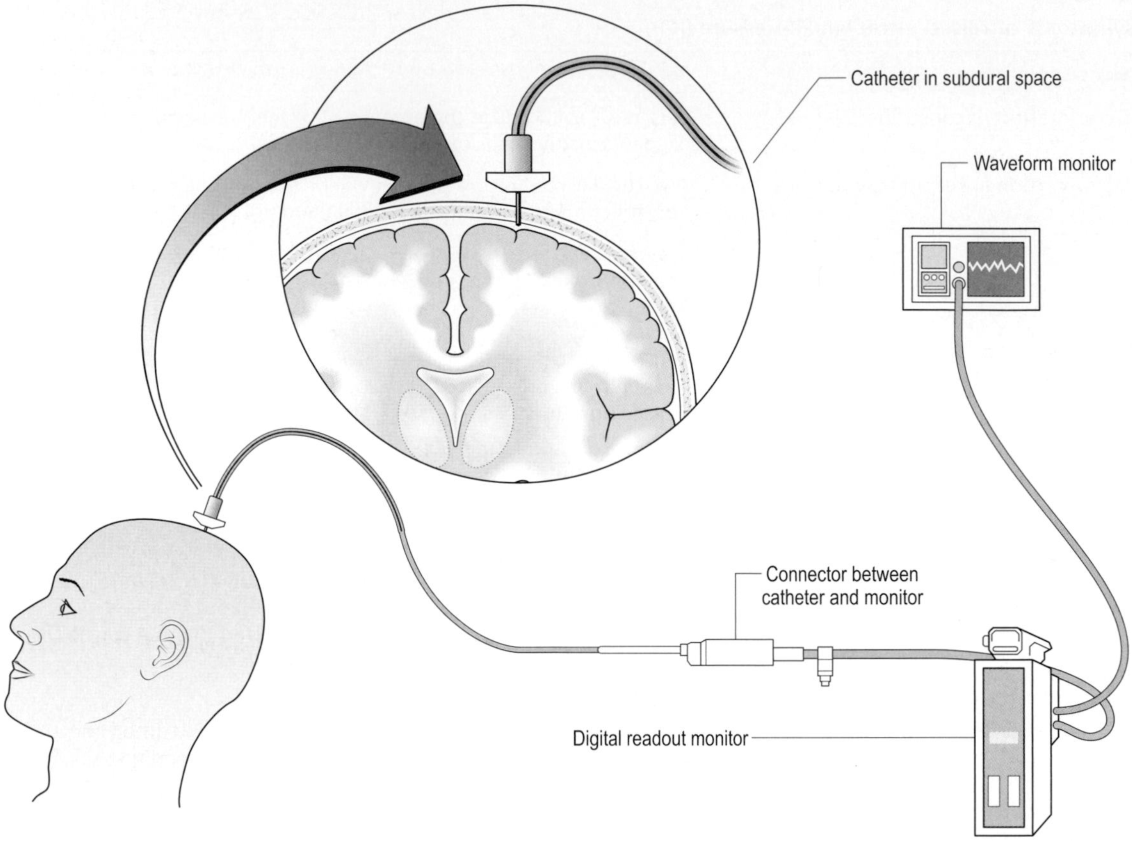

Fig. 9.20 The fibreoptic transducer-tipped catheter system for monitoring intracranial pressure (Camino system). (Adapted from Hickey 2002.)

Box 9.5

Neurosurgical approaches

Burr hole
A burr hole is a hole drilled through the cranium to allow access to the brain, usually to obtain a biopsy of tumour tissue.

Craniotomy
Access is gained to the brain via the formation of a bone flap, which is fashioned by several burr holes in a circular formation. The bone between the burr holes is cut with a wire saw and usually replaced at the close of surgery.

Craniectomy
This is a hole made in the skull by chipping away the bone, which means that it cannot be replaced. Usually used in the posterior fossa approach where the bone is particularly thick.

Trans-sphenoidal approach
This approach gains access to the pituitary gland and the incision is upper submucosa. This allows easier access to the pituitary gland (Hickey 2002).

An additional surgical technique is the transoral route. To gain access to the base of the brain and upper cervical spinal cord, an approach via the patient's mouth has been successfully used. This particular approach is not usually indicated for tumour removal.

NURSING PRIORITIES AND MANAGEMENT: Head injury

Head-injured patients with raised ICP can present in different ways on admission to hospital. The person may initially appear not to have sustained an injury, but can progress to become drowsy or confused, or develop speech problems or limb deficits. Seizure activity may occur.

Immediate priorities

The immediate nursing aim is to prevent further damaging rises in ICP and the first priority is to identify any alteration in respiratory function due to an obstructed airway or an absent cough or gag reflex. The appropriate interventions are described in Box 9.6.

The nurse should be aware of the presence of other injuries, e.g. multiple injuries, if the patient has been in a road traffic accident. Elaboration of the assessment and appropriate interventions for this can be found in Chapters 18 and 27.

Assessment of neurological status

This is performed in order to:

- make an initial assessment of the patient, which may influence any immediate action that needs to be taken
- have a baseline with which to compare the patient's condition and detect any changes in their condition.

> **Box 9.6**
>
> **Respiratory care priorities in a patient with raised intracranial pressure**
>
> 1. Assess the rate, depth and pattern of respirations to indicate the patency of the airway. Report if the rate is less than 14 and more than 24, and any irregularities in rate or rhythm, as these would indicate a rise in ICP.
> 2. Assess the skin for cyanosis, which would indicate inadequate respiration.
> 3. Apply oropharyngeal and tracheal suctioning only as required to remove secretions. Suction for no more than 15 s and consider pre-oxygenation prior to suctioning with 100% oxygen to prevent a build-up of carbon dioxide in the blood, resulting in further elevation of ICP.
> 4. Institute measures to achieve optimal respiratory status including insertion of a Guedel airway, positioning the patient on their side with a 30° head-up tilt, and administer oxygen as prescribed.
> 5. Assist with monitoring arterial blood gases and mechanical ventilation as required.

Any deterioration in neurological status may be an early indication that ICP is rising further, thus increasing the likelihood of herniation. Neurological assessment is important, as this may be the only indication that the patient's condition is deteriorating and a standardised method of monitoring neurological status will enhance this process. One commonly used method is the Glasgow Coma Scale (Fischer & Mathieson 2001). This is described in detail in Chapter 28.

The frequency of observations is determined by the patient's condition, ranging from intervals of 15 min to 4 h. Medical staff should be promptly informed of any pertinent changes in the patient's neurological status.

The nurse, as the health care professional who normally spends most time with the patient, should learn to observe changes in the patient's behaviour which may herald an impending change in neurological status. These may include the patient who does not answer questions so readily or who is becoming agitated and restless.

The expert neurosurgical nurse will be alert to the early warning signs which must be reported so that either surgical or conservative treatment can be carried out as soon as possible (see p. 409). Quite subtle changes in the patient's condition may be the only initial indication that ICP is rising.

STOP THINK **9.4** Consider the experience of caring for a patient with raised ICP. What range of signs and symptoms might occur?

Cardiovascular assessment

The final life-threatening concern in a patient with a rising ICP is the effect of alterations to systemic and cerebral circulation, due to shock and cardiovascular instability. Unless requested by medical staff to do otherwise, the nurse should always report if:

- systolic pressure is less than 90 or more than 170 mmHg
- diastolic pressure is less than 50 or more than 100 mmHg
- the pulse rate is less than 50 or more than 100 beats/min.

Readings which are outwith these parameters will render the patient more susceptible to brain damage as a result of raised ICP and lowered cerebral perfusion pressure. The recognition of the vulnerable patient has been greatly facilitated by the use of the early warning system chart.

Surgery

Preoperative care Urgent surgery may be indicated on admission or in response to subsequent deterioration. The nurse may need to prepare the patient in a very short time and also provide adequate explanation and reassurance (see Ch. 26).

The approaches used in surgery are outlined in Box 9.5.

Postoperative care The overall priorities for patients following neurosurgery are:

- continuous assessment of neurological status (see Ch. 28, p. 970)
- instituting measures to avoid secondary brain damage
- administration of appropriate therapies.

The main complications of neurosurgery are outlined in Table 9.3.

As the patient progresses, their needs will require to be reassessed and the nursing interventions adjusted accordingly. Each patient will progress at a different rate, so continuing assessment and meeting the identified needs on an individual basis are important. The aim of care is to ensure optimum function and the early detection of complications.

Subsequent considerations

All of the nursing interventions identified in Chapter 26 will apply. Only those interventions specific to the patient who is unconscious due to raised ICP are included here. The main aim of care remains that of preventing further rises in ICP.

STOP THINK **9.5** Using the information on care of the head-injured patient, select an approach to care that you are not familiar with and reflect on the care required for the first postoperative day following craniotomy (see also Ch. 28).

The patient care outlined in the following sections uses the Roper et al (2000) framework of the activities of living model.

Communicating

Unpleasant stimuli are known to cause a rise in ICP, so the nurse should take a calm, reassuring approach. Relatives should be encouraged to talk to the patient and, although they may feel rather foolish at first, they will be encouraged if they see the nurse doing this. They should, however, be warned to avoid discussing potentially upsetting topics. Everyone should be made aware that the unconscious patient may still be able to hear (Hickey 2002) and that they should therefore be sensitive to what they discuss in the patient's presence.

Non-verbal communication, particularly touch, has been shown to decrease ICP, so relatives should be encouraged to touch the patient, e.g. by holding hands or gently stroking

Table 9.3 Complications of neurosurgery

Complications	Cause	Interventions
Altered conscious level	Increased ICP due to cerebral haemorrhage/oedema	Frequent assessment of neurological status
Onset of seizures	Cerebral irritation	Observation of seizures. Appropriate interventions if they occur (see p. 427)
Limb weakness	Increased ICP due to cerebral haemorrhage/oedema	Frequent assessment of limb movements
Speech problems	Increased ICP due to cerebral haemorrhage/oedema	Frequent assessment of verbal responses
Respiratory problems	Increased ICP due to cerebral haemorrhage/oedema	Frequent assessment of respiratory status
Loss of swallowing reflex	Increased ICP due to cerebral haemorrhage/oedema	Frequent assessment of swallowing reflex
Loss of corneal reflex	Increased ICP due to cerebral haemorrhage/oedema	Frequent assessment of corneal reflex
Periorbital oedema	Direct result of surgery	Observe for swollen/bruised periorbital tissues

the patient's arm, despite the extensive equipment which may surround them.

Any investigations that are to be performed should be explained to the patient and their family, who will be anxious and distressed at this time, particularly as outcomes may be uncertain.

Breathing

Respiratory assessment and appropriate intervention, as outlined in the previous section, will continue as long as the ICP remains elevated. The patient's position should be changed every 2 h or as the need arises, and chest physiotherapy should be instituted as this helps prevent pooling of secretions in the lungs and atelectasis. The patient, if able, should be encouraged to undertake deep-breathing exercises. There is evidence to demonstrate the benefits of adopting the prone position to improve respiratory status; however, this is not recommended in this instance as it may lead to a further rise in ICP (Sullivan 2000) (see Ch. 29, p. 995).

Maintaining a safe environment

The patient's bed should be positioned where they can be easily observed. If the patient is restless or agitated, the nurse should attempt to find out why. Adequate non-narcotic analgesics, such as codeine phosphate and dihydrocodeine, can relieve a headache and are the analgesics of choice, as they do not mask conscious level and will minimise the risk of raising ICP. If the patient is confused, they may attempt to climb out of bed, despite explanations as to why they should not do so. They may not appreciate their limb deficit and may attempt to walk, thus endangering themselves. If appropriate, relatives can help persuade the patient to stay in bed and, as a last resort, sedation may be necessary. The use of side rails should be considered, but the correct precautions must be taken. If the patient proves very difficult to manage, it may be necessary to replace the bed with a mattress on the floor or to care for the patient sitting in a chair, possibly with a table secured in front. Such situations should be fully explained to relatives beforehand.

The nurse should always be aware of the possibility of a seizure and appropriate interventions carried out should this occur (see p. 427).

Controlling body temperature

Each 1°C rise in body temperature increases the metabolic demand of the brain by 10% (Hickey 2002). This increases blood pressure and encourages vasodilatation, which will increase ICP. Body temperature should be recorded at least 4-hourly, as pyrexia may indicate hypothalamic damage or the presence of infection. Any source of potential infection, such as leakage of CSF from the patient's ears (otorrhoea) or nose (rhinorrhoea) from a base-of-skull or anterior-fossa fracture must be identified and reported. Confirmation of this is obtained by testing the fluid for the presence of glucose, using a reagent strip. A positive result, although not absolutely conclusive, is indicative of the presence of CSF. The identification of a fracture on the skull X-ray will confirm the evidence. CSF leakage left undetected increases the risk of developing meningitis.

Necessary measures to reduce the patient's temperature include tepid sponging, cool fanning or medication, such as paracetamol suppositories.

Mobility

The patient will require frequent positional changes to avoid developing pressure ulcers. Semi-prone and lateral positions are both suitable. Moving the patient also encourages expansion of the lungs and prevents pooling of secretions. A slight head-up tilt of 30° will not only reduce ICP but also aid lung expansion and prevent chest infection. The patient's body should be maintained in neutral alignment, avoiding neck flexion and rotation. The hips should be carefully positioned, avoiding flexion over 90°. These positions aid venous drainage as they minimise intra-abdominal and intrathoracic pressure, which will help to decrease ICP.

Passive movement exercises, which are joint movements undertaken without effort on the part of the patient, should be performed to prevent muscle wasting and limb contractures as these will hinder rehabilitation. However, isometric exercising (see Ch. 10) should be avoided as this raises ICP. Thromboembolism deterrent (TED) stockings should be used to minimise the risk of deep venous thrombosis.

As the patient's condition improves, further movement should be encouraged. The physiotherapist will provide specialised exercises if there is a limb deficit (Hickey 2002). Sitting out of bed in a chair will help to reduce respiratory complications and encourage limb movements. It may also act as an important psychological boost for the patient and their family as they will view this as progress.

Eating and drinking

As soon as the patient is able, oral food and fluid intake should be encouraged. Intravenous fluids may be required, however, and fluid restrictions should be carefully monitored and recorded to avoid inadvertent increases in ICP due to worsening cerebral oedema. Some patients may require enteral feeding, and the nurse should observe all the usual precautions, as detailed in Chapters 4 and 21. The patient with a basal skull fracture must not have the tube passed nasally as there is a danger of further damage and infection and therefore passing the tube orally is suggested.

Eliminating

Observation of urinary output should be monitored, in line with any restricted intake, and some patients require urinary catheterisation. The precautions and associated nursing care for this can be found in Chapter 8. As consciousness is regained, the patient may attempt to remove the catheter, an indication that normal functioning is returning. Constipation should be avoided to minimise rises in ICP caused by straining at stool (see Ch. 4).

STOP THINK **9.6** Discuss with your mentor the approaches to care you have seen in practice with the care of the unconscious patient. Consider the appropriateness of these approaches and whether there might be better alternatives.

Rehabilitation

This forms a crucial part of the recovery process and the principles outlined in Chapter 34 apply. The aim is to maintain and promote function, and prevent further deterioration and occurrence of complications. The neurological deficits which can impede progress during the rehabilitation process are described in Box 9.7.

The patient with a head injury may experience neurological deficits including limb weaknesses and speech and visual problems. They may also experience changes in personality, memory and intellect, and a combination of all these factors makes full rehabilitation very difficult to achieve.

> **Box 9.7**
>
> **Neurological deficits that can impede rehabilitation**
>
> - Motor impairment, e.g. spasticity or ataxia
> - Sensory impairment, e.g. loss of sense of pain or touch
> - Communication disability, e.g. dysphasia
> - Psychological disability
>   - — cognitive intelligence, e.g. memory loss
>   - — perceptual, e.g. eye–hand coordination
>   - — emotional, e.g. irritability
>   - — behaviour or personality, e.g. poor self-image
> - Social disability, e.g. social withdrawal
> - Educational or vocational disability
>
> All the above have an effect on the patient's ability to resume educational or vocational activities.

The ward team, in partnership with the patient's family and friends, should aim to assess the patient's needs and provide optimal care and support. Realistic goals should be set as the rehabilitative process may take months or years to achieve. Some patients may remain in a persistent vegetative state requiring constant nursing in a care facility (see Ch. 28, p. 970).

In some circumstances, the patient's role within the family changes. They may previously have been the provider within a family and may now have to revert to being dependent on others. Employment prospects may alter and, for some, a return to work is impossible. This can affect both the family's short- and long-term plans and may also have financial implications. An alteration to the patient's personality may affect relationships within a family, resulting in stress and discord. Indeed, some families will report that the person has completely changed and is now different from the person they knew before (see also Ch. 34). Often, due to the distress caused by such changes, repeated explanations are required and the reactions of the family can range from apparent calm acceptance to rudeness and even verbal aggression towards nursing staff. This should be accepted and seen as part of the family's way of coming to terms with the reality of the situation.

The multidisciplinary approach

Early and close liaison between the many health care professionals involved in hospital and community work is essential. The resources of the voluntary sector and self-help groups should be brought in, as well as the patient's family and friends. Sinnakaruppan and Williams (2001) reviewed the perceived needs of family carers and identified that information giving and emotional support were the two most important.

Preparation for discharge

Many patients and their families will be particularly anxious as the time for discharge approaches. Much of this anxiety can be allayed by appropriate preparation and reassurance and an effective plan for discharge. The residual problems that may persist vary widely, ranging from headache to major behavioural changes, with or without neurological deficits. The degree of residual deficits will determine what intervention is required in the discharge plan. Other factors may include whether the patient requires further surgery or other therapies, necessitating attendance at a hospital or rehabilitation centre. A home assessment may be performed jointly by the occupational therapist and community nurse. Pre-discharge visits home may be considered and will help to identify potential problems. If appropriate, referral to a community liaison nurse and/or to the primary health care team should be made to enable optimal assessment and support within the community setting.

Despite these preparations, it is not usually until the patient is at home that the family members fully appreciate the difficulties that may be before them. Home routines may require to be adjusted, and whilst this may be easy in the early stages, it becomes more difficult to accept in the long term. Other members of the family will often view the disruption to their personal lives negatively and eventually much of the early support gradually disappears. If the patient is still at a stage in which they require support, this withdrawal can be catastrophic. Often the patient's partner may be left to shoulder the burden alone, and in this situation, a support group such as Headway (see 'Useful websites') may help. This organisation seeks to provide help and assistance to patients and their families. Regular meetings and other special outings are arranged, along with helpful literature. Relatives are provided with a forum for discussion of the problems they face and many appreciate sharing their problems with others who are similarly placed. Some families acknowledge a sense of failure should the patient require to be admitted for long-term care. They may feel that they have let their loved one down and do not like to admit that they are unable to cope.

CEREBROVASCULAR DISEASE

'Cerebrovascular disease' can be defined as brain disease occurring as a result of a pathological disorder of the blood vessels or of the blood supply. This section considers:

- stroke, the most common cerebrovascular disorder
- subarachnoid haemorrhage, an uncommon but major life-threatening situation that demands acute neurosurgical intervention.

Stroke

A stroke, uncommon in children, can occur at any time during adult life. Thrombotic stroke tends to be seen in the 60–90 year age group, and embolic and haemorrhagic stroke in the 25–60 year age group.

Stroke is the third most common cause of death in developed countries: 200 per 100 000 will have a stroke each year. Age increases the risk. Most strokes occur in the 65–75 year age group and are more common in men. In the UK, 100 000–120 000 strokes occur per annum, of which 70 000 result in death. The mortality rate rises in proportion to the length of time the patient is unconscious. Of patients unconscious for 48 h or more, 98% will die, compared with 12% where there is no loss of consciousness (Lindsay & Bone 2004).

Subarachnoid haemorrhage

Subarachnoid haemorrhage is often wrongly referred to as 'cerebral' or 'brain haemorrhage'. A subarachnoid haemorrhage is experienced by 10 000–15 000 people per year, with 15% dying before they reach hospital. It has a male bias in the under-40s, but this reverts to a female bias in the over-40s (Lindsay & Bone 2004).

PATHOPHYSIOLOGY

Causes of stroke

There are three main causes of stroke:

- cerebral thrombosis
- cerebral embolus
- cerebral haemorrhage.

As a result of the rise in substance abuse, an increasing cause of stroke in the under-45s is the pharmacological action of drugs such as crack and crack cocaine (see Ch. 36).

Cerebral thrombosis This is the most common cause of stroke, in which atherosclerosis causes narrowing of the lumen of the affected blood vessels (Lindsay & Bone 2004) (see Ch. 2). It occurs either during sleep or shortly after waking and is thought to be due to the older person's poorer reflex response to changes in position (postural hypotension). As the atheroma builds up, it initially only partially occludes the blood vessel until the blood supply is suddenly disrupted. During the 24–48 h following this, neurological deficits frequently worsen.

Cerebral embolus An embolus may lodge in the narrowed lumen of a bifurcation in the cerebral circulation. The usual origin of the embolus is a cardiac thrombus, in the presence of cardiac disease such as myocardial infarction. Air or fat, the latter for example from a fractured femur, can also act as an embolus. Embolic stroke can occur at any time.

Cerebral haemorrhage Haemorrhage can occur into:

- the cerebral tissues — intracerebral haemorrhage
- the subarachnoid space — subarachnoid haemorrhage.

The most common cause of subarachnoid haemorrhage is a weakness in the wall of a cerebral blood vessel, which causes a dilatation (an 'aneurysm'). Other causes include arteriovenous malformations (AVMs), but in some patients no cause is identified. Hypertension, although seen in some patients, is not always present, but damage caused by arteriosclerotic changes is common. Cerebral aneurysms may be described eponymously as 'Berry' or as 'saccular'. Most aneurysms form on the anterior part of the circle of Willis (see Ch. 2) and some patients have multiple aneurysms.

The exact cause of aneurysm formation remains unknown and some remain silent, causing no symptoms. Some bleeding can occur through the very thin aneurysmal wall and produce mild signs and symptoms of subarachnoid haemorrhage without rupture occurring.

Risk factors

Certain predisposing contributory factors increase the likelihood of cerebrovascular disease (see p. 14).

The effects of a stroke

The occurrence of a stroke, for whatever reason, will result in an interruption of the cerebral blood supply, diminishing the essential oxygen and glucose levels of the brain. Within hours, oedema occurs at the site of the main lesion as a result of the changes to the cell membranes, allowing fluid to leak into the extracellular space. This gradually worsens, peaking between the fifth and seventh day and then gradually resolving.

A classification system for stroke is given in Box 9.8.

The damage caused by a stroke is due largely to the extent of ischaemia that occurs. It has been established that there is a reduction in global cerebral blood flow following stroke. In and around the immediate area of the infarction, more subtle changes are detected in regional cerebral blood

Box 9.8

Classification of stroke

Transient ischaemic attacks
- Onset and disappearance of a neurological deficit within 24 h due to temporary disturbance of blood supply to the brain
- No residual neurological deficit
- Symptoms commonly last from several minutes to 2–3 h, but may last up to 24 h

Reversible ischaemic neurological deficit
- Neurological deficit persists longer than 12–24 h
- Symptoms may last days or weeks
- Minimal, partial or no residual neurological deficit

Stroke in evolution
- Symptoms persist beyond 24 h with an associated progressive deterioration of neurological status
- Residual neurological deficits
- Probably due to a failure of collateral circulation

Completed stroke
- Condition stabilises and neurological deficit remains

flow. These comprise areas of reduced blood flow bordered by areas of increased flow due to vasodilatation of the arteriolar bed. Progression from reversible ischaemia to infarction depends on the degree and duration of the reduced blood flow (Lindsay & Bone 2004). The affected area of the brain loses its ability to carry out its function, e.g.:

- controlling movement in a specific part of the body
- controlling cognitive or emotional processes, speech or language
- experiencing sight, sound, taste or touch.

Another influence on the course of events is the occurrence of cerebral oedema. As the oedema starts to subside, cells begin to function again, explaining the rapid progress potentially made in the first 2–3 weeks.

After this initial period, recovery is slower, partly due to other cells taking over the functions of the permanently damaged cells. At this stage, the patient begins to learn ways of handling their disability and regains their self-confidence and interest in general affairs.

Generally speaking, if a patient shows a marked improvement within the first week, then minimal deficit will result. Conversely, if little or no improvement is made during this time, the outcome is likely to be poorer. The most common types of residual disability are listed in Box 9.9.

Common presenting symptoms The onset of cerebrovascular disease can be difficult to pinpoint. In thrombotic and embolic stroke, minor symptoms are often dismissed by patients and it is not until a significant symptom presents that the patient seeks medical help. Earlier symptoms, e.g. tingling and weakness of a limb, are the result of mild transient interruptions of neurological function. Major episodes requiring medical intervention include loss of consciousness, speech difficulties and hemiplegia, which may be accompanied by loss of vision on the affected side.

Box 9.9

Common types of disability caused by stroke

Motor deficits
- Movement deficits
  - loss of movement in the limbs on one side of the body (hemiplegia)
  - weakness in the arms and legs (hemiparesis)
- Speech difficulties, such as:
  - dysarthria, where the patient has distorted and indistinct speech but is able to understand what is said and can still read and write
  - dysphasia, i.e. loss of the ability to talk, read and write
- Facial paralysis on the affected side, causing drooling, indistinct speech and difficulty in chewing and swallowing

Sensory deficits
- Visual deficits
  - partial loss of the visual field
  - double vision
  - poorer vision than previously
- Poor response to superficial sensation, e.g. heat and cold
- Perceptual deficits, such as incorrect perception of the environment or loss of sense of smell
- Lack of awareness of the disabled part of the body

Loss of consciousness
- From mild impairment to coma
- Loss of memory or shortened attention span

Emotional deficits
- Emotional disturbances, e.g. change of personality, from quiet and pleasant to surly and aggressive, or vice versa
- Loss of self-control or inhibitions
- Confusion
- Depression

Bladder/bowel dysfunction
- Loss of bladder and/or bowel control (incontinence)
- Frequency
- Urgency

Subarachnoid haemorrhage typically causes sudden, severe headache, often accompanied by vomiting. The patient may be alert and orientated and may feel intense fear at what they are experiencing. Alternatively, there may be loss of consciousness, seizures and evidence of neurological deficits such as IIIrd nerve palsy, hemiplegia or hemiparesis (Lindsay & Bone 2004). Many of these symptoms are related to the effects of raised ICP (see p. 408).

The patient may still have a residual headache and neck stiffness which may be confirmed by passive neck flexion. This indicates meningism, caused by the presence of blood in the subarachnoid space irritating the sensitive tissue of the meninges. Kernig's sign, demonstrated by extending the knee to stretch the nerve roots, will cause the patient some pain and is an indicator of meningism.

Conscious level may be depressed and there may be evidence of seizures. Other findings will include hypertension and pyrexia. Signs and symptoms will depend on a variety of factors and can occur according to the area of the brain affected (see Fig. 9.5).

STOP THINK **9.7** Think of two patients you have cared for, who have had a stroke. For each patient, write a short word picture of how you recall them, then compare your notes with the common presenting symptoms you have just read about. How similar were they?

MEDICAL MANAGEMENT

Investigations will be as follows:

A CT scan may be performed to determine the location and type of stroke and to ensure that there is no other, potentially treatable, lesion to account for the stroke. If a subarachnoid haemorrhage is diagnosed and the patient is alert, obeying commands and has no focal neurological deficits, a lumbar puncture is indicated (Jamieson et al 2002). Confirmation of the subarachnoid haemorrhage will result when examination of the CSF reveals uniform bloodstaining or, if 6 h have elapsed since the original bleed, straw-coloured CSF, called 'xanthachromia', is apparent. This colour is due to the breakdown of haemoglobin.

If the patient is displaying signs of raised ICP, e.g. is in coma or has a neurological deficit, lumbar puncture is contraindicated because of the risk of coning (see p. 407). The safe alternative of CT is used, which may reveal the presence of blood in a variety of locations such as the surface of the cerebral hemispheres or in the ventricular system.

Angiography If blood is detected, either by lumbar puncture or CT scan, angiography is indicated (see Appendix 1). The presence and location of aneurysms and other blood vessel anomalies such as stenosis will be demonstrated. Angiography is not without risk and its performance may be delayed if the patient is in a vulnerable clinical condition. Electrocardiography may be performed to exclude or confirm cardiac disease.

Treatment Approaches to stroke management vary widely because of the variety of presentations. They will depend on:

- the site of the occlusion or aneurysmal rupture
- the degree and extent of the ischaemia or haemorrhage
- the effectiveness of medical and nursing intervention
- the patient's response.

The aims are to prevent further brain damage, reduce the risk factors, provide supportive care and regain functional independence.

Treatment can be conservative or surgical.

Conservative management is as follows.

- Anticoagulant therapy is often used in an attempt to halt further deterioration and to improve the patient's recovery. However, some doubt has now been cast on its usefulness, as a risk of further haemorrhage into the infarcted brain has been identified (Lindsay & Bone 2004). One example of an anticoagulant is warfarin.
- The use of thrombolytic agents, especially recombinant tissue plasminogen activator (rTPA), has been investigated. Early indications are that its use within a few hours of infarction produces a sustained, significant neurological improvement (Lindsay & Bone 2004).
- Calcium antagonists, e.g. nimodipine, have been used in patients following subarachnoid haemorrhage and their use has been shown to reduce the incidence of cerebral infarction.
- Antiplatelet agents. The use of aspirin as an antiplatelet agent is now well established practice, with the recognition that the sooner treatment is commenced the better. Other factors. Pre-existing contributory disorders may be treated with medication, e.g. antihypertensive agents and diuretics may be used in the patient with raised blood pressure.

Surgical management uses two techniques (Lindsay & Bone 2004):

- carotid endarterectomy, which involves the removal of stenosing or ulcerating atheromatous lesions at the bifurcation of the common carotid arteries
- a superficial temporal to middle-cerebral artery anastomosis (ST–MCA bypass), which provides an artificial collateral blood supply to the affected part of the brain.

Aims of treatment in subarachnoid haemorrhage The main aim of treatment is to avoid a potentially fatal recurrence of bleeding. In untreated patients, 30% will bleed again within 28 days, and 70% of these will die.

Preventing rebleeding An effective way to prevent rebleeding is to place a metal clip across the neck of the aneurysm. This entails a craniotomy, a major neurosurgical procedure. This procedure is not suitable for all patients, either due to their general condition or to the location of the aneurysm. Alternative surgical procedures include wrapping, which involves the application of muslin gauze around the fundus of the aneurysm. Wrapping may be combined with clipping in some patients. A third technique, known as 'trapping', may be indicated. This involves clipping the feeding vessels supplying a large aneurysm. Another technique involves the insertion of helical platinum coils into the aneurysmal sac to induce thrombosis (Nichols et al 2002).

The timing of surgery is crucial and opinions vary with regard to this. When surgery is carried out as soon as possible to avoid the risk of rebleeding, there are higher morbidity and mortality rates during the operation. Delayed surgery decreases the operative risks but increases the risk of rebleeding. Antifibrinolytic therapy may be used in an attempt to prevent this (Lindsay & Bone 2004).

There are now well-established grading systems to identify the patient most at risk from deterioration after subarachnoid haemorrhage. The best known of these is the Hunt and Hess scale which is described in Hickey (2002). A critical review of scales is provided by Cavanagh and Gordon (2002).

Complications of subarachnoid haemorrhage that may influence treatment are as follows.

Rebleed This is a risk which peaks between days 7 and 10 following the original bleed, due to the process of fibrinolysis, which dissolves the clot that formed over the ruptured vessel (Lindsay & Bone 2004).

Cerebral ischaemia Reduction of the blood supply to any part of the brain can have serious consequences for the patient. The extent of its effects will depend on the site and extent of the ischaemia. About half of the patients who develop ischaemia will be left with a permanent deficit.

Box 9.10

Hydrocephalus

This is a condition in which there is a progressive dilatation of the cerebral ventricular system due to a production of CSF which exceeds the absorption rate. This may be brought about by an obstruction of one of the pathways by, for example, a tumour. Other causes include congenital stenosis and infection.

It can occur at all ages; it may be congenital in the newborn or secondary to some other intracranial pathology in the older child and adult.

Treatment is by insertion of a ventriculoperitoneal shunt. This is a long narrow plastic tubing, valve and reservoir device. One end is inserted into the lateral ventricle and the other end is sutured into the patient's peritoneum via a subcutaneous route. The excess CSF is now 'shunted' from the ventricles into the peritoneum, from where it then returns to the bloodstream.

Arterial narrowing (vasospasm) is common following subarachnoid haemorrhage and can have similar results (Kirkness et al 2002). A case study on the use of drugs to control vasospasm is provided by Le Strange (2003).

Hydrocephalus The normal drainage of cerebrospinal fluid may be impaired by the presence of a haematoma pressing on the narrow pathways or by haemorrhage into the CSF impeding the flow of the normally clear fluid. About one-fifth of patients are affected, although only one-third require treatment (see Box 9.10).

Intracerebral haematoma Bleeding during a subarachnoid haemorrhage may result in a localised collection or haematoma. This will contribute to a rise in ICP and may demand treatment.

Epilepsy Seizures may occur, necessitating treatment with anticonvulsants (see p. 427).

NURSING PRIORITIES AND MANAGEMENT: Stroke

Prevention

One of the most important aspects of stroke management is prevention, by identifying at-risk individuals and dealing with early predisposing factors such as hypertension.

Transient ischaemic attack (TIA)

A TIA is caused by insufficient blood reaching the brain, for a brief period. It is similar to a stroke but the pathology is transient, symptoms lasting for only a few minutes. These are:

- weakness of one side of the body
- tingling and twisting of the mouth
- loss of speech
- disturbance of vision (www.stroke.org.uk).

If an individual or their relative notices the symptoms of a mild TIA, they should contact a doctor immediately, as TIAs can be treated.

Reducing the risk of stroke

Although action can be taken to reduce the likelihood of stroke occurring, the following factors put people at greater risk.

High blood pressure Using medication to reduce high blood pressure does reduce the risk of a stroke. Ideally blood pressure should be checked periodically, e.g. every 4 years until the age of 40, and every 2 years after that. Drinking alcohol raises blood pressure. The consistent consumption of four or more units of alcohol per day for men and three or more for women is not advised (NHS Health Scotland 2003).

Cigarette smoking In people who smoke 20 cigarettes a day or more, the risk of having a stroke is three times greater than that for people who do not smoke (www.stroke.org.uk). Smokers should therefore be encouraged to stop smoking, and young people discouraged from starting to smoke (see Ch. 3).

High blood cholesterol may lead to coronary heart disease. Patients with high blood cholesterol can reduce the amount of cholesterol-rich foods they take, by the following measures:

- using spread which is high in polyunsaturates rather than saturates, and using vegetable oil for cooking
- using skimmed milk, rather than full-cream milk
- avoiding cream and cheese, and cutting down on the number of eggs eaten
- choosing lean cuts of meat or removing the fat.

Being overweight may increase the likelihood of high blood pressure, so at-risk patients should try to control their weight.

Diabetic patients are more likely to have a stroke, so the level of glucose in the blood and urine should be checked regularly (see Ch. 5, Part 2).

The contraceptive pill increases the risk of stroke in younger women, particularly if there is a family history of arterial disease. Other forms of contraception should therefore be recommended.

Nursing care following a stroke

Often the immediate priorities and follow-up care overlap, and they are separated here for the purposes of explanation only. An optimal outcome is more likely when appropriate techniques and resources are utilised, encompassing every member of the multidisciplinary team, and when the rehabilitation process commences as soon as possible. NHS Education for Scotland (2005) provide a framework of core competencies for all health care professionals involved in the care of individuals with or at risk of a stroke, in acute and primary care settings.

Immediate priorities

Airway Techniques for maintaining a patent airway and adequate ventilation, outlined in Box 9.6, are a priority (see Ch. 28).

Safety and comfort Hemiplegia often results from stroke, so the care of paralysed limbs and avoiding the hazards of immobility are axiomatic.

Similarly, the patient with a decreased level of consciousness will require to have their safety needs met (see Ch. 28). Raised intracranial pressure will pose a number of dangers for the patient (see interventions outlined on p. 412 for care of a patient with a head injury).

The patient who has experienced a haemorrhage will be assessed for headache and an analgesic such as codeine phosphate or dihydrocodeine, which do not mask conscious level, prescribed. Patients often have a stiff neck which can be alleviated by cold packs and a position in bed which avoids extreme flexion or sudden movement of the neck. A quiet darkened room will also relieve discomfort, particularly if the patient is photophobic. An antiemetic may also be prescribed for nausea and vomiting.

Patient safety and comfort are greatly enhanced when consideration is given to the patient's ability to communicate and to their emotional well-being, as well as that of their family.

Communicating Speech impairment or loss can be a frightening experience for the patient and their family. Early referral to a speech and language therapist (SALT) is important, so that an expert assessment can be performed and an appropriate strategy identified. It is crucial to ascertain the type and nature of the speech deficit, e.g. whether the patient's difficulties are related to expression or to comprehension. The nurse should encourage and help the patient to perform the exercises prescribed by the speech and language therapist.

Powerful emotions are often displayed by the patient following stroke (Hickey 2002). Many of these patients display anger at or frustration with the frightening situation in which they find themselves. This can be vented onto the nurse and can manifest itself as lack of cooperation or physical abuse. Patients who are unable to communicate their feelings verbally may feel trapped inside a body that refuses to do as they want. Some patients are convinced that their words are properly formed and fail to realise that what the nurse or family is hearing is indistinct or jumbled. The patient needs to be repeatedly reminded of what has happened to them and why they feel the way they do, in order to try to reassure them. Patients and their friends and family can become very distressed when they meet and this needs to be handled with sensitivity. Some patients experience denial (see Research Abstract 9.1).

Mobility Patients with mobility difficulties require a clutter-free environment. The nurse should ensure that any obstacles likely to pose a danger are removed and that the patient is wearing appropriate clothing and footwear, e.g. outdoor shoes rather than loose-fitting slippers.

Visual impairment may also be dangerous for the patient (see Box 9.9). Simple interventions that may help include providing an eye patch to eliminate double vision and approaching the patient with homonymous hemianopia, i.e. loss of vision in the same half (right or left) of the visual field in both eyes, from the side with the intact field of vision. These interventions should also be explained to the patient's family, who should be advised about basic safety precautions at home following discharge, e.g. removal of loose rugs and any necessary rearrangement of furniture.

RESEARCH ABSTRACT 9.1

During the first few months after a stroke, family caregivers must learn how to care for the stroke survivor in the home setting. Although there are some studies that address the needs and concerns of stroke caregivers during the early post-stroke period, there are very few caregiver studies that report strategies used by caregivers to deal with their needs and concerns. Studies are also lacking that report the advice that caregivers would offer to others. The purpose of this study was to determine the self-reported needs, concerns, strategies and advice of family caregivers of stroke survivors during the first 6 months after hospital discharge. Using open-ended questions, 14 female family caregivers of stroke survivors (8 African–American, 6 white) were interviewed to identify their needs and concerns, strategies they used to deal with stroke and advice they would offer to other stroke caregivers. Findings revealed five major categories of caregiver needs and concerns: information, emotions and behaviours, physical care, instrumental care and personal responses to caregiving. Based on the findings, an initial needs and concerns checklist was developed. This checklist, as well as the list of strategies and advice, may help to identify relevant areas for caregiver intervention.

Bakas T, Austin J K, Okonkwo K F, Lewis R R, Chadwick L 2002 Needs, concerns, strategies and advice of stroke caregivers the first 6 months after discharge. Journal of Neuroscience Nursing 34(5): 242–251

Differences of opinion exist with regard to mobility following subarachnoid haemorrhage. One approach advocates that patients should have strict bed rest and that their visitors should be restricted; however, this approach can heighten the patient's anxiety, particularly when they feel well. An alternative approach is to allow the patient up to the toilet provided they are symptom-free (Hickey 2002). The patient with a neurological deficit or alteration in conscious level should be nursed in an easily observable bed with side rails as required. Seizure precautions should also be adopted as outlined on page 427.

Eating and drinking Initially the patient's fluid intake is likely to be via an intravenous infusion and the nurse will be responsible for maintaining this accurately. A patient who has had a subarachnoid haemorrhage may be prescribed a fluid regimen of 2.5–3 L/day. This helps to maintain arterial blood pressure, which encourages adequate cerebral perfusion and, in turn, prevents cerebral ischaemia and infarction. As the patient progresses, an oral diet may be introduced gradually, providing that swallowing and cough reflexes are intact. The patient may need help with feeding, or can be given adapted eating utensils which allow them to feed themselves. Being spoon-fed can be embarrassing and sensitivity is required to preserve the patient's dignity and self-esteem. The nurse should determine the patient's capability; for example, hemiplegia may prevent them from cutting up their own food but, once this is done, they can feed themselves. The patient with a facial paralysis should be encouraged to chew food on the unaffected side only.

Dysphagia may hinder progress. If the patient experiences swallowing difficulties, these should be assessed to determine the extent of the difficulty before attempting oral feeding. A combined assessment may be performed by the dietitian and speech and language therapist. Recommendations may include the use of nasogastric feeding with a prescribed proprietary liquid diet, and the use of specialised exercises and techniques to aid swallowing. Increased oral hygiene is important in both instances. The patient with dysphagia receiving nasogastric feeding will be more prone to a dry mouth and the patient who is managing to take an oral diet may leave food debris in the affected side of their mouth. Regular oral inspection and oral hygiene are essential (see Ch. 15).

Eliminating Interruption of the patient's usual elimination pattern is due to loss of consciousness and enforced immobility. Urinary incontinence is best resolved by retraining the patient to use bedpans or urinals at specified intervals, rather than resorting to catheterisation. Condom-type urinary appliances may be suitable for male patients, but these are not without practical problems. No successful female equivalent is yet available.

Kwan et al (2004), in a before-and-after study, evaluated the introduction of an integrated care pathway for acute stroke, and found evidence that the use of the pathway improved the quality of documentation and process of care, and reduced the risk of certain post-stroke complications; for example urinary tract infections were significantly less frequent.

CASE HISTORY 9.1

Mrs F

Mrs F had her stroke on May 21st. She was completely paralysed on the right side and had lost all power of speech. A CT scan on May 22nd showed a large area of ischaemic damage on the left side. By June 1st her speech was normal, but she still could not walk at all or use her right arm. She took her first steps on June 21st, and 1 month later was walking alone using a tripod. A little movement returned in her right arm 6 weeks after her stroke. She was discharged on July 16th, and by early November she was walking to the local shops, talking normally and was able to use her right hand and arm for holding cans.

Mrs F's story is not unusual, and illustrates several points:

- There was a rapid recovery over the first month, when her speech returned and leg movements started
- Her recovery continued, although slowly, for about 6 months
- This happened despite the fact that the scan appeared to suggest that Mrs F had lost a lot of brain function.

Processes of recovery

1. Reduction of brain swelling around the stroke area
2. Possible growth of nerve axons
3. Use of other parts of the brain
4. Learning new ways of coping
5. Adaptation in behaviour by others towards the person who has had a stroke.

Behind this success story must be close collaboration between community nurses and other members of the health care professions.

Rehabilitation

The overall aim of rehabilitation, as outlined in Chapter 34, is the active promotion and restoration of independence, and this applies equally to all patients following a stroke, whether they are at home, in hospital or in a rehabilitation centre (see Case History 9.1).

Lindsay & Bone (2004) describe the common complications following a stroke and provide advice on how to deal with these.

Therapy Different types of therapy can aid rehabilitation. These are not necessary immediately, as many people recover spontaneously, but can be of help once it is apparent that specific problems remain. Clear evidence exists of the value of a multidisciplinary approach to managing the patient.

Physiotherapists can assist people to walk again and suggest suitable aids such as canes, Zimmer frames or foot splints. They can also help the patient to regain movement in paralysed arms.

Occupational therapists can help patients learn adaptive ways to dress and cook for themselves, and can suggest suitable home aids.

Speech and language therapists (SALTs) help patients to overcome problems with speech, often involving the patient in attending speech therapy sessions at the hospital.

The nursing interventions identified during the acute period will often be continued during the rehabilitative phase, e.g. care of the paralysed limbs must be maintained. Other areas of nursing will include attention to speech difficulties and sensory deficits and preparing the patient for discharge home with adequate support and advice as reflected within a well-constructed care package. Involvement of the patient's family in the recovery phase is crucial as their cooperation can result in the increased likelihood of success (see Box 9.11).

The patient will have been referred to the local primary health care team for assessment and support. Once home, the patient's ability to live independently can be enhanced by aids such as hand rails in the bathroom and adapted cutlery. Advice on rearranging the patient's furniture at home may facilitate easier mobility and reduce the likelihood of an accident. The use of information from the Stroke Association (see 'Useful websites') should be considered along with help and support from appropriate community groups.

Box 9.11

Some do's and don'ts for home carers of individuals recovering from stroke

- Do not overprotect the individual
- Do encourage them to exercise
- Do not accuse them of 'not trying'
- Do not pull their weak arm
- Do encourage friends to visit
- Do not become gloomy and pessimistic
- Do think twice before selling the double bed
- Do continue a normal sex life

9.8 With the help of your community nurse mentor, try to find an example of such a multidisciplinary approach in support of a patient and their family from your own placement experience of nursing in the community.

9.9 How many people in the UK suffer from stroke every year? Have you looked after a stroke patient with severe physical and behavioural problems? If not, ask a fellow student to help you with this question. How many different members of the hospital and primary care teams do you think were involved in the patient's care? Consider each team member's role, then try to draw a circle with the patient and their spouse, partner or main carer in the middle, surrounded by each team member. What might be their feelings about having to meet so many people?

INTRACRANIAL TUMOURS

Approximately 2250 people in the UK die from a brain tumour every year. The cause of primary brain tumours is unknown, but they are the most commonly known disorders affecting the nervous system, and occur in 6 per 100 000 of the population (Lindsay & Bone 2004).

Astrocytoma, a malignant tumour of star-shaped astrocytes, occurs twice as often in males as in females and is most common in the 40–60 year age group. Up to 50% of brain tumours occur in more than one location. Some appear to be congenital in origin while others are related to hereditary factors (Hickey 2002).

There are two age peaks for intracranial tumours: the first decade of life, and the 50s and 60s. There is a slight male preponderance, except for meningiomas and neurilemmomas (Lindsay & Bone 2004).

PATHOPHYSIOLOGY

Intracranial tumours can be classified according to their pathology, as outlined in Table 9.4, but the presence of a benign tumour in a crucial location, such as a confined space, can prove equally serious. Intracranial tumours can grow in one of two ways: they may encapsulate, or spread and infiltrate surrounding tissue. Their rate of growth can be very slow or extremely rapid.

The pathological features of tumours are:

- cerebral oedema
- raised ICP
- focal neurological deficits
- seizures
- altered pituitary function
- hydrocephalus.

Common presenting symptoms are extremely variable. Presentation will be determined by the location, type, size and speed of growth of the tumour and its effect on surrounding structures.

The neurological symptoms of brain tumours may occur alone or in combination. There may be general symptoms, e.g. epilepsy, focal symptoms, dependent on location, such as hemiparesis or cranial nerve deficits, and signs of raised ICP such as headache.

MEDICAL MANAGEMENT

Investigations CT scanning is likely to be the investigation of first choice. Other investigations may include MRI scanning and cerebral angiography. Additional investigations include measuring the ESR and taking a chest X-ray to establish the possible presence of metastases. If a pituitary tumour is suspected, endocrine studies and visual field testing will be performed. If acoustic neuroma is suspected, audiometric studies will be performed.

Exploratory surgical procedure Burr hole biopsy, in which a small piece of tissue is removed for pathological examination, may confirm the diagnosis. This technique relies upon the ability of the operator to remove a specimen of tumour tissue which reflects the true extent and pathology of the growth.

Treatment This may be with surgery, radiotherapy and/or chemotherapy.

Surgery The tumour is removed (if possible) using one of four different approaches, as outlined in Box 9.5, and a combination of radiotherapy and surgery may be indicated where surgery alone cannot remove all of the tumour.

Chemotherapy has been used for some time, but the clinical benefits remain uncertain (Lindsay & Bone 2004). Armstrong and Gilbert (2002) provide an update on new approaches in chemotherapy (see Ch. 31).

NURSING PRIORITIES AND MANAGEMENT: Intracranial tumours

As a priority, assessment should be made of the patient's and family's understanding of the reason for admission. Someone with an intracranial tumour can usually carry out their normal daily activities, unless there is a rise in ICP caused by swelling or by tumour enlargement. The onset of symptoms can be slow and progressive or almost immediate, in which case the person's condition deteriorates rapidly.

Immediate priorities

The patient should be assessed for increasing ICP, primarily through the assessment of conscious level, and the nurse should observe for any deterioration in the patient's condition. If the patient has experienced seizures before admission, this should be carefully noted and the nurse should be prepared should a seizure occur.

If the patient has speech problems, e.g. dysphasia, time should be taken to ensure they have communicated their needs, possibly drawing on information from relatives.

Subsequent considerations

After physical and neurological assessment, the speech and language therapist, physiotherapist and occupational therapist should be involved in assessing the patient, offering advice and assistance.

Support during investigations

The patient will be anxious to know the results of investigations and worried about the diagnosis. The investigations can confirm the diagnosis and/or identify the type of

Table 9.4 Classification of tumours

Tumour	Description	Usual site	Incidence (% of total)	Remarks
Tumours of neuroepithelial tissue				
Astrocytoma Grade I Intermediate astrocytoma Grades II & III	Well differentiated, insidiously invasive, relatively benign Will possess some of the characteristics of grade I astrocytomas but cell differentiation less well defined	Cerebral hemispheres of adults; most commonly the frontal lobes followed by the temporal and parietal sites (occipital lobe astrocytoma is rare)	10	A cystic type of astrocytoma is sometimes located in the cerebellum. A childhood tumour of the first decade of life
Glioblastoma multiforme (anaplastic astrocytoma) Grade IV	Rapidly growing, undifferentiated cells, extremely malignant and highly vascular. Infiltrates brain tissue extensively. Peak age is 48–52 years with a male bias. Can produce extensive brain swelling while still relatively small in size	Grade IV shown to spread into the white matter of both hemispheres via the anterior corpus callosum	18	
Oligodendroglioma	Rare, slow-growing tumour, age of onset 40 years. Relatively benign — minor signs and symptoms can be present for a number of years before diagnosis is confirmed. Shows a marked tendency to calcify (may be seen on skull X-ray)	Demonstrates a predilection to grow in close proximity to the ventricular wall and commissural midline structures in the frontal region of the cerebral hemispheres. Can also be found in the temporal lobes	4	Can 'mimic' a meningioma upon presentation. Unlike many tumours, raised ICP is a late sign in the patient with an oligodendroglioma. Sudden deterioration can occur, thought to be due to spontaneous haemorrhage and cystic degeneration within the tumour body
Ependymoma	Rare, undifferentiated, slow-growing glioma. Often seen in childhood and young adult	Arises from the ependymal layer of the ventricular system; therefore may be found in any of four lobes	5	Due to involvement of the CSF pathways, hydrocephalus and raised ICP are early common features
Optic nerve glioma	Occurs mainly before the age of 20 years. Follows a relatively benign course, remaining localised to the optic nerve and chiasma	Optic nerve and chiasma	4	Approximately 60% of patients have an associated neurofibromatosis called a spongioblastoma
Medulloblastoma	Rapidly growing, malignant tumour of childhood. Composed of round, undifferentiated cells. Commonest intracranial neoplasm of childhood. Usually occurs before the age of 10 years	Cerebellar vermis or fourth ventricle roof	3	Can 'seed' throughout the subarachnoid space. Slight male bias. Hydrocephalus is common
Tumours of nerve sheath cells				
Neurilemma/ Schwannoma	Slow-growing, benign tumour. Well encapsulated. Usually unilateral, predilection for females, occurs in the middle years of life	The Schwann cell sheath of cranial nerves VIII, V and VII located within the confined cerebellopontine angle		A tumour of the sheath of the VIIIth nerve. Referred to as an acoustic neuroma. Other tumour types may be seen in this location, e.g. meningioma, but a differential diagnosis may not be made until surgery
Neuroma (neurofibroma)	A complex familial disorder characterised by widespread benign tumours throughout the nervous system. Inherited as an autosomal dominant trait. Known as Recklinghausen's disease. Manifests itself in young adulthood	The neurilemma of nerves; therefore tumours may appear intracranially, i.e. VIIth nerve, acoustic neuroma, or extracranially, i.e. spinal roots and peripheral nerves	10	Patient will present with cutaneous pigmentation of the skin termed 'café au lait' spots. Some of these patients will also have a meningioma or glioma

Continued

Table 9.4 Classification of tumours *(Continued)*

Tumour	Description	Usual site	Incidence (% of total)	Remarks
Tumours of meningeal and related tissues				
Meningioma	Benign, slow-growing tumour arising from the arachnoid cells of the arachnoid villi. An irregular single mass usually well encapsulated	Intracranial venous sinuses — most common, superior sagittal sinus known as a parasagittal meningioma. Other sites include sphenoid ridge convexity of hemispheres and suprasellar region and olfactory groove	15	Can become very large before signs and symptoms appear. Predilection for females in 40–60 year age group. Do not show any malignant change
Tumours of blood vessel origin				
Haemangioblastoma	Slow-growing, vascular tumour of developmental origin. Single or multiple lesions occur. Manifests in children and young adults, male bias. May be familial	Cerebellar hemisphere	2	May be associated angiomatosis of the retina or abnormal organs. von Hippel–Lindau disease
Germ cell tumours				
Teratoma	Rare tumour of childhood and young adulthood	Pineal parenchymal cells; therefore located around the pineal gland		The terms pinealoma and teratoma are often interchanged
Local extensions from regional tumours				
Chordoma	Soft tumour with a jelly-like consistency	Arise extradurally at the base of the skull		
Metastatic tumours				
Metastatic tumour	Well defined, usually multiple secondary deposits of a primary growth elsewhere in the body. Common primary sites are bronchus and breast	As lesions are often multiple, can occur anywhere in the cerebrum or cerebellum	12	The symptoms and signs of a secondary intracranial growth may precede those of the original growth
Other malformative tumours				
Craniopharyngioma	A tumour of developmental origin, may be cystic or solid. Does not usually present until adolescence. May calcify	Arises from embryological remnants of the craniopharyngeal duct (Rathke's pouch) into the suprasellar region and the posterior fossa	3	Sometimes referred to as cholesteatoma
Epidermoid cyst	Congenital fluid-filled cyst of the ectodermal layer. May contain keratin and cholesterol. Occurs in childhood	Posterior fossa		
Dermoid cyst	Similar to epidermoid cyst; arises from the ectodermal layer but contains more solid material such as hair, sebaceous glands or even teeth	Posterior fossa		Difficult to differentiate from other posterior fossa tumours until direct visualisation at surgery
Colloid cyst of the third ventricle	Rounded cystic tumour of childhood	Choroid plexus within the third ventricle		Often presents with an acute, sometimes intermittent hydrocephalus
Vascular malformations				
Angioma	Arterial and/or venous congenital abnormality comprising enlarged and tortuous vessels. Usually have a 'feeder' artery and a 'draining' vein	Anywhere in the cerebral cortex, most commonly in the region of the middle cerebral artery		A unilateral capillary-venous malformation and the presence of a facial naevus is termed the Sturge–Weber syndrome. Hamartomas are small vascular malformations

Table 9.4 Classification of tumours *(Continued)*

Tumour	Description	Usual site	Incidence (% of total)	Remarks
Angioblastoma	Cystic tumour comprised of angioblasts	Cerebellum		The patient may also exhibit an angioblastoma of the retina
Tumour of the anterior pituitary				
Pituitary adenoma	Benign, slow-growing, well encapsulated tumour. Classified by the clinical syndrome, i.e. the hormone produced. Three types of hypersecreting adenomas: prolactin-secreting (prolactinoma); excess growth hormone (acromegaly); ACTH-secreting (Cushing's disease). Hyposecreting tumours are very rare	Anterior lobe of the pituitary gland	8	Hyposecreting tumours will produce panhypopituitarism and chiasmal compression

Adapted from Hickey (2002).

tumour, and the patient should be encouraged to discuss their fears and anxieties. An excellent account of the problems encountered by patients can be found at news.bbc.co.uk/1/hi/health/3636697.stm and news.bbc.co.uk/1/hi/health/4193093.stm. This diary was maintained by Ivan Noble, a BBC reporter who had a malignant tumour and in it he spoke honestly of his feelings and concerns. He died, aged 37, early in 2005, but his account of his personal journey and comments from people worldwide who read the diary provide a remarkable insight into one person's experience of cancer and the impact his sharing of the experience has had for people in several countries (see Research Abstract 9.2). The nurse should be aware of the reality of a grieving process should the diagnosis be life limiting and accept the patient's reactions. Some fears and anxieties may be unfounded and can be alleviated by sensitive nursing interactions.

RESEARCH ABSTRACT 9.2

The purpose of this study was to describe the experience of being a patient with a brain tumour in the neurosurgery clinic of a university hospital. Eight brain tumour patients volunteered to participate. The data were collected by interviewing the participants on the day preceding brain surgery and 3–7 days postoperatively. The interviews used open-ended questions and the responses were analysed according to themes.

Preoperatively, some patients had a fearless and calm attitude towards their illness, whereas others were fearful and depressed. Postoperatively, the patients' body images changed, and they were concerned about the future. They perceived their care as matter-of-fact and friendly, both before and after the surgery, and they thought their basic needs were met. Some patients would have wanted more psychological support, especially after the surgery, whereas others found the psychological support adequate.

The patients were willing to participate in decision making about their care, and they trusted the professional skill and competence of the nurses. Suggested improvements in care were to minimise the atmosphere of urgency and hurry, appoint a primary nurse for each patient, and give more attention to after-care.

Lepola I, Toljamo M, Aho R, Louet T 2001 Being a brain tumor patient: a descriptive study of patients' experiences. Journal of Neuroscience Nursing 33(3): 143–147

Non-surgical interventions

Medication Steroids, particularly dexamethasone, are prescribed once a tumour is diagnosed, to reduce swelling around the tumour, and therefore ICP. The patient can feel better almost immediately after commencing steroids, finding relief from headache, nausea, vomiting and the effect of neurological deficits. However, there are established side-effects from steroid medication:

- irritation of the lining of the stomach — H_2 antagonists, e.g. cimetidine and ranitidine, are routinely prescribed to counteract this
- glycosuria — urine is routinely tested for glucose and ketones
- adrenal insufficiency, which will occur if medication is withdrawn suddenly (see Ch. 5).

Radiotherapy The radiotherapist can assess the patient in the ward or as an outpatient. If the patient requires urgent radiotherapy, this will be discussed by the radiotherapist, and the nurse should also be available to discuss with the patient their feelings and reactions to the treatment (see Ch. 31).

Inoperable tumours

A tumour may be inoperable due to inaccessibility or because of its type and size. Surgery could involve great risk of neurological deficits postoperatively. This situation offers a considerable challenge to all members of the multidisciplinary team to be able to communicate effectively and offer adequate support (see Chs 31 and 33). Sherwood et al (2004) highlight the needs of bereaved caregivers and identify the work of caring, informal and formal support, information and dealing with symptoms as key issues in achieving optimal end of life care.

Ongoing care

Major deficits

The provision of care at this stage will be dependent upon the patient's condition. Advice from specialists in palliation may be sought and the involvement of relatives will be crucial, as evidenced by the findings of Sherwood's work outlined above.

Preparation for discharge

The patient may have no neurological deficits or only slight deficits, such as limb weakness. If this is so, they should be encouraged to maintain their previous lifestyle.

If the patient has severe neurological deficits and requires considerable assistance with daily living, the situation should be discussed with both patient and family.

If the family members are anxious to have the patient at home, their wishes should be discussed with the ward team, community nurses and the patient's GP in order to ensure adequate support is available and in place prior to the patient's discharge. A home visit by the occupational therapist or physiotherapist may be advisable to assess the patient's requirements when at home.

Hospice care should be discussed prior to discharge and, if the patient and family wish, further information can be obtained from the palliative care team.

EPILEPSY

Epilepsy can be a symptom of an identifiable cause, such as head injury, or a disorder with no identifiable cause. Five per cent of the population will have a seizure in their lifetime, but with recurrence in only 0.5% (Lindsay & Bone 2004). The occurrence of an isolated seizure does not mean that the person is 'epileptic'. Box 9.12 shows causes at different stages of life. For some the cause will prove to be psychogenic, i.e. not of organic origin. Epileptic seizures can occur at any age, although the age of onset can often provide a clue as to the cause, e.g. in early childhood it may be due to pyrexia, whereas in the middle years of life, a brain tumour is more likely (Hickey 2002). Thomas (2002) describes the particular problems of epilepsy in older people.

PATHOPHYSIOLOGY

An intermittent, uncontrolled discharge of neurones within the central nervous system results in a seizure. It can range from a major motor convulsion to a brief period of lack of awareness and can occur in any individual at any time, even in an apparently healthy nervous system. Each individual is susceptible to seizure if the threshold level, which is different for everyone, is breached. In some instances, the cause is obvious, e.g. a seizure can be secondary to structural damage to the brain; in others, no apparent cause can be detected and it is described as an 'idiopathic' or 'primary' seizure.

Box 9.12

Causes of epilepsy at different stages of life

Newborn
- Hypocalcaemia
- Hypoglycaemia
- Asphyxia
- Hyperbilirubinaemia
- Water intoxication
- Inborn errors of metabolism
- Trauma
- Intracranial haemorrhage (vitamin K deficiency, thrombocytopenia)

Infancy
- Febrile convulsions
- Inborn errors of metabolism
- Congenital defects
- CNS infection

Childhood
- Trauma
- Congenital defects
- Arteriovenous malformation
- CNS infection

Adolescence and adulthood
- Trauma
- Neoplasm
- Withdrawal from drugs or alcohol
- Arteriovenous malformation
- CNS infection

Late adult
- Trauma
- Neoplasm
- Drug/alcohol withdrawal
- Vascular disease
- Degenerative disease
- CNS infection

Common presenting symptoms depend on when the person is examined. During certain types of seizure, the patient may be unconscious, apnoeic and incontinent of urine, whilst in others, changes are barely noticeable. Between seizures, the patient may show no neurological impairment or deficit. Seizures are classified as outlined in Box 9.13.

MEDICAL MANAGEMENT

Investigations Electroencephalography (EEG) will be performed (Louden 2004). Other investigations such as CT scanning and MRI may also be considered in order to identify possible organic causes.

The most dependable diagnostic tool is a reliable eyewitness account of the seizure.

Treatment The mainstay of therapy is medication, which is effective in keeping many people free from seizures. A range of anti-epileptic medication is available and guidance is provided by NICE (2004) on their use.

Box 9.13

Classification of seizures

I. Partial (focal, local) seizures
- A. Simple partial seizures (consciousness is not impaired)
  1. With motor symptoms
  2. With somatosensory or special sensory symptoms
  3. With autonomic symptoms
  4. With psychic symptoms
- B. Complex partial seizures (with impairment of consciousness)
  1. Beginning as simple partial seizures and progressing to impairment of consciousness
     — with no other features
     — with features as in I.A.1–4
     — with automatisms
  2. With impairment of consciousness at the start
     — with no other features
     — with features as in I.A.1–4
     — with automatisms
- C. Partial seizures evolving to secondarily generalised seizures
  1. Simple partial seizures evolving to generalised seizures
  2. Complex partial seizures evolving to generalised seizures
  3. Simple partial seizures evolving to complex partial seizures to generalised seizures

II. Generalised seizures (convulsive or non-convulsive)
- A. Absence seizure
  1. Absence seizures
  2. Atypical absence seizures
- B. Myoclonic seizures
- C. Clonic seizures
- D. Tonic seizures
- E. Tonic-clonic seizures
- F. Atonic seizures

III. Unclassified epileptic seizures
Includes all seizures that cannot be classified because of inadequate or incomplete data.

For those patients who have an identifiable focus amenable to surgery, this option will be offered. The most commonly employed technique is resection of the specific cortical area, e.g. temporal resection. Over half of the patients treated become free from seizure or acquire easier control.

NURSING PRIORITIES AND MANAGEMENT: Epileptic seizures

Most individuals with seizures live independently, with regular monitoring by their GP or at an epilepsy outpatient clinic. However, occasionally treatment loses its efficacy and the patient requires to be admitted to hospital for reassessment.

Immediate priorities

Once notification is received at the ward that a patient is to be admitted due to a worsening of seizures, the following essential equipment should be assembled and be readily available:

- oxygen and suction in good working order
- a selection of various sizes of artificial airways
- charts for recording neurological status, vital signs and seizures
- side rails should be in place and may be padded for additional safety
- anticonvulsant medication, particularly in the intravenous or intramuscular form.

If the patient is having a seizure, the following actions must always be carried out:

- ensure privacy is provided for the patient
- use suction if necessary to prevent aspiration of secretions
- ensure side rails are in place, using pillows as padding if required
- ensure safety by removing any objects or furniture likely to cause harm
- loosen any restrictive clothing
- insert an airway only when teeth have unclenched (after the tonic stage); any attempts to insert objects into the patient's mouth prior to this serve no purpose and may cause harm to the nurse (bitten fingers) or to the patient (broken teeth)
- record pupillary activity — pupils will begin to react as the patient recovers.

Immediately following a seizure the nurse should:

- place the patient in the recovery position, to facilitate the drainage of secretions
- allow the patient to sleep with minimal disturbance
- allow time for the patient to wake up and provide gentle reassurance and assistance to encourage reorientation
- record a description of what happened on the seizure observation chart.

The nurse should record:

- the time at which the seizure occurred
- what the patient was doing at the time
- any aura or crying out prior to the seizure
- any loss of consciousness
- which parts of the body were affected
- any stiffening or jerky movements
- any urinary or faecal incontinence
- the length of each phase
- the length of the recovery period
- the patient's behaviour after the seizure
- any weakness in part of the limbs.

Prescribed anticonvulsant medication should be administered and, where appropriate, medical staff informed.

For further helpful information on caring for patients at risk of seizure, see Lanfear (2002), Pena (2003) and Wehrle (2003).

Further considerations

The patient should be allowed to express their feelings and fears and they and their family should be given adequate explanations and support. Explanation about the medication, its effects and side-effects, will encourage the patient's adherence to prescribed regimens. Monitoring of medication serum levels should be carried out, as this test will indicate if there is an adequate or inadequate dosage of the medication, or if the blood levels are too high. If too high, the patient may experience side-effects; if too low, seizures may recur. Common side-effects of anticonvulsant medications are:

- drowsiness
- dizziness
- gastric upset
- diplopia
- ataxia.

The patient must be allowed time to come to terms with the diagnosis of epilepsy. They may experience feelings of anger, grief and/or disbelief, and the nurse should discuss with both the patient and family the realities of epilepsy, but encourage a positive outlook. This should stress the full life that can be led, despite the diagnosis.

The patient may note the experience of an aura prior to a seizure and the nurse can advise how to use the time available to ensure personal safety. Advice should be given prior to discharge about safety in the home (see Box 9.14) and the possible involvement of the primary care team (Bingham 2004).

STOP THINK **9.10** What information does your local library have about self-help groups for people with epilepsy?

Equally, 'triggers' that may induce a seizure should be discussed, such as:

- lack of food and sleep
- excessive heat
- constipation
- menstruation
- alcohol
- anxiety or stress.

Medical opinion varies as to whether someone with epilepsy should drink alcohol, as it can interfere with anti-epileptic medications, preventing them from effecting the intended seizure control. Large amounts of any liquid are known to trigger a seizure, but significant alcohol intake is also often associated with late night, irregular eating habits and forgotten tablets. However, whether or not to drink alcohol is an individual decision, bearing in mind medical advice on the particular case.

It may be suggested to the patient that they carry a card or wear a MedicAlert to inform about their condition should a seizure occur.

Employment

The patient's employment situation should be discussed, especially if it entails driving or operating machinery. The patient must be told of the requirement to inform the DVLA of their liability to have seizures and should be advised to stop driving in the meantime. This may present major problems to the patient, who may have to look for alternative employment; this may affect self-esteem or outlook for the future.

It must be recognised that some employers may not be prepared to employ someone with epilepsy and that their current position may have to be reviewed. Epilepsy is common in adolescents. They may experience a change in outlook for the future and have to consider a change to their hoped-for career structure.

Physical activity

The patient should be encouraged to continue normal physical activities, with some emphasis being placed on the need to take adequate precautions, e.g. when swimming. It should be suggested that the patient lets someone know or takes a friend who could deal with a potential seizure.

Involving the patient's family

The patient's family should be given time and the opportunity to express their perceptions and concerns, and the nurse should be prepared to provide advice and explanations. The nurse should explain about the type of seizure the patient is experiencing, e.g. a generalised seizure, and family members should be told what to expect if a seizure occurs, e.g. that the patient will have sudden uncontrolled movements and will appear to be holding their breath. They should know exactly what to do and why they are doing it. Epilepsy Action provides helpful advice through their website (see 'Useful websites'). Consideration must be

Box 9.14

Safety measures at home

- Fireguards are essential and should be securely fixed to the wall.
- Smokers should consider and understand the dangers of smoking in an armchair or in bed.
- Cordless kettles and irons are safer than trailing flexes.
- Pot handles should point to the back of the cooker. Hot food or liquid should not be carried.
- Sharp corners can be covered by rounded plastic pieces; these are available from supermarkets, children's departments and ironmongers.
- Glass doors should either use safety glass or be covered in safety film; available from children's departments.
- If seizures are frequent and unpredictable, the patient should let someone know when they are taking a bath or shower. The water should not be very hot and the depth should only be a few inches. The patient should turn the taps off before getting in. A shower is more suitable, particularly if the patient can sit, unless the shower tray has a high lip where water can gather.
- If the toilet door can be hung to open outwards, the person will not block it if they fall. Locks should not be used, except for special safety locks that can be opened in an emergency. An 'engaged' sign can be used instead.
- Soft pillows can be dangerous. It is best to avoid pillows or to obtain special safety pillows.
- In a small proportion of people with epilepsy, a seizure may be triggered by flickering light. These people should place the television set at eye level, at least 3 m away, with a small, lit lamp on top.
- An epileptic parent should ensure that garden gates have locks, so that, should the parent have a seizure, their children cannot wander off.

CASE HISTORY 9.2

Miss S

I am 22 years of age, and was diagnosed with epilepsy 4 months ago. I had previously thought epilepsy was something that became apparent at birth or in early childhood. Now I understand that the particular type of epilepsy that I have, juvenile myoclonic epilepsy, is commonly diagnosed in the late teens and early twenties.

At first the diagnosis did not seem to worry me. It was a novelty, both to me and to my family and friends. However, 2 or 3 months later, the novelty wore off, and the long-term aspects of epilepsy became more apparent. It was only then that the reality of having epilepsy began to sink in.

Being a student and living away from home has meant that my friends have carried most of the burden of supporting me. It has been of immense comfort to know that I can trust those around me and I have not encountered many negative reactions. On the contrary, my family and friends have shown an interest in all aspects of epilepsy, not only in what they should do if someone has a seizure. I have also found, however, that living away from my parents has made it difficult for them. Whilst they have supported me completely, they have never seen me have a seizure. I think that this has made it difficult for them to accept that I do have epilepsy.

I have found that there are a number of ways in which epilepsy impacts upon my life. It has become necessary for me to lead an organised life, so that I get enough sleep and am able to take my medication at the appropriate times. The biggest impact I have found involves challenging the stigma that, for some people, still surrounds epilepsy. It is sometimes difficult to combine maintaining my privacy with informing the appropriate people. I feel that if I am not open about having epilepsy, then I am contributing to a belief that epilepsy is something which should not be talked about, or that people should be ashamed of being associated with. For this reason I decided to be entirely open about having epilepsy from the start.

I have found that there is a very fine line between being sensible and letting epilepsy take over my life. In reality there are very few restrictions placed upon me, but at the same time, this does not mean that epilepsy is not always at the back of my mind.

With thanks to Sarah Canning, student nurse, Edinburgh University, for her Case History 9.2.

RESEARCH ABSTRACT 9.3

A feasibility study of a psycho-educational family intervention — 'Be Seizure Smart' — aimed at improving attitudes and increasing family functioning was conducted. The intervention was individually tailored for each family member by:

- providing information about epilepsy, treatment and seizure management according to the individual's knowledge base
- addressing unique concerns and fears
- providing emotional support.

Participants were 10 families of children with epilepsy, aged 7–13 years. Data were collected about 2 weeks before and after the intervention, which was delivered over 3–4 months, by using structured interviews. One-tailed paired t tests were used to determine changes from pre-test to post-test. Participants were also asked to evaluate the intervention and make suggestions about how the intervention could better meet their needs. Results generally indicated that the intervention had the anticipated effects. Knowledge scores increased for both parents and children. Children had fewer concerns and were more satisfied with family relationships.

Information and support needs decreased for both children and their parents. Information need reductions were statistically significant for both parents and children; support need reductions were significantly reduced only for parents. Although child and parent attitudes were more positive after the intervention, this finding was not statistically significant. Moreover, parents indicated overall satisfaction with the programme and appreciated the convenience of in-home telephone interactions with the nurse and receiving information specific to their needs in the mail. It was concluded that the 'Be Seizure Smart' intervention had strong potential to help children with epilepsy and their families and that the intervention should be developed further and piloted on a larger sample.

Austin J K, McNelis A M, Shore C P, Dunn D W, Musick B 2002 A feasibility study of a family seizure management programme: Be Seizure Smart. Journal of Neuroscience Nursing 34(1): 30–37

given to meeting the needs of children whose parents have epilepsy. Advice should include the following:

- Ensure the safety of the individual, which can involve removing harmful objects and ensuring that all restrictive clothing is loosened
- After the seizure, place them on their side, in the recovery position, and allow them to sleep, giving them adequate time to wake up and reorientate to time and place
- Ensure that the family knows to seek medical advice if a seizure lasts longer than usual or if seizures continue without time for the individual to recover
- Ensure that the family is aware that the individual may have feelings of shock, anger and lack of self-esteem and that time should be allowed for them to come to terms with these feelings (see Case History 9.2).

Greenhill and Betts (2003) provide useful advice on the lifelong care of women with epilepsy.

The multidisciplinary team should work together to give the individual and their family encouragement and advice about being at home. Bingham (2004) highlights the provision of support for people in the community who have epilepsy. It may be helpful to explain that one person in every 200 has epilepsy, so that they can recognise that they are not alone. Involvement in groups for people with epilepsy provides advice and support (see Research Abstract 9.3).

STOP THINK **9.11** Discuss with your fellow students what may be some of the social implications of epilepsy (see Case History 9.2). Try to find out whether someone with epilepsy is permitted to drive a car.

MULTIPLE SCLEROSIS

Multiple sclerosis is a chronic neurological disorder and is the most common cause of neurological disability in young adults in the UK (MacLean 2004). The age of onset is 20–50 years and it is slightly more common in females. The cause is unknown and the disorder typically follows a pattern of relapses or exacerbations and remissions (Lindsay & Bone 2004).

The occurrence of multiple sclerosis varies significantly in different parts of the world. Its incidence in the Orkney and Shetland Islands of the UK is 309 per 100 000, whereas in Italy it is 13 per 100 000 (Lindsay & Bone 2004). It is therefore described as a disorder of temperate climates. However, those who move from an area of high risk to one of low risk do not lessen the chance of the disease occurring. Multiple sclerosis is not hereditary, but the risk of a child developing multiple sclerosis where a parent is afflicted is approximately 15 times greater than in the unaffected population (Lindsay & Bone 2004).

A definitive diagnosis is usually difficult because demyelination develops over a varying period of time. To be conclusive, there must be dissemination over a period of time and in several locations within the nervous system.

PATHOPHYSIOLOGY

According to Lindsay and Bone (2004), it is thought that a viral infection affects the white matter of the brain and spinal cord, producing demyelinated lesions that prevent normal conduction of nerve impulses. The demyelination results in scarring or sclerotic patches, and the remission, typical in multiple sclerosis, is the result of healing of these areas. However, in time, these lesions degenerate to a point where recovery is unlikely and the resultant disruption of function becomes permanent.

Common presenting symptoms Clinical features vary considerably, depending on which nerves are affected, but may include:

- blurring of vision or double vision — an early and common symptom; a patient presenting to their GP or practice nurse with this particular symptom is always investigated with a view to diagnosis of multiple sclerosis
- weakness and dragging of limbs and extreme fatigue
- slurred speech
- nystagmus — a disturbance in the normal balance of the eye in which a slow drift in one direction is followed by a fast corrective movement
- loss of sensation in a specific area of the body, e.g. part of the arm
- difficulty in determining the position of limbs in space
- 'stiff limbs'
- intention tremor
- clumsiness/difficulty with movement
- incontinence/retention of urine or hesitancy with urinary flow.

Sometimes fatigue will override all these symptoms.

MEDICAL MANAGEMENT

Investigations

Lumbar puncture Examination of the CSF may reveal:

- a mild rise in cell count
- an elevated total protein and gamma globulin fraction (in 60% of cases)
- oligoclonal bands in the gamma globulin in 80% of cases (Lindsay & Bone 2004).

Visual evoked responses A delay in conduction is noted in the pathways.

RESEARCH ABSTRACT 9.4

The purpose of this study was to describe the experiences of patients with relapsing multiple sclerosis (MS) who are being treated with interferon beta-1a. MS patients often experience fear and uncertainty about their future and derive benefit from understanding their diagnosis, as well as learning about their anticipated disease course. Interferon beta-1a treatment can delay the accumulation of physical disability that naturally occurs over time in patients with untreated relapsing MS and thus offer hope for their future. However, patients may be afraid to start interferon beta-1a because they do not know what to expect.

To answer the question, 'What is the patient's experience on interferon beta-1a', we used Heideggerian phenomenological and Colaizzi's qualitative data analysis techniques to interpret serial interviews of 15 patients with relapsing MS. Interviews were audiotaped, transcribed verbatim and analysed using the Martin qualitative data analysis computer program. The theme clusters that emerged were learning, feelings, adaptation and interferon beta-1a issues.

An exhaustive description of the phenomena that were derived illustrates the patients' process of learning about their illness and adapting to changes in their lives. Starting a new treatment requires coping and challenges use of resources. Social support is vital to patients, particularly those who have difficulty injecting themselves. Most of the patients expressed a sense of improvement in their condition since starting on interferon beta-1a treatment and considered it crucial to their hope for the future.

Miller C, Jezewski M A 2001 A phenomenologic assessment of relapsing MS patients' experiences during treatment with interferon beta-1a. Journal of Neuroscience Nursing 33(5): 240–244

MRI identifies areas of demyelination.

CT scan may be required to exclude other disorders (see Appendix 1).

Treatment There is still no specific treatment. Steroid therapy may be helpful in acute exacerbations to manage symptoms and physiotherapy is helpful in the rehabilitation of numb, affected limbs. The use of interferon has been tried in some patients; however, clinical outcomes have not conclusively proved its usefulness. Outcomes continue to be assessed as part of a national surveillance scheme (Lindsay & Bone 2004) (see Research Abstract 9.4). Many complementary therapies exist and are used with varying degrees of success, e.g. special diets and hyperbaric oxygen.

Essentially, care consists of supporting the patient and their family and alleviating symptoms.

NURSING PRIORITIES AND MANAGEMENT: Multiple sclerosis

The extensive tests involved in obtaining a diagnosis may necessitate admission to hospital or attendance at an investigation unit on an outpatient basis.

Many patients with multiple sclerosis lead a normal life at home, requiring admission to hospital only if they

CASE HISTORY 9.3

Multiple sclerosis: a carer's view

'It's the "not knowing" what I'll be like tomorrow that I find so difficult to cope with,' was the heartfelt cry of one MS sufferer. Caught up in the turmoil of wanting desperately to make plans for the following day, she was weary of the continual conflict between her desire to be independent and her body's limitations. The uncertainty and unpredictability of MS make it particularly wearing and difficult to come to terms with. As both a nurse and the relative of an MS sufferer, it would appear to me that coping with frustration becomes a major part of everyday life:

- frustration at having to rely heavily on family and friends
- frustration at loss of bodily function
- frustration at some members of society who don't seem to understand
- frustration at feeling a burden.

Coming to terms with limitations is only one aspect of living with MS; making the most of life within the confines of such restrictions is another. When caring for someone with MS, whether in hospital or in the community, the most important part we can play is in helping the patient to maintain their integrity and to adapt to changes imposed by further degeneration.

experience deterioration in their condition. Lisak (2001) provides an overview of the symptomatic management of multiple sclerosis, and comprehensive guidelines on the management of patients in both primary and secondary care have been issued by NICE (2003b).

For the patient who is experiencing difficulties, hospitalisation will not only provide an opportunity for nursing and other health care staff to help the patient and their family to deal with problems that are disrupting the patient's daily life, but also enable the nurse to learn more from the patient about the experience of living with multiple sclerosis (see Case History 9.3). Courts et al (2004), in a small qualitative study, explored both the lived experience of multiple sclerosis and their participants' perspective of their needs, the most poignant of which was the need for someone to listen and to help them to learn about their condition. Williams (2004) reviews the evidence for current practice in the management of patients during a relapse or exacerbation of their condition and evaluates how the evidence can be incorporated into patient care.

Immediate priorities

Communicating

The patient admitted for investigations is likely to be fearful and will require adequate explanation about the tests and examinations to be carried out. Frequently, the nurse is asked about these tests and should be prepared to answer questions or, if unable to do so, should find the answer for the patient. It is important that there is an awareness of the patient's knowledge regarding the condition, as the patient will either fear the worst, often with only a partial understanding of what the diagnosis may be, or may not be aware of the possibility of having multiple sclerosis until the diagnosis is confirmed. Increasingly, patients are well informed from use of the internet.

It is advisable for the nurse to be present when the doctor is speaking to the patient, so that the nurse knows what information the patient has received. Often the patient wishes to discuss certain points and will find it reassuring to seek supporting advice and information from the nurse after the doctor has left.

The patient will need time to consider the condition and what effects it will have on their outlook for the future. Patients often experience a range of feelings and emotions related to the loss of self-esteem and body image and may worry about how the condition will eventually affect them. Expressed feelings may include shock, denial, depression and anger. The nurse must accept these feelings and provide adequate support to facilitate the patient's coping mechanisms. Providing information about support groups, e.g. the Multiple Sclerosis Society (see 'Useful websites') is often helpful. Normally, the patient's family should be included and they will require explanations about their relative's condition. They too should be provided with opportunities to discuss their feelings and fears.

Deterioration in the patient's physical condition can cause major psychological and social problems. Family members and/or carers may experience difficulties in coping and may require help and advice.

Admission to hospital during the course of the disease progression can cause considerable stress, especially for the patient who has a set routine at home that allows maintenance of independence. The nurse should encourage the patient to continue to be independent and to follow their daily routine as far as possible when in hospital. People often have well-developed coping mechanisms, and if nurses indicate that they think they know best, this may cause patients frustration and anger (Hickey 2002). They can then seem difficult to look after and a vicious circle develops, where patients dread even more having to come into hospital.

Subsequent considerations

Problems with communication

Communication impairment in the patient with multiple sclerosis can include difficulties in pronouncing words, slow and/or slurred speech and poor concentration. This can create major problems with everyday communication for the patient. People may not understand that, although the patient has speech problems, their intellectual capabilities are not affected, and reactions towards the patient may cause them to lose confidence in their ability to communicate.

The speech and language therapist should be involved and can give advice on how to improve the patient's ability to communicate. Useful techniques to help the patient include:

- ensure that an erect posture is maintained, as this aids breathing and assists with speech
- reduce background noise as much as possible
- encourage the patient to express the most important points at the beginning of a sentence, when energy and concentration are greatest
- use communication aids such as picture boards or computer boards.

Maintaining a safe environment

The patient with multiple sclerosis can experience difficulties with:

- movement, e.g. ataxia, unintentional tremors or paralysis
- vision, e.g. diplopia
- sensory disturbance, e.g. detection of pain and temperature.

Account needs to be taken of the patient's immediate environment, both at home and in hospital, in order to avoid accidents. The patient may already be aware of the potential dangers at home and may take care to avoid them, or may be experiencing a deterioration and realise that adaptations are required in order to maintain safety.

Some patients may be unable to accept that their condition is deteriorating and that they are not able to perform certain tasks safely. When in hospital, an accurate assessment of the patient's condition, level of understanding and, if necessary, home conditions should be made. This will involve assessments by the community team, including the community nurse, occupational therapist, physiotherapist and social worker.

In hospital, the nurse should involve the patient in making any necessary changes to their new surroundings, as they will know best what suits them, e.g. the location and height of the bed, depending on their mobility. Ensure there is adequate space to manoeuvre a wheelchair properly. The nurse-call system should be within easy reach and the patient should be instructed in its use. The patient with clumsiness of movement or tremor may require assistance with some activities, e.g. at mealtimes, when there is a risk of spilling liquid and food, possibly risking a burn.

Mobility

Maintaining mobility plays a large part in being independent. A problem for the patient with multiple sclerosis is the uncertainty of the rate at which deterioration in mobility will occur. The patient's family should be aware of any limitations that are necessary and also encourage the proper use of any mobility aids required when at home.

The attitude of the ward team is very important; the members should work together to encourage a positive outlook for the patient, while making time to understand the patient's and family's feelings and fears.

If the patient uses mobility aids at home, they should also be used when admission to hospital is required. This enables the patient to maintain independence and also allows the physiotherapist to assess the effectiveness of any aids. For example, if the patient's mobility is deteriorating, is use of a walking stick sufficient to maintain safety? Common problems may include ataxia, limb weakness and lack of coordination. Techniques which may be useful in helping these problems are:

- maintaining a good posture
- when walking, making contact with the ground with the heel of the foot first
- taking care to place feet firmly in the direction of travel
- looking straight ahead rather than down at the ground
- relaxing and trying not to feel self-conscious.

The physiotherapist may suggest exercises to maintain the function of a limb and to prevent muscle wastage, and the nurse and the patient's family can give encouragement for the exercises to be practised. Rietberg et al (2005), in a systematic review of exercise therapy, concluded that, for those patients not experiencing a relapse, exercise can be beneficial.

Skin care

The patient and family should be taught the importance of regular skin inspection, e.g. to observe the sacrum and heels closely and to look for redness or blanching of the skin. If this occurs, the patient should be aware of the importance of relieving the pressure from the problem area, e.g. by lying on their side in bed.

Using a wheelchair

The physiotherapist and occupational therapist may advise that the patient requires a wheelchair in order to maintain mobility. It can be very distressing for the patient to realise that this stage has been reached. It must be emphasised that this does not mean that the patient becomes totally reliant on the wheelchair and is unable to maintain independence. The patient may need to use the wheelchair outside the house only if required to walk a long distance, or around the house only when feeling tired.

The patient may have become unable to stand and be able to weight-bear for short periods only. In this case, they are dependent on the wheelchair for mobility, but should be encouraged to continue to perform tasks involving their hands, e.g. shaving and washing, in order to maintain a degree of independence.

If the patient requires physiotherapy when at home, advice and support can be obtained from the community physiotherapist. Some local multiple sclerosis societies also offer a physiotherapy service.

Advice should be given to the patient about when to use the wheelchair, what in particular to look for, and why:

- The wheelchair should be used only when necessary, so that the patient utilises any residual walking ability, thus helping to prevent muscle weakness.
- The importance of relieving pressure, especially on the sacral area, should be discussed, as the immobile patient may lie or sit in the same position for a period of time.
- Careful positioning of limbs should be ensured, taking into account any weakness or paraesthesia.
- The footrest on the wheelchair should always be used; care should also be taken that no part of the foot or ankle is rubbing against the footrest or wheel.
- The legs should be placed in proper alignment and the patient should check regularly that the limbs are safely in position on the footrest (www.mssociety.org.uk).

Balance of rest and exercise

The patient should be advised about the importance of rest periods to avoid becoming overtired or overstressed, which will exacerbate the condition. Relaxation techniques and a specific rest/exercise programme may be beneficial and should be discussed with the patient and their family.

Fatigue is a significant symptom of multiple sclerosis and can enforce changes in the patient's lifestyle. The patient may have to learn to ask for help when feeling tired and this can be difficult for someone who may normally have led an active, independent life. Although rest is very important, exercise is also vital to maintain muscle strength and help reduce the risk of spasticity. It will also improve circulation and prevent pressure ulcers and joint stiffness. Exercise will contribute to maintaining the patient's independence.

Employment

If the patient's current employment involves physical exertion, this may prove problematic with regard to returning to work. The patient may have to consider how their disorder will affect current employment and think about finding alternative work, although in many cases this may prove impossible.

Eliminating

The patient may experience bladder dysfunction, which can vary in severity, including incontinence, urinary frequency or urine retention. Problems with constipation are also of concern. The urinary problems are due to the reflex action of the bladder having been disturbed due to sites of demyelination in the lower spine, particularly the cauda equina.

The social implications of incontinence can be enormous and some patients will avoid going out for fear of embarrassment (see Ch. 24). The patient should be encouraged to take time when passing urine and to ensure that the bladder is completely empty. Journeys can be planned to take account of the availability of toilets and this will reassure the patient. If a urine infection is suspected, a specimen should be sent to bacteriology for culture and sensitivity. It may be necessary to use aids such as protective pants and pads (see Ch. 24).

Urinary catheterisation may be required if persistent urinary retention is experienced. Some patients will prefer self-catheterisation at set intervals and many become very competent at performing this procedure. Adequate instruction on hygienic technique can facilitate this (see Ch. 8). Advice from a continence advisor may also be useful (see Ch. 24).

Some patients will require an indwelling catheter, and support should be provided to enable them to come to terms with this alteration to body image.

The importance of an adequate fluid intake of 2.5–3 L/day should be stressed. Many patients mistakenly think that if they stop drinking they will no longer be incontinent.

The immobile patient will be especially prone to constipation, which will aggravate coexisting urinary problems. The patient and the family should be advised as to how constipation can be avoided by taking an appropriate diet, an adequate fluid intake and maintaining as much mobility as possible. Regular aperients may be required and the occasional use of enemas and suppositories may be indicated.

Expressing sexuality

The patient may experience a change in body image, and the nurse should try to encourage a positive attitude in order to improve the patient's self-esteem.

Sexual counselling may be beneficial for both partners.

Men may experience impotence and women diminished libido, due to neurological damage. The patient may be too embarrassed or worried to discuss such difficulties with a nurse or doctor, and external services such as Outsiders (see 'Useful websites') and marriage guidance services may be a helpful alternative (see also Ch. 34).

Advice on contraception may be required, especially by women, as some oral contraceptives may interfere with existing medication. Pregnancy should be avoided during active stages of the disease as this may exacerbate the symptoms, although successful pregnancy may be achieved.

STOP THINK **9.12** Find out where the marriage guidance and sexual health counselling services are in your area.

Eating and drinking

There has been some research into the link between diet and multiple sclerosis, and a number of specialised diets have been identified (www.mssociety.org.uk). It has been demonstrated that people with multiple sclerosis have higher levels of saturated fats and lower levels of polyunsaturated fats in the myelin sheath and the dietary advice outlined below may be useful to patients. They should:

- decrease the intake of saturated fats and increase the intake of unsaturated fats
- try to include more chicken and white fish in the diet
- ensure that when cooking red meat, visible fat is trimmed off prior to cooking
- note that liver contains vitamin B_{12} and arachidonic acid, an essential fatty acid (see Ch. 21)
- use semi-skimmed or skimmed milk
- ensure a high-fibre content, i.e. wholemeal and wheaten bread, pulses and cereals, and eat plenty of fruit and fresh vegetables.

The speech and language therapist and dietitian may be able to offer assistance and advice if the patient has swallowing difficulties. The nurse can assist by encouraging the patient to:

- sit up straight with the head supported, if necessary
- eat in a quiet, relaxed atmosphere and not speak while eating
- take time when eating, to avoid choking
- eat certain types of food that are easier to swallow, e.g. semi-solid or liquidised foods.

Personal cleansing and dressing

In hospital and at home, the patient should be encouraged to maintain independence with regard to washing and dressing. It may seem to the patient, and at times to the nurse or to the patient's family, that it would be quicker and easier for the nurse to do these activities for the patient. The patient may feel under stress to hurry in order to release the nurse to go and attend to other patients. The nurse should explain that there is no hurry to have everything finished for a set time.

The carer should be encouraged to allow the patient to perform these activities at home, so that they have some degree of independence. The occupational therapist can assess the patient when in hospital and give advice regarding washing and dressing, offer a range of dressing aids and suggest specially adapted clothing, e.g. with Velcro instead of buttons and zips. The patient can be referred to the community occupational therapist if further difficulties are anticipated, due to the possible deterioration in the patient's condition.

STOP THINK **9.13** Many people with multiple sclerosis develop particular patterns of behaviour over the years. Have you or any of your fellow students observed this in such patients, either at home or in hospital? If so, can you describe them? How did you adapt your work to fit in with these routines?

Patient education

The patient and the family should be as well informed as possible about the diagnosis of multiple sclerosis and should be aware of the most successful methods of maintaining independence. They should know their primary care team and understand that they can increasingly call on the community services, e.g. the community nurse, physiotherapist, GP, as the patient's condition worsens. They should also be aware of the possibility of the occurrence of behavioural and mood changes. Euphoria, depression, apathy and emotional lability are common.

Preparation for discharge

Episodic hospitalisation may become necessary as the multiple sclerosis condition becomes more widespread, and the patient and family should be given the opportunity to voice any worries or fears to allow adequate preparation for discharge on each occasion. A comprehensive assessment of the patient's home situation should be performed, if possible well before there is any mobility problem, and should involve all members of the multidisciplinary team in order to gauge the suitability and likely success of discharge.

In cases where there is decreasing ability to perform activities of living, a home visit for the patient involving the nurse, occupational therapist, social worker and physiotherapist may be indicated. Assessment of the home situation, layout and the patient's ability to adapt, while maintaining safety and maximal independence, can be carried out. Some adjustments may be required in the house, e.g. bath aids and rearrangement of furniture. If the patient depends on a wheelchair for mobility, the doorways may have to be widened, cupboards lowered, and a shower may be required instead of a bath.

The patient may have to be rehoused at ground floor level in order to accommodate access to and from the house in a wheelchair. This involves major changes not only for the patient but also for the family and can be very traumatic, especially if they have to leave a district they have lived in for a long time, and to leave good friends and neighbours.

Advice regarding income and benefits available, e.g. mobility and attendance allowance, can be given by the social worker. Outpatient appointments can be arranged for physiotherapy, occupational or speech therapy, if necessary.

Some doctors advocate discussing the possibility of relapse so that the patient is better prepared when it occurs. On the other hand, some patients may not have a period of relapse for up to 20 years and may worry unnecessarily if the subject is broached too soon. As indicated, some patients may benefit from being informed of the availability of support groups, and it may be possible for the patient to be seen by a member of a support group prior to discharge. Such groups offer a range of services, including general advice, physiotherapy and ongoing counselling.

For further information on the experiences and health concerns of people with multiple sclerosis as they grow older, see Finlayson et al (2004).

PARKINSON'S DISEASE

Parkinson's disease is a chronic neurodegenerative disorder of the basal nuclei, with a slow onset that progresses gradually, often resulting in premature death (Lindsay & Bone 2004). It has an annual incidence of approximately 0.2/1000 and a prevalence of 1.5/1000 in the UK (Haslett et al 2002). Both incidence and prevalence increase with age, with the majority of those diagnosed aged over 60, and it affects both genders; however, McCall (2003) observes that one in seven will be under 50 years. A syndrome indistinguishable from Parkinson's disease is seen in some substance abusers. Some 'designer' drugs contain a substance called MPTP (1-methyl-4-phenyl-1,2,3,6,tetrahydrapyridine) which can cause typical Parkinsonian features. It is thought that research which seeks to understand this syndrome may lead to further developments in the treatment of Parkinson's disease (Lindsay & Bone 2004).

PATHOPHYSIOLOGY

The patient with Parkinson's disease (or syndrome) is known to have degenerative changes in the substantia nigra which forms part of the basal nuclei. Depletion of the dopaminergic neurones in the substantia nigra results in a decrease in the levels of the neurotransmitter, dopamine, essential for the control of movement, coordination and posture. As a result, the balance between dopamine and acetylcholine is lost and the acetylcholine effects exaggerated. Several forms of Parkinson's disease have been identified, including medication-induced Parkinsonism. For example, the use of phenothiazines such as chlorpromazine in mental health disorders may lead to the development of tardive dyskinesia (Cortese et al 2004, Houltram & Scanlan 2004). Another unusual form was an outbreak of encephalitis lethargica in 1916–28, and those afflicted, now in their late 80s or 90s, developed Parkinson's disease. No new such outbreaks have occurred in the UK. However, although viral, ischaemic and ageing processes have been implicated, for most of those who have Parkinson's disease, no specific cause can be identified.

Common presenting symptoms The clinical features may include:

- a triad of symptoms: tremor, muscle rigidity and dyskinesia, including slowness in initiating or repeating movements and impairment of fine movements; in addition, there are the excessive cholinergic effects, e.g. excessive gastrointestinal secretions
- cramps
- expressionless face
- disturbance in free-flowing movement, particularly on initiating movement or changing direction (see p. 436)
- loss of postural reflexes
- autonomic manifestations, e.g. excessive perspiration
- general weakness and increased fatigue.

For further information, see Haslett et al (2002).

9.14 With reference to your chosen physiology text, e.g. Marieb (2004), consider how the basal nuclei regulate the groundwork for the fine control of movement, not under voluntary control. Think how any disturbance of the function of the basal nuclei in general, and the substantia nigra in particular, can result in the symptoms seen in disorders known as the dyskinesias, such as Parkinson's disease/ syndrome.

MEDICAL MANAGEMENT

Investigations such as CT scanning may be considered in order to eliminate other disorders. There is no specific diagnostic test for Parkinson's disease. Diagnosis is usually based on clinical presentation.

Treatment Medication is the mainstay of treatment and the aim is to maintain the patient at the lowest effective level of medication (McGuire 1997). Treatment is symptomatic and does not halt the pathological process. Medicines can be divided into different categories and their prescription and use in particular combinations, or on their own, requires careful management and monitoring.

Dopaminergic preparations such as levodopa are administered to replace the depleted dopamine. In older people, levodopa with a decarboxylase inhibitor is often used; however, it is only used once the symptoms of the disease compromise the individual's normal functioning. In younger patients, dopa-agonists, e.g. pergolide, are given to stimulate the surviving dopamine receptors in the basal ganglia. Anticholinergic agents such as trihexyphenidyl may be considered to treat the cramps, tremor and rigidity associated with Parkinsonism, but their use does appear to be receding (McGuire 1997). The enzymes monoamine oxidase A and B play a key role in the breakdown of dopamine. Selegiline is a medication which inhibits this process and appears to have a symptomatic effect. Amantadine acts by allowing the dopamine to stay longer at its site of action without being used up by other cells. It may be useful in the control of tremor but helps only a small proportion of patients.

Patients who experience sudden fluctuations in their symptoms in spite of careful management of their medications may be prescribed apomorphine. This is a potent dopa-agonist and is sometimes given as a 'rescue' medicine in advanced states. It produces a direct effect at the sites where dopamine is active in the brain. It is usually given by intermittent subcutaneous injection, but continuous infusion may be considered (Hagell & Odin 2001).

Many of the medications have variable side-effects and accurate titration usually necessitates admission to hospital. Another curious aspect is an 'on–off' phenomenon, whereby, at certain times of the day, the patient loses the benefit of the dopamine and becomes rigid and immobile for a period of time. It is important to recognise this, as alteration to the medication regimen can reduce the likelihood of this happening.

Surgery may be indicated for some patients. This comprises, for example, bilateral subthalamic nucleus stimulation (Eriksen et al 2003) or specific neurosurgery for movement disorders (Tornqvist 2001).

NURSING PRIORITIES AND MANAGEMENT: Parkinson's disease

Parkinson's disease has an insidious onset. Some of its effects may be attributed by the patient and their family to old age. The progressive nature of the disease, combined with the potential embarrassment of many of its symptoms, can result in a patient who is aware of what is happening but at a loss to know how to obtain help (see Case History 9.4).

The importance of the role of the patient's family or carer, and of the community nurse and primary health care team in supporting them, cannot be overstressed. The family's or carer's ability to cope with the mobility and other problems associated with Parkinson's disease can make the difference between a level of independence, with the patient living in their own home, and enforced, frequent hospitalisation or long-term care with total dependence on others for everything. Mobility aids may be of limited use. The use of self-assessment in the earlier stages of the disease, while the patient is still able to articulate their needs, is helpful, both for the accurate evaluation of needs and to facilitate empowerment of the patient in sharing in decision-making about their care.

Immediate priorities

Typically, many of the early symptoms of Parkinson's disease may be treated by the family doctor, with the patient and their family making necessary adjustments to their home, e.g. removal of rugs and other obstacles over which the patient may trip.

The progress of the disease can vary, but should the patient's condition worsen, admission to hospital may become necessary. Hospitalisation will provide an opportunity for nursing and other health care staff, such as the physiotherapist, speech and language therapist and occupational therapist, to advise the patient and the family on how to deal with the problems which are interfering with the patient's daily life.

CASE HISTORY 9.4

Parkinson's disease: the family's perspective

We are 7 years into living with father's Parkinson's disease. There have been so many challenges for him and for us over the years, and the challenges keep changing as the disease progresses. Here are just three of them:

- *'They didn't know him as he was.'*
  With each new admission to care, we are having to work harder to make sure that staff understand that the painfully slow speech from an expressionless face still conveys humour, awareness of world events, kindness and insight.
- *'Food goes everywhere, from face to shoelaces.'*
  It is hard to accept that it is probably now right to use that large bib at mealtimes. It lets him enjoy his meals independently and keeps his clothes clean, which matters a lot to him … but I still don't like it.
- *'He's changing.'*
  We knew it would happen, but it's been a shock to watch the first signs of mental change. It is painful to listen patiently to his attempts to sort out delusion from reality.

Once stabilised, and if the home circumstances permit, the patient will be discharged. Re-admission to hospital will only become necessary should further problems arise, such as worsening of symptoms. Much of the care and advice which the patient receives while in hospital is directed towards maintaining independence, dignity and self-esteem in what is a profoundly distressing disorder.

Mobility

Problems can include difficulty in starting to walk or stopping walking, shuffling, tottering, impaired balance when turning and ongoing stiffness, interrupted by a 'freezing' of movement. Many of the techniques employed to assist the patient can be used by the relatives in the patient's home. The patient's strength and range of motion need to be improved in conjunction with the medication therapy programme. Warm relaxing baths and passive and active range of movement exercises are a good starting point. Relatives should be advised to continue this activity at home. Effort should also be directed towards improving the patient's gait, with the assistance of the physiotherapist. Useful tips to consider are given in Box 9.15.

If the patient experiences difficulty in rolling over in bed or getting in and out of bed, they can be advised to use a low bed with a firm mattress or to place a board under their existing mattress. Additional techniques are given in Box 9.15 and additional suggestions inspired by patients themselves can be found at www.parkinsons.org.uk (see 'Useful websites').

Exercise

Some patients may benefit from an exercise programme to assist mobility and improve posture. It is important that this programme is performed under supervision initially, until the patient and their helper are conversant with the techniques. Again, the importance of continuing these at home should be stressed to both patient and family.

Eating and drinking

The person with Parkinson's disease may have difficulty with eating and drinking due to abnormal posture, tremor, poor swallowing and excessive saliva. There may be embarrassment about their untidiness when eating, and the length of time it takes to eat often results in food going cold. People will often choose to eat alone rather than endure the social embarrassment of seeing others watching them eat. Families may adapt mealtimes creatively; for example, two small servings may mean that food stays hot and portion

Box 9.15

Useful tips for the nurse or carer to encourage a frail older man with Parkinson's disease to move

General tips

- Gently rocking the patient to and fro encourages initiation of walking when he 'freezes'.
- Advise the patient to consciously lift each foot as he is walking and to place his heel on the ground first. To encourage this, tell the patient to think that he has a series of imaginary steps to climb. These techniques help to counteract the usual propulsive movement.
- Remind the patient to swing his arms when walking.
- Teach the patient to broaden his stance to provide a more stable base.
- Remind the patient to think about his posture and to stand erect.
- If the patient starts to shuffle, tell him to stop and start again.
- Tell the patient to adopt the habit of taking small steps when he is turning and to turn only in a forward direction.

Rolling over in bed

1. The patient is advised to bend his knees so that his feet are flat on the mattress and then swing the knees in the direction that he wishes to turn.
2. The next move involves the patient clasping their hands and lifting them straight up, straightening the elbows as they do so, then turning the head and swinging the arms in the same direction as the legs.
3. The patient then grips the edge of the mattress and adjusts his position until comfortable.

To turn in the opposite direction, the process is reversed.

Some patients find a 'monkey pole' helpful. Whilst this is easy to attach to a hospital bed, it is not usually possible in the home; however, an alternative the patient may consider is tying a stout rope to the bottom of the bed and ensuring that the free end of the rope is within reach. This may allow the patient to alter his position in bed without help.

Getting into and out of bed independently

1. To get into bed, the patient sits on the edge of the bed near the pillow so that when he lies down, his head is in the correct position on the pillow.
2. Once this manoeuvre has been mastered, the patient only has to lift his legs onto the bed and then adjust himself into a comfortable position.

Finding the correct spot to sit on the mattress may take some practice, but once mastered the patient will find this a convenient way to get into bed.

Getting out of bed is more complicated and several techniques can be suggested. One example is as follows:

1. The patient lies on his back with his arms at his side.
2. He then lifts his head, tucking his chin into his chest, and sits up supported by the elbows.
3. The patient then sits up, pushing the trunk so that he is leaning forward, bent at the hips.
4. Support is now achieved by using his outstretched arms behind him.
5. He should now move his legs towards the edge of the bed until he is sitting up and ready to stand up.

Rising from a chair

The patient should avoid low chairs, choosing instead firm, high-backed chairs. In the home, the height of a low chair can be increased with blocks under the legs and it will help to raise the back of the chair slightly higher than the front. Cushions or a spring-ejector seat will also help. Placing a sturdy armchair in a frequently used location within the home is ideal. The patient can use the arms of the chair to assist him to rise from it.

size is less daunting. Staff in some restaurants, following discussion, may be sensitive to such difficulties and very helpful.

The speech and language therapist may be asked to assess the patient's swallowing ability and to draw up a programme of swallowing management. This could include facial exercises and techniques to encourage swallowing, e.g. taking a sip of iced water to stimulate the swallowing reflex.

The dietitian's advice should also be sought. It is usual to establish what kind of foods the patient likes best. A review of their current dietary intake will alert the nurse to any deficiencies or inappropriate foods; for example, it is easier to swallow semi-solid food than lumpy food. If tremor is a problem, the patient can be taught to hold their arm close in to their body, using their elbow as a pivot. Bendable straws could be used and cups containing hot liquids should only be filled halfway to avoid spillage or scalding.

It is important for the patient's self-esteem to resist the temptation to feed them before this is absolutely necessary. Many patients may still be able to feed themselves if their food is cut up for them. Feeding the patient for the convenience of speed is unacceptable.

Some of the swallowing difficulties which may be experienced are as follows:

- coughing within a few seconds of the act of swallowing
- food sticking in the throat
- nasal regurgitation
- fear of swallowing
- drooling
- food which remains in the mouth once the meal is completed.

If the patient wears dentures, these should be checked frequently to ensure that they fit properly. The importance of good oral hygiene should be emphasised. Patients should check their body weight weekly and keep a record of this, as weight loss may occur. Some hospitalised patients need to have suctioning equipment readily available while they are eating, in case they choke.

STOP THINK **9.15** Work out how many day-to-day abilities need to be considered in helping a person with advanced Parkinson's disease to continue to enjoy watching television.

Communication

The communication impairment seen in the patient with Parkinson's disease includes a loss of facial expression, which may lead to the assumption that the patient is cognitively impaired and, due to the abnormal stooping posture, there may be loss of normal eye contact and body language. The speech and language therapist should be involved in the care of the patient at an early stage and, should communication problems arise, a programme of exercises and therapy will be instituted. Facial exercises encourage the patient to pronounce sounds more clearly, e.g. by mouthing words slowly and clearly. Imagining that someone else is trying to lip read their words can often help the patient. There are also exercises for breathing, strengthening the voice and controlling the speed of speech, many of which can be continued in the patient's home. Other simple measures include reading out loud or singing, for example in the bath. Alternatively, the patient can stand in front of a mirror, watching their lips as they talk.

Eventually the voice may become so weak that meaningful communication is impossible and an alternative means of communication becomes necessary. Communication aids must be appropriate to the patient's needs, and advice regarding their use should be taken from the speech and language therapist. Aids can range from using a simple picture board through to sophisticated computer devices.

More simply, it may be possible for the patient to write down messages using pen and paper. However, the ability to write also deteriorates progressively and the writing becomes smaller and smaller (micrographia) as muscle stiffness increases. An alternative device, which may be useful for some patients, is a portable amplifier which will make a weak voice sound louder. However, this will not improve slurred speech. Reading books and newspapers also becomes difficult when muscle rigidity interferes with the ability to hold them and to turn pages.

For further advice and support for patients with Parkinson's disease, see www.parkinsons.org.uk.

Elimination

The impairment of mobility in conjunction with urinary frequency or hesitancy can lead to embarrassing episodes of incontinence. This can be difficult to deal with and initially the patient is encouraged to visit the toilet regularly. The use of continence aids may be indicated (see Ch. 24) and the advice of a continence advisor should be sought. It is important that patients are encouraged to maintain a fluid intake of 2.5–3 L/day.

Eventually catheterisation of the bladder may be unavoidable. Many patients and their families reach a stage where they would prefer to have a catheter inserted rather than suffer the continual embarrassment of incontinence and odour. For some, the increasing expense associated with laundering clothes and sheets may become overwhelming.

Constipation is a common problem in Parkinson's disease, so the patient and family should be taught preventive action. A high-fibre diet and plenty of fluids will encourage regular bowel motions. Failing this, it will be necessary to administer faecal softeners or bulking agents regularly and, when required, an enema.

Personal cleansing and dressing

The oily skin and excessive perspiration seen in patients with Parkinson's disease, due to excess parasympathetic activity, demand more frequent washing and bathing. If tremor is present, men will find an electric or battery-operated shaver easier to use.

Slowness in performing voluntary movement (bradykinesia) can make daily activities such as dressing difficult for the patient. For example, buttoning clothes and tying shoelaces may become impossible. Adaptations to clothing, e.g. replacing buttons and other types of fastening with Velcro, and the use of appropriate aids will allow the patient to continue to dress independently for as long as possible, thus maintaining independence. Cardigans are sometimes easier to take off and on than pullovers.

A change of clothing style may be indicated, e.g. pull-on tracksuit trousers, slip-on shoes, elastic shoelaces and front-opening skirts with an elasticated waistband are also easier to manage.

Discharge

Every opportunity should be taken to advise the patient and family about the best way to manage the disorder at home. Each of the areas already outlined should be included in the discharge plan.

Additional points to consider following discharge from hospital are as follows:

- The names and times of the medicines to be taken should be written down. The importance of maintaining the correct dosage is emphasised and some indication of the medicine's action and possible side-effects should be given.
- A daily exercise programme should be devised for the patient, along with instructions about how much the patient should do.
- Contact should be established with the appropriate community services, such as nursing, social services, physiotherapy, occupational therapy and speech and language therapy, who may be providing the patient and family with support at home.
- Advice on dietary aspects along with sample menus should be provided.
- Advice on safety should be provided. The removal of loose rugs and identification of other similar dangers in the home should be highlighted.

The patient should be encouraged to remain as active as possible for as long as possible, but should also be warned to pace their activity. Each individual will approach this situation in their own unique way and this has to be taken into account when proffering advice. The attitude and approach of the family, where appropriate, can be crucial to the patient's progress towards maintaining independence for as long as possible. A helpful account of the psychosocial impact of late stages of the disease is provided by Calne (2003).

For further information on palliative care for people with Parkinson's disease, see Thomas & MacMahon (2004a,b).

INFECTIONS OF THE CENTRAL NERVOUS SYSTEM

There are many infections of the central nervous system, of which the following are considered: bacterial meningitis, i.e. infection of the meninges, viral encephalitis, i.e. infection of the cerebral tissue, and cerebral abscess.

A serious outbreak of bacterial meningitis occurred in Stroud, Gloucestershire, in 1985 (Cartwright et al 1986) and since then sporadic outbreaks have occurred in other parts of the UK. Many of the victims are young children and teenagers. It is estimated that there are about 5000 cases per year in England and Wales, with 500 deaths and approximately 1000 patients being left permanently disabled (Lindsay & Bone 2004). Approximately 10 000 people contract viral meningitis annually. As a result of this, the Meningitis Trust (see 'Useful websites') was set up with the following aims:

- to raise funds for research into all aspects of meningitis
- to provide help and support for the victims and families
- to educate the public about the disease and its symptoms in the hope that awareness and early diagnosis will save lives.

PATHOPHYSIOLOGY

In bacterial meningitis, purulent exudate is found in the subarachnoid space. The most likely route of entry is via the bloodstream, which can carry microorganisms from, for example, an infected middle ear. Other routes of entry include direct extension from a skull or facial fracture, via the CSF, and extensions along cranial and spinal nerves. The circulating CSF acts as an effective means of spreading the microorganisms. Causative organisms in adults include *Streptococcus pneumoniae*, *Haemophilus influenzae* and *Neisseria meningitidis*.

Viral encephalitis may accompany viral infections elsewhere in the body, e.g. the respiratory tract. The commonest virus in the UK is the herpes simplex virus. Some viruses, such as in Creutzfeldt–Jakob disease, appear to be latent for many years and are called 'slow viruses' (Lindsay & Bone 2004).

Cerebral abscess most commonly occurs following middle ear and mastoid infections. Pus accumulates in the cerebral tissue, its location depending on the source and method of spread of infection. Other related conditions are extradural abscess, where pus accumulates in the extradural space, and subdural empyema, where pus accumulates in the subdural space. The offending organisms include the *Streptococcus* and *Staphylococcus aureus*. Once formed, the abscess comprises a mature capsule containing necrotic tissue, inflammatory cells and necrotic debris. The presence of an intracranial abscess can result in raised ICP (Lindsay & Bone 2004).

Common presenting symptoms Infections of the central nervous system affect all age groups. Common symptoms are described in Box 9.16. A patient with meningitis may have had some predisposing infection and be receiving treatment for it, e.g. antibiotics and ear drops for an ear infection, or may have experienced a head injury and have a compound skull fracture, a fractured base of skull or a facial fracture (see 'Head injury', p. 406). In the last case, the patient may not have realised the extent of the injury, initially deferring medical attention after the accident, but may begin to feel unwell over a period of time. Their GP may suspect a serious problem as the patient's condition deteriorates. Admission to hospital will be necessary and, if the patient's condition is serious, referral to a neurosurgeon will be made, as the condition can rapidly become fatal, especially in children.

MEDICAL MANAGEMENT

Examination Typically, the patient is pyrexial, complains of headache and may be disorientated and drowsy. They find all external environmental stimuli, such as strong light (photophobia), painful (see Box 9.16) and their reaction to interference is often aggressive.

Investigations The patient with any focal neurological signs, or presenting with a Glasgow Coma Scale of <7, should have a CT scan performed to exclude an intracranial mass,

Box 9.16

Features of presentation in CNS infections

Bacterial meningitis (abrupt onset)

Infants

Non-specific:
- Drowsiness
- Irritability
- Off feeds
- Distress on handling
- Vomiting or diarrhoea
- Fever

More specific:
- Neck stiffness
- Tense or bulging fontanelle
- Purpuric or petechial rash that does not blanch under pressure

Late:
- High-pitched or moaning cry
- Coma
- Neck retraction
- Shock
- Widespread haemorrhagic rash

Older children and adults

Non-specific:
- Vomiting
- Fever
- Back or joint pains
- Headache

More specific:
- Neck stiffness
- Photophobia
- Confusion
- Purpuric or petechial rash that does not blanch under pressure

Late:
- Coma
- Neck retraction (in severe cases this, in combination with spasm, causing the heels to bend backwards, produces opisthotonos)
- Shock
- Widespread haemorrhagic rash

Viral encephalitis (insidious onset)
- Headache and fever are both present
- Conscious level deteriorates gradually. Confusion is common
- Moderate neck stiffness
- Seizures can occur
- ICP may be elevated as a result of cerebral oedema
- Cranial nerve deficits and focal neurological signs may be present.

Cerebral abscess (insidious onset, 2–3 weeks or more)
- Headache is recurrent and fever is usually present
- Patient becomes confused and drowsy
- Neck stiffness is indicative of circulating CSF infection
- Partial or generalised seizures occur in 30% of patients
- ICP is elevated as abscess expands
- Cranial nerve deficits occur and focal neurological signs include speech disorders, motor and sensory deficits and ataxia

such as an abscess. A lumbar puncture may be performed to identify the offending organism. A moderate increase in lumbar CSF pressure may be noted. The changes seen in the CSF are outlined in Table 9.5.

Other investigations include blood cultures and X-rays to detect the source of infection. In the patient with a cerebral abscess, there may be a rise in the ESR. This may be confirmed by the identification of the organism on CSF analysis, or of a lesion, such as an abscess, on CT scanning. Brain biopsy guided by CT scan may be helpful. When an abscess is suspected, the CT scan should be enhanced with contrast medium to highlight small lesions which may otherwise be missed.

Treatment The patient with bacterial meningitis or a cerebral abscess should commence antibiotics as soon as possible. Penicillin is the antibiotic of choice and is usually given intravenously in high doses, such as penicillin 24 million units over 24 h, but it should be remembered that a significant proportion of the population is allergic to penicillin and so other antibiotics may be used.

Surgery will be performed if the presence of a cerebral abscess is confirmed and adequate explanations should be given to the patient and family of what is involved in this course of treatment (see Hickey 2002 for complications). This may involve burr hole aspiration (repeated, if necessary), primary excision of the whole abscess or evacuation of the abscess contents leaving the capsule intact. This avoids damaging the surrounding brain.

When there are signs of high ICP, the patient requires immediate surgical intervention to drain the abscess. This will relieve the ICP and will prevent coning and herniation of cerebral contents (see 'Head injury', p. 407). The patient may have a focal neurological deficit or be in a coma (see Ch. 28).

NURSING PRIORITIES AND MANAGEMENT: Infections

For those patients who require surgery, the general pre- and postoperative care is as given in Chapter 26. The nurse should observe the patient for signs of the abscess recollecting: this will present as raised ICP. The patient's family will require explanations, support and comfort.

Immediate priorities

Neurological status and vital signs

Because the patient with an intracranial infection may have a decreased conscious level and because this may deteriorate rapidly, observations should be recorded and any change in condition reported immediately. Vital signs are very important as the patient may be pyrexial, and as the infection continues, the patient's temperature can increase further. Pulse, blood pressure and respirations may be high when recorded, owing to infection: any changes in these observations should be reported. There may be signs of raised ICP (see p. 408).

Breathing

The respiratory pattern should be observed for rate, depth and frequency, as a change may indicate a rising ICP.

Any respiratory distress should be reported immediately. Oxygen may already have been prescribed and the nurse should encourage the patient to tolerate it, giving explanations when necessary. Nursing the patient in a bed with a head-up tilt of 30° will not only help to decrease ICP, but also encourage lung expansion. The nurse should be aware of the risk of a chest infection developing.

Controlling body temperature

In order to reduce pyrexia, the patient's temperature should be recorded frequently and any further rise reported immediately, as this may indicate that the antibiotics are not controlling the infection and that the patient's condition could deteriorate. Each 1°C increase in temperature increases the body's demand for oxygen by 10%, which encourages vasodilatation and increases ICP. Nursing measures to reduce pyrexia may include tepid sponging, use of a fan and the administration of paracetamol, either per rectum or orally. The effects of these measures should be evaluated.

Seizure activity

If seizures are observed, they should be recorded, noting the type of seizure, its duration and exactly what happened (see section on 'Seizures', p. 427). An airway, oxygen and suction should be at hand.

Communication

Communication can be difficult, as the patient may be experiencing severe headache, nausea and vomiting, have photophobia and be disorientated and drowsy. A calm darkened environment will comfort the patient, who will be distressed about their condition and what is happening to them.

Explanations should be given to the patient about what is happening and why, and the patient should be given time to ask questions and express their feelings.

The family will also require reassurance and explanations, but they should be advised not to overstimulate the patient, although touch could be suggested as this can be comforting.

Maintaining a safe environment

Side rails should be placed in position to prevent the patient falling out of bed due to restlessness or confusion.

Medication

In order to give the patient adequate relief from pain, analgesics should be administered.

The nurse should ensure that prescribed antibiotics are given or taken at the correct time by the patient, to ensure maintenance of the medication at a therapeutic level in the bloodstream. An accurate fluid balance chart should be maintained as the patient can become dehydrated due to pyrexia, nausea and vomiting. Signs of dehydration include dry skin or mouth or a diminishing urinary output and these should be reported. Intravenous fluids will be prescribed until the patient is able to tolerate adequate oral fluids.

Personal cleansing and dressing

Once an assessment of the patient's needs has been carried out, assistance should be given with personal cleansing and dressing. If the patient has a decreased conscious level, care should be exercised in meeting their needs and, as their condition improves, independence should be encouraged.

Mobility

The patient should be as mobile as their condition allows. Initially, bed rest may be necessary and all care should be taken to ensure that their position is changed 2-hourly. Examination of the skin should be carried out at frequent intervals in order to detect signs of pressure, such as redness.

Preparation for discharge home

If the source of the infection has been identified, it will be treated or, if necessary, further investigations carried out. If it has been treated successfully, e.g. in sinusitis or an ear infection, the patient should be advised to contact their GP if there is a recurrence of the infection. The need to continue medication on discharge should be fully explained, with emphasis on the importance of completion of the course of antibiotics.

If the reason for the introduction of the infection was an injury, such as a skull or facial fracture, further investigations may be required to ensure proper healing. While rehabilitating in the ward, the patient will have been assessed by the ward team. Maintenance of optimum function of the patient is a priority, both physically and mentally, and

Table 9.5 Changes in cerebrospinal fluid which is infected

CSF	Acute bacterial meningitis	Viral encephalitis
Appearance	Yellow	Clear
Cells	Polymorphs 1000–2000 per cubic mm or more	Mononuclear 50–1500 per cubic mm
Protein	Increased 1.0–5.0 g/L	Mildly elevated
Chloride	110–115 mmol/L	Normal
Glucose	Much reduced or absent	Normal
Organisms	Present on culture	Absent on culture. Require specialist virological testing to identify
Pressure	Increased	Increased

outpatient appointments may be required, e.g. for physiotherapy. The patient's family should be involved in the patient's planned discharge and rehabilitation programme at home. Advice and encouragement for this should be given by the ward team. Advice should also be given about employment, driving and other activities, especially if the patient has experienced seizures (see p. 428).

Coping after meningitis

The Meningitis Trust (see 'Useful websites') offers a comprehensive support system for those affected by meningitis. This includes a 24-h support and information line, home and hospital emotional support visits, provision of financial support, grant funding and a rehabilitation advisory service. The Trust emphasises that complete recovery takes time and they provide guidance on how to deal with a range of minor after-effects, e.g. general tiredness, headaches and difficulty in concentration.

Care of the dying patient

The patient's condition may deteriorate rapidly after admission, if medication and surgery have not treated the cause of the infection successfully. In these circumstances, all of the patient's needs should be attended to. Adequate pain relief should be given and the patient should be comforted (see Ch. 28).

REFERENCES

Armstrong T S, Gilbert M R 2002 Glial tumours: new approaches in chemotherapy. Journal of Neuroscience Nursing 34(6): 326–330

Austin J K, McNelis A M, Shore C P, Dunn D W, Musick B 2002 A feasibility study of a family seizure management programme: Be Seizure Smart. Journal of Neuroscience Nursing 34(1): 30–37

Bakas T, Austin J K, Okonkwo K F, Lewis R R, Chadwick L 2002 Needs, concerns, strategies and advice of stroke caregivers the first 6 months after discharge. Journal of Neuroscience Nursing 34(5): 242–251

Bingham E 2004 Diagnosis and support for people with epilepsy. Practice Nursing 15(2): 64–70

Calne S M 2003 The psychosocial impact of late stage Parkinson's disease. Journal of Neuroscience Nursing 35(6): 306–313

Cartwright K A V, Stuart S M, Noah N D 1986 An outbreak of meningococcal diseases in Gloucestershire. Lancet 2: 558–561

Cavanagh S J, Gordon V L 2002 Grading scales used in the management of aneurysmal subarachnoid haemorrhage: a critical review. Journal of Neuroscience Nursing 34(6): 288–295

Cortese L, Jog M, McAuley T J et al 2004 Assessing and monitoring antipsychotic-induced movement disorders in hospitalized patients: a cautionary study. Canadian Journal of Psychiatry 49(1): 31–36

Courts N F, Buchanan E M, Werstlein P O 2004 Focus groups: the lived experience of participants with multiple sclerosis. Journal of Neuroscience Nursing 36(1): 42–47

Department of Health 2000/2001 Hospital episode statistics. DH, London

Eriksen S K, Tuite P J, Maxwell R E et al 2003 Bilateral subthalamic nucleus stimulation for the treatment of Parkinson's disease: results of six patients. Journal of Neuroscience Nursing 35(4): 223–231

Fischer J, Mathieson C 2001 The history of the Glasgow Coma Scale: implications for practice. Critical Care Nursing Quarterly 23(4): 52–58

Greenhill L, Betts T 2003 The lifelong care needs of women with epilepsy. Practice Nursing 14(7): 302, 304–306, 308–309

Hagell P, Odin P 2001 Apomorphine in the treatment of Parkinson's disease. Journal of Neuroscience Nursing 33(1): 21–34, 37–38

Haslett C, Chilvers E R, Boon N A, Colledge N R 2002 Davidson's principles and practice of medicine, 19th edn. Churchill Livingstone, Edinburgh

Headway 2004 Prevention and safety (head injury). Online. Available: www.headway.org.uk

Hickey J V 2002 The clinical practice of neurological and neurosurgical nursing, 5th edn. Lippincott, Philadelphia

Houltram B, Scanlan M 2004 Extrapyramidal side effects. Nursing Standard 18(43): 39–41

Jamieson E M, McCall J M, Whyte L A 2002 Guidelines for clinical nursing practice, 4th edn. Churchill Livingstone, Edinburgh

Kirkness C J, Thompson J M, Ricker B A et al 2002 The impact of aneurysmal subarachnoid hemorrhage on functional outcome. Journal of Neuroscience Nursing 34(3): 134–141

Kwan J, Hand P, Dennis M, Sandercock P 2004 Effects of introducing an integrated care pathway in an acute stroke unit. Age and Ageing 33(4): 362–367

Le Strange D G 2003 The pharmacologic treatment of vasospasm after subarachnoid haemorrhage: a case study. Journal of Neuroscience Nursing 35(6): 332–335

Lepola I, Toljamo M, Aho R, Louet T 2001 Being a brain tumor patient: a descriptive study of patients' experiences. Journal of Neuroscience Nursing 33(3): 143–147

Lindsay K, Bone I 2004 Neurology and neurosurgery illustrated, 4th edn. Churchill Livingstone, Edinburgh

Lisak D 2001 Overview of symptomatic management of multiple sclerosis. Journal of Neuroscience Nursing 33(5): 224–230

Louden W 2004 The role of EEGs in the treatment and prognosis of epilepsy. Nursing Times 100(4): 36–38

MacLean R 2004 The challenge of managing patients with multiple sclerosis. Nursing Times 100(4): 42–44

McCall B 2003 Young-onset Parkinson's disease: a guide to care and support. Nursing Times 99(30): 28–29

McGuire R 1997 Parkinson's disease. Professional Nurse 13(1): 33–37

Miller C, Jezewski M A 2001 A phenomenologic assessment of relapsing MS patients' experiences during treatment with interferon beta-1a. Journal of Neuroscience Nursing 33(5): 240–244

Montague S E, Watson R, Herbert R 2005 Physiology for nursing practice, 3rd edn. Baillière Tindall, London

National Institute for Clinical Excellence (NICE) 2003a Head injury: triage, assessment, investigation and early management of head injury in infants, children and adults. NICE, London

National Institute for Clinical Excellence (NICE) 2003b Management of multiple sclerosis in primary and secondary care. NICE, London

National Institute for Clinical Excellence (NICE) 2004 Newer drugs for epilepsy in adults. NICE, London

news.bbc.co.uk/1/hi/health/3636697.stm

news.bbc.co.uk/1/hi/health/4193093.stm

NHS Education for Scotland 2005 Stroke: core competencies for healthcare staff. NHS Education for Scotland, Edinburgh

NHS Health Scotland 2003 Alcofacts. NHS Health Scotland, Edinburgh

Nichols D A, Brown R D, Meyer F B 2002 Coils or clips in subarachnoid haemorrhage? Lancet 360(9342): 1262

Rietberg M B, Brooks D, Uitdehaag B M J, Kwakkel G 2005 Exercise therapy for multiple sclerosis. The Cochrane Library, Oxford

Roper N, Logan W, Tierney A J 2000 The Roper–Logan–Tierney model of nursing. The activities of living model. Elsevier, Edinburgh

Sherwood P R, Given B A, Doorenbos A Z et al 2004 Forgotten voices: lessons from bereaved caregivers of persons with a brain tumour. International Journal of Palliative Nursing 10(2): 67–75

Sinnakaruppan I, Williams D M 2001 Family carers and the adult head injured: a critical review of carers' needs. Brain Injury 15(8): 653–672

Sullivan J 2000 Positioning of patients with severe traumatic brain injury: research-based practice. Journal of Neuroscience Nursing 32(4): 204–209

Swann I J, Teasdale G M 1999 Current concepts in the management of patients with so-called 'minor' or 'mild' head injury. Trauma 1: 143–145

Thomas S 2002 Epilepsy and services for older people. Nursing Older People 14(4): 23–29
Tornqvist A L 2001 Neurosurgery for movement disorders. Journal of Neuroscience Nursing 33(2): 79–82
Tortora G, Grabowski S R 2003 Principles of anatomy and physiology, 10th edn. Wiley, London
Waugh A, Grant A 2001 Ross and Wilson's anatomy and physiology in health and illness, 9th edn. Churchill Livingstone, Edinburgh
Williams G 2004 Management of patients who have relapses in multiple sclerosis. British Journal of Nursing 13(17): 1012–1016
www.mssociety.org.uk
www.parkinsons.org.uk
www.stroke.org.uk

FURTHER READING

Armstrong T S, Gilbert M R 2002 Glial tumours: new approaches in chemo therapy. Journal of Neuroscience Nursing 34(6): 326–330
Barker E 2002 Neuroscience nursing: a spectrum of care, 2nd edn. Mosby, St Louis
Calne S M, Kumar A 2003 Nursing care of patients with late stage Parkinson's disease. Journal of Neuroscience Nursing 25(6): 242–251
Cheung J, Hocking P 2004 The experience of spousal carers of people with multiple sclerosis. Qualitative Health Research 14(2): 153–166
Cook A, Sheikh A 2003 Trends in serious head injuries among English cyclists and pedestrians. Injury Prevention 9(3): 266–267
Finlayson M, Van Denend T, Hudson E 2004 Aging with multiple sclerosis. Journal of Neuroscience Nursing 36(5): 245–251, 259
Gimenez R 2000 My experience with a second brain aneurysm. Clinical Nurse Specialist 14(6): 253–255
Greenhill L, Betts T 2003 The lifelong needs of women with epilepsy. Practice Nursing 14(7): 302, 304–306, 308–309
Haslett C, Chilvers E R, Boon N A, Colledge N R 2002 Davidson's principles and practice of medicine, 19th edn. Churchill Livingstone, Edinburgh
Hickey J V 2002 The clinical practice of neurological and neurosurgical nursing, 5th edn. Lippincott, Philadelphia
Lanfear J 2002 The individual with epilepsy. Nursing Standard 16(46): 43–53
Marieb E N 2004 Human anatomy and physiology, 6th edn. Benjamin Cummings, San Francisco
Mhor D C, Hart S L, Julian L et al 2004 Association between stressful life events and exacerbation in multiple sclerosis: a meta-analysis. British Medical Journal 328(7442): 731–733
Montague S E, Watson R, Herbert R 2005 Physiology for nursing practice, 3rd edn. Baillière Tindall, London
Pena C 2003 Seizure. American Journal of Nursing 103(11): 73–81
Pfohman M, Criddle L M 2001 Epidemiology of intracranial aneurysm and subarachnoid haemorrhage. Journal of Neuroscience Nursing 33(1): 39–41
Price A M, Collins T J, Gallacher A 2003 Nursing care of the acute head injury: a review of the evidence. Nursing in Critical Care 8(3): 126–133
Roberts I, Schierhout G 2004 Hyperventilation therapy for acute traumatic brain injury. Cochrane Library, Oxford
Thomas S, MacMahon D 2004a Parkinson's disease, palliative care and older people: part 1. Nursing Older People 16(1): 22–27
Thomas S, MacMahon D 2004b Parkinson's disease, palliative care and older people: part 2. Nursing Older People 16(2): 22–26
Tortora G J, Derrickson B 2006 Principles of anatomy and physiology, 11th edn. Wiley, London
Waugh A, Grant A 2001 Ross and Wilson's anatomy and physiology in health and illness, 9th edn. Churchill Livingstone, Edinburgh
Wehrle L 2003 Epilepsy: its presentation and nursing management. Nursing Times 99(20): 30–33
www.parkinsons.org.uk
Yang J, Wang K, Chiang Y et al 2003 Effects of head elevation on cerebral blood flow velocity in post-cerebral operation patients. Journal of Nursing Research 11(2): 129–136

USEFUL WEBSITES

Epilepsy Action
www.epilepsy.org.uk

Headway – the brain injury association
www.headway.org.uk
Freephone helpline 0808 800 2244

Meningitis Trust
www.meningitis-trust.org.uk

Multiple Sclerosis Society
www.mssociety.org.uk

Parkinson's Disease Society
www.parkinsons.org.uk

Stroke Association
www.stroke.org.uk

The Outsiders
www.outsiders.org.uk

DISORDERS OF THE MUSCULOSKELETAL SYSTEM

10

Brian Lucas

INTRODUCTION

A fully functioning musculoskeletal system is fundamental to optimal health in the normal active human being. Injury or disease involving this system can have a profound effect on an individual's ability to perform the activities of daily living and can result in either temporary or permanent disability, one of the main problems usually being the degree of decreased mobility. The overall aim of nursing care is to prevent further injury, reduce the risk of complications, promote healing, maximise independence within individual constraints of the existing condition and promote optimal rehabilitation.

This chapter will describe some of the more common disorders of the musculoskeletal system that are caused by either trauma or disease and will outline relevant principles of nursing management.

Epidemiology

The main causes of musculoskeletal trauma or disease in the UK include road traffic collisions (RTCs), industrial and other work-related accidents, sporting accidents and damage due to underlying disease.

Road traffic collisions

In 2002 there were 314 519 road casualties in the UK (National Statistics 2004) and many of these will have sustained musculoskeletal injuries. It should be emphasised that it is often the immediate treatment of injury or suspected fracture that determines the ultimate outcome of an RTC; this applies particularly to injuries of the spinal column and fractures of major long bones.

Work-related injuries

In the UK in 2001/2002, 251 workers died as a result of injuries sustained at work, 28 940 sustained major injuries and 130 572 sustained injuries which resulted in sickness of more than 3 days' duration (National Statistics 2004). As with RTCs, many work-related injuries result in broken bones, damaged joints or torn ligaments/tendons.

In many countries low back pain is the most common cause of long-term disability in middle age (Guzmán et al 2004). Repetitive strain injuries (RSI) or cumulative trauma disorders (CTD) are also increasing, possibly due to the increased use of computers in the workplace (Winzeler & Rosenstein 1997).

Sporting injuries

With increased leisure time and facilities and the many health campaigns promoting the benefits of exercise, more time is being spent in sporting activities, with a resultant increase in sporting injuries. In many cases these are minor, but they can also be serious and result in permanent disability: diving into shallow water can cause serious injury to the cervical spine; knee and lower limb injuries are common in football and skiing; and shoulder, upper limb and spinal injuries often result from horse riding accidents.

Damage due to underlying disease

Relatively minor trauma may also highlight a previously undiagnosed underlying disease process. For example, osteoporosis in a postmenopausal woman may only be diagnosed when she presents with a fractured wrist or neck of femur (see p. 460).

Osteoarthritis, i.e. degenerative arthritis, is the commonest condition to affect joints in humans (Hakim & Clunie 2002) and is mainly due to wear and tear on the articular cartilage of the larger weight-bearing joints and to the degenerative changes associated with the ageing process.

Rheumatoid arthritis is a chronic or subacute disease of the musculoskeletal joints and affects 34/100 000 women and 14/100 000 men (Hakim & Clunie 2002). It usually affects more than one joint (polyarthritic) and can be extremely disabling.

The contribution of the science of bioengineering

Musculoskeletal conditions involve, or are caused by, disruption of the mechanics of the human body. Through research, bioengineers are making vital contributions to the understanding of these mechanics and, with the availability of more biologically compatible materials, are able to design a wider and more refined range of replacement joints and limbs. Joint replacement surgery is now a common procedure and has revolutionised the quality of life for thousands of post-injured or older people. This chapter provides examples of these and other bioengineering developments such as endoprosthetics following bone tumour excision.

ANATOMY AND PHYSIOLOGY OF THE MUSCULOSKELETAL SYSTEM

This section gives a brief overview of the anatomy and physiology of the musculoskeletal system. For detailed information, refer to anatomy and physiology textbooks and become familiar with the model skeleton in your classroom.

For further information, see Marieb (2004).

The skeletal system

The skeleton can be divided into the axial skeleton (the bones of the head and trunk, excluding the pectoral and pelvic girdles) and the appendicular skeleton (the bones of the limbs, including the bones of pectoral and pelvic girdles).

The main functions of the skeleton are:

- support for the body
- protection for internal organs
- movement — bones and muscles act as levers to produce movement through joints
- mineral storage — minerals such as calcium and phosphorus
- blood cell formation — red bone marrow produces red and white blood cells and platelets (Knight et al 2004).

Structurally, the skeletal system consists of two types of connective tissue: bone and cartilage.

Bone

STOP THINK **10.1** Look up the factors involved in the development and growth of healthy bone. Describe them.

Unlike other connective tissue, bone contains large amounts of mineral salts, mainly tricalcium phosphate and calcium carbonate, which, when deposited on the collagen fibres, results in hardening. There are two types of bone tissue: compact and cancellous.

The hard outer layer of a bone is compact bone tissue, cortical bone, while cancellous tissue fills the inside. Cancellous tissue is spongier in appearance and the larger spaces contain the highly vascular red bone marrow and the fatty yellow bone marrow. The thickness of each type of tissue varies, depending on the type and function of the particular bone. In long bones such as the femur, the shaft, diaphysis, is enclosed by a thick layer of cortical tissue which gives strength for weight-bearing, while at each end, the epiphyses, the cortical tissue is thinner and encloses a greater mass of cancellous tissue.

Flat bones, such as the sternum and the pelvis, have a thinner layer of cortical tissue and a relatively greater amount of cancellous tissue. This is the reason why they are chosen for bone marrow biopsy.

Tissue renewal

Like the skin, bone tissue is constantly being replaced, but at variable rates in different parts of the body. The cancellous bone at the epiphyses, e.g. in the upper end of the femur, is replaced about every 4 months in an adult, in contrast to the compact bone in the shaft of the femur which will never be completely replaced during a lifetime. This process of growth and repair is dependent on balanced activity between the three types of bone cell: osteoblasts, osteocytes and osteoclasts (see Fig. 10.1).

STOP THINK **10.2** Referring to an anatomy and physiology text, define the function of each type of bone cell.

For further information on bone, see Knight et al (2004).

Cartilage

This is a form of connective tissue which is tough, flexible, avascular and devoid of nerve fibres. It forms part of the support mechanism of the body.

There are three types of cartilage:

- hyaline cartilage — firm yet pliable and forms the articular cartilage that covers the articulating surfaces of synovial joints

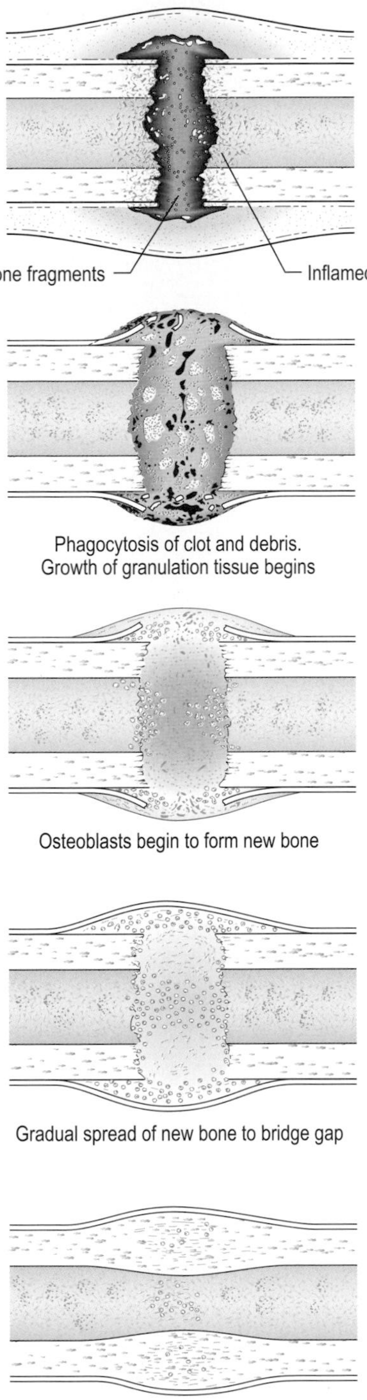

Fig. 10.1 Stages in bone healing.

- fibrocartilage — strong, compressible and tension-resistant and is found in areas such as the intervertebral discs
- elastic cartilage — contains more elastin fibres than the others and therefore has a greater ability to stretch whilst retaining its strength; it is found in the external ear and the epiglottis.

The axial skeletal system

The skull and vertebral column form the central axis of the skeletal system. It is a strong, flexible column of 33 bones,

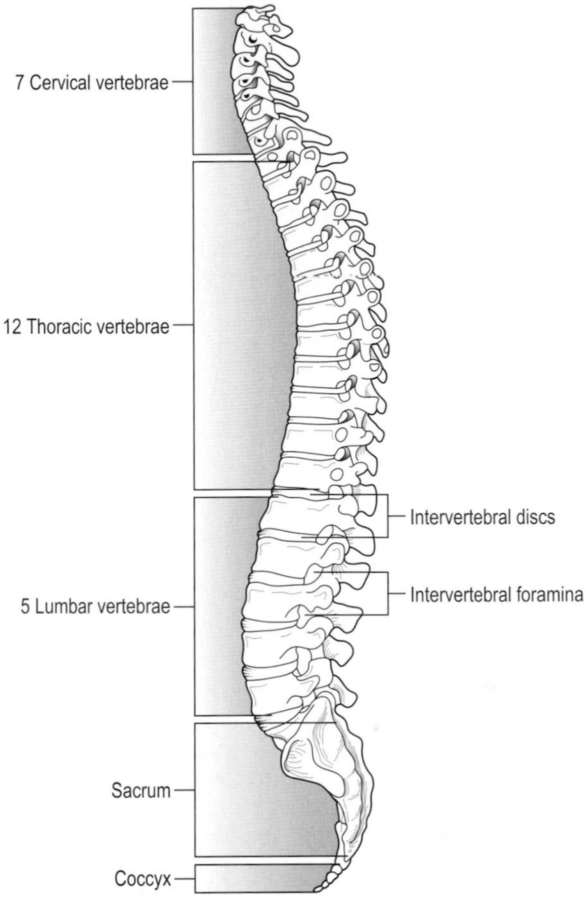

Fig. 10.2 The vertebral column — lateral view.

24 of which are 'true' vertebrae — the cervical, thoracic and lumbar — the remainder being fused to form the sacrum and coccyx (see Fig. 10.2). Between each of the vertebrae from C2 to S1 is a strong joint created by the fibrocartilaginous intervertebral discs, which allow flexibility and act as shock absorbers when the spine is exposed to vertical forces.

The spinal column functions to protect the spinal cord, to support the skull and to act as a point of attachment for the ribs and muscles of the back.

The appendicular skeletal system

The bones of the upper and lower limbs and their girdles are the main parts of the appendicular skeletal system and are characterised by the presence of synovial joints which connect the articular surfaces of adjoining bones (see Fig. 10.3). The bones that make up the joint are held within a fibrous capsule, which consists of two layers:

- an outer layer of dense connective tissue which allows movement but resists dislocation
- an inner layer lined with synovial membrane which secretes synovial fluid; this provides nourishment and lubrication.

The articular surfaces of the bones involved are covered in hyaline cartilage — articular cartilage.

Ligaments

Ligaments attach bone to bone and are vital in maintaining the stability of a joint. They are made of dense connective

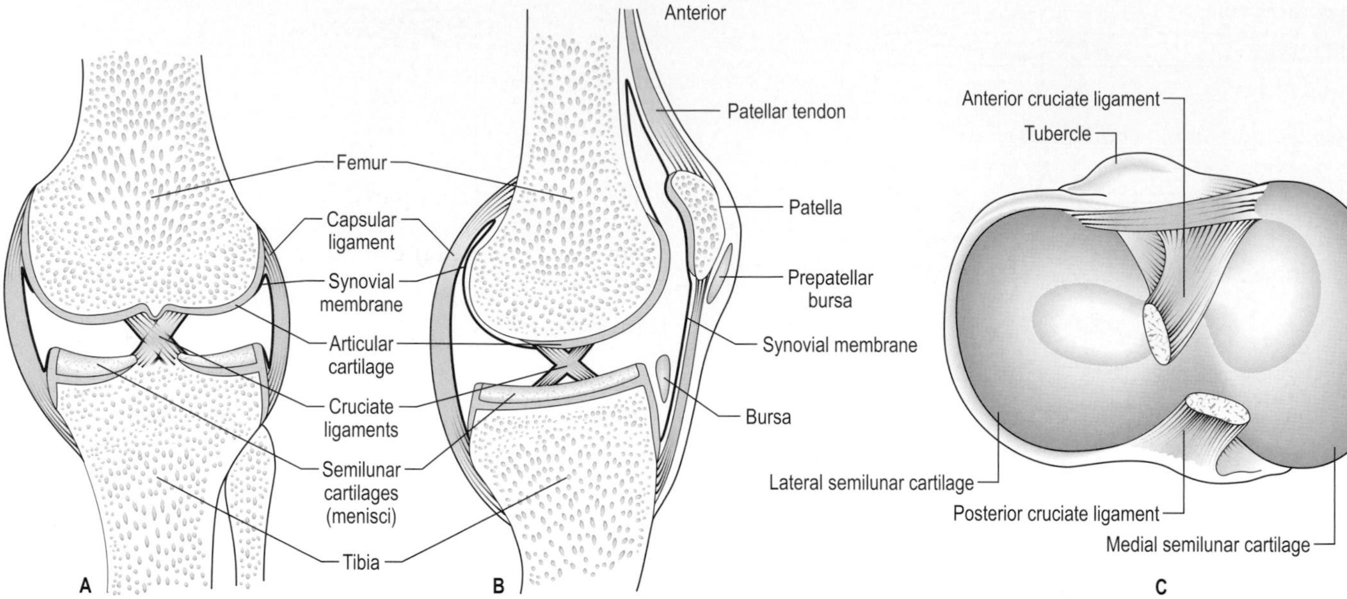

Fig. 10.3 The knee joint. A: Section viewed from front. B: Section viewed from side. C: Superior surface of the tibia showing the semilunar cartilages and cruciate ligaments.

tissue and have a relatively poor blood supply. A joint may have many ligaments, such as the knee which has the cruciate ligaments to prevent the femur and tibia moving forwards on each other and the medial and lateral collateral ligaments which prevent side to side movement (see Fig. 10.3). Damage to ligaments can result in an unstable and painful joint, common in football injuries.

The muscular system

Skeletal muscle tissue is composed of multinucleated muscle cells which are long and cylindrical in appearance. Each muscle is made up of muscle fibres and connective tissue. A good blood and nerve supply is essential for muscle function and the mechanics of movement.

STOP THINK **10.3** Find a chart or model of the muscular system. Identify and name the main muscle groups.

For further information, see Kneale & Davis (2004).

Tendons

Tendons attach muscle to bone and allow movement of joints to take place. As with ligaments, tendons too have a relatively poor blood supply. Damage to tendons can therefore be as serious as bony injury and prevent movement in an individual.

GENERAL PRINCIPLES OF NURSING MANAGEMENT OF MUSCULOSKELETAL DISORDERS

Nursing assessment

This will involve a holistic assessment of the patient, as musculoskeletal disorders can have profound effects on a patient physically, psychologically and socially. In addition, visual inspection, palpation, measurement, and other investigations such as radiological/imaging studies (see Box 10.1) and blood tests in rheumatoid arthritis for example, are necessary.

In particular the nurse should assess for:

- the patient's description of pain and other symptoms
- abnormal position or appearance of limbs or affected part, with loss of function (compare with contralateral side)
- abnormal posture or gait
- use of walking aids or prostheses
- concurrent health problems, allergies and medications
- the patient's perception of the cause of the primary problem
- the patient's knowledge and understanding of the condition
- the impact on activities of living (ALs) (Roper et al 2000), especially relating to impaired mobility
- the patient's and the family's expectations and coping strategies.

Problems and strengths (actual and potential) are identified in the following categories:

- life-threatening problems such as shock
- pain
- impaired mobility
- knowledge deficit
- potential for further injury — physical safety and neurovascular complications, especially compartment syndrome (see p. 450) and deep vein thrombosis (DVT)
- psychosocial consequences
- rehabilitation
- patient and family strengths — these should be defined and used constructively.

Box 10.1

Investigations for musculoskeletal abnormalities

Radiological and imaging studies
- X-ray — to detect abnormal position, fractures, bone density and presence of fluid or abnormalities in joint capsules
- Computed tomogram (CT scan) — makes use of the fact that different tissues have varying radiodensities. A series of radiographs are made at different angles and planes and the computer integrates the information to produce pictorial slices (sometimes 3D) which can be used to detect soft tissue injuries or tumours and inflammatory or metastatic skeletal disease or fracture
- Magnetic resonance imaging (MRI) — magnetic fields used to show the difference in hydrogen density of various muscle and soft tissues, indicating the presence of abnormalities
- Dual energy X-ray absorptiometry (DEXA) scan — scan for bone density
- Arthrogram — injection of a radio-opaque substance or air into a joint followed by X-ray to identify abnormalities of joint structures. Largely superseded by arthroscopy and MRI scan, where available
- Myelogram — a contrast medium is injected into the subarachnoid space of the lumbar spine in order to visualise disc herniation or tumours. Largely superseded by MRI scan, where available

Joint examination
- Arthroscopy — endoscopic visualisation of structures inside a joint. May also involve withdrawal of synovial fluid for analysis, and treatments such as washout of the joint to remove debris or the trimming of any damaged structures, e.g. the menisci in the knee joint

Muscle and nerve studies
- Electromyography (EMG) — measures electrical potential of muscle during rest and activity
- Nerve conduction velocities (NCVs) — measures speed of nerve impulse conduction

Other tests
- These include bone biopsy, densimetry, total body calcium and various haematological studies for hormone and mineral levels

Nursing interventions

- Treat life-threatening problems — ABC of resuscitation (see Chs 2 and 27) and treatment of shock (see Ch. 18)
- Relieve pain
- Maintain an appropriate degree of therapeutic restriction and mobility
- Constantly monitor and reduce the risk of neurovascular complications such as compartment syndrome and DVT
- Maintain a safe environment
- Explore the patient's and family's understanding of the condition and provide support and education based on individual needs
- Coordinate multidisciplinary intervention for psychosocial problems
- Facilitate rehabilitation

SKELETAL DISORDERS

FRACTURES

PATHOPHYSIOLOGY

Fractures, which patients often refer to as a 'broken bone', are a break in the continuity of a bone (Langstaff 2000) as a result of direct or indirect trauma, underlying disease (pathological fracture) or repeated stress on a bone (stress fracture).

Classification of fractures A simple or closed fracture is one where there is no communication between the external environment and the fracture site. When direct contact between the fracture site and the external environment occurs, it is known as a compound or open fracture.

A fracture may be described as 'stable' when the bone ends are lying in a position from which they are unlikely to move, or as 'unstable' when the bone ends are displaced or have the potential to be displaced.

Common fracture patterns are shown in Figure 10.4.

MEDICAL MANAGEMENT

Priorities of treatment If a fracture has been sustained following trauma it is important to follow the principles of trauma treatment (see Ch. 27). Once the patient's physical condition has been stabilised, specific treatment for the fracture will continue. For all fractures there is a risk of the edges of the broken bones damaging soft tissues or blood vessels/nerves, either at the time of injury or subsequently, due to poor handling of the affected limb.

Whether the fracture is a major life-threatening injury, such as an open shaft of femur fracture, or one where the physical damage is relatively slight, such as a phalangeal fracture, the principles of treatment remain the same, i.e. reduction of the fracture, maintenance of the reduced position, and restoration of function (rehabilitation).

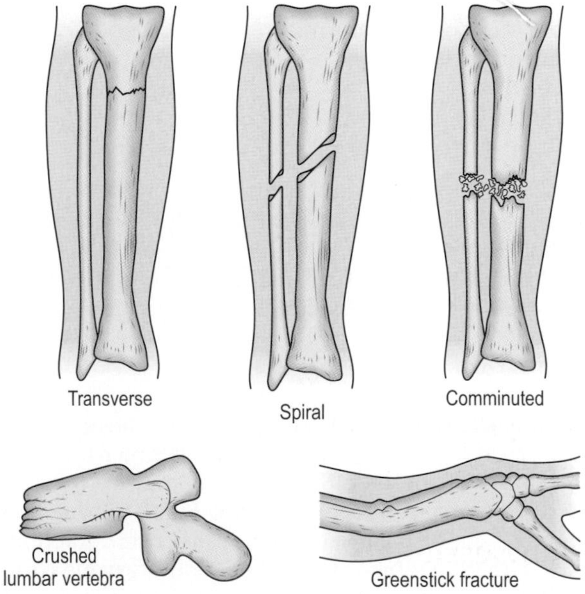

Fig. 10.4 Patterns of fracture.

Reduction of fractures Fractures are said to be reduced when displaced bone fragments are pulled into their normal anatomical position. In many cases, a general anaesthetic will be necessary to overcome the protective muscle spasm and severe pain.

Maintenance of position It is important, following reduction, that the fracture is held in the correct anatomical position until bony union occurs. Various methods are used, depending on the site and the type of fracture. These include external splintage using an orthosis, i.e. a removable splint, plaster of Paris (POP) or synthetic (resin/plastic based) casts, skin or skeletal traction, or an external fixator frame. Operative reduction with internal fixation by metal pins, plates, screws or nails may also be used to hold the bony fragments in position. When the blood supply is grossly affected, it may be necessary to implant a prosthesis to replace the affected bone, e.g. in some cases of fractured neck of femur.

Restoration of function When one part of a limb is immobilised, there is a tendency for related joints and muscles to become stiff and weak; for example, during splintage of a wrist fracture, the finger and shoulder joints can be affected. Appropriate physiotherapy is therefore essential.

Patients require varying degrees of rehabilitation, involving a multidisciplinary team approach (see Ch. 34). It should be remembered that even when the physical damage is slight, the psychosocial impact may be considerable.

Traction

Orthopaedic traction occurs when a pulling force is applied to a part or parts of the body, and counter-traction, a pulling force in the opposite direction, is also applied (Lucas & Davis 2004). Counter-traction is most usually supplied by the body weight of the patient. It is used in the following circumstances:

- to reduce and immobilise fractures/dislocations and maintain normal alignment of all injured tissues
- to prevent and correct deformity
- to reduce muscle spasm
- to relieve pain
- to immobilise an injured or inflamed joint
- to keep joint surfaces apart.

Traction is less used than in the past as alternative methods, in particular internal fixation, enable patients to become mobile more quickly and therefore avoid the problems of bed rest. However, it still has its place in treatment and nurses must know the principles of its use.

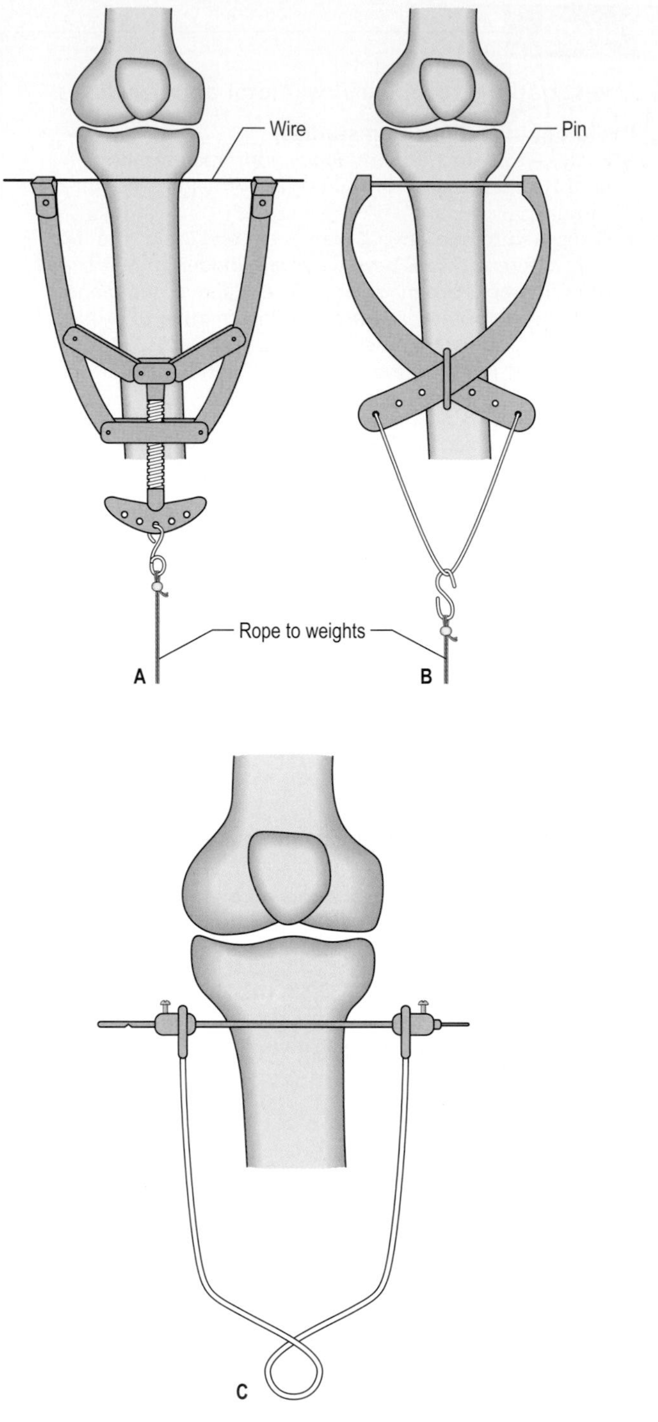

Fig. 10.5 Skeletal traction may be applied by — A: a Kirschner wire and traction stirrup; B: a Steinmann pin and traction stirrup; or C: Steinmann pin and Böhler stirrup.

Types of traction

Balanced or sliding traction This relies on the patient's own body weight to produce the necessary counter-traction, usually by tilting of the bed. Skeletal pins may be used to provide a firm point of attachment (see Fig. 10.5), but the most common type of balanced traction uses skin traction. This is Buck's traction which is used as a temporary measure for pain relief in patients with a fractured neck of femur (see Fig. 10.6). However, a Cochrane Review (Parker & Handoll 2004) could find no evidence which conclusively demonstrated the benefit of such traction for the outcome measures of pain relief or ease of fracture reduction at the time of surgery.

Fixed traction This is the application of counter-traction acting through an appliance which obtains purchase on a part of the body. The most common is a Thomas splint,

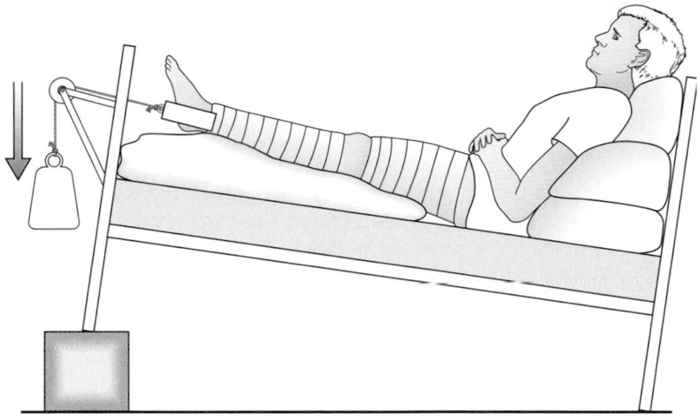

Fig. 10.6 Buck's traction for femoral neck fractures.

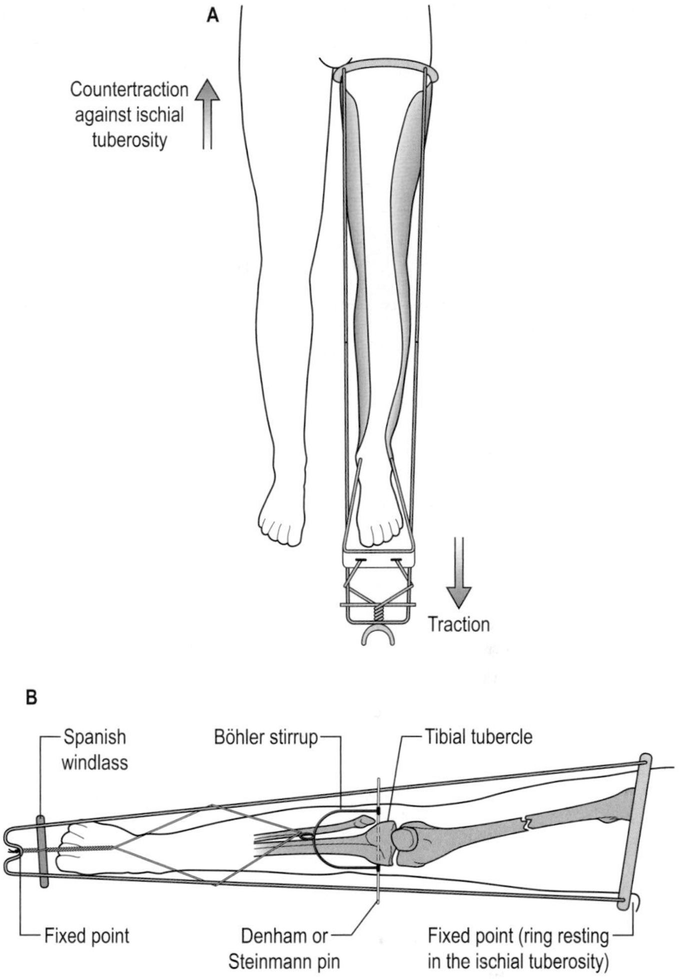

Fig. 10.7 A: Fixed traction using skin traction and Thomas' splint. B: Fixed traction using skeletal pin and Thomas' splint.

used for restricting movement of a fractured shaft of femur when transferring a patient, e.g. between hospitals, or in the treatment of fractures of the shaft of femur in children (Lucas & Davis 2004). Skin or skeletal traction may be used (see Fig. 10.7). Methods used to apply skin traction for balanced or fixed traction are outlined in Box 10.2.

For further information, see Kneale & Davis (2004).

PRINCIPLES OF NURSING MANAGEMENT: Traction

In addition to the general principles outlined earlier for management of musculoskeletal injuries, the following are specific to a patient in traction.

Traction equipment and purpose

The nurse should have a thorough understanding of the type and purpose of the particular traction in use and explain these simply and clearly to the patient in order to obtain their active participation in overall treatment, rehabilitation and prevention of complications. All patients in traction should be assessed by the nurse for their moving and handling needs with particular reference to the equipment required. Patients are taught how to lift themselves up using the overhead lifting aid and also which movements are safe.

All parts of frames, pulleys, ropes and slings should be inspected at regular intervals every day to ensure that they are correctly positioned and in good working order; this is especially important when the patient has been moved, e.g. after using a bedpan.

Observation of neurovascular status and prevention of complications

Observation of colour, sensation and movement (CSM) of the injured limb must be carried out throughout the patient's stay in hospital. The patient should be helped and encouraged to describe changes in sensation and levels of pain, and any complaint of discomfort, pain or paraesthesia must be thoroughly investigated (Lucas & Davis 2004).

Box 10.2

Application of skin traction

Skin traction can be applied using a ready-prepared skin traction kit made of either Venfoam (non-adhesive) or Elastoplast (adhesive). Elastoplast is very rarely used, both because of its potential for damaging skin and also because skin traction is nowadays used only in the short term, before surgery or application of external fixation. Non-adhesive skin traction is adequate for short-term use.

Venfoam kit

Made of non-adhesive, soft foam padding, this can be applied directly to the skin and held in position with a crepe bandage. It will take approximately 2–3 kg of weight. It must be reapplied twice a day because of loss of bandage pressure. Avoid bandaging over the joint, such as the knee, and ensure that the foot of the bed is elevated to provide traction counterbalance.

External pressure can come from any part of the traction or be caused by restricted movement; internal pressure may be the result of tissue damage and swelling.

Nursing staff must be alert for:

- increased risk of pressure ulcers and skin reactions due to the patient's reduced mobility and/or the traction equipment
- drop foot caused by excessive pressure on the common peroneal nerve located around the head of the fibula
- compartment syndrome (CS) — a compartment consists of muscles surrounded by inelastic fascial tissue. CS occurs when there is increased tissue pressure resulting in inadequate tissue perfusion and anoxia within the compartment (Tucker 1998). This results in tissue death and permanent loss of function can occur within 6–8 h.

It is vital to be aware that compartment syndrome is a hazard of the complex nature of musculoskeletal trauma, surgery and immobilisation (Maher et al 2002) that can occur even when a pulse is present and there is capillary refill (see Box 10.3).

Box 10.3

Impending compartment syndrome — dialogue between student (S) and mentor (M)

S You've explained what compartment syndrome is but how do I know that it is actually happening, especially when I can still feel a pulse and the capillary refill appears to be normal?

M Well, the first thing to keep in mind is that there is always a possibility of it happening where there is fairly extensive musculoskeletal trauma and constricting devices or traction are in use. Also, don't depend solely on observation of capillary refill and pulse — they can give a false sense of security. Obviously, degree of swelling, colour, pulse and capillary refill are very important and you may be able to feel a tight and tense muscle mass on palpation — but what the patient feels and can describe to you will be the deciding factor.

S I've noticed that you spend a lot of time talking to the patients about how things feel and really pursuing their answers — but what are the critical clues that you're looking for?

M I get red alerts when they describe deep throbbing pain inappropriate to the injury and a persistent sensation of pressure or pain on stretch, or if they complain of abnormal sensations such as numbness, tingling, loss of sensation, increased sensitivity or weakness.

S How can we prevent compartment syndrome?

M Attention to all the basic principles of treatment such as correct tissue alignment, splinting the affected part but encouraging normal movement of other parts, elevation, keen and constant observation of neurovascular status, assessment of major nerve function such as in the peroneal, ulnar and median nerves, prompt action to relieve constriction from bandages, slings and plaster casts, educating the patient to detect adverse signs and symptoms and possibly anticipating fasciectomy, i.e. surgically opening the skin and fascia to allow the tissues to expand and relieve pressure.

S What action should we take if we suspect impending compartment syndrome?

M Report signs and symptoms immediately to a member of the surgical team and take any necessary nursing action, such as reassuring the patient and stopping elevation, which can increase the compartment pressure, checking and possibly reapplying the traction, relieving the constriction and continuing to monitor changes. It is possible to measure tissue pressure with a direct needle measurement device — and anything above 30 mmHg needs action.

Prevention of infection at skeletal pin sites

A Cochrane Review (Temple & Santy 2004) concluded that there is little evidence as to which pin site care regimen best reduces infection rates. However, a consensus conference has produced best practice guidelines based on the available literature and expert opinion (Lee-Smith et al 2001). These indicate that:

- pin sites do not need to be cleaned if there is no exudate present. However, when necessary, cleaning should be done using normal saline
- pin-site crusts should be removed as it allows visualisation of the wound and free drainage of exudate
- pin sites may be left exposed if there is no exudate, otherwise woven gauze should be used.

Purulent discharge, redness or inflammation suggests infection and a wound swab should be taken to identify the causative organisms. The appropriate antibiotics should be commenced and the pin sites cleaned with normal saline and dressed with woven gauze, the frequency of dressing change depending on the amount of exudate (Lee-Smith et al 2001).

Maintaining normal body system functions

Traction, with its accompanying degree of restriction on movement and positioning, can create particular problems and the following interventions are important:

- Assessment and planning of care together with a physiotherapist, to coordinate and encourage breathing exercises, active and passive exercises to maintain joint mobility and prevent muscle wasting and deep vein thrombosis (DVT). In particular, regular dorsiflexion of the foot to counteract foot drop should be carried out. Local policy may determine the prophylactic measures to be implemented with the aim of preventing the complication of DVT.
- Ensure adequate fluid intake (2 L or more daily) and a balanced diet with plenty of fibre.
- Assess and plan care to prevent constipation; treat if present.
- Deal sympathetically with the awkwardness of using bedpans and urinals and fear of soiling the bed.
- As normal sleep position and pattern will be disturbed, every attempt should be made to make the patient

comfortable and relaxed before resorting to the use of hypnotic medication.
- Often patients are in traction for a long time and will feel the need for close physical contact with their partners. Ensure undisturbed privacy for them.
- Be creative in finding ways to alleviate boredom which is a hazard of lengthy hospitalisation, particularly when movement is restricted.

STOP THINK

10.4 Discuss ways in which you can help relieve the boredom of a patient who is in traction. Which other health professionals could you call upon to help in this respect?

10.5 Ask the physiotherapist in your clinical area to show you how to measure a patient for crutches and how to use them. Try walking with crutches yourself.

10.6 How many different kinds of walking aids can you identify in your clinical area? Discuss each with the physiotherapist.

Casts

A cast is a splinting device consisting of layers of bandages impregnated with plaster of Paris (POP), fibreglass or resin, some of which are applied wet and solidify as they dry out. Their main uses are to immobilise and hold bone fragments in reduction and to support and stabilise weak joints.

The advantages and disadvantages of the main categories of casting types are summarised below.

Plaster of Paris POP has better moulding properties, can be split or windowed if tension increases due to swelling and is cheaper. However, it takes 48 h to dry, and interferes with visualisation of bony detail on X-ray, making it more difficult to assess if a fracture is healing. It can be heavy and deforms permanently when it becomes wet. It is usually used for new injuries as a backslab, i.e. half a plaster held in place with a bandage, which allows for any potential swelling to take place. It has been suggested, however, that backslabs are no better than a full cast in allowing for pressure due to swelling in an acute injury (Younger et al 1990).

Synthetic casts These casts set within 20 min and allow early weight-bearing. They are stronger than POP due to the fibreglass content; thus, fewer layers are required and they are lighter. As they do not accommodate swelling, this material is infrequently used as the initial method of cast immobilisation following trauma, but if used, regular assessment of the neurovascular status of the limb is required. Synthetic casts are ideal for use in older patients, because they are lightweight and allow early mobilisation. A disadvantage is that they are more expensive than POP.

Adjustable focused rigidity primary casts These were developed in the 1990s and are adjustable to accommodate swelling or atrophy (wasting), reducing the risk of neurovascular impairment or insufficient support for a limb (Petty & Wardman 1998).

Cast bracing

A cast brace is applied closely to the limb and fitted with hinges to allow joint movement; this stimulates articular cartilage nutrition (Dandy & Edwards 2003). It allows early weight-bearing but needs specialist skills to apply correctly.

PRINCIPLES OF NURSING MANAGEMENT: Casts

In addition to the general principles of nursing management for musculoskeletal disorders (p. 446), the following will also apply.

Potential for neurovascular problems

Although padding such as Velband will allow for some swelling within the restricting cast, tissue pressure may build up and result in pain, tingling and discoloration. Unexplained pain is an important indicator that something is wrong, and therefore careful assessment and investigation of the cause, while alleviating the patient's discomfort, are essential. If not attended to immediately, pressure could lead to tissue necrosis and nerve palsy, the signs and symptoms of which include severe pain, odour and discoloration on the cast.

Prevention of neurovascular complications

- Elevate the limb above the level of the heart on cloth-covered pillows, unless compartment syndrome is suspected when elevation can exacerbate the condition and should be stopped (Love 1998).
- Avoid denting a moist cast by handling it only with the palms of the hands and not allowing it to rest on a flat, hard or sharp surface.
- Ensure that physiotherapy is carried out regularly.
- Have plaster cutting equipment ready and bivalve the cast, i.e. split it down both sides into two halves if signs and symptoms of neurovascular compromise do occur. Spread it enough to relieve pressure and remember to cut the padding, which may have shrunk due to drying blood and exudate.
- Cut an inspection and treatment window if pressure ulcer symptoms occur. The window must be replaced so that swelling does not rise into the space and cause more problems.
- Use an appropriate bed aid, such as a bed cage, to allow adequate air circulation, which aids in the drying process.

Care of the cast

Avoid getting the cast wet. Do not cover a plaster for any prolonged period with plastic or, in the case of a leg plaster, with rubber boots, because of condensation; however, synthetic protective covers can be used to permit the patient to take a shower. Teach the patient how to protect the cast when washing and when using bedpans and urinals. Casts can be cleaned by wiping with a damp cloth.

Many patients will go home wearing casts, so be sure to give them clear verbal and written instructions specific to their cast (see Box 10.4).

Removal of a cast

Application of a cast should be carried out only by experienced nurses or other health professionals, but all nurses

Box 10.4

Advice to patient with hand to elbow plaster

The plaster holds all the broken bones firmly in place to allow them to heal in the correct position. To prevent your fingers swelling, support your arm in the sling provided during the day and on pillows at night. It is important that you exercise the finger, elbow and shoulder joints of your injured arm at regular intervals, otherwise they will become stiff and painful to move.

The following exercises should be carried out at least four times each day:

- make a firm fist then stretch the fingers as wide as possible
- try to touch each fingertip with the thumb of that hand
- bend and stretch the elbow joint
- lift your arm high above your head — use the other arm to help
- move your arm behind your back as if you wanted to scratch between your shoulder blades.

Do not wet, heat or otherwise interfere with the plaster and do not insert sharp objects between the plaster and the skin to scratch — this could cause skin damage and infection.

Report to the doctor or Emergency Department AT ONCE if:

- the plaster cracks, becomes loose or uncomfortable
- there is pain
- the fingers become numb or difficult to move
- the fingers become more swollen, blue or very pale
- there is discharge
- you have any other problems.

need to be aware of the procedure for removal of a cast, to be familiar with the equipment used and to know where it is located.

Casts may need to be removed and renewed if they become loose or are damaged in any way. Where serious signs and symptoms of neurovascular complications have developed, splitting and removal will be required as an emergency procedure.

Guidelines for removal of a cast are given in Box 10.5.

External fixation

Bone fragments are held in position by skeletal pins inserted into the bone on either side of the fracture and held in alignment by a scaffold or a ring fixator (see Fig. 10.8). They are used for the treatment of some closed fractures, e.g. the pelvis, to stabilise open fractures with extensive soft tissue loss until the soft tissue has healed, for fractures that have not united by other methods, and for reconstructive surgery such as leg lengthening. Depending on the reason for their use they can be in place for as little as 6 weeks, e.g. for treatment of a closed fracture, or up to 1 year, e.g. in non-union of a tibial fracture.

PRINCIPLES OF NURSING MANAGEMENT: External fixation

In addition to the general principles relating to altered neurovascular status, positioning and potential for pin site

Box 10.5

Guidelines for removal of a cast

Equipment

- Plaster cutter — a small electric saw with a circular oscillating blade (with an integral dust extractor)
- Plaster spreader
- Large flat-bladed bandage scissors
- Plaster shears
- Plaster knife
- Protective eyewear such as goggles

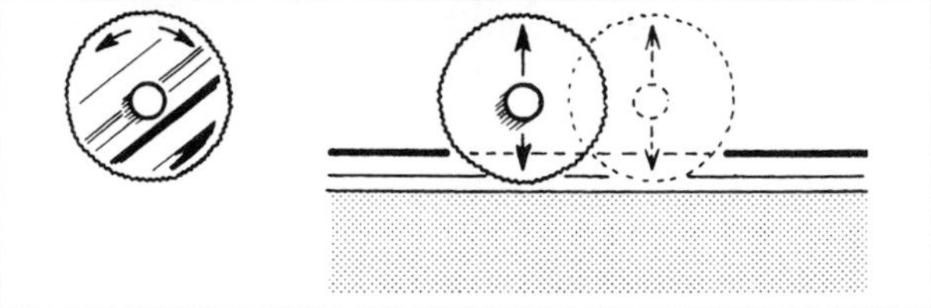

Procedure

- Explain to the patient what the procedure entails and, if the cast is padded, demonstrate the plaster cutter by turning it on and explaining its action (the electric cutter is not used on plasters that are not padded). Shears will be used on unpadded casts. Instruct the patient to shield the eyes as the saw could throw off fragments of plaster. Give reassurance that the saw will not cut the skin because of its oscillating action and the depth of padding.
- Mark where the cutting line will be with a felt pen and dampen it to reduce plaster dust. This line should avoid bony prominences; it is usually in front of the lateral malleolus and behind the medial malleolus in the lower limb, and along the ulnar or flexor surface in the upper limb.
- Grasp the electric cutter.
- Dust extractor apparatus and goggles should be used by plaster room personnel to comply with health and safety regulations.
- Turn on the cutter and push the blade firmly and gently through the cast, at the same time allowing the thumb to contact the cast as the blade oscillates. When you feel a 'give' or lack of resistance, you know you are through.
- Lift the cutter blade up a degree but not out of the groove and repeat until the line of cut is complete. The movement is one of alternating pressure on the oscillating blade and lifting slightly, at right angles to the plaster within the groove of the cut. It is wise to get the 'feel' of this by practical experience with discarded plasters and then in actual practice under the guidance of an expert.
- Cut the cast down both sides.
- Insert the blades of the plaster spreader at several sites along the line of cut then separate the cast with the hands.
- Cut the padding with the bandage scissors.
- Lift the limb carefully out of the posterior portion of the cast, maintaining the same position.
- After removal of the cast, wash the skin gently with pure soap and water, pat dry and apply skin cream. Expect a scaly appearance, some muscle atrophy, pain and stiffness, but reassure the patient that prescribed exercise will help to regain normal feeling, appearance and function in a relatively short period of time.

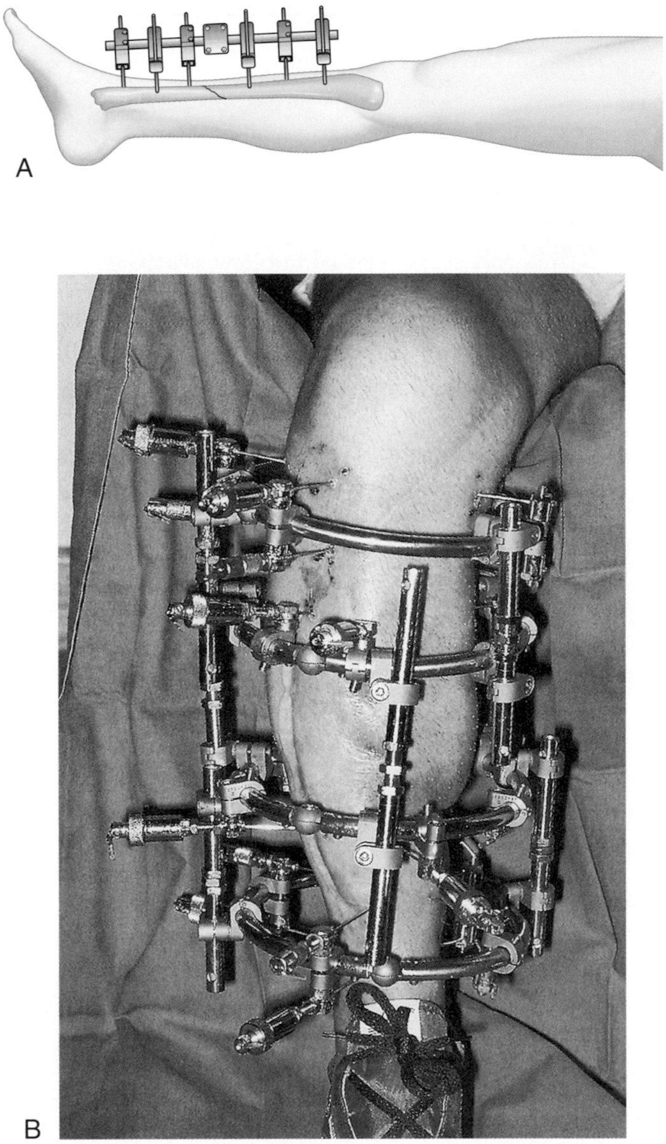

Fig. 10.8 Types of external fixation. A: External fixation of the tibia. B: External ring fixator in position on the tibia.

infection that have already been discussed, the following is specific to external fixation. As this device allows for early discharge of a patient, the nurse must ensure that the patient, carers and community staff are familiar with and confident in the care required (Sims et al 1999).

Appearance

The appearance of the appliance may cause the patient concern. In hospital, patients with an external fixator may be nursed with other patients having the same treatment and may therefore feel comfortable. On discharge, however, they may be exposed to the gaze and curiosity of the public. Limb (2004), in a survey of 60 patients with external fixators, found that they had below-average mean scores on a self-concept scale, with particularly low scores related to body image. He suggests that individual or group discussions may help patients through the process of treatment.

For further information, see Dandy & Edwards (2003).

Internal fixation

Fractures may also be stabilised by surgical intervention where nails, plates, wires, screws or rods hold the bone fragments in place (see Fig. 10.9). Again this permits earlier mobilisation and reduces the potential for complications. All perioperative principles of nursing management apply in this instance (see Ch. 26).

FRACTURES OF SPECIFIC SITES

Fracture of the femoral shaft

Femoral shaft fractures are most commonly seen in young people following motorcycle or car accidents.

MEDICAL MANAGEMENT

Following X-ray to confirm the diagnosis:

- operative treatment may consist of either internal fixation, usually the preferred option, or rarely, external fixation.
- the fracture may be reduced under general anaesthetic and skeletal traction applied. Any accompanying wounds are debrided or sutured at the same time. If there is adequate callus formation within 2–6 weeks, a cast brace may be applied.

NURSING PRIORITIES AND MANAGEMENT: Fracture of the femoral shaft

In addition to the principles of management relating to a fracture, operative intervention and traction, the following are specific to fracture of the shaft of femur.

Haemorrhage

An early complication may be damage to the femoral artery from bone fragments, in addition to bleeding from other

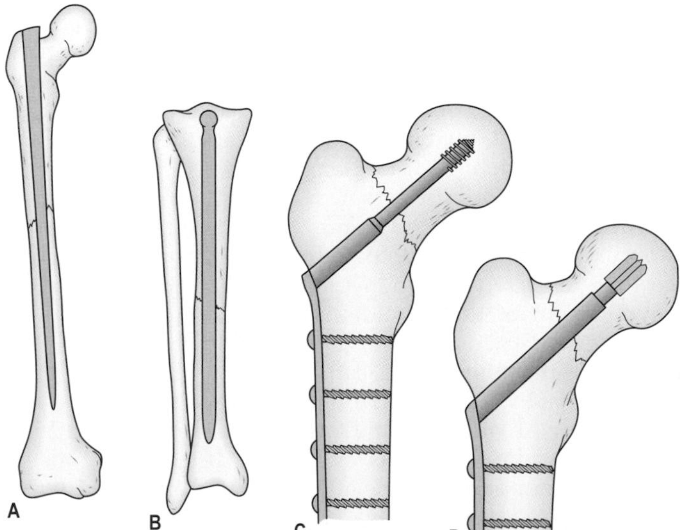

Fig. 10.9 Types of internal fixation. A, B: Intramedullary nails. C: Compression nail for fixation of femoral neck. D: Sliding nail fixation of the femoral neck.

damaged tissues and the bone marrow. As much as a litre of blood can be contained within the thigh, and this hidden haemorrhage can result in hypovolaemic shock (see Ch. 18).

The nurse must be alert for signs of haemorrhage and shock and ensure that i.v. replacement therapy is ready and that blood is sent for cross-matching.

Fat emboli

Fat emboli are a particular hazard following fracture of the shaft of the femur but can also occur following fracture of any long bone. There are two theories relating to the cause: one is that fat cells from damaged tissue migrate into ruptured veins; the other is that catecholamines released through the stress of trauma mobilise lipids from fatty tissue. In the lung, these droplets are converted into free fatty acids which are toxic to lung tissue and disrupt alveolar function. Additionally, the droplets may become enmeshed in the capillary network of the alveoli and disrupt gas exchange. This can lead to cerebral hypoxia and, if large vessels in the pulmonary system are involved, to respiratory failure and death. Early signs of fatty emboli are increased respiratory rate, anxiety, transient petechial haemorrhage and confusion. The last two are the classic and most important clinical signs.

The nurse must be alert for early signs of altered mental status — anxiety, irritability and especially confusion. Report this immediately and be prepared to deal with respiratory failure and arrest and to transfer the patient to intensive care. Equipment should be ready for immediate blood gas analysis.

Collaborative care

The nurse has an important role in coordinating the care provided to ensure that all physical and psychosocial issues are addressed.

Fracture of neck of femur

There are over 69 000 fractures of the femoral neck, commonly known as a hip fracture or fractured neck of femur, in the UK each year (Shire Pharmaceuticals 1998) and 1.66 million worldwide (Santy 1998). They are most common in older people, particularly women who may have osteoporotic bones. There is much evidence to show that preventive methods can be useful in reducing the risk (see Research Abstract 10.1).

It is also recognised that successful care of a patient with a fractured neck of femur depends on a coordinated approach throughout the patient journey from initial injury to long-term rehabilitation (SIGN 2002a). This means the involvement of the multidisciplinary team as well as the nursing and medical staff. The physiotherapist will help to ensure that the patient can walk and get out of a chair and bed safely. The occupational therapist will ensure that the patient can manage activities such as eating and bathing, providing adaptations as necessary. If a patient needs additional support at home after discharge, or needs to find alternative accommodation, the social worker can help. Other health care professionals will be involved following individual patient assessment; for example, some patients may require a chiropodist if they cannot bend to attend to their pedicure.

RESEARCH ABSTRACT 10.1

Hip fracture: the SIGN guidelines

The Scottish Intercollegiate Guidelines Network have examined the evidence for the prevention and treatment of hip fractures, and graded this to provide nurses and other health care workers with a basis for evidence-based practice. Included in their recommendations are:

- Assessment of the risk of hip fractures and falls should be carried out and those at increased risk should be offered multiple interventions — an exercise programme, balance training, modification of identified hazards, treatment with calcium and vitamin D, and hip protectors.
- For patients who have sustained a hip fracture the routine use of traction preoperatively is not recommended.
- Prophylaxis against deep vein thrombosis should be considered; mechanical means (foot pumps or intermittent pneumatic compression) and aspirin, and heparin for high-risk patients.
- Discharge planning should begin within 48 h of admission and is a multidisciplinary team effort.

Scottish Intercollegiate Guidelines Network (SIGN) 2002a Prevention and management of hip fractures in older people No. 56. Online. Available: www.sign.ac.uk

MEDICAL MANAGEMENT

History and examination The patient may have been found on the floor following a fall and, if living alone, could have been there for some time and be suffering from hypothermia and dehydration. Careful assessment to identify other reasons which may have led to the fall, such as a cerebrovascular accident or myocardial infarction, should be made. The patient will complain of severe pain in the hip or knee and there will be visible shortening and external rotation of the affected leg. Diagnosis will be confirmed by X-ray.

Treatment Depending on the site of the fracture, and the age and condition of the patient, the treatment will be either internal fixation with a plate and screws or replacement of the head of femur with a metal prosthesis. Intracapsular fractures high in the neck of the femur have a serious effect on the blood supply to the femoral head (see Fig. 10.10) which would certainly need operative replacement.

NURSING PRIORITIES AND MANAGEMENT: Fracture of neck of femur

In addition to the general principles relating to musculoskeletal injury and fractures, the following priorities need to be addressed.

Potential complications As a result of age and general physical condition when found, the patient may be confused and fearful and need a great deal of comfort and reassurance. Measures will be taken to reverse any hypothermia and dehydration. Risk assessment of the patient for skin

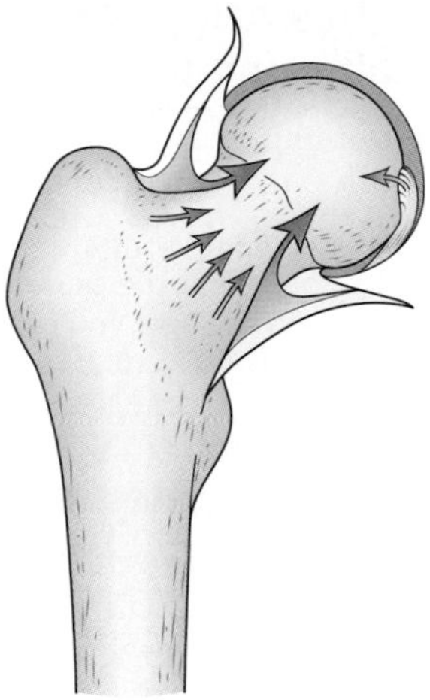

Fig. 10.10 Blood supply of the femoral head via the capsule. Intramedullary vessels and ligamentum teres.

breakdown using an approved scale such as the Waterlow scale (see Ch. 23) should be recorded and the patient may be nursed on a therapeutic bed. Vital signs will be monitored at 4-hourly intervals to detect early signs of complications.

Pain With an extracapsular fracture there is often extensive bruising which adds to the severe pain. When the cause has been established, this may be treated by repositioning and supporting the body and limbs, and administering prescribed analgesics. Pain assessment and pain relief measures should be implemented (see Ch. 19).

Increased risk of multisystem complications For an older patient, such acute trauma and associated surgery may lead to multisystem failure (see Ch. 18).

Rehabilitation Discharge planning should commence within 48 h of admission (SIGN 2002a). The use of an integrated care pathway (ICP) can help to improve the standard of overall care by ensuring that each member of the multidisciplinary team knows the best available evidence for care and when that care should be carried out (Tarling et al 2002) (see Table 10.1). Early supported discharge schemes, often led by nurses, can help to ensure that patients are discharged rapidly but safely to their home environment (Renton & Brown 2001).

STOP THINK **10.7** Discuss with your mentor how an ICP differs from a nursing care plan, and what are the advantages and disadvantages of each.

Fracture of the tibia and fibula

Fracture of the tibia and fibula is one of the most common injuries dealt with by orthopaedic surgeons. These fractures usually result from direct impact to the limb, and extensive skin and soft tissue damage may be present. RTCs and sports injuries are common causes.

MEDICAL MANAGEMENT

Treatment There are three choices of treatment.

Cast immobilisation This is the treatment of choice for closed, stable injuries. If the fracture requires manipulation, the patient will receive a general anaesthetic which will necessitate a stay in hospital; otherwise the patient may be discharged home from the Emergency Department. Following reduction of the fracture, a long leg plaster cast will be applied and plain radiographs taken to confirm the position of the fracture. Repeat X-rays will be taken at 1 week, 2 weeks and then at monthly intervals following reduction. The patient will not be allowed to bear weight on the injured leg for at least 1 month following injury. At this stage a Sarmiento type plaster, patellar tendon bearing, may be applied (McRae & Esser 2002) and the patient allowed to bear weight through the injured limb. The average length of stay in plaster for this type of injury is 12–16 weeks.

Internal fixation Fractures which are closed but unstable will benefit from internal fixation using a nail, but some patients may be placed in a plaster cast for 6–8 weeks

Table 10.1 Extract from the integrated care pathway of a patient with a fractured neck of femur — postoperative day 1 (nursing part only)

Patient problem/need	Nursing intervention	Expected outcome
Recovery from anaesthetic	4-hourly monitoring of vital signs	Vital signs within normal limits
Wound care	Check wound site dressing Check and record wound drainage	Dressing dry and intact Drain to be removed at 24 h after surgery as further drainage minimal
Neurovascular status of limb	Monitor neurovascular status of affected limb	No neurovascular deficit
Relief of pain	Use pain score with patient 4-hourly Administer analgesics as prescribed	Pain relief at level acceptable to patient
Risk of deep vein thrombosis (DVT)	Ensure anti-embolic stocking in situ Thromboprophylaxis injection as prescribed Monitor for signs of DVT	Reduction in risk and early detection of problem
Reduced mobility	Ensure patient understands correct way to transfer and mobilise	Patient to sit in chair Patient to walk to end of bed with aid of Zimmer frame

following surgery. Routine postoperative care as discussed in Chapter 26, and cast care (see p. 451) will be required. The patient will be able to use crutches once fully recovered from the effects of surgery.

External fixation If there is skin loss or a contaminated wound at the fracture site, the choice of treatment is more commonly an external fixator. This enables frequent observation of the wounds and easy access for wound dressing changes. An external fixator is applied under a general anaesthetic in an operating theatre.

This type of fixator holds the fracture in position and the patient can be walking, weight-bearing or not, dependent on the injury and the stability of the fixation of the injured limb, and discharged home to allow the community nurse and general practitioner (GP) to attend to the wounds. The patient is reviewed at regular intervals at the outpatient clinic (see Case History 10.1).

CASE HISTORY 10.1

Mr K

Mr K is a 40-year-old man who lives alone. He sustained a compound fracture to his left tibia and fibula while skiing with friends in the Highlands of Scotland. One friend stayed with him on the mountainside while the other alerted the emergency services, who arrived within an hour. The paramedical team applied a clean dressing over the open wound and splinted his leg.

On arrival at the hospital, Mr K was in obvious pain, although he had been using the analgesic gas Entonox, so the doctor administered an intravenous analgesic.

In the Emergency Department, the named nurse, Bill, noted Mr K's temperature, pulse, blood pressure and respirations, and the colour, sensation and movement of the injured limb, all of which were within normal limits. A clean sterile dressing was applied to the wound following inspection by the doctor.

Confirmation of the diagnosis was made by radiography and it was decided to take Mr K to the operating theatre for application of an external fixator to his left leg. This was explained to him and a picture of an external fixator in position was shown to him and the two friends who had accompanied him. His first reaction was revulsion at all the metal pins and scaffolding, but as his friends joked about his 'bionic parts' his anxiety subsided.

After an uneventful postoperative period, Mr K was allowed to sit in an armchair on day 1 with his leg elevated on a stool to reduce the swelling. The wound had been dressed in theatre following the local dressing policy of the institution. The physiotherapist gradually assisted Mr K to walk with the help of crutches without bearing weight on his left leg, and showed him how to manage the awkward appliance to avoid injuring himself. He was helped to widen two pairs of trousers below the knee so that he could cover the external fixator.

As Mr K lived on his own, the social worker made arrangements for a home help to be provided on discharge. His two friends agreed to visit him and provide him with food and other provisions at the weekends. Mr K was shown how to dress the pin sites himself and educated to be aware of the warning signs of infection or other complications. It was arranged that a community nurse would visit weekly to bring fresh supplies of dressings and to check the pin sites. He was given a contact name and number if he required advice between visits.

Mr K was discharged home 6 days after his accident with a return appointment for 2 weeks later.

NURSING PRIORITIES AND MANAGEMENT: Fracture of the tibia and fibula

The principles of nursing management for each type of treatment are given on pages 451, 452 and 453.

STOP THINK **10.8** Jot down the complications associated with fractures. Discuss with colleagues the causes of each complication and say how you can prevent it. Check your findings with Table 10.2.

Fracture of neck of humerus

Fracture of the neck of the humerus commonly occurs in older adults with osteoporosis after a fall on an outstretched hand. Often the bone is not displaced or badly impacted and normally heals well, depending on its stability. The major complication is of shoulder and elbow stiffness.

MEDICAL MANAGEMENT

Treatment This injury can usually be treated at home following the initial visit to the Emergency Department, providing there is no gross displacement or neurovascular complications. The arm is supported in a shoulder immobiliser, broad arm sling or collar and cuff for approximately 2 weeks. Movement is gradually introduced, followed by outpatient physiotherapy, in order to avoid the major complication — development of a stiff shoulder joint. If the fracture does not heal, internal fixation may be required.

NURSING PRIORITIES AND MANAGEMENT: Fracture of neck of humerus

Assessment of ability to carry out normal activities of daily living This is done before the patient is discharged home from the Emergency Department. Home nursing and home help are arranged accordingly, or a supported discharge scheme may be in place (Renton & Brown 2001).

Skin care of injured arm If a supported discharge scheme is not available, it is wise to have the community nurse attend to washing the injured arm two or three times a week, taking particular care of the axilla. The sling is reapplied and neurovascular status and degree of mobility monitored. Case History 10.2 outlines the continuing care of an older lady with fractured neck of humerus.

STOP THINK **10.9** After initial instruction from your tutor or mentor and with a fellow student, practise applying a broad arm sling, a high sling and a collar and cuff.

Colles' fracture

This is one of the most common fractures seen at the Emergency Department and usually involves the lower end of the radius within 2.5 cm of the wrist joint. There may be an associated fracture of the ulnar styloid. The obvious feature of a Colles' fracture is the classic 'dinner fork' deformity (see Fig. 10.11). It is commonly found in middle-aged and older women after a fall on an outstretched hand.

Table 10.2 Prevention of complications of fractures

Complication	Cause	Prevention
Damage to soft tissue — neurovascular compromise	Trauma Sharp fragments/edge of bone	Monitor neurovascular function regularly — report abnormalities
Complications associated with immobility:		
Diminished function of all body systems	Decreased physical stimulation	Encourage active and passive exercise
Muscle atrophy — decreased range of movement — contractures	Lack of normal exercise	Coordinate physiotherapy programme
Altered psychological processes	Decreased social stimulation	Provide social and mental stimulation
Pressure ulcers	Casts — prolonged pressure	Regular pressure area care and position change
Infection	Open wound postoperatively Skeletal pin sites	Apply principles of infection control
Malunion	Mal-apposition of bony fragments Inadequate mobilisation (e.g. swelling subsides — cast becomes loose)	Meticulous and regular monitoring of cast fit and traction alignment
Delayed union	Unstable fracture Poor blood supply	Maintain adequate circulation and splintage
Non-union	Infection Soft tissue intrusion	Infection control
Fat embolus — emergency	Fat globules released into circulation from bone marrow at fracture site — usually associated with fractured femur or multiple fractures	Early reduction and splintage Report confusion, chest pain, dyspnoea immediately (see p. 454)

CASE HISTORY 10.2

Mrs L

Mrs L is a 70-year-old lady living alone in sheltered housing. She was admitted to the Emergency Department following a fractured neck of humerus, which was treated with a sling. The supported discharge scheme sister undertook a multidisciplinary assessment of Mrs L, who was discharged home after a stay of 2 h in the Emergency Department. The social worker within the supported discharge team arranged a suitable social care package to provide the support Mrs L would require.

The supported discharge scheme staff nurse visited Mrs L at home to wash and dry the skin around her injured shoulder, inspecting it for any signs of friction or pressure. Extensive bruising was noted over the shoulder region. The sling was reapplied. The nurse checked that Mrs L was moving her joints as advised and that no joint stiffness was present. It was established that no neurovascular deficit was present and Mrs L was educated to look for any developing signs of tingling or numbness of the fingers, change in finger colour or warmth, and/or reduced ability to move the arm.

The team's occupational therapist carried out an assessment and suggested changes to the environment, such as removing the bath mat on which Mrs L had slipped and replacing it with a non-slip one. Mrs L attended the hospital outpatient department 10 days later where she was seen by an orthopaedic specialist. The supported discharge team completed their package of care at this point, but social services continued to provide social care, including help with hygiene needs.

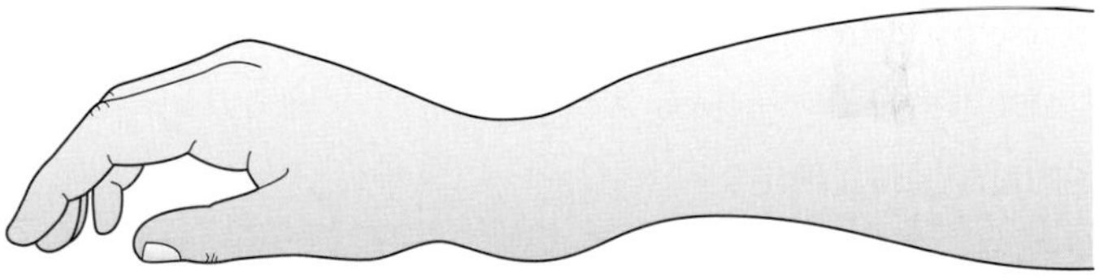

Fig. 10.11 The 'dinner fork' deformity of Colles' fracture.

MEDICAL MANAGEMENT

Examination Diagnosis will be confirmed by the appearance of the patient's wrist and by plain X-rays.

Treatment Manipulation of the joint is required to reduce the fracture and for this anaesthesia is required. This may be a haematoma block, i.e. the blood clot around the fracture is injected with a local anaesthetic, intravenous regional anaesthesia, i.e. Bier's block, or general anaesthesia. A Cochrane Review (Handoll et al 2004) concluded that there was insufficient evidence to establish the relative effectiveness of different methods of anaesthesia but that a haematoma block provides poorer analgesia than intravenous regional anaesthesia. After successful reduction, the position is maintained by a backslab for 2–3 days to allow for any swelling, and then by a complete hand to below elbow cast. Internal or external fixation may be necessary if closed reduction is unsuccessful.

Prevention This fracture is more often seen in the winter months, and older people should be advised to avoid slippery surfaces. Osteoporosis investigation and advice should also be initiated, to ensure that the risk of future fractures is minimised (see p. 461).

NURSING PRIORITIES AND MANAGEMENT: Colles' fracture

In addition to the management principles already discussed which relate to musculoskeletal trauma, fractures and plaster casts, the following priorities should be noted.

Removal of rings Marked swelling of the fingers is likely to occur and it is important to remove all rings and bracelets from the injured hand as soon as possible. If swelling has already made this impossible, it will be necessary to obtain the patient's permission to cut the rings off using the special ring cutter found in all Emergency Departments. The arm should be kept elevated to reduce swelling.

Advice Ensure that the patient is given written and verbal advice for a hand to elbow plaster as described in Box 10.4 (p. 452). Advice is equally as important after the plaster cast has been removed, usually after 6–8 weeks, as the wrist joint will be stiff and weak due to lack of use. Nursing staff in fracture clinics should educate patients about the rehabilitation exercises they should perform and encourage them to do these regularly. A removable splint, futura splint, can be provided to give some support. In some areas, nurse-led clinics are being developed so that this patient group can receive holistic care from an experienced orthopaedic nurse practitioner (Wardman 2002).

SPINAL INJURIES

Injury or damage to the vertebral column which protects the spinal cord may be confined to bony and/or ligament injury or may be accompanied by damage to the cord itself. This spinal cord damage can happen at the time of injury or be the result of poor handling of the patient by health care professionals. It is estimated that 500–700 people per year in the UK sustain traumatic injury to the spinal cord (Harrison 2000) but many more sustain vertebral fractures or ligament damage with no spinal cord damage. Common reasons for spinal cord injury (Smith 2004a) are:

- road traffic collisions
- falls, such as falling downstairs
- industrial injuries, mainly building site falls
- sports injuries, e.g. rugby, skiing and diving.

PATHOPHYSIOLOGY

The resultant damage can involve transection, compression, contusion or interference to the spinal cord, accompanied by varying degrees of paralysis and sensory deficit below the level of the lesion (see Fig. 10.12). There is hope, however, that research can find ways of reversing this damage (see Research Abstract 10.2).

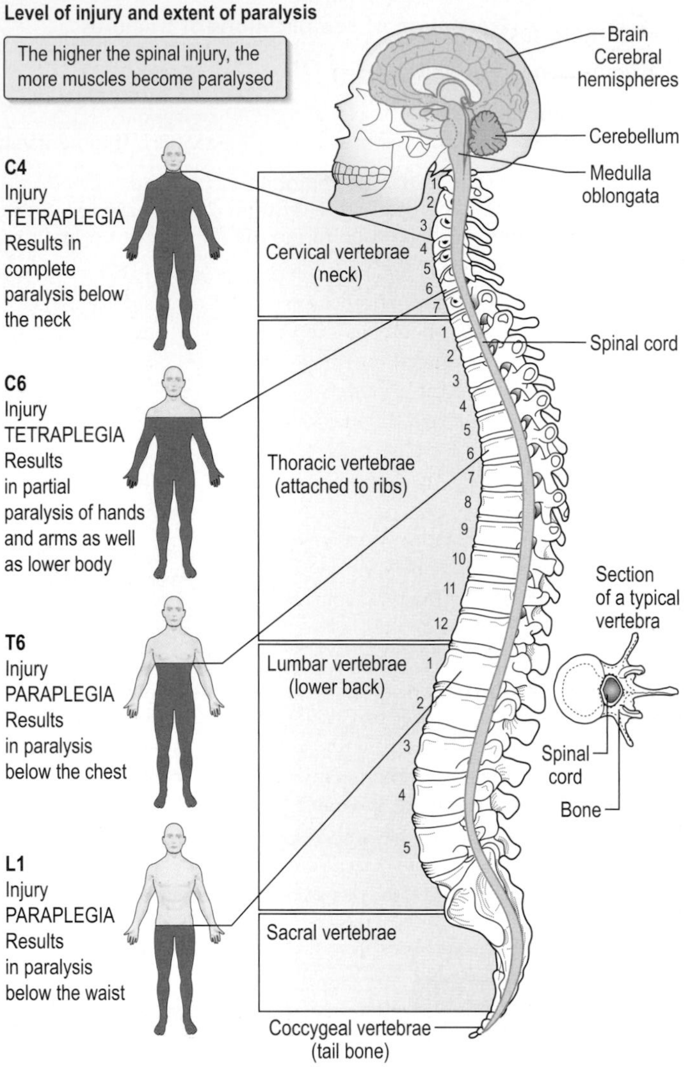

Fig. 10.12 Level of injury and extent of paralysis. (Reproduced with permission from the Spinal Injuries Association 2000; see 'Useful websites' and addresses.)

MEDICAL MANAGEMENT

The three principles of management (Smith 2004a) are:

- *Preserving existing neurological function*, which includes correct moving and handling of the patient. Vertebral fractures may be stabilised with halo traction (see Fig. 10.13) which facilitates early mobilisation in patients with intact neurological function. Some stable fractures, especially lower thoracic and lumbar fractures, can be treated by bed rest on a firm base.
- *Physiological resuscitation*, i.e. attending to the potential life-threatening respiratory and cardiovascular effects related to spinal cord injury, e.g.:
  — ineffective airway clearance
  — ineffective breathing pattern
  — hypotension
  — bradycardia
  — hypothermia.

RESEARCH ABSTRACT 10.2

International Spinal Research — the 4 cm future

A registered charity, Spinal Research, is working on research trials with the hope of finding ways of regenerating 4 cm of spinal cord in a paralysed person. These 4 cm could potentially help a seriously paralysed person to breathe unaided or to regain use of the arms. A number of possibilities are being explored.

- *Neuroprotection.* Most spinal injuries do not completely sever the spinal cord but the neurones that do die send out signals to nearby uninjured neurones and these also die a few hours after the original injury. Research is examining how this early secondary damage can be reduced.
- *Chondroitinase treatment.* Chondroitinase is an enzyme that partially removes the barrier formed by scar tissue around a spinal cord injury, thus allowing regenerating nerve fibres to pass through.
- *Combating blockers.* Antibodies have been developed to counteract the effects of Nogo, a family of protein molecules that prevent the regrowth of spinal cord nerve fibres.
- *Filling the gap.* Biocompatible materials have been developed which can form a bridge across the damaged region so that nerve fibres, blood vessels and supporting tissues can regrow.
- *Nurturing regrowth.* Olfactory glia are cells that guide and protect newly forming nerve fibres. They are present in the olfactory system but researchers have transplanted them into spinal cord injuries in the laboratory and some regenerative effect has occurred.
- *Replacing stem cells.* Stem cells have the potential to develop into any type of cell in the body and thus could replace all the damaged tissue in the spinal cord. Stem cell research using embryonic stem cells has ethical issues and is still in its early stages. Scientists do not yet understand how to control stem cells and make them turn into the required cell types, and those transplanted into spinal injuries tend to turn into cells that make cell tissue.

A combination of some or all of these methods could mean that spinal cord injuries may be successfully reversed, or at least the patient's clinical condition improved.

Spinal Research 2004 Spinal cord repair. Online. Available: www.spinal-research.org

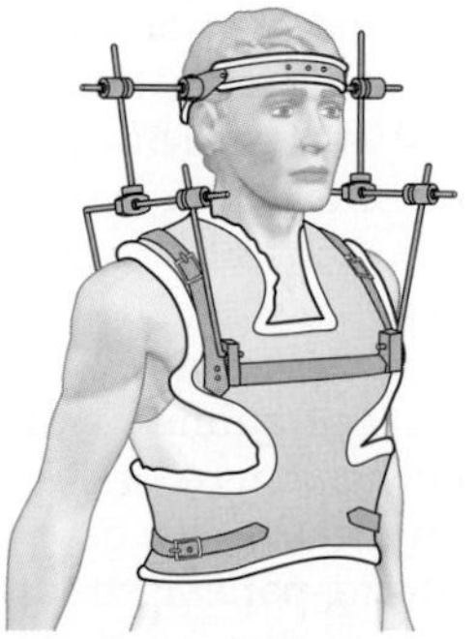

Fig. 10.13 'Halo-vest' traction. A halo fixed to the skull — attached to bars mounted on the chest.

The last three are caused by spinal shock, i.e. the cessation of conduction within the spinal cord neurones. This results in a loss of voluntary movement and sensation below the level of the injury and progressive loss of sympathetic and parasympathetic activity, which can last for up to 6 weeks.

- *Prevention of secondary complications*, which may be physical or psychological (see p. 460).

It is accepted practice in the UK and Eire that any patient with an actual or potential spinal cord injury is transferred to one of 12 specialist spinal injury units (SIUs) (Harrison 2000). Ideally this should occur immediately but may be delayed due to patients being unfit to travel or a bed not being available. All nurses in general hospitals should therefore understand the principles of caring for a patient with a confirmed spinal cord injury, and that every patient with spinal trauma should be treated as a potential spinal cord injury patient until investigations such as MRI or X-rays have provided a firm diagnosis. Patients who have damaged the ligaments supporting the vertebral column (see Fig. 10.14) may have a potentially dangerous unstable spine.

NURSING PRIORITIES AND MANAGEMENT: Spinal injuries

Basic principles of positioning and moving patients with spinal injury All nurses should be aware of the importance of maintaining anatomical alignment of the vertebral column in patients with suspected spinal cord injury, both before patients reach hospital and once they are admitted, to avoid scenarios such as that outlined in Case History 10.3. Manoeuvres such as log rolling the patient (see p. 951) (for thoracolumbar injuries), pelvic twists (for cervical injuries) and using special beds (e.g. an electric turning bed) are carried out under the guidance of an experienced nurse.

STOP THINK **10.10** What do you suspect are the main reasons for such different outcomes for the accident victims described in Case History 10.3?

CASE HISTORY 10.3

First aid for accident victims — the effect on outcome

Two 18-year-old men were brought into the Emergency Department on the same night. They had both sustained multiple injuries to the head and body in similar road traffic collisions — P had been moved from his overturned vehicle by well-meaning people at the scene of the accident whilst waiting for the ambulance to arrive, whereas T was supported in the position in which he was found until the ambulance team arrived. They applied a neck collar and maintained skeletal alignment whilst transferring him to the ambulance and at all times subsequently. Spinal X-rays showed that the men had identical injuries to the cervical spine.

Two months later, T walked out of the spinal injuries unit; many months later, P was wheeled out of the same unit as a quadriplegic.

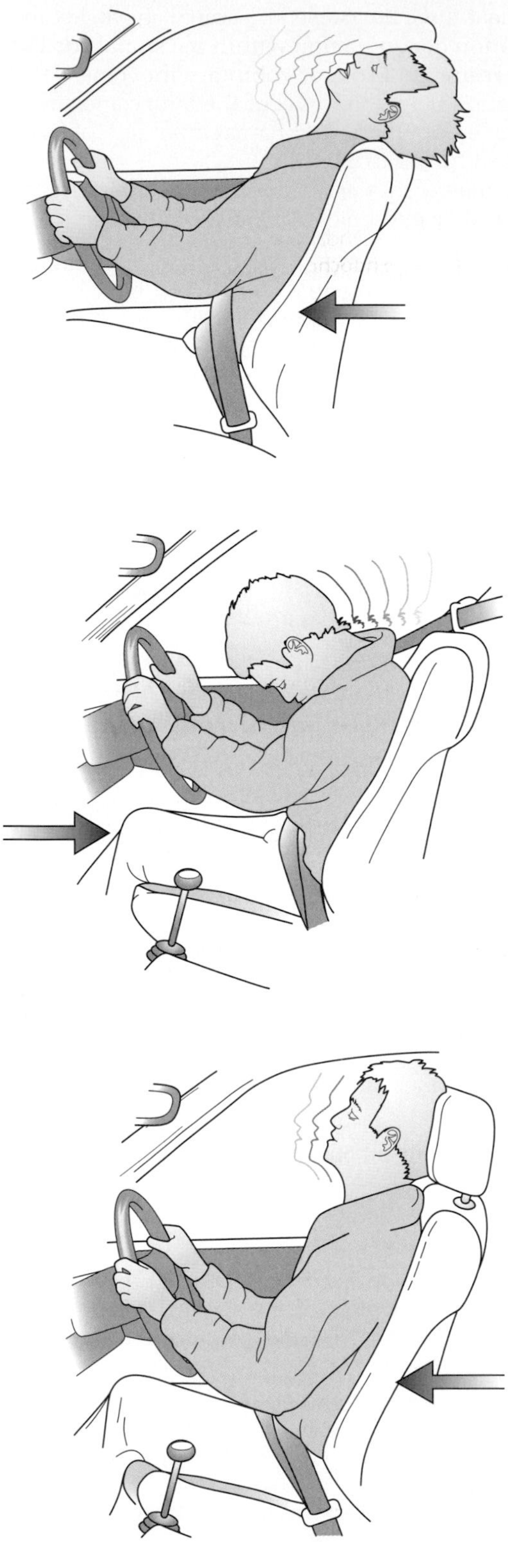

Fig. 10.14 Combined flexion/extension (whiplash) injury of the cervical spine. Movement of the head is limited by a head restraint.

Respiratory and cardiovascular monitoring This is a vital nursing responsibility, to detect any deterioration in the functioning of these systems. Depending on the level of injury, patients may be ventilated. Deep vein thrombosis is a potential complication and prophylaxis should be carried out according to local policy.

Additional physical care Patients with a spinal cord injury have the potential to develop additional physical problems, in particular paralytic ileus, gastric ulceration and pressure ulcers. During the acute stage the patient will have a flaccid bowel and bladder, and therefore urinary catheterisation will be necessary and manual evacuation of faeces will be undertaken by a suitably qualified practitioner.

Psychological care Spinal cord injury is a life-changing event, not only for the patient but also for the family. The experience of SIU staff is that two of the most important interventions nurses can perform are to be truthful at all times, ensuring all staff are providing the same information, and to reduce the effects of sensory deprivation through the use of therapeutic touch and aids such as mirrors (Harrison 2000). Long-term support and adaptation will be necessary and organisations such as the Spinal Injuries Association (see 'Useful websites and addresses') are vital in this.

10.11 You are on placement with a community nurse who has been asked to teach the principles of first aid in spinal injury. Ask if you can accompany her to the teaching session or, if this is not possible, ask her to share her teaching plan with you.

OSTEOPOROSIS

Osteoporosis is 'a progressive systemic skeletal disease characterised by low bone mass and microarchitectural deterioration of bone tissue, with a consequent increase in bone fragility and susceptibility to fracture' (World Health Organization 1994). It is estimated that 1 in 3 women and 1 in 12 men in the UK will develop clinically significant osteoporosis (Allsworth 2004).

PATHOPHYSIOLOGY

The characteristic overall reduction in bone mineral density (BMD) is caused by both uncontrollable and modifiable factors (Howard 2001). Eighty per cent of BMD is determined by genetically determined risk factors such as race, gender and stature. The remaining 20% is influenced by non-genetic factors which can be modified to enhance BMD (see below). Patients become susceptible to fractures, with the wrist, e.g. Colles' fracture, vertebrae and neck of femur as the most common sites.

MEDICAL MANAGEMENT

Prevention is aimed at ensuring that patients have as high a BMD as possible. Modifications to diet, e.g. increased calcium, and exercise, ensuring sufficient weight-bearing exercise, are key in this. Peak BMD is reached during a person's mid-30s and therefore such modifications should ideally be made before this, although there are benefits in all age groups.

Early identification is also key. It has long been recognised that a low-impact or fragility fracture, i.e. one sustained by falling from standing height or less, especially a distal radial fracture, is suggestive of osteoporosis and merits further investigation and patient education (Royal College of Physicians 1999). In particular, women under 50 with a low-impact Colles' fracture should have their bone density measured and appropriate treatment initiated by their GP or local osteoporosis unit (Royal College of Physicians 1999).

In the presence of osteoporosis, medication therapy is instituted to inhibit bone resorption by osteoclasts and therefore slow down the rate of bone loss. A group of drugs known as the bisphosphonates are widely prescribed and are designed to bind calcium to bone; in the UK, etidronate, alendronate and risedronate are licensed for use (Allsworth 2004). Vitamin D and calcium supplements are also prescribed, as vitamin D is required for the absorption of calcium, and calcium supplementation is vital in the prevention and treatment of postmenopausal osteoporosis (James 2000).

Hormone replacement therapy (HRT) was widely prescribed for the prevention and treatment of osteoporosis but questions about long-term safety, in particular the increased risk of breast cancer, have led to a change in thinking. A review of the evidence (Lookinland & Beckstrand 2003) concludes that HRT should not be used for the primary prevention of chronic diseases such as osteoporosis, and if it is used to control menopausal symptoms it should be limited to 2–3 years at the lowest dose (see Ch. 7).

NURSING PRIORITIES AND MANAGEMENT: Osteoporosis

Prevention Nurses can play a key role in education of the population about the importance of diet and exercise in the prevention of bone problems later in life. Community nurses, school nurses and health visitors are specific groups that can contribute, but all nurses can use time spent with patients as a health promotion opportunity.

Early detection and treatment A number of hospitals are developing schemes whereby patients identified as at risk of osteoporosis, especially patients who have had a Colles' or femoral neck fracture, are screened for osteoporosis and treated appropriately. Many of these schemes are nurse led (Content et al 2003).

BONE TUMOURS

A patient with a bone tumour usually requires complex care which is interprofessional, multi-agency and comprises many types of treatment. A key nursing role is therefore the coordination of care and specialist nurses with a knowledge of orthopaedic and oncology care are invaluable in this and in supporting patients through their journey.

Primary bone tumours can be benign or malignant, although some benign tumours may become malignant. Bone tumours are usually classified according to the cell type from which they originate (see Table 10.3). Metastatic bone disease is malignant bone disease due to secondary deposits in bone tissue from a primary neoplastic site elsewhere (see Ch. 31).

For further information, see Kneale & Davis (2004).

Table 10.3 A classification of bone tumours

Tissue of origin	Benign tumour	Malignant tumour
Bone	Osteoid osteoma Osteoblastoma Aneurysmal bone cysts	Osteosarcoma
Cartilage	Osteochondroma Chondroma Endochondroma	Chondrosarcoma
Fibrous marrow	Fibroma	Fibrosarcoma Myeloma
Uncertain	Giant cell tumour Benign fibrous histiocytoma	Ewing's sarcoma Malignant fibrous histiocytoma

Reproduced with permission from Henry (2004).

PATHOPHYSIOLOGY

Primary bone tumours are known to occur in specific age groups and in certain sites of bone tissue. Osteosarcoma, for example, is most often seen in people under the age of 30 and usually occurs in the metaphyseal region of the distal femur, proximal tibia and proximal humerus.

As the bone tumour grows, eruption into the surrounding tissues can occur which may be noted as a warm swelling of the affected area. The tumour will originate from a specific cell type within the bone tissue, but may then involve a variety of bone cells.

Approximately 30–70% of all new cancers develop skeletal metastases and, of these, 80% arise from carcinomas of the breast, prostate and lung, with those of the kidney and thyroid to a lesser degree (Dupuy & Goldberg 2001). Bony metastases are usually transmitted by the blood and tend to occur in sites where red bone marrow is present, the commonest sites being the femur, humerus and acetabulum.

MEDICAL MANAGEMENT

History Patients most commonly present with pain, due to stretching of the surrounding tissue by the tumour and/or its impingement on nerves and blood vessels. Pain at night and pain not relieved by rest are indications of malignant tumours. Other symptoms include swelling, reduction in movement of the affected limb and reduced sensation (Henry 2004).

Investigations There are three main investigations:

- Blood tests — raised serum alkaline phosphatase may be present, due to increased osteoblastic activity, and a raised ESR or white cell count can occur in certain tumours due to the necrotic nature of the tumour (Henry 2004)
- Imaging — plain X-ray may reveal the presence of a tumour, but other forms of imaging may be used to provide more detail, especially MRI and CT scans
- Biopsy — in order to determine histopathology and microbiology.

Treatment is usually dependent on the type of bone tumour.

Benign bone tumours Osteochondroma, the most common type, is managed by wide excision. Osteoclastoma, common in the femur and tibia, may require excision and

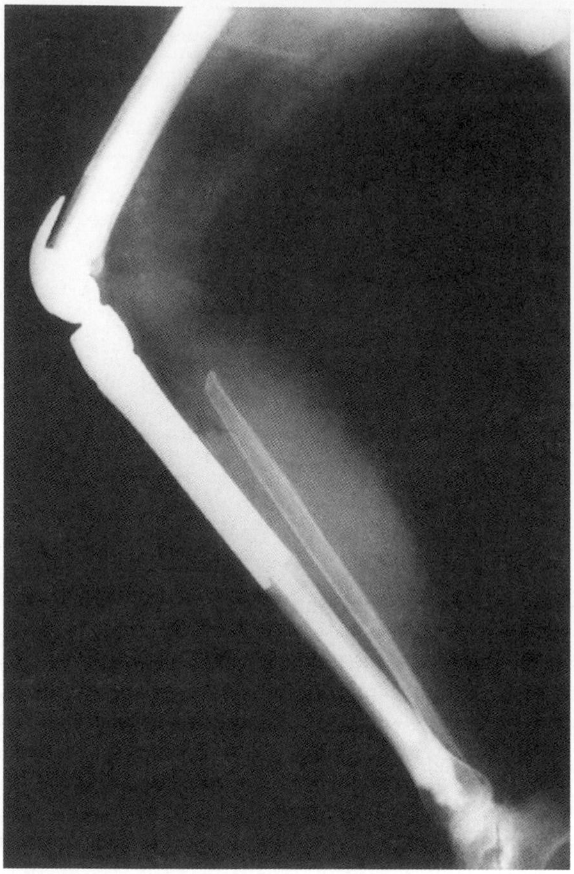

Fig. 10.15 Endoprosthetic replacement of the proximal tibia (lateral view) with distal femoral component and excision of head of fibula.

insertion of an endoprosthesis (see Fig. 10.15). Prostheses are now being used which are extendable, allowing for growth in skeletally immature patients.

Malignant bone tumours The most common type, osteosarcoma, which affects young people up to 30 years of age, is usually treated with chemotherapy followed by surgery, either limb sparing, with endoprosthesis, or amputation. The second most common, chondrosarcoma, occurs in people aged 40–60 and is usually treated by wide excision (with endoprosthesis) or amputation.

Metastatic bone disease The treatment of a patient with metastatic bone disease tends to be symptomatic. The major problem for the patient is pain, which can be severe and debilitating. Pain assessment is crucial in facilitating good pain control which may be achieved by analgesics, radiotherapy, chemotherapy and/or surgery (see Ch. 31).

NURSING PRIORITIES AND MANAGEMENT: Primary bone tumours

Once the patient has seen their GP, immediate hospitalisation will ensue. The care of a patient undergoing chemotherapy and/or radiotherapy is described on pages 1041–1059.

The care of a patient who has a custom-built prosthetic implant will be specific to the implant but the principles of postoperative care are similar to the care of a patient following joint arthroplasty (see p. 472).

Psychological care is paramount for patients with bone tumours, as treatment can last for several months and be very debilitating, e.g. chemotherapy followed by major surgery. Concerns about body image may arise and there will be many fears, including fear of the unknown and of dependence (Henry 2004).

AMPUTATION OF A LIMB

With the development of new treatments amputation is becoming less common, but can still be necessary in some instances. The most common reasons are:

- primary malignant bone tumour, where limb salvage is not possible
- trauma, such as a crushing injury
- vascular insufficiency, such as peripheral vascular disease
- congenital anomaly
- severe infection, such as chronic osteomyelitis with systemic manifestations.

It has been estimated that a large number of the patients who undergo amputation of a limb, or part of a limb, in the Western world do so due to the effects of peripheral vascular disease, while trauma remains the most common reason in the developing countries.

NURSING PRIORITIES AND MANAGEMENT: Amputation of a limb

Coping with loss Loss of a limb through amputation is like any other major loss. As the majority of amputations are carried out as elective procedures, the nurse will be able to make physiological, psychological and social assessments of the patient, and therefore plan care which will assist in the adjustment and adaptation process for the patient (Donohue 1997). This may include arranging for the patient to visit the local prosthetic department or to meet a patient who has had an amputation and is coping successfully.

Occasionally a patient may undergo an amputation as an emergency procedure following a severe crushing injury. In this case, the psychological preparation of the patient and family can only be very limited. They are very likely to require extra support and understanding during the postoperative period.

Wound dressing A stump bandage is used for the first few days and then replaced with a special shrinker sock, which has better elastic properties and is lighter than a crepe bandage. It maintains uniform compression on the wound, thereby reducing oedema, promoting wound healing and beginning to shape the stump, which eases the fitting of the prosthesis.

Phantom sensation (phantom limb) is the name given to the painful sensation experienced by some patients following an amputation and can develop into a form of non-malignant pain, the causal mechanism of which is still not fully understood (McCaffery & Pasero 1999). If it becomes a chronic problem, treatment in the form of transcutaneous electrical nerve stimulation (TENS), ultrasound, local nerve blocks, relaxation therapy or medication, such as the adjuvant analgesic carbamazepine, has been shown to be effective (Judd 1997).

For further information, see Ramachandran & Hirsten (1998).

Pneumatic post-amputation mobility aid Some centres use a prosthesis known as a pneumatic post-amputation mobility (PPAM) aid to help the patient regain balance, reduce oedema of the stump and encourage early walking after lower limb amputation. The aid consists of an inflatable plastic tube which is placed around the patient's stump. The tube is encased in a metal frame with a rocker foot. The use of the PPAM aid can help the patient adjust to the change in body image as the time without an artificial limb is reduced.

BONE INFECTIONS

Over the last century there have been dramatic reductions in the numbers of bone infections, largely due to the development of antibiotics and improved infection control. However, antibiotic resistance, the re-emergence of tuberculosis (TB) in Western countries, and the increased use of metallic implants in orthopaedic surgery all mean that the potential for orthopaedic infections is ever present. This section will outline the three most common types: osteomyelitis, septic arthritis and TB.

Osteomyelitis

PATHOPHYSIOLOGY

Acute osteomyelitis is most commonly caused by *Staphylococcus aureus* and the bacteria usually accumulate in the metaphyseal plate where they proliferate (Burden & Kneale 2004). As the infection spreads, the patient develops pyrexia and severe pain and the affected part is hot and swollen (Dandy & Edwards 2003). If untreated, the infection spreads through the marrow, erodes the cortex and the periosteum and an abscess forms, which will eventually discharge through the skin. By this stage it has become chronic osteomyelitis. If the infection is close to a joint it may track into the joint, causing septic arthritis; this most commonly occurs at the hip, knee, shoulder, elbow and wrist joints (Dandy & Edwards 2003).

MEDICAL MANAGEMENT

History Patients may have had recent trauma affecting the bone or an infection elsewhere in the body. Local signs of infection will be pain, heat and redness, and systemic symptoms of pyrexia, nausea, sweating and malaise may also be present.

Investigations Blood cultures, wound swabs or needle biopsy samples are taken to identify the causative organism and thus ensure the appropriate antibiotic is prescribed. White cell count, erythrocyte sedimentation rate (ESR) and C-reactive protein (CRP) (see Appendix 1) will all be raised in the presence of infection.

A plain X-ray will exclude any other causes for the symptoms, and a CT scan will highlight bony abscesses or sinus tracks. An MRI scan may also be carried out to detect any soft tissue or bone marrow involvement.

Treatment Antibiotic therapy is the first line of treatment. This can include instillation of the antibiotics directly into the medullary canal of the bone via an irrigation tube (Sims et al 2001). If this is not successful surgical intervention, involving removal of infected material and clearing of the area, may be necessary. This may result in wide excision requiring bone grafting or external fixation in order to remedy the resulting bone deficit. In severe cases amputation may be necessary.

NURSING PRIORITIES AND MANAGEMENT: Osteomyelitis

Early detection All nurses need to be alert to the condition so that early referral and treatment can be instituted to prevent progression.

Elevation of the affected part This will reduce pain and may be accompanied by the use of traction, splints or casts to rest the affected area.

Pain and comfort Rest, gentle handling, use of bed cradles to relieve pressure of bedclothes, prompt administration of analgesics and antipyretics, reassurance and distracting activity will all help to relieve pain to some extent.

Antibiotic therapy Initially, antibiotics will be administered intravenously. Increasingly this is being carried out in the community by appropriately skilled nurses, thereby reducing the need for prolonged inpatient stay. If antibiotics are instilled directly into the bone the patient will remain in hospital (Sims et al 2001).

Chronic osteomyelitis Patients with chronic infection may have many hospital admissions and treatments and be anxious about the long-term prognosis. Nurses can help by ensuring patients are kept fully informed of their condition and its treatments, and by referring them to appropriate agencies such as social services or occupational therapy.

Joint infection

Septic arthritis

PATHOPHYSIOLOGY

Septic arthritis can be caused by osteomyelitis, infection from a penetrating wound or bacteraemia from a distant focus of infection. Most commonly the organism is *Staphylococcus aureus*, but gonorrhoea infections affect sexually active teenagers and young adults (ARC 2004). It should be suspected in systemic conditions, especially diabetes mellitus, which may present with swollen and painful joints.

MEDICAL MANAGEMENT

History Septic arthritis usually presents as a hot, swollen, red and painful joint which the patient is reluctant to move.

Investigations Blood cultures, blood tests and aspiration of the joint will confirm the presence of infection and identify the causative organism. Imaging, such as X-rays, CT and MRI, will help to identify the extent of the problem.

Treatment The joint is drained by needle aspiration, arthroscopic washout or open surgery, depending on the joint involved. Antibiotic therapy is instituted, usually intravenously at first. If treatment is not successful, patients may be left with long-term arthritic changes and reduced mobility.

NURSING PRIORITIES AND MANAGEMENT: Septic arthritis

The priorities are similar to those for patients with osteomyelitis. Infection in a joint can be exquisitely painful and patients with lower limb infections may require a walking aid as it will be too uncomfortable to weight-bear.

Tuberculosis

Rates of tuberculosis (TB) declined during the 20th century in developed countries due to improved living conditions and the availability of specific medication, but towards the end of the century the incidence increased for a number of reasons, including movement of unvaccinated people between countries and susceptibility to infection of immunosuppressed patients such as those with HIV (see Ch. 16).

PATHOPHYSIOLOGY

TB usually occurs in the lungs and may spread to the skeletal system, especially the vertebral column, where half of all cases of skeletal infection occur (Burden & Kneale 2004). The course of the disease is similar to that of osteomyelitis, although the pace is much slower. It can cause vertebral fractures and in some cases paraplegia. Surgical treatment may be necessary once the active disease has been controlled, including vertebral fusion to prevent further collapse of vertebrae, or joint replacement.

MEDICAL MANAGEMENT

History Symptoms usually develop slowly with little redness or heat initially. Localised tenderness sometimes occurs.

Investigations Blood tests, sputum/urine tests, X-rays and MRI are all used to aid diagnosis.

Treatment is by antitubercular drugs, such as rifampicin, and by addressing the symptoms.

NURSING PRIORITIES AND MANAGEMENT: Tuberculosis

Management involves implementation of the principles of infection control (see Ch. 16), health education and comfort measures to alleviate symptoms. It may take up to 2 years to successfully treat skeletal TB and patients require support, for example, regular supervision and monitoring of medication regimen for side-effects to ensure completion of the treatment. In some areas specialist TB teams have been set up for this reason.

The journal *Tuberculosis* is a useful source of additional information.

DISORDERS OF JOINTS

This section gives examples of the management of disorders of the lumbar spine, osteoarthritis and rheumatoid arthritis.

DISORDERS OF THE LUMBAR SPINE — BACK PAIN

Lumbar spine disorders or 'back pain' account for more lost working hours than any other medical condition and up to 25% of referrals to some orthopaedic clinics are for this condition (Dandy & Edwards 2003).

PATHOPHYSIOLOGY

Damage or trauma to the vertebrae, ligaments or intervertebral discs can result in instability and potential impingement on the spinal cord. Figure 10.16 highlights the major causes of low back pain. In the lumbar spine mechanical causes are the most common, i.e. abuse, overuse or underuse of the back (Smith 2004b). This section will focus on management of acute back strain, recurrent back strain and management of prolapsed intervertebral disc.

Acute back pain/strain

This is associated with a sudden sharp movement or an attempt to lift a heavy object from an extended position, or it may occur when people with sedentary occupations indulge in bursts of excessive exercise. It may be manifest by sudden severe pain in the lumbar region, due to an acute muscle or ligament strain in the lumbar spine.

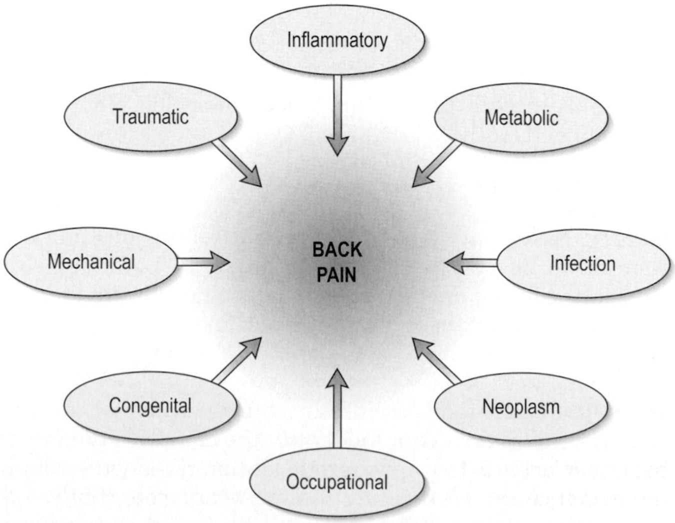

Fig. 10.16 Causes of back pain.

MEDICAL MANAGEMENT

Treatment

- Rest for 24 h maximum in the most comfortable position and then resume activity (Hilde et al 2004)
- Analgesics, non-steroidal anti-inflammatory drugs (NSAIDs) and/or antispasmodic medication (Van Tulder et al 2004).

NURSING PRIORITIES AND MANAGEMENT: Acute back pain/strain

Prevention through health education

Nurses have many opportunities in the workplace, community and hospital to teach people how to organise their environment and activities in order to avoid acute back strain. Much research has gone into the ergonomics of correct lifting techniques and many teaching aids such as videos and leaflets are available (see Disabled Living Foundation in 'Useful websites and addresses').

Nurses are themselves a high-risk group for back injury and a code of practice has been published by the RCN Advisory Panel for Back Pain in Nurses (2002). Both employer and employee responsibilities are set out and there are specific guidelines for assessment and planning of patient care (see Box 10.6).

For information about lifting practices, see Jamieson et al (2002) and Royal College of Nursing (2002).

10.12 Find out what moving and handling aids are available in the clinical area to which you are currently attached. How often are they used? What different techniques for moving and handling patients have you personally used?

Box 10.6

Moving and handling of patients/clients

Assessment and planning

1. Particularly heavy patients, or helpless patients with no ability to assist nurses, need to be individually assessed by a competent patient handling team. Student nurses and support workers should not be expected to undertake these assessments without competent supervision.
2. The care plan or profile should include the following information:
   - The current weight of the patient
   - The extent of the patient's ability to assist and weight-bear, and any other relevant information
   - The technique to be employed to handle that particular patient which should be consistent with the activity undertaken. This should be based upon:
     — the task
     — the patient
     — the environment
     — the equipment
     — the patient handlers.
3. The Manual Handling Operations Regulations and Guidance (UK Government Health and Safety Executive 1992) do not contain any weight limits and state that there is no threshold below which handling may be regarded as safe. All patient handling should be assessed looking at all risk factors, not just weight.
4. Mechanical handling devices or equipment should be used for moving totally dependent patients from bed to chair, trolley, toilet, etc. Sliding equipment should be used for moving totally dependent patients in bed.

From the RCN Advisory Panel for Back Pain in Nurses (2002).

Recurrent back pain/strain

A patient who suffers recurrent back pain or strain should be fully investigated to rule out any other causes, such as a spinal tumour or a prolapsed intervertebral disc.

MEDICAL MANAGEMENT

Treatment Physiotherapy, medication and strategies for dealing with chronic pain are the mainstays of treatment. Specific medication may include tricyclic antidepressants and gabapentin (see Ch. 19). Patients are often referred to a chronic pain clinic where an interprofessional team aims both to relieve pain and to enable patients to live with their pain (Hansson et al 2001). This involves supporting the patient's ability to manage pain by improving self-efficacy, a measure of how confident an individual is to engage in a specific behaviour (Oliver & Ryan 2004). This is achieved by helping patients to understand the reason for their pain, and by teaching behavioural techniques that can help to reduce it, such as pacing activities over time and learning to use relaxation techniques (Oliver & Ryan 2004).

Osteopathy or chiropractic treatment may also be of benefit (Currie 2000), although a systematic review found no evidence on the short- or long-term effectiveness of osteopathy, chiropractic or spinal manipulation for people with non-specific chronic low back pain (Patterson 2004).

NURSING PRIORITIES AND MANAGEMENT: Chronic back pain/strain

The nursing role within a chronic back pain management programme can encompass case management, administration and monitoring of analgesics, education and, with an appropriate qualification, counselling (Smith 2004b).

Prolapsed intervertebral disc

PATHOPHYSIOLOGY

The intervertebral discs consist of a firm nucleus pulposus surrounded by a ring of fibrocartilage and fibrous tissue which links two vertebrae together. Age-related loss of water content and an increase in collagen content leads to stiffening of the discs (Smith 2004b). The disc space becomes narrowed and distorted, leading to increased stress on the spine and intervertebral discs. Eventually the disc may rupture and the soft contents, the pulposus, will prolapse, causing compression and stretching of nerve roots or fibres. Dandy and Edwards (2003) state that 90% of lumbar disc protrusions involve L4–5 or L5–S1 (see Fig. 10.17).

MEDICAL MANAGEMENT

History The classic presentation is of a patient with acute lumbar pain radiating down the thigh and lower leg;

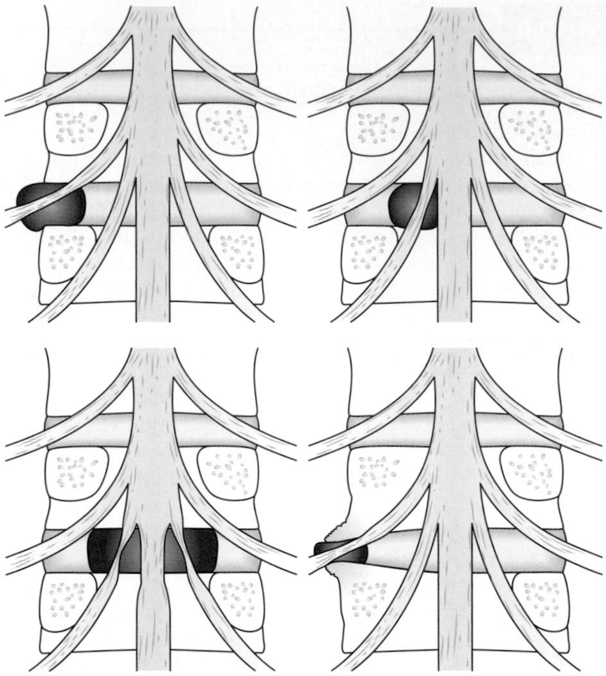

Fig. 10.17 Disc prolapse and root compression in the lumbar spine. A laterally placed prolapse may compress the L4 root, a more central prolapse will compress L5, and a central prolapse will compress the cauda equina. Osteophytes in the lateral canal will also produce root compression.

the precise position is dependent on the spinal nerve root affected, but a few patients may present with only leg symptoms. The patient may also be 'locked' in the classic bent position. There may be a history of dull lower back pain.

Examination Muscle spasm and an intense focal area of pain may be identified. The straight leg raising test will indicate restriction of movement well below 90° of hip flexion and there may be neurological signs such as numbness, tingling or diminished motor function. If necessary, an MRI scan will confirm the diagnosis.

Treatment Conservative treatment for acute back pain as outlined above should be tried first, although manipulation of a spine with acute disc prolapse is said to be dangerous as it could lead to a spinal cord injury (Dandy & Edwards 2003). Localised epidural steroid injections may prove beneficial (Smith 2004b).

The indication for disc excision is when there is proven disc protrusion with accompanying neurological signs and no improvement after 6 weeks of conservative treatment, or if any neurological deficit worsens. Intervention will comprise either of the following:

- Disc excision involves excision of the ligamentum flavum and inferior portion of the lamina (laminectomy) overlying the affected nerve root. The herniated portion of the disc and all disc material is excised, relieving the pressure on the nerve root. Surgery can also be performed in the day case procedure of a microdiscectomy (Cox & Boswell 2000).
- Chemonucleolysis is injection of an enzyme (chymopapain) into the prolapsed disc which breaks down the disc material, thus relieving pressure on the nerve root. This procedure is performed under image intensifier control and appropriate analgesic cover to prevent/relieve the accompanying pain which can be severe.

A Cochrane Review of surgery for lumbar disc prolapse (Gibson et al 2004) found that chemonucleolysis is more effective than placebo but less effective than surgical discectomy. As in both procedures some disc tissue will have been removed, there will be a reduction in its shock-absorbing function, and unnatural stresses may trigger degenerative reactions, with the result that between 30 and 60% of patients may suffer permanent, though varying, degrees of stiffness and back pain (Dandy & Edwards 2003).

NURSING PRIORITIES AND MANAGEMENT: Prolapsed intervertebral disc

A patient who presents with a central disc prolapse is an orthopaedic emergency as the prolapsed disc causes pressure directly on the spinal cord. Without prompt surgical decompression, the presenting neurological manifestations will result in permanent disability. For all patients it is important that they are part of the decision-making process with regard to their treatment — see Case History 10.4 for an example of this.

CASE STUDY 10.4

A patient with a prolapsed intervertebral disc

Ms G, a 54-year-old lady, sustained an injury to her back whilst carrying concrete blocks during home renovation. For 2 months she had pain but attempted to continue with her normal activities, including full-time work as a nurse lecturer. Eventually, when the symptoms did not improve, she saw her GP. He suggested an MRI scan and told her that she probably had a herniated disc which would require surgery.

Ms G did not accept this and refused the MRI scan; instead she arranged to see a chiropractor. However, this did not help and she asked her GP to refer her for physiotherapy; she also agreed to have the MRI scan. This revealed herniation and rupture of the intervertebral disc at L5/S1. Ms G was still 'afraid of undergoing the knife' and decided to persevere with physiotherapy. However, by 4 months after the original injury, her symptoms had worsened and she agreed to see a neurosurgeon. Conventional surgery would require up to 5 days in hospital, but Ms G was adamant that she did not want a general anaesthetic or to stay in hospital. It was agreed therefore that she would have a microdiscectomy as a day case with an epidural anaesthetic, a new treatment at the time. After this was performed Ms G used a number of complementary therapies, including aromatherapy, herbal medicine and meditation, to manage her postoperative care and she returned to work 8 days after surgery.

Cox C L, Boswell G M 2000 Integrating complementary health care in outpatient surgery for discectomy: the patient's perspective. Journal of Orthopaedic Nursing 4(4): 179–184

Conservative treatment

As most of the conservative treatment can be carried out at home, it is the community nurse who will have responsibility for advising and supporting the patient and family in all comfort measures. The care that might be given by the community nurse is described in Nursing Care Plan 10.1. Case History 10.5 provides background information about the patient.

Operative treatment

In addition to the general principles for perioperative care, the following points are specific to postoperative management of patients having a discectomy/laminectomy and chemonucleolysis.

Pain This can be expected to be severe following chemonucleolysis, but it may be complicated by the development

Nursing Care Plan 10.1 Community nursing care of patient with prolapsed intervertebral disc (see Case History 10.5)

Problem A, actual; P, potential	Goal	Nursing intervention	Evaluation
Communication			
• **Pain (A) related to disc prolapse**	Improvement and control	Advise on: • Self-administering medication • Self-assessment on pain chart	Significant reduction in level of experienced pain
• **Anxiety (A) related to children's welfare and reduced mother role**	Reduce anxiety by addressing causes	• Define problems – discuss with Mrs S and husband • Neighbour willing to help Mon./Wed./Fri., husband at weekend • Arrange nursery care for Emma Tues. and Thur. (social worker)	Mrs S will report satisfaction with arrangements Enquire daily Children and husband adapting and appear happy
Reduced mobility related to rest (A)	Maintain Mrs S in limited mobility – ensure comfort	• When lying in bed, advise to lie supine on a well supported mattress • Mr S to assist with shower • Ensure radio, TV, telephone, magazines available	Mrs S states she is more comfortable Adequate diversional therapy observed
Maintaining a safe environment (P)	Prevent accidental ingestion of Mrs S's medication by children Prevent other accidents	• Discuss problem with Mrs S, husband and neighbour • Locate safe place • Ensure child-proof medication cap • Discuss potential home accidents – give Royal Society for Prevention of Accidents (RoSPA) leaflet	There are no preventable incidents or accidents Family and friends demonstrate raised awareness of safety – discuss leaflet
Nutrition (P)	Maintain balanced diet to prevent constipation	• Arrange friend to assist with food preparation • Home help Tuesdays and Thursdays • Mrs S to sit well supported when eating	Mrs S will report no constipation
Neurological impairment (P)	Early detection and reduction in risk	• Educate Mrs S and her husband in signs and symptoms of deterioration in colour, warmth, sensation, movement of lower limbs. • Provide advice about what to do if deterioration occurs	Any neurological deterioration will be detected and dealt with promptly and appropriately

CASE HISTORY 10.5

Mrs S

Mrs S is 30 years old and married to a builder. The couple have two children, 7-year-old Tim and 4-year-old Emma. Mrs S is being treated at home for a prolapsed intervertebral disc, her prescribed treatment being pain control and neurological assessment. The community nurse plans to visit Mrs S until her condition begins to improve. She has already ascertained that Mrs S's next door neighbour is also a friend.

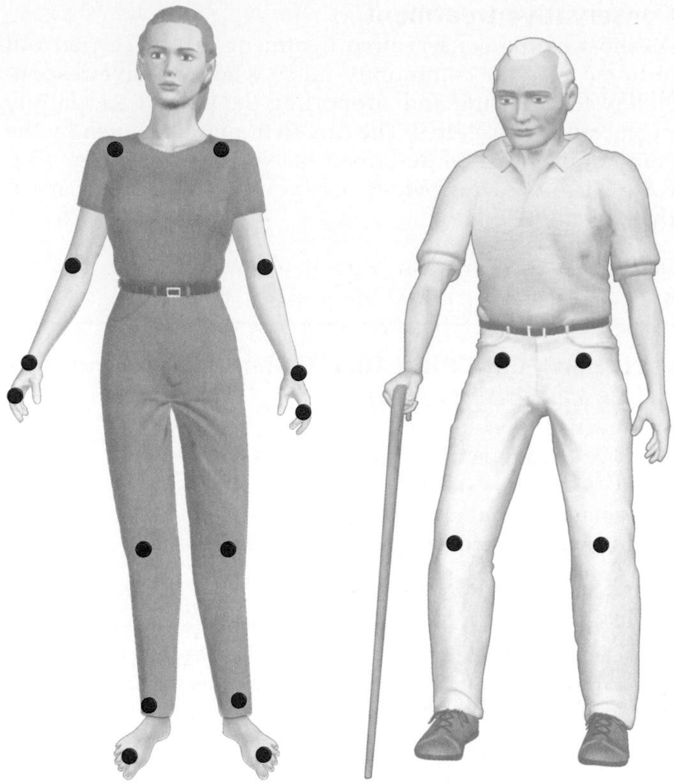

Fig. 10.18 Some differences between rheumatoid arthritis and osteoarthritis. Rheumatoid arthritis affects small joints, is symmetrical and is more common in young women. Osteoarthritis mainly affects the weight-bearing joints and is more common in older and heavyweight people.

of neurological deficit. Neurological status should therefore be monitored carefully. The use of patient controlled analgesia (PCA) or of epidural analgesia following spinal surgery will help to ensure that the patient's pain is well controlled.

Positioning and mobilising Frequent position changes should be encouraged, always maintaining spinal alignment. Normal movements can be gradually resumed as soon as the patient's general condition permits. Minimal flexion of the knees, using the knee rest or a pillow for support while in the supine position, will allow spinal muscles to relax. A pillow between the knees will provide comfortable alignment when in the lateral position.

Early mobilisation is usually prescribed. The bed should be lowered and the patient taught to roll to the edge, swing the legs to the floor and stand up in one smooth movement.

DEGENERATIVE AND INFLAMMATORY JOINT DISORDERS

There are over 200 conditions that can affect synovial joints and tissues. This section focuses on two common joint diseases: osteoarthritis and rheumatoid arthritis (see Fig. 10.18).

Rheumatoid arthritis

PATHOPHYSIOLOGY

Rheumatoid arthritis (RA) is a systemic disease of connective tissue which affects approximately one million people in the UK (Hill & Ryan 2000). It is an autoimmune disease, i.e. the body's immune system attacks its own tissues and becomes self-destructive. The cause of this is not yet known and research continues, but it is thought that factors such as infection, stress and trauma might act as initiating factors in people with a genetic disposition (Ryan & Oliver 2002). The joints are acutely inflamed due to inflammatory changes in the synovial membrane. The synovium becomes thicker, very vascular and the site of increased cell infiltration which may cause an effusion within the joint that manifests as a swollen joint. As the proliferative tissue spreads as a 'pannus' over the articular cartilage, the cartilage is slowly eroded.

Systemic inflammatory changes can affect many of the body's organs and lead to pericarditis, pleuritis and bowel vasculitis, as well as general malaise and anaemia. It is therefore potentially a very debilitating chronic disease. Life expectancy is reduced by approximately 7 years in men and 3 years in women, mainly due to infections, renal or respiratory disease, or the RA itself (Hakim & Clunie 2002). However, there is no one path of RA progression and some patients have permanent remission whilst others have severe relentless deterioration in symptoms; each patient must therefore be assessed individually.

MEDICAL MANAGEMENT

History The disease most commonly starts when a person is in her 30s or 40s with a gradual onset of pain and stiffness, particularly in the morning, affecting the small joints of the hands and feet. The person may also present to their GP complaining of loss of appetite and weight, mild pyrexia, and characteristics of anaemia. As the RA progresses, other joints may become involved, with inflammation, swelling and progressive loss of function. Commonly the wrists, elbows, shoulders, cervical spine, temporomandibular joints, knees and ankles are affected.

For some patients the onset of RA is acute, with multiple joint involvement from the onset, with rapid progress to loss of function.

Examination The affected joints will appear swollen, be warm to the touch, and the patient will complain of pain when the normal range of movement is attempted. If the joint is severely affected, some crepitus may be heard. With time, joints often become deformed, especially in the hands and feet.

Investigations X-rays of both hands and feet will usually be sufficient to confirm the diagnosis. A blood specimen will be taken for assessment of the level of haemoglobin, number of white blood cells, ESR, CRP and the presence of rheumatoid factor.

Diagnosis The American Rheumatism Association criteria for classification of RA provide a diagnostic guideline (Arnett et al 1988). The seven criteria are:

- morning stiffness
- arthritis in three or more joints with swelling
- arthritis of the hand joints
- symmetrical arthritis
- subcutaneous nodules
- presence of rheumatoid factor
- joint changes on X-ray.

The first four criteria must have been present for at least 6 weeks and a patient must have four or more of the seven criteria to be diagnosed as having RA.

Treatment There is no known cure for RA, and therefore intervention is directed towards relieving pain, modifying the level of disease activity and maintaining optimal functional ability for each individual (Ryan & Oliver 2002).

The aims of medical treatment are to:

- reduce the patient's pain with the use of analgesics, e.g. NSAIDs
- reduce joint destruction with the use of disease-modifying antirheumatic drugs (DMARDs) such as methotrexate, and/or early short-term use of local or systemic steroid therapy. Newer treatments, 'biologics', are being tested. These alter the normal immune response by blocking the normal inflammatory process. They are administered intravenously (infliximab) or subcutaneously (etanercept) (Ryan & Oliver 2002)
- prevent or minimise deformity of a joint by splinting damaged or painful joints (see Fig. 10.19)
- assist the patient to adapt their lifestyle
- correct anaemia.

The main surgical treatments are:

- synovectomy — removal of excess synovial membrane from within the joint capsule of the affected joint. This is less frequently performed because the synovial inflammation recurs. However, tenosynovectomy, removal of synovial membrane from around tendons within joints, is a quick and safe method of relieving nerve entrapment (Hakim & Clunie 2002)
- osteotomy — division of a bone and removal of a piece so that the joint can be realigned. This alters the weight distribution within a joint, most commonly of the metatarsal bones of the feet
- arthroplasty — remodelling of an affected joint using synthetic materials and/or metal, most commonly of the hip and knee joint
- arthrodesis — surgical fusion of a joint, which will reduce or eliminate the joint pain but create a stiff immovable joint, most commonly performed on the ankle.

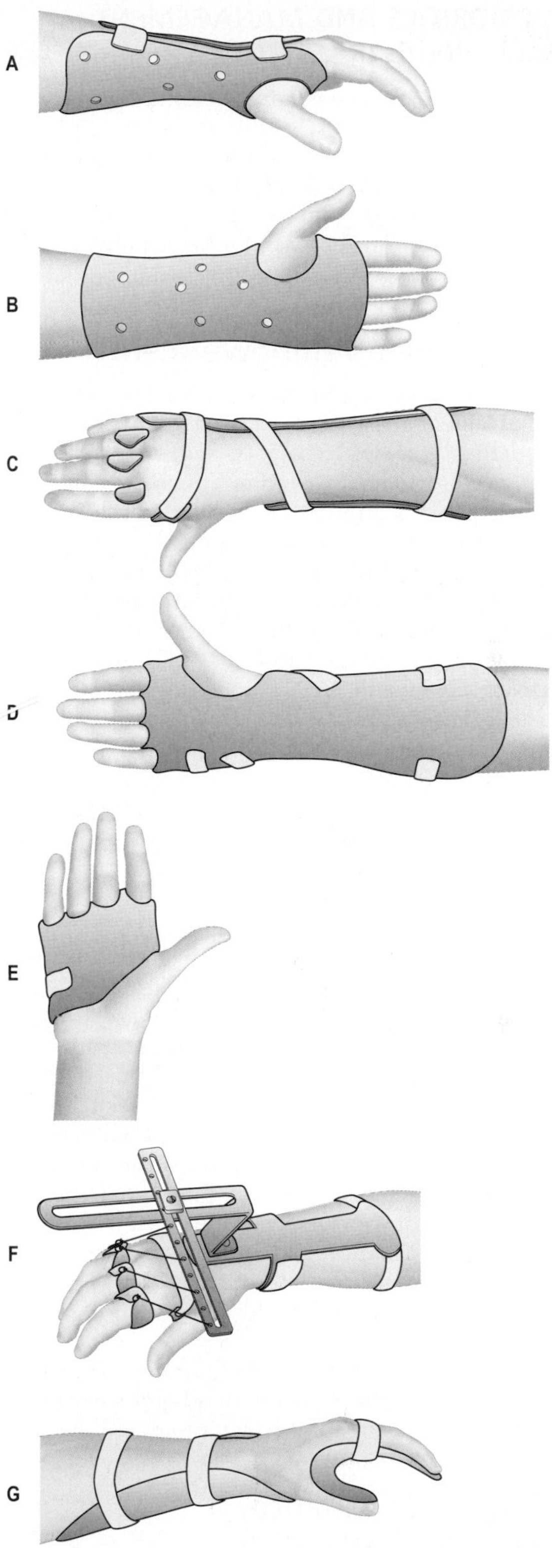

Fig. 10.19 Different types of splint. A–E: Resting splints. F: Functional splint used to stabilise a joint during activity. G: Corrective splint to immobilise a joint, realign soft tissue or correct contracture or deformities.

NURSING PRIORITIES AND MANAGEMENT: Rheumatoid arthritis (RA)

The aim of care is to relieve symptoms and to maintain and, if possible, improve quality of life. A multidisciplinary approach is essential, but coordination of care and therapeutic interventions such as joint injections often fall within the remit of rheumatology nurse specialists. Nurse-led clinics have been shown to be popular with patients (Hill 1997).

Patient involvement/empowerment

As a chronic disease, the key to successful treatment of RA is patient involvement and empowerment, as these increase the likelihood that a person will cope with the treatment regimen and necessary lifestyle adaptations (Mulligan & Newman 2003). There is an increased focus on the concept of the expert patient and on self-management programmes. The Chronic Disease Self-Management Program (CDSMP) is a generic programme which has been adapted for rheumatoid arthritis patients and, in the UK, the Expert Patient Programme, which is being funded and implemented through the National Health Service, includes RA (Mulligan & Newman 2003). These programmes address crucial issues such as family and personal relationships, adaptation of the home, and work and leisure activities.

Controlling pain

A range of analgesics may need to be considered, from paracetamol/aspirin, compound analgesics such as co-codamol, to NSAIDs. NSAIDs can cause gastrointestinal side-effects and the National Institute for Clinical Excellence (2001) advocates the use of the cyclo-oxygenase (Cox) II group of NSAIDs, such as celecoxib, as these reduce the risk of side-effects. Corticosteroids are usually used in the short term in acute episodes of pain/inflammation. When they are used for long-term therapy, abrupt withdrawal must be avoided as the body may not have sufficient glucocorticoids to deal with stress (see Ch. 5). Herbal therapy is tried by many patients and a Cochrane Review (Little & Parsons 2004) suggests that one herbal therapy — gamma-linolenic acid (GLA) — may potentially relieve pain, morning stiffness and joint tenderness, although the evidence is not conclusive.

Local pain control can be achieved in some joints by other methods, such as splints for the hand and wrist joints (see Fig. 10.19).

Maintaining independence and fostering well-being

Exercise and mobility The principles of joint protection should be explained to the patient, such as respecting pain and not being fearful or ignoring it, balancing work and rest, using the larger or stronger joints rather than small ones, and reducing the effort to a joint (Maher et al 2002).

Adaptation of living space The muscle power of the patient with RA is reduced, and therefore the use of aids such as a variable-height bed, raised or ejector chair and raised toilet seat may be of assistance.

Walking aids, such as a stick or elbow crutches, may help to retain the patient's level of mobility by reducing the weight load placed on specific joints. The hand pieces of the aids may need to be adapted to accommodate the finger and wrist deformities that are common features of the disease.

Diet The patient with RA may require assistance in maintaining nutritional status due to anorexia and/or difficulty in using eating and drinking utensils. Frequent, light, appetising meals should be served. The occupational therapist can supply a variety of utensils, such as large-handled cutlery and a tilting kettle stand, which will help the patient to retain independence. A patient with RA is likely to develop anaemia due to the chronic inflammatory process of the disease and medication therapy and iron supplements may be prescribed.

Sexual activity Counselling regarding sexual activity may be required. The Arthritis and Rheumatism Council and the Association to Aid the Sexual and Personal Relationships of People with a Disability (SPOD) have both produced booklets containing useful information for RA patients and their partners (see 'Useful websites and addresses').

Osteoarthritis

PATHOPHYSIOLOGY

Osteoarthritis (OA) is by far the most prevalent joint disorder, with knee and hip OA together affecting up to 10–25% of people in retirement (Doherty & Dougados 2001). It is characterised by a relatively slow deterioration of the articular cartilage that covers the joint surfaces. Although not primarily an inflammatory disease, there is some inflammation in the joint due to the presence of cartilage debris and some synovitis (Maher et al 2002). The disease may be classified as primary or secondary, the former being a progressive condition of unknown origin, more common in the older person, especially females. Secondary osteoarthritis can affect people of any age or gender and is usually associated with a previous injury/condition of the joint, such as a previous fracture or a childhood hip condition such as Perthes disease. It can also develop following repeated high impact joint movements in sport or occupation, e.g. professional footballers are particularly prone to hip and knee OA.

MEDICAL MANAGEMENT

History and examination Pain on movement and stiffness at rest are the most common early symptoms, and may have been present for up to a year before a patient consults a health professional (Peat et al 2001), who will confirm that the normal range of movement of a joint is reduced.

Investigations Plain radiographs of the affected joint will be taken, although the degree of destruction of the joint space does not always correlate to the degree of pain and disability a patient is experiencing.

Diagnosis is confirmed by the patient history and the appearance of the joint on the X-ray, showing narrowing of

Box 10.7

Treatment of the patient with osteoarthritis

Non-operative
- Education
- Glucosamine sulphate, analgesics and NSAIDs
- Physiotherapy
- Walking aids
- Occupational therapy
- Shoe raise
- Modification of activities

Surgical (see Fig. 10.20)
- Debridement/joint washout — removal of osteophytes and washing out of joint debris
- Osteotomy — removing parts of a bone to correct line of weight-bearing
- Arthrodesis — fusion of a joint
- Arthroplasty — creation of a joint
- Total joint replacement — creation of a joint

the joint space and possible formation of bony outgrowths at the bony margins, known as osteophytes.

Treatment The goals of care are pain control, improvement of function and health-related quality of life, and avoidance of side-effects where possible (Barlow 2001). Treatment can be classified as non-operative or surgical (see Box 10.7).

Non-operative treatment Many patients do not require, or want, surgical intervention and for these patients education and support are vital — interventions that nurses are ideally placed to provide. These may be formal OA education and support groups or more informal support for individuals or groups given by practice or community nurses. Arthritis Self-Management Programme (ASMP) Groups may be led by health professionals or by people who themselves have OA (Barlow 2001). These programmes combine advice about medication and lifestyle changes, including appropriate physical exercise such as walking or swimming. Research Abstract 10.3 considers the experience of patients living with OA.

As well as prescription medication, patients should be advised to try glucosamine sulphate, a biological compound which is said to have pain-reducing effects and may also slow down the rate of cartilage damage; a Cochrane Review concluded that it was safe and effective in OA (Towheed et al 2004). For knee arthritis, intra-articular injections of hyaluronic acid or steroids have been shown to be effective in relieving symptoms (Ayral 2001).

Surgical treatment Patients with knee OA may benefit from arthroscopic washout and removal of osteophytes. There is some evidence that drilling exposed bone in the knee joint to make it bleed will cause a clot to form, and that from this a fibrocartilaginous tissue will develop which mimics to some extent the destroyed articular cartilage. This procedure is available in a few centres only (Esteve-de-Miguel 2003). Other operative procedures are shown in Figure 10.20. Of these, joint replacement, particularly of the hip and knee joints, is now the most common.

RESEARCH ABSTRACT 10.3

Living with osteoarthritis: insiders' views

A small-scale American study (Kee 1998) examined 20 patients' individual perspectives and experiences of living with osteoarthritis (OA). The patients were over the age of 60, living in the community and had had OA for at least 1 year.

Four themes emerged — refusing to give up, pragmatism towards treatment strategies, staying in charge, and tangible caring:

- 'Refusing to give up' was attempting to limit the negative effects of OA by emphasising the more positive aspects of lives and lifestyles.
- 'Pragmatism towards treatment strategies' was concerned with receiving advice about treatment for OA from various sources and trying them but stopping if they were not effective; this included advice from health professionals.
- 'Pragmatism' was linked to the third theme 'Staying in charge' where patients reported adjusting medication dosages, such as 'My doctor told me to take aspirin regularly but I only take it when I need it because of what I've been reading about stomach ulcers'. The patients used the conventional health care system on their own terms so that they could continue to maintain control of their lives.
- 'Tangible caring' referred to caring demonstrated by friends and families, such as providing helpful devices ordered from catalogues.

The research suggests that nurses can play an important part in helping OA patients to view their illness as something with which they can live, to recognise that they do have ultimate control over their treatment, and to know that others care for them and are sources of practical assistance. In order to do this, nurses need extensive knowledge of important matters such as appropriate self-help organisations, assistive devices and gadgets, and therapy options, including alternative therapies.

Kee C C 1998 Living with osteoarthritis: insiders' views. Applied Nursing Research 11(1): 19–26

Joint replacement Figure 10.21 illustrates types of prostheses used in hip replacement (see Case History 10.6). Joint replacements are very successful and it is not uncommon for research studies to report 95% survivorship of the prosthesis at 10 years (e.g. Font-Rodriguez et al 1997).

A new type of surgery is hip resurfacing, where the arthritic surfaces are debrided and a short stem metal prosthesis to cover the femoral head is inserted, preserving the femoral neck; at the same time a metal cup is inserted into the acetabulum. The femoral head prosthesis and cup are usually made of cobalt chrome. These are used in younger patients and those who are particularly active. The theory is that when the prostheses wear out it will be easier to replace them with a conventional hip replacement, because more bone has been left intact; however, as yet, there is a lack of long-term follow-up studies to support the theory (Vale et al 2002).

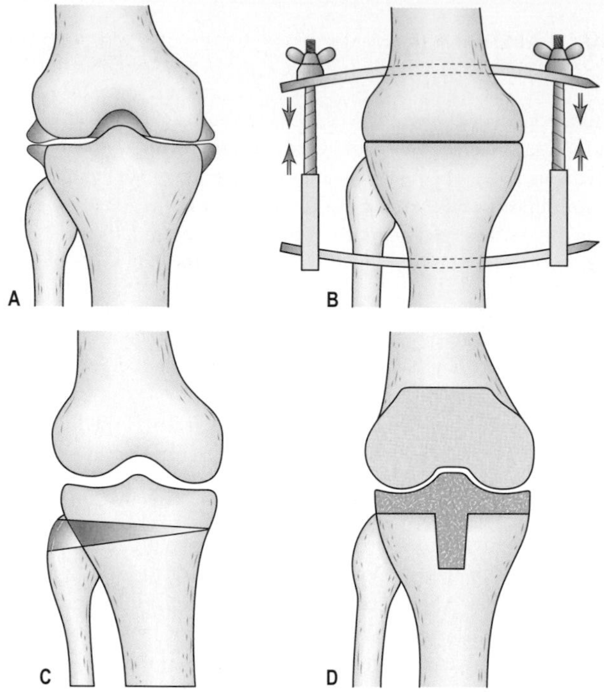

Fig. 10.20 Operations for osteoarthritis. A: Debridement and removal of osteophytes. B: Arthrodesis. C: Osteotomy to correct alignment. D: Total joint replacement.

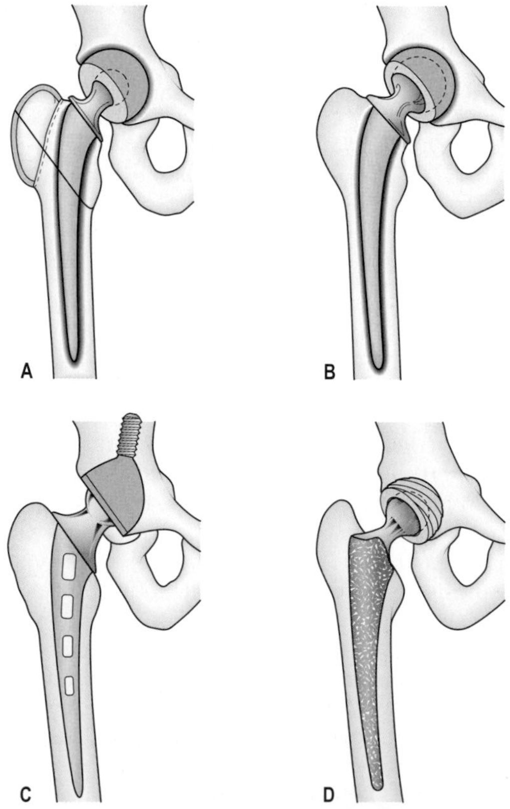

Fig. 10.21 Types of total hip replacement. A: Charnley hip replacement with greater trochanter reattachment. B: Müller-type replacement with larger femoral head. C: Ring-type replacement using a long threaded acetabular component, without cement. D: Uncemented prosthesis with sintered surfaces and screw-in acetabular prosthesis.

Postoperative complications — total hip replacement (THR)

Dislocation of the femoral component One of the risks of a THR is dislocation of the prosthesis, i.e. the femoral component comes out of the acetabular cup. It is common for patients to have to follow certain restrictions for the first 6 weeks postoperatively to reduce this risk, namely not crossing their legs, sleeping on their back, and not getting into a bath, although a study examined 499 patients on whom no restrictions on postoperative mobilisation were imposed and only three suffered dislocation (Talbot et al 2002). To help prevent dislocation during the inpatient stay, some orthopaedic surgeons request that the patient is nursed sitting with no more than 45° of flexion at the hip joint. A Charnley wedge or foam troughs in which the patient's lower legs rest may also be used to reduce excessive adduction which can increase the incidence of dislocation of the hip joint replacement. The femoral bone tissue has an excellent blood supply; therefore, compared with other forms of surgery, blood drainage can be excessive. Accurate recording of the drainage volume is essential and, if excessive, the patient may need a blood transfusion. If a wound drain is used the nurse must ensure that contamination of the drainage system does not occur when emptying the collecting chamber(s). Autotransfusion is becoming a more frequent practice within orthopaedic surgery (see Ch. 18).

NURSING PRIORITIES AND MANAGEMENT: Joint replacement

Preoperative care

As with any surgery, the key to success is planning and early patient involvement. It is increasingly being advocated that such planning should begin as soon as a patient is listed for surgery, with an initial health check to ensure that the patient does not have surgery postponed at preoperative assessment due to ill health (DH 2002). Patients may also attend a group information session where they can find out more about the surgery and rehabilitation ('Hip and Knee Club'). Preparing patients for surgery is an ideal role for an orthopaedic nurse practitioner.

Postoperative care

Postoperative care will follow the basic principles outlined in Chapter 26 with the following additions.

Prevention of infection Bacterial infection of the bone around the prosthesis can have a severe debilitating effect and, if this occurs, the prosthesis may have to be removed, leaving a grossly unstable joint; therefore prophylactic therapy is essential. In addition to basic attention to infection control, especially when undertaking invasive procedures, and attention to clearing up any septic foci, i.v. antibiotic therapy is commenced perioperatively and continued postoperatively, i.e. one dose perioperatively and two doses postoperatively.

Deep vein thrombosis (DVT) Hip and pelvic surgery have the highest incidence of DVT, and therefore local policy to

CASE HISTORY 10.6

A patient's perceptions of an experience surrounding total hip replacement

Two months after an operation for hip replacement I am trying to record my experiences, but one thought predominates to such an extent that everything else fades into insignificance. I can think of nothing other than the fact that I have no pain: no pain walking, no pain sitting, no pain lying in bed, no pain at all. Two ideas arise from this: one, that it does not seem at all healthy to be so conscious of the absence of pain. The hope must be that sooner or later being pain-free will become the normal unobserved fact of life. The other is a retrospective awareness of the debilitating effect of continuous chronic pain, the insidious way in which everything developed. People now keep exclaiming that I look so well, that my colour has improved so much. They never in the past told me that I looked old and grey. This must have been as unremarkable to others as the experience of continuous pain was to me.

There were many different kinds of pain. The worst in intensity was probably the pain on weight-bearing, but somehow it did not bother me so very much. I felt I could anticipate it, control it by leaning on a stick or furniture, or by refraining from walking altogether. There were sudden and very acute bouts of pain, sharp like toothache, on sudden movements or jolts, but these passed and did not matter much. There was the impossibility of ever sitting or lying in comfort — much less severe pain, but the most difficult to bear. It was when that particular pain suddenly got much worse that I first told the GP how I felt. When, in spite of anti-inflammatory painkillers, even the weight of the sheet became intolerable and lack of sleep became difficult to cope with, an appointment was made with the orthopaedic specialist services. The nature of the worst of the continuous pain, however, was none of these; it was almost not experienced as pain at all. It was a deep nagging, dragging, twisting sensation which was nauseating and depressing, not responding to analgesics at all, analgesics which I took in maximal dosage and which added to the feeling of nausea, depression and apathy. Neither the GP nor I myself was keen on the thought of surgery: the GP no doubt because he was conscious of obesity being a contraindication for surgical intervention; I myself because I knew of many cases when no great improvement followed hip replacement. As soon as my friends had heard that I had been put on the waiting list, example after example was related to me of how wonderful Mr or Mrs X, Y or Z was as a result of this operation — 'a new lease of life', 'years younger', 'never looked back'. But my own attention focused, not on their reassurance, but on those people I had met who had developed infections, whose prosthesis had broken down, who had to have a second operation. It was no help to see a television programme and read a newspaper article about the inferior quality of the prostheses which were coming on the market at that time.

Now, after the operation, I have joined the ranks of those who extol its virtue, but even the most enthusiastic supporters had not prepared me for the speed with which it would be possible to lead a normal life: walking within 48 h, discharged from hospital within 2 weeks, fully independent by the time of the follow-up outpatient appointment 6 weeks after operation. Here, in summary, are the events which I now believe made the whole experience entirely positive: on first appointment at the orthopaedic outpatient clinic the thorough examination, the fact that the surgeon appeared to understand how much pain I had — perhaps even better than I did — and did not belittle what I was saying. The fact that he arranged immediately, before the operation, to start physiotherapy and that he promised an operation as soon as possible. I was on the waiting list for only 6 months. A week before the operation there was a day of tests and examinations in the ward to which I was to be admitted, giving a good opportunity to allay anxiety. I was glad that I had explanations of the operation, the anaesthetic and the possible risks. I appreciated the time taken to answer my questions and the sensitivity of the staff, though I do not think I could have entered into any decision making in spite of the explanations. My anxiety about the postoperative phase, about living alone, upstairs, in a relatively large flat was well understood and arrangements were made by the occupational therapist, at that early stage, for various pieces of helpful equipment to be delivered to the house. I was assured that I would be fully rehabilitated by the time of discharge which was anticipated to be after about 7 days, but I found this difficult to believe.

On admission I was immediately aware of the cordiality and friendliness of the nursing staff and of the community spirit of the patients who made me feel welcome and who augmented the very adequate information given to me by the staff, both in print and in discussion.

Preoperative relief of anxiety and postoperative pain control were superb; after the initial intravenous analgesic cover, painkillers were offered every 4 h, but not really needed, except before physiotherapy, after the first few days. It was interesting to observe that all patients who had hip operations went through the same progression of skill acquisition and setbacks, learning how to get in and out of bed, how to turn in bed, how to walk, first with a Zimmer frame, then with two sticks, and later one stick, how to pick things up off the floor, to put on stockings and shoes, to shower independently, to dress and undress, to climb stairs and to get in and out of a car. It was evident that all the nurses knew exactly what each patient was capable of doing. All were willing to help but clearly expected and encouraged independence. The nurses' awareness of patients' progress and the supervision of the activities of less highly qualified staff were always in evidence. It was reassuring to notice that there was vigilance in case deep vein thrombosis arose and to see the speed with which one patient was advised to go to bed, the foot of which was raised, and how speedily support stockings were offered. With the emphasis throughout on what one can do by oneself and encouragement to get moving, it was a boost to self-confidence to know that nurses were vigilant for complications and setbacks. I found it helpful to have been shown the X-ray of the new hip as it makes it possible to visualise what the joint is doing during various activities, and to understand why one is advised never to cross the legs, to get on all fours or to pick things up off the floor from the sitting position. A pillow between the legs during sleep helps prevent crossing the legs accidentally.

There were 12 women in the ward, most of them in for hip or knee operations. The impression gained on admission of a friendly, supportive group spirit was reinforced throughout. What a wealth of experience, what a reservoir of knowledge, what abundance of empathy, goodwill and helpfulness. There was also a tremendous amount of fun and humour, perhaps enhanced by the experience all had of being pain-free all of a sudden. On discharge I was part of a supported discharge scheme, which meant that a physiotherapist and nurses visited me during my first few weeks at home to check that I was continuing to make progress. It was reassuring to have this support when I got home.

I learned a lot, not only about health and illness, but also about emotional, social and economic stress, and about coping strategies. The importance of the patient community and its therapeutic potential is seldom recognised in general nursing but it should never be underestimated.

prevent this complication should be implemented (SIGN 2002b, Davis 2004). There is much debate as to the most appropriate method of prevention and the evidence is controversial (Love 1999). Common methods used are thrombotic/embolic deterrent (TED) stockings, foot pumps, which reduce venous stasis, and chemical prophylaxis using heparin injections.

Urinary retention is a potential problem. If all nursing measures, such as helping patients to the toilet or commode rather than using a urinal or bedpan, fail then intermittent catheterisation may be advised. The insertion of a self-retaining catheter should be avoided because of the risk of creating a septic focus (see Ch. 8). In some orthopaedic centres, oral or i.v. antibiotics may be administered prior to and after catheterisation, but the research evidence to support this is inconclusive.

Mobility and rehabilitation The patient may begin to mobilise as soon as their condition permits, which is usually on the first day postoperatively. This will be supervised by the physiotherapist and the nurse. A hydraulic bed is essential for correct manoeuvring, as care must be taken not to flex the hip more than 45° when helping the patient out of bed or while sitting; therefore a high armchair should be used.

A walking frame may be used at first and the physiotherapist will re-educate the patient to use a normal walking gait. Depending on progress, the patient should practise using crutches or walking sticks before discharge.

Aids to living The occupational therapist will provide aids for dressing, such as a stocking applicator, and any other aids found to be necessary after an assessment of the home environment and the patient's capabilities.

Discharge planning

Discharge planning should begin preoperatively, and in some centres patients will be identified as suitable for an early supported discharge scheme where a hospital at home environment is provided. It is essential, however, that the patient accepts this and is not forced into early discharge (Jester 2003). Support after discharge may be continued by a telephone helpline and nursing advice service (O'Brien et al 1999). Where such services do not exist, the community nurse will provide care, such as wound suture removal, and will liaise with the hospital team as necessary.

STOP THINK **10.13** From the information provided above, write a concise discharge plan for a patient who has undergone an uncomplicated total hip replacement.

SOFT TISSUE INJURIES

LIGAMENT INJURIES

PATHOPHYSIOLOGY

Excessive extension, flexion and/or rotation of a joint may result in a partial or complete rupture of a ligament. Whiplash injury is the term used to describe a ligamentous injury to the cervical spine area often occurring after a RTC (see Fig. 10.14, p. 460). This injury is due to excessive flexion and extension movements to the neck. The knee is heavily dependent on its ligaments for stability and they are susceptible to injury, particularly the anterior cruciate ligament which limits forward movement of the tibia on the femur. Injured ligaments never heal soundly or regain their former strength as the scar tissue that forms at the site is never as strong as the original tissue (Dandy & Edwards 2003).

MEDICAL MANAGEMENT

History and examination People who suffer these injuries are often young and will complain of severe pain around the injured area after feeling or hearing something snap or tear. Pain may be increased when the person's body weight is exerted through the injured limb. Limitation of normal joint movement may be found with swelling of the injured part. Joint instability may be noted during the physical examination.

Investigations Plain radiographs are taken to rule out a bony injury to the area. An MRI scan or examination of the joint under general anaesthesia may be undertaken.

Treatment If bleeding into the injured joint (haemarthrosis) has occurred, this may be aspirated under local anaesthesia. The injured area will be supported, e.g. using a cervical collar for a whiplash injury (see Fig. 10.22) or a POP cylinder/knee brace for a knee injury. Physiotherapy is instituted in order to build up muscle groups that surround the joint which the injured ligament normally supports. Surgical intervention is usually needed only when the injury affects the knee joint or where there is damage to more than one ligament and/or gross instability of the joint. Repairing ruptured ligaments is generally not successful, because the repaired ligament will not have the same 'stretchiness' as the original, and therefore they are usually replaced with a length of tendon or prosthetic material (Dandy & Edwards 2003).

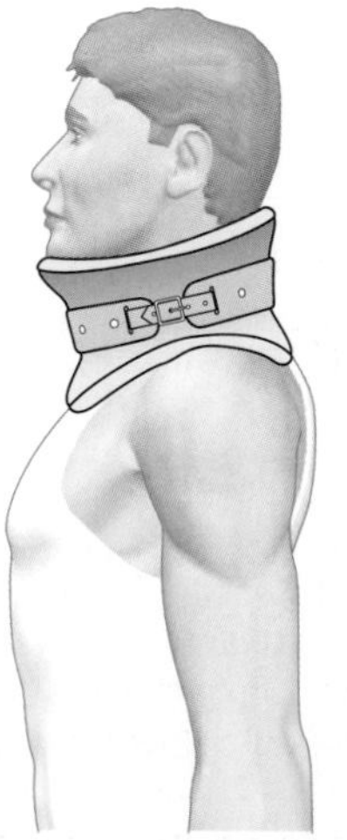

Fig. 10.22 Cervical collar.

NURSING PRIORITIES AND MANAGEMENT: Ligament injuries

The patient may arrive at the Emergency Department within a few hours of injury (see Ch. 27). In other cases, the patient may present 12–24 h after injury when the pain and swelling have greatly increased. If no other injury has been sustained, the patient may be treated and discharged to attend as an outpatient.

Pain This will be the major patient problem on presentation at hospital. Such pain should be assessed (see Ch. 19, p. 745) and an effective analgesic prescribed. As ligamentous injuries are sustained following severe trauma to the body part, the surrounding soft tissues will also be involved, causing further bleeding which will increase the swelling and irritate the surrounding tissues, thus increasing the patient's pain. The use of NSAIDs will be of value to reduce the inflammatory process.

Muscle spasm This is a common sign of soft tissue irritation and, if severe, the patient may need to be prescribed a mild antispasmodic as well as an analgesic.

Support/immobilisation Refer to priorities and management of patients in casts (see p. 451). In addition, when a cervical collar is worn, it can usually be removed to allow daily skin care. Following anterior cruciate ligament repair a patient usually wears a knee brace for the first 6–8 weeks, which prevents flexion greater than 90°, and nurses should ensure that the patient can correctly apply the device.

Psychosocial care Ligamentous injury may take up to a year to heal completely, and work and financial status, as well as social interaction, can be affected (Smith 2004c).

MUSCLE AND TENDON INJURIES

PATHOPHYSIOLOGY

These injuries are most often caused either by direct trauma at the site of the injury, i.e. an in-site injury, or by a sudden sharp movement of the joint associated with sports such as tennis and squash, i.e. a shearing injury. The large tendons and muscles of the lower limbs, such as the Achilles tendon, are the most common sites of injury, with a reported incidence of 18 per 100 000 persons (Bhandari et al 2002).

MEDICAL MANAGEMENT

History and examination The patient will experience a distressing tearing sensation or a kick at the site of the injury and possibly an inability to put the foot down. Swelling and tenderness will develop within a few hours following the injury. Bruising will appear later and may be extensive and alarming for the patient. On examination, a gap between the ends of the muscle or tendon may be felt in superficial muscle injuries. MRI or ultrasound may be used to determine the extent of the injury.

Treatment For muscle injuries the principles of RICE — Rest, Ice, Compression and Elevation — should be followed in order to control haemorrhage and haematoma. Early mobilisation within pain limits is important, as muscle healing occurs through aerobic metabolic pathways and therefore needs adequate circulation. Surgery may be necessary if there is a large intramuscular haematoma or if there is a large muscle tear affecting movement of a joint.

Tendon injuries are usually treated conservatively, with a cast or splint holding the ends together until healed. Surgery may be required for a complete tendon rupture, particularly of the Achilles tendon; however, a systematic review of surgical versus conservative treatment of Achilles tendon injury concluded that whilst surgery reduced the risk of re-rupture, it significantly increased the risk of infection (Bhandari et al 2002).

NURSING PRIORITIES AND MANAGEMENT: Muscle and tendon injuries

Comfort The nurse has a key role in helping the patient to institute and maintain RICE.

Mobility Once activity is commenced, the physiotherapist will teach the patient to use the most appropriate walking aid, usually a pair of crutches. Assessment of the patient's home circumstances with regard to mobility will be required.

Following surgery, routine postoperative care will be necessary. The use of a cast or brace will necessitate education of the patient in their care and management.

PERIPHERAL NERVE INJURIES

Nerves can be damaged due to underlying disease or following trauma. In this section, the focus will be on injuries following trauma.

PATHOPHYSIOLOGY

A single nerve or group of nerves may be damaged depending on the site of injury. Nerve injuries can be due to either direct or indirect force and can be divided into three types (Wellington 2004).

- Neuropraxia — intact nerves with temporary damage usually due to compression
- Axonotmesis — divided axons with maintenance of the endoneural tubes, usually due to severe blow or traction, a pulling injury; prognosis is good
- Neurotmesis — the whole nerve is divided, usually from a penetrating wound such as a stabbing. No recovery is possible without surgical repair.

MEDICAL MANAGEMENT

History and examination Following an accident, a patient may become aware of tingling (paraesthesia), numbness and/or loss of movement of the affected part. Examination of the distribution of the loss of sensation and movement will aid diagnosis as to the extent of the injury.

Investigations Plain radiographs are useful to assess bony injury and for the presence of any foreign material, such as glass fragments, which may have caused the injury.

Diagnosis is confirmed by the absence or alteration of neurological function and sensation of the affected part. Nerve conduction studies, which involve stimulating a nerve with a wave pulse to evaluate the sensory and motor responses along the course of the peripheral nerve, may be carried out (Dandy & Edwards 2003). Electromyography (EMG), which records motor activity at rest and on attempted muscle contraction, may also be used (Wellington 2004).

Treatment Primary surgical repair is indicated only when a nerve has been cleanly divided. Secondary repair may include suturing and grafting of nerve tissue from a less important nerve within the patient's body. Non-operative management involves immobilisation of the affected part in the anatomical position, using a lightweight cast or splint. Peripheral nerves are capable of regenerating at a rate of 1–2 mm/day (Wellington 2004). It is possible to calculate roughly the length of time to recovery although there is no guarantee that each nerve cell will heal.

NURSING PRIORITIES AND MANAGEMENT: Peripheral nerve injuries

Complete recovery may occur but take a few weeks, months or years. However, the patient may need to adapt to permanent and severely disabling physical, psychological and social changes (Wellington 2004).

In the short term, as the patient will have been involved in some form of trauma, nursing care as outlined in Chapter 27 will apply.

Should the patient require surgery, general perioperative care will be as described in Chapter 26.

Preventing further injury

The patient will have partial or complete loss of the protective mechanisms of touch and pain, and care must be taken to prevent further injury to the affected part. Movement of the injured limb must be through the normal range of passive joint movements, otherwise joints, muscles, tendons, ligaments and other nerves could be damaged further. To prevent the development of joint contracture and deformity, the patient may be fitted with a lightweight splint which holds the joints in their anatomical position. This may be needed for a long period. Exposure to extremes of temperature should be avoided, to prevent a skin burn.

Subsequent considerations

Pain Sharp shooting pain and a constant tingling sensation can be very troublesome and the patient may need prolonged use of analgesics. Antidepressant medication, such as amitriptyline and adjuvant analgesics, are known to be beneficial as a supplementary medication in the relief of neuropathic pain (see Ch. 19). The nurse may also wish to suggest, as an adjunct, the use of one of the many complementary therapies that are widely available (Wellington 2004).

Washing and dressing The patient will need advice and information to assist in adapting their usual mode of personal cleansing and dressing. For example, a patient with a median nerve injury due to a laceration of the wrist of the dominant hand may have difficulty in brushing their teeth or combing their hair. The occupational therapist can provide advice and appropriate aids.

Splints If a splint is used, the patient will need information and advice about the correct method of application and removal. The patient with sensitive skin has to be taught to inspect it for signs of pressure by removing the splint at regular intervals throughout the day.

Exercise The physiotherapist will exercise the joints of the injured limb passively to prevent stiffness and muscle wasting. The patient may be able to use their own hands to exercise the joints, or a relative can be taught the skill of passive exercises. Not only will this assist physical recovery but it can also be of psychological benefit.

Support As recovery from a peripheral nerve injury may be prolonged, the patient will require support and understanding from family, friends and the members of the health care team to relieve boredom and prevent the development of depression. Group sessions for patients with similar injuries who are receiving physiotherapy, occupational therapy and/or diversional therapy can be an excellent psychological support mechanism. The social worker can assist with social and/or financial problems which may develop due to the possible lengthy absence from employment.

Permanent disability If the nerve injury prevents return to the previous occupation, it will be necessary to ensure that the patient has access to specialist advice about retraining and new employment opportunities. In some instances, alteration to body image could have a severe psychological effect. Nurses should be aware of this and provide support and counselling as needed by the patient.

CONCLUSION

This chapter has outlined the basic principles of nursing management that relate to the more common musculoskeletal disorders and has focused on some of the critical factors that influence management and care in specific disorders. It has stressed that the focus of care is the patient and family, and that the challenge to nursing increases with changing trends in therapeutic interventions, early supported discharge schemes, care in the community, and an ageing population whose lifestyle has been revolutionised by joint replacement surgery and multidisciplinary care and support.

Trauma is a constant in human societies and musculoskeletal injuries will always be a fact of life. However, continuing research and more attention to health screening and health promotion have shown that many accidents and conditions are preventable and many diseases amenable to treatment.

A wide knowledge of musculoskeletal disorders is essential for both hospital- and community-based nurses, to enable them to respond to the needs of patients and their families, to work actively to prevent accidents and complications, and to give appropriate information, advice and care.

REFERENCES

Allan D 1988 Nursing and the neurosciences. Churchill Livingstone, Edinburgh

Allsworth A 2004 Osteoporosis: nursing implications. In: Kneale J, Davis P (eds) Orthopaedic and trauma nursing, 2nd edn. Churchill Livingstone, Edinburgh, p 380–389

Arnett F C, Edsworth S M, Block D A 1988 The American Rheumatism Association 1987 revised criteria for the classification of rheumatoid arthritis. Arthritis and Rheumatism 31(3): 315–324

Arthritis Research Council (ARC) 2004 Infection and arthritis: rheumatic disease: topical reviews. Online. Available: www.arc.org.uk/about_arth/med_reports/

Ayral X 2001 Injections in the treatment of osteoarthritis. Best Practice and Research Clinical Rheumatology 15(4): 609–626

Barlow J 2001 How to use education as an intervention in osteoarthritis. Best Practice and Research Clinical Rheumatology 15(4): 545–558

Bhandari M, Guyatt G H, Siddiqui F et al 2002 Treatment of acute Achilles tendon ruptures: a systematic overview and meta analysis. Clinical Orthopaedics and Related Research 400: 190–200

Burden J, Kneale J D 2004 Orthopaedic infections. In: Kneale J, Davis P (eds) Orthopaedic and trauma nursing, 2nd edn. Churchill Livingstone, Edinburgh, p 215–236

Content G, Hajela V, Lucas B 2003 Osteoporosis screening and education following distal radial fracture: an expanding role for fracture clinic nurses. Journal of Orthopaedic Nursing 7(3): 137–140

Cox C L, Boswell G M 2000 Integrating complementary health care in outpatient surgery for discectomy: the patient's perspective. Journal of Orthopaedic Nursing 4(4): 179–184

Currie H 2000 A critical analysis of the evidence for chiropractice treatment of low back pain. Journal of Orthopaedic Nursing 5(1): 4–8

Dandy D J, Edwards D J 2003 Essential orthopaedics and trauma, 4th edn. Churchill Livingstone, Edinburgh

Davis P 2004 Why move? In: Kneale J, Davis P (eds) Orthopaedic and trauma nursing, 2nd edn. Churchill Livingstone, Edinburgh, p 76–104

Department of Health 2002 Improving orthopaedic services – a guide for clinicians, managers and service commissioners. DH, London

Doherty M, Dougados M 2001 Evidence-based management of osteoarthritis: practical issues relating to the data. Best Practice and Research Clinical Rheumatology 15(4): 517–525

Donohue S 1997 Lower limb amputation 3: the role of the nurse. British Journal of Nursing 6(20): 1171–1174, 1187–1191

Dupuy D, Goldberg N 2001 Image-guided radiofrequency tumour ablation: challenges and opportunities – part II. Journal of Vascular and Interventional Radiology 12(10): 1135–1148

Esteve-de-Miguel C 2003 The arthroscopic treatment of knee osteoarthritis. Current Orthopaedics 17: 63–69

Font-Rodriguez D E, Scuderi G R, Insall J N 1997 Survivorship of cemented total knee arthroplasty. Clinical Orthopaedics and Related Research 345: 79–86

Gibson J N A, Grant I C, Waddell G 2004 Surgery for lumbar disc prolapse (Cochrane Review). In: The Cochrane Library, Issue 2. Wiley, Chichester

Guzmán J, Esmail R, Karjalainen K et al 2004 Multidisciplinary bio-psycho-social rehabilitation for chronic low-back pain (Cochrane Review). In: The Cochrane Library, Issue 3. Wiley, Chichester

Hakim A, Clunie G 2002 Oxford handbook of rheumatology. Oxford University Press, Oxford

Handoll H H G, Madhok R, Dodds C 2004 Anaesthesia for treating distal radial fracture in adults (Cochrane Review). In: The Cochrane Library, Issue 3. Wiley, Chichester

Hansson M, Bostrom C, Harms-Ringdahl K 2001 Living with spine-related pain in a changing society: a qualitative study. Disability and Rehabilitation 23(7): 286–295

Harrison P 2000 Managing spinal injury: critical care. Spinal Injuries Association, London

Henry C 2004 Care of patients with bone tumours. In: Kneale J, Davis P (eds) Orthopaedic and trauma nursing, 2nd edn. Churchill Livingstone, Edinburgh

Hilde G, Hagen K B, Jamtveldt G et al 2004 Advice to stay active as a single treatment for low-back pain and sciatica (Cochrane Review). In: The Cochrane Library, Issue 3. Wiley, Chichester

Hill J 1997 Patient satisfaction in a nurse led rheumatology clinic. Journal of Advanced Nursing 25: 347–354

Hill J, Ryan S (eds) 2000 Rheumatology: a handbook for community nurses. Whurr, London

Howard W J 2001 A critical review of the role of targeted education for osteoporosis prevention. Journal of Orthopaedic Nursing 5(3): 131–135

James A 2000 Osteoporosis: cause and treatment. Nursing Times 96(22): 36–37

Jester R 2003 Early discharge to hospital at home: should it be a matter of choice? Journal of Orthopaedic Nursing 7(2): 64–69

Judd M 1997 Caring for the patient with musculoskeletal trauma. In: Walsh M (ed) Watson's clinical nursing and related sciences, 5th edn. Baillière Tindall, London

Kee C C 1998 Living with osteoarthritis: insiders' views. Applied Nursing Research 11(1): 19–26

Kneale J, Davis P (eds) 2004 Nursing the orthopaedic patient. Churchill Livingstone, Edinburgh

Knight C, Mathew A, Muir J K 2004 The locomotor system. In: Kneale J, Davis P (eds) Orthopaedic and trauma nursing, 2nd edn. Churchill Livingstone, Edinburgh, p 47–75

Langstaff R 2000 Fracture healing and principles of fracture management. In: Langstaff D, Christie J (eds) Trauma care: a team approach. Butterworth-Heinemann, Oxford, p 13–25

Lee-Smith J, Santy J, Davis P et al 2001 Pin site management. Towards a consensus: part 1. Journal of Orthopaedic Nursing 5: 37–42

Limb M K 2004 An evaluation survey of self-concept issue in adult patients undergoing limb reconstruction procedures. Journal of Orthopaedic Nursing 8(1): 34–40

Little C, Parsons T 2004 Herbal therapy for treating rheumatoid arthritis (Cochrane Review). In: The Cochrane Library, Issue 2. Wiley, Chichester

Lookinland S, Beckstrand R L 2003 HRT: decide based on the evidence. Nurse Practitioner 28(9): 46–54

Love C 1998 A discussion and analysis of nurse-led pain assessment for the early detection of compartment syndrome. Journal of Orthopaedic Nursing 2: 160–167

Love C 1999 A focused review of nursing and the effectiveness of preventative measures for deep vein thrombosis. Journal of Orthopaedic Nursing 3(2): 73–80

Lucas B, Davis P S 2004 Why restricting movement is important. In: Kneale J, Davis P (eds) Orthopaedic and trauma nursing, 2nd edn. Churchill Livingstone, Edinburgh, p 105–139

Maher A B, Salmond S W, Pelino T A 2002 Orthopaedic nursing, 3rd edn. Saunders, Philadelphia

McCaffery M, Pasero C 1999 Pain: clinical manual, 2nd edn. Mosby, London

McRae R, Esser R 2002 Practical fracture treatment, 4th edn. Churchill Livingstone, Edinburgh

Mulligan K, Newman S 2003 Psycho-educational interventions in rheumatic diseases: a review of papers published from September 2001 to August 2002. Current Opinion in Rheumatology 15: 156–159

National Institute for Clinical Excellence 2001 Guidance on the use of cyclo-oxygenase (Cox) II selective inhibitors, celecoxib, rofecoxib, meloxicam and etodolac, for osteoarthritis and rheumatoid arthritis. NICE, London

National Statistics 2004 Mortality statistics 2002, injury and poisoning. Online. Available: www.statistics.gov.uk

O'Brien S, Dennison J, Breslin E et al 1999 A review of an orthopaedic outcome assessment telephone follow-up helpline and nursing advice service. Journal of Orthopaedic Nursing 3(1): 18–23

Oliver S, Ryan S 2004 Effective pain management for patients with arthritis. Nursing Standard 18(50): 43–52

Parker M J, Handoll H H G 2004 Pre-operative traction for fractures of the proximal femur. The Cochrane Library, Issue 2, 2004. Wiley, Chichester

Patterson J 2004 Spinal manipulation for chronic low back pain. Bazian Ltd, Wessex Institute for Health Research and Development, University of Southampton

Peat G, Croft P, Hay E 2001 Clinical assessment of the osteoarthritis patient. Best Practice and Research Clinical Rheumatology 15(4): 527–544

Petty A C, Wardman C 1998 A randomized, controlled comparison of adjustable focused rigidity primary casting technique with standard plaster of Paris/synthetic casting technique in the management of fractures and other injuries. Journal of Orthopaedic Nursing 2: 95–102
Renton S, Brown J 2001 An evaluation of an orthopaedic supported discharge service. Journal of Orthopaedic Nursing 5(3): 120–124
Roper N, Logan W W, Tierney A J 2000 The Roper Logan Tierney model of nursing. Churchill Livingstone, Edinburgh
Royal College of Nursing Advisory Panel for Back Pain in Nurses 2002 Code of practice for patient handling. RCN, London
Royal College of Physicians 1999 Osteoporosis – clinical guidelines for prevention and treatment. RCP, London
Ryan S, Oliver S 2002 Rheumatoid arthritis. Nursing Standard 16(20): 45–52
Santy J 1998 Rehabilitation of the patient with a hip fracture: facing the challenge. Journal of Orthopaedic Nursing 2(1): 11–15
Scottish Intercollegiate Guidelines Network (SIGN) 2002a Prevention and management of hip fractures in older people No. 56. Online. Available: www.sign.ac.uk
Scottish Intercollegiate Guidelines Network (SIGN) 2002b Prophylaxis of venous thromboembolism. No. 62, Section 5. Online. Available: www.sign.ac.uk
Shire Pharmaceuticals 1998 Accidents and hip fractures in the elderly. Shire Pharmaceuticals, Hampshire
Sims M, Bennett N, Broadley L et al 1999 External fixation: part 1. Journal of Orthopaedic Nursing 3: 203–209
Sims M, Trent J-C, Lake S et al 2001 The Lautenbach method for chronic osteomyelitis: nursing roles, responsibilities and challenges. Journal of Orthopaedic Nursing 5(4): 198–205
Smith M 2004a Care of patients with acute spinal cord injuries. In: Kneale J, Davis P (eds) Orthopaedic and trauma nursing, 2nd edn. Churchill Livingstone, Edinburgh, p 390–410
Smith M 2004b Care of patients with spinal conditions and injuries. In: Kneale J, Davis P (eds) Orthopaedic and trauma nursing, 2nd edn. Churchill Livingstone, Edinburgh, p 359–379
Smith M 2004c Sports injuries. In: Kneale J, Davis P (eds) Orthopaedic and trauma nursing, 2nd edn. Churchill Livingstone, Edinburgh, p 495–512
Spinal Research 2004 Spinal cord repair. Online. Available: www.spinal-research.org
Talbot N J, Brown J H M, Treble N J 2002 Early dislocation after total hip arthroplasty. Journal of Arthroplasty 17(8): 1006–1008
Tarling M, Aitken E, Lahoti O et al 2002 Closing the audit loop: the role of a pilot in the development of a fractured neck of femur integrated care pathway. Journal of Orthopaedic Nursing 6(3): 130–134
Temple J, Santy J 2004 Pin site care for preventing infections associated with external bone fixators and pins (Cochrane Review). In: The Cochrane Library, Issue 2. Wiley, Chichester
Towheed T E, Anastassiades T P, Shea B et al 2004 Glucosamine therapy for treating osteoarthritis (Cochrane Review). In: The Cochrane Library, Issue 2. Wiley, Chichester
Tucker K 1998 Compartment syndrome: the orthopaedic nurse's vital role. Journal of Orthopaedic Nursing 2(1): 33–36
UK Government Health and Safety Executive 1992 Manual handling operations regulations 1992: guidance on regulations. HSE Books, Suffolk
Vale L, Wyness L, McCormack K et al 2002 A systematic review of the effectiveness and cost-effectiveness of metal-on-metal hip resurfacing arthroplasty for treatment of hip disease. Health Technology Assessment 6(15): 1–109
Van Tulder M W, Scholten R J P M, Koes B W et al 2004 Non-steroidal anti-inflammatory drugs for low back pain (Cochrane Review). In: The Cochrane Library, Issue 2. Wiley, Chichester
Wardman C 2002 Nurse led fracture review clinic: an innovation in practice. Journal of Orthopaedic Nursing 6(2): 90–94
Wellington B 2004 Peripheral nerve injuries. In: Kneale J, Davis P (eds) Orthopaedic and trauma nursing, 2nd edn. Churchill Livingstone, Edinburgh, p 436–449
Winzeler S, Rosenstein B D 1997 Orthopaedic problems of the upper extremities. American Association of Occupational Health Nurses (AAOHN) Journal 45(4): 189–200
World Health Organization 1994 Assessment of fracture risk and its application to screening for postmenopausal osteoporosis. Report series 843. WHO, Geneva
Younger A S E, Curran P, McQueen M M 1990 Backslabs and plaster casts: which will best accommodate increasing intra-compartmental pressures. Injury 21: 179–181

FURTHER READING

Dandy D J, Edwards D J 2003 Essential orthopaedics and trauma, 4th edn. Churchill Livingstone, Edinburgh
Jamieson E M, McCall J M, Whyte L A 2002 Guidelines for clinical nursing practice, 4th edn. Churchill Livingstone, Edinburgh
Kneale J, Davis P (eds) 2004 Orthopaedic and trauma nursing, 2nd edn. Churchill Livingstone, Edinburgh
Knight C, Mathew A, Muir J K 2004 The locomotor system. In: Kneale J, Davis P (eds) Orthopaedic and trauma nursing, 2nd edn. Churchill Livingstone, Edinburgh, p 47–75
Langstaff D, Christie J (2000) Trauma care: a team approach. Butterworth-Heinemann, Oxford
Maher A B, Salmond S W, Pellino T A 2002 Orthopaedic nursing, 3rd edn. Saunders, Philadelphia
Marieb E 2004 Human anatomy and physiology, 6th edn. Benjamin Cummings, California
Ramachandran V S, Hirsten W 1998 The perception of phantom limbs: the D.O. Hebb lecture. Brain 121(9): 1603–1630
Royal College of Nursing Advisory Panel for Back Pain in Nurses 2002 Code of practice for patient handling. RCN, London
Scottish Intercollegiate Guidelines Network (SIGN) 2002 Prevention and management of hip fractures in older people No. 56. Online. Available: www.sign.ac.uk
Walsh M (ed) 2002 Watson's clinical nursing and related sciences, 6th edn. Baillière Tindall, London
Waugh A, Grant A 2001 Ross and Wilson's anatomy and physiology in health and illness, 9th edn. Churchill Livingstone, Edinburgh

USEFUL WEBSITES AND ADDRESSES

Arthritis Care
www.arthritiscare.org.uk

Arthritis Research Campaign
www.arc.org.uk

The Association to Aid the Sexual and Personal Relationships of People with a Disability (SPOD)
286 Camden Road
London N7 0BJ

Disabled Living Foundation
www.dlf.org.uk

National Osteoporosis Society
www.nos.org.uk

RCN Society of Orthopaedic and Trauma Nursing
20 Cavendish Square
London W1M 0AB

Spinal Injuries Association
www.spinal.co.uk

BLOOD DISORDERS

11

Fiona M. Duke
Catherine Paton

INTRODUCTION

Blood is a vital body fluid which, via the cardiovascular system, reaches all body organs and tissues. It has three primary functions:

- to transport oxygen, nutrients and other substances
- to protect the body against microorganisms and other foreign materials
- to regulate homeostatic systems.

Disorders of the blood are diverse and may be acute or chronic. All age groups may be affected, although some disorders are more common in certain age ranges than in others. Some disorders, such as haemophilia, are sex-linked; others, such as sickle cell disease and thalassaemia, are more prevalent among certain ethnic groups. Still others, such as nutritional anaemia, occur worldwide.

Causes of blood disorders

Contributing factors in the development of blood disorders can be divided into nine types:

- *Developmental*. Infants and older people can be predisposed to anaemia, the former group because of increased nutritional requirements for growth and development, and the latter because of poor nutrition resulting from factors such as depression or inability to get out to shops.
- *Genetic*. Inherited disorders include:
  — abnormalities of the red blood cells, e.g. spherocytosis
  — haemoglobin abnormalities, e.g. thalassaemia and sickle cell anaemia
  — lack of a clotting factor, e.g. haemophilia and von Willebrand's disease.
- *Dietary*. Nutritional deficiencies can be related to poverty, lack of knowledge about nutrition and healthy cooking methods, and to overriding political and economic circumstances.
- *Sociocultural*. Dietary habits leading to nutritional deficiency may be related to values and beliefs. Strict vegetarians, for example, may develop vitamin B_{12} deficiency anaemia. Lifestyle factors, such as a reliance on fast foods or a habit of skipping meals, can also lead to nutritional anaemias. Other social factors such as homelessness and unemployment can contribute to poor nutrition, leading to the development of blood disorders.
- *Environmental*. Exposure to industrial chemicals — benzene, lead, sodium chlorate — and to ionising radiation has been linked to the development of blood disorders such as aplastic anaemia, agranulocytosis and leukaemia.

- *Pharmacological*. Some over-the-counter and prescription drugs are known to cause specific blood disorders (Craig et al 2002). Agranulocytosis can be caused by dapsone, used to treat leprosy, and by some medications to reduce excessive thyroxine production, e.g. carbimazole. Quinine, quinidine and heparin can cause thrombocytopenia by damaging the platelets. Prolonged use of aspirin and non-steroidal anti-inflammatory drugs (NSAIDs) can lead to iron deficiency anaemia. Most cancer chemotherapy agents cause myelosuppression and thus anaemia, neutropenia and thrombocytopenia.
- *Iatrogenic*. Surgical interventions that cause blood disorders include the use of prosthetic heart valves, which can damage red blood cells, and total gastrectomy which, through the resulting lack of intrinsic factor, leads to vitamin B_{12} anaemia, i.e. pernicious anaemia.
- *Pathological*. Diseases which can cause blood disorders, particularly anaemia, include inflammatory diseases, malabsorption syndromes, cancers and infections.
- *Idiopathic*. In some cases of anaemia, especially aplastic anaemia, no cause may be identified.

The nurse's role in the treatment of blood disorders

The nurse's role in caring for patients with blood disorders in a community, hospital or occupational setting will include the following functions:

- promoting health, e.g. by encouraging good dietary habits
- detecting early signs of illness such as pallor, fatigue and frequent absence from work
- assisting with medical investigations, e.g. bone marrow aspiration, dietary history-taking
- explaining tests, diagnoses, treatments and prognoses to patients
- educating patients about lifestyle, diet and medication
- providing emotional support to patients and their families
- referring patients to other professionals such as genetic counsellors.

Depending upon their work setting and specialism, nurses will play a variety of roles in the care of patients with blood disorders. Primary health care nurses may be involved in health screening and may be the individual's first point of contact with the health care team. Hospital nurses may care for anaemic patients in all types of wards and units. Specialist nurses may work as sickle cell disease counsellors or in a haemophilia centre. Macmillan nurses may provide care at home for patients with malignant haematological disorders.

The particular needs of patients with blood disorders will vary in accordance with the nature of their illness. Some patients may present with one very acute episode of illness, e.g. massive haemorrhage because of, for example, trauma or disseminated intravascular coagulation (DIC), and then return to full health after treatment. More commonly, patients are diagnosed with blood disorders after a prolonged period of malaise.

ANATOMY AND PHYSIOLOGY

Blood is red viscous fluid which is pumped from the heart via the arteries to the capillaries in the tissues and returns via the veins to the heart. Its central role is to help maintain an optimal environment for the functioning of the body cells. It fulfils this role by performing the following functions:

- transporting oxygen, essential nutrients and other important substances, e.g. hormones, enzymes, chemicals to all cells
- removing carbon dioxide and other waste products from the cell
- haemostasis
- protecting the body from microorganisms and antigens
- regulating water, electrolyte and acid–base balance
- regulating body temperature.

The total volume of blood circulating in an average 70 kg male adult is 5 L. Blood consists of cellular and fluid components. The main constituents of plasma, the fluid component, are:

- water
- plasma proteins
- electrolytes
- nutrients
- hormones
- enzymes
- waste products.

Cellular components of blood

There are three different cellular components of blood:

- erythrocytes
- leucocytes
- thrombocytes.

These cellular components are developed in the active bone marrow found in the medullary cavity of certain bones in the adult. The sites of the active bone marrow are:

- ends of the long bones, e.g. humerus
- ilia of the pelvis
- vertebrae
- ribs
- skull
- sternum.

These sites can be extended when there is an increased demand for blood cells. All types of blood cell are derived from a common pluripotent stem cell.

Erythrocytes (red blood cells)

Red blood cells are biconcave discs. Haemoglobin, the oxygen carrying molecule within the erythrocyte, makes up 33% of the red cell weight and gives blood its characteristic red colour. The thin cell membrane allows gaseous exchange between the cell and surrounding tissues. The cell is also soft and pliable, allowing it to pass along the capillary lumen easily. During maturation, the red blood cell extrudes its nucleus. The mature cell therefore has no capacity to reproduce, repair, grow or make haemoglobin.

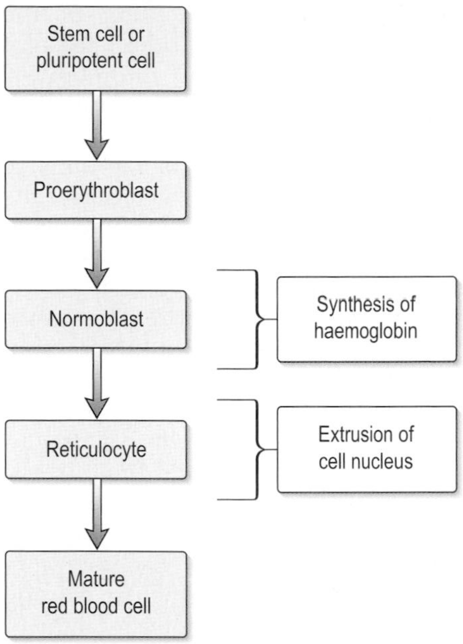

Fig. 11.1 Maturation of red blood cell.

Function Oxygen is carried in the form of oxyhaemoglobin by the red blood cells from the lungs to the tissues. Carbon dioxide, as carboxyhaemoglobin, is transported from the tissues to the lungs.

Maturation (see Fig. 11.1) The total number of circulating red blood cells remains fairly constant at $3.9–6.5 \times 10^{12}$ cells/L (there is a slight variation between men and women) to ensure that the optimum amount of oxygen is available to the tissues. To ensure this number, the body has to maintain a balance between the number of cells produced and the number broken down.

The reticulocyte numbers are increased when there is a greater demand for red blood cells. Therefore, a reticulocyte count can be used as a measure of response to treatment for anaemia (a deficiency of haemoglobin in the blood due to a lack of red blood cells and/or haemoglobin content). Treatment should stimulate production of more reticulocytes.

The essential factors required for red cell production are:

- erythropoietin produced by the kidney
- iron — part of the haemoglobin molecule (see below)
- amino acids
- vitamins B_{12} and folic acid (both for DNA synthesis)
- vitamins B_6, thiamine, riboflavin, C and E
- intrinsic factor — for absorption of vitamin B_{12} from the gut
- thyroxine
- androgens
- adrenocortical steroids
- human growth hormone.

Haemoglobin is a complex molecule of haem and globin. The haem fraction is a combination of porphyrin and iron. The globin complex is composed of four polypeptide chains.

Life span The average life span of a red blood cell is 120 days. At the end of its life span, the cell is broken down in the bone marrow, spleen and liver by macrophages. The haemoglobin molecule is split into its major components: haem and globin. The globin is further split into amino acids, which are then stored in the body's amino acid pool. The haem is split into iron (which is stored in the liver and reused by the marrow) and porphyrin (which is converted to bilirubin). The bilirubin (insoluble in water and bound to albumin) is transported to the liver, converted into soluble bilirubin and excreted into the small intestine as a constituent of bile. From there, some is reabsorbed and excreted by the kidneys as urobilinogen. The majority of the bilirubin is excreted in the faeces as stercobilirubin.

Leucocytes (white blood cells)

There are three types of white blood cell:

- granulocytes
- lymphocytes
- monocytes.

Granulocytes are characterised by the presence of granules in the cytoplasm and are divided into three subtypes: neutrophils, eosinophils and basophils. Lymphocytes are subdivided into T lymphocytes and B lymphocytes.

Normal numbers and percentages of each type and subtype are given in Table 11.1.

Function White blood cells are involved in the defence of the body against microbes and other foreign antigens (see Ch. 16).

Maturation All white blood cells develop from the pluripotent stem cell in the bone marrow and mature

Table 11.1 Normal number of different subtypes of white blood cells

Type	Subtype	Normal value (cells/L)	Percentage of total	
Granulocytes		$2.5–8.0 \times 10^9$	40–75	
	Neutrophils	$2.0–7.5 \times 10^9$	40–70	Percentage of total white blood cell count
	Eosinophils	Up to 0.4×10^9	1–6	
	Basophils	$<0.1 \times 10^9$	<1	
Lymphocytes		$1.5–4.0 \times 10^9$	20–50	
	B lymphocytes		15–30	Percentage of total lymphocytes
	T lymphocytes		40–80	
Monocytes		$0.2–0.8 \times 10^9$	2–10	

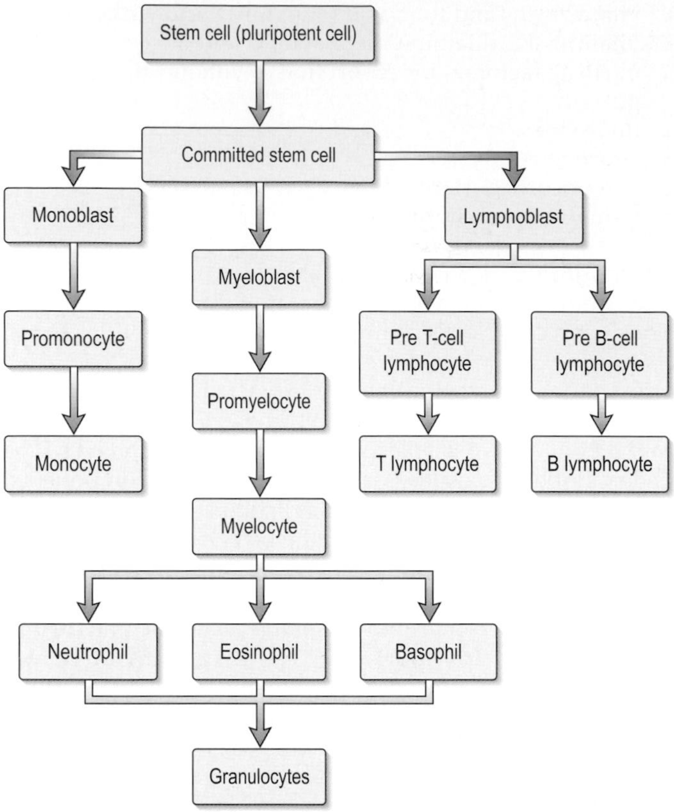

Fig. 11.2 Development of different types of leucocyte, each stage controlled by a specific growth factor.

through several stages as illustrated in Figure 11.2. Maturation is regulated by specific haemopoietic growth factors, e.g. granulocyte colony stimulating factor (GCSF), at each stage of maturation. Lymphocytes mature in either bone marrow (B lymphocytes) or the thymus (T lymphocytes) (see Ch. 16). Monocytes enter the tissues from the blood and mature into macrophages (scavenger cells in different tissues).

Life span The different types of white blood cell have variable life spans. Neutrophils, once they enter the blood, circulate for about 7 h and then migrate into the tissues, where they die after a few days. Lymphocytes have a variable life span, ranging from 100 days to several years. Monocytes, as macrophages, can survive for many years.

Thrombocytes (platelets)

Platelets are small, granular, non-nucleated blood cells that play a vital role in haemostasis (the arrest of bleeding). The normal concentration of platelets is 140–400 × 10^9/L.

Function Platelets are involved in the first three phases of haemostasis:

- phase 1 — vasoconstriction of an injured vessel
- phase 2 — formation of platelet plug
- phase 3 — formation of fibrin clot.

The fourth and final stage — fibrinolysis, the dissolution of the fibrin clot — does not involve platelets.

During phase 1 of haemostasis, narrowing of the damaged blood vessel occurs in response to the release of powerful vasoconstrictors — serotonin and thromboxane A — by the platelets. This reduces blood flow and thus decreases the likelihood of the platelet plug being sloughed off. In phase 2, platelets adhere to the site of the damage and release adenosine diphosphate (ADP), which causes the platelets to adopt a spherical shape conducive to aggregation. In phase 3, a fibrin clot is formed. This involves the conversion of prothrombin to thrombin, which then acts on the plasma protein fibrinogen to form fibrin. This fibrin clot is soluble at first but becomes insoluble in the presence of calcium and clotting factor XIII (fibrin-stabilising factor).

The formation of fibrin in phase 3 is made possible by two cascades of events known as the extrinsic pathway, events outside the damaged blood vessel, and the intrinsic pathway, events inside the vessel (see Fig. 11.3). The extrinsic pathway is activated by the tissue damage. The intrinsic pathway is activated by exposed collagen. Each stage in the intrinsic pathway is regulated by a particular clotting factor. Together, the two cascades act on clotting factor X, which then activates the prothrombin.

Vitamin K, a fat-soluble vitamin, is required for the synthesis in the liver of the following clotting factors (Summerton et al 2002):

- factor II (prothrombin)
- factor VII
- factor IX (Christmas factor)
- factor X (Stuart factor).

Maturation Platelets arise from the pluripotent stem cell and mature into megakaryocytes, mainly regulated by thrombopoietin. The megakaryocyte then fragments into many platelets.

Life span Platelets circulate for 7–10 days before being destroyed.

Plasma

Plasma is the straw-coloured fluid part of the blood which is left after the cellular components are removed. It contains blood clotting factors. Serum is the term for the fluid which separates from blood when it coagulates. It contains none of the blood clotting factors. The main constituents of plasma are shown in Figure 11.4.

For further reading on the anatomy and physiology of blood see Waugh & Grant (2001) and Tortora & Derrickson (2006).

Blood groups

ABO blood groups

Red blood cells have specific antigens, agglutinogens, on the red cell membrane. These agglutinogens are referred to in terms of the ABO blood group system. A person can have either the A or B agglutinogen on the red blood membrane, or neither, or both. Agglutinogens are inherited and are present from birth.

The importance of these agglutinogens is apparent when one person is given blood from another person. A person

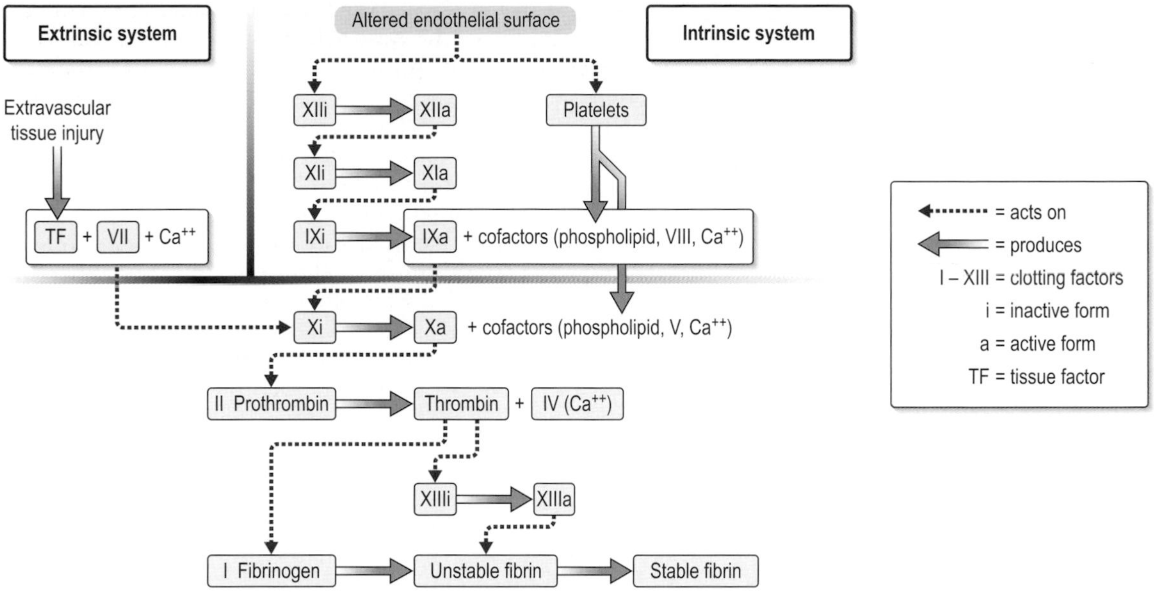

Fig. 11.3 Blood coagulation.

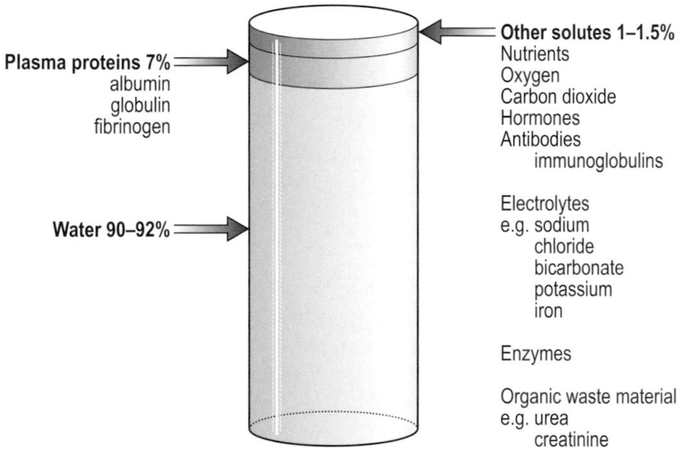

Fig. 11.4 The main constituents of plasma.

with the agglutinogen A (blood group A) has anti-B antibodies in the serum (antibodies are substances that cause clumping to occur when attached to particular antigens). A person with agglutinogen B (blood group B) has the anti-A agglutinin (or antibody). A person with both agglutinogens A and B (blood group AB) has no agglutinins, whilst a person with neither A nor B agglutinogens (blood group O) has both anti-A and anti-B agglutinins (see Table 11.2). Therefore, if a person is given a transfusion of blood from a different group, the red cells will clump together and haemolyse (break down). In a blood transfusion, it is the reaction between the donor's red cells and the recipient's serum, i.e. between the introduced agglutinogen and the agglutinin already present, which causes an adverse reaction which can be fatal. Thus, if the recipient's serum has anti-B agglutinin present, the donor's cells must be either blood group A or O.

Not only the red cells but also the white blood cells and platelets have ABO agglutinogens. Therefore, if a patient is to receive a transfusion of other cellular components, the correct blood group should be used.

Table 11.2 Antigens and antibodies present in different blood groups

Blood group	Agglutinogen present on red cell membrane	Agglutinin present in serum
A	A	Anti-B
B	B	Anti-A
AB	AB	None
O	O	Anti-A and anti-B

The Rhesus factor

In the UK, 85% of the population have a second important class of antigen present on their red cells: the Rhesus (Rh) factor (Craig et al 2002). A person is either Rh-positive or Rh-negative. The antibody, anti-D, does not occur naturally in the plasma of Rh-negative blood, but stimulation to produce it can occur if a person receives a Rh-positive blood transfusion or if, during childbirth, red blood cells from a Rh-positive baby cross the placental barrier into the circulation of a Rh-negative mother. If the person is later exposed to Rh-positive red blood cells, agglutination and haemolysis of the red blood cells will occur. Blood to be transfused must therefore be carefully cross-matched for the Rh factor.

The Rh factor is only carried on the red blood cells.

Other blood groups

The ABO and Rh factor blood groupings are the most important blood classifications, but there are more than 12 other blood group systems which normally do not cause agglutination unless the patient requires multiple blood

Box 11.1

The importance of checking blood component compatibility

SHOT (Serious Hazards of Transfusion) annual report 2001/2002 warns that 71.7% of incidents reported involved the transfusion of wrong blood; 35% of these incidents occurred during bedside administration (SHOT 2003).

transfusions, e.g. patients who have had a massive haemorrhage or who have leukaemia; in such cases it may be necessary to ensure the donor's blood is compatible with other known antibodies in the recipient's serum.

Blood transfusion

A blood transfusion is the administration to one individual of blood donated by another individual. The practice of blood transfusion makes it possible to save lives when severe haemorrhage has occurred, when major surgery is required or when there is failure of the bone marrow to produce blood cells. Transfusion does, however, expose patients to the risk of potentially fatal complications, e.g. infection, haemolytic reactions (see p. 491) or receiving a mismatched unit of blood (see Box 11.1).

For further guidelines about safe transfusion of blood, see Gray & Illingworth (2004).

Under some circumstances, patients may need blood products to be cytomegalovirus (CMV) negative. CMV is a herpes viral infection which causes few symptoms in the healthy person. However, for patients who are immunocompromised, and especially those undergoing bone marrow/stem cell transplantation, exposure to the virus may lead to potentially fatal complications such as pneumonitis, liver dysfunction and graft failure.

Transfusion of blood products carries the risk of transfusion-associated graft-versus-host disease (TA-GVHD) whereby transfused lymphocytes engraft in the recipient — a very rare possibility in immunocompetent patients, but may occur in the immunocompromised patient, especially those with haematological diseases. Irradiating blood products will prevent this potential complication.

For further information and guidelines to indicate which patients should receive irradiated blood products, see Wilkins (2000).

Blood transfusion products readily available are given in Table 11.3.

Cross-matching

Before a unit of blood or blood component is transfused into another person, the blood from the donated unit must be cross-matched with that of the recipient's serum, i.e. the blood from the donated unit is mixed in the laboratory with a sample of the recipient's serum. The donor's blood should be of the same ABO blood group to prevent a potentially fatal agglutination reaction.

A Rh-negative recipient should receive Rh-negative blood. Details of the results of the cross-matching are recorded along with the blood unit number on the documentation sent with the unit of blood when the blood transfusion is given. This documentation is retained after the unit of blood has been used in case of any transfusion reaction (see p. 491 for the nursing care of patients receiving transfusions). Patients may be able to donate their own red cells prior to elective surgery, i.e. autologous transfusion, to avoid the risk of receiving an allogeneic blood transfusion.

STOP THINK **11.1** Attend a blood donor session to find out about:

(a) the categories of people who are allowed to donate blood
(b) the screening process for blood donations
(c) the process of donating a unit of blood
(d) the care of the donor before, during and after the procedure
(e) how the blood is stored after donation.

DISORDERS OF RED BLOOD CELLS

These disorders can be divided into:

- disorders in which there is a deficiency of haemoglobin in the blood due to lack of red cells and/or reduced haemoglobin content
- disorders due to blood loss
- disorders due to excessive production of red blood cells.

ANAEMIAS

Anaemias are those disorders in which there is a reduction in the haemoglobin concentration in the blood. There are three main types of anaemia (see Fig. 11.5):

- anaemia due to decreased red cell production, resulting from:
  - — reduced bone marrow function
  - — lack of essential factors for cell maturation
- anaemia due to blood loss
- haemolytic anaemia — due to excessive destruction of the red cells.

Anaemia is extremely common worldwide; the overall incidence of iron deficiency affects 30% of the world population (Parker-Williams 2000). Anaemia is defined as a haemoglobin level of less than 13.5 g/dL blood for men and less than 11.5 g/dL for women (Hoffbrand et al 2001).

The anaemias are a complex group of red blood cell disorders, which may be:

- primary, i.e. the presenting illness
- secondary to another disease, e.g. infection, cancer, gastrointestinal malabsorption syndrome, chronic renal failure, or an inherited disorder of haemoglobin synthesis or formation
- acquired:
  - — iatrogenic, e.g. medication-induced
  - — environmental, e.g. benzene exposure
  - — nutritional, e.g. iron, protein, vitamin B_{12} or folate deficiency.

Table 11.3 **Blood transfusion products available**

Product	Indications for use	Special points
Whole blood	Acute, severe bleeding requiring replacement of red blood cells and plasma and clotting factors	Stored at 4°C Remains viable for 35 days Platelets and clotting factors have much reduced viability
Fresh whole blood	As above	Blood <24 h old, therefore more likely to contain viable clotting factors
Red cell concentrate	Replacement of red blood cells only. Therefore used when haemoglobin level is low	Up to 200 mL plasma removed per 500 mL blood
Washed red cells	As for red cell concentrate. Specially prepared to remove antigens	Prevents anaphylactic transfusion reactions
Frozen red cells	As for red cell concentrate	Storage life span lengthened, therefore useful for rare blood groups
Platelet concentrate	Patients with platelet count $<20 \times 10^9$ cells/L but not actively bleeding	Platelet units from blood banks contain platelets from many units of blood, therefore there are frequent reactions. Patient may require i.v. hydrocortisone + i.v. chlorphenamine prior to transfusion. Stored at 20°C. Viability of platelet concentrate only 24 h. Never place in fridge
Other blood components:		
Fresh frozen plasma	Hereditary or acquired bleeding disorder Volume replacement Liver disease Disseminated intravascular coagulation	Frozen within 6 h of cell separation and viable for 1 year. Once thawed, use within 30 min
Cryoprecipitate (factor VIII, fibrinogen)	Haemophilia	From fresh frozen plasma. Last part to thaw is cryoprecipitate
Factor VIII	Haemophilia A	From fresh frozen powder (half-life 12 h)
Factor IX	Christmas disease	
Human immunoglobulin	Passive immunity, especially immunosuppressed patients	
Albumin solution	Hypoproteinaemic oedema, ascites, acute volume replacement	

Anaemia is found in all age groups. At each developmental stage there are potential dietary reasons for the occurrence of anaemia, as follows (Craig et al 2002):

- In infancy, anaemia can occur if a poor diet is provided, especially at the time of weaning
- In adolescence, a growth spurt may cause anaemia, particularly if during this period 'fad eating' leads to an inadequate intake of the essential nutrients for red cell formation (see Ch. 21)
- Women of child-bearing age may become anaemic due to menstrual blood loss for which inadequate dietary compensation is made
- In pregnant women, extra demands for red cell synthesis may lead to the development of anaemia
- In older people, poor eating habits resulting from difficulty in shopping, reduction in income, depression, poor dental hygiene or badly fitting dentures can all lead to a reduced intake of essential nutrients for red blood cell formation.

Many people are diagnosed as anaemic only by chance when they seek medical advice for an unrelated symptom or attend a health clinic, e.g. antenatal or occupational health, for a routine medical examination. It is therefore likely that nurses working in any area of community or hospital nursing will care for people with anaemia.

STOP THINK **11.2** In a group, discuss the social, cultural and environmental factors which might contribute to the development of anaemia.

PATHOPHYSIOLOGY

Anaemia occurs when the oxygen-carrying capacity of the red blood cells is reduced. Its symptoms all stem from a lack of oxygen in the tissues. Their severity depends on two main factors:

- haemoglobin concentration, i.e. oxygen-carrying capacity of the red blood cell
- ability of the person to adapt to lower oxygen concentration. Some patients with chronic anaemia live

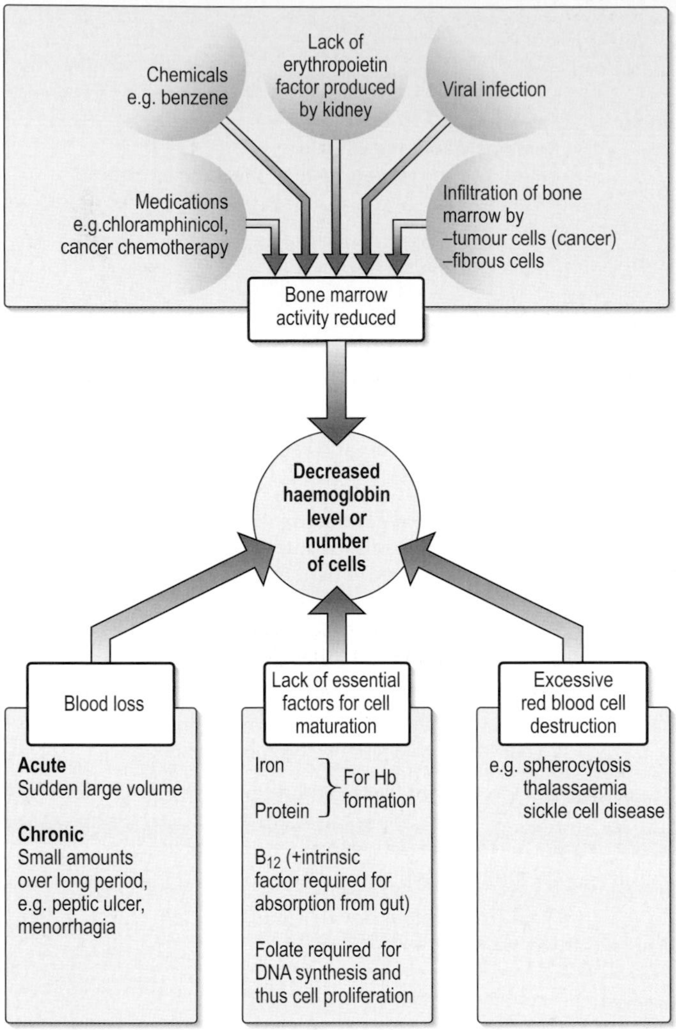

Fig. 11.5 Main types of anaemia.

very active lives with a haemoglobin level that in other people would cause severe symptoms.

Common presenting symptoms The clinical features of anaemia are diverse and may depend on other factors, e.g. the underlying cause of the anaemia. Each type of anaemia has specific clinical features but there are common presenting symptoms, as follows:

- *Tiredness and lethargy* — a very subjective symptom for which the person is unlikely to consult a general practitioner (GP). Some people have a variety of explanations for tiredness, e.g. the season, social life, stress and workload
- *Breathlessness* — a compensatory mechanism to overcome low oxygen concentration, which may be present only on exertion. The person may dismiss this symptom, thinking they are just 'not fit'
- *Palpitations* — due to the heart increasing its rate to increase blood flow to tissues
- *Loss of appetite* — often an unexplained feature but may be due to dysphagia, sore mouth due to epithelial lining fragility, or sheer fatigue
- *Dysphagia* — difficulty in swallowing, and sore mouth
- *Oedema* of ankles, especially at the end of the day — due to a degree of heart failure
- *Dizziness, fainting and dimness of vision* — due to lack of oxygen to the brain
- *Headache and lack of concentration* — resulting from insufficient oxygen supply to the brain
- *Angina and/or intermittent claudication* — because of impaired blood flow to peripheral and/or coronary arteries; this is especially likely in older people
- *Bleeding* — rectal bleeding, haematuria, haemoptysis or menorrhagia.

MEDICAL MANAGEMENT

To diagnose anaemia and establish its cause, it is necessary to clarify the patient's symptoms and discover if there are any other symptoms that the person may not consider significant or may not wish to volunteer.

History and examination Careful questioning about the patient's state of health in the present and recent past and about the use of medication, e.g. aspirin, which may cause bleeding, or phenytoin, which causes folate deficiency, may help to uncover the cause of the anaemia. A determination of the person's social circumstances and dietary intake may also be important.

An accurate and detailed dietary history is often difficult to obtain but may reveal deficiencies in iron, folic acid or vitamin B_{12}. This history may be taken by the GP, practice nurse or dietitian. Questioning about social background should include consideration of:

- financial circumstances
- home circumstances
- work environment, including exposure to harmful substances.

Clinical examination may reveal:

- paleness of skin which may be difficult to assess as many people are pale but not anaemic
- paleness of mucous membranes, e.g. conjunctiva, palms of hands, buccal cavity
- signs of underlying disease, e.g. cancer, hypothyroidism or infection
- signs of complications of anaemia, e.g. cardiac failure, glossitis, stomatitis, jaundice due to haemolytic breakdown (see p. 497)
- signs of pregnancy.

Investigations used in the diagnosis of anaemia include the following:

Blood tests Not all of the following will be relevant for all patients:

- *Full blood count* — to establish total number of red cells, white cells and platelets. The result is compared with normal values (see Appendix 2)
- *Haemoglobin concentration* — a level 10% below normal is usually considered a sign of anaemia
- *Haematocrit or packed cell volume (PCV)* — proportion of total blood volume which consists of red cells. Dehydrated patients have a high PCV as the plasma volume is reduced

- *Reticulocyte count* — a small percentage of reticulocytes are normally present in blood. A larger percentage may indicate increased bone marrow activity if the red blood cell count is low (see p. 481 on maturation of red cells)
- *Mean corpuscular volume (MCV)* — measures the average red cell volume
- *Mean cell haemoglobin (MCH)* — measures the average concentration of haemoglobin. A low MCH may be found when haemoglobin is low
- *Blood film* — examination of blood cells under the microscope to detect any abnormality in size or shape
- *Erythrocyte sedimentation rate (ESR)* — measures the speed at which red cells settle in uncoagulated blood left standing for 1 h. The height of the plasma column above the sedimented blood cells is measured (in mm) and compared with normal height. ESR may be raised because of an underlying problem causing the anaemia, e.g. infection.

Bone marrow aspiration This is the removal with a special needle of a small quantity of bone marrow which can then be mounted on slides and stained for examination under a microscope. This is not done routinely but is indicated if the anaemia is severe or has no apparent cause, or if there is evidence of another blood disorder such as aplastic anaemia or leukaemia (see Box 11.2).

Treatment The type of treatment given for anaemia will depend on the cause and severity of the condition. A few patients will need to be hospitalised but most can be treated in the community by their GP. The treatment may involve medication and health education. Blood transfusions may be needed either initially or repeatedly over a period of time. Intervention will also include treatment of the underlying cause of the anaemia.

Treatment may be short term (a few weeks), long term (months or years) or, as in the case of pernicious anaemia, lifelong. Follow-up care for all anaemic patients is important to encourage adherence to the medication regimen and to prevent recurrence and long-term effects. This care may be provided by the GP or at an outpatient clinic.

NURSING PRIORITIES AND MANAGEMENT: Anaemias

As the anaemias are such a diverse group of disorders, nursing intervention can take a variety of forms. It is vital that the patient is considered as an individual and that psychological, social and environmental concerns are taken into account along with the medical considerations pertinent to the specific form of anaemia.

Certain nursing interventions will be common to all patients. The first task to be carried out is an assessment of the patient's background, illness, needs and goals. Following assessment, a treatment plan will be agreed between the patient and the health care team.

Life-threatening complications

The patient may present with any of the following potentially life-threatening problems:

- cardiac failure
- breathlessness
- shock.

These complications may arise if there has been severe blood loss over a short period of time or if a chronic condition suddenly enters an acute phase. This is more likely to occur in individuals who have other conditions such as hypertension, chronic obstructive airways disease (COAD) and/or pre-existing chronic blood loss (see Chs 2, 3 and 18).

Box 11.2

Bone marrow aspiration

Purposes
- Diagnosis — to examine cell populations and thus determine type of anaemia, leukaemia or lymphoma
- Monitoring — to assess progress of disease and response to treatment

Sites
Red bone marrow is found in the cavities of the flat bones of the adult, e.g. skull, clavicle, scapula and iliac crest. The site usually chosen (for ease of access to minimise trauma to nearby structures) is the iliac crest — left and right, anterior and posterior.

The nurse's role
The patient may be anxious about this investigation, especially if there is awareness that the results may show a malignant condition. This anxiety may be heightened if the patient has been talking with others who have undergone the procedure.

Providing the patient with information on all aspects of the test — the use of premedication and local anaesthetic, the site to be used, the degree of discomfort to be expected, the time that it will take, and when the results will be reported — will help to reduce anxiety.

It is the policy of some doctors, especially where repeated aspiration will be required, to give a sedative such as lorazepam or a light general anaesthetic.
The individual may undergo the procedure as an outpatient, inpatient or in a day ward. Whatever the setting, the nurse's role will include:

- Assessing the patient's understanding of the test and providing more information if necessary
- Preparing the equipment
- Ensuring that the patient is comfortable and is positioned correctly
- Observing the patient throughout the procedure and drawing attention to any change in condition
- Assisting the doctor
- Applying a pressure dressing and making the patient comfortable after the procedure
- Inspecting the aspiration site frequently for haemorrhage or haematoma formation
- Documenting the patient's response to the procedure
- Preparing the patient for discharge by explaining care of puncture site, what discomfort may be expected, who to contact if ill-effects arise, when results will be available and timing of the next appointment.

Possible complications
- Haemorrhage — patient's platelet count should be checked before aspiration
- Infection

Major problems of nursing anaemic patients

Tiredness

Anaemic patients will tire easily because of poor oxygenation of cells and tissues. Patients with severe anaemia will be exhausted after even the slightest exertion. It is important that their daily routine in hospital or at home ensures periods of rest. If cardiac failure is evident, they may need to be nursed in bed or in a chair. The nurse should be aware of the potential problems of immobility, paying particular attention to pressure areas. Such patients may require assistance with personal hygiene and dressing. They should be reassured that their tiredness is not imaginary but is part of the anaemia and that it will lessen as treatment progresses.

Breathlessness (see Ch. 3)

The breathlessness may be mild, arising only on exertion, or it may be a major problem causing great distress. The most important aspects of nursing the breathless patient are to ensure maximum perfusion of oxygen to the tissues and to reduce the patient's distress. This can be achieved by nursing the patient in an upright position (to allow maximum lung expansion and use of accessory respiratory muscles), administering oxygen as prescribed, explaining to the patient the reason for the breathlessness and giving reassurance that it will lessen as the anaemia improves.

Breathlessness, if incapacitating, will require the nurse to assist the patient with personal hygiene, changing position in bed and mobilisation.

Nutrition

The anaemic patient will require a high-protein diet which includes all the nutrients necessary for red cell production (see p. 481). Breathlessness, a lack of energy to shop and prepare food, a sore mouth and dysphagia may all contribute to anorexia. A sore mouth can be especially distressing and the nurse will need to carry out an initial evaluation using an assessment tool such as that described in Beretta (2003). Care should include not only that which will improve and heal the mouth but also relevant health education about oral hygiene and care of dentures, e.g. use of a soft toothbrush, regular mouthwashes and prevention of dry and cracking lips (Jamieson et al 2002) (see Ch. 15).

It will be necessary for anaemic patients who have a low income and/or a poor understanding of nutrition to receive guidance in budgeting and the components of a balanced diet as well as advice about social security allowances. The multidisciplinary team may therefore include a dietitian and a social worker.

Other important considerations include dietary restrictions deriving from the patient's cultural background and/or spiritual beliefs. Dietary restrictions may also be imposed by a pre-existing medical disorder such as diabetes mellitus. Older patients may have ill-fitting dentures which may lead to reliance on a poorly balanced 'soft' diet. In such cases, referral to a dentist may be appropriate.

Safety

Giddiness, faintness, light-headedness and sensitivity to cold may make the anaemic patient prone to injury. Since the body responds to poor oxygenation by preserving the blood supply to the essential organs, anaemic patients will have poor peripheral circulation and, consequently, fragile skin. The reduced attention span typical of anaemic patients will also make them vulnerable to falls, minor injuries and hypothermia. Anaemic patients should be warned against changing position suddenly, especially from lying to standing, and should be given instruction on first aid for minor injuries and on the prevention of hypothermia (see Ch. 22).

Skin integrity (see Chs 12 and 23)

The anaemic patient's reduced oxygen and nutrient supply to the skin increases the risk of pressure ulcers. Hypoxic skin will not necessarily break down quickly, but if damaged it will take longer than usual to heal. When the patient's mobility has been impaired, either as a result of the anaemia or because of a concurrent condition, e.g. arthritis, the nurse must be alert to the importance of maintaining skin integrity. An initial and continuing assessment of all pressure points should be made using such tools as the Waterlow scale (see p. 851). Once the patient's level of risk of developing pressure ulcers has been determined, an appropriate intervention should be planned. Prevention of pressure ulcers is likely to include ensuring that the patient's position is changed 2-hourly, the use of appropriate pressure-relieving devices and instructing the patient about the importance of regularly changing position.

Communication

Anxiety and fear may present a barrier to communication by preventing the patient from asking for information about diagnosis, prognosis and treatment. The patient's physical condition, e.g. breathlessness and sore mouth, may also impede communication. The nurse caring for anaemic patients must be aware of these potential difficulties and of the effect that they can have upon patient–staff relationships.

The nurse should assess actual and potential communication difficulties and help the patient and the health care team to anticipate and overcome obstacles. The patient should be encouraged to voice fears and should be given the appropriate reassurance and information. Here, the nurse should try to involve other relevant members of the team. The nurse should be receptive to the patient's non-verbal as well as verbal messages and, in doing so, anticipate those times when support and reassurance will be needed.

Anxiety

Prior to diagnosis, the anaemic patient may fear the presence of a life-threatening illness, particularly if symptoms such as breathlessness, palpitations and chronic headaches have been experienced. The disorientation, confusion and general slowing of intellectual responses arising from cerebral hypoxia can be especially distressing. Explanation of the causes of these symptoms and reassurance that they should improve as the anaemia responds to treatment will help to reduce the anxiety suffered by both the patient and the family.

Iron deficiency anaemia

Iron deficiency anaemia is the most common anaemia worldwide. It affects an estimated 600 million people (Craig et al 2002) and is recognised as one of the most prevalent diseases of nutritional origin in developing countries (Mehta & Hoffbrand 2000). The onset of this form of anaemia is usually insidious, taking place over a period of months. This is explained by the fact that iron stored in the body is usually reused after the breakdown of red blood cells and only a very small proportion is lost (less than 1 mg/day) through hair, urine, faeces and sweat (Mehta & Hoffbrand 2000).

PATHOPHYSIOLOGY

Iron is part of the haem component of the haemoglobin molecule: each haemoglobin molecule is composed of four molecules of haem with one ferrous ion, which is the oxygen carrier that transports oxygen from the lungs to the tissues (Tortora & Derrickson 2006).

A typical Western diet contains 10–15 mg of iron/day, but only 5–10% is absorbed (Mehta & Hoffbrand 2000). The ferrous form is more soluble than the ferric form; a low pH in the duodenum maintains iron in ferrous form, the form in which it can be absorbed from the gut. Vitamin C, present in fresh fruit and vegetables, enhances absorption.

Iron deficiency anaemia may be caused by:

- inadequate intake, i.e. poor diet
- increased iron requirement, e.g. in pregnancy
- lack of gastric acid, e.g. following total gastrectomy or gastric atrophy
- duodenal or jejunal malabsorption.

Common presenting symptoms As the onset of iron deficiency anaemia is usually very gradual, the patient may not consult their doctor until some time after symptoms have begun to appear. The most common presenting symptoms are tiredness and pallor, but any of the other general symptoms of anaemia (see p. 486) may be apparent. Symptoms specific to iron deficiency anaemia may include:

- painless glossitis — smooth, raw tongue
- angular stomatitis
- koilonychia — brittle, spoon-shaped nails
- dysphagia and glossitis; with the formation of a pharyngeal web (5–15% of cases), also called Paterson–Kelly syndrome (Palmer & Penman 2002)
- atrophic gastritis and achlorhydria
- pica — a strong desire to eat unusual substances, e.g. coal.

MEDICAL MANAGEMENT

History and examination The patient may give a history suggestive of chronic blood loss, e.g. menorrhagia, and examination may reveal general signs of anaemia.

Investigations Blood samples will be taken for such tests as full blood count, haemoglobin level, blood film, MCV, MCH, serum iron and total iron-binding capacity (TIBC) (see Appendix 1). Estimates of ferritin, an iron storage protein, distinguish iron deficiency anaemia from that caused by chronic blood loss. These tests can be done in a GP's surgery. Other investigations, e.g. faecal occult blood and endoscopy, may be undertaken to establish the cause of the deficiency. Such tests will be selected according to the patient's symptoms and medical history. Bone marrow aspiration is rarely performed if iron deficiency anaemia is present, but will show a bone marrow with no iron stores (see p. 487).

Treatment If dietary adjustment is insufficient to correct the anaemia, medication is given and, in very severe cases, blood transfusion is carried out.

Medication Iron supplements will be prescribed, usually in the following forms:

- *Oral iron supplements* — usually ferrous sulphate 200 mg three times a day before food. Medication should be continued for 3–6 months after the haemoglobin level has returned to normal to build up iron stores (Craig et al 2002). Side-effects, which include constipation, nausea, abdominal pain and diarrhoea, often lead to poor compliance. Alternative iron preparations which may be better tolerated, but which are more expensive, include ferrous gluconate and ferrous fumarate.
- *Intramuscular iron injections*. These are given only where there is proven malabsorption syndrome or poor compliance. Administration of i.m. iron via the 'Z track' technique prevents or minimises back-tracking of iron and skin discoloration (Skinner 1998).

Blood transfusion If the anaemia is very severe (less than 7 g/dL), a slow infusion of red cell concentrate will be administered. However, there is a danger, particularly in older or very young patients, of blood volume overload leading to cardiac failure.

NURSING PRIORITIES AND MANAGEMENT: Iron deficiency anaemia

Many of the general nursing considerations for the care of anaemic patients (see pp. 487–488) are relevant to the treatment of iron deficiency anaemia. Patients with this condition will most likely be cared for by a community nurse.

Nursing considerations

Blood transfusions

A few patients with iron deficiency anaemia will require a blood transfusion (see Case History 11.1). This measure may be interpreted by the patient and family as a sign that the condition is very grave; therefore, it is important that the nurse clarifies the reason for the transfusion, explains what is involved, and gives reassurance that the procedure is safe. Many people fear being infected with a transmittable disease, especially AIDS, or hepatitis C, and it may be necessary to explain the screening procedures performed on all blood donations. Practising Jehovah's Witnesses will refuse blood transfusions (see Box 11.3). Some Muslims may be reluctant to accept a blood transfusion and may wish to consult their families or a religious leader before agreeing to the procedure.

The nurse must be familiar with local policies for prescribing and checking blood products prior to transfusion to minimise the risk of administering incompatible blood. Any doubt about the unit of blood to be given should be referred to the haematology laboratory medical staff.

CASE HISTORY 11.1

Mrs B

Mrs B, a frail lady aged 82 years, has been admitted to hospital as an emergency after collapsing at home. She used to enjoy an active social life until her husband died a year ago. Since then her family and friends have noticed that she has become withdrawn and depressed and rarely goes out except to shop.

Mrs B has always enjoyed good health, until recently. On admission to hospital she admitted that over the past few months she has become increasingly tired and breathless when she climbs stairs or walks uphill. She has noticed that her ankles tend to swell, especially in the evening. She also finds that she has become forgetful; her neighbours have noticed that she appears confused at times.

A blood test has revealed that Mrs B has a haemoglobin level of 7 g/dL blood, and other blood test results have proved that she has an iron deficiency anaemia. Mrs B has been prescribed three units of red cell concentrate to be given prior to any further investigations of the iron deficiency anaemia. Her nursing care is outlined in Nursing Care Plan 11.1.

Box 11.3

Jehovah's Witnesses and blood transfusions

Devout Jehovah's Witnesses believe that it is against God's law to receive transfusions of blood or blood products. This belief is based on three biblical references: Genesis 9: 4; Leviticus 17: 14; and Acts 15: 28–29 (Jehovah's Witness 2003).

If a Jehovah's Witness requires a blood transfusion as an urgent or essential part of treatment, they or their next of kin will need to be approached by the medical practitioners and informed of the gravity of the situation. If the treatment is refused, this must be documented. Alternative ways of supporting the patient should be considered, e.g. autologous transfusion or drugs.

Each unit of blood must be administered at the prescribed rate and correct temperature. Close observation of the patient in the first 15 min of each unit is essential as this is when transfusion reactions are most likely to occur (see Nursing Care Plan 11.1).

Patient education

By helping the patient to understand the nature of the disorder and come to terms with the fact that, although the anaemia is not a life-threatening illness, it may become very severe if left untreated, the nurse will encourage acceptance of treatment.

The patient will need to learn which foods are rich in iron and may need advice on budgeting for a well-balanced diet. By assessing the patient's perception of the problem, level of knowledge and sociocultural background, the nurse can ensure that the advice offered is relevant and comprehensible. Referral to a social worker, e.g. for advice about social security benefits, may be appropriate.

Careful and clear instruction should be given to reinforce the doctor's and pharmacist's directions regarding medication. Important points to emphasise are:

- how frequently the medication should be taken
- that it is to be taken before food
- the possible side-effects of constipation and indigestion and how to overcome them; to avoid undue alarm, the patient should be warned that oral iron supplements will turn the stools black
- safe storage
- the importance of the continuation of medication and the importance of follow-up.

In certain circumstances when the patient is unable to take oral iron preparations, daily administration of i.m. iron may be necessary for a period of about a week. The patient needs to trust both the value of this short-term therapy and the skill of the practitioner, as the possible side-effects of an unpleasant taste in the mouth, palpitations and potential pain on administration could easily result in reluctance to continue treatment.

Discharge planning

If the person has been hospitalised for treatment, the following considerations should be discussed before discharge:

- socioeconomic conditions at home
- social services available, e.g. home care assistants and lunch clubs, if family members are unable to help
- the importance of a follow-up appointment with the consultant or GP
- the importance of taking the prescribed medication.

In older people, there is often a link between recent bereavement (i.e. in the last 6–12 months) and the onset of iron deficiency anaemia, as loneliness, grief and depression may lead to self-neglect. This problem may be accentuated if the bereaved person also has difficulty with personal care. Care needs to be taken that such patients are not returned to their former social circumstances without the necessary follow-up and support by the GP, health visitor, social worker or grief counsellor.

STOP THINK

11.3 A 72-year-old widower is admitted to hospital with general tiredness, breathlessness and mild congestive heart failure. He is diagnosed as having iron deficiency anaemia. His wife died 6 months ago and his only daughter, who is married and has two young children, lives a considerable distance away.

With regard to the patient's discharge:

(a) identify potential problems
(b) discuss how these might be resolved
(c) identify what community services might be required.

Megaloblastic anaemias

These anaemias stem from a lack of one or more of the essential factors for the synthesis of DNA, resulting in a reduction in red blood cell proliferation. There are two types of megaloblastic anaemia (see Table 11.4):

- folate deficiency
- vitamin B_{12} deficiency.

Nursing Care Plan 11.1 Care of Mrs B during blood transfusion (see Case History 11.1)

Nursing considerations	Action	Rationale	Expected outcome
1. Anxiety (a) About cause of anaemia	• Reduce anxiety and stress of receiving blood transfusion by explaining and clarifying information given	Information given about procedures and care reduces anxiety and discomfort	Appear calm, not anxious
(b) About safety of blood transfusion	• Reassure Mrs B by explaining screening and cross-matching of blood	Mrs B may fear receiving infection from donor, especially HIV, AIDS or hepatitis B virus. Fear of receiving wrong blood group	Accept blood transfusion
(c) About possibility of complications	• Reassure Mrs B she will be observed and monitored frequently for any signs of complications. Tell her she must inform nurses of any new symptoms		
2. Correct blood given to correct patient	• Check blood unit details against blood transfusion cross-matching form, prescription and patient's details with a registered nurse as per local policy. Document blood unit transfused	Prevention of wrong blood being given to wrong patient, with possible incompatible reaction	Correct blood given to correct patient as detailed on prescription sheet
3. Condition of blood to be transfused is optimal	• Ensure blood stored at correct temperature prior to commencing transfusion. Blood transfusion is commenced within 30 min of removal from special refrigerator. Blood is not artificially warmed (unless directed by doctor because of special antibodies)	Blood not stored at correct temperature may undergo haemolysis (red cell breakdown) Risk of microorganism contamination increased	Blood is given at correct temperature
4. Early detection of acute haemolytic transfusion reaction	• Record Mrs B's temperature, pulse and BP *before* starting and 15 min after start of each unit of blood and then as per local policy until completion of each unit	Signs and symptoms of blood transfusion incompatibility usually occur within 15 min of starting the unit of blood	Any symptoms or signs of incompatibility are detected immediately
	• Observe Mrs B for any restlessness		
	• Record and report any nausea or vomiting		
	• Observe and record any complaints of: – flushing – burning sensation in arm above cannula – chest tightness, headache or pain – dyspnoea – loin pain – lumbar pain		

Continued ▶

Nursing Care Plan 11.1 Care of Mrs B during blood transfusion (see Case History 11.1) *(Continued)*

Nursing considerations	Action	Rationale	Expected outcome
4. Early detection of acute haemolytic transfusion reaction (*Continued*)	• Report any signs or symptoms to doctor	Symptoms of pain in arm, chest, lumbar region and loin and dyspnoea are due to agglutination of red blood cells in blood vessels, causing obstruction to blood flow	
	• Summon doctor immediately if Mrs B develops circulatory collapse		
	• Stop blood transfusion if any signs or symptoms of incompatibility occur	Incompatible blood transfusion rarely causes sudden collapse	
	• Keep unit of blood and infusion-giving set if incompatibility occurs		
	• Return both to haematology laboratory	Blood will be further tested for cause of incompatibility. Mrs B's unit of blood may have been wrongly cross-matched or labelled or her red blood cells may have other rare antibodies which require special cross-matching	
5. Circulatory overload	• Monitor Mrs B's pulse, respiratory rate and blood pressure. Report any abnormal measurements		
	• Observe and report to medical staff any dyspnoea or wheezing		
	• Ensure transfusion is regulated at prescribed rate		
	• Measure urinary output		
	• Give furosemide as prescribed and monitor urinary output	Mrs B has developed some cardiac failure due to her anaemia and the transfusion could increase her blood volume to a level at which the cardiac failure deteriorates. It is important that signs of cardiac failure and pulmonary oedema are detected early. Furosemide, as a diuretic, will increase fluid output and thus reduce circulatory volume	Any signs of cardiac overload are detected immediately

Continued ▶

Nursing Care Plan 11.1 Care of Mrs B during blood transfusion (see Case History 11.1) *(Continued)*

Nursing considerations	Action	Rationale	Expected outcome
6. Pyrexia	• Monitor temperature and pulse as in 4		
	• Report any abnormal temperature and pulse recordings to doctor	Fever can occur for unknown cause at start of each unit. Temperature falls if transfusion slowed. May occur 1.0–1.5 h after transfusion. Subnormal temperature which rises later may be a sign of infection	All episodes of abnormal temperature are recorded and reported. Any further action requested by doctor is implemented immediately
	• Report any chest pain or sign of infections		
	• Ensure blood used has been out of special blood fridge for maximum 30 min	To prevent blood temperature rise with the increased risk of growth of organisms. Greater risk of contamination by microorganisms	Blood unit always commenced within 30 min of removal from special blood fridge
	• Do not continue transfusion of a unit of blood after 4 h		
	• Report if transfusion rate becomes slow		
	• Administer any medications as prescribed, e.g. antipyretics, antibiotics		
7. Allergic reactions	• Observations of temperature and pulse as in 4	Allergic response to protein in the plasma	Any signs of allergic reaction are detected immediately and the appropriate action implemented
	• Observe for any skin rashes		
	• Observe for any oedema around eyes		
	• Observe for any signs of laryngeal oedema (see Ch. 3)		
	• Observe for shortness of breath		
	• Record and report any of above signs to doctor immediately. If symptoms are mild, slow transfusion. If severe, stop transfusion, treat patient for shock (see Ch. 18)		

Table 11.4 Causes of the megaloblastic anaemias

Type	Causes
Folate deficiency	Inadequate dietary intake Disease of upper small bowel, malabsorption or extensive surgical resection of small bowel Increasing body demands because of: • very active cell proliferation, e.g. in haemolytic anaemia or leukaemia (see pp. 496 and 501) • pregnancy Interference with folate metabolism by medications, e.g. methotrexate (see Ch. 31) Unexplained mechanisms, e.g. ingestion of alcohol and anti-epileptic medications, e.g. phenytoin and primidone
Vitamin B_{12} deficiency	Inadequate vitamin B_{12} in diet (especially vegans), pernicious anaemia Gastric surgery, gastric atrophy or intrinsic factor deficiency Disease of terminal ileum where vitamin B_{12} is absorbed, e.g. Crohn's disease (see Ch. 4)

Deficiencies of these two vitamins account for most cases of this type of anaemia. Vegans are at particular risk of vitamin B_{12} deficiency as B_{12} is only found in meat products. However, the commonest cause of vitamin B_{12} deficiency (80%) is pernicious anaemia (Hoffbrand & Provan 1997) due to a lack of intrinsic factor in gastric parietal cells. One in 100 people over the age of 60 have pernicious anaemia.

PATHOPHYSIOLOGY

Red blood cells are produced continually and have a life span of approximately 120 days (see p. 481). Folate and vitamin B_{12} are essential factors for the synthesis of DNA required by each cell (see Figs 11.6 and 11.7). If DNA synthesis is reduced (because of lack of folate or vitamin B_{12}), the cell nucleus is abnormal and this results in the normoblasts (see Fig. 11.1) becoming larger than normal (macrocytic). While macrocytes may contain a greater amount of haemoglobin than normal red cells, the total amount of haemoglobin will be reduced as the total number of red blood cells is reduced. There may also be large, primitive nucleated red cells (megaloblasts) in the peripheral blood.

For further reading on the role of folate in health, see Fox & Cameron (1995).

Common presenting symptoms Vitamin B_{12} and folic acid are required by all dividing cells. Therefore a deficiency of these factors not only affects red blood cells but also the gastrointestinal epithelium, giving rise to glossitis, anorexia, diarrhoea and malabsorption. It also causes spinal cord and peripheral nerve damage which can give rise to the following symptoms:

- paraesthesia (pins and needles or tingling)
- coldness or numbness in limbs
- ataxia (lack of coordination of movement, staggering)
- paralysis.

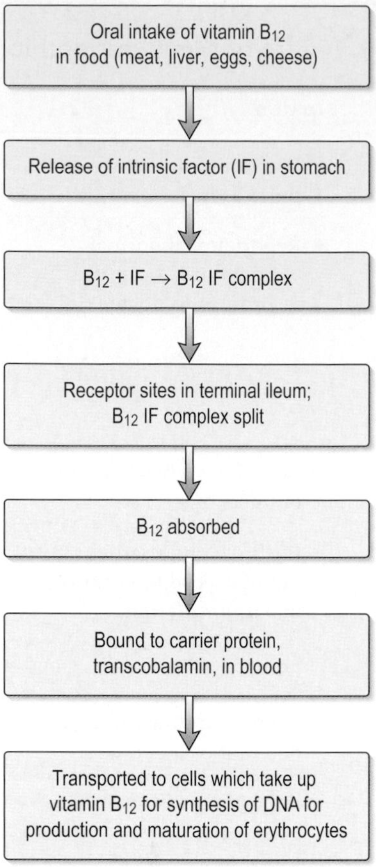

Fig. 11.6 Vitamin B_{12} absorption and transport.

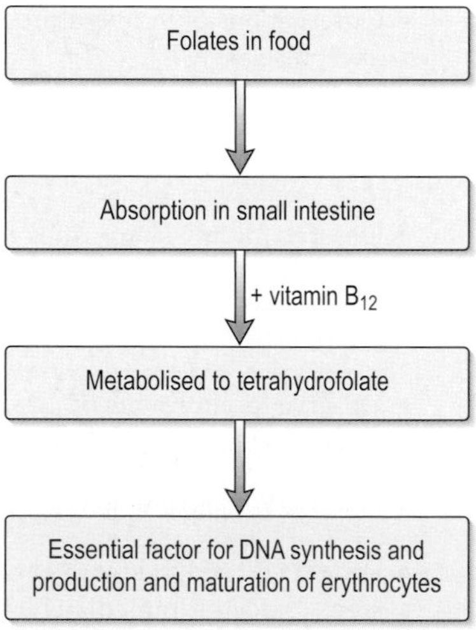

Fig. 11.7 Absorption and utilisation of folates.

For further reading on role of folate in prevention of neural tube defects in pregnancy, see Hoffbrand et al (2001).

MEDICAL MANAGEMENT

History and examination Medical investigation is similar to that for anaemia (see p. 486). However, in suspected megaloblastic anaemia the doctor will be alert to the following specific features:

- glossitis
- angular stomatitis
- mild jaundice (lemon yellow skin pallor because of increased fragility of red cells)
- excess urobilinogen (due to excessive red cell breakdown)
- mild symptoms of malabsorption and weight loss
- evidence of possible increased need for either factor, e.g. pregnancy or vegan diet.

If a lack of vitamin B_{12} intrinsic factor (pernicious anaemia) is suspected, patients may present with the following neurological symptoms:

- paraesthesia, especially in toes
- symptoms of subacute combined degeneration of the spinal cord causing muscular weakness, loss of muscular coordination and paralysis. These symptoms are apparent in approximately 10% of all cases of pernicious anaemia and these neurological features may arise before other symptoms.

Investigations Specific diagnostic blood tests for megaloblastic anaemia include serum B_{12} levels and red cell folate level. Other investigations include:

- assessment of gastric parietal cell antibodies
- Schilling test (see Appendix 1)
- endoscopy
- bone marrow aspiration (see p. 487)
- neurological examination (see Ch. 9)
- past medical history for gastric or intestinal surgery, alcohol abuse or epilepsy
- possible pregnancy.

Treatment for megaloblastic anaemia is as follows:

- Folate deficiency — 5 mg folic acid daily for 4 months
- Vitamin B_{12} and intrinsic factor deficiency:
  - — injection of hydroxycobalamin 1000 mcg (1 mg) i.m. twice during the first week, then weekly until blood count is normal
  - — maintenance dose of hydroxycobalamin 1000 mcg (1 mg) i.m. every 3 months for life.

STOP THINK **11.4** Reflect on the implications for the patient of the lifelong necessity for 3-monthly injections.

NURSING PRIORITIES AND MANAGEMENT: Megaloblastic anaemias

Folate deficiency

Individuals with folate deficiency are usually diagnosed and treated by a GP or at an antenatal clinic and are referred to a haematology outpatient department only if further tests are necessary, e.g. bone marrow aspiration. The setting for nursing intervention will therefore be a community health centre or the patient's home. Patient education with regard to diet and acceptance of medication will be the most important aspect of nursing care.

A patient with folate anaemia will need to know which foods contain folic acid, how to budget for these if income is low and how to avoid destroying folic acid in food preparation. The patient will also need to understand how to take folic acid supplements correctly. The nurse should also emphasise the importance of follow-up checks with the consultant or GP.

Nurses must be on the alert for patients who may be susceptible to folic acid deficiency, i.e. those whose diet is inadequate, those with extensive disease of the small intestine and those with increased folic acid requirements, and advise them as to how to prevent its occurrence.

Vitamin B_{12} and intrinsic factor deficiency

Patients may need to be admitted to hospital for diagnosis and treatment in the initial stages but most will be diagnosed by their GP. If the anaemia is not yet acute, treatment can be started immediately by a community or practice nurse, who will administer prescribed vitamin B_{12} injections. The nurse should bear in mind that the patient may be very breathless at first and will need some degree of assistance with personal care tasks (see p. 488) and support in adjusting to a regimen of regular injections. The patient and family should be encouraged to participate in the management of the anaemia, possibly by learning how to administer the hydroxycobalamin injections themselves.

Patients in the advanced stages of pernicious anaemia are rarely seen today. If cardiac failure and severe neurological problems do develop, major nursing interventions will be required (see Chs 2 and 9).

Aplastic anaemia

This form of anaemia results from the failure of bone marrow stem cells to mature and proliferate. In 20–50% of all cases of this very rare disease, onset can be connected with exposure to one of the following:

- chemical compounds, i.e. industrial chemicals, especially benzene
- medications, for example chloramphenicol and certain cytotoxic chemotherapeutic agents, e.g. busulfan, phenothiazines and anti-epileptic medication
- ionising radiation, whether therapeutic or industrial
- viral infection, notably hepatitis
- rarely bone marrow infiltration by disease, e.g. multiple myeloma, metastases from primary tumours.

The remaining 50–70% of cases are idiopathic, having no detectable cause.

PATHOPHYSIOLOGY

There is considerable reduction in the number of blood stem cells causing:

- lack of red blood cells: anaemia
- lack of white cells: leucopenia
- lack of platelets: thrombocytopenia.

These three conditions together are referred to as pancytopenia. In aplastic anaemia, the degree of anaemia, leucopenia and thrombocytopenia, and therefore the severity of the disorder, is variable.

Common presenting symptoms The onset of aplastic anaemia is often insidious: 1 or 2 months may elapse between the individual's exposure to the causal agent and the development of symptoms. The presenting symptoms are the result of pancytopenia and include:

- general symptoms of anaemia
- infections, e.g. throat, upper respiratory tract
- bleeding, e.g. in the skin and mucous membranes, especially the gums.

MEDICAL MANAGEMENT

History and examination Medical investigation may uncover no abnormality other than the presenting symptoms; for example, careful examination may reveal no enlarged liver or spleen. However, questioning might bring to light the patient's exposure to chemicals or the use of over-the-counter medication. It may require very careful and extensive questioning to uncover the causative factor, which may have seemed trivial to the patient at the time. The recollections of family and friends may be of help.

Investigations will include:

- blood film and blood count to reveal pancytopenia
- bone marrow aspiration to reveal the degree of stem cell failure. This procedure gives a definitive diagnosis.

Treatment If the patient is not admitted to hospital on presentation, immediate admission to hospital occurs once a diagnosis of aplastic anaemia is made.

In mild to moderately severe cases, supportive therapy with blood and platelet transfusion may be given. Antibiotic therapy will be essential to treat any infections. Androgens are thought to stimulate bone marrow cell synthesis, e.g. oxymetholone orally or high-dose methylprednisolone, and may be tried (see Ch. 5). Other possible medications are antilymphocyte or antithymocyte globulin, ciclosporin and haemopoietic growth factors. However, the side-effects of these medications may cause problems, e.g. pyrexia, rashes, hypo- or hypertension, and nephrotoxicity (Howard & Hamilton 1997).

If the aplastic anaemia is severe or the above treatment is unsuccessful, allogeneic bone marrow transplantation will be considered as an urgent treatment.

NURSING PRIORITIES AND MANAGEMENT: Aplastic anaemia

Life-threatening complications

The nurse must be on the alert for the development of grave complications of aplastic anaemia. The nurse's role will therefore include:

- prevention of infections
- early detection of infections
- immediate implementation of nursing care of septic patients when infection is confirmed
- prevention and early treatment of bleeding.

Nursing considerations

Psychological state

The patient, the family and friends may experience feelings of guilt if and when the causative agent of the anaemia is identified; they may believe that they were to blame for the patient's contact with the toxin. The nurse must be sensitive to the patient's concerns as information is assimilated about diagnosis and prognosis and as the need for sudden transfer to hospital and, possibly, being nursed in protective isolation becomes evident (see Ch. 16). Some patients will not survive a year.

Patient education

It is vital to inform the patient how to prevent overexertion and to detect the signs of injury, bleeding and infection. The teaching programme will depend on the severity of the disorder and the patient's response to treatment and should include the family, friends and carers.

The nurse should also assess the patient's understanding of the reason for and importance of all medication, what action to take if medication is accidentally omitted and how to get new supplies in good time. A patient prescribed steroids, e.g. prednisolone, should understand that it is most important to continue taking them even if feeling ill. The patient should also be advised to inform any doctor or dentist about prescribed steroids and always to carry a card giving details of their medication.

The nurse will also need to advise the patient, family and any members of staff unfamiliar with caring for pancytopenic patients about reducing the risk of infection and haemorrhage. Information leaflets are invaluable in reinforcing all details given, as patients and carers will find it hard to remember everything.

Test coordination

The nurse will act as coordinator in the programme of diagnostic tests and will prepare the patient for stem cell bone marrow graft if this is to be performed. Further details on caring for profoundly pancytopenic patients are given in the section on nursing management of acute leukaemia (p. 505).

Rehabilitation

Rehabilitation begins even before the patient's discharge from hospital and must be planned in response to the potential for recovery, motivation and needs (see Ch. 34). The multidisciplinary team involved may include a physiotherapist, occupational therapist, dietitian, social worker, district nurse, health visitor, counsellor and psychologist.

Realistic goals must be set in discussion with the patient. Consideration must be given to avoiding the causative agent of the anaemia in the future. It may be necessary for the patient to change their job. This may require liaison between medical staff, the patient's employer and a social worker.

Discharge planning

Before discharge it will be important to discuss with the patient any fears or apprehensions to clarify details of who to contact if there are any further episodes of illness and to go over any written information provided.

Haemolytic anaemias

These anaemias result from the premature destruction of red blood cells, in response to either an inherited or an acquired

Box 11.4

Causes of haemolytic anaemias

Inherited
- Red cell membrane fragility, e.g. spherocytosis
- Haemoglobin defects
  - — structure: sickle cell
  - — synthesis: thalassaemia
- Red cell metabolism defect, e.g. glucose-6-phosphate dehydrogenase deficiency

Acquired
- Antibody attack, e.g. mismatched blood transfusion
- Direct cell injury
  - — traumatic, e.g. prosthetic heart valve
  - — chemical or medication-induced, e.g. sodium chlorate, vitamin K analogues, sulfasalazine (Salazopyrin), nitrates
  - — infection, e.g. bacterial, disseminated intravascular coagulation
- Paroxysmal nocturnal haemoglobinuria

defect. Many of the haemolytic anaemias are rare or very rare. The most common inherited anaemias are sickle cell disease and thalassaemia. The most common acquired forms result from direct cell injury following infection or medical treatment. Causes of haemolytic anaemias are listed in Box 11.4.

PATHOPHYSIOLOGY

In this type of anaemia, the life span of the red blood cells is reduced because of red blood cell fragility, leading to excessive breakdown. This results in a reduced oxygen-carrying capacity in the blood and thus hypoxia in the tissues. This causes stimulation of the production of erythropoietin, a growth factor which stimulates the bone marrow to increase erythropoiesis (see p. 481). A healthy person with mild haemolytic anaemia will not experience symptoms. However, if the red cell life span is greatly reduced (<15 days) the bone marrow will not be able to compensate adequately and the person will experience symptoms of haemolytic anaemia. This will occur more quickly if for any reason the bone marrow is not healthy. The resulting haemolytic anaemia gives rise to increased bilirubin and urobilinogen (see Fig. 11.8).

MEDICAL AND NURSING MANAGEMENT

The medical and nursing care provided will vary according to the specific type of haemolytic anaemia. This chapter will discuss only the management of sickle cell anaemia.

STOP THINK **11.5** (a) What is the difference between sickle cell disease and b-thalassaemia?
(b) How is b-thalassaemia treated?
(c) What are the possible complications of this disorder and how can these complications be minimised?

Sickle cell anaemia

The sickle cell anaemias are a group of haemolytic anaemias in which there is an inherited structural abnormality in the haemoglobin molecule (HbS). This abnormality is the result of the substitution of one amino acid in the globin molecule for another in the haemoglobin. The abnormal haemoglobin causes a characteristic sickle-like shaping of the red blood cell when it is in the deoxygenated state (Mehta & Hoffbrand 2000). It is a recessively inherited blood disorder of which there is a homozygous and a heterozygous variant (see Ch. 6). In the heterozygous variant, the person inherits the abnormal haemoglobin gene (HbS) from one parent and the normal (HbA) gene from the other parent. This person has the sickle cell trait (HbSA) and usually will be unaware of the abnormality unless tested for the trait or develops symptoms when exposed to hypoxic conditions, e.g. anaesthesia or unpressurised aircraft. The trait will be passed on to any children. In the homozygous variant, the abnormal gene is inherited from both parents and the person will suffer from sickle cell anaemia.

A crucial factor in diagnosing this haemolytic anaemia is a knowledge of the patient's racial origin and family history. This inherited sickle cell trait or sickle cell anaemia

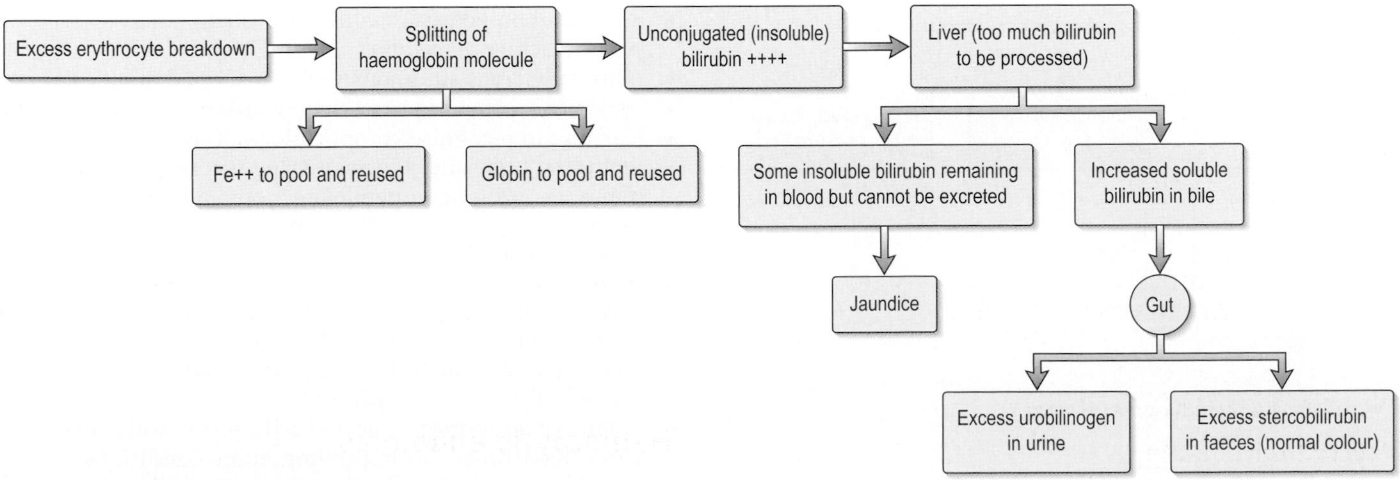

Fig. 11.8 Development of symptoms of haemolytic anaemia.

occurs more commonly among people of African, Caribbean, East Mediterranean, Middle Eastern, Indian and Pakistani origin. It is thought that this geographical distribution might be explained by the fact that sickle cell trait (not sickle cell anaemia) offers some protection against malaria (Hoffbrand et al 2001).

PATHOPHYSIOLOGY

The normal pattern of the amino acids in the beta chains of the globin part of haemoglobin (see p. 481) is altered in sickle cell haemoglobin by the substitution of a different amino acid for the normal one (HbS). HbS has certain properties which distinguish it from normal HbA haemoglobin. It is less soluble, especially when in a deoxygenated state and when the blood pH is below normal. Under these conditions crystals are formed within the red blood cell, making it more rigid and distorting it into a sickle shape (Hoffbrand et al 2001). The effects of this abnormal cell are shown in Figure 11.9.

Common presenting symptoms Sickle cell anaemia normally presents in childhood but might not become apparent until adulthood. Often the presenting symptoms are those of haemolytic anaemia (see Fig. 11.8) or of a painful 'sickle cell crisis' in response to a triggering factor (see Box 11.5). The clinical features of a crisis are:

- Pain caused by the obstruction of small blood vessels in the tissues. Characteristics of the pain are the acuteness of onset and its unresponsiveness to mild analgesics.

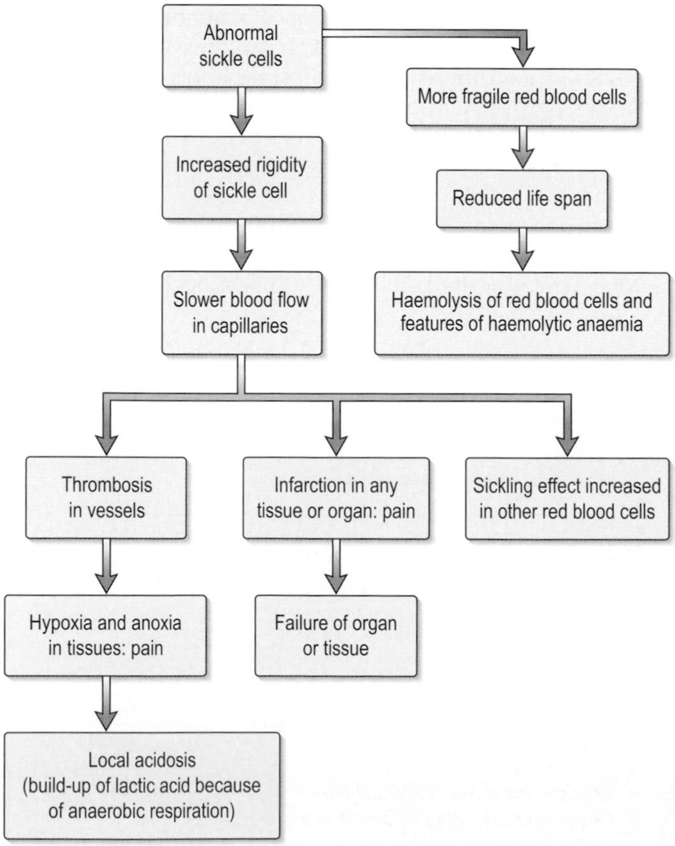

 Fig. 11.9 Pathophysiology of sickle cell anaemia.

Box 11.5

Trigger factors in sickle cell anaemia

- Reduced oxygen, e.g. during strenuous exercise
- Anaesthesia
- Dehydration
- Infection
- Fever
- Pregnancy
- Sudden change in temperature
- Alcohol — possibly because of dehydration
- Emotional stress
- Extreme fatigue

The location of the pain depends on the location of the obstruction.

- Anaemia — although these patients are usually anaemic, the body often compensates so that the symptoms of anaemia occur only as the result of a very severe crisis.
- Infection — there is an increased incidence of minor infections, septicaemia, pneumococcal meningitis and osteomyelitis.

MEDICAL MANAGEMENT

Investigations A blood film will demonstrate the presence of the sickle-shaped red blood cells. The presence of HbS can be demonstrated when the red blood cells are mixed with a special solution of sodium metabisulphite. The screening test for sickle cell anaemia and sickle cell trait uses electrophoretic analysis to measure the rates of movement of the different haemoglobins in an electrical field.

Treatment There is no cure for sickle cell disease. Management is based on alleviation of symptoms and promotion of a lifestyle that minimises crisis events and includes the following elements:

- avoiding situations that may trigger a crisis (see Box 11.5)
- early treatment of any infections, even minor ones
- prophylactic penicillin and pneumococcal vaccination
- education on general health and nutrition and prophylactic use of folic acid 5 mg daily
- managing crisis situations with prescribed analgesics, opiates are often required during crises
- learning to recognise complications of sickle cell disease, including bone and joint pains, leg ulcers, priapism in males, i.e. prolonged penile erection, gallstones, blurred vision, kidney disease in patients over 50 years of age, and peptic ulcers
- frequent follow-up in special clinics to monitor disease
- genetic counselling
- good antenatal care
- alerting other practitioners, e.g. surgeons and anaesthetists, to the condition
- obtaining support from sickle cell centres and social work departments in improving home conditions
- possible treatment with allogeneic stem cell transplant
- possible trial of hydroxyurea, a cytotoxic medication.

NURSING PRIORITIES AND MANAGEMENT: Sickle cell anaemia

Life-threatening concerns

Patients in sickle cell crisis admitted as emergencies to hospital may be very frightened. The nurse needs to appreciate the severity of the pain and the possible need for the administration of opiates. These should not be withheld and addiction problems rarely occur. The severe pain of a crisis does not respond to mild analgesics. Some hospitals within areas with a population in which sickle cell anaemia is relatively common have set up protocols for the management of patients admitted with sickle cell anaemia crisis in order to minimise the trauma of admission and to ensure the appropriate management of care.

Of equal importance to the alleviation of pain in sickle cell crisis is the management of the underlying cause of the crisis. An i.v. infusion may be commenced to maintain good hydration and to administer medications, e.g. antibiotics.

Patients admitted in a crisis require vigilant observation and monitoring. The underlying cause may not be apparent at first and therefore monitoring of the patient may alert nurses to signs and symptoms of the cause as well as to changes in the patient's condition.

Oxygen therapy (see Ch. 3) and blood transfusion (see p. 484) may be necessary.

Nursing considerations

Because these patients are often frightened, the nurse should listen carefully to their concerns. Since they may have had several previous episodes, such patients often know the best way that they should be treated when in a crisis.

Men may be admitted with a particularly embarrassing condition — priapism due to thrombosis in the corpus cavernosa. This requires not only the administration of analgesics, but also i.v. hydration and possibly exchange blood transfusion to reduce the percentage of sickle cells. Chronic priapism can occur and the patient's sexual function may be impaired (Midence & Elander 1996).

Before discharge from hospital, the patient should be made aware of the importance of recognising and avoiding situations that may cause a sickle cell crisis and of the need to seek medical advice at the onset of a painful episode, especially if it is accompanied by symptoms of another illness, including minor ailments.

A newly diagnosed patient will require a comprehensive education programme about the disorder, the ways to minimise complications, and any adaptations to be made to lifestyle. Arrangements should be made for the screening of all members of the family if this has not been done previously. Genetic counselling should be offered. Some areas with a high incidence of sickle cell disease employ special nurse counsellors to carry out screening and to advise patients and their families about the disorder and its consequences (see Ch. 6).

The emphasis in caring for a person with sickle cell anaemia is on promoting health and minimising ill-health.

STOP THINK **11.6** It may not always be appropriate to ask a family member to act as an interpreter. Why?

Anaemia resulting from blood loss

The blood loss responsible for these anaemias may be:

- acute — loss of a large volume of blood over a short period of time, as in haemorrhage (for pathophysiology, medical management, and nursing priorities and management, see Chs 18, 20 and 27)
- chronic — loss of a small, even microscopic, amount of blood over a long period of time.

Chronic blood loss is very common and is the form that will be considered here.

There are a number of disorders in which there is a constant or intermittent loss of small amounts of blood. Thus, this type of anaemia is secondary to another disorder, although it may be the presenting illness. Frequently, it is only when a diagnosis of anaemia has been established that the causative illness is suspected. The most common causes of chronic blood loss are listed in Box 11.6. Some patients realise that they have been bleeding but are too afraid to seek advice and discover its cause.

PATHOPHYSIOLOGY

No ill-effects will be felt until the blood loss has caused depletion of the body's iron stores. Thus the pathophysiology is similar to that of iron deficiency anaemia.

Common presenting symptoms are as for iron deficiency anaemia (p. 489). There may be additional symptoms according to the underlying disorder, e.g. stomach pains, heavy menstruation, weight loss, or blood in stools — either fresh or digested — resulting in black tarry stools known as melaena. The patient may be known to have an underlying illness, e.g. peptic ulceration.

MEDICAL MANAGEMENT

History and examination are as for the diagnosis of iron deficiency anaemia. Detailed and careful questioning may uncover symptoms that the patient considers insignificant or is afraid to report.

Investigations are as for the diagnosis of iron deficiency anaemia. Other tests may be required according to clinical features presented. Common investigations include barium meal and barium enema, rectal examination and endoscopy.

Box 11.6

Common causes of chronic blood loss

- Peptic ulceration, including side-effects of steroid therapy
- Gastric irritation — side-effect of alcohol and some medications, e.g. aspirin
- Menorrhagia — excessive regular menstrual flow
- Genitourinary bleeding, e.g. with bladder carcinoma
- Liver disease
- Chronic inflammatory disease
- Oesophageal varices (blood loss may be acute)
- Malignancy

Treatment will depend on the specific cause of the blood loss. Possibilities for treatment include oral iron therapy and blood transfusion.

NURSING PRIORITIES AND MANAGEMENT: Anaemias resulting from blood loss

Life-threatening concerns

If anaemia is very severe, nursing care will be implemented according to the complications that arise (see Chs 2, 3 and 18). If immediate transfusion is required, nursing care will be as described on page 491. The nurse must monitor the patient very closely for possible cardiac failure and pulmonary oedema.

Nursing considerations

In the initial interactions with a patient who presents with unexplained bleeding, the nurse should bear in mind that the patient may be feeling apprehensive about receiving a diagnosis, and possibly guilty about not seeking medical advice earlier. Giving the patient clear information about necessary tests and investigations will help to allay anxiety. If the patient is to undergo tests at an outpatient department, a clear explanation should be given about any pre-investigative preparation, how long the tests will take and what they will involve, and about whether the patient will be fit to return home unaccompanied afterwards.

Thorough nursing assessment can be invaluable in establishing the cause of bleeding and will include questioning, observation, monitoring of vital signs and discussion with the patient's family and friends.

The patient should be informed about the implications of the diagnosis and the proposed treatment. In planning care, the nurse must attempt to prioritise the patient's needs and problems and be sensitive to individual values and perceptions. Counselling may help the patient, especially if the diagnosis is cancer or any other chronic disorder that will affect the patient's lifestyle. Counselling may also be appropriate if the patient has a self-inflicted disorder, e.g. alcohol-induced gastritis.

The patient with anaemia caused by blood loss may be treated in hospital, in an outpatient clinic or health centre, or at home. Good liaison among all staff involved in the various stages of treatment is vital in ensuring continuity of care. Whether the patient's care is long or short term, follow-up must be emphasised to ensure that the disorder has been cured or is being adequately monitored.

DISORDERS CAUSED BY OVERPRODUCTION OF RED BLOOD CELLS: ERYTHROCYTOSIS

A raised haemoglobin level usually indicates an absolute increase in the number of circulating red blood cells. This may be a false finding if the plasma volume is reduced, as in dehydration.

There are three situations in which the number of red blood cells is increased:

- Pathological proliferation of red blood cells with no erythropoietin stimulus — this is called primary proliferative polycythaemia or polycythaemia rubra vera
- Physiological response due to hypoxia, e.g. at high altitudes or with pulmonary disease — a secondary polycythaemia
- Inappropriate production of erythropoietin, or similar substance, in certain pathological conditions, e.g. malignant tumours — causing a secondary polycythaemia.

Polycythaemia vera

This disease, often characterised by high facial colour and suffused conjunctiva, occurs most commonly in men over the age of 40 years. If the disorder is well controlled, survival for 20 years is possible. There is usually an increased white cell and platelet count as well as a high red cell count.

PATHOPHYSIOLOGY

The raised red blood cell, leucocyte and platelet count and haemoglobin level have a number of consequences, including hyperviscosity of the blood, thrombosis and hypertension, all of which could precipitate cardiac failure. Thrombosis and sluggish circulation may precipitate peripheral vascular disease. Splenomegaly develops in 75% of all patients due to the increase in the number of red blood cells to be broken down.

Common presenting symptoms Hyperviscosity of the blood can give rise to symptoms associated with a sluggish circulation and arterial and venous thrombosis. The patient may therefore present with symptoms of:

- cerebral vascular disease, e.g. headaches, dizziness, blackouts, stroke and lack of concentration
- peripheral vascular disease, e.g. intermittent claudication
- hypertension, e.g. headaches, epistaxis, dyspnoea
- angina and cardiac failure.

Gout may also be a feature due to the increased cell turnover and raised uric acid levels. Excess histamine production released from basophils can cause gastric ulceration and pruritus, especially on exposure to extremes of temperature.

MEDICAL MANAGEMENT

History and examination The patient may not present to the doctor with any symptoms but may attend for a health check-up and be found to have hypertension. He may have a ruddy complexion and the palms of the hands and the oral mucosal membrane may be a deep red colour. An enlarged spleen is found in 75% of patients.

Investigations Blood analysis will include full blood count, haemoglobin level, PCV and blood viscosity. Estimation of the red blood cell mass will be made using radioactive chromium-51. Bone marrow aspiration will be performed and usually demonstrates a hypercellular state and an increased number of megakaryocytes, large nucleated cells of the marrow that produce platelets.

Treatment Venesection (the removal of whole blood) is the simplest form of treatment. It is repeated until the PCV is reduced to below 50% and leads to a dramatic alleviation of symptoms.

Once the diagnosis is established, radioactive phosphorus (^{32}P) may be given by i.v. injection. This treatment is given in an outpatient department, as the radioactive level within the body will not be high enough to present a risk to other people within the community provided the patient follows certain guidelines. This treatment takes up to 3 months to be effective.

Myelosuppressive medications, e.g. busulfan and melphalan, may be given orally until the disorder is controlled (see Ch. 31).

All patients will require frequent monitoring to minimise the effects of the disorder. Possible complications are thrombosis, haemorrhage, myelofibrosis (fibrosis of bone marrow tissue which interferes with all blood cell production) and acute leukaemia.

NURSING PRIORITIES AND MANAGEMENT: Polycythaemia vera

The main aims of nursing care are:

- to support the patient during diagnostic tests
- to help the patient understand the diagnosis, treatment and possible long-term effects
- to advise the patient how to detect the onset of complications.

Nursing considerations

Both the patient and the family will need to come to terms with a chronic disorder that may alter lifestyle and shorten life. The patient will probably undergo tests as an outpatient or day patient and the nurse should provide information about all investigations. The nurse will be required to assist the doctor in performing a bone marrow aspiration (see p. 487).

The patient undergoing venesection, commenced by the doctor, must be monitored for signs and symptoms of shock (see Ch. 18). One complication of venesection in patients with polycythaemia vera is difficulty in maintaining flow because of the hyperviscosity of the blood.

Patient education

Before receiving radioactive phosphorus the patient must be given, preferably in writing, clear instructions regarding limitations of activities or contact with people, e.g. children or pregnant women, in view of the fact they are radioactive. If this care is impossible at home, arrangements will have to be made to admit the patient to a single room in a ward. If admission is required, the need for isolation to protect other patients, visitors and staff must be tactfully explained to the patient (see Ch. 31).

Once treatment has begun, it is important to teach the patient how to monitor for any signs of thrombosis, e.g. pain. If medication has been prescribed, detailed instructions about taking oral cytotoxins will be given (see Ch. 31). The importance of continued monitoring via blood tests and outpatient appointments should be emphasised.

DISORDERS OF WHITE BLOOD CELLS AND LYMPHOID TISSUE

The following sections will consider the nurse's role in the treatment of:

- leukaemia
- lymphoma
- multiple myeloma
- myelodysplastic syndromes.

LEUKAEMIA

The leukaemias are a group of malignant disorders in which there is an abnormal and excessive proliferation of immature, and therefore ineffective, blood cells. When these cells are examined microscopically it is usually possible to identify the specific subtype of blood cell that is affected, e.g. granulocyte, lymphocyte or monocyte.

Leukaemia is divided into two types: acute and chronic. Acute leukaemia is characterised by the malignant proliferation occurring at the 'blast' level of cell maturity (see p. 482); in the chronic form, the predominant malignant cell appears to mature but function is usually abnormal.

Leukaemia is uncommon but occurs in all ages, in both sexes and in all races. The total number of new cases of leukaemia per year in the UK is approximately 180 per million population (Mehta & Hoffbrand 2000).

Within the UK, the incidence of leukaemia varies from region to region. This variance may, in part, be explained by the aetiological factors listed below.

Aetiology

The aetiology of leukaemia is not fully understood but exposure to certain factors which may affect the genetic makeup of the cell are associated with increased incidence. These factors include exposure to:

- radiation
- viruses
- chemicals, especially petroleum derivatives such as benzene
- some cytotoxic medications.

Congenital factors or genetic disorders such as Down's syndrome are also associated with chromosomal abnormalities and implicated in the development of leukaemic disease.

Acute leukaemia

PATHOPHYSIOLOGY

Acute leukaemia is thought to arise from a genetic alteration in a single bone marrow cell which then proliferates to produce a clone of identical cells. As these abnormal cells proliferate, they gradually crowd out the bone marrow. This affects the production of normal blood cells — red cells, platelets and white cells — so that fewer and fewer normal cells are produced, which leads to anaemia, thrombocytopenia and leucopenia, especially neutropenia.

Acute leukaemia is subdivided into acute myeloid leukaemia (AML), beginning in the myeloid stem cell, and acute lymphoblastic leukaemia (ALL), beginning in the lymphoid stem cell. In adults, AML is three times more common than ALL, while in children ALL accounts for most cases (Treleaven & Mellor 2000). Though distinct, AML and ALL can coexist. They are classified by morphological differences according to an internationally recognised system, devised by French, American and British haematologists, known as the FAB classification. The World Health Organization has devised a more recent classification which is undergoing consideration (Viele 2003).

For further information on the FAB classification of acute leukaemia, see Bratt-Wyton (2000).

Common presenting symptoms Common symptoms, which derive from the effects of the disease on bone marrow function are:

- acute infection, associated with fever — with more than one infection coexisting, or recurrent episodes of infection occurring over a period of weeks, e.g. upper respiratory tract, oral *Candida albicans* or skin infections
- bleeding of the gums, epistaxis, purpura
- anaemia (see p. 486).

STOP THINK **11.7** How can these symptoms be explained in terms of the function of the different blood cells?

Other symptoms may occur because leukaemic cells infiltrate tissues and organs:

- bones causing bone pain
- liver and spleen leading to hepatosplenomegaly causing abdominal pain
- gums causing gum swelling.

Less commonly affected are:

- meninges causing headaches
- testes causing swelling and pain.

In cases where there are high circulating counts of blast cells, symptoms of hyperviscosity will be manifested, e.g. headaches, blurred vision.

MEDICAL MANAGEMENT

History and examination The patient may describe either:

- an acute onset of symptoms occurring over the last 72 h and appear pale, pyrexial, tachycardic and exhibiting other signs and symptoms of acute infection, *or*
- a 2–3 month history of relatively minor recurrent infections.

On examination, evidence may be found of lymphadenopathy, petechiae, purpura and bruising (see Case History 11.2).

Investigations Diagnosis can be established by blood counts and microscopic examination of a blood film which together usually show a picture of:

- high white blood cell count (mainly blast cells)
- low red cell count
- low haemoglobin
- low platelet count.

CASE HISTORY 11.2

Mrs D

Mrs D, aged 40 years, is a housewife. She and her husband have two sons, aged 12 and 14. Mrs D's husband often works overtime so she is kept busy looking after the household. She enjoys gardening, keep-fit classes and reading.

Over the past 2 or 3 months she has been excessively tired. Although she sleeps well at night, she does not feel rested in the morning. She has had mouth ulcers, cold sores and a persistent sore throat. At first, she attributed these symptoms to being run down. Finally, she sought her GP's opinion about the sore throat. He prescribed antibiotics but, because of her other symptoms, took a blood sample for a full blood count in case she was anaemic. He advised her to contact the surgery in a few days for the blood test results and to return to see him if the sore throat continued.

Mrs D was very shocked when later that day the GP telephoned to tell her she was very anaemic and that he had arranged an emergency appointment at the local hospital for her to see the haematology consultant that evening. Mrs D was advised by the haematologist that she needed urgent investigation into her abnormal blood count; arrangements were made for her immediate admission.

Further investigation confirmed a diagnosis of acute myeloid leukaemia. After further discussion with the consultant and her husband, Mrs D has consented to chemotherapy.

A central venous access device, e.g. Hickman catheter, has been inserted to provide long-term access for drug administration, blood sampling, blood product transfusion and possible parenteral nutrition. Mrs D has received a blood transfusion so that her haemoglobin level immediately prior to the first course of treatment is 11 g/dL. She is neutropenic and thrombocytopenic.

Her nursing care for day 2 of her first course of chemotherapy is given in Nursing Care Plan 11.2. The chemotherapy medications she is receiving are i.v. daunorubicin and cytarabine.

This diagnosis will be confirmed by examination of a bone marrow aspirate and biopsy (see p. 487). Under the microscope, at least 30% of the bone marrow will have been replaced by leukaemic cells. Further laboratory testing of the marrow using cytochemistry, immunophenotyping, cytogenetic analysis and molecular studies will lead to a precise diagnosis of a particular subtype of acute leukaemia, often indicating prognosis.

For further information on bone marrow examination in acute leukaemia, see Mehta & Hoffbrand (2000).

Further aspirations of bone marrow are taken and examined during and after the completion of treatment to assess the response of the disease and help to indicate the prognosis.

If the patient has ALL, two further diagnostic investigations will be carried out:

- a lumbar puncture, as there is a high risk of central nervous system involvement, especially in the cerebrospinal fluid
- examination of the testes, as this is a region to which leukaemia may spread.

Treatment

Treatment is aimed at controlling and eliminating the disease with a long-term view of giving the patient months or many years of disease-free survival. This is often achieved through the administration of chemotherapeutic agents and in some cases bone marrow or stem cell transplantation. Ongoing research into the use of therapies that target malignant cells without significantly affecting normal cells is also being examined (Stull 2003).

Before treatment commences several issues need to be considered.

- Assessment of the patient's general state of health, e.g. cardiac, renal and pulmonary function
- Assessment of CMV status through blood sampling. Blood products will be required during treatment and CMV negative patients are at risk of developing complications if given CMV positive blood (see p. 484)
- The insertion of a long-term central venous access device preventing the need for repeated venepuncture, e.g. Hickman line for blood sampling and the administration of medication
- Referral for the fitting of a wig
- The discussion of fertility issues with patients of child-bearing age whose fertility may well be compromised by treatment. Male patients should be offered sperm banking facilities and female patients the opportunity to review the strategies available to them to maintain the possibility of future fertility (Foster 2002).

STOP THINK **11.8** Reflect on the benefits, complications and long-term care of central venous access devices. Refer to Hamilton (2000).

Chemotherapy (see Ch. 31)

Chemotherapy refers to the use of chemical agents in the treatment of malignant disease. It aims to cure disease by eradicating and suppressing abnormal cell production. As these medications are relatively non-selective, normal cells which are undergoing cell division are invariably damaged, giving rise to potentially life-threatening complications, such as infection and haemorrhage caused by bone marrow suppression and side-effects such as nausea and vomiting, mucositis, alopecia and infertility. Treatment is often a fine balance between maximal destruction of malignant cells with minimal damage to normal cells.

The chemotherapy regimens used to treat acute leukaemia are based on national protocols of treatment devised by the Medical Research Council (MRC) (1995, 2001) which change over time in the light of ongoing research. Several courses of treatment are usually administered, each course lasting several days, using a variety of different chemotherapy medication combinations that affect cell death by different means.

Initial treatment (the induction phase) is aimed at achieving remission, indicated by a reduction of blast cells to <5% of the total white cell count in the bone marrow. Remission is then consolidated by further chemotherapy (the consolidation phase) with the aim of eliminating any remaining leukaemic cells. Maintenance therapy is administered to patients with ALL for a further year after the completion of consolidation chemotherapy.

The classification of chemotherapy medications is discussed in detail in Chapter 31. Table 11.5 outlines some of the combinations of medications commonly used in the treatment of AML (MRC 2001). All are administered i.v. except for thioguanine which is taken orally.

As can be seen, regimens of treatment are complex and are reviewed for individual patients prior to the administration of each course. Other combination options may be offered according to guidelines indicated by the MRC (2001).

Treatment regimens for ALL are more complex (see Table 11.6) and include an intensification phase between induction, which is split into two phases, and consolidation therapy. Once induction therapy is completed, patients may go on to undergo bone marrow or stem cell transplantation. This may be allogeneic or autologous (see Table 11.7) or consolidation chemotherapy. Maintenance therapy follows consolidation chemotherapy for patients with ALL using some of the medications already given by a variety of routes of administration.

Table 11.5 A possible treatment option for acute myeloid leukaemia (AML)

Phase of treatment	Course number	Drugs	Action
Induction chemotherapy	Course 1	Daunorubicin Cytarabine Tioguanine	Cytotoxic antibiotic Antimetabolite Antimetabolite
	Course 2	Daunorubicin Cytarabine Tioguanine	Cytotoxic antibiotic Antimetabolite Antimetabolite
Consolidation chemotherapy	Course 3	Amsacrine Cytarabine Etoposide	Dye derivative that intercalates with DNA Antimetabolite Plant alkaloid
	Course 4	Mitoxantrone Cytarabine	Dye derivative that intercalates with DNA Antimetabolite
	Course 5 (administered in some cases only)	Cytarabine	Antimetabolite

Adapted from MRC (2001).

Table 11.6 A possible treatment option for acute lymphoblastic leukaemia (ALL)

Phase of treatment	Drugs	Method of administration	Action
Induction chemotherapy: Phase 1	Vincristine	IV	Vinca alkaloid
	Daunorubicin	IV	Cytotoxic antibiotic
	Prednisolone	Oral	Steroid
	L-Asparaginase	IM	Protein synthesis inhibitor
	Methotrexate	IT	Antimetabolite
Phase 2	Cyclophosphamide	IV	Alkylating agent
	Cytarabine	IV	Antimetabolite
	6-Mercaptopurine	Oral	Antimetabolite
	Methotrexate	IT	Antimetabolite
Intensification	Methotrexate	IV	Antimetabolite
	L-Asparaginase	IM	Protein synthesis inhibitor
Consolidation therapy with either transplantation	Fractionated total body irradiation over 4 days		
or	followed by Etoposide	IV	Plant alkaloid
four cycles of chemotherapy using different combinations of drugs	Vincristine	IV	Vinca alkaloid
	Cytarabine	IV	Antimetabolite
	Etoposide	IV	Plant alkaloid
	Dexamethasone	Oral	Steroid
	Daunorubicin	IV	Cytotoxic antibiotic
	Cyclophosphamide	IV	Alkylating agent
	Tioguanine	Oral	Antimetabolite

Adapted from MRC (1995).
IV, intravenous; IM, intramuscular; IT, intrathecal.

Table 11.7 Transplantation for malignant haematological disease

Type of transplant	Explanation
Bone marrow transplantation	This involves the transfer of bone marrow, which contains 90% of haematopoietic progenitor cells, into someone whose bone marrow has been destroyed by high dose therapy, to re-establish haematopoiesis. Marrow is harvested by multiple aspirations from the pelvis under general anaesthetic and infused intravenously
Stem cell transplantation	This involves the transfer of immature blood cells, known as stem cells, to re-establish haematopoiesis for someone whose bone marrow has been destroyed by high dose therapy. Stem cells may be obtained from peripheral blood or the umbilical cord and are infused intravenously
Syngeneic transplant	This refers to the transplantation of bone marrow or stem cells between identical twins
Allogeneic sibling transplant	This involves the use of bone marrow or stem cells from a matched sibling donor obtained from a bone marrow harvest or peripheral blood stem cell collection
Matched unrelated donor transplant (MUD)	Where a matched sibling donor is not available, a volunteer donor of bone marrow or stem cells may be found from national or international donor registries
Autologous transplant	This involves the use of a patient's own bone marrow or stem cells following high dose therapy to reduce the period of pancytopenia. The cells are usually taken during a period of remission, preserved and returned at a later date

Blood growth factors (see p. 482)
To reduce the period of neutropenia for certain patients, granulocytic colony stimulating factor (GCSF) can be given by s.c. injection. GCSF may also be given to promote the production of granulocytes:

- for patients about to undergo stem cell collection prior to storage
- for related or unrelated donors of stem cells for transplantation

(see Table 11.7 and Ch. 31).

Bone marrow or stem cell transplantation (see Table 11.7)
Transplantation involves the transfer of healthy bone marrow or stem cells into someone whose own bone

marrow has been destroyed by high dose chemotherapy. This may involve the use of the patient's own bone marrow or stem cells, or donor products. The bone marrow or stem cells engraft into the patient's marrow and restore normal marrow function. When bone marrow is used, engraftment may take 4–6 weeks. This is reduced to 2 weeks if stem cells are used. Bone marrow or stem cells may be 'harvested' from:

- the patient, as blood counts are recovering immediately after a course of chemotherapy
- a related or unrelated donor with a matching tissue type.

As there are many potential life-threatening complications and side-effects associated with transplantation, guidelines indicate which patients are most likely to benefit from this procedure.

For further information on stem cell/bone marrow transplantation, see Outhwaite (2000) and Provan et al (2004).

Research has shown that allogeneic transplantation offers a survival benefit for selected patients with acute leukaemia who are under 60 years of age (MRC 1995, 2001). The following protocols of selection are currently used.

For AML After the first course of induction chemotherapy, microscopic and cytogenetic analysis of a bone marrow aspirate will reveal the percentage of blast (leukaemic) cells present and their cytogenetic makeup. These results enable the patient to be assigned to a 'good', 'standard' or 'poor' risk group as defined by the MRC (2001) which will determine treatment thereafter. For patients assigned to the 'good' risk group, transplantation has not been shown to offer a survival benefit as compared to the use of chemotherapy alone. If an adult patient is assigned to the 'standard' or 'poor' risk group, then depending on age and availability of a donor, allogeneic transplantation from a matched sibling is recommended several weeks after the completion of chemotherapy.

Autologous stem cells may be collected after course 2 for use at a later stage.

For ALL All suitable patients less than 50 years of age who have a matched sibling donor are recommended to proceed to allogeneic transplantation in first remission. Patients who have poor cytogenetic indicators are recommended for unrelated donor transplantation in the event of a sibling donor being unavailable. Autologous transplantation may be recommended if a donor cannot be identified for the patient.

Prognosis

Over the last 40 years, 5-year survival for younger patients with AML has risen from 0% to approximately 45% although this varies according to age and prognostic factors (MRC 2001). The prognosis for patients with ALL is similar but also varies considerably depending on adverse factors such as age, speed of achieving remission and the presence of genetic abnormalities (MRC 1995).

Other medical interventions

As has been shown, leukaemic disease and treatment leads to the suppression of normal blood cell production. This predisposes the patient to thrombocytopenia, anaemia and neutropenia, all of which require medical intervention as the patient becomes symptomatic.

Thrombocytopenia Platelet transfusion will be required if the platelet count falls below 10×10^9 cells/L. Platelets will also be required with higher counts in other specific instances, e.g. bleeding gums. In some circumstances patients may need these to be CMV negative and/or irradiated (see p. 484).

Anaemia Red cell transfusion to minimise the effects of anaemia may be needed if counts drop below 10×10^9 cells/L. As for platelet transfusions, some patients may require CMV negative and/or irradiated blood products (see p. 484).

Neutropenia To reduce the incidence of infection, prophylactic antibiotics such as ciprofloxacin are often administered from the start of chemotherapy and for some time after the completion of treatment.

Antifungal and antiviral agents, e.g. itraconazole and acyclovir, are also administered to minimise the incidence of infections such as *Candida albicans* and those caused by the herpes virus. These agents will also be used as part of an oral hygiene regimen.

Neutropenic patients are extremely susceptible to infection and a pyrexia of ≥38°C for more than 1 h can indicate possible septicaemia. Treatment protocols for the management of neutropenic sepsis are specific to individual haematology units. Such protocols may vary from time to time and from hospital to hospital and include the taking of blood cultures and swabs, e.g. axilla and mouth, medical examination, chest X-ray and the administration of broad spectrum i.v. antibiotics.

Prevention of tumour lysis syndrome

Tumour lysis syndrome occurs as a result of the rapid breakdown of tumour cells during the induction phase of treatment. This leads to metabolic disturbances which include the excessive production of uric acid which is excreted via the renal system. If abnormally high levels are produced, crystals of uric acid may be deposited in the kidneys and lead to renal failure. In order to prevent this, oral allopurinol is administered from the start of treatment which slows the production of uric acid.

NURSING PRIORITIES AND MANAGEMENT: Acute leukaemia (see Nursing Care Plan 11.2)

The aim of nursing care for the patient undergoing treatment for acute leukaemia is to support the patient physically and psychologically through diagnosis, treatment and possibly relapse. The nurse should be present at any consultation taking place between medical staff and patient to reinforce and explain information given and should take time to inform the patient about pretreatment investigations and procedures. The nurse will also administer prescribed treatment and supportive care, offering psychological support throughout to patients and their loved ones.

Nursing Care Plan 11.2 Care of Mrs D during chemotherapy for myeloid leukaemia (see Case History 11.2)

Nursing considerations	Action	Rationale	Evaluation
1. **Risk of infection (because of neutropenia and chemotherapy)**	• Use a single room with separate toilet and washing facilities	To reduce contact with staff and other patients	All symptoms and signs of infection are noted and reported immediately and thus treatment for any infection commences early
	• Wash hands using antiseptic solution before giving any nursing care, with scrupulous attention to wrists and between fingers and careful drying	To remove commensal bacterial skin flora that may cause infection in patient; single most important preventive action against cross-infection	
	• Instruct and assist with personal hygiene using antiseptic solution	To reduce skin bacterial flora and risk of endogenous septicaemia	
	• Inspect skin daily for infection, especially folds of buttocks, axilla, perineum, breasts, puncture sites, skin breakdown, skin lesions and rashes	To detect any skin infection early	
	• Explain mouth care regimen: – use of chlorhexidine 0.4% solution after meals and at bedtime – use of antifungal agent in mouth care as prescribed by doctor (after all meals and at bedtime) – gentle brushing of teeth using a soft toothbrush	To prevent bacterial and fungal infections of mouth and reduce risk of septicaemia. To reduce risk of bacterial infection	
	• Inspect mouth daily for signs of infection using Oral Assessment Guide (see p. 513). Take swabs from any new lesions	Early detection of mouth infection	
	• Record axillary temperature, pulse and BP 4-hourly (unless patient is receiving blood products)	Early detection of infection. Axillary route used because of sore mouth and risk of infection	
	• Report any elevation of temperature to doctor immediately	To ensure any infection is treated appropriately and immediately	
	• Take blood cultures from vascular access device and peripherally as a baseline and at onset of pyrexia		

Continued

Nursing Care Plan 11.2 Care of Mrs D during chemotherapy for myeloid leukaemia (see Case History 11.2) *(Continued)*

Nursing considerations	Action	Rationale	Evaluation
1. Risk of infection (because of neutropenia and chemotherapy) *(Continued)*	• Take nasal, throat and skin swabs from axilla, groin	To detect any microorganisms that might cause skin infections and septicaemia	
	• Inform patient and visitors of the restrictions re. plants and flowers	Earth is a source of *Serratia marcescens*, stagnant water a medium for *Pseudomonas aeruginosa*	
	• Advise Mrs D about dietary restrictions: no raw unpeeled fruit or raw vegetables	Raw, unpeeled fruit and raw vegetables may be contaminated with *Pseudomonas aeruginosa*, *Klebsiella* species and *Escherichia coli* and cause septicaemia	
	• Administer no medications rectally or evacuant enemas or suppositories	Can cause rectal abscesses and septicaemia in immunosuppressed patient	
	• Report any symptoms, e.g. dysuria, to doctor immediately.	To commence appropriate antibacterial/antifungal or antiviral treatment immediately	
	Report any change in patient's condition, especially increased drowsiness, headache, irritability or restlessness	Changes in central nervous system may be first indication of septicaemia	
	• Access vascular access device according to local protocol and observe exit site daily for signs of infection	To detect complications and ensure care of device and exit site dressing is appropriate	
2. Inadequate oxygenation of tissues due to anaemia	• Assist with all activities of living as appropriate	To conserve energy and reduce oxygen requirements	Patient is not unduly tired
	• Observe pressure areas twice daily	To detect any skin breakdown due to hypoxia of skin	Any pressure ulcer is detected at first sign, if not prevented
	• Organise nursing care or assistance to allow periods of rest	To conserve energy	
	• Use Spenco mattress on bed	To reduce risk of pressure ulcers	
3. Easy bleeding due to thrombocytopenia	• Inspect skin daily for signs of new bruises, petechiae, purpura	To detect any bleeding immediately	Bleeding is detected early and prompt treatment is given

Continued

Nursing Care Plan 11.2 Care of Mrs D during chemotherapy for myeloid leukaemia (see Case History 11.2) *(Continued)*

Nursing considerations	Action	Rationale	Evaluation
3. Easy bleeding due to thrombocytopenia *(Continued)*	• Inspect mouth daily for bleeding		
	• Test urine daily for protein and blood • Test and inspect all stools for blood		
	• Observe any vomit for blood		
	• Observe any headache and/or change in conscious level		
	• Observe any other overt episodes of bleeding, e.g. epistaxis		
	• Report to doctor immediately any signs or symptoms of bleeding	To ensure treatment is given as soon as possible	
	• Record pulse and BP 4-hourly	To detect any hidden bleeding suspected because of tachycardia and hypotension	
	• Administer platelets as prescribed, ensuring compatibility of donor blood, observing and monitoring for any allergic or other reaction by recording quarter-hourly pulse and BP and asking patient about any complaints	To ensure platelets are given safely	
4. Side-effects of chemotherapy (a) Bone marrow suppression (b) Extravasation of chemotherapeutic agents, especially daunorubicin	See 1, 2, 3 • Administer chemotherapy according to protocol • Access vascular access device according to protocol	To ensure safe administration of chemotherapy To reduce the risk of damage to the vascular access device	All side-effects of chemotherapy agents are observed and prompt relevant nursing care is implemented so that Mrs D experiences as few side-effects as possible
	• Observe exit site of vascular access device and surrounding area vigilantly for extravasation	To ensure that extravasation is detected as soon as possible	
	• Report promptly to medical staff any signs of swelling, tenderness or inability to access vascular access device	To ensure that extravasation is dealt with promptly and appropriately	

Continued ▶

Nursing Care Plan 11.2 Care of Mrs D during chemotherapy for myeloid leukaemia (see Case History 11.2) *(Continued)*

Nursing considerations	Action	Rationale	Evaluation
4. Side-effects of chemotherapy (*Continued*) (c) Nausea and vomiting	• Administer antiemetics according to prescription	To prevent or minimise nausea and vomiting	
	• Report to doctor nausea and vomiting not controlled by antiemetics	So that antiemetic regimen can be reviewed	
	• Encourage patient to try alternative measures of controlling nausea and vomiting, e.g. relaxation tapes	To prevent or minimise episodes of nausea and vomiting	
	• Record all episodes of and measure all vomit	To assess possibility of dehydration and possible electrolyte imbalance	
	• Reassure patient that nausea will stop when chemotherapy course has been completed	Patient already aware of possibility but symptoms can be very depressing	
(d) Stomatitis	• As for mouth regimen in 1		
(e) Flu-like symptoms due to cytarabine	• Observe and report any symptoms to doctor immediately of shivering, headache or pyrexia	Early detection	
	• Monitor temperature 4-hourly		
(f) Red urine after i.v. daunorubicin	• Reassure patient that red urine is temporary consequence of i.v. daunorubicin		
	• Test all urine for blood during and immediately after bolus injection of daunorubicin	Difficult to differentiate between red colouring and bleeding due to thrombocytopenia	
(h) Hyperuricaemia because of rapid breakdown of tumour cells following chemotherapy	• Test urinary pH and measure output. Encourage oral fluid intake especially between administration of chemotherapy medications		
	• Administer allopurinol as prescribed	To reduce uric acid crystal formation and possible renal failure; to prevent or minimise high uric acid levels	
5. Anxiety about diagnosis, treatment, side-effects, prognosis	• Be prepared to listen to any anxieties		Mrs D feels able to talk with staff and feels she fully understands as much as she wishes to know about her disorder, its treatment and the consequences

Continued

Nursing Care Plan 11.2 Care of Mrs D during chemotherapy for myeloid leukaemia (see Case History 11.2) *(Continued)*

Nursing considerations	Action	Rationale	Evaluation
5. Anxiety about diagnosis, treatment, side-effects, prognosis (*Continued*)	• Answer questions honestly and ensure, by reporting in writing, that all members of the multidisciplinary team know what information was given and what anxieties Mrs D is voicing		
	• Request further discussion with doctor or registered nurse as required		
	• Arrange for support from other relevant personnel if appropriate, e.g. social worker, chaplain, special organisations, e.g. CancerBACUP, Cancerlink	May require reiteration of information previously given by doctors, nurses or other members of the team, because of mental adjustment to diagnosis	
6. Altered body image (a) Alopecia	• Reassure Mrs D that hair loss is temporary: reinforce information given about when hair loss will occur, likely duration and rate of regrowth	To try to reduce emotional trauma of alopecia. Accurate information will help her to adjust and explain to her husband and her children	Mrs D is able to feel she is still attractive to her husband and that her appearance is acceptable to her children
	• Advise Mrs D to reduce handling of hair but encourage her to keep hairstyle attractive	To reduce trauma to weak hair and minimise loss	
	• Discuss ways of enhancing her appearance once hair loss starts, e.g. wearing a wig, turban or scarf	To help her to feel as attractive as possible when alopecia is complete	
(b) Herpes	• Give written information to read	To help her understand information given and a basis to ask further questions	Mrs D will feel staff understand the disfigurement of the herpes and that she is helping herself
	• Advise and assist Mrs D to carry out mouth care regimen as in 1		
(c) Sexuality	• Be sensitive to possible worries about sexuality	To help her explore feelings about changes in sexual function and body image, and to help her discuss this with her husband when she feels able	Mrs D will feel she received relevant information and is able to discuss this topic
	• Listen to worries; give truthful answers to any questions about sexual functioning		

Continued

Nursing Care Plan 11.2 Care of Mrs D during chemotherapy for myeloid leukaemia (see Case History 11.2) *(Continued)*

Nursing considerations	Action	Rationale	Evaluation
6. Altered body image (c) Sexuality (*Continued*)	• Offer written information for her to read		
	• Listen to feelings and concerns about having a vascular access device in situ for a considerable period of time		
7. Inadequate nutrition and hydration (a) Anorexia	• Ensure oral hygiene regimen continued as in 1	To maintain infection-free mouth and because absence of blood improves taste	Weigh weekly: Mrs D should maintain admission weight
(b) Nausea and vomiting	• Administer antiemetics as prescribed by doctor	To prevent or minimise nausea and vomiting	
(c) Hypermetabolic state	• Help her choose a high-protein/high-carbohydrate diet from menu	To reduce or minimise effects of malnutrition, minimise weight loss and maintain protein intake	
	• Arrange for dietitian to talk to her daily to help meet dietary needs		
	• Discuss with Mrs D and her husband the possibility of him bringing certain foods she particularly wishes within restrictions (see 1)		
	• Encourage high-protein/high-energy drinks between meals		
	• Ensure meals are attractively served and in small portions if appropriate	To improve or minimise effects of malnutrition and immunosuppression	
	• Ensure 2–3 L fluid intake (see 4)	To prevent hyperuricaemia	Fluid balance assessed daily: Mrs D does not develop negative fluid balance

Nursing considerations

Prevention of infection

The most important aspect of nursing care of patients undergoing chemotherapy for leukaemic disease is assessing the risk and minimising the incidence of infection. Therefore, the nurse must be aware of the potential sources of infection, routes of transmission, sites of entry and common organisms involved.

Sources of infection may be exogenous (environmental) or endogenous (internal) to the patient. Protective isolation is discussed in Chapter 16 and involves nursing the patient in a single room, with en-suite facilities if possible, to reduce contact with environmental microorganisms.

Prevention of exogenous infection

This will be achieved by:

- all staff undertaking strict hand hygiene using bactericidal solutions prior to patient contact and between tasks performed for the same patient
- wearing protective clothing such as disposable plastic aprons when undertaking invasive procedures, disposing of excretory products or assisting in the personal hygiene of patients
- wearing sterile gloves for invasive procedures
- restricting the number of visitors
- encouraging the patient to avoid raw and uncooked foods
- restricting items taken into the single room
- avoiding stagnant water in humidification equipment or flower vases as these potentially harbour *Pseudomonas*.

For research findings and discussion about handwashing techniques and aseptic i.v. management, see Dougherty & Lister (2004) and Chapter 16.

Protection from endogenous sources of infection

The patient's own microflora pose more of a threat to the immunosuppressed patient than exogenous sources. Organisms that normally live with the patient during health and offer protection, take advantage of the immunosuppressed patient and cause opportunistic infection (Hart 2000).

Infection caused in this way may be prevented by:

- regular and vigilant observation of the patient, e.g. 4-hourly recordings of temperature, pulse and blood pressure
- regular observation and care of the mouth using bactericidal solutions (see p. 506 and Ch. 15)
- teaching the patient to pay particular attention to personal hygiene and handwashing practices
- consistent care of any vascular access device according to local protocol.

Prevention of haemorrhage

The nurse should carefully observe and monitor the patient to detect any bleeding. This should include:

- reporting all signs and symptoms of bleeding immediately to medical staff
- administering platelet transfusions promptly once prescribed by medical staff
- taking pulse and blood pressure readings at least 4-hourly, being aware of the risk of bruising from the sphygmomanometer cuff in thrombocytopenic patients, possibly necessitating a reduction in the frequency of recordings
- undertaking daily urinalysis for visible or occult blood
- testing all stools for visible or occult blood
- observing for changes in levels of consciousness or development of headaches which may indicate cerebral haemorrhage
- observing sputum and vomit for blood
- inspecting skin daily for purpura
- assessing pain, especially in the abdomen, as this may be an indication of haemorrhage
- avoiding i.m. injections and the use of aspirin-based medications, wet razors or harsh tooth brushes.

Minimising the side-effects of chemotherapy

General side-effects of chemotherapy are discussed in Chapter 31. Common short-term side-effects experienced by patients receiving chemotherapy for leukaemic disease are discussed here.

Nausea and vomiting

Nausea and vomiting may result in reluctance to accept treatment and, if left untreated, may lead to dehydration and electrolyte imbalance. However, control is possible through the use of antiemetic medications given prior to, and at regular intervals after, the administration of treatment. A wide range of medications is currently available so that alternatives can be used if first line medications are ineffective. The use of relaxation techniques may also help.

Compromised nutritional intake

Loss of appetite is common during and post chemotherapy. Several factors may influence the patient's inability to eat, such as nausea and vomiting, stomatitis and neutropenia, necessitating a restricted diet, usually avoiding raw and uncooked foods which are likely to cause infection in the immunocompromised patient. Advice should be sought from the dietitian about the best foods and supplementary drinks to take. Occasionally it may be necessary to give the patient parenteral nutrition for a period of time. If this is the case the patient will require careful monitoring to ensure electrolyte balance is maintained. Daily or weekly weighing of the patient will assess any weight loss.

Mucositis

Chemotherapy inhibits cell replication in the oral cavity and leads to inflammation of the oral mucosa known as mucositis. The production of saliva is also reduced, leading to changes in the normal microflora of the mouth, thus increasing the possibility of infection. Ulcers which develop within the mouth allow infection to enter the circulation, compromise nutrition and cause considerable pain, sometimes severe enough to merit the administration of continuous s.c. opioids. Daily oral assessment using a specialist tool (see Table 11.8) will help to ensure that oral hygiene is undertaken and evaluated regularly. Patients may be encouraged to use a bactericidal mouthwash several times a day, often in conjunction with an antifungal agent.

Table 11.8 Oral assessment guide

Category	Tools for assessment	Methods of measurement	Numerical and descriptive ratings 1	2	3
Voice	Auditory	Converse with patient	Normal	Deeper or raspy	Difficulty talking or painful
Swallow	Observation	Ask patient to swallow	Normal swallowing	Some pain on swallowing	Unable to swallow
Lips	Visual/palpatory	Observe and feel tissue	Smooth, pink and moist	Dry or cracked	Ulcerated or bleeding
Tongue	Visual/palpatory	Feel and observe appearance of tissue	Pink and moist; papillae present	Coated or loss of papillae with a shiny appearance with or without redness	Blistered or cracked
Saliva	Tongue blade	Insert blade into mouth, touching the centre of the tongue and the floor of the mouth	Watery	Thick or ropey	Absent
Mucous membranes	Visual	Observe appearance of tissue	Pink and moist	Reddened or coated (increased whiteness) without ulcerations	Ulceration with or without bleeding
Gingiva	Tongue blade and visual	Gently press tissue with tip of blade	Pink, stippled and firm	Oedematous with or without redness	Spontaneous bleeding or bleeding with pressure
Teeth or dentures (or denture-bearing area)	Visual	Observe appearance of teeth or denture-bearing area	Clean and no debris	Plaque or debris in localised areas between teeth (if present)	Plaque or debris generalised along gumline or denture-bearing area

Reproduced with permission from Eilers et al (1988).
This assessment tool, based on clinical experience and research, requires the nurse to score, on a scale of 1–3, eight different indicators of mouth hygiene and health, thus obtaining a total score of between 8 and 24. If a score of 8–10 is obtained, assessment should be repeated morning and evening. For scores >10, assessment should be carried out 8-hourly.

Communication (see Ch. 31)

Communication may be difficult for the patient because of changes in mood, sore mouth and feelings of lethargy. It is important for staff to listen to anxieties, fears and wishes.

Psychological care (see Ch. 31)

Patients with haematological disease may experience several factors which can affect them psychologically. For example, treatment involves repeated admission to hospital for courses of chemotherapy; having successfully completed one course, followed by a break at home, patients may find it difficult to face further hospitalisation and therapy. Periods of isolation cut the patient off from the outside world and may lead to sensory deprivation. Once discharged, after a period in isolation, patients may be so overwhelmed by a fear of the possibility of life-threatening infection that this takes over their lives.

Patient education

Helping patients to understand their illness and its management may allow them to retain a sense of control, even when very ill. Clear information will also help them to cope during periods at home between courses of treatment.

The active involvement of the family should be encouraged as the patient is given guidance in the following areas:

- monitoring body temperature
- recognising and responding to the symptoms of infection and haemorrhage
- maintaining a high standard of personal hygiene and oral care
- recognising and responding to complications associated with a vascular access device
- adhering to the oral medication regimen
- emergency contact details.

Discharge planning

On discharge, whether between courses or on completion of treatment, patients should receive a date for an outpatient appointment. The patient's GP and community nurse will be informed of discharge and arrangements made regarding continuing care. It is also important that patients receive information about who to contact in the event of an emergency.

Other professionals who may be involved in discharge planning include:

- the social worker — for help with housing and social security benefit claims
- the occupational therapist — to assess both the patient's ability to cope with everyday activities and the need for any adaptations to the home environment
- the physiotherapist — to assess the patient's mobility and assist in the achievement and maintenance of optimal fitness
- the dietitian — to advise on nutrition and supplementary foods.

Many patients achieve remission from their disease for varying lengths of time. However, many relapse and require re-admission for further treatment.

STOP THINK **11.9** A 21-year-old woman who is engaged to be married in 6 months is diagnosed as having acute leukaemia. She has undergone chemotherapy and is in remission, i.e. there is no evidence of leukaemic cells in the peripheral blood film or in the bone marrow. She has been in hospital for 3 months and is now about to be discharged. She has experienced a degree of alopecia, has lost a great deal of weight and is sensitive about her appearance. Reflect on the following:

(a) What do you think her main fears and anxieties might be?
(b) How could you help her to enhance her appearance?
(c) What support services are available in the community for the patient, her fiancé and her family?
(d) What practical advice should she be given prior to discharge?

Chronic leukaemia

PATHOPHYSIOLOGY

Unlike that of acute leukaemia, the onset of chronic leukaemia is insidious and the disease may be present for some time before the patient seeks medical attention. A proportion of patients are diagnosed as the result of incidental blood testing for some other condition.

Chronic leukaemia is subdivided into chronic myeloid leukaemia (CML) and chronic lymphocytic leukaemia (CLL). CML seems to be a disease of the pluripotent stem cells leading to an increase in neutrophils and their precursor cells in the peripheral blood (Mehta & Hoffbrand 2000, Treleaven 2000). Ninety-five per cent of the leukaemic cells have an abnormal chromosome known as the Philadelphia chromosome (chromosome 22) which results from a reciprocal translocation of part of the long arms of chromosomes 9 and 22 (Mehta & Hoffbrand 2000).

After a chronic phase of 2–3 years the disease enters an accelerated stage and finally transforms into acute leukaemia which is the main cause of death in patients with CML.

CLL is a malignant disorder of the B lymphocytes which proliferate and accumulate in the blood, bone marrow, lymph nodes and spleen. Most cases occur in adults aged between 60 and 80 years of age with men more often affected than women (Matutes & Dearden 2000). It is the commonest type of leukaemia in Western countries (Mehta & Hoffbrand 2000).

Common presenting symptoms These may be similar to those of acute leukaemia and include:

- fatigue
- anaemia
- weight loss
- infection
- painless lymphadenopathy (CLL)
- problems secondary to splenomegaly, e.g. abdominal discomfort.

MEDICAL MANAGEMENT

History and examination The patient may describe any of the above symptoms. Of patients with suspected CML, 90% will have splenomegaly and 50% will have hepatomegaly. For patients with suspected CLL, more than 66% of them will present with painless lymphadenopathy, infection and symptoms derived from bone marrow failure, e.g. anaemia, thrombocytopenia.

Investigations Diagnosis of either of these diseases will be confirmed by further investigations including peripheral blood count results, examination of a bone marrow aspirate, biochemistry results, CT scans and chest radiography.

Results of these tests indicating the presence of chronic leukaemia include:

- low haemoglobin
- abnormal white cell count which may be extremely high, e.g. $100 \times 10^9/L$
- low platelet count
- hypercellular bone marrow (CML)
- marrow infiltrated by lymphocytes (CLL)
- hyperuricaemia.

Treatment

CML For some time, the first line treatment for CML has been interferon which has been shown to have an anti-cancer effect, reduce white cell counts and induce remission in some patients although its mode of action is poorly understood (Howard & Hamilton 1997). For patients who fail to respond to interferon, a new medication called imatinib, which works by causing disruption to specific aspects of malignant cellular growth, has been found to give a progression free survival with fewer side-effects (Provan et al 2004). However, revised guidelines from the National Institute for Clinical Excellence (NICE) have now recommended imatinib as first line treatment for all patients with Philadelphia chromosome CML in the chronic phase (Campbell 2003).

Allogeneic transplantation is a potentially curative option and is recommended for younger patients that have a sibling donor. If undertaken when the patient is in chronic phase during first year of diagnosis, there is a 70% chance of cure (Mehta & Hoffbrand 2000). For those who do not have a sibling donor, matched unrelated donor stem cells or bone marrow will also provide the possibility of a cure, though the results are less encouraging (Treleaven 2000).

For patients whose disease transforms into acute leukaemia, treatment is highly problematic and may not be successful.

CLL Although there is no curative treatment for CLL, the administration of chemotherapy will control the disease. However, research suggests that treatment is harmful if administered in the early stage of the disease. Due to the older age of patients on presentation, approximately 50% will die of causes unrelated to CLL. When the disease does progress, treatment should be started. This may include splenectomy, leucopheresis and supportive care alongside the administration of chemotherapy and possibly allogeneic transplantation for a very limited number of patients (Breed 2003).

Examples of first line chemotherapy (Matutes & Dearden 2000) include:

- chlorambucil, an alkylating agent, *or*
- fludarabine, a purine analogue and cyclophosphamide
- a combination of cyclophosphamide, vincristine, doxorubicin (cytotoxic antibiotic) and prednisolone for its antitumour effect

followed, for younger patients, by autologous stem cell transplantation once remission has been achieved.

If these fail, second line treatment includes:

- a combination of fludarabine, cyclophosphamide and mitoxantrone (see Ch. 31)
- methylprednisolone alone.

The above medications are known for their antitumour effect in CLL if previous combinations are unsuccessful.

Supportive care may include the administration of intravenous immunoglobulin and antibiotics for patients experiencing recurrent infections, allopurinol to control hyperuricaemia, and radiotherapy.

Prognosis

The average survival for CML is 3–4 years, with transplantation offering a curative option for some patients.

CLL has a variable clinical course. Some patients may require little or no treatment for many years whereas others experience rapid disease progression.

NURSING PRIORITIES AND MANAGEMENT: Chronic leukaemia

Unless requiring intensive treatment, many patients remain at home. Some need little nursing care at home while others require considerable support as they cope with the reality of a life-threatening disease.

Hospital-based nurses may be involved in assisting with diagnostic procedures and investigations and the administration of supportive therapies such as antibiotic administration. However, if more intensive treatment or transplantation is pursued as a potentially curative option, nursing care will be more intensive and long term.

The nursing care required will include:

- giving information about tests, diagnosis and treatment options
- assisting in the administration of treatment
- providing psychological support to help the patient come to terms with a chronic and potentially life-threatening illness
- educating the patient about medication, including the importance of continuing with intermittent courses of chemotherapy, perhaps over several years
- supporting the patient who experiences concurrent symptoms, e.g. tiredness and abdominal discomfort
- giving advice about the level of work and activity that can realistically be attempted
- stressing the importance of follow-up in outpatient clinics.

LYMPHOMA

The lymphomas are a group of malignant disorders characterised by a proliferation of lymphoid cells originating in the lymph nodes or lymphoid tissue. Most often the disease is of B cell origin, more rarely of T cell origin.

Lymphoma is divided into:

- Hodgkin's lymphoma (Hodgkin's disease, HD)
- non-Hodgkin's lymphoma (NHL).

The incidence of HD is approximately 4–5 new cases per 100 000 of the population per year. It is most common among people between 20 and 30 or over 50 years of age and more common among men than women in the ratio of 1.5:1 (Pettengall 2000).

NHL is the more common of the lymphomas with approximately 11 new cases per 100 000 of the population per year (Dearden & Matutes 2000). Incidence increases with age and, as with HD, it seems to be more common in men than in women. The incidence of the disease has increased over the last 50 years, probably due to the incidence of HIV-related lymphoma.

Aetiology

Though the risk factors for HD and NHL remain unclear, several predisposing conditions have been identified including those related to genetic factors and exposure to viral infections and certain chemicals.

For further information see Dearden & Matutes (2000), Grundy (2000) and Pettengall (2000).

PATHOPHYSIOLOGY

In both HD and NHL, cells in the affected lymph tissue (usually lymph nodes) reveal a disruption of normal structure.

HD is characterised by the presence of large, multinucleated cells known as Reed–Sternberg cells within the lymphoma tumour mass. However, these are usually outnumbered by non-malignant cells such as lymphocytes, granulocytes, fibroblasts and plasma cells which are involved in mounting an immune response against the malignant cells. HD is classified according to a system known as the Revised European American Lymphoma classification (or the REAL classification) which uses morphological, immunological and genetic techniques to distinguish differences in the disease.

For further information, see Mehta & Hoffbrand (2000).

NHL is much harder to classify, which may explain why at least six different classifications have been devised over the years. Currently, the most commonly used system is the REAL classification (see above). In spite of the complications of classification, some generalisations can be made to divide NHL into 'high grade', 'intermediate grade' or 'low grade'. 'Low grade' lymphomas have the best prognosis, running an indolent course, whereas 'high grade' lymphomas are aggressive with an acute clinical onset. Paradoxically, 'high grade' lymphoma may be cured by and respond better to treatment than indolent disease, where relapse is common.

Common presenting symptoms

Hodgkin's disease For 80–90% of patients with HD, the most common manifestation of the disease is a painless enlarged lymph gland, often described as 'rubbery'. Such glands are found in the neck and supraclavicular fossae, axillae or inguinal regions. These may grow slowly or rapidly and compromise other organs by compression or obstruction.

Other symptoms include infection, pruritus and pain in the diseased lymph nodes on consuming alcohol. The reasons for this are unclear.

Non-Hodgkin's disease Patients with NHL may present similarly as for HD with painless lymphadenopathy. However, as extra-nodal disease is more common, a wider range of presenting symptoms may be seen such as:

- breathlessness — due to enlarged mediastinal lymph nodes or obstruction of the superior vena cava, affecting respiratory function
- oedema — especially of the limbs, due to lymph node obstruction
- backache — due to retroperitoneal lymph node enlargement
- acute or subacute bowel obstruction — due to small bowel lymphoma
- nausea, anorexia and upper abdominal discomfort — due to lymphoma of the stomach
- bone pain — due to bone involvement
- symptoms of anaemia — due to bone marrow involvement
- weakness or paralysis of one or more limbs (often involving both legs) — due to compression of spinal nerve roots
- infection caused by defective humoral and/or cell-mediated immunity (see Ch. 16).

Some patients, more commonly those with HD, also present with systemic symptoms medically known as B symptoms which may include one or more of the following:

- persistent unexplained fever of 38°C
- drenching night sweats requiring the patient to change bed linen and night clothes
- weight loss >10% of body weight.

These symptoms are significant when staging the disease and give some indication of prognosis.

MEDICAL MANAGEMENT

History and examination It can be very difficult to palpate certain lymph nodes and so clinical examination, which may also detect other signs of the disease, must be thorough.

Investigations Diagnosis is by means of:

- lymph node biopsy — undertaken as day case treatment, performed under local anaesthetic
- blood tests including full blood count, ESR and urea and electrolytes
- bone marrow aspiration (see p. 487)
- CT scan of chest, abdomen and pelvis
- Chest X-ray.

Staging of the disease After clinical examination and the results of investigations are known, the disease can be staged. This is done for both HD and NHL but is of more importance in HD. Staging establishes the extent of the disease by looking at the number and location of involved lymph nodes or extralymphatic sites and takes into account the presence or absence of B symptoms. This is known as the Cotswold Classification (see Box 11.7). Staging the disease in this way influences treatment options and prognosis.

Treatment

Hodgkin's disease Treatment depends on the stage of the disease. For early stage disease the following options are available.

- Radiotherapy alone may be used, localised on one side of the diaphragm (see Ch. 31). A mantle-shaped field is used to treat disease localised above the diaphragm and an inverted-Y field is used to treat disease localised below the diaphragm; however, approximately 30% of patients thus treated relapse.
- More often, the best choice of treatment for 'non-bulky' (i.e. small diseased lymph nodes) stage IA and IIA Hodgkin's disease is a short course of chemotherapy, aiming to eliminate disease outside the area targeted by radiotherapy, followed by localised radiotherapy.

Advanced stage disease is treated with combination chemotherapy, the most common combination used being ABVD, i.e. adriamycin (now known as doxorubicin), bleomycin (a cytotoxic antibiotic), vincristine, and dacarbazine

Box 11.7

Staging of lymphomas — the Cotswold Classification

Stage I	One lymph node involved or one extralymphatic site, e.g. stomach, Peyer's patches, thyroid
Stage II	Two or more lymph nodes involved but on the same side of the diaphragm or an extralymphatic site plus lymph nodes on the same side
Stage III	Lymph node involvement on both sides of the diaphragm with or without extralymphatic sites
Stage IV	Diffuse involvement of extralymphatic sites, e.g. bone marrow, liver

Associated with each stage will be either A (no symptoms) or B (fever, night sweats, >10% weight loss in preceding 6 months).

(an alkylating agent). The medications are usually given in 2-week pulses every 28 days for a total of six courses of treatment. If there is no response or the patient relapses, the combination of medications is changed.

Patients with 'bulky' (i.e. large diseased lymph nodes) mediastinal disease may be given chemotherapy followed by deep X-ray therapy.

Most of these treatments can be given on a day patient basis with no need for hospital admission unless side-effects of treatment occur, or the patient lives too far away to attend hospital on a day patient basis.

Patients who relapse post radiotherapy will be offered chemotherapy. Patients who relapse post chemotherapy for advanced disease may be offered high dose chemotherapy with autologous stem cell transplantation.

Non-Hodgkin's lymphoma Specific chemotherapy regimens are prescribed according to the type of lymphoma and the stage of the disease. Regimens are continually being refined as clinical understanding improves. A few examples of treatment are given here.

For further information, see Dearden & Matutes (2000).

- *'Low grade' NHL.* Patients who are asymptomatic with 'low grade' NHL are generally followed closely without treatment until symptoms, such as those listed previously (see p. 516) indicate the need. When required, chemotherapy will be administered either as single agents, e.g. chlorambucil, cyclophosphamide, fludarabine, or in combination, e.g. cyclophosphamide, doxorubicin, vincristine and prednisolone. Relapsed patients may respond to the same treatment that induced remission.
- *'High grade' NHL.* In the early stages of the disease combination chemotherapy is used with CHOP — i.e. **C**yclophosphamide, doxorubicin **H**ydrochloride (adriamycin), vincristine (**O**ncovin), **P**rednisolone — being the gold standard of treatment to date. For patients who relapse, further chemotherapy followed by autologous or allogeneic stem cell transplantation may be offered. Current research involving the use of monoclonal antibodies, e.g. rituximab, which target specific cells is being evaluated (Provan et al 2004).

Prognosis

Prognosis for HD depends on the stage of the disease. There is a >90% cure rate for patients with stage I and II disease but this falls to 50% for patients with stage IV disease (Mehta & Hoffbrand 2000).

For patients with NHL prognosis depends on the type of disease. Average survival rates for advanced 'low grade' NHL are 8–10 years. For advanced 'high grade' NHL, though remission rates are high at 80%, relapse occurs in 50% of patients within the first 5 years post treatment (Grundy 2000).

NURSING PRIORITIES AND MANAGEMENT: Lymphoma

Many patients with lymphoma are cared for in day bed units where they undergo diagnostic investigations and staging and receive subsequent treatment and follow-up. However, some patients will require admission to hospital, especially if they:

- live too far away from hospital to attend as a day patient
- are experiencing side-effects of radiotherapy treatment such as nausea, diarrhoea and fatigue which require medical intervention
- develop a significant infection after chemotherapy and require i.v. antibiotic therapy
- require high-dose chemotherapy and stem cell transplantation.

Nursing considerations

As lymphoma comprises such a diverse group of blood disorders and treatment is so varied, nursing care cannot be prescriptive. Some patients will remain independent of any nursing assistance, whereas others will be hospitalised throughout the course of treatment for their disease. Whether the patient is hospitalised or not, some generalisations can be made about nursing care offered. These include:

- explanation of diagnostic and staging investigations
- providing information about the disease itself
- administering specific treatment and managing side-effects with care and skill
- offering psychological support to patients who may be shocked by the possibility of serious illness
- enabling family and friends to care appropriately for their loved one.

After the course of treatment, nursing care may be required continually or intermittently. Patients should be given detailed information about post-radiotherapy/chemotherapy care. This should include the following information:

- a contact number when in need of advice
- the signs of infection or bleeding and who to contact should either of these occur
- medication and details about how and when to take it
- dietary advice
- level of activity and when to return to employment
- the importance of attendance at follow-up clinics
- appropriate self-help groups
- sexual counselling as appropriate
- referral to community nurse, social worker and GP.

Whatever the outcome of treatment, patients with HD or NHL require high-quality physical and psychological care from nursing staff who are able to recognise and meet their individual needs, values and concerns.

MYELOMA

Myeloma is an uncommon malignant disorder characterised by an abnormal and unregulated proliferation of plasma cells which develop from mature B lymphocytes. There are approximately 50 new cases per million population per year in the UK (Mehta & Hoffbrand 2000), the incidence increasing over the age of 40. It is a disease that is twice as common in people of Afro-Caribbean descent, less common in Asians (Provan et al 2004) and more prevalent in men than in women.

Aetiology

Though the cause of myeloma is unknown there appears to be some connection with occupational exposure to certain products, e.g. rubber, wood, textiles, petroleum and radiation (Dowling 2000).

PATHOPHYSIOLOGY

Normal plasma cells are present in bone marrow and develop from B lymphocytes following antigen stimulation. Each plasma cell produces a specific immunoglobulin with a specific immune function. In myeloma there is a malignant proliferation of one clone of plasma cells, which produce an immunoglobulin known as a paraprotein, which is incapable of normal function. Depending on the type secreted, the abnormal paraprotein may be detected in the serum and/or urine where it is referred to as Bence–Jones protein.

The plasma cells may form multiple tumours, plasmacytomas, in the bone — hence multiple myeloma — which have osteolytic properties and eventually erode the bone, resulting in lytic lesions.

Proliferation of the plasma cells and the production of an abnormal paraprotein lead to:

- infiltration of the bone marrow
- skeletal destruction
- high levels of the abnormal proteins in the blood, kidneys and other tissues
- depression in the production of immunoglobulins.

Each of these has pathological consequences as follows:

- Bone marrow infiltration will lead to pancytopenia
- Skeletal destruction will cause pain, hypercalcaemia (see Ch. 31) and pathological fractures
- Deposition of the abnormal proteins within the renal tubules may cause renal failure
- Abnormal proteins may lead to hyperviscosity of the blood, bleeding disorders and the presence of cryoglobulins, abnormal proteins which are insoluble at low temperatures and cause obstruction of the small blood vessels, and amyloidosis. Amyloidosis occurs when the abnormal protein accumulates, forming amyloid tissue which, if deposited in an organ, may lead to failure of function
- A reduction in immunoglobulin levels will immunocompromise the patient and increase the risk of infection.

Common presenting symptoms The most common presenting symptoms are:

- bone pain, especially in the lower back region, and pathological fractures
- spinal cord compression due to vertebral collapse
- anaemia, mediated by cytokines rather than by marrow replacement
- renal failure
- hypercalcaemia
- infection
- amyloidosis affecting the kidney and leading to proteinuria and nephrotic syndrome (see Ch. 8).

MEDICAL MANAGEMENT

History and examination The patient may have experienced symptoms for a number of months but may not have considered them significant enough to seek medical advice, e.g. back pain is often not reported until it becomes incapacitating. Alternatively, the patient may have been receiving treatment by a GP and/or physiotherapist for a condition which did not improve or even became worse.

Some patients have a history of 'sudden onset' bone pain caused by pathological fracture or experience extreme bone tenderness throughout the body. Others present with pneumonia due to neutropenia and lowered immunoglobulin levels, and yet others may present with clinical features of renal failure and/or hypercalcaemia.

Investigations To confirm a diagnosis of myeloma and determine its stage, evidence of two of the following three features is required:

- the presence of paraprotein
- lytic bone lesions
- infiltration of the bone marrow by excess plasma cells.

Evidence of the above will be determined by the following investigations:

- electrophoresis of the blood and urine
- skeletal survey and isotope bone scan (see Appendix 1)
- bone marrow aspiration and trephine biopsy.

To establish the systemic effect of myeloma on the body, the following tests are performed:

- full blood count
- serum urea and electrolytes
- serum calcium and alkaline phosphatase levels
- uric acid levels
- plasma viscosity.

Treatment Initial treatment for myeloma is aimed at controlling symptoms of the disease, particularly the presence of pain. Thereafter, although chemotherapy, radiotherapy and occasionally surgery are used, myeloma remains, with the rare exception of transplantation (see Box 11.7), an incurable disease (Dowling 2000).

Chemotherapy The most common chemotherapeutic agent used is the alkylating medication melphalan, usually given orally for a few days every month together with prednisolone, a steroid which potentiates the action of melphalan and appears to depress myeloma activity. Cyclophosphamide is also useful. However, none of these provides a long-term response and most patients experience a progression of their disease.

Younger patients able to tolerate more intensive treatment are offered vincristine and doxorubicin as a 4-day infusion together with a high dose of the steroid dexamethasone. This treatment has been shown to produce a rapid response for more than 75% of patients and is widely used prior to autologous transplantation.

Radiotherapy Radiotherapy is useful in the treatment of myeloma because it is a particularly radio-responsive disease. Specific bony lesions can be targeted, thus reducing bone deposits which will prevent fractures and reduce pain.

Surgery Internal fixation of fractured bones or areas of lytic lesions that are liable to fracture may be necessary to stabilise bones which are diseased.

Transplantation Allogeneic transplantation (see Box 11.7) offers a curative option for a small number of patients.

Younger patients under 55 years of age may be given intensive chemotherapy followed by a stem cell transplantation from an allogeneic sibling donor. Though relapses occur and transplant mortality is high, affecting approximately 30% of patients, more than 50% achieve complete remission (Samson 2000).

Autologous transplantation (see Box 11.7) can be given to patients under 65 years of age. Although this offers a survival benefit over conventional chemotherapy, it is not curative and all patients eventually relapse.

Plasmapheresis Plasmapheresis may be used to reduce a high blood viscosity, as the removal of the patient's plasma will also reduce the paraprotein level. This is done only as a temporary measure whilst other treatment is given.

Prognosis

Currently myeloma is an incurable disease, except perhaps for patients who have undergone transplantation when the median survival may be 3–4 years.

NURSING PRIORITIES AND MANAGEMENT: Myeloma

Myeloma is a serious disorder with multisystem effects, some of which are potentially life threatening. In order to plan and implement care, it is important that the nurse has a thorough knowledge of the disease and its effects on the patient.

Nursing considerations

Pain management

The most distressing symptom for the patient is often pain, which may have been present for some time. Assessment of pain must take this into account as the patient may well be exhausted and depressed by chronic pain (see Ch. 19). Pain management strategies will depend on the cause and level of distress associated with the pain. Strategies include the use of:

- radiotherapy to local bone lesions
- analgesics — opioids and non-steroidal anti-inflammatory drugs, the latter used with care as they have been associated with renal failure in older myeloma patients
- chemotherapy, which often alleviates pain soon after commencement
- lightweight braces which provide support for the spine for patients with multiple myeloma lesions.

Maintaining mobility whilst preventing fractures

Whilst prolonged periods of bed rest should be avoided, to prevent the increased risk of hypercalcaemia and pulmonary embolism, so too should too much activity which increases the risk of fracturing weak bones. Management should include:

- ensuring pain is controlled prior to attempting exercise and movement and being aware that increased activity may increase the level of pain and the need for analgesics
- working alongside the physiotherapist and occupational therapist in helping the patient attain an optimal level of activity
- maintaining a safe environment
- ensuring that a home assessment has been carried out prior to discharge for any adaptations that may be needed to facilitate access within the patient's home
- referring, if assessed as beneficial, to home care nursing staff when the patient is discharged.

The prevention of renal failure (see Ch. 8)

As renal failure is a common complication of myeloma caused by uric acid, calcium and Bence–Jones proteins, it is important that the patient is adequately hydrated. Since an intake of 3–4 litres of fluid a day is recommended, patients need to understand the need for this and be advised about strategies to maintain the high fluid intake, especially when they are at home.

When patients are in hospital receiving symptom control or chemotherapy, i.v. fluids may be necessary to ensure an adequate fluid intake.

Prevention of infection

Infection may be debilitating and occur frequently, most commonly affecting the respiratory and urinary tracts. Management strategies include:

- monitoring the patient for signs and symptoms of infection
- treating any infection promptly by i.v. antibiotics
- ensuring adequate hydration is maintained
- avoiding urinary catheterisation to prevent the possibility of infection
- maintaining a diet high in calories and protein to enable skeletal repair and to support the immune system.

Anaemia

Anaemia, causing fatigue, will be corrected by regular blood transfusion. Patients may need reassurance about the frequency of transfusion and to be assisted in establishing strategies to maximise their energy by ensuring adequate rest and minimising feelings of fatigue.

Prevention of hypercalcaemia (see Ch. 31)

Destruction of bone, leading to the liberation of excessive amounts of calcium, predisposes the patient to hypercalcaemia. This may be prevented by:

- encouraging an oral/i.v. intake of at least 3 litres of fluid daily
- encouraging physical activity which reduces the liberation of calcium
- observing the patient for signs and symptoms of hypercalcaemia, e.g. dehydration, confusion
- administering i.v. pamidronate promptly, if prescribed, to control the hypercalcaemia.

Prevention of spinal cord compression

This is regarded as an oncological emergency and occurs in 10–15% of patients with myeloma (Dowling 1997). Nurses need to know the signs and symptoms of this, commonly pain and sensorimotor impairment, and alert medical staff quickly as treatment *must* be prompt.

Communication
Good communication skills are vital to effective nursing intervention. On admission, in addition to coping with distressing and debilitating symptoms, the patient faces a diagnosis of a malignant disease which is probably incurable. Whether patients are young or old, the stress of ill-health and coming to terms with life-threatening illness will be keenly felt. Nursing management strategies include listening to the patient's anxieties — which may range from anxieties about their illness to financial worries or family issues — and answering questions honestly, in a way that is appropriate for the patient, bearing in mind that this may need to be repeated, further explained and/or written down.

Patient education
Acquiring knowledge about the disease and its management potentially helps the patient to feel more in control. In preparation for discharge, the patient should receive information about:

- the side-effects of treatment and how to self-monitor for these
- how to prevent or minimise complications, e.g. maintaining oral fluid and dietary intake
- safe techniques for moving and handling
- methods of reducing muscle weakness
- the importance of follow-up with the GP and attendance at outpatient clinics
- the availability of self-help groups (see Useful websites, p. 523).

Discharge planning
The nature of arrangements for discharge will depend on the patient's physical and psychological state, the type of treatment received and the availability of carers at home or in the community. Important aspects to consider in planning are:

- the level of dependency of the patient
- the availability of home carers and the type and degree of support needed by them, e.g. from Macmillan Nurses
- the skills to be learned by carers, e.g. safe moving and handling of the patient.

MYELODYSPLASTIC SYNDROMES (MDS)

These are a group of clonal disorders derived from an abnormal stem cell which retains the capacity to differentiate into end-stage cells. However, this differentiation is disordered and ineffective and leads to hypercellular bone marrow but cytopenic peripheral blood. Morphological abnormalities of red blood cells, white blood cells and platelets are common and these form the basis for diagnosis. During the course of MDS, the abnormal clone is prone to lose its ability to differentiate, with the disease transforming into acute leukaemia as occurs in approximately 10–40% of cases.

MDS is more common in men than women, and tends to be a disease affecting adults over 60 years of age. The annual incidence has been reported as four new cases per 100 000 population (Hamblin 2000), but as many cases remain undiagnosed, actual incidence is probably higher.

Aetiology
MDS occurs most often as a primary condition with an idiopathic cause, but it may also develop secondary to exposure to:

- cytotoxic medications, e.g. alkylating agents
- certain chemicals, e.g. benzene
- radiation.

PATHOPHYSIOLOGY
MDS occurs as a result of chromosomal damage, e.g. deletions on chromosomes 5 and 7, and genetic abnormalities which lead to more rapid cell division in the abnormal clone of cells as compared to normal cells. The disease is divided into five subgroups according to the FAB classification (Provan et al 2004).

For further information, see Mehta & Hoffbrand (2000).

Common presenting symptoms While some patients may present with symptoms of one or more of the cytopenic disorders, e.g. fatigue caused by anaemia or infection caused by neutropenia, others may be detected accidentally through routine blood tests carried out for other reasons.

MEDICAL MANAGEMENT

History and examination On presentation most patients are asymptomatic; the remainder may show signs and symptoms of bone marrow failure, infection, bruising or fatigue. In some cases hepatosplenomegaly may be present with occasional cases of gum hypertrophy, pleural and pericardial effusion, and painful, swollen joints.

Investigations Diagnosis is made on the basis of results from the following investigations:

- bone marrow aspiration and trephine biopsy, where morphological abnormalities and the degree of cellularity, e.g. hypercellular, will be detected
- full blood count revealing anaemia, neutropenia or thrombocytopenia
- MCV which is often raised
- vitamin B_{12} and folate levels to eliminate any deficiency that would affect the blood picture
- cytogenetic analysis, looking for chromosomal abnormalities.

Treatment Treatment is most often aimed at symptom relief. Interventions include:

- regular blood transfusion
- platelet transfusion administered prophylactically and when spontaneous bleeding occurs
- infection prevention strategies and prompt treatment in the event of infection
- the administration of colony stimulating factors such as GCSF and erythropoietin
- the administration of low dose or intensive chemotherapy, although neither of these proffers long-term survival
- allogeneic bone marrow transplantation, considered only for patients under 65 years due to the mortality and morbidity risks associated with this treatment

- autologous stem cell transplantation may be a future possibility for some patients with high risk MDS though further research is needed to determine the benefits of this (Burgoyne & Knight 2000).

Prognosis

The course and prognosis of MDS is variable, with some patients remaining stable for many years, whilst others experience rapid progression to AML. The majority of patients die within 2 years of diagnosis, the cause of death being more or less equally divided between:

- leukaemia occurring as a result of disease transformation
- complications of cytopenia
- unrelated causes such as cardiovascular disorders.

For younger patients who have undergone transplantation, cure rates of 40–45% have been quoted (Hamblin 2000) though treatment mortality increases with age.

Nursing management

The nursing priorities when caring for patients with MDS include:

- an understanding of the manifestation of the disease and its progression
- knowledge of treatment and supportive therapies
- the ability to educate the patient regarding treatment, nursing care and self-care
- the ability to support the patient through life-threatening illness.

As the care of patients with MDS is often shared between outpatient and inpatient services, it is essential that nursing staff in both areas share information about individual patients in order that they receive consistent care.

DISORDERS OF PLATELETS AND COAGULATION

Disorders of coagulation can be subdivided into three types:

- disorders due to lack of clotting factors
- platelet disorders
- disorders due to another cause, e.g. liver disorders.

These disorders may be inherited or acquired. All age groups are affected, but some coagulation disorders are sex-linked; for example, haemophilia occurs only in males but is genetically carried by females.

CLOTTING FACTOR DISORDERS

These disorders involve a deficiency in one or more of the blood factors required for haemostasis: inherited clotting disorders result from the lack of specific clotting factors; the acquired disorders involve the failure of certain clotting factors to be activated usually as a result of vitamin K deficiency or liver disease.

Haemophilia

The haemophilias are a group of inherited disorders in which there is a lifelong deficiency of one of the substances necessary to blood clotting. These deficiencies include (see Ch. 6):

- haemophilia A — lack of factor VIII
- haemophilia B or Christmas disease — lack of factor IX
- von Willebrand's disease — lack of von Willebrand factor, which is necessary for normal platelet adhesion and factor VII production; it is not sex-linked.

PLATELET DISORDERS

Thrombocytopenic purpura (TCP)

Any disturbance in the number or function of circulating platelets will affect the normal coagulation process (see p. 483). The condition thrombocytopenia implies a reduction in the number of platelets and may be either inherited or acquired.

PATHOPHYSIOLOGY

Inherited TCP is fortunately rare. Acquired TCP may occur as a result of factors which either decrease normal platelet production or increase platelet destruction (see Box 11.8). Decreased production is usually caused by drugs or some other agent whereby the bone marrow is suppressed. The most common form of TCP due to increased platelet destruction is idiopathic thrombocytopenic purpura (ITCP). This commonly affects individuals in their teens or early 20s and is thought to be autoimmune in origin. Whatever the cause, TCP will result in a prolonged bleeding time, which may give rise to bruising, purpura or petechiae. Less obviously, visceral bleeding can also occur.

Common presenting symptoms include a history of bleeding episodes, e.g. bleeding gums, epistaxis, melaena

Box 11.8

Causes of acquired thrombocytopenia

- Decrease in platelet production
- Aplastic anaemia
- Vitamin B_{12}, folic acid deficiency
- Bone marrow infiltration
  - — leukaemia and lymphoma
  - — carcinoma
  - — myelofibrosis: formation of fibrous tissue within the bone marrow cavity
- Other disorders
  - — viral infection
  - — bacterial infection
- Platelet destruction
- Idiopathic autoimmune disorder
- Idiopathic thrombocytopenic purpura (ITCP)
- Large-volume blood transfusion — due to the short life span of platelets, there may be no viable platelets in the blood transfusion units and the patient will, if requiring a large volume of blood, have insufficient platelets
- Disseminated intravascular coagulation (DIC) (see Ch. 29)

and haematuria. In contrast to haemophilia, if pressure is applied to the bleeding point, bleeding will stop and not recur unless further trauma occurs. As with leukaemia, symptoms of anaemia may be presenting features in chronic thrombocytopenia.

MEDICAL MANAGEMENT

History and examination A careful clinical history is required, especially to pinpoint any recent minor illness or drug therapy, including over-the-counter medicines. Thorough clinical examination is carried out to detect any signs of bruising, petechiae, purpura or any underlying disorder.

Investigations include:

- full blood count to identify low platelet count or anaemia and to exclude any other blood disorder
- coagulation screen to exclude other coagulation disorders.

Treatment Some cases of TCP resolve spontaneously, possibly because the formation of antibodies against the person's own platelet membrane antigens is transient. However, TCP usually becomes a chronic condition. In cases where an exacerbating factor such as a medication or chemical is withdrawn, spontaneous remission may also occur.

Steroid therapy may be given until resolution occurs, as steroids improve platelet survival. Response to steroid therapy is usually seen within days or weeks; however, thrombocytopenia may recur when the steroids are withdrawn.

Immunoglobulin G i.v. may be given for 3–5 days (see Ch. 16). Splenectomy may be required, as the spleen is a major site of platelet destruction. Platelet transfusions are given if bleeding is severe.

NURSING PRIORITIES AND MANAGEMENT: Thrombocytopenic purpura (TCP)

Nursing considerations

In hospital

Nursing priorities during the patient's stay in hospital include the following:

- Controlling superficial bleeding by application of external pressure. The bleeding tendency is not generally life threatening.
- Observing the patient for evidence of bleeding, and determining severity of bleeding by means of:
  - regular monitoring of patient's pulse during diagnostic stage and initial treatment. Blood pressure is not usually measured as this may cause bruising and petechiae
  - daily inspection of the skin for petechiae, purpura and bruises, and of the mouth for bleeding and infection. Precautions must be taken to minimise the occurrence of infection in soft tissue which has been damaged
  - regular testing of urine, stools and vomit for less obvious sources of blood loss.
- Being alert to complaints of headaches and drowsiness, as these may indicate cerebral bleeding.
- Ensuring that the patient is protected from injury by advising on environmental hazards and that feelings of faintness may indicate anaemia or low blood pressure.
- Giving explanations and support during tests and treatment, and looking and listening for indications of anxiety.

Discharge planning

The aim of discharge planning is to enable the patient to make the transition from dependence upon the nurse to monitor the condition to becoming competent and confident in self-monitoring. The importance of monitoring all bleeding episodes must be stressed, along with the need for regular follow-up to assess platelet levels.

Precautions which the patient should be advised to take include:

- taking medicines as prescribed
- avoiding aspirin preparations
- avoiding i.m. injections
- carrying identification, e.g. Medic-Alert bracelet
- minimising potential for soft tissue injury
- avoiding contact sports.

The family should be included in the patient's education programme to ensure that all members of the household understand the necessity of certain restrictions upon lifestyle. However, it should also be stressed that it is important for the patient to maintain a balance between being overcautious on the one hand and taking unnecessary risks on the other.

The aim of rehabilitation is to allow the patient to achieve an optimal level of function until spontaneous recovery or throughout the remainder of life.

REFERENCES

Beretta R 2003 Assessment: the foundation of good practice. In: Hinchcliffe S, Norman S, Schrober J (eds) Nursing practice and health care, 4th edn. Arnold, London
Breed C D 2003 Diagnosis, treatment and nursing care of patients with chronic leukaemia. Seminars in Oncology Nursing 19(2): 109–117
Burgoyne T, Knight A 2000 Myelodysplastic syndromes. In: Grundy M (ed) Nursing in haematological oncology. Baillière Tindall, Edinburgh
Campbell K 2003 Revised advice on use of imatinib for chronic myeloid leukaemia. Nursing Times 99(41): 20–21
Craig J I, Haynes A P, McClelland D B L et al 2002 Blood disorders. In: Haslett C, Chilvers E R, Boon N A et al (eds) Davidson's principles and practice of medicine, 19th edn. Churchill Livingstone, Edinburgh
Dearden C, Matutes E 2000 Non-Hodgkin's lymphoma. Medicine 28(3): 71–78
Dowling M 1997 Multiple myeloma. Professional Nurse 12(5): 354–357
Dowling M 2000 Myeloma. In: Grundy M (ed) Nursing in haematological oncology. Baillière Tindall, Edinburgh
Eilers J, Berger A M, Peterson M C 1988 Development, testing and application of the oral assessment guide. Oncology Nursing Forum 15(3): 325–330
Foster R 2002 Fertility issues in patients with cancer. Cancer Nursing Practice 1(1): 26–30
Grundy M (ed) 2000 The lymphomas. In: Nursing in haematological oncology. Baillière Tindall, Edinburgh

Hamblin T J 2000 Myelodysplastic disorders. Medicine 28(3): 54–57
Hamilton H 2000 Venous access. In: Grundy M (ed) Nursing in haematological oncology. Baillière Tindall, Edinburgh
Hart S 2000 Prevention of infection. In: Grundy M (ed) Nursing in haematological oncology. Baillière Tindall, Edinburgh
Hoffbrand A, Provan D 1997 ABC of clinical haematology macrocytic anaemias. British Medical Journal 314: 430–455
Hoffbrand A, Pettit J E, Moss P A H 2001 Essential haematology, 4th edn. Blackwell Scientific, London
Howard M R, Hamilton P J 1997 Haematology. Churchill Livingstone, Edinburgh
Jamieson E M, McCall J M, Whyte C A 2002 Clinical nursing practices, 4th edn. Churchill Livingstone, Edinburgh
Jehovah's Witness 2003 Showing respect for life and blood. www.watchtower.org/library/rq/article_12.htm
Matutes E, Dearden C 2000 Chronic lymphocytic leukaemia. Medicine 28(3): 65–67
Medical Research Council Working Party on Leukaemias in Adults 1995 UKALL XII protocol for adult patients with acute lymphoblastic leukaemia under 56 years of age. MRC, London
Medical Research Council Working Party on Leukaemias in Adults 2001 AML 15 protocol for adults with acute myeloblastic leukaemia under 60 years of age. MRC, London
Mehta A, Hoffbrand V 2000 Haematology at a glance. Blackwell, Oxford
Midence K, Elander J 1996 Adjustment and coping in adults with sickle cell disease: an assessment of research evidence. British Journal of Health Psychology 1: 95–111
Palmer K R, Penman I D 2002 Alimentary tract and pancreatic diseases. In: Haslett C, Chilvers E R, Boon N A et al (eds) Davidson's principles and practice of medicine, 19th edn. Churchill Livingstone, Edinburgh
Parker-Williams E J 2000 Investigation and management of anaemia. Medicine 28(2): 14–20
Pettengall R 2000 Hodgkin's disease. Medicine 28(3): 68–71
Provan D, Singer C R J, Baglin T et al 2004 Oxford handbook of clinical haematology. Oxford University Press, Oxford
Samson D 2000 Multiple myeloma. Medicine 28(3): 78–81
Serious Hazards of Transfusion 2003 SHOT report 2001/2002 www.shot uk.org
Skinner S 1998 Understanding drug therapies: a handbook for nursing practice. Baillière Tindall, London
Stull D M 2003 Targeted therapies for the treatment of leukaemia. Seminars in Oncology Nursing 19(2): 90–97
Summerton C, Shetty P, Sandle L N et al 2002 Nutritional, metabolic and environmental disease. In: Haslett C, Chilvers E R, Boon N A et al (eds) Davidson's principles and practice of medicine, 19th edn. Churchill Livingstone, Edinburgh
Tortora G J, Derrickson B 2006 Principles of anatomy and physiology, 11th edn. John Wiley, New York
Treleaven J 2000 Chronic myeloid leukaemia. Medicine 28(3): 63–67
Treleaven J, Mellor S 2000 Acute leukaemia. Medicine 28(3): 58–62
Viele C S 2003 Diagnosis, treatment and nursing care of acute leukaemia. Seminars in Oncology Nursing 19(2): 98–108
Waugh A, Grant A 2001 Ross and Wilson's anatomy and physiology in health and illness, 9th edn. Churchill Livingstone, Edinburgh

FURTHER READING

Bratt-Wyton B 2000 The leukaemias. In: Grundy M (ed) Nursing in haematological oncology. Baillière Tindall, Edinburgh
Dearden C, Matutes E 2000 Non-Hodgkin's lymphoma. Medicine 28(3): 71–78
Dougherty L, Lister S 2004 The Royal Marsden NHS Trust manual of clinical nursing procedures, 6th edn. Blackwell, Oxford
Fox B A, Cameron A G 1995 Food science, nutrition and health, 6th edn. Edward Arnold, London
Gray A, Illingworth J 2004 Right blood, right patient, right time. RCN guidance for improving transfusion practice. Royal College of Nursing, London. Online. Available: www.rcn.org.uk/members/downloads/rightblood.pdf
Grundy M (ed) 2000 Nursing in haematological oncology. Baillière Tindall, Edinburgh
Hoffbrand A, Pettit J E, Moss P A H 2001 Essential haematology, 4th edn. Blackwell Scientific, London
Kirschbaum M 1998 Neutropenia: more than a low neutrophil count. European Journal of Oncology Nursing 2(2): 115–122
Mehta A, Hoffbrand V 2000 Haematology at a glance. Blackwell, Oxford
Outhwaite H 2000 Blood and bone marrow transplantation. In: Grundy M (ed) Nursing in haematological oncology. Baillière Tindall, Edinburgh
Pettengall R 2000 Hodgkin's disease. Medicine 28(3): 68–71
Provan D, Singer C R J, Baglin T et al 2004 Oxford handbook of clinical haematology. Oxford University Press, Oxford
Tortora G J, Derrickson B 2006 Principles of anatomy and physiology, 11th edn. John Wiley, New York
UK MAGIC Project IMF UK www.ukmf.org.uk/guidelines/gdmm.shtml
Waters J, Thomas V 1995 Pain from sickle cell crisis. Nursing Times 91(16): 29–31
Waugh A, Grant A 2001 Ross and Wilson's anatomy and physiology in health and illness, 9th edn. Churchill Livingstone, Edinburgh
Wilkins P 2000 Blood component support. In: Grundy M (ed) Nursing in haematological oncology. Baillière Tindall, Edinburgh
Workman M L, Ellerhost-Ryan J, Hargrave-Koertge V 1993 Nursing care of the immunocompromised patient. Saunders, London

USEFUL WEBSITES

CancerBACUP
www.cancerbacup.org.uk

Leukaemia Research Fund
www.lrf.org.uk

Leukaemia Care Society
www.leukaemiacare.org.uk

Lymphoma Association
www.lymphoma.org.uk

Myeloma Society
www.myeloma.org.uk

Sickle Cell Society
www.sicklecellsociety.org.uk

SKIN DISORDERS

12

Barbara E. Page

INTRODUCTION

Intact skin is vital to health and well-being. As the largest organ in the body, weighing approximately 4 kg, containing over a million nerve endings and having a surface area of 2 m^2, the skin has many vital functions (Hughes & Van Onselen 2001):

- sensation
- temperature regulation
- synthesis of vitamin D
- insulation and protection of internal organs
- barrier to harmful external factors.

Skin disorders range from minor conditions, resolved with over-the-counter (OTC) preparations, to potentially life-threatening skin conditions requiring intensive treatment in specialist units. Many conditions are of a cyclical long-term nature with patients requiring care in different settings: ward, outpatient treatment centre and community. This chapter aims to introduce dermatology nursing by discussing the most common conditions encountered. Dermatology as a visual specialty may require the reader to consult a colour atlas (Graham-Brown & Bourke 1998, White 2003).

Nurses in every specialty encounter individuals with skin disorders, creating opportunities to detect early disease, give knowledgeable treatment advice and provide emotional support to patients and family members coping with chronic conditions. A good knowledge base helps the nurse to dispel myths about the contagious nature of skin disorders, as the social and psychological implications of skin disease should not be dismissed lightly. Success, power and achievement are often dependent on appearance and 'image'. The media support images of the soft-skinned baby, blemish-free teenager, the smooth sophisticated adult and such images are reflected in money spent by both genders to achieve cosmetic perfection. Dermatology research has investigated the quality of life of patients with skin disorders and has recorded the impact of skin disease on an individual's life. The experience of skin disease may restrict social, professional and personal activities and impact on careers and relationships. Problems with sexuality and relationships can be linked to low self-esteem and the self-concept of an altered body image associated with having a skin condition (Marks 2003). The psychological morbidity of skin disease is often unrecognised by professionals (Lewis-Jones 1999) despite patients actively reporting their experiences of ostracism, stigmatisation and isolation — the 'unclean' leper status of having a skin disorder. The person with a skin disorder has to cope with the physical problem and its associated complex therapies while being confronted with psychological, social and cultural rejection.

STOP THINK **12.1** Before reading further, try this exercise. You are in a communal changing room in a busy clothes shop when you realise the person trying on clothes next to you has a generalised rash. It appears to be very itchy, and as the person scratches, numerous flakes of skin are shed. Stop now and write down your immediate reaction to this scenario. Ask your colleagues to join you in this exercise.

Repeat this exercise when you have read through this chapter. Evaluate any changes in your answer.

Epidemiology

Skin disease is common and its prevalence is such that approximately 20% of the UK population have a skin disorder meriting medical management. The type, incidence and prevalence of skin disorders depend on social, economic, geographical, racial and cultural factors (Gawkrodger 2003). Internal and external factors contributing to skin disorders are summarised in Figure 12.1. The economic implications of skin disease can be considerable for individuals, families and employers. Skin diseases are the most common group of occupational health problems leading to absence from work. Industrial-acquired dermatoses lead to lost working time and often to compensation claims as work-induced disorders.

Age is an important factor in diagnosing disorders, with some conditions being exclusive to a particular age group, and others persisting throughout life. Atopic eczema, for example, is most common in infancy, while acne develops in adolescence and normally wanes by the late 20s. Middle age brings pemphigus and malignant melanoma. Older people show expected degenerative skin changes, with 27% having malignant skin lesions. Psoriasis and eczema occur in all age groups and can be cyclical in nature throughout life.

Research confirms malignant melanoma as a significant health problem in white adults, affecting 3% of that population and accounting for two-thirds of deaths from skin cancer (p. 549). In 1992, in response to the rise in skin cancer, the government defined a target and key actions to be taken to 'halt the year on year increase in the incidence of skin cancer by the year 2005' (DH 1992). Current UK campaigns aim to change social behaviour in relation to sunlight by educating the public that a suntan is a sign of damaged skin rather than a desirable fashion statement. The SunSmart Campaign (Cancer Research UK 2003) encourages people to protect themselves and their children from the sun's harmful rays and so reduce their risk of skin cancer. They stress the importance of the individual being aware of the appearance of their own moles, emphasising the fact that all moles change slowly over the years. People should be alert for specific changes, a vital factor in early detection of melanoma (see p. 550). Travel leaflets now promote sunscreens and avoidance of sunburn.

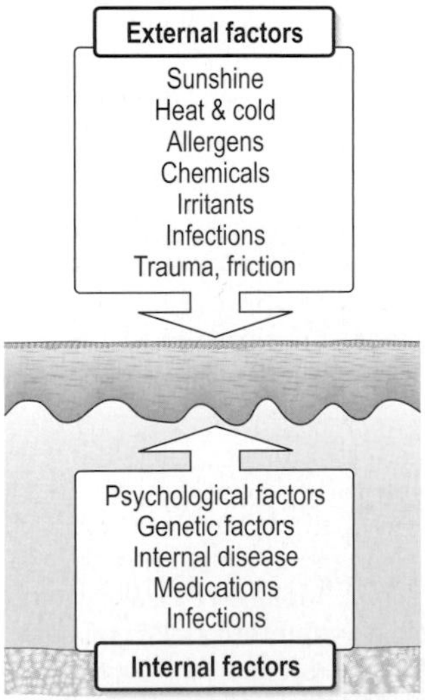

Fig. 12.1 Internal and external factors causing skin disease. (Adapted from Hunter et al 2002, with permission from Blackwell Science Ltd.)

Genetic or hereditary factors can be relevant to the diagnosis, and a family history should be part of the assessment. Patients with skin disorders report stress as a contributory factor in creating or exacerbating their condition, e.g. divorce, trauma, bereavement, exams. Psychological stress is common, but while psychological problems can make conditions worse, most skin disorders are stressful conditions in their own right. Certain skin disorders are recognised as being entirely of psychogenic origin, e.g. dermatitis artefacta, trichotillomania and dysmorphobia.

Social factors are relevant to skin disorders, and improvements in standards of living, personal hygiene and nutrition have reduced the rate of certain skin disorders (Gawkrodger 2003). The current rise in the number of patients with asthma and eczema appears to be associated with increasing affluence and these might now be considered as diseases of the advantaged. Unemployment and low wages restrict job mobility and the patient with acquired industrial skin disease may have difficulty in making appropriate job changes to alleviate the condition. Continuing rises in prescription charges may force patients into decisions about which of the prescribed medications they can afford. Skin care prescriptions often involve combinations of preparations, and anecdotal evidence suggests that patients choose those parts of the prescription they can best afford, thus preventing full management of a skin disorder. Homelessness and poor housing create problems in maintaining skin care, the former often resulting in limited access to medical care. Nurses working with vulnerable client groups need to be aware of such issues.

The nurse's role

Since publication of the Patients' Charter (DH 1991), patients with skin disorders and associated support groups have asserted their right to access specialist staff and be nursed in specialist areas (DH 2004). Inpatient hospital management is an effective method of targeting, educating and training the patient in skin management techniques. Cure is not a word widely used in dermatology due to the cyclical nature of many conditions, so nurses involved in care often forge long-term relationships with patients. Nurses with dermatology experience of chronic skin disease can, through holistic practice, help patients who require sympathy, empathy and guidance from specialist practitioners who have the time, knowledge and willingness to share clinical skills with this motivated client group. Kurwa and Finlay (1995) reported inpatient management as improving quality of life for dermatology patients, while peer group interaction between patients in dermatology wards is recognised as a beneficial adjunct to therapy.

The role of the dermatology liaison nurse is now well established (Lawton 2004). The liaison role focuses on the sharing of specialist knowledge and skills, resulting in a seamless transition of care and the removal of arbitrary barriers that used to coexist between care settings (Ruane-Morris et al 1995). The supportive role of nurses in primary care is vital. Patients referred to dermatologists reflect a small minority of people with skin disorders. Self-medication, OTC therapies (Nathan 1996) and nurse prescribing mean that, for many, community pharmacists and community teams are the first point of contact for most patients. The liaison nurse uses educational input to support the primary care team in providing information and therapies that are valid, accurate and up to date and, in an advisory and consultative capacity, helps sustain continuity of care (Stone 1997a). This independent role means availability to visit patients' homes, nursing homes, schools and places of work and provides expertise to reduce the fragmented care that sometimes exists in primary care settings. The NMC *Code of Professional Conduct* (2004) supports dermatology nurse practitioners in extending nurse-led initiatives in many areas of clinical practice (Legge 1997) including:

- nurse-led clinics for chronic disease management (eczema, psoriasis, acne), leg ulcers, cryosurgery (local freezing with liquid nitrogen), skin biopsy, iontophoresis (treatment for excessive sweating)
- laser therapy
- nurse counselling
- nurse-led phototherapy
- patient education programmes
- nurse prescribing.

Nurses are therefore an important group within the dermatology team, playing a vital role in the provision of direct specialised care.

ANATOMY AND PHYSIOLOGY

Structure of the skin

Originally formed from the embryonic ectoderm and mesoderm, skin is composed of two layers: epidermis and dermis. Beneath these layers, a bed of subcutaneous fat protects and insulates the underlying organs.

The epidermis

The epidermis is composed of stratified epithelium and varies in thickness between different parts of the body, e.g. the skin on the palms and soles is thicker than that on the face or back. There are no blood vessels in the epidermis, the cells being nourished by means of diffusion of materials. Structures tracking through the epidermis include hair follicles and sweat and sebaceous glands (see Fig. 12.2A). The epidermis is composed of several layers, its health depending on three factors involving these layers (Waugh & Grant 2001):

- regular division and migration of epidermal cells to the skin surface
- gradual keratinisation of these cells
- desquamation or rubbing away of these cells.

The layers of the epidermis are as follows (see Fig. 12.2B):

Basal layer (stratum basale) The cells lying nearest the dermis form the germinative layer where cell division occurs. Cells migrate upwards from this layer, becoming keratinised over a period of 21–28 days before being shed.

Prickle cell layer (stratum spinosum) Cells in this layer appear to be connected by fine processes or prickles. These intercellular connections act as protection against shearing forces or trauma to the skin.

Granular layer (stratum granulosum) Within this layer, fine granules form in the cells. This granular substance, keratohyalin, is a precursor of keratin, which gradually replaces the cytoplasm of the cells.

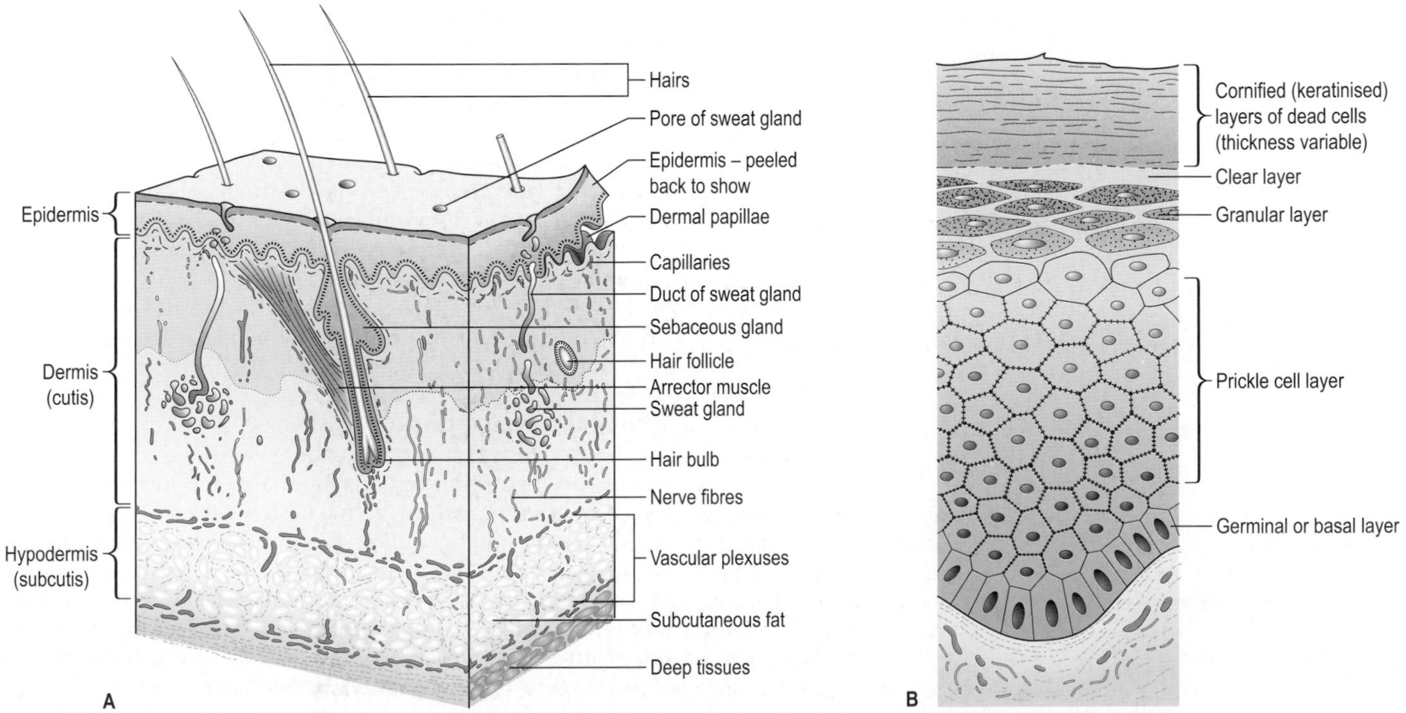

Fig. 12.2 A: The structure of the skin. B: The layers of the epidermis.

Clear cell layer (stratum lucidum) This layer is present only where the skin is thickened, e.g. the soles of feet. The cells exhibit nuclear degeneration and contain large amounts of keratin. Injury or friction to the skin increases the production of these cells, resulting in a callus or corn.

Horny layer (stratum corneum) This layer is composed of thin, flat, non-nucleated cells, the cytoplasm of which has been totally replaced by keratin.

The epidermal/dermal junction is convoluted into dips and ridges called rete pegs, which help to prevent damage to the skin from shearing forces. The configuration of these ridges is visible at the epidermal surface as corresponding characteristic, individualised patterns, e.g. at the fingertips.

The dermis

The dermis is composed of fibrous connective tissue providing a supportive meshwork for the structures and organs within. The papillary layer has many capillaries and lies next to the basal layer of the epidermis. The reticular layer, lying above the subcutaneous fat layer, has fewer blood vessels and is less reactive.

The ground substance of the dermis is a jelly-like material acting as a support and a transport medium. It functions as a water reservoir which may be utilised by the body in an emergency, e.g. during haemorrhage (see Ch. 18).

Tissue mast cells are often found near hair follicles and blood vessels, producing heparin and histamine when damaged.

Tissue macrophages have the protective function of engulfing foreign particles within the dermis.

Collagen fibres Ascorbic acid (vitamin C) is required by fibroblasts to generate these strong fibres, which bind with water molecules to give skin its tight, 'plump' appearance; 40–80% of the total body water is thought to be accommodated within the dermis. Wrinkling is thought to occur when collagen fibres lose their water-binding properties. They may also rupture during growth spurts, pregnancy or obesity, leaving fine white scar-like striae, recognised as abdominal stretch marks in pregnant women.

Elastin fibres These yellow fibres, also formed by fibroblasts, are bound loosely around bundles of collagen and, in combination with the ground substance and collagen, help the dermis to maintain its characteristic properties.

Lymph vessels play a major role in draining excess tissue fluid and plasma proteins from the dermis, thereby maintaining correct volume and composition of tissue fluids.

Nerve endings Specialised sensory receptors present in the dermis and basal layer of the epidermis detect mechanical and thermal changes (see Ch. 22).

Glands

Sweat glands are coiled tubes of epithelial tissue opening as pores onto the skin surface. They have individual nerve and blood supplies and secrete a slightly acid fluid containing excess excretory products (water and salts). Sweat also helps to keep keratin supple. Sweat glands are of two types: eccrine and apocrine. Eccrine glands are controlled by the sympathetic nervous system, producing secretions in response to temperature elevation or fear. Release of latent heat by the evaporation of sweat helps to lower body temperature. Apocrine glands in the pubic and axillary areas are not functional until puberty. They are thought to secrete pheromones, chemical signals released into the external environment.

The sebaceous glands are lined with epidermal tissue, secreting sebum, a greasy, slightly acid substance which helps to form a waterproof covering over the skin and, like sweat, to keep the keratin supple. The acid sebum has antibacterial and antifungal properties. Most sebaceous glands open into hair follicles. Sebum production is influenced by sex hormone levels.

Functions of the skin

Protection

The skin has several protective properties. The greasy horny layer forms a waterproof seal against undue entry or loss of water. The skin surface protects against microorganisms (through its acidity) and acts as a barrier to chemicals, gases and gamma and beta rays. Internal organs are shielded by the skin from minor mechanical blows, and repeated pressure or friction stimulates an increase in cell division, producing thickened areas of skin, e.g. corns and calluses. Melanin produced in the basal layer of the epidermis screens the dermis from ultraviolet rays.

Sensation

Nerve endings present throughout the dermis and basal epidermis continually monitor the environment and are most highly concentrated in areas such as the fingertips and lips. Innervated hair follicles help the individual to avoid injury by stimulating reflex action in response to touch.

Formation of vitamin D

Epidermal cells synthesise 7-dehydrocholesterol, which is slowly converted to vitamin D when skin is exposed to ultraviolet rays. Circulatory vitamin D, in combination with phosphorus and calcium, is essential to the formation of healthy bone. Deficiencies can lead to the development of disorders such as rickets and osteomalacia. Excess vitamin D, a fat soluble vitamin, is stored in the liver.

Temperature regulation (see Ch. 22)

Core body temperature is usually static at around 37°C. Heat is produced in the body by the metabolic processes of the liver, muscles and digestive system. Temperature is controlled by the heat-regulating centre in the hypothalamus, which responds to changes in the temperature of circulating blood and influences cardiovascular centres in the medulla oblongata. These centres control the size of the lumen of the arteries and arterioles and thereby control the rate of blood flow through the capillary beds in the dermis.

In cold conditions heat is retained by vasoconstriction and generated by the involuntary muscular action of shivering. During overheating, sweating is induced and vasodilatation occurs. As sweat evaporates from the skin, latent heat is lost from the skin surface, causing it to cool. Vasodilatation allows large quantities of blood to circulate in the uppermost layers of the dermis. Heat is then lost through convection, radiation and conduction. Blood flow is controlled by precapillary sphincters via constriction or relaxation, directing blood either to the capillary bed closer to the skin surface (resulting in maximum heat loss) or to the deeper tissues of the skin (minimising heat loss).

Other functions

During starvation, subcutaneous fat is utilised both as an energy source and as a water reserve. Water can also be mobilised from the dermis during haemorrhage or shock. The skin also has an excretory function, with urea and salts being excreted in small amounts through sweat.

SKIN ASSESSMENT

In completing a comprehensive skin assessment, it is important to obtain a full history, which should include:

- onset, initial site and duration of the condition
- associated symptoms, e.g. itch, redness
- actions that worsen the condition, e.g. sunlight exposure
- family history, e.g. genetic predisposition, allergies
- associated systemic disorders, e.g. asthma, hay fever
- current medication — oral and topical therapies, prescribed and OTC
- social history — occupation, hobbies, housing, alcohol/drug intake
- impact of the disorder on daily life — personal coping strategies, self-esteem and self-image.

The history should reveal the person's description and understanding of the disorder as well as their perception of living with it. An effective assessment should determine the impact of the skin disorder on those around the patient. Skin disease, with all its social implications, has a major cultural impact that varies tremendously within our multicultural society. For example, in Asian society, skin disease may impact negatively on arranged marriages or payment of dowries for brides (Barker 1995). Cultural beliefs need to be identified if treatment programmes are to be adapted to acknowledge such issues. It is important to ask patients what they have already used to treat their skin disorder. Many OTC preparations or treatments, borrowed from well-meaning friends, can exacerbate an existing skin condition. When examining skin, the nurse must have a knowledge of 'normal' skin to be able to identify the abnormal. The entire skin surface is examined to determine the extent of the disorder. Palpation of skin lesions will determine changes in skin texture with associated crusting or scaling.

Refer to Gawkrodger (2003), pp. 14–15, for a diagrammatic representation of, and terminology associated with, dermatological lesions.

In skin disorders, the term 'lesion' describes a small area of disease, while an 'eruption' or 'rash' describes widespread skin involvement. Skin assessment includes routine examination of the hair and nails as changes can aid diagnosis, e.g. nail changes in psoriasis or fungal infection. The distribution of lesions can vary. Psoriasis tends to localise on the outer aspects of elbows and knees, while eczema is most common in the skin flexures.

During assessment, the nurse should recognise that skin changes can be a manifestation of systemic disorders, e.g. T-cell lymphoma (see Ch. 11). Peters (2001) reminds the nurse to recognise the wide diversity of skin colour and differences in pigmentation in our multiracial society. The physiology of the disorder will be the same, but differences in pigmentation can influence skin changes during illness. Skin assessment methods must be pertinent to racial groups. Communication with patients is important for accurate assessment, as a patient's description of symptoms is relevant to diagnosis and management. Initial nursing management involves alleviation of distressing symptoms while awaiting diagnosis.

The nurse should also recognise that the effect of the physical appearance of a skin disorder on quality of life is often viewed by the patient as being of greater importance than the discomfort of having abnormal skin (Lewis-Jones 1999).

PRINCIPLES OF THERAPY IN SKIN DISORDERS

This section looks briefly at the available therapies and the basic principles of application.

Topical therapy

The skin as the target organ of treatment is readily accessible and the pathology of many skin disorders requires topical therapy as the first line of management. Topical therapy describes all treatments applied directly to skin. The classification of topical preparations is outlined in Box 12.1, and the advantages and disadvantages in using topical therapies are outlined in Box 12.2.

Emollients — agents which moisturise and lubricate the skin — are the mainstay of dermatology treatment. They can be used in skin maintenance programmes and are vital in preparing the skin for the specific therapies available for different disorders, e.g. tar, steroids. The choice of emollient depends on the disorder:

- dry, hyperkeratotic skin — use oily occlusive ointments
- flaky rough excoriated skin — use grease-based preparations

Box 12.1

Classification of topical preparations

- Creams — have a light effect due to high water content. They rub in easily and cool the skin
- Lotions — used if skin is 'weeping'. Good for scalp treatment as they are not greasy to apply
- Ointments — greasy preparations used as a base for the drug being applied. They last for 6–8 h on the skin, encouraging absorption by a barrier effect
- Pastes — ointments applied to medicated bandages for occlusive use or used in combination as a stiffer paste to apply treatment directly to lesions. This permits a slower, more effective absorption on the target sites

Box 12.2

Advantages and disadvantages of topical therapy

Advantages
- Drug delivered directly to target area
- Reduces systemic absorption
- Patient can view improvement
- Side-effects easily identified

Disadvantages
- Time-consuming
- Messy
- Preparations smell or stain the skin
- Patient can see deterioration or lack of improvement

- erythematous, inflamed skin — benefits from the cooling effect of water-soluble creams.

Patients may use a combination of emollients for different areas, e.g. cream for the face and ointment for the body.

For further reading on the application of emollients, see Dawkes (1997).

The commitment needed to maintain treatment cannot be underestimated as topical therapies can be messy, time-consuming and smelly. Treatment programmes often have to be customised because of the unique therapeutic response of each patient.

Regular nursing assessment will identify any improvement or deterioration and allow treatment to be amended appropriately. In order to achieve the desired outcome, the skilled practitioner needs a sound knowledge of dermatology therapies balanced with clinical nursing abilities to educate, support and motivate the patient to complete lengthy treatment programmes.

Phototherapy (ultraviolet light B)

Patients with certain skin disorders, most commonly psoriasis and eczema, can be treated with ultraviolet light B (UVB) in measured doses. UVB is the wavelength in natural sunlight responsible for sunburn. Treatment requires outpatient attendance two to three times weekly over a period of weeks. A test dose administered to the patient's back determines a safe starting dose. This dose is gradually increased over the treatment period. Phototherapy is given in a cabinet with fluorescent lamps emitting UVB.

Photochemotherapy (psoralen and ultraviolet light A)

The treatment combination of psoralen and ultraviolet light A (PUVA) requires the patient to take oral psoralen (a natural plant extract) in tablet form 2 h before exposure to UVA. Photochemotherapy is given in a cabinet with fluorescent lamps emitting UVA. Bath PUVA (methoxypsoralen lotion) is a treatment in which a measured amount of psoralen is added to 150 L of bath water. Patients soak for a specific time, pat the skin dry and then treatment is given in a UVA light cabinet. Again, psoriasis and eczema can both be treated with PUVA. A test dose is administered to determine a safe starting dose and treatment is given in twice weekly sessions.

Patients having light therapy wear protective goggles during UVB/PUVA exposure. After PUVA they must also wear dark glasses for 24 h to protect the lens of the eye. UVB/PUVA is administered in specialist units to ensure accurate recording of the amount of light therapy given, as guidelines exist that restrict the amount a patient may receive. Patient education prior to initiating treatment, combined with effective nursing support during therapy, empowers the patient with the skills and knowledge needed to undergo therapy and to participate actively in it (Rathmell 2003).

Complementary therapies

The increasing interest in complementary therapies to treat skin disorders reflects a rise in public awareness of non-traditional approaches to treatment, perhaps stimulated by the failure of orthodox medicine to provide 'cures'. The nurse is ideally placed to discuss both the orthodox and complementary options available. Discussion should focus on the safe use of complementary therapies initiated by referral to a licensed practitioner who has undergone accredited training. A House of Lords Report (2000) stressed that complementary therapy should be viewed as a useful adjunct and not as a full alternative to routine therapies. Patients may wish to use such therapies as positive adjuncts to conventional management.

DISORDERS OF THE SKIN

PSORIASIS

Psoriasis is a chronic, non-infectious inflammatory skin disorder characterised by well-demarcated erythematous plaques with adherent silver scales. The epidermal cell proliferation rate increases greatly, while epidermal turnover time is reduced. During normal skin production, epidermal cells mature in transit through the skin layers and are eventually shed as keratin. In psoriasis, increased cell production and transit time mean that cells do not keratinise completely and so cannot be shed. This causes the build-up of a white, waxy silver scale as immature skin cells remain adherent to the skin. Psoriasis is prevalent in 2% of the UK population, yet the cause remains unknown. It can occur in any age group and is an unpredictable skin disorder with exacerbations and remissions. Genetic influences predispose to the condition, with 35% of patients showing a family history.

Precipitating/aggravating factors include:

- infection — streptococcal throat infection
- medications — can exacerbate or trigger psoriasis
- sunlight — in some patients, psoriasis improves during the summer and relapses during the winter; however, others report that sunlight aggravates the condition
- hormonal — psoriasis can get better or worse during pregnancy or menopause
- psychological stress — can exacerbate psoriasis, but the condition itself is recognised as stressful

- trauma — creates the 'Koebner effect' where psoriasis is triggered in damaged skin, e.g. the site of an injury or surgical scar.

Psoriasis varies from mild forms, with plaques localised to the knees and elbows, to severe forms which are potentially life threatening. Classification of psoriasis is made on clinical presentation (Hunter et al 2002).

Guttate psoriasis (see Fig. 12.3) presents as drop-like symmetrical lesions on the trunk and limbs. It is most common in adolescents and young adults and is often triggered by a streptococcal throat infection. It responds well to therapy.

Plaque psoriasis (see Fig. 12.4) presents as well-demarcated, erythematous plaques covered in dry, white waxy scale often localised to the knees and elbows. Removal of this build-up of keratin leaves small bleeding points. Plaques vary considerably in size and can extend to cover the trunk and scalp. Plaque psoriasis tends to be chronic, with exacerbations and periods of remission.

Flexural psoriasis affects the axillae, submammary and anogenital areas and looks different from typical psoriasis. Plaques are sharply defined but the skin has a thin glistening redness, often with painful fissures in the skin folds.

Pustular psoriasis (palmoplantar pustulosis) is a localised form of psoriasis affecting the hands and feet. It is characterised by yellow/brown pustules which dry into brown scaly macules. It is a painful condition, difficult to treat.

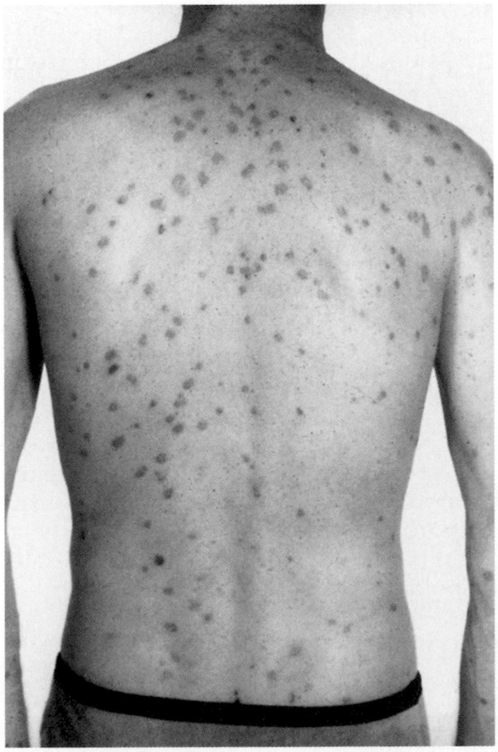

Fig. 12.3 Guttate psoriasis. (Reproduced with kind permission from Dr Graham Lowe, Ninewells Hospital, Dundee.)

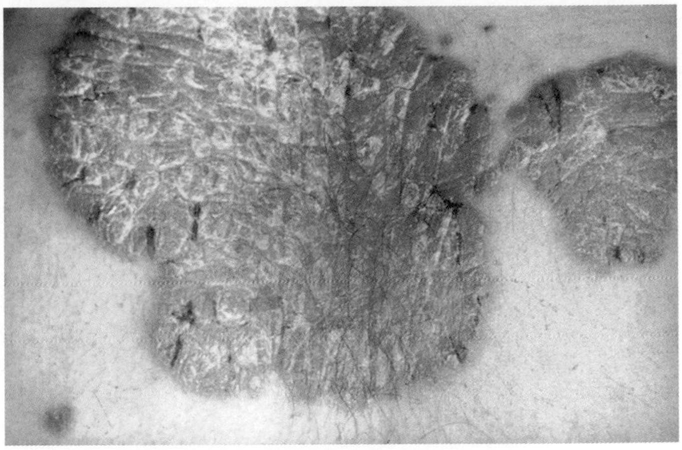

Fig. 12.4 Plaque psoriasis. (Reproduced with kind permission from Dr Graham Lowe, Ninewells Hospital, Dundee.)

Generalised pustular psoriasis is a rare yet serious form of the disease. Sheets of sterile pustules develop, merging on an erythematous background. These areas of skin shear and the patient will present with pyrexia, malaise and require hospital admission. It is often triggered when attempts are made to withdraw oral or topical steroids, or may just reflect the instability of the condition.

Scalp psoriasis can often be the sole manifestation of the disorder. Thick scale adheres to the scalp and can extend to the edges of the scalp margin and behind the ears.

Nail changes in psoriasis can involve pitting of nails and onycholysis, where the distal edge of the nail separates from the nail bed. There is no effective topical treatment for psoriatic nail changes.

Erythrodermic psoriasis is a rare but severe form. The skin becomes uniformly red with high blood volume flushing it. The patient feels unwell and maintaining body temperature is difficult. It can be triggered by the irritant effects of therapies, e.g. dithranol, tars, by withdrawal of oral/systemic steroids or by a medication reaction. Erythrodermic psoriasis is an unstable state that is potentially life threatening and warrants urgent hospital admission. The condition can progress to a generalised pustular psoriasis.

Psoriatic arthropathy Psoriasis can be complicated by psoriatic arthropathy, a 'rheumatoid-like arthritis' affecting about 5% of psoriatic patients. Joint changes occur in hands, feet, spine and sacroiliac joints. This 'rheumatoid-like arthritis' mimics rheumatoid disease but notably the rheumatoid factor test is negative. Psoriatic arthropathy is a difficult combination to treat, meriting the combined expertise of a rheumatologist and a dermatologist.

PATHOPHYSIOLOGY

The pathophysiology of psoriasis is characterised by certain general processes (see Fig. 12.5). The epidermis thickens, with an associated increased blood flow to the skin, and becomes raised to accommodate skin changes (parakeratosis).

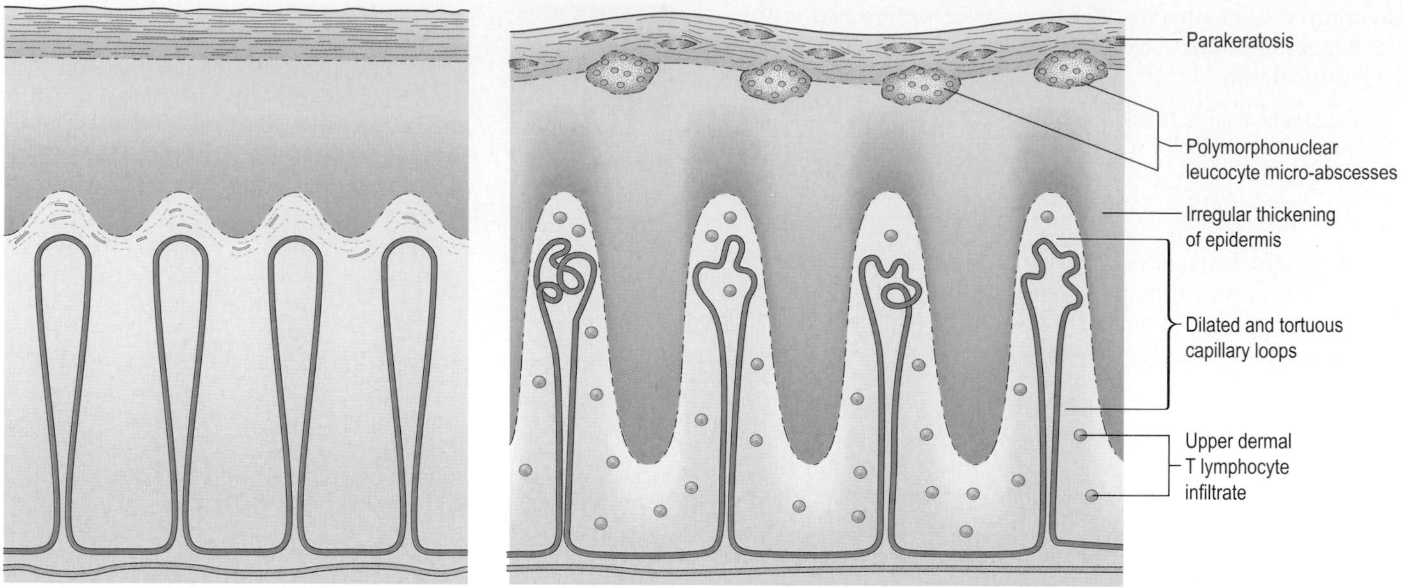

Fig. 12.5 Histology of psoriasis (right) compared with normal skin (left). (Reproduced from Hunter et al 2002, with permission from Blackwell Science Ltd.)

The epidermal cell proliferation rate increases. The transit time of epidermal cells maturing through normal skin is approximately 27 days, whereas in psoriasis it is 4 days. This suggests that psoriasis results from an increase in activity of dividing cells associated with an increase in their rate of reproduction, with trigger factors as yet unidentified.

Common presenting symptoms are as follows:

- *Pain*. Fissures form, particularly on hands and feet, because of loss of flexibility in the thickened epidermis.
- *Erythema*. Within the dermis, blood vessels dilate and increase blood flow to skin, causing generalised redness and heat loss.
- *Scaling*. The horny layer of the epidermis sheds easily in normal skin, but in psoriasis the cells become 'sticky' and build up, creating the silver-scale appearance diagnostic of psoriasis.
- *Pustules*. In inflammatory conditions, an infiltration of white blood cells is normal. Increased infiltration in pustular psoriasis accumulates as microabscesses in the outer layer of the skin.
- *Pruritus (itch)*. Many textbooks describe psoriasis as non-itchy, but patients often report itch to be troublesome.
- *Sore throat*. Streptococcal throat infection is a common precipitating factor in guttate psoriasis.

MEDICAL MANAGEMENT

Where possible, psoriasis is managed on an outpatient basis, but the severity of activity in erythrodermic/pustular psoriasis will result in hospital admission to prevent potential life-threatening complications of an unstable psoriatic state (see p. 534).

Investigations Diagnosis can be made from the clinical picture and relevant history. Diagnosis and subsequent management may require all or a combination of the following examinations and tests:

- skin biopsy
- skin swab for flexural psoriasis
- throat swab
- Auspitz sign — gentle removal of the silvery scale from a plaque reveals pinpoint bleeding from the dilated superficial capillaries
- routine blood tests — viral check and full blood count.

Treatment may involve topical and systemic medication and phototherapy. PUVA/UVB are effective therapies for psoriasis (see p. 530). The combination of therapies chosen depends on diagnosis and severity of the disorder, topical prescribed therapies being the mainstay of psoriasis treatment (see p. 529).

Medication Combined systemic and topical medication is useful in the management of psoriasis. Systematic medications used include:

- antihistamines — to alleviate itch and promote sleep and rest
- analgesics — to reduce the pain and discomfort of inflamed skin
- antibiotics — to treat streptococcal throat infections.

The majority of psoriatic patients respond to topical therapies, but the more extensive forms of psoriasis may require a systemic approach (Hunter et al 2002). Medications that are particularly important in this regard are methotrexate, ciclosporin and retinoids (see p. 534).

NURSING PRIORITIES AND MANAGEMENT: Psoriasis

General nursing considerations

The goals of nursing management will vary depending on the type and severity of the psoriasis. For example, erythrodermic or pustular psoriasis will merit skilful clinical inpatient management. However, many psoriatic patients will be treated as outpatients in a combination of settings, e.g. a specialist centre, the GP practice or at home. Education, support and empathy are vital to underpin the practical management of psoriasis. The nurse involved in outpatient management should have specialist dermatology knowledge and skills to support the patient through treatment regimens which can be messy and long-term. Decision-making regarding appropriate therapies should involve the patient and establish a partnership addressing the physical, social and emotional rehabilitation inherent in a successful outcome. Treatment sessions provide ideal opportunities for the nurse to explain the rationale for using topical therapies, to listen to concerns and to answer questions.

Psychological support

During skin assessment and nursing review, it often becomes apparent that the patient's psoriasis is affecting quality of life. The patient with a skin disorder is vulnerable and treatment sessions provide a private time between nurse and patient during which routine conversation can often reveal the true effect of the impact of the skin disorder on daily life (see Box 12.3). Psoriasis is a condition requiring long-term management, and it is through the collaboration of patient, carer and professional that the right blend of therapies for effective treatment can be found. Clinical psychologists in dermatology units work closely with the patient, as body image, sexuality, quality of life and personal coping strategies are all management considerations, and effective counselling can enhance the therapeutic effect. The Psoriasis Association (see 'Useful websites', p. 552) is a nationwide patient support group with local groups highly active in raising public awareness, supporting the patient and family, and raising funds for research.

Box 12.3

Problems reported by patients with skin disorders

Emotional problems

- Low self-esteem
- Feel body is 'unclean'
- Relationships can be problematic
- Feel people stare — real and imagined
- Regarded as infectious or contagious

Clothing restrictions

- Avoid short sleeves
- Avoid dark clothes due to skin shedding
- Avoid summer clothes where skin is exposed
- Clothes get stained or ruined due to messy creams

Social restrictions

- Skin gets itchy in hot pubs/clubs
- Avoid swimming or sports as people stare
- Avoid communal changing rooms when shopping

Financial implications

- Routine prescriptions are expensive but essential
- No allowances available to replace clothing or bedding
- No allowances available for fuel bills due to extra laundering and bathing

Nursing considerations in outpatient treatment

Management of topical therapy

A range of topical therapies is used in the outpatient management of psoriasis (see Box 12.4). The nurse should encourage patients to attend regularly for treatment, stressing the importance of meticulous adherence to prescribed treatment regimens. The nurse should also explain the different preparations used, giving advice on correct application and potential side-effects. Many prescribed topical therapies are not appropriate for use on the face. By providing clear information and ongoing psychological support, the nurse can help to ensure the patient perseveres with treatment. Specific considerations in using topical preparations are as follows:

Emollients The application of emollients is fundamental in the management of psoriasis. Bland emollients moisturise and lubricate the skin, helping to ease scaling and promote patient comfort. Regular applications seal the stratum corneum, thus reducing transdermal heat and fluid loss, which is particularly relevant in erythrodermic psoriasis (see p. 531). Patients with erythrodermic or generalised pustular psoriasis are often treated with emollients initially to allow fiery skin to 'settle' before the next line of treatment is introduced.

Coal tar ointments are distilled from coal in the production of gas. They are usually blended with white soft paraffin and have an antipruritic, anti-inflammatory and keratolytic effect. Treatment starts with low concentrations, which are gradually increased according to the tolerance of the skin. Tar applications are messy and smelly and they stain, so tend to be used for inpatient treatment. Proprietary blends of cleaner tar creams are available for outpatient therapy.

Tar is never applied to the face or to flexures. Patients must be advised that if ointment irritates or burns the skin,

Box 12.4

Examples of topical therapies used in psoriasis management

- Emollients — emulsifying ointment, 50/50 (white soft paraffin/liquid paraffin)
- Bath additives — Aveeno, Dermol 600, Hydromol, Oilatum
- Soap substitute — aqueous cream, emulsifying ointment, Epaderm
- Coal tar ointments — Alphosyl HC, coal tar solution, crude coal tar solution, Carbo-Dome
- Dithranol — Micanol, Dithrocream, Dithranol in Lassar's paste
- Vitamin D analogues – calcipotriol, tacalcitol, calcitriol
- Scalp therapy — olive oil, Cocois scalp application, Capasal shampoo, Polytar liquid, Alphosyl shampoo
- Phototherapy — ultraviolet light B (UVB)
- Photochemotherapy
  - — oral: psoralen tablets + ultraviolet light A (UVA)
  - — bath: trimethylpsoralen + UVA

it should be removed immediately in an emollient bath and advice sought.

Dithranol, originally obtained from the Goa tree in India and now made synthetically, suppresses cell proliferation (Buxton 2003). It is available in many forms, but patients must be informed that it can stain skin and clothes; staining can last for 10–14 days after treatment has finished. Dithranol is applied by spatula to affected skin and then covered with stockinette gauze to prevent the ointment spreading to surrounding skin. This procedure is time consuming and messy but effective. For outpatient therapy, short-contact treatment is available. Cream is applied to the plaque after protecting the surrounding skin with petroleum jelly and removed 30 min later.

Vitamin D analogues such as calcipotriol, tacalcitol and calcitriol are applied as a cream or ointment directly to plaques. They are non-messy, non-staining and well tolerated. Calcipotriol inhibits cell proliferation and stimulates epidermal cell differentiation, correcting the increased cell turnover time associated with psoriasis. Due to potential systemic absorption, there is a restriction on the quantities prescribed. The restriction will relate to the extent and severity of the psoriasis and it is important that patients are aware of the prescriptive guidelines.

PUVA/UVB (see p. 530) Both therapies are available to patients on an inpatient and outpatient basis. The treatment programme varies for each individual depending on identification of skin type and tolerance of sunlight. In PUVA therapy, 8-methoxypsoralen is taken orally 2 h before ultraviolet exposure is photoactivated, causing cross-linkage between DNA and inhibiting cell division. Retinoids (see p. 535) can be given with PUVA to stimulate more rapid skin clearance at lower total doses of ultraviolet light. Phototherapy is a pleasant treatment, the patient acquiring a gentle tan.

Goeckerman regimen This is a long-established and effective combination treatment in which the patient takes tar baths prior to exposure to ultraviolet light (Hughes & Van Onselen 2001).

Ingram regimen This is a combination therapy involving tar baths, ultraviolet exposure and dithranol applications.

Cocois ointment is a blend of tar, emulsifying ointment and salicylic acid used to treat scalp psoriasis. It is gently massaged into the scalp, left overnight and removed with shampoo of the patient's choice.

Olive oil can be used in maintenance therapy to reduce the build-up of scale on the scalp. For maximum benefit, patients are advised to warm the oil before applying it to the scalp.

Nursing considerations in inpatient care

Generalised pustular psoriasis and erythrodermic psoriasis can be life-threatening conditions requiring skilled nursing management.

Monitoring vital signs

Body temperature The patient will have difficulty in adapting to changes in environmental temperature. Body temperature must be monitored regularly, as skin temperature will fluctuate and may mask subnormal core temperature (see Ch. 22).

Blood pressure should be checked regularly. Hypotension may develop due to the shunt of blood to the peripheral circulation, leading to reduced cardiac output and potential cardiac and renal failure.

Maintaining fluid balance

Rehydration is important to correct the insensible fluid loss from the skin. The majority of patients will maintain a balance if encouraged to supplement their oral intake. The liberal use of topical emollients will help to reduce fluid loss.

For further reading on the management of erythroderma, see Gawkrodger (2003).

Other fundamentals of care

Basic hygiene Soothing emollient baths are ideal in psoriatic conditions to lubricate the skin and prevent further heat and fluid loss. In severe cases, however, bathing may be prohibited due to the disruption in the patient's thermoregulatory control caused by a high blood volume flushing the skin. Regular and liberal use of emollients will suffice until the patient's condition is stable enough to permit bathing (Hughes & Van Onselen 2001).

Rest This is of paramount importance to the patient's recovery.

Diet Because of the possibility of protein loss through the skin, dietitians should advise the patient on appropriate food choices, ensuring that foods are high in protein and have sufficient calories to counteract loss and promote healing. Supplementary protein drinks may also be indicated.

Physiotherapy This will help to minimise the side-effects of bed rest. Patients with psoriatic arthropathy will benefit from gentle exercise to maintain mobility and flexibility.

Systemic medication therapy

The severe nature of pustular and erythrodermic psoriasis usually merits systemic medication therapy, e.g. methotrexate and acitretin.

Methotrexate This cytotoxic medication, often used in the treatment of cancer (see Ch. 31), is a folic acid antagonist with an anti-inflammatory effect inhibiting mitosis. It is given once weekly via the oral, intramuscular or intravenous route. Careful monitoring of liver and bone marrow function is carried out and the patient on long-term methotrexate may require a liver biopsy to monitor the potential side-effect of liver fibrosis or cirrhosis. Improvement can usually be seen in 2–4 weeks. The patient should be advised to avoid alcohol and certain drugs that can interact with methotrexate, e.g. aspirin. As nausea is a side-effect of methotrexate, patients are advised to take medication with food and an antiemetic should be prescribed.

Acitretin This retinoid is a vitamin A derivative which is very effective in pustular and plaque psoriasis. The medication is given on a daily basis in a dosage related to body weight. Acitretin influences the activity of the epidermis, normalising the plaques by thinning down hyperkeratotic lesions. A fasting blood lipid level is checked before starting acitretin and the patient is monitored for hyperlipidaemia during therapy, with referral to a dietitian for advice on a low-cholesterol diet if necessary. Patients may report side-effects persisting until the dose is reduced (as the psoriasis improves). Dryness of the mouth, lips and nose are common and unpleasant side-effects. Patients should be advised to use basic emollients and lip salves to ease discomfort. Reassurance that side-effects will abate once treatment is reduced or discontinued may help the patient to persevere with treatment.

Female patients taking acitretin require advice regarding adequate contraceptive measures during treatment and for 2 years after discontinuing, as this drug can be harmful to a developing fetus.

Complementary therapies

Many 'cures' are offered in psoriasis. For example, treatment programmes involving holidays in Israel are advertised, where therapy takes the form of skin exfoliation with Dead Sea salt during natural exposure to sunlight. Acupuncture, hypnotherapy and aromatherapy are also treatment options which have varying degrees of success. The best advice the nurse can offer is that the patient considering complementary therapy consults a recognised licensed practitioner. Combined complementary and conventional therapies can provide an active and beneficial treatment programme. Complementary therapies are becoming more widely available within GP surgeries (Ernst & White 2000).

The contribution of the nurse

The nurse's role in assisting the patient to manage their psoriasis will be varied and invaluable. Education, empathy and skilful clinical nursing must underpin practical management and psychological support (Penzer 1996). Psoriasis can have a major impact on quality of life. In a survey by Gupta et al (1993), of 127 patients with psoriasis, 10% reported a wish to die and 6% reported active suicidal intent. This study reinforces the importance of assessing the psychological impact of the skin disorder. The range of topical therapies can be bewildering, so the nurse must utilise clinical skills, supported by information leaflets, to ensure that the patient fully understands the treatment and methods of application. This practical support can enhance adherence with treatment and have a major impact on its success.

ECZEMA

The word 'eczema' comes from the ancient Greek 'to boil out of' and is the term applied to a range of inflammatory skin disorders. The aetiology of eczema is unknown. Most classifications of eczematous skin disorders use the term 'eczema' synonymously with 'dermatitis', as both terms apply to the inflammatory skin changes provoked by either internal (endogenous) or external (exogenous) factors. Eczema may occur as a result of one or both types of factor (Gawkrodger 2003).

Priorities of medical and nursing management are similar for all classifications of eczema.

Endogenous eczema

Atopic eczema (see Fig. 12.6)

Atopic eczema is a common inflammatory cutaneous skin disorder affecting 20% of infants in the UK; there are associated genetic and environmental factors. The word 'atopy' covers the classification of related disorders, e.g. asthma, eczema and hay fever. Atopic eczema can be a chronic itchy distressing disorder, having a major impact on a child's behaviour and quality of life and causing severe disruption to family life. Infantile eczema can resolve spontaneously but sometimes progresses to a chronic pattern of episodic exacerbations. Commonly affected sites are the flexural aspects of knees and elbows with involvement of the face and wrists. The prevalence of atopic eczema continues to rise and although this has been linked with increasing affluence in the UK population, it remains unclear how the two factors are related (Hay & Rustin 2004).

For further information on the impact of atopic eczema on the family, see Lawson et al (1998).

Pompholyx eczema

This blistering eczema is localised to palms and soles. It develops rapidly, causes acute discomfort on the hands and feet and can become secondarily infected. The cause is unknown and outbreaks do not appear to be related to any external factors.

Discoid eczema

This is an eczema of unknown aetiology, characterised by symmetrical coin-shaped lesions that affect the limbs and can be intensely itchy. It is more common in middle-aged and older people and may only last for a few weeks.

Asteatotic eczema

This condition mainly affects older people, commonly on the lower legs. It appears to be associated with a deficiency

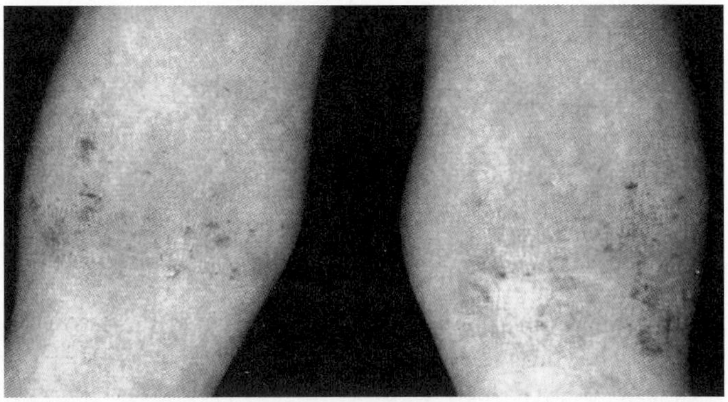

Fig. 12.6 Atopic eczema. (Reproduced with kind permission from Dr Graham Lowe, Ninewells Hospital, Dundee.)

of sebaceous secreting glands, resulting in excessive dryness and scaling of the skin. Central heating, diuretic therapy and over-frequent washing are also implicated as possible causes. The stratum corneum develops a 'crazy paving' appearance due to a network of fine red superficial fissures. Asteatotic eczema is readily treatable in the early stages with liberal use of emollients and bath oils. Scratching of a persistent itch creates a more resistant eczema which may merit topical steroid therapy.

Varicose eczema

This usually presents as chronic patchy eczema of the legs, with or without the presence of a varicose ulcer (see Ch. 23). The eczema arises due to associated chronic venous stasis and the area involved may become itchy. The eczema is often accompanied by the presence of varicose veins, oedema and pigmentation of the skin, the last occurring due to haemosiderin from the blood leaking through capillary vessels under elevated venous pressure (Gawkrodger 2003). Patients often develop a secondary response to this initial area of eczema and may produce associated eczematous areas on other parts of the body.

Exogenous eczema

Irritant contact eczema is very common, especially in industrial settings. The eczema usually erupts at the maximum point of contact. Presentation varies according to the nature of the irritant contact. The epidermis may be damaged by abrasion, and the effect of the irritant, e.g. coal dust, cement, is exacerbated by rubbing against clothing. Epidermal necrosis may occur within hours of contact with strong chemicals, while eczema triggered by milder substances, e.g. detergents, may take longer to evolve. Many patients with atopic eczema appear prone to irritant contact eczema and should be advised to avoid work where exposure to irritants could be problematic.

Allergic contact dermatitis

Allergic contact dermatitis is a condition in which the skin develops a specific immunological hypersensitivity. The most common allergic response of this type, particularly amongst women, is to nickel as found in inexpensive jewellery. Continued exposure to the allergen will result in an eczematous response, ranging from mild to severe. Allergic contact dermatitis may be triggered by, for example, rubber, certain plants and cosmetics; in many cases a change of job or avoidance of the allergen may be necessary (Hunter et al 2002). The most difficult cases to treat are those in which allergic contact dermatitis is suspected but no definitive triggering factor can be proven.

PATHOPHYSIOLOGY (see Fig. 12.7)

Acute eczema presents with redness and swelling caused by increased vasodilatation and generalised oedema of the skin. The erythema may be generalised over the body. Acute eczema exacerbated by scratching will extend to an exudative, scaling and crusting phase.

In chronic eczema involving recurrent exacerbations, the skin is scaly, excoriated, thickened and pigmented. The eczematous areas will be localised to more defined parts of the body and lichenification will be apparent. Lichenification is a skin response to repeated scratching in which the affected areas become thickened and toughened and show a marked exaggeration of normal skin markings. Chronic scratching and thickened skin in combination allow deep, painful fissures to develop as the skin loses its normal elasticity.

Common presenting symptoms are as follows:

Itch (pruritus), which accompanies most eczematous conditions, can be acute and distressing. The itch–scratch–itch cycle quickly becomes established. The skin is well supplied with sensory nerves that respond quickly to the mechanical stimulation of scratching or any external stimulation. Because of the manner in which sensory impulses are transported, itch has two components: a quick, localised prickly sensation, followed by a slow and diffuse burning itch.

Redness Blood supply to the skin is prolific and is normally only required to function at low volume. Inflammatory skin diseases alter this balance by causing dilatation of blood vessels feeding the skin, leading to a generalised total body redness (erythroderma). In atopic eczema, white dermographism can be evoked due to the abnormal response of the skin's vascular change. Firm strokes of the skin normally produce a 'weal and flare' response, a pink raised weal lasting about 30 min, but in atopic patients a simple white line arises, leaving the pressure site with no erythema.

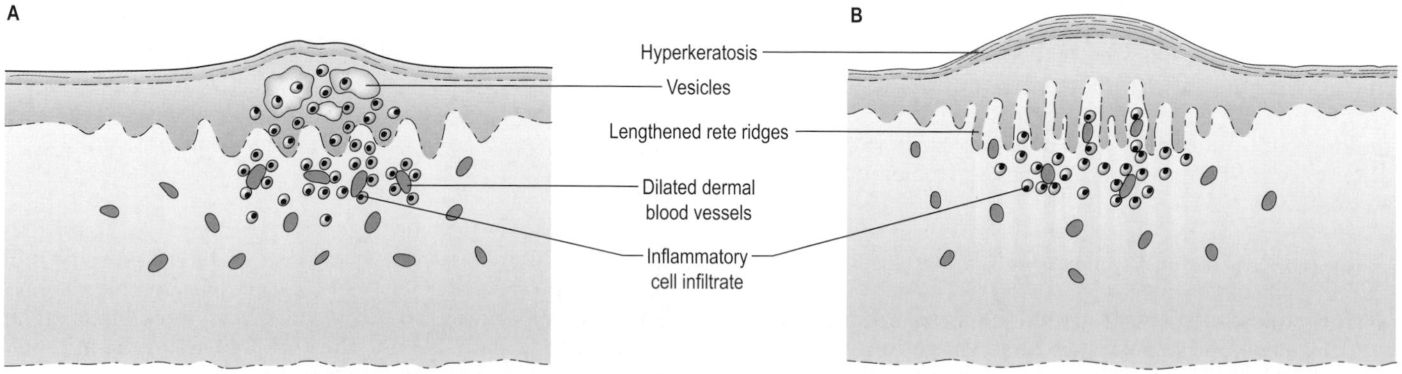

 Fig. 12.7 The histology of acute (A) and chronic (B) dermatitis.

Fissures/lichenification Chronic stages of eczema create a thickening of skin over flexures or any area traumatised by scratching. Open fissures are painful and slow to heal. In the chronic stages, there is also a generalised thickening of the prickle cell and horny layers of the skin.

Summary Eczematous conditions present with varying degrees of severity. An acute phase of eczema may present as a weeping, inflamed response, while a chronic condition gives rise to fissures and clearly defined excoriated areas. Patients will describe itch, pain and tenderness. Loss of the normal barrier of intact skin has associated fluid and heat loss. Excoriations may lead to secondary infections, which contribute to keeping the eczema active, and patients with atopic eczema tend to be more susceptible to viral infections, e.g. herpes simplex virus and eczema herpeticum (see p. 543).

MEDICAL MANAGEMENT

Diagnosis is made from the clinical picture of the disease process and the patient's history. Many of the exogenous conditions are managed in an outpatient setting; however, severe exacerbations warrant hospital admission.

Investigations Precise diagnosis may require all or a combination of the following.

Laboratory investigations will include:

- skin swabs — excoriated lesions may result in secondary infection
- skin scrapings — to exclude fungal infection
- skin biopsy — for immunohistological examination when the diagnosis is in doubt.

Patch testing may be carried out to confirm allergic contact dermatitis. A range of patch tests is available in which suspected allergens, e.g. nickel, fragrance, hairdressing products, plant material and rubber, are made up in a concentration which would normally produce no reaction unless the patient is sensitive to them. Allergens are applied to the back, left in situ for 48 h and then removed. The site of the test is 'read' at 96 h. Positive results vary from mild erythema to small blisters. Patch tests should not be carried out while the patient is in the acute phase of eczema or using a topical steroid to avoid exacerbating the condition or obtaining misleading results.

For further reading on patch testing, see Ratcliffe (1998).

Blood tests may indicate the presence of specific antibodies to external factors, e.g. dust mite, cat/dog hair or pollens, supportive of a diagnosis of atopic (exogenous) eczema.

Treatment is either systemic or topical.

Systemic medication therapy includes the use of:

- antihistamines — to reduce itch by blocking histamine receptors; although drowsiness is a side-effect, it may aid sleep and rest
- antibiotics — to treat bacterial infection, specifically *Staphylococcus aureus*, caused by excoriation
- analgesics, e.g. paracetamol — to ease heat, tenderness and localised pain.

Box 12.5

Examples of topical therapies used in the management of eczematous conditions

- Emollients — 50/50 (white soft paraffin/liquid paraffin), Dermol 500, Doublebase, Diprobase cream, Epaderm, Oilatum cream
- Bath additives — Aveeno, Cetraben, Dermol 600, Hydromol, Oilatum, Oilatum Plus
- Soap substitute — aqueous cream, emulsifying ointment, Epaderm
- Corticosteroids — very potent, potent, moderate, mild
- Corticosteroids/antibiotics — Dermovate-NN, Betnovate-C, FuciBET, Locoid C, Fucidin H
- Bandages — Ichthopaste, Quinaband, wet wrap dressings

Topical therapies are a priority in the management of eczema (see Box 12.5). Eczema also improves in some patients on exposure to natural sunlight.

NURSING PRIORITIES AND MANAGEMENT: Eczema

General nursing considerations

Nursing management is of central importance in the treatment of eczema, and patients and their families must be involved in setting goals for care. The short-term priority of management is to alleviate discomfort. A tired, hot, itchy patient is not in an ideal state to absorb information and learn self-care techniques, and therefore an immediate and sympathetic approach to care is important (Hughes & Van Onselen 2001). Ongoing support and reassurance are fundamental to achieving long-term goals. Informing the patient about eczema creates greater understanding of the condition and its outlook. Treatment sessions present the ideal opportunity to familiarise the patient with topical therapies, their effects and the rationale for their use.

Giving psychological support

Collaboration of patient, carer and health professional is vital to a successful treatment outcome. Substantial time and effort can be required to motivate, educate and empower the patient to share the process of managing the condition. The National Eczema Society is an active patient support group offering a wide range of information, skin education road shows and peer group support essential to raising self-awareness and self-esteem (Jeyasingham 1997).

Nursing considerations in topical therapy

Emollients

These moisturisers, used to make dry and scaly skin smoother, take the form of bath oils, creams and ointments and are the mainstay of treatment. Itch, heat and dryness all respond promptly to lubrication. Many emollients create a barrier for inflamed skin, preventing further fluid and heat loss. Eczema is a condition in which the skin is chronically dry, so long-term use of emollients maintains good skin moisture. Patients should be advised to avoid perfumed products and use prescribed bath oils and soap substitutes. Continued use of emollients throughout the day is a major adjunct to therapy. In hospital, the patient will use very greasy moisturisers and emollients, but these products may be unsuitable for use at home or in the workplace. For community use, there are bland emollients such as Aveeno, Cetraben, Diprobase, Doublebase, Oilatum or Hydromol which are effective, non-messy and non-staining. Many of these are available in pump dispensers and are attractively packaged to encourage use.

Steroids

The application of steroid creams and ointments constitutes the next line of management in inflammatory skin disorders. These preparations are absorbed into the skin to dampen down the inflammatory response mechanism. Because steroid therapy will have a major impact on the eczematous skin, it is important that the patient understands the correct methods of application. Absorption of topical steroid and the volume of cream used will be greater if the skin is dry and excoriated (Morris 1998). Thus the skin must be regularly moisturised with emollient as an adjunct to steroid therapy, and steroids should be applied to freshly bathed skin or at least 20 min after the application of an emollient. Using the 'fingertip method', measured amounts of cream (see Fig. 12.8) are gently massaged into the affected areas for maximum effect (Hunter et al 2002).

Although the best treatment advice is to start with the lowest strength of steroid possible to treat the skin, many eczematous conditions require a potent steroid to switch off the inflammatory process. Treatment programmes involve starting with a medium to strong steroid applied twice daily, gradually reducing the strength of the creams used as the condition improves. Many patients are aware of the side-effects of topical steroids, e.g. systemic absorption, striae, loss of subcutaneous fat and fragile skin. The nurse must emphasise that it is prolonged use of strong topical steroids with inadequate use of emollients that produces chronic side-effects. In eczema, secondary bacterial infection may be present and treatment may include a combined steroid and antibiotic cream.

Bandaging

A variety of occlusive, medicated bandages is available for dermatological therapy (see Box 12.5). Applied overnight, they provide a cooling effect and their occlusive action creates a moist environment which aids the absorption of topical therapy. They also provide a mechanical barrier, preventing damage to the skin from scratching. The use of wet wrap dressings is a well-established therapy in managing the child or adult with eczema. The technique involves the initial application of emollient, or steroid and emollient, followed by covering with, first, a wet layer of Tubifast, a tubular conforming bandage, and then a dry layer of Tubifast. Water in the moist bandages evaporates, creating a cooling effect that markedly reduces pruritus (Page 2003). This is a simple procedure that is quick to apply, well tolerated and effective. The skilled community nurse who can teach bandaging techniques to parents can help to restore harmony to a family when a child with eczema is distressed by itch, particularly during the night. Tubifast garments for children have recently been introduced in the form of vest top, tights and leggings.

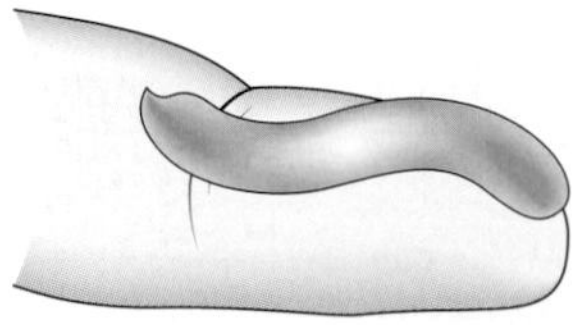

Fig. 12.8 Fingertip unit measures about 0.5 g of ointment. (Reproduced from Hunter et al 2002, with permission from Blackwell Science Ltd.)

Other considerations

Rest

Rest is imperative for recovery in more severe eczematous conditions. In hospital, the patient is afforded the opportunity to suspend activities of socialisation, taking time out to allow the skin to heal. In the home or school, disruptive, manipulative behaviour is often described in the child with atopic eczema, who may merely be distraught by itch and inadequate sleep (Titman 2003). The nurse must give clear information and reassurance on the safe use of antihistamine medications in children. Many parents are not keen to give their child medicines, but the judicious use of antihistamines will provide rest and relief for the eczema sufferer and the family (Bysshe 1996).

Diet

Diet is implicated in some forms of infantile eczema where the child is allergic or intolerant to milk or milk products. The best advice to give to patients is to maintain a well-balanced diet while avoiding foods known to cause irritation (Hughes & Van Onselen 2001). Exclusion diets to identify food allergy are difficult and should be attempted only under the supervision of a dietitian.

Complementary therapies

The stress of having a skin disorder applies particularly to eczema, where patients can be distraught with physical symptoms and altered body image. When conventional medicine, with its potential side-effects, cannot offer a cure, the nurse working with patients with skin disorders should also be aware of the diverse range of complementary therapies available.

These include:

- evening primrose oil
- homeopathy
- herbal therapy
- aromatherapy
- reflexology.

Complementary therapy should not be viewed as a total alternative to conventional medicine and referral to a qualified practitioner is essential for safe management. Traditional Chinese medicine using self-help tools from energy-based therapies, e.g. Dru Yoga, Shiatsu and Chi

Kung, can blend with Western techniques to reduce stress and boost the body's natural healing capacity. Habit reversal methods are available that focus on breaking the itch–scratch–itch cycle of eczema (Bridgett 1996). The main aim of habit reversal is to create awareness in patients of when and how often they scratch their skin. Treatment methods vary for each age group so specialist help must be sought before undertaking such techniques.

The contribution of the nurse

The specific role of the nurse depends on the severity of the condition and the treatment setting. Current policy to maximise outpatient management places the primary care team at the forefront of skin care, and therefore their clinical skills and educational abilities must address the identified need. Much of dermatology nursing focuses on the child with atopic eczema and their family, due to the acknowledged impact this condition has on quality of life. Co-ordinated care and holistic practice can be achieved through a multidisciplinary team approach (Lynn et al 1997).

School nurses can support and motivate the child to maintain skin care at school while educating teachers about the physical and psychosocial impact of eczema (National Eczema Society 2003). Health visitors should be involved in regular monitoring to ensure therapies are not inhibiting the child's development.

In the workplace, the occupational health nurse advises on changes in work practice to reduce risk factors and the incidence of industrial-acquired skin disorders (Payling 1996). In every setting, the nurse practitioner should utilise all available resources and refer patients appropriately to the relevant agencies and support groups.

STOP THINK **12.2** Ms H is the single parent of three children aged 1, 3 and 5 years. She is unemployed and lives in rented one-bedroom accommodation while on a council house waiting list. Her 3-year-old son has severe eczema. He is kept awake at night by severe itch and disrupts the household.

Discuss with a health visitor how this mother might be helped to cope with this situation.

SKIN INFECTIONS AND INFESTATIONS

This section describes infections and infestations commonly encountered in the community; awareness of them is particularly relevant to the community practitioner. Many of these conditions cause consternation among sufferers because of their real or perceived social implications. Sound common sense, the ability to dispel myths, and practical skill in identifying, assessing and treating the conditions described are fundamental to care (Docherty 2001).

Fungal infections

The most common fungal infections are caused by the dermatophytes *Trichophyton* and the yeast-like fungus *Candida albicans*, which are responsible for superficial infections confined to the skin and mucous membranes. Deep fungal infections can remain localised or cause systemic disease.

Dermatophyte infections

Dermatophytes are botanically related fungi responsible for superficial fungal infection. Some dermatophyte infections are confined to humans, while others principally affect animals, although transfer of fungal infections from animal to human does occur, causing severe inflammatory skin reactions. Dermatophytes grow in keratin, i.e. stratum corneum, hair and nails, and these superficial infections are usually indirectly acquired by contact with keratin debris carrying fungal hyphae (Gawkrodger 2003). The term 'tinea' is the generic description given to these fungal infections.

Tinea pedis or athlete's foot is the most common of the dermatophyte infections. The patient complains of itchy, scaling skin between the toe webs, commonly acquired through contact with infected keratin on the floors of swimming pools or showers.

Tinea cruris affects young males, presenting as scaly erythematous lesions on the inner thighs and spreading to the perineum and buttocks. The source of infection is usually athlete's foot and the fungus is transferred to the groins on fingers or towels.

Tinea unguium is the term for fungal dystrophy of the toenails in which the nail thickens, discolours and becomes very friable.

Cattle ringworm (tinea corporis) is common amongst farm workers or visitors to farms. The fungus is picked up from gates or fences where cattle have left keratin debris containing the organism. The face and forearm tend to be affected and the fungus provokes a severe inflammatory reaction.

MEDICAL MANAGEMENT

Skin scrapings taken for examination under the microscope and fungal culture are used to confirm the diagnosis. Topical treatments are broad-spectrum antifungal creams, e.g. miconazole (Daktarin) and clotrimazole (Canestan), which are available over the counter. Topical therapy for dystrophic nails is ineffective. Oral therapy is available for scalp, nails and skin ringworm.

NURSING PRIORITIES AND MANAGEMENT: Dermatophyte infections

Nursing management focuses on containment of infection and promotion of basic hygiene (Hughes & Van Onselen 2001). Avoidance of shared face cloths/towels prevents further spread. The nurse can advise on prescribed and OTC therapies and their correct method of application. Treatment programmes may involve combined oral and topical therapies, and patients should be advised to persevere where therapies take time to resolve the condition. Conditions can recur, so educating the patient in management of the condition is beneficial in preventing this.

Candida infection

Candidiasis (thrush) is the term applied to infections of the skin and mucous membranes by *Candida albicans*. This fungus is a normal commensal of the human digestive system, only becoming pathogenic if the opportunity presents itself. Immunosuppressed patients, people with diabetes, patients on broad-spectrum antibiotics or on topical and systemic steroid therapies are all at risk from this opportunistic infection.

Buccal mucosal candidiasis refers to oral thrush presenting as milky curd-like spots on the tongue and inner cheeks. It often affects babies, older people and patients on broad-spectrum antibiotics (see Ch. 15).

Candida vulvovaginitis describes vaginal thrush, which presents with a creamy vaginal discharge and itchy erythema of the vulva. This condition tends to be associated with pregnancy, use of oral contraceptives, antibiotics and diabetes.

Candida balanitis is a thrush infection of the foreskin and glans. It tends to be more common in uncircumcised males and may be associated with poor hygiene or diabetes. It can recur if a sexual partner also has vaginal thrush.

Chronic paronychia is a candidal infection of the nail plate which is common in people whose occupation involves repeated immersion of the hands in water, e.g. hairdressers, nurses, bartenders. The nails become distorted and the nail base is painful, red and swollen.

Intertrigo is the term given to candidal infection of the skin folds. Where two skin folds are in opposition, such as the groins, axillae and submammary regions, there is increased heat and humidity and thrush infections are common, e.g. nappy rash. Obesity and poor hygiene exacerbate the problem. The skin displays erythematous, well-demarcated erosive lesions and is tender, moist and painful in these areas.

Angular cheilitis is a common condition of older people where the deep grooves at the side of the mouth tend to be moist with saliva; a *Candida* infection exacerbates the problem. It is common in denture wearers but can also be a feature of iron or vitamin B_{12} deficiency.

MEDICAL MANAGEMENT

Skin swabs, scrapings or nail clippings are taken to confirm diagnosis. Urinalysis should be performed to exclude diabetes. A full blood count must be carried out in older people with angular cheilitis.

Treatment is specific to the area affected. Antifungals in the form of creams, ointments and pessaries are very effective. Oral antifungal drugs are indicated in the treatment of nail infections. A combined mild steroid/antifungal, e.g. clobetasone butyrate (Trimovate), is appropriate to treat intertrigo, reducing both inflammation and infection. Combination packs of vaginal pessary and cream are available for vaginal thrush, e.g. clotrimazole, and these are usually single applications, depending on the dose/strength of the preparation. Newer OTC preparations include a single dose of the antifungal drug fluconazole (Diflucan).

NURSING PRIORITIES AND MANAGEMENT: Candida infection

Providing advice on basic skin hygiene and information about therapies available, whether prescribed or OTC, is an important nursing role. The nurse must be able to identify those at risk of opportunistic infection, e.g. older people, babies and patients having chemotherapy. The nurse's role as counsellor is vital in the treatment of genital thrush and confidential information should be respected when sexual partners are treated concurrently to prevent reinfection.

Infestations

Scabies

Scabies is a skin infestation caused by the mite *Sarcoptes scabei* and acquired by prolonged close physical contact with the mite. The female scabies mite burrows approximately 1 cm into the stratum corneum, is fertilised by the male mite and begins to lay eggs along the burrow. For the first 4–6 weeks after infestation there may be no itching, but thereafter, pruritus dominates the picture, especially at night. This is thought to be due to a hypersensitive response to the mite (Hunter et al 2002). Skin examination usually reveals burrows, principally on the hands and feet, the sides of fingers/toes, between finger and toe webs, the wrists and the insteps. Facial burrows are only seen in babies. Burrows can also present on the genitalia of males. A scabies 'rash' may be present in the axillae, umbilicus and thighs. Excoriation can cause burrows to become eczematised and infected, which can often confuse diagnosis.

Norwegian scabies is the term given to the form of scabies presenting in patients who have sensory deficits where the sensation of itch is absent, e.g. in spinal injuries, or in patients who are immunosuppressed either because of disease or treatment of disease, e.g. AIDS, lymphoma, systemic steroids or transplantation. Absence of scratching leads to large numbers of mites remaining on the skin in crusted lesions. During skin shedding, mites are shed into the environment, and therefore any person in contact is at considerable risk of developing scabies from the patient with Norwegian scabies.

MEDICAL MANAGEMENT

Diagnosis can be confirmed by using a needle to remove a mite from a burrow and examining it microscopically. Current topical therapies are permethrin and malathion (see Box 12.6 for treatment advice and guidelines for application). Once the infestation is treated, further therapy with a combined steroid/antibiotic cream may be necessary to reduce itch and treat excoriated lesions until the skin is fully healed. Antihistamine tablets are appropriate if itch disturbs sleep. Soothing topical preparations, e.g. Eurax cream, can be useful until residual itch disappears.

NURSING PRIORITIES AND MANAGEMENT: Scabies

The priority is to treat the patient and identify close contacts requiring treatment. The nurse combines practical advice with psychological support, recognising the social

Box 12.6

Patient advice sheet for the self-treatment of scabies

How to apply a scabicide

1. Read the advice leaflet thoroughly before starting treatment
2. The skin should be cool and dry. Avoid bathing immediately before applying cream
3. Apply the cream as prescribed from the neck down — avoid the face
4. Pay particular attention to finger/toe webs, the soles, skin folds (axillae/groin), under finger- and toenails
5. Put on clean nightwear and change bed linen — normal laundering is adequate
6. Leave the cream for 8–12 h as the prescription states (overnight is ideal)
7. Bathe or shower at the end of the 8–12 h period

Points to note

- It is important that all family members/contacts are treated at exactly the same time. If there is any delay in treatment, avoid further contact with the person until they are treated
- If hands are washed during the treatment period of 8–12 h ensure cream is reapplied to the hands
- Weaker strengths of cream are available for pregnant women or infants
- Treatment can be repeated but your doctor will decide if this is needed
- Scalp treatment may be required in infants and older people

embarrassment that infestation can create. Outpatient management is ideal and the nurse must identify current treatments and their correct method of application. As recurrent scabies is often due to poorly applied treatments, both patient and nurse should read carefully the advice leaflets provided with topical scabicides. The patient may require repeated applications of scabicide until the condition resolves. Transient contact with the patient is unlikely to cause transmission and the nurse can be reassured and can reassure colleagues about this. However, the patient with Norwegian scabies is highly contagious and should be isolated while treatment is ongoing. Local infection control policies must be followed. Normal washing of linen and clothes is adequate.

STOP THINK **12.3** A family of five (two adults and three children, aged 15, 6 and 3 years) have to treat themselves for a scabies infestation. Their GP suggests that a leaflet could be given to them to ensure they follow the correct advice. Review existing printed leaflets. How would you guide the family in obtaining information from the world wide web?

Head lice (pediculosis capitis)

Head lice are transmitted by close contact. The adult female louse lays eggs which are cemented to the hair approximately 0.5 cm from the root. Scalp irritation and itch are due to the saliva produced as the louse bites the scalp. The 'nit' is the empty case left once the larvae have hatched — the case becomes white and is more easily detected. Head lice is an emotive topic, as it continues to be endemic amongst schoolchildren and causes great consternation to parents.

NURSING PRIORITIES AND MANAGEMENT: Head lice

The initial priority is to treat the patient and appropriate contacts. Treatment usually consists of a lotion applied to the scalp, e.g. malathion (Prioderm), which is left on for a number of hours and then shampooed out. Treatment may need to be repeated. Gently combing with a fine-tooth comb assists in the final removal of nits. Department of Health (2001) guidelines rotate scalp therapies to prevent the development of treatment-resistant head lice.

Carbonyl, a product found in head lice treatments, was highlighted as carcinogenic in animals and many scalp preparations were restricted to prescription-only availability. Department of Health guidelines also identified a theoretical risk to humans and acted in response to public alarm. At present the nurse should continue to reassure parents that adherence to treatment is preferable to an uncontrollable rise in head lice infestation. Current scalp therapies are constantly reviewed and their safe use is encouraged, following the treatment guidelines issued with each product. These preparations cannot be used as prophylactic treatment to prevent infestation. The school nurse is ideally placed to target and educate students, teachers and parents in the treatment, preventive strategies and environmental measures that will assist in the reduction and control of head lice.

Bacterial infections

Staphylococcal and streptococcal infection: cellulitis

Cellulitis is an acute, spreading and potentially serious infection of dermal and subcutaneous tissue, characterised by red, tender skin at the site of bacterial entry. Organisms isolated in cellulitis include *Staphylococcus aureus* and *Streptococcus pyogenes*. Cellulitis is a common condition in older people, who tend to suffer from lower limb oedema (see Ch. 2). Infection enters the skin in a variety of ways, including surgical wounds, stasis eczema or leg ulcers, minor abrasions and i.v. drug injection sites. Erysipelas is the name given to a superficial streptococcal infection of the skin.

In adults, the most common presentation is cellulitis of the lower limbs, with the point of entry of infection usually being a fissure between the toes which may be secondary to tinea pedis (athlete's foot). The site affected will be oedematous, red, hot and painful. An associated general malaise with rigors and fever develops. Enlarged local lymph nodes may be present.

MEDICAL MANAGEMENT

Management involves isolation of the organism by blood cultures and treatment with appropriate oral or i.v. antibiotic therapy. Analgesics reduce the pain of inflammation.

NURSING PRIORITIES AND MANAGEMENT: Cellulitis

Bed rest, monitoring of temperature and appropriate action if rigors occur are the first line of nursing management. Pain assessment and administration of regular analgesics will ease discomfort.

Cellulitis of the lower limbs requires bed rest and elevation of the affected limb to reduce oedema. Exercising reduces the complications of prolonged bed rest and should be encouraged. Once the condition resolves, general advice on basic skin care and avoidance of predisposing factors is helpful. Patients can have recurrent cellulitis and may be prescribed prophylactic antibiotic therapy to prevent future episodes.

Staphylococcal infections

Impetigo

Impetigo is a superficial bacterial infection of the skin caused by *Staphylococcus aureus*, sometimes combined with haemolytic streptococci. The head and neck are the most common sites. The condition starts as a small but gradually enlarging pustule that ruptures to leave a raw exuding surface. The exudate dries and forms the yellow golden crust typical of impetigo. It can occur as a secondary infection, e.g. associated with eczema and scabies.

Folliculitis

Folliculitis, an infection of superficial hair follicles by *Staphylococcus aureus*, presents as a small pustule on an erythematous base centred around the follicle. In dermatological conditions, folliculitis may be exacerbated by the use of greasy ointments, occlusive bandages and tar therapies.

MEDICAL MANAGEMENT

In all bacterial infections, treatment is by the use of topical and oral antibiotic therapies (Gawkrodger 2003).

NURSING PRIORITIES AND MANAGEMENT: Bacterial infections

The nurse should give guidance about each infection and its transmission. Guidelines on personal hygiene and the avoidance of communal use of towels/cloths can reduce the spread of infection. Practical management includes the gentle application of mild topical antiseptics to remove crusted lesions. Correctly applying creams and ointments in the direction of the hair growth can reduce the incidence of folliculitis and patients should be advised to complete their course of systemic or topical antibiotics to ensure treatment efficacy. The nurse must recognise and acknowledge the profound psychological impact of having a skin infection, as the social stigma of impetigo and the public perception that these conditions are associated with poor hygiene create major worries for both patient and family. Good clinical practice, enhanced with practical information and sympathetic support, will help to address the patient's physical and psychological needs.

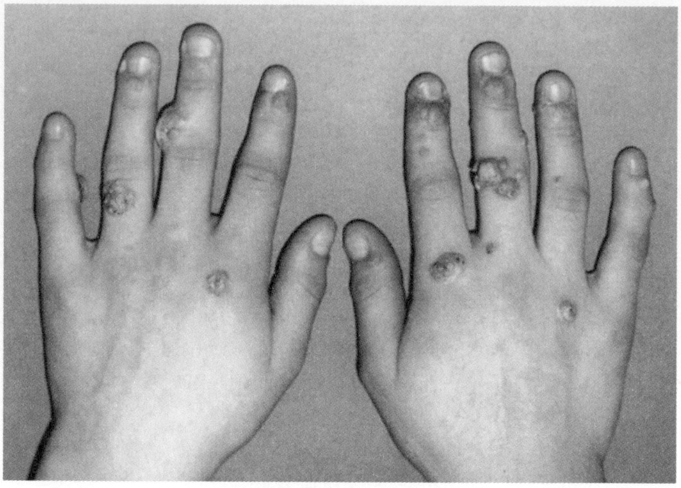

Fig. 12.9 Hand warts. (Reproduced with kind permission from Dr Graham Lowe, Ninewells Hospital, Dundee.)

Viral infections

Warts (see Fig. 12.9)

Infection by the human papilloma virus affects the DNA in epidermal cells, creating warts. Different clinical manifestations are specific to different viruses (Gawkrodger 2003).

Warts are benign, highly contagious and can be cosmetically unacceptable. Group transmission is the mode of contact, e.g. in gyms, swimming baths or schools. The classification of warts is outlined in Box 12.7.

MEDICAL MANAGEMENT

Diagnosis is based on history and clinical appearance. Treatment may involve topical application of ointments or premedicated plasters containing salicylic acid to soften and remove the wart, or cryosurgery.

The nurse should explain virus transmission and encourage the meticulous continuation of treatment. Many patients become disheartened by the slow resolution of the problem and discontinue treatment. Regular assessment by the practice nurse may encourage adherence to recommended treatment.

Box 12.7

Classification of warts

- Common warts — hyperkeratotic nodules occurring on the hands and feet of children. These often resolve spontaneously
- Plane warts — smooth flat-topped warts appearing on the face and hands
- Plantar warts — commonly known as verrucae where the papilloma virus is pressured into the dermis, creating a callus. The most common site is the feet
- Genital warts — a mass of warts with a cauliflower-like appearance present on the perianal and genital areas

Molluscum contagiosum

This is a pox virus producing solid, skin-coloured or pearly-white papules on the skin. It affects adults but is more common in children, arising over a period of 2–3 months. The lesions may be single or multiple, occurring on the neck and trunk.

MEDICAL MANAGEMENT

Initial diagnosis is based on history and clinical appearance but if the condition does not resolve spontaneously, freezing the papules with local applications of liquid nitrogen can be carried out. When the condition occurs in children, parents require explanation and reassurance that the condition tends to be self-limiting. Normal basic hygiene rules prevent further spread.

Herpes simplex virus (HSV)

There are two types of herpes simplex virus: type 1 causes cold sores on the lip and face; type 2 is associated with genital herpes. Initial contact with the herpes simplex virus is usually in childhood and often goes unnoticed. However, development of primary cutaneous herpes simplex can occur and, in a child with atopic eczema, can be a severe life-threatening condition. Following primary infection, the virus can establish itself in sensory ganglia and be reactivated by, for example, sunlight, stress and colds. Reactivation of the virus is preceded by a tingling sensation before a cluster of small vesicles develops. The vesicles burst and lesions then crust, usually resolving in 10–14 days. Genital herpes is a sexually transmitted disease affecting the penis, vulva, perianal area and rectum. Following the primary episode, the virus persists in the presacral ganglion and can recur. This can be a serious condition in pregnant women because of the risk of transmitting the virus to the baby during labour and delivery.

MEDICAL MANAGEMENT

Recurrent herpes simplex is treated with topical aciclovir (Zovirax) which is now available over the counter. It must be used immediately on awareness of the tingling sensation, and applied five times daily for 5 days to inhibit vesicle eruption. Patients with genital herpes should be referred to genitourinary medicine for further investigation, appropriate management and expert counselling.

NURSING PRIORITIES AND MANAGEMENT: Herpes simplex

The nurse can advise patients at risk of recurrent episodes of primary herpes simplex on the use of topical aciclovir and should recommend its continued use until course completion. The patient should be reminded of basic hygiene standards to avoid further transmission of the virus during the active phase. The patient with genital herpes may require support and counselling from specialist genitourinary services. The pregnant woman with genital herpes requires good liaison between the woman and her obstetrician and midwife, to acknowledge the condition and its potential complications and to initiate appropriate action to minimise virus transfer during delivery (Gawkrodger 2003).

Eczema herpeticum (complication of HSV)

Eczema herpeticum is a widespread cutaneous herpes simplex infection occurring in patients with atopic eczema. In children it can be life threatening and the patient will be systemically unwell and febrile. Vesicles erupt rapidly over the face and neck and can extend over the rest of the body. The skin is taut, red and painful. As vesicles erupt and rupture, the patient becomes susceptible to secondary bacterial infection, e.g. impetigo (see p. 542).

MEDICAL MANAGEMENT

Treatment depends on the severity of illness and is a combination of antiviral and antibiotic therapies. The patient who is pyrexial and systemically unwell should be hospitalised. A side room to ensure source isolation is ideal, but good infection control procedures using standard infection control will reduce the infection risk to other susceptible patients (see Ch. 16). Oral aciclovir is adequate in minor cases, but if the patient is unwell then aciclovir is given by the i.v. route. The patient with eczema using topical steroids must discontinue these immediately until the virus resolves. Any secondary bacterial infection should be treated with topical antibiotic cream and oral antibiotic therapy. Analgesics may also be required, e.g. paracetamol.

NURSING MANAGEMENT AND PRIORITIES: Eczema herpeticum

The nurse's role in hospital is to maintain infection control policies in order to reduce the transmission of infection. The patient who is systemically unwell requires regular observations of temperature, fluid intake and rest until infection resolves. The nurse should assist in topical applications of prescribed creams as the patient may feel too unwell or too distressed by pain to manage this independently. Once the viral infection resolves, the nurse can advise the patient on restarting topical steroids for the eczema. Patients who are at risk of cold sores should keep aciclovir in reserve to use promptly if a cold sore develops. As aciclovir is now an OTC preparation, effective treatment is easier to achieve. A few days' delay in getting an appointment with a GP can be detrimental as this condition erupts quickly.

Herpes zoster (shingles)

Herpes zoster is caused by the varicella zoster virus. After an attack of childhood chickenpox, the virus remains dormant in the dorsal root ganglia of the spinal cord but can be reactivated later in life as shingles. The trigger factor is unknown, but the condition is common in immunosuppressed or stressed patients (see Ch. 16) and tends more commonly to affect middle-aged and older people.

PATHOPHYSIOLOGY

Once reactivated, the virus multiplies by invading host cells and utilising the replicatory mechanisms of the host cell to produce new DNA. The cell is lysed and virus particles are released to invade another cell. The virus particles migrate along the nerve fibres towards the skin surface, causing nerve damage and consequent pain. Balloon degeneration of the prickle cell layer of the epidermis results in the formation of fluid-filled vesicles (Gawkrodger 2003), which erupt across the thoracic and/or cranial dermatome with a characteristic unilateral band-like distribution. Fluid taken from vesicles will contain virus particles.

Pain and tenderness often precede the vesicular erosions, and patients may have fever and will feel generally unwell. As the vesicles crust over, the infective risk resolves over a period of 2–3 weeks. The lesions can be erosive and may take longer to heal in older people.

MEDICAL MANAGEMENT

Diagnosis is confirmed by clinical history and viral culture. Treatment is by topical antiviral agent if lesions are still erupting, e.g. aciclovir. Oral or i.v. aciclovir is essential management in immunosuppressed patients. The potential complications of herpes zoster are:

- herpes zoster ophthalmicus
- postherpetic neuralgia — this merits the attention of the specialist pain team.

NURSING PRIORITIES AND MANAGEMENT: Shingles

In an acute attack of shingles, the patient may require hospitalisation. Standard infection control policies provide guidelines for isolation of the patient until the infectious stage resolves. The patient should be nursed by staff who have had chickenpox to reduce the contact problem, as there is a risk that contact with a patient suffering from shingles may cause chickenpox to anyone without immunity to that disease. In the early stages of shingles, topical applications of antiviral cream, e.g. aciclovir, can shorten the duration of the illness. The more seriously ill patient will require oral or i.v. aciclovir. Prompt referral to an ophthalmologist is vital for the patient with any eye involvement (see Ch. 13).

Certain groups of people are particularly susceptible to the transmission of herpes zoster, e.g. patients having radiotherapy and/or chemotherapy, and immunocompromised patients on oral or topical steroids. Community nursing staff should be aware of the long-term problems associated with shingles. A small proportion of patients report persistent pain (postherpetic neuralgia) continuing for many years. Chronic pain has a major impact on daily living and requires full assessment. Treatment options available for postherpetic neuralgia include transcutaneous electrical nerve stimulation (TENS), ultrasound, antidepressants and/or anticonvulsant therapy. Referral to a pain control clinic is advisable for the patient with intractable pain (see Ch. 19).

For further reading on skin infections, see Gawkrodger (2003), pp. 44–59, 64–65.

BULLOUS DISORDERS

The term 'bullous disorders' covers those skin conditions in which large watery blisters (bullae) arising within or immediately under the epidermis are a presenting feature (Hunter et al 2002). There are many causes of bullae (see Fig. 12.10) and histological location influences the classification of the disorder.

Early detection and treatment are essential, as many of the bullous conditions are severe and potentially life threatening.

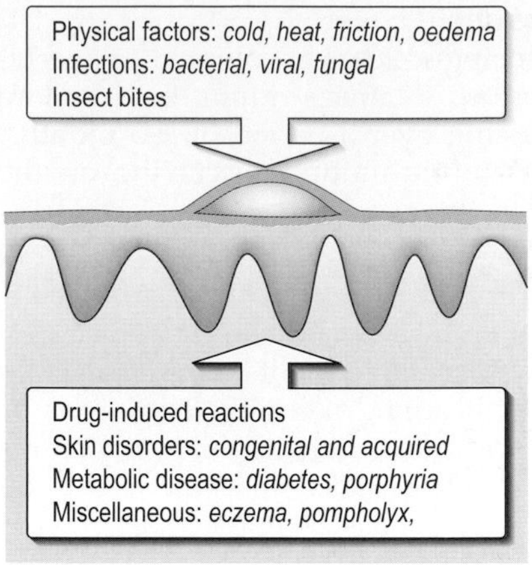

Fig. 12.10 Causes of blisters (bullae).

Pemphigus (intraepidermal bullae)

PATHOPHYSIOLOGY

This is an autoimmune disease occurring in adults. It is characterised by the development of autoantibodies against epidermal cell surface molecules creating superficial erosions and blisters on epidermal and mucosal surfaces.

Common presenting symptoms The main presenting feature is the presence of superficial fluid-filled blisters within the epidermis. These blisters are flaccid, thin-roofed and offer little resistance; consequently they shear, leaving raw, denuded skin. Pain from the exposed sites is a major factor in management. Oral lesions are common.

Clinical diagnosis is confirmed by a positive Nikolsky's sign, such that when lateral pressure is applied to the skin surface with a thumb, the epidermis shears and appears to slide over the dermis (Buxton 2003).

Pemphigoid (subepidermal bullae)

PATHOPHYSIOLOGY

This is more common in older people; 80% of patients are usually aged 60 and over (Marks 2003). Like pemphigus, pemphigoid is an autoimmune disease. Antibodies bind to the junction between dermis and epidermis, and blisters are formed in response to enzymes released from inflammatory cells.

Common presenting symptoms The patient reports generalised intense itch, followed by erythematous plaques on the skin (pre-pemphigoid stage), followed by the development of tense blisters affecting any area of the body. Nikolsky's sign is negative.

Toxic epidermal necrolysis (subepidermal)

PATHOPHYSIOLOGY

This condition presents as a dermatological emergency and is often precipitated by a drug hypersensitivity. The skin split is subepidermal and the entire epidermis shears off in layers, leaving raw, denuded areas. A review of the patient's medication and removal of the causative factor(s) are essential to management.

Common presenting symptoms The skin is erythrodermic and painful, with the skin shearing off in sheets. Nikolsky's sign is positive. The patient will be distressed by pain and may have erosions in the mouth, oesophagus and bronchus.

MEDICAL MANAGEMENT

Early diagnosis is imperative due to the life-threatening potential of bullous disorders. Hospitalisation is a major aspect of treatment and management.

Investigations will include the following:

- Skin biopsy — to identify the type of skin split and exclude other bullous disorders
- Blood tests — to monitor urea and electrolytes in view of the associated fluid loss from eroded skin. In pemphigus the serum contains antibodies binding to the intracellular areas of the epidermis; titration of these antibodies is relevant to building a picture of the disease activity
- Skin swab — to define the bacteriological status of skin exposed to secondary infection.

Treatment will involve medication with the following:

- Antibiotics — to treat secondary infection
- Corticosteroids — in pemphigus and pemphigoid, high-dose oral steroids, e.g. prednisolone 60–100 mg/day, are the first line of management and are maintained until blistering stops. A gradual reduction in dosage is then commenced, aiming for low-dose maintenance therapy
- Analgesics — to alleviate pain from eroded skin lesions; choice is dependent on patient need and disease activity
- Antihistamines — to reduce itch and aid rest
- Immunosuppressants, e.g. cyclophosphamide, azathioprine — used in combination with oral steroids to control the disease process of pemphigus and pemphigoid.

Plasmapheresis is considered in severe cases and allows monitoring of circulating pemphigus antibodies. Topical therapy is non-specific, aiming for patient comfort.

NURSING PRIORITIES AND MANAGEMENT: Bullous disorders

This section focuses on general nursing care of the three disorders described. Although rare, they are more commonly seen in dermatology units. It may help the reader to understand the rationale behind nursing priorities to note that these patients have similar needs to patients with severe burn injuries (see Ch. 30).

Major nursing considerations

Analgesia

Analgesia must be effective and consistent. Pemphigus and toxic epidermal necrolysis are distressing, painful conditions when shearing of the skin is active. Pain assessment tools (see Ch. 19) permit the nurse and patient to determine pain control needs, ensure accurate delivery of analgesics, and evaluate their efficacy, which is particularly relevant prior to dressing changes. Pain clinics are a specialist service to assist in prescribing appropriate analgesics by the most effective route for this type of pain.

Bed rest

Patients must rest to avoid further trauma to the skin. Pressure-relieving beds are available which are helpful in nursing patients with these conditions.

Hygiene

The maintenance of good personal hygiene and the prevention of cross-infection are extremely important. Gentle washing or the application of soaks, i.e. potassium permanganate, for their mild antiseptic/antipruritic effect can be soothing and help to minimise further trauma.

Isolation may be necessary due to skin loss. The patient will be susceptible to infection and the use of immunosuppressants will increase this susceptibility. In severe cases, barrier nursing may be required (see Ch. 16).

Diet

Approximately 20% of an adult's dietary protein is used for skin repair and growth in normal health. Therefore, an increased intake of dietary protein is advisable in bullous conditions. Referral to a hospital dietitian will ensure the prescription of any necessary supplements. Constipation induced by fluid loss, or as a side-effect of analgesics, is an associated problem. Mild laxatives may be indicated to prevent added discomfort.

Monitoring vital signs

Temperature Regular observation of body temperature is required, as fluctuations may occur due to fluid and heat loss from the skin. Variations in environmental temperature can be reduced by nursing the patient in a side room.

Blood pressure is checked regularly if there is associated fluid loss, steroid-induced hypertension or rehydration by i.v. fluids.

Monitoring electrolyte and fluid balance

This is imperative in any condition associated with skin loss. Rehydration may initially be achievable by increasing the patient's oral intake and monitoring output. An i.v. infusion may be necessary in severe cases. If skin loss presents problems in siting a peripheral infusion, a central line may be required, with monitoring of central venous pressure providing an accurate assessment of fluid requirements.

Urinalysis should be monitored for a potential diabetic state induced by oral steroid therapy.

Dressings and topical therapy

A dressing procedure provides the best opportunity to complete a skin assessment and evaluate disease activity. In pemphigus and toxic epidermal necrolysis, raw areas are recorded and dressed. The tense bullae of pemphigoid are identified and left intact to permit reabsorption of blister fluid, thereby minimising further trauma. Blisters restricting movement are uncomfortable for the patient and can be aspirated using a sterile alcohol swab, syringe and needle, leaving the blister roof intact (Hughes & Van Onselen 2001). Administration of analgesics prior to the application of topical therapy is important to reduce the patient's apprehension about dressing changes. Each patient's needs and disease severity determine dressing requirements, but the main aims of management are to:

- keep dressing changes to a minimum
- maximise patient comfort
- ensure dressings are easily removable.

By following these guidelines, the nurse minimises further trauma and promotes skin healing. Simple applications of soothing emollients or a non-adherent dressing secured by gauze stockinette will possibly be all that is tolerated. Heavier pads and bandaging create constriction and pain. The skilled practitioner will be guided by the patient's comments and will adjust dressings appropriately.

Special care beds/pressure-relieving equipment

Facilitating rest and comfort is a primary aim in care. The use of low-pressure, air-fluidised beds enhances comfort and reduces the need for positional changes which contribute to shearing forces on the skin. The temperature regulator in these beds maintains an appropriately warm environment, helping the patient to maintain body temperature. This warm environment also increases the amount of insensible fluid loss, so the patient's fluid intake must be increased to compensate. Most patients achieve this by increasing oral intake, but i.v. fluid supplements are a consideration. Dressings are kept to a minimum and remain moist with the use of these beds, and so tend to be easily removed.

Care in the community

Although these conditions are rare, as our older population increases, the incidence will rise. The community nurse has a dual role: firstly, in identifying disorders and coordinating referral for specialist help; and secondly, after discharge from hospital, in ensuring the patient understands the rationale behind long-term maintenance medication, encouraging adherence to and monitoring side-effects of systemic therapies.

ACNE

Acne is a disorder of the pilosebaceous glands. It is a common condition, usually developing during adolescence, between 11 and 14 years. It reaches a peak between 17 and 21 years, gradually improving and disappearing around 21 years in most cases. However, 6% of adults between 25 and 40 years still experience acne (Cunliffe & Gollnick 2001). The psychological impact of acne should not be underestimated, as its onset during the years when visual impact is important to developing new relationships can have a devastating effect on the young adult. Dermatologists are very aware of the impact that acne can have on quality of life.

PATHOPHYSIOLOGY (Fig. 12.11)

During puberty, circulating androgens stimulate sebum production. Hyperkeratosis occurs at the mouth of the hair follicle and the dilated chamber fills with sebum. The organism *Propionibacterium acnes*, commonly referred to as *P. acnes*, grows in large numbers, creating the comedone. *P. acnes* breaks down the sebum into inflammatory chemicals which leak into the surrounding dermis or pour out through a rupture in the follicle wall (Gawkrodger 2003).

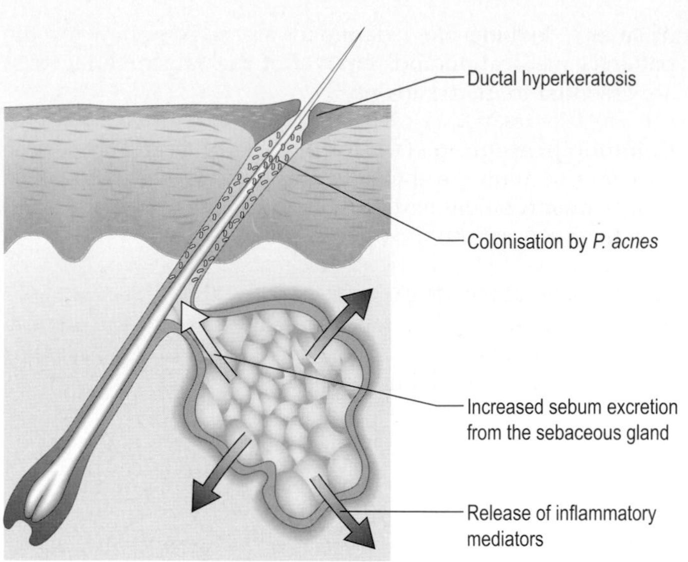

Fig. 12.11 Aetiopathogenesis of acne.

Common presenting symptoms Acne affects the face, neck, upper back and front of the chest. In more severe cases, these lesions may spread further. Lesions can include comedones, papules, pustules, nodules, cysts and residual scars.

MEDICAL MANAGEMENT

Treatment relates to the severity of the condition. Mild acne should respond to topical therapies, antiseptic washes and antibiotic preparations, while moderate/severe acne will merit combined topical and systemic therapies (Layton 1995), as follows:

- Antibiotics — oral tetracyclines given over a 6-month period reduce the inflammatory process. Side-effects of and contraindications to tetracycline should be noted (British National Formulary 2006). If the patient is intolerant of tetracyclines, the drug of choice would be erythromycin.
- Isotretinoin — a medication derived from vitamin A that reduces sebum production. It does have side-effects and careful monitoring of liver function and blood fat levels is indicated. The medication is teratogenic and female patients must use effective contraception. Isotretinoin has been shown to clear acne in 90% of patients with no recurrence. At present it is only available by prescription from hospital dermatology departments (Cunliffe & Gollnick 2001).

NURSING PRIORITIES AND MANAGEMENT: Acne

The role of the nurse is to educate and dispel the many myths of acne (Boston & Preston 2001). The patient should be reassured that acne is not linked to poor diet, an excess of sweets or chocolate, or poor hygiene. Indeed, most acne sufferers are overzealous in personal hygiene. The nurse should encourage continuation of topical and oral therapies for the full treatment course. The female patient starting isotretinoin needs referral to family planning services to ensure adequate contraceptive measures are established from 1 month before starting treatment until 3 months after completion.

The nurse must respond sympathetically to the acne sufferer. The degree of distress may not always equate with the severity of disease, and care must address the social and psychological impact of acne. Skin disease has been known to provoke suicide, and the nurse working with acne patients should recognise that individuals can become so disturbed by their perceived problem that they are pushed to this extreme (Cotteril & Cunliffe 1997). It is imperative that the impact of acne is not underestimated, and prompt referral to a dermatologist will initiate effective treatment.

STOP THINK **12.4** You are asked to provide a series of health talks for a group of school students. Acne is one of the topics requested. Devise a plan for your talk with relevant aims for this age group. Consider answers to the questions you may be asked on diet, cosmetics, infection and social impact.

PHOTODERMATOSES

This term applies to skin disorders that are induced or aggravated by sunlight. These disorders are relatively common and can impose severe limitations on daily life. This section will highlight specific disorders and briefly describe diagnostic techniques and treatment options. The discussion on nursing management focuses on assisting the patient to maintain independent living within the limitations imposed by photosensitivity.

Sunlight

Sunlight is composed of different wavelengths of ultraviolet light, divided into ultraviolet A (UVA), ultraviolet B (UVB) and visible light. UVA in larger doses can produce erythema, passes through window glass and is less variable in intensity. UVB is well recognised as the cause of sunburn. Visible light consists of longer wavelengths and easily penetrates the epidermis with minimal significance. Some conditions, however, demonstrate an abnormal sensitivity to visible light. Certain factors affect the intensity of sunlight:

- time of day — strongest between 11.00 and 15.00 h
- geography — weaker in northern latitudes
- season — UVB less intensive in winter months
- reflective effect of snow, water and sand.

Note that clouds do not protect against sunburn as UVB penetrates cloud cover.

Types of photodermatosis

PATHOPHYSIOLOGY

Polymorphic light eruption (PLE) is the most common of the photodermatoses, with women being affected twice as frequently as men (Gawkrodger 2003). It affects patients in early spring, disappearing in autumn. Several hours after exposure to sunlight, the patient develops an itchy papular, pruritic rash, which persists for 7–10 days. The rash can be provoked by UVB or UVA wavelengths, and it should be remembered that UVA also penetrates window glass and thin clothing.

Solar urticaria is very rare and appears as itchy red patches which may be swollen and resemble nettle rash or weals. This reaction occurs almost immediately, within 10 min after sunlight exposure, and subsides within 1 h of sunlight avoidance, with no residual damage to skin.

Photo-aggravated dermatoses Some pre-existing skin conditions, e.g. atopic eczema, psoriasis, rosacea (a chronic inflammatory facial skin condition) and herpes simplex, can be exacerbated by sunlight exposure.

Photo-contact dermatitis refers to disorders in which direct contact of the skin with a substance, e.g. tars, sunscreens, followed by exposure to ultraviolet light provokes a dermatitis. Certain genetic disorders, e.g. xeroderma pigmentosum, also produce a photosensitive reaction.

Chronic actinic dermatitis This condition particularly affects men over the age of 50 years but can also occur in women (Gawkrodger 2003). Patients are sensitive to sunlight (UVB, UVA, visible light) and artificial light sources and have many allergies to substances in direct contact with their skin, e.g. plants, flowers, wood, perfumes, sunscreens and rubber. Sparing of the shaded skin can be present, e.g. behind ears, eyelids, under a watch strap, and there may be marked differences between skin covered by clothing and exposed skin, particularly the neck and arms. The condition presents with marked erythema, eczema and thickening of the skin of the face, neck and hands. Skin changes may be evident in areas covered by clothing, e.g. the arms.

MEDICAL MANAGEMENT

Management begins with a full history and assessment of related factors and presenting symptoms (see Box 12.8).

Investigations required are as follows:

Phototesting provides an objective assessment of photosensitivity disorders and is available in specialist photobiology/dermatology units. Phototesting is performed with the use of a monochromator (Ferguson 2004) to identify if abnormal light sensitivity is present and establish which wavelengths are responsible, i.e. UVA, UVB or visible light. The patient's back is the test site used. Varying doses at different wavelengths are irradiated to small areas and delayed erythema is noted at 7 and 24 h. These responses are compared with known responses of a control group, thus helping to determine the degree of photosensitivity and wavelengths responsible.

Patch testing is used to identify contact allergies causing an exacerbation of the disorder. Patients may have multiple allergies which are relevant to diagnosis and subsequent management.

Treatment involves systemic and topical therapy and sometimes UVB and PUVA therapy (see p. 530). Drug therapy

Box 12.8

Influencing factors and common presenting symptoms of photosensitive conditions

Influencing factors
- Drug history
- Family history
- Hobbies
- Allergies
- Occupation
- Sites involved
- Skin type

Common presenting symptoms
- Eczema
- Erythema
- Heat
- Itch
- Oedema
- Pain
- Urticaria

may include antihistamines, immunosuppressants and oral and topical steroids. Sunscreens offer a sun protection factor (SPF) either by chemically absorbing and filtering ultraviolet light or by physically reflecting and scattering ultraviolet rays to protect the skin. A combination sunscreen creates a more effective sun block. Some light-sensitive conditions, e.g. PLE (see p. 547), can be treated with a course of phototherapy (UVB/PUVA) desensitisation and patients should be encouraged to continue exposure to maintain their new tolerance level. Unfortunately, this is lost during winter and the phototherapy has to be repeated the following spring.

NURSING PRIORITIES AND MANAGEMENT: Photodermatoses

Patients with diagnosed photosensitive disorders require practical help and support from nursing staff trained in the management of photodermatology. Many patients are relieved that investigations have produced a diagnosis rather than a dismissal of symptoms as merely 'a bit of sunburn'. Factual information from nursing staff is vital if the patient is to cope with lifestyle changes imposed by the diagnosis. General advice includes:

- regular use of emollients
- meticulous, regular (every 2 h) application of prescribed sunscreens to exposed sites
- treatment with a steroid ointment/cream if the condition flares
- sun avoidance between 11.00 and 15.00 h
- protective, closely woven clothing, to provide a further effective barrier to sunlight; in severe cases, a wide brimmed hat, scarf and gloves may prove helpful
- use of clear museum film, which blocks out ultraviolet light, applied to house windows and car windows (Dawe et al 1996).

Giving psychological support

Social isolation is a major problem for individuals with severe photosensitive disorders. Many patients, distressed by their diagnosis and the restrictions it entails, reject management regimens which would lead to a life indoors or only leaving home after sundown. They often find maintenance of topical therapies to be time consuming, messy and cosmetically unacceptable. Others stoically accept the limitations and persevere with the use of sunscreens to permit them freedom to continue a restricted form of daily living.

The nurse must display a sympathetic understanding of the psychological trauma associated with the restrictions imposed by such a diagnosis. The overall aim of nursing support should be for the patient to control skin management in an informed and motivated manner, with instant access to professional help as needed.

URTICARIA, ALLERGY AND ANAPHYLAXIS

Urticaria is a common condition and lesions are described as 'hives' or nettle rash. The skin feels irritable and produces white raised weals that turn pink with a bordered edge. The weals can be extensive over the body. There are many causes, but the condition often resolves spontaneously. In some cases the condition can extend, creating swelling around the eyes, mouth and throat known as angioedema (see Ch. 16). In severe attacks, breathing can be compromised, so angioedema must be treated promptly (Mygind et al 1996).

PATHOPHYSIOLOGY

In response to the initial trigger factor, the dermis becomes oedematous with dilatation of blood vessels and degranulation of mast cells and the release of histamine. The weal of urticaria is oedema of the dermis, which can extend rapidly into the subcutaneous tissues causing angioedema.

Classification of urticaria (see Box 12.9) Acute contact urticaria can be related to contact factors, e.g. animal fur, plants, insect stings. Extensive urticaria associated with

Box 12.9

Classification of urticaria

- Chronic — idiopathic
- Acute — IgE-mediated, e.g. food allergy, drug reaction
- Physical — dermographism, cholinergic, cold, solar, heat, delayed pressure
- Contact — immune (e.g. animal saliva) or non-immune (e.g. nettle sting)
- Pharmacological — aspirin, opiates, non-steroidal medications, food additives
- Systemic cause — systemic lupus erythematosus, lymphoma, thyrotoxicosis, infection, infestation
- Inherited — hereditary angioedema
- Other — urticarial vasculitis, papular (insect bites), mastocytosis, pregnancy

Reproduced with permission from Gawkrodger (2003).

angioedema is usually idiopathic but can be related to the ingestion of food or drugs, such as strawberries, nuts, aspirin and penicillin. Urticaria is more common in individuals with atopic eczema. Cold, heat, sun, pressure and water can all induce physical urticaria. Sweating in response to physical exercise or eating spicy food may also induce urticaria with isolated facial swelling. Hereditary angioedema is a rare and potentially fatal autosomal dominant condition. It presents in childhood and requires skilful long-term management during acute attacks and in establishing prophylactic therapy (Gawkrodger 2003).

MEDICAL MANAGEMENT

Clinical history and skin examination will help to determine the provoking factors. Antihistamines are essential in the management of urticaria. These H_1 antagonists block histamine release and the newer preparations, e.g. cetirizine, desloratadine, are non-sedating. In acute attacks, the patient requires oral antihistamines until the condition resolves, usually in a few days. In chronic urticaria, the patient may require maintenance antihistamines for several months. In an acute attack of angioedema, the use of i.v. antihistamines may be necessary. Urticaria can be associated with anaphylaxis (see Ch. 16) and, in this situation, adrenaline and antihistamine drugs will be used in combination. Severe urticaria may also require short-term use of systemic steroids. Patients with identified severe reactions to foodstuffs are trained to administer i.m. or s.c. adrenaline at the onset of attacks (Lawlor 1998).

NURSING PRIORITIES AND MANAGEMENT: Urticaria, allergy and anaphylaxis

The nurse in every setting will encounter the patient with allergies. Angioedema and anaphylactic reaction can prove fatal, so professionals must recognise the urgency of the situation and be fully trained in initiating emergency action (McGeary 1997). The role of the nurse during an acute attack is to assist with medical management until the acute phase stabilises. Afterwards, the nurse's role as provider of factual information and management of the condition begins.

Dietitians provide dietary advice to assist in the avoidance of foods that trigger urticaria. Dietary exclusion is difficult, as food labelling is not always helpful. Public pressure has persuaded food companies and supermarkets to focus on the importance of accurate food labelling, as the incidence of food allergy, and in particular peanut allergy, seems to be increasing (Ministry of Agriculture, Fisheries and Food 1996). Peanut allergy and sensitisation can lead to severe anaphylactic shock and death, so accurate food labelling is vital. Expectant mothers are advised to avoid eating nuts to prevent sensitisation in children. However, as knowledge of the mechanisms of food allergy improves, diagnosis and management will also improve. The link between breast feeding, weaning and allergy continues to be researched (Stabell Benn et al 2004).

The patient who has severe allergic reactions should be trained in the use of adrenaline pens (EpiPen). The nurse can help the patient and family in relation to all aspects of the allergy, in particular to recognise warning symptoms and to use the EpiPen promptly whilst seeking medical assistance. It will be necessary for those involved in caring for the child with an allergy, e.g. school teachers, to be aware of potential problems and to be given instruction on using the EpiPen (Keen & Comer 1995).

The nurse has a positive role in raising awareness of allergies, giving informed advice to patients, carers and fellow professionals, and providing the empathy and support required to improve and maintain patients' quality of life.

SKIN TUMOURS

The skin, as a complex organ system, can produce many tumours, both benign and malignant, within the epidermis and dermis. The reader should refer to a colour atlas of dermatology to fully appreciate the wide diversity of skin tumours (White 2003). Skin biopsy for histology is necessary in the diagnosis, prognosis and management of skin tumours.

Malignant melanoma is the most serious of the skin tumours and its incidence is rising. Melanoma accounts for less than 10% of cutaneous tumours but is responsible for 80% of skin cancer deaths – over 1600 each year in the UK (Cancer Research UK 2003). Figures in the UK suggest that 65% of patients with melanoma have a survival rate of 5 years (Cancer Research UK 2003). Melanoma commonly arises in a naevus (mole), involves the pigment-producing melanocytes and can metastasise rapidly via the circulatory and lymphatic systems. This differentiates it from other skin tumours. Prognosis depends on tumour thickness (Breslow 1970). Early detection and excision of thin tumours (less than 1 mm thick) carries an excellent prognosis and potential cure. Late-stage untreated melanoma with secondary deposits has a poorer outcome and treatment is often palliative, e.g. radiotherapy, chemotherapy, laser therapy (see Ch. 31).

Research suggests that excessive childhood sun exposure is an important factor in the aetiology of melanoma. Current campaigns such as Cancer Research UK (2003) and Scotland's 'Keep Yer Shirt On' are targeting the early years. In Scotland, the incidence of skin cancer has doubled in the last 20 years; approximately 6000 people are diagnosed with non-melanoma skin cancer and approximately 600 with malignant melanoma (Scottish Executive 1999). The aim is to significantly reduce the incidence of skin cancer in those under 75 years by the year 2010. The 'Keep Yer Shirt On' campaign, funded for 3 years by a New Opportunities Grant, has a coordinated partnership approach involving health promotion, education services, childcare partnerships and dermatology.

Overall, the aims of the campaign are to increase public awareness of the dangers of excessive sun exposure and the importance of regular skin checks to ascertain changes in moles at an early stage (see Box 12.10), and to promote 'safe sun' and encourage behavioural and social changes that might prevent or reduce the incidence of melanoma. Advice includes:

- avoidance of direct sun between 11.00 and 15.00 h
- use of high sun protection factor (SPF) creams
- use of T-shirts/sun hats.

Nurses in contact with any group of people can encourage regular checking of 'moles' as a preventive strategy which

Box 12.10

Mole watching — warning signs of melanoma

- Are new or existing moles getting larger?
- Changes in the normal smooth edge of the mole to a more irregular shape
- Changes in colour of the mole
- Is the mole itchy or painful?
- Is there any surrounding or underlying inflammation?
- Is there any bleeding, oozing or crusting?

could have a profound impact on the early detection, incidence and mortality rates of malignant melanoma (see Research Abstract 12.1).

For further reading, see Van Der Weyden (1996), Buchanan (2001) and Chapter 31.

A DEVELOPING SPECIALISM

This chapter has focused on some of the more common skin disorders encountered in hospital and in the community, but there are many more that could have been included. Further reference to a specialist textbook will reveal the full scope of dermatology as a major specialty. It is recognised that the majority of patients with a skin disorder are managed in primary care and that sound knowledge and skills in dermatology are important for community nurses. This is particularly important for nurses who are nurse prescribers (Bowman 1998).

The British Dermatological Nursing Group (BDNG) was established in 1989 as an independent specialty group for nurses and health care professionals with an interest in dermatology. It continues to develop educational initiatives, guidelines and protocols, addressing the needs of nurses working with patients with skin disorders. The Royal College of Nursing document *Standards of Care for Dermatology Nursing* (RCN 1995) was developed to provide an established level of requirement on which to base specialist practice (Stone 1997b). In 2002, a group of specialist dermatology nurses, together with NHS Education for Scotland, prepared a competency framework for dermatology nursing to support continuing professional development, and a core curriculum for caring for people with dermatological conditions has now been published (NHS Education for Scotland 2003).

There is also value in practice initiatives such as:

- the development of care systems (Gradwell & Haynes 1999) to enhance communication with patients, thus empowering them to be involved in care delivery
- the incorporation of quality of life indices into nursing assessment, providing subjective measurement of the impact skin disorders have on life (Thoms 1997)
- the role of the named nurse in assessing and ensuring that care plans are patient focused and need centred
- the education, counselling and sharing of clinical skills to underpin a supportive partnership that will enhance treatment concordance

RESEARCH ABSTRACT 12.1

It is known that individuals can make a significant impact on identifying early melanoma, when still curable, by conducting periodic skin self-examination (SSE), thus detecting new lesions or significant changes in pre-existing lesions. Providing patients with photographs as a baseline measure may encourage them to carefully watch lesions, detect changes or perform SSE more regularly.

A study conducted in New York (Oliviera et al 2004) set out to assess the impact of a brief nurse-delivered intervention, using digital photographs, on patients' adherence to performing SSE. Patients (n = 100) at high risk for melanoma skin cancer (five or more dysplastic naevi) had whole-body digital photography as part of their clinical evaluation. Patients were randomized: Group A (n = 49) received a teaching intervention (physician and nurse education module) with a photo book (personal whole-body photographs compiled in the form of a booklet, with nurse instruction on how to use the photographs); Group B (n = 51) received the teaching intervention only. Self-administration questionnaires were provided at three intervals: baseline, post-teaching intervention and at the 4-month post-baseline visit. To assess adherence with SSE, patients were asked, 'How many times in the past 4 months did you or someone else thoroughly examine your skin?'. In Group A, 10.2% of patients at baseline reported skin examination three or more times during the past 4 months, while 61.2% reported skin examination three or more times at the 4-month follow-up. In Group B the respective figures at baseline and 4-month follow-up were 19.6% and 37.2%. The increase in reported skin examination was compared between the two groups (>51% v >17.6%, P = 0.001).

The results suggest that a brief nurse-delivered intervention is effective at increasing patient adherence with SSE. The effect of the intervention was further enhanced with the use of digital photographs as an adjunct to SSE.

Oliviera S A, Stephen S W, Dusza M P H et al 2004 Patient adherence to self-examination. Effect of nurse intervention with photographs. American Journal of Preventive Medicine 26(2): 152–155

- the development of advice leaflets, reinforcing verbal instructions. Simple to prepare, these are beneficial to patients who may be overwhelmed by the bewildering array of ointments and lotions prescribed for their skin disorder.

The development of dermatological nursing in the UK over the last decade has been considerable in relation to service innovation, educational initiatives, growing involvement in research and the shaping of policy. Major changes have also taken place in the patterns of care delivery, the role of the patient and family in disease management and the collaboration between all health care professionals. Nurses must continue to develop their knowledge and skills as they are a key resource for dermatological clients in both hospital and home.

REFERENCES

Barker D 1995 More than skin deep. Practice Nurse 8(13): 761–767
Boston M, Preston D 2001 Acne and rosacea. In: Hughes E, Van Onselen J (eds) Dermatology nursing: a practical guide. Churchill Livingstone, Edinburgh
Bowman J 1998 Changing roles – should nurses prescribe? Dermatology in Practice 6(3): 14–16
Breslow A 1970 Thickness, cross sectional area and depth of invasion in the prognosis of cutaneous melanoma. Annals of Surgery 172: 902–908
Bridgett C 1996 Behavioural approaches to treating atopic eczema. Health Visitor 69(7): 284–285
British National Formulary 2006 British Medical Association and Royal Pharmaceutical Society of Great Britain, London
Buxton P K 2003 ABC of dermatology. BMJ Publishing, London
Bysshe J 1996 Eczema: making an unpleasant condition more bearable. Professional Care of Mother and Child 6(3): 59–61
Cancer Research UK 2003 SunSmart guidelines. London
Cotterill J A, Cunliffe W J 1997 Suicide in dermatology patients. British Journal of Dermatology 137: 246–250
Cunliffe W J, Gollnick H P M 2001 Acne diagnosis and management. Martin Dunitz, London
Dawe R J, Russell S, Ferguson J 1996 Borrowing from museum and industry – two photoprotective devices. British Journal of Dermatology 135: 1016–1017
Department of Health 1991 The patient's charter. HMSO, London
Department of Health 1992 Health of the nation. HMSO, London
Department of Health 2001 The prevention and treatment of head lice. TSO, London
Department of Health 2004 The NHS improvement plan. Offering a better service. www.dh.gov.uk
Docherty C 2001 Infections and infestations. In: Hughes E, Van Onselen J (eds) Dermatology nursing: a practical guide. Churchill Livingstone, Edinburgh
Ernst E, White A 2000 The BBC survey of complementary medicine use in the UK, complementary medicine on the NHS. www.bbc.co.uk/health
Ferguson J 2004 Chronic actinic dermatitis. Journal of the European Academy of Dermatology and Venereology 18(Suppl 1)
Gawkrodger D J 2003 Dermatology: an illustrated colour text, 3rd edn. Churchill Livingstone, Edinburgh
Gradwell C, Haynes M 1999 Developing a care system for dermatology patients. Professional Nurse 14(12): 821–823
Graham-Brown R, Bourke J 1998 Mosby's color atlas and text of dermatology. Mosby, London
Gupta M A, Schork N J, Gupta A K et al 1993 Suicidal ideation in psoriasis. International Journal of Dermatology 32: 188–190
Hay R J, Rustin M H A 2004 Key advances in the clinical management of atopic eczema. Royal Society of Medicine Publication, London
House of Lords 2000 Regulation of complementary therapies in medicine. Select Committee on Science and Technology, 6th edn. TSO, London
Hughes E, Van Onselen J (eds) 2001 Dermatology nursing: a practical guide. Churchill Livingstone, Edinburgh
Hunter J, Savin J, Dahl M 2002 Clinical dermatology, 3rd edn. Blackwell Science, Oxford
Jeyasingham M 1997 National Eczema Society – 21 years of patient advice and support. British Journal of Dermatology Nursing 1(1): 10–12
Keen S, Comer L 1995 Subcutaneous administration of adrenaline for anaphylaxis. Nursing Times 5(91): 36–37
Kurwa H A, Finlay A Y 1995 Dermatology inpatient management greatly improves life quality. British Journal of Dermatology 113: 575–578
Lawlor F 1998 Diagnosing and treating common urticaria. Dermatology in Practice 6(3): 18–20
Lawton S 2004 Dermatology. Developing the nurse led role. Nursing Times 100(17): 20–22
Layton A 1995 Acne: assessment and treatment. Community 1(7): 36
Legge A 1997 Skin care: take three experts. Nursing Times 93(44): 70–71
Lewis-Jones S 1999 Quality of life – skin disease and disability. Dermatology in Practice 7(3): 8–10
Lynn S, Lawton S, Newham S 1997 Managing atopic eczema: the needs of children. Professional Nurse 12(9): 622–625
Marks R 2003 Roxburgh's common skin diseases. Arnold, London
McGeary T 1997 Fatal reaction. Nursing Times 20(93): 26
Ministry of Agriculture, Fisheries and Food 1996 Food Safety Information Bulletin 78: 1–2
Morris A 1998 Effects of long-term topical corticosteroids. Dermatology in Practice 6(3): 5–8
Mygind N, Dahl R, Pederson S et al 1996 Essential allergy. Blackwell Science, Oxford
Nathan A 1996 Over the counter treatments. Primary Health Care 6(5): 16–17
National Eczema Society 2003 Schools packs. NES, London
NHS Education for Scotland 2003 Caring for people with dermatological conditions: a core curriculum. NHS Education for Scotland, Edinburgh
Nursing and Midwifery Council 2004 Code of professional conduct: standards for conduct, performance and ethics. NMC, London
Oliviera S A, Stephen S W, Dusza M P H et al 2004 Patient adherence to skin self-examination. Effect of nurse intervention with photographs. American Journal of Preventive Medicine 26(2): 152–155
Page B E 2003 Wet wraps. Nursing Scotland March/April: 22
Payling K J 1996 Occupational skin disorders. Professional Nurse 11(6): 393–395
Penzer R 1996 Psoriasis. Nursing Standard 10(29): 49–55
Peters J 2001 Assessment of the dermatology patient. In: Hughes E, Van Onselen J (eds) Dermatology nursing: a practical guide. Churchill Livingstone, Edinburgh
Rathmell B 2003 What I tell my patients about PUVA. British Journal of Dermatology Nursing 7(3): 12–13
Royal College of Nursing 1995 Standards of care for dermatology nursing. Scutari Press, Middlesex
Ruane-Morris M, Thomson G, Lawton S 1995 Community liaison in dermatology. Professional Nurse 10(11): 687–688
Scottish Executive 1999 Towards a healthier Scotland. TSO, Edinburgh
Stabell Benn C, Wohlfahrt J, Aaby P et al 2004 Breastfeeding and risk of atopic dermatitis, by parental history of allergy during the first 18 months of life. American Journal of Epidemiology 160(3): 217–223
Stone L 1997a Dermatology nursing: planning for the future. Nursing Standard 11(49): 39–41
Stone L 1997b Education and training in dermatology nursing. British Journal of Dermatology Nursing 1(1): 5–7
Thoms H 1997 Quality of life in psoriasis. British Journal of Dermatology Nursing 1(3): 5–7
Titman P 2003 Understanding childhood eczema. Wiley, Chichester
Waugh A, Grant A (eds) 2001 Ross and Wilson's anatomy, physiology in health and illness, 9th edn. Churchill Livingstone, Edinburgh
White G 2003 Color atlas of dermatology, 3rd edn. Mosby, London

FURTHER READING

Absolon C M, Cottrell D, Eldridge S M et al 1997 Psychological disturbance in atopic eczema: the extent of the problem in school aged children. British Journal of Dermatology 137: 241–245
Bridgett C, Noren P, Staughton R 1996 Atopic skin disease – a manual for practitioners. Wrightson Biomedical, Petersfield
Buchanan P J 2001 Skin cancer. Nursing Standard 15(45): 45–52, 54–55
Cork M J, Britton J, Butler L et al 2003 Comparison of parent knowledge, therapy utilization and severity of atopic eczema before and after explanation and demonstration of topical therapies by a specialist dermatology nurse. British Journal of Dermatology 149(3): 582–589

Cox N, Walton Y, Bowan J 1995 Evaluation of nurse prescribing in a dermatology unit. British Journal of Dermatology 133(2): 340–341
Dawkes K 1997 How to apply emollients effectively. British Journal of Dermatology Nursing 1(2): 8–9
Gawkrodger D J 2003 Dermatology: an illustrated colour text, 3rd edn. Churchill Livingstone, Edinburgh
Gill S 2003 Children and dermatology: the implications of recent findings for dermatology departments. Dermatological Nursing 2(4): 12–15
Lawson V, Lewis-Jones M, Finlay A et al 1998 The family impact of childhood atopic dermatitis: the dermatitis family questionnaire. British Journal of Dermatology 138(1): 107–113
Mateos M 2002 The health visitor's role in setting up a nurse led clinic. Dermatological Nursing 1(4): 6–8
MacKie R M 1997 Clinical dermatology: an illustrated textbook, 4th edn. Oxford Medical, Oxford
Peters J 2004 Adult eczema and behaviour modification. Dermatological Nursing 3(2): 8–10
Ratcliffe J 1998 How to conduct a patch test. British Journal of Dermatology Nursing 2(4): 8–9
Robertson S 2003 Treatment options for managing hyperhidrosis: a case study. Dermatological Nursing 2(1): 10–11
Rolfe G 2002 Nursing role for acne in primary care. British Journal of Dermatology Nursing 6(3): 9–11
Sarkany R 1999 World wide web – the impact of the internet on dermatology. Dermatology in Practice 7(3): 16–18
Talbot L, Curtis L 1996 The challenges of assessing skin indicators in people of color. Home Healthcare Nurse 14(3): 167–173
Van Der Weyden R 1996 Changing attitudes to sun exposure. British Journal of Nursing 3(5): 765–769
Walsh D 1996 Aromatherapy in the management of psoriasis. Nursing Standard 11(13): 53–56

USEFUL WEBSITES

Acne Support Group
www.stopspots.org

British Dermatological Nursing Group
www.bdng.org.uk

National Eczema Society
www.eczema.org

Shingles Support Society
www.herpes.org.uk

Skin Care Campaign
www.skincarecampaign.org

The Psoriasis Association
www.psoriasis-association.org.uk

DISORDERS OF THE EYE

13

Christine Thom
Allyson Sanderson

INTRODUCTION

The principal aims of this chapter are to present the knowledge and specialised care required for the ophthalmic patient, to raise awareness pertaining to visual impairment (VI) and how VI impacts upon the social, physical and psychological aspects of daily living, and to consider the implications for practice of a range of disability-related legislation such as the Disability Discrimination Act (DDA 1996) (Casserley 2001). Changes in patient care management, including the trend towards a decrease in the length of hospital stay and the increasingly 'normal' practice of day case or short-stay regimens, has led to a greater need for partnerships between hospital and community teams. As life expectancy increases in the UK, there is a higher incidence of cataract, age-related maculopathy and diabetic eye disease and it is increasingly important, therefore, for health care professionals to recognise adverse ocular signs and symptoms and to ensure prompt referral for specialised care. Not all ocular conditions cause VI, and many clinical conditions are successfully treated with medical and surgical interventions. The ocular conditions and diseases presented in this chapter will provide the reader with a sound knowledge base related to causes, diagnoses, treatments and related nursing care. The nurse, in all environments, has a duty of care to be up-to-date in practice, and to facilitate health promotion and screening in primary and secondary care settings (McSherry & Pearce 2002, Tingle & Cribb 2002, NMC 2004).

Incidence of visual impairment and blindness

The World Health Organization (WHO) estimates that, globally, 180 million people are visually impaired and, of this number, 40–45 million are blind (www.who.int). It is thought that with appropriate resources, improved environmental conditions and timely intervention, 80% of the global incidence of blindness could be avoided either by treatment, e.g. cataract surgery, or by prevention programmes, e.g. for trachoma. The developing countries account for 9 out of 10 of the world's blind population. It is predicted that the global burden of blindness will double by 2020 (www.who.int) due to an increase in the population and longer life expectancy (Thylefors 1998).

The main causes of blindness globally are:

- cataract — opacity of the lens — the leading cause, responsible for 50% of all blindness, but readily treatable with surgery
- trachoma — ocular inflammation and corneal opacity caused by repeated infection of the cornea and conjunctiva by *Chlamydia trachomatis*. This is the most

common preventable condition and accounts for 12.5% of all blindness
- xerophthalmia — dryness and ulceration of the cornea associated with vitamin A deficiency. This preventable condition, which accounts for 6% of all blindness, can be eradicated with vitamin A supplementation
- glaucoma — raised intraocular pressure (IOP), causing optic nerve damage with associated visual field loss. Although the condition itself, which accounts for 15% of all blindness, is not preventable, the threat to sight can be reduced by screening, topical medication and surgery
- onchocerciasis — river blindness — caused by a microfilarial (parasitic worm) infestation transmitted by bites of the black fly. The parasitic worms invade the eye, destroying all structures. It is estimated that there are 18 million people infected worldwide and that Africa has the highest prevalence, with the disease being endemic in 30 African countries. This disease can be prevented by controlling the black fly population and can be treated by the drug ivermectin. WHO assists with funding and supports both trachoma and onchocerciasis programmes which have established health education and promotional work in progress.

WHO is also at the forefront of 'Vision 2020 – The Right to Sight: A Global Initiative for the Elimination of Avoidable Blindness'. The aim is to eliminate avoidable blindness as a public health problem by the year 2020.

For further information, see www.who.int and www.v2020.org.

In developed countries such as the UK, resources are more readily available and government-led initiatives such as 'Action on Cataract' (NHS Executive 2000) have been targeted to streamline clinical services and reduce the number of people with cataract. The main causes of VI and blindness are cataract and glaucoma (see p. 553), with age-related maculopathy (see p. 584) and diabetic eye disease (see p. 585) accounting for most of the remaining VI and blindness. Although none of these conditions is preventable, modern drug, laser and surgical treatments mean that there is more opportunity for controlling the course of the disease and thus reducing the potential for VI and blindness. The Royal College of Ophthalmologists (RCO) estimate that 4.3 million people over 65 years of age in the UK have a VI in one or both eyes (see 'Useful websites'). The cost to the government is estimated at greater than £120 million per annum for cataract treatment alone.

STOP THINK **13.1** Using associated websites (see 'Useful websites') and library resources such as CD-ROM, investigate epidemiological trends in relation to blindness and its causes.

ANATOMY AND PHYSIOLOGY

The components of the sensory mechanisms responsible for sight are the eyes, the optic nerves and tracts, and the visual cortex and association areas of the brain.

Accessory structures play a vital role in enabling the eyes to scan and focus on objects in the environment and in protecting and maintaining the optical properties of the eyes.

The eye

The eyeball (see Fig. 13.1)

With minor individual variations, the eyeball is spherical in shape, with the cornea on the anterior aspect being slightly more steeply curved. The length of an adult eye is approximately 24 mm.

The eyeball or globe has three main layers of tissue:

- *The outer layer* of the globe consists of the fibrous white sclera posteriorly and the transparent cornea anteriorly. The junction of the two is called the limbus. The cornea

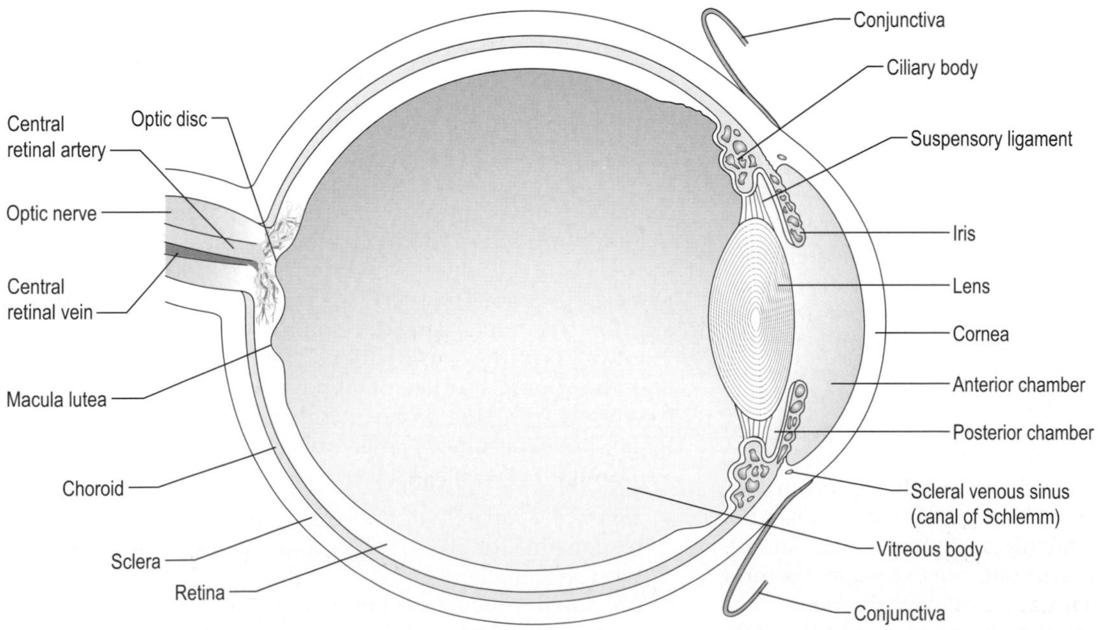

 Fig. 13.1 Section of the eye.

is transparent due to its avascularity and the regular arrangement of its fibres. It is well supplied with nerve endings from the trigeminal nerve.

- *The middle vascular layer*, known as the uveal tract, consists of the choroid, the ciliary body and the iris. The choroid lines the sclera in the posterior compartment of the eye and continues into the muscular ciliary body, into which are inserted the suspensory ligaments. These ligaments extend to the lens and hold it in position. This diaphragm-like ligamentous structure is known as the zonule. The contraction or relaxation of the ciliary body changes the shape of the lens and controls its refractive and focusing power. The iris is the pigmented anterior portion of the uveal tract. It contains both circular and radial muscle fibres which control the size of the pupil.
- *The inner layer* of the eyeball is the retina. It contains several million photoreceptive cells which are responsible for converting light into electrical impulses. The retina arises just behind the equator of the eyeball in an area known as the ora serrata. This leaves a small anterior section of the choroid — the pars plana — exposed. This is important because it allows surgical access without retinal damage.

The retina consists of two layers: the pigmented outer layer, which lines the choroid, and the innermost neural layer, which is in contact with the vitreous humor. Rod cells predominate in the periphery and function best in dim light. Cone cells predominate near the centre of the retina and are adapted for bright light and colour vision. The greatest concentration of cone cells is at the macula, a small area in the centre of the retina which has as its midpoint the fovea centralis, the most vital part of the retina for high-definition vision. These photoreceptor cells are linked through a series of synapses to ganglion cells whose axons run together to form the optic nerve.

The two compartments and three chambers of the eye

Inside the globe, the lens, suspended by the zonule, divides the eye into two main compartments. The anterior compartment is itself divided into two chambers, the anterior chamber in front of the iris and the posterior chamber behind the iris. The compartment behind the lens is sometimes referred to as the vitreous chamber, as it contains the clear jelly-like substance called the vitreous humor.

Internal environment and intraocular pressure (IOP)

The anterior compartment is bathed in a clear fluid called aqueous or aqueous humor, which is produced by the ciliary body and which provides nutrients to the lens and cornea. Aqueous flows from the posterior chamber through the pupil to the anterior chamber and drains away through the sieve-like fibrous trabecular meshwork located in the angle between the iris and cornea around the circumference of the eye (see Fig. 13.2). This in turn drains into the vascular canal of Schlemm and thereby into the systemic venous circulation. The production and drainage of aqueous must be constant in order to maintain a normal IOP, which is variable over a 24-h period, within the range of 10–20 mmHg (Waugh & Grant 2001).

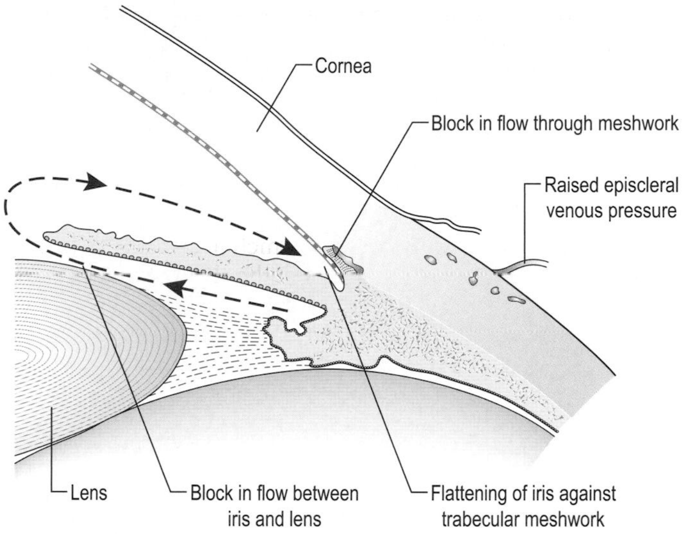

Fig. 13.2 Normal aqueous drainage and possible sites of obstruction. (Adapted from Khaw et al 2004, with permission from the BMJ Publishing Group.)

Box 13.1

Terms associated with visual acuity and refractive errors

- Emmetropia — normal sight; light rays focus on the retina
- Ametropia — defective sight due to refractive error
- Myopia — short-sightedness; light rays focus in front of the retina
- Hypermetropia — long-sightedness; light rays focus behind the retina
- Presbyopia — loss of focused reading/near-vision capacity, resulting from loss of lens elasticity due to ageing
- Astigmatism — irregular curvature of the cornea which prevents light rays from focusing at a single point

The shape of the eye can, by determining the depth of the anterior chamber and the angle between the cornea and iris, affect the functioning of the drainage system. The larger, elongated eye of the myope (short-sighted person) has a naturally occurring deep anterior chamber with an open angle, whereas the small eye of the hypermetrope (long-sighted person) has a shallow anterior chamber with a narrow angle (see Box 13.1). Any interference with normal drainage of the aqueous humor raises the IOP, leading to the decreased blood supply, pain and impaired vision associated with conditions such as glaucoma and postoperative or traumatic complications.

The visual pathways and interpretative centres

The optic nerve runs from the posterior aspect of the globe and enters the cranial cavity via the optic foramen. The

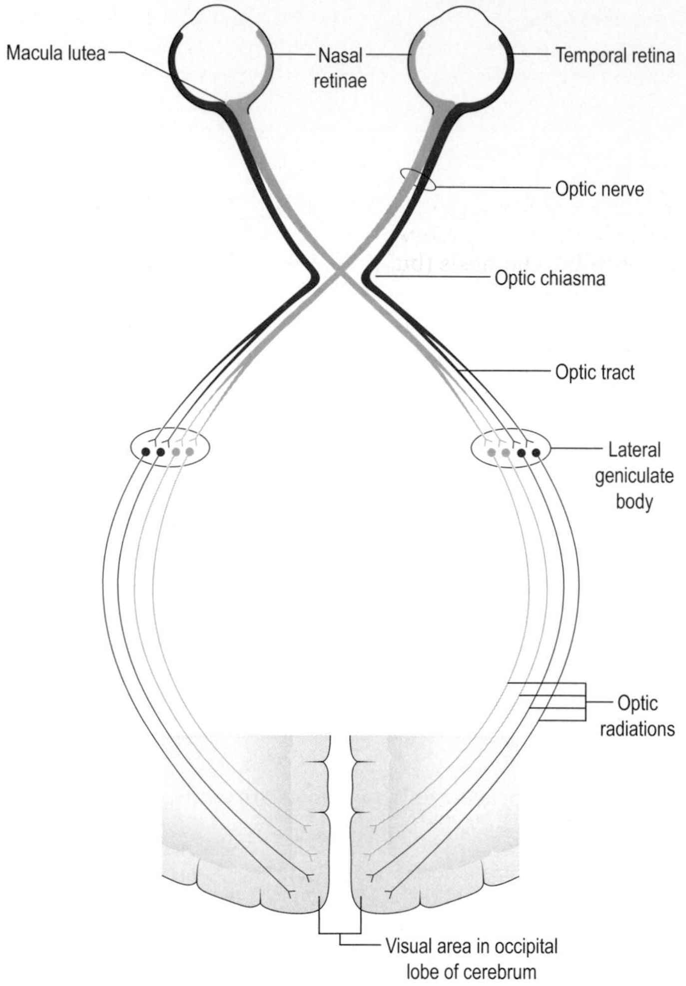

Fig. 13.3 The optic nerves and their pathways.

medial nerve fibres cross over to the opposite side at the optic chiasma (see Fig. 13.3) to join with the lateral fibres and form the optic tract before synapsing in the lateral geniculate body of the thalamus. From the lateral geniculate body, the fibres run in the optic radiations to the occipital lobe of the cerebrum.

The main blood supply to the eye is via the ophthalmic artery, a branch of the internal carotid artery, which runs alongside the optic nerve.

Accessory structures

The exposed anterior aspect of the eyeball is protected by the eyebrow, eyelids and eyelashes. The conjunctiva, a mucous membrane, lines the eyelids (palpebral conjunctiva) and reflects back on itself to cover the exposed sclera. This fold forms the conjunctival sac or fornix and is an ideal site for the instillation of topical drugs. At the limbus, the conjunctiva is modified to form the epithelial layer of the cornea. The conjunctiva facilitates free movement of the globe.

The exposed surface of the eye is also covered by a three-layered film of tear fluid. Mucous secretion from conjunctival goblet cells forms the first layer of the tear film and

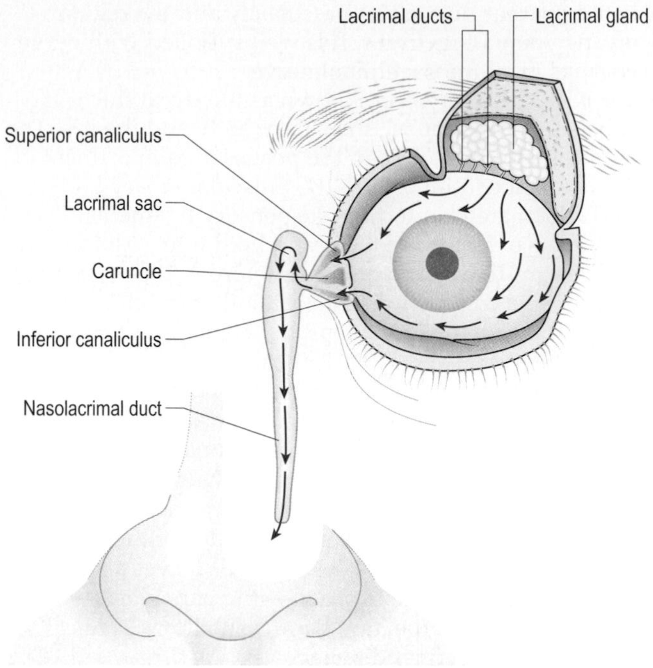

Fig. 13.4 The lacrimal apparatus. Arrows show the direction of the flow of tears.

ensures an even spread of tears over the cornea. The second (middle) layer of the tear film is the watery fluid secreted by the lacrimal glands, situated under the outer aspect of the upper orbital rim, and by the accessory glands in the conjunctiva. The third (outer) lipid layer of tear film is secreted by the Meibomian glands of the lids. This is thought to reduce the evaporation rate of tears and to prevent the lids sticking together during sleep. The main functions of tear fluid are to lubricate the eye, to facilitate O_2 and CO_2 exchange, to provide an optically smooth corneal surface and to cleanse the eye with the bacteriostatic enzyme, lysozyme.

Excess tears are drained from the eye via the lacrimal apparatus at the inner canthus at the nasal end of the lid margins, into the lacrimal sac and thence into the nose through the nasolacrimal duct (see Fig. 13.4).

Posteriorly and laterally the globe is protected by the bony orbit, the extraocular recti and oblique muscles, responsible for tracking movements, and by orbital fat.

The physiology of vision

Light rays are bent (refracted) as they pass through the varying densities of the clear media of the cornea, aqueous, lens and vitreous to focus on the retina. The cornea is responsible for approximately two-thirds of the refractive power of the eye and is relatively constant. However, by virtue of its elasticity, the lens has the ability to change shape and thereby vary the amount of refraction for clarity of focus. This is known as accommodation and is necessary in order for objects at different distances to be visualised with equal clarity.

The normal eye in its relaxed state brings rays of light from distant objects into sharp focus. However, for clear focusing on near objects, an autonomic reflex known as the synkinetic near reflex comes into play. This reflex involves accommodation, miosis and convergence, as follows:

- *Accommodation* — the ciliary body contracts and changes shape, thus releasing tension on the zonular fibres and allowing the lens to thicken and increase its refractive power
- *Miosis* — constriction of the pupil — accompanies accommodation and ensures that light rays are concentrated to pass through the centre of the lens and focus on the macula
- *Convergence* — in-turning of the eyes — seeks out the object to be focused on.

Failure to focus may be described as ametropia, or refractive error (see Box 13.1).

Once the rays of light are focused on the retina, their energy is converted into neuroelectrical energy by the photoreceptor cells. These nerve impulses are transmitted via other neural cells in the retina to the optic nerve and so by the visual pathway to the visual cortex. Here, they are interpreted as sensations of light, form and colour and are processed into images of objects which are given meaning by other cerebral areas through correlation with information stored as memory in the association areas of the brain (see also Ch. 9).

ASSESSING THE EYE AND VISUAL FUNCTION

Examination of structure

It is vital for nurses working with ophthalmic patients to learn to examine the eye in a systematic way and to recognise abnormalities and their significance. In order to do so, it is necessary to know what a normal eye looks like and what normal expectations are for an eye recovering from surgery or disease. It is essential to work in good light using a pen torch and to proceed systematically, examining all ocular structures from outermost to innermost as follows:

- lids — observe position, closure, bruising, discharge
- conjunctiva — observe degree of injection (visible blood vessels), chemosis (bulging effect due to oedema), discharge, wounds
- cornea — observe clarity, type and extent of any opacity, shape, suture lines, wounds
- anterior chamber (AC) — observe depth, clarity, presence of hyphaema (blood in AC), hypopyon (pus in AC)
- iris — observe colour, position, appearance
- pupil — observe size, shape, position, colour of reflection from lens
- intraocular lens (IOL) — if appropriate, observe position and reflection
- retina — examine through dilated pupil using ophthalmoscope.

The possible implications of clinical features that may be found in the course of an eye examination are listed in Table 13.1.

Testing visual function

Visual acuity

Visual acuity (VA) assessment is generally carried out by nurses and is the mathematical estimation of visual function for different distances.

Table 13.1 Significance of clinical features found on eye examination

Structure	Clinical features	Possible significance
Lids	Bruising (ecchymosis) Swelling Drooping Increased lacrimation Discharge	Surgical handling Trauma Infection
Conjunctiva	Redness (injection) Swelling (chemosis)	Surgical handling Trauma Allergy Infection
Cornea	Cloudy Crinkled Fluorescein staining Suture line not intact Penetrating injury	Increased IOP Infection Loss of AC Ulceration
Anterior chamber (AC)	Hyphaema (blood in AC) Hypopyon (pus in AC) Shallow AC	Hyphaema due to surgery should gradually resolve Increasing IOP = bleeding/inflammation Hypopyon = infection Shallow = ? aqueous loss
Iris	Muddy	Inflammation
Pupil	Irregular shape	Iris prolapse Adhesions Trauma

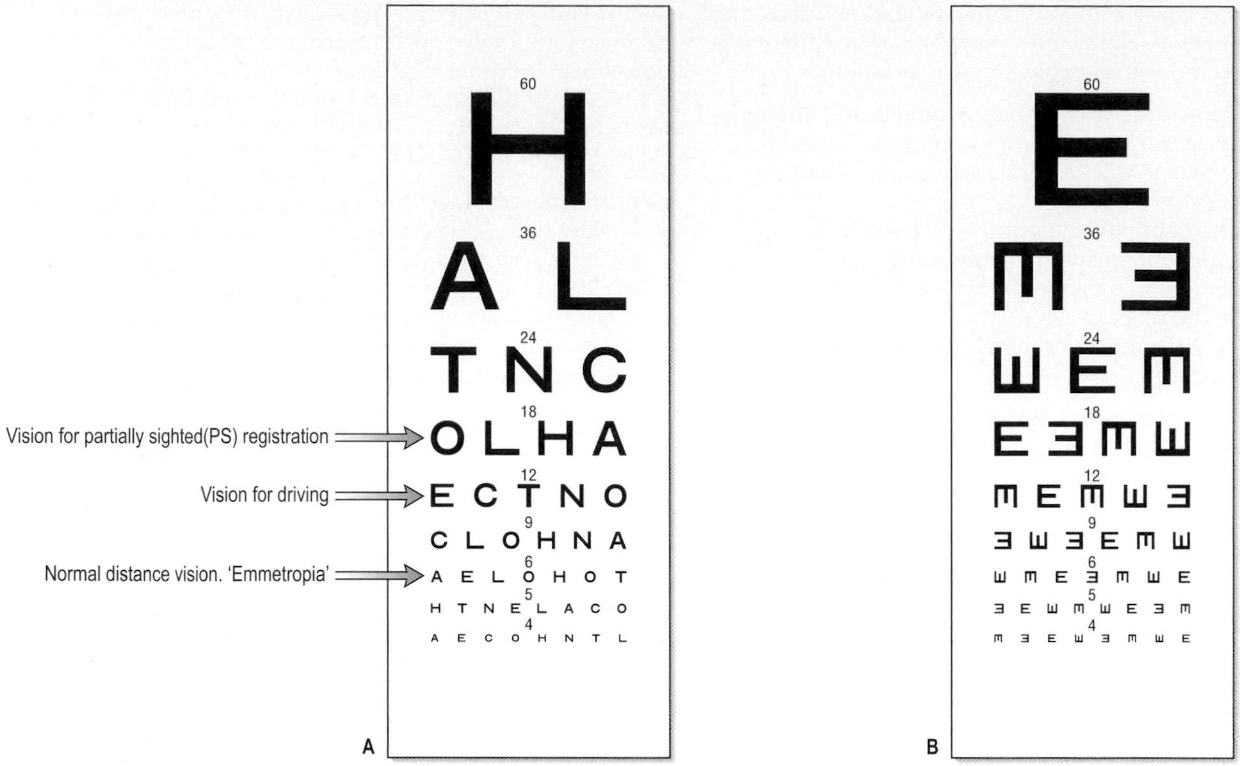

Fig. 13.5 Eye testing charts. A: Snellen test-type chart; the standard method for testing visual acuity in the UK. B: 'E' chart for non-English speakers. The patient is given a wooden or plastic E and is asked to make it indicate the positions in which it appears on the chart.

Distance vision This is tested using Snellen test-type charts. These charts display letters or pictures arranged in rows of precise and diminishing size (see Fig. 13.5). Each eye should be tested separately, with the benefit of any spectacles or contact lenses, if the patient normally wears these, to ensure that what is being checked is 'best corrected vision'. The eye not being tested must be completely occluded. In normal testing, the patient is positioned 6 m away from the chart and asked to read each line aloud until they can no longer make out the letters. The result is recorded as a fraction of the distance from the chart in metres over the normal reading distance of the last complete line read, plus the number of extra letters read from the line below or minus the number of letters read incorrectly, e.g. 6/9 – 2 with correction (i/c) (see Fig 13.5). If glasses or contact lenses are worn, this is recorded as i/c gls. or i/c CL, respectively.

Normal distance acuity is accepted as 6/6, although the expectation of what the patient is likely to achieve will vary with age. If the result is 6/9 or less (see Fig. 13.5), the patient may be asked to read the chart again, looking through a pinhole (PH). A pure refractive error should improve with this simple method of sharpening focus. The improved acuity would be recorded as 6/9 i/c PH.

If the patient cannot read the top letter, recorded as 6/60, then ability to count fingers (CF) at 1 m, detect hand movements (HM) or perceive light (PL) is tested. Awareness of direction of a light source may also be noted (projection). Testing in more complicated situations, such as when the patient cannot read or understand English, can be facilitated by using a Snellen 'E' chart (see Fig. 13.5B). If the patient has learning difficulties, poor concentration or expressive dysphasia (see p. 417), then testing of visual acuity can be carried out using a Sheridan Gardiner singles booklet in which single letters or pictures of varying size are presented one at a time for the patient to identify or match.

Near vision is tested in a similar fashion by asking the patient to read text in various sizes of standard print, which are prefixed with the letter N. N5 is accepted as normal reading acuity. Near vision should be checked in conditions of good illumination.

Binocular vision involves simultaneous perception of an image by both eyes and fusion of the two images in the visual cortex to form a single image. Binocular vision is thought to play a role in depth perception. Having two eyes also widens the field of vision and counters gaps in the visual field caused by natural blind spots.

STOP THINK **13.2** Look carefully straight ahead and note what you see. Now close one eye. What do you not see? Now repeat with the other eye. What do you no longer see?

The visual field The range of what the eye can see with respect to angle of view, rather than distance, is called the visual field. Normally this is about 60° nasally, 90° temporally, 50° superiorly and 70° inferiorly. Assessment of the integrity of the visual field is an important aid to diagnosis of retinal detachment and neurological disease and is essential in the management of open-angle glaucoma. Visual field testing can be carried out in the following ways:

- *Simple confrontation test* — the examiner compares the patient's field of vision with their own. Facing the patient, who is asked to maintain a fixed gaze on the examiner's face, the examiner moves a finger from various points on their own periphery of vision and asks the patient to indicate when it appears in their field of vision.
- *Perimetry*, using basic to increasingly more sophisticated field analyser systems, e.g. the Henson, Friedmann, Goldmann or Humphrey systems, gives accurate measurements of visual field defects known as scotoma.

For examples of perimetry printouts, see Kanski (2003).

Colour blindness

Colour vision depends on the normal functioning of the retinal cones. A colour-blind person is unable to distinguish between some colours — usually red and green. While approximately 10% of the male population are born with defective colour vision, this problem is estimated at only 1% in females (Chong 1996). Colour blindness can also be acquired; it is characteristic of certain disease processes such as optic neuritis and some macular disorders, and may develop in people with a drug dependency.

The most common method of testing for colour blindness is by means of Ishihara colour plates. These are a series of cards on which numbers, composed of red and green dots, have been printed against a background of different coloured dots. A person with defective colour vision would be unable to distinguish the numbers from the surrounding background.

Some occupations require normal colour vision, usually for reasons of safety. For example, an electrician needs to be able to distinguish between coloured wires, and an airline pilot between the coloured lights on the aircraft's instrument panel. Applicants for positions such as these will be tested for colour vision. There are no restrictions on driving cars, lorries or buses, as traffic lights have a fixed sequence and can be recognised by position rather than colour.

STOP THINK **13.3** What other occupations can you think of that require normal colour vision?

Eye changes with ageing

By age 70, most people will need some form of visual aid, since, with advancing years, the ability of the lens to accommodate decreases as it becomes less elastic. Focusing is affected as the cornea flattens, causing astigmatism (see Box 13.1). A decrease in pupil size reduces the amount of light entering the eye, and retinal cells become less efficient due to deposits laid down by ageing pigment epithelial cells. Tear film is reduced in volume and altered in structure, with the result that tears evaporate more quickly, leading to dryness and irritation of the eye. However, some older patients complain of watering eyes, e.g. due to malposition of eyelids (see 'Entropion'/'Ectropion', p. 584). The corneal periphery often develops a marked grey ring at its junction with the sclera — known as arcus senilis.

For further information on caring for older people with visual impairment, see Chivers (2003).

PRESERVATION OF VISION

Nurses can do a great deal through health education and active intervention to help people preserve their vision (Milligan 2002). The following list highlights methods which all nurses should use to contribute to health education and promotion:

- Promote the maintenance of good health through regular exercise, not smoking and a balanced diet. It is believed, although not proven, that these actions will reduce the risk of ocular degeneration, especially in people with diabetes mellitus.

For further information, see www.diabeticretinopathy.org.uk/prevention

- Observe individual behaviour and general appearance; missed appointments, unkempt clothes and a reluctance to go out may suggest ocular problems. Should any changes be noted, prompt action and referral to ensure early screening and accurate diagnosis are vital. The community nurse's observation of changes in appearance or behaviour in patients can often bring ophthalmic problems to light and result in early diagnosis and treatment. Prompt referral to the appropriate health professional is essential.

STOP THINK **13.4** Take 5 minutes to consider changes in behaviour or appearance that may be indicative of deteriorating vision.

- Encourage regular eye examination — especially in children, people over 40 years of age and individuals in high-risk groups, e.g. those with diabetes mellitus or hypertension. Free sight testing is available for people over 60 years of age, those in high-risk groups, lower income groups and people over 40 years of age who have a family history of glaucoma.

For further information on free sight testing and benefits available, see www.rnib.org.uk

- Provide advice and ensure the correct use, storage and cleaning of glasses and contact lenses. It is vital that contact lenses are properly maintained and used according to optometrists' and manufacturers' guidelines. If guidelines are not followed, there is a risk of long-term, possibly permanent damage to the cornea, due to infection, ulceration or abrasion.
- Monitor carefully oxygen therapy in babies to prevent retinal damage.
- Treat promptly any eye infections, in order to prevent ocular damage.
- Encourage the use of eye protection where required. Both work- and leisure-related eye injuries can be prevented by wearing eye protection (see Box 13.2). Milligan (2002) reviewed the causes and measures for the prevention of ocular injuries: 85% occur in males aged 20–40 and approximately 70% result from industrial accidents. While statutory and health and safety regulations and better supervision by occupational health nurses have helped to reduce the number of industrial eye injuries, lack of eye protection remains a problem. The occupational health nurse and the prison nurse (in those custodial settings with work

Box 13.2

Preventing eye injury

Protective eyewear should always be worn during any prolonged exposure to strong sunlight or snow, as well as for the following activities:

- Chipping masonry
- Chopping wood
- Drilling
- Laying insulation
- Playing squash
- Pruning trees or shrubbery
- Stripping paint
- Sunbed bathing
- Welding
- Working under the chassis of a car.

programmes) are in a prime position not only to instruct on first aid irrigation for chemical eye injuries, but, just as importantly, to encourage the use of eye protection, through promoting attitude change and participating proactively in risk assessment of work which requires eye protection. Although the wearing of eye protection is mandatory in certain work environments, e.g. chemical laboratories and any area where grinding of metal occurs — Health and Safety at Work Act (1974) and Personal Protective Equipment at Work Regulations (1992) — nurses should be aware that some people are reluctant to wear eye protection as it may be uncomfortable and can obscure vision.

- Advocate the correct and safe labelling of chemical products, and ensure first aid, e.g. eye irrigation, is available for emergency use. Individuals should be urged in the workplace and at home to heed the labels on chemical products indicating whether they are harmful to the eyes: careful note should also be taken of first aid instructions in case of accidental splashing.
- Ensure that visual display units (VDUs) are used in accordance with the Health and Safety Executive (2003) recommendations for short, frequent rest periods to prevent eye fatigue. Employers must provide an annual sight test for all VDU users.
- Promote the wearing of sunglasses. Exactly what type of ocular damage exposure to sunlight can cause is not known, but it is believed to contribute to long-term ocular changes, i.e. cataract, macular degeneration.

For further information, see www.afbp.org.

THE VISUALLY IMPAIRED PERSON

It is difficult for sighted individuals to appreciate fully the value and importance of vision in everyday life.

STOP THINK **13.5** Using a structured model of activities of daily living (AL) such as Orem (2001) or Holland et al (2003), discuss and list how being VI would impact upon these. Working through this may help you to gain some understanding of the daily experience of the visually impaired person (VIP). To experience a 'temporary VI' ask a colleague to blindfold you, using a sleep shade, and then to guide (see Fig. 13.6) and assist you through as many of the ALs as possible. Include eating a meal, going into a busy room, buying an item with the correct money and travelling on public transport. Reflect on this experience by asking yourself how it affected the essential 'you'. Did you feel any less intelligent? Did you feel anxious or vulnerable? Did it change the way others reacted to you? Share your experiences and insights with your colleagues.

Registration of blindness, i.e. severely sight impaired, and partial sight, i.e. sight impaired

There are few totally blind people, as most visually impaired people have some residual sight. An ophthalmologist will certify the degree of impairment, using a certificate of vision impairment form (CVI in England) or blind person form (BP1 in Scotland). Rehabilitation support can be obtained without registration.

For further information on Wales and Northern Ireland, see www.rnib.org.uk.

Registration, which is completely voluntary, entitles the individual to many local and national benefits. These will be explained by the social worker, who visits individuals in their homes and helps to arrange for appropriate support. Some areas also have the benefit of a mobility or rehabilitation officer, who is specially trained to help newly registered individuals to relearn certain daily living skills, and to move about safely in their own environment. This may involve the use of special canes or guide dogs (see 'Useful websites'). Rehabilitation officers also teach communication and information technology (IT) skills and advise on retraining for employment. Their overall aim is to enable the VIP to function as independently as possible.

People with impaired vision may be referred to a low-vision clinic and assessed by an optometrist or specialist nurse, to determine whether a variety of low visual aids (LVAs), for distance or near vision, can help individuals to make best use of their residual sight. These professionals may also provide information and advice on adaptation or retraining for employment. Employers can also be advised by various agencies, including Action for Blind People (afbp) and the Royal National Institute of the Blind (RNIB) (see 'Useful websites') about the sophisticated electronic equipment now available for VI employees. The introduction of the Disability Discrimination Act (DDA) (1996) made it unlawful to treat disabled individuals in a discriminatory way (Brading & Curtis 2000). Employers and service providers, including the NHS, must make reasonable adjustments to their services, ensuring, for example, equal access for disabled persons (Thomas & Ryan 1997).

Considering the needs of the visually impaired person

All nursing care should be planned using a structured approach to assessment and implemented using an agreed care pathway. This approach facilitates accountability and audit mechanisms.

Orem's model for nursing (Orem 2001) takes account of universal needs but focuses on specific areas of self-care deficit, builds on the individual's strengths and promotes personal responsibility for health maintenance. Education and counselling are also essential components of this model.

Some general principles of care for the VIP are outlined below:

- *Orientation to place* — if the person is at home, the environment is familiar and it is therefore important to keep things in their usual place. Every assistance should be given to help the person to move around the community and workplace until confident to do so independently. Appropriate visual aids should be used. If the person is admitted to hospital, it is the nurse's responsibility to provide adequate orientation, based on individual needs. Older people can become confused in this situation and need constant reassurance and support.
- *Maintaining a safe environment* — it is essential to remove any hazardous objects in the person's environment. Doors should be either fully open or properly closed. Fires should have guards. Loose flooring must be secured.

STOP THINK **13.6** Examine the hospital or home environment to identify problems that the VIP may encounter. How could you reduce or eliminate these problems?

- *Communication* — a VIP will need to utilise other senses, especially hearing and touch, as approximately 80% of sensory information is obtained visually. Perception, through focused use of these other senses, will therefore be heightened (www.rnib.org.uk). Ensure the VIP has access to radio, talking books/newspapers, information in large print, Braille or on audiotape, and other more sophisticated means of communication as required. When approaching, address the person by name and identify yourself. Describe what you are doing so that the VIP feels involved. Remember also to say when you are leaving the room, as otherwise the VIP may not be aware of this.
- *Eating and drinking* — in hospital and community care settings it is best practice that food should be placed close to the VIP, bearing in mind their functioning visual field. The content and position of food on the plate should be described using a clock-face analogy. Plate guards, non-slip mats, and using crockery which contrasts with the food colour can be helpful for those with severe visual impairment. Many safety devices are available for use in the home to help with cooking.

For further information, see www.rnib.org.uk

- *Personal hygiene and grooming* — after initial orientation and help, the VIP should be encouraged to be as independent as possible, within the realms of safety.
- *Mobility* — early mobilisation should be encouraged in the home and hospital and all appropriate assistance given. The preferred method of guiding a person with visual impairment is illustrated in Figure 13.6.

The *Getting On – Services for People with VI* booklet offers valuable advice and in-depth information; see www.afbp.org.

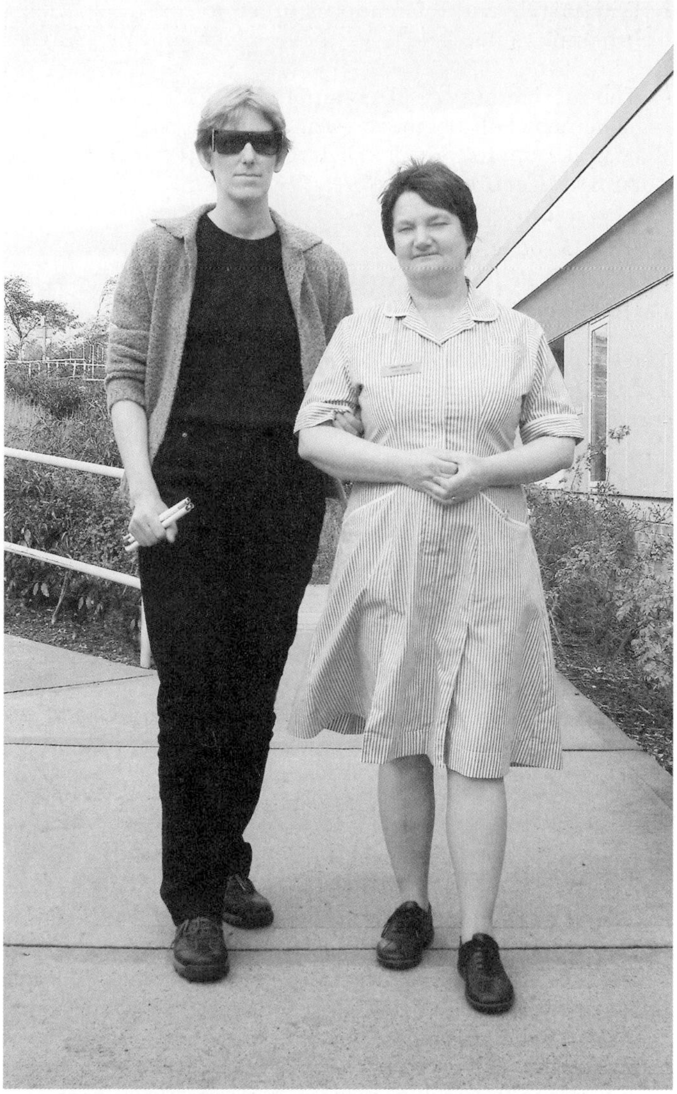

Fig. 13.6 Guiding a VIP. Before you set off, offer your arm to the VIP. Ask which side is preferred. The VIP should hold your arm just above the elbow. Check that the VIP is ready to go. Always walk one pace in front and at the same pace as the person. Describe the environment and warn the VIP of any obstacles or changes in the journey, e.g. stairs (up or down), doors, kerbs. In this way, the VIP can sense any manoeuvre or turning of the guide's body and can walk more confidently. The 'collapsible' cane or the guide dog is in the VIP's 'free' hand. (Reproduced with permission from Medical Photography Department, St. John's Hospital, West Lothian.)

With good rehabilitation training and family support, the VIP should be able to get around in their environment safely and effectively. It will take confidence, time and patience to achieve this level of ability, and the VIP will require understanding and ongoing support. Scullion (2001) believes that if impairment is badly managed or met with hostility, then disability will occur.

DISORDERS OF THE EYE

The more common eye disorders and their management are described in the sections which follow. The coverage is not exhaustive and the reader is urged to consult specialist ophthalmic texts, such as those given in the Further Reading list.

The present survey of common eye disorders and their management will begin by setting out the basic principles that must be followed when carrying out ophthalmic nursing procedures.

NURSING PRIORITIES AND MANAGEMENT: General ophthalmic procedures

The eye is a delicate organ which can be easily damaged — even in the course of treatment. In providing care, the nurse must therefore at all times observe the following principles.

Asepsis

Asepsis should be observed by the nurse and the underlying principles taught to patients and relatives. The nurse must, however, be realistic in the assessment of how and what the patient and relatives will manage in the home setting. Each eye should be treated separately. Drops and ointments should only be used in the eye for which they are prescribed. In hospital, topical medication should be dated upon opening and discarded after 1 week (after 4 weeks in the community). These precautions will reduce the risk of eye infection, which can pose a threat to vision.

Handling

Gentle handling is essential. Pressure on the eyeball must be avoided. This applies particularly to the cleansing of the upper eyelids. A sterile, moist, non-woven swab, dental roll or cotton wool ball is used to wipe from inner to outer canthus along the eyelash line and is discarded after a single use. Cotton wool balls can be used with the proviso that they have been thoroughly soaked and then squeezed out to ensure that no dry fibres are protruding. Patients should be cautioned against rubbing their eyes. The cornea is particularly vulnerable to abrasion injuries.

Irrigation

When irrigating the eye, the warmed solution should be directed across the skin of the lateral cheek so as to prepare the patient for the solution coming into contact with the eye. After this the irrigating motion should be directed away from the nasal side of the sclera. This will wash harmful foreign material away from the lacrimal duct to the side of the cheek, where it can be received in a kidney dish (see Box 13.5, p. 580).

Examination

Both eyes should be examined systematically (see p. 557) before and after any treatment, using a pen torch. Any abnormality or significant change in visual acuity must be reported. The patient should be asked to describe how each eye feels. Any pain must be reported immediately. As eye complications can develop rapidly, it is vital to refer patients immediately to avoid permanent damage. Both eyes should be examined, because the unaffected eye may react in sympathy with the affected one (sympathetic ophthalmitis). Photophobia is to be expected postoperatively and following trauma.

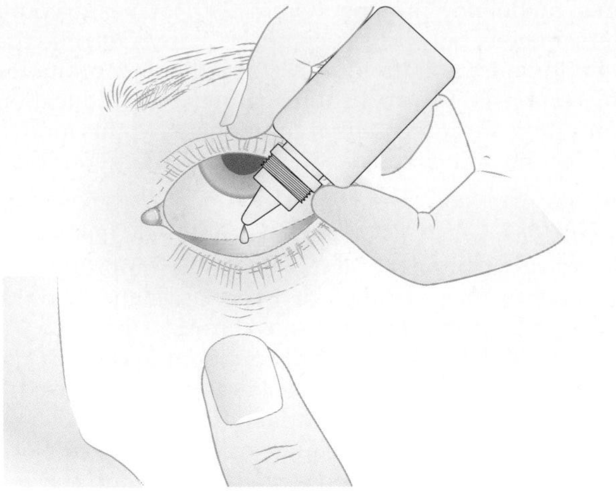

Fig. 13.7 Instilling eye drops into the lower central fornix.

Instilling eye drops and ointments

Eye drops are inserted into the middle of the lower conjunctival sac. To facilitate this, the patient is asked to tilt their head back and look up, while the lower lid is gently pulled down (see Fig. 13.7). Dropping the solution onto the sensitive cornea will cause discomfort and trigger a reflexive squeezing shut of the eye. After drop instillation the patient is asked to close the eyes gently for 30 s to maximise absorption.

Eye ointment is instilled into the lower conjunctival sac with the patient's head tilted back as described above. Contact of the tube with the eye should be avoided.

Topical drugs used in ophthalmology are listed in Table 13.2.

Padding the eye

Eye pads are applied to promote healing or to apply pressure to the eye and occasionally for comfort, when photophobia or lacrimation is excessive. It is important to appreciate that the term 'double padding' does not mean that both eyes are covered but that two pads are applied to the treated eye.

Eye pads are applied after eyes have been cleansed (if required), examined and treatment instilled. Ensure that the eye is closed underneath the pad at all times to prevent corneal damage.

The eye pad is held in position and non-allergenic tape is applied by first attaching one end lightly to the forehead, then diagonally across the eye pad towards the lateral aspect of the cheek, before the end is secured with light pressure. The downward movement maintains lid closure. The diagonal position of the tape facilitates comfort, permitting facial muscle movement. To facilitate removal a tab should be made at the top of the tape. This is grasped and with a gentle, even pressure the tape is removed. The skin on the forehead and cheek are supported as this is being done in order to reduce any dragging movement on the eyeball. The eye is examined when a pad is removed and the pad must be inspected for signs of infection or haemorrhage before discarding.

When the eye cannot be closed voluntarily, e.g. in the unconscious patient, care should be taken to avoid corneal

Table 13.2 Classification by usage of topical drugs utilised in ophthalmology

Drug	Strength	Specific action and usage
Dilatation of the pupil Drugs in this group act on the autonomic nervous system to induce mydriasis (dilatation of the pupil by acting on the iris muscles) or cycloplegia (contraction of the ciliary muscles). Some drugs (*) have a combined mydriatic cycloplegic action. All examples given have rapid onset (within 20 min) and short duration of action (4–24 h). They are frequently used in combination to facilitate refraction (cycloplegia required), ophthalmoscopy, fundal photography, cataract and retinal surgery, and the laser treatment of diabetic retinopathy.		
Cyclopentolate (G)*	0.5% and 1%	Treatment of anterior uveitis
Tropicamide (G)*	0.5% and 1%	
Phenylephrine (G)	2.5%	
Glaucoma medication There are now topical drugs which combine a beta-blocker with a prostaglandin analogue or a carbonic anhydrase inhibitor.		
Pilocarpine (G)	0.5–4%	Constricts the ciliary muscle and increases the aqueous outflow via the trabecular meshwork (action is accompanied by pupil constriction — miosis) More commonly used in the management of acute glaucoma or as an adjunct treatment for chronic glaucoma
Timolol (G)	0.25% and 0.5%	A non-selective beta-blocker which reduces aqueous production Used for the treatment of chronic and secondary glaucoma
Brimonidine (G)	0.2%	An α_2-blocker which reduces aqueous production and increases aqueous outflow via the uveoscleral outflow system Used for the treatment of chronic and secondary glaucoma
Latanoprost (G)	0.005%	A prostaglandin analogue which increases aqueous outflow via the uveoscleral outflow system Used as an adjunct treatment for chronic glaucoma
Dorzolamide (G)	2%	A carbonic anhydrase inhibitor which reduces the production of aqueous Used for the treatment of chronic and secondary glaucoma
Anti-inflammatory		
Betamethazone (G) or (Oc)	1%	Steroid Used to treat anterior segment inflammations May be combined with the antibiotic neomycin
Flurbiprofen (G)	0.03%	Non-steroidal Used to inhibit intraoperative pupil miosis
Antibacterial		
Chloramphenicol (G) or (Oc)	0.5%	Broad-spectrum bacteriostat
Fusidic acid (G)	1% viscous eye drop	Broad-spectrum bactericidal
Antiviral		
Aciclovir (Oc)	3%	Disrupts the synthesis of viral DNA in the treatment of herpes simplex keratitis
Anaesthetic agents Surface active anaesthetics which have rapid onset (30 s) and short duration of action (20 min). Used to facilitate the removal of conjunctival and corneal foreign bodies, investigative procedures which require surface anaesthesia, and selectively as pain relief.		
Oxybuprocaine (G)	0.4%	Used in combination with G fluorescein for tonometry
Tetracaine (amethocaine) (G)	1%	Commonly used for minor surgical procedures
Proxymetacaine (G)	0.5%	Causes less initial stinging which makes it useful for children
Staining agents		
Fluorescein (G)	1% and 2%	Stains damaged living tissue Facilitates the detection of corneal surface damage, i.e. abrasions and leaking corneal wounds

Continued

Table 13.2 **Classification by usage of topical drugs utilised in ophthalmology** *(Continued)*

Drug	Strength	Specific action and usage
Staining agents *(Continued)*		
Rose Bengal (G)	1%	Stains dead devitalised tissue Facilitates the diagnosis of keratoconjunctivitis sicca (xerophthalmia)
Lubricating agents		
Tear replacement solutions — surface contact time is improved by the choice of generic viscous bases		
Liquifilm (G)	1.4%	Viscosity from polyvinyl alcohol
Viscotears (G)	0.2%	Viscosity from polyacrylic acid
Lacri-Lube (Oc)		Viscosity from white soft paraffin Useful overnight

G, guttae — drops; Oc, occulentum — ointment.
Based on data from Kaiser et al (2004) and Riordan-Eva & Whitcher (2004).

abrasion from bedclothes or other articles when turning or otherwise attending to the patient. The cornea can be kept moist by the instillation of lubricants and lid closure can sometimes be improved with the application of a paraffin gauze dressing, as in the case of a sedated and ventilated patient.

NURSING PRIORITIES AND MANAGEMENT: Conditions requiring surgical intervention

The term 'intraocular surgery' describes procedures that are carried out inside the globe of the eye and which may involve structures in the anterior, posterior or vitreous chambers. Although there are many ophthalmic conditions which require operative intervention, the present discussion will focus on cataract, retinal detachment, glaucoma and perforating injuries. These conditions will have in common certain general priorities for ophthalmic and perioperative nursing management along with specific priorities relating to each condition. The general principles of perioperative ophthalmic nursing care are outlined below, followed by a discussion of nursing care specific to particular conditions. To facilitate shorter patient admission periods, patient assessment and education are increasingly undertaken in pre-assessment clinics which are frequently nurse-run. The reader is also referred to Chapter 26 for the principles of pre- and postoperative nursing management.

General nursing considerations

Assessing visual status

The patient's visual acuity and functional status are determined at the pre-assessment clinic through formal testing and interview. It is important to establish normal visual status so that the patient is not demeaned by inappropriate restrictions. It is equally important to determine any risks to ensure that a safe environment is maintained. The patient should be orientated to the ward or day bed area with a view to maintaining as normal a degree of independence as possible. Dependency level will fluctuate during the perioperative period, e.g. owing to anaesthesia, treatment and/or padding. The potential difficulties should be discussed fully with the patient.

Alleviating stress

Anxiety levels are normally high for patients admitted to hospital and this may be exacerbated in ophthalmic patients by fear of blindness and loss of independence. The patient should be given the opportunity to discuss particular fears and should be provided with clear and realistic information. Care should be taken not to raise false expectations about operative results. The patient may have practical concerns about managing everyday activities following the operation. These should be addressed and the patient should be reassured that continuing guidance and support will be available from the health care team and community organisations.

Giving information

Most patients are anxious to know the time of their surgery and how long it will take. If a local anaesthetic is to be used, they may be concerned about their level of awareness during the procedure and about whether they will be able to cooperate (see Research Abstract 13.1). Depending on the patient's visual acuity, it is often helpful to discuss the operation using a model of the eye. It is important to anticipate and dispel any misconceptions that the patient may have about eye surgery. However, not everyone will want to know the details of the surgery and the appropriate amount of information for each individual should be provided and their wishes respected.

Procedures for preoperative eye preparation should be explained. If the patient is able to carry out self-medication, instruction in the instillation of drops can provide a good opportunity to begin a teaching programme for postoperative self-care.

For further information on the nurse's role in promoting the correct administration of topical eye treatment, see Marsden & Shaw (2003).

RESEARCH ABSTRACT 13.1

The effects of handholding on anxiety in cataract surgery patients under local anaesthesia

This Korean study by Moon and Cho (2001) aimed to assess the effectiveness of handholding on the anxiety levels of patients undergoing elective local anaesthetic cataract surgery in a country where over 100 000 cataract patients undergo this type of surgery annually.

An experimental and control group design was used pre- and post-test involving visual analogue scales, interviews and physiological measures of pulse and blood pressure. Blood was also taken pre-handholding and before the end of handholding to assess a variety of body chemicals associated in the immune system's response to stress.

The results showed a significant decrease in anxiety levels during operation in the handholding group (n = 30) compared to the control group (n = 32). Epinephrine levels in the handholding group were also significantly lower. This suggests that handholding has the potential to reduce anxiety in patients having cataract extraction under local anaesthesia.

Moon J S, Cho K S 2001 The effects of handholding on anxiety in cataract surgery patients under local anaesthetic. Journal of Advanced Nursing 35(3): 407–415

Managing positioning and activity

As a general rule, any position or activity that markedly increases venous pressure in the head should be avoided in ophthalmic patients. It is usually recommended, though sometimes not feasible, that they are nursed with the head slightly raised, with the patient either semi-recumbent or lying on the unoperated side. Exceptions to this are:

- in cases of retinal detachment — the surgeon will prescribe both pre- and postoperative positions, depending on the site of the detachment
- following vitrectomy — the surgeon may prescribe the position.

It is vital that such instructions for positioning are followed precisely.

Postoperative vomiting should be prevented by ensuring that an antiemetic is prescribed and given promptly if the patient complains of nausea. Increased blood flow caused by a head-down position or straining will raise IOP and can result in damage to optical structures or suture lines. The majority of patients go home shortly after surgery and some restrictions on activity and positioning may be applicable. The reason for these activity and positioning regimens, and for their duration, should be explained to the patient and encouragement to follow these recommendations should be given.

Examining the eye

The eye should be examined systematically, both pre- and postoperatively, using a pen torch, to check for signs of infection, and to ensure that normal healing occurs. Early recognition of abnormalities reduces the risk of potential damage which might result in loss of sight. It is helpful to use the non-affected eye as a baseline against which to compare the operated or injured eye.

Subconjunctival haemorrhage is not abnormal, particularly in patients who have had cataract surgery under local anaesthetic. Often a localised subconjunctival bleed may be noted in the area of the anaesthetic infiltration or in the postoperative antibiotic injection site, if the needle or cannula has disrupted a small blood vessel. If bleeding into the anterior chamber (hyphaema) is present, it should be recorded and a diagram indicating size relative to the anterior chamber entered in the medical and nursing notes. Postoperative expectations may include some degree of lid bruising and swelling, especially following local anaesthesia. Conjunctival redness (injection) and oedema (chemosis) are sometimes noted to spread out from the postoperative antibiotic injection site. The cornea and anterior chamber (AC) should be clear. A fine suture line may be evident, although cataract wound size is often so small and the wound tunnelled in such a way that it is self-sealing and therefore does not require sutures. The wound is concealed under the top lid and examined by asking the patient to look downwards and then gently retracting the top lid. The depth and shape of the AC should be noted, as a shallow AC, i.e. one in which there appears to be a decreased space between the cornea and the iris, may indicate that aqueous from the AC is leaking from the site of the wound.

Managing dressings

The eye is protected by a plastic Cartella shield at night for up to 1 week postoperatively. Dark glasses may be worn during the day to reduce the discomfort of glare. The patient should be taught to put the glasses on over the forehead to avoid accidentally poking the earpieces into the eye.

PAINLESS LOSS OF VISION

Cataract

Any opacity of the lens can be defined as a cataract. Cataracts can develop as part of the ageing process. They can also be congenital or develop following trauma, as sequelae to inflammatory and degenerative disease, or as a result of the prolonged use of some medications, e.g. corticosteroids.

For further information, see Yanoff (1998).

PATHOPHYSIOLOGY

The lens of the eye is normally transparent due to the regular arrangement of its crystalline fibres and the nature of the proteins inside them. These fibres, which originate in the epithelium of the lens capsule, continue to be laid down throughout life. This results in thickening and a loss of elasticity. Opacity will eventually develop with ageing.

Clinical features The main feature of a mature cataract is that it reflects as a grey or milky white lens behind the pupil, which normally appears black.

Common presenting symptoms of age-related cataract are as follows:

- gradually decreasing acuity affecting distance vision more than near vision

- general dimming of vision because of the reduced amount of light reaching the retina
- more frequent refractive errors because of reduced elasticity of the lens
- increased dazzle and glare in bright light and appearance of haloes around lights at night
- monocular diplopia — double vision or a 'ghosting' effect in one eye
- alteration in colour and depth perception.

STOP THINK **13.7** Wrap several layers of clear adhesive tape around both lenses of a pair of glasses. Alternatively, smear both lenses with petroleum jelly. Wear them for a while to experience something of what it feels like to have bilateral cataracts. Then try this with vision totally occluded in one lens and the other lens wrapped in just a few layers of tape or smeared with a thin film of jelly. How would this affect your daily activities? Discuss the experience with your colleagues.

MEDICAL MANAGEMENT

During the developmental stages of cataract, spectacles may provide a degree of improvement in visual acuity. It is impossible, however, to reverse the opacification process. Surgical removal of the cataract will ultimately be the only effective treatment. The National Cataract Survey (Desai et al 1999) indicated that 70% of all cataract procedures in the NHS were performed as day cases and this is recognised as the preferred form of care (Royal College of Ophthalmologists 2001). The NHS Executive (2000) reported that, in the late 1990s, 86% of cataract surgery was being done under local anaesthetic. This trend towards local anaesthetic day care is likely to remain popular, as it offers the least disruption to the patient's daily routine and makes effective economic use of health resources.

The retinal function is examined and, although there may be age-related maculopathy or other coexisting ocular pathology, cataract removal will still be considered, albeit with a guarded prognosis.

Surgical procedures Cataract removal is performed when the cataract interferes with activities of living (ALs).

Before the operation, the pupil is dilated to facilitate lens delivery and to reduce the risk of damage to the iris. An incision is then made into the globe at the limbus in the 12 o'clock section of the eye. The principal methods of lens removal are:

- phacoemulsification — ultrasonic fragmentation to break up the nucleus and aspirate soft lens material, leaving the posterior capsule intact
- extracapsular extraction — removal of the entire nucleus and cortex through a large incision, leaving the posterior capsule intact. This procedure is carried out more often in developing countries as it is not dependent on the availability of sophisticated phacoemulsification equipment and of the necessary technical maintenance.

Intraocular lens implantation The best visual correction is achieved by the insertion of an intraocular lens (IOL) positioned in front of the posterior capsule at the time of cataract removal. This is possible in the majority of cases. Unforeseen surgical complication, e.g. severe posterior capsular rupture with the release of a large amount of vitreous into the anterior chamber, is the main contraindication to insertion of an IOL. In the UK, the strength of lens is calculated for each patient based on a combination of:

- biometry — measurement of the axial length of the eye along the visual axis
- keratometry — measurement of the corneal curvature
- the patient's previous optical history.

The nurse must not only be able to carry out the tests, but also to interpret them proactively with a view to obtaining the best postoperative vision.

IOLs may be inserted as a secondary procedure. It is important to know which kind of lens is in situ in order to ensure appropriate postoperative care. In the rare situation when no IOL is inserted, a contact lens or corrective spectacle may be issued.

Postoperative medication The inflammatory response, which accompanies all healing, is controlled postoperatively by a combination of topical steroids and antibiotics. It is vital that the patient understands the reasons for the prescribed postoperative instillation of drops and why treatment must not be stopped before completing the course.

NURSING PRIORITIES AND MANAGEMENT: Cataract extraction and implantation of an intraocular lens

As day case cataract surgery has become the norm, most ophthalmic units will have developed care pathways using local or national clinical guidelines such as those of the Scottish Intercollegiate Guidelines Network (SIGN 2001). The evolution of cataract documentation relates to the rapid and safe throughput of patients and to the associated need to incorporate multidisciplinary notes that reduce duplication while promoting individualised care. The principles of perioperative management are covered in Chapter 26 and those relating to intraocular surgery in Nursing Care Plan 13.1. The following points specific to cataract extraction and IOL implantation should be noted.

Major nursing considerations

IOL management

It is important for the nurse to find out which method has been used for extraction and whether or not an IOL has been implanted. If an IOL is in situ, its position must be checked at each eye examination.

Problems which may arise following IOL implantation include:

- a secondary rise in intraocular pressure, usually accompanied by severe one-sided headache above the brow of the operated eye
- cystoid macular oedema which results in the patient noting reduction and distortion of vision
- infection, with the rare, but sight-threatening possibility of endophthalmitis.

Should any of these signs and symptoms be present, the patient and relatives should know who to contact promptly so that action can be taken to prevent permanent eye damage.

Nursing Care Plan 13.1 A patient undergoing intraocular surgery

Nursing considerations	Action	Rationale	Expected outcome
Preoperative preparation **1. Anxiety relating to local anaesthetic; being awake during the procedure; draping procedure in theatre; communication with staff during procedure**	• Explain that local anaesthetic ensures painless procedure, reduces postoperative discomfort of general anaesthetic, and enables earlier discharge • Explain that draping and skin cleansing are carried out to reduce the risk of infection • Explain that the unoperated eye needs to be closed to protect the cornea from accidental damage and reduce eye movement	Information given about procedures reduces patient anxiety and discomfort	Patient is able to recall details of preparation and appears more relaxed
	• Explain that whilst the eye is anaesthetised it is possible to overcome muscle activity and position the eye in the orbit so as to permit easy access to most surgical sites • Explain that some patients may experience periods of 'seeing lights' during the procedure	Patients commonly express a fear that the eye will be placed on the cheek to facilitate surgery. Placing the eye on the cheek is impossible without total destruction of the optic nerve, which, together with the extraocular muscles and cheek ligaments, tethers the eye securely within the orbital cavity	
	• Explain that throughout the time in theatre one nurse will hold the patient's hand and they will agree on a signalling system so that if the patient has any discomfort or pain this can be communicated; remedial measures will be taken immediately	An agreed communication system reduces anxiety and increases well-being the operation well	Patient communicates appropriately during the procedure and tolerates
Discharge considerations **1. Anxiety about visual function following surgery**	• Explain that visual recovery is not complete until the eye is fully healed • Visual function is to be assessed at first dressing within 48 h • Explain that 'floaters', which occur following discharge, and the experiencing of flashing lights may precede the development of complications and urgent review in the OPD should be sought	Improved knowledge reduces anxiety	Patient is able to recall information given Patient can demonstrate procedure used Patient outlines procedure to obtain urgent OPD review

Continued ▶

Nursing Care Plan 13.1 A patient undergoing intraocular surgery *(Continued)*

Nursing considerations	Action	Rationale	Expected outcome
Discharge considerations (Continued)			
2. The patient has a parkinsonian tremor and is unable to instil the eye drops	• Teach carer(s) to instil eye drops prior to surgery. If there is no carer (or neighbour), the community nurse should visit and instil eye ointment twice daily	Rehabilitation and discharge planning should begin at pre-admission clinic or first hospital attendance. Early liaison with the community nurse will help to ensure that treatment continues and that the nurse is fully informed of individual aspects of the case. It will also reassure the patient that a supportive health care team exists	

OPD, outpatient department.

It should be explained to the patient and the family that during the healing process there will be a period of adaptation, as the brain adjusts to changes in visual perception. The patient should be told to take care with moving about during this period, especially if there are pre-existing conditions that affect balance.

Premature cessation of treatment by patients, or failure to ensure regular instillation of the eye drops, is a recognised risk following eye surgery, and particularly so in day case cataract surgery, which accounts for the majority of ophthalmic day care. This is thought to be linked to the professionals' concerted drive to shorten and normalise this surgical event to a 2–3 h visit, with no fasting requirements (for patients having a local anaesthetic) or need for the patient to remove clothing and change into a hospital gown, thus possibly leading patients to misinterpret this situation and equate what appears to them to be 'low level care' with 'no care'. As a result, they may view the postoperative eye drop administration as an optional extra, rather than an essential part of their total care package. Education must therefore be clear and consistent and the nurse should check that the patient and the family or carers understand the instructions and the importance of following these precisely.

Refractive laser treatments

Individuals with myopia, hypermetropia or astigmatism have become dissatisfied with the inability to obtain their best vision with either spectacles or contact lens. This consumer demand has led to the current practice of laser surgery to correct their refractive errors.

Current excimer laser techniques include photorefractive keratectomy (PRK), which alters corneal curvature by ablating surface corneal tissue and results in a reduction of refractive power. Laser in situ keratomileusis (LASIK) consists of cutting a hinged flap of cornea under very precise conditions, performing the laser ablation in the corneal bed and then replacing the flap. This is thought to reduce discomfort and promote faster visual recovery (Riordan-Eva & Whitcher 2004).

Prior to undertaking any treatments, it is essential to seek advice from an ophthalmologist, as complications can occur, including over- or undercorrection, and loss of best corrected VA.

For further details, see www.moorfields.org.uk.

STOP THINK **13.8** One of your patients has undergone a cataract extraction and IOL implantation. As you systematically examine the eye, you note the following clinical signs:

- eyelids — slightly bruised and swollen
- conjunctiva — pink
- cornea — cloudy, suture line intact
- anterior chamber — formed, hyphaema noted and more extensive than at previous dressing
- iris — muddy
- pupil — dilated and round
- posterior chamber IOL — in situ and reflecting.

Which clinical signs are within normal expectations and which would alert you to a problem that demands immediate attention? What could this problem be? What action will you take?

Glaucoma

Glaucoma can be defined as a disease process with a characteristic pattern of cupping of the optic disc and reproducible field loss. The IOP may be raised or normal. The condition may be acquired or genetic in origin. Acquired glaucoma can be further classified as primary open-angle glaucoma (POAG), primary closed-angle glaucoma (PCAG — both acute and chronic), and glaucoma secondary to pathological processes (secondary glaucoma).

STOP THINK **13.9** Revise your knowledge of aqueous dynamics within the eye.

Primary open-angle glaucoma

This type of glaucoma, also known as chronic simple glaucoma, causes progressive and irreversible loss of the peripheral visual field, with the central 10% being spared until a later stage. It is initially symptomless.

PATHOPHYSIOLOGY

The normal range of IOP is 12–20 mmHg and this varies throughout the 24-h period. In POAG, the pressure is generally elevated and the diurnal variation may show considerable fluctuation, i.e. IOP is lower in the morning, peaks during the day and lowers again in the evening (Kanski 2003).

Raised IOP decreases the blood flow in the optic disc capillaries with resultant excavation and atrophy of the optic nerve head and subsequent loss of nerve fibres passing through it (cupping). A progressive loss of the visual field results from damage to nerve fibre bundles as they enter the optic disc.

Clinical features The outward appearance of the eye is normal. On examination, if there is cupping of the optic disc, peripheral visual field loss and possible raised IOP, a diagnosis of glaucoma may be made.

Common presenting symptoms There is usually a gradual and painless loss of peripheral vision. The patient rarely notices this deterioration until considerable damage has been done. This loss of vision is irreversible. The glaucoma is often detected by an optometrist during a routine eye examination.

MEDICAL MANAGEMENT

The main aim of treatment is to reduce IOP to allow better capillary perfusion at the optic nerve head. This involves improving the aqueous drainage system or decreasing the production of aqueous, or a combination of both. Medical treatment is the mainstay in the majority of cases (European Glaucoma Society 2003), although there is a growing trend towards early surgical or laser intervention.

Tests and investigations Diagnosis and medical assessment of the nature and severity of the condition will rely on the following:

- tonometry — measurement of IOP with instruments that allow for corneal contact
- visual field analysis
- ophthalmoscopy to examine the optic nerve head and estimate the degree of cupping
- gonioscopy — examination of the state and depth of the angle of the eye
- phasing — measurement of IOP by tonometry at different times of the day.

Treatment Whether the medical regimen is implemented alone or in combination with a surgical procedure, it is important to maintain monitoring of the efficiency of treatment indefinitely. The regimen may include the administration of some combination of the following medications:

- Topical beta-blockers, and topical carbonic anhydrase inhibitors to reduce aqueous production (see Table 13.2). Topical regimens may be prescribed for long-term continuous use; systemic drugs are generally prescribed for short-term or intermittent use
- Topical prostaglandin analogues to increase uveoscleral outflow are increasingly being used in the initial treatment of POAG
- Topical miotic drops to constrict the pupil and stretch open the trabecular meshwork, thus facilitating aqueous drainage.

Surgical treatment for POAG is usually performed when conservative management has failed, indicated by progression of visual field loss and persistent elevation of IOP, or when the patient's social situation or health prevents adherence to the recommended eye drop regimen.

The principle of surgery is to create a fistula between the anterior chamber and the subconjunctival space in order to bypass the existing drainage system and increase the outflow of aqueous. The most commonly used procedure is trabeculectomy.

Postoperatively, a small bleb under the conjunctival flap will be visible. A small V-shaped hole in the iris may be noted if a peripheral iridectomy has been performed.

The success of surgery is measured by whether the IOP remains within normal limits, but there can be no actual improvement in visual acuity. If a trabeculectomy drains well, topical treatment may be discontinued.

Laser treatment involves applying short bursts of a laser beam through a lens resembling a gonioscopy lens, targeting selected areas of the trabecular meshwork. Application of argon laser burns to the trabecular meshwork (argon laser trabeculoplasty) has been found to be effective in selected cases in reducing IOP. The scarring caused by the laser burns appears to stretch the tissues between the burns, thus opening up spaces in the trabecular meshwork and facilitating drainage of aqueous.

NURSING PRIORITIES AND MANAGEMENT: Primary open-angle glaucoma (POAG)

Major nursing considerations

Screening

Measurement of IOP and visual field testing may be carried out in the community by the optometry service as part of a 'shared care' scheme or in hospital-based screening clinics. More hospitals are providing nurse-led screening clinics. These present ophthalmic nurses with the challenge of expanding and extending their roles, enabling them to combine patient education with new skills such as optic disc photography and disc assessment using a slit lamp and lenses.

Patient adherence to treatment recommendations

This is a major concern, especially in the outpatient department and the community setting where most patients with glaucoma will be seen. It is a nursing responsibility to assess the patient's understanding of the condition as well as the rationale for treatment, together with the patient's ability to instil the drops and continue with other aspects of treatment, such as punctal occlusion after topical beta-blockers.

Self-administration of drops may be difficult and requires arm and neck flexibility and hand dexterity to manage the drop dispenser bottle successfully. Various appliances are available to help with the procedure but it still requires skilful demonstration to patients and carers to ensure success. In some cases, the community nurse may be best placed to know how to encourage particular patients who have good hand dexterity, but low confidence, to be more active in their own eye drop instillation.

STOP THINK **13.10** How could you encourage a patient who is prescribed topical antiglaucoma treatment to adhere to the regimen?

Postoperative observation and monitoring

Depth of AC Postoperatively, the depth of the AC in the operated eye should be compared to that of the unoperated eye and variations must be reported. It is possible for overdrainage to result in a shallow AC or for underdrainage to result in a deeper AC.

Signs of raised IOP Severe postoperative pain, accompanied by a cloudy cornea and flat AC, is abnormal and must be investigated.

Administering laser treatment

Fully explaining what is involved and reassuring the patient of support throughout the procedure, and monitoring afterwards, will be helpful in allowing the treatment to be administered precisely and safely. Protective goggles are mandatory for all staff in attendance.

During application of laser treatment, it is necessary for the nurse to understand the potential hazards to the patient and to staff (see Nursing Care Plan 13.2).

For further information, see Batterbury & Bowling (1999) and Al-Husainy et al (2001).

Retinal detachment

Retinal detachment describes a separation between the neural and pigmented layers of the retina.

PATHOPHYSIOLOGY

The light-sensitive cells in the neural layer are detached from the essential pigments in the pigment layer as fluid effusion between the layers gradually causes more separation. Retinal detachments are most frequently associated with holes or tears in the retina. These occur as a consequence of vitreous traction, degenerative disease or vitreous loss, which may be traumatic or postoperative. Predisposing factors include myopia, aphakia, trauma or retinal/choroidal tumour. If one eye is affected, the other is also at risk.

Common presenting symptoms The patient may present at various stages with painless visual disturbances or loss of vision. The external appearance of the eye is unchanged, unless recent traumatic injury or surgical intervention has taken place. During the early stages, the rods and cones are falsely activated, causing sensations of flashing light. As flakes of pigment are shed into the vitreous, the patient may see showers of floating shapes and strands in the vitreous field. Later, the patient may describe an impression of a curtain coming down or across the line of vision.

MEDICAL MANAGEMENT

Treatment The exact nature and extent of the retinal detachment and the presence of retinal fluid will dictate the specific procedure for repair that is used. An internal approach, i.e. a vitrectomy, in which some of the vitreous humor is removed and the volume replaced with expansile gas or silicone oil, will almost inevitably induce a cataract within a 1–2 year period. Depending on the precise location of the detachment, an alternative external approach, with use of a scleral band, may be possible. This procedure does not carry the same sequelae, but may not be appropriate, due to the position of the detachment.

Surgical procedures The aim of surgery is to produce a controlled inflammatory response to seal the detachment, release the subretinal fluid and bring the retinal layers into normal apposition. Surgery should be undertaken at the earliest opportunity to give the best possible visual outcome, especially in those situations where the macula is still attached or has been detached for less than 1 week.

External cryotherapy in the form of a carbon dioxide (CO_2) freezing probe can be applied to the sclera behind the detached retina or an internal laser can be targeted at the appropriate area of the retina: both of these treatments will cause an inflammation of the choroid and retina and lead to adhesion of the detached neurosensory and pigment epithelium layers. Draining of subretinal fluid aids repositioning of the layers, which may be supported by internal tamponade, created by intravitreal air, silicone oil or volume-expanding gases. A silicone explant may be sutured onto the outer surface of the sclera. Once it is seen to be in the correct position and of the correct size and provides the surgeon with the appropriate retinal indentation, it is permanently tied with non-absorbable sutures, in order that the compressive effect is not lost over time. The explant is not normally visible.

Outpatient treatment with argon laser and volume-expanding gases may be satisfactory in cases of dry retinal detachments. Here, the inflammatory response is controlled by mydriatic and steroid eye drops.

For further information, see Chignell & Wong (1999).

NURSING PRIORITIES AND MANAGEMENT: Retinal detachment

Major nursing considerations

Patient positioning

Correct positioning is a vital component of the management of retinal detachment. Individualised regimens determined by the surgeon must be strictly observed. The positioning prescribed will depend on the site and the nature of the surgical repair. The patient must be fully informed of the reasons for positioning, as adherence to the regimen is very important to the success of the treatment. If the outcome of the surgery is simply re-attachment with no predicted improvement in vision, the patient may decide against surgery and the associated positioning, which can prove

Nursing Care Plan 13.2 Ensuring patient cooperation in laser treatment associated with glaucoma

Nursing considerations	Action	Rationale	Expected outcome
Anxiety due to: • **Lack of understanding of laser treatment** • **Fear of pain and discomfort during procedure**	• Explain to the patient about sitting during the procedure as for gonioscopy and that a similar lens will be applied to the eye	The patient will have experienced gonioscopy as part of the earlier examination and will therefore be familiar with the procedure	The patient can demonstrate awareness of what the procedure entails and has confidence in the medical and nursing team
	• Describe the anatomy of the eye, how the laser beam is targeted on the problem areas and what the expected outcome will be	Expectations of a positive outcome will reduce anxiety	
	• Explain the importance of maintaining a steady position and gaze	The patient's cooperation is necessary to ensure that only targeted areas are exposed to the laser	The patient is cooperative during the treatment, keeps a steady direction of gaze and does not appear unduly anxious. Accidental burns are avoided
	• Reassure the patient that the treatment may be uncomfortable but should not be painful. Patient will experience bright flashes of light and there may be a slight headache afterwards • Reassure the patient that the procedure is well controlled and that there will be careful follow-up	Information given about procedures reduces patient anxiety and discomfort	

arduous for those with musculoskeletal and respiratory conditions. Normal functional positions are usually allowed at mealtimes and for toilet purposes. Complete bed rest is seldom necessary for longer than 24 h postoperatively, after which mobilisation is permitted with the patient following an individualised regimen of head positioning if intravitreal air or gas is used (see Nursing Care Plan 13.3).

The overall aim is to enable the detached area to fall back into position preoperatively and to maintain normal apposition postoperatively. Generally, if the detachment is superior, the patient will be nursed lying flat with one pillow; if the detachment is inferior, nursing will be with the patient sitting upright in bed or in a chair. In the case of a temporal or nasal detachment, the patient will be nursed lying on the opposite side to the affected area. These positions are reversed postoperatively if surgery has included internal tamponade, i.e. intravitreal air. This surgery is more likely to be performed under general anaesthetic.

Patient education and counselling

The patient should be made aware that vision may be temporarily poorer than before surgery due to the manipulation of the eye, administration of mydriatic eye drops and the alterations to the focusing power of the eye resulting from any explant, e.g. scleral band, which might be present. Visual improvement, unless there is an already existing eye condition such as macular degeneration, will be a gradual process.

Postoperative pain

Postoperative pain can be expected to be fairly severe, depending on the complexity and the duration of the surgery. If severe pain persists despite the use of narcotic analgesics, an acute rise in IOP, possibly precipitated by retinal surgery, should be suspected and reported. If severe pain persists and the IOP is within normal limits, some problem with the explant must be suspected.

Postoperative appearance of the eye

In retinal surgery, the conjunctival incision is encircling, there is extensive handling of the globe and, if vitrectomy instruments have been used, there may be considerable trauma to the conjunctiva. The nurse can therefore expect to observe marked chemosis with bruising and swelling of the eyelids. Pressure dressings or regular cold compresses

Nursing Care Plan 13.3 Positioning of a patient with retinal detachment

Nursing considerations	Action	Rationale	Expected outcome
The patient has knowledge deficit about enforced positional bed rest to prevent further detachment of retina and help postoperative recovery	• Establish knowledge base by preparing and presenting a teaching session using a model of an eye. Include a family member if patient has significant visual loss. Include: – description of normal retina and its function – possible cause of detachment – description of surgical procedure – positioning before and after surgery to help retina fall back into place. Explain that this will be prescribed by the specialist and that every attempt must be made to observe it	Misconceptions about eye surgery are often lurid and frightening. Understanding what really happens will reduce fear and make cooperation with instructions more likely. The informed patient experiences a significant reduction in anxiety levels and is more likely to cooperate	The patient is able to describe what happens in retinal detachment, how it can be repaired, and asks questions which indicate an acceptable level of knowledge Patient appears more relaxed about the need for positioning and is very cooperative
	• Encourage questions	Given time and encouragement, patients may express a variety of questions and individual concerns	
	• Reinforce explanations frequently	Due to the blocking effect of anxiety, patients do not always absorb information and it may be necessary to repeat or rephrase it	

may be applied postoperatively. The eye must be monitored closely to ensure that the conjunctival incision heals cleanly and that there is no evidence of rejection or extrusion of the silicone explant.

Corneal transplant (keratoplasty)

Indications for corneal transplant include destruction of the cornea by injury or disease, some cases of advanced keratoconus (conical cornea) and corneal opacity. Transplants may be full or partial thickness. Keratoplasty is primarily an elective procedure with donor material supplied principally by the Corneal Transplant Service Eye Banks in Bristol and Manchester. The donor eyes and donor blood are screened thoroughly (Armitage & Easty 1998) to minimise the risk of using donor material where underlying infection or corneal disorder is present. The donor material should be harvested within 24 h of death.

NURSING PRIORITIES AND MANAGEMENT: Corneal transplant

The perioperative period is managed as for other intraocular surgery.

Special considerations

The use of donated tissue

Recipients rarely ask questions regarding the source of a donated cornea, but nurses must be ready to give reassurance and support, as the use of donor corneas can be an emotive issue. Sometimes the donor's relatives ask if the tissue has been used. If the nurse is involved in giving confirmation, care should be taken not to violate confidentiality whilst still providing adequate information. The entire team caring for the patient must invest time in preparing and delivering consistent, individualised information.

Postoperative examination

Following surgery, any conjunctival redness (injection) should gradually lessen. If the conjunctiva does not soon return to the 'white eye' state, the cause may be raised IOP or transplant rejection. These possibilities must also be considered when inspection of the cornea reveals a loss of clarity, a finding which must be reported immediately. The wound should be examined to ensure the suture line remains intact and the corneal disc (transplant) has stayed in position, as disruption of either may affect the optical power of the transplant.

Patient involvement and cooperation

Both the patient and the family should be made aware that corneal transplant requires a lengthy follow-up period. The cornea is an avascular structure, and therefore healing will be slow. The corneal sutures will remain in situ for several months. If a good optical result has been obtained, it may be decided to leave the sutures in indefinitely, rather than risk disturbing the transplant.

It must also be emphasised that any topical medication prescribed must be continued, to avoid rejection of the transplant and prevent infection. The patient should be warned that optimal visual recovery cannot be expected for some months, or even up to 2 years after surgery. Some may be disappointed by the initial outcome, when vision may seem to be poorer than before transplant.

Prior to discharge, patient and carer teaching should ensure that the need for attending review appointments is understood, as early rejection may be asymptomatic, and that they are aware of the importance of early recognition of symptoms of transplant rejection. Such symptoms may include:

- increased redness of the conjunctiva
- cloudiness of the cornea
- reduction of visual function, and/or
- discomfort in the operated eye.

Temporal arteritis (giant cell arteritis, cranial arteritis)

This is a progressive disease process affecting the over-60 age group, in which the middle layer of medium-sized arteries becomes inflamed. When the external carotid system is involved, ocular damage results with sudden loss of vision, which may be preceded by, or accompany, polymyalgia rheumatica (stiff aching muscles, especially around the shoulders).

PATHOPHYSIOLOGY

There is degeneration of the retina, which results from thrombosis or occlusion of the ophthalmic artery, secondary to necrotic inflammatory changes in the middle layer of the temporal and cranial arteries. The cells in the destroyed middle layer are replaced by collagen. During the active phase of this process, there is a raised erythrocyte sedimentation rate (ESR) (see Ch. 11).

Clinical features Patients often complain of general malaise, loss of weight and lethargy, or a 'flu-like' illness which may last for a few days or weeks and which precedes a sustained visual disturbance. This is in contrast to the prodromal phase, in which fleeting episodes of blurred vision may occur, accompanied by unilateral temporal or occipital headache. On presentation, the patient may complain of scalp tenderness and jaw claudication. The loss of vision is sudden in onset, usually affecting one eye before the other. The length of time between both eyes being affected is extremely variable, ranging from several hours to several days.

MEDICAL MANAGEMENT

Diagnosis is made following ophthalmoscopy and the identification of a raised ESR. The ESR may not be high in the early stages of the disease and repeat tests may be necessary. The diagnosis may be confirmed by carrying out a temporal artery biopsy.

Treatment may be instigated in the community or in hospital and consists of systemic corticosteroid therapy which lowers the ESR to within normal limits. The initial dose may be given i.m. to achieve the effective therapeutic level. The starting high-dosage rate, i.e. 80–120 mg/day, is reduced to a maintenance oral dose, which may be administered for up to 2 years. Topical treatment is not usually prescribed unless a secondary condition, e.g. iritis, develops.

NURSING PRIORITIES AND MANAGEMENT: Temporal arteritis

Nursing intervention is directed towards the care of a patient undergoing corticosteroid therapy. In particular, monitoring and recording regimens, e.g. of blood pressure, urinalysis and body weight, will be required to give warning of any complication arising from the therapy. If vision deficit is severe, help and support will be necessary and registration as a blind or partially sighted person may be required.

RED EYE

Primary acute closed-angle glaucoma (PCAG/ACAG)

Closed-angle glaucoma presents as an acute episode of severe raised IOP, usually unilateral. It is an ophthalmic emergency and requires immediate intervention from a specialist department, as permanent ocular damage occurs if untreated or treated incorrectly. Prophylactic treatment is required for the unaffected eye.

PATHOPHYSIOLOGY

Raised IOP develops as a result of disruption of the circulation of aqueous humor in the anterior chamber, which can be associated with hypermetropia. Pupil dilatation is accompanied by forward displacement of the iris, which blocks the trabecular meshwork, reducing or stopping the flow of aqueous to the canal of Schlemm. The pupillary margin of the iris also comes into contact with the lens, causing the pupil to become semi-dilated and fixed, further impeding the flow of aqueous and increasing forward displacement of the iris. Aqueous build-up results in corneal oedema and disturbance of sensory nerve fibres.

Common presenting symptoms are as follows:

- Sudden onset, with severe pain in one eye accompanied by frontotemporal headache on the affected side
- Nausea and possible vomiting; these symptoms can sometimes lead to a misdiagnosis of gastric or abdominal problems
- Blurred and reduced vision
- Photophobia and increased lacrimation

- Red eye, especially around the limbal area (due to marked ciliary injection)
- Corneal haze due to oedema
- Semi-dilated pupil, unreactive to light
- Poorly defined iris details (muddy in appearance)
- On palpation over a closed lid, the eye feels hard because of raised IOP.

MEDICAL MANAGEMENT

Tests and investigations include the following:

- A full history (see Table 13.3)
- Systematic ocular examination using slit lamp
- Gonioscopy — examination of the angle of the eye (see Fig 13.2)
- Measurement of IOP.

Acute signs and symptoms should be managed as follows:

- Pain relief by analgesics, including i.m. opiates
- Control of nausea and vomiting with i.m. antiemetics
- Increase in outflow of aqueous humor by freeing the iris angle. To achieve this, a regimen of intensive topical miotic therapy is commenced to constrict the pupil rapidly and draw the iris away from the angle. Prophylactic therapy is also prescribed for the other eye to prevent an acute attack
- Reduction in production of aqueous humor by administration of carbonic anhydrase inhibitors such as acetazolamide (Diamox), either orally or intravenously. If the response to this is unsatisfactory, osmotic diuretics such as oral glycerol or i.v. mannitol can be used.

Surgical intervention Once the acute signs and symptoms have been managed, surgical intervention may be contemplated. The method depends on the appearance of the angle and may be any of the following:

- Argon laser trabeculoplasty (ALT) — small holes are created in the peripheral iris of the affected eye
- Surgical procedures, including iridectomy or trabeculectomy (see 'Glaucoma', p. 568)
- Post ALT, topical steroid treatment and possible long-term antiglaucoma therapy (see Table 13.2) to reduce inflammation and stabilise IOP.

For surgical procedures, the preparation and perioperative care are as for Nursing Care Plan 13.1 (see p. 567).

NURSING PRIORITIES AND MANAGEMENT: Primary acute closed-angle glaucoma (PCAG)

Screening

It is essential to acknowledge that the patient may experience severe pain and fear at the potential loss of vision. Reassurance and support are vital at this time.

The experienced ophthalmic nurse requires the skills to assess the ocular condition through a knowledge of clinical signs and symptoms (see p. 557). This will aid possible diagnosis and prompt referral for specialist intervention. Nursing priorities and management are as for POAG (see p. 569) and a patient undergoing laser treatment (see Nursing Care Plan 13.2). Further tests, for example of visual fields and of IOP, should be delayed until acute signs and symptoms have resolved.

Table 13.3 Systematic approach to history-taking

Assessment	Question	Rationale
History of injury	How did the accident occur? When did the accident occur? Where did the accident occur? Which eye is affected? Is the injury unilateral/bilateral? Were safety goggles worn?	To aid diagnosis For medicolegal reasons
Ophthalmic history	Are glasses or contact lenses worn? Has a similar accident occurred before? Has patient had a previous eye injury or operation?	To ascertain if preventive lessons are learnt To aid clinical examination and diagnosis
Medical history	Does patient have any general health problems? Has patient had previous surgery?	Some systemic disorders may affect the eye, e.g. diabetes mellitus, hypertension, altered thyroid activity Patient may require surgery and may have had a reaction to an anaesthetic previously
Medications	Is patient taking medication at present?	Some medications may affect the eye, e.g. aspirin and the contraceptive pill Patient may have an allergy to a medication To ensure safe prescribing and avoidance of any contraindications to use
Allergies	Is patient allergic to any substance, e.g. medications, Sellotape, Elastoplast?	A substance may inadvertently be given to which the patient is allergic, complicating the condition

Uveitis

PATHOPHYSIOLOGY

Uveitis is inflammation of the uveal tract. Anterior uveitis (or iritis) can involve the iris or the ciliary body, or both. Posterior uveitis involves the choroid (choroiditis). It is an acute condition, the exact cause of which may be unknown, although it is often associated with rheumatoid conditions, irritable bowel syndrome (IBS), ankylosing spondylitis and sarcoidosis (Kunimoto et al 2004). Recurrent episodes are expected; they usually respond to prompt treatment and carry a fairly good prognosis. Secondary iritis may accompany other eye infections or trauma.

Clinical features are as follows:

- Mild to severe pain, due to ciliary body spasm
- Red eye, due to vascular congestion in the conjunctival vessels at the limbus
- Photophobia
- Cloudy aqueous, due to the increase in aqueous protein content and presence of white blood cells (the debris floating in the aqueous is known as 'flare and cells')
- Reduced vision, dependent on the severity of the attack and degree of inflammation
- Cellular exudates, i.e. keratic precipitates (KPs), may be present on the posterior surface of the cornea
- Loss of iris details (muddy iris)
- Inflammation of the iris may cause it to adhere to the anterior surface of the lens (synechiae formation); this will interfere with aqueous flow
- Possible raised IOP, which, if untreated, may progress to secondary glaucoma.

MEDICAL MANAGEMENT

- Patients should be investigated to determine the cause of recurrent uveitis via blood tests, the most commonly used being HLA-B27 and ESR. The aetiology is most commonly idiopathic or autoimmune (Kunimoto et al 2004).
- Outpatient review is usual, but in severe cases hospital admission may be required.
- Usual treatment is with topical steroids and cycloplegics, eye drops which dilate the pupil and paralyse the ciliary muscle; however, in severe cases, these may be given via subconjunctival injection.
- Raised IOP must be treated, as described in the PCAG section (see p. 573).
- Ocular pain must be managed, and the wearing of dark glasses can alleviate photophobia.
- Treatment will be long term if attacks are frequent with acute flare-ups.

NURSING PRIORITIES AND MANAGEMENT: Uveitis

Major nursing considerations

Setting priorities (triage)

Screening for potential health problems and prioritising patients' needs are two interrelated aspects of the nurse's role in the community. It is vital that community nurses are able to recognise ophthalmic conditions which need urgent medical attention. Uveitis is one such condition, as raised IOP and/or severe inflammation will quickly cause irreparable damage if treatment is delayed.

STOP THINK **13.11** List the ophthalmic conditions that require emergency treatment.

Education

Once the diagnosis is confirmed and treatment has been commenced, the nurse's role will include providing guidance and support for both the patient and the family to ensure adherence to the treatment regimen, recognition of signs and symptoms, and prompt self-referral if the condition recurs. These actions will serve to reduce the severity of the attack and the risk of complications.

Ensuring a safe environment

Dilated pupils allow an increased amount of light to enter the eye, causing photophobia. Patients experience dazzle when in bright sunlight or when facing car headlights from oncoming traffic at night. Appropriate adjustments to lifestyle, such as not driving or working heavy machinery whilst on cycloplegics, is a medicolegal requirement for the duration of the treatment (Ayres & Shaw 2001).

Keratitis

Keratitis refers to inflammatory conditions of the cornea. These may be caused by certain bacteria, viruses or fungi resulting in corneal ulceration. They may also be associated with trauma, external eye disease, dry eye and extensive contact lens wear (Kunimoto et al 2004). If the superficial layer, the epithelium, alone is affected, there is minimal damage with little visual loss. If the middle portion (stroma) is involved, loss of transparency and altered corneal curvature may lead to significant loss of vision. Severe inflammation may result in inflammatory debris being shed into the anterior chamber and settling as a collection of cells (hypopyon).

PATHOPHYSIOLOGY

Clinical features are as follows; the severity of signs and symptoms will vary dependent upon the actual cause:

- Red, inflamed eye
- Photophobia with spasm of the eyelid (blepharospasm)
- Lacrimation/profuse tears, although there are some instances of dry eye presentation
- Reduced vision
- Possible discharge and 'sticky' eye.

Bacterial keratitis

The most common causative agents are *Pneumococcus*, *Streptococcus* and *Pseudomonas*. These invade the cornea, resulting in an inflammatory reaction. The condition tends to recur, may range from superficial to severe and may result in corneal thinning and, in rare cases, perforation.

Viral keratitis

The most common form is dendritic (herpetic) ulcer, which is caused by the herpes simplex virus. Its distinguishing feature is the branching, tree-like pattern it forms on the cornea, which is visible only on corneal staining with fluorescein.

Fungal keratitis

Fungal infections of the eye are an increasing problem. The damage they cause is severe, and specific antifungal treatment agents are limited, making clinical management complex. Complications can develop rapidly. The distinguishing feature of this kind of ulceration is that it appears as feathery extensions over the cornea. It can be associated with minor trauma from vegetation, e.g. plants, or with contact lenses.

Acanthamoeba

This form of keratitis is associated with acanthamoeba, an organism which inhabits polluted water and swimming pools. Although rare, it is serious and is linked with certain features of contact lens wear, e.g. use of soft, disposable lenses, poor hygiene levels and excessive contact lens wear which breaches the manufacturer's guidance (Kunimoto et al 2004). Clinical features include ring abscess formation and corneal melt, as well as typical keratitis signs and symptoms previously mentioned (see p. 575). Treatment is medical and intensive, but poor response to treatment can result in severe visual impairment.

For further information, see www.revoptom.com/handbook/default.htm and select 'keratitis'.

MEDICAL MANAGEMENT

Conjunctival and corneal swabs, and fluorescein staining can confirm the diagnosis. The fluorescein fixes to damaged corneal tissue and turns the affected area a bright fluorescent green, indicating the extent of the damage. Topical antibiotic, antiviral or antifungal therapy is usually commenced immediately to avoid rapid development of complications. Differential diagnosis must be sought, by:

- obtaining a thorough patient history
- taking corneal scrapings
- slit lamp examination
- sending contact lens/lenses for culture and sensitivity.

Possible secondary ocular complications of raised IOP or iritis must be treated as necessary. Steroids are generally contraindicated for keratitis. Patients should be managed, wherever possible, by an ophthalmic corneal consultant.

NURSING PRIORITIES AND MANAGEMENT: Keratitis

Patients are generally cared for on an outpatient basis, unless they present in an acute state and require intensive topical treatment day and night. The principles for uveitis (see p. 575) should be followed with these additions:

- The patient should be taught not to touch or rub the eye as this may extend the ulceration.
- Careful hygiene is essential to prevent cross-infection. Tears should be wiped from the cheek only, using a clean disposable tissue on each occasion. Principles of isolation and infection control will be observed in the hospital situation (see Ch. 16).
- With regard to dendritic ulcer, anyone who has an outbreak of herpes simplex, commonly known as 'cold sores', should be advised to guard against touching the sores and then rubbing their eyes. Nursing staff with active sores should not have contact with ophthalmic patients.
- Re-education regarding contact lens wear. Long-term use may be contraindicated. The principles of contact lens care are as follows:
  - — Maintain strict hygienic practice
  - — Do not exceed the recommended wearing time
  - — Do not clean with saliva or tap water
  - — Remove lenses if the eyes become inflamed or sore
  - — Remove soft lenses whilst administering drops containing preservatives (Batterbury & Bowling 1999).

Conjunctivitis

Conjunctivitis, i.e. inflammation of the conjunctiva, is a common condition, which may be acute, subacute or chronic. It can be unilateral or bilateral in presentation, the latter form often being due to cross-infection. Causative agents are bacteria, viruses, fungi, parasites, toxins, chemicals, foreign bodies and allergies.

PATHOPHYSIOLOGY

The activating agent causes vascular dilatation of both the palpebral conjunctiva (lining the eyelid), and the bulbar conjunctiva (covering the eyeball), cellular infiltration leading to formation of papillae and follicles, and serous exudation. In severe cases, oedema of the conjunctiva (chemosis) may occur.

Clinical features include:

- Brick-red appearance of the conjunctiva
- Gritty feeling as of a foreign body in the eye
- Mucopurulent discharge, common in bacterial conjunctivitis, the eyelids sticking together at night
- Varying degrees of pain.

The patient may be photophobic, but visual acuity is not necessarily affected. Eversion of the lids may reveal follicle formation, i.e. cellular structures within the conjunctiva are inflamed and raised, which is the cause of the gritty sensation.

MEDICAL AND NURSING MANAGEMENT

Accurate diagnosis is made through slit lamp examination, conjunctival swabs or taking corneal scrapings to obtain cells, in order to detect accurately the cause of the infection, so that appropriate treatment can commence. As well as educating the patient in eye hygiene and self-medication, the nurse must monitor for complications such as secondary corneal inflammation (keratoconjunctivitis), which would cause visual reduction. Conjunctivitis is highly infectious and family members, peers and other patients should be advised about the prevention of cross-infection. Scrupulous hand washing and the use of individual towels should be emphasised.

For further information, see Khaw et al (2004).

Herpes zoster ophthalmicus (ophthalmic shingles)

This is an acute unilateral infection of the trigeminal ganglion, which extends from the scalp to the nose and includes the eye. It is caused by the chickenpox virus and is fairly common in people over 50 years of age (see Ch. 16).

PATHOPHYSIOLOGY

Common presenting signs and symptoms, all on the affected side, are as follows:

- Pain and tingling sensation
- Swollen eyelids
- Skin rash of the forehead and around the eye
- Characteristic vesicular eruptions over the course of the nerve
- Potential serious ocular complications, including uveitis, keratitis and conjunctivitis
- Regional adenopathy and general malaise of the patient.

MEDICAL MANAGEMENT

- Prevention of cross-infection
- Immediate administration of systemic antiviral agents, usually commenced by the GP
- Topical antiviral agents, usually commenced by the ophthalmologist
- Analgesics for associated pain
- Ocular lubricants if required to relieve ocular discomfort
- Regular eye-bathing if ocular discharge.

Allergy to topical medication

Allergic reaction to topical eye medication manifests as inflammation of the eyelids extending to the cheeks. The lids become red and oedematous and may be moist in the acute stage, drying to form light crusts later. There is intense itching, which may result in excoriation. Common causative agents are atropine, neomycin and preservatives in eye drops.

Management consists of reviewing medication, suspending all medication for 24 h if possible and substituting an alternative agent. Cortisone lotion and cool bathing may be prescribed for the affected skin area to relieve itching and oedema.

EXTERNAL EYE DISEASES

These are common and easily treated, once accurately diagnosed. Nurse specialists in many ophthalmic units manage patients with such diseases and it is advisable for community and nursing home staff to contact the local ophthalmic unit to confirm best practice and to obtain advice.

Blepharitis

This is a chronic inflammatory condition of the eyelids and eyelashes, resulting in redness, crusting and itchiness. Blepharitis may predispose the patient to stye or chalazion and may recur, requiring long-term management using:

- lid hygiene (see Box 13.3) and application of warm flannel compresses
- topical antibiotics
- ocular lubricants, if associated with dry eye (see 'Age-related conditions', p. 584)
- systemic antibiotics.

If there is acne rosacea, psoriasis or eczema and if treatment is ineffective, referral to a dermatologist should be considered (Khaw et al 2004) (see Ch. 12).

Stye

This is an infection of an eyelash follicle, which should be treated with warm compresses and topical antibiotics.

Chalazion or meibomian cyst

This is a blocked duct from the meibomian 'lipid secreting' glands. Treatment is as for blepharitis in the first instance, progressing to 'incision and curettage' if the condition persists. This procedure is performed under a local anaesthetic by an ophthalmic nurse practitioner in the ophthalmic outpatient department. Biopsy of the cyst contents is necessary should the cyst recur.

Cysts and lesions of the eyelids can have a similar clinical appearance; careful history of the duration and pathology are therefore essential. Referral to an ophthalmic consultant is advised to exclude any possible malignancies.

For further information, see www.revoptom.com/handbook/default.htm.

Box 13.3

Lid hygiene

This is a method of cleaning the eyelids to remove excess oily secretions from the meibomian glands. It is an effective therapeutic treatment in the prevention and management of external eye disease. Requirements are:

- any type of mild baby shampoo. Do not use other types of shampoo as these are too harsh and will irritate the eyelids
- some cotton buds
- a quarter of a teacup of cooled, boiled water.

Method

The procedure is explained to the patient. Add a few drops of baby shampoo to the water and mix well. Wet the end of the cotton bud and gently rub the bud along the root of the eyelashes on the external lid. Ask the patient to look down when bathing the top lid and up when bathing the bottom lid. Use separate cotton buds for each eyelid. The process is continued for 5–10 min and is usually carried out four times daily. It should be continued long term, and at least once or twice daily as part of general hygiene. Frail and handicapped people may require assistance in order to prevent them from sustaining a conjunctival or corneal abrasion in the course of self-care. Lid hygiene with cotton buds is unsuitable for children, as they are more inclined to move during the procedure and acquire an abrasion.

DIPLOPIA (DOUBLE VISION)

Diplopia refers to a person's experience of seeing the same object in two different areas of their visual field. Diplopia can be either monocular — 'with one eye only' — associated with cataract, refractive error, macular disease and retinal detachment, or binocular — 'present with both eyes' — usually associated with nerve palsies, squint, trauma or myasthenia gravis. Different factors are involved in childhood squints and for further information reference should be made to paediatric texts.

NURSING PRIORITIES AND MANAGEMENT: Diplopia

The cause of diplopia should be established prior to any intervention or long-term treatment to alleviate symptoms. Nurses should reassure their patients and attention should be given to maintaining a safe environment in case of dizziness or nausea. Advice must be sought from the local ophthalmic unit. One eye may be occluded to make the patient more comfortable during the investigation period which may last days or weeks and may on occasion involve neurological tests and a brain scan. Binocular diplopia of sudden onset must be referred promptly to rule out any underlying life-threatening cause such as a cerebral space-occupying lesion.

MEDICAL MANAGEMENT

Following diagnosis, treatment includes:

- occlusion of one eye after assessment by an orthoptist and ophthalmologist
- use of prisms on the patient's glasses
- injection of botulinum toxin to overactive muscle — this results in temporary paralysis, for approximately 3 months, and encourages increased function of the underactive muscle. The botulinum blocks the transmission of the nerve impulses at the neuromuscular junction by interfering with release of the neurotransmitter acetylcholine (see Ch. 9)
- surgical intervention to correct squint, either by 'recession' or 'resection'. This is not considered until other treatments have been implemented.

EYE INJURIES

It is vital to record an accurate history (see Table 13.3) to rule out any non-visible injury, such as an intraocular foreign body (IOFB). The visual acuity (VA) must be measured and a systematic eye examination (see Table 13.1) conducted to establish a diagnosis and for medicolegal reasons. The only exception to this practice is in the case of chemical injury, when the main priority is irrigation. A triage system (see Box 13.4) must be utilised in clinical practice which, together with the nurse's professional judgement, aims to facilitate the preservation of vision. Some of the more common types of eye injury are described below.

Box 13.4

Ophthalmic triage

Patients attending an ophthalmic emergency department are placed in one of three categories depending on the severity of their clinical condition.

Emergency
True emergencies requiring immediate specialist attention:

- Chemical burns (initiate first aid immediately)
- Penetrating injuries
- Intraocular foreign body
- Acute glaucoma
- Retinal detachment
- Sudden loss of vision in one eye
- Blunt trauma

Urgent
Specialist attention required as soon as possible:

- Hyphaema
- Corneal foreign body, abrasion or ulcer
- Radiation and welding burns
- All acute infections or allergies
- Suspected postoperative complications

Non-urgent
Minor ocular irritations, such as chalazion and long-standing visual disturbances

Hyphaema

This refers to a haemorrhage in the anterior chamber of the eye.

PATHOPHYSIOLOGY

A direct blow to the eye, e.g. a clenched fist, golf ball or champagne cork, causing rupture of the small iris blood vessels, usually results in a primary hyphaema. It may be microscopic, with diffuse red cells visible only with the aid of a slit lamp, or severe, with a level of blood seen in the anterior chamber (AC) of the eye. Occasionally, the blood can completely fill the AC. The degree of pain and the reduction in vision depend upon the severity of the bleeding. A secondary hyphaema may occur after intraocular surgery.

MEDICAL MANAGEMENT

A patient with a microscopic or moderate hyphaema will not require admission, but will be advised to rest at home for several days. These hyphaemas rarely re-bleed.

A patient with a severe hyphaema may be admitted for observation, as there could be an associated rise in IOP or further bleeding. Quiet activity will be allowed. Investigations will include B-scan, fundal examination, blood tests to estimate clotting time and possible CT scan to determine cause. Topical drops will be prescribed, including antibiotics, cycloplegics and steroids (see Table 13.2).

NURSING PRIORITIES AND MANAGEMENT: Hyphaema

Observation of the level of hyphaema is made according to the ophthalmologist's instruction. Any increase in pain or discomfort may be caused by raised IOP or a re-bleed.

In order to reduce the risk of increased bleeding, or dislodging the hyphaema into the posterior chamber of the eye, the patient is advised to bend at the knees to reach things from below waist height and not to bend over, lift or strain.

On discharge, the patient will be advised to avoid active or contact sports until the first follow-up appointment and to assess visual function in the injured eye daily to detect possible complications, e.g. retinal detachment (see p. 570 and Nursing Care Plan 13.1). Protective eyewear will be necessary in the future, e.g. whilst playing squash, to prevent recurrence of a similar injury (see Box 13.2).

Penetrating injuries

Whatever the apparent extent of a penetrating injury, these must always be treated as an emergency and thoroughly investigated. Depending on the results of history taking and examination, X-rays and ultrasound scanning may be necessary to confirm the presence, location and type of any foreign body.

MEDICAL MANAGEMENT

Treatment is dependent on the cause of the injury and on the extent of involvement of ocular structures. It may include the administration of mydriatic, steroid and antibiotic eye drops, and possibly of systemic antibiotics to reduce the risk of complications from inflammation and infection. In addition, the measures described below will be taken.

Perforating injuries The patient will be admitted to hospital for surgical repair of the wound and possible excision of iris prolapse. If the lens is damaged it may be removed at the same time. If facial or other injuries are present, these will be reviewed and treated by the appropriate specialists (see Ch. 15).

Small puncture wounds These may seal themselves, but the patient is admitted to ensure that the wound stays closed and that intraocular infection does not develop. If the wound is not completely sealed, a cyanoacrylate glue or 'bioadhesive' may be instilled onto the affected cornea and a 'bandage' contact lens placed over this site to seal the wound and hold the lens in place, until such time as the wound has healed. The glue gradually dissolves to allow for removal of the surface lens.

Intraocular foreign bodies Admission is essential for surgical removal of the foreign body, which could be embedded in the iris, vitreous humor or lens. If the foreign body is metallic, it may be removed with the aid of a magnet. If it is found in the lens, a lens extraction is carried out (see p. 566). Vitrectomy may be necessary if there has been vitreous haemorrhage.

Complications following penetrating injury The most common complications are corneal scarring, raised IOP, haemorrhage, hypopyon, iris prolapse and retinal tears/detachments.

Severe infections can occur following any injury, making intensive treatment with antibiotic eye drops and systemic antibiotics necessary.

It is always important to examine the uninjured eye for signs of 'sympathetic ophthalmitis', a rare complication which presents as a low-grade iritis. The cause of the sympathetic inflammatory process is thought to involve an immune response to damaged uveal tissue. The use of topical steroids has reduced the occurrence of this potentially sight-threatening condition, which was formerly managed by enucleating the injured eye.

A severely damaged eye with no prospect of useful vision may become very painful and unresponsive to analgesics. It may be necessary to enucleate the eye to give relief to the patient.

Following repair of large penetrating injuries, or severe infections, the eye may collapse entirely and become a shrunken mass in the orbit. This wasting of the globe (phthisis bulbi) can be unsightly and the patient may wish the eye to be enucleated.

NURSING PRIORITIES AND MANAGEMENT: Penetrating injuries

Anxiety

The patient and relatives will be highly distressed at the possibility or reality of severe injury and permanent sight loss, therefore the nurse's key responsibility is to comfort and offer support. The patient's main concerns are the degree of visual impairment, the altered body image and changes in working life and everyday lifestyle. Effective communication is vital to prevent any misunderstandings. Any questions and concerns must be answered honestly. A process of grieving is normal when any degree of vision is lost.

Return to the community

If the eye is damaged to the extent that no useful vision is retained, the patient will need continuing support in the community. Patients in this situation are particularly susceptible to depression when they return home and begin to grapple with the full implications of their disability (Karlson 1998). They will need practical and psychological support through the grieving and adaptation period. Assessment of the level of support required should be carried out prior to discharge and with regard to the patient's home and work environment. The community nurse should be advised of immediate practical measures regarding dressings and wound care but also how further support and information can be accessed on behalf of the patient, e.g. from a psychologist or orbital prosthetist. Liaison with support groups and counselling options should be discussed. Where possible patients should be encouraged to meet their own eye care needs.

For further information, see Nursing Times (2003).

Chemical burns

These must be treated as emergencies and irrigation (see Box 13.5) must be started immediately (Khaw et al 2004), prior to prompt referral to an ophthalmic emergency department. Many chemical substances have antidotes, so the chemical label or details on the container should be taken to the emergency department along with the patient.

PATHOPHYSIOLOGY

The burn may be caused by an acid or an alkali, e.g. substances such as antifreeze, car battery acid, household

Box 13.5

Irrigation of an eye

Copious irrigation of the affected eye(s) should be carried out with 1 litre of sodium chloride 0.9% via an i.v. giving set; alternatively, non-sterile water can be used in an emergency. Ensure the patient is comfortable, reclining on their back with the head and neck supported. Clothing should be protected by a waterproof cape and towels. Ask the patient to hold the receiver dish and to turn their head slightly to the affected side. Instil topical anaesthetic drops (e.g. tetracaine 1.0% or proxymetacaine, 1 or 2 drops). Gently pull down the lower eyelid and irrigate with a steady flow of fluid, while asking the patient to move the eye around and to evert the upper lid to ensure thorough irrigation. Continue irrigation for at least 15 min, re-instilling local anaesthetic drops as required. Remove particles or foreign bodies with a moistened cotton bud or forceps. Wait 5 min prior to checking pH levels of the tear film, which should be 7.4 or below. Continue irrigation until this neutral pH is indicated when reading the colour reaction of a strip of universal pH paper when it touches the tear film in the lower fornix of the eye.

cleaning agents, cement and superglue. In general, acids cause only superficial burns because coagulation of the tissues prevents further penetration. The structures involved are usually the palpebral and bulbar conjunctivae and the cornea. Alkalis penetrate the eye structures more deeply and, as well as severely damaging the eyelids, conjunctivae, cornea and sclera, readily penetrate the internal eye.

The patient will complain of severe, burning pain due to the exposure of the pain receptors of the trigeminal nerve. Absence of pain or a white eye, 'blanching', does not mean the burn is mild: it may be so severe that it has destroyed the nerve endings. There will be extreme watering of the eyes due to reflex action and the lids will be very swollen and red. Burns to the surrounding skin may also be evident.

MEDICAL MANAGEMENT

On arrival in the emergency department the patient is taken for immediate irrigation of the eye (see Box 13.5). This is one time when visual acuity is not assessed before treatment. Anaesthetic eye drops are instilled to reduce the pain and ensure the patient's cooperation with irrigation. The irrigating fluid will be either sodium chloride 0.9% or a solution of trisodium edetate — a neutralising fluid used specifically for lime burns. Once the nurse is sure that all traces of the chemical have been removed, a full history can be taken and visual acuity assessed.

Following irrigation, ocular examination will be carried out using a slit lamp to assess the extent of the injury. Chemical injuries are usually successfully treated without causing any long-term damage. Occasionally, however, the burn can cause extensive damage to the cornea and conjunctiva.

Treatment for minor burns An antibiotic ointment is prescribed, and possibly cycloplegics to relieve iris spasm,

Box 13.6

Rodding of fornices

Local anaesthetic eye drops are instilled and a glass rod lubricated with antibiotic ointment is inserted under the upper eyelid. The patient is asked to look down and the rod is passed gently but firmly from side to side several times whilst outward pressure is exerted. This breaks down any adhesions already formed and leaves a film of ointment in the fornix to prevent any recurrence.

This process is repeated under the lower eyelid with the patient looking up.

prior to an eye pad being applied for 6 h. If both eyes require padding, the better eye is left exposed until the patient arrives home, when the other eye should be padded. The topical treatment is prescribed for several days but the patient may be asked to return for review the day after commencement of treatment.

Treatment for severe burns Admission to the ward for intensive treatment and observation is usual. Depending on the severity of the pain, i.m. analgesics are given for at least the first 24 h. An antibiotic ointment is applied at least four times daily to lubricate the fornices, and mydriatic eye drops are instilled to relieve accompanying iris spasm and iritis. Usually topical steroids are administered. To prevent the development of conjunctival adhesions (symblepharon), rodding of the fornices may be required (see Box 13.6). Monitoring of IOP is required in the event that uveitis occurs and leads to a secondary glaucoma.

NURSING PRIORITIES AND MANAGEMENT: Chemical burns

Anxiety

Suffering chemical burns causes high levels of anxiety, and the nurse's role is to provide reassurance and emotional support by explaining the procedures, answering questions, ensuring adequate pain relief and contacting the patient's family. Eye pads or dark glasses are used to reduce the photophobia caused by iris spasm and pupil dilatation.

Return to the community

It is essential to maintain prescribed treatment and to attend follow-up outpatient appointments. It is also important for the nurse to educate the patient about the severe risk to sight (and to livelihood) posed by such burns, and to stress the necessity for wearing eye protection in DIY, manual work and when using strong cleaning agents, in order to reduce or prevent further sight-threatening accidents (see Box 13.2). If there is permanent damage to one or both corneas, a keratoplasty may be carried out (see p. 572).

It may be necessary, in cases of significant sight loss, to ensure that the patient and carers are fully supported and are offered appropriate advice by special community services for the visually impaired person (see 'Penetrating eye injury', p. 579).

Radiation injuries

Irradiation from ultraviolet, infrared or laser light can cause eye damage.

PATHOPHYSIOLOGY

Ultraviolet radiation causes corneal epithelial damage (arc eye, welders' flash) and most commonly occurs when approved eye goggles with protective sides are not worn during welding or when the individual is using a sun bed or sunlamp (see Box 13.2). Usually the signs and symptoms do not appear until several hours after exposure, when the patient presents with photophobia, pain and excessive lacrimation. The reason that there is this latent period is not fully understood. Fluorescein drops show dot-like staining of the cornea. Treatment is symptomatic and includes pain relief and the use of eye pads or dark glasses. The corneal healing is variable but there should be no long-term effects.

Infrared radiation penetrates the eye through the cornea and can cause cataract.

Laser radiation can cause irreversible damage to the retina.

NURSING PRIORITIES AND MANAGEMENT: Radiation injuries

Prevention

Health education and accident prevention are major parts of the nurse's role. The need for those at risk to use protective eyewear must be stressed. Nurses working in occupational health, general practice, in the community and in emergency and outpatient departments with laser equipment should implement a programme of health education which focuses on this topic. It is also important to stress that other people working in the immediate environment of the radiation source may sustain injuries. Nurses must be aware of relevant legislation (Al-Husainy et al 2001).

STOP THINK **13.12** Can you think of reasons why people might fail to use appropriate eye protection? Is there any legislation governing the provision of protective eyewear? Discuss this issue with your lecturer, mentor and colleagues and reflect on how it applies to your own workplace.

Central retinal artery occlusion (CRAO)

This condition is an ophthalmic emergency. The patient will experience sudden, complete and painless loss of vision in one eye, due to an obstruction of the central retinal artery. It is associated with emboli, thrombosis, diabetes mellitus, hypertension, giant cell arteritis and trauma (Kaiser et al 2004). The retinal artery and some of its branches may be obliterated. The damage to retinal cells is irreparable.

MEDICAL MANAGEMENT

Emergency intervention Treatment must begin within minutes if any degree of visual recovery is to be achieved. Vital time is often lost as the patient may think that the visual loss is transitory and therefore may not seek help immediately. The aim of treatment is to reduce the normal IOP rapidly by massage of the globe, administration of osmotic medication, e.g. i.v. mannitol, to draw fluid from the eye by osmosis and/or paracentesis to release aqueous from the anterior chamber. This should allow the retinal artery to dilate and the clot may be flushed along to a peripheral arterial branch.

Continuing management Once the emergency stage has passed the patient is given a full examination. Any underlying medical condition, e.g. hypertension, is diagnosed and treated appropriately, often by the GP. Residual visual impairment is assessed and the patient given all necessary support in terms of health education and maintaining independent living when back in the community.

Minor eye injuries

Corneal foreign body

There is usually a history of something entering the eye. The eye will be extremely painful, especially on blinking. On examination, a foreign body will be visible on the anterior surface of the cornea. Anaesthetic eye drops are instilled and the foreign body is removed with a moistened cotton bud or a 10G needle. This can be carried out by the doctor or an experienced ophthalmic nurse (see Box 13.7 for additional information).

Subtarsal foreign body

The nurse should suspect the presence of a foreign body when, despite the patient's complaint of something entering the eye, nothing can be seen on normal inspection. There will be discomfort, especially on blinking. The upper lid should be everted and the foreign body, if present, removed with a moistened cotton bud (see Box 13.8). The nurse should check for a possible corneal abrasion.

Box 13.7

Rust ring

If a metallic foreign body is left in contact with the cornea for more than 4 h, a rust ring may develop around its perimeter.

It can be easily removed after 1 day of the application of antibiotic ointment. This is done with a 10G needle or a small battery-powered instrument called a burr.

Box 13.8

Eversion of an eyelid

This procedure is carried out if the presence of a foreign body is suspected under the upper eyelid. With the patient's eyes open and looking down, the upper lid lashes are grasped. At the same time, the upper edge of the tarsal plate (at the crease of the eyelid) is depressed, using a glass rod or cotton bud. This allows the lid to be turned over to expose the subtarsal conjunctiva and facilitates inspection, irrigation and foreign body removal.

Corneal abrasion

Usually caused by a fingernail, a twig or other sharp object, this is an extremely painful condition, with profuse lacrimation. Fluorescein eye drops should be instilled in order to determine the extent of the abrasion.

An eye pad is not always required after treatment for abrasion or removal of a foreign body. Need depends upon the severity and location, i.e. if the abrasion is central and large. If the patient feels more comfortable with the eye closed, a pad may be worn for about 6 h. Antibiotic ointment may be prescribed to prevent infection, as well as mydriatics if pain is severe.

A follow-up appointment may be given depending on the severity of the abrasion or the depth at which the foreign body was embedded.

SURGICAL REMOVAL OF AN EYE

There are three methods of removing an eye:

- *Enucleation* — surgical removal of the globe. The extraocular muscles are cut at their insertion and the optic nerve severed.
- *Evisceration* — removal of the contents of the globe, leaving the scleral shell.
- *Exenteration* — a more extensive operation involving removal of the eye and surrounding tissues.

Special considerations

The choice of operation is dependent upon the diagnosis which has necessitated the removal of an eye. A badly injured eye may be enucleated (see Nursing Care Plan 13.4) whilst an infected eye would require to be eviscerated. Exenteration would be required when a malignant tumour extended beyond the globe.

Maintenance of a good cosmetic appearance post-surgery has led to the development of a range of socket and orbital implants, which may reduce the psychological trauma experienced.

Management is as for extensive penetrating injuries. The nurse may find that if a patient has suffered severe pain and blindness in an eye, the relief from pain after it has been removed is often so great that this helps in coping with the loss. Contact with others who have had an eye removed may help to reassure the patient that it is possible to adapt and to live a full life following this traumatic experience. Many areas throughout the country have support groups which allow the patient the opportunity to share and discuss feelings and coping mechanisms with others who have gone through the same experience.

Artificial eye fitting

The National Artificial Eye Service (NAES) (1998) in Blackpool provides training to enable personnel to make and fit artificial eyes. Patient education, support and follow-up services are also provided by technicians in local ocular prosthetic departments.

An artificial eye is individually designed to fit the socket and implant exactly and is painted by an ocular artist to match the patient's other eye. The prosthesis is shell-like in shape and form and not, as anticipated, ball-shaped. If an orbital implant has been inserted, the artificial eye will move in unison with the natural eye because the extraocular muscles have been preserved and attached to the implant.

Unfortunately, lack of information about artificial eyes can cause a great deal of anxiety and often a degree of revulsion. This is usually dispelled by explaining that the appearance of the socket is similar to the inside of the mouth. Anxiety is further reduced by contact with people who have adapted successfully to living with an artificial eye and by an opportunity to see and handle an artificial eye before surgery and thereby gain reassurance that they look quite natural (see Nursing Care Plan 13.4).

Principles of artificial eye care

Nurses should be prepared to assist or advise on the care of an artificial eye. Principles of daily management are as follows.

Removal of an artificial eye

A special extractor is provided by the ocular prosthetic department. The eyelids are opened with the thumb and forefinger, and the lower edge of the eye is gently levered out with the aid of the extractor. If an extractor is not available, then a finger will suffice (see Fig. 13.8A).

Insertion of an artificial eye

The eyelids are opened with the thumb and forefinger. The eye is inserted under the upper lid with the curve of the eye towards the nose. The lower lid is depressed slightly. The eye can then be slipped into position (see Fig. 13.8B).

Care of the artificial eye

An artificial eye should be cleaned at least once a day with ordinary soap in cold or lukewarm water. It should be thoroughly rinsed afterwards under running water. Chemical cleansers or disinfectants must not be used.

The patient is encouraged to wear the eye both day and night. If they prefer not to, the eye should be placed in cold water or a saline solution in a clean, labelled receptacle.

When not in regular use, the eye should be stored in cotton wool or tissue to prevent scratching. Through normal wear the eye may lose its high polish. In this case it can be sent to the nearest ocular prosthetic department for repolishing, free of charge. Replacements can be obtained cost-free (NHS patients) from the same department. The community nurse may need to prompt older patients in particular to take advantage of this service, and they may need to approach their GP for initial referral to a consultant.

Care of the socket

The socket should remain healthy if the artificial eye is kept clean in the recommended way. Occasionally, infection or irritation may result from scratches on the eye and lead to ulceration.

The socket can be irrigated with normal saline and treated with an antibiotic ointment for a short period. The artificial eye should not be inserted until the infection or irritation has cleared up.

Nursing Care Plan 13.4 A patient undergoing enucleation: postoperative

Nursing considerations	Action	Rationale	Expected outcome
Anxiety/distress • **Due to having eye removed**	• Reassure and spend time with the patient. Encourage the patient to express feelings and talk about fears. Reassure the patient that it is normal to grieve over the loss of an eye	Giving information reduces anxiety and aids recovery	The patient will come to terms with the necessity of having the eye removed
• **Due to altered body image**	• Discuss what the wound and socket will look like after surgery, likening it to the inside of the mouth. Discuss aftercare of socket and show an artificial eye, allowing the patient and family to handle it, if they wish • Arrange for someone who has had similar surgery to come and talk with the patient. Suggest dark glasses can be worn until the patient is fitted with an artificial eye	Reduces fear about the after-effects of the operation	The patient will be adjusted to altered body image and will accept the situation of wearing an artificial eye
• **Due to fear of having wrong eye removed**	• Eye to be removed is identified and checked with patient, doctor and case notes (some units mark the forehead with an arrow to identify correct eye) • Reassure patient that many checks are made prior to the operation to ensure correct eye is removed	Relieves anxiety and reassures the patient	Correct eye will be removed. Patient will be reassured of this

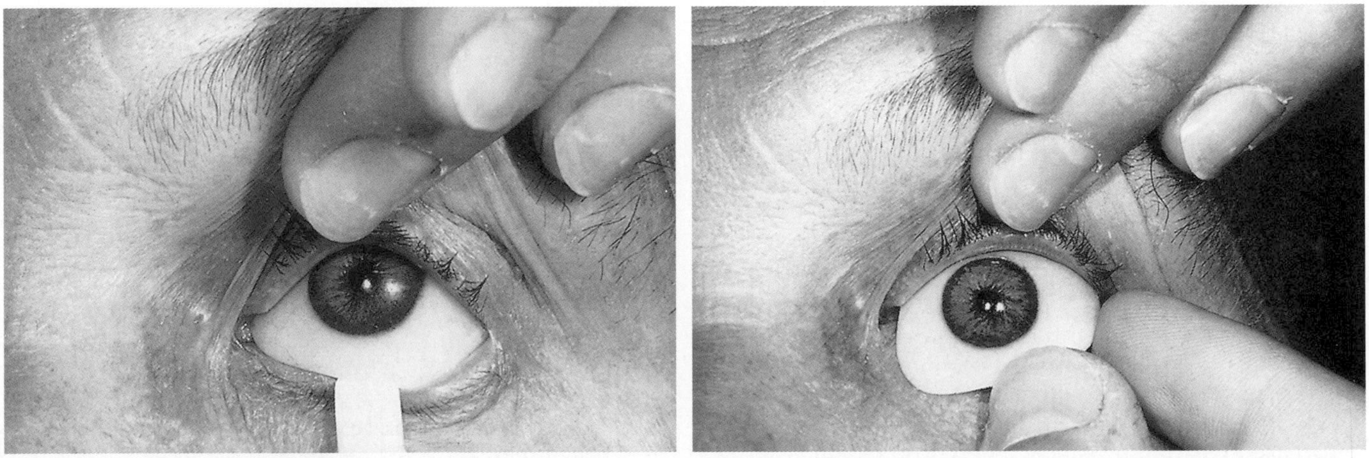

A B

Fig. 13.8 A: Removing an artificial eye. B: Inserting an artificial eye. (Reproduced with permission from The National Artificial Eye Service 1998.)

It is not advisable to leave the eye out for long periods as shrinkage of the socket can occur, causing difficulty and discomfort on re-insertion of the eye.

AGE-RELATED CONDITIONS

Age-related maculopathy (AMD)

Macular degeneration is the major cause of blindness in older people in developed countries. It accounts for 50% of individuals on the blind (severely sight impaired) or partially sighted (sight impaired) register and the incidence is increasing. Central 'fine detail and focus' vision is affected, with peripheral vision maintained.

PATHOPHYSIOLOGY

Retinal pigment epithelial cells (RPEs) wear out with age and are never replaced. As they degenerate they deposit material on the underlying membrane, which accumulates to form yellowish white spots on the retina. Initially this process does not affect vision, but eventually the cell loss will result in atrophy of the RPE layer, which may then disperse pigment into the macula. It affects form and colour vision primarily and the patient notices difficulty with activities such as reading and sewing, and problems in identifying faces and coins.

In some cases, a new blood vessel membrane may develop and cause lifting of the central retina. This results in distorted and blurred central vision.

AMD can occur in the presence of other eye conditions such as cataract and glaucoma, complicating the diagnosis and treatment of the other disorder.

MEDICAL MANAGEMENT

There is limited treatment available, with research ongoing. Any underlying disease should be accurately diagnosed through assessment of visual acuity (reading and distance), Amsler grid, colour vision, clinical examination and possible fundal fluorescein angiogram (FFA) (see 'Diabetic retinopathy', p. 585) and treated. New developments include the following:

- *Argon laser treatment* — this could be beneficial if there are early symptoms of new blood vessel membrane formation. In some cases a degree of vision can be regained following this, although if there is foveal damage there will be a persistent central scotoma (blind spot).
- *Photodynamic therapy (PDT)* — this treatment is the process of i.v. injection of verteporfin, 'a light sensitive drug', circulated into the retinal vessels to allow photodynamic treatment (laser) of the degenerated tissue (Murphy & Nesbitt 2001).
- *Vitamin and mineral supplements in high dosage* (www.icapsinfo.co.uk) — prior to the patient starting treatment, discussion with the GP is essential, as the supplements, including lutein, selenium, copper and zinc, have been linked with certain systemic side-effects, e.g. high dose beta carotene has been linked to an increased risk of lung cancer. High dose vitamins and minerals are believed to reduce the progression in advanced AMD, but not in early AMD (Bartlett & Eperjesi 2003, Kaiser et al 2004). Many ophthalmologists believe a well-balanced diet with a daily intake of fruit and vegetables (see Ch. 21) is as effective and that these supplements are not required.
- *Low visual aids (LVA) and referral to welfare advisor* — to discuss registration (see p. 560), available support, local and national organisations such as the Macular Disease Society (see 'Useful websites').

Nursing intervention is that of a supportive and educational role, especially at the point of diagnosis and possible registration, as grief, fear and depression are common (McBride 2001). Liaison with the multidisciplinary team and social services is needed to ensure the VIP is fully supported and empowered to live as full and independent a life as possible.

STOP THINK **13.13** You are a community nurse who visits Mr S (see Case History 13.1) daily to give him his insulin injection. Mrs S breaks down whilst you are there. What advice would you offer her and where would you advise her to go for assistance?

For further details, see www.maculardisease.org and Kanski (2003).

Entropion

Defined as a malposition of the eyelid with the lid margin turned towards the globe, this condition most commonly affects the lower lid and is caused by reduced elasticity of the connective tissue, which may be a result of the ageing process, of trauma or of a badly applied eye pad. The inturned eyelashes irritate the cornea and can cause discomfort and ulceration.

Nursing and medical management Discomfort can be relieved in the following ways:

- Short-term intervention by the application of tape to the affected lid margin, usually the lower one, to retract it in such a way that downward traction of the tape, when applied to the cheek, restores the normal position
- Botulinum toxin injection, as a short-term measure and alternative to taping
- Ocular lubricants, either ointment or drops, to lubricate the eye

CASE HISTORY 13.1

Mrs S

Mr and Mrs S are both 70 years old and live in a bungalow on the outskirts of a large town. Over the past 2 months, Mrs S has noticed a marked reduction in her near vision. Increasingly, she has noticed that she requires help to identify shopping items and to clean the house. Her enjoyment of completing the crosswords and reading has been lost. After a visit to her optician and GP she is referred to the eye hospital. At her appointment, the consultant tells her she has age-related macular degeneration and that, although she will not go blind, her sight will not improve. He recommends that she should consider becoming registered as partially sighted. Mrs S is distressed by this and goes home to think about it.

- Topical antibiotics if the cornea is damaged by infection or abrasion
- Repositioning of the lid by a simple surgical procedure or eversion sutures.

For further details, see www.revoptom.com/default.htm and select 'entropion' and www.eyelidsurgery.co.uk/treatments/blb-coralimplant.htm.

Ectropion

Defined as a malposition of the eyelid when the lid margin is turned away from the globe, mainly affecting the lower lid, this condition is associated with atonic tissue around the eyes. Due to malposition of the lid and punctum, tears overflow and run down the cheeks. The individual constantly wipes the eye, drawing the lid even further down and exacerbating the condition.

Nursing and medical management The use of ocular lubricants may be required if the eye is infected or sore. Topical cream to the skin is soothing if excessive tearing (epiphora) is causing excoriation. Cautery to the inner eyelid contracts the tarsal conjunctiva and inverts the lid. Minor oculoplastic surgery may be required to reposition the eyelid.

Dry eye syndrome (keratitis sicca)

This is a common, chronic and bilateral condition, requiring prompt assessment, diagnosis and management.

PATHOPHYSIOLOGY

Either a reduced quantity of tear production, poor quality of tear film, or both, result in symptoms of dry, burning and gritty eyes, occasionally with excessive epiphora which is exacerbated by humidity, wind and cigarette smoke. The diagnosis can be complex as the condition is associated with systemic disease such as rheumatoid arthritis and Sjögren's syndrome.

Nursing and medical management and nursing priorities
These are dependent upon the severity and actual cause of the condition, but consist of one or more of the following:

- Instillation of ocular lubricants four times a day or when required and at night — the ophthalmologist may recommend a preservative-free preparation
- Punctal occlusion — inserting collagen or silicone plugs into the upper and lower punctum, preventing drainage of tears
- Punctal cautery to seal puncta
- Corrective surgery, e.g. tarsorrhaphy, which involves partial closure of the lids, thereby decreasing the surface area of the cornea from which the tear film evaporates (Kanski 2003).

Entropion, ectropion and dry eyes are common conditions in older people, who may not always realise that a simple treatment such as the instillation of ocular lubricants or minor lid surgery is often effective in treating the great discomfort associated with the conditions. It is often the community nurse who is best placed to detect, assess and refer for further advice, as well as to provide encouragement to those patients to attend the ophthalmic unit.

SYSTEMIC DISEASE AND DISORDERS OF THE EYE

The eye is a sensitive indicator of systemic disease. Visual disturbance or abnormal appearance of the retina or optic disc may be the first manifestation of health breakdown. In this section, ophthalmic conditions associated with some of the more common systemic diseases will be described. Other conditions are described in Table 13.4.

Nursing priorities and management should be based on the general principles of ophthalmic management as well as the specific principles that pertain to the disease process in question. The reader should refer to relevant chapters in the present text as well as to more specialised ophthalmic texts.

For further information, see Blaustein (1994).

Diabetes mellitus

Diabetes mellitus is a common disorder in developed countries and its incidence is increasing markedly in both developed and developing countries worldwide as diets include more processed foods and refined sugars (see Ch. 5). Poorly controlled diabetes can lead to retinopathy, early cataract development, vascularisation of the iris (rubeosis) and a high incidence of minor eye conditions such as chalazion.

Diabetic retinopathy

PATHOPHYSIOLOGY

Elevated blood sugar levels, associated with prolonged poor diabetic control, damage the blood vessel basement membrane. In the retina, this leads to leakage and the formation of fatty and haemorrhagic lesions. These changes are given the term 'retinopathy'. The patient will usually complain of gradual and painless loss of vision — unless there is bleeding into the vitreous humor, in which case loss of vision may be sudden and very frightening (Hall & Waterman 1997). The diagnosis and progression of the disease can be confirmed by fluorescein angiography. Diabetic retinopathy is the leading cause of preventable blindness in the working population in developed countries (Vafidis 2000).

There are two forms of the condition: background and proliferative.

Background retinopathy The small retinal vessels become fragile, aneurysms form and leakage occurs, causing localised oedema and haemorrhage. Background retinopathy can cause loss of central vision if macular oedema occurs and the hard exudates encroach on the fovea. Peripheral vision will be retained.

Proliferative retinopathy In this condition there is further deterioration as new blood vessels and fibrous bands form in response to breakdown and occlusion of the normal circulation. The main complications that can arise from this are bleeding into the vitreous humor and tractional retinal detachment. Eventually, proliferative vascularisation

Table 13.4 Further eye problems secondary to systemic diseases

Disorder	Main ophthalmic clinical features	Cause	Treatment
Thyroid function imbalance (Graves' disease)	Upper lid retraction	Sympathetic nerve innervation	Lubricating drops during day and antibiotic ointment nightly
	Exposure keratitis	Exposure of eyeball	As above
	Swelling of lids and conjunctiva	Infiltration of lymphocytes in orbital tissue and associated oedema	Partial tarsorrhaphy
	Exophthalmos		Systemic steroids
	Compression of optic nerve		Surgical decompression
	Diplopia	Infiltration of lymphocytes in muscle tissue leading to fibrosis	Prism spectacles Botulinum A neurotoxin injection into the appropriate lid muscle Strabismus surgery
Migraine	Headache with visual disturbances Characteristic aura: multicoloured, jagged shape, firework-like	Idiopathic; possibly chemical changes in the brain caused by various triggers, e.g. stress, or dietary, e.g. eating oranges or chocolate	Feverfew herbal remedy Ergotamine Rest
Multiple sclerosis	Uniocular	Localised demyelinating lesion to the cranial nerves III IV VI	Symptoms may recover spontaneously but will always recur
	Small unequal pupils: do not react to light but do with accommodation, unable to dilate with atropine		
	Optic neuritis Rapid reduction of central vision Sudden onset of pain especially when looking upwards		Systemic painkillers
	Central scotoma		
	Diplopia		Prism spectacles Botulinum A neurotoxin injection Strabismus surgery
Intracranial aneurysm	Uniocular/binocular Diplopia Blurred vision Ptosis Visual field defects	Pressure on visual pathway Pressure on cranial nerves III IV VI	Detection and clipping of aneurysm Botulinum A neurotoxin injection Strabismus surgery
Nephritis	Blurred vision Papilloedema Retinal haemorrhage Retinal detachment	Hypertension	Reduce hypertension Laser treatment Vitrectomy Surgical repair of detachment

can affect the angle of the eye by blocking the trabecular meshwork and causing glaucoma.

MEDICAL MANAGEMENT

Early diagnosis is critical, as is good control of blood sugar levels and regular monitoring of ophthalmic status. Complications are treated as they arise. Laser treatment may be used to delay the progress of proliferative retinopathy. This involves treating the peripheral retina with multiple laser burns, panretinal ablation, so that the oxygen requirement of retinal tissue is reduced. This in turn reduces the stimulus for new vessel formation. Focal burns may also be used to seal off leaking blood vessels. Small 'grid pattern' burns may be used to aid the absorption of the fluid from vessel leakage.

Severe vitreous haemorrhage or tractional retinal detachment may be treated by removing the vitreous humor (vitrectomy) and replacing it with clear infusional fluid, gas or silicone oil.

NURSING PRIORITIES AND MANAGEMENT: Diabetic retinopathy

Patient education

Ongoing education and encouragement to adhere to diabetic regimens are important in the attempt to delay the onset or progression of complications and to encourage early awareness of visual changes. The community nurse or diabetic specialist nurse has a key role to play by reinforcing the connection between maintaining good blood sugar levels and reducing the risk of ophthalmic complications. Explanation and support during laser treatment will be particularly important to encourage the patient's cooperation so as to prevent accidental burns (see p. 571).

Vitrectomy management

Perioperative care for patients undergoing vitrectomy procedures is as for other retinal detachment surgery (see p. 570), with a particular emphasis on ensuring that the prescribed postoperative position is maintained. Outpatient care and education are aimed at encouraging active patient participation and attendance for review so that this problematic sight-threatening scenario is carefully monitored.

Cerebrovascular accident (CVA)

A CVA involves an interruption of the blood supply to a part of the brain and may be caused by blockage or rupture of a blood vessel. CVA results in ischaemia of the affected part and development of neurological defects. If the visual pathways are involved, vision will be affected and the damage may be permanent. When a patient suffers a transient ischaemic attack (TIA), vision may be temporarily affected, but will usually be restored when the attack subsides (see Ch. 9).

NURSING PRIORITIES AND MANAGEMENT: Cerebrovascular accident (CVA)

The extent of the visual deficit must be assessed to facilitate rehabilitation and maintain patient safety. This may be difficult if the patient's ability to communicate has been affected by the CVA. The accuracy of the assessment is dependent upon the nurse's skilled observation and on the patient's health status at the time of assessment.

STOP THINK **13.14** You have a patient who has recently suffered a right-sided CVA. He is aphasic (unable to speak) and has left hemiplegia (paralysis of the left side). Discuss how you might go about detecting visual field loss just by observing his activity. Having done this, describe how your findings would affect your care plan.

Hypertension

Fundal examination of the eye is part of the screening process for hypertension (see Ch. 2).

Hypertensive retinopathy in a young adult appears as widespread narrowing of the retinal arteries caused by spasm of the arterial walls. In an older person with arteriosclerosis, the arteries are narrow and rigid. As hypertension increases in severity, haemorrhages and exudates become visible. The haemorrhages are flame-like in appearance and are found close to the disc. The exudates are due to lipids and occur around the macula. Oedema of the retina occurs in malignant hypertension and may also be present in some cases of mild hypertension. The optic disc is swollen and hyperaemic. The patient will complain of varying degrees of visual disturbance. The condition is painless. The outward appearance of the eye remains normal.

The eye condition improves as hypertension is brought under control by appropriate treatment (see Ch. 2).

Acquired immune deficiency syndrome (AIDS)

Ophthalmic complications affecting both the anterior segment of the eye and the retina develop in about 30% of patients with AIDS. They are caused by HIV infection, opportunistic infections and AIDS-related neoplasms, and may affect any part of the eye (Riordan-Eva & Whitcher 2004). (For further information on HIV and AIDS, see Ch. 37.)

HIV retinopathy

Clinical signs are yellowish-grey, cotton wool-like spots, dot-like haemorrhages and microaneurysms over the retina. Vision remains normal unless the macula is involved. Some patients respond to antiviral agents.

HIV encephalopathy nystagmus

In central nervous system involvement, nystagmus, gaze palsies and visual field defects may occur. No treatment is available at present.

Opportunistic infections

HIV/AIDS patients are prone to all types of eye infection. The most common infections include severe herpes zoster ophthalmicus, herpes simplex, *Candida* retinitis, *Toxoplasma* choroidoretinitis and cytomegalovirus (CMV) retinitis. Some of these infections may respond to prolonged administration of systemic antiviral agents.

CMV retinitis, the most common retinal infection in AIDS, is seen in 15–46% of patients, in particular when the CD4 count is <50 cells/mm^3 (see Ch. 37) (Kaiser et al 2004). Fear of blindness is often more distressing for the patient than fear of dying. CMV retinitis, with intraretinal haemorrhages and retinal necrosis, leads to retinal detachments and progressive loss of vision, but the use of highly active antiretroviral therapy (HAART) has dramatically reduced the incidence of this infection in developed countries (Khaw et al 2004). Palliative treatment by antiviral agents, e.g. ganciclovir, may be offered in an attempt to prevent blindness in the last few months of life. This can be given intravenously or by intravitreal implant.

AIDS-related neoplasms

Kaposi's sarcoma may involve any of the ocular structures. Treatment may include cryotherapy, radiotherapy or the administration of cytotoxic drugs.

NURSING PRIORITIES AND MANAGEMENT: Aids-related eye diseases

The general principles of nursing a patient with AIDS (see Ch. 37), together with the principles of nursing a patient with eye infections, apply in all of the above conditions. Full care and support facilities should be made available to both the patient and the family/partner.

CONCLUSION

This chapter has demonstrated the specialised care required for ophthalmic patients and visually impaired people. It is a dynamic field of health care, therefore nursing roles and responsibilities are evolving in response to the influence of technological, statutory and organisational changes (Lee & Waterman 2003). Nursing roles within this specialty include nurse practitioners, nurse consultants and clinical nurse specialists (Conway 1996). These experienced nurses have been educated and empowered to develop and enhance clinical practice and to provide expert care, which includes, for example, performing incision and curettage, neodymium:yttrium-aluminium-garnet (Nd:YAG) laser treatment, emergency eye care, glaucoma monitoring and cataract pre-assessment care. These advances in nursing roles can in part be attributed to the effect of the European working time directives (McSherry & Pearce 2002) and reduction in junior doctors' hours (Harris & Redshaw 1998). However, eye disorders may be encountered in a wide range of contexts. It is therefore vital that general and community nurses should have a working knowledge of basic ophthalmic nursing care so that they are competent to prepare the individual and the family and/or carers for the necessary procedures, and to monitor progress and aftercare when the patient has returned home, thus working in partnership with the ophthalmic unit team. They must also be able to recognise when it is necessary to seek further advice and prompt referral, if appropriate, either to an ophthalmologist or to an experienced ophthalmic nurse. Staff education and effective dialogue should be established through ophthalmic in-service study days and visual impairment awareness programmes.

The impact of visual impairment on everyday life must never be underestimated. This chapter has stressed the importance of recognising the significance of adverse signs and symptoms and the fact that delay can result in irreparable damage and permanent loss of sight. It has emphasised the nurse's responsibility in helping to preserve sight and in supporting the patient and the family and/or carers as they meet the practical and emotional challenges of visual impairment. Ophthalmic nursing care should be 'seamless' and address not only the clinical aspects but also the psychosocial aspects of patient need, especially for those for whom sight loss cannot be remedied by medicine or surgery.

REFERENCES

Al-Husainy S S, Kritzinger E, Tsalmoumas M D 2001 Accidental laser injuries. Eye News 8(1): 18–22

Armitage W J, Easty D L 1998 Corneal transplantation 1: the storage and supply of corneas for transplantation. Eye News 4(5): 9–10

Ayres N, Shaw M 2001 Driving with a visual impairment: informing patients about safety and legal requirements: part 2. Ophthalmic Nursing 5(1): 8–11

Bartlett H, Eperjesi F 2003 Age-related eye disease study (AREDS): the conclusions. Optician 225(5886): 22–26

Batterbury M, Bowling B 1999 Ophthalmology – an illustrated coloured text. Churchill Livingstone, Edinburgh

Brading J, Curtis J 2000 Disability discrimination: a practical guide to the law, 2nd edn. Kogan Page, London

Casserley C 2001 DDA matters – human rights and disability. New Beacon, London

Chong, N V H 1996 Clinical ocular physiology: an introductory text. Butterworth-Heinemann, Oxford

Conway J 1996 Nursing expertise and advanced practice. Mark Allen, Dinton

Desai P, Misassian D C, Reidy A 1999 The National Cataract Survey 1997/98: a report of the results of the clinical outcomes. British Journal of Ophthalmology 83: 1336–1340

Disability Discrimination Act 1996 HMSO, London

European Glaucoma Society 2003 Terminology and guidelines for glaucoma, 11th edn. European Glaucoma Society, Savona, Italy

Hall B, Waterman H 1997 The psychosocial aspects of visual impairment in diabetes. Nursing Standard 11(39): 40–43, 45–46

Harris A, Redshaw M 1998 Professional issues facing nurse practitioners and nursing. British Journal of Nursing 7(22): 1381–1385

Health and Safety at Work Act 1974 HMSO, London

Health and Safety Executive 2003 The law on VDUs: an easy guide. Health and Safety Executive Books, Sudbury

Holland K, Jenkins J, Solomon J, Whittam S 2003 Applying the Roper, Logan and Tierney model in practice. Churchill Livingstone, Edinburgh

Kaiser P K, Freidman N J, Pineda R 2004 The Massachusetts Eye and Ear Infirmary illustrated manual of ophthalmology. Elsevier Science, Philadelphia

Kanski J J 2003 Clinical ophthalmoscopy: a systematic approach, 5th edn. Butterworth-Heinemann, Edinburgh

Karlson J S 1998 Self-reports of psychological distress in connection with various degrees of visual impairment. Journal of Visual Impairment and Blindness 92: 483–490

Khaw P T, Shah P, Elkington A R 2004 ABC of eyes, 4th edn. BMJ Books, London

Kunimoto D Y, Kuntakor D, Makar M S 2004 The Wills eye manual: office and emergency room diagnosis and treatment of eye disease, 4th edn. Lippincott Williams and Wilkins, Philadelphia

Lee A, Waterman H 2003 Specialisation within ophthalmic nursing: the experience of ophthalmic nurses. Part 2. Ophthalmic Nursing 6(4): 18–23

McBride S 2001 Patients talking 2: the eye clinic journey experienced by blind and partially sighted adults. RNIB, London

McSherry R, Pearce P 2002 Clinical governance: a guide to implementation for health care professionals. Blackwell Science, Oxford

Milligan H 2002 The aetiology of ocular trauma and the ophthalmic nurse's role in its prevention. Ophthalmic Nursing 5(4): 14–18

Moon J S, Cho K S 2001 The effects of handholding on anxiety in cataract surgery patients under local anaesthetic. Journal of Advanced Nursing 35(3): 407–415

Murphy S, Nesbitt P 2001 Advances in management of age-related macular degeneration. Ophthalmic Nursing 5(3): 20–23

National Artificial Eye Service (NAES) 1998 The use and care of artificial eyes. NAES, Blackpool

NHS Executive 2000 Action on cataract: good practice guidance. DH, London

Nursing and Midwifery Council (NMC) 2004 NMC code of professional conduct: standards for conduct, performance and ethics. NMC, London

Orem D 2001 Nursing: concepts of practice, 6th edn. Mosby, New York

Personal Protective Equipment at Work Regulations 1992 HMSO, London

Riordan-Eva P, Whitcher J P 2004 Vaughan and Ashbury's general ophthalmology, 16th edn. McGraw-Hill, New York

Royal College of Ophthalmologists 2001 Cataract surgery guidelines. RCO, London

Scottish Intercollegiate Guidelines Network (SIGN) 2001 Day case cataract surgery guideline No. 53. A national clinical guideline. SIGN, Edinburgh

Scullion P 2001 Models of disability. Primary Health Care 11(4): 28–29

Thomas A, Ryan B 1997 Being informed: the Disability Discrimination Act. Ophthalmic Nursing 1(2): 31–33

Thylefors B 1998 A global initiative for the elimination of avoidable blindness. Journal of Community Eye Health 11(25). Online. Available: www.jceh.co.uk/journal/25_1.asp

Tingle J, Cribb A 2002 Nursing law and ethics, 2nd edn. Blackwell Science, Oxford
Vafidis G C 2000 Epidemiology of diabetic eye disease. In: Rudnicka A R, Birch J (eds) Diabetic eye disease: identification and co-management. Butterworth-Heinemann, Oxford
Waugh A, Grant A 2001 Ross and Wilson's anatomy and physiology in health and illness, 9th edn. Churchill Livingstone, Edinburgh
Yanoff M 1998 Ophthalmic diagnosis and treatment. Butterworth-Heinemann, Boston

FURTHER READING

Al-Husainy S S, Kritzinger E, Tsalmoumas M D 2001 Accidental laser injuries. Eye News 8(1): 18–22
Batterbury M, Bowling B 1999 Ophthalmology – an illustrated coloured text. Churchill Livingstone, Edinburgh
Blaustein B H (ed) 1994 Ocular manifestations of systemic diseases. Churchill Livingstone, New York
Chawla H B 1999 Ophthalmology: a symptom-based approach. Butterworth-Heinemann, London
Chern K C 2002 Emergency ophthalmology. McGraw-Hill Education, Maidenhead
Chignell A H, Wong D 1999 Management of vitreo-retinal disease: a surgical approach. Springer, London
Chivers J 2003 Care of older people with visual impairment. Nursing Older People 15(1): 22–26
Freeney M, Cook R, Hali B, Duckworth S 1999 Working in partnership to implement Section 21 of the Disability Discrimination Act across the National Health Service. NHS Executive, London
Holz F G 2003 Age-related macular degeneration – diagnostic and therapy. Springer-Verlag, Berlin
James B 2003 Lecture notes on ophthalmology. Blackwell Science, Oxford
Kanski J J 2003 Clinical ophthalmoscopy: a systematic approach. Butterworth-Heinemann, London
Khaw P T, Shah P, Elkington A R 2004 ABC of eyes, 4th edn. BMJ Books, London
Knox K A 2001 Nurse management and treatment of acute recurrent anterior uveitis. Ophthalmic Nursing 5(1): 27–30
Kunimoto D Y, Kuntakor D, Makar M S 2004 The Wills eye manual: office and emergency room diagnosis and treatment of eye disease, 4th edn. Lippincott Williams and Wilkins, Philadelphia
Marsden J 1999 The role of the ophthalmic nurse practitioner (ONP) in the Ophthalmic A and E Department. Ophthalmic Nursing 3(1): 4–6
Marsden J, Shaw M 2003 Correct administration of topical eye treatment. Nursing Standard 17(30): 42–44
McBride S 2000 Patients talking. Hospital outpatient eye services – the sight-impaired user's view: a pilot study. RNIB, London
McBride S 2001 Patients talking 2: the eye clinic journey experienced by blind and partially sighted adults. RNIB, London
Newton A 2002 What a difference a visual impairment training programme makes. Ophthalmic Nursing 6(1): 7–9
Nursing Times 2003 Clinical skills: eye care. Nursing Times 99(8): 29
Pavan-Langston D 2003 Manual of ocular diagnosis and therapy, 5th edn. Little, Brown, Boston
Rendall J 1998 Discharge instructions after cataract surgery. Ophthalmic Nursing 2(1): 10–16
Schoofs N 2000 How to treat a patient with Sjögren's syndrome. Ophthalmic Nursing 3(4): 8–9
Scullion P 2000 Equity of access for disabled people. Professional Nurse 15(10): 667–670
Vernon S 2001 Differential diagnosis in ophthalmology. Manson Publishing, London
Watkinson S 2005 Visual impairment in older people: the nurse's role. Nursing Standard 19(17): 45–52
Williams B 2000 Corneal pain and its management after corneal trauma. Ophthalmic Nursing 4(1): 6–8
Yanoff M 1998 Ophthalmic diagnosis and treatment. Butterworth-Heinemann, Boston

USEFUL WEBSITES

Action for Blind People (afbp)
www.afbp.org

AMD (Age-related Macular Degeneration) Alliance International
www.amdalliance.org

Calibre Tape Library
www.calibre.org.uk

Department of Health
www.dh.gov.uk

Glaucoma Australia Inc
www.glaucoma.org.au

Glaucoma Service Foundation to Prevent Blindness
www.wills-glaucoma.org

Guide Dogs for the Blind Association
www.guidedogs.org.uk

International Glaucoma Association
www.iga.org.uk

Macular Disease Society
www.maculardisease.org

Moorfields Eye Hospital NHS Foundation Trust
www.moorfields.org.uk/home

Royal College of Ophthalmologists (RCO)
www.rcophth.ac.uk

Royal National Institute of the Blind (RNIB)
www.rnib.org.uk

Specific Eye Conditions (SPECS)
www.eyeconditions.org.uk

Talking Newspaper Association of the UK (TNAUK)
www.tnauk.org.uk

World Health Organization
www.who.int (*see Fact sheets 95, 142 and 143*)

Informative websites for nurses and patients
www.diabeticretinopathy.org.uk/prevention (*patient information site on retinopathy*)
www.eyecasualty.co.uk (*eye casualty at Oxford eye hospitals*)
www.eyelidsurgery.co.uk (*information on eye lid surgery*)
www.eyenet.org (*national eye care outcomes network*)
www.mdsupport.org (*support for macular degeneration sufferers and families*)
www.nurseseyesite.nhs.uk (*national ophthalmic website*)
www.revoptom.com (*clinical ophthalmic website*)
www.sightsavers.org.uk (*charity combating blindness in developing countries*)

USEFUL ADDRESSES

In Touch
Room 6084, BBC Broadcasting House
London W1A 1AA
Radio 4 Action line 0800 044 044

Weekly Radio 4 programme featuring news, views and information of interest to those with visual impairment

Partially Sighted Society
Queens Road
Doncaster DN1 2NX
01302 323132
E-mail info@partsight.org.uk

DISORDERS OF THE EAR, NOSE AND THROAT

14

Anna M. Serra
Angela J. Griggs

INTRODUCTION

Some problems of the ear, nose and throat (ENT) are very common. Most people at some time in their lives suffer from nosebleeds, sore throats or earache. Many of these problems will be dealt with successfully at home, often with the advice of a pharmacist or general practitioner (GP). Some ENT problems, however, can be life threatening, requiring an immediate visit to an emergency department (ED), surgery and, in some cases, a period of nursing care at home following discharge.

To nurse ENT patients effectively in a home or hospital setting, a basic knowledge of the anatomy and physiology of the relevant structures, along with a thorough understanding of the clinical features of common disorders, is essential. The health visitor, district nurse, practice nurse, school nurse or occupational health nurse is often in a position to detect problems before the medical practitioner or even the patient is aware of them.

This chapter will describe, in turn, the basic structure and functioning of the ear, nose and throat, describing the most commonly encountered disorders of each, and outlining appropriate medical and nursing interventions. As in every area of nursing care, one of the most important contributions that nurses can make is in the area of communication and education as they provide support and reassurance to the patient and family, and convey information about the causes of the patient's condition, its treatment and measures to prevent its recurrence.

THE EAR

ANATOMY AND PHYSIOLOGY OF THE EAR

The ear can be divided into three sections: the external ear, the middle ear and the inner ear. The external and middle ears are primarily involved with the transmission of sound. The inner ear contains the organ of hearing as well as structures concerned with body balance (see Fig. 14.1).

The external ear comprises the cartilaginous pinna and the external auditory canal (or external meatus), the inner two-thirds of which is composed of bone rather than cartilage. The purpose of the pinna and canal is to capture sound waves and funnel them to the tympanic membrane,

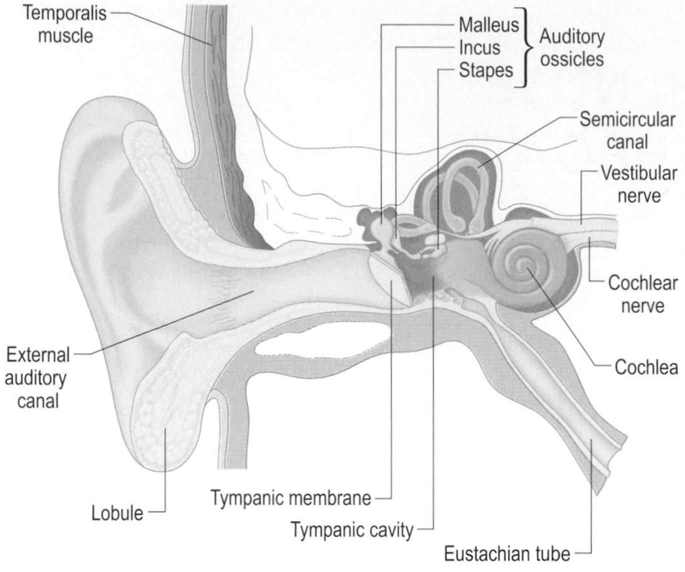

Fig. 14.1 Sagittal section of the ear.

which is located at the end of the external canal and divides the external from the middle ear. The healthy membrane has a pearly sheen and reflects light.

The middle ear is ventilated by the eustachian tube, which communicates with the nasopharynx. Three small bones, called the auditory ossicles or ossicular chain, pass on sound vibrations received by the tympanic membrane to the inner ear. The first of these, the malleus, i.e. 'hammer', is attached to the tympanic membrane and joins with the incus, i.e. 'anvil' or middle ossicle. The incus in turn is attached to the stapes, i.e. 'stirrup', the 'footplate' of which lies against the membranous oval window or fenestra of the inner ear.

The inner ear houses the cochlea, which is shaped like a snail shell and is the organ of hearing. The cochlea contains the organ of Corti, which consists of cells with hair-like projections on a membranous layer and connects with the terminal ends of the auditory nerve. The canals of the cochlea and the organ of Corti are bathed in endolymph. Perilymph is the fluid contained within the bony (osseous) cavities of the inner ear, whereas endolymph is the fluid within membranous cavities. As sound waves are transmitted by the ossicles they travel along this fluid and disturb the hair cells. This disturbance changes to impulses, which travel along the auditory nerve to the brain stem and cortex, where they are interpreted as meaningful sound.

The posterior part of the inner ear is formed by three semicircular canals and by the vestibular apparatus. These assist in the perception of body position against gravity and in the maintenance of balance. The vestibular apparatus consists of the utricle and saccule and is sensitive to linear acceleration. The semicircular canals are sensitive to rotatory acceleration. Balance is maintained by the adjustment of muscles, joints, tendons and ligaments in response to information gathered by the vestibular apparatus and the canals as well as that received by the eyes.

For further information, see Becker et al (1993).

DISORDERS OF THE EXTERNAL EAR

Otitis externa

PATHOPHYSIOLOGY

The most common causes of otitis externa, or inflammation of the external ear, are infection and allergy. Infection may be caused by scratching the ear with contaminated fingernails or other sharp objects. Instruments such as auriscopes or hearing aid earpieces placed in the meatus may cause minor injuries, giving rise to infection if they have been inadequately disinfected (see Ch. 16). Itching is an early symptom of allergy and may be caused by cosmetics or antibiotic preparations. In otitis externa, multiple bacteriological flora are usually present. The condition most commonly occurs in hot, humid climates, where it tends to be recurrent and may be severe.

Common presenting symptoms The patient usually presents with a history of pain and itching localised to the ear and a burning sensation followed by discharge, which initially may be watery and then becomes thicker. If there is gross oedema of the meatus and a large amount of debris is present, the patient may suffer from conductive deafness (see p. 593).

MEDICAL MANAGEMENT

If a discharge is present in otitis externa, a swab is obtained for culture and sensitivity. Cleansing of the external meatus is performed so that a full inspection can be carried out and to ensure good skin contact for any topical treatments.

NURSING PRIORITIES AND MANAGEMENT: Otitis externa

The first priority of the nursing staff is to clean the external meatus so that an examination can be carried out and any prescribed treatment administered effectively. This procedure is called aural toilet and should only be carried out by an appropriately qualified ENT nurse. Cotton wool dressed carriers can be used. Care must be taken not to damage the skin. Gentle pulling of the pinna will straighten the canal and allow easier access. The best light source is a Bulls' eye lamp and head mirror or an operating microscope. Large amounts of discharge and debris are best removed by an appropriately qualified nurse or doctor using microsuction via a fine-bore tube under an operating microscope in the outpatient department.

It may be necessary to administer an oral analgesic before the external auditory canal can be properly examined, as often any movement of the pinna is painful.

Since the vast majority of patients are seen in the community or outpatient department, the nurse's involvement will range from the total management of ear conditions in a nurse-led clinic to demonstrating how to administer topical preparations effectively. The nurse should also teach the patient safe techniques for cleansing the external ear and stress the importance of frequent, thorough cleansing of any appliances, including hearing aids, that are put in the ear.

For further information on nurse-led aural care clinics, see Zeitoun et al (1997).

Cerumen excess

PATHOPHYSIOLOGY

Cerumen is the normal waxy secretion of special glands in the external auditory canal. Along with shed skin scales and hair, the cerumen normally migrates to the external meatus but can be hindered by coarse hair, particularly in the older male, or if the individual impacts the material by attempting to clean the ears with cotton wool buds or other instruments. Nurses should provide patients with health education information regarding the normal cleansing mechanism and avoiding the use of cotton buds and other foreign bodies (Reynolds 2004).

Common presenting symptoms The patient usually presents with dulled hearing. Tinnitus may develop, causing the patient distress (see p. 600), and disturbance of balance may result from pressure of the hard material on the tympanic membrane.

MEDICAL MANAGEMENT

Sometimes small amounts of soft wax can be removed by instruments or suction under a microscope. If there is an excessive amount, the doctor, district nurse, practice nurse or outpatient nurse will need to remove the material by irrigating the external canal. Often, however, the wax is too hard and compacted for this to be carried out immediately and a course of drops, containing sodium bicarbonate in glycerol or warmed olive oil, has first to be prescribed for several days to soften the wax. At this stage, written information on the procedure can be taken home by the patient to aid understanding.

NURSING PRIORITIES AND MANAGEMENT: Cerumen excess

Individuals with cerumen excess are usually seen in the doctor's surgery or, more rarely, in the outpatient department, for removal of the impacted wax. Ear syringing with a metal syringe is now obsolete and impacted wax is removed by ear irrigation or microsuction (Price 1997).

The nurse will have to teach the patient how to insert the eardrops at home over the required period before the irrigation is carried out. The doctor or nurse who performs the irrigation should first take a full history to eliminate the presence of a weakened tympanic membrane and should examine the ear for any infection, inflammation or perforation in order to determine that the tympanic membrane is intact, thus eliminating the danger of the solution being introduced into the middle ear and causing infection and damage. During the procedure the patient sits upright with clothing protected by a waterproof covering. It is helpful if the patient can cooperate by holding a container under the ear to receive the returning fluid. Various types of ear irrigator are available. Unless a special solution has been prescribed, tap water or an isotonic solution such as normal saline may be used to irrigate the canal.

It is important that the solution is at 37°C, i.e. body temperature, as variations in temperature may cause the patient to experience vertigo (see p. 601).

Before starting, ask the patient to inform you if any discomfort is experienced. The pinna is pulled gently upwards and backwards to straighten the canal while the solution is introduced from the irrigator in an upwards direction so that the wax will be washed out with the return flow. It is important that the flow of water is not aimed directly at the tympanic membrane as this could cause damage. When the canal is clean or when 2 min have passed (Harkin 2002), the procedure is discontinued and the canal gently dried and re-examined. To avoid vertigo the patient should be encouraged to remain seated for a few minutes to recover.

Patients should also be advised that, following effective wax removal, they may be hypersensitive to even quite normal sounds for a short time.

For further information on ear irrigation, see Price (1997) and Harkin (2002).

Foreign bodies in the ear

Small objects may become lodged in the ear by some mishap or, as frequently occurs among children, by accident during play (Reynolds 2004). Such objects may lie undetected for years unless they have damaged the tympanic membrane. Sometimes gentle irrigation will wash out the foreign body, but if it has become impacted it may be necessary for the patient to be admitted to hospital as a day case and for the object to be removed under general anaesthetic.

Only objects that will not expand when in contact with water should be irrigated.

DEAFNESS AND HEARING LOSS

Although total deafness is comparatively rare, many people suffer hearing loss to varying degrees. Deafness can affect both adults and children. Many children who are deaf continue to be so for all of their lives, but some can be helped to maximise auditory function. This chapter will concentrate on hearing problems among adults. There are estimated to be 9 million deaf and hard of hearing adults in the UK. This figure is rising as the number of those over 60 increases, with 698 000 of this age group being severely or profoundly deaf (RNID 2003).

PATHOPHYSIOLOGY AND MEDICAL MANAGEMENT

Deafness is usually classified into conductive and sensorineural disorders, as follows.

Diagnosis of the type of hearing loss from which an individual is suffering will be by examination and audiometry (see Box 14.1). Conductive deafness can often be helped by removing any obstruction (cerumen or a foreign body) or by amplifying sounds by means of a hearing aid. Because the external and middle ear are fairly accessible, surgical intervention may also be an option. By contrast, in sensorineural deafness, where the damage is to the organ of Corti or the cochlear portion of the VIIIth cranial nerve, surgery does not usually have much effect.

Conductive deafness results from a reduced ability of the sound waves to reach the fluid in the cochlea. The sound is quieter but not distorted. This can be due to:

- congenital abnormality
- otitis externa
- foreign bodies

Box 14.1

Hearing tests

Tuning fork tests
These tests are a simple means of determining a patient's basic auditory status. They may be performed in a clinical or home environment.

Rinne test
Air conduction is tested by holding a vibrating tuning fork first to the front of the ear and then by placing the tuning fork footplate against the mastoid bone. Patients should hear sound clearer to the front of the ear. Result = Rinne positive. Normal hearing.

Weber test
Bone conduction is tested by placing the vibrating footplate of a tuning fork to the middle of the forehead. This sound should be heard centrally. If conductive hearing loss is present, sound will be lateralised. If sensorineural hearing loss is present then sound will localise to the good ear.

Audiometry
Audiometric tests measure hearing acuity. Relatively simple tests, which include delivering tones of variable frequency and intensity, the spoken word and measuring middle ear pressures, are amongst the methods used to determine the type and source of any hearing loss. Electric response audiometry measures the patient's response to an acoustic stimulus by way of an electroencephalogram and can provide reliable and exact information on the site of a disorder, e.g. the cochlea, auditory nerve tract or brain stem.

Detailed descriptions of these tests can be found in Becker et al (1993).

- excessive cerumen
- otitis media (secretory and suppurative)
- damage to the tympanic membrane, incus, malleus or stapes.

Sensorineural deafness is caused by a defect of the cochlea or its connecting nerves. The sound heard is quieter and is also distorted. This is a result of the loss of the high frequencies, which register consonant sounds. In severe cases, patients may not be able to hear the sound of their own voice. This can be due to:

- ageing
- medication
- trauma, including head injury and noise
- infection
- Ménière's disease
- congenital malformation.

Presbycusis, the most common type of sensorineural deafness, develops as a consequence of ageing and is becoming increasingly prevalent in Western society. In the UK, 55% of people over 60 are deaf or hard of hearing (RNID 2003). Audiometry initially shows loss of ability to hear high tones, but there is gradual deterioration of lower tone hearing as well. Degeneration of the nervous tissue leads to loss of intelligibility in the sounds that are heard. Hearing loss in this disorder is symmetrical, i.e. it affects both ears. A hearing aid may be of slight advantage, but distortion and poor discrimination may cancel out any benefit from amplification. When communicating with these patients, it is important to speak a little slower and distinctly and to try to eliminate any background noise. Because the high tones are affected first, the individual may have trouble hearing consonants, as these are usually of higher tone than vowels.

Medication It has been recognised for some time that salicylates and quinine can cause deafness, but this can be reversed by discontinuing these medications. Other drugs, such as antibiotics of the aminoglycoside group, some diuretics, such as i.v. furosemide, and cytotoxic agents of the nitrogen mustard group can cause irreparable damage.

Trauma Noise-induced hearing loss is well documented and has become recognised as an industrial disease. Socioacusis, the term used to describe the hearing loss caused by sources of noise outside work, can be as great a risk as loud noise in the workplace (RNID 1999). A single exposure to a loud noise such as an explosion or gunshot can cause permanent deafness, or the injury may be temporary. Tinnitus usually accompanies this injury and often takes longer to resolve than any deafness (see p. 600). Exposure to loud noise over a period of time leads to destruction of the hair cells in the organ of Corti. The Noise at Work Regulations (HMSO 1989) laid down strict standards of noise control and protection for employers, who are liable to be prosecuted if they do not comply (see 'Useful websites' for more information). Occupational health nurses have a role to play in monitoring noise levels and encouraging auditory health through education. Unfortunately many people, particularly the young, willingly subject themselves to high levels of noise, e.g. at rock concerts and clubs, where the music is usually amplified, and also when listening to their personal stereos or car radios. Although personal stereos present less of a risk than rock concerts, it is recommended that only those with a mechanism to limit the volume be used, and children should be prevented from playing with toys that make a loud sound close to their ears (RNID 1999). On audiometry, early changes in hearing caused by exposure to noise are seen as a dip that gradually deepens and involves adjacent frequencies.

Head injuries or trauma resulting in deafness usually involve fractures or penetrating injuries of the temporal bone. Occasionally, concussion (see Ch. 9) can cause deafness due to haemorrhage into the middle ear or cochlea. These injuries are often accompanied by severe vertigo, nausea and vomiting.

Infection leading to deafness is usually viral in origin. The causative viruses are those associated with mumps, measles, meningitis, chickenpox and rubella.

Ménière's disease See page 601.

NURSING PRIORITIES AND MANAGEMENT: Deafness and hearing loss

In the case of conductive deafness, the nurse's role may be to prepare the patient for surgery and facilitate postoperative recovery. Some of the surgical procedures that may benefit patients are myringoplasty, ossiculoplasty and stapedectomy. A patient for whom surgery is not feasible may be fitted with a hearing aid and educated in its use by members of the audiology department, including the hearing therapist. In this case the nurse, as a member of the multiprofessional team, should also explain how to obtain the greatest benefit from the aid. Most patients in this situation also benefit from learning how to lip-read. Lip-reading sessions are available as a day or evening class at the audiology department or a local college. It can take many months to become proficient at lip-reading, so the earlier the patient starts the better. Slow progress, combined with deteriorating hearing, can be very demotivating.

Communicating effectively with a hearing-impaired patient is a very important nursing priority. In the assessment, the nurse should obtain and record information about the patient's preferred method of communicating, e.g. lip-reading, finger-spelling or sign language. For a less profoundly deaf patient, it may be that speaking face to face in a distinct voice and eliminating background noise are adequate (see Box 14.2). A study by the RNID (2004) suggested that deaf adults who used sign language were dissatisfied with and disadvantaged in their communication with health care staff, including nurses (see Research Abstract 14.1).

It is now recognised that deafness can have a profound psychological impact and that hearing-impaired individuals may require support to help resolve problems. Many deaf people would prefer to have counselling from a counsellor who is deaf, and attempts should be made to find such a professional if preferred (via BACP if necessary; see 'Useful websites'). According to Ratna (1994), the problems deaf clients bring to counselling include isolation, frustration, discrimination and physical and sexual abuse.

Box 14.2

Talking with someone who has a hearing deficit

- Do not speak until you have the person's attention and they can see your full face
- Never turn your back on the person when you are speaking or cover your mouth
- Ask the person if they can lip-read
- Do not exaggerate your lip movements
- Direct your voice to one ear if it has better hearing than the other
- Speak slowly, enunciate clearly and do not shout
- Remember that vowels are heard more easily than consonants
- Check that the person has understood what you have said
- If the person has difficulty in understanding, try rephrasing the sentence
- Do not laugh at misinterpretations
- Have patience. Give the person time to adjust their hearing aid if necessary
- Encourage the person to participate in group conversations when the occasion arises
- If verbal communication is impossible, explore alternative means, e.g. sign language

For information on the experience of deafness, see Taylor & Bishop (1991).

Chan (1997) confirmed this when describing a service he and his team of hearing and deaf health care professionals have developed for deaf people with mental health problems.

Nurses can make a valuable contribution by recognising the problems faced by patients with hearing loss and helping them to obtain the appropriate help.

STOP THINK **14.1** How might a person with a severe hearing deficit know that the telephone or doorbell is ringing?

Community nurses can provide tremendous help and support for patients and their relatives when sensorineural deafness is a problem. They should be able to assist their patients to obtain many of the aids available, including a hearing dog for the deaf, which can help to overcome communication difficulties in everyday life. There are many associations, both voluntary and professional, which can provide support and help. The nurse working in the community should be a resource person for patients and guide them to the support that is available (see 'Useful websites').

STOP THINK **14.2** Find out which professional or voluntary support groups there are for deaf people in your area. What services do they offer? Compile a resource list.

Hearing aids

It is estimated that there are 2 million hearing aid users in the UK. In addition, there are thought to be another 3 million people who would benefit from the use of a hearing aid (RNID 2003).

All electronic hearing aids have a microphone, which picks up the sound; the sound is processed electronically either by analogue or digital circuits to make it more audible. This is then delivered to the receiver, converted back to sound and reaches the ear via an ear mould. As there are many models on the market, it is important that the most appropriate one is chosen for each person's needs and lifestyle. While most hearing aids enclose all the components in a neat package on or near the ear, they differ in such aspects as frequency response, output and ability to reduce the effects of sudden, loud noise. Hearing aids conduct sound either through air or via the bone behind the ear.

After the most appropriate model of hearing aid has been identified, the patient will require some training in order to be able to receive maximum benefit from it. The fact that most aids make all sounds, including background noise, louder, means that the patient will have to develop the skill of picking out sounds essential to communication. Social interaction may be difficult until this skill is mastered, and if the individual is not given enough information and support, the aid may be abandoned as useless. Digital aids are designed to overcome this problem as they can customise how sound is processed.

STOP THINK **14.3** Find out how many patients in your ward or on your community caseload have a hearing aid. How much training and support regarding their use did they receive? How many use them? How useful do they find their hearing aids to be? What would you do if you were visiting an older person in their own home, and they responded to your questions by showing you a drawer containing several hearing aids and saying, 'None of these are any use'?

RESEARCH ABSTRACT 14.1

Are we being heard?

The RNID decided to commission this report because of the frequency with which they received examples of poor communication experienced by deaf and hard of hearing people when attempting to use the NHS. The study took place within the context of the Disability Discrimination Act (1995), which came into force in 2004, and places a legal obligation on the NHS to meet the needs of disabled people. The NHS in England, Wales and Scotland have acknowledged defects in their services which affect disabled people, including difficulties in communication with staff and in finding their way around premises. There are thought to be approximately 9 million deaf and hard of hearing people in the UK. As one in every seven people in the UK has some level of hearing loss, and it is known that the average GP will have up to four patients with hearing loss in their surgery daily, it is important that health care professionals in all care settings are aware of the particular needs for effective communication of those who have reduced hearing.

The RNID and the UK Council on Deafness conducted this research in collaboration with 21 UK-based deaf and hard of hearing groups and charities; a total of 866 participants completed the survey.

The main findings reported by deaf and hard of hearing people when using GP services concluded that 35% had experienced difficulty communicating with their GP or practice nurse and 15% avoided going to see their GP because of communication problems. Making and keeping appointments was another problematic area, with 28% reporting that they found their hearing loss made it difficult for them to make an appointment and of 24% who stated they had missed an appointment, 19% had missed more than five. Of those who did see their GP or nurse, 35% reported being unclear about their condition because of communication problems. Of those who used British Sign Language (BSL), 33% were either unsure about medication instructions or had taken inaccurate doses.

The situation in NHS hospitals is equally disturbing, as 42% of the deaf and hard of hearing who had visited a hospital for non-emergency treatment found it difficult to communicate with staff. BSL users experienced even more difficulties, with 77% of this group reporting communication problems for emergency and non-emergency overnight stays and 70% of those admitted to emergency departments were not provided with a BSL/English interpreter to facilitate effective communication.

Overall, the picture is one of poor communication, resulting in people having inadequate access to health care and insufficient information about their health condition and treatment, thus limiting their ability to make informed choices, and being placed in higher risk situations than their hearing counterparts. It is also unacceptable that family, including young children, and friends have to act as interpreters and on occasion convey critical health information. The financial cost to the NHS of missed appointments is put at approximately £20 million a year. The financial and non-financial costs to the patient, family and friends will never be known.

The report notes that NHS staff do wish to deliver a better and more equitable service to the deaf and hard of hearing but that often the necessary resources and infrastructure are not available. Solutions recommended include increasing the number of BSL/English interpreters, using video phones, providing improved written information, installing loop systems to allow better use of hearing aids in noisy environments, providing visual displays in appointment areas and clear lighting, and providing deaf awareness education, including communication skills, for all health care staff, whether working in hospital or community settings. Deaf awareness seminars should be provided for appropriate hospital departments and GP surgery staff, so that these areas have at least one formally trained 'front line' staff member.

RNID 2004 A simple cure. A national report into deaf and hard of hearing people's experiences of the National Health Service. RNID, London (see also 'Useful websites')

All hearing aid models are battery powered and have an on/off switch which is sometimes combined with the volume control. Many models also have a switch marked 'T' which is for use with telephone and other systems fitted with an induction loop. This loop eliminates some background noise and clarifies incoming speech.

STOP THINK **14.4** Where in your area are induction loops fitted? How can you tell?

The ear moulds are individually made to fit each user's ear. They can be disconnected from the aid for cleaning, which should be done frequently. The tube that connects the earpiece to the main aid can also be detached and washed and any blockage removed with a pipe cleaner. If a hearing aid is not working, make sure that:

- the switch is in the 'on' position
- the battery is still good and is of the right type
- the mould is clean and fits properly (check for excessive cerumen)
- the connecting tube is pliable and patent.

If all of the above are in order and the aid is still not working, it should be returned to the hearing aid clinic for maintenance. All hearing aids and batteries supplied by the NHS are maintained and replaced free of charge.

DISORDERS OF THE MIDDLE EAR

Secretory otitis media (glue ear)

Glue ear is the most common cause of hearing impairment and the most common reason for elective surgery in children. Approximately 80% of children will suffer from glue ear before they are 4 years old (Scottish Intercollegiate Guidelines Network 2003).

PATHOPHYSIOLOGY

This disorder is known as glue ear because it is characterised by a thick, tenacious fluid, which collects in the middle ear. Normally, the mucosal secretions of the middle ear drain down the eustachian tube into the nasopharynx. It is not certain whether the abnormal accumulation of this fluid is caused by the viscosity of the fluid, congestion of the eustachian tubes or obstruction caused by enlarged adenoids or a tumour.

Common presenting symptoms Pain is rarely associated with this condition. The adult patient usually comes to the medical practitioner complaining of hearing loss. A child might never complain, and their condition might be discovered only upon investigation into poor performance at school or during routine screening of hearing at school.

MEDICAL MANAGEMENT

Examination of the tympanic membrane by auriscope usually confirms the diagnosis, as in this disorder the membrane has a characteristic dull grey or orange appearance. It will also lose its normal translucence and become retracted.

Treatment

Conservative treatment is to prescribe a decongestant, or antihistamines, to reduce oedema of the nasal mucosa. Mucolytics, which liquefy the mucus, have been shown to have no effect on the condition (Scottish Intercollegiate Guidelines Network 2003).

Surgical intervention involves performing a myringotomy, incising the tympanic membrane and suctioning of the glue. If a grommet is not inserted, the delicate tympanic membrane heals within a few days. The fluid may, of course, accumulate again. The insertion of a grommet (see Fig. 14.2) is sometimes considered appropriate, although some specialists think this can lead to scar formation in later years which will impair hearing. If a grommet is inserted, it usually gradually slides out of the membrane over 9–12 months; patients sometimes find it on their pillow when they waken one morning. A grommet allows aeration of the middle ear, thus restoring middle ear air pressure. There is usually a marked improvement in hearing after this procedure, which is maintained in about 75% of patients.

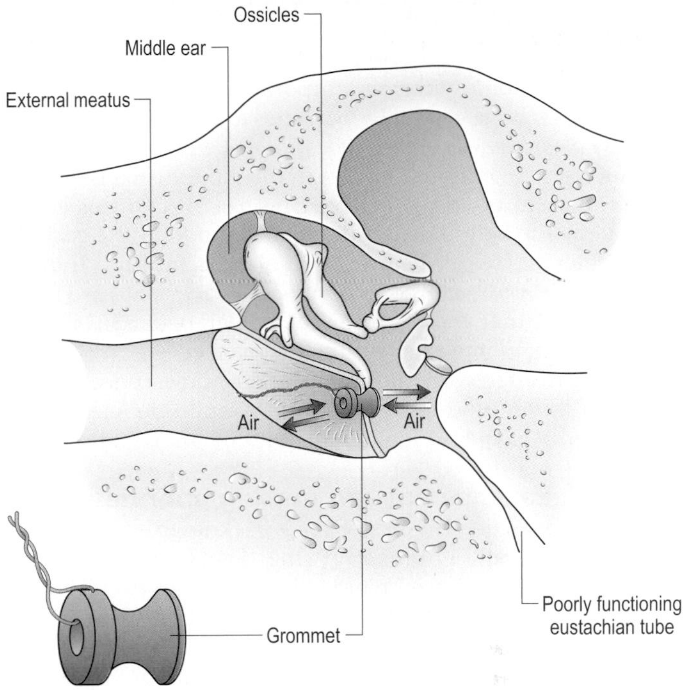

Fig. 14.2 Grommet and grommet in situ.

NURSING PRIORITIES AND MANAGEMENT: Secretory otitis media (glue ear)

Only care specific to ENT patients is outlined in this chapter. The reader is referred to Chapter 26 for details of perioperative care.

Preoperative care

Most of this surgery is carried out on a day case basis, and the nurse must ensure that the patient and family are adequately informed about what the surgical procedure will entail. This may involve the use of diagrams and it may be helpful to show a grommet to them if one is to be inserted. As grommet insertion is usually performed on children and young people, it is vital that the appropriate emotional and psychological support is given by suitably qualified staff in a specialist area. When communicating with the patient preoperatively, the nurse should make allowances for hearing loss (see Box 14.2).

Postoperative care

The anaesthetic for this operation is very light. Measures to prevent the spread of infection, e.g. washing the hands before and after touching the affected ear, how to change and dispose of cotton wool plugs in the external auditory canal, and specific instructions about whether and when it is safe to allow water to enter the ear must be discussed with the patient. When a grommet is in place, some surgeons allow swimming, as long as the patient does not dive or swim underwater. Others prefer their patients not to swim until it has been expelled. Usually, a cotton wool plug moistened with petroleum jelly is inserted in the external canal when the hair is being washed or when taking a shower. The nurse must ensure that the patient and family understand this advice and that information booklets or advice sheets are given. The importance of attending the clinic for a follow-up visit, even if the hearing has improved dramatically, should be stressed. This visit is to ensure that the membrane is healing satisfactorily, to check the position of the grommet and to check for signs of infection. Patients should be told to go to their GP if they experience any pain or if there is a bloodstained discharge from the ear. Most of these precautions apply to all patients who have undergone aural surgery.

Sigler & Schuring (1993) give information which the nurse should explain to the patient in relation to postoperative self-care at home.

Otosclerosis

Otosclerosis is a condition in which the ossicles in the middle ear, along with the temporal bone, begin to soften. This spongy bone gradually becomes a dense sclerotic mass; the ossicles may become fixed and less effective in passing on auditory vibrations. The individual with this condition will complain of increasing hearing loss. While this loss is conductive in origin, if the damage extends to the cochlea, sensorineural loss of hearing will also occur. Mild tinnitus (see p. 600) may also be experienced, in which case some people find that they can actually hear better in a noisy environment where their tinnitus is masked.

This disorder commonly begins in adolescence and its cause is as yet unknown. Heredity, vitamin deficiency and otitis media have all been cited as significant factors.

Medical management and nursing priorities

Although no cure for otosclerosis is known, surgery can often dramatically improve hearing. The surgery of choice, stapedectomy, involves freeing the stapes and replacing it with a prosthesis. This restores the vibration necessary to permit the transmission of sound waves. The procedure is a very delicate one requiring the use of an operating microscope, as the stapes is one of the smallest bones in the body. Surgery may be performed under local anaesthetic and hospital admission may be no more than 24 h (Ayache et al 2003).

Great care must be taken in the early postoperative period, as the patient may take a little while to regain their sense of balance. This short-term vertigo, if discussed and explained in the preoperative period, should cause minimal distress to the patient. Prior to discharge, advice should be given on the prevention of aural infection, the importance of preventing the entry of water into the ear and the need to guard against blowing the nose until the operative site is completely healed. Violent nose blowing can force air up the eustachian tube, increasing middle ear pressure, which can affect the operated area and prosthesis. Follow-up appointments in the outpatient department and appropriate community support by the GP will ensure optimal progress and recovery.

For those for whom the symptoms of otosclerosis are not too severe, or for whom surgery is inappropriate, a hearing aid may restore and maintain satisfactory hearing. For others, neither surgery nor a hearing aid will have long-term effectiveness and varying degrees of deafness will result.

Acute suppurative otitis media (ASOM)

PATHOPHYSIOLOGY

This is an acute bacterial infection of the middle ear which is especially common in childhood. The most common causative organisms are *Streptococcus pneumoniae, Haemophilus influenzae, Streptococcus pyogenes* and *Staphylococcus aureus.* Onset usually follows acute tonsillitis, the common cold or influenza, when infection travels up the eustachian tube to the middle ear. The whole middle ear may be affected, including the mastoid air cells, small air spaces in the posterior portion of the temporal bone, behind the middle ear (see Fig. 14.1).

Common presenting symptoms The patient usually presents with acute ear pain. There may be deafness, general malaise and pyrexia. On examination, the eardrum is red and bulging due to the collection of pus in the middle ear. The tympanic membrane may rupture, releasing the discharge and dramatically and instantaneously relieving the pain.

MEDICAL MANAGEMENT

Treatment The patient with ASOM is usually seen and treated by a GP. The exact treatment given will depend on the stage of the infection, as follows.

Early stage At this stage the tympanic membrane will still look normal. A broad-spectrum antibiotic effective against the most common organisms is usually prescribed. Antipyretic analgesics such as paracetamol will be necessary to relieve pain and reduce fever. Vasoconstricting nasal sprays may also be helpful in keeping the eustachian tubes patent, thereby allowing escape of fluid from the middle ear. In severe cases, admission for i.v. antibiotics and pain control may be necessary (Scottish Intercollegiate Guidelines Network 2003).

Bulging eardrum If the infection has reached this stage, a myringotomy may be performed. This involves applying a local anaesthetic before making an incision in the tympanic membrane to allow the pus to escape. If a myringotomy is performed in preference to allowing the eardrum to rupture, the membrane will heal with less scarring and hearing should not be impaired. During this procedure a swab of the discharge will be taken for culture and sensitivity so that the appropriate antibiotic can be prescribed.

Discharging ear By this stage the tympanic membrane will already have ruptured. A swab of the discharge will be taken and the ear carefully mopped out and then dressed with a small plug of cotton wool. Broad-spectrum antibiotics will be prescribed in the first instance while the results of bacteriology are awaited.

The patient will have to visit the GP regularly so that healing of the membrane can be monitored. If necessary, a myringoplasty (reconstruction of the eardrum) will be performed.

NURSING PRIORITIES AND MANAGEMENT: Acute suppurative otitis media (ASOM)

Early stage

If at this stage a nurse, possibly a practice nurse, is involved, their role will be to ensure that the prescribed course of antibiotics is completed in order to eradicate all the organisms. It may be necessary to teach the patient or a relative how to administer a nasal spray.

Discharging ear

If the disease has reached this stage, the nurse's role will include mopping out the external ear as often as required and carrying out microsuction clearance of the debris.

If appropriate treatment is given early enough, ASOM should resolve and hearing return to normal. Occasionally, complications do occur, including chronic suppurative otitis media and acute mastoiditis, which are described below.

Chronic suppurative otitis media (CSOM)

PATHOPHYSIOLOGY

Common presenting symptoms This condition follows unresolved ASOM. The patient will present with a perforated tympanic membrane, a discharging ear and some degree of conductive deafness. Pain is not usually a complaint. The discharge may be intermittent and is mucoid, becoming purulent in the presence of secondary infection.

MEDICAL MANAGEMENT

The recommended treatment is to keep the ear dry by the use of topical medication before correcting the hearing loss by performing a tympanoplasty.

For further information on middle ear reconstructive procedures and care, see Waddington et al (1997).

Tympanoplasty Following removal of diseased tissue, an attempt may be made to re-establish the sound transmission mechanism in the middle ear by reconstructing the tympanic membrane (myringoplasty) using a connective tissue graft taken from the fascia covering the temporal bone and reconstructing the ossicular chain (ossiculoplasty). This combined reconstruction is known as a tympanoplasty (Brackman et al 2001).

NURSING PRIORITIES AND MANAGEMENT: Tympanoplasty

Preoperative care

The patient is usually admitted on the day of surgery. In view of their obvious hearing deficit, the establishment of good communication is very important. To help avoid complications, the ear must be dry and free from infection. Hearing tests will be carried out to confirm the degree of hearing loss.

If some of the patient's hair has to be removed, this will be done in the operating theatre. To help alleviate anxiety, the nurse should give the patient information about the procedure and warn about sensations that may be experienced afterwards, such as dizziness and tinnitus (see p. 600). It is also helpful to describe the very bulky bandage that will be present around the head and affected ear so that this does not alarm the patient and family. Hearing aids should be worn to the operating theatre.

For patients who are having surgery on the ear in which they normally wear a hearing aid, a temporary aid may be fitted to their other ear if appropriate.

Postoperative care

General postoperative care is as described in Chapter 26. The majority of patients undergoing ear surgery are given a hypotensive anaesthetic in order to reduce bleeding and thereby allow the surgeon a clearer view of the tiny operative field. This involves the i.v. administration of a hypotensive agent such as pentolonium. Frequent blood pressure readings are therefore required until the preoperative baseline levels are regained.

Following the operation, the patient should be encouraged to lie with the affected area uppermost and should be observed for nausea, vomiting and vertigo, all of which might be present due to possible interference with the semicircular canals during surgery. The aim of the pressure dressing and bandage is to prevent bleeding and haematoma formation, but the nurse should always observe the patient's bandages and pillows for bloodstains.

Following this type of surgery, the patient should be asked to smile, wrinkle their nose and shut their eyes tightly. The ability to perform these movements indicates that there has been no damage to the facial nerve. A record of the time of checking and level of function of the nerve should always be kept for medical and legal reasons. Because of its location, the VIIth cranial (facial) nerve is at risk of damage during surgery to the middle or inner ear.

Most patients are able to be up on the evening of surgery and return home the next day. They should be advised that they may experience dizziness during the following 2 or 3 weeks and should avoid sudden movements such as quickly turning the head. Sutures should be removed in 5–7 days, either at the GP's surgery or on the ward. Packing is usually present in the external meatus for between 1 and 3 weeks following surgery. The patient will be shown how to change the piece of cotton wool at the entrance to the meatus as required, without disturbing the packing.

Patients will naturally be very anxious to know if the graft has taken and if the infection has been completely removed. Offering accurate information and giving specific answers to questions will help to alleviate these anxieties (Gerber et al 2000).

CSOM with choleastoma

PATHOPHYSIOLOGY

This potentially dangerous condition is sometimes called attico-antral disease, because it is found in the attic (upper) area of the middle ear. On examination it may be possible to see the choleastoma, an ingrowth of keratinising squamous epithelium from the external ear into the middle ear, usually from the site of a previous perforation. The squamous epithelium growing within the middle ear produces keratin, which has the ability to erode the bony ossicles and may even spread into the inner ear.

Common presenting symptoms The patient will complain of a foul-smelling discharge from the ear and of deafness.

MEDICAL MANAGEMENT

The treatment of choice is mastoidectomy (see below).

Acute mastoiditis

This condition arises from acute otitis media and is caused by the infection spreading to the bony walls of the cells of the mastoid process.

MEDICAL MANAGEMENT

Conservative medical management is by administration of antibiotics; surgical management is a cortical mastoidectomy.

Mastoidectomy A cortical mastoidectomy involves incision, drainage and removal of unhealthy mucosa and bone cells from the mastoid process of the temporal bone, leaving the middle ear structures intact. A modified mastoidectomy may be performed if the disease is confined to the attic or upper area and the patient has good hearing. This is currently the most common surgical procedure for middle ear infection. It involves removal of most of the air cell system within the mastoid cavity, especially in the attic area, and preservation of the remnants of the tympanic membrane and the ossicles, although these are not usually functioning. Every effort is made to preserve the ossicular chain and tympanic membrane in order to retain hearing. The procedure involves exenterating (clearing out) the mastoid cells and removing the outer attic and posterior wall, thus leaving a large cavity to allow air from the meatus to circulate and dry up secretions.

NURSING PRIORITIES AND MANAGEMENT: Mastoidectomy

Nursing care is as for patients undergoing tympanoplasty (see p. 599).

> **Box 14.3**
>
> **An experience of tinnitus**
>
> I shall never forget the first time I experienced tinnitus. It was in the dead of night when I heard a high-pitched whine in my left ear. I was so taken aback that I got up out of bed and went in search of the source of the noise. Before long, however, I realised that the noise was being carried with me.
>
> The tinnitus had been preceded about a month beforehand by nausea and severe vertigo which I had accepted as transitory. To find that I was left with this noise made me feel very anxious indeed. I had difficulty in coming to terms with the fact that it might always be present. My reaction was 'It can't be! There must be something to combat it and make the noise go away!'.
>
> When it became clear to me that I was now a 'tinnitus sufferer' I experienced a phase of reactive depression and felt that life was not worthwhile. Naturally, I searched for a cure and eventually joined the local branch of the Tinnitus Association. This was a move which I made by myself, but the Association proved to be an invaluable source of emotional and practical support and information.
> A hearing therapist and a clinic psychologist have now joined the team at my audiology clinic and they are giving tinnitus sufferers like me a great deal of help in many ways.

Other complications of middle ear infection

Less common complications of middle ear infection are facial nerve paralysis, meningitis, extradural or subdural abscess, labyrinthitis, lateral sinus thrombosis and brain abscess.

DISORDERS OF THE INNER EAR

Tinnitus

Tinnitus is a little understood but most distressing feature of some ear diseases and disorders. It may also occur spontaneously or as a postoperative complication. Possibly because it is so puzzling, has no known cause and is not a visible symptom, sufferers often feel that they receive very little sympathy and understanding.

PATHOPHYSIOLOGY

Tinnitus is usually a subjective sensation of sound in the ear. It is a relatively common complaint which may arise in association with a wide range of conditions, including inner and middle ear disease, overuse of medications such as aspirin and quinine, abnormalities of the auditory nerve, renal problems, cardiac problems and anaemia. It is often accompanied by vertigo and/or deafness.

The Tinnitus Association produces an excellent range of factsheets and a free newsletter for interested professionals, as well as helping sufferers (see 'Useful websites').

Common presenting symptoms Tinnitus can vary in severity from an intermittent mild ringing sensation in the ear to an incessant noise, loud enough to make life unbearable. The perceived sound varies in volume and character from one individual to another. Some patients are aware of the sound only during their waking hours, while others are aware of it mainly at night or when they are somewhere very quiet. Tinnitus may cause difficulty in sleeping, with irritability, tiredness and lack of concentration following restless nights. The persistent symptoms cause many tinnitus sufferers to feel anxious and depressed (see Box 14.3). The feelings are exacerbated in some by fears that the tinnitus is an indication of a more serious underlying disease or that it will cause an increase in hearing loss.

In the worst cases, individuals with tinnitus may suffer total deafness because the noise in their ear eliminates all other sounds.

MEDICAL MANAGEMENT

To aid diagnosis, a careful history must be taken, including information about all other symptoms and any medications. This should be done in a tinnitus clinic within an ENT department. A hearing test and careful examination of the ear (including radiography) may help determine the cause. Unfortunately, in many instances, no treatable cause will be found. In certain patients, a hearing aid can give some relief by reducing or masking the tinnitus. A noise generator that looks like a hearing aid can help to cancel out the undesirable sound and can be of help to some. Tinnitus retraining therapy (TRT) aims to reduce the brain's perception of tinnitus and so reduce the problem it is causing. TRT may include counselling, relaxation therapy, the appropriate use of hearing aids, noise alleviators and medication, as well as the treatment of any stress and anxiety.

For an overview of the issues surrounding the use of this therapy, see Sizer (1998).

NURSING PRIORITIES AND MANAGEMENT: Tinnitus

Very few tinnitus sufferers will be patients in hospital, unless their condition has arisen as an early postoperative complication. The majority will attend their GP's surgery or their nearest ENT outpatient department. Wherever nursing staff encounter these patients, high priority should be given to allowing them to express their fears and to recognising and relieving their anxiety and possible depression. Once an ENT specialist has carried out all the tests required to determine a diagnosis, any prescribed treatment and training can be commenced. Where there is no medical treatment, a planned programme of care, including TRT, counselling, explanations and information giving, such as details of support groups, will be necessary to help the patient adapt and to relieve any worries. There are more than 100 tinnitus support groups in the UK and they can be of enormous help to sufferers by providing ongoing emotional support (see 'Useful websites').

For further information on tinnitus and health anxiety, see Heath (1994).

STOP THINK **14.5** Find out if there is a tinnitus support group in your area. If there is, try to arrange to attend one of their meetings.

Vertigo

PATHOPHYSIOLOGY

Vertigo is a disturbance of equilibrium in the absence of an external cause which creates a sensation of rotating motion of oneself or one's surroundings. It is usually caused by irritation of the vestibular apparatus and is most frequently associated with disorders of the bony labyrinth and with Ménière's disease. Cardiac, neurological or viral infections and therapeutic medications such as streptomycin can also cause vertigo.

Common presenting symptoms Vertigo is a disabling and often frightening sensation that may be transient or recurring. It is not the same as dizziness and may be relatively mild or quite severe. The motion perceived is often described as a whirling sensation, but rocking and swaying sensations are also reported. Severe attacks of vertigo may be sudden and dramatic, accompanied by pallor, nausea and vomiting.

For more information on vertigo management, see Lauder (1993).

MEDICAL MANAGEMENT

A careful history is required from the patient and must include any precipitating factors such as head and neck movements. Any other symptoms such as tinnitus or deafness should be ascertained. It is also helpful to know how long the periods of vertigo last. Details of medication and any recent trauma can also aid diagnosis. A neurological and cardiovascular examination and perhaps radiography, hearing tests and blood tests may be advisable.

Occasionally, surgery will be required to treat the particular disorder of which vertigo is a symptom, but treatment is more commonly pharmacological, or using the Eplay manoeuvre or Cooksey Cawthorne head and neck exercises, which are taught by a physiotherapist (Lauder 1993). An occupational therapy assessment of home safety may also be beneficial.

NURSING PRIORITIES AND MANAGEMENT: Vertigo

As is the case with tinnitus sufferers, the majority of individuals who experience vertigo will be distressed and incapacitated by their condition. They will usually be seen in their homes, as they are likely to feel unsafe venturing out. The first nursing priority for these patients is safety. The attacks of vertigo may be unpredictable, or may be associated with a particular head movement. For example, for one individual, a precipitating circumstance might be standing on a stepladder with their head back and to one side in order to change a light bulb; for another, it may be simply a quick movement to bend down and pick up a baby from its cot. The nurse should discuss with the patient and family how to avoid the particular head and/or other movements in order to eliminate attacks, if this is possible.

Ménière's disease

PATHOPHYSIOLOGY

In Ménière's disease, the membranous labyrinth is distended by an increase in the endolymph, at the expense of the perilymph, and the organ of Corti degenerates. The most widely held theory of its cause is that it arises as a result of local ischaemia, although it has been suggested that it may be due to viral infection, biochemical disturbance, vitamin deficiency or local physiological faults.

Common presenting symptoms Ménière's disease is characterised by four disabling features:

- vertigo
- tinnitus
- sensorineural hearing loss
- nausea and vomiting.

It may arise at any age but is most common among individuals aged 30–50. As it runs its course over a period of many years, deafness increases. Although this hearing loss may initially affect only one ear, it will, in 10% of patients, eventually affect the other as well (Becker et al 1993, McAllen 1996). Many patients have a warning that an attack is imminent, e.g. there is a feeling of fullness in the ear or the character of the tinnitus changes.

During an attack the patient will have vertigo, nausea and vomiting and will want to lie down and remain as still as possible, in order to relieve these distressing symptoms. Nystagmus may be present and, as a consequence of vagal stimulation, sweating, bradycardia and diarrhoea may occur.

MEDICAL MANAGEMENT

It may be difficult to arrive at a conclusive diagnosis of Ménière's disease, as many other disorders, e.g. labyrinthitis, intracranial disease and acoustic neuroma, display similar symptoms. Given that, between attacks, clinical examination may prove negative, diagnosis will rely heavily on careful history taking and audiological investigations.

Treatment The most common treatment for the symptoms of Ménière's disease is the prescription of medication, e.g. a labyrinthine sedative, such as cinnarizine, and diuretics. A vasodilator such as nicotinic acid or moxisylyte may be prescribed to alleviate local ischaemia. The majority of patients respond well to medication therapy and may have long periods of respite from severe symptoms. Adherence to a low-salt diet may be advised to reduce the volume of endolymph.

Surgery may occasionally help to relieve symptoms. This may take the form of decompression of the endolymphatic sac, the creation of a fistula between the endolymph and perilymph reservoirs, or a vestibular neurectomy.

NURSING PRIORITIES AND MANAGEMENT: Ménière's disease

The main nursing priority in case of an attack of Ménière's disease is to ensure the patient's safety. Attacks are often so severe that the patient needs to lie as still as possible, and, if in hospital, may gain a sense of security if the side rails on the bed are raised. Vomiting can be so severe as to cause dehydration. If the patient cannot take fluids orally, i.v. fluids and antiemetic drugs will be necessary until oral medication and feeding can be tolerated.

Patients suffering from Ménière's disease often have to make lifestyle changes in order to cope with some of the symptoms of the disorder. The nurse should be prepared to offer advice on lifestyle adaptations. As an individual faced with the problems associated with Ménière's disease is likely to feel anxiety, it is vital that the nurse provides clear information and explanations, particularly with regard to prognosis.

The involvement of the primary health care team and of the occupational health nurse will be especially important, as it is often not until the patient is back at home following diagnosis that many questions with regard to participation in sport, driving, safety at home and in the workplace begin to be considered.

THE NOSE

ANATOMY AND PHYSIOLOGY OF THE NOSE

The principal function of the nose is to provide a passageway for air entering and leaving the respiratory tract (see Fig. 14.3). In so doing, it acts as an 'air conditioner', ensuring that inspired air is humidified, sufficiently warm and free from particulate matter.

The terminal fibres of the olfactory nerve are located in the roof of the nasal cavity. The lower two-thirds of the nose are supported by cartilage and the upper third is enclosed by bone. The cavity is divided in half by the septum which consists of cartilage anteriorly and bone posteriorly. The entrance is lined with stratified squamous epithelium and coarse hairs (termed vibrissae) and the passages are lined with a mucous membrane of ciliated columnar epithelium. These passages are highly vascularised. A branch of the maxillary artery supplies the lower posterior section of the cavity, and the anterior and posterior ethmoidal arteries supply the mucous membrane. All these vessels join at Little's area on each side of the septum (see Fig. 14.4).

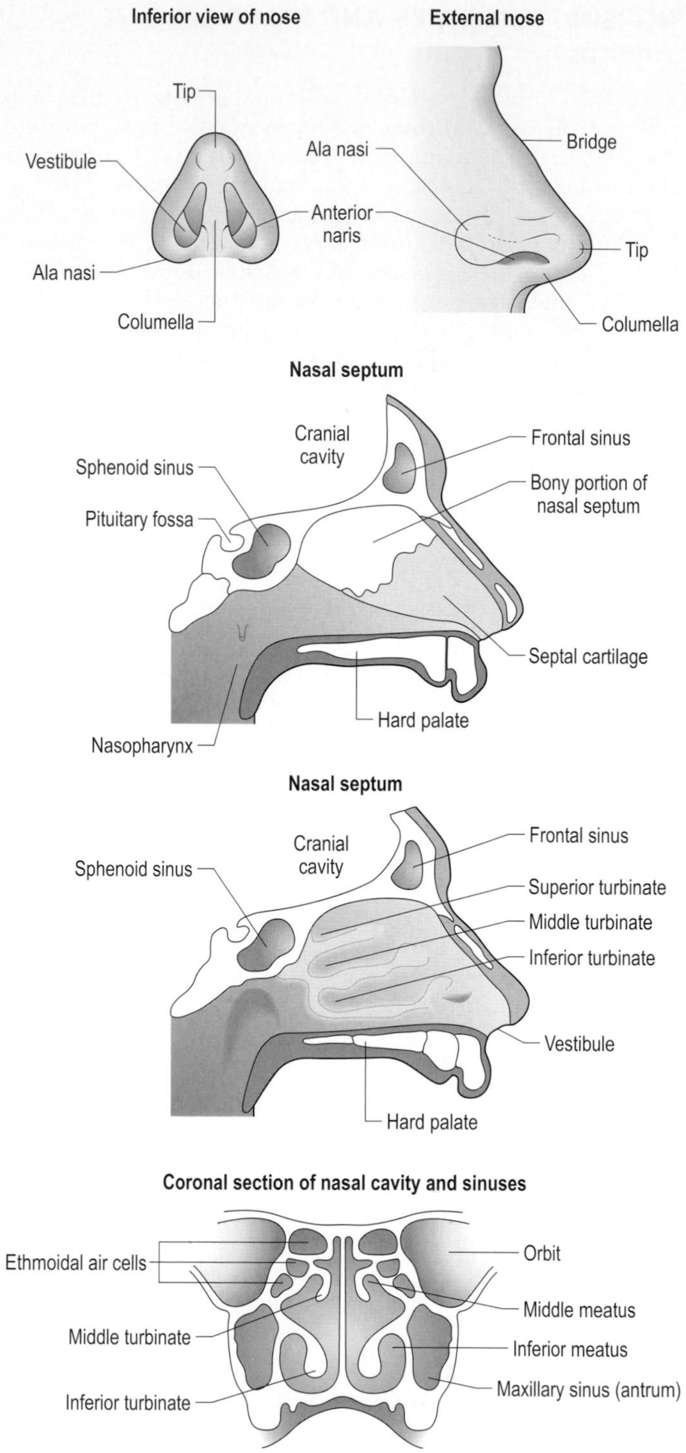

Fig. 14.3 The nose and paranasal sinuses.

For further information, see Becker et al (1993).

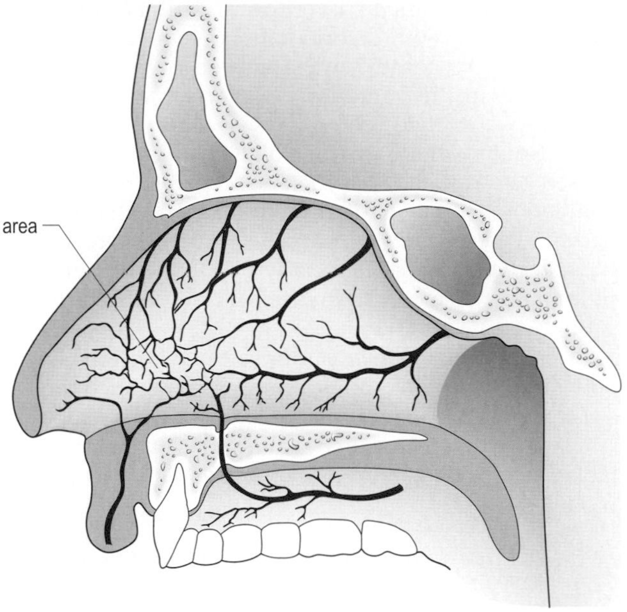

Fig. 14.4 Blood supply to nose (sagittal section).

DISORDERS OF THE NOSE

Epistaxis

PATHOPHYSIOLOGY

Epistaxis is bleeding from the nose. It is not a disease in itself but a symptom of some other disorder, which may be of a local or general nature. Local causative disorders include idiopathic, trauma caused by nose-picking, foreign bodies, a blow to the nose or surgery. More generalised disorders that sometimes give rise to nosebleeds can be:

- vascular, e.g. hypertension and cardiac failure
- congenital, e.g. haemophilia and hereditary haemorrhagic telangiectasia
- neoplastic, e.g. leukaemia
- medication-induced, e.g. a side-effect of anticoagulant therapy
- infections, e.g. influenza, rhinitis, sinusitis and the common cold.

Common presenting symptoms Epistaxis can affect males and females equally and can occur at any age but is most common in childhood and early adolescence, when it usually occurs in Little's area (see Fig. 14.4) and is often the result of trauma or infection. In middle-aged or older individuals, the bleeding is more likely to occur in the posterior part of the nose and may be associated with hypertension. This form of epistaxis may be very frightening and can be life threatening if it proves difficult to control.

Patients may refer themselves to the local emergency department when they have an active epistaxis. They may then either be admitted to the appropriate hospital ward or, if the bleeding has stopped, given an outpatient clinic appointment. One patient's experience of epistaxis is recounted in Box 14.4.

Patients often present at clinics with a history of recurrent epistaxis, but are rarely actually bleeding at that time. On examination, dilated blood vessels may be apparent. The best treatment to prevent the bleeding recurring is cautery by the use of a chemical, such as silver nitrate, electrocautery or diathermy.

Box 14.4

An experience of epistaxis

It first started on a Saturday morning. I bent down to pick up my bag from the floor and realised my nose was running. On wiping it, I saw fresh blood. Going into the bathroom, I could still feel it running and the tissue was getting soggy with blood. Remembering some first aid, I squeezed the soft front of my nose, sat down and leaned forward. At least it stopped the blood coming out of my nose, although I could taste some in my mouth now. After 10 min I stopped squeezing and the bleeding stopped. I cleaned around the front of my nose, but spent the rest of the day not daring to blow my nose in case the bleeding started again.

All was well until Wednesday evening. I'd just had a bath and was watching TV, when I felt my nose running. Again, there was blood on the tissue and dripping from my nose. Like the previous time, I squeezed my nose, but after 10 min, when I released the pressure, the blood started dripping and I squeezed again. Again, on releasing the pressure, the blood continued to drip and I now had a pile of bloodstained tissues in the bin and patches of blood all over the bathroom floor as I tried stuffing tissues up my nose as well. By now an hour had passed and still the blood dripped. I didn't think it was ever going to stop and wasn't sure what to do.

My flatmate suggested contacting my GP. She phoned and we were advised to go to the emergency department of our local hospital. So my flatmate drove me to the hospital and I took the washing up bowl to catch the blood, as I didn't want to mess up the car!

On arriving at the emergency department, my flatmate booked me in and I was seen very quickly by a nurse. On releasing the squeeze on my nose, the blood still continued to drip out and the nurse said I would see a doctor. The nurse then squeezed my nose for me. I was glad as my arms were aching from all the squeezing I had done. My blood pressure was taken and the doctor saw me.

Despite all the blood coming out of my nose the doctor sprayed it with a local anaesthetic and had a look inside. They could see a blood vessel at the front of my nose that was bleeding, so they put a stick on it, to cauterise the vessel and the bleeding stopped. It was a great relief and after an hour of no further bleeding I was allowed to go home with some nasal cream and an outpatient's appointment for 4 weeks' time.

MEDICAL MANAGEMENT

The management of epistaxis can be divided into resuscitation of the patient, arrest of the haemorrhage and diagnosis and treatment of any underlying cause (Ell & Parker 1992).

A patient with a severe active epistaxis is usually admitted to hospital as an emergency. Vital signs are recorded to monitor for shock, as bleeding may be severe enough to necessitate blood transfusion. Treatment is by insertion of a nasal pack. This usually takes the form of a nasal tampon or pneumatic packing with an inflatable balloon. Nasal packs are usually left in place for 24–72 h. Antibiotics are given if the packs are in longer than 24 h, to prevent any risk of infection developing and spreading to the middle ear. Occasionally, when these measures fail to control the bleeding, arterial ligation is necessary. If the bleed is the result of some underlying medical condition, this will need to be investigated and treated at the same time.

NURSING PRIORITIES AND MANAGEMENT: Epistaxis

Nursing intervention will vary, depending on the site, severity and cause of the epistaxis, as well as the patient's age.

Anterior nosebleeds

Most patients with anterior nosebleeds will be children or adolescents and will be treated as outpatients in their GP's surgery or at the hospital.

NURSING PRIORITIES AND MANAGEMENT: Anterior nosebleeds

The first priority of nursing intervention will be to stop the bleeding, whilst providing psychological support. The patient should be helped to sit upright with the head slightly forward and asked to mouth breathe and spit out all blood. This helps to estimate the blood loss and prevents the blood from being swallowed and causing nausea. Digital pressure with the thumb and forefinger should be applied to the cartilaginous part of the nose and ice packs to the area above it, i.e. Little's area (see Fig. 14.4). This area has many surface arterioles which may have weakened walls. Ten continuous minutes of this pressure is usually sufficient to control an anterior nosebleed. If these first aid measures fail, or if there are recurrent nosebleeds, the patient will probably be transferred to hospital for insertion of a nasal pack or cautery of the area.

Once the bleeding is under control, the nurse should explain to the patient and, where appropriate, to the parents, how to prevent nosebleeds from recurring. Advice should be given about blowing the nose gently, avoiding picking the nose and trying to keep the nasal mucosa slightly moist by using soft petroleum jelly. An explanation of how to cope with and control a nosebleed should also be given.

Hospital treatment

This will be necessary for severe epistaxis that cannot be controlled by the above measures. By providing clear and concise information, the nurse can help alleviate the patient's anxiety and aid recovery. A specialist nurse can pack the nasal cavity or assist the medical practitioner to do so. When a nasal pack is in place, the patient will only be able to breathe through the mouth and may be afraid of suffocation. Frequent oral hygiene and plenty of oral fluids should be offered to prevent the oral mucosa becoming dry. These drinks must not be hot, as this can cause local dilatation of blood vessels and exacerbate the problem. Eye care may be necessary as the packing may obstruct the nasolacrimal duct, causing tears to overflow. Nasal packing can also cause hypoxia, with disorientation as well as alterations to vital signs. Oxygen therapy and blood gas monitoring will be needed in this situation. The systemic effects of nasal packing were investigated by Ogretmenoglu et al (2002). Their results suggested that bilateral anterior nasal packs caused hypoxia, tachycardia and hypercapnia due to hypoventilation. This led them to recommend that nasal packs be removed as early as possible, and that oxygen therapy be given routinely, especially for patients with cardiopulmonary disease, with appropriate monitoring of O_2 saturation.

Areas that have been cauterised may become encrusted. Soft petroleum jelly should be applied to such areas twice a day for a few weeks until the mucosa has healed.

Some patients admitted as emergencies with uncontrollable nosebleeds will be in hypovolaemic shock (see Ch. 18, p. 718).

For further information on first aid, read Malem & Butler (1993).

STOP THINK **14.6** Revise the signs and symptoms of shock so that you can visualise the likely appearance of a patient admitted with severe, uncontrollable epistaxis.

Although anxieties can be reduced by answering the patient's questions and giving information, sedatives may also be prescribed. Following an epistaxis, patients are usually nursed propped up in bed to aid venous return from the area and to make it easier for them to spit out any blood. Ice packs may be applied to the nose to help constrict the vessels and control bleeding. The nurse should explain to the patient how to breathe through the mouth and an emesis basin or sputum carton should be to hand. Again, it is important to offer frequent oral hygiene, plenty of cool drinks and eye care as necessary. As these patients often have dysphagia because of the pressure of the nasal pack on the soft palate, a nutritious soft or even liquid diet may be appropriate. Bed rest is usually advised, although patients should be allowed to use the commode at the side of the bed to ease the strain of elimination.

Packing is usually removed in 2 or 3 days. If the bleeding has not been controlled, the patient will have the appropriate arteries ligated in theatre. If a deviated nasal septum (see p. 606) has been a contributory cause, corrective surgery may be performed.

If hypertension or another medical disorder has caused the nosebleed, an appropriate specialist medical opinion is sought and treatment commenced. The nurse may, in the meantime, obtain appropriate patient education booklets or information sheets in relation to the relevant disorder from colleagues working in the ward(s) specialising in the care of such patients, so that the patient can be given appropriate advice (see Ch. 2).

Community care

To prevent the recurrence of epistaxis, support should continue after the patient has returned home and resumed normal activities. If the patient is at home, the GP and practice nurse will be informed of their condition so

CASE HISTORY 14.1

Mrs E

Mrs E is 58 years old and lives with her husband, who suffers from chronic obstructive airways disease and is unemployed. They have a son and a daughter, both of whom are married and have children. Mrs E works in a television assembly factory and enjoys watching TV, going to bingo and participating in the factory social club. She smokes 20 cigarettes a day and drinks about 14 units of alcohol a week, mainly at the weekend. She often baby-sits for her son and daughter. She has to do all the housework, cooking and shopping as her husband's breathing problems leave him with little energy.

For the past few months Mrs E has been suffering from nosebleeds, but today's was very severe and could not be controlled, even with the help of the occupational health nurse at the factory. She was brought to the local hospital's emergency department (ED) by ambulance. By the time she arrived her blood pressure was 90/50 and her pulse 105; she was pale and shivering. She was also very anxious and frightened.

In the ED an Epistat catheter was inserted and an intravenous infusion commenced. Mrs E was then transferred to the ward where the staff nurse welcomed her and took her to the bed she had prepared. The staff nurse was given a report by the ED nurse and after helping Mrs E to transfer from the trolley to bed she planned to observe her infusion closely and to monitor the bleeding and her blood pressure.

On admission, Mrs E was still anxious and distressed. She was a very fastidious lady and the mess her nosebleed had made concerned her. She was also very worried about what her husband would do for his meal and how he would be kept informed of her condition.

In prioritising Mrs E's needs, the staff nurse took into account the details of her medical condition as well as other concerns that the patient herself felt to be important. She helped Mrs E into a hospital nightgown after washing the blood from her skin and put her blouse into cold water to soak. She checked the infusion and Mrs E's blood pressure, then brought the ward phone to the bedside and telephoned Mrs E's husband. As Mrs E had difficulty talking, because of the nasal catheter, the nurse assisted in a three-way conversation in which Mrs E was reassured that her husband was all right. A neighbour had made his tea for him, and Mrs E's daughter was on her way to the hospital, bringing her mother's toiletries and nightclothes. This conversation reassured Mrs E and allowed her to feel more relaxed. This in turn helped the staff nurse to concentrate on monitoring Mrs E's condition and helping to alleviate her problems.

For further information, see Becker et al (1993).

that they can encourage the patient to implement the advice received in hospital and can monitor hypertension if present.

For information on epistaxis in older people, see Ell & Parker (1992).

STOP THINK **14.7** Using a nursing model familiar to you, prioritise and plan the nursing interventions you think Mrs E (see Case History 14.1) will require over the next 24 h and say how you would evaluate her care. Discuss the plan with your teacher and/or with a qualified member of your nursing team.

DISORDERS OF THE PARANASAL SINUSES

The paranasal sinuses are a group of air spaces surrounding the nose which, it is said, make the skull lighter and add resonance to the voice. They consist of two frontal, two maxillary and two ethmoid sinuses and a single sphenoid sinus divided by a septum. These sinuses all drain into the nose (see Fig. 14.3).

Acute sinusitis

PATHOPHYSIOLOGY

Acute sinusitis is the inflammation of one or more of the paranasal sinuses. It usually develops as an infection secondary to an upper respiratory tract infection or dental disease. Because of the close anatomical connection of the sinuses with the nose, sinus infection is common. It may be acute or chronic.

Common presenting symptoms Pain is a symptom, and it may be facial, supraorbital or interocular, depending on the sinus involved. Tenderness in the area of pain and nasal obstruction may also be features, and nasal discharge may be present. The patient usually complains of general malaise and is pyrexial.

MEDICAL MANAGEMENT

A nasal swab may be taken for culture and sensitivity. Sinus radiography may also be performed to determine which sinuses are affected. Medical treatment usually consists of the prescription of mild analgesics, antibiotics and nasal decongestant drops.

NURSING PRIORITIES AND MANAGEMENT: Acute sinusitis

The patient with acute sinusitis is usually nursed at home, and will be advised to rest in bed, to drink plenty of fluids, to take mild analgesics such as paracetamol and to self-administer any prescribed nasal drops. Oral hygiene is also important as the individual will probably be mouth breathing because of the nasal obstruction. Moist steam inhalations can also bring some relief and help to loosen crusting in the nasal cavities. Many sufferers find inhalations very soothing first thing in the morning and last thing at night. After 2 or 3 days the person should have improved sufficiently to be fully active again.

Chronic sinusitis

PATHOPHYSIOLOGY

Chronic sinusitis is common and can be quite debilitating. It can develop for several reasons, including:

- inadequate treatment of an acute episode
- septal deviation or nasal polyps preventing adequate drainage of the sinuses
- pollution, e.g. cigarette smoke
- allergic nasal disease.

Common presenting symptoms The main symptoms of chronic sinusitis are purulent nasal discharge, postnasal drip, facial pain, headache and recurrent throat infections.

MEDICAL MANAGEMENT

Treatment is initially conservative, consisting of treating any infection with prescribed antibiotics and nasal decongestant sprays. Surgery may be necessary to remove all of the diseased mucosal lining and widen the opening to the nasal passage to allow more effective drainage.

This is functional endoscopic sinus surgery (FESS). FESS is the most recent advance in the surgical management of nasal and paranasal sinus disease. By means of nasal endoscopes, the surgeon is able to visualise, diagnose and treat any disease or deformity. CT and/or MRI scans are vital for both diagnostic and intraoperative use. Meticulous postoperative management and follow-up are essential in achieving effective results.

Possible complications of FESS are:

- haemorrhage
- cerebrospinal fluid leak
- visual disturbance/blindness
- periorbital haematoma.

NURSING PRIORITIES AND MANAGEMENT: Chronic sinusitis

Nursing priorities when caring for these patients are:

- to prepare the patient for surgery and to observe for any possible complications, including haemorrhage and infection
- removal of nasal packing as per the surgeon's instructions
- administration of prescribed analgesics and antibiotics.

On discharge, the patient must be advised on the correct method for instillation of nasal drops and the importance of steam inhalations.

For fuller details of FESS, see Krouse et al (1997).

14.8 Discuss with a patient the experience of nasal packing and its removal.

Nasal injury

PATHOPHYSIOLOGY

Injuries to the nose are fairly common and usually occur in sporting activities, falls, accidents and assaults. A blow to one side of the nose may fracture and displace the bone, causing deviation on the other side. A direct blow to the front of the nose can splay out the nasal bones, resulting in a depressed bridge. An injury that is sufficiently severe to fracture the nasal bones will also cause soft tissue swelling and may cause epistaxis.

MEDICAL MANAGEMENT

Investigations will involve a radiographic examination, although this does not always reveal the fracture or may simply reveal a previously undetected fracture. An examination of the nose using a nasal speculum will allow the practitioner to see if the airways are patent and if there is any damage to the septum. Palpation of the nasal bones must be carried out very gently, as they will be very tender and painful for up to 3 weeks following a fracture.

Treatment of a broken nose involves manipulating the fractured bones. Occasionally this can be done at the time of the accident, but more commonly it is done a few days later, when the oedema has subsided, usually as a day case procedure. The manipulation must be performed within 10 days of injury to prevent calcification of the nasal bones. If the corrected fracture is unstable, a plaster of Paris cast is usually taped in position over the nose for about 10 days to allow the fracture to set correctly.

NURSING PRIORITIES AND MANAGEMENT: Nasal injury

If nursing attention is available immediately, treatment of a fractured nose will probably involve first aid measures to stop any epistaxis and to limit the oedema. This involves compressing the end of the nostrils gently between the thumb and forefinger, which unfortunately will be very painful for the patient, and encouraging the patient to sit with the head slightly forward and to spit out any blood. If ice is available, an ice pack applied to the bridge of the nose can help to control bleeding and swelling. Any epistaxis which results from a blow to the nose is usually short lived.

DISORDERS OF THE NASAL SEPTUM

Deviation of the nasal septum

The nasal septum separates the nostrils. It is usually thin and quite straight. The upper part is composed of bone and the lower part of cartilage. Deviations of the nasal septum can range from a simple bulge to a marked S-shaped deformity. Most people have some degree of deviation; hence, when introducing a nasogastric tube, the patient should always be asked which nostril is easier to breathe through.

PATHOPHYSIOLOGY

Developmental problems or trauma may result in a deviated nasal septum. Patients usually complain of nasal obstruction, infection of the sinuses or chronic otitis media due to the inability of the eustachian tubes to function properly. Any combination of these symptoms may be present, or there may be no symptoms. Simply having a septal deviation is not a reason to operate on it.

MEDICAL MANAGEMENT

An assessment by the medical practitioner of the symptoms, correlated with the degree of the deformity, should be carried out before a treatment plan is agreed. Inspection of the nose with a nasal speculum should reveal the extent of the deviation.

If surgery is the chosen treatment, this is likely to be either a submucous resection or a septoplasty. There is often some confusion as to what these procedures involve. In both operations, access to the bony and cartilaginous parts of the septum is gained by stripping off the nasal mucosa. In a submucous resection, the affected parts of the septum are removed; during a septoplasty the septum is freed, allowing it to be repositioned along the midline of the nose. A nasal pack is usually inserted following these procedures to prevent haemorrhage.

NURSING PRIORITIES AND MANAGEMENT: Deviation of the nasal septum

Septal surgery is often carried out as a day case and packs can be in place from 4 to 24 h. Nursing care in hospital will be similar to that given for epistaxis (see p. 604). Patients are usually discharged 2–4 h after the nasal packing has been removed. There will be a degree of nasal obstruction for 2 or 3 weeks after surgery, until the post-surgical swelling has subsided. Patients are usually advised to stay away from work or crowded places for 10–14 days after surgery to minimise the risk of infection. They are also advised to follow the surgeon's instructions with regard to steam inhalations, nasal douches or decongestant sprays.

Septal haematoma

This usually results from trauma, including surgery, and is a collection of blood beneath the mucoperichondrium of the septum. The patient complains of nasal obstruction and pain. Examination usually reveals a bilateral swelling in the nasal cavities. Antibiotics are given to prevent infection and it is often necessary to incise and drain the haematoma.

Septal perforation

Trauma or snorted illegal drugs are usually the cause of a hole in the septum. Although the patient is often symptom-free, excessive crusting or epistaxis may occur. Occasionally the patient complains of whistling on inspiration. If symptoms are troublesome, surgical closure may be attempted.

NASAL OBSTRUCTION

Obstruction of the nasal cavities can result from a number of causes but patients usually present with similar symptoms, the most common being obstructed breathing and increased nasal discharge. Some of the most common causes are:

- infection
- allergy
- deviated nasal septum
- foreign bodies
- polyps
- neoplasms.

Nasal obstruction resulting from the first two causes does not usually require hospital treatment. Deviated nasal septum is described above; the other causes are described below.

Foreign bodies in the nose

PATHOPHYSIOLOGY

It is usually very young children, aged 2–4 years, or those with learning difficulties, who insert foreign bodies into the nasal cavity. These objects may be organic or inorganic. Inorganic bodies include buttons, beads and small plastic or metal objects which may lie undetected for a long time, only to be found during a routine examination, sometimes as late as when the child reaches adolescence or adulthood. Organic bodies such as peas, wood, paper, cotton wool or sweets cause a local inflammatory reaction which will eventually lead to the formation of granulation tissue. The resulting nasal discharge will eventually become purulent, foul-smelling and bloodstained. Characteristically, the discharge is from only one cavity.

MEDICAL MANAGEMENT

Following a thorough examination, the foreign body is usually removed in the outpatient department. Occasionally it has been in place for such a long time that a general anaesthetic is needed for smooth and safe removal.

NURSING PRIORITIES AND MANAGEMENT: Foreign bodies in the nose

Support will be given to both the patient and the family as removal can be frightening. Epistaxis is a possible complication following removal, irrespective of the type of anaesthetic used.

Nasal polyps

PATHOPHYSIOLOGY

Nasal polyps are projections of oedematous mucous membrane and may look like bunches of grapes. They result from prolonged infection or allergy and are usually bilateral and multiple. They occur more commonly in adult males than in females.

Common presenting symptoms Patients usually complain of nasal obstruction and discharge. Occasionally the size of the polyps may cause broadening of the external nose. The patient may complain of headaches if there is sinus involvement and there may be loss of smell and taste.

MEDICAL MANAGEMENT

On examination, a characteristic glossy, greyish swelling will be visible. If probed, it will be found to be soft, insensitive and mobile. Surgical removal is the treatment of choice. This may be carried out under local or general anaesthetic. The patient who is given a local anaesthetic will require less time in hospital, but the decongestant that the local anaesthetic contains shrinks the polyps and makes them more difficult to identify and remove. With a general anaesthetic, the polyps can be removed at a less hurried pace but bleeding may be more profuse and might therefore obscure some of the smaller polyps. Recurrences are common and an attempt should be made to treat any underlying infection or allergy.

NURSING PRIORITIES AND MANAGEMENT: Nasal polyps

Nursing staff should be alert to epistaxis, which is the main postoperative complication of polyp removal. Given that polyps can be associated with allergies, many patients may also suffer from asthma and should be closely observed in this regard.

A nasal pack is usually inserted after the procedure. Appropriate nursing care is detailed on page 604. As it is fairly common for polyps to recur, the importance of attending the outpatient department for follow-up should be explained to the patient.

Common problems during nasal surgery

- *Bleeding* — this occurs because the nasal mucosa has such a rich blood supply. It can be controlled by the use of ice packs. If the surgeon suspects that the bleeding might be severe, a nasal pack may be inserted.
- *Oedema* — oedema of the mucosa is likely to occur as a consequence of manipulation. Ice packs may help to minimise swelling.
- *Watery discharge* — the irritation of the mucosa, which results from surgery, will cause the production of an excessive amount of watery discharge known as rhinorrhoea. The nurse should provide an adequate supply of tissues or apply a nasal bolster made of gauze to absorb discharge. This helps to make the problem more manageable.
- *Pain* — as the nose is blocked after surgery, the patient may experience frontal headaches, which should be alleviated by means of prescribed analgesics, e.g. paracetamol.

Neoplasms

Nasal and sinus tumours are rare. When they occur, they are usually unilateral. Malignant tumours are often infected and ulcerated, in which case they usually produce epistaxis or a profuse purulent discharge. Headache may also be a feature if there is sinus involvement.

Treatment may consist of surgery, radiotherapy, chemotherapy or a combination of these. Patients receiving radiotherapy or chemotherapy are usually treated as outpatients and may be visited by community nurses, including Macmillan nurses, if they experience any side-effects of treatment requiring nursing intervention.

For further information on nasal and sinus neoplasms and treatments, see Sigler & Schuring (1993).

THE THROAT

ANATOMY AND PHYSIOLOGY OF THE THROAT

The throat is usually considered to consist of the pharynx and the larynx. The pharynx may be divided into the nasopharynx and the oropharynx.

The nasopharynx extends from the nasal septum to the eustachian tubes and rests behind and above the soft palate. The oropharynx extends from the posterior boundary of the hard palate to the hyoid bone; it contains the uvula and the tonsils and is surrounded by lymphoid tissue.

The larynx is the organ of voice production and airway protection. It is composed mainly of cartilage and muscle and is lined with a mucosa of stratified squamous epithelium (upper part) and ciliated pseudostratified columnar epithelium (lower part).

DISORDERS OF THE THROAT

Benign tumours

These generally arise as a result of voice abuse or overuse and the patient usually presents with continued hoarseness. The tumours are usually attached to the vocal cords and vary greatly in size. Resolution of small nodules may be achieved by voice rest and appropriate speech therapy. Larger nodules may require surgical removal.

For further information on benign and malignant tumours, see Sigler & Schuring (1993).

Carcinoma of the larynx

PATHOPHYSIOLOGY

Carcinoma of the larynx is classified according to its location and extent, i.e. supraglottic (above the vocal cords), glottic (confined to the vocal cords) or subglottic (below the vocal cords) (see Fig. 14.5). It accounts for 1% of all malignant disease and is more common in males than in females. The majority of patients have a history of heavy smoking, although the disorder does occasionally occur in non-smokers. High levels of alcohol consumption can be an influencing factor. The most common form of the disease is squamous cell carcinoma. About 10% of all patients with carcinoma of the larynx have a coexisting carcinoma of the bronchus.

Common presenting symptoms Some patients with laryngeal carcinoma do not seek medical help until the disease is advanced, having ignored the symptom of hoarseness for some time. Occasionally patients are treated initially for laryngitis and by the time a tumour has been diagnosed it is advanced. Otalgia, dyspnoea, dysphagia, neck lumps and weight loss are all symptoms of advanced laryngeal carcinoma. The impact of the diagnosis and the community care needs of a patient newly diagnosed with cancer are discussed by Glover and Cameron (2004).

MEDICAL MANAGEMENT

Carcinoma of the larynx has a high rate of cure if detected early. The form of treatment offered will depend on the site of the tumour and how early it has been detected. If the tumour is confined to the vocal cords it is usually diagnosed as a result of the patient consulting their GP with a history of hoarseness. Patients who have suffered from hoarseness for more than 3 weeks should have a mirror examination of their larynx (indirect laryngoscopy) to investigate the possibility of carcinoma. Diagnosis is confirmed by an examination of the patient's larynx under general anaesthesia (direct laryngoscopy) and a histological examination of a biopsy of the tumour.

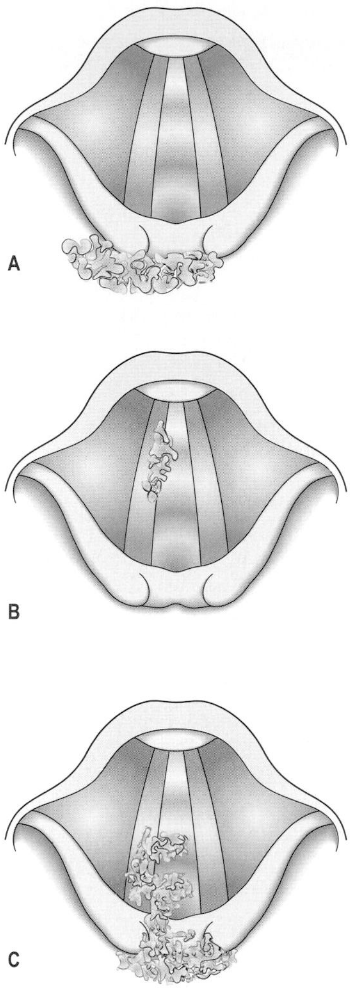

Fig. 14.5 Tumours of the larynx. A: Supraglottic tumour. B: Glottic tumour. C: Subglottic tumour — extensive spread to supraglottic area.

In recent years, in some centres in the UK, there has been increasing use of the CO_2 laser to remove laryngeal tumours, ranging from very small vocal cord (glottic) tumours to larger tumours requiring partial or hemilaryngectomy. When using the laser, it is possible effectively to remove all of the tumour but less of the normal healthy tissue, and so preserve more function. Otherwise, the treatment of choice for a glottic tumour is radiotherapy. If the disease is more extensive and/or invasive, treatment may be radiotherapy, chemoradiation or total laryngectomy.

- In chemoradiation, chemotherapy is given at various points during the radiotherapy course, for example on days 1, 22 and 43. The aim is to provide an effective treatment for the disease, while preserving the larynx.
- Total laryngectomy involves removal of the larynx and the creation of a permanent end tracheostome (see pp. 610–615).

Hanna et al (2004) undertook a non-randomised retrospective study of 42 patients, 23 of whom had had a total laryngectomy and postoperative radiotherapy, and 19 who had concurrent chemoradiation, with the aim of comparing quality of life between the two groups. Overall, the scores for both groups were similar, with no statistically significant differences noted. However, there were differences between patient experiences; for example, the surgical group reported greater difficulties with social functioning, while the chemoradiation patients reported greater difficulty coping with a dry mouth.

Laryngeal surgery may also have to be performed on patients who have a residual or recurrent tumour following radiotherapy. Nursing interventions appropriate to this procedure are outlined in the next section.

The lymphatic nodes in the neck are the most likely site for metastatic spread from a laryngeal tumour. If the nodes are involved they are treated by removal, i.e. a selective neck dissection, either as a separate surgical procedure, if the primary site is being treated by radiotherapy or laser excision, or at the same time as total laryngectomy.

Very advanced tumours of the larynx may be considered inoperable, in which case the patient may be given palliative radiotherapy and/or chemotherapy to relieve some of the more distressing symptoms of the disease (see Ch. 31). In addition, a tracheostomy is sometimes performed to relieve any respiratory obstruction and a percutaneous endoscopic gastrostomy (PEG) tube inserted to aid nutrition, hydration, administration of medications and patient comfort.

A study undertaken by Forbes (1997) indicated that the most frequent symptoms and problems experienced by head and neck cancer patients, in a palliative care situation, are pain, weight loss, feeding difficulties, respiratory problems and communication difficulties.

Laryngectomy

Preoperative preparation

Various members of the multidisciplinary team (MDT) will spend some time with the patient and family prior to surgery to explain the operation and its after-effects. This team will consist of medical and nursing staff, including the clinical nurse specialist (CNS), speech and language therapist (SALT), physiotherapist, medical social worker, dietitian and, often, former patients who have had a laryngectomy. Most centres have written information that can be used to supplement oral information. NHS policy (DH 2000) has emphasised the need for good communication between health professionals and patients. The provision of high quality information is an essential part of care.

The role of the head and neck oncology CNS is fully discussed in Semple (2002). For further details on creating information for patients with head and neck cancer, see Semple & McGowan (2002), and for laryngectomy see the NALC website (see 'Useful websites').

Physical preparation Diagnostic radiography of the neck and chest is performed and CT scan or MRI carried out. A full blood analysis is made. Total laryngectomy may also include a partial thyroidectomy, so thyroid function must be checked pre- and postoperatively (see Ch. 5).

An electrocardiograph (ECG) is ordered to check heart function (see Ch. 2). The patient will also be given a dental check-up and receive any necessary dental treatment to help circumvent the risk of pathogenic organisms in the oral cavity. Local preparation of the skin may be required, for example if the patient has a beard.

NURSING PRIORITIES AND MANAGEMENT: Total laryngectomy

Preoperative priorities

The nurse's priorities at this stage will centre on providing support and information for both the patient and the family and preparing the patient physically and psychologically for the operation (see Ch. 26; see also Research Abstract 14.2).

STOP THINK **14.9** Consider Case History 14.2. What information would you consider it important to obtain during an initial chat with Mr G to help you plan his nursing care?

Discuss this with your colleagues and check your ideas with your teacher or a qualified member of the nursing team.

The patient is usually admitted at least one day before surgery. It is important for the patient to get to know the team members at this stage, and in some units it is possible to meet the community nurse who will be helping the patient on returning home.

RESEARCH ABSTRACT 14.2

Laryngectomy: the patient's view

This study of laryngectomy, which looked at the incidence of disability and acceptability, was carried out in Wolverhampton. Data were collected using a 10-question questionnaire. Of the 82 patients approached, 65 replied, giving a response rate of 79%. Of the 65 who responded, 54 had undergone a total laryngectomy and 11 had this operation combined with a partial pharyngectomy. The average age was 68 years, the male:female ratio was 3:1, and the time since surgery ranged from 6 months to 35 years.

Respondents had experienced a substantial number and range of problems. These included having a worse sense of smell, being unable to blow their nose, experiencing difficulties in swallowing, an increase in chest infections, and stomal crusting or bleeding. None of the respondents reported weight loss and a majority were satisfied with their voice rehabilitation. Communication methods did not include voice prosthesis so one could reasonably expect this satisfaction rate to be higher now. Generally, respondents who felt they had achieved satisfactory rehabilitation indicated no reduction in their social acceptability. Of the 54 people who replied to the question about their sexual activity, 34 said there was no restriction. Most of those who had enjoyed swimming prior to surgery (29%) expressed their unhappiness at being unable to continue. The availability of stoma swimming aids may help those anxious to swim again. A disappointing 9% of respondents continued to smoke, most having changed from cigarettes to pipe or cigars.

Despite their problems, 91% of respondents considered the operation to have been worthwhile and 78% had found a laryngectomy club to be useful.

These findings can and should be used to better inform patients preoperatively and to act as a focus for postoperative problem identification and education.

Jay S, Ruddy J, Cullen R J 1991 Laryngectomy: the patients' view. Journal of Laryngology and Otology 105: 934–938

CASE HISTORY 14.2

Mr G

Mr G is a 64-year-old retired labourer. A widower, with a married daughter Ann, who lives in Canada with her husband and two young children, he has no other family. He lives alone, but has helpful neighbours. He is a keen bowler and enjoys the social side of the bowling club. He also reads a lot and listens to music.

Mr G has been diagnosed as having a subglottic tumour with extensive spread and is to be admitted to hospital for a total laryngectomy and selective neck dissection of left lymph nodes. Ann and her family have made plans to come home and spend 2 weeks with Mr G in his own home following his expected discharge from hospital in 3 weeks' time.

Mr G arrives at the ward with his friend Mr J and is welcomed by the staff nurse, who takes Mr G to a four-bed room and explains that he will be there until his operation, after which he will be in a high dependency unit for one or two nights before returning to the ward. The nurse leaves Mr G and his friend to unpack his bag and then returns with a cup of tea for them both. She asks about his activities of living with a view to planning his nursing care. Whilst discussing his social situation and lifestyle, Mr G tells the staff nurse he smokes 20 cigarettes a day and consumes about 30 units of alcohol a week and has continued with this pattern for many years. She takes this opportunity to discuss the advantages of stopping smoking with him and, with his consent, refers him to the smoking cessation advisor with a view to him stopping smoking and starting nicotine replacement therapy the next day. Since Mr G's nearest relative is his wife's sister, who lives 200 miles away, he gives her name and that of his friend as next of kin. His friend tells the staff nurse that he and his wife will visit and do Mr G's washing for him.

For further information on helping people stop smoking, see Haw (2002).

The patient and family will need support in adjusting to the diagnosis of cancer and the altered body image which will result from this type of surgery (Price 1998) (see Case History 14.2).

Patients undergoing total laryngectomy will need to be prepared for the fact that they will have a permanent 'hole' in the neck through which they breathe. They will be unable to talk initially. They will be able to swim only under supervision and after receiving advice and guidance on the use of special stoma devices. They will lose their sense of smell because they take in air through the mouth and stoma rather than the nose. In view of these after-effects, some patients will refuse surgery altogether, a decision which may be very difficult for families and members of the health care team to accept.

To aid observation, the patient is usually nursed in a single room, being admitted into this room in order to become familiar with the surroundings. A nasogastric or stomagastric tube will be present postoperatively for feeding, as well as i.v. infusions, oxygen and wound drains. These, along with tracheal suction, humidification and practical aspects of care, need to be demonstrated and discussed preoperatively to help reduce anxiety and thereby aid recovery (Feber 1998).

An appropriate means of communication, which works for the patient, the family and the members of the multidisciplinary team (MDT), should be arranged before surgery. For example, a pad and pencil would usually be kept close to hand, but if the patient has literacy difficulties or problems with sight, other means of communication must be sought. The establishment of a good communication scheme preoperatively will help the patient to regain confidence postoperatively and should minimise frustration.

The SALT will visit the patient preoperatively to explain their role, and may suggest that a visit from a previous laryngectomy patient would be of benefit. This visitor must be someone who has developed good speech, is an effective communicator and is well integrated back into the community. During this visit it may be suggested that the patient look at the visitor's stoma, but this issue is not forced. If well planned, these visits can be very reassuring to the patient and family. Some people refuse the offer of such a visitor and their choice must be respected.

The physiotherapist will also assess the patient prior to surgery, explaining their role in the patient's postoperative care and teaching them deep breathing and leg exercises.

In the period leading up to surgery, it is important that any malnourishment is corrected by enteral or parenteral supplements. The dietitian or nursing staff will assess the patient's nutritional state preoperatively and will explain to the patient how they will be fed postoperatively. A study by Lennie et al (2001) indicates that more preoperative information and education on what to expect postoperatively is needed (see Research Abstract 14.3). Kelsey (1997) describes a successful nutritional assessment tool. The duration of parenteral feeding is dependent on the type of surgery performed and the state of the wound.

Postoperative priorities

Immediately following surgery the main nursing priorities will be maintenance of a clear airway (see Box 14.5), observation of the tracheostome, management of pain, establishment of good communication with the patient, and reassurance and support of the patient and family.

The patient will be nursed in the semi-recumbent position initially and then gradually encouraged to sit more upright to aid respiration and neck drainage. It is important that the patient's head is flexed slightly forward to ease tension on the suture lines. When the patient is being moved, the head should always be supported.

Initially the patient's vital signs should be recorded at half-hourly intervals; as these become stable within the normal range, recordings can be reduced to 4-hourly. In the immediate postoperative period the naso/stomagastric tube should be on free drainage to prevent vomiting. This allows the pharyngeal repair to heal and prevents fistula

RESEARCH ABSTRACT 14.3

Are we preparing laryngectomy patients adequately for changes in eating habits?

This descriptive study obtained its sample from a national internet-based laryngectomy support group in the United States. There were 34 returned questionnaires (an 83% response rate); 85% of the respondents were male. The mean age was 62 years (range 47–76) with an average of 5 years since laryngectomy had been performed. The participants completed a Food Eating Experiences and Diet Questionnaire which was designed by the researchers to provide qualitative and quantitative data.

A pilot study which tested the questionnaire on five laryngectomees resulted in some modifications to content and clarity. There were five sections to the questionnaire with the first three focusing on potential changes related to different aspects of eating. The fourth section measured perception of hunger and appetite. The last section obtained perception of information given by health care professionals on potential changes in eating following laryngectomy. In each section data were collected by either or both Likert and visual analogue scales, with an area for free text to make comments or give explanations.

Ninety per cent of the participants experienced some change. Most frequently noted were decreases in smell, taste, the overall enjoyment of eating and desire to try new foods and an increase in the time it took to eat meals. Fifty per cent of the participants found they took at least 10 min longer to eat a meal. For the majority, laryngectomy did not affect their perception of hunger and appetite and the number of meals eaten each day. A large number indicated their lack of satisfaction with the information related to eating and nutrition which they had received prior to surgery. Comments indicated that the information was either insufficient or incomplete, with the loss of taste and smell in particular needing more attention. Some respondents felt the information received focused primarily on speech changes. Most participants found themselves looking for information on eating and nutrition from a variety of non-health care sources including laryngectomee support groups and websites.

The results indicated that, as well as increasing the amount and detail of preoperative information and teaching on alterations following laryngectomy, facilitating access to laryngectomy information sources and support groups was a worthwhile intervention. Solving these problems can be made easier by discussing them with those who have experienced the same or similar problems.

Lennie T A, Christman S K, Jadack R A 2001 Educational needs and altered eating habits following a total laryngectomy. Oncology Nursing Forum 28(4): 667–674

Box 14.5

Resuscitation of a 'neck breathing' patient

The principles of resuscitation of a 'neck breathing' patient are the same as those for any other patient, although a few alterations of technique apply. The ABCs of first aid — airway, breathing and circulation — are given top priority.

Initially, the stoma would be covered by the resuscitator's mouth, but as soon as possible a cuffed tracheal tube should be inserted, and inflated to prevent any leakage of the air which is being introduced by the resuscitator. The tube should then be connected to an Ambu bag and resuscitation continued as normal. The National Association of Laryngectomee Clubs has a video, *LIFE*, which demonstrates the correct methods (see 'Useful websites').

Box 14.6

Potential complications of laryngectomy

Psychosocial distress
Laryngectomy can be viewed as a series of losses which present enormous challenges and require a great deal of adaptation. It can result in psychological morbidity, including depression, low self-esteem, poor sleep, fears of isolation and rejection. Feber (2000) makes the point that, when measuring the success of their surgery, patients include social, economic and cultural as well as medical factors.

Blockage of the trachea
This potentially life-threatening complication can occur if the trachea has not been sufficiently humidified and the stoma cleaned. The potential for tracheal blockage should be stressed during the educational preparation of the patient for discharge, as it tends to occur when patients have returned to the community and have not cared for their stoma, in particular the humidification and cleansing aspects of care, as taught in hospital. As a result, mucus will have been allowed to accumulate in and around the stoma where it has dried to produce a crust which can become large enough to cause an obstruction to the airway. Postoperative radiotherapy which includes the trachea in the fields can cause mucositis of the tracheal lining and viscous secretions which can produce a similar result.

Stenosis of the tracheostome
Like tracheal blockage, this complication is potentially life threatening and may occur when the patient has returned to the community. It may be the result of fibrosis occurring as healing takes place, in which case wearing a stoma button or tube for part or all of the time can be an effective preventive method. The patient should have been made aware of this potential problem and taught that observation of stoma size, using a stoma gauge if necessary, is an essential part of daily stoma care and that help should be sought if there is any reduction in size or difficulty in breathing. Some patients may need a stomaplasty, a refashioning procedure which will increase the size of the stoma.

Failure to produce voice
Coltart (1998) discusses why, despite advances including surgical voice restoration and the use of voice prostheses, not all patients learn to speak again but become dependent on non-verbal communication.

Fistula formation
If the pharyngeal repair breaks down, a fistula may form which allows saliva and food to leak from the incision, causing excoriation of the skin and possibly leading to infection. This is usually treated by inserting a feeding tube, if one is not already in place, and ensuring that the patient does not take any oral fluids until healing has taken place. Reilly (1998) gives a comprehensive overview of enteral feeding, including techniques which can be used in this situation. Healing may take several weeks and antibiotics may be prescribed if infection is present. If the fistula does not heal spontaneously, surgical closure may be necessary.

Wound breakdown
This is most likely to occur in patients who have had radiotherapy prior to surgery. Careful wound care can help to prevent its occurrence.

formation (see Box 14.6). A stomagastric tube is inserted through a created tracheo-oesophageal fistula, which is later used for a voice prosthesis.

Once bowel sounds have been detected, usually 24 h postoperatively, the patient can commence fluids. Water is given first, then full-strength feeding is gradually established. This gradual progression is necessary to avoid the problems of vomiting and diarrhoea. The nurse must check that the naso/stomagastric tube is in the correct position. Once naso/stomagastric feeding has been established, the i.v. infusion will be discontinued.

STOP THINK **14.10** What are the methods for confirming that the naso/stomagastric tubes are correctly positioned in the stomach? (See Ch. 21.)

Humidified oxygen is administered to the patient during the immediate postoperative period to help keep the lining of the tracheal mucosa and the inspired gases moist (Baxter et al 1993). The patient may have a cuffed (preferably with a low-pressure cuff) tracheostomy tube in position (see Fig. 14.7, p. 616). The cuff pressure must be recorded and released as soon as possible to prevent damage to the tracheal lining. The tube is usually removed 24–48 h after surgery. Some patients return from theatre without a tube in position; here careful observation of the stoma for swelling or obstruction will be necessary. Normally, excessive secretions are moved into the trachea by ciliary action and expelled by coughing. For the new laryngectomy patient, this can be difficult, and tracheal suction is necessary in the immediate postoperative period as these secretions can be excessive and the patient is able to make only limited coughing movements.

A drain will be present on each side of the neck. These drains must be patent at all times. The colour, nature and amount of drainage must be recorded. The wound is closed with fine sutures or clips and may be covered by a clear plastic dressing to aid observation. Stoma care is performed as necessary and usually at least twice daily postoperatively to prevent crusting and infection.

Good pressure area care is necessary in the first 24 h, but care must be taken when moving the patient due to the neck wound. A 2-hourly change of position should be carried out and full use made of special mattresses.

The immediate postoperative period can be very difficult for the patient and family as they realise the full implications of the surgery. Often the patient is very agitated the first time they are sufficiently awake to ask for something and discover that they have no voice. The communication skills of the ENT nurse are especially important at this time. The nurse should remind the patient of the prearranged communication plan and display patience and understanding (see Box 14.7). The patient should never be left without any means of communication or help such as a buzzer or bell. This is very important for the patient's confidence to avoid the very natural fear of requiring tracheal suction and not being able to attract attention.

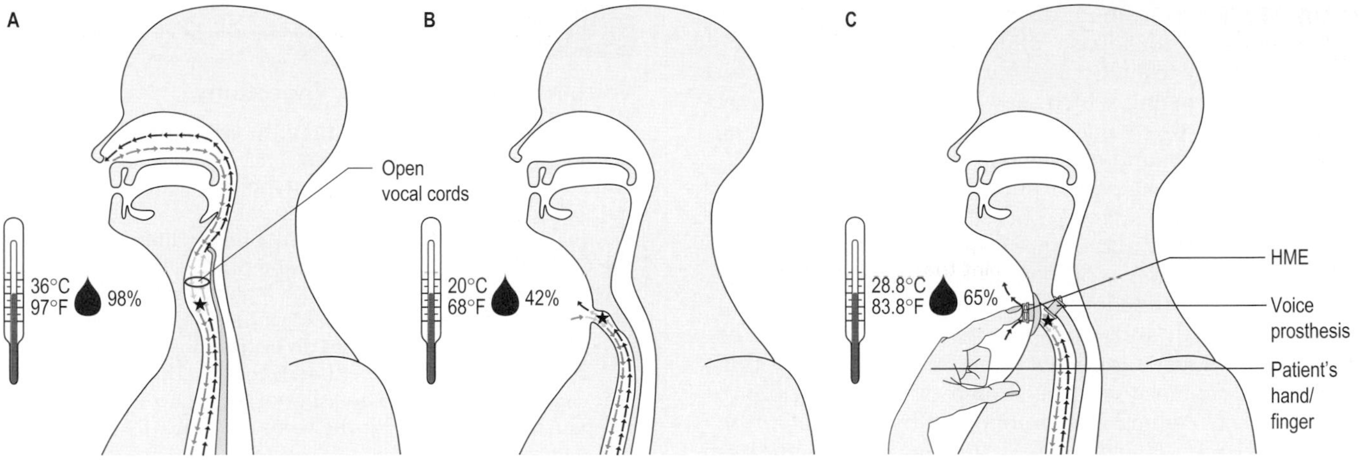

Fig. 14.6 Pre- and post-laryngectomy humidification and temperature levels, with HME and voice prosthesis in place. A: Before laryngectomy the humidification and temperature are at high levels. B: After laryngectomy they drop drastically, leading to excessive mucus production and coughing. C: With an HME a significant improvement in the humidity and temperature is obtained, reducing physical and psychological problems. The HME is being used in combination with a Provo voice prosthesis. (Adapted with kind permission from Platon Medical Ltd.)

Box 14.7

Communication with a person who has lost the ability to speak following head and neck surgery

- As much preoperative explanation and information as possible should be given in the time available.
- Adequate materials, e.g. pen, paper, picture cards or 'magic' slate, should be available, and be seen by the patient to be available, before surgery and subsequently at all times.
- Be patient, and maintain a calm and unhurried atmosphere.
- Always give encouragement and praise.
- Remember that previous hearing levels have not been altered. There is no need for you to raise your voice or write down information.
- Pay extra special attention to non-verbal communication such as facial expression, hand and body positions and movements.
- Stress that the inability to communicate is temporary; skill levels will considerably improve in almost all patients.
- Communicating by writing only is difficult for most. The following points are worth remembering:
  — some people are unable to read or write, i.e. they are illiterate
  — writing takes much longer than speaking
  — writing can be disruptive of thought processes
  — for most people it is difficult to communicate depth of emotions and feelings by the written word
  — lack of privacy (? use 'magic' slate which can be immediately erased)
  — never read a previously written communication unless invited to do so.
- Do not ask two questions at once.
- On occasions, ask questions that only require a yes or no answer.
- Develop your own lip-reading skills.
- Do not finish sentences for the person.
- If the person is only able to say the first few words or part of a sentence, repeat what you have understood and ask them to fill in on what you have missed.

Mouth care is particularly important while the nasogastric tube is in position. The specific mouth care given to each patient will be determined by individual assessment.

STOP THINK **14.11** Try not speaking for a minimum of 1 h during an average non-working day. Record how you felt during this time, indicating the number of times you went to speak and the times you actually were unable to stop yourself automatically speaking. Discuss your findings with your mentor or personal tutor.

On the first or second postoperative day, the patient is usually well enough to be helped out of bed and begin walking. Over the following days the patient should be encouraged to increase activity until fully ambulant.

Naso/stomagastric feeding is continued until the patient's pharyngeal repair is fully healed, usually 10–14 days after surgery. This is tested by a SALT, who administers a swallowing assessment, which involves giving the patient a drink of dye and observing the wound for any signs of leakage. If the wound appears to have healed, the naso/stomagastric tube is removed at the surgeon's discretion and the patient is allowed to commence a soft diet. Foods should be of a gradually increasing consistency until a normal diet for that person is tolerated. However, Lennie et al (2001) found that many have significant long-term alterations to eating habits (see Research Abstract 14.3).

Wound drains are removed when drainage is minimal (approximately 3–4 days after surgery). The neck sutures may be removed around the seventh day, or later if the patient has had previous radiotherapy. Stoma sutures are usually removed after 10 days.

Tracheal suction is given when necessary, but the need for this should gradually diminish as the patient's cough reflexes become stronger. Stoma care is continuous; the nurse should encourage the patient to participate in this. Mechanical humidification may still be required at certain times (see Fig. 14.6); alternatively, a Buchanan laryngectomy protector or similar other lightweight protector may be worn. A heat moisture exchanger (HME) is a highly effective and increasingly popular means of providing humidification (see Fig. 14.6c). It is a small, disposable, lightweight device which can fit on to a base plate over the stoma or be connected directly to a tube. The patient must be taught how to remove any crusting which may form around the stoma. Patients needing to wear a tube or stoma button must be shown how to clean and change it.

Rehabilitation of the patient should start as soon as possible; ideally, this will involve the supportive participation of the patient's family and of the community nurse. Dropkin (1989), in her seminal work on the relationship between disfigurement, dysfunction and coping ability, found that between the fourth and sixth postoperative days could be considered the most significant time in terms of accepting the defect. Acceptance may be shown by the performance of self-care tasks, which is then followed by re-socialisation behaviours. Lack of achievement in these areas indicates a need for increased nursing intervention. The patient will first need to become accustomed to their altered appearance. If appropriate, they could be given a hand mirror, perhaps on the second postoperative day, after the nurse has explained what they should expect. The presence of family members at this time might be helpful but the patient should make the decision about this. Progress in wound healing and a decrease in face and neck swelling over a period of days can be encouraging for the patient. Once accustomed to looking in a mirror, the patient should be encouraged to wipe away secretions from the stoma, gradually progressing to performing stoma care and changing the stoma tube or button by themselves. The patient must be made aware of the importance of wearing a protector for humidification purposes to prevent the formation of crusts which can cause obstruction as well as a predisposition to chest infections.

Voice rehabilitation

Coltart (1998) considers what forms of operative planning will be most appropriate to achieve the best results for the patient. The surgeon, with the SALT and other members of the MDT, will have discussed voice rehabilitation with the patient preoperatively. In selecting the most appropriate voice aid, they will have addressed the physical, social and psychological needs of the patient, as not every voice aid is suited to all patients.

Following laryngectomy, voice rehabilitation will begin when the surgeon and SALT are satisfied that the wounds are adequately healed. Some patients will be reviewed in outpatient departments for fitting of a prosthesis. The SALT will see patients on a regular basis to teach the use of the aid. It is important to advise patients that it can take time to achieve coherent speech again.

Once the naso/stomagastric tube has been removed, the SALT can begin to start voice rehabilitation by means of speaking valves or oesophageal speech. If the patient has mastered a few simple words prior to discharge, their confidence may be increased tremendously. Motivation and support are important factors in the acquisition of speech; again, the participation of the patient's family can be of enormous benefit. Following discharge the patient will continue to attend for speech therapy. Voice restoration methods available for individuals who have undergone laryngectomy are described in Box 14.8.

Box 14.8

Voice restoration after laryngectomy

Tracheo-oesophageal puncture with voice prosthesis
The voice prosthesis is a valve which can be inserted into a puncture created at the time of laryngectomy (primary puncture) or later (secondary puncture). The patient breathes in, covers their stoma with a finger, thus forcing the expired air through the valve and producing voice. Alternatively, a special housing and 'hands free' system incorporating a heat moisture exchanger (HME), which opens on inspiration and closes on expiration, can be used instead of the patient's finger (see Fig. 14.6). The speech and language therapist (SALT) and specialist nursing staff teach the patient how to care for the valve and other devices.

Oesophageal speech
Oesophageal speech was formerly the only method available to restore voice after laryngectomy. In order to master this technique, the patient should have regular sessions with a specialised SALT over a period of months at least. Success rates are very variable. If a valve has been inserted, most SALTs will still teach this method alongside the techniques used with valves, as no single method can guarantee success.

Electronic vibrator or artificial larynx
This device, when applied to the soft tissues of the neck, produces a tone, so that, when the patient articulates, sound is produced. Initially, it can take some time to find the exact place on the neck which gives the best result. The sound produced is monotonous and somewhat mechanical, and for these reasons it is unacceptable to some. It can also be of limited use if the neck is tender or painful.

Pen and paper, hand-held computer
Either of these methods is used by some people, from preference or if all of the above approaches have been unsuccessful.

Preparation for discharge

By demonstrating patience and understanding and sensitively implementing a planned rehabilitation programme, the MDT can help to build up the patient's confidence prior to discharge, to try to ensure that the patient will be able to cope with any problem that may arise. The patient should feel at ease with the stoma and be confident in caring for it and for any voice prosthesis. They should be encouraged to socialise with other patients, perhaps by moving to a multi-bed room. Most centres use a staged discharge plan with the patient going home for at least one overnight stay or weekend before discharge.

Mason et al (1992) describe a stepwise method for teaching self-care to laryngectomy patients prior to discharge, called the Nottingham system. The aim is to identify problems early, assess progress continuously and provide extra support when needed. Tracheostome care is divided into 10 different aspects of care, e.g. removing the tube, cleaning the stoma and skin care. Each element of care is then broken down into five teaching phases, commencing with the professional performing the task and ending when the patient is totally self-caring. The date of successful completion of each phase is recorded. Before starting the teaching plan an agreement is reached between patient and professionals on the anticipated number of days required to reach competence. If a patient is found to require a considerably longer time to gain competence in any aspect of self-care, the GP is informed of the likely need for extra support. Although the Nottingham system was devised for laryngectomy patients, it can just as easily be used for those who have had a tracheostomy.

The community nursing services will be involved in preparations for the patient's return home. They will be contacted by ward staff as soon as a discharge date has been decided. The community nurse's main role is one of support and they will withdraw services slowly as the patient becomes increasingly confident at home. It is important to support the patient's partner and family as they also have just experienced challenging situations. Vickery et al (2003) found some partners experienced more distress than the patients.

A social worker is often required to help patients and their families with practical difficulties before, during and following surgery. Some individuals who have undergone a laryngectomy may be unable to return to their former employment. For example, those who were previously employed doing heavy manual labour will be unable to resume such work because, following laryngectomy, they are unable to hold their breath and increase intrathoracic pressure. Negotiation between the social worker and the employer to try to find a feasible job reallocation may allow such a patient to continue working. However, if continued employment is impossible, the social worker and/or a benefits advisor will assist patients to receive all the social security benefits to which they are entitled. The social worker or CNS may also be able to help patients and their families with travelling expenses during the treatment programme by obtaining a cancer charity grant.

Patients will attend the ENT or head and neck oncology outpatient clinic after discharge to ensure that no problems arise with which they feel unable to cope. The National Association of Laryngectomee Clubs (NALC) circulates a regular newsletter and has branches in most areas of the UK (see 'Useful websites'). The support that this Association can give is invaluable to many patients, who greatly benefit from the opportunity to share experiences and talk about problems with others in a similar situation. Many patients also form lasting friendships with those laryngectomy patient(s) who visited them preoperatively. NALC holds regular national study days for nurses and other health care professionals.

For further information on coping with dysfunction and disfigurement after head and neck cancer surgery, see Dropkin (1989, 1997). For information on promoting self-esteem after laryngectomy, see Feber (1996). More information on rehabilitation is to be found in Clarke (1998) and on post-discharge care in the community on the NALC website (see 'Useful websites').

Tracheostomy

The surgical procedure of tracheostomy involves making an opening through the skin and structures of the neck into the trachea. It is one of the earliest operations described; there is evidence that it was performed by the Egyptians in biblical times.

A tracheostomy may be short or long term and may be planned as elective surgery or performed as an emergency procedure.

Indications

The indications for a tracheostomy are as follows:

- *Airway obstruction* — this may be caused by the inhalation and impaction of a foreign body in the larynx. Severe inflammation may also cause obstruction, as might laryngeal cancer which is being treated by radiotherapy.
- *Bronchial toilet* — after head injury, drug overdose, cerebrovascular accident, coma or certain neurological disorders, the patient may require assistance with respiration and removal of bronchial secretions.
- *Need to improve respiratory efficiency* — when patients with impaired respiration are relying on their own efforts rather than assisted ventilation, the performance of a tracheostomy cuts down dead space and improves respiratory efficiency by 30–50% (Serra 1998).
- *Artificial ventilation* — if artificial ventilation is required for more than 72 h, a tracheostomy may be indicated, as it has been shown that endotracheal intubation for 72 h or longer can cause laryngotracheal damage.
- *Major head and neck surgery* — a tracheostomy will maintain the airway and protect it from haemorrhage and obstruction due to oedema both during and after surgery (see also Ch. 28).

Box 14.9 lists some of the indications for short- and long-term tracheostomies.

MEDICAL MANAGEMENT

Prior to performing a tracheostomy, the medical staff must explain to the conscious patient what is involved and the effect the procedure will have. In an emergency situation, such as when the patient presents with stridor or is unconscious, the medical and nursing staff will have minimal opportunity or time to prepare the patient pre-operatively. Consequently, a planned programme of support and explanation will be required afterwards.

Box 14.9

Indications for tracheostomy

Short-term tracheostomy
- Assisted ventilation
- Burns and scalds
- Foreign body lodged in trachea
- Major head and neck surgery
- Severe infection
- Trauma to larynx, face, mouth or oropharynx
- Vocal cord paralysis

Long-term tracheostomy
- Congenital deformity
- Trauma causing permanent damage
- Untreatable tumours, causing airway obstruction
- Vocal cord paralysis

Tracheostomy is usually carried out with the patient under a general anaesthetic, but in emergencies a local anaesthetic may be used. Tracheostomy involves making an incision into the trachea through the third and fourth tracheal rings. The percutaneous or mini-tracheostomy is infrequently used in the ENT situation.

For further information on this, see Fisher & Howard (1992).

An appropriately sized tracheostomy tube is then inserted. For the first 24–48 h, a cuffed tracheostomy tube (see Fig. 14.7) is normally used to prevent blood from the wound being aspirated and aspiration pneumonia developing. A permanent tract usually forms 2–3 days postoperatively, at which time it is possible to change the tube. Tracheal dilators must always be to hand in case the tube is expelled accidentally and it is necessary to keep the stoma open. Most hospitals have a policy regarding the first tube change, which is likely to be performed by medical staff or experienced nursing staff with medical back-up.

There are several types of tracheostomy tube available, and the most appropriate one will be chosen for each patient. As mentioned above, a cuffed tube, preferably with a low-pressure cuff, may be inserted during the operation. Single-use disposable tubes are usually employed and may be cuffed or plain. All tubes have an introducer, which is removed immediately on insertion, and an inner tube, which can be removed for cleaning without necessitating removal of the whole tube. Most tubes are made of polyvinyl chloride (PVC) and silicone, although silver tubes are occasionally used.

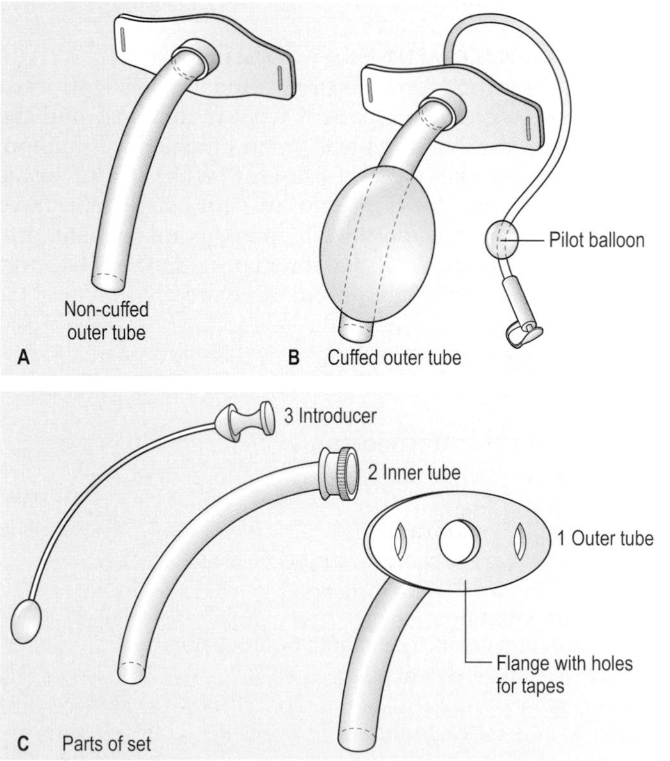

Fig. 14.7 Tracheostomy tubes in common use. A: Non-cuffed outer tube. B: Cuffed outer tube. C: Parts of tracheostomy tube set.

NURSING PRIORITIES AND MANAGEMENT: Tracheostomy

Preoperative priorities

Physical and psychological preparation of the individual for a tracheostomy is a priority of preoperative nursing care as the procedure can cause many difficulties. If the tracheostomy is short term, these problems will be of limited duration, but if it is to be long term, the patient and family will require additional information and education. They may need help in coming to terms not only with the problems presented by the stoma but also with the diagnosis, e.g. cancer, that necessitated surgery. Patients who have been well prepared for a tracheostomy tend to cope better than those who have not. Unprepared patients may become insecure, withdrawn and depressed. The main problems in the immediate postoperative period, for which the patient has to be prepared prior to surgery, are as follows:

Temporary loss of voice Air will bypass the vocal cords following the tracheostomy, making speech impossible unless a tube with a speaking valve is inserted. A system of communication whereby the patient can make themselves understood by staff and family members should be worked out beforehand (see p. 611 and Box 14.7).

Altered body image Body image is concerned with the control and function as well as physical appearance of the body. The very thought of coughing out sputum, which most people usually go to great lengths to hide, but which in the case of the patient who has a tracheostomy must be done through an open hole and tube in their neck, as well as their need for suction, is not easy to understand and accept. High quality information and education must be offered to help the patient and family adjust to the presence of a tube in the neck. A visit from a patient who has adjusted well to having a tracheostomy may help.

Increased secretions These are produced because of the irritation caused by the tube and air bypassing the nose. This should be explained to the patient along with the need for suction. It is helpful, if possible, to show the equipment required for this prior to surgery.

Ideally, a patient undergoing tracheostomy should be nursed in a single room initially and care assigned to one nurse who can gain the confidence of the patient and family.

Postoperative priorities

Maintenance of the airway

On return to the ward the patient should be nursed in a sitting position with the neck well supported; the tapes around the neck, which are fixed to the flange of the tracheostomy tube, must be tied securely in position.

Suction should be carried out when necessary. To prevent infection, it is necessary to perform this procedure with a clean technique, according to Harris (1984) and Harris and Hyman (1984), whose research has not yet been superseded (see also Ch. 28). A sterile catheter should be used each time and should touch only the inside of the tracheostomy tube. The catheter diameter should be no more than half that of the tube to allow adequate flow of gases around it. If it is too wide, it will draw air out of the lungs more quickly than it can be replaced, which can cause atelectasis. Griggs (1998) gives a formula and chart to allow calculation of the correct catheter size.

Suction should be applied only as the catheter is being removed. Thumb-control catheters are ideal for this. Since the patient is unable to breathe during suction, it should be performed for no longer than 10–15 s; the patient should be allowed enough time to recover before it is repeated. The amount and type of secretions should be observed and recorded. A study on tracheal suction by Day et al (2002) indicated poor levels of knowledge and potentially unsafe practice among the nurses studied.

The physiotherapist will teach the patient how to cough into a tissue; as the patient becomes competent at this, the need for suction will gradually be eliminated.

Continuous humidification is given immediately post-operatively via a mechanical humidifier. When the patient begins to be up and about, a protector over the stoma will humidify inhaled air, act as a filter and have a cosmetic effect by covering the tube.

Care of the wound

The stoma into which the tube is inserted will require regular cleansing to prevent crusting and infection. A dressing beneath the tracheostomy tube can aid comfort and help to prevent sores caused by the tube and hard flanges as well as excoriation of the skin from tracheal secretions. However, these dressings can be a source of infection (Bond et al 2003). Skin can be protected with a barrier cream or film. If sutures are present, these will be removed according to local policy (see Ch. 23, p. 856).

For further information on adult tracheostomy care, see Serra (2000); for a pictorial guide, see Harkin & Russell (2001a).

Complications

The following complications may occur after tracheostomy. Hackeling et al (1998) describe a 7-year audit of complications that brought tracheostomy patients to the Emergency Department.

Blockage of tracheostomy tube Tracheal dilators and a spare cuffed tracheostomy tube must always be kept to hand in case this problem arises. Sometimes the blockage can be relieved by suction or by changing the inner tube. At other times it will be necessary to change the whole tube.

Displacement of the tube The tube can become displaced into the pre-tracheal tissue or completely out of the stoma if the tapes holding it in place have not been secured adequately. Dilators should be used to keep the stoma open until the tube can be replaced. Tapes should be checked for correct fit at least twice daily. Assessment and management of a patient in this situation are described by Seay and Gay (1997).

Surgical emphysema Emphysema is the abnormal presence of air in the tissues. Surgical emphysema is iatrogenic in origin, being a result of faulty suturing, and can be corrected by releasing the sutures.

Haemorrhage The insertion of a cuffed tracheostomy tube can help to control bleeding and prevent aspiration of blood. It is possible, however, for a major blood vessel to be eroded by a badly placed or poorly managed tube, causing a massive haemorrhage.

Dysphagia, nausea, vomiting If the tracheostomy tube is the wrong shape for the type of tracheostomy and the size of the patient, it may also tether the larynx and exert excess pressure on the posterior wall of the trachea and oesophagus, resulting in nausea, dysphagia and vomiting. These effects can be relieved by the insertion of a different type of tube.

Damage to the tracheal mucosa This can result from poor suctioning technique, badly chosen or improperly inserted tubes, or prolonged and/or overinflation of the tube cuff. Ulceration of the anterior wall or a tracheo-oesophageal fistula may result and can lead to tracheal stenosis.

Infection A wound or respiratory tract infection can result from poor technique when performing stoma toilet, changing the tube or applying suction, or from inadequate maintenance of respiratory status.

Changing the tracheostomy tube

The first tube change should be performed by experienced medical or nursing staff, as it takes 2–3 days for a tract to form and there is a danger of the tube being displaced or inserted into the pre-tracheal tissues. Two people should always be present for this procedure. One will remove the old tube and the other will immediately insert the new one. The tapes are then securely tied.

Decannulation or removal of the tube

The tube can be removed without any preliminaries, but usually the patient is gradually reintroduced to breathing through the nose and mouth. A tube with a speaking valve allows the patient to breathe in through the tube and out through the larynx. Once the patient has become accustomed to this, the tube can be replaced by a 'blocker' so that the patient has to breathe in through the nose and mouth. Once able to tolerate this continuously for 24 h and oxygen saturation levels are satisfactory day and night, the tracheostomy tube can be removed. Another method of achieving decannulation is to insert a smaller tube each time it is changed.

Whichever method is used, after removal of the tube a dressing must be applied to allow the tracheostomy site to heal. This can be a very anxious time for patients and support and encouragement are necessary. The stoma should shrink rapidly and close off in a short time.

Humidification

Humidification will prevent the tracheostomy patient breathing in cold dry air, which could cause the secretions of the trachea to become dry and difficult to remove and eventually lead to infection and blockage of the tube. A selection of aesthetically pleasing covers, which humidify and filter the air, are available and the patient should be introduced to these before discharge. A HME can be worn under these covers.

Preparation for discharge

Before discharge can take place, the patient and family must be well prepared for all foreseeable difficulties and should be proficient in total care of the tracheostomy tube. The teaching of self-care techniques can begin with the nurse demonstrating procedures while the patient watches in a mirror. Rudy and McCullagh (2001) describe a nurse teaching programme initiated in order to help non-specialist nurses develop skills and confidence in identifying barriers to learning and motivation when teaching tracheostomy care to their patients. It is wise to teach not only the patient but also the family how to care for the tracheostomy in case the occasion arises when the patient is unable to do this themselves (Mason et al 1992). However, some surgeons do prefer their patients to report to the ward or unit for a weekly tube change.

For an outline of outpatient nursing care, see Minsley & Wrenn (1996).

The community nurse will be actively involved in the patient's discharge and reintegration into the community. Ideally, they will visit the patient in hospital and arrange for suction apparatus to be installed in the home if necessary. After discharge, they should visit the home regularly to ensure that the patient is coping with the stoma and altered body image. Barnett (2005) gives an overview of the care needed by a patient living with a tracheostomy in the community.

Tonsillitis

The tonsils are composed of lymphoid tissue and lie between the faucial pillars (see Fig. 14.8). During early childhood they enlarge in response to upper respiratory tract infections and in adulthood should become reduced in size. In old age they normally atrophy. It is generally agreed that tonsils have a role to play in the body's defence system against infection.

Each year an average of 12 000 people in the UK undergo the surgical procedure of tonsillectomy. The majority of these patients are 14 years of age or younger. Among people aged 15–25, more females seem to require this surgery than males. Among the older population the tonsils are usually removed as a treatment for tumour.

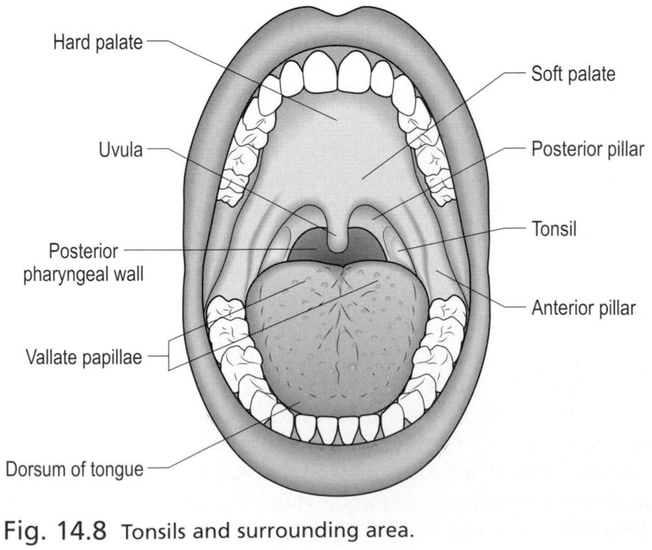

Fig. 14.8 Tonsils and surrounding area.

PATHOPHYSIOLOGY

Common presenting symptoms Patients usually present with a sore throat. Tonsil pain increases with swallowing and is often referred to the ear because of the involvement of the trigeminal nerve, which supplies both sites. They may also present with pyrexia, inflamed tonsils with exudate, lethargy and the absence of a cough (Scottish Intercollegiate Guidelines Network 1999).

Recurrent bouts of infection are the most common reason for the removal of tonsils. Infection may take the form of acute tonsillitis, acute otitis media (see p. 598) or a peritonsillar abscess (see p. 619). Streptococci, staphylococci and *Haemophilus influenzae* are the organisms most commonly present.

Patients with tonsillar tumours normally present with dysphagia. These patients usually also complain of weight loss and may have speech problems. They may also suffer from facial pain and deafness because of the involvement of cranial nerves. Tonsillar tumours are rare.

MEDICAL MANAGEMENT

There is some controversy among medical practitioners about when tonsil infections should be treated conservatively and when tonsillectomy, with or without adenoidectomy, should be performed. The size of the tonsils is not usually the main criterion, but rather the history of the effect of repeated infections on the general health of the patient. Consideration is also given to absence from school or work, loss of appetite, speech defects, nasal catarrh or colds, hearing loss, breathing problems and abdominal pain, the last a sign of mesenteric adenitis, which occurs because of transmission of infection through the lymphatic system (Scottish Intercollegiate Guidelines Network 1999).

Tonsillectomy is an elective operation and is not considered in the presence of respiratory tract infections, during the incubation period after contact with an infectious disease, or if there is tonsillar inflammation. Tonsils are removed by dissection and any bleeding vessels are ligated or diathermy is applied. There remains a debate about the use of disposable instruments for tonsillectomy.

NURSING PRIORITIES AND MANAGEMENT: Tonsillectomy

Postoperative priorities

Airway

On returning from theatre, patients should be positioned in the post-tonsillectomy position, i.e. semi-prone, as this allows any blood or saliva to flow out of the mouth and helps keep the airway clear.

Haemorrhage

Half-hourly recordings of pulse and blood pressure and observations of breathing, pallor, restlessness and frequent swallowing are carried out to ensure early diagnosis of haemorrhage. Frequent swallowing is one of the first signs of tonsil haemorrhage and can go unnoticed unless the patient is closely observed. Particular attention must be paid to the sleeping patient.

Chewing and swallowing

Encouraging the patient to eat regularly (Cook et al 1992) and to swallow is important, as the exercising of the throat muscles seems to help keep the tonsil bed free from infection and to prevent the occurrence of secondary haemorrhage.

Infection

Pyrexia is not uncommon on the first postoperative day, as part of the general metabolic response to the trauma of surgery, but if it continues, antibiotics should be prescribed and the source of infection sought.

Analgesics

Prescribed analgesics should be administered and their effectiveness observed. They should be administered before meals, before going to sleep and first thing in the morning. Good pain management is vital in ensuring the patient has a comfortable and uncomplicated postoperative recovery.

Preparation for discharge

Patients are usually discharged from hospital within 24 h. They are advised to avoid dirty, dusty atmospheres for approximately 2 weeks and to take a similar amount of time away from work or school/college. An advice sheet should be given on discharge with a contact number to ring should any difficulties be experienced at home, including bleeding, pyrexia and otalgia (earache). Research Abstract 14.4 discusses post-tonsillectomy morbidity after discharge.

Post-tonsillectomy pain control and pain relief following discharge and the adequacy and accuracy of preoperative information and advice were the topics of a study by Stone (1996).

Peritonsillar abscess (quinsy)

PATHOPHYSIOLOGY

This is a very painful condition and can be life threatening. It usually occurs as a complication of acute tonsillitis. Pus forms in the space behind the capsule of the tonsil. The abscess is usually unilateral and affects males more than females.

The patient presents with a pyrexia high enough to cause a rigor. There is usually a history of an episode of acute tonsillitis which has subsided, only to return on one side. There is acute pain radiating to the ear on the affected side, trismus (spasm of the jaw muscles) is present and swallowing is so difficult that saliva dribbles out of the mouth. The voice becomes muffled because of the large swelling which affects the function of the palate. The neck glands on the affected side will be enlarged and tender.

MEDICAL MANAGEMENT

Antibiotic cover must be prescribed and the abscess may need to be incised and drained. Usually it is necessary to administer i.v. fluids, and antibiotics are always given parenterally for the first 24 h. Analgesics will be required when the pain is severe. Very rarely the swelling will be so severe that it will obstruct the airway; it may then be necessary to perform a tracheostomy to allow the patient to breathe.

RESEARCH ABSTRACT 14.4

Early post-tonsillectomy morbidity

This prospective study was undertaken to assess the amount and nature of post-tonsillectomy morbidity within 2 weeks of discharge from hospital. Complete follow-up data were obtained from 149 patients (103 children under 16 years and 46 adults) when they attended a follow-up review with one of the authors. All patients were admitted on the day of surgery, had their tonsils removed by dissection and, with two exceptions, were discharged within 24 h. The two exceptions were discharged within 36 h when pyrexia had subsided and oral antibiotics had been commenced.

Following verbal advice from medical and nursing staff, all patients were discharged with oral analgesics and a written information sheet, which advised different actions for specific problems. In spite of this, a surprisingly large number of patients contacted their GP. Whether these patients were adults or children is not stated. Forty patients (27%) were responsible for a total of 53 GP consultations, 23 were prescribed antibiotics and two were prescribed mouthwashes. Throat pain was the commonest reason for consultation. Two out of five patients who consulted for otalgia were inappropriately prescribed a topical steroid and antibiotic. The responses to secondary haemorrhage were particularly worrying. Nineteen patients had this potentially fatal complication. Despite clear advice to the contrary, only seven patients sought advice or care.

The inability to recognise expected symptoms, such as throat pain, or to seek advice for haemorrhage, despite the information given, led the authors to suggest that all patients who experienced any operation-related problems should telephone the ward in the first instance. The need to improve or reinforce information was recognised, as well as the very real increase in workload for GPs and increase in antibiotic prescriptions. Other suggestions for improvement included routine assessment by a nurse practitioner and giving patients a review appointment which could be cancelled if all was well.

As the number of day case patients and early discharges continue to rise, the need to provide patients with information which can be clearly understood, remembered and accepted, so as to enable patients to recognise problems and act appropriately when they do occur, is essential. General practitioners must also become familiar with normal symptoms and responses to tonsillectomy.

Kuo M, Hegarty D, Johnson A, Stevenson S 1995 Early post-tonsillectomy morbidity following hospital discharge: do patients and GPs know what to expect? Health Trends 27(3): 98 –100

NURSING PRIORITIES AND MANAGEMENT: Peritonsillar abscess

Nursing care of the patient with peritonsillar abscess will include:

- physical and psychological support of the patient
- administration of analgesics, antipyretics and antibiotics
- administration of prescribed i.v. fluids
- ensuring good oral hygiene
- observation and recording of the patient's airway, temperature, pulse, blood pressure, fluid intake and output
- care of the tracheostomy if this has been performed (see p. 616).

Patients who require admission to hospital will be very anxious, agitated and in pain. They will require explanations, reassurance and swift administration of analgesics. As many will be unable to swallow, observations must be made for signs of dehydration; if dehydration is present, it will be necessary to administer i.v. fluids as prescribed by medical staff.

Good oral hygiene is important, especially once the abscess has been drained, as the patient will have had to spit out pus and will have a foul taste in the mouth. Once the pain has been relieved by analgesics and drainage of the abscess, the patient will be able to commence oral fluids and gradually begin taking a normal diet. Oral antibiotics will be substituted for the i.v. administration.

The patient is usually discharged once able to eat and drink normally and has been apyrexial for 24 h. If the abscess has been severe enough to require a tracheostomy, this would be removed and the patient would be discharged only when the wound had healed. Patients are often sent home before they have finished their course of antibiotics; the importance of completing the course must therefore be clearly explained to them. Most patients who have a previous history of tonsillitis are re-admitted in 6–8 weeks to have a tonsillectomy performed as peritonsillar abscesses have a habit of recurring.

For further details of the management and care of a patient with a peritonsillar abscess, see McCall (1993).

Snoring/obstructive sleep apnoea (OSA)

Over the last few years, the issue of snoring in association with OSA has been addressed as it has been recognised that these individuals may have a contributing anatomical defect.

PATHOPHYSIOLOGY

The patient may show signs of chronic sleep deprivation. The patient's partner and/or family may complain of loud snoring and periods of breath-holding when the patient is asleep. This may be as a result of the tissues of the soft palate and pharynx collapsing and causing a temporary obstruction of the oropharynx. When the patient breathes, this tissue, including the uvula and possibly large tonsils, may vibrate, resulting in loud snoring. Patients may hold their breath due to this obstructing tissue. This condition can be dangerous, due to the possible development of severe hypoxaemia and systemic and pulmonary hypertension (Shenwell & Wilson 1994).

MEDICAL MANAGEMENT

Investigations Admission to hospital for a sedation nasendoscopy will be necessary. By means of a nasendoscope the medical staff can view the oropharynx of the sleeping patient and observe the activity and position of the tissues and structures. At this time monitoring of oxygen saturation levels is also possible.

Many centres now carry out sleep studies, which record the patient's breathing, snoring and pattern of electrical activity during overnight sleep.

Treatment A variety of treatments is available. These include weight loss in overweight people, change of sleeping position, mandibular advancement splints and the use of nasal decongestants. Continuous positive airway pressure may also be used (see below).

If it is obvious that there is collapse of excess tissues in the oropharynx, then the surgical technique of uvulopalatopharyngoplasty, with or without tonsillectomy, may be performed at a later date. This involves tightening of the soft palate and pharyngeal tissue, removal of the uvula and possible tonsillectomy. Correction using a laser or punctate diathermy is an alternative procedure (Macdougald 1994, Whinney et al 1995).

Lasers are used for a wide range of problems in ENT, not only sleep apnoea. For fuller details, see McKennis & Waddington (1993).

NURSING PRIORITIES AND MANAGEMENT: Obstructive sleep apnoea (OSA)

Uvulopalatopharyngoplasty

The priorities and management are the same as for tonsillectomy (see p. 618). Patients may experience nasal regurgitation on swallowing. This will usually resolve over a short period of time.

Continuous positive airway pressure (CPAP)

This treatment avoids surgery and can be carried out by the patient at home each night. The patient requires a considerable amount of education and supervision during the initial stages and continuous ongoing support. This education and support are usually provided by a specialist nurse who plays a key role in coordinating and implementing continuity of care from the initial sleep investigation stage and throughout.

Nasal CPAP works as a pneumatic splint, as the continuous positive pressure stops the pharynx collapsing and vibrating. At night the patient wears a well-fitting nasal mask which is connected via tubing to a small machine which delivers the positive pressure airflow. The mouth is left uncovered. The nasal cavity needs to be free of obstruction.

Most patients tolerate CPAP well, despite occasional problems with nasal and face irritation. It is most commonly used for moderate to severe OSA.

For further information on sleep apnoea, see Macdougald (1994), Shenwell & Wilson (1994) and Kendrick (1995).

CONCLUSION

The specialty of ENT care is a continually evolving one that presents many challenges to the nurse, who will encounter patients of various ages and backgrounds, each with specific needs in regard to the intensity, duration and setting of treatment. The ENT nurse is likely to encounter a wide range of disorders, some of which will have profound implications for the patient's ability to function within family, work and social spheres and which will require thorough assessment and individualised care planning. As always, the nurse's ability as communicator will do much to determine the effectiveness of these interventions. In this specialty, in which many patients will suffer from disorders that will impair hearing and/or the ability to speak, the need for skill and inventiveness in communication is especially important.

Nurses in various fields can make an important contribution to health education and preventive care as these relate to, for example, smoking and potential and existing ENT disorders. By helping to implement programmes for vaccinations, community and school nurses help to prevent the hearing impairment often seen in children whose mothers contracted rubella during the early months of their pregnancy. A knowledge of how to evaluate noise levels can help occupational health nurses to protect workers from noise-induced hearing loss, and school nurses can alert young people to the fact that personal stereos are capable of producing the same volume of sound as a pneumatic drill, and thus present a serious risk of hearing impairment. For patients with a chronic condition, such as Ménière's disease or tinnitus, hospital and community nurses can provide ongoing psychological support, practical advice on day-to-day coping and information about local support groups. As the causes of certain ENT disorders become better understood, and as pharmacological and surgical treatments make further strides forward, ENT nursing will continue to offer challenges and rewards for nurses in a variety of care settings.

Most large ENT units also care for patients suffering from head and neck cancer. The implementation of the recommendations for cancer units and centres made by Drs Calman and Hine in *A Policy Framework for Commissioning Cancer Services* (HMSO 1995) and the NICE Guidance on commissioning cancer services (NICE 2004) have implications not only for where these patients should receive their care but also for the education and training needs of the nurses who care for them.

REFERENCES

Ayache D, Corre A, Van Prooyen S, Elbaz P 2003 Surgical treatment of otosclerosis in elderly patients. Otolaryngology – Head and Neck Surgery 129(6): 674–677

Barnett M 2005 Tracheostomy management and care. Journal of Community Nursing 19(1): 4, 6–8

Baxter K, Nolan K, Winyard J et al 1993 Are they getting enough? Meeting the oxygen therapy needs of postoperative patients. Professional Nurse 8(5): 310–312

Becker W, Naumann H H, Pfaltz C R 1993 Ear, nose and throat diseases, 2nd edn. Thieme, New York

Bond P, Grant F, Coltart L, Elder F 2003 Best practice in the care of patients with a tracheostomy. Nursing Times 99(30): 24–25

Brackman D E, Shelton C, Arriaga M A (eds) 2001 Otologic surgery, 2nd edn. Elsevier, Philadelphia

Chan E 1997 A talent for listening. Nursing Times 51(93): 36–37

Coltart L 1998 Voice restoration after laryngectomy. Nursing Standard 13(12): 36–40

Cook J A, Murrant N J, Evans K L, Lavelle R J 1992 A randomised comparison of three post tonsillectomy diets. Clinical Otolaryngology 17: 28–31

Day T, Farnell S, Haynes S, Wainwright S, Wilson-Barnett J 2002 Tracheal suctioning: an exploration of nurses' knowledge and competence in acute and high dependency ward areas. Journal of Advanced Nursing 39(11): 35–45

Department of Health 2000 The NHS cancer plan. TSO, London

Dropkin M J 1989 Coping with disfigurement and dysfunction after head and neck cancer surgery: a conceptual framework. Seminars in Oncology Nursing 5(3): 213–219

Ell S R, Parker A J 1992 A study of epistaxis in the elderly. Care of the Elderly 4(2): 80–83

Feber T 1998 Design and evaluation of a strategy to provide support and information for people with cancer of the larynx. European Journal of Oncology Nursing 2(2): 106–114

Feber T 2000 Head and neck oncology nursing. Whurr, London

Forbes K 1997 Palliative care in patients with head and neck cancer. Clinical Otolaryngology 22: 117–122

Gerber M J, Mason J C, Lambert P R 2000 Hearing results after primary cartilage tympanoplasty. Laryngoscope 111(12): 1994–1999

Glover E, Cameron S 2004 Support in the community. Cancer Nursing Practice 3(10): 34–39

Griggs A 1998 Tracheostomy: suctioning and humidification. Nursing Standard Continuing Education Reader. RCN, London

Hackeling T, Triana R, Ma O J, Shockley W 1998 Emergency care of patients with tracheostomies: a 7 year review. American Journal of Emergency Medicine 16(7): 681–685

Hanna E, Sherman A, Cash D et al 2004 Quality of life for patients following total laryngectomy vs chemoradiation for laryngeal preservation. Archives of Otolaryngology – Head and Neck Surgery 130(7): 875–879

Harkin H 2002 Action on ENT: ear care guidance. NHS Modernisation Agency, London

Harris R B 1984 National survey of aseptic tracheostomy care techniques in hospitals with head and neck/ENT surgical departments. Cancer Nursing 7(1): 23–32

Harris R H, Hyman R B 1984 Clean vs. sterile tracheostomy care and level of pulmonary infection. Nursing Research 33(2): 80–85

HMSO 1989 The Noise at Work Regulations. Statutory Instrument 1989 No 790. HMSO, London

HMSO 1995 A policy framework for commissioning cancer services. A report by the expert advisory group on comments by the Chief Medical Officers of England and Wales, April 1995. HMSO, London

Jamieson E M, McCall J M, Blythe R, Whyte L A 2003 Guidelines for clinical nursing practices, 4th edn. Churchill Livingstone, Edinburgh

Jay S, Ruddy J, Cullen R J 1991 Laryngectomy: the patients' view. Journal of Laryngology and Otology 105: 934–938

Kelsey A 1997 A nutritional assessment tool for patients with cancer. Journal of Cancer Nursing 2: 95–97

Kuo M, Hegarty D, Johnson A, Stevenson S 1995 Early post-tonsillectomy morbidity following hospital discharge: do patients and GPs know what to expect? Health Trends 27(3): 98–100

Lauder W 1993 Preventative measures to maintain control: management and treatment of vertigo. Professional Nurse 8(8): 506–508

Lennie T A, Christman S K, Jadack R A 2001 Educational needs and altered eating habits following a total laryngectomy. Oncology Nursing Forum 28(4): 667–674

Macdougald I 1994 Laser therapy for OSAS. Nursing Times 90(19): 32–34

Mason J, Murty G, Foster H, Bradley P C 1992 Tracheostomy self-care: the Nottingham system. Journal of Laryngology and Otology 106: 723–724

McAllen P A 1996 Managing Ménière's

disease. American Journal of Nursing 96(6): 16E–16H
National Centre for Clinical Excellence (NICE) 2004 Improving outcomes in head and neck cancers. NICE, London. (www.nice.org.uk)
Ogretmenoglu O, Yilmaz T, Rahimi K, Aksoyek S 2002 The effect on arterial blood gases and heart rate of bilateral nasal packing. European Archives of Otorhinolaryngology 259(2): 63–66
Price B 1998 Cancer: altered body image. Nursing Standard 12(21): 49–55
Price J 1997 Problems of ear syringing. Practice Nurse 14: 126–128
Ratna H 1994 Counselling deaf and hard of hearing clients. Counselling 5(2): 128–131
Reilly H 1998 Enteral feeding: an overview of indications and techniques. British Journal of Nursing 7(9): 510–512, 514–516, 518
Reynolds T 2004 Ear, nose and throat problems in Accident & Emergency. Nursing Standard 18(26): 47–53, 55
RNID 1999 Noise exposure and hearing loss. Royal National Institute for Deaf People, Policy Division, London
RNID 2003 Facts and figures on deafness and tinnitus. Royal National Institute for Deaf People, London
RNID 2004 A simple cure. A national report into deaf and hard of hearing people's experiences of the National Health Service. Royal National Institute for Deaf People, London
Rudy S F, McCullagh L 2001 Overcoming the top 10 tracheostomy self-care learning barriers. ORL – Head and Neck Nursing 19(2): 8–14
Scottish Intercollegiate Guidelines Network (SIGN) 1999 Management of sore throat and indications for tonsillectomy. Publication No 34. SIGN, Edinburgh
Scottish Intercollegiate Guidelines Network (SIGN) 2003 Diagnosis and management of childhood otitis media in primary care. Publication No 66. SIGN, Edinburgh
Seay S J, Gay S L 1997 Problem in tracheostomy patient care: recognising the patient with a displaced tracheostomy tube. ORL – Head and Neck Nursing 15(2): 10–11
Serra A M 1998 Tracheostomy care: part one. Nursing Standard Continuing Education Reader. RCN, London
Shenwell A, Wilson P 1994 Rest and respiration during obstructive sleep apnoea. Nursing Times 90(19): 30–32
Vickery L E, Latchford G, Hewison J et al 2003 The impact of head and neck cancer and facial disfigurement on the quality of life of patients and their partners. Head and Neck 25: 289–296
Whinney D J, Williamson P A, Bickwell P G 1995 Punctate diathermy of the soft palate: a new approach in the surgical management of snoring. Journal of Laryngology and Otology 109: 849–852

FURTHER READING

Becker W, Naumann H H, Pfaltz C R 1993 Ear, nose and throat diseases, 2nd edn. Thieme, New York
Clarke L K 1998 Rehabilitation for the head and neck cancer patient. Oncology 12(1): 81–94
Cochrane M A 2002 Establishment of a nurse-run acupuncture treatment for hayfever. Complementary Therapies in Nursing and Midwifery 8: 17–20
Davis R, Roberts D 1999 Nursing care of the patient with head and neck cancer. Oncology Nurses Today 4(1): 9–15
Dixson R K 2000 The why, what, and how of endoscopic sinus surgery. Seminars in Perioperative Nursing 9(4):163–167
Dobbins M, Gunson J, Bale S et al 2005 Improving patient care and quality of life ofter laryngectomy/glossectomy. British Journal of Nursing 14(12): 634–640
Docherty B, Bench S 2002 Tracheostomy management for patients in general ward settings. Professional Nurse 18(2): 100–104
Dropkin M J 1989 Coping with disfigurement and dysfunction after head and neck cancer surgery: a conceptual framework. Seminars in Oncology Nursing 5(3): 213–219
Dropkin M J 1997 Coping with disfigurement/dysfunction and length of hospital stay after head and neck cancer surgery. ORL – Head and Neck Nursing 15(1): 22–26
Edward D 1997 Face to face. Patient, family and professional perspectives of head and neck cancer care. King's Fund, London
Edwards M, Feber T 2003 Working with anxiety in cancer: psycho-oncological care. Cancer Nursing Practice 2(1): 19–26
Ell S R, Parker A J 1992 A study of epistaxis in the elderly. Care of the Elderly 4(2): 80–83
Epstein O, Perkin G D, deBono D P, Cookson J 2003 Clinical examination, 3rd edn. Elsevier, London
Feber T 1996 Promoting self-esteem after laryngectomy. Nursing Times 92(30): 37–39
Fisher E W, Howard D J 1992 Percutaneous tracheostomy in a head and neck unit. Journal of Laryngology and Otology 106: 625–627
Gibson A R, McCombe A W 1999 Psychological morbidity following laryngectomy: a pilot study. Journal of Laryngology and Otology 113: 349–352
Harkin H 2002 Action on ENT: ear care guidance. NHS Modernisation Agency, London
Harkin H, Russell C 2001a A guide to tracheostomy patient care. Nursing Times 97(25): 34–36
Harkin H, Russell C 2001b Preparing the patient for tracheostomy tube removal. Nursing Times 97(26): 34–36
Haw S 2002 Providing support to stop smoking. Professional Nurse 17(8): 458–459
Heath I 1994 Tinnitus and health anxiety. British Journal of Nursing 3(10): 502–505
Jamieson E M, McCall J M, Whyte L 2003 Guidelines for clinical nursing practices, 4th edn. Churchill Livingstone, Edinburgh
Kendrick A H 1995 Sleep apnoea. Professional Nurse 10(10): 624–628
Krouse H J 2003 Efficacy of video education for patients and caregivers. ORL – Head and Neck Nursing 21(1): 15–20
Krouse H J, Krouse J H, Christmas D A 1997 Endoscopic sinus surgery in otolaryngology nursing using powered instrumentation. ORL – Head and Neck Nursing 15(2): 22–26
Lauder W 1993 Preventative measures to maintain control: management and treatment of vertigo. Professional Nurse 8(8): 506–508
Macdougald I 1994 Laser therapy for OSAS. Nursing Times 90(19): 32–34
Malem F, Butler K 1993 Nurse-aid management of ear and nose emergencies 2. British Journal of Nursing 2(18): 926–928
McCall M E 1993 It killed George – or managing the peritonsillar abscess patient effectively. ORL – Head and Neck Nursing 11(1): 10–12
McKennis A, Waddington C 1993 Lasers: uses in otolaryngology – lighting the way to the future. ORL – Head and Neck Nursing 11(1): 26–32
Minsley M A, Wrenn S 1996 Long-term care of the tracheostomy patient from an outpatient nursing perspective. ORL – Head and Neck Nursing 14(4): 18–22
Mooney W 2002 Lasers in laryngeal malignancy. ENT News 11(4): 50–52
NHS Quality Improvement Scotland 2003 Caring for the patient with a tracheostomy. Best Practice Statement. NHS Quality Improvement Scotland, Edinburgh. Online. Available: www.nhshealthquality.org
Phillips S 1997 Obstructive sleep apnoea: diagnosis and management. Nursing Standard 11(17): 43–46
Price J 1997 Problems of ear syringing. Practice Nurse 14: 126–128
Semple C J 2002 The role of the CNS in head and neck oncology. Nursing Standard 15(23): 39–42
Semple C J, McGowan B 2002 Need for appropriate written information for patients with particular reference to head and neck cancer. Journal of Clinical Nursing 11: 585–593
Serra A 2000 Tracheostomy care. Nursing Standard 14(42): 45–52
Shenwell A, Wilson P 1994 Rest and respiration during obstructive sleep apnoea. Nursing Times 90(19): 30–32
Sigler B A, Schuring L T 1993 Ear, nose and throat disorders. Mosby's Clinical Nursing Series. Mosby, St Louis
Sizer D 1998 How TRT got NBM-ed [editorial]. RNID Tinnitus Helpline Newsletter 19: 1–5
St George's Healthcare Trust 2000 Guidelines for the care of patients with tracheostomy tubes. Portex Ltd, Hythe, Kent
Stone C 1996 Post-tonsillectomy pain relief following discharge from hospital. NT Research 1(1): 57–65
Taylor G, Bishop J (eds) 1991 Being deaf: the experience of deafness. Open University, Milton Keynes
Thurgood K, Thurgood G 1995 Ear syringing: a clinical skill. British Journal of Nursing 4(12): 682–687
Waddington C, McKennis A, Goodlett A 1997

Treatment of conductive hearing loss with ossicular chain reconstruction procedures. Association of Peri-operative Registered Nurses (AORN) Journal 65(3): 511–525
Wilson P, Roesser R 1997 Cerumen management: professional issues and techniques. Journal of the American Academy of Audiology 8: 421–430
Wright D 1993 Deaf people's perceptions of communication with nurses. British Journal of Nursing 2(11): 567–571
Wright D 2002 Swallowing difficulties protocol: medication administration. Nursing Standard 17(14–15): 43–45
Zeitoun H, Demajunder R, Hemmings C, Lee W 1997 Developing a nurse-led aural care clinic. Nursing Times 93(45): 45–46

USEFUL WEBSITES

Association of Teachers of Lipreading to Adults (ATLA)
www.lipreading.org.uk

British Association of Head and Neck Oncology Nurses
www.bahnon.co.uk

British Deaf Association
www.britishdeafassociation.org.uk

British Association for Counselling and Psychotherapy (BACP)
www.bacp.co.uk

Hearing Concern
www.hearingconcern.org.uk

Hearing Dogs for Deaf People
www.hearing-dogs.co.uk

Let's Face It
(A national and international group for the facially disfigured, including cancer sufferers)
www.letsfaceit.force9.co.uk

National Association of Laryngectomee Clubs (NALC)
(For laryngectomy patients, but tracheostomy and head and neck cancer patients are also welcome)
www.nalc.ik.com

National Deaf Children's Society
www.ndcs.org.uk

Royal College of Nursing ENT/Maxillofacial Nursing Forum
www.rcn.org.uk/ent

Royal National Institute for Deaf People (RNID)
www.rnid.org.uk

Scottish Council on Deafness
www.scod.org.uk

Tinnitus Helpline
Contact via the RNID — www.rnid.org.uk

DISORDERS OF THE MOUTH

15

Rosemary Kelly

INTRODUCTION

The mouth is central to many activities of daily living which we often take for granted until some minor but painful problem such as toothache or an aphthous ulcer reminds us of the importance of the condition of the mouth to our general feeling of well-being. The mouth is the source of the infant's first pleasurable activity, the sucking reflex being present at birth and perhaps, during teething, of the first experience of *dis*-ease. For individuals approaching the end of life, or for anyone who is acutely ill, good mouth care can give much comfort and relief and help to preserve dignity.

Oral health is defined as:

> *... a standard of health of the oral cavity and related tissues without active disease. This state should enable the individual to eat, speak and socialise without discomfort or embarrassment and contribute to general well-being.*
>
> *Scottish Office Department of Health (1995).*

Although this book addresses adult health, it is important to realise that good oral health practices laid down in childhood can only influence adult health in a positive way, and the nurse can help to encourage these (see Box 15.1, p. 629). Nurses can also contribute to prevention and detection of oral cancer (Macpherson et al 2003) and alleviate the misery caused by iatrogenic mucositis. However, McGuire (2002) notes that: '… there are a number of barriers that prevent patients from receiving needed care. These barriers range from a lack of knowledge, to inconsistent practice, to administrative and environmental issues. Indeed, a remarkable number of individuals and settings do not appear to regard this problem as significant.' She highlights the financial implications of mucositis in cancer care. Miller and Kearney (2001) suggest that 'unfortunately, mouth care has become a ritualistic and banal activity, a topic of conflicting advice and subjective conclusions from sporadic research'.

Mouth care should not be regarded as a standard procedure, but must be adapted to meet the needs of individuals in various care settings throughout life, and at various points on the health–illness continuum. The mouth is often the first indicator of generalised systemic disease or disease in adjacent structures. In addition, its immediate visibility gives any dysfunction a particular significance for the individual, who may be acutely aware of any disfigurement, whether cosmetic or functional. This can give rise to many difficulties affecting the person's self-perception and quality of life.

STOP THINK **15.1** From your own experience, how many activities of daily living (see Roper et al 2000) are affected, and in what ways, after a dental procedure, e.g. a filling or extraction requiring local anaesthesia? Now consider how much worse it would be for a patient if any of these activities were affected in the long term or even permanently.

ANATOMY AND PHYSIOLOGY

The mouth or oral cavity has evolved as a 'workshop', where much activity associated with chewing (mastication), drinking and speaking takes place (see Fig. 15.1):

- Entrance is between the lips (red, muscular and sensitive) through the vestibule, a small space immediately before the inner entrance which consists of gums (gingivae) covering alveolar ridges of maxillae and mandible, into which are set teeth.
- The opening (parotid duct) from the parotid gland, one of the salivary glands, is into the vestibule.

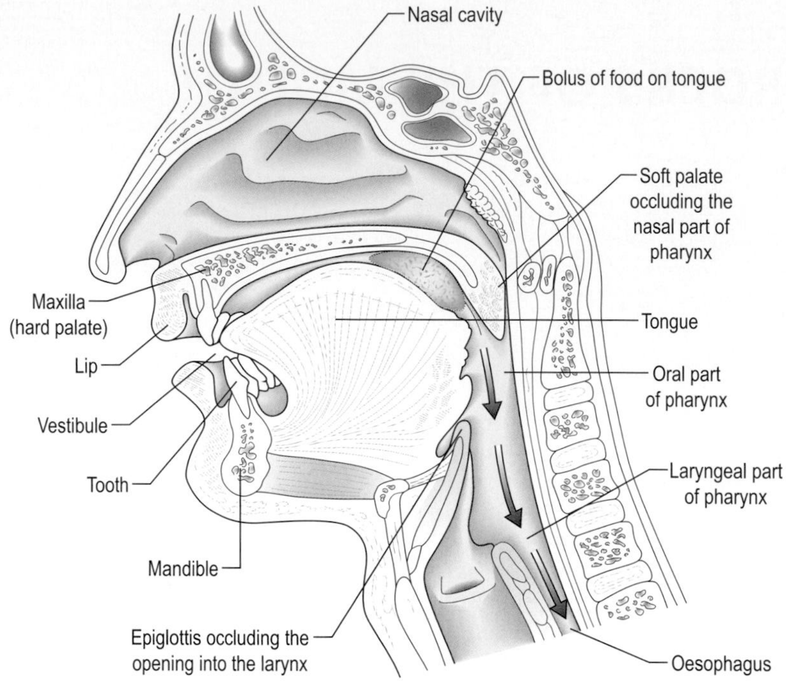
1(A) Oral stage: preparatory phase
(Time taken varies)
Lips open; saliva is stimulated
Liquid or portion of food is taken
↓
Solid material is broken down by teeth, moistened by saliva
↓
Strenuous movements of jaw and cheek muscles and mobile tongue against the hard palate, teeth and alveolar ridges form food into bolus
↓
Tongue tip gathers stray food particles from between lips and teeth and from the floor of the mouth and incorporates them into bolus
↓
The lips must be closed. The soft palate is lowered and bolus or liquid is propelled backwards by strong humping movements and funnelling of the tongue
Nasal cavity
Bolus of food on tongue
Soft palate occluding the nasal part of pharynx
Maxilla (hard palate)
Tongue
Lip
Oral part of pharynx
Vestibule
Tooth
Laryngeal part of pharynx
Mandible
Epiglottis occluding the opening into the larynx
Oesophagus
1(B) Oral stage: executive phase
(Time taken should not exceed 1 s)
The bolus of food on the tongue is propelled towards the oropharynx. The soft palate rises to close the nasopharynx and so prevent nasal regurgitation
↓
The bolus must contact pillars of fauces and the posterior oropharyngeal wall to trigger the swallow 'reflex' and initiate:
↓
2 The pharyngeal stage
(Normally lasts 0.75 s)
↓
The bolus passes the laryngeal part of the pharynx, through the open cricopharyngeal sphincter, and so to:
↓
3 The oesophageal stage
(2 s)

Fig. 15.1 The importance of oral competence to the process of feeding, chewing and swallowing.

- The roof of the mouth is formed by bony hard palate (maxilla) and muscular soft palate.
- Lateral walls are formed by the muscles of the cheeks.
- The floor of the mouth is almost entirely filled by the muscular tongue, which is very mobile and sensitive. Tiny projections on it, called papillae, contain nerve endings of taste. There are also openings from two pairs of salivary glands: submandibular and sublingual.
- The rear exit to the oropharynx is under the border of the soft palate, through two archways (palatoglossal and palatopharyngeal) which enclose the palatine tonsil. The area posterior to the molar teeth is known as the retromolar trigone.
- The entire oral cavity is lined with mucous membrane, much of which is stratified epithelium to cope with 'wear and tear'.

The mouth is situated close to many other structures, and disease or injury of the mouth may also affect, for example, the eye, ear, nose, maxillary sinuses, pharynx, larynx and neck. The face and neck are richly supplied with arteries, veins, nerves, muscles, lymph vessels and nodes, and knowledge of all these is important to understanding the effects of trauma or disease arising in, or affecting, the mouth.

The stages of normal swallowing

Only in the mouth is there normally any voluntary control over the process of digestion. The first stage (oral) must be accomplished (see Fig. 15.1) so that the swallowing reflex is triggered when the bolus reaches the posterior pharyngeal wall, and the second stage (pharyngeal) then commences. During this and the third stage (oesophageal), swallowing is involuntary.

A deficiency in the mouth may cause difficulty in the later stages of the swallowing mechanism.

Several cranial nerves (CNs) are involved in the acts of swallowing and voice production (see Table 15.1).

Normal swallowing is discussed in detail by Langley (1989).

A means of communication

The lips, tongue, hard and soft palate and teeth, together with throat and facial muscles, all manipulate sound to give quality and resonance to speech. The mouth also contributes to other expressions of emotion, e.g. smiling, laughing, whistling and kissing. Thus any disturbance to the norm caused by trauma, cerebrovascular accident or surgery can cause diminution or failure of these very basic functions and so reduce quality of life. Understanding some of the changes that may occur will help the nurse to assist the patient's recovery (see 'Orofacial trauma', p. 635, 'Tumours', p. 641, and Ch. 4).

Saliva

This is formed by a combination of secretions from the parotid, submandibular and sublingual glands and from the mucous membrane. Saliva keeps the mouth moist; without it, oral functions are very difficult. Salivary amylase is the enzyme that assists with digestion of food.

For a discussion of the physiology of salivation, see Holmes (1998).

Teeth

Teeth are important structures for biting and chewing food. Children have 20 temporary or deciduous teeth, which are gradually replaced by 32 permanent teeth between the ages

Table 15.1 Cranial nerves involved in stages of swallowing. Damage to any of these nerves may affect the ability to eat

Nerve	Type	Function
CN I	Olfactory	Sense of smell
CN V	Trigeminal	Sensory to gums, cheek, lower jaw and muscles of mastication; motor to muscles of mastication
CN VII	Facial	Taste from anterior two-thirds of the tongue; motor to muscles of face
CN IX	Glossopharyngeal	Secretion of saliva; sensory to posterior one-third of tongue, soft palate, pillars of fauces and pharynx; taste from posterior tongue; motor to pharynx
CN X	Vagus	Sensory to larynx; motor to palate, pharynx and larynx
CN XI	Accessory	Motor to laryngeal and pharyngeal muscles, and muscles of head control
CN XII	Hypoglossal	Motor to muscles of tongue

Note: CN II, CN III, CN IV, CN VI and CN VIII are not involved in motor or sensory functions of swallowing.
Adapted from Langley (1989) and Waugh & Grant (2001).

of approximately 6 and 24 years. Time of eruption can be a measure of developmental age.

Overcrowding of teeth may necessitate extraction of third molars (wisdom teeth) during young adulthood. However, impaction of wisdom teeth is now more commonly seen at a later age because fewer molars are now extracted (Scottish Intercollegiate Guidelines Network 2000a).

The importance of good orodental health throughout life is discussed later in the chapter.

See Chapter 4, Waugh & Grant (2001) and, for a more detailed account, Johnson & Moore (1997).

Bones of the face (see Fig. 15.2)

Many of these bones are complex and fragile, and hence trauma to the mouth may result in a complicated injury (see 'Orofacial trauma', p. 635).

DISORDERS OF THE MOUTH

Disorders of the mouth can be broadly classified into five categories:

- derangement of orofacial tissues
- orodental disease
- infections and inflammatory conditions (localised or systemic)
- traumatic injury
- tumours.

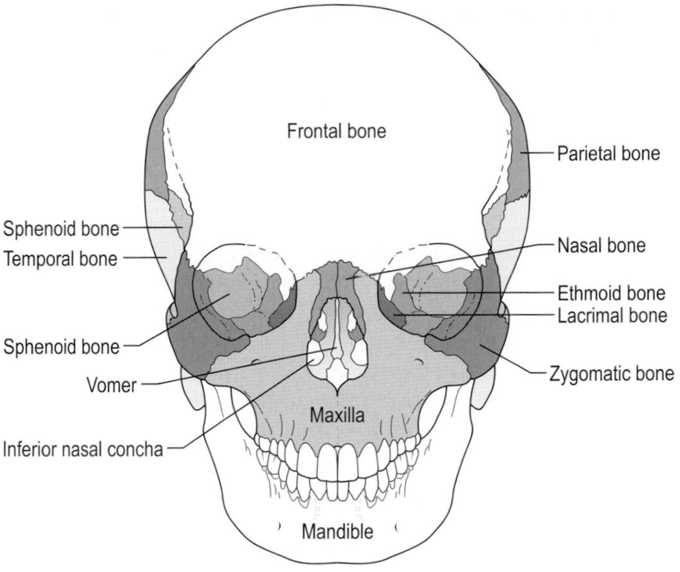

Fig. 15.2 The bones of the face.

DERANGEMENT OF OROFACIAL TISSUES

Defects involving the mouth may require a series of corrective procedures and may present the individual with physical, social and emotional problems in childhood, young adulthood and maturity (Cheng et al 1998). The most commonly occurring congenital malformations of the mouth are dental and jaw disproportion. Cleft lip and cleft palate together have an incidence of approximately 1 in 700–1000 live births. Of this number, roughly one-third are cleft lip, one-third cleft palate, and the remaining third cleft lip and cleft palate. Other deformities of the face and mouth are comparatively rare, but can be devastating for both child and parents, and may involve dilemmas for parents if diagnosed prenatally (Moss 2001).

Problems associated with dental/jaw disproportion, cleft lip/palate and other deformities of the face or mouth may concern:

- appearance
- dentition/occlusion
- eating and drinking
- speech
- hearing
- mid-face growth
- psychosocial adjustment.

PATHOPHYSIOLOGY

Cleft lip and palate result from an embryonic developmental failure 6–12 weeks after conception (Waugh & Grant 2001). Cleft lip may be unilateral or bilateral and can vary in severity from a slight notch to complete division of lip and gum. Cleft palate can result in inability of the soft palate to meet the posterior pharyngeal wall, and close off the nasopharynx. If uncorrected, speech is affected, producing a typically 'nasal' delivery in which certain consonants, particularly C, D, K, P, S and T, cannot be properly enunciated.

For information on rarer deformities of the mouth and face, see Wray et al (2003).

MEDICAL MANAGEMENT

Treatment The medical management of oral defects requires a multidisciplinary approach extending from infancy to adulthood. Treatment protocol will depend on the extent of the deformity and on the age of the child.

For management of cleft lip/palate, see Ray (2003) and Table 15.2.

Orthognathic surgery, i.e. surgery to correct major facial deformities, is an important and developing area of maxillofacial work and is carried out in only a few units in the UK. It requires a team approach involving neuro-, maxillofacial, plastic and ophthalmic surgeons, and assessment and correction take place throughout life (Moos 2003).

NURSING PRIORITIES AND MANAGEMENT: Congenital orofacial derangement

Nursing considerations

Referral Although any deformity may be discovered by prenatal screening, nevertheless the experience for parents of such a newborn child may be very traumatic, and the provision of sensitive and supportive counselling should not be delayed. Parents should be referred within a few days of their child's birth to the relevant specialist professionals, e.g. specialist nurse, orofacial consultant, orthodontist, speech therapist, genetic specialist (see Ch. 6), and should be given information on their local branch of the Cleft Lip and Palate Association (CLAPA) (see 'Useful websites', p. 651) or other appropriate self-help group. Professional psychological support may also be required as there can be great family stress (Martin 1995, 1998).

Oral hygiene Nurses should emphasise to parents the importance of good dental hygiene as there is a higher risk of caries and infection, and parents may mistakenly feel that, compared with gross abnormality, the loss of a few teeth due to dental caries is inconsequential.

Table 15.2 Treatment of cleft lip and palate

Procedure	Timing/patient's age
Lip repair	0–6 months
Palate repair	4–24 months
Bone graft to alveolus	9–11 years
Osteotomy (for correction of defect of hard palate) Rhinoplasty (for nasal defect)	Around 18 years
Pharyngoplasty (to correct the pharynx) Myringotomy revision procedures	As and when necessary
Orthodontic treatment	Throughout childhood and into adulthood
Speech therapy	As and when necessary

Pre- and postoperative nursing care of patients undergoing major corrective surgery will take into account the general considerations discussed in Chapter 26, incorporating the specialised skills and techniques demanded by each procedure; Chapter 6 provides a discussion of genetic disorders and their management.

ORAL HEALTH AND ORODENTAL DISEASE

Dental and periodontal disease affects about 95% of the population of the UK in varying degrees and accounts for the largest proportion of disorders of the mouth (Morris et al 2001). Because most of this disease is preventable, this discussion of orodental disease will begin with a consideration of dental health, first with respect to recent trends and then with regard to the promotion of orodental care.

Changing patterns of dental health

Incidence of dental caries can be measured in terms of the number of decayed, missing and filled teeth; dmft indicates the status of deciduous teeth and DMFT that of permanent teeth. From the early 1970s, there was a substantial improvement in dental health in the UK. More people retained their natural teeth into later life, and there was a marked decrease in dental caries in children. By 1998, dentate adults had fewer missing teeth and more sound, untreated teeth on average than in 1978. However, improvement in children's dental health appears to be falling off and there was no improvement in 2001/2002 compared to the two previous years. Moreover, dental caries appears to increase as the child grows older (Nunn et al 2003). In the UK, 40% of children have dental decay, but there is wide regional variation ranging from dmft = 0.94 in the West Midlands to dmft = 2.55 in Scotland (Pitts et al 2003). There is also a direct correlation between dental caries and social deprivation. There are serious implications for health in later years if dental disease remains untreated in childhood (Fayle et al 2001).

STOP THINK **15.2** Consider why regional variations might exist.

Promoting oral health

Nurses in all spheres of practice (see Box 15.1) can help with early education in the simple preventive measures that are the key to oral health. A nurse-led initiative described by Black (2000) is aimed at educating children and their parents to improve their diet and dental health, and to identify orodental problems early (Scottish Intercollegiate Guidelines Network 2000b, Scottish Executive 2003).

See Wray & Gibson (1997) and Scully & Cawson (1999) for illustrations of oral soft tissue disease, and Sweeney & Bagg (1997) for an interactive programme on the mouth.

Oral hygiene Parents should introduce a dental hygiene routine as soon as their child's first teeth appear, using a soft, baby toothbrush. Most children will require supervision until they are 7 or 8 years old.

The teeth should be brushed last thing at night and, ideally, after every meal. The toothbrush should be held

Box 15.1

Contribution of nurses and midwives to orodental health

Health visitors and public health nurses
Encourage oral hygiene in childhood and visits to dentist and orthodontist. This is a primary preventive function of the health visitor, school nurse and public health nurse. Educate on oral cancer prevention (smoking, alcohol and other substance abuse). Demonstrate dental hygiene. Alert parents to the need for children's visits to the dentist. Encourage healthy eating principles (Scottish Executive Health Department 2001).

Occupational health nurses and practice nurses
Educate on adverse effects of smoking and excessive alcohol. Raise awareness of symptoms of intraoral cancer. Advise on good handwashing practices and healthy eating.

District nurses
Identify potential problems in older people. Advise on continued dental examination. Raise awareness of oral cancer.

Nurses caring for older people
As above. Increase mouth comfort and self-esteem.

Nurses working with those with learning disability
Supervise early and continued dental care and thus minimise need for restorative dentistry.

Midwives
Give dental care advice in pregnancy.

All nurses
Encourage and/or assist with oral hygiene for patients' comfort and health. Have dental/oral health literature available (Scottish Executive Health Department 2001).

at an angle of 45° and the teeth brushed horizontally to avoid damage to the gums. All exposed surfaces of the teeth should be brushed.

Toothbrushes should be renewed every 3 months, and hard brushes should be avoided as they can damage tooth enamel and gums.

Toothpaste with added fluoride is recommended, except in areas with fluoridated water. Current advice is that it is unnecessary to rinse, thus leaving a film of fluoride toothpaste (Park & Ross 2002). Toothpaste with sugar added to improve flavour should be avoided. Sensitivities to certain toothpaste ingredients, e.g. cinnamon-aldehyde, menthol and peppermint occur occasionally and will resolve spontaneously when use is discontinued (Francalanci et al 2000).

Dental floss with or without added fluoride may be used to clean between the teeth. Overzealous use can damage the gums and it is best not used by children. Similar care should be taken in the use of toothpicks.

Disclosing tablets can be useful to demonstrate how plaque is left after inadequate brushing. Chewed after cleansing, the tablet produces a stain on any teeth still covered with plaque. Correct brushing should then remove the plaque.

Common misconceptions Chewing gum after meals to increase saliva is of limited value in reducing decay. To be of any benefit, sugar-free gum must be chewed for 20 min and be backed up by other forms of dental care.

Chewing an apple after a meal does not clean the teeth. Rather, it leaves an acidic deposit, which encourages development of plaque.

Diet There is a direct correlation between the incidence of caries and availability of sucrose. There appears to be a vicious circle of deprivation in which poor diet, i.e. high in sugar and fat, combined with inadequate intake of fruit and vegetables, predisposes to dental decay in children. Eventually, as people age, poor dental status may affect nutrition and as a result may contribute to the risk of vascular disease, which appears to follow the north/south axis of deprivation (Bates et al 2001). Continued health promotion is needed to improve the diet of schoolchildren, especially in Scotland. It may be that adults, whose dental health is now on average better than adults of 20 years ago, are unaware of the need to reinforce good eating habits for the future. Nurses could contribute to health education in this area, and emphasise the cariogenic action of non-milk sugars, which include fruit juices, honey and table sugar, especially when consumed by young children last thing at night (Levine 2001).

For information on diet and a list of resources, see Oral Health Group (2003) and Scottish Executive (2003).

STOP THINK **15.3** Examine the contents labels of the prepared foods you normally buy. Do any of these products contain more sugar than you had realised?

Access to dental care Often, the dental surgery is the first remembered clinical setting for health care. If these first visits are reasonably pleasant, then a positive attitude may be created towards future regular dental check-ups, and subsequent serious disease can then be diagnosed early (Fayle et al 2001).

Early access to orthodontic services, particularly for those with congenital abnormalities, will help to minimise problems in later life.

In the adult population, changes from institutional living to community-based housing for those with learning difficulties may be associated with reduction in dental attendance and treatment (Stanfield et al 2003). Older housebound people face similar problems (Simons 2003), especially those with a depressive illness (Friedlander et al 2003).

However, the future dental health of the nation may be affected by factors including regional variation in accessibility of NHS dentistry, increased treatment charges and changes in funding of dental services (McGrath & Bedi 2003, Tickle et al 2003). Seventy-five per cent of British adults consider oral health as being important to quality of life (McGrath & Bedi 2002). However, Nuttall et al (2001) found that only 59% of adults were likely to attend for regular dental check-ups, while younger adults (16–24 years) were less likely to do so than 5 years previously.

STOP THINK **15.4** Consider why young adults are less likely to attend a dentist regularly. How could nurses influence this?

Fluoride is a substance naturally present in some areas in water. It is taken up by growing teeth and makes enamel harder and more resistant to the development of caries. There is strong evidence that caries is considerably reduced in areas of naturally occurring fluoridated water (Stephen et al 2002). However, much controversy still continues over the practice of adding fluoride to the water supply (Cross & Carton 2003).

Fluoride supplements can be given to children from the age of 6 months. Dentists, pharmacists and health visitors should be able to advise on the correct amount required locally. Overdosing causes fluorosis, which can cause 'mottling' of teeth, i.e. brown spots with white opacities.

For further information on dental health education, see Levine (1996a,b).

Dental and periodontal disease

PATHOPHYSIOLOGY

Plaque is a firmly adherent, non-calcified deposit of bacteria, mucus, food particles and cellular debris which accumulates on the surface of a tooth, particularly at the base. It forms rapidly in the absence of good oral hygiene and reacts immediately with sugar to form an acid which can attack and erode tooth enamel, leading, if unchecked by adequate saliva combined with good dental hygiene, to gum disease and dental caries.

Calculus is hard mineralised plaque which requires removal by a dental surgeon or dental hygienist.

Caries is progressive, localised decay of teeth caused by bacterial action. It is characterised by demineralisation of the inorganic portion and destruction of the organic substance of the tooth.

Gingivitis — inflammation of the gums Normal gums are pink, e.g. in Caucasians, or brown, e.g. in Asian or African people, and are firm. In gingivitis, the gums are purple–red, soft and puffy, tender, and may bleed easily. Regular oral hygiene and dental care reduce this reversible stage of gum disease.

Untreated, gingivitis can lead to gum recession and the formation of pockets (found in 75% of dentate adults) around the base of teeth, in which plaque and calculus can collect. Further infection from bacteria in plaque may lead to periodontitis.

Periodontitis is characterised by gradual loss of the supporting membrane of the teeth and erosion of supporting bone. Membrane and bone, once destroyed, cannot be replaced and subsequent loosening of teeth occurs.

Acute ulcerative gingivitis is an uncommon condition caused by a mixed infection of a bacillus and spirochaetes, associated with poor oral hygiene, smoking, throat infections, stress and HIV infection. The gums are sore and bleed easily and ulcers develop which may spread more deeply. There is foul-smelling halitosis, and cervical or neck lymph glands may be enlarged.

Common presenting symptoms The patient commonly presents to the general practitioner (GP) or dentist with a combination of symptoms which may include toothache, bleeding gums and emission of pus from the gums (pyorrhoea). If oral hygiene has been habitually poor, the patient is more likely to wait until pain is severe before presenting. Many people fear going to the dentist and delay for as long as possible.

MEDICAL MANAGEMENT

Investigations include X-rays, sialograms (see Appendix 1) and relevant blood tests.

Dental surgery or outpatient procedures Most orodental problems are treated in dental surgeries (NHS or private practice). Treatments such as extractions, fillings, root treatment for dental abscess, and restorative work such as fitting crowns and dentures are carried out with the patient under a local anaesthetic administered by the dentist. Some procedures necessitate general anaesthesia, which is administered by an anaesthetist. Treatment of gingivitis is with mouthwashes and metronidazole or penicillin. Scaling, i.e. removal of plaque and calculus, is carried out when swelling has subsided.

Inpatient or day-case procedures Procedures which can be classed as minor oral surgery but which may require hospital treatment include:

- removal of impacted wisdom teeth
- removal of dental cysts
- removal of salivary glands or ducts
- apicectomy — excision of apex of tooth root
- pre-prosthetic surgery
- placement of implants.

Patients may be referred to a dental hospital/school or to an oral/maxillofacial unit.

Patients with certain conditions or who are taking certain types of medication will require hospital admission and special monitoring as follows (Stenhouse & Wray 2003):

- Diabetes mellitus — insulin dosage must be monitored; there is a risk of delayed healing
- Heart valve disease — monitoring is very important as infection can lead to bacterial endocarditis (see Ch. 2)
- Corticosteroid medication — must be monitored; healing may be delayed
- Anticoagulants — must be monitored; there is increased risk of haemorrhage.

NURSING PRIORITIES AND MANAGEMENT: Orodental disease

Nursing considerations

Outpatient care Individuals treated in dental surgeries or as hospital outpatients will require reassurance and advice on aftercare at home. The nurse should make available written information such as that presented in Box 15.2 and ensure that the patient understands and can carry out instructions for self-care and knows where to call for advice should problems arise.

Box 15.2

Information for patients having minor oral surgery

Following surgery to your mouth, you can expect some swelling and discomfort. This may last for some days. The following information will help you in the postoperative period.

On the day of treatment

1. Rest for a few hours. You do not necessarily have to lie down, however.
2. Avoid strenuous exercise for 24 h.
3. Avoid rinsing your mouth for 24 h, even if it tastes unpleasant. Rinsing may disturb any blood clots and start up bleeding.
4. Your lips and/or tongue may be numb. Be careful not to bite or burn them inadvertently.
5. Avoid hot fluids, alcohol, hard foods and cigarettes.
6. Pain or soreness can be relieved with a mild painkiller, e.g. co-codamol or paracetamol (no more than eight tablets in 24 h for an adult).
7. Should the wound begin to bleed, apply a compress (a clean cotton handkerchief rolled up is ideal). Place this on the bleeding point and bite firmly on it for 10 min, or longer if necessary.
8. If you are at all worried, or if anything untoward occurs, such as prolonged bleeding, excessive pain or swelling, please telephone the oral surgery department where you received treatment.

On the day after treatment

A mouthwash can now be used to cleanse the mouth. It is not necessary to purchase a proprietary mouthwash, although you can if you wish. It is the mechanical action of washing out the mouth which is of importance, rather than the substance used.

Warm salty water is very effective to cleanse and freshen the mouth. Dissolve half a teaspoon of salt in a tumbler of warm water. Hold a mouthful of the solution in the mouth for a minute or two and then spit it out. Finish the tumbler in the same way. Repeat the procedure several times a day for 5 days.

Follow-up

You will have been given another appointment if further treatment is necessary. If you have any problems please contact the oral surgery department for advice.

Inpatient care Many patients are treated as day cases. However, stay may be longer if any of the above conditions apply.

The preparation of patients for anaesthesia is described in Chapter 26. Because of 'dentist phobia', patients undergoing dental surgery often experience anxiety which may seem disproportionate to the size of the procedure, and need much reassurance.

Postoperatively, the patient may experience considerable pain, swelling and bruising. Nursing Care Plan 15.1 gives an example of the care that is required following a wisdom tooth extraction.

On discharge, the patient should be given clear, adequate information on self-care and a number to call should further advice be needed.

Promoting oral health and comfort in special client groups

Most people are able to maintain good oral hygiene independently throughout much of their lives. Others, for reasons of physical or cognitive disability, or infirmity due to illness or advanced age, will need supervision and assistance in carrying out dental and periodontal care routines. The importance of this aspect of daily care must not be minimised, as poor orodental health can seriously compromise the individual's well-being, both functionally and socially.

Physically disadvantaged and those with learning difficulties

Individuals with limited motor control or manual dexterity may require help with brushing teeth. Toothbrushes with adapted handles are available to aid gripping and the nurse should be aware of how these can be obtained, often from an occupational therapist. Many people with limited movement depend on the mouth and teeth to hold or control equipment; it is thus especially important that their teeth are kept in good condition. Occasionally, it is difficult to gain the cooperation of a disadvantaged person who needs dental treatment; in such cases, general anaesthesia may be required even for a simple procedure. The practice of good oral hygiene is obviously preferable to repeated general anaesthesia.

The older person

Adequate dental care for older people can greatly enhance quality of life with regard to comfort, self-image and social interaction (Fiske et al 1990). However, Holmes (1996) commented that 'much of the care is not supported by research, and oral-care practices have remained unchanged for many years' (see p. 636 for a review of mouth care products).

Many older people now retain their natural teeth and regular dental check-ups should be encouraged by community nurses. Good oral hygiene and regular assessment of oral/dental health for older people in hospital should form part of any nursing care plan. However, Samaranayake et al (1995) found considerable unmet dental need among a group of 147 older people in five long-stay wards.

Older people in general have specific problems relating to oral health as follows (the figures in parentheses are from Samaranayake et al 1995):

- Gum retraction/resorption — this occurs naturally, causing root surfaces to be exposed, and with natural wear of the teeth can necessitate repair work.
- Dry mouth (35%) — this can lead to a coated tongue (56%) and increases the risk of decay.
- Ill-fitting dentures (45%) — as a result of the natural resorption of the alveoli when teeth are lost. Continuous wearing of dentures can lead to the development of *Candida*-associated denture stomatitis (19%) (see 'Infections and inflammatory conditions of the mouth', p. 632). Dentures should therefore be removed at night, cleaned and kept in water or a weak solution of Milton or other proprietary cleanser. Dentures left dry for any length of time can shrink.
- Angular cheilitis (25%).

Nursing Care Plan 15.1 Care of a patient following removal of impacted wisdom teeth

Nursing considerations	Action/intervention	Expected outcome
1. Pain due to manipulation of jaw	• Administer adequate analgesics and monitor their effect	Patient is free of pain
2. Risk of haemorrhage	• Withhold mouthwashing overnight	Blood clot left undisturbed; bleeding minimised
3. Vomiting because of swallowed blood from tooth socket	• Give constant reassurance; stay with the patient or allow privacy according to patient's wishes	Patient is comforted; dignity and self-esteem respected
4. Personal hygiene	• Provide frequent sponging, especially of face and hands	Comfort maintained
5. Oral hygiene	• Provide gentle, warm saline mouthwashes the morning after; gentle brushing, avoiding socket	Mouth is freshened; debris removed; haemorrhage avoided
6. Risk of infection	• Administer antibiotics if prescribed • Implement special precautions for patients at risk	Infection avoided; normal healing takes place
7. Discharge	• Evaluate outcome of treatment and postoperative care • If the patient is fit for discharge: give aftercare information; refer to community nurse and hygienist; arrange return appointment	Patient is confident about performing self-care; professional supervision is continued

- Loss of appetite — older people who have lost interest in meals should be examined for any of the above and for early indications of intraoral cancer. Specialist opinion should always be sought for any ulcer which does not heal within 2–3 weeks (Macpherson et al 2003).
- Reduced manual dexterity and general weakness.

STOP THINK **15.5** Consider the nursing care of older patients. Is the same quality of care given to teeth as to washing face and hands and combing hair? Carry out a thorough examination of the oral cavity (see Macpherson et al 2003).

Jamieson et al (2002) describe mouth care in detail; Macpherson et al (2003) give a detailed, illustrated description of examination of the oral cavity. See also Sweeney & Bagg (1997), Wray & Gibson (1997) and Scully & Cawson (1999) for illustrations of oral disease which the nurse might encounter during routine oral inspection and which would warrant seeking specialist advice.

Acutely ill people

During the acute phase of any illness, the patient may require assistance or supervision in carrying out oral hygiene, but the objective should be to encourage optimum independence as far as possible.

Many acutely ill people suffer from stomatitis (mucositis) and/or candidosis and will require special measures. These are further discussed in the following section.

INFECTIONS AND INFLAMMATORY CONDITIONS OF THE MOUTH

These can give rise to considerable pain and discomfort, and the individual, already often ill, debilitated and poorly nourished, can become more so if the oral condition is not reversed. The mouth may be affected by the following:

- local and systemic infections (see Table 15.3)
- oral manifestations of a generalised systemic disease:
  - — gastrointestinal and nutritional disorders (see Chs 4, 20 and 21, and Table 15.4)
  - — blood (haemopoietic) and endocrine disorders (see Chs 5 and 11)
  - — dermatological disorders (see Ch. 12).

For further information and illustrations of the above conditions, see Wray & Gibson (1997) and Scully & Cawson (1999).

Stomatitis

PATHOPHYSIOLOGY

Stomatitis, or inflammation of the mouth (stoma), is also called mucositis and can be caused by:

- vitamin deficiency (B_{12}, folic acid)
- viral infection, including HIV
- radiotherapy to head and neck
- chemotherapy

Table 15.3 Common local and systemic infections affecting the mouth

Infection/organism	Oral presentation	Cause/effect
Candidosis is an opportunistic oral infection most commonly caused by *Candida albicans;* can be broadly divided into three types (Wray & Bagg 1997)	Different presentations are recognised and may be found at the same time, especially in terminal illness, and when associated with HIV and AIDS. Anorexia is common (Ventifridda et al 1998)	Destruction of normal oral flora due to immunosuppression caused by, e.g. antibiotics, cytotoxic drugs, radiotherapy to head and neck, HIV, severe debilitation post-surgery, anaemia and other blood disorders, diabetes mellitus, terminal illness (identified in 75–89% of patients) (Ventifridda et al 1998)
(a) Pseudomembranous candidosis ('thrush')	White–yellow plaques like milk curds, easily wiped off, leaving painful, bleeding surface; patient may complain mucosa feels rough and tender, and of dryness and a metallic taste	May also occur in oropharynx (? a cause of anorexia); in infants (poor hygiene) is highly infectious; and in advanced HIV (Palmer et al 1996)
(b) Erythematous candidosis	Minimal white plaques, painful erosion of dorsum of tongue, generalised erythema and oedema	Often related to use of broad-spectrum antibiotics (antibiotic stomatitis)
	There may be clear demarcation from normal tissue; may be asymptomatic and thus undiagnosed	May be seen in areas in contact with dentures (denture stomatitis, and associated with poor oral hygiene, xerostomia, smoking. Occurs in 50% of denture wearers
	Erythema with no obvious predisposing factors	May indicate HIV infection
(c) Hyperplastic candidosis or candidal leukoplakia	Firm adherent white patches or tiny nodules on erythematous base	Have potential to become malignant
	Hairy leukoplakia has corrugated appearance	Usually associated with HIV
Candidal cheilosis (often found with chronic candidosis)	Soreness, redness and cracks at corner of mouth	Habitual licking, nutritional deficiencies, diabetes mellitus
Chickenpox (varicella)	Occasionally vesicles develop on oral mucosa, similar to characteristic vesicles on skin	May result in loss of appetite and nutritional deficiencies
Herpes labialis (cold sore), herpes simplex virus type 1	Vesicular eruption on lip; patient is not always aware of infective nature — virus present in saliva	Often follows primary herpetic infection, stress, fever, local irritation. Exposure to sunlight may reactivate the virus
Herpes zoster (shingles), varicella-zoster virus	Affects one or more branches of trigeminal nerve (CN V), usually unilaterally	Mainly affects older or immunocompromised people
Herpangina, Coxsackie virus group A	Multiple ulcers and erythema affecting palate and fauces	Mild, short-lasting
HIV infections/AIDS (see also candidosis, particularly pseudomembranous)	Oral disease present in 80% of patients with AIDS and 50% of patients with HIV (Palmer et al 1996). Oral manifestation may be first clinical sign; may present as hairy leukoplakia (Epstein–Barr virus has been isolated)	Early management is advised so as to avoid serious complications when immune system is further suppressed, and to maintain quality of life (Scully & Cawson 1999)
Kaposi's sarcoma (KS)	Red–blue or purple patches on skin of cheek or oral mucosa, especially palate (Palmer et al 1996)	50% of patients with KS have oral lesions
Bell's palsy — usually a viral infection of facial nerve (CN VII)	Drooping of mouth, unable to close eye or wrinkle forehead	Very disfiguring; patient feels stigmatised

Illustrations and further information on treatment of these and other oral conditions can be found in Wray & Gibson (1997) and Scully & Cawson (1999)

- bone marrow transplantation (BMT) and graft-versus-host disease (GVHD)
- liver failure
- renal failure.

Common presenting symptoms In this condition, cell regeneration in the epithelium of the mucous membrane cannot keep pace with the rate of destruction which occurs as a result of any of the above. The mucosa becomes thin and there is erythema and some loss of taste. Later, oedema develops and the mucosa breaks down at the slightest trauma, giving rise to haemorrhage and ulceration (Wells 2003).

The pain caused by stomatitis can be excruciating. One patient described drinking water as 'like swallowing

Table 15.4 Gastrointestinal and nutritional disorders affecting the mouth

Disorder	Oral presentation	Cause/effect
Bulimia nervosa	Erosion of teeth due to exposure to gastric acid from self-induced vomiting	Tooth erosion may be first indication of disorder
Crohn's disease	Irregular swelling of lower lip, angular cheilitis and folded thickening of oral mucosa	Mainly due to lymphoedema Sensitivity to foods, flavouring, dyes and preservatives
Coeliac disease	Recurrent oral ulceration	Caused by folic acid deficiency
Pernicious anaemia	Generalised papillary loss with mucosal atrophy	Caused by vitamin B_{12} deficiency
Iron deficiency anaemia	Atrophic glossitis	Less severe than that due to folic acid or vitamin B_{12} deficiency

Illustrations and further information on treatment of these oral conditions can be found in Wray & Gibson (1997) and Scully & Cawson (1999).

broken glass'. A sore mouth is one of the side-effects that makes chemotherapy, radiotherapy to the head and neck area or preparation for bone marrow transplantation (BMT) an unhappy experience for many people (Coleman 1995, Wells 1998, and see Ch. 31). In health, saliva normally helps to clear the mouth of harmful pathogens; however, in these patients saliva becomes increasingly viscoid, resulting in xerostomia (dry mouth) which upsets the normal pH balance (Holmes 1998), creating an ideal environment for invasion by *Candida albicans*.

Candidosis (thrush)

PATHOPHYSIOLOGY

Candidosis, candidiasis, or moniliasis is caused by infection with *Candida (Monilia) albicans*, a yeast-like fungus normally found in the respiratory, alimentary and (in females) genital tracts of healthy people. Oral candidosis is very common in people who are ill, debilitated, older or terminally ill. Presentation and predisposing factors are summarised in Table 15.3.

Systemic diseases showing oral manifestations

These include blood disorders such as leukaemia (bleeding gums), polycythaemia vera (bright red oral mucosa) and thrombocytopenic purpura (petechiae on tongue). For greater detail on these conditions, see Chapter 11. In dermatological conditions (see Ch. 12), examples of oral symptoms are Koplik's spots in measles and oral vesicles in chickenpox (varicella).

Burning mouth syndrome

Although this condition is neither inflammatory nor infective, it is relatively common, particularly among older women. The oral mucosa appears entirely normal, but the sufferer complains of a continuous or intermittent burning sensation on tongue, palate, lips and lower alveolus.

Aetiological factors include vitamin deficiency, allergies, haematological disorders, undiagnosed diabetes, xerostomia and cancer phobia, the last, in particular, causing much anxiety. Although Scala et al (2003) contend there is no consensus on the diagnosis and there is no definitive cure, Lamey (1996) considers the problem can usually be readily managed and patients should be advised to seek specialist advice.

MEDICAL MANAGEMENT OF INFECTIONS AND INFLAMMATORY CONDITIONS

Treatment begins with the identification of the pathogen by culture swab or saliva washings. An appropriate antibiotic or antifungal agent is prescribed. All patients having radiotherapy, chemotherapy or preparation for BMT should be referred for dental assessment before treatment starts (Ali 2003). If being treated for a systemic disease, the patient's medication should be reviewed, with appropriate consideration of drug interactions. Only if the symptoms become severe will causative treatments such as radiotherapy be withdrawn temporarily.

Appropriate mouthwashes may be prescribed; again, drug interactions should be avoided (Barkvoll & Attramadal 1989).

NURSING PRIORITIES AND MANAGEMENT: Infections and inflammatory conditions of the mouth

Many patients with these conditions are already ill people; to have to cope with an excruciatingly painful mouth can often overwhelm them completely and lead to total demoralisation. Nurses write frequently about oral care, but despite that, Miller and Kearney (2001) comment, 'Rarely do experts teach it, and it frequently is delegated to the most junior (inexperienced) members of the nursing staff'.

Nursing responsibilities for oral care

Much of the traditional ritual of oral care is unsuited to a sick person with xerostomia, acute stomatitis (mucositis) and/or candidosis, and it is difficult to encompass the many aspects of care in a limited text, but the student should consider the following when caring for individuals and challenge inappropriate practice.

Self-care should be encouraged whenever possible as patients know what their own mouths will tolerate (Little 1996) and are more likely to cooperate.

Assessment The condition of the oral cavity may change from day to day; frequent assessment is vital, using a tool and chart to record changes. Thorough examination (Macpherson et al 2003) is necessary and although the patient may find it intrusive, it can be used as an opportunity to supervise and offer encouragement. Holmes and Mountain (1993), Coleman (1995) and Wells (2003) evaluate oral assessment tools which have benefits in different care settings.

Frequency There is general agreement that care should be regular, but opinions vary as to frequency. Four times daily may be adequate for some patients, but those able to tolerate only rinsing or even just moistening, may benefit from half-hourly care. This may be an opportunity for relatives to contribute to care (Watson 1989). Cleaning before meals may improve appetite (Roberts 1990).

Regimen A simple regimen is advocated. If possible, dentate patients should continue using toothbrush and toothpaste; a soft brush and toothpaste with added fluoride are recommended (Park & Ross 2002). If there is fragile mucosa, foam sticks may remove debris but will not remove plaque. Gauze swabs held in forceps or wrapped around a finger are too rough and may remove a layer of regenerating epithelium. Irrigation with a syringe may be appropriate in some circumstances, but forceful use may damage mucosa. Following intraoral surgery, a patient may find it difficult to adapt to the changes inside the mouth because of alteration to contour and presence of insensate flaps (Little 1996), so supervision may be necessary to ensure removal of debris.

Oral care preparations A mouth with acute stomatitis can be regarded as an open wound, and the nurse must consider whether or not some traditionally used oral care products are appropriate treatment.

Evidence for and against some oral care equipment and preparations described over almost three decades is summarised in Table 15.5.

Other esoteric recommendations for oral care in a palliative care setting include pineapple chunks, cider and soda mouthwash for a 'dirty' mouth, and semi-frozen tonic water and gin (1:1), or fruit juice (Regnard et al 1997). There is no evidence to support use of any of these for radiation-induced mucositis or xerostomia.

From the information contained in Table 15.5, it can be seen that there is considerable variation in the opinions of practitioners and researchers, but in the absence of compelling evidence, Park and Ross (2002) consider best practice to include brushing with fluoride toothpaste for natural teeth, use of chlorhexidine mouthwash to prevent plaque and Biotene Oral Balance system for xerostomia.

For a discussion of related research, see Wells (2003).

Temperature is important. Ice cubes may seem soothing if a mouth feels inflamed, but may delay the healing process. Warm solution is recommended for wound irrigation (Hollinworth 1997); it should assist in healing a damaged mouth and is often preferred by patients.

Analgesics must always be adequate and timed appropriately, e.g. to give maximum benefit at mealtimes and to cover periods away from the ward or home when receiving treatment. Opioids may be appropriate; topical anaesthetic agents including benzydamine mouthwash, Mucaine or lozenges containing local anaesthetic may be used (Regnard et al 1997, Wells 2003).

Dignity and self-esteem Consideration should be given at all times to the importance to the patient of maintaining dignity and self-esteem. A sore mouth can be a further demoralising factor for a patient already under stress. All nursing care plans for oral care must form part of holistic care and must consider any therapeutic measures being implemented by other members of the multidisciplinary team.

Reference should also be made to oral hygiene as described earlier in this chapter, in Chapters 26–33 and in Jamieson et al (2002), considering each individual's needs.

OROFACIAL TRAUMA

Traumatic injury to the mouth or face typically gives rise to much anxiety concerning disfigurement. Moreover, because of the high vascularity of this area, blood loss at the time of injury may be considerable and the patient, together with companions or relatives, are likely to be very alarmed.

A national survey (Hutchison et al 1998) estimated that about 500 000 people in the UK suffer facial injuries, with a decrease in those from road traffic collisions (RCAs) being offset by a marked increase in assaults (Magennis et al 1998). Soft tissue injuries to the face range from simple lacerations, knife wounds and bites to multiple injuries resulting in tissue loss. Bone injuries include fracture of the mandible and fracture of the maxillae, malar (zygomatic) and nasal bones (middle third fracture). The signs and symptoms of different types of fracture are summarised in Table 15.6.

Causes

Violence

Approximately 125 000 people in the UK suffer facial injury annually as a result of assault (Magennis et al 1998). Many of these are teenagers and young adults where alcohol is often associated with either victim or assailant. Figures for 1995–98 show 75% of assaults were on men, but there is a rising trend in assaults on women and those of both genders aged 18–30 (Sivarajasingam & Shepherd 2001). It is now thought that in the past there has been considerable under-reporting by the police of offences. Injury data now being supplied by emergency departments show an increase of between 25 and 50% compared to previous police statistics (Sutherland et al 2002). Emergency department data are now being used to monitor violence prevention initiatives such as closed circuit television and the use of strengthened glass in bar glasses.

Table 15.5 Mouth care equipment and preparations: evidence for and against

Preparation/strength of evidence	Evidence	Observations from clinical practice
Toothbrush, hand or electric, with soft head (strong evidence for)	Familiar to patients and recommended by several authors since Howarth (1977), removes plaque (Pearson & Hutton 2002, Sadler et al 2003)	Hard brush will damage fragile mucosa, small soft brush recommended (Miller & Kearney 2001)
Foam sticks (some evidence for)	Less effective than brushing, but will reduce plaque and control gingivitis (Pearson & Hutton 2002)	Used with chlorhexidine for fragile mucosa, or for edentulous patients
Toothpaste/dentifrice with added fluoride (strong evidence for)	Fluoride is proven to reduce caries (Mouatt 2003)	
Chlorhexidine mouthwash (strong evidence for)	Recommended by Ferretti et al (1987); said to be the 'gold standard' of antiplaque and gingivitis agents by Moshrefi (2002); antimicrobial, prevents plaque formation, decreases incidence of mucositis	'Burning' of mucosa and staining of teeth (Roberts 1990) can be reduced by dilution with water 1:1 (Park & Ross 2002). Some proprietary mouthwashes such as Corsodyl contain alcohol and are not recommended for radiation-induced mucositis (Miller & Kearney 2001)
Fluoride mouthwash, topical gel (strong evidence for dentate patients)	Fluoride is proven to reduce caries (Mouatt 2003)	Frequent use needed; requires time to be absorbed by tooth enamel
Benzydamine hydrochloride (Difflam) mouthwash (evidence equivocal)	Studies, including Epstein et al (2001) and Cheng & Chang (2003), have reported varying benefits	Can relieve mucosal pain, but may cause initial stinging and may require dilution 1:1 with water
Fluconazole (Diflucan) — antifungal (strong evidence for) not to be confused with Difflam (benzydamine hydrochloride)	Effective in treating oral *Candida albicans* and more efficacious than amphotericin (Finlay et al 1996)	One daily dose leads to better patient cooperation with treatment
Nystatin suspension — antifungal (some evidence for)	Efficacy reduced by chlorhexidine (Barkvoll & Attramadal 1989), so 1 h should elapse between taking these to allow each to be effective	Poor patient cooperation; to be effective, at least 20 min should elapse after application before eating or drinking
Water mouthwashes (some evidence for)	Recommended by Howarth (1977), Feber (1995). Increased intake will maintain hydration and help xerostomia (Wells 2003)	Patients can acceptably carry a bottle and use frequently (Sadler et al 2003)
Saliva replacement, range of commercial preparations, e.g. Biotene Oral Balance system, BioXtra, Saliva Orthana (some evidence for)	Varying reports of efficacy (Miller & Kearney 2001, Meyer-Leuckel & Kielbassa 2002); optimal substitute for saliva not yet discovered (Sadler et al 2003); Biotene Oral Balance found to be superior to other agents (Epstein et al 1999)	Mucin-based preparations are said to be better tolerated (Davies et al 2001) but mucin is derived from porcine gastric mucosa, so is unsuitable for Jews, Muslims and other groups (Miller & Kearney 2001)
Pilocarpine (Salagen) (some evidence for)	Increases salivary flow only if some salivary gland function remains (Taylor 2003)	Side-effects include sweating; often discontinued for this reason (Miller & Kearney 2001)
Ascorbic acid (insufficient evidence)	Used in palliative care settings (Milligan et al 2001) No evidence of benefit for radiation xerostomia or mucositis	
Sodium bicarbonate mouthwash (insufficient evidence)	Used traditionally but no confirmatory controlled studies (Sadler et al 2003). Is not antimicrobial Said to remove crusted mucosa (Roberts 1990); Tombes & Gallucci (1993) advise against its use	
Saline mouthwash (insufficient evidence)	Used traditionally but no confirmatory controlled studies (Sadler et al 2003) Recommended for patients having oral radiation (Feber 1995)	
Lemon and glycerine (evidence against)	Causes demineralisation of teeth (Meurman et al 1996) Being anhydrous, will aggravate xerostomia (Sadler et al 2003)	
Hydrogen peroxide (evidence against)	No scientific or clinical evidence (Krishnasamay 1995) Astringent, exacerbates xerostomia, unpleasant taste (Davies et al 2001)	

Table 15.6 Characteristics and management of maxillofacial fractures

Fracture	Signs and symptoms	Management
Fractured nasal bones	Nasal deviation or flattening; bruising Septal haematoma causing obstructed breathing	Manipulation of nasal bones and septum; nasal pack and plaster of Paris for 1–2 weeks Drainage of haematoma
Fractured malar bone	Black eye; swelling over cheek, sometimes flattening; anaesthesia of areas supplied by injured nerves (infraorbital and superior dental); inability to open mouth; diplopia	Elevation of malar bone through incision in temporal region. May require fixation by wiring of bone
'Blow-out' fracture of malar	Periorbital haematoma; diplopia	Insertion of implant to orbital floor to stop eye dropping
Fractured maxilla/middle third fracture	Grossly swollen face; failure of teeth to occlude properly; bilateral periorbital haematoma; fractured nasal bones; teeth may be loosened; CSF rhinorrhoea	Intermaxillary fixation (IMF) eyelet wires, Gunning splints, etc. Open reduction and internal fixation (ORIF) using wires, screws, plates
Fractured mandible with/without other fractured facial bones	Displaced or undisplaced; local pain and swelling; severe pain on opening mouth, sublingual haematoma	Undisplaced: usually no treatment Displaced: reduction with wires, splints or plate depending on site of fracture

NB: there will be considerable variation in presentation and in the timing of manipulative procedures, in accordance with the exact site and combination of fractures.

Domestic violence is often unreported by the victim, and Lydon (1996) suggests the following reasons for this:

- fear due to repeated psychological abuse
- fear of reprisals
- fear for their children's safety or that they will be taken into care
- financial dependence on the assailant.

Lydon comments that domestic violence is often trivialised and challenges nurses to be proactive in trying to bring to the fore this serious issue in our society. The Zero Tolerance campaign (theme: 'Violence against women and children is a crime'), which started in Edinburgh and spread country-wide, is a very successful example of raising awareness of this issue (see Women's Aid, 'Useful websites', p. 651).

STOP THINK **15.6** Discuss how you would react if you suspected that someone presenting to the Emergency Department had been assaulted by someone they know well.

Road traffic collisions (RCAs)

Incidence of facial injuries was reduced following the introduction of seat belt legislation (Department of Health and Social Security 1978), and the more recent introduction of airbags has reduced fatalities and severity of injuries to the head (Frampton et al 2002).

Industrial injuries

Accidents in the workplace involving machinery or equipment are often followed by claims for compensation. Nurses should therefore not comment on the circumstances of any incident, either in person or by telephone, other than by using standard statements agreed by hospital policy (Nursing and Midwifery Council 2004).

Sports injuries

These are usually the result of a collision or fall and are most commonly soft tissue injuries (Hill et al 1998). Wearing helmets or gum shields may reduce the severity of injury.

Accidents

Accidental falls are common among older people, often resulting in facial injury. The underlying cause of the fall may require investigation (Chew & Edmondson 1996).

Burns

The treatment of burn injuries is discussed in detail in Chapter 30. It is emphasised here, however, that to assist in the prevention of contractures of the mouth and subsequent difficulty in function or administration of a general anaesthetic, patients with burns should be encouraged to drink from a cup as early as possible and to avoid the use of straws.

STOP THINK **15.7** Take a few sips of a drink directly from a cup and then with a straw. What do you observe about the maxillofacial movement required for these two actions?

MEDICAL MANAGEMENT

Immediate intervention Emergency treatment will involve whatever resuscitative measures are required to maintain the patient's airway, breathing and circulation and to prevent the development of clinical shock (see Chs 18 and 27). Priorities for intervention will have to be set, as cerebral and pulmonary injuries are often associated with maxillofacial injuries in severely injured trauma patients (Alvi et al 2003, National Institute for Clinical Excellence 2003). A full physical examination will involve neurological observations and X-rays as appropriate, and will be followed by referral to the appropriate specialists, e.g. maxillofacial, orthopaedic or ophthalmic surgeons. Cannell et al (1996) state that, in using an injury assessment tool (Ali & Shepherd 1994) when assessing multiply injured patients, maxillofacial injuries often tend to be underscored and that a maxillofacial surgeon should be involved as soon as possible to minimise facial deformity. However, the person with a maxillofacial injury with minimal displacement of bone and no symptoms of head injury may delay attending for treatment until, eventually, swelling and bruising make the injury appear more alarming.

Treatment of maxillofacial injuries The signs and symptoms of maxillofacial injuries, together with appropriate treatments, are summarised in Table 15.6.

Soft-tissue injuries require thorough cleansing. This may entail scrubbing of the wound under general anaesthesia, to remove glass, debris, gravel or dirt. Failure to clean the injury adequately will lead to 'tattoo scarring', i.e. a permanent blue–grey scar. Facial suturing should adhere to plastic surgery techniques (McGregor & McGregor 2000).

Bone injuries The objectives of treatment are to restore pre-existing anatomy, functional occlusion of teeth and facial appearance. The most common method of immobilisation now employed is open reduction and internal fixation (ORIF) when the fracture is exposed, reduced (i.e. repositioned) and fixed with wires, screws, a rigid plate or mini-plates. Plates (see Fig. 15.3) may be left in situ permanently or removed after 3 months. However, other methods of fixation using the patient's bite, known as intermaxillary fixation (IMF), may still be used successfully, for example:

- *Eyelet wiring* — wires are twisted around the upper and lower teeth, leaving a loop (eyelet). The teeth are then brought into proper occlusion and wired together (see Fig. 15.4).
- *Arch bar wiring* — this technique is similar to eyelet wiring but is used when fewer teeth exist.
- Gunning splint and cast cap splints are other methods of IMF and are described in Wray et al (2003).

Undisplaced fractures of the mandible generally require no surgical treatment.

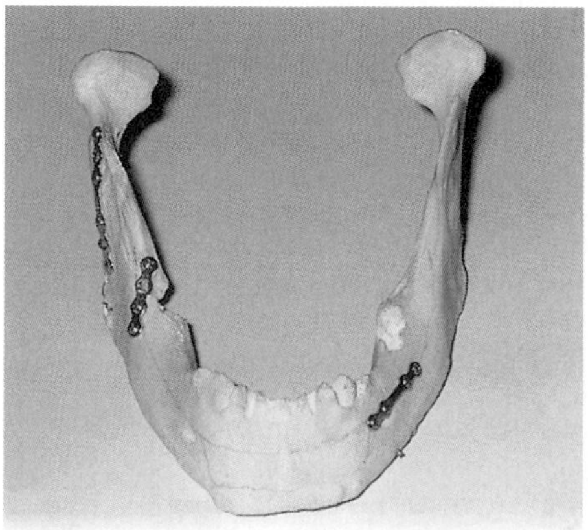

Fig. 15.3 Interosseous plating.

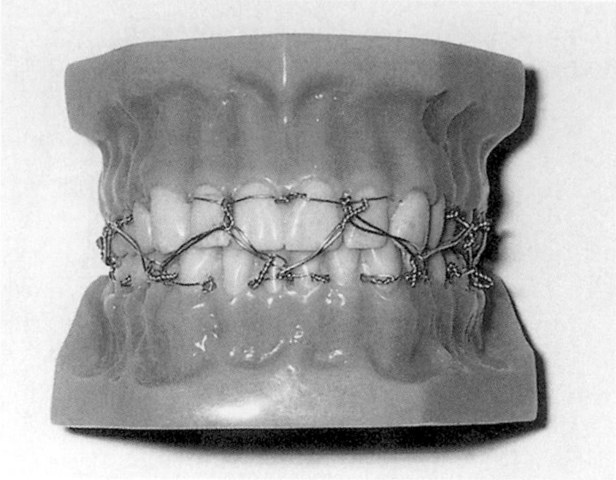

Fig. 15.4 Eyelet wiring.

A fractured maxilla can be immobilised internally (ORIF) or externally (IMF), depending on the precise nature of the injury. Internal fixation can be achieved by means of metal plates or with internal suspension wires. The latter hold the maxilla and mandible in occlusion and are fixed to the malar or frontal bone.

External fixation is now less commonly seen but may be achieved by inserting rigid pins into the bones via the skin. These are then secured externally with rods and joints. This method may be used for more complicated injuries.

Treatment of a fractured malar (zygoma) may take the following forms:

- Elevation through incision in the temporal region
- Wiring or plating of the fracture
- Kirschner wires (K-wires) — rigid wires which may be inserted into the bone in one or more directions, and the ends cut just clear of the skin
- An implant may be necessary to repair a shattered orbital floor.

Fractured nasal bones may also form part of a compound facial injury. Here, the fracture is reduced by manipulation of the nasal bones and may be immobilised by a plaster of Paris splint.

For further information on orofacial trauma, see Wray et al (2003).

NURSING PRIORITIES AND MANAGEMENT: Orofacial trauma

Orofacial injuries vary widely both in presentation and in their impact upon the individual's lifestyle and psychological well-being. Case Histories 15.1 and 15.2 outline the experiences of two patients admitted to hospital after receiving blows to the face. Each has different needs, priorities and concerns, and hence different requirements for nursing care. While the treatment of individuals who have suffered orofacial trauma must take into account a range of physical and emotional considerations, only that care which is specific to the mouth and face will be described here. General pre- and postoperative care is discussed in Chapter 26; reference to other chapters will be made as appropriate.

CASE HISTORY 15.1

Ms Y

Ms Y, aged 23, was brought to the Emergency Department by a neighbour who heard a disturbance and found her dazed. She was found to be suffering from concussion, a fractured malar bone and facial lacerations, and was admitted to the ward. Ms Y explained that she received these injuries when she tripped and fell against a door.

Ms Y was advised that she would have to have the fractured malar reduced and stabilised under anaesthetic. She was assured that the operation was not a major procedure, but that the fracture would simply be fixed by means of wires. She was also given general information on preoperative procedures and postoperative care. She was advised not to use a mouthwash too vigorously.

She was able to take a soft diet, however, and was advised to continue with soft foods for 7–10 days and to take as much protein as possible to promote healing.

After the incident, Ms Y was also suffering from diplopia (double vision) as a result of a slight displacement of one eye. This persisted and she was later referred for orthoptic exercises.

While she was on the ward, Ms Y began to disclose some of her domestic problems, first to her primary nurse and then to the medical social worker who, with Ms Y's agreement, had become involved. Ms Y indicated that she would consider accepting assistance from a women's support group. The social worker arranged for Ms Y's children to be cared for until she was ready for discharge.

Ms Y's discharge was planned well in advance. Through liaison with women's support agencies, she was assisted in reviewing her home circumstances and was offered alternative accommodation with her children.

Life-threatening concerns

Harrahill and Eastes (2000) discuss the risk of injuries which may be missed, and the importance of skilled nursing observation. For patients who have suffered maxillofacial injury, the immediate priority of intervention is likely to be to maintain the airway. Respiratory difficulty and haemorrhage will require immediate care.

Respiratory difficulty

This problem can vary in severity and may be due to swelling of the tongue caused by oedema or haematoma, or to the patient's inability to control the tongue because of disturbance of the muscle attachments. If conscious, the patient should be sat up and propped forward as soon as possible, if other injuries allow. The airway must be kept clear. If the maxilla is fractured, it may be necessary to insert two fingers into the patient's mouth and hook behind the hard palate to re-establish the airway. In severe cases, early intubation or tracheostomy may be necessary.

Haemorrhage

There may be significant haemorrhage from middle third fractures resulting in cheek swelling, and nasal packing may be required. Bleeding may also be profuse when soft tissue injury has occurred, and immediate measures may be necessary, e.g. applying pressure on a bleeding point or pressure point until ligation of the damaged vessel can be performed. Bleeding can also be controlled by holding the skin edges together with Steri-strips until suturing can be carried out.

Shock

Nursing and medical staff must be alert to the warning signs of shock and should be prepared to take urgent action (see Ch. 18).

Major nursing considerations

Observation and monitoring

Vital signs Temperature, pulse, pulse oximetry, respiration, blood pressure and pain should be recorded at regular intervals. Neurological observations may be appropriate (see Ch. 9).

Rhinorrhoea The nurse should also watch for the presence of rhinorrhoea (nasal discharge) caused by leakage of cerebrospinal fluid (CSF). This can occur in fracture of the maxilla if the cribriform plate of the ethmoid bone is disturbed. CSF gives a positive reaction to Dextrostix.

Eye integrity/vision (see Ch. 13). The nurse should check for abnormal pupil reactions, proptosis and acute pain. Vision should be checked hourly at first, especially if the patient cannot open the eyes because of oedema. The nurse should gently open the eyes and check pupil reaction. Any rapid decrease in visual acuity can indicate retrobulbar haemorrhage, which can lead to blindness and requires urgent action. Double vision can indicate a fracture of the orbital floor.

Major patient problems

Pain

Pain must be assessed (see Ch. 19) but is not normally a major early problem. It is important, however, not to underestimate the patient's pain and to explain why analgesics may have to be withheld initially while investigations are carried out (see Ch. 27).

Anxiety

Anxiety caused by fear of disfigurement and scarring may be the first concern of many patients and relatives. An injury to the eye will be a source of further anxiety.

Patients and relatives should be given the opportunity to talk about their fears, particularly in the early stages when profuse bleeding may make the injury look horrific. Nurses should offer the reassurance that healing is usually rapid and that as much as possible will be done to minimise scarring. However, it is equally important not to raise expectations unduly. Some people have unrealistic ideas about the results that surgery can produce, and it is unfair to allow them to imagine that what existed before can always be fully restored. Scars can fade and may be camouflaged, but it is not always possible to disguise the disfigurement caused by major tissue loss or bone displacement and it may be appropriate to introduce psychological support at an early stage (Rumsey et al 2002).

Other considerations

Every effort should be made to clean blood and debris from the patient before relatives arrive, in order to avoid unnecessary distress. Dirty clothing should be removed, observing local policy for the care of patients' property.

Oral hygiene should be carried out within the limitations of the patient's condition. For example, a blood clot should be left undisturbed as far as possible to minimise further bleeding, but broken teeth, debris and so on should be removed if this has not already been done. Gentle irrigation with warm saline may be helpful.

Nursing care in surgical interventions

Patients who have soft tissue injury without bone damage will have suturing and/or reconstruction carried out as soon as possible.

Many patients with maxillofacial fractures will require surgical intervention to reduce and stabilise the fracture. The timing of this surgery will vary according to the patient's overall condition and the amount of localised swelling which may make assessment of the fracture difficult. In many cases, fixation is best left for a few days; if the general condition permits, the patient may be discharged home for the interim. Alternatively, direct transfer to a specialised unit may be arranged.

Postoperative management

The overall aim of postoperative management is to assist as necessary with the activities of daily living and to help the patient achieve independence in these activities as soon as possible.

Monitoring vital signs In the initial postoperative period, the patient's vital signs should be recorded every 15 min. As the condition stabilises, the patient can gradually be raised to a sitting position to aid respiration, help drainage and minimise oedema. The patient should be encouraged to maintain an upright position even at night. Moving and handling advisors now counsel against pillows placed in armchair fashion. A reclining armchair, if available, can be useful later if other injuries permit.

Respiration The patient may have a nasal airway in situ to assist breathing and this will need occasional suction to ensure it remains patent. The mouth may also need gentle suction if the patient is afraid to swallow saliva for fear of choking. The patient should be encouraged to relax and to practise gentle swallowing movements.

Oral hygiene It is very important to help the patient maintain good oral hygiene. If the jaws have been wired, a soft toothbrush or Q-tips can be used to keep the anterior surface of the teeth and splints clean. The inside of the mouth can be cleansed with mouthwash taken through a straw (or a feeding cup with a spout) and squeezed out between the teeth. An alternative method is to have the patient lean forward and to irrigate the mouth through gaps between the teeth, using a monojet syringe, letting the fluid run out.

Preventing wound infection The skin entry points of external fixation should be kept free of crusting by cleaning with normal saline. An ointment such as sterile petroleum jelly may be applied.

Sutures to facial lacerations can be kept clean with normal saline and removed in 3–4 days to minimise scarring. Supporting Steri-strips may then be applied over the wound for a further 3–4 days. Any intraoral lacerations are usually repaired using catgut, which will be absorbed, but the mouth should be checked in case any non-absorbent sutures have been used, e.g. inside the lip.

Maintenance of fixation The guiding principle of the treatment of maxillofacial fractures is, as for any other types of fracture, to obtain healing in the optimal position, e.g. that which maintains proper occlusion. In order for callus to form, and thus for healing to take place, the bone must remain immobile. Many patients will have fractures fixed with internal metal plates. However, if the jaw is immobilised by other means, appropriate instruments for releasing the fixation, i.e. wire cutters, or scissors for elastic bands, must always be available at the patient's bedside for immediate use should any danger of airway obstruction arise.

Instruments for tightening screws should also be at hand, and the fixation checked at regular intervals. Most patients will be aware if it becomes loose, but older people or those with head injury may not be. To avoid confusion, only those instruments appropriate for loosening or tightening the individual's particular type of fixation should be available at the bedside.

Nutrition (see also Ch. 21). A nasogastric tube may be inserted to allow for postoperative aspiration and/or drainage of old blood. Oral feeding should be encouraged as soon as possible, and there are particular problems if the jaws must be kept wired for several weeks. A liquid diet must be taken, which may make it difficult for the patient to consume sufficient calories to maintain body weight. All food must be liquidised and supplemented with 'sip feeds', of which a wide variety is now available. Frequent, small meals should be taken throughout the day.

The dietitian should be consulted, ideally before the surgery takes place, to assess the patient's dietary requirements. Older patients with a low body mass index (BMI) will require special monitoring and encouragement. This is especially important if food is served by non-nursing personnel who may not appreciate the significance of unfinished meals.

STOP THINK **15.8** How can a calorie intake adequate to promote healing be provided within the constraints of a hospital setting for Ms Y (Case History 15.1), who has no interest in food, and Mr J (Case History 15.2), whose injuries prevent him from eating solid food?

Allaying fears Nursing staff should bear in mind that the patient is likely to be very alarmed on recovery from anaesthesia to find that interdental or external fixation is in place, even if previously informed that this would be necessary. It is important that the patient is given some means of expressing feelings and concerns and is briefed fully on how to manage basic functions such as eating and how to avoid choking if coughing up phlegm or vomiting.

Communication will be frustrating for the patient initially if the jaws have been fixed, but most difficulties will be

CASE HISTORY 15.2
Mr J

Mr J, aged 30, was assaulted while returning from an evening out with friends. He was unconscious for a short time after the incident. He was brought to the Emergency Department in the recovery position to prevent blood from inside his mouth trickling down the pharynx (and potentially the trachea) and causing respiratory distress. Fortunately, he had not suffered pneumothorax, in which case he might not have been able to lie in this position. It was difficult to restrain him as he was restless from the combined effects of blows to the head and the alcohol he had taken. He was found to be suffering from a middle third fracture, a fractured mandible, fractured ribs and facial lacerations.

Mr J was advised that his jaws would have to be wired together and external fixation applied, but he had difficulty concentrating and absorbing information. His wife was present during the discussion. She was very anxious and mentioned that she had been concerned by the fact that her husband had been drinking more lately.

When he awoke from the anaesthetic, Mr J was quite frightened, as he did not remember much of what had been explained to him preoperatively. The nurse in the recovery ward told Mr J to breathe deeply and encouraged him to relax. She then explained again what had happened and what was preventing him from opening his mouth. She explained why it was important for him not to disturb the fixation, but also assured him that if it ever became urgent for him to release his jaw, the necessary equipment was at hand. She then stayed with Mr J until the feeling of the wires became more familiar to him, and ensured that adequate analgesics and sedation were being administered (see Ch. 19).

Mr J had some problems in the first few postoperative days when he turned in bed and accidentally knocked his frame. He was somewhat apprehensive about having a visit from his active 2-year-old daughter.

He was able to take only a liquid diet, and so liquidised meals were provided with supplementary drinks. He was advised that he could obtain a prescription from his GP for high-calorie drinks during the time when the wiring was in place.

Mr J was surprised at how quickly the appearance of his injury improved. His facial wounds healed quite rapidly and he was encouraged that within a few months the scars would fade and become less noticeable.

While he was still in hospital, he was encouraged to review his alcohol intake and was given information on the effects of alcohol abuse and on local self-help groups from whom he and his family could obtain support as he addressed his dependency problem (see Ch. 36).

overcome by otherwise healthy people, given sufficient encouragement and reassurance in the early stages. Writing pads, 'magic' slates, picture cards and other aids may be used to facilitate communication. Special care will be needed for patients with learning difficulties.

Mobility When and how well the patient will be able to return to normal activity will depend on the nature of any other injuries incurred. Patients with facial injuries can be up on the day following surgery, but there are obvious restrictions if a maxillocranial frame is in place.

STOP THINK **15.9** Stop and reflect on how your own activities would be affected if you had metal rods protruding from your head.

Body image Disfigurement caused by facial injuries is of great concern to most patients, and for the majority scarring will be a source of continuing anxiety.

Many people will be reluctant to look at themselves in a mirror following surgery and should not be forced to do so (see Case History 15.2). It might help for the nurse to ask the patient if he would like her to describe how his face looks to her; if her account is matter-of-fact and accepting, he may be more willing to look at himself. Unfortunately, for many people, disfigurement will give rise to deep feelings of grief and loss which may never be completely resolved, and specialist help may be needed (Robinson et al 1996).

Alcohol Smith et al (2003) showed the benefit of a nurse-led psychological intervention on alcohol consumption and misuse in young males following alcohol-related facial injury (Scottish Intercollegiate Guidelines Network 2003).

Discharge planning

Patients who are fit and who can maintain adequate self-care can be discharged when postoperative swelling has subsided. They should be provided with written instructions on diet and oral hygiene, and given a telephone number to call in case of emergency. Referral to the community nurse should be made for care of wounds, checking of fixation and assessment of diet. A follow-up appointment should be made for the patient to return after 4–6 weeks to have the fixation removed.

Post-traumatic stress disorder (PTSD)

There is growing awareness of the psychological impact of a traumatic event (Joy et al 2000, Sen et al 2001), and of the need to address the long-term psychological problems which many trauma patients, regardless of age, experience. In particular, older patients who are already frail may never recover fully from maxillofacial injury and surgery. Some who are fit to go home may well be too afraid or self-conscious to go out of their house. The community nurse is in an ideal position to encourage such individuals to venture into the outside world again. Some may require long-term care, whether within the family, in sheltered housing or in an appropriate care home.

TUMOURS OF THE MOUTH

Oral cancer is more common than is often realised, the mortality rates being comparable with malignant melanoma and cervical cancer (Soutar 2003), and attempts are being made to raise awareness (www.mouthcancerawareness.org.uk). The mortality rates could be much reduced, as early diagnosis should lead to cure (Macpherson et al 2003), and nurses in their role as health educators can make a significant contribution to this reduction (see Box 15.1, p. 629).

Treatment of intraoral tumours is frequently carried out in specialised units. However, as the use of advanced reconstructive techniques becomes more widespread and patients are discharged into the community at an earlier stage, often to continue treatment as outpatients, nurses in more general areas of practice are likely to encounter these patients. To help to ensure continuity of care from hospital to the community, it is important for general nurses to have an understanding of the long-term problems faced by these patients (Espie et al 1989, Freedlander et al 1989, Rogers et al 2002, Kelly 2003).

Treatment plans vary from centre to centre and there are different schools of thought within the medical profession as to which treatment schedule best promotes survival and, also important, a good quality of life (Robertson et al 2001). However treated, it is likely that many patients will suffer some disruption of several basic mechanisms which control the functions of eating and speaking. Patients may be left with short-term, long-term or permanent malfunction, which will vary greatly from patient to patient and is dependent on many factors. Table 15.7 indicates some of the malfunctions following surgery and/or radiotherapy.

It must be stressed that each patient is very much an individual whose needs and priorities will differ significantly from those of another patient with a seemingly similar problem. There can therefore be no set plan of care, and nurses must be ready and equipped to modify their ideas, working in conjunction with the other members of the multidisciplinary team and with the patient, to meet that individual's needs. As rehabilitation may take many months or years, it is often necessary for this multidisciplinary liaison to continue for some considerable time to ensure the best possible quality of care (Kelly 2003).

The pathophysiology and common presenting symptoms of tumours of the mouth are described under the following headings:

- tumours of the lips
- tumours of the floor of the mouth and tongue
- tumours of the palate
- tumours of the salivary glands.

However, because the separate functions of the mouth, e.g. speaking, chewing and swallowing, are frequently interdependent, medical and nursing management will be discussed with reference to the whole mouth.

Tumours of the lips

PATHOPHYSIOLOGY

Benign tumours, including granulomata, are treated by simple excision.

Malignant disease may take the form of basal cell carcinoma (BCC, often called 'rodent ulcer' because of its pattern of 'eating' or 'gnawing into' tissue) or squamous cell carcinoma (SCC). Malignant melanomas may also rarely occur on the lips (see Ch. 12).

Predisposing factors include prolonged, unprotected exposure to sunlight, e.g. among outdoor workers, fair skin and pipe smoking. The lower incidence of lip cancers among women may possibly be due to the barrier effect of cosmetics.

Common presenting symptoms Basal cell carcinoma may appear as a nodule or as a small, unstable ulcerating area with persistent crusting. It may also be diffuse and invasive. The patient often reports: 'I thought it had healed up, but I kept knocking the top off it.' The ulcer may have 'pearlised' rolled edges. These tumours are generally slow

Table 15.7 The effects of intraoral disease and treatment on the mechanisms of eating

Normal mechanism and cranial nerves involved	Disruption caused by intervention	Effects
Teeth bite and chew food, powered by muscles of jaw and supplied by trigeminal nerve (CN V)	Teeth may be extracted due to caries or to give access to tumour	Soft food only can be taken until fitting of dentures, if this is possible
Saliva secreted by parotid gland (CN IX), submandibular and sublingual glands mixes with food	Glands may be excised during surgery or damaged by radiotherapy	Dry mouth (xerostomia) Stomatitis Thrush
Tongue and teeth powered by muscles of jaw break down food and form it into bolus	Muscles damaged or weakened by surgery and trauma	Re-education of eating skills will be needed
Mouth kept closed by superficial facial muscles (supplied by CN V and CN VII); buccinator prevents food gathering in cheek pouches	Internal contours of mouth are altered; lack of control Temporomandibular joint malfunction	Drooling Food gathers in mouth Trismus — mouth cannot open
Tongue helps propel food to back of mouth and into contact with oral part of pharynx	Excision of part or whole tongue Tongue becomes fixed or insensate	Patient needs to push food to oropharynx
Simultaneously with above, muscles of soft palate elevate and tighten, straightening out to close off nasal cavity and preventing food from entering it	Damage to palate and nerves allows food to enter nasal space	Food, liquids come down nose unless obturator (see Box 15.3) can be fitted
Larynx rises under shelter of epiglottis to close off airway, preventing entry of food	CN IX damage causes paralysis of pharyngeal muscles	Aspiration of fluid to lungs necessitates permanent tracheostomy and gastrostomy

growing and do not metastasise, although occasionally a tendency to multiple BCC is seen.

Squamous cell carcinoma is more aggressive and, if untreated, may assume the 'cauliflower' look of a malignant ulcer and will eventually fungate and cause severe pain.

Tumours of the floor of the mouth and tongue

PATHOPHYSIOLOGY

Tumours of the tongue account for approximately one-third of all intraoral tumours in the UK. Others included in the category of the floor of the mouth are found on the lower alveolus, tonsillar fossae and retromolar trigones, and about 90% are of the SCC type (Lewis 2003). Fifty years ago the male to female ratio was 5:1; it is now 2:1 in Scotland and incidence and mortality are also rising in almost all EU countries (Soutar 2003).

Spread usually involves the local lymph nodes, e.g. cervical, submandibular and submental. Distant metastases occur rarely in the lung.

Predisposing factors Heavy smoking combined with excessive alcohol consumption is associated with these cancers. However, there is an increase in younger people with no history of smoking or excess alcohol consumption (Llewellyn et al 2003), and it is now accepted that oral cancer may occur in any age group. Other risk factors are deprivation and diets poor in fruit and vegetables. There are also connections with anaemia, vitamin deficiencies and chronic oral infections, e.g. syphilis, herpes simplex virus, human papilloma virus and HIV (Soutar 2003).

Common presenting symptoms These cancers may become apparent in a variety of ways. In the early stages, intraoral SCC is easily mistaken for infection, irritation from dentures or a simple aphthous ulcer. Dysplasia, i.e. abnormal mucosa which presents as white patches (leukoplakia) or red patches (erythroplakia), is a precancerous condition which can revert to normal if the individual stops smoking. Unchecked, this condition will often become malignant. More advanced tumours are usually unmistakable, but many patients present late for various reasons, including fear, misdiagnosis and self-neglect (Lewis 2003).

Tumours of the hard and soft palate

PATHOPHYSIOLOGY

These tumours may arise from the epithelium of the mucous membrane (SCC), in the maxillary sinuses, in the maxilla or in the minor salivary glands in the palate. They are less common than tumours of the floor of the mouth, but are potentially more disfiguring, as spread may occur locally to the floor of the orbit or to the eye.

Common presenting symptoms Onset may be insidious. The patient may notice a dull ache for some time and may complain of 'sinusitis'. The pain will eventually increase and swelling may develop over the cheek. There may be some displacement of the eye (proptosis) in advanced cases. Rarely, a malignant melanoma appears as a pigmented lesion of the palate and goes unnoticed until the individual presents with a secondary tumour of the cheek or neck.

Tumours of the salivary glands

PATHOPHYSIOLOGY

The most common cause of swelling of the parotid gland is mumps (acute parotitis), an infectious, inflammatory condition that usually resolves without treatment. Mumps may, however, be relatively severe in adults and lead to pancreatitis or orchitis.

Benign (pleomorphic salivary adenomas, PSAs) or malignant tumours may develop in the parotid, submandibular, sublingual and other minor salivary glands. Salivary gland ducts may become blocked by small accretions (see 'Orodental disease', p. 630).

Common presenting symptoms The patient presents with a swelling, which is often asymptomatic and therefore sometimes long-standing, in the area of the affected gland. If left untreated, a parotid gland tumour may involve the facial nerve (CN VII), resulting in facial palsy, a severe disfigurement.

MEDICAL MANAGEMENT OF TUMOURS OF THE MOUTH

Tests and investigations A treatment plan for malignant tumours will be devised on the basis of careful staging of the cancer (see Table 15.8 and Ch. 31). Investigation may include the following:

- history
- physical examination — visual and by palpation
- blood tests
- diagnostic X-rays — face and jaw, chest and spine as appropriate
- orthopantomogram (OPT or OPG; see Appendix 1)
- sialogram (see Appendix 1)
- computed tomography (CT) scan
- magnetic resonance imaging (MRI); see Chapter 31
- positron emission tomography (PET) scan, if available
- examination under anaesthetic (EUA)

Table 15.8 TNM classification for lip and oral cavity

T: Primary tumour	
T1	Tumour ≤2 cm
T2	Tumour >2–4 cm
T3	Tumour >4 cm
T4	Tumour invading adjacent structures
N: lymph nodes (neck)	
N1	Ipsilateral single node ≤3 cm
N2	Ipsilateral single node >3–6 cm
	Ipsilateral, multiple nodes ≤6 cm
	Bilateral, contralateral nodes ≤6 cm
N3	Node >6 cm
M: distant metastases	
M0	No distant metastases
M1	Distant metastases

Adapted with permission from Sobin & Wittekind (2002).

- videofluoroscopy
- fine needle aspiration
- biopsy — results are essential for staging disease and planning treatment
- sentinel node biopsy (SNB) to evaluate spread of cancer to the neck (Ross et al 2002) (see Appendix 1).

The patient's age, general physical condition and mental outlook will also be taken into consideration.

Treatment Patients are often seen at a combined clinic, where many medical and other professional personnel may be present, and this can be very stressful (Telfer & Shepherd 1993). At this clinic different specialist consultants, e.g. surgeons and oncologists, liaise to plan treatment, which may be radical, i.e. intended to effect a cure, or conservative, i.e. intended to alleviate pain, prevent fungating tumours and subsequent haemorrhage. Radical treatment may involve extremely difficult adjustments for patients and, for some, a significant reduction in the quality of life (Espie et al 1989, Freedlander et al 1989, Rogers et al 2002).

The treatment options for oral tumours are radiotherapy, surgery and, less commonly as first-line treatment, chemotherapy. These treatment modes may be used singly or in combination; sequence and timing vary from one centre to another (McMahon 2003).

Chemotherapy is usually given concurrently with other treatment. It may be used to reduce the bulk of some tumours prior to surgery or in cases of recurrent tumours (see also Ch. 31).

Radiotherapy can be given as the sole treatment, or pre- or postoperatively. It may take either of the following forms:

- teletherapy (external radiation) by means of megavoltage machines or supervoltage machines
- brachytherapy, in which a radioactive source is placed in or near the tumour, e.g. interstitial needles to tumours of the lip or oral cavity. This treatment is being used increasingly in tongue cancer to try to maximise quality of life (Sandhu et al 1999).

Many tumours, e.g. SCC, are highly curable by radiotherapy. Sarcoma and malignant melanoma, on the other hand, are less radiosensitive (Holmes 1997, and see Ch. 31).

Surgical excision Treatment by this method ranges from small local excisions with direct closure, to major operations with full reconstruction. Benign tumours are usually excised.

Some centres carry out excision of tumours initially, with secondary reconstruction later; others carry out immediate reconstruction (Hislop & Soutar 2003). Table 15.9 summarises current surgical procedures.

Both radiotherapy and surgery treat SCC successfully, either independently or in combination, but there is lack of agreement among medical practitioners as to the best timing of each. Gene, viral oncolytic and antibody therapies are being researched (Ganly 2003).

Nurses should be aware of the effect of radiation on the epithelium (Little 1996, Holmes 1997, Wells 2003, and see Ch. 31). Following radical radiotherapy, healing after surgery may be delayed; occasionally, orocutaneous (between mouth and skin) fistulae may develop. A late effect may be bone necrosis (osteoradionecrosis).

Follow-up and aftercare will require outpatient appointments at regular intervals for at least 5 years. Dental and/or prosthetic provision may include dentures, obturators (see Box 15.3) and other prostheses provided by members of the multidisciplinary team as and when necessary. Referral to other consultants, e.g. ENT, ophthalmic, thoracic and neurological specialists, will be made as

Box 15.3

Obturators

Obturators are prostheses which are designed to fill a defect in the palate after maxillectomy. They are fitted in three stages:

1. *Surgical splint* — fitted during surgery to hold a skin graft in place and/or avoid collapse of the cheek and upper lip. After about 2 weeks, it is replaced by a temporary obturator.
2. *Temporary obturator* — used throughout radiotherapy. This allows the patient to become accustomed to wearing and handling an obturator.
3. *Definitive obturator* — fitted after shrinkage of defect. It may be composed of a soft malleable 'bung' which fills the defect, and a denture which fits over the bung.

Without the obturator, the patient will be unable to speak or eat properly, and fluid will run into the nasal cavity. With a well-fitting obturator, the patient can eat and speak normally.

The obturator must be removed after meals and cleaned by brushing or by immersion in a proprietary cleaning solution (if the obturator has been 'built up', cleanser should not be used). The mouth must be rinsed after all food to prevent accumulation of plaque, debris, etc.

Table 15.9 Surgery for tumours of the mouth

Site	Excision	Reconstruction
Superficial lesion of lip, leukoplakia	Shaving	None
Lip, parotid gland, T1 tumour of mouth	Simple excision	None: direct (primary) closure
Lip	Wedge excision	Direct closure
Tongue	Local excision	Split-skin graft
Lip, alveolus, tongue	Local excision	Local flap: many varieties — Abbé, tongue, buccal, nasolabial, etc. (see Soutar & Tiwari 1996)
Mouth/pharynx (all sites), cheek, neck	Local/wide excision ± neck dissection	Free flap common in many centres
As above (especially for recurrent tumour as palliative procedure)	As above	Pedicled flap (deltopectoral, pectoralis major)

appropriate. Speech therapy and dietary advice will be essential for many patients.

NURSING PRIORITIES AND MANAGEMENT: Tumours of the mouth

The presence of an oral tumour may not give rise to immediate life-threatening concerns, except where a long-neglected tumour causes respiratory distress or haemorrhage.

Patients will vary widely in the symptoms with which they present, and usually require much reassurance when a biopsy confirms the diagnosis. They will be admitted as soon as appropriate treatment has been arranged, or immediately if the disease is advanced. A gastrostomy (see Ch. 21) may be planned if swallowing difficulties are anticipated. The nurse may require to be the patient's advocate, to ensure adequate understanding before consent to treatment. Referral to the primary care team and/or Macmillan or Marie Curie home care nurses will be beneficial to many patients for support before definitive treatment starts.

Immediate nursing priorities

Nursing intervention in the early stages of treatment will focus on controlling pain (see Ch. 19), relieving anxiety, encouraging self-care in oral hygiene, and nutritional assessment (see Ch. 21). Supplementary feeding may be necessary, as weight loss is common among this group of patients. Existing physical conditions must be taken into account in any nursing plan. An additional concern may be the assessment and control of alcoholism. Excessive consumption of alcohol is a causative factor in many cases of oral cancer, and advice and information on limiting the intake of alcohol may be given by nurses (Scottish Intercollegiate Guidelines Network 2003, Smith et al 2003, and see Ch. 36).

Preoperative preparation

Giving information

All patients will require adequate and honest information about the proposed treatment and its implications (see Ch. 31). In view of the many variations in procedures, and the diverse presentations and responses to treatment that are possible, nurses should be wary of giving information based on limited knowledge of apparently similar cases. What is feasible for one person may not be possible for another, and expectations or anxieties should not be raised unduly.

The patient should, however, be allowed to voice any concerns about the disease and its implications for normal functioning, e.g. speaking and eating, and for appearance. Many patients also have a deep fear of cancer and may have misconceptions about prognosis and the likely course of the disease. It is important for their needs to be recognised and any unfounded anxiety relieved.

Information giving is discussed by Ream (2000).

A multidisciplinary approach

A successful outcome will depend in part on the continuity of care provided by the multidisciplinary team. Along with medical staff, the nursing team will include ward, theatre and high dependency unit nurses, specialist nurses, community nurses and possibly Macmillan and Marie Curie nurses. The following professionals also contribute to care, and the nurse must be aware of each team member's role and facilitate liaison wherever appropriate:

- Dietitian — assesses dietary intake and advises staff and patient on maintaining adequate nutrition; liaises with pharmacy, the nutritional support person in the commercial companies and the community dietitian for provision of enteral feeding equipment (Dawson et al 2001)
- Speech and language therapist — advises patient on pre- and postoperative exercises to assist with speech and swallowing difficulties; advises on alternative means of communicating if loss of voice is permanent (Jackson et al 1999) (see Ch. 14)
- Physiotherapist — gives instruction and assistance with pre- and postoperative exercises to assist breathing, expectoration, limb and shoulder movements
- Dentist (associate specialist) or prosthodontist — assesses need for dental care, especially when radiotherapy is part of treatment, and fits obturator and/or dentures (Ali 2003)
- Dental hygienist — advises patient on care of teeth and oral hygiene, especially during radiotherapy and/or chemotherapy
- Maxillofacial technician — advises on whether provision of a prosthesis is realistically possible; designs, constructs and fits this when appropriate for each individual patient
- Medical social worker — gives information and advice on availability of grants for special needs; arranges home help, day care
- Hospital chaplain or other religious counsellor — gives spiritual comfort and practical help
- Voluntary support agencies — provide emotional and practical support for patient and family.

STOP THINK **15.10** Discuss the ways in which each member of the team would be able to contribute to the care of the patient described in Case History 15.3 while in hospital and in the community.

Postoperative care

The postoperative nursing care of individuals who have undergone major surgery for intraoral cancer is highly specialised and combines the skills of many specialties. There will be variations in procedures and approaches among centres, and each patient will require a highly individualised plan for care.

Many centres reconstruct facial defects using free tissue transfer. Figure 15.5 outlines nursing procedures for the monitoring of free flaps.

Soutar & Tiwari (1996) describe free flaps. See also Coull & Wylie (1990), Coull (1992) and Haskins (1998) for discussions of nursing responsibility for monitoring free flaps.

Participation of relatives

Oral tumours and the effects of treatment may have far-reaching consequences not only for the patients concerned

CASE HISTORY 15.3
Mrs C

Mrs C, a 45-year-old housewife with two teenage children, was referred to an oncology unit from a dental hospital after she reported that she had had a lump in her mouth for some weeks. No lymphatic nodes were palpable in her neck and Mrs C was not too concerned that she might have cancer because she had never smoked and rarely took alcohol. She and her husband were consequently very shocked when they were given the result of a biopsy which showed squamous cell carcinoma.

Mrs C was assured that the disease was treatable and was advised to have surgical excision in the first instance, possibly followed by radiotherapy. Liaison was immediately set up with a Macmillan nurse, who visited her at home and discussed with Mrs C and her family their fears about cancer.

Mrs C felt that she did not want her husband to visit her until 3 or 4 days after the surgery. Her husband, however, felt anxious at not seeing her and came to visit of his own accord on the first postoperative day. The nurse prepared him for how his wife would look, and although he was initially shocked by her appearance, he felt that the result was not as bad as he had anticipated. He was also able to appreciate the rapid improvement which had taken place by the second day.

For herself, Mrs C was glad that he had visited. She felt more alert than she had believed possible. She also noticed the relief on her husband's face on his second visit and was able to believe him when he said she looked much better. On the third day, having prepared them, he brought their two children.

Three years later, Mrs C is attending the outpatient clinic for regular follow-up appointments. She has upper and lower dentures, which she wears all day, and is able to chew, swallow and speak well. She is socially very active and has adjusted well to the effects of her surgery, although she feels anxious every time she visits the clinic. Even after 3 years, she admits, 'I worry in case they find anything'.

but also for their families (Espie et al 1989, Freedlander et al 1989, Diamond 1999, Walton 2003). Relatives must often provide care for the patient after discharge. They are likely to experience much anxiety and to need maximum support. Nurses must help them through this very stressful time (see also Nicholson & Wells 2003).

Relatives will need constant reassurance, especially during the early postoperative days, and should be counselled before the first postoperative visit, which is usually very stressful (see Case History 15.3). It is advisable to reinforce and supplement verbal advice with written information, particularly with regard to oral hygiene, diet, radiotherapy, chemotherapy and local support groups. Local written information is now often available and general information booklets are also available, e.g. BACUP, Macmillan Cancerline (see 'Useful websites').

Altered body image

The impact of surgery to the face and mouth upon day-to-day function is visible to everyone. Basic activities such as breathing, eating and drinking may have to be performed with some loss of dignity. This, together with the disfiguring effects of the surgery, will require the patient to accept an altered body image, which can be a very difficult adjustment to make. Below, a patient describes, in a diary shared with the author (Kelly 1987), how she feels about her swollen face:

> *He said I was 'round the corner' — but I don't really feel like it. I asked about my face which is freakish and he said when I start walking about, gravity would reduce it. I feel a bit shy about it. I feel a freak especially when I see in a mirror — avoid mirrors meantime!*

This patient also refers to being 'unleashed' from drainage and feeding tubes —another assault on body image.

Another patient who had undergone several operations, commented: 'Each time, I feel I am a little less of the person I once was.' Remarks such as 'Of course, until I get my teeth, I can't go anywhere' are also frequently heard. It is worth noting that for many patients, after this type of surgery, dentures (if they can be worn) may be purely cosmetic rather than functional (Ali 2003). Many patients, e.g. those who have had a tracheostomy, will be temporarily unable to speak following their surgery. It is important for nurses to bear in mind that it may be difficult for these individuals to convey their emotions in writing and that it may be necessary to 'read between the lines' in order to fully appreciate the extent of their emotional pain. The effects of a permanent tracheostomy are discussed in Chapter 14.

STOP THINK **15.11** Consider how Mrs C in Case History 15.3 is likely to feel about her condition and the consequences of treatment. How is her body image likely to be affected?

Robinson (1997) describes research into coping with disfigurement. For vivid descriptions of the impact of oral cancer on life, read Diamond (1999).

Discharge planning

Prior to the patient's discharge, liaison should be established with the GP and community nurse and appropriate appointments and home visits arranged. In many cases a Macmillan nurse will visit the patient in the ward and will continue to give support at home. Each of these professionals will coordinate subsequent visits through the local health centre according to assessment of the patient's needs and should be encouraged to contact any member of the hospital team for help and support at any time.

Particular advance planning will be required if the patient's social circumstances are less than optimum; for example, many patients live alone or in hostel accommodation, and early liaison with social workers will ensure that the best possible social support is provided.

Rehabilitation

Following discharge after major oral surgery and radiotherapy, the process of rehabilitation may not be complete for a period of some months or even years. Patients will need ongoing support as they learn to cope with changes in lifestyle and in the activities of daily living (see Ch. 34). Planning for rehabilitation should start from the day of admission and must take into account the following considerations:

- *Living arrangements* — the patient may need to live with relatives temporarily or permanently, or may need rehousing if they are to live alone. Long-term nursing support, e.g. from Macmillan and Marie Curie nurses,

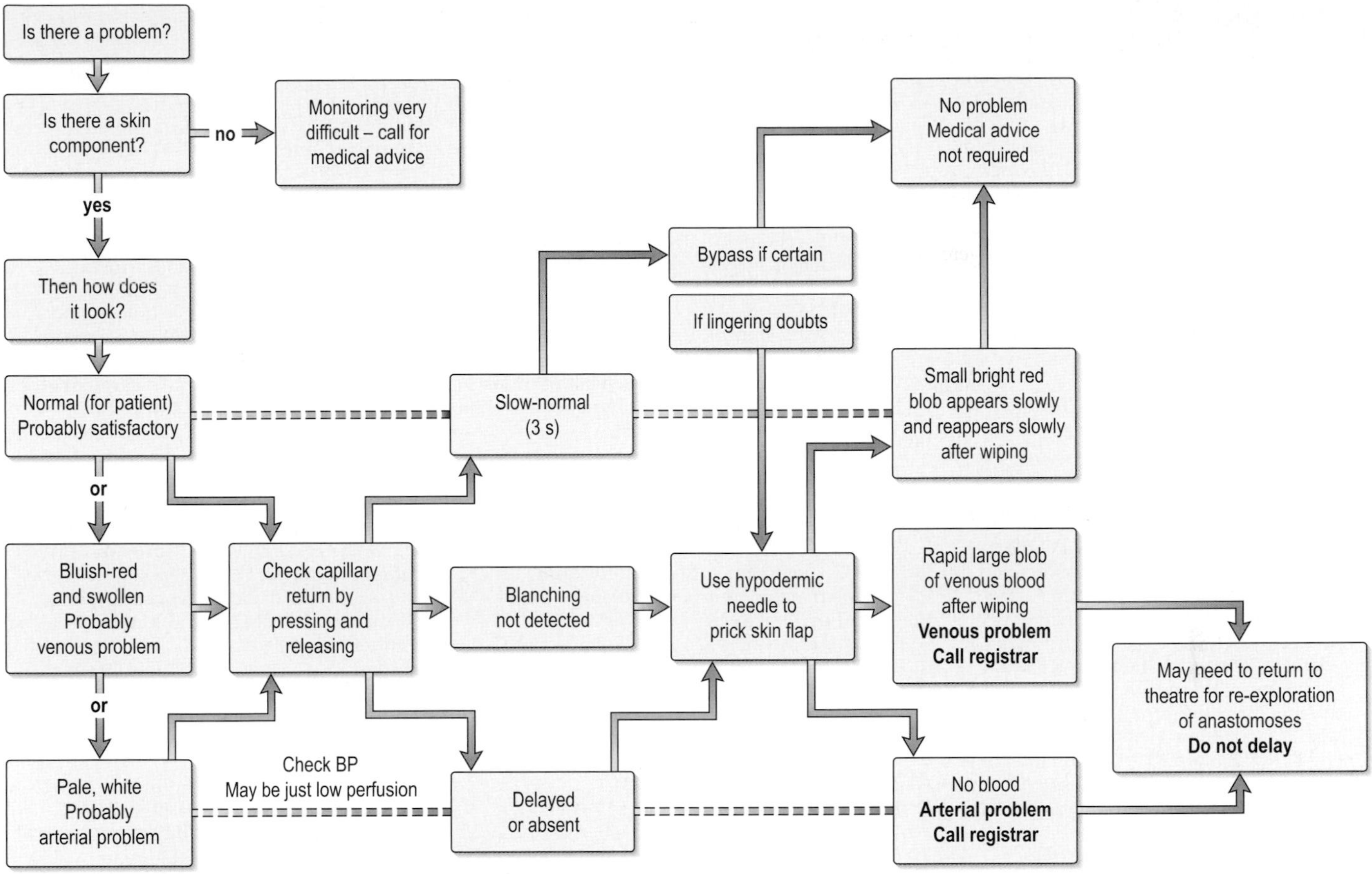

Fig. 15.5 An algorithm for monitoring free flaps.

and community-based services, e.g. Meals-on-Wheels, may need to be arranged.

- *Breathing* — patients with a tracheal stoma will need to be instructed in its management and will need support in adjusting to their altered appearance.
- *Oral hygiene; eating and drinking* — the patient (or carer) will need to be proficient in maintaining oral hygiene and using special equipment for giving enteral feeds if necessary.
- *Communication* — training in alternative forms of communication will be needed to compensate for a loss in speech.
- *Psychological support* — the patient should receive pre-discharge counselling to help in adjusting to an altered body image. Ongoing professional support may be needed for some time after discharge as the patient readjusts to life in the community (Robinson et al 1996), and both the patient and family should be able to contact members of the hospital team for support and advice.
- *Work* — the patient will need help in adjusting to new employment circumstances, whether changing jobs, stopping working or returning to a previous job, and in learning to cope with a changed appearance and function and with the reactions of colleagues.
- *Education* — the patient may need information on such matters as nutrition, giving up smoking and reducing alcohol intake (Scottish Intercollegiate Guidelines Network 2003).

The patient and family should be informed about local self-help groups where they can obtain practical and psychological support.

STOP THINK **15.12** Consider how you might go about planning the long-term rehabilitation of Mrs C in Case History 15.3.

Nursing and stress

Caring for patients with intraoral tumours can give rise to considerable stress and nurses may find this area of care quite harrowing. Unfortunately, ward nurses frequently see patients return with a recurrence of the cancer, and some may question whether radical treatment has in fact been justified. Liaison with outpatient clinics will make it apparent, however, that many patients do in fact survive to lead fulfilling lives for many years after treatment.

For a discussion of staff support in cancer nursing, see Magnusson & Robinson (2000) (see also Chs 17 and 31).

Palliative care

In cases of advanced disease, only approximately 10% of patients with oral cancer survive over 5 years; there is therefore a need to address issues of palliation, often from time of diagnosis (Scottish Intercollegiate Guidelines Network 2000c, McDougall 2003; see also Ch. 33).

STOP THINK **15.13** After reading this chapter, consider the different priorities you may have to set in delivering effective oral care throughout different stages of the health–illness continuum.

REFERENCES

Ali A 2003 Restorative dentistry in head and neck oncology. In: Bagg J, McFarlane T W, McCann M, Soutar D S (eds) The A–Z of oral cancer – an holistic route. The Royal Society of Edinburgh, p 31–33. Online. Available: www.royalsoced.org.uk/events/reports/oral_health2002.pdf

Ali T, Shepherd J P 1994 The measurement of injury severity. British Journal of Oral and Maxillofacial Surgery 32(1): 13–18

Alvi A, Doherty T, Lewen G 2003 Facial fractures and concomitant injuries in trauma patients. Laryngoscope 113(1): 102–106

Barkvoll P, Attramadal A 1989 Effect of nystatin and chlorhexidine digluconate on Candida albicans. Oral Surgery 67: 279–281

Bates C J, Cole T J, Mansoor M A et al 2001 Geographical variations in nutrition-related vascular risk factors in the UK: National Diet and Nutrition Survey of People Aged 65 years and Over. Journal of Nutrition, Health and Aging 5(4): 220–225

Black S 2000 Teething troubles. Nursing Standard 15(1): 22–23

Cannell H, Paterson A, Loukota R 1996 Maxillofacial injuries in multiply injured patients. British Journal of Oral and Maxillofacial Surgery 34: 303–308

Cheng K K, Chang A M 2003 Palliation of oral mucositis symptoms in pediatric patients treated with cancer chemotherapy. Cancer Nursing 26(6): 476–484

Cheng L H, Roles D, Telfer M R 1998 Orthognathic surgery: the patient's perspective. British Journal of Oral and Maxillofacial Surgery 36(4): 261–263

Chew D J, Edmondson H D 1996 A study of maxillofacial injuries in the elderly resulting from falls. Journal of Oral Rehabilitation 23(7): 505–509

Coleman S 1995 An overview of the oral complications of adult patients with malignant haematological conditions who have undergone radiotherapy or chemotherapy. Journal of Advanced Nursing 22(6): 1085–1091

Cross D N, Carton R J 2003 Fluoridation: a violation of medical ethics and human rights. International Journal of Occupational and Environmental Health 9(1): 24–29

Davies A N, Broadley K, Beighton D 2001 Xerostomia in patients with advanced cancer. Journal of Pain and Symptom Management 22(4): 820–825

Dawson E R, Morley S E, Robertson A G et al 2001 Increasing dietary supervision can reduce weight loss in oral cancer patients. Nutrition and Cancer 41(1–2): 70–74

Department of Health and Social Security 1978 Road accident statistics. HMSO, London

Diamond J 1999 C: because cowards get cancer too. Vermillion, London, p 193–195

Epstein J B, Emerton S, Le N D et al 1999 A double-blind crossover trial of Oral Balance gel and Biotene toothpaste versus placebo in patients with xerostomia following radiation therapy. European Journal of Cancer 35(2): 132–137

Epstein J B, Silverman S Jr, Paggiarino D A et al 2001 Benzydamine HCl for prophylaxis of radiation-induced oral mucositis: results from a multicenter, randomized, double-blind, placebo-controlled clinical trial. Cancer 92(4): 875–885

Espie C A, Freedlander E, Campsie L M et al 1989 Psychological distress at follow-up after major surgery for intraoral cancer. Journal of Psychosomatic Research 33(4): 441–448

Fayle S A, Welbury R R, Roberts J F 2001 British Society of Paediatric Dentistry: a policy document on management of caries in the primary dentition. International Journal of Paediatric Dentistry 11(2): 153–157

Feber T 1995 Mouthcare for patients receiving oral irradiation. Professional Nurse 10(10): 666–670

Ferretti G A, Hansen I A, Whittenburg K et al 1987 Therapeutic use of chlorhexidine in bone marrow transplant patients: case studies. Oral Surgery 63(6): 683–687

Finlay P M, Richardson M D, Robertson A G 1996 A comparative study of the efficacy of fluconazole and amphotericin B in the treatment of oropharyngeal candidiasis in patients undergoing radiotherapy for head and neck tumours. British Journal of Oral and Maxillofacial Surgery 34(1): 23–25

Fiske J, Gelbier S, Watson R M 1990 The benefit of dental care to an elderly population assessed using a sociodental measure of oral handicap. British Dental Journal 168: 153–156

Frampton R, Welsh R, Thomas P 2002 Belted driver protection in frontal impact – what has been achieved and where do future priorities lie? Annual Proceedings/Association for the Advancement of Automotive Medicine 46: 93–109

Francalanci S, Sertoli A, Giorgini S et al 2000 Multicentre study of allergic contact cheilitis from toothpaste. Contact Dermatitis 43(4): 216–222

Freedlander E, Espie C A, Campsie L M et al 1989 Functional implications of major surgery for intraoral cancer. British Journal of Plastic Surgery 42: 266–269

Friedlander A H, Friedlander I K, Gallas M et al 2003 Late-life depression: its oral health significance. International Dental Journal 53(1): 41–50

Ganly I 2003 Novel and experimental treatments. In: Bagg J, McFarlane T W, McCann M, Soutar D S (eds) The A–Z of oral cancer – an holistic route. The Royal Society of Edinburgh, p 17–20. Online. Available: www.royalsoced.org.uk/events/reports/oral_health2002.pdf

Harrahill M, Eastes L 2000 Seven strategies to decrease the risk of missed injuries. Journal of Emergency Nursing 26(3): 276–277

Hill C M, Burford K, Martin A et al 1998 A one-year review of maxillofacial sports injuries treated at an accident and emergency department. British Journal of Oral and Maxillofacial Surgery 36(1): 44–47

Hislop W, Soutar D S 2003 Management of orofacial malignancy. In: Wray D, Stenhouse D, Lee D, Clark A (eds) Textbook of general and oral surgery. Churchill Livingstone, Edinburgh, Ch. 17

Hollinworth H 1997 Less pain, more gain. Nursing Times 93(46): 89–91

Holmes S 1996 Nursing management of oral care in older patients. Nursing Times 92(9): 37–39

Holmes S 1997 Radiotherapy, 2nd edn. Lisa Sainsbury Foundation Series. Austin Cornish, London

Holmes S 1998 Xerostomia: aetiology and management in cancer patients. Support Care Cancer 6: 348–355

Holmes S, Mountain E 1993 Assessment of oral status: evaluation of three oral assessment guides. Journal of Clinical Nursing 2(1): 35–40

Howarth H 1977 Mouth care procedures for the very ill. Nursing Times 73(10): 354–355

Hutchison I, Magennis P, Shepherd J P et al 1998 The BAOMS United Kingdom survey of facial injuries. Part 1: aetiology and the association with alcohol consumption. British Journal of Oral and Maxillofacial Surgery 36: 4–14

Jackson M S, Wrench A A, Soutar D S et al 1999 Carcinoma of the tongue: the speech therapist's perspective. British Journal of Oral and Maxillofacial Surgery 37(3): 200–204

Jamieson E M, McCall J M, Whyte L A 2002 Clinical nursing practices, 4th edn. Churchill Livingstone, Edinburgh

Johnson D R, Moore W J 1997 Anatomy for dental students, 3rd edn. Oxford University Press, Oxford

Joy D, Probert R, Bisson J I et al 2000 Post-traumatic stress after injury. Journal of Trauma Injury, Infection and Critical Care 48(30): 490–494

Kelly R 1987 A study of patients who have undergone surgery for cancer in the head and neck region. Unpublished paper (accessible from author)

Kelly R 2003 Patients' pathways – coordinating care. In: Bagg J, McFarlane T W, McCann M, Soutar D S (eds) The A–Z of oral cancer – an holistic route. The Royal Society of Edinburgh, p 14–16. Online. Available: www.royalsoced.org.uk/events/reports/oral_health2002.pdf

Krishnasamay M 1995 Oral problems in advanced cancer. European Journal of Cancer Care 4: 173–177

Lamey P-J 1996 Burning mouth syndrome. Dermatological Clinics 14(2): 339–354

Langley J 1989 Working with swallowing disorders. Winslow Press, Bicester

Levine R S 2001 Caries experience and bedtime consumption of sugar-sweetened food and drinks – a survey of 600 children. Community Dental Health 18(4): 228–231

Lewis M 2003 Presentation and diagnosis – the clinician's view. In: Bagg J, McFarlane T W, McCann M, Soutar D S (eds) The A–Z of oral cancer – an holistic route. The Royal Society of Edinburgh, p 9–13. Online. Available: www.royalsoced.org.uk/events/reports/oral_health2002.pdf

Little J 1996 Head and neck cancer: oral care during radiotherapy. Nursing Standard 10(22): 39–42

Llewellyn C D, Linklater K, Bell J et al 2003 Squamous cell carcinoma of the oral cavity in patients aged 45 years and under: a descriptive analysis of 116 cases diagnosed in the South East of England from 1990 to 1997. Oral Oncology 39(2): 106–114

Lydon C 1996 Too slap happy. Nursing Times 92(45): 48–49

Macpherson L M D, Gibson J, Binnie V, Conway D I 2003 Oral cancer prevention and detection for the primary health care team. The Oral Cancer Awareness Group, University of Glasgow Dental School, Glasgow. Online. Available: www.hebs.scot.nhs.uk/services/pubs/pdf/oralbook.pdf

Magennis P, Shepherd J P, Hutchison I et al 1998 Trends in facial injury: increasing violence more than compensates for decreasing road trauma. British Medical Journal 316(7128): 325–326

Martin V 1995 Helping parents cope: cleft lip, cleft palate. Nursing Times 29(31): 38–40

Martin V 1998 Cleft care. Paediatric Nursing 10(7): 6

McDougall H 2003 Palliative care for head and neck cancer. In: Bagg J, McFarlane T W, McCann M, Soutar D S (eds) The A–Z of oral cancer – an holistic route The Royal Society of Edinburgh, p 29–30. Online. Available: www.royalsoced.org.uk/events/reports/oral_health2002.pdf

McGrath C, Bedi R 2002 Understanding the value of oral health to people in Britain – importance to life quality. Community Dental Health 19(4): 211–214

McGrath C, Bedi R 2003 Dental services and perceived oral health: are patients better off going private? Journal of Dentistry 31(3): 217–221

McGregor A D, McGregor I A 2000 Fundamental techniques of plastic surgery and their surgical applications, 10th edn. Churchill Livingstone, Edinburgh

McGuire D B 2002 Mucosal tissue injury in cancer therapy: more than mucositis and mouthwash. Cancer Practice 10(4): 179–191

McMahon J 2003 Current treatment of oral cancer – an overview. In: Bagg J, McFarlane T W, McCann M, Soutar D S (eds) The A–Z of oral cancer – an holistic route. The Royal Society of Edinburgh, p 10–13. Online. Available: www.royalsoced.org.uk/events/reports/oral_health2002.pdf

Meurman J H, Sovari R, Pelttari A et al 1996 Hospital mouth-cleaning aids may cause dental erosion. Special Care in Dentistry 16(6): 247–250

Meyer-Leuckel H, Kielbassa A M 2002 Use of saliva substitutes in patients with xerostomia. Schweizer Monatsschrift fur Zahnmedzin 112(10): 1037–1058

Miller M, Kearney N 2001 Oral care for patients with cancer: a review of the literature. Cancer Nursing 24(4): 241–254

Milligan S, McGill M, Sweeney M P et al 2001 Oral care for people with advanced cancer: an evidence-based protocol. International Journal of Palliative Nursing 7(9): 418–426

Moos K F 2003 Orthognathic surgery. In: Wray D, Stenhouse D, Lee D, Clark A (eds) Textbook of general and oral surgery. Churchill Livingstone, Edinburgh, Ch. 13

Morris A J, Steele J, White D A 2001 The oral cleanliness and periodontal health of UK adults in 1998. British Dental Journal 191(4): 186–192

Moshrefi A 2002 Chlorhexidine. Journal of the Western Society of Periodontology – Periodontal Abstracts 50(1): 5–9

Moss A 2001 Controversies in cleft lip and palate management. Ultrasound in Obstetrics and Gynaecology 8(5): 420–421

Mouatt B 2003 Dental decay and the case for fluoride. Journal of Family Health Care 13(2): 34–36

National Institute for Clinical Excellence (NICE) 2003 Guideline No CG4. Head injury: triage, assessment, investigation and early management of head injury in infants, children and adults. NICE, London

Nicholson C, Wells M 2003 After treatment is over. In: Faithfull S, Wells M 2003 (eds) Supportive care in radiotherapy. Churchill Livingstone, Edinburgh, Ch. 4

Nunn J, Gordon P, Morris A et al 2003 Dental erosion – changing prevalence? A review of British national children's surveys. International Journal of Paediatric Dentistry 13(2): 98–105

Nursing and Midwifery Council (NMC) 2004 Code of professional conduct: standards for conduct, performance and ethics. NMC, London

Nuttall N M, Bradnock G, White D et al 2001 Dental attendance in 1998 and implications for the future. British Dental Journal 190(4): 177–182

Palmer G D, Robinson P G, Challacombe S J et al 1996 Aetiological factors for oral manifestations of HIV. Oral Diseases 2(3): 193–197

Park O, Ross M 2002 Caring for your mouth. Beatson Oncology Centre, Glasgow. Online. Available: www.show.scot.nhs.uk/beatson

Pearson L S, Hutton J L 2002 A controlled trial to compare the ability of foam swabs and toothbrushes to remove dental plaque. Journal of Advanced Nursing 39(5): 480–489

Pitts N B, Boyles J, Nugent Z J et al 2003 The dental caries experience of 5-year-old children in England and Wales. Surveys co-ordinated by the British Association for the Study of Community Dentistry in 2001/2002. Community Dental Health 20(1): 45–54

Ray A 2003 Clefts of lip and palate. In: Wray D, Stenhouse D, Lee D, Clark A (eds) Textbook of general and oral surgery. Churchill Livingstone, Edinburgh, Ch. 16

Ream E 2000 Information and education for patients and families. In: Kearney N, Richardson A, Giullio P (eds) Cancer nursing practice. Churchill Livingstone, Edinburgh, Ch. 7

Regnard C, Allport S, Stephenson L 1997 ABC of palliative care: mouthcare, skin care and lymphoedema. British Journal of Medicine 315: 1002–1005

Roberts H 1990 Mouthcare in oral cavity cancer. Nursing Standard 4(19): 26–29

Robertson A G, Robertson C, Soutar D S et al 2001 Treatment of oral cancer: the need for defined protocols and specialist centres: variations in the treatment of oral cancer. Clinical Oncology (Royal College of Radiologists) 13(6): 409–415

Robinson E, Rumsey N, Partridge J 1996 An evaluation of the impact of social interaction skills for facially disfigured people. British Journal of Plastic Surgery 49(5): 281–289

Rogers S N, Lowe D, Fisher S E et al 2002 Health-related quality of life and clinical function after primary surgery for oral cancer. British Journal of Oral and Maxillofacial Surgery 40(1): 11–18

Roper N, Logan W W, Tierney A J 2000 The elements of nursing: a model for nursing based on a model of living, 5th edn. Churchill Livingstone, Edinburgh

Ross G, Soutar D S, Shoaib T et al 2002 The ability of lymphoscintigraphy to direct sentinel node biopsy in the clinically N0 (node-negative) neck for patients with head and neck squamous cell carcinoma. British Journal of Radiology 75(900): 950–958

Rumsey N, Clarke A, Musa M 2002 Altered body image: the psychosocial needs of patients. British Journal of Community Nursing 7: 563–566

Sadler G R, Stoudt A, Fullerton J T et al 2003 Managing the oral sequelae of cancer therapy. MedSurg Nursing 12(1): 28–36

Samaranayake L P, Wilkieson C A, Lamey P-J et al 1995 Oral disease in the elderly in long-term hospital care. Oral Diseases 1(3): 147–151

Sandhu A P, Robertson A G, Soutar D S et al 1999 Interstitial iridium-192 implantation for recurrent and/or locally advanced head and neck cancer. Clinical Oncology (Royal College of Radiologists) 11(6): 371–378

Scala A, Checchi L, Montevecchi M et al 2003 Update on burning mouth syndrome: overview and patient management. Critical Reviews in Oral Biology and Medicine 14(4): 275–291

Scottish Executive 2003 Towards better oral health in children: a consultation document on children's oral health. TSO, Edinburgh

Scottish Executive Health Department 2001 Nursing for health: a review of the contribution of nurses, midwives and health visitors to improving the public's health in Scotland. TSO, Edinburgh

Scottish Intercollegiate Guidelines Network (SIGN) 2000a Guideline No 43. Management of unerupted and impacted third molar teeth. SIGN, Edinburgh

Scottish Intercollegiate Guidelines Network (SIGN) 2000b Guideline No 47. Preventing dental caries in children at high caries risk. SIGN, Edinburgh

Scottish Intercollegiate Guidelines Network (SIGN) 2000c Guideline No 44. Control of pain in patients with cancer. SIGN, Edinburgh

Scottish Intercollegiate Guidelines Network (SIGN) 2003 Guideline No 74. Management of harmful drinking and alcohol dependence in primary care. SIGN, Edinburgh

Scottish Office Department of Health 1995 The oral health strategy for Scotland. Scottish Office Department of Health, Edinburgh

Scully C, Cawson R A 1999 Oral disease, 2nd edn. Churchill Livingstone, Edinburgh

Sen P, Ross N, Rogers S 2001 Recovering maxillofacial trauma patients: the hidden problems. Journal of Wound Care 10(3): 53–57

Simons D 2003 Who will provide dental care for housebound people with oral problems? British Dental Journal 194(3): 137–138

Sivarajasingam V, Shepherd J P 2001 Trends in community violence in England and Wales 1995–1998: an accident and emergency department perspective. Emergency Medicine Journal 18(2): 105–109
Smith A J, Hodgson R J, Bridgeman K et al 2003 A randomized controlled trial of a brief intervention after alcohol-related facial injury. Addiction 98(1): 43–52
Sobin L H, Wittekind C (eds) 2002 UICC TNM classification of malignant tumours, 6th edn. Wiley-Liss, New York
Soutar D S 2003 Epidemiology – the extent of the problem. In: Bagg J, McFarlane T W, McCann M, Soutar D S (eds) The A–Z of oral cancer – an holistic route. The Royal Society of Edinburgh, p 7–8. Online. Available: www.royalsoced.org.uk/events/reports/oral_health2002.pdf
Soutar D S, Tiwari R (eds) 1996 Excision and reconstruction in head and neck cancer. Churchill Livingstone, Edinburgh
Stanfield M, Stanfield M, Scully C et al 2003 Oral healthcare of clients with learning disability: changes following relocation from hospital to community. British Dental Journal 194(5): 271–277
Stenhouse D, Wray D 2003 Oral surgery in medically compromised patients In: Wray D, Stenhouse D, Lee D, Clark A (eds) Textbook of general and oral surgery. Churchill Livingstone, Edinburgh, Ch. 35
Stephen K, Macpherson L, Gilmour W et al 2002 A blind caries and fluorosis prevalence study of school-children in naturally fluoridated and nonfluoridated townships of Morayshire, Scotland. Community Dentistry and Oral Epidemiology 30(1): 70–79
Sutherland I, Sivarajasingam V, Shepherd J P 2002 Recording of community violence by medical and police services. Injury Prevention 8(3): 246–247
Taylor S E 2003 Efficacy and economic evaluation of pilocarpine in treating radiation-induced xerostomia. Expert Opinion on Pharmacology 44(9): 1489–1497
Telfer M R, Shepherd J P 1993 Psychological distress in patients attending an oncology clinic after definitive treatment for maxillofacial malignant neoplasia. International Journal of Oral and Maxillofacial Surgery 22(6): 3347–3349
Tickle M, Milsom K M, King D et al 2003 The influences on preventive care provided to children who frequently attend the UK General Dental Service. British Dental Journal 194(6): 329–332
Tombes M B, Gallucci B 1993 The effects of hydrogen peroxide rinses on the normal oral mucosa. Nursing Research 42(6): 332–337
Ventafridda V, Ripamonte C, Sbanotto A et al 1998 Mouth care. In: Doyle D, Hanks G W C, MacDonald N (eds) Oxford textbook of palliative medicine, 2nd edn. Oxford University Press, Oxford, Ch. 9.10
Walton M 2003 The patient's perspective. In: Bagg J, McFarlane T W, McCann M, Soutar D S (eds) The A–Z of oral cancer – an holistic route. The Royal Society of Edinburgh, p 25–27. Online. Available: www.royalsoced.org.uk/events/reports/oral_health2002.pdf
Watson R 1989 Care of the mouth. Nursing 3(11): 20–24
Waugh A, Grant A 2001 Ross and Wilson's anatomy and physiology in health and illness, 9th edn. Churchill Livingstone, Edinburgh
Wells M 1998 The hidden experience of radiotherapy to the head and neck: a qualitative study of patients after completion of treatment. Journal of Advanced Nursing 28(4): 840–848
Wells M 2003 Oropharyngeal effects of radiotherapy. In: Faithfull S, Wells M (eds) Supportive care in radiotherapy. Churchill Livingstone, Edinburgh, Ch. 10
Wray D, Bagg J 1997 Pocket reference to oral candidosis. Science Press, London
Wray D, Gibson J 1997 Oral medicine. Churchill Livingstone, Edinburgh
Wray D, Stenhouse D, Lee D, Clark A 2003 (eds) Textbook of general and oral surgery. Churchill Livingstone, Edinburgh

FURTHER READING

Bagg J, McFarlane T W, McCann M, Soutar D S (eds) 2003 The A–Z of oral cancer – an holistic route. The Royal Society of Edinburgh. Online. Available: www.royalsoced.org.uk/events/reports/oral_health2002.pdf
Coull A 1992 Making sense of surgical flaps. Nursing Times 88(1): 32–34
Coull A, Wylie K 1990 Regular monitoring: the way to ensure flap healing. Nursing priorities following flap repair and reconstruction surgery. Professional Nurse 6(1): 18–21
Diamond J 1999 C: because cowards get cancer too. Vermillion, London
Faithfull S, Wells M 2003 (eds) Supportive care in radiotherapy. Churchill Livingstone, Edinburgh
Haskins N 1998 Intensive nursing care of patients with a microvascular free flap after maxillofacial surgery. Intensive and Critical Care Nursing 14(5): 225–230
Holmes S 1997 Radiotherapy, 2nd edn. Lisa Sainsbury Foundation Series. Austin Cornish, London
Holmes S 1998 Xerostomia: aetiology and management in cancer patients. Support Care Cancer 6: 348–355
Jamieson E M, McCall J M, Whyte L A 2002 Clinical nursing practices, 4th edn. Churchill Livingstone, Edinburgh
Johnson D R, Moore W J 1997 Anatomy for dental students, 3rd edn. Oxford University Press, Oxford
Langley J 1989 Working with swallowing disorders. Winslow Press, Bicester
Levine R S (ed) 1996a A handbook of dental health for health visitors, midwives and nurses. Health Education Authority, London
Levine R S (ed) 1996b The scientific basis of dental health education, 4th edn. Health Education Authority, London
Macpherson L M D, Gibson J, Binnie V, Conway D I 2003 Oral cancer prevention and detection for the primary health care team. The Oral Cancer Awareness Group, University of Glasgow Dental School, Glasgow. Online. Available: www.hebs.scot.nhs.uk/services/pubs/pdf/oralbook.pdf
Magnusson K, Robinson L 2000 The practice base of cancer nursing. In: Kearney N, Richardson A, Giullio P (eds) Cancer nursing practice. Churchill Livingstone, Edinburgh, Ch. 2
Oral Health Group 2003 Online. Available: www.ncl.ac.uk/dental/research/diet
Ray A 2003 Clefts of lip and palate. In: Wray D, Stenhouse D, Lee D, Clark A (eds) Textbook of general and oral surgery. Churchill Livingstone, Edinburgh, Ch. 16
Ream E 2000 Information and education for patients and families. In: Kearney N, Richardson A, Giullio P (eds) Cancer nursing practice. Churchill Livingstone, Edinburgh, Ch. 7
Robinson E 1997 Psychological research on visible differences in adults. In: Lansdown R, Rumsey N, Bradbury E et al (eds) Visibly different: coping with disfigurement. Butterworth-Heinemann, London
Scottish Executive 2003 Towards better oral health in children: a consultation document on children's oral health. Scottish Executive, Edinburgh
Scully C, Cawson R A 1999 Oral disease, 2nd edn. Churchill Livingstone, Edinburgh
Soutar D S, Tiwari R (eds) 1996 Excision and reconstruction in head and neck cancer. Churchill Livingstone, Edinburgh
Sweeney M P, Bagg J 1997 Making sense of the mouth (video and CD-ROM). Partnership in Oral Care, Glasgow
Waugh A, Grant A 2001 Ross and Wilson's anatomy and physiology in health and illness, 9th edn. Churchill Livingstone, Edinburgh
Wells M 2003 Oropharyngeal effects of radiotherapy. In: Faithfull S, Wells M (eds) Supportive care in radiotherapy. Churchill Livingstone, Edinburgh, Ch. 10
Wray D, Bagg J 1997 Pocket reference to oral candidosis. Science Press, London
Wray D, Gibson J 1997 Oral medicine. Churchill Livingstone, Edinburgh
Wray D, Stenhouse D, Lee D, Clark A 2003 (eds) Textbook of general and oral surgery. Churchill Livingstone, Edinburgh

USEFUL WEBSITES

British Dental Health Foundation
www.dentalhealth.org.uk

CancerBACUP online
www.cancerbacup.org.uk

Changing Faces
www.changingfaces.org.uk

CLAPA (Cleft Lip and Palate Association)
www.clapa.com

Craniofacial Support Group
http://headlines.org.uk

Disfigurement Guidance Centre
www.timewarp.demon.co.uk

Let's Face It
www.letsfaceit.force9.co.uk

Macmillan Cancerline
www.macmillan.org.uk

Mouth Cancer Foundation
www.mouthcancerawareness.org.uk

The Centre for Women's Health
www.show.scot.nhs.uk

Women's Aid
www.womensaid.org.uk
www.scottishwomensaid.co.uk
(*see also local telephone directory for nearest centre*)

DISORDERS OF THE IMMUNE SYSTEM, INFECTION CONTROL AND INFECTIOUS DISEASES

16

Mary Henry
Claire Kilpatrick

INTRODUCTION

The immune system is a complex and fascinating network of cells and proteins which is programmed to respond to the many challenges presented to it by foreign particles, microorganisms such as bacteria, viruses, fungi and protozoa, and tumour cells. Its function is to protect the body from anything that could be harmful. In order to carry out this function, it has to be able to recognise 'self' from 'non-self', which it attacks and attempts to eliminate or destroy.

Human beings and animals have a number of non-specific barriers to foreign substances; for example, the intact skin protects the body from invasion and substances in some body fluids help to kill microorganisms (see Fig. 16.1). It is when these barriers fail or are compromised that the specific immune responses come into play.

Healthy individuals can fight off infection by immune mechanisms, and in many cases immunity to a disease occurs after a single encounter with the infectious organism. Sometimes, the system is unable to function normally because of an immune deficiency or a functional disorder. When a large number of microorganisms enter the body, the immune system may function normally but still be too slow to prevent the person from developing the infectious disease. Immune suppression can occur as result of other disease; it can also be iatrogenic, resulting from medication, including chemotherapy, or radiotherapy.

Health care-associated infection (HAI) and infectious diseases

There is heightened concern and activity in the UK, and globally, in relation to health care-associated infection in particular and to the prevention and control of all infectious diseases. Health care-associated infection (HAI or HCAI), previously known as hospital-acquired infection and in some countries as nosocomial infection, is the term used to refer to infection acquired during receipt of some form of health care. New infections such as Legionnaire's disease, human immunodeficiency virus (HIV) and severe acute respiratory syndrome (SARS) and long-standing infectious diseases such as *Mycobacterium tuberculosis* and influenza continually pose challenges to public health as well as to health care settings, as do more commonly occurring infections, such as methicillin-resistant *Staphylococcus aureus* (MRSA). For the purposes of this chapter, health care settings where HAI must be controlled include hospitals, care homes and primary care facilities; however, the guidance given applies also to patients who are being cared for in their own homes.

Measures developed and applied at local settings and national levels aim to reduce the burden of HAI, and other infectious or communicable diseases, on individuals, health care organisations, and within the National Health Service as a whole. The Health Protection Agency, Health Protection Scotland and Departments of Health in all UK countries

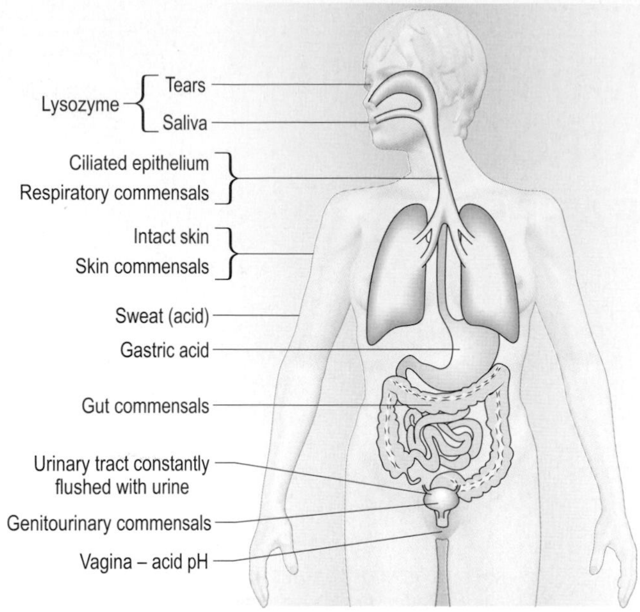

Fig. 16.1 Barriers to infection.

coordinate many activities, such as national surveillance and control programmes, in order to highlight and act upon the actual burden in specific settings (see 'Useful websites', p. 689).

For further information on the national burden of HAI, see Plowman et al (1999), National Audit Office (2000, 2004) and the UK Health Department websites (see 'Useful websites', p. 689).

It is thought that up to one-third of all HAI is preventable. Nurses must consider not only how they can address infection prevention, control and management within health care settings, but also how they might influence the wider public health arena.

Epidemiology

Epidemiology is the study of disease in relation to populations, e.g. who is being affected by MRSA, or by SARS, and when and where they are being affected. A population considered at risk, for example from MRSA, could be monitored using epidemiological methods to gather information which relates the disease to the population by studying both ill and healthy individuals. Epidemiology is closely linked with risk assessment and management, and results of studies can help to influence structures, processes and outcomes, including control measures and action plans.

In order to identify infectious diseases including HAI, methods must be in place to gather the appropriate information to inform knowledge of the distribution of such diseases. There are various ways to monitor disease.

- *Incidence* is the number of new cases in a defined period within a specific population, e.g. incidence of wound infections postoperatively in all patients undergoing surgery in the next financial year.
- *Prevalence* is the number of cases that occur either at a particular time (point prevalence) or over a defined period of time (period prevalence), e.g. the number of patients with urinary tract infections at any one time within a hospital.
- *Surveillance* is 'the ongoing systematic collection, collation, analysis and interpretation of health data essential to the planning, implementation and evaluation of public health practice, closely integrated with the timely dissemination of these data to those who need to know. The final link of the surveillance chain is the application of these data to prevention and control' (Centers for Disease Control 1998).

Data collected over time show the changing patterns of infectious diseases in our society, providing information on newly emerging diseases and identifying specific problem areas, e.g. outbreaks and seasonality of diseases. Risk management not only contributes to the prevention of infection but also assists in the control of outbreaks of infection. To fully appreciate infection control principles, including immunology, the relevant anatomy and physiology must be understood.

ANATOMY AND PHYSIOLOGY

The lymphoid system

The lymphoid (or lymphatic) system consists of organs and tissues made up of cells which are involved in the immune response. These structures may be described as being either primary or secondary, as follows.

Primary lymphoid organs

The thymus gland and the bone marrow are known as primary lymphoid organs. Lymphocytes develop in the bone marrow (see Ch. 11): T lymphocytes differentiate in the thymus gland; B lymphocytes differentiate in the bone marrow. It is in the organ where they differentiate that lymphocytes acquire the surface receptors which enable them to recognise antigens.

Secondary lymphoid organs

The spleen and lymph nodes are known as secondary lymphoid organs, as are other areas of lymphoid tissue which are associated with mucosal surfaces in the body, such as in the respiratory, gastrointestinal and genitourinary systems. The spleen contains white blood cells, or leucocytes (see Chs 4 and 11), and is involved in the breakdown of erythrocytes, leucocytes and platelets. The lymph nodes are small collections of lymphoid tissue (1–25 mm in diameter) which are found all over the body, often where lymphatic vessels branch. Lymph nodes act as filters, trapping any foreign materials or antigens so that they can be attacked and destroyed by specialised white blood cells which accumulate there in large numbers.

For further information, see Waugh & Grant (2001).

Types of immune response

Two types of immune response are involved in recognising and eliminating any 'foreign' material which enters the body:

- *Non-specific or innate immunity* — by which any foreign cell or particle is identified as such and attacked. Even tumour cells which arise in the body's own tissues can be recognised as foreign and may be destroyed. This response is non-specific in that it is the same whether the foreign particle or antigen is a bacterium, a particle of asbestos or other agent. The response occurs as soon as the antigen is encountered. No 'memory' is involved and a second contact with the same antigen will produce the same response at the same rate.

- *Specific or adaptive immunity* — in which special cells (B and T lymphocytes) are programmed to respond to recognised antigens. This response is highly specific: each lymphocyte is equipped to recognise only one antigen. Once contact has been made with that antigen and it has been destroyed, some 'memory' cells (see p. 657) remain in the body. If the same antigen is encountered again, these cells are stimulated to reproduce, and the response is both faster and greater.

Cells and chemicals involved

Cells

The cells involved in the immune response are white blood cells (leucocytes) (see Box 16.1). These may be granular (granulocytes or polymorphonuclear leucocytes) — neutrophils, basophils and eosinophils, or non-granular (agranulocytes) — mononuclear phagocytes, i.e. monocytes and macrophages, and lymphocytes. In this section these cells will be described according to their function.

Phagocytes

have the ability to recognise foreign material and to engulf and digest microorganisms by a process called phagocytosis. Three cells are classed as phagocytes: neutrophils, monocytes and macrophages.

Neutrophils

are small cells and live only for a few days. They originate in the bone marrow and circulate in the blood.

Box 16.1

Components of the immune system

Cells

Leucocytes (white blood cells)

- Granular (granulocytes or polymorphonuclear leucocytes)
  - — neutrophils
  - — basophils and mast cells
  - — eosinophils
- Non-granular (agranulocytes)
  - — Mononuclear phagocytes (monocytes and macrophages)
  - — Lymphocytes
    B lymphocytes
    T lymphocytes

Chemicals

Complement
Cytokines, e.g. interferons
Inflammatory mediators, e.g. histamine
Antibodies (immunoglobulins)

Monocytes

are approximately the same size as neutrophils. They also originate in the bone marrow and circulate in the blood, but they may enter the tissues, where they become macrophages.

Macrophages

are larger than neutrophils and monocytes. They are long lived and are found in the tissues, principally in the liver, spleen, lymph nodes and lungs. Mainly involved in non-specific immunity, they are also activated by lymphokines, which are produced by T cells in the cell-mediated immune response (see p. 658). Phagocytosis can take place only if the invading cell becomes adherent to the surface of the phagocyte. This occurs by a chemical attraction between the surface of the phagocyte and antigen. The process can be assisted by complement (see p. 656) and by antibodies.

Accessory cells

function by releasing chemicals which are harmful to invading organisms. This group of cells comprises basophils, eosinophils and mast cells.

Basophils and mast cells contain histamine and other chemicals which give rise to an inflammatory response when released. They are important in allergies, e.g. hay fever. Basophils circulate in the bloodstream. Mast cells, although similar in function, are located in connective tissues and mucous membranes.

Eosinophils are capable of phagocytosis, but their main function is to attach themselves to larger parasites such as helminths (worms) and destroy them by releasing harmful substances. They may also help to control the inflammatory response by breaking down histamine. There is an increase in the number of eosinophils in people suffering from allergic conditions and parasitic infections.

Lymphocytes

originate in the bone marrow as stem cells and subsequently differentiate into B and T cells.

B cells are the lymphocytes which produce antibodies. They differentiate in the bone marrow and then mature in the secondary lymphoid tissues. The antigen receptor on their surface is specific for one antigen only. B lymphocytes are capable of 'memory' and are specialised to deal with microorganisms which do not, of their own accord, enter host cells, e.g. circulating bacteria.

T cells have various functions. They originate in the bone marrow and then mature and differentiate in the thymus gland. They are also antigen-specific and have an antigen receptor which is similar in structure and function to that of the B cells. T lymphocytes are capable of 'memory' and are specialised to deal mainly with microorganisms which invade host cells, e.g. viruses.

T cells can be broadly divided into two groups:

- T-helper cells
- T-cytotoxic cells.

T-helper cells are subdivided into the cells which interact with B cells, helping them to produce antibody, and the cells which assist the mononuclear phagocytes, helping them to destroy intracellular pathogens.

T-cytotoxic cells destroy host cells which are infected by viruses or other intracellular pathogens.

Chemicals

Complement

is the collective name for a group of proteins which induce chemical reactions and are involved in the control of inflammation. Their three main functions are:

- To coat microorganisms with a substance which phagocytic cells can recognise. This ensures that the microorganism adheres to the surface of the phagocytic cell.
- To activate the destruction of the microorganism inside the phagocyte once ingestion has taken place. Complement also participates in the acute inflammatory response by inducing vasodilatation and increasing the permeability of the capillary endothelium.
- To assist in the lysis of invading cells.

Cytokines

are molecules of mainly proteins, whose function is to signal between cells during the immune response. Interferons are one example. There are many different interferons and they protect cells of the same species from viral attack. They are synthesised by virally infected cells and secreted into the extracellular fluid. Here they bind to specific receptors on other, non-infected cells, which 'surround' the infected cell and prevent the spread of virus.

Histamine

is released by mast cells when they degranulate after adhering to a microorganism. This gives rise to increased vascular permeability, arteriolar dilatation, smooth muscle contraction in the respiratory and alimentary tracts, and increased secretion of respiratory mucus.

Antibodies

are the principal substances involved in the adaptive or specific immune response. Collectively known as immunoglobulins, they are proteins capable of recognising and binding to their own specific antigen, usually a microorganism.

Antibodies are produced by B lymphocytes and, once formed, circulate in the plasma. They have three functions:

- to bind to antigens
- to bind to phagocytes
- to activate the complement pathway.

There are five classes of antibody: immunoglobulin G (IgG), IgA, IgM, IgD and IgE. Each of the five classes may be produced with specificity for a single antigen. Their structure varies according to function and they are present in different amounts in the bloodstream (see Box 16.2).

Box 16.2

Immunoglobulins

Immunoglobulins are proteins with known antibody activity. They form the central component of the immune system and are synthesised by lymphocytes and plasma cells. The five classes of immunoglobulins are as follows:

- IgM — the first immunoglobulin to appear in the bloodstream in the primary response to infection. Since it disappears fairly quickly after the antigen disappears, it is an indicator of current or very recent infection.
- IgG — produced in large quantities in both the primary and secondary responses to infection. It is also important as a defence against infection in the first few weeks of life, being the only immunoglobulin which crosses the placenta to the fetus.
- IgA — secreted onto the luminal surface of the respiratory, alimentary and genitourinary tracts and present in saliva, tracheobronchial and genitourinary secretions as well as in the serum. It is important in preventing the entry of microorganisms from the external orifices of the body.
- IgE — normally found on the surface membrane of basophils and mast cells. It is associated with allergic reactions such as hay fever.
- IgD — present in small quantities bound to B cells where it aids in the 'memory' function.

Immunoglobulins can be taken from a donor by plasmapheresis and given:

- to someone who has been exposed to a pathogen and is not immune, e.g. antitetanus immunoglobulin (Humotet)
- as short-term prophylaxis, when exposure is anticipated and there is not time for vaccine to take effect, e.g. tickborne encephalitis
- to someone who is heavily immunosuppressed, following exposure to a pathogen which could cause serious infection because of an inadequate immune response.

Passive immunisation with immunoglobulins does not confer long-term protection: this requires vaccination (see p. 657).

The non-specific immune response

When a foreign substance enters the body, the first line of defence is the non-specific immune response, which comprises the following components:

- mechanical barriers, e.g. the skin, cilia in the upper respiratory tract
- phagocytes
- chemicals, e.g. complement, the interferons
- substances found in body secretions, e.g. lysozyme, gastric acid.

These defences can be effective on their own, but help is sometimes needed from adaptive or specific immune response mechanisms.

Disadvantages of the non-specific response are as follows:

- The cells can differentiate between 'self' and 'non-self' but cannot recognise specific antigens.
- Adaptation does not occur after exposure, i.e. the same level of response is produced for each exposure to an antigen.
- There is no 'memory' and so developing the same infection a second time cannot be prevented.

The specific immune response: natural immunity

The specific immune response involves the lymphocytes and comprises the humoral or antibody-mediated response, initiated by B lymphocytes, and the cell-mediated response, initiated by T lymphocytes. These responses are described separately here, but they interact with each other as well as with non-specific factors. The humoral response deals mainly with extracellular organisms, and the antibodies which it produces are present in the serum. The cell-mediated response is important for dealing with intracellular organisms.

Specificity

When first exposed to an antigen, the circulating lymphocytes differentiate to recognise and bind to that one particular antigen. This recognition and binding is like a lock and key mechanism on a door. Many different keys may go into the same lock, but only one will fit closely enough to turn in the lock and open the door, the primary response.

On re-exposure to the antigen, perhaps many years later, the remaining progeny of that cell (memory cells) will be stimulated to replicate as a secondary response.

Antibody-mediated immune response

This response may be described in terms of its primary and secondary phases.

Primary response The first time an antigen is encountered in the body it takes approximately 2 weeks for a corresponding antibody to be detected in the blood. The production of this antibody is called the primary response. Although the immune system reacts immediately to antigens, the synthesis of antibodies takes some time.

An antigen binds to its specific receptor on the surface of the B lymphocyte, triggering the following sequence of events:

- The B lymphocyte is stimulated to develop into a plasma cell and to undergo multiple divisions so that identical plasma cells are formed.
- The plasma cells synthesise antibodies.
- Some B lymphocytes differentiate to become memory cells, which persist and replicate in the body long after the invading antigen has been dealt with (see Fig. 16.2).
- Once sufficient quantities of an antibody have been produced to destroy all the antigen, the plasma cells die, leaving memory cells ready to respond to a future attack by that antigen.
- Antibodies bind to the antigen, activating the complement system (see p. 656).
- When several antibodies bind to one antigen, the complex thus formed is chemically attracted to the surface of phagocytic cells, resulting in the formation of an antigen–antibody–phagocyte complex.
- The presence of antibodies triggers the phagocyte into action, resulting in ingestion and digestion of the bacterium.

The time interval between contact with the antigen and the production of antibodies (IgM), however, may allow disease to develop in the individual due to the effects of the antigen, e.g. infection from microorganisms.

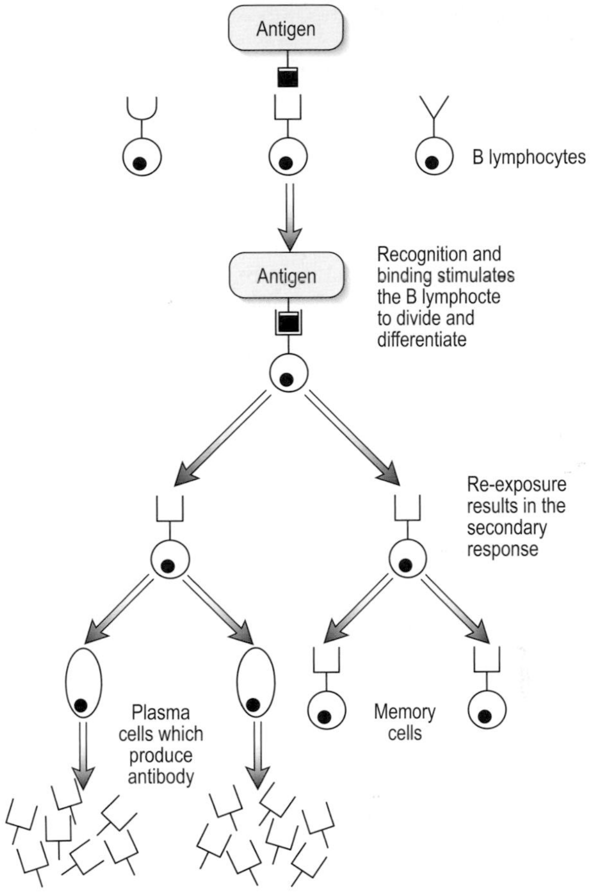

Fig. 16.2 The primary immune response.

Secondary response When the body encounters an antigen for the second time, the memory cells respond rapidly by producing plasma cells, which then produce antibodies. This response occurs within a few days and, together with any residual antibody from the primary response, usually prevents disease from developing. In other words, the individual has developed an immunity.

Immunisation: artificial immunity

Vaccination or immunisation is a means of artificially invoking a primary immune response to a particular microorganism (antigen) so that when the antigen is subsequently encountered, the individual will be immune to it. The principle of immunisation is to introduce altered microorganisms or toxins into the body so that the individual does not develop the disease, but does mount an immune response. In other words, it mimics the natural response to infectious disease. Booster doses may be required months or years after the first dose of a vaccine in order to maintain an adequate level of memory cells. There are three types of vaccine:

- *Live attenuated vaccines*. Laboratory cultures of virulent strains of some organisms lose their virulence. These are then capable of inducing immunity without causing disease. The bacille Calmette–Guérin (BCG:

tuberculosis) and rubella vaccines are of this type. However, live attenuated vaccines should not be given to someone who is immunocompromised or taking long-term corticosteroid medication, as their immune system cannot mount the appropriate response.
- *Toxoids.* The toxin produced by the bacterium is chemically modified by the use of formalin so that its toxicity is lost, but its antigenicity is retained, and is therefore capable of producing an immune response. The tetanus toxoid is an example of a toxoid.
- *Killed vaccines.* These are preparations in which the organisms have been killed by heat or chemicals; the whooping cough vaccine is one example.

Immunity can therefore be natural, i.e. acquired in utero or after infectious disease, or artificial, i.e. acquired after immunisation. Figure 16.3 illustrates the processes involved in natural and artificial immunity.

Cell-mediated immune response

As it is not possible for antibodies to reach microorganisms which live inside host cells, for example viruses, a different system, known as the cell-mediated immune response, carries out this function. In order that a T lymphocyte recognises an infected cell, a major histocompatibility complex (MHC) is involved. The MHC is a group of molecules which are important in interactions between cells in the immune system, in particular in the recognition of infected cells. One of these molecules is present on the surface of the cell in association with antigen, and the T cells recognise and bind to this on the surface of the macrophages, producing cytokines (see p. 656) which activate the macrophage and kill the intracellular microorganism. Cytotoxic T cells are also antigen-specific, having acquired a specific antigen receptor during their maturation in the thymus gland. They recognise antigen in association with the MHC on virally infected cells, which they destroy.

Once all the antigen has been destroyed, the immune response is 'switched off' until the next time. The involvement of other cells (e.g. mast cells) in the immune response has been discussed on page 655.

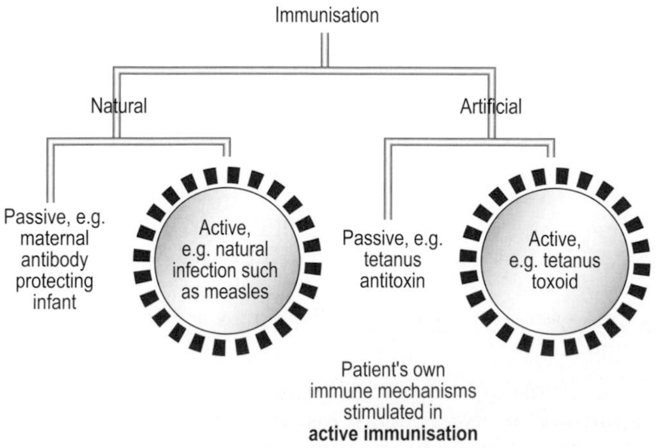

Fig. 16.3 Natural and artificial immunity.

Understanding of all immunology processes will help to ensure that patients and clients are assisted in fighting infection, particularly while receiving health care.

PREVENTION, CONTROL AND MANAGEMENT OF INFECTION

History

Infection control measures have been adopted to help prevent the spread of infection for centuries. In the 14th century, the Venetians applied quarantine to ships arriving at their port in order to contain diseases such as the bubonic plague. In the 19th century, Semmelweiss, a Hungarian obstetrician, realised that infection was being passed on the hands of health care workers to patients and showed that mortality rates could be greatly reduced by handwashing. Equally, Florence Nightingale emphasised the importance of cleanliness and hygiene in preventing and controlling illness. Also in the 19th century, separate hospitals for infectious diseases were first established.

Developments in the understanding of the microorganisms which cause disease are landmarks in the history of health care. The invention of the microscope allowed the study of minute organisms, invisible to the naked eye. In 1676, van Leeuwenhoek designed a primitive version of this piece of now indispensable equipment, whereby bacteria could be seen. Since then many advances have been made in analysing and studying the structure of bacteria. Modern techniques are attributed primarily to Pasteur, Lister and Koch for their work on microorganism activity, the prevention of bacterial invasion in tissues and techniques for diagnostic bacteriology.

Infection control measures are essential in everyday clinical practice today. The occurrence of antibiotic-resistant organisms, such as MRSA, vancomycin-resistant enterococci (VRE) and multidrug-resistant tuberculosis (MDRTB), thought to be attributed to many years of use and misuse of antibiotics, has greatly increased and is of concern internationally.

Jenner introduced vaccination in 1796 but it was not until the 20th century that it became routine. Vaccination has controlled 10 major diseases throughout the world: smallpox, diphtheria, tetanus, yellow fever, pertussis, *Haemophilus influenzae* type b, poliomyelitis, measles, mumps and rubella. However, in an age when there is heightened awareness of the risks from bioterrorism, the threat of infections familiar only to older generations, for example smallpox, is again causing great concern. The threat from disease spread through accidental or deliberate release of microorganisms raises the issue of herd immunity in populations that have not had to consider the protection they enjoy through acquired immunity, i.e. vaccination. Governments internationally are preparing both for the re-emergence of diseases that have previously been eradicated or controlled and for the emergence of new diseases.

STOP THINK **16.1** All health care workers receive hepatitis B vaccination. If, after a primary course of three injections over a period of 6 months, the antibody titre is inadequate, what course of action will be taken?

For further information on hepatitis B immunity, see www.who.int/vaccines/en/hepatitisb.shtml.

The threat from microorganisms continues in the 21st century. As new species are identified, existing ones genetically mutate to ensure their survival in a changing environment. These minute organisms continue to cause significant disruption to our health. Influenza and norovirus (winter vomiting and diarrhoeal disease) are prime examples of infections that have been in existence for many years and cause major disruption most winters. Concern continues that a world pandemic of influenza will occur, as it did in 1918, when it killed millions.

The understanding of microorganisms must continue to develop as they themselves develop, particularly if nurses are to be alert to such threats in the environment.

The infection control team

Health care workers, patients, relatives and carers together have a contribution to make in the prevention, control and management of the spread of infection. Those involved include nurses, doctors and dentists, allied health professionals, health care assistants, domestic and catering services, estates management, sterile services staff, administrative and management staff, education and training staff. The role of the infection control team is well defined and includes the utilisation of the risk management approach (see p. 661) to ensure that appropriate measures and action plans are in place. The structure for infection prevention and control programmes of work at organisation level is guided by national and local requirements. The infection control doctor and infection control nurse have clear responsibilities within this structure.

The microbiology laboratory is an important partner. Laboratory staff are a key resource in the process of obtaining, analysing and reporting on samples from patients.

Many settings also have infection control link nurses/personnel to enhance the effectiveness of the work of the team. The link person in a ward, department or community team will have received additional education to improve the communication between infection control teams and the clinical setting and may assist with clinical audit and awareness of clinical staff in relation to standard infection control precautions (see p. 664). The work of the team is guided by the Control of Infection Committee which is responsible for strategic and operational decisions about infection control.

The nurse's role in infection control

Nurses can contribute to the application of all aspects of prevention measures by acting as role models and by educating others. Nurses have a pivotal role in managing infection in acute or primary care settings by:

- containing and controlling the sources of microorganisms
- preventing infection and the potential spread of microorganisms that can cause harm
- treating and managing identified infections
- promoting the most fundamental aspects of patient care.

Nurses have a duty of care as stated in the Health and Safety at Work Act (1974) to prevent, control and manage infection. Nurses, as the largest staff group in health care, have a responsibility to prevent the spread of infection and act accordingly to ensure they do not put themselves and others at unnecessary risk from infection (NMC 2004). Nurses must therefore understand physiology, immunology, fundamental infection control measures and how a risk management approach operates within the field of infection prevention, control and management, an approach that has become increasingly popular in health care overall.

Nursing assessment is vital to health and control of infection, whether the health care setting is the home, the hospital, the clinic or the care home, as it can reveal crucial information about patients, their surroundings and their behaviours. Nursing models and processes must incorporate approaches to prevention, control and management of infection, for example within care plans and pathways.

The health of the nurse while at work is also important. The nurse should:

- stay away from work if unwell, particularly if the illness could be communicated to others, e.g. influenza
- be aware of their immune status regarding infectious diseases such as rubella, chickenpox, measles, tuberculosis, tetanus, hepatitis B and poliomyelitis. Nurses can obtain advice from their general practitioner (GP) or from their employer's Occupational Health Department
- discuss other health concerns that may have an impact upon the ability to work, or upon others, with the Occupational Health Department, e.g. skin conditions that may be caused by supplies used during work and that may harbour and spread microorganisms.

How infection spreads

The terms 'infection process', 'cycle of infection' or 'chain of infection' are often used to describe the circumstances that can lead to patients or others acquiring HAI or any infectious disease. The rationale for application of recommended precaution measures to prevent spread is based on this chain of events. It is crucial to understand how microorganisms spread and infection occurs. The infection process is related to:

- the presence of an infectious agent, i.e. microorganisms that are capable of causing infection
- a reservoir or source where microorganisms can be found. Within health care settings this may include the environment, e.g. dust, bedding, equipment, furniture, sinks, washbasins, bedpans and surfaces; and humans, e.g. patients, staff and visitors, especially on hands
- the potential for microorganisms to be transmitted from sources. These are often called portals of exit and include the means by which microorganisms might spread, such as exhalation, aerosolisation, secretion and excretion
- a means or route of transmission for microorganisms, categorised as blood borne, droplet, airborne, contact, food and water borne (common vehicle) and vector borne

- portals of entry — for microorganisms to enter susceptible sites, commonly through a variety of invasive devices, e.g. intravenous lines, urinary catheters, respiratory devices or any device that breaches the normal immune defences (see Fig. 16.1), as well as wound sites, open skin lesions, mucous membranes and ingestion
- a susceptible host — anyone who, for whatever reason, is at risk from microorganisms that would not normally cause them harm. Factors that affect the body's natural ability to fight infection include:
  - — the presence of underlying disease, e.g. diabetes mellitus
  - — immunocompromised status, e.g. HIV, chemotherapy treatment
  - — poor nutritional status
  - — extremes of age, i.e. the very young and the very old.

The principles of all precautions and measures taken in order to prevent and control infection are based on the interruption of this process. If measures are not taken, a cycle will continue and patients, staff and others may be exposed to potentially pathogenic (disease-causing) microorganisms.

Microbiology

Microbiology is the study of microorganisms such as bacteria, fungi, protozoa, viruses and helminths. In recent years, minute protein particles called prions have also been identified that cause transmissible spongiform encephalopathies (TSEs), e.g. variant Creutzfeldt–Jakob disease (vCJD).

Bacteria

Bacteria, including variations of the microscopic beings such as mycoplasmas, rickettsiae and chlamydiae, are small microorganisms of simple primitive form. Bacteria are commonly found living within our bodies and in our environment, for example in soil and water. Bacteria constitute the normal commensal flora within the body (see Table 16.1). However, such bacteria can become disease-producing organisms (see p. 662).

Viruses

Viruses are a group of parasitic infective agents so small that they are visible only through electron microscopy. Viruses have no independent metabolic activity and may replicate only within the cell of a living plant or animal.

Fungi

Fungi are simple plants that are parasitic on other plants, animals and humans. A few can cause fatal disease and illness in humans. They are classically opportunistic, e.g. in a postoperative patient, where antibiotic therapy may not only eradicate the infective organism, but also protective normal flora. Fungi can proliferate and cause infection such as *Candida albicans* (see Ch. 15).

Protozoa

These are the smallest single-cell organisms, many species of which can cause human disease. Most are harmless; however, some cause particular problems in hot climates, e.g. *Plasmodium*, the protozoa which causes malaria.

Table 16.1 Normal commensal microorganisms

Site	Organism
Skin	*Staphylococcus epidermidis* Diphtheroids *Corynebacterium* sp.
Mouth and throat	Staphylococci Streptococci Anaerobes *Neisseria* sp.
Nose	Staphylococci Diphtheroids
Gut	*Escherichia coli* *Klebsiella* sp. *Proteus* sp. *Streptococcus faecalis* *Clostridium perfringens* Yeasts *(Candida)*
Kidneys and bladder	Normally sterile
Vagina	Lactobacilli Streptococci Staphylococci Anaerobes

Helminths

These are large parasites — worms — which can be a major cause of morbidity, mainly in developing countries.

For further information, see Gould & Brooker (2000) and Humphreys & Irving (2004).

Routes of transmission

Clear understanding of the most common routes or means of transmission can ensure that no matter what the microorganism, the spread can be controlled:

- *Blood borne* — through sexual transmission, injury or inoculation. The main concern within health care settings or for health care workers in the community is the transmission of HIV and hepatitis B and C through sharps injuries or blood splashes. Many different organisms besides blood-borne viruses can be spread unwittingly by health care staff while caring for patients, e.g. through blood and body fluids, secretions, excretions, non-intact skin or mucous membranes. Standard infection control precautions, which have superseded Universal Precautions, apply at all times in all health care settings (see p. 664).
- *Airborne* — through inhalation. Airborne transmission is by small particles that can remain suspended in the air for long periods of time and can be widely dispersed by air currents.
- *Droplet* — through inhalation. Droplet transmission differs from airborne as the particles are larger and therefore do not remain suspended in the air. Spread is therefore through close contact with infected persons who may be sneezing, coughing, talking or undergoing airway procedures such as intubation or bronchoscopy.

The droplets can settle in the environment close to where they have originated, e.g. within 1 metre of an infected coughing patient.

- *Contact* — direct or indirect. This is regarded as the most common route of transmission related to HAI. Direct is the transfer of organisms by contact with people, primarily contaminated hands. Indirect is the transfer of organisms through the environment and the items within it, e.g. fomites (any inanimate object that can carry disease-causing organisms), and patient care equipment.
- *Food and water borne* (also known as common vehicle) — food and water can be the most common reservoirs for microorganisms, but the term 'common vehicle' also includes transmission through medication, blood or other solutions.
- *Vector borne* — usually spread via insects such as mosquitoes and ticks but cockroaches, ants and flies can also transmit infection. This mode of transmission is not common in the UK but should be considered in pest control policies.

Certain organisms can be transmitted through more than one of these routes and all modes of spread must be considered when carrying out risk assessments and providing care. Bacteria tend to cause the most concern while health care is being provided as they can often be avoided (see Table 16.2).

Diagnostic sampling

Sample taking is an important element of a nurse's role. Sampling provides identification of microorganisms for diagnosis, relevant treatment and screening purposes, e.g. on admission, transfer or discharge; preoperative or other pre-procedure screening; for 'clearance' purposes, e.g. to exclude previous known infections; and in contact tracing, e.g. to identify or exclude transmission of infection often in unsuspecting, otherwise healthy individuals. Health care settings will have a screening policy, e.g. some settings will screen on admission when patients are having elective orthopaedic surgery, due to the high risks related to such surgery and the implications of joint replacement failures due to infection. There are various sources and types of sample. For example, samples may be taken from the respiratory tract including the ear, nose and throat and the eye using a swab, a fluid (including sputum) aspirate or a tissue, or from the gastrointestinal tract and biliary system by sampling faeces, fluid or tissue (samples of vomit are not normally sent for testing as the results are of limited analytical value).

In order to avoid false-positive and false-negative results, it is important to ensure that there is no contamination from other microorganisms while obtaining samples, that an adequate amount of a sample is taken and that it is sent promptly to the laboratory. The value of swab sampling is frequently questioned, but it is a common, convenient and inexpensive option in clinical practice. If contamination occurs, for example from intact skin surrounding a suspected infected surgical wound (false positive), or not enough sample is sent to the laboratory, for example a dry swab is used to sample a small patch of dry skin for microbiological screening purposes (false negative), analysis will be limited and results will not be meaningful. Accurate completion of laboratory forms is also essential.

THE RISK MANAGEMENT APPROACH

The risk to health from infection is one of many risks to be managed in health care settings. The risk management approach to HAI was developed during the 1970s as part of the growing health and safety agenda around the developed world. The World Health Organization (WHO) definitions provide a basis for the risk management approach in relation to infection control:

- *Hazard* — a biological, chemical or physical agent with the potential to cause an adverse health effect
- *Risk* — a function of the probability of an adverse health effect and the severity of that effect associated with exposure to a hazard.

Hazards and risks from microorganisms are present in our environment at all times. Once they are identified, appropriate control measures and action plans must be adopted to ensure that the greatest time and resource is spent in the areas with the greatest risks of infection. For example, a risk assessment is carried out when a chemical disinfectant must be used to decontaminate a piece of equipment. Guidance on how to use and handle safely the disinfectant and the equipment is provided for the health and safety of both patients and staff. A review of the decisions made must be undertaken within a defined timescale as the use of the disinfectant may change over time and the risks may change, requiring updated guidance on control measures for staff.

For further information, see www.hse.gov.uk/coshh — Care of Substances Hazardous to Health Regulations produced by the Health and Safety Executive.

In summary, the correct systems, management and culture must be in place to ensure that actions are effective in preventing, controlling and managing HAI:

- *Systems* include structures and processes at national, organisational and individual practitioner level, e.g. guidance given through policies and procedures, education and training, and frequent planned monitoring of outcome through audit, surveillance and research.
- *Management* includes the appropriate support being available and a clear commitment towards addressing the risks of infection, considering these alongside the many other pressures faced within health care. Ensuring that the correct processes are in place to achieve this must be a management priority and education on this is mandatory in many areas.
- *Culture* includes the continuous improvement of quality through individual behaviour, whereby nurses can be seen as role models, aware of the systems and processes to manage hazards and risks from infection. Good infection control practice by health care and associated staff helps maintain an overall culture of good practice, making it easier for all to comply, especially during periods of stress.

Table 16.2 Examples of common bacteria encountered while providing health care

Organism	Main sources	Main mode of spread and means of entry	Examples of resulting disease/conditions
Staphylococcus aureus including MRSA	People, skin, wounds, and at times in sputum Environmental dust	Direct and indirect contact with persons carrying the organism or from the environment. Entry through e.g. open wounds	Wound and skin infection Bacteraemia, endocarditis Osteomyelitis and septic arthritis
Clostridium difficile	In the animal and human lower bowel, therefore faeces and any faecally contaminated areas. Especially found in hospitalised patients who have received antibiotic therapy that has disturbed their normal bowel flora Also soil	Direct and indirect contact with persons carrying the organism or from the environment, especially as it can form spores that survive for long periods in the environment. Often also called faecal–oral spread if ingestion occurs resulting in further GI upset/infection	GI infection, characterised by loose, foul-smelling green stools and abdominal pain The most common cause of HAI diarrhoea Can lead to pseudomembranous colitis
Streptococcal infections	Found in humans, at various sites, and in the environment	Direct and indirect contact with persons carrying the organism or from the environment Through droplets from infected respiratory tracts	Pharyngitis Wound infection, rarely necrotising fasciitis Septicaemia Toxin-mediated disease, e.g. scarlet fever, toxic shock syndrome Pneumonia and associated bacteraemia
Enterococci, including vancomycin-resistant enterococci (VRE) *Pseudomonas aeruginosa*	Mainly environmental sources but also in the human GI tract. In the lower bowel of animals and humans, most commonly in hospitalised patients who have received antibiotic therapy Moist sites in the environment, but especially poorly draining shower areas and open fluid containers Also soil	Direct and indirect contact with persons carrying the organism or from the environment	Urinary tract infection Wound infection Endocarditis Eye and ear infections Wound infections, e.g. in burns Septicaemia Respiratory infections, especially in the immunocompromised, e.g. cystic fibrosis patients
Mycobacterium tuberculosis (TB)	Found in humans, animals and in the environment	Through the airborne route when respiratory infection is present Through direct contact when other systems are infected	Respiratory or pulmonary TB; can be termed as open TB Closed TB, where another system or site of the body is infected. It can infect any organ in the body (see Ch. 3)
Escherichia coli	Found in humans, particularly the GI tract, and in the environment	Direct and indirect contact with persons carrying the organism From the environment or from food From poor hand hygiene	GI infection Urinary tract infection

Policies and procedures

Underpinning much of the work undertaken in clinical practice are the policies and procedures that guide best practice, for example related to hand hygiene, isolation of infectious patients, aseptic technique and insertion of urinary catheters. These must be current and have planned timescales for review. Many nurses are involved in framing policies, including those at management, specialist and general level. However, it is not enough to have an infection control policy manual; the recommended practices must be learned, applied and monitored with feedback given to ensure continuous quality improvement for up-to-date patient care. It is part of accountable practice that each member of the multidisciplinary team adheres to policies and procedures; failure to do so is considered breach of the Health and Safety at Work Act (1974).

STOP THINK **16.2** Locate the infection control policy manual in your area of work and familiarise yourself with the guidance it provides, related to your nursing duties. How do you contact the local infection control team for further guidance if needed?

Antibiotic prescribing and use

Another important area of practice in which policy should be available to guide many health care practitioners is antibiotic prescribing and use. This is now of particular concern to those nurses who have a role in prescribing, as antibiotic resistance (see Box 16.3) is increasing and strategies and recommendations have been published by WHO and in many countries to combat the problem. There have recently been cases around the developed world where patients have died from infections that could not be treated, as the causative microorganism was resistant to all the available antibiotics. This is of great concern in a world that has relied heavily upon the benefits of antibiotics.

For further information, see Department of Health (2000).

Box 16.3

Antibiotic use and resistance

- Antibiotics can work in different ways to treat infections. They can be bacteriostatic — stopping bacteria from multiplying, or they can be bactericidal — interfering with the cell wall of bacteria, thus killing them.
- Bacteria mutate and change to protect their cell structure against antibiotics, thus becoming resistant. Drug-resistant organisms can not only spread and cause further harm but can also transfer their resistance to other organisms. As new antibiotics are developed it is anticipated that bacteria will continue to protect themselves by mutating and again become resistant.
- Misuse and overuse of antibiotics are thought to have contributed to the problem. Pressure from patients to be given antibiotics, the contribution of topical antibiotics to antibiotic resistance and over-the-counter availability of antibiotics in many countries outside the UK are all considerations. Some resistance, however, will be inevitable.
- Policies should include guidance on the appropriate use of antibiotics for treatment in all clinical eventualities, including the use of 'broad spectrum' and 'narrow spectrum' antibiotics, and the length of time antibiotics should be taken. Guidance on use of antibiotics for prophylaxis is equally important, e.g. the use of antibiotics before, during and after surgery to prevent rather than treat infection (Scottish Intercollegiate Guidelines Network 2000).
- Nurse prescribing and its role in antibiotic resistance is important at this time when nurse prescribing is being extended. Points for consideration include the difficulties associated with diagnosing infection accurately, awareness of allergies to and toxic effects of antibiotics, the potential side-effects and the reduction in effectiveness of other medications when taking antibiotics, e.g. the oral contraceptive pill. Patient education is also important, e.g. there is often no point in taking antibiotics for viral complaints such as a sore throat, and completing an entire course of antibiotics as prescribed is essential.
- Antibiotic resistance has a major impact upon demands for services within health care as additional elements are required to care for those affected, e.g. isolation facilities.

Outbreak management

When an outbreak of any infectious disease occurs, at times even when guidance has been followed, a well-coordinated, multidisciplinary response will minimise the impact of the outbreak by controlling and managing the impact and ongoing risks. Outbreaks may have minimal impact or major, widespread implications, including death or serious illness. Local infection control policies state the response that will be mounted when an outbreak is suspected or confirmed, with the definition of what is considered an outbreak within the area also being clearly stated, as this can vary between settings. Policies should include details of the people involved and their roles during the incident, the communication processes and the actions to be taken, including risk assessments. Communication is crucial in these situations, as it is within all health care provision. Meetings are established during these times to facilitate the response and this might include extraordinary meetings of the Control of Infection Committee.

Outbreaks may happen in health care facilities as well as in the community, but those within health care settings receive most attention, particularly in the media. Outbreaks in the community often spread to health care settings, where more immunocompromised patients are present in an environment already conducive to spread of infection (see Box 16.4).

Food hygiene

Infection spread via the food-borne route can have a major impact upon health care and the community. The Stanley Royd Hospital outbreak in 1984, in which a number of older

Box 16.4

Examples of microorganisms causing outbreaks

Norovirus infection

- This is a commonly occurring gastrointestinal infection that usually causes seasonal outbreaks of vomiting and/or diarrhoea.
- Although the illness tends to be short lived and less severe than other forms of gastroenteritis, the disruption caused in hospitals and long-term care facilities is extensive if a ward or department has to be closed to further admissions or if the occurrence of symptoms among staff results in staff shortages.

MRSA

- Outbreaks of MRSA are frequently encountered, often not causing significant harm but certainly causing disruption. The impact upon patients, staff, resources and budgets, both locally and on the NHS as a whole, can be significant.
- In large outbreaks, wards or areas may be closed to admissions, surgery may be cancelled and patients and staff may be affected, directly or indirectly.
- If the outbreak is significant, staff may be screened for the microorganism to prevent further spread, depending on the local screening policy.
- There are many strains of MRSA, but if microbiology reference laboratories identify the strain, specific risk assessments can be carried out and actions taken.

people died and many staff and patients became ill, led to Crown immunity being removed from health care settings in order that they could be monitored and instructed on best practice in relation to food hygiene; previously, they had been exempt from prosecution if they were deemed to be at fault. The *Escherichia coli* outbreak, spread through meat in a butcher's shop in Wishaw, Lanarkshire, in 1996, resulted in the death of many people in that community and attracted much media interest over hygiene controls in food premises.

In hospitals and care facilities, guidance on effective food preparation, production and distribution techniques is vital for effective infection control. Major outbreaks of food-borne illness have led to the incorporation of the Hazard Analysis and Critical Control Point (HACCP) risk management system as a preventive mechanism for the safety of foodstuffs. The system identifies possible safety risks in a food production facility and attempts to control that risk at critical points.

The nurse's role in food hygiene often involves basic measures such as the care of fridges, microwaves and eating utensils. However, awareness of the importance of food hygiene overall, as well as the other elements of best practice, is essential.

For information about those infectious diseases that require to be 'notified' for monitoring purposes, whether an isolated case or during an outbreak situation, see www.hpa.org.uk/infections and www.isdscotland.org.

STANDARD INFECTION CONTROL PRECAUTIONS

Standard infection control precautions (SICPs), first recommended in the USA, incorporate fundamental infection prevention and control measures that help to interrupt the chain of events that can lead to infection, whether the risk management approach has been adopted or not. Elements of these precautions should always be included in guidance, policies and procedures. Before the introduction of SICPs, published recommendations on elements of infection control had become more common following the introduction of health and safety legislation, and had specifically featured general infection control guidance under such terms as 'safe working practice' and 'body substance isolation', but most widely under the heading of 'universal precautions'. Universal precautions were first introduced during the initial HIV epidemic in the 1980s, to protect patients against exposure to blood and body fluids regardless of their blood-borne viral status. These precautions appeared to motivate and greatly improve compliance with general infection control measures and ultimately had a major impact on health care, for example, the increased use of gloves in practical care procedures. During the 1990s, however, wide variation in the interpretation and implementation of universal precautions became apparent and steps were taken to outline practical, feasible recommendations for preventing cross-infection at all times and to further encourage standardisation of precautions throughout all health care settings. Universal precautions were at this point replaced with standard precautions, which throughout this chapter are referred to as standard infection control precautions (SICPs), in order to take into account the many micro-organisms that can be spread while providing care and not only blood-borne viruses such as HIV.

SICPs are a set of recommendations for the care of all patients regardless of their infection status, when exposed to any:

- blood
- body fluids, e.g. serous fluid, lymph fluid
- secretions or excretions (except sweat), e.g. sputum, urine
- non-intact skin
- mucous membranes.

There are nine elements to standard infection control precautions (see Table 16.3).

Hand hygiene

People's hands are considered the most common vehicle by which microorganisms might be transported and cause infection to those who are susceptible. Therefore, all of the steps that lead to adequate hand decontamination must be considered and applied in practice in all settings (see Table 16.4). Guidance related to hand hygiene for the very specific work carried out in specialised areas such as theatres should additionally be available at local and national level. The terms hand hygiene, hand decontamination and hand washing are used interchangeably in today's health care (Gould 2004, Rickard 2004).

For recommended hand washing technique, see Gould (2004), NHS Education for Scotland (2004) and Royal College of Nursing (2004a).

Environmental prevention, control and management of infection

A clean environment contributes to the prevention of infection. It is common sense and good practice to ensure that the environment is clean so that infection is not spread and patients are reassured that standards of cleanliness and hygiene are high.

In hospital

The responsibilities for ensuring the patient's environment is clean must be made clear to all. Cleaning is usually conducted using a general purpose detergent, warm water in a clean receptacle and clean or disposable cloths or mops. Drying is also important, although large surfaces, e.g. floors, may have to be 'air-dried'. Wet environments are not acceptable for patients who are at particular risk, e.g. in transplant units, intensive care units and burns units. Stagnant moisture or fluid can be a focus for micro-organisms and lead to HAI, e.g. *Pseudomonas aeruginosa* from eye- and mouth-care solutions left next to intensive-care patients. Disinfectants may be used when particular risks are known, under guidance from infection control teams and from policies and procedures.

If any contamination of the environment is observed, decontamination must take place immediately. Particular attention must be given to horizontal surfaces, e.g. bedrails, bedside cabinets, chair arms, tables, floors or health care equipment such as pumps, especially those that are

Table 16.3 Standard infection control precautions

Element	Action/timing	Rationale
1. Hand hygiene	At the right times In the most appropriate way for the situation (see Table 16.4)	Frequently called the single most important action to prevent, control and manage infection
2. Personal protective equipment (PPE)*	Gloves (powder-free): — non-latex alternatives should be available and their use is being increasingly encouraged due to the adverse affects of latex Aprons, gowns, footwear Eye and mouth protection	To protect mouth and eyes in particular, and the skin of the face, hands and the rest of the body with the use of clothing and equipment in order to avoid contamination/soiling/ splashing and potential exposure to harmful microorganisms, originating from patients, the environment or even live vaccinations The use of gloves does not negate the need for hand decontamination and all PPE must be disposed of safely and properly immediately after being removed Often this is into clinical waste
3. Prevention of occupational exposure to infection	Cover all breaks in skin Avoid sharps injuries: — never resheath sharps such as needles — utilise sharps receptacles close to the point of use — never try to retrieve any items from sharps receptacles Avoid splashes with blood or body fluids by using PPE when exposure is anticipated Report any exposure incidents following local policies (see www.riddor.gov.uk/info.html)	To additionally protect health care workers, carers and others from exposure to microorganisms that cause infection, e.g. hepatitis B, C, HIV, MRSA
4. Management of blood and body fluid spillages	Utilise cleaning products and disinfectants (often found in 'spillage kits') immediately spillages occur, following local policies	To protect all of those in the surrounding area from exposure to microorganisms found within spillages that could cause harm and to protect the environment from contamination
5. Management of equipment utilised during care	Prevent reuse of single-use devices Prevent single-patient use devices being used on other patients Ensure reusable devices are handled safely and decontaminated between use on the same patient and before use on others, following local policies: — basic cleaning measures are a vital part of health care and should also be performed before any required disinfection processes	To ensure that items used during care are not a factor in the spread of potentially infectious microorganisms directly to patients or a factor in the contamination of patients' environment leading to indirect spread of infection
6. Environment control	At the right times and in the most appropriate way for the situation Cleanliness and maintenance must be kept at the optimum level	To ensure that the care setting, its fixtures and fittings and other items within it are adequately decontaminated and maintained to prevent cross-infection occurring through this route
7. Safe disposal of waste, including sharps	Waste is categorised by regulations so that it will be segregated and subsequently destroyed safely and effectively: — clinical waste generated in the home and community is often dealt with differently from that generated in hospital settings; local policies reflecting current regulations must be followed — the area around the opening of clinical waste bags and sharps containers is often the most contaminated in health care settings and should never be touched. 'Hands-free' waste sack holders, e.g.foot-operated, must always be in place	To prevent the risk of inappropriate, avoidable exposure to the microorganisms found contaminating clinical waste in particular, thus protecting all health care workers and others The use of PPE when handling waste is essential

Continued

Table 16.3 Standard infection control precautions *(Continued)*

Element	Action/timing	Rationale
7. Safe disposal of waste, including sharps *(Continued)*	Attaching waste bags to other pieces of furniture, e.g. trolleys, is not generally acceptable, nor is overfilling of bags	
8. Linen	Safe handling, transport and processing of bags: — linen should never be held against the body or shaken, even if protective clothing is worn — linen should always be disposed of into appropriate receptacles immediately after being removed and never placed on the floor	To prevent the risk of inappropriate, avoidable exposure to microorganisms when linen is being handled or reused, thus protecting health care workers and others and preventing contamination of the environment Linen can be heavily contaminated with potentially pathogenic microorganisms; items such as urinary catheters, needles, etc. are often found in linen by laundry staff, putting them at unnecessary risk Use of PPE when handling used linen is essential
9. Appropriate patient placement	Choosing the most appropriate site/area to care for a patient must be considered using a risk management approach at all times, e.g. consider the route of transmission of any known or suspected infections/colonisation, how these might then spread to others, the potential outcomes of this spread, the availability of resources to site patients in the best place	To prevent exposure of others and the environment to potentially infectious microorganisms and to protect the patient as far as possible

*Also known as protective clothing.

Table 16.4 Hand hygiene

	Action	Rationale
Provision of hand decontamination facilities	Access to adequate hand hygiene facilities and supplies is an essential element of SICPs in all settings where exposure to microorganisms might occur The use of 'hands-free' tap systems, e.g. elbow taps, is recommended wherever possible in health care as this ensures that hands are not contaminated during the process of turning taps on or off and potentially becoming a source for further contamination of patients or the environment Also important is the use of mixer taps to ensure water of the right temperature can be provided as well as the absence of plugs to discourage washing in filled sinks where microorganisms can harbour Where running water cannot be accessed, the use of alcohol hand decontamination products, e.g. gels, is a useful alternative	By providing adequate facilities, hand decontamination should be carried out in the correct manner at the correct times to prevent cross-infection from occurring Alcohol gel is appropriate if hands are not soiled; it is inactivated by organic matter

	Level 1 Social handwash	Level 2 Hygienic handwash	Level 3 Surgical scrub
When **to wash or decontaminate**	**Before** commencing/leaving work, eating/handling of food/drinks, preparing/giving medications, general patient/client contact	**Before** aseptic procedures, contact during all patients'/clients' care procedures, leaving isolation rooms (all levels of transmission-based precautions)	**Before** surgical/other invasive procedures **Between/within** the above described procedures if any contamination occurs

Continued

Table 16.4 Hand hygiene *(Continued)*

	Level 1 Social handwash	Level 2 Hygienic handwash	Level 3 Surgical scrub
When **to wash or decontaminate** *(Continued)*	**After** visiting the toilet; patient/client contact, handling laundry/equipment/waste, blowing/wiping/touching nose *NB* even if gloves have been worn	**After** contact with isolated patients/clients, any potential contact with body fluids/ excretions/secretions, etc. *NB* even if gloves have been worn **Between/within** the above described procedures if any contamination occurs **In high-risk areas at all times:** infant nurseries/special care baby units, infectious disease units/ intensive care/therapy units, wards/ departments during outbreaks of infection	
Why **decontaminate**	To render the hands physically clean and to remove microorganisms picked up during activities (transient microorganisms)	To remove or destroy transient microorganisms and to provide residual effect	To remove or destroy transient microorganisms and also to substantially reduce those which normally live on the skin (resident microorganisms)
How **to decontaminate** When washing hands for whatever purpose, the tap should first be turned on and the hands wet before applying the soap. A good lather should be evident for undertaking the steps, with all areas of the hands being covered (and forearms when surgical scrub is being undertaken). Following this, hands should be rinsed well Cleansing solutions' instructions should give guidance as to the volume of solution to be used; this also applies to alcohol hand products.	Using soap, preferably liquid, wash hands Alternatively, where hands are not soiled, utilise alcohol hand products using the same steps	Using an approved antiseptic hand cleanser or soap, wash hands If hands have any contact before or during a procedure, but are not soiled with any body fluids and, therefore, do not require hand washing with soap or an antiseptic hand cleanser, alcohol hand-rub can be used, using the same technique. Any soilage can inactivate the activity of alcohol and therefore hand washing in these circumstances is essential *NB* Alcohol hand-rubs/gels can also be used following hand washing, e.g. when performing aseptic techniques	Using an antiseptic hand cleanser carry out Level 2 hygienic hand wash for 2 to 3 min, ensuring all areas of hands and arms are covered (The time used for surgical scrub is often debated and local policies must be followed)

	Action	Rationale
How **to dry**	Using clean disposable towels, dry each area of the hand thoroughly each time after washing. This should be done by drying each part of the hand, remembering all of the steps included in the hand washing process If 'hands-free' taps are not available, the disposable towels should then be used to turn off the tap	Hand drying is an important process in removing any remaining transient microorganisms on the hands and hands that are not dried properly can become dry and cracked, leading to problems Recontamination of the hands following drying should be avoided as far as possible Other forms of hand drying, e.g. hot air driers or reusable towels, are available but are not considered acceptable in ensuring that the whole hand decontamination process is effective Reusable towels that are freshly laundered are sometimes acceptable in the home
Additional points Gloves	It may be necessary to change gloves and decontaminate hands between tasks on the same patient	To ensure that contamination of gloves/hands does not lead to microorganisms coming into contact with an area/site of the body where they would not normally be present and might cause infection

Continued

Table 16.4 Hand hygiene *(Continued)*

	Action	Rationale
Cuts and abrasions	Cover all cuts and abrasions with a waterproof dressing, even when gloves are being worn	To prevent inadvertent exposure to blood or body fluids and to protect the patient from exposure to the blood or body fluids of the health care worker
Soap	Liquid soap dispensers should be kept clean and the 'topping up' of solutions into bottles should not take place If bar soap must be used in home care settings, it should be kept on a rack that facilitates drainage	To prevent microorganisms from harbouring in dispensers and spreading to those using them and subsequently to patients Liquid soap solutions can become contaminated when a 'topping up' system is used
Nail brushes	Do not use nail brushes to scrub nails or any part of the hands during social or hygienic hand washing	Most microorganisms can be easily removed by hand washing and scrubbing can break the skin, leading to increased risk of picking up microorganisms or dispersing skin scales that may cause harm to others
Nails	Nails must be kept short and clean Nail polish or artificial nails should not be worn	To prevent the harbouring of microorganisms which may then be spread It has been shown that nails and chipped nail polish can harbour potentially harmful bacteria
Hand creams	Communal hand creams should not be used unless in a wall-mounted pump dispenser that undergoes a maintenance and cleaning regimen If a particular skin problem is experienced, advice should be sought from your GP or Occupational Health Department	To protect skin from drying and cracking, where bacteria can harbour Communal tubes or tubs of hand cream can become contaminated with microorganisms from the hands of those using them, therefore only individual tubes of hand cream should be used or those that are in contained dispensers Hand skin problems should be appropriately treated to try to ensure broken skin is not a problem when being potentially exposed to microorganisms in the workplace
Jewellery	Wrist and hand jewellery should be removed at the start of each shift if there will be close personal contact with patients during this time	To prevent contamination of jewellery, particularly those with intricate parts such as stones, with microorganisms and subsequent spread to health care workers or patients

SICPs, standard infection control precautions.

frequently touched or are used for eating. Other surfaces frequently touched by health care workers, e.g. hand rails, telephones, keyboards and door handles, are also important, and while recent media headlines have implicated items such as lift buttons, those items closer to patient care are probably more crucial in environment control and protection of patients.

Cleaning schedules must reflect specific risks, e.g. the volume of activity, the condition of the patients and the procedures being undertaken. This applies to clinical areas as well as local or central storage areas for supplies such as personal protective equipment (PPE), waste and linen. PPE or other clean or sterile equipment must never be stored in sluice areas, unless they are specifically for use there, and cleaning equipment must never be stored in communal areas, e.g. bathrooms. Supplies must always also be stored off the ground. Items used for cleaning must also have a schedule so they do not harbour microorganisms. Cleaning of soft furnishings such as curtains, chairs and carpets should include vacuuming. Increasing the frequency of cleaning and of reviewing methods of cleaning is essential during outbreaks or when there is increased risk of cross-infection, e.g. from incontinent patients or the presence of multidrug-resistant organisms.

Schedules for the pick-up of linen and waste bags are also important and must be agreed, recorded and monitored. If waste bags are not picked up frequently, this can lead to increased contamination of the environment, and storage of waste bags in communal areas such as corridors is not acceptable.

New items, such as invasive scopes, and large areas/items such as flooring or furniture, must be given specific decontamination attention with the involvement of the infection control team.

Schedules should also be drawn up for care of ventilation (air) systems, particularly in high-risk areas such as theatres and transplant units, and for water- and ice-dispensing machines, which can be a focus for microorganisms.

At home

In the home environment, risk assessments must be carried out and the most appropriate and common-sense approach used; for example, asking a patient's partner to wear full PPE when cleaning up a urine or vomit spillage may be unrealistic. Education and support from the community nurse are essential to provide people at home with the information necessary to prevent the spread of infection.

Many disciplines are involved in environment control and service level agreements can ensure that all are aware of the standards to be achieved and tasks to be undertaken. Many reports have been published (Auditor General 2000, 2003) about the lack of cleanliness and hygiene in health care, often focusing on the reduced numbers of dedicated cleaning staff, particularly in acute areas. Roles such as the modern matron, directors for infection prevention and control, and infection control managers, as well as infection control teams, can create a positive culture towards cleaning.

SICPs and respiratory infection

The spread of respiratory infection worldwide, e.g. SARS and influenza, has put respiratory hygiene and cough etiquette on the health agenda. Health care workers and patients need standard procedures, especially during seasons when outbreaks are more common, such as:

- covering the mouth and nose when coughing or sneezing
- using disposable tissues and disposing of them directly into bins
- performing hand hygiene after any contact with respiratory secretions or used tissues.

The proximity of patients to one another in areas such as waiting rooms is also a consideration for the spread of respiratory infections and regularly updated guidance will be made available to address such ongoing concerns, particularly from the Health Protection Agency and Health Protection Scotland.

Key points representing good practice in preventing infection are shown in Box 16.5.

STOP THINK **16.3** Think about a patient you have cared for recently. Identify how you considered their risks for infection during provision of routine daily care, bearing in mind the steps in the cycle of infection. Also think about which SICPs you applied, or should have applied, and why you did or did not apply them.

Box 16.5

Good practice in preventing infection

- A good standard of personal hygiene
- Appropriate wearing of uniforms, e.g. those working in hospital should change clothing before leaving and follow local policies on the best way to launder uniforms
- Appropriate placement of flowers in clinical areas, especially high-risk areas, where microorganisms may breed and spread infection (particularly harmful to immunocompromised patients)
- Appropriate care of animals when patients are present; animals may spread infections to patients — and vice versa, as it is thought that animals too may now harbour MRSA
- Avoiding sitting on or placing clinical items on patients' beds as beds may be contaminated with microorganisms and therefore can easily contaminate items placed on them, including uniforms and intravenous equipment
- Appropriate wearing of jewellery, as it may lead to cross-infection
- Long hair should be tied back away from the face and neck
- Appropriate use of white coats and other overcoats which, if not properly laundered, can be a source of microorganisms. Many doctors have stopped wearing white coats as they do not serve any personal protective equipment (PPE) purpose
- Ensuring reusable, communal items, e.g. stethoscopes and tape, are stored in a clean area and decontaminated where appropriate after use. Keeping items such as tape and scissors in uniform pockets poses an unacceptable infection risk

Decontamination of reusable medical devices

Health care workers require specific guidance on decontamination of reusable medical devices, such as surgical instruments (see Fig. 16.4). Decontamination encompasses cleaning, disinfection and sterilisation. The main areas to consider when undertaking decontamination include:

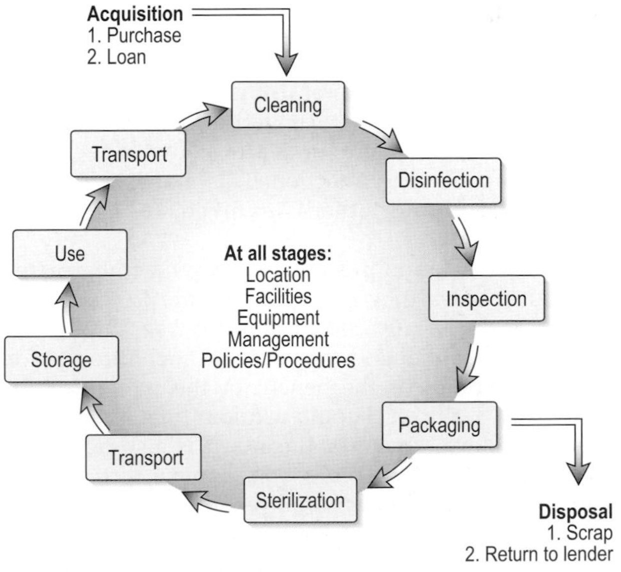

Fig. 16.4 Decontamination cycle.

- the risk of HAI from a reusable device and the most appropriate technique to protect patients from infection. Transmissible spongiform encephalopathies (TSEs), including CJD and vCJD, present a serious risk and need particular guidance
- general patient and staff safety to protect them from potentially infective microorganisms where devices are in use and to ensure that devices are safe to be handled and only used following decontamination, e.g. free of potentially harmful chemicals used during disinfection

- recognition of the symbols that guide health care workers handling and reprocessing medical devices, e.g. the symbols for 'do not reuse', 'single use only' and 'sterile', which can be found on the packaging of all items.

Many health care workers, including nurses, are responsible for handling and packaging items before sending them to a reprocessing department, e.g. central sterilising unit, returning them to stores for redistribution or sending them for repair. Training on sterilising unit policies is essential for those responsible for reprocessing surgical instruments to avoid decontamination failures that can lead to HAI. Automatic washer disinfectors and ultrasonic cleaners should be used. If cleaning is not carried out correctly, failures will occur, even in sterilised items. Cleaning prior to sterilisation is as important as sterilisation itself. Manual cleaning is discouraged, both to protect health care workers from cross-infection and also because the automated process is often more efficient. Where manual cleaning of instruments is essential, guidance must be sought from the infection control team and from the most up-to-date policies, including the use of appropriate PPE. Items with hollow bores and areas that are hard to reach are particular harbours of microorganisms.

Additional precautions

Transmission-based or expanded precautions, incorporating isolation procedures, previously often known as barrier nursing, should be applied when highly transmissible or antibiotic-resistant microorganisms are present in a patient. The procedures are commonly categorised by the organism's route of transmission, the most common being:

- droplet
- airborne
- contact.

Knowledge of the route of transmission will make the precautions to be taken clear and easy to understand without the need for more in-depth knowledge of the specific microorganism or infection. This makes it possible for all disciplines and others involved to apply the appropriate precautions.

People under isolation precautions may be embarrassed or depressed because they feel that they are in some way 'dirty'. Nurses are legally responsible for keeping patient information confidential and may divulge such information only if it is essential for the benefit of the patient or the safety of others. Nurses should explain this to patients to minimise embarrassment or unease. It is also helpful to inform the patient about infection control procedures. Maintaining patient confidentiality should not hinder measures such as isolation. Patients in circumstances such as isolation often require increased psychological support.

Full details of the measures to be adopted in addition to SICPs should be available within local infection control policies and from infection control teams. Although the recommendations, accepted internationally, are specific with regards to measures to prevent and control the spread of infection through identified routes of transmission, slight variations may occur due to local situations and facilities.

Table 16.5 shows examples of infectious diseases, their means of spread and precautions to be employed.

For further information, see Garner (1996).

How to set up and maintain isolation for MRSA

(see Fig. 16.5 and Box 16.6)

Appropriate equipment for effective isolation care in single side-rooms must be provided at the door to the room, i.e. gloves, aprons and other PPE, alcohol hand products and waste disposal receptacles. When isolation facilities are limited or not available, patients with the same infectious disease should be cohorted following a risk management approach. This practice is sometimes necessary within health care settings to contain a specific infection, for example when numerous patients are infected with norovirus and there are not enough single rooms. During and following isolation of a patient, cleaning of their environment often causes anxiety among those involved in this process. Keeping such areas — whether at home, in hospital or in care homes — clutter free is essential, so that cleaning can be carried out efficiently. Thorough terminal cleaning of all areas, including soft furnishings, e.g. curtains, may be required, following local policies and procedures or a risk assessment, usually aided by the infection control team. Specific cleaning equipment must be dedicated to isolation rooms/areas and not used for other areas. Linen and waste are often 'double-bagged' to avoid any further contamination when they are removed and linen should be sent to laundries in water soluble bags.

Anxiety again can occur over delivery of meals and care of utensils and crockery when patients are known to have specific infections and reassurance and guidance will be needed. Guidance states that patients should be treated the same whatever the infection and that adherence to SICPs and appropriate additional measures should generally be adequate. Risk assessments may be carried out by infection control teams in some circumstances and specific guidance given if required. Visitors, whether they be other health or social care workers or relatives or friends, including children, can be as anxious as the patients they are visiting in isolation or at home with a specific infection. They must be advised about appropriate contact with the patient and their environment and good hygiene in order to avoid becoming contaminated during visits and to ensure cross-infection does not occur. Often infection control teams will provide staff with supporting information and guidance, including information for children.

Where patients with airborne infections such as pulmonary TB are being cared for, it is recommended that they are placed in a negative-pressure isolation room which has the necessary ventilation to aid the prevention of spread. The converse is a positive-pressure ventilation room which is used when trying to protect immunosuppressed patients from circulating air which may harm them in their compromised state, e.g. those who are neutropenic.

Aseptic and clean techniques

Aseptic and clean techniques can prevent the entry of microorganisms into susceptible sites, for example surgical sites and insertion sites of invasive devices.

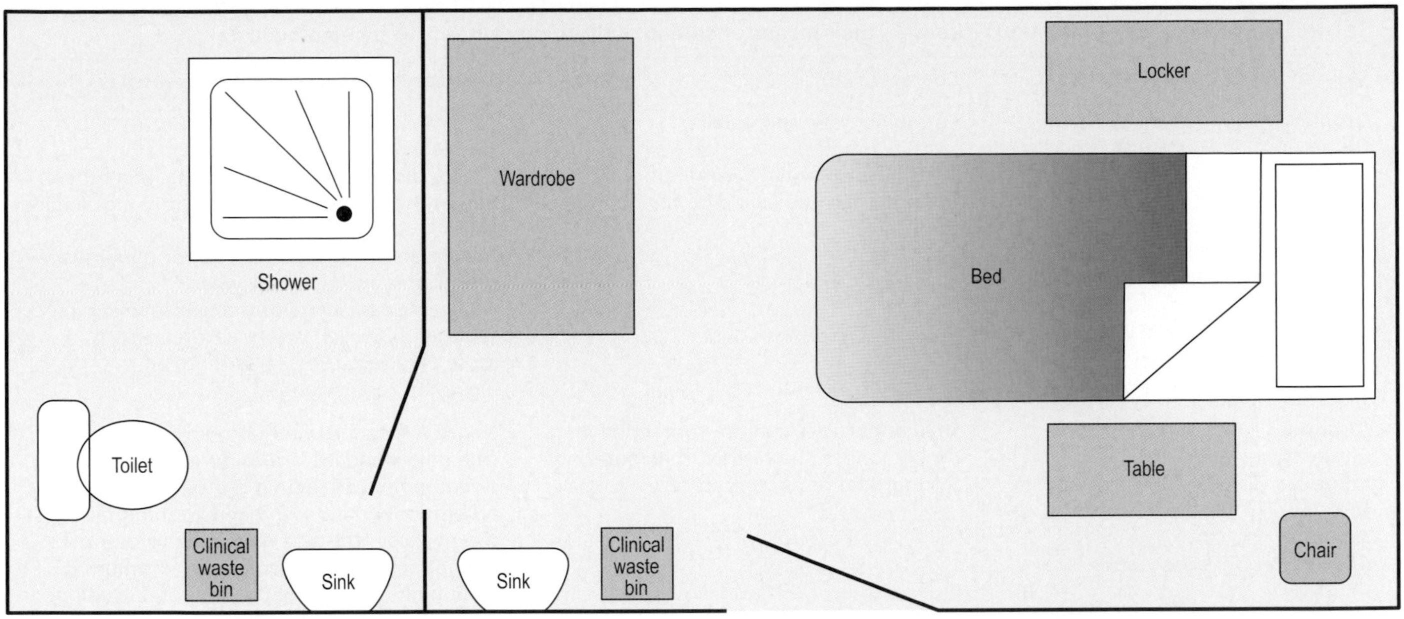

Fig. 16.5 Accommodating a patient with MRSA — room, equipment and appropriate arrangement. (See also Box 16.6.)

Box 16.6

Accommodating a patient with MRSA

Single room with closable door and attached bathroom

- Minimal belongings and equipment in the room
- Handbasin with liquid soap and alcohol rub/gel and disposable hand towels both inside and outside the room door
- Aprons and gloves available outside the door
- Foot-operated clinical waste bin next to the sink, in the cubicle by the door
- Table/trolley on the door-side of the bed, kept clean and clutter-free
- Own vital signs machine or blood pressure cuff and thermometer if possible
- Red water soluble linen bags outside the door
- Sign on the door making it clear to adopt contact precautions (see p. 670). NB: Also recorded on report sheet and reiterated at the nursing handover report
- Sign on the door advising visitors to ask a nurse before entering
- Advice from nurse re MRSA, gloves, aprons and hand washing, given without breaching confidentiality or causing anxiety to those who do not understand such infections

Bathroom

- Own washbasin
- Soap, alcohol rub/gel and disposable hand towels available
- Gloves and aprons available
- Foot-operated clinical waste bin

Informing the patient

- Advise the patient about MRSA and why they are being isolated; provide reassurance and ensure they understand
- Explain they can still have visitors and that they also will receive advice
- Make sure the patient understands any treatments for MRSA, e.g. nasal cream, and the importance of adhering to the regimen
- Information leaflets should be used

Actions when nursing the patient

Before entering

- Collect all necessary equipment
- Wash and dry hands, put on gloves and apron
- Open the door using outside handle

Whilst in the room

- Make sure only gloves and apron surface make contact with the patient or the environment

Leaving the room

- Open the door with inside handle. As you reverse out and before exiting, remove apron first, then gloves and put them in the clinical waste bin within the cubicle, using the foot pedal
- Leave without touching anything further
- Close door with outside handle
- Decontaminate hands

NB

- If any equipment has been brought out of the cubicle it must be washed/wiped appropriately immediately
- If the general ward's observation equipment is being used for this patient, their observations should be done last and the equipment always cleaned after it has been used
- Catering staff must be advised as to appropriate measures when delivering meals

With thanks to Hannah O'Regan, Student Nurse, University of Edinburgh for her contribution to Fig. 16.5, and Box 16.6.

Table 16.5 Examples of infectious diseases, their means of spread and the precautions to be employed

Main mode of transmission	Characteristics	Summary of main prevention measures
Droplet Diphtheria Influenza virus *Legionella* Meningococcal disease MRSA (occasionally) Respiratory syncytial virus Rotavirus Small round structured virus *Streptococcus pyogenes*	Coughing, sneezing, talking (within 1 metre) Splashing, potential aerosolisation during procedure (could be further than 3 feet)	Surgical mask for patients and health care workers Ensure distance between patients and others and utilise barriers to facilitate this, e.g. single room Remember importance of PPE for patient care procedures, including eyewear *NB* eyeglasses can be protective against direct splashes; however, where aerosol occurs, more extensive eyewear is required, e.g. wrap-round goggles
Airborne Chickenpox (varicella) Influenza virus Measles Smallpox *Mycobacterium tuberculosis*	Smaller particles that are suspended in the air longer and further, then entering through the respiratory tract	Negative pressure ventilation rooms (the gold standard is considered to be a single room, with adjoining toilet and anteroom with its own hand washing facilities) Use of respirator-type devices (surgical masks are not considered adequate) and other PPE Limit high-risk aerosol procedures, including avoidance of nebuliser use
Contact Chickenpox (varicella) Food poisoning, e.g. *Salmonella, Campylobacter* Hepatitis A Influenza virus MRSA Poliomyelitis Rotavirus Shingles (varicella) Small round structured virus *Streptococcus pyogenes* Vancomycin-resistant *Enterococcus*	Hands as the main vehicle of transmission Environmental contamination is also common	Utilisation of barriers to prevent spread, e.g use of single rooms Hand hygiene critical Frequent environmental decontamination (as per local policies) Remember importance of PPE for patient care procedures

PPE, personal protective equipment.

Aseptic technique

Asepsis involves ensuring that:

- all equipment used is sterile
- the setting, e.g. the dressing trolley, is prepared by washing it with detergent and water and drying it. A disinfectant wipe with 70% alcohol is then recommended for the surface
- SICPs are adopted by personnel involved
- the patient is prepared for the procedure. Skin cleansing is a major factor in the prevention of infection and up-to-date guidance on this should be available within local policies
- items are disposed of or reprocessed appropriately following the procedure
- appropriate documentation is completed to describe the procedure and any findings.

Aseptic technique should be employed for:

- wounds healing by primary intention, e.g. surgical incisions, fresh breaks in the skin or burns
- insertion of cardiovascular invasive devices, e.g. central venous catheters, peripheral venous catheters
- insertion of indwelling urinary catheters
- percutaneous endoscopic gastrostomy and jejunostomy tubes
- tracheostomy tubes and chest drains
- vaginal examination using instruments.

Clean technique

This is a modified aseptic technique that can be employed when managing certain wounds healing by secondary intention, for example chronic leg ulcers, which are often heavily colonised with microorganisms in the first instance. Avoiding the unnecessary entry of other microorganisms into the site is still essential, although on certain occasions sterile equipment such as gloves may not be necessary; clean gloves may be adequate. A non-touch technique is vital to ensure that no non-sterile items come into contact with the site. A risk management approach will determine the appropriateness of adopting a clean as opposed to an aseptic technique. Liaison with the infection control team or other nurse specialists, for example tissue viability nurses, before proceeding may be advisable.

Dressings also prevent invasion of microorganisms in susceptible sites, as does appropriate maintenance and care of invasive lines and tubes. Dressings should keep a wound or insertion site free from potential contamination and infection and be impermeable to bacteria. Dressings used on wounds where slough or necrotic tissue is present should minimise or remove this dead tissue (see Ch. 23).

Guidelines for care: key areas of concern in relation to HAI

Evidence-based or best practice guidelines, derived from systematic or critical reviews, are a fundamental part of nursing care. Guidelines often focus on the highest risk areas, such as intensive care units, burns units and long-term care homes, as well as on specific priority diseases such as MRSA. If clear guidance is not available, a common-sense approach is important, for example continuing to provide high quality standards of care until further, more specific evidence is available.

High-risk procedures have become a focus for the production of guidelines, applicable in all settings. HAI can be prevented by managing high-risk procedures appropriately. A review (Harbarth et al 2003) suggests that emphasis should be placed on key areas with HAI reduction potential (see Table 16.6).

The prevention of urinary tract infections

Urinary tract infections are known to account for approximately 30–40% of all HAIs and are considered the most common.

For further information, see Chapter 8 (this volume) and Department of Health/Hospital Infection Society (2001a,b).

The prevention of surgical site infections

For further information, see Chapters 23 and 26 (this volume), Mangram et al (1999) and Dougherty & Lister (2004).

The prevention of cardiovascular line infections

Insertion of cardiovascular lines invades the epithelial barrier, which protects the skin from potential invasion. Bacteraemia (bacterial blood infection) caused by these devices contributes significantly to HAI.

Risks present from many sources while cardiovascular lines are in situ. These include:

- contamination of the device itself while it is being inserted or manipulated
- contamination of the dressing used to cover the device. Preferred dressings are semi-permeable polyurethane, which allows visual inspection and prevents unnecessary disturbance, e.g. it can be left in place for bathing, and minimises the risk of bacteria at the invasive site
- microorganisms present in stopcocks, extension sets, taps, filters — these adjuncts should be used only where appropriate and the use of stopcocks and taps in particular should be avoided
- contamination during attachment of administration sets, and any of the above adjuncts, to the device and/or to the infusion container
- contamination of additives to infusion fluids
- contamination that may present in pre-packaged infusion fluids, administration equipment, or even infusion devices or dressings themselves.

Patients who require a cardiovascular device are often already compromised in their health, which is a risk factor. The use of multilumen catheters, the type of catheter and the insertion site are also risk areas. For example, insertion of lines into the internal jugular vein or the femoral artery poses a higher risk due to their position near a hair line and in the groin, which are ideal environments for bacterial growth. Disturbance of devices and their attachments must be kept to a minimum and they should be replaced at optimum times.

For further information, see Department of Health/Hospital Infection Society (2001c).

The prevention of respiratory tract infections, particularly those associated with artificial adjuncts

Reducing the incidence of HAI pneumonia within health care settings is also being considered. The use of devices to facilitate artificial breathing and support respiratory distress is a key factor in the potential for HAI. Areas for consideration, particularly related to nursing care, include:

- care and dressing of insertion sites such as tracheostomies and chest drain tubes
- the correct technique for suctioning of respiratory secretions
- the correct use and care of nebulisers when administering saline or water for loosening secretions, or medications (see Box 16.7)
- humidification systems
- artificial respirator bags
- intubation with endotracheal tubes — some nurses trained and competent in advanced life support may insert endotracheal tubes

Table 16.6 The preventable potential for key HAI areas

HAI type	Reduction potential (%)	Setting details
Catheter-associated urinary tract infections	46–60	All specialties
Surgical site infections	24–34	Surgical specialties
Central venous catheters associated with bloodstream infection	14–71	70% neonatals 56% adult critical care
Ventilator assisted pneumonias	38–70	Intensive care units

Box 16.7

The use of nebulisers and associated risks

A newspaper article revealed that a patient had acquired *Legionella* following a hospital stay. Following investigation of the source of this infection, an alert was distributed from the Medicines and Healthcare Products Regulatory Agency in England and Wales and Scottish Healthcare Supplies in Scotland, stating the importance of the care of nebulisers, in particular cleaning them after use. Manufacturers' instructions should be followed and recent reviews have highlighted sufficient evidence to recommend cleaning them with sterile water rather than tap water to avoid contamination from microorganisms such as *Legionella*. *Legionella* can cause disease in humans following inhalation from contaminated water vapour. If water sources are adequately treated and managed for home and health care setting consumption, *Legionella* should be avoided. Immediate drying and storage of nebulisers are equally as important so that they do not become a source of infection between uses on the same patient; nebulisers are considered single-patient use items.

- breathing circuit tubing
- anaesthetic machine tubing and connections.

All the above points must be considered in the community setting, although the focus for infection rate reduction programmes is frequently on acute settings.

For further information, see Chapters 3, 13 and 29 (this volume), Tablan et al (2003) and www.devices.mhra.gov.uk.

A common feature of all guidelines is the use of antiseptics to prepare sites prior to insertion of devices or breaches in the skin (see Box 16.8).

Box 16.8

The use of antiseptics

- The use of antiseptics is often debated, particularly in relation to wound care and preoperative skin preparation. Many studies have shown the benefits of using them appropriately
- Like antibiotics, not all antiseptics will kill or inhibit all microorganisms
- Resistance to antiseptics may occur as it has with antibiotics
- Antiseptics, whether in fluid, lotion, cream or dressing format, should be used after a risk assessment; misuse must be prevented as, like any medicine, they can have adverse effects
- Patients can have allergies to certain antiseptics or contraindications to their use, for example povidone–iodine
- 'Topping-up' of bottles that contain fluids or lotions, such as antiseptic solutions, rather than disposing of the used bottle and replacing it completely, can allow microorganisms to build up within the solution, which can be a source of infection when used on the skin of health care workers or patients

Guidelines for the prevention of sexually transmitted infections and for the prevention of gastrointestinal infections, including the introduction of feeding systems such as nasogastric tubes, are also important and available.

Transition from home to hospital and hospital to home

Effective communication between staff working within primary and acute care settings is vital if infections that might be introduced to the home from hospital or to the hospital from home are to be prevented, controlled and managed appropriately. Nurses should liaise between settings, disciplines and agencies to influence and inform decision making in relation to infection control. Whether working in the NHS, in education as a school nurse or lecturer, in the prison service, general practices, independent hospitals or care homes, or with commercial companies providing health care products, nurses must consider ways in which the potential for infection can be managed across the spectrum of health care services. Communication in all its forms is core to this.

STOP THINK **16.4** Discuss with a community nurse how the control of infection can be achieved in the patient's home, e.g. hand hygiene, use of protective clothing, aseptic techniques and disinfection of equipment.

INFECTIOUS DISEASES

'Infectious' (or 'communicable') diseases are illnesses caused by microorganisms which are not normally present in or on the body, such as salmonellosis, hepatitis B and tuberculosis. Such infections contrast markedly with those which are acquired as a result of poor asepsis in invasive techniques or as a consequence of antibiotic therapy, immunosuppressive drugs or inadequate hand washing, normally thought to be HAI. Infectious diseases can be caught by anyone, at any time, in any place, and do not usually result from a particular nursing or medical procedure. This does not mean, however, that they cannot be spread from person to person; this presents a particular danger when patients with infectious disease are nursed in hospital.

Causes

Infectious diseases are generally caused by:

- bacteria, e.g. salmonellosis, meningococcal meningitis
- viruses, e.g. hepatitis, chickenpox
- protozoa, e.g. malaria, toxoplasmosis, amoebic dysentery.

Knowledge of the organism that is causing the disease is important in the planning of care.

Transmission

Most infectious diseases are ingested (e.g. hepatitis A), inhaled (e.g. tuberculosis) or inoculated (e.g. hepatitis B). Inoculation in this context refers to blood or body fluid entering a cut or skin abrasion or being splashed onto mucous membranes; it can also occur following needlestick injury. The organisms can be transmitted directly, i.e. straight from one person to another through direct contact with the infectious body substance, or indirectly, i.e. deposited on hands or surfaces where they can be picked up by touch.

Some infectious diseases are so common in the population that only general care is needed. Many people suffer from cold sores (herpes simplex), but the common-sense precautions of avoiding mucous membrane contact until the sores have healed, careful handwashing and washing of cutlery and cups, and not sharing toothbrushes, razors or face cloths are usually enough to prevent transmission.

Diseases such as chickenpox are so common and so easily transmitted through inhalation, particularly in children, that special precautions to prevent their spread in the community are rarely necessary, although these may need to be enforced in settings such as hospitals where there are particularly susceptible individuals. Other common diseases are prevent-able by an active immunisation programme; for example, immunisation against diphtheria, pertussis (whooping cough) and tetanus; poliomyelitis; measles, mumps and rubella and *Haemophilus influenzae* type B is now offered for all infants. It is still advisable, however, for pregnant women because of the risk of damage to and/or infection in the fetus during pregnancy, and for people who are immunosuppressed to keep away from anyone known to have an infectious disease.

Immunity to infectious diseases

Immunisation against many diseases is carried out during childhood, with booster doses being required only in later life. A booster dose is a smaller dose of a vaccine which boosts the level of memory cells, specific to the given antigen, circulating in the bloodstream (see Fig. 16.2).

Nurses and health visitors have an important role to play in encouraging parents to have their children vaccinated. Vaccination should be carried out by staff that are aware of the risks and the benefits. Some parents are afraid that their child might develop an adverse reaction to a vaccine; however, this is an uncommon occurrence and few of the children so affected have developed serious complications. In the late 1970s in England and Wales, the percentage of infants vaccinated against whooping cough fell dramatically due to public concern about vaccine-damaged children, although such cases were very rare. There was a concurrent rise in the number of whooping cough cases reported, a proportion of whom had serious systemic complications.

STOP THINK **16.5** Identify recent trends for vaccination uptake for measles, mumps and rubella.

SALMONELLOSIS

PATHOPHYSIOLOGY

Salmonellosis is caused by one of about 200 serotypes of the genus *Salmonella* which cause disease in humans and animals (Payne 2000). Only a few of these are commonly encountered in the UK. The organism is ingested; common sources are contaminated meat and poultry products and untreated milk. The incubation period is 12–72 h (Heymann 2004). Some salmonellae, e.g. *S. typhi* and *S. paratyphi*, can cause enteric fever.

Common presenting symptoms

are highly variable, ranging from mild symptoms to life-threatening septicaemia. Normally, the effects of infection are acute enterocolitis with diarrhoea, blood in the stools, abdominal pain and nausea; less frequently, they include vomiting, fever, headache and toxaemia. Rarely, arthritis, cholecystitis, endocarditis, pyelonephritis, acute renal failure, meningitis or pneumonia occur.

MEDICAL MANAGEMENT

Investigations

Diagnostic investigation includes stool bacterial culture while diarrhoea persists. If enteric fever, septicaemia or a focal infection is suspected, blood cultures during the acute stage of the illness are done. Serological tests are of little value except in the detection of a 'carrier'.

Treatment

Rehydration and electrolyte replacement may be necessary in the treatment of severe enterocolitis. Antibiotics are not generally given in uncomplicated intestinal infection as they tend to prolong the excretion of the organism. They are given if the disease is severe with evidence of systemic spread and/or a vulnerable patient, e.g. a frail or older person. Antibiotics are absolutely indicated in enteric fever caused by *S. typhi* and *S. paratyphi*. Ciprofloxacin is exceedingly active and is the drug of choice in all cases of salmonellosis and enteric fever. It is not licensed, however, for use in pregnancy or in those under 18 years of age. Chloramphenicol is a useful alternative, although it can be associated with side-effects such as severe haematological disorders.

NURSING PRIORITIES AND MANAGEMENT: Salmonellosis

Many people with salmonellosis become ill at home, often after eating an undercooked meal or after eating infected poultry. Eggs may also be contaminated. Most people will wait to see if the symptoms subside before contacting their GP, but if a particular item of food is suspect they may seek help earlier.

Institutional outbreaks can and do occur and are usually a result of defects in food hygiene, either at kitchen or at ward level. Cross-infection in the ward can occur, either directly from a patient with salmonellosis to another person, or via nurses' hands if hygiene is poor. However, the exact cause of such outbreaks is not always identified.

The nurse is unlikely to be involved in caring for a patient at home with acute salmonellosis, unless there are concurrent problems. The community nurse or health visitor may be involved in helping to obtain faecal specimens from other members of the family and in trying to trace the source of infection, in conjunction with, in England and Wales, the Environmental Health Officer and the Consultant in Communicable Disease Control (CCDC) and, in Scotland, with the Consultant in Public Health Medicine (CPHM Communicable Diseases and Environmental Health). Such visits are an excellent opportunity for health education in general and about food hygiene as part of a planned programme which takes into account family needs. SICPs must be applied and patients should be advised that the prescribed course of antibiotics must be completed.

Life-threatening concerns

Those that may arise are septicaemia, focal sepsis, severe fluid and electrolyte imbalance, dehydration and acute renal failure.

Major patient problems

These include skin excoriation from severe diarrhoea, fever, abdominal pain, nausea, loss of appetite and weakness because of constant diarrhoea.

Further considerations

Specific ongoing nursing care

Ongoing care comprises the following aspects:

- Preventing the spread of infection through the adoption of SICPs and provision of guidance about hand washing. Care with faeces will be needed in hospital and in the home, with particular attention paid to surfaces which may be contaminated; regular cleaning regimens should be in place. Contact precautions may also be applied in health care settings.
- In hospital, designating one nurse on each shift to look after the patient. It is important for nurses to spend time with the patient giving information and reassurance about isolation procedures to counteract the loneliness of isolation.
- Ensuring that fluid intake is adequate (see Ch. 20).
- Ensuring that nutrition is adequate (see Ch. 21), while trying to accommodate the patient's wishes; this can be difficult in hospital, where there is central catering and where meals are delivered at specific times.
- Keeping the anal region clean and dry and applying a 'for use by this patient only' barrier cream to prevent excoriation.
- Ensuring that the patient can get to the toilet or has a commode at the bedside and has the opportunity to wash their hands afterwards.
- Trying to ensure privacy as far as possible.
- Being sensitive to any odour problem; discussing this with the patient might help.
- Encouraging visitors to visit at different times of the day and providing guidance about hand washing.
- Identifying key carers at home and providing guidance about infection control.
- Encouraging self-care and independence.

HEPATITIS B

Hepatitis B is a viral infection which is transmitted from mother to child mostly at birth, sexually, by blood contact, especially injecting drug users (see Chs 36 and 37) and needlestick injury. It is endemic in some parts of the world. The virus, HBV, has been found in most body secretions and excretions, but only blood, saliva, semen and vaginal secretions have been shown to be infectious (Heymann 2004). Hepatitis B was formerly seen in people who had received blood and blood products and in people who had been given injections with contaminated needles. These risks have largely been eliminated in the developed countries by the screening of blood donors, the testing of donor blood and the single use of sterile syringes and needles. The main risk to health care workers is that of inoculation with infected blood, either through needlestick injury with a contaminated needle or by being splashed with infected blood on skin abrasions or mucous membranes.

PATHOPHYSIOLOGY

The virus is made up of several components, each of which is capable of inducing an immune response. HBsAg (hepatitis B surface antigen) is the first antigen to appear in the blood after infection. The presence of anti-HBs antibodies in the blood is the best measure of immunity to the virus.

Acute hepatitis B may have one of four outcomes:

- complete recovery
- fulminant hepatitis — rare but frequently fatal
- carrier state — HBsAg-positive
- chronic hepatitis — may lead to cirrhosis of the liver and to hepatocellular carcinoma (see Ch. 4).

Some people become infected with the hepatitis B virus without developing the acute disease. This is known as subclinical infection and such individuals are more likely to develop the carrier state. These individuals may be unaware of the infection and of their potential for transmitting the virus to others.

The incubation period for hepatitis B is 45–180 days (Heymann 2004). Onset is insidious.

Common presenting symptoms
are highly variable, ranging from unapparent infection or malaise, with abnormal liver function tests, to cases of fatal acute hepatic necrosis. Normally, anorexia, nausea, vomiting, abdominal discomfort and fever occur, followed perhaps by arthralgia, urticaria or glomerulonephritis caused by antigen–antibody complexes, progressing to jaundice.

MEDICAL MANAGEMENT

Investigations
are serological. HBsAg is indicative of infection and infectivity and occurs both before and during the acute illness. This finding must be interpreted with caution, however, as HBsAg may still be present in carriers and the chronically infected who have become jaundiced from some other cause. Carriers are of high infectivity when HBeAg is present (a marker of replication in the liver) and of low infectivity when anti-HBeAg is present. HBV DNA is a more sophisticated measure of replication, infectivity and the progression to chronic liver disease. IgM anti-HBc is an antibody to the 'c' or 'core' antigen which may be present during the diagnostically difficult 'window' when HBsAg and anti-HBs are in equivalence and neither is detectable in the serum. Serial estimation of these, other antigens/antibodies, other viruses such as hepatitis D and the liver

enzymes may be necessary to establish the stage and progression of the disease.

Treatment

There is no effective treatment for the acute disease. Bed rest is not of proven value. Chronic hepatitis B may be treated by immunosuppression with a tapering course of corticosteroids such as prednisolone for 6 weeks, but now recombinant interferon or interleukin-2 is favoured. Liver transplantation, however, may still be the last recourse for a patient with advancing chronic disease.

Effective vaccines are available and are recommended for health care personnel working with patients, particularly high-risk patients, and those in contact with blood, particularly when handling sharp instruments. Prophylaxis (vaccination and/or specific immunoglobulin) is also given after inoculation accidents and other significant exposure accidents and to sexual contacts of HbsAg-positive persons as well as to infants born to HbsAg-positive mothers.

Some health care staff, e.g. surgeons and midwives, are required to demonstrate their immunity to hepatitis B virus before they are allowed to perform 'exposure-prone procedures' (EPP) where their gloved hands may be in contact with sharp objects such as needles, instruments or spicules of bone, inside a body cavity or wound and where their hands are not always completely visible.

For up-to-date information on immunisation against infectious disease, see the most recent version of The Green Book published by the Department of Health (www.dh.gov.uk/publicationsandstatistics).

NURSING PRIORITIES AND MANAGEMENT: Hepatitis B

Since there is no treatment for acute hepatitis B, nursing priorities are to alleviate symptoms and to support the patient until the disease has run its course. People with acute hepatitis B may stay at home, requiring admission to hospital only when they are too ill to be looked after at home or when they require specific medical intervention (Chislett 2003, Christopher 2003). SICPs must be applied.

Life-threatening concerns

Fulminant hepatitis will lead to gross liver failure and all of the associated problems (see Ch. 4).

Major patient problems

These include lethargy, weakness, nausea, vomiting and anxiety about transmission.

Further considerations

Specific ongoing care

This includes the following interventions:

- preventing the spread of infection through the adoption of SICPs
- encouraging the patient to rest; lethargy and weakness are often the first symptoms to arise and the last to go away
- ensuring that fluid intake is adequate (see Ch. 20)
- accurate recording of fluid balance
- ensuring that nutrition is adequate (see Ch. 21)
- providing skin care and regular change of position
- ensuring that the patient can get to the toilet or has a commode at the bedside
- ensuring that the patient does not share razors and toothbrushes with others
- designating one nurse per shift to look after the patient in hospital; loneliness and dejection can be minimised by ensuring that time is taken to talk with the patient and to discuss their needs — access to a telephone, television and other diversions may be important
- encouraging relatives and friends to be flexible about their visiting times
- encouraging self-care and independence.

PULMONARY TUBERCULOSIS

Pulmonary tuberculosis is now the most common form of tuberculosis infection, although other systems are sometimes affected, e.g. the genitourinary or skeletal systems. It is more common in immigrants from countries which have a higher prevalence of tuberculosis than the UK (Baker 2001). This disease is notifiable in the UK.

PATHOPHYSIOLOGY

Pulmonary tuberculosis is a bacterial infection caused by *Mycobacterium tuberculosis*, also known as the tubercle bacillus. The bacteria enter the body by being inhaled; once they reach the epithelial surface of the alveolus, they cause swelling of the epithelial cells and local capillary dilatation. Although some organisms will be engulfed by alveolar macrophages (see p. 655), they will not be destroyed and will continue to multiply; some will escape and may enter the bloodstream, with the potential to infect any other organ in the body (miliary TB). Lymph nodes are often infected.

Invasion of the lung tissue gives rise to an inflammatory reaction in which the infected alveoli fill with fluid, macrophages and bacteria. The resultant lung damage eventually leads to fibrosis, which will be visible on a chest X-ray. The primary lesion in the lung is often asymptomatic and confined to one area. Healing of the lung tissue occurs, sometimes leaving an area of calcification.

The patient becomes Mantoux-positive 4–6 weeks after primary infection and also following immunisation, i.e. they will develop a hypersensitivity reaction to an injection of tuberculin. A chronic cough with bloodstained mucopurulent sputum develops as the disease becomes more advanced.

Dormant bacilli may be reactivated by an alteration in immunity resulting from advancing age, malnutrition or other diseases. People with HIV (see Ch. 37) are prone to developing tuberculosis. People with pulmonary tuberculosis are considered to be infectious until they have had 2 weeks of appropriate medication.

Common presenting symptoms

Normally the initial infection is unapparent. Pulmonary disease is characterised by cough, fever, fatigue and weight loss, and less frequently by haemoptysis, chest pain or erythema nodosum. Extrapulmonary disease is less common but can involve most organs of the body, causing, for example, meningitis, lymphadenitis, pericarditis, pleurisy, nephritis, cystitis, osteomyelitis, arthritis, laryngitis or peritonitis.

MEDICAL MANAGEMENT

Investigations

Diagnostic investigation includes chest X-ray, often with tomograms and CT scans. Microscopy and culture of sputum, gastric washings, urine, CSF, aspirate or biopsy material are performed as appropriate. Histology of biopsy material is undertaken. Skin testing with tuberculin may be performed, especially in the young.

Treatment

Normally, pulmonary tuberculosis is initially treated with a combination of isoniazid, rifampicin, ethambutol and pyrazinamide to avoid emergence of bacterial resistance. If the isolate is shown to be sensitive, one or two of the medications may be discontinued after 2 months. Other antibiotics may be used when resistance is present or likely to be a problem, and particularly in patients from abroad. Ethambutol is not normally given to patients under 5 years of age or to very old people. Therapy continues for at least 6 months.

NURSING PRIORITIES AND MANAGEMENT: Pulmonary tuberculosis

The main aims in nursing patients with pulmonary tuberculosis are to establish medication and to encourage adherence to the treatment regimen. The underlying health of these patients may not be good and their nutritional status is often poor. The prospect of having to take a large number of tablets regularly over a long period of time is daunting and the side-effects of some medications mean that some people stop taking them. A great deal of support and encouragement will be needed.

Once a person is diagnosed as having pulmonary tuberculosis, it is important that they are kept away from anyone who is immunosuppressed until no longer infectious. Contacts may require follow-up; in the case of staff, this is done by the occupational health department. Non-staff contacts such as family members can be referred to a TB liaison nurse or a chest physician.

A sputum specimen sent to bacteriology will be examined directly under the microscope for the presence of tubercle bacilli. If these bacilli are seen, the report will state 'AAFB (acid alcohol fast bacilli) seen on direct film', 'film positive', 'smear positive' or 'ZN (Ziehl–Neelsen) positive', and the patient will be considered to have 'open' pulmonary tuberculosis. This means that there are enough bacilli in the sputum for them to be seen easily in a small sample, and therefore that the sputum is infectious to others. Culture of the organism may take 6–8 weeks and is necessary to make a firm diagnosis; there are mycobacteria other than *M. tuberculosis*. Infectivity also depends on whether or not the person is 'productive'; a person who is highly productive of sputum and is film-positive is much more likely to infect others than someone who is film-positive and not coughing up any sputum at all (King 2001, Negus et al 2004).

Life-threatening concerns

Respiratory failure may develop if the patient is too weak to cough. Tuberculosis in people who are immunocompromised, such as those with HIV, can result in serious illness.

Major patient problems

These include difficulty in maintaining the medication regimen and in learning how to prevent the spread of droplet infection when coughing.

Further considerations

Specific ongoing care

Nursing care and physiotherapy for people with pulmonary tuberculosis are similar to those for patients with any other respiratory infection (see Ch. 3). The dietitian may be asked to advise on appropriate diet.

The risk of spreading the infection to others is greatly reduced when the person remains at home, in which case care with sputum is usually all that is necessary. Isolation precautions are required for patients with pulmonary tuberculosis in hospital. Recent advice from the British Thoracic Society (see 'Useful websites') recommends that the patient who is smear-positive should be segregated in a single room, preferably with negative pressure, as such patients are infectious. Because of this, in addition to SICPs, airborne precautions should be taken, e.g. wearing a specific type of mask as respiratory protection when caring for the patient. Masks should be carefully removed and discarded, and the hands washed afterwards.

Staff who have been in close respiratory contact with patients with open pulmonary tuberculosis may be screened by Mantoux and Heaf tests and, if necessary, by chest X-ray. Other staff contacts may receive TB contact cards.

Patients are sometimes found to have pulmonary tuberculosis when they are being investigated in hospital for chest disease. Other patients who have been cared for in the same area may be notified through their GP or the TB liaison nurse.

There may be difficulties in explaining the importance of medication, particularly if English is not the patient's first language. Tracing and follow-up of contacts of people with pulmonary tuberculosis is important. Those relatives and friends of the patient who have been in close respiratory contact are generally referred to an infectious diseases physician for examination and follow-up. The British Thoracic Society recommends that there should be trained tuberculosis health visitors or nurses to provide support in implementing policies for screening, follow-up and contact tracing (Oxtoby 2003).

STOP THINK **16.6** Miss A is a 78-year-old woman who has lived alone since her sister's death a year ago. Recently, she lost her appetite and developed a persistent cough. A sputum specimen was taken and open pulmonary tuberculosis diagnosed. Normally a pleasant, cooperative person, Miss A was grumpy and resentful when the nurse visited her at home, and there were soiled tissues strewn all over the bed and floor. Devise a care plan to prevent the spread of infection from sputum and saliva.

MENINGOCOCCAL INFECTION

Infections caused by a Gram-negative bacterium, *Neisseria meningitidis*, are commonly known as meningococcal infections. There are five common serotypes: A, B, C, W-135 and Y. In the UK, vaccination against meningococcal serogroup C is recommended and available for all under 25 years. Meningococcal disease is an important medical emergency demanding early diagnosis and prompt treatment (Boyne 2001). Meningitis may also be of viral origin, usually presenting in a less severe form.

PATHOPHYSIOLOGY

The organism is frequently inhaled and carried in the nasopharynx. More rarely, it then enters the bloodstream, giving rise to meningitis and/or septicaemia. Meningococcal group B is the most common cause of bacterial meningitis in the UK (Haslett et al 2002).

Common presenting symptoms

are highly variable. Early recognition is essential. Meningitis may present with severe headache, neck stiffness, photophobia, fever, vomiting, drowsiness and non-blanching rash. Seizures may also be seen. Septicaemia may present with a non-blanching rash, fever, vomiting, cold hands and feet, shivering, rapid or unusual breathing, stomach/joint pains and drowsiness. Late signs of septicaemia in meningitis are impaired consciousness, hypertension, cyanosis and raised intracranial pressure. Fulminating cases may present with sudden shock, extensive purpura and disseminated intravascular coagulation (see Ch. 18). Delirium and coma may supervene.

MEDICAL MANAGEMENT

Investigations

Blood, CSF (if the patient is stable) and pharyngeal swab samples should be taken, in addition to aspirates from other sterile sites, if appropriate. Molecular methods of polymerase chain reaction (PCR) testing are becoming increasingly important.

Treatment

The medication of choice in the treatment of meningococcal infections in the UK is benzyl penicillin, given in high dosage parenterally, commenced as soon as the diagnosis is suspected. If the bacteriological diagnosis cannot be established with certainty, or when there is allergy to penicillin, then broad-spectrum treatment is often given to cover other bacterial pathogens; this usually consists of a high-dose injectable cephalosporin such as cefotaxime. Close household and respiratory secretions/salivary contacts are given a short course of rifampicin or ciprofloxacin to eradicate nasopharyngeal carriage. This is also given to the index case, as penicillin does not eradicate carriage. MenC vaccine should be offered to all cases and unimmunised close contacts where serotype group C is confirmed. Vaccines can also be offered for close contacts of cases with A, W-135 and Y cases. SICPs and droplet/contact precautions apply.

NURSING PRIORITIES AND MANAGEMENT: Meningococcal infection

Life-threatening concerns

The meningococcus bacteria invade the bloodstream and endotoxins initiate the release of a complex cascade of chemical mediators which may lead to the manifestations of septic shock — hypotension, hypovolaemia, vasodilatation and severe capillary leak and metabolic acidosis. This leads ultimately to multiorgan failure and, if all life support interventions fail, death (see Ch. 18).

STOP THINK **16.7** The initial flu-like symptoms of meningococcal meningitis can quickly progress to septicaemia, even when detected early. What are the clinical indicators that would alert you to this potentially mortal progression? What is the pathophysiological significance of the haemorrhagic rash that develops in some, but not all, cases of meningitis?

Major patient problems

Meningeal irritation may result in neck stiffness. Vomiting and sweating may lead to dehydration and electrolyte imbalance (see Ch. 20).

For further useful information, see the Meningitis Research Foundation and the Meningitis Trust (see 'Useful websites').

CHICKENPOX AND SHINGLES

Chickenpox and shingles are caused by the same virus, known as the varicella zoster virus (VZV). Primary infection causes chickenpox (varicella), and most people have chickenpox only once, since infection usually confers lifelong immunity. The virus remains latent, however, and recurrence in a different form — shingles (herpes zoster) — can occur months or many years after the initial infection and on more than one occasion.

Chickenpox is highly infectious, from both respiratory droplets and skin lesions. Although common in children, susceptible adults can also be infected, sometimes causing more complications. Disease is more severe and sometimes fatal in the immunocompromised, in unborn babies before 20 weeks' gestation and in neonates infected in the perinatal period. Shingles is usually seen in older people (50–80 years of age) and only the skin lesions are infectious. People can develop chickenpox after contact with someone suffering from shingles; but shingles cannot be contracted from a person suffering from chickenpox. This is because shingles occurs as a result of reactivation of the VZV, whereas primary infection results in chickenpox (which may be subclinical). Contact with chickenpox or shingles, in someone who is not already immune, can result in primary infection.

Vaccination against varicella is now recommended for all non-immune health care workers who have direct patient contact. This is to protect susceptible health care workers and also to protect vulnerable patients from acquiring chickenpox from an infected member of staff.

Chickenpox

PATHOPHYSIOLOGY

The incubation period of chickenpox is 2–3 weeks, commonly 14–16 days. A case is infectious for at most 5 days (usually only 1–2 days) before the onset of the rash and until all vesicles have crusted over, usually about 5 days after the last crop.

Common presenting symptoms

Initial symptoms are usually a slight fever and the development of a skin rash which is maculopapular at first, becomes vesicular and then forms a scab. The lesions do not all occur at the same time but in succession, so that on different parts of the body they may be at different stages. Areas of the body that are normally covered by clothing often have more lesions than exposed parts.

MEDICAL MANAGEMENT

Treatment

There is specific treatment for chickenpox with aciclovir but this is usually not recommended for uncomplicated disease. Antibiotics may be given for secondary infection of vesicles. Zoster immunoglobulin can be given to those at special risk (e.g. the immunocompromised) who have been in contact with the disease and have not had it themselves.

NURSING PRIORITIES AND MANAGEMENT: Chickenpox

Life-threatening concerns

Rarely, chickenpox can cause severe illness. The most common cause of death in adults with the disease is primary viral pneumonia, which is treated with parenteral antiviral agents. Children may develop septic complications or encephalitis. The disease can be severe or even fatal in the immunocompromised.

Major patient problems

The rash may cause irritation and discomfort, and secondary bacterial infection of lesions can occur.

Further considerations

Chickenpox is highly infectious, both from respiratory secretions and from skin discharges. Strict isolation, following airborne and contact precautions as well as SICPs will be required until the period of communicability is over. PPE must be worn for every entry to the room, the door must be kept closed and negative ventilation used if available. Decontamination of the room is also essential.

Shingles

PATHOPHYSIOLOGY

Common presenting symptoms

The first symptoms the person notices are often pain and paraesthesia in the affected area; this is usually the trunk but can be the face or a limb. A rash appears, starting with a macule on which vesicles develop over several days. The vesicles, which are a grey colour, dry up and crust over, usually in a week or so. The rash is characteristically restricted to the area supplied by the sensory nerves of one or an associated group of dorsal root ganglia. Subsequent healing may take several weeks, and residual or prolonged pain occurs in about 10% of cases.

MEDICAL MANAGEMENT

Treatment

involves administering analgesics, aciclovir and sometimes applying idoxuridine paint to the vesicles in the early stages. Early aciclovir treatment may prevent development of severe disease.

NURSING PRIORITIES AND MANAGEMENT: Shingles

Shingles can flare up spontaneously or may follow treatment for another disease, e.g. radiotherapy, where the patient is immunocompromised.

Major patient problems

Pain and discomfort may result from the lesions, which may persist for a long time. The patient may experience anxiety and depression if the condition fails to improve; this is especially common among older patients. A sympathetic and optimistic attitude can do a lot to make the symptoms more bearable (Williams 2002).

Further considerations

Care of the skin condition is similar to that for other skin disorders (see Ch. 12); it should be borne in mind that the lesions will be susceptible to secondary bacterial infection. SICPs must be applied.

If the person is in hospital, they should be kept apart from other vulnerable patients. Isolation precautions may be necessary until the lesions have crusted over, especially if lesions cannot be adequately covered to prevent contamination of outer clothing or bed linen. Only immune staff should nurse patients with shingles (see Box 16.9).

DISORDERS OF IMMUNITY

Four types of immunity disorder can be identified:

- immunodeficiency
- hypersensitivity
- autoimmune disease
- graft rejection after transplantation.

In this chapter, only the first three are addressed.

IMMUNODEFICIENCY

Immunodeficiency may be primary or secondary in nature.

Box 16.9

Staff contact with infectious diseases of childhood

The following questions should be posed in determining which staff members should provide nursing care for patients with diseases such as measles, mumps, rubella and chickenpox:

1. Are the staff members known to be immune (e.g. rubella antibody-positive) or have they been immunised? In the case of a disease that produces lasting immunity, have they had the disease themselves?
2. Are they working with susceptible patients, e.g. neonates, young children, the seriously ill or the immunosuppressed?

If the answer to '1' is 'yes', it is usually all right for the staff members to work as usual.

If the answer to '1' is 'no' and to '2' is 'yes', the staff members should be reassigned to a non-susceptible area until the incubation period is over.

In circumstances where there is any doubt, the control of infection or occupational health department should be consulted.

Primary immunodeficiency

Primary immunodeficiency states are very rare, but may arise under either of the following two conditions:

- there are not enough cells available
- the number of cells is adequate but they have a functional defect.

These problems will be discussed in relation to the cells and proteins involved, i.e. impairment of phagocytes, B lymphocytes or T lymphocytes.

STOP THINK **16.8** Recall the cells and proteins that are involved in the immune response.

Impairment of phagocytes

Phagocyte impairment may occur in the following forms:

- *Neutropenia* — a low number of neutrophils (see p. 655). This condition can be congenital (very rare), secondary to drug or radiation therapy (see Ch. 31) or overwhelming infection, or associated with the autoimmune diseases (see p. 683).
- *Functional defects* — abnormalities in phagocyte structure or function. These can result in the inability of phagocytes to localise in an inflammatory site, or in their inability to ingest and digest microorganisms.
- *Failure of complement activation.* There are many steps in the complement pathway, and many components are involved or created during complement activation. Some appear to be more important than others (Roitt & Delves 2001). Absence of one of the complement components can make phagocytosis difficult, as it is easier for the granular leucocytes to ingest microorganisms if their outer surface is coated with complement.

STOP THINK **16.9** Recall the function of B lymphocytes and try to work out what will happen if they are deficient.

Impairment of B lymphocytes

Occasionally B lymphocytes fail to mature properly in the bone marrow, resulting in B-cell deficiency and therefore diminished antibody production. People with B-cell deficiency are particularly prone to bacterial infections, e.g. *Staphylococcus aureus* (Roitt & Delves 2001).

Impairment of T lymphocytes

T-cell deficiency occasionally occurs in children in whom absence of the thymus gland means that the cells cannot differentiate to become T lymphocytes. People with T-cell deficiency are particularly prone to some viral infections, e.g. varicella (Roitt & Delves 2001).

Secondary immunodeficiency

This occurs as a result of some other condition; an individual suffering from secondary immunodeficiency is sometimes called a 'compromised host'. This term simply means that the person's immune defences are in some way reduced or compromised, making them particularly susceptible to infection.

The commonest clinical situations in which this happens are AIDS (see Ch. 37), chemotherapy, intercurrent infection (such as HIV infection, TB, chickenpox) and in people who are post-transplant.

Other factors that contribute to patients being more susceptible include extremes of age, general health status, nutritional state, underlying conditions such as diabetes mellitus, immunosuppressive medication and previous exposure to infection.

HYPERSENSITIVITY

An excessive immune response, hypersensitivity, can result in damage to normal tissue. This response may be immediate or delayed. Four types of hypersensitivity reaction have been described: types I, II and III are antibody-mediated; type IV is mediated mainly by T cells and macrophages (Roitt & Delves 2001).

Type I: anaphylactic or immediate hypersensitivity

In this type of immune response, excessive IgE production results in IgE binding to mast cells which, when the antigen is encountered, release histamine, giving rise to an acute inflammatory reaction. This type of response usually develops within minutes of exposure to the antigen and will recur on subsequent encounters.

The reaction can be local, as in asthma (see Ch. 3), hay fever and eczema, or systemic, as in anaphylactic shock. Typical antigens are the house dust mite, pollen, latex and foodstuffs such as shellfish, eggs and nuts; the increasing number of people with allergy to nuts has resulted in many food labels indicating whether the product contains nuts. The nature of the symptoms will depend on whether the antigen is encountered locally or systemically, or absorbed via the intestine.

Atopy is a term used to describe the tendency of 10–15% of the population to suffer from allergic diseases such as asthma, eczema, hay fever, urticaria and food allergy. There is often a familial (genetic) disposition to this condition.

Type II: antibody-dependent cytotoxic hypersensitivity

In this type of response, antibodies react to normal tissue cells, which then bind to complement or to phagocytes, resulting in lysis or phagocytosis of the cell. This can occur as a result of 'foreign' antigens entering the body, e.g. a mismatched blood transfusion (see Ch. 11) or a transplant, or can be induced by medications or infections which appear to alter cell surface antigens such that an attack by native antibodies ensues.

Type III: immune-complex-mediated hypersensitivity

In this form of hypersensitivity, large immune complexes, i.e. antigens bound to antibodies (see p. 657), form in excess and are deposited in the capillary endothelium of the kidney, joints, skin and other sites. They may activate complement and attract phagocytes, resulting in mast cell degranulation and local or general inflammation. The inflammation may be acute, as in serum sickness; chronic, as in glomerulonephritis; or both, as in farmer's lung. This type of hypersensitivity resembles an anaphylactic reaction, but takes longer (several hours or more) to develop.

Type IV: cell-mediated or delayed hypersensitivity

In this type of immune reaction, sensitised T cells, on repeat contact with an allergen (antigen), release cytokines (soluble chemicals) which attract phagocytes and function without the presence of antibodies. These reactions cause chronic and sometimes extensive inflammation and are apparent a few hours after exposure to the antigen.

This type of immune response is the basis of the Mantoux test (see p. 677), which is given to find out whether a person has tuberculosis, has developed immunity to tuberculosis or is not immune. It also gives rise to contact dermatitis (see Ch. 12) and sarcoidosis (see p. 683), and contributes to graft rejection.

Anaphylactic shock (type I)

Anaphylactic shock is a sudden and severe form of type I hypersensitivity reaction, where there is an inappropriate or excessive response to some foreign material such as an antibiotic or other medication, a vaccine or a bee sting (Ferns & Chojnacka 2003, Reading 2004).

PATHOPHYSIOLOGY

IgE antibodies are the mediators of this reaction. The mechanism is similar to that of hay fever, except that the response is systemic rather than localised.

Common presenting symptoms

The characteristic feature of anaphylactic shock is collapse within seconds or minutes after exposure to the offending allergen. Usually this follows an injection or, less commonly, ingestion of the offending antigen. Laryngeal oedema manifests as swelling in the throat, hoarseness or stridor. Examination of the patient may show an urticarial skin rash which may be localised or widespread. The rash is itchy and can coalesce to form giant hives. In anaphylaxis, urticaria is part of a life-threatening condition. However, urticaria can present independently as a mild type I hypersensitivity and can be alleviated by the application of antihistamine creams.

Angioedema resulting from a sudden increase in vascular permeability can lead to oedema of the skin, respiratory obstruction and severe hypotension, the result of which may be fatal.

MEDICAL MANAGEMENT

There is not usually time for investigations in patients with anaphylactic shock. The diagnosis must be made rapidly. Treatment in mild cases is with subcutaneous adrenaline to restore blood pressure and relax the airways. This can be repeated at 3-min intervals. Severe cases require intensive cardiovascular and respiratory support with adrenaline given intravenously.

Antihistamines may also be given to counter the harmful effects of the histamine released by mast cells. Corticosteroids are sometimes given but have a delayed effect, as they act on the immune system and do not counter the chemicals already released.

NURSING PRIORITIES AND MANAGEMENT: Anaphylactic shock

Life-threatening concerns

Anaphylactic shock may occur suddenly and unexpectedly and is life threatening, especially in circumstances where emergency facilities are not available. Death may ensue if prompt action is not taken. Maintenance of airway, breathing and circulation is paramount. Emergency procedures are as follows (see also Ch. 18):

1. To help restore blood pressure, place the patient flat in the left lateral position and insert an airway to prevent respiratory obstruction.
2. Give adrenaline intramuscularly, unless the patient's condition is good and there is a strong central pulse.
3. Give oxygen by face mask if it is available.
4. Send for medical aid (GP or hospital doctor) or ambulance (dial 999); ask a relative, if present, to stay with the patient while you do this.
5. Be prepared to institute cardiopulmonary resuscitation.
6. Check pulse and blood pressure regularly and after any medication.

Major patient problems

Should the patient survive, severe anxiety after the event is likely. The question of how to prevent a similar occurrence will need to be explored and the cause of the reaction investigated. People with frequent unpreventable attacks should have a MedicAlert card or bracelet, and the patient and relatives should be supplied with, and taught how to administer, adrenaline using, for example, the autoinjector pre-filled adrenaline 'pens'.

For further information on emergency medical treatment of anaphylactic reactions for first medical responders and community nurses, see the Resuscitation Council (UK) guidelines (www.resus.org.uk/pages/guide.htm).

Transfusion reaction (type II)

This is a type II antibody-dependent cytotoxic hypersensitivity. An adverse reaction to a blood transfusion can occur when the immune system mounts an antibody response to the transfused blood. For details of this kind of reaction and the associated medical and nursing care, see Chapter 11.

Serum sickness (type III)

This condition is a type III immune-complex-mediated hypersensitivity reaction to foreign antigens, i.e. that of another species. It occurs when the immune system recognises the proteins in an introduced serum as foreign and produces antibodies against them. Antigen–antibody complexes, known as immune complexes, form and may be deposited in the skin, joints, heart and kidneys, resulting in a temperature rise, urticarial skin rash, swollen lymph glands/nodes and swollen and painful joints. Serum sickness was common in the days when horse serum was used as a source of immunoglobulin (Roitt & Delves 2001). Its occurrence led to the development of blood transfusion-derived products such as Humotet (human antitetanus immunoglobulin). Insulins used in diabetes mellitus are now produced by genetic engineering to avoid allergic reactions to non-human insulin components (see Ch. 5).

Sarcoidosis (type IV)

This is a type IV hypersensitivity reaction, the cause of which is as yet unknown.

PATHOPHYSIOLOGY

This disease may take a subacute or chronic form and is characterised by disturbances in cell-mediated immunity in which the balance between the different types of T lymphocyte is altered. Lesions or granulomas may develop in the lungs, liver, spleen, parotid glands, joints, skin, eyes, mediastinal and superficial lymph nodes, and phalangeal bones. In the subacute form, often discovered incidentally on routine chest X-ray, the lesions usually resolve spontaneously without treatment; however, in chronic sarcoidosis they may lead to the production of fibrous tissue causing permanent damage, e.g. interstitial fibrosis in the lungs, myocardial damage leading to cardiac arrhythmias, skin rashes and damage to the iris, possibly leading to blindness. Although the disease may involve other organs, the severity of their involvement is variable. The disease is primarily pulmonary (Baughman et al 2003).

Common presenting symptoms

Most patients have pulmonary symptoms, i.e. dyspnoea on exertion and unproductive cough, in addition to general malaise, weakness, loss of appetite, fever and weight loss. Lymph node enlargement may also be detected on examination.

MEDICAL MANAGEMENT

Investigations

Diagnostic investigation includes chest X-ray and lung function tests (see Ch. 3). Biopsy of the lung or other tissue can confirm the diagnosis. In some cases, a Kveim test is used to confirm the diagnosis. Intradermal infection of sarcoid tissue produces a characteristic microscopic appearance on biopsy 4–6 weeks later (typical of type IV).

Treatment

of chronic sarcoidosis occasionally involves the administration of corticosteroids to suppress the immune (type IV) reaction, often for several years. Oxygen may be given in acute or severe cases involving the heart and lungs.

For further information on sarcoidosis, see the British Lung Foundation (www.lunguk.org/sarcoidosis).

NURSING PRIORITIES AND MANAGEMENT: Sarcoidosis

The priorities in nursing care will depend on the level of impairment caused by the granulomatous lesions. Commonly, there is respiratory impairment and occasionally a potential for cardiac arrhythmias. Vision may be affected and liver function disturbed. Sarcoidosis may not be the prime reason for admission to hospital but must not be neglected in setting priorities for care.

AUTOIMMUNE DISEASES

These disorders occur when the body's tolerance to 'self' breaks down and autoantibodies, i.e. antibodies against 'self' antigens, are formed. Autoimmune disorders may be:

- organ-specific, focusing on one tissue
  —Hashimoto's thyroiditis
  —pernicious anaemia (see Ch. 11)
- generalised
  — rheumatoid arthritis (see Ch. 10)
  — systemic lupus erythematosus (SLE)
  — sarcoidosis.

Why autoantibodies sometimes cause disease is not yet completely understood. Their production may be initiated by minor changes in cells or by the exposure of previously 'hidden' cells as a result of damage, infection or genetic mutation, resulting in 'new' surface antigens being presented to the immune system. Autoimmune diseases may also involve a hypersensitivity reaction, whether immediate or delayed.

Goodpasture's syndrome (anti-GBM disease)

PATHOPHYSIOLOGY

People with this rare disorder develop antibodies to their own kidney glomerular basement membrane (GBM). These antibodies bind to the glomerular membrane, fix complement and cause glomerulonephritis. They may also be deposited in the basement membranes of the lung alveoli. The cause of this disease is not known. It is potentially fatal and is commoner in young men. Fortunately, it is rare.

Common presenting symptoms,
which may be acute and severe, include:

- haematuria, mild or severe
- haemoptysis, dyspnoea, cough.

MEDICAL MANAGEMENT

History and examination
The onset can be rapid, with symptoms of nephritis and pulmonary haemorrhage.

Investigations
Urinalysis will confirm haematuria and proteinuria, and a chest X-ray will determine the degree of lung involvement. The diagnosis is confirmed if serology or kidney or lung biopsy reveals the presence of anti-GBM antibodies. Blood chemistry shows raised serum creatinine and blood urea nitrogen. Urine collection will demonstrate reduced creatinine clearance, indicating some degree of kidney failure.

Treatment
This disease must be treated urgently, as renal and respiratory failure can occur. High-dose parenteral corticosteroids, e.g. prednisolone, are given, sometimes in conjunction with a cytotoxic medication such as azathioprine or cyclophosphamide. Plasmapheresis may be carried out to remove circulating anti-GBM antibodies. If renal failure develops, dialysis will be undertaken. Kidney transplant may be required but can be attempted only after intensive plasmapheresis to ensure that no circulating anti-GBM antibodies remain. Oxygen therapy and assisted ventilation (see Ch. 29) may be required if respiratory failure develops.

NURSING PRIORITIES AND MANAGEMENT: Goodpasture's syndrome

Patients with Goodpasture's syndrome will present with both respiratory and renal failure which may require intensive nursing support (Fox & Swann 2001).

Myasthenia gravis

This rare autoimmune disease is thought to be caused by a disorder of the thymus gland, whereby it produces defective T lymphocytes. It usually occurs in individuals aged between 15 and 50 years, and is more common in females than in males.

PATHOPHYSIOLOGY
The defective T cells stimulate B cells to produce antibodies to the acetylcholine receptors in the neuromuscular junction. Acetylcholine allows the normal transmission of impulses from the motor nerves to voluntary muscle (see Chs 9 and 10).

The autoantibodies react with the acetylcholine receptor, blocking the attachment of the acetylcholine neurotransmitter and thus impairing or preventing normal muscular activity.

Complement fixation may also result in destruction of the receptors.

Common presenting symptoms
The classic symptom of myasthenia gravis is that some muscle groups tire quickly (Kittiwatanapaisan et al 2003). Movement may be strong at first but rapidly weakens. Localised symptoms include diplopia or ptosis (see Ch. 13) due to weakness of the extraocular muscles, as well as weakness in chewing, swallowing, talking and moving the limbs. The muscles around the shoulder girdle are those most commonly affected.

Symptoms are often worse at the end of the day or after exercising. Double vision or progressively quieter speech may be early symptoms. Respiratory muscles may be affected, resulting in a weakened cough. Relapses sometimes occur after infections or following emotional disturbance.

MEDICAL MANAGEMENT

History and examination
The patient presents with a history of muscle weakness and inability to sustain muscle power, e.g. difficulty in brushing hair. Anti-acetylcholine receptor antibodies can be detected in the serum.

Investigations
Diagnosis is assisted by giving an intravenous injection of the short-acting anticholinesterase, edrophonium, allowing acetylcholine to accumulate. Muscle power improves within 30 s of the injection and often persists for 2–3 min as a result of the temporary increase in acetylcholine at the damaged neuromuscular junction.

Treatment
Therapy usually begins with cholinesterase inhibitors, e.g. pyridostigmine. If necessary, immune-directed treatment is added, beginning with either thymectomy or high-dose corticosteroids. Short-term therapies, e.g. i.v. immunoglobulin or plasmapheresis, may be effective in the early stages of treatment or later during an exacerbation (Richman & Agius 2003).

NURSING PRIORITIES AND MANAGEMENT: Myasthenia gravis

Life-threatening concerns

There are two potential crisis situations: a myasthenic crisis reflects an acute exacerbation of the condition; a 'cholinergic crisis' may occur as a consequence of a toxic response to medication. The patient becomes paralysed, pale and sweaty, salivates excessively and has persistently small pupils. This occurs as a result of excessive acetylcholine, which causes hyperstimulation of the acetylcholine receptors. It requires urgent medical attention. The consequences of a myasthenic or cholinergic crisis are life threatening. Paralysis of the respiratory muscles can rapidly lead to severe hypoxia; consequently, the patient may require resuscitation and ventilation (see Ch. 29). Baseline and repeat peak flow monitoring may be necessary. Some drugs, including common antibiotics, can cause deterioration.

Major patient problems

These include fatigue and muscle weakness. Patients may need help with eating, drinking, washing and dressing. Difficulty with swallowing can lead to choking and reduced mobility may lead to pressure ulcers (see Ch. 23).

Further considerations

Most people suffering from myasthenia gravis live independently at home for as long as possible. Their nursing care, when required, will depend on the severity of symptoms. The potential seriousness of their condition may not be obvious. The educational aspect of community care for family and friends will be a priority. Advice on a nutritious diet is particularly important where chewing and swallowing are impaired. Small mouthfuls of food should be chewed slowly before swallowing. Soft, moist food is usually easiest to manage. Choking is a danger, but can often be avoided by helping the patient to concentrate on chewing and then swallowing. Eye care may be required if blinking is impaired; this may include the use of eye drops to prevent dryness of the cornea (see Ch. 13). If breathing is made difficult by respiratory muscle fatigue, the patient may be more comfortable sitting up or propped up in bed.

Useful advice is available from the Myasthenia Gravis Association (see 'Useful websites').

Systemic lupus erythematosus

Systemic lupus erythematosus (SLE) is an uncommon multisystem disorder in which autoantibodies against a variety of cellular antigens are produced. Thus any cell or tissue can be affected. Women are more often affected than men, and onset usually occurs in young adulthood. It is commoner in people of Afro-Asian and Chinese origin.

PATHOPHYSIOLOGY

The cause of this disease is not yet known, although both genetic and environmental factors, e.g. the effect of sunlight, medications, hormone levels or viral infections, have been suggested. Damage is caused by the deposition of immune complexes in the tissues (a type III hypersensitivity reaction) and by the autoantibodies reacting directly with normal tissue cells (a type II hypersensitivity reaction).

Common presenting symptoms

are often vague and non-specific, so that other illnesses or psychological problems may be considered responsible. Joint symptoms, e.g. arthritis, polyarthralgia, and fever, rashes and Raynaud's phenomena are common features. Fatigue is a common non-specific symptom, and skin rash, usually on areas which are exposed to sunlight such as the face, neck and scalp, may occur; characteristically, this is a 'butterfly rash' across the nose and cheeks. Nephritis is common, along with decreased urine output.

Vasculitis, especially in the smaller blood vessels, can give rise to skin rash or ulceration, nephritis, neuropathy or stroke. There may be poor peripheral perfusion, due to inflammation and consequent occlusion of small blood vessels. There may also be cardiopulmonary symptoms, including decreased cardiac output due to pericarditis, myocarditis, endocarditis and pulmonary infarction.

Occasionally there is cerebral inflammation leading to confusion, epilepsy or psychiatric symptoms.

MEDICAL MANAGEMENT

History and examination

As the symptoms of SLE are diverse, and their severity highly variable, a thorough history will be required. There may be external signs of tissue damage such as skin rash, which will assist the doctor in making a diagnosis. Some patients will have lymphadenopathy and an enlarged spleen. Other features will depend on the specific organs involved.

Investigations

In the course of diagnostic investigation, the erythrocyte sedimentation rate will usually be found to be raised. Antinuclear antibodies will be found in the serum of most patients with this disease. Some patients will have detectable anti-DNA antibodies and circulating immune complexes. Anaemia, leucopenia and thrombocytopenia (see Ch. 11) may be present on haematological examination. Depending on the organs involved, renal, cardiac or respiratory function may be altered.

Treatment

is aimed at relieving symptoms and preventing organ damage. Non-steroidal anti-inflammatory drugs (NSAIDs) such as ibuprofen may help to alleviate joint pain and other symptoms. Antimalarial drugs are sometimes used, as they can reduce the frequency of exacerbations of skin and joint lesions. Corticosteroids, e.g. prednisolone, are given when major organs such as the heart, lung, kidney and brain are involved.

NURSING PRIORITIES AND MANAGEMENT: Systemic lupus erythematosus

The specific care of patients with SLE depends very much on the stage of the disease and on the organs involved. In any event, the aim is to alleviate symptoms as they present (Sohng 2003, Tretheway 2004).

Life-threatening concerns

Depending on the nature and severity of organ involvement, myocardial infarction, respiratory failure and renal failure may ensue. Appropriate resuscitative measures are described in Chapters 2, 3 and 8.

Major patient problems

As fatigue is common, the patient should be encouraged to have adequate rest. For patients who have experienced alteration in bowel habit, dietary advice may help. Patients may experience confusion, depression due to CNS involvement or fears about prognosis. Epilepsy may also occur.

Poor peripheral circulation leading to cold hands and feet may develop. Patients are also likely to become susceptible to infection due to the debilitating effects of the disease process and the immunosuppressive effects of treatment.

Further considerations

Both pregnancy and the contraceptive pill have exacerbating effects on this disease. Patients suffering from photosensitivity should be encouraged to minimise exposure to sunlight and to protect the skin when exposure is unavoidable. Emotional support will be needed as this is a chronic disease of uncertain progression. Patient information is available from www.rheumatology.org/public/factsheets.

CONCLUSION

This chapter has introduced the immune system, disorders of immunity and infectious diseases. Infectious diseases, including those that cause HAI, affect patients in many ways and health care staff and carers must take account of patient susceptibility, sources of microorganisms, their routes of transmission and the many measures available to prevent, control and manage all of these. Nurses are in a key position to rise to the many challenges infectious diseases and HAI present today. They must be effective role models and demonstrate strict adherence to SICPs and other recommended practice at all times. All nurses, including those with a specialist qualification in infection control, should seek to enhance local infection control practice and to influence nationally, even globally, the prevention and control of infection in hospital and in community settings. In order to do this, nurses must have a sound understanding of immunology, the infection process, ways of preventing, monitoring and controlling infection and of risk management, and be able to contribute effectively to multidisciplinary teams within this rapidly developing field of health care.

CASE HISTORY 16.1

Mr B

The following condition is commonly encountered both in the community and hospital settings. Recognising the susceptibility of this patient to infection from the information available, and considering how his immune system will cope with further interventions while in hospital, is the first step in a scenario that will challenge your thinking on prevention and control of infection.

Mr B arrives in the ward for total hip replacement surgery. He is 62 years old with type 2 diabetes, on hypoglycaemics. He is assessed on admission and worked up for surgery. The significant factors noted are: he is overweight and is a smoker, he states that he eats well and controls his diabetes, his skin is dry in places and he is a social drinker.

His wife is in attendance with him and is recovering from a hysterectomy, for which she was discharged from hospital 4 weeks ago. It later transpires that she is continuing to see the practice nurse for an ongoing postoperative wound problem.

Mr B is found to have a foot ulcer and his diabetic control is examined more closely. During further examination of Mr B's foot ulcer, samples are taken and sent to the microbiology laboratory. This decision was taken as signs and symptoms of infection were present around the site on the foot, e.g. erythema (redness), swelling and heat, with evidence of scanty serous exudate. He is experiencing no pain from this wound site as his ability to sense pain is impaired by his diabetes and it is established that this is why the ulcer has developed thus far without being identified. The multidisciplinary team are eager to manage and treat the ulcer appropriately in order to progress with Mr B's proposed hip surgery and are considering antibiotic therapy on results of the samples taken.

Dressings are applied to the wound in order to protect it and encourage healing but also to prevent any potential spread of microorganisms to the environment and other patients, especially as there are many patients with exposed postoperative wounds in his ward.

STOP THINK

16.10 What do you think are the risks to Mr B from his existing foot ulcer and how might this wound pose a risk to others around him at this stage?

The results from Mr B's admission screen and foot ulcer yielded a moderate growth of MRSA. The infection control team visit the ward to discuss this information. They enquire as to Mr B's background situation, advise on his isolation care and give further explanation, including a patient information leaflet, to Mr B and his wife.

STOP THINK

16.11 What do you think the advice for patient care would be and why, taking into account Mr B's and the other patients' risks as discussed earlier, particularly considering the risks from MRSA?

16.12 What further information do you think the team would collect to try to ascertain the epidemiology of the MRSA infection? Do you think any specific discussions would take place with Mrs B?

16.13 Think about a situation where you have or should have isolated a patient and applied additional precautionary measures to ensure the spread of infection was minimised. Were the facilities and resources available to enable you to do this? Did everyone involved appear to adhere to the same high standards of infection control measures?

Treatment for Mr B's foot ulcer leads to some improvement and the surgical team decide to operate, especially as MRSA is not isolated from any other sites on his body.

Mr B is anxious and asks many questions about the 'additional' measures that are being taken during his care. The infection control nurse visits the ward again and clarifies the control measures for MRSA and similar infections, prior to, during and after surgery, including:

- being cared for in an isolation room, with the door closed and a sign on the door
- all staff who enter wearing plastic aprons and, when performing care, gloves
- staff removing their gloves and aprons before they leave the room and decontaminating their hands at the sink or with alcohol gel from the containers mounted by the door

Continued

CASE HISTORY 16.1
Mr B *(cont'd)*

- being taken straight into the theatre and not spending time in the pre- and postoperative areas
- certain items for care remaining in his room at all times for his use alone, but other items being removed to keep the room clutter-free.

While discussing these infection control measures with Mr B, Mrs B comments on her recent hospital admission and that she had heard someone in her ward had MRSA. On further discussion, the infection control nurse learns about Mrs B's ongoing problems with her surgical wound and suggests that, as healing is delayed, she talk to her practice nurse about screening for MRSA, if this has not already been done.

Mr B's surgery is successful and his foot wound is almost healed when he is told he will be discharged. At this time Mrs B receives word from her general practice that she does indeed have a light growth of MRSA within her wound and she will get further advice when she attends.

The ward staff and the infection control team provide Mr and Mrs B with advice for discharge:

- that their family can visit them as normal
- that hand hygiene and environmental cleanliness are the most important points
- that their laundry can be washed in their own washing machine at as high a temperature as possible, separating towels and bedding from other clothing, as these items are often where MRSA is most likely to harbour
- that their cooking utensils and crockery can be washed as normal in a dishwasher or with hot, soapy water.

They also provide a discharge letter including a summary of the infection control instructions to Mr B and an additional letter containing guidance given to Mrs B to be passed onto their general practice, especially as they will both continue to have dressing changes to foot and abdomen respectively.

STOP THINK

16.14 What measures do you think would be taken to ensure Mr B's room is safe to be used by the next patient? Do you think, given today's pressures upon health care, enough time is dedicated to preparing rooms or bed spaces before a new patient goes into them?

16.15 What measures do you think the practice nurse would take to ensure Mrs B's MRSA does not spread through the practice?

16.16 Think about the fact that Mrs B has no information about how she first acquired the MRSA in her wound. How might she feel and what could be done about this situation to try to ensure that those involved have learned and acted upon this information?

REFERENCES

Auditor General 2000 A clean bill of health? A review of domestic services in Scottish hospitals. Audit Scotland, Edinburgh

Auditor General 2003 Performance audit. Hospital cleaning. Audit Scotland, Edinburgh

Baker T 2001 Tuberculosis returns. Nursing Times 97(26): 56–57

Baughman R P, Lower E E, duBois R M 2003 Sarcoidosis. Lancet 361(9363): 1111–1118

Boyne L 2001 Meningococcal infection. Nursing Standard 16(7): 47–55

Centers for Disease Control 1998 CDC surveillance update. CDC, Atlanta

Chislett L 2003 Infection control. The delivery of hepatitis B vaccine. Nursing Times 99(7): 50–52

Christopher L 2003 Hepatitis B – a deadly virus. Practice Nurse 25(5): 48–51

Ferns T, Chojnacka I 2003 The causes of anaphylaxis. British Journal of Nursing 12(17): 1006–1012

Fox H L, Swann D 2001 Goodpasture syndrome: pathophysiology, diagnosis, and management. Nephrology Nursing Journal 28(3): 305–312

Gould D 2004 Systematic observation of hand decontamination. Nursing Standard 18(47): 39–44

Harbarth S, Sax H, Gastmeirer P 2003 The preventable proportion of nosocomial infections: an overview of published reports. Journal of Hospital Infection 54: 258–266

Haslett C, Chilvers E R, Boon N A et al (eds) 2002 Davidson's principles and practice of medicine, 19th edn. Churchill Livingstone, Edinburgh

Health and Safety at Work Act 1974 (Application outside Great Britain Order) 2001. TSO, London

Heymann D 2004 Control of communicable diseases manual, 18th edn. American Public Health Association, Washington, DC

King L 2001 Minimising the risk of hospital transmission of pulmonary TB. Nursing Standard 16(4): 45–52

Kittiwatanapaisan W, Gauthier D K, Williams A M, Oh S J 2003 Fatigue in myasthenia gravis patients. Journal of Neuroscience Nursing 35(2): 87–93

Negus J, Vinney K, Bothamley G 2004 The ethics of legally detaining a patient who has tuberculosis. Nursing Times 100(36): 52–55

Nursing and Midwifery Council (NMC) 2004 The NMC code of professional conduct: standards for conduct, performance and ethics. NMC, London

Oxtoby K 2003 Raising the profile of the forgotten disease. Nursing Times 99(22): 38–39

Payne D 2000 Deadly risk from exotic pets. Nursing Times 96(24): 13

Reading D 2004 Managing anaphylaxis. Practice Nurse 28(3): 28–31

Richman D P, Agius M A 2003 Treatment of autoimmune myasthenia gravis. Neurology 61(12): 1652–1661

Rickard N A S 2004 Hand hygiene: promoting compliance among nurses and health workers. British Journal of Nursing 13(7): 404–410

Roitt I, Delves P J 2001 Essential immunology. Blackwell, Oxford

Scottish Intercollegiate Guidelines Network (SIGN) 2000 Antibiotic prophylaxis in surgery. A national clinical guideline. SIGN Publication No. 45. SIGN, Edinburgh

Sohng K Y 2003 Effects of a self-management course for patients with systemic lupus erythematosus. Journal of Advanced Nursing 42(5): 479–486

Tretheway P 2004 Systemic lupus erythematosus. Dimensions of Critical Care Nursing 23(3): 111–115

Williams H 2002 Life after shingles: the management of postherpetic neuralgia. British Journal of Community Nursing 7(6): 290–291

www.riddor.gov.uk/info.html Reporting of Injuries, Diseases and Dangerous Occurrences Regulations

FURTHER READING

Ayliffe G A J, Fraise A P, Geddes A M et al 2000 Control of hospital infection. A practical handbook, 4th edn. Arnold, London

Boyce J M, Pitter D 2002 Guideline for hand hygiene in health-care settings. Recommendations of the Health care Infection Control Practices Advisory Committee and the HICPAC/SHEA/APIC/IDSA Hand Hygiene Task Force. MMWR 51(RR16): 1–44

Department of Health/Hospital Infection Society 2001a Standard principles for preventing hospital-acquired infections. Journal of Hospital Infection 47(Suppl): S21–S37. Online. Available: www.needlestickforum.net

Department of Health/Hospital Infection Society 2001b Guidelines for preventing infections associated with the insertion and maintenance of short-term indwelling urethral catheters in acute care. Journal of Hospital Infection 47(Suppl): S39–S46

Department of Health/Hospital Infection Society 2001c Guidelines for preventing infections associated with the insertion and maintenance of central venous catheters. Journal of Hospital Infection 47(Suppl): S47–S67

Department of Health 2000 UK Antimicrobial resistance strategy and action plan. DH, London

Department of Health 2002 Getting ahead of the curve – a strategy for combating infectious diseases (including other aspects of health protection). A report by the Chief Medical Officer. DH, London. Online. Available: www.dh.gov.uk

Department of Health 2003 Winning ways: working together to reduce health care associated infection in England. Report from the Chief Medical Officer. DH, London. Online. Available: www.dh.gov.uk

Department of Health 2004 A matron's charter. An action plan for cleaner hospitals. DH, London

Department of Health 2004 Towards cleaner hospitals and lower rates of infection: a summary of action. DH, London. Online. Available: www.dh.gov.uk

Department of Health 2005 The Green Book. Immunisation against infectious disease. DH, London. Online. Available: www.dh.gov.uk/publicationsandstatistics

Department of Health Standing Medical Advisory Committee (SMAC) 1998 The path of least resistance. DH, London

Dougherty L, Lister S (eds) 2004 The Royal Marsden manual of clinical nursing procedures, 6th edn. Blackwell, Oxford

Emslie S 2004 Why risk management is taking greater prominence at board level. Health Care Risk Report (Feb): 20–21

Garner J S 1996 Guideline for isolation precautions in hospitals. Infection Control Hospital Epidemiology 17: 53–80. Online. Available: www.cdc.gov/ncidod/hip/INFECT/isolation.htm

Gould D 2004 Systematic observation of hand decontamination. Nursing Standard 18(47): 39–44

Gould D, Brooker C 2000 Applied microbiology for nurses. Macmillan, London

Harbarth S, Sax H, Gastmeirer P 2003 The preventable proportion of nosocomial infections: an overview of published reports. Journal of Hospital Infection 54: 258–266

House of Lords Select Committee on Science and Technology 1998 Seventh Report: Resistance to antibiotics and other antimicrobial agents. TSO, London

Humphreys H, Irving W L 2004 Problem oriented clinical microbiology and infection. Oxford University Press, Oxford

Mangram A, Horan T, Perason M et al 1999 Guideline for prevention of surgical site infection. American Journal of Infection Control 27(2): 96–134

National Audit Office 2000 Report by the Comptroller and Auditor General: The management and control of hospital acquired infection in acute NHS trusts in England. NAO, London

National Audit Office 2004 Report by the Comptroller and Auditor General: Improving patient care by reducing the risk of hospital acquired infection: a progress report. NAO, London

National Institute for Clinical Excellence (NICE) 2003 Infection control: prevention of health care-associated infections in primary and community care. NICE, London. Online. Available: www.nice.org.uk/pdf/infection_control_fullguideline.pdf

NHS Education for Scotland 2004 Promoting the prevention and control of infection through cleanliness champions. Unit 3B: How to wash hands properly. NHS Education for Scotland, Edinburgh

Plowman R, Graves N, Griffin M et al 1999 Socio-economic burden of hospital acquired infection. Public Health Laboratory Service, London

Reilly J 2001 Clinical governance in the real world. Nursing Times 97(50): 36–37

Reilly J, Twaddle S, McIntosh J et al 2001 An economic analysis of surgical wound infection. Journal of Hospital Infection 49(4): 245–249

Roberts C, Casey D 2004 Link nursing. An infection control link nurse network in the care home setting. British Journal of Nursing 13(3): 166–170

Royal College of Nursing (RCN) 2004a Good practice in infection control. RCN, London

Royal College of Nursing (RCN) 2004b Methicillin resistant staphylococcus aureus (MRSA). RCN, London

Scottish Executive Health Department (SEHD) 2002 Preventing infections acquired while receiving health care. The Scottish Executive's Action Plan to reduce the risk to patients, staff, and visitors, 2002–2005. SEHD, Edinburgh. Online. Available: www.scotland.gov.uk/library5/health/preventinfect.pdf

Scottish Executive Health Department, Health care Associated Infection Task Force 2004 The NHS Scotland code of practice for the local management of hygiene and health care associated infection (HAI). SEHD, Edinburgh. Online. Available: www.scotland.gov.uk/library5/health/lmhhai-00.asp

Tablan O, Anderson L, Besser R et al 2003 Guidelines for preventing health-care associated pneumonia. Recommendations of CDC and the Health care Infection Control Practices Advisory Committee. MMWR 53(RR03): 1–36

UK Guidance on Best Practice in Vaccine Administration 2001 The Vaccine Administration Taskforce, Shire Hall Communications, London

Watterson L 2004 Monitoring sharps injuries: EPINet™ surveillance results. Nursing Standard 19(3): 33–38

Waugh A, Grant A 2001 Ross and Wilson's anatomy and physiology in health and illness, 9th edn. Churchill Livingstone, Edinburgh

Wilson J 2001 Infection control in clinical practice, 2nd edn. Baillière Tindall, Edinburgh

www.dh.gov.uk/publicationsandstatistics for up-to-date information on immunisation against infectious disease in The Green Book

www.hpa.org.uk/infections for notification of infectious diseases in England

www.hse.gov.uk/coshh for the Health and Safety Executive Care of Substances Hazardous to Health Regulations

www.isdscotland.org for notification of infectious diseases in Scotland

www.lunguk.org/sarcoidosis for the British Lung Foundation data on sarcoidosis

www.mhra.gov.uk for the Medicines and Health care Products Regulatory Agency

www.resus.org.uk for the Resuscitation Council (UK) guidelines

www.who.int/vaccines/en/hepatitisb.shtml for information about vaccines and hepatitis B

USEFUL WEBSITES

Advisory Committee on Dangerous Pathogens
www.advisorybodies.doh.gov.uk/acdp

American College of Rheumatology
www.rheumatology.org/public/factsheets
For information about systemic lupus erythematosus

British Thoracic Society
www.brit-thoracic.org.uk

Centers for Disease Control and Prevention
www.cdc.gov

Clinical Negligence and Other Risks Scheme (CNORIS)
www.cnoris.com
CNORIS is a risk management scheme for the NHS in Scotland developed by the Scottish Executive Health Department in partnership with Willis Ltd

Defra
www.defra.gov.uk/environment/waste
Clinical waste regulations

Department of Health, Social Services and Public Safety
www.dhsspsni.gov.uk/hss/governance/archived_standards.asp
Infection control — assurance standards

Health Protection Scotland (formerly Scottish Centre for Infection and Environmental Health)
www.show.scot.nhs.uk/scieh
www.hps.scot.nhs.uk

Hospital Infection Society
www.his.org.uk

Infection Control Nurses Association
www.icna.co.uk

Meningitis Research Foundation
www.meningitis.org

Meningitis Trust
www.meningitis-trust.org

Myasthenia Gravis Association
www.mgauk.org

NHS Scotland (Fit for Travel)
www.fitfortravel.nhs.uk
Travel advice for the public on infectious diseases around the world, maintained and updated by Health Protection Scotland

World Health Organization
www.who.int

SECTION TWO

COMMON PATIENT PROBLEMS AND RELATED NURSING CARE

STRESS

17

Graeme D. Smith
Josephine (Tonks) N. Fawcett

INTRODUCTION

'Stress' is a word that frequently enters into everyday conversation as people remark on the difficulties and challenges of life. Most people would probably describe themselves as being 'stressed' from time to time, but what does this really mean? Is stress something that resides within the environment, in situations that are threatening, harmful or unpleasant, or is it essentially an internal state, an effect of the individual's perception of what is happening to them. Benner and Wrubel (1989), in their seminal text, defined stress as 'the disruption of meanings, understanding and smooth functioning so that harm, loss or challenge is experienced and sorrow, interpretation, or new skill acquisition is required'.

Stress may have physiological or psychological origins and research into stress is a highly complex field involving a number of sciences, including biology, physiology, psychology and sociology. These disciplines take different approaches to the definition, observation and measurement of stress. When biologists and physiologists talk of sources of stress, they are referring to empirical phenomena. Their interest is in examining identifiable events and their measurable effects upon the organism or system being stressed. Anything which affects the equilibrium of the organism may be described as a stressor; this would include bacterial or viral infections, dehydration, excessive cold or heat, inadequate food, and so on. Therefore stress can be viewed as a disturbed homeostasis that manifests itself via certain physiological and psychological imbalances (Watson & Fawcett 2003). The impact of stress occurs only when the cumulative effects of stressors surpass the individual's ability easily to return to equilibrium. However, despite the popular connotations, not all stress is a bad thing. Stress comes in two types, described as eustress or distress. Having the optimum amount of pressure to keep us happy and performing at our best is called eustress. Distress means that our functional capability is impaired in some way; this can take many forms, such as anxiety, depression or physical illness. Some of the most commonly associated triggers related to stress are listed in Box 17.1.

Social scientists view stress in terms of the pressures upon the individual to conform (or not) to societal norms. The inherent values expressed in a society's organisation and functioning may themselves be a source of stress to the individual. Modern industrial society, for example, provides

Box 17.1

Common triggers of stress

- Bereavement
- Illness, injury or trauma
- Interpersonal conflict
- Environmental factors
- Financial issues
- Uncertainty/change
- Work overload

Adapted from the Stress Management Society.

food, safety and shelter for its members in return for a commitment to work, often at some sacrifice to personal interests, leisure and family life.

Psychologists view stress from the perspective of the interaction of individuals and groups with the environment, describing the effects of stress on cognition, emotional well-being and behaviour.

It is important for nurses to have a clear understanding of the concept of stress as they endeavour to provide the best possible care for their patients. It is essential to appreciate why patients might be feeling stressed and how their stress might be alleviated. In relation to the nurse's own well-being, an understanding of stress and its effects is equally important. Nursing is physically and emotionally strenuous work, and it is vital for nurses to be able to recognise the signs of stress in themselves and to know how to go about managing stress in their daily work.

This chapter begins by outlining some definitions of stress as a type of stimulus, as a response, or as an interaction between an individual and their environment and the effects of stress upon physiological systems. The second section of the chapter introduces some of the more influential models that seek to describe and explain stress. This provides a basis for the third section, which examines the relationship between stress and disease.

The discussion then turns to the concept of coping, and various cognitive and behavioural mechanisms which people commonly employ to deal with stress. A description of the therapeutic strategies that are available to assist the individual in managing stress is then given.

PHYSIOLOGICAL RESPONSES TO STRESS

The physiological response to stress is normally seen in response to stressors such as illness, perceived danger or trauma. The stress response enables the individual to meet the challenges set by these situations and involves:

- activation of the sympathetic nervous system
- increased secretion of several hormones.

The stress response

In 1935, Cannon summarised the response of an individual, or animal, to external threat as the 'flight, fight or fright' reaction, often referred to as the 'acute stress response'. Real and imagined psychosocial stressors are an essential component of living and, when present to a moderate degree, have been described as 'eustress' since they optimise performance and improve learning. It is when a threat is perceived to be of an order which endangers either a person's sense of self-worth or even life itself, that the full manifestations of the acute stress response are seen. After events such as a car crash, bomb explosion or unexpected physical attack, rapid physiological adaptations of the acute stress response are activated. This can, in some circumstances, be life saving. Consider, for example, the situation in which smoke suddenly appears in a room and, all too soon, the first flames begin to spread; a person will often find a sudden unexpected ability for rapid action to deal with such an emergency. Along with a surge of physical strength, there will be an increased ability to tackle the flames and a marked enhancement in the ability to run and thereby escape the danger. Such a response is enabled by a release of hormones brought about by activation of the sympathetic nervous system and the adrenal medulla.

An alarm reaction of lesser magnitude is a common occurrence in the more ordinary trials of life. This occurs, for example, in such circumstances as running out of petrol on the motorway en route to an important engagement, losing one's front door keys, or being with someone who unexpectedly becomes acutely ill. The severity of the alarm reaction varies considerably between different individuals and also between different occurrences of a similar situation. Thus, when a person's car breaks down on the motorway for a second time, they may feel even more distressed than on the first occasion. Alternatively, they may be more confident in their ability to deal with the event and consequently be less 'stressed'.

The manifestation of stress is derived not merely from external problems or dangers but from the way in which people attempt to manage these problems. Ostell (1991), amongst others, described stress as the state of affairs that exists when the way in which people attempt to manage problems taxes or exceeds their coping resources. When the response to a stressor is severe, normal social relationships can be affected, as aspects of the 'flight, fight or fright' response potentially impinge upon rational behaviour.

As indicated, aversive physical stimuli that provoke stress events include excessive noise, cold or heat, and physiological imbalances such as those associated with sleep deprivation, lack of food or chronic pain. Such stressors not only act to bring about hormonal changes associated with the acute stress response, but also have their own selective effects on physiological functioning.

An example of such a selective effect can be seen in the body's response to cold, as it strives to maintain homeostasis. In cold conditions, the blood supply is redistributed to less exposed areas in order to limit heat loss and, via the mechanical act of shivering, the body temperature can be increased (see Ch. 22). In addition, the secretion of thyrotrophin-releasing hormone from the hypothalamus is increased, thereby stimulating the pituitary gland to secrete thyroid-stimulating hormone (TSH). This in turn causes enhanced release of the thyroid hormones thyroxine and triiodothyronine, which raise basal metabolic rate and hence increase heat production and core temperature.

To maintain homeostasis when threatened by a stressor, the body employs a range of physiological mechanisms. Some stressors are short lived, in which case the body may be able to react to the situation and quickly resolve the disturbance evoked by the stressor. Other stressors may last for days, months or even years. There are many examples of this chronic form of stress, for example when people must live with chronic disease or social disharmony. Where there has been repeated exposure to a particularly stressful or aversive event, there can be a further reaction, characterised by a conditioned fear response to any neutral stimulus experienced at the same time as the previous stressor. This effect is responsible for many of the anxiety reactions or acts of avoidance some people show in response to specific harmless objects.

The general adaptation syndrome (GAS)

Hans Selye, in his seminal work on the response-based model of stress, noted that the diverse noxious stimuli which challenged the ability of the body to maintain homeostasis induced a common pattern of effects (Selye 1936, 1976).

Selye deduced that, whatever the nature of the stressor, it resulted in a pattern of non-specific responses that formed part of what he described as a general adaptation syndrome (GAS). These responses, providing they were not overwhelming, enabled a physiological adaptation to take place (Selye 1976).

The syndrome is considered to have three phases. In the first phase 'the alarm reaction', the sympathetic nervous system and the adrenal glands are activated. Together they prepare the body for flight or fight. If the stressor continues, the triggering of neural and endocrine responses in the alarm reaction is followed by the second phase of 'resistance'. Stimulation of the hypothalamo-pituitary–adrenal axis results in increased secretion of corticosteroids, the endocrine response. In this phase, the internal responses of the body mobilise resources and enable tissue defences to achieve the maximum adaptation possible. The third and final phase of the general adaptation syndrome is 'exhaustion', in which the body may succumb to the stressor.

The general adaptation syndrome is criticised for providing a somewhat simplistic, stereotypical model of the responses of the body and failing to take full account of the individual variations of psychological and physiological responses. Lazarus (1966) argued that there is a circularity about Selye's model, in so far as something about the stimulus elicits a particular stress response while something about the response indicates the presence of a stressor.

STOP THINK

17.1 Identify five stressors in each of the following categories:
(a) emotional
(b) physical
(c) environmental
(d) societal.

The acute stress response

During the alarm reaction to stress, a series of physiological responses involving limbic and brain stem structures are triggered (Fox 2004). Neural pathways from the amygdaloid nuclei in the limbic system mediate responses to emotional stress, and pathways from the reticular formation in the brain stem mediate responses to physiological stressors such as pain and injury. This activates the hypothalamo-pituitary–adrenal axis and results in the secretion of a range of hormones.

An immediate response to threat or stress involves the neural connections from the hypothalamus to the sympathetic outflow, activating both postganglionic and preganglionic sympathetic nerves passing to the adrenal medulla. This is the emergency reaction which was first described by Cannon (1935). In the adrenal medulla, acetylcholine released at preganglionic sympathetic nerve terminals activates the chromaffin cells to secrete adrenaline and noradrenaline. In humans, adrenaline is secreted in greater amounts than noradrenaline. The release of these hormones takes place in a matter of seconds or minutes.

The hormones liberated from the adrenal medulla have many effects which facilitate emergency reactions. For example, adrenaline and noradrenaline improve cardiac and respiratory function. Heart rate and force of contraction are increased. Bronchioles are dilated and the depth and rate of respiration are increased. Blood flow is redistributed to areas of need, i.e. the heart and skeletal muscles. Blood glucose and basal metabolism are raised and blood clotting facilitated. The increase of blood glucose is due mainly to the actions of adrenaline on the liver to promote glycogen breakdown and enhance gluconeogenesis from fatty acids and proteins. Adrenaline also acts on the pancreas to inhibit insulin secretion. The piloerection and pupillary dilatation, so characteristic of the behaviour of fighting cats, represent yet another physiological consequence of hormone release from the adrenal medulla. Sweating by the eccrine glands is increased. In the meantime, functioning of the digestive tract is reduced and urinary sphincters are closed.

The physiological effects of adrenaline and noradrenaline are explained in Chapter 5. Adrenaline acts on α- and β-adrenoceptors, whereas noradrenaline acts predominantly on α-adrenoceptors.

In the more long-term responses to stress described by Selye, the centre of activity passes from the adrenal medulla to the adrenal cortex, and to the hypothalamus and pituitary, which are responsible for activating the adrenal cortex. Corticotrophin-releasing hormone (CRH) is secreted by the hypothalamus as well as by extrahypothalamic sites in the brain. CRH acts on the anterior pituitary gland, stimulating the secretion of adrenocorticotrophic hormone (ACTH) and beta-endorphin. Beta-endorphin is produced by the pituitary gland and hypothalamus of vertebrates.

Beta-endorphin reduces susceptibility to pain and is probably one of the means by which stress and the stimuli of conditioned fear give rise to endogenous analgesia. Opiates act in a similar way to endorphins, but are not rapidly degraded by the body, as natural endorphins are, and thus have a long-lasting effect on pain perception and mood (Pert 1997).

Other factors influence the release of ACTH, including antidiuretic hormone (ADH) and hypothalamic vasoactive intestinal peptide (VIP). The ACTH liberated by the anterior pituitary acts to stimulate cells in the adrenal cortex to secrete corticosteroids.

Glucocorticoids secreted by the adrenal cortex play a key role in adaptation to stress (Bowman & Rand 1996). Cortisol (hydrocortisone) accounts for approximately 95% of the glucocorticoid activity of the adrenal cortex. Glucocorticoids modify metabolism so as to increase blood glucose concentrations. They do this by mobilising tissue protein and amino acids and by these actions may induce a negative nitrogen balance. Glucocorticoids are needed to enable other hormones to bring about mobilisation and metabolism of fat. These metabolic effects of glucocorticoids ensure the supply of adequate fuel to the cells when the body is under stress, and in this respect the adrenal cortex provides an important back-up system for the adrenal medulla. In addition, glucocorticoids play important roles in the proper functioning of many organ systems and tissues in the body, including the cardiovascular system, the nervous system, lymphoid tissue and skeletal muscle.

Glucocorticoids, such as cortisol and corticosteroid, possess appreciable mineralocorticoid activity, retaining sodium chloride and indirectly increasing extracellular fluid volume, although they are much less potent in this respect than aldosterone. The secretion of aldosterone is not regulated by ACTH, and so its release is independent of the stress response. Mineralocorticoid activity by hormones such as cortisol may in part underlie important, though poorly understood, actions on the cardiovascular system. An increase of extracellular fluid volume can be of great importance under circumstances when stressors induce shock or when there is loss of body fluids after haemorrhage or burn injury.

Additionally, glucocorticoids can decrease the number of circulating lymphocytes, eosinophils and basophils and, at pharmacological concentrations, suppress the immune response. In addition to their direct effects, the corticosteroids exert an enabling influence on the actions of several other hormones and are necessary for the body to show a full response to the adrenaline and noradrenaline released from the adrenal medulla. As a result of its wide-ranging functions, especially in the maintenance of fluid and electrolyte balance, the adrenal cortex is essential to life (see Box 17.2).

Box 17.2

Hormonal mediators and effects of short- and long-term stress

Short-term stress

Mediated by the catecholamine release of adrenaline and noradrenaline from the adrenal medulla, short-term stress leads to:

- increased heart rate
- bronchodilatation
- increased blood pressure
- liver conversion of glycogen stores to glucose for release into the bloodstream
- altered blood flow patterns to increase arousal and decrease digestive and urinary activity via selective vasoconstriction
- increased platelet aggregation
- pupil dilatation and piloerection
- increased metabolic rate
- sweating from eccrine glands.

Long-term stress

Mediated by the release of glucocorticoids and mineralocorticoids from the adrenal cortex, long-term stress leads to:

- gluconeogenesis whereby proteins and fats are broken down to form glucose
- increased blood glucose levels
- retention of sodium and water by the kidneys (aldosterone effect)
- increased blood volume and blood pressure via the above plus vasoconstriction and reduced fluid shift
- increased coagulability and viscosity of the blood
- suppression of the immune system and inflammatory response
- altered blood biochemistry, e.g. in serotonin, endorphin and dopamine levels.

The chronic stress response

Clearly, as Selye (1976) established, there are limits to the body's ability to maintain its phase of resistance and adaptation in the face of continuing stress; environmental stressors can be toxic and physiologically overwhelming. Where the person is physiologically challenged but not overwhelmed, in conditions of prolonged stress, enlargement of the adrenal glands and thymicolymphatic atrophy will occur. When stress persists beyond a certain period of time, disturbances occur in the homeostatic balance of the body and there is an ever-increasing danger that disease processes will be precipitated.

An important part of the body's defence mechanism in the phase of resistance is the pituitary secretion of ACTH, which in turn stimulates the adrenal cortex to release corticosteroids. One of the early signs of the body's inability to meet the demands of unremitting stress is a blunting of the amounts of ACTH released by the anterior pituitary in response to that stress. Under these circumstances, the adrenal cortex frequently shows hyperplasia, which persists despite the reduced secretion of ACTH. This blunting of the ACTH response to stress also occurs in long-standing timidity, which is possibly due to high arousal together with slow habituation to the stressors. This is coupled with an associated enlargement of the adrenal glands and hypersecretion of adrenal steroids under comparatively non-threatening circumstances. Likewise, blunting of the ACTH responses to stressors is seen in depressive illness and in many forms of anxiety. In depressed individuals, there is frequently a high corticosteroid excretion associated with enlargement of the adrenal glands and an increase in the concentrations of CRH in cerebrospinal fluid.

Emotional as well as hormonal changes characterise chronic stress. These include emotional exhaustion, a decreased sensitivity to rewards and a withdrawal from decision making, which is characteristic of fatigue. This can progress to the condition known as 'burnout', a complex phenomenon involving extreme physical and emotional distress which, for the individual, is often linked to organisational factors (Hall 2004). In burnout, the physical and emotional fatigue may be manifest as a lack of involvement with, or sympathy or respect for, colleagues and clients. At its final stage, chronic stress may result in total collapse. Long-lasting stress in which there is a poor coping strategy is correlated with increased occurrence of a variety of diseases (Levi 1971, Cooper 2004, Hesselink et al 2004). These may be described as diseases of adaptation and are related to deranged secretion of adaptive hormones in the phase of resistance. These conditions include digestive disturbances, hypertension, myocardial infarction, allergies and sleep disturbances. Such chronic stress may also lead to anxiety, depression or behavioural disturbances, such as appetite disorders or increased usage of alcohol, tobacco, caffeine or even illegal substances.

Due to the prevalence of cardiovascular disease in Western society, particular attention has been paid in recent years to the relationship of stress to hypertension, myocardial dysfunction leading to unexpected sudden death, and to coronary atherosclerosis and myocardial infarctions (Cooper 2004, Critchley et al 2004).

Unexpected sudden death arising from cardiac failure has been found frequently to follow emotional upheaval or shock. It may be caused either by adrenosympathetically induced ventricular fibrillation or by apparent vagal stimulation and cardiac standstill. The increase in blood concentrations of glucocorticoids, mineralocorticoids and catecholamines as a result of stress can derange the vital myocardial electrolyte equilibrium. In a series of unexpected sudden deaths, the postmortem catecholamine concentrations in the blood were found to be excessively high, almost as high as in fatal adrenaline poisoning.

Increase in the blood concentrations of adrenaline, by its enhancement of platelet aggregation (see Box 17.2), can promote thrombus formation in atherosclerotic coronary arteries and thus lead to myocardial infarction. Statistical data show a close correlation between the high incidence of ischaemic heart disease in professional persons exposed to demanding occupational stress and in the 'Type A' individual, characterised by time consciousness, irritability and driving ambition (Yousfi et al 2004).

Based on the evidence of the serious consequences of excessive or prolonged stress, in combination with poor coping strategies, it can be seen that improvements to the working environment and social milieu, together with 'stress education' to lessen reactivity to adverse circumstances, should be encouraged. These measures may have as profound an impact on the health of a community as did the improvements to diet and sanitation in the mid-19th century.

MODELS OF STRESS

The physicist Robert Hooke (1635–1703) used the word 'stress' in the 17th century to refer to the ratio of an external force (created by a load) to the area over which that force was exerted. The resultant strain created a deformation or distortion of the object by what became known as Hooke's Law.

There is an interesting similarity between this use of the word stress and its modern application in the realm of human emotion and behaviour; indeed, people frequently use words such as 'weight' and 'strain' when describing their feelings of anxiety and stress.

During the 20th century, the adoption of the concept of stress by the biological and behavioural sciences resulted in the formulation of a number of models to describe stress and its effects, including the:

- stimulus-based model
- response-based model
- systems model
- general adaptation syndrome
- transactional model
- phenomenological approach.

Each of these models and its implications for nursing practice will be described in the following sections.

The stimulus-based model

In this model the person is viewed as being constantly exposed to external or environmental 'stressors' in their daily life, e.g. the demands of work, family responsibilities, bereavement or disablement, or to more specific stressors such as smells or poor lighting. These stressors have the potential, however, to cause distressing feelings and/or physical symptoms and to undermine well-being.

In the stimulus-based model, stress is a state that can generally be empirically observed, measured and evaluated, and which can potentially be removed or altered to reduce the individual's stress: it is possible, in theory, to persuade noisy neighbours to be quieter, make a cold working environment warmer, or poor lighting conditions more satisfactory. As an approach to identifying areas that might be improved in order to increase productivity, this model has some appeal for industrial planners and managers (Sutherland & Cooper 2000).

Limitations of the model In many situations, such as a bereavement or disablement, the original stressor cannot be changed or adapted to reduce distressing feelings. Even in relatively simple situations such as that illustrated in Case History 17.1, removing the stressor is not necessarily a straightforward matter. It quickly becomes apparent that the stimulus-based model has substantial shortcomings when considered in relation to the breadth of human experience (Sutherland & Cooper 2000).

Whilst it has some application in limited contexts, such as certain working environments, it does not explain why some people experience stress in certain situations while others, in similar circumstances, do not. Nor does it explain why a given situation may be stressful for a person at one time but not at another. Moreover, this model offers no explanation as to why a person may be stressed in response to apparently neutral stimuli such as birds, spiders or aeroplanes. Lazarus (1966), in a seminal text, argued that it is not possible to evaluate the human experience of stress objectively; only a personal account of feelings and experiences can adequately convey the nature of an individual's stress.

The response-based model

In this model, the word 'stress' is used to describe the experience of a person who feels they are in a threatening or difficult situation. Stress is thus a person's response to threat which, as in the stimulus-based model, is not

CASE HISTORY 17.1

J

A health visitor could not understand initially why her client, J, an unsupported mother of two, appeared to be tense and unhappy when they met at the child surveillance clinic. She asked how J was feeling, and J described how she had new neighbours in the flat above her who played loud music until early in the morning, preventing her and her two children from getting enough sleep. She had tried to talk with them but they had been hostile towards her and made her feel apprehensive. She didn't dare complain to them again. The lack of sleep was affecting J and her children.

J had difficulty concentrating at work and felt like crying frequently during the day; the children were overtired and generally irritable, making it even more difficult for her to cope.

The health visitor asked J if she could intervene by contacting the housing department on her behalf, but J said that she was afraid that this would make matters worse.

necessarily inherent in the environment or situation. By using the response-based model, it is possible to make sense of an individual's unique stress responses and even of responses that might seem, within the stimulus-based model, to be irrational, such as a fear of birds, spiders or of flying.

The systems model

A response-based model that considers the human stress response as 'a multifactorial, interactive, dynamic, phenomenon' is the systems model described in seminal work by Everly and Sobelman (1987). In this model the stress response is defined as consisting of six components:

1. Environmental stimuli Some environmental stimuli, or stressors, activate the stress response as a direct consequence of their physical or biochemical properties, i.e. their effects are not mediated by cognitive–affective evaluation. Examples of such stressors are caffeine, nicotine and extremes of heat and cold. Many environmental stimuli are not, however, intrinsically harmful but are perceived as such by the individual and, in this way, set the stage for activation of the stress response.

2. Cognitive–affective domain Everly and Sobelman (1987) described this as 'the critical "causal" phase in most stress responses', in that it is the individual's interpretation of the environment that gives rise to most stress reactions. The perspective that the individual takes towards their environment will be determined by 'biological predispositions', 'personality patterns', 'learning history' and 'available resources'. Everly and Sobelman (1987) argued that cognitive appraisal precedes emotional response.

3. Neurological triggering mechanisms The locus coeruleus, limbic system and hypothalamic nuclei are the anatomical sites for 'the integration of sensory, cognitive, affective, and visceral activity' (Everly & Sobelman 1987). In response to cognitive–affective appraisal, these structures trigger neurological and endocrine reactions. They also seem to be involved in a feedback system in which visceral and somatic efferent messages are relayed in response to emotional arousal. Everly and Sobelman suggested that 'these centers seem capable of establishing an endogenously-determined neurological tone that is potentially self-perpetuating' and which 'may, over time, serve as the basis for a host of psychiatric and psychophysiologic disorders'.

4. The physiological stress response axis The stress response itself occurs sequentially along the neurological, neuroendocrine and endocrine axes and results in neural and hormonal activity directed at target organs.

Neurological axis Neurological activity is especially evident in reactions to sudden acute stress and results in direct activation of the sympathetic nervous system, seen as raised heart rate and blood pressure, and the parasympathetic nervous system, seen as constricted pupils, increased salivation and urinary bladder contraction, and in the transmission of messages to skeletal muscle, resulting in contraction.

Neuroendocrine axis This is based in the adrenal medulla and plays an important role in longer-term arousal. Release of the catecholamines noradrenaline and adrenaline by the adrenal medullae results in such sympathetic responses as increased cardiac output and diminished blood flow to the skin and gastrointestinal system.

Endocrine axis This axis also plays an important role in chronic arousal. The hypothalamus, pituitary gland, adrenal cortex and thyroid gland are stimulated serially to release into the circulatory system the range of hormones described earlier in this chapter.

5. Coping In this final phase of the stress response, the individual attempts to reduce their level of arousal by manipulating the environment or making cognitive adjustments.

6. Target-organ effects If coping is unsuccessful and arousal is either excessive or prolonged, the physiological processes of the stress response are likely to lead to target organ dysfunction or disease.

Limitations of the model. One of the problems in viewing stress purely as a response is that this can lead to the assumption that the occurrence of stress in the life of the individual is solely their own responsibility. The descriptive term 'coping', used in a technical sense by stress researchers to describe physiological and psychological ways of adapting to stress, can also be used in an emotive way in everyday discourse to describe an individual's lack of mastery in stressful circumstances. Thus, someone who 'copes' with stress masters a situation in a positive way, whilst someone who does not 'cope' is seen to be lacking in this ability. Such judgements on self or others can have a harmful emotional effect on the individual.

Hans Selye's general adaptation syndrome

Hans Selye's extensive physiological research as an endocrinologist (Selye 1936, 1946a,b, 1976) was largely based upon the response-based model of stress.

The transactional model

A behavioural model of stress that incorporates a dynamic view of the individual and their interaction with the stress in their environment is called a transactional model. The person appraises, or seeks meaning in, what is perceived to be a potentially threatening situation in an attempt to respond in a way that minimises the distress. The process of appraisal is highly individual; each person will perceive a threatening situation differently and attach their own meanings to it (Lazarus & Folkman 1984). Moreover, the relationship between the individual and their environment is a dynamic one which constantly changes as the process of appraisal continues.

Nursing application. Case History 17.2 highlights how the transactional model of stress has clear advantages for the clinical nurse. Although Mr P's feeling of terror was related to the stressor of being in hospital and the prospect of surgery, these circumstances in themselves did not fully account for his state of mind. His feeling of stress derived from his appraisal of the situation, and this appraisal reflected his childhood experience. The transactional model

CASE HISTORY 17.2
Mr P

Nurse T was asked to interview Mr P on his admission to the ward for minor dental surgery the following day. Mr P, a 30-year-old engineer, was married and had two children, a girl and a boy. He lived with his family near the hospital and worked in a factory in a nearby town. During the interview, Nurse T noticed that while Mr P appeared to be in good health and to have a clear understanding of the surgery he was about to undergo, he seemed uneasy. Knowing that many patients feel apprehensive before having surgery, she asked him how he was feeling. Mr P replied: 'I feel silly, stupid and embarrassed about it but I am very scared — have been since I got the appointment in the post — can't understand why! I haven't been able to sleep for the past week and when I do I have awful dreams.'

The nurse talked further with Mr P about his feeling of fear. She asked him if he had ever been in hospital before and he recalled with some difficulty how, as a small child, he had been admitted as an emergency for a circumcision. As he talked he realised how frightened he had been at that time and that when he had been readmitted for an inflamed wound, his fear had become even greater. He remembered that his mother had been unable to stay with him.

The following day Mr P had his surgery. Before leaving the ward he said to Nurse T that he had felt better after talking with her. He had still felt afraid but the powerful feeling of terror had gone.

of stress recognises that a person such as Mr P, rather than being a passive recipient of stress, interacts actively with a situation.

Cox's man–environment model

Cox et al (2002) defined five stages within a man–environment model:

1. Source of demand where a situation is perceived as threatening
2. The individual's perception of demand, and coping based upon personality and early experiences
3. Psychophysiological changes in response to the perceived threat
4. Coping responses and consequences, i.e. how the individual sets about dealing with the threat
5. Feedback, both physiological and psychological.

The 'demand' is described as arising from the individual's psychological and physiological needs. The individual attempts to understand the demand and their ability to do this determines the way they set about coping. Stress may occur at a time of hopelessness, when the person understands the nature of the threat but is unable to respond in a way that diminishes or removes it. At this time, physiological responses also become active as methods of coping with stress. At each stage of the model, the individual receives evaluative feedback.

Limitations of the model. Given the complexity of individual experiences and coping strategies, it is extremely difficult to subject transactional models of stress, such as Cox's man–environment model, to empirical evaluation.

STOP THINK **17.2** Discuss with your lecturer or mentor how the terms 'stress' and 'stressor' are used differently within various models of stress.

The role of appraisal

How individuals appraise, or find meaning in adversity, is crucial to how they withstand it. The concept of resilience (see p. 700) may explain why some people, e.g. patients with cancer or AIDS (Polk 1997), can withstand and survive the adversity whilst others cannot. Appraisal is crucial to the individual's ability to continue a healthy life after catastrophe or illness, and, as with resilience, the personal traits of the individual will influence their ability to find meaning in what is happening to them.

Appraisal then becomes an interpretative process involving perception, intuition and reason, by which the person feeling stressed distinguishes between safe and threatening situations. While not all situations involving feelings of stress are severe, it is worth remembering that people experiencing stress may be 'in extremis' or very seriously ill. The cognitive process of appraisal as described here may, in fact, be a spontaneous emotional reaction rather than a well thought-out process.

People are unique in their experiences and personalities, and because no two people, and no two situations, are exactly the same, the appraisal will be about the meaning that the person finds within the circumstances.

The phenomenological approach

Phenomenological approaches to knowledge emphasise the importance of the object as it appears within a context, rather than the object in itself. Thus a phenomenological approach to stress rests largely upon the description given by the individual of their own experience of stress. The writings of phenomenological philosophers such as Merleau-Ponty and Heidegger describe human experience as 'being-in-the-world' whereby each person is defined by their own thoughts, feelings, memories, relationships and social settings. Mind and body are not described as separate but as one integral whole (Benner & Wrubel 1989). This topic is further examined under psychosomatic problems (see p. 701). The body is the physical means of knowing and sensing the world and, with disablement or disease, the experience of the person will be impaired (Benner & Wrubel 1989). Whether the impairment is of the mind or the body, the whole experience of the person will be affected.

This view of human experience invites the nurse to use an intuitive approach when working with people who are distressed, because it acknowledges the complexity of individual responses, and recognises that providing the right kind of help is, similarly, a complex and subtle task.

Case History 17.3 underlines the fact that a solution to a problem which may seem reasonable to one person may present insuperable difficulties to another. In order to understand Nurse R's rejection of the suggested option, Nurse D would need to know more about why R overeats. If it were possible to ask R about her feelings, she might offer one or more reasons for her behaviour. For instance:

- she may feel anxious and unhappy as a student and feel reassured when she eats sweet foods

CASE HISTORY 17.3

D and R

D, a student nurse, notices at mealtimes that her colleague R often mentions her distressed feelings about her weight. Knowing that she frequently eats sweets and cakes, D suggests to her that all she would need to do to lose weight would be to stop eating between meals. R, however, rejects this option as being too difficult to carry through.

- she may have started overeating as a child at a time of family distress
- she may have been abused as a child
- she may feel sexually unattractive and find eating a means of gaining consolation
- she may feel constantly hungry.

Nursing application The description of human experience from a phenomenological viewpoint attributes to the person a wisdom about themselves and their problems that cannot easily be gained from an 'objective' position (Benner & Wrubel 1989). But does this mean that the nurse is merely a passive observer when working with distressed people? If suggestions and advice cannot be offered in any but the most uncomplicated situations, then what help can be offered?

The most effective help that can be given by the clinical nurse is support in enabling the person to identify what is causing their stress and to deal with it in their own way. This does not entail the nurse, however subtly, suggesting what they think the patient should do. Rather, it involves being aware and respectful of the person's right to choose what they feel is appropriate for them. This is not a passive position for the nurse to take but is a highly interactive and enabling one (Rogers 1974, Egan 1997, Kennedy & Charles 2002).

In Case History 17.4, L, a health visitor, does not attempt to deal with the situation by taking action or giving suggestions, even though her concern that Mrs H had not eaten or moved for some time might have prompted her to do so. L's support and concern do, however, enable Mrs H to talk about how she feels and then to accept help in dealing with the body of her cat.

This example also underlines a further facet of stress, i.e. that people often experience stress when they are not themselves being threatened. Stress can arise as an empathic response through the perception of the stress experienced by another. When L perceives the intense distress of her client, she too may experience that distress.

Phenomenology, appraisal and the role of stress

In a sense, all appraisal is phenomenological, because it rests upon the individual's own attribution of meaning to a situation (Lazarus & Folkman 1984). Personality can, however, play a large part in determining what features of their environment an individual attends to, and what they attend to is a feature of the meaning that a situation has for them (Lazarus & Folkman 1984, Benner & Wrubel 1989). Rather than describing the individual as 'appraising' a situation, however, Benner and Wrubel (1989) prefer to speak of the person 'being in' a situation. They emphasise that the

CASE HISTORY 17.4

Mrs H

L has been an experienced health visitor for a number of years, working with a general practice in a rural area. She had been visiting Mrs H for a year or two and had been alerted by the home help to the possibility that Mrs H was not eating as regularly as she ought. Mrs H was 84 years old and had lived alone for 20 years, since her husband died. She had always been fiercely independent, but her home help telephoned on Thursday morning to ask if Mrs H could be visited urgently.

When L arrived she found Mrs H sitting in her kitchen with her elderly cat on her lap. It was apparent that the cat had died. Mrs H's home help thought that she had been sitting with her cat throughout the night and was worried that she had not eaten or moved. L did not know what to do and so sat quietly beside Mrs H for some time. She felt it would somehow be wrong to try to separate her from her lifelong friend.

After a while, Mrs H and L talked quietly about her cat and how he had become ill and died during the night. Mrs H said that she did not know whether she would be able to live without him. Much later, however, she agreed to put the cat out in the garden and allowed a neighbour to come and bury him. When the village heard what had occurred, many people came forward to give Mrs H sympathetic support and to keep her company.

attribution of meaning to a situation is unique for every individual, even though many people's interpretations appear to coincide. Taking this even further, they argue that there are no situations with an objective reality beyond the highly individual interpretations that are put upon them.

For Benner and Wrubel (1989), stress is woven into the fabric of our 'being in the world' and is not 'out there' to be dealt with. From this point of view, it would be harmful to suppress painful emotions, as these assist us in our interpretations of the world. Emotions such as anger or guilt give guidance to people about what is happening to them in the world. To teach people to relax may give them some short respite from painful tension until they are ready to confront their problems again and may be useful for this reason, but to teach relaxation as a way of dealing with problems may be misguided. Stress is part of the person's self, their concerns, thoughts, feelings about the past and future, memories and relationships to others and to objects.

The concept of resilience

An interesting and developing concept for nurses is that of resilience in individuals, which enables them to 'spring back' following distressing events (Jacelon 1997). The research indicates that people who can spring back have a constellation of personality traits such as above-average intelligence, interest in life, a positive outlook and flexibility. Those who can visualise their own future are also more likely to be resilient.

The notion of resilience as a process is less well researched, although nurses will recognise the individual learning and change described by Polk (1997) as 'survival, recovery and rehabilitation'. Those able to undergo this process are more likely to be members of social groups, to have friends and family, hope and the ability to find meaning and purpose in their experience of life.

Box 17.3

Physical and mental factors associated with stress

- Headaches
- Altered bowel function
- Insomnia
- Recurrent fatigue
- Depression
- Anxiety
- Reduced self-esteem
- Poor concentration

The important thing to be learned from this research for nurses working clinically is how to identify ways to enable those without the personality traits or social systems in place (Dewar & Morse 1995) to be helped towards rehabilitation, education and consolation.

STOP THINK **17.3** What are the developmental aspects of a person's life that create a more resilient personality?

For further information on the concept of resilience, see Jacelon (1997).

STRESS AND DISEASE

Research has shown that stress can be a contributory factor in disease presentation. There are several physical and mental factors which are commonly associated with stress. These are listed in Box 17.3.

A relatively new area of behavioural medicine, psychoimmunology, looks at how the body's immune system is affected by psychological factors, such as stress. It is well recognised that heart disease and duodenal ulcer may result from excessive stress and psychoimmunologists believe that many other diseases may result from an impaired immune system's ability to deal with stress. These include inflammatory bowel disease, cancer, allergies and arthritic disorders, all of which may be related in some way to the body's inability to defend itself from stress.

In the following section the role of stress in several common disorders is examined.

PSYCHOSOMATIC PROBLEMS

The term psychosomatic means mind ('psyche') and body ('soma'). A psychosomatic disorder is one which therefore involves both mind and body. Most disorders do involve both the mind and the body; however, the term psychosomatic disorder is mainly used to mean 'a physical disease which is thought to be caused, or made worse, by psychological factors'. Some physical diseases are thought to be particularly prone to be worsened by factors such as stress, e.g. irritable bowel syndrome (IBS), psoriasis, eczema, peptic ulcer, hypertension and heart disease. It is thought that the physical element of the illness, e.g. the extent of a rash, the level of the blood pressure, can be affected by psychological factors.

It is well known that the mind can cause physical symptoms. For example, when we are afraid or anxious we may develop a fast heart rate, a tremor, nausea, fast breathing, sweating, dry mouth, chest pain, headaches and a 'knot in the stomach'. These physical symptoms are due to an 'overdrive' of nervous impulses sent from the brain to various parts of the body, and to the release of adrenaline into the bloodstream. When physical symptoms are caused by mental or emotional stress it is called 'somatisation'. For example, many people have occasional headaches caused by mental stress. The tension headache is due to increased tone of muscles of the neck and the scalp. However, stress can cause many other physical symptoms such as tiredness, dizziness, back pain, diarrhoea and, in women, dysmenorrhoea. The somatic symptoms due to anxiety result from enhanced activity of the autonomic nervous system. Psychogenic factors may produce muscle tension and pain. This autonomic nervous overactivity may manifest itself in several bodily systems, including, as illustrated below, the gastrointestinal system.

Anxiety attacks

As previously noted, a certain amount of anxiety and stress is a vital and healthy adaptation mechanism. In a moderate and appropriate degree, stress arouses and alerts us, improving mental and physical activity and helping us to perform better, for example in interviews, or enabling us to avoid dangerous situations.

Anxiety or panic attacks are characterised by severe sympathetic arousal, often in the absence of any obvious or immediate stressor. Panic attacks are a common presenting problem in those visiting their general practitioner (GP) with feelings of stress. During an attack, the person often experiences intense fear, accompanied by physiological signs such as palpitations, sweating, trembling, rapid respiration and pallor. The fear may be associated with a fear of collapse, death or a need to escape. Sufferers often explain they feel that their heart might burst.

By explaining the nature of these attacks, the nurse can sometimes bring an element of relief to the sufferer. It is true that the circularity of being afraid of the fear often intensifies the symptoms. Practical advice on the management of attacks is also helpful (see Case History 17.5).

Anxiety attacks are symptomatic of underlying distress. They can be acute and of rapid onset, occurring perhaps only once or twice, or can develop into a chronic symptom. Attacks may occur at any time, causing intense feelings of fear where there is no obvious cause, such as fear or discomfort in a centre seat at the cinema or on a bus. The stressor causing the attack may only become apparent, if at all, upon later introspection or therapy.

There is increasing evidence that complementary and alternative therapies can be helpful for stress-related symptoms and anxiety and depression. They can be used either alongside conventional medication-based treatment, i.e. complementary therapy, or instead of it, i.e. alternative therapy. Many of these therapies arguably have fewer side-effects than medication (Kessler et al 2001).

Post-traumatic stress disorder

This condition, which has been recognised for many years, can affect people who have experienced any serious

CASE HISTORY 17.5

Midwifery Sister B

Midwifery Sister B had been working very hard in her new post in the labour suite and she discussed with her colleagues her feeling of apprehension that she might make a mistake or be unable to deal with the management responsibility that her new post entailed. The suite was often understaffed, and although she realised that this was not her responsibility, she felt guilty about the demands it placed upon her colleagues. On her night off she went with one or two friends to a pub and, although she had not drunk a great deal, she knew that she had exceeded her usual limit.

The following morning she awoke with a feeling of unease that she found difficult to describe. She experienced something like a feeling of agitation but her skin also felt as if it were 'crawling'. She had planned to go for a walk with her friends but, when she reached the park where she was to meet them, the feeling she had experienced throughout the morning became much more intense. She became sweaty, had great difficulty in breathing and felt very afraid. Feeling her pulse, she realised that her heart was beating very fast. Sister B later described her fear that she might collapse and die during this attack. This feeling lasted for 10 min. Her friends took her home, and later she contacted her family doctor.

This episode was described by the doctor, following some routine investigations, as an anxiety attack. He explained what had happened physiologically and was able to offer reassurance. He suggested that she either attend a stress reduction workshop or talk to a counsellor, and reduce her coffee and alcohol consumption. After Sister B had taken the opportunity to talk about her fears and problems with a counsellor, she felt more able to deal with her new job. She noticed, however, that when she began to feel tired and worried, the physical signs of sweating and palpitation would re-emerge. She used this as an indication that she needed a rest. Sister B also noticed that alcohol exacerbated the problem, as it had during her first attack.

Box 17.4

Migraine phases

Migraine attacks follow a pattern consisting of the five phases described below (Blau 1987). The third and fourth phases are prerequisites of a diagnosis of classical migraine.

1. **Prodrome**
   - Subtle symptoms; may not be noticed
   - Craving to eat sweet food
   - Mood variations
   - Tiredness
   - Mild photophobia
   - Heightened visual perception
2. **Aura**
   - Multicoloured visual disturbances
   - Scotoma with flickering, scintillating edge
   - Tingling of face, sometimes one sided
   - Numbness of face
3. **Headache**
   - Slowly developing throbbing pain
   - Lasts 2–72 h
4. **Resolution**
   - Sleep is major resolving mechanism
   - Vomiting
5. **Postdromal phase**
   - 'Washed-out' or drained feeling
   - Euphoria
   - Impaired concentration
   - Irritability
   - Cerebral flow observations indicate that anomalies can outlast headache by 24 h

accident or trauma outside the range of their normal experience, such as a severe road traffic accident, rape, physical attack, 'plane crash, bomb blast, war or terrorist attack. The disorder can follow one or more of such events and can occur not only in those directly involved but also in those called to assist, such as emergency workers or onlookers. The greater the scale of the incident, the more likely it is for post-traumatic stress disorder to arise.

The person, having escaped adversity and perhaps having a sense of relief at having escaped relatively unharmed, can be very perplexed at the occurrence of distressing symptoms, sometimes a considerable time after the event. There may be a loss of memory and total amnesia and sufferers often report feeling mentally numbed (Mckinley & Brooks 1991, Fagan & Freme 2004). Symptoms may include:

- mood swings and feelings of aggression
- feelings of alarm, anxiety and irritability
- feeling jumpy
- flashbacks to the original trauma that leave the person feeling as though they were back in the traumatic situation
- loss of interest in pleasurable events
- phobic and depressed feelings, panic
- sleep disturbances, e.g.
  — waking in alarm and unable to return to sleep
  — difficulty in getting to sleep
  — early morning waking
  — distressing nightmares
  — night sweats.

Migraine/headache

Migraine headaches have been known about for well over 2000 years and it is estimated that they are experienced by 10% of the population. Changes in the size of blood vessels and the levels of neurotransmitter substances are thought to be responsible for migraine headaches. It is recognised that they are not caused solely by stress but have a number of precipitating factors such as menstrual cycle, diet, dehydration and certain sounds and smells which, in conjunction with a feeling of stress, may trigger an attack. Many people report that the attack, paradoxically, occurs after the cessation of the stressful event.

For many people, migraine is a very debilitating and distressing condition. An analogy is of a storm building up and causing, instead of lightning, wind and rain, intense pain, nausea and vomiting, often lasting for several hours. The person is often prevented from continuing with normal activities. The phases of an attack are outlined in Box 17.4.

Physiologically, the hypothesis put forward to explain migraine (Blau 1987) is that stress causes cerebral hypoxia through increased activity in catecholamine pathways. This suggestion is supported by the observation that cerebral

Box 17.5

Symptoms associated with chronic fatigue syndrome

- Substantial impairment in short-term memory or concentration
- Sore throat
- Tender lymph nodes
- Muscle pain
- Multi-joint pain without swelling or redness
- Headaches of a new type, pattern or severity
- Poor sleep
- Post-exertional malaise lasting more than 24 h

Based on data from Sharpe & Wilks (2002) and Aylett & Fawcett (2003).

oxygen consumption rises when the individual is stressed. The role of the catecholamines — adrenaline, noradrenaline and dopamine — is to activate the cerebral metabolism. If the nerve fibres penetrate deeply enough into the brain, the sympathetic nervous system could release noradrenaline and increase neuronal metabolism in the surrounding tissue. In this hypothesis, stress increases cerebral metabolism, thereby increasing the risk of migraine.

Interventions

The person should, if possible, identify any trigger factors of their migraine attacks and avoid them. The pain can be treated with analgesics in conjunction with metoclopramide for the nausea; the latter will also improve the uptake of the analgesic from the intestine. Complementary therapies commonly used for the management of migraine/headache include acupuncture, osteopathy, relaxation therapy and homeopathy.

For further information, see Cunningham (1999).

Chronic fatigue syndrome (myalgic encephalomyelitis)

Chronic fatigue syndrome (CFS) is characterised by protracted periods of fatigue associated with a wide range of accompanying symptoms (see Box 17.5).

The symptoms of this puzzling illness, which is also referred to as myalgic encephalomyelitis, include extreme muscle fatigue, poor memory and concentration and slips of the tongue (Aylett & Fawcett 2003). This condition can cause considerable distress and disability over a period of months and sometimes years. The individual may, with devastating consequences, be unable to continue full- or even part-time work or may be forced to take frequent periods of sick leave. This and other implications of the illness can cause stress to loved ones and adversely affect the well-being of the family as a whole.

Fatigue and depression as sequelae to infection have long been recognised, particularly in relation to Epstein–Barr, Coxsackie and other enteroviruses. It is important, however, that postviral fatigue syndrome is not mistaken for psychiatric illness (Sharpe & Wilks 2002). Even today, not all GPs recognise postviral fatigue as a medical condition (CFS/ME Working Group 2002).

Some health professionals advise rest, while others, recognising the adverse effects of long-term inactivity, advise exercise. Good emotional support is vital, and it is most important that depression, where present, is treated. Other treatments are aimed at the detection of possible allergies and/or candidiasis and at maintaining a good diet.

Many patients who are able to undertake a modest amount of exercise report some improvement in symptoms. Conventional treatment approaches to CSF/ME include the prescription of antidepressant medication to promote sleep, and anti-inflammatory medication, i.e. aspirin and ibuprofen, may be prescribed to reduce muscular aches and pains. Complementary therapies are sought by many patients who do not find improvement or look to enhance the improvement from conventional medicines. Despite limited scientific evidence, herbal remedies, acupuncture, osteopathy and aromatherapy are widely used for the management of chronic fatigue syndrome.

Irritable bowel syndrome (IBS)

Stressful life events have long been associated with the development of IBS. IBS is a common functional disorder characterised by abdominal pain and altered bowel function. Although IBS is not life threatening, for many patients it can have a serious impact upon their daily activities and health-related quality of life. There are several factors which can trigger attacks of IBS in some people, e.g. work stress and examinations.

People with anxious (neurotic) personality traits may find symptoms difficult to control. The relationship between the mind, brain, nervous impulses and overactivity of internal organs such as the gut is complex (Lea & Whorwell 2003). Some patients have reported relaxation techniques, stress counselling, cognitive therapy and psychotherapy useful in controlling symptoms. Complementary therapies are also commonly employed in the management of IBS, for example gut-directed hypnotherapy, acupuncture and homeopathy are all used with good effect (see Case History 17.6). Reducing chronic stress is an appropriate and highly achievable therapeutic goal in the management of IBS (Smith 2003).

CASE HISTORY 17.6

K

K is a 24-year-old primary school teacher who was diagnosed with irritable bowel syndrome (IBS) 3 years ago. On attending a gastrointestinal clinic she reports that important life-changing events, e.g. the recent breakdown of a relationship, have made her symptoms much worse. The anxiety over IBS symptoms causes stress, which worsens the symptoms and creates a vicious circle. K states, 'Because I have IBS, I spend a lot of my time worrying about whether or not the symptoms will affect me each day' and 'I am sure the stress of my boyfriend leaving me has made my IBS much worse!'. K is encouraged by the nurse to practise stress management techniques and has been referred for gut-directed hypnotherapy.

Depression

Depression is a psychological state of melancholy and dejection that can have physical symptoms. It is not the case that everyone who feels stressed also has depression or anxiety, but the illness can be the outcome of feelings of stress; conversely, people experiencing depression can also become stressed (Herbert 1997).

It is difficult to formulate an exact definition of depression and its relationship to stress. The experience of depression seems to range from unpleasant but normal feelings of being 'fed up' to severe states of mental ill-health requiring psychiatric intervention. It is important to recognise that clinical depression, which is a serious mental illness, can be life threatening, as suicide and self-harm are frequent outcomes in severe depression. It is vital for health professionals to be alert to this possibility.

Houston et al (2003) argue that the GP, in particular, can play a major role in the detection and treatment of depression and in the after-care of patients who deliberately self-harm, as can the community psychiatric nurse (CPN).

Symptoms of depression

The presence of depression is often not obvious to the nurse, as observable signs do not always indicate the unpleasantness of the feelings that the individual is experiencing. Some symptoms, however, particularly when they occur in combination, strongly indicate the presence of depression, for example early morning wakening, a feeling of grinding tiredness, loss of energy, loss of interest in sexual relationships, loss of appetite, feeling 'down' and a feeling of bad temper. The link between anxiety and depression is debatable, but if this division is dispensed with, the list of potential symptoms of depression might, arguably, be expanded to include panic or anxiety attacks.

Feelings associated with depression

The relationship between stress and depression is an extremely close one. Some people experiencing depression feel stressed by, amongst other things, their inability to continue with day-to-day activities. Others, who are burdened by overwhelming demands, respond by becoming depressed. What is not understood is why some people respond to stress by becoming depressed whilst others show other emotions such as anger.

People experiencing depression often describe their circumstances in terms that denote an ongoing feeling of oppression, as of being under a cloud, of everything looking black or grey, or of being in a tunnel without an end. Feelings of hope diminish, to be replaced by feelings of hopelessness. They often feel uncared for and alone even when this is not the case. Undertaking tasks or projects often becomes impossible as inertia takes the place of activity. Depressed individuals often blame themselves for problems in their relationships or daily lives, where others who are not depressed might show anger. This leads to the hypothesis that depression is anger turned in on itself when for some reason it cannot be expressed openly (Freud 1917, Worden 2002).

Causes of depression

Depression can occur at any time in life and may follow on from any painful event or loss, such as the death of a loved one or the loss of a job. Depression which, when it occurs in adulthood, does not have an obvious cause, may be the result of early childhood loss or distress. Individuals who have been the victims of sexual, physical or emotional abuse as children may suffer depression as adults in a delayed response to the loss associated with abuse, which is triggered by a more recent experience of distress. Early unresolved loss has been suggested as a possible explanation for the distressing symptoms of depression following childbirth. Depression may also be triggered by the lack of light and sunlight exposure during the winter months, known as seasonal affective disorder (SAD). Conventional medical approaches for moderate to severe depression often require anti-depressant medication. In milder cases of depression, counselling and psychotherapy may be helpful, in conjunction with lifestyle, exercise and dietary advice. Complementary therapies can be used in the treatment and prevention of depression (see Box 17.6).

COPING

The concept of coping

Used in a neutral sense, the term 'coping' refers to the way in which the individual responds to a stressful situation or to the perception of threat, by attempting consciously and unconsciously to maintain an equilibrium. It is revealing, however, to reflect upon everyday usage of the word, as it can be a value-laden term, used in intrinsically judgemental descriptions of an individual's degree of mastery over a situation or environment. Consider the degree of approval or disapproval that might be implied in the following statements:

- 'She coped well in her first managerial position.'
- 'She cannot cope.'

Box 17.6

Complementary therapies used in the treatment of depression

- *Psychological therapies* — cognitive behavioural therapy and relaxation training.
- *Acupuncture* — traditional acupuncture treatment or electroacupuncture can ease depression. Some studies found this to be superior to antidepressant medication and with fewer side-effects.
- *Homeopathy* — various remedies may help. The remedy ignatia is often used to ease grief, pulsatilla may relieve tearfulness, sulphur is often indicated for despair and aurum metallicum, a natural mineral derived from gold, is used for suicidal feelings.
- *Herbal medicine* — the herb St John's wort (*Hypericum perforatum*) has been clinically proven to relieve mild or moderate depression.
- *Reflexology, meditation and yoga* — these have also been used in the treatment of depression but have not yet been tested by research.
- *Light therapy* — exposure to bright light and the use of light boxes can help people suffering from seasonal affective disorder (SAD).

- 'He finds it difficult to cope with exams.'
- 'He couldn't cope with the patient's relatives.'

The association of 'coping' with mastery and of 'failure to cope' with weakness should not be automatic. It may be the case that the individual who succumbs to feelings of stress is more able to sense tension in a situation than the person who gives the appearance of coping well. The person who effects their removal from a situation may in fact be 'coping' with it, by acknowledging that distancing or disengagement is the best way, in the circumstances, to preserve emotional health or physical safety. In some situations, the determination to persevere or to achieve mastery may be a damaging choice, ending in disease.

Different situations demand different strategies for coping. In some cases the individual may need to confront a difficulty or overcome an obstacle. In other circumstances, the person must learn how to carry on with their life in the face of an ongoing situation such as bereavement, disability or unemployment. What 'coping' entails will depend upon the individual's unique circumstances and needs, and various models such as resilience and hardiness have been put forward in an attempt to identify the factors that contribute to an individual's style of coping.

Models of coping

An understanding of the models of coping can enhance the ability of the nurse to care compassionately for patients who are experiencing stress.

One of the well-known approaches to the concept of coping focuses on the role of personality in the individual's response to stressful events and identifies 'Type A' behaviour (see below) which characterises the individual as being particularly susceptible to the health risks associated with stress. An alternative and influential approach which discusses coping within the context of stress, burnout, support and hardiness, is found in Kobasa's (1979) seminal attempts to identify those who are particularly resilient, i.e. who exhibit hardiness under stress (Duquette et al 1995). Those with hardiness have a sense of personal achievement and are less likely to have physical or psychological symptoms, and are less likely to become emotionally exhausted (Dillard 1990). This concept has many similarities to that of resilience.

Some models describe coping in terms of palliation strategies. For example, strategies that may be sought by those experiencing the early stages of burnout are exercise, relaxation, prescribed medication, drug abuse, smoking and alcohol consumption. Other models describe coping in terms of problem solving, or, as in Lazarus' (1966) approach, in terms of a dynamic process by which the individual engages with the source of the stress. It is also possible to discuss coping in terms of defence mechanisms that individuals employ to preserve themselves from a perceived threat.

Coping and personality

Some people appear to be relatively unaffected by traumatic events, while others seem to be quite unable to withstand what might appear to the onlooker to be minor upheavals. Researchers have attempted to identify individuals who are more likely than others to cope effectively with stress, by isolating relatively stable and highly consistent inborn dispositions or traits which enable the individual to function well in difficult situations. Such traits may be related to, for example, conformity or non-conformity, conscientiousness, compulsive behaviour, or the ability to suppress, repress or sublimate feelings.

Type A behaviour patterns. Extensive research into the question of whether there are certain people who experience stress more acutely than others, and who are more likely to succumb to cardiac or circulatory disease as a result, has identified a 'Type A' individual who is at particular risk from the effects of stress. Type A behaviour is not, strictly speaking, a trait; traits are by definition inborn, whereas Type A behaviour appears to be learned by social modelling. Those with Type A behaviour both wish to achieve and are high achievers (Westra & Kuiper 1997) and are more likely to have a job-centred lifestyle than one based upon interpersonal contacts with others (Fukunishi & Hattori 1997). Type A behaviour seems to have very positive short-term consequences; for example, in business or other organisations, people who show involvement, drive and initiative are often highly valued. However, O'Connor et al (1995) and Miller et al (1996) consider that this behaviour may be linked to suppressed feelings of hostility and anger, which confer different cardiovascular disease risks. The long-term consequences of Type A behaviour, however, are often negative. The Type A person is typically observed engaged in polyphasic activity, concurrently undertaking a number of tasks. Other characteristics associated with Type A individuals include time urgency, impatience, desire for control and aggression. The following interrelated elements are present in Type A behaviour patterns:

- a set of beliefs about oneself in relation to the world
- a set of values which merge with motivation and commitment
- a set of beliefs about lifestyle that are focused upon achievement and control.

Type A individuals invest a great deal of themselves in their lifestyle and expend a great deal of energy in maintaining control. When challenged, their response is often highly emotional and this is likely to stimulate frequent surges of catecholamine secretion, which can induce, in the physically unhealthy person, coronary heart disease. They often show signs of raised serum cholesterol levels, raised serum fats and diabetic-like traits; at the same time they are frequently smokers who do not have time for regular exercise. Understandably, Type A behaviour is often destructive to relationships with family members, friends or colleagues.

It is important to bear in mind that people can change their learned behaviours and improve their ability to cope with certain experiences. In addition, there can be some degree of habituation to stressors such that they seem less stressful over time.

Personality and health Kobasa (1979) examined the mediating effects of personality, not in relation to stress and disease, but in relation to stress and health. Whilst much research effort had been directed towards understanding the role of mediators such as early childhood influences, physiological predisposition and social resources in relation to the onset of disease, Kobasa (1979) asked why some people can be under considerable stress but not become ill. Using the social readjustment rating scale (Holmes & Rahe 1967), she tested the following hypotheses:

- People who have a greater sense of control over their own lives will remain healthier than those with a sense of powerlessness.
- People who have a sense of commitment to various areas of their lives will be healthier than those who have a sense of alienation.
- People who view change as a challenge will remain healthier than those who view change as a threat.

Kobasa (1979) postulated a state of hardiness in the personalities of those who can be stressed without becoming ill. The hardy person has certain characteristics, including:

- a clear sense of self and of personal meaning
- an understanding of values, goals and capabilities and a belief in their importance
- a vigorous involvement in and commitment to their own environment
- an internal locus of control
- active involvement in change.

Klag & Bradley (2004) critique Kobasa's findings and examine the concept of hardiness in stress and illness.

The process model of coping

Lazarus and Folkman (1984) described coping in terms of a dynamic process involving movement, force and energy within the individual and their relationship with the source of stress. An important feature of the process approach is that it reflects the fact, often observed in clinical settings, that an individual's response to their situation changes and evolves over time. This response is highly complex and unique to each individual and might be described as occurring in stages, although these stages are not sequential or predictable.

Worden (2002), for example, describes four tasks of mourning that the individual must complete in order to emerge from a state of grief:

- accepting the reality of the loss
- experiencing the pain of grief
- adjusting to an environment from which the deceased is missing
- withdrawing emotional energy and reinvesting it in another relationship.

For the individual, these tasks of mourning may not be sequential, but may be experienced instead as an 'ebb and flow' of feelings. For the nurse, Worden's definition of the tasks of grieving will give an indication of the direction that a person might take in their mourning. For the individual concerned, the stages passed through might be recognised only in hindsight.

The process approach emphasises that the individual copes with stress in a unique way that is governed by both childhood and adult experiences. The ability to cope is shaped by the developmental processes that the individual undergoes from birth to death. The individual's perspective will change continually, and situations that may be stressful at one time may be viewed differently at another stage of life.

PSYCHOLOGICAL DEFENCES

While it is possible to think of defence mechanisms as both conscious and unconscious strategies of self-protection against perceived threat, these mechanisms may seriously compromise the effective functioning of the individual. Defence mechanisms operate essentially by restricting situations which are seen as threatening, narrowing down the individual's field of action to one that is manageable. They enable the individual, often against overwhelming odds, to maintain an equilibrium of feelings, thoughts and actions in daily life.

Problems arise when they feature inappropriately, as when a defence mechanism first acquired to combat severe or terrifying feelings in one domain becomes active without cause in another, perpetuating the emotional disturbance that gave rise to the mechanism in the first place. This may occur some time after the original experience, and the content of that experience may not be accessible to the person even after therapy. While it is useful for the clinician to bear in mind that unresolved conflict may exist, the detailed and often long-term task of helping the person to understand the extent of their defences is best left to therapists and counsellors.

Defences may be compared to a sea wall, in that the magnitude of the original intense fear and distress will determine the height, breadth and depth of the defence. These defences are not always infallible, however; they can be breached during sleep, under the influence of alcohol and other medications, and in conditions of stress.

A number of defence mechanisms have been identified, the most common of which are listed in Box 17.7.

MANAGEMENT OF STRESS

Effective stress management techniques can prevent stress-related ailments, boost vitality and improve quality of life. The management of stress can be approached in a number of ways (see Box 17.8).

One stress management technique often employed is to offer the individual the opportunity to examine the sources of their stress in present or past experience and to consider ways of modifying their responses to that stress. This therapy can be provided by a psychotherapist, clinical psychologist or qualified counsellor who may also be a nurse.

Some individuals suffering from acute anxiety or depression may find it impossible to confront the source of their difficulty and to make constructive changes without first being given some relief from their distressing feelings. Here, the carefully monitored use of appropriate medication, described on pages 708–709, can facilitate recovery and change. The individual suffering from stress can also learn a number of techniques that will assist them to reduce or manage their stress in day-to-day life. The role of complementary therapies in stress management is examined in the next section.

Techniques such as relaxation, yoga, biofeedback, visualisation and meditation have all gained in credibility and

Box 17.7

Defence mechanisms

Repression
Unconsciously keeping unacceptable feelings out of awareness. Not acknowledging angry or jealous feelings towards others.

Disavowal or denial
Blocking a perception from memory. Someone whose father left the family at birth may unconsciously think of him as having died rather than confront the feelings of loss and anger.

Projection
Unconsciously attributing to others their own aggressive or angry feelings. The feeling that one is being 'got at' by a colleague may be a projection of one's own angry negative feelings towards the colleague.

Introjection
Accepting another's values and opinions as one's own. A young person living with a domineering parent may unconsciously accept the attitudes of the parent rather than risk confrontation.

Reversal
Detaching a feeling from the person or object to which it should be directed and directing it to oneself instead. A wish to physically harm another may instead become a process of self-harm.

Displacement
Directing strong feelings about another person towards someone less dangerous than the original source of the feeling, e.g. a child experiencing powerful and angry feelings towards a mother may punish a favourite doll instead.

Isolation
Detaching a feeling from a thought in order to deprive the thought of emotional significance. Nurses sometimes describe helping at the scene of an accident without being in touch with the experience of the associated feelings.

Reaction formation
Disguising feelings by repression of the real feeling and reinforcement of the opposite feeling. A husband caring for a disabled wife may feel angry at her dependence, but instead shower her with loving attention.

Rationalisation
Finding false reasons to justify unacceptable attitudes. Following the termination of an employment contract, a person might claim to be pleased to be no longer employed, rather than acknowledge painful feelings of worthlessness.

Conversion
Converting a psychological disturbance into a physical disorder. A feeling of panic or fear accompanied by physical symptoms may be regarded as physical symptoms alone by the person to unconsciously avoid confronting the cause.

Box 17.8

Stress management techniques

- *Deep breathing* — this means taking a long, slow breath in, and very slowly breathing out. If you do this a few times, and concentrate fully on breathing, you may find it quite relaxing.
- *Muscular tensing and stretching* — try twisting your neck around each way as far as is comfortable, and then relax. Try fully tensing your shoulder and back muscles for several seconds, and then relax completely.
- *Improve your diet* — reduce caffeine, nicotine, junk foods and sugar, and increase whole grains, vegetables, fruit and water.
- *Vitamins and minerals* — stress puts added strain on the liver and nervous system. To strengthen these, boost intake of B vitamins, vitamin C, zinc and magnesium.
- *List major stresses* and consider solutions or lifestyle changes for each. Prioritise, practise time management and learn to delegate and say, 'No'.
- *Make time for rest and relaxation* and time for yourself on a regular basis.
- *Take regular exercise* to relieve stress and stimulate endorphin production, which has a relaxing effect.

Adapted from the Stress Management Society.

popularity in recent years. When taught well and followed up with continuing support, courses in such techniques can help people to adopt a new approach to the problem of stress. Moreover, learning a new skill such as deep relaxation can impart to the individual a feeling of well-being which may facilitate positive change in various areas of their life. However, it is important to note that if stress lies in the interaction between the person and their environment, or in the meaning they attribute to their situation, then clearly a short workshop on relaxation, for example, cannot hope to seriously address the source of their stress. Indeed, it should be borne in mind that there is a potential for courses in stress reduction to exacerbate the problem, if the individual is made to feel that any stress that is not helped by the techniques offered is intractable or somehow abnormal.

Counselling in stress

Counselling and psychotherapy aim to assist people to overcome the emotional barriers or psychological problems caused by stress and enable them to address their problems and make the life changes needed to improve their health and well-being.

Finding and choosing therapeutic help

There are a number of ways to find therapeutic help and various professional bodies for counselling and psychotherapy will give suggestions (see 'Useful websites', p. 713), although the availability of some types of psychotherapy will depend upon where in the UK the person seeking help lives. Whilst many people travel long distances to see a counsellor or psychotherapist, the regular nature of the consultations, which may be weekly, may cause an added burden if extensive travel is required.

If psychotherapeutic help is sought through the NHS, a referral can be made by the GP. Many departments of clinical psychology will accept self-referrals, but will ask the person if they may contact their GP. Where the therapy being sought is through the private sector, the person pays a fee for each consultation.

For therapy to be effective, it must respond to the person within their own frame of reference and be relevant to their own life from their own unique perspective. Finding an appropriate form of therapy can be very difficult for the individual, and many people are reluctant to approach a professional agency or voluntary organisation for assistance with personal problems. Many people think about it and wait for long periods before plucking up the courage to seek help, and often their first point of contact is with a member of the primary care team at their local surgery; this may be the GP, the practice nurse or another member of the primary care team, such as the health visitor or community psychiatric nurse. The practice nurse, or nurse practitioner undertaking screening programmes, is well placed to be able to listen to patients who are distressed (Cunningham 1996). Often, merely discussing the problem with a member of the practice team can provide considerable relief. However, when further help is required, the patient can be referred to the community mental health team, including, for example:

- the practice counsellor
- the community psychiatric nurse (CPN)
- a clinical psychologist
- the community psychiatrist.

The GP may also wish to discuss with the patient the possibility of prescribing antidepressants, but first will investigate whether the patient is suffering from a physical illness such as hyper- or hypothyroidism or anaemia which can cause symptoms similar to depression. Reassurance can be given that panic attacks are not life threatening and advice given on how to deal with them. The GP can also authorise official sick leave to enable the patient to rest.

The therapist–client relationship

People are highly individual in their feelings, experiences, backgrounds and personalities. A model of therapy which is helpful to one person may not suit another, and a therapist who is helpful to one person may fail to establish a good rapport with another. For this reason it is important for therapists to be clear with their clients about the way in which they work, what the work involves, its likely duration and, if private consultation is sought, its cost. It is possible for the client to change therapists if the therapy does not seem to be helpful, although there is one major proviso to this. For personal change to take place, therapist and client must work closely in a relationship of trust. This will enable the therapist to reflect back and challenge the behaviour that is causing the client distress. The fact that this can be an unsettling experience for the client may not be the right reason for them to abandon therapy. Nevertheless, the therapist should be willing to discuss any feeling on the client's part that the therapy is proving detrimental or unhelpful and, if appropriate, to give guidance on finding an alternative therapist.

The person wishing to become a therapist must undertake appropriate education, which involves the study of theory as well as undertaking supervised work with clients. Nurses working in clinical settings may undertake shortened courses which will help them to develop the necessary skills to listen in a therapeutic way to people in their daily work. An example of therapeutic listening is given in Case History 17.7.

CASE HISTORY 17.7

Mrs A

Mrs A cares for her cognitively and physically handicapped son, S, at home, with the help of the community nursing service and the local social work department. She is 68 years old and a widow; her son is 29. He is visually impaired and unable to communicate easily by speaking. He is always incontinent. Although he can walk, Mrs A always has to guide him. Getting him out of bed and dressed in the morning is very heavy work for her.

Mrs A has known her community nurse, N, for a number of years. N feels a sense of despair that Mrs A never has any freedom from S and has rarely had any time to herself in the years she has known her. N has tried repeatedly, both by herself and in conjunction with social work colleagues, to plan some respite care for S. This planning has taken the form of a provision for day care at a local day centre and periods of respite care at a local residential unit. But somehow, when the time came for S to attend, Mrs A managed to avoid sending him. The only assistance she will accept is from the local care attendant team; one helper, who has become a friend, sits with S for 2 hours while Mrs A does her shopping.

One day N was able to sit and talk with Mrs A whilst S was asleep. By listening carefully to her, N realised that Mrs A felt extremely guilty about S's handicap. She felt that she had caused S's condition by not taking sufficient rest during her pregnancy, and she relieved her feelings of guilt by caring for him all the time. She was also extremely fearful of what would happen to S after she died.

N continued to listen carefully to Mrs A as she talked about her painful feelings, and was aware that she had not been able to share these feelings with anyone before. She did not try to make Mrs A feel better by taking away her feelings of guilt, nor did she try to reassure her. Instead, she simply listened carefully and attentively.

They did not talk again about this problem, although N was ready to listen if Mrs A wished to raise the subject again. Some time later, however, Mrs A asked N if she could help her organise some day care for S, as it would help him to get used to other people. N was then able to arrange respite care for S, which Mrs A accepted and which also enabled her to get some rest.

Medication

The personal experience of stress can be so severe and overwhelming that the individual becomes unable to take any action to alleviate their feelings. Severe anxiety or depression, perhaps in combination with an overpowering feeling that a serious physical illness is lurking, can have an immobilising effect on the person so that even the prospect of action to alleviate symptoms is daunting. When people feel as severely distressed as this, they may begin to entertain thoughts of suicide.

Medication can help to alleviate severe distress by relieving its most acute symptoms and thus enabling emotional rest to take place. Some medications are intended to help with sleeplessness, while others which do not have a tranquillising effect will permit those taking them to continue to work, to problem-solve, to drive, and so on. Medication should always be supplemented by continued monitoring and support by the medical practitioner. The following provides a brief overview of the main types of medication used in the treatment of stress-related conditions.

Tricyclic and related antidepressants

The most common antidepressant medications used in severe stress and depression are the tricyclic and related groups. These are usually prescribed to people suffering from moderate to severe depression, although it is important to realise that they work by alleviating symptoms. This can be useful; for instance, the person who is debilitated by anxiety might be able to find ways of living that are more constructive once their feelings of anxiety are lifted. These medications may not be helpful, however, when the depression is related to bereavement, an unhappy working environment, overwhelming family responsibilities or disturbing memories of abuse or neglect, for it is only when the underlying cause of depression can be understood, and appropriately treated, that the person is likely to obtain any lasting benefit.

Management The person prescribed tricyclic antidepressants must be seen frequently following prescription as they may take 2–4 weeks before having an effect; during this time the patient may feel isolated and helpless. Side-effects include the following:

- constipation
- sleepiness
- dry mouth
- blurred vision
- urinary retention
- sweating.

Tolerance seems to develop over time and some of the side-effects become less apparent.

If the individual's depression is severe, they may feel suicidal. Careful support and perhaps hospitalisation may be essential at this time. Treatment with this group of medications should be continued for at least 1 month (BMA 2005). Reduction or withdrawal should be carried out very slowly to avoid severe symptoms such as strange, fragmented dreams, headaches, recurrence of anxiety, depression or restlessness.

Selective serotonin reuptake inhibitors (SSRIs)

Serotonin, also known as 5-hydroxytryptamine, is a substance widely distributed in body tissue. Serotonin participates in the transmission of nerve impulses and has a function in controlling mood. SSRIs block the reuptake of serotonin, producing an increase in the amount of the neurotransmitter at central synapses. Examples of commonly prescribed SSRIs for stress-related conditions are fluoxetine and paroxetine. In contrast to the tricyclic antidepressants, SSRIs have few antimuscarinic and anticholinergic effects, and cause little sedation or weight gain. They may, however, cause nausea, diarrhoea, insomnia and anorexia.

Benzodiazepines

The benzodiazepines are 'anxiolytics'. They act at a specific central nervous system receptor or by potentiating the action of inhibitory neurotransmitters to help calm patients and promote rest and sleep. They are therefore used to help treat, but not cure, the symptoms of anxiety, such as tension, tremor, sweating and disturbed thought processes.

However, this class of medication fell into disrepute when individuals who were taking the medication for extended periods of time found that their original symptoms were intensified and that the medication was addictive. It is now recommended that benzodiazepines are prescribed for periods not exceeding 2 or 3 weeks and under careful supervision (BMA 2005).

Monoamine oxidase inhibitors

Monoamine oxidase inhibitors (MAOIs) prevent the breakdown of monoamine neurotransmitters, thereby prolonging their action. Monoamines, which include noradrenaline and tyramine, play an important role in the metabolism of the brain. MAOIs are recommended for people with depression, anxiety and somatic complaints, for patients who do not respond to tricyclics and patients with agoraphobia. They are used less commonly than tricyclic antidepressants or SSRIs because of dangers of dietary and medication interactions.

Trazodone hydrochloride

This medication exhibits antiserotonin and α-receptor antagonist properties. Its sedative properties are useful in the treatment of anxiety.

Beta-adrenoceptor-blocking drugs

Beta-adrenoceptor-blocking drugs, also called beta-blockers, act by blocking the stimulation of beta-adrenergic receptors by the neurotransmitters adrenaline and noradrenaline. These are produced at the nerve endings of that part of the sympathetic nervous system which facilitates the body's reaction to anxiety, stress and exercise. Beta-blockers act to reduce anxiety and some physical symptoms, such as trembling, which are caused by a stress reaction. They are particularly useful for situational anxiety. For example, some musicians who become stressed take a beta-blocker to ease their shakiness before a concert performance.

Alcohol and stress

It is commonly believed that one way to cope with stress is to use alcohol. However, although alcohol may give short-term relief of stress, in the long run, it does not and drinking alcohol to 'calm nerves' is often a slippery slope to heavier and problem drinking. For most people who stay within the recommended drinking levels (see Ch. 36), alcohol can be an enjoyable aid to relaxation. However, the more an individual uses alcohol to relieve stress, the less effective it becomes. Eventually, more and more alcohol is required to achieve the desired effect of relaxation. The after-effects of alcohol may also increase feelings of anxiety and depression.

Other means of stress reduction

Complementary therapies

There is an increasing interest in complementary therapies in stress management. The five main complementary therapies are:

- acupuncture
- osteopathy
- chiropractice
- homeopathy
- herbal medicine.

Other well-known therapies include hypnotherapy, aromatherapy and massage, all of which are increasingly used in stress management. Complementary therapies focus on the whole person, with lifestyle, environment, diet, mental, emotional and spiritual health being considered alongside physical symptoms. Many complementary therapies are based on the belief that the body naturally strives to maintain homeostasis. Interventions aim to stimulate this natural healing ability. Taking responsibility for one's own health is regarded as an important part of healing, so clients are often actively involved in their own treatment. For example, self-hypnosis techniques are employed in hypnotherapy (Gonsalkorale et al 2002).

Exercise

Although there is strong research-based and anecdotal evidence that regular vigorous exercise has a positive effect upon the individual's ability to deal with feelings of depression and stress, the effects of exercise are not generally accepted or understood; for instance, those taking physical exercise may have considerable exposure to light and this may have a therapeutic effect upon feelings of depression (Groom & O'Connor 1996). There is, however, evidence that aerobic exercise may trigger panic attacks in those already experiencing them (Reif & Hermanutz 1996). Proponents of exercise, as a means of stress reduction, argue that exercise may be essential for psychological, physiological and social development, having a direct effect upon feelings of self-esteem (Segar et al 1998). However, in the treatment of depression, aerobic exercise in particular is efficacious (Beesley & Mutrie 1997, Moore & Blumenthal 1998). Physical fitness is seen as a positive aid towards emotional stability. Guidelines for exercise as a means towards stress reduction are given in Box 17.9.

Exercise works in a paradoxical manner in reducing stress. It is itself a physical stressor causing an acute stress response but nonetheless functions as a relaxant. The physiological effects of exercise include increased blood flow and oxygen consumption, as well as changes in blood pressure, heart rate, respiration and metabolic rate.

Physical exercise acts as a relaxant for a number of reasons:

- Most exercise involves effort and concentration and thus it can be difficult to sustain anxious thoughts whilst engaged in physical exercise.
- Meeting a physical challenge can give the individual a sense of achievement.
- During strenuous exercise the body produces noradrenaline and endorphins; these substances help to alleviate depression and arguably bring about feelings of happiness and tranquillity (Pert 1997).
- Exercise can be taken in the company of other people and so can diminish feelings of social isolation.

Box 17.9

Guidelines for exercise

- Any exercise is good
- Set aside a specific time for exercise. Treat that time as sacrosanct, but do not feel worried if it is necessary for some reason to miss a session
- Exercise at least three times a week if possible, for at least half an hour
- Exercise should be gentle but vigorous; build up slowly to a good exercise level
- If in doubt, have a health check and talk over your exercise programme with your general practitioner prior to starting

Relaxation

Relaxation has long been known to help alleviate feelings of stress and to enhance health-seeking behaviour (Vines 1994). Relaxation may take various forms, including relieving muscle tension, e.g. through exercise, taking time off, either on a daily or weekly basis or as a scheduled holiday, and meditation. Everly and Benson (1989) and Knight (1995) discussed the response elicited physiologically and psychologically by certain types of meditative relaxation. They identify two components of these meditation techniques which cause the relaxation response and a reduction in feelings of stress:

- the repetition of a word, sound, phrase, liturgical prayer
- the positive disregard of everyday thoughts when they come to mind.

There are six types of activity which specifically foster this type of meditative relaxation:

- meditation
- autogenic training
- pre-suggestion hypnosis
- prayer (repetitive or liturgical)
- yoga exercises
- t'ai chi chu'an.

For many people, these techniques produce a sense of well-being as well as an increase in concentration and energy. They also produce the following physiological changes (Everly & Benson 1989):

- decreased oxygen consumption and carbon dioxide elimination with no change in the respiratory quotient
- reduced heart and respiratory rates and lowered blood level of lactate
- reduced blood pressure.

Everly and Benson (1989) argue that, during relaxation, there are physiological alterations consistent with a decrease in central and peripheral adrenergic excitation, and that people who undertake regular meditative relaxation (see

Box 17.10) recover faster from stressful events than those who do not relax in this way.

For further information, see Fontana (2002).

CONCLUSION

Stress is not in itself a pathological or abnormal phenomenon. Indeed, it is hard to imagine how any individual might go through life without being faced with stressful situations. For some individuals, stress can, to a significant degree, be treated as a challenge and as a spur to personal growth and maturation. Why it is that certain people seem better able than others to withstand stressful conditions has been the subject of a great deal of debate as researchers have attempted to identify the physiological, psychological and social factors that mediate the experience of stress.

The fact that the word 'stress' is used freely in daily conversation without invoking the negative connotations of 'mental illness' perhaps indicates how the potentially grave effects of stress can be underestimated or obscured. As this chapter has shown, stress can be closely associated with serious physical, emotional or psychiatric illness, including heart disease and depression. Stress can also give rise to detrimental coping behaviours such as drug, alcohol and other forms of substance abuse (see Ch. 36). For this reason it is vital that stress is taken seriously by health professionals and that its mechanisms and effects are clearly understood.

From the nurse's perspective, perhaps the most important aspect of the experience of stress is its uniqueness for each individual. The experience of stress, like the experience of pain, must be assessed in each patient, and approaches to stress management must be congruent with the individual's personality, experiences and values. It is hoped that this chapter has assisted the nurse in formulating a practical understanding of stress and its effects, and will enable a positive contribution to be made to the treatment and management of stress and stress-related disorders in their patients. It is also hoped that the reader will be able to meet with greater confidence the challenge of recognising and coming to terms with the effects of stress in their own professional and personal life.

Box 17.10

Guidelines for meditative relaxation

Setting the scene

- Find a quiet, warm, comfortable room where you are unlikely to be disturbed (try to exclude children, pets, ticking clocks or telephones).
- Meditate sitting upright and well supported in a comfortable chair. Rest the feet flat on the floor and the hands loosely in your lap.
- Have a watch or clock in clear view. The session lasts 20 minutes. If you feel that you are likely to fall asleep, set an alarm.
- Loosen any tight clothing; slip off your shoes if this makes you more comfortable.
- Meditate whilst neither too hungry nor too full.
- Try to meditate twice each day for 20 minutes. Because you may feel deeply relaxed, it is better not to meditate close to bedtime, as this might interfere with your sleep patterns

The process

- During the process of meditation you will remain completely conscious.
- You may prefer to meditate with your eyes closed. Begin the process by taking one or two deep, relaxing breaths.
- Gently begin to count, either on each inhalation or exhalation, with the number one, then two, then three ... Every time you become aware of a thought, any thought, calmly return to number one. It is unlikely, though, that after a number of years of regular meditating you will go beyond the number one; indeed, the principle of this sort of meditation is not one of mastery, but of the gentle pushing aside of thoughts to enable the body and the mind to achieve complete rest.
- You may find that you have spent the whole session thinking over a problem. If so, do not worry; before you finish the session gently return to the counting, for 1 or 2 minutes.
- If you find that you have fallen asleep, do not worry about this. It may be that you are very tired and your body needs sleep. Before finishing the relaxation, gently return to the counting for 1 or 2 minutes. If you find that during the meditation, you have solved a major problem, written a poem or worked out a solution, before finishing the session, gently return to your counting.
- At the end of the session, before moving, stretch gently and sit with the eyes closed for a few moments.

REFERENCES

Aylett E, Fawcett T N 2003 Chronic fatigue syndrome: the nurse's role. Nursing Standard 17(35): 33–37

Beesley S, Mutrie N 1997 Exercise is beneficial adjunctive treatment in depression [letter; comment]. British Medical Journal 315(7121): 1542–1543

Benner P, Wrubel J 1989 The primacy of caring. Addison Wesley, London

Blau J N (ed) 1987 Migraine: clinical, therapeutic, conceptual and research aspects. Chapman and Hall, London, Ch 11, p 185–204

Bowman W C, Rand M J 1996 Textbook of pharmacology, 3rd edn. Blackwell Science, Oxford

British Medical Association and Royal Pharmaceutical Society of Great Britain 2005 British National Formulary. BMA, London. Online. Available: http://bnf.org/bnf

Cannon W B 1935 Stresses and strains of homeostasis. American Journal of Medical Science 189: 1

CFS/ME Working Group 2002 Report of the Chief Medical Officer of an independent working group. DH, London

Cooper C L 2004 Handbook of stress, medicine and health, 2nd edn. CRC Press, London

Cox T, Randall R, Griffiths A 2002 Interventions to control stress at work in hospital-based staff. HSE Books, Sudbury

Critchley H D, Taggart P, Sutton P M, Holdright D R 2004 Mental stress and sudden cardiac death: asymmetric midbrain activity as a linking mechanism. Brain 128(1): 75–85

Cunningham J 1996 For better or for worse. Practice Nurse 12(10): 624–627

Dewar A L, Morse J M 1995 Unbearable incidents: failure to endure the experience

of illness. Journal of Advanced Nursing 22: 957–964
Dillard N L 1990 Hardiness and academic achievement. Indiana University School of Nursing, Bloomington, IN
Duquette A, Kerouac S, Sandhu B K, Ducharme F, Saulnier P 1995 Psychosocial determinants of burnout in geriatric nursing. International Journal of Nursing Studies 32(5): 443–456
Egan G 1997 The skilled helper: a systematic approach to effective helping. Brooks/Cole, Pacific Grove, CA
Everly G S, Benson H 1989 Disorders of arousal and the relaxation response: speculations on the nature and treatment of stress related diseases. International Journal of Psychosomatics 36(1–4): 15–21
Everly G S, Sobelman S H 1987 The assessment of the human stress response: neurological, biochemical and psychological foundations. AMS Press, New York
Fagan N, Freme K 2004 Confronting post traumatic stress disorder. Nursing 34(2): 52–53
Fontana D 2002 The meditator's handbook: a complete guide to Eastern and Western techniques. HarperCollins, London
Fox S I 2004 Human physiology, 8th edn. McGraw-Hill, Boston
Freud S 1917 Mourning and melancholia. Standard edition, Vol XIV. Hogarth Press, London
Fukunishi I, Hattori M 1997 Mood states and type A behaviour in Japanese male patients with myocardial infarction. Psychotherapy and Psychosomatics 66(6): 314–318
Gonsalkorale W M, Houghton L A, Whorwell P J 2002 Hypnotherapy in irritable bowel syndrome: a large scale audit of a clinical service with examination of factors influencing responsiveness. American Journal of Gastroenterology 94: 954–961
Groom K N, O'Connor M E 1996 Relation of light and exercise to seasonal depressive symptoms: preliminary development of a scale. Perceptual and Motor Skills 83(2): 379–383
Hall D S 2004 Work-related stress of registered nurses in a hospital setting. Journal for Nurses in Staff Development 20(1): 6–14
Herbert J 1997 Stress, the brain and mental illness. British Medical Journal 315: 530–535
Hesselink A E, Penninx B W, Schlosser M A, Wijnhoven H A 2004 The role of coping resources and coping style in quality of life of patients with asthma and COPD. Quality of Life Research 13(2): 509–518
Holmes T H, Rahe R H 1967 The social readjustment rating scale. Journal of Psychosomatic Research 11: 213–218
Houston K, Haw D, Townsend E, Hawton K 2003 General practitioner contacts with patients before and after deliberate self harm. British Journal of General Practitioners 53(490): 365–370
Jacelon C S 1997 The trait and process of resilience. Journal of Advanced Nursing 25(1): 123–129
Kennedy E, Charles S C 2002 On becoming a counsellor: a basic guide for non-professional counsellors. Newleaf Publications, London
Kessler R C, Soukup J, Davis R B et al 2001 The use of complementary and alternative therapies to treat anxiety and depression in the United States. American Journal of Psychiatry 158(2): 289–294
Klag S, Bradley G 2004 The role of hardiness in stress and illness: an exploration of the effect of negativity, affectivity and gender. British Journal of Health Psychology 9(Pt 20): 137–161
Knight S 1995 Use of transcendental meditation to relieve stress and promote health. British Journal of Nursing 4(6): 315–318
Kobasa S C 1979 Stressful life events, personality and health: an inquiry into hardiness. Journal of Personality and Social Psychology 37(1): 1–11
Lazarus R S 1966 Psychological stress and the coping process. McGraw-Hill, New York
Lazarus R S, Folkman S 1984 Stress, appraisal, and coping. Springer, New York
Lea R, Whorwell P J 2003 New insights into the psychosocial aspects of irritable bowel syndrome. Current Gastroenterology Reports 5: 343–350
Levi L (ed) 1971 Society, stress and disease, Vol 1. Oxford University Press, Oxford, p 280–366
Mckinley B, Brooks N 1991 Post traumatic stress disorder explained. Nursing Standard 5(19): 35–38
Miller S B, Dolgoy L, Friese M, Sita A 1996 Dimensions of hostility and cardiovascular response to interpersonal stress. Journal of Psychosomatic Research 41(1): 81–95
Moore K A, Blumenthal J A 1998 Exercise training as an alternative treatment for depression among older adults. Alternative Therapies in Health and Medicine 4(1): 48–56
O'Connor N J, Manson J E, O'Connor G T, Buring J E 1995 Psychosocial risk factors and nonfatal myocardial infarction. Circulation 92(6): 1458–1464
Ostell A 1991 Coping, problem solving and stress: a framework for intervention strategies. British Journal of Medical Psychology 64: 11–24
Pert C 1997 Molecules of emotion. Simon and Schuster, London
Polk L V 1997 Towards a middle-range theory of resilience. Advanced Nursing Science 19(3): 1–13
Reif W, Hermanutz M 1996 Responses to activation and rest in patients with panic disorder and major depression. British Journal of Clinical Psychology 35(Pt 4): 605–616
Rogers C R 1974 On becoming a person. Constable, London
Segar M L, Katch V L, Roth R S et al 1998 The effect of aerobic exercise on self-esteem and depressive and anxiety symptoms among breast cancer survivors. Oncology Nursing Forum 25(1): 107–113
Selye H 1936 Syndrome produced by diverse nocuous agents. Nature (London) 138: 32
Selye H 1946a The general adaptation syndrome and the diseases of adaptation. Journal of Clinical Endocrinology 6: 117
Selye H 1946b What is stress? Metabolism 5: 525
Selye H 1976 The stress of life. McGraw-Hill, New York
Sharpe M, Wilks D 2002 ABC of psychological medicine: fatigue. British Medical Journal 325(7362): 480–483
Smith G D 2003 IBS: nursing management and psychological therapies. Gastrointestinal Nursing 1(7): 24–29
Stress Management Society. Online. Available: www.stress.org.uk
Sutherland V J, Cooper C L 2000 Strategic stress management. Macmillan, London
Vines S W 1994 Relaxation with guided imagery: effects on employees' psychological distress and health seeking behaviors. American Association of Occupational Health Nursing Journal 42(5): 206–213
Watson R, Fawcett T N 2003 Pathophysiology, homeostasis and nursing. Routledge, London
Westra H A, Kuiper N A 1997 Cognitive content specificity in selective attention across four domains of maladjustment. Behaviour Research and Therapy 35(4): 349–365
Worden J W 2002 Grief counselling and grief therapy: a handbook for the mental health practitioner, 3rd edn. Routledge, London
Yousfi S, Matthews G, Amelang M, Schmidt-Rathjens C 2004 Personality and disease: correlations of multiple trait scores with various illnesses. Journal of Health Psychology 9(5): 627–647

FURTHER READING

Bowlby J 1980 Attachment and loss: loss, sadness and depression. Vol 3. Tavistock, London
Cunningham S M 1999 Migraine: helping clients choose the right treatment and identify triggers. British Journal of Nursing 8(22): 1515–1523
Diamond S, Franklin M A 2001 Conquering your migraine. Simon and Schuster, London
Dryden W 1990 Individual therapy. Open University Press, Milton Keynes
Healy D 2004 Psychiatric drugs explained, 4th edn. Churchill Livingstone, Edinburgh
Jacelon C S 1997 The trait and process of resilience. Journal of Advanced Nursing 25(1): 123–129
Klag S, Bradley G 2004 The role of hardiness in stress and illness: an exploration of the effect of negativity, affectivity and gender. British Journal of Health Psychology 9(Pt 20): 137–161
Palmer J A, Palmer L K, Michiels K, Thigpen B

1995 Effects of type of exercise on depression in recovering substance abusers. Perceptual and Motor Skills 80(2): 523–530
Parkes C M 1972 Bereavement. Tavistock, London
Parkes C M 1972 Determinants of outcome following bereavement. Omega 6: 303–323
Segar M L, Katch V L, Roth R S et al 1998 The effect of aerobic exercise on self-esteem and depressive and anxiety symptoms among breast cancer survivors. Oncology Nursing Forum 25(1): 107–113

USEFUL WEBSITES

International Stress Management Association (UK)
www.isma.org.uk

Migraines.net
http://migraines.net

Mind Tools
www.mindtools.com

Stressbusting.co.uk
www.stressbusting.co.uk

Stress Coping (Counselling, Strategies & Management Advice)
www.stress-counselling.co.uk

Stress Management Society
http://stress.org.uk

UK National Work-Stress Network
www.workstress.net

18 SHOCK

Dorothy J. Armstrong

INTRODUCTION

Despite advances in diagnosis, treatment and management, shock remains one of the leading causes of death in the critically ill patient. It is important that nurses from all areas of clinical practice have the knowledge required to identify patients at risk and ensure timely and appropriate intervention is carried out.

The aim of this chapter is to facilitate the understanding of the pathophysiology of shock and the nursing care required.

In any environment, awareness of the predisposing factors which may lead to shock, early detection and prompt action are vital for a good prognosis. Caring for patients who are suffering from shock requires not only an understanding of the pathophysiology of shock and the principles of its treatment and management, but also an awareness of the devastating psychological and social impact such a sudden change from health to illness can have on patients and their families.

THE PATHOPHYSIOLOGY OF SHOCK

Circulatory homeostasis exists when the circulating blood volume and the vascular tone of blood vessels are in dynamic equilibrium. Shock is a state in which tissue perfusion is inadequate to maintain the supply of oxygen and nutrients necessary for normal cellular function and disequilibrium ensues. The cells may also be unable to extract and utilise normally the reduced supply of substrates and oxygen which is delivered.

Shock is categorised according to the underlying cause (Haslett et al 2002), namely:

- Hypovolaemic — due to reduction of blood volume
- Cardiogenic — due to myocardial dysfunction
- Obstructive — due to obstruction to blood flow in the circulation
- Distributive — due to altered vascular resistance. This category includes septic shock, neurogenic shock, spinal shock and anaphylactic shock.

The stages of shock

Before considering specific types of shock it is necessary to understand the basic pathophysiological processes which produce the clinical picture typically observed in shock. These processes can be divided into four stages (Hand 2001):

1. *Initial stage* — there are no signs and symptoms but cellular changes begin to occur in response to a disturbance in cell perfusion and oxygenation. This disturbance progresses to a change from aerobic to anaerobic cellular metabolism, in which production of lactic acid and pyruvic acid leads to metabolic acidosis.

2. *Compensatory stage* — physiological adaptations occur in an attempt to overcome the original problem, e.g. hypovolaemia.
3. *Progressive stage* — compensatory mechanisms begin to fail and produce adverse effects.
4. *Refractory stage* — pathophysiological processes set in motion cannot be arrested or reversed. Death is imminent.

It is important to understand that the stages of shock comprise continuous and complex processes and that there is usually no sudden transition from one stage to the next.

The compensatory stage

When circulation becomes inadequate due to reduction of circulating fluid, pump failure or massive vasodilatation, various mechanisms are activated in response to hypotension, hypoxaemia or acidosis, or a combination of these. These mechanisms are neural, hormonal and chemical, but since the body functions as a whole system they are closely interlinked.

Neural mechanisms Hypotension leads to decreased stimulation of the aortic and carotid sinus baroreceptors, which in turn reduces impulses to the vasomotor centre and thus reduces inhibition of the vasoconstrictor centre. This stimulates the sympathetic nervous system, resulting in the activation of the stress response. This response includes the discharge of the catecholamines, namely adrenaline and noradrenaline, resulting in vasoconstriction in the skin, kidneys, gastrointestinal tract and other organs while blood supply to the heart and brain is preserved. Vasoconstriction and increased heart rate may initially restore the arterial blood pressure to normal, but peripheral resistance will be raised, making the myocardium work harder to maintain cardiac output. Urinary output and peristalsis will decrease, and the individual's skin will become pale and cool. Sympathetic nervous system stimula-tion will also result in increased respiratory rate and depth, dilated pupils and increased sweat gland activity, causing the 'clammy' skin typically found in all forms of shock, other than early septic shock.

Hormonal mechanisms Adrenaline secreted by the adrenal medulla stimulates the anterior pituitary gland to release adrenocorticotrophic hormone (ACTH), which causes the adrenal cortex to release glucocorticoids such as hydrocortisone and mineralocorticoids such as aldosterone.

Glucocorticoids raise blood sugar by increasing gluconeogenesis and thereby the availability of glucose for energy. In addition, the glucocorticoids mobilise amino acids from the tissues and decrease protein synthesis. They also reduce glucose uptake by the cells and mobilise fatty acids from the adipose tissue into the plasma. Cortisol shifts cell metabolism from glucose to fatty acids for energy, enhancing fatty acid oxidation, and also reduces tissue destruction by stabilising lysosomal membranes (Guyton & Hall 2000).

Aldosterone decreases excretion by increased reabsorption of sodium and chloride by the kidney, and increases excretion of potassium and hydrogen ions. Thus metabolic acidosis and hypokalaemia can occur. The high serum osmolality resulting from a high concentration of sodium chloride stimulates the hypothalamic osmoreceptors to release antidiuretic hormone (ADH) from the posterior pituitary gland.

ADH stimulates an increase in renal water reabsorption, in an attempt to restore normal serum osmolality and thus increase circulating fluid and blood pressure.

Noradrenaline secretion by the adrenal medulla results in renal artery vasoconstriction, which in turn stimulates secretion of renin by the kidney. In the circulation, renin reacts with angiotensinogen, producing angiotensin I. This is converted by an enzyme in the lungs to angiotensin II, which causes venous constriction and increases aldosterone release, thus leading to increased fluid and sodium retention, increased blood volume and therefore increased venous return, blood pressure and renal perfusion.

Thyroxine secreted by the thyroid gland sensitises the beta-receptors in the heart to noradrenaline and so increases heart rate, systolic pressure, stroke volume and cardiac output.

Chemical mechanisms Poor lung perfusion leads to ventilation–perfusion mismatch and decreased oxygen tension in the circulating blood. This is detected by chemoreceptors in the aorta and carotid bodies. The carbon dioxide concentration falls as the respiratory rate increases and the amount of carbon dioxide is 'blown off', thus producing a respiratory alkalosis. Cerebral blood vessels constrict in response to decreased carbon dioxide tension leading to cerebral hypoxia. Subsequently, the acid–base balance is further complicated by a metabolic acidosis resulting from the anaerobic metabolism of glucose to lactic acid.

These mechanisms may initially combine to compensate for the initial problem, but unless the latter is promptly and successfully overcome, more clinical signs will become evident. The typical clinical picture at this stage of shock is of a patient with cool, pale, clammy skin, decreased urinary output, increased heart rate and decreased bowel sounds. The patient may be anxious, restless or confused due to the cerebral effects of hypoxia, hypocapnia and sympathetic nervous system stimulation.

Anxiety will intensify the physiological responses to stress and thus it is very important for the nurse to provide much needed reassurance to both the patient and any relatives during a major life crisis.

The progressive stage

Although the compensatory mechanisms may at first appear to reverse the effects of shock, if the cause is not treated appropriately then the next stage of shock becomes evident.

With decreased perfusion, the supply of oxygen and nutrients to the cells will be inadequate to produce sufficient adenosine triphosphate (ATP) (see Fig. 18.1). The sodium pump will fail and sodium will increase inside the cells while potassium leaks out (see Fig. 18.2). This can result in hyperkalaemia, which may in turn cause cardiac arrest. The anaerobic metabolism which results from an inadequate oxygen supply will increase the production of lactic acid, resulting in a metabolic acidosis.

The consequences of the increasing acidosis and hypoxia are that the precapillary sphincters become fatigued, causing collapse of the microcirculation and increasing hydrostatic

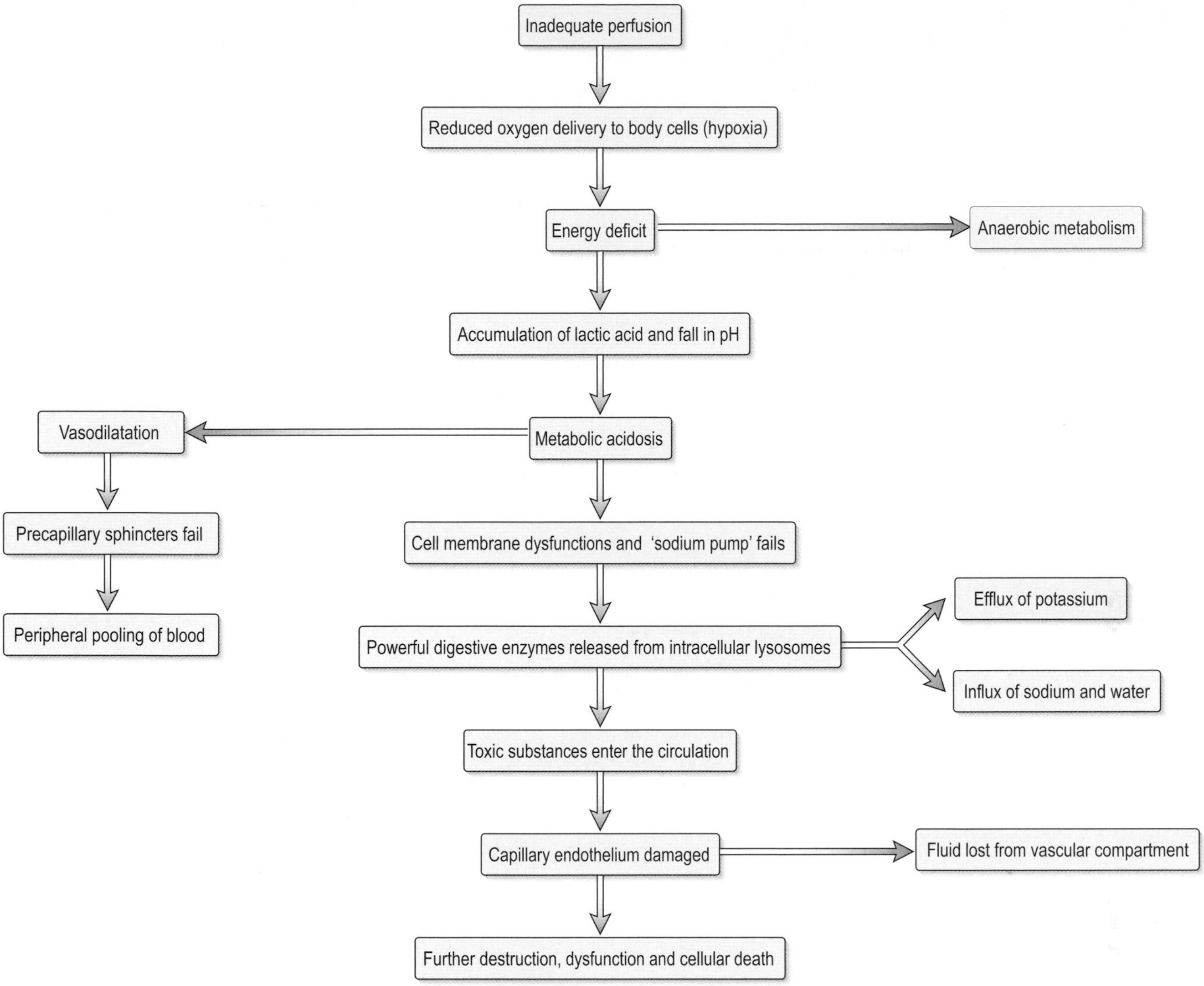

Fig. 18.1 Effects of inadequate perfusion on cell function.

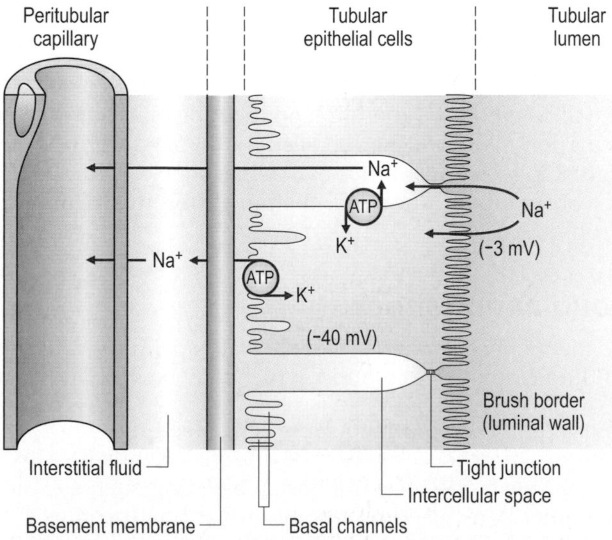

Fig. 18.2 The sodium–potassium pump. (Reproduced with permission from Guyton & Hall 2000.)

pressure and capillary leakage. Haemoconcentration and viscosity will increase. Sludging in the microcirculation may lead to disseminated intravascular coagulation (DIC; see p. 732), one of the complications of shock. Figure 18.3 illustrates the vicious cycle of shock.

Prolonged vasoconstriction and its impact on cell function will soon compromise the functioning of the vital organs, as follows:

- The kidneys will be unable to filter, reabsorb and excrete fluid normally. Urinary osmolality will fall, and output will be reduced to below 20 mL/h. Acute tubular necrosis may occur, causing a marked rise in blood urea and creatinine.
- Pancreatic cells will release the enzymes amylase and lipase into the circulation, contributing to the formation of myocardial depressant factor (MDF), which decreases myocardial contractility.
- The lungs will become less compliant as fluid and plasma proteins leak into the alveoli, altering osmotic pressure and leading to pulmonary oedema. This in turn reduces gaseous exchange and may result in adult

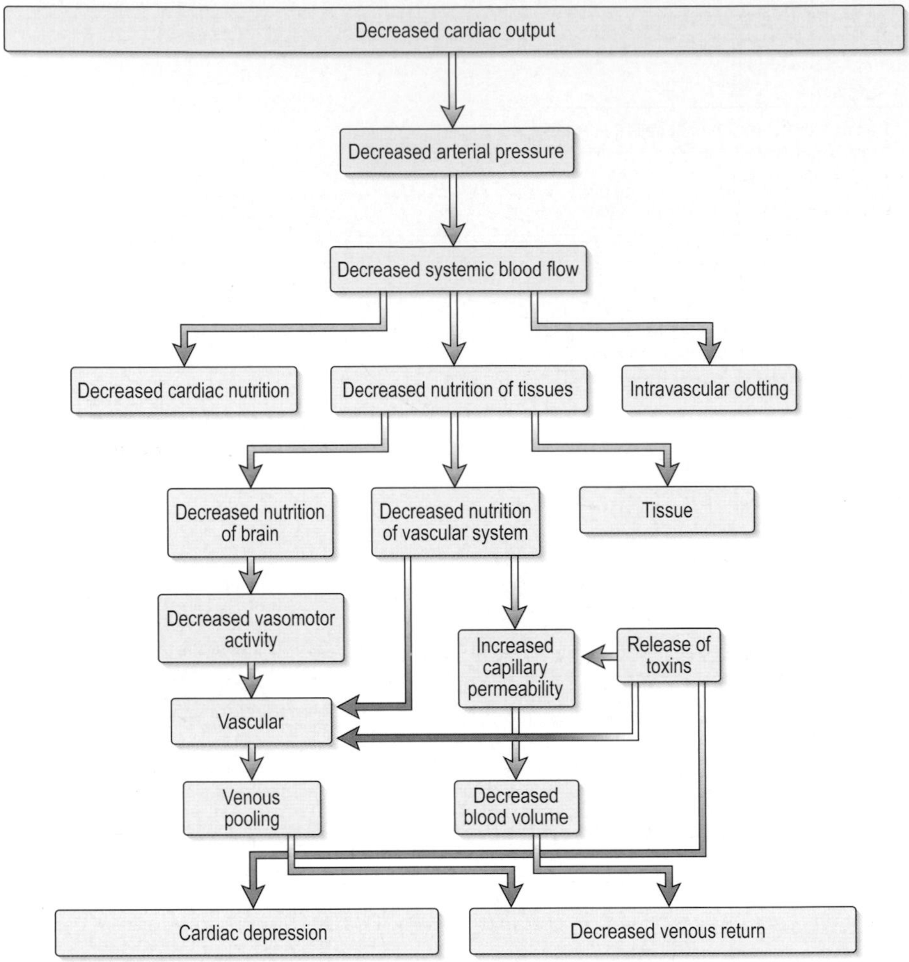

Fig. 18.3 The vicious cycle of shock. (Reproduced with permission from Guyton & Hall 2000.)

respiratory distress syndrome (ARDS; see p. 732). Hydrostatic or cardiac pulmonary oedema may occur as the heart fails. All of these changes will increase hypoxia and acidosis.

- The heart will eventually fail as coronary perfusion and oxygen supply become inadequate to meet the demands of the myocardium, which will be working hard to maintain blood flow by pumping rapidly against high resistance and disadvantaged by the effect of MDF.
- Ischaemic damage to the intestinal mucosa will result in the release of bacteria and toxins from the gut into the circulation.
- Alteration in cerebral function may have a number of effects, ranging from a dulling of responses to major behavioural changes.

The refractory stage

Continuing circulatory collapse, increasing acidosis, sludging of red cells and platelets due to decreased intravascular volume will all contribute to decreasing perfusion of tissues. Massive bleeding due to DIC may also exacerbate this effect. Inadequate ventilation will lead to increasingly inadequate oxygenation. Renal failure will contribute to increasing metabolic abnormalities, and vital centres in the brain will eventually cease to function due to ischaemia and hypoxia. If the refractory stage is reached, the shock is irreversible and death will occur.

TYPES OF SHOCK

Specific aspects of the pathophysiological processes of shock will be evident depending on the type of shock which is occurring. The following sections will describe the distinguishing features of hypovolaemic shock, cardiogenic shock, obstructive shock and the different forms of distributive shock.

Hypovolaemic shock

This is the most common type of shock. Its primary cause is loss of fluid from the circulation, which may be described as:

- *external fluid loss* — due to superficial bleeding, vomiting, diarrhoea, overuse of diuretics or burns
- *internal fluid loss* — due to internal bleeding such as haemothorax or bleeding into tissues at fracture sites after injuries, paralytic ileus, intestinal obstruction or acute dilatation of the stomach.

While internal conditions may not be an obvious cause of fluid loss, their effect can be very serious. For example, 1 L — around 20% of the blood volume of an average man — or more of fluid may be sequestered in the gastrointestinal tract during paralytic ileus and/or acute dilatation of the stomach, and the same volume or more of blood may escape into the tissues and/or thorax as a result of multiple injuries.

The physiological implications of hypovolaemia are:

- reduced blood volume
  ↓
- decreased venous return
  ↓
- decreased cardiac output
  ↓
- reduced tissue perfusion.

In early hypovolaemic shock, the compensatory mechanisms described (see p. 725) are activated when the blood pressure starts to fall. These mechanisms will compensate for up to 10% reduction of the circulating volume of a healthy person without the development of marked symptoms. However, if a greater volume of fluid is lost and is not replaced quickly, the compensatory mechanisms may fail quite suddenly, in which case the patient's condition will deteriorate rapidly. It should be recognised that, in older people, the cardiovascular system is often less able to cope with haemodynamic changes, and the heart may be less able to pump faster and harder in order to maintain cardiac output against high peripheral resistance.

Recognising hypovolaemic shock

The following signs and symptoms of hypovolaemic shock are reliable only if they are considered in relation to one another and the patient's previous, stable, condition. Nevertheless, whenever several of these indicators occur together, the possibility of shock should be considered, as a successful outcome depends upon early intervention. The nurse should therefore be alert to the following:

- rapid and deep respirations in response to sympathetic nervous system stimulation, hypoxia and acidosis
- a rapid, weak, thready pulse, due to low blood flow despite a rapid heart rate
- narrowing of the pulse pressure, i.e. a reduced difference between systolic and diastolic pressures due to decreased stroke volume and increased peripheral resistance indicating vasoconstriction of the skin and viscera, reflecting decreased blood flow (Guyton & Hall 2000)
- anxiety, restlessness and confusion, which may indicate decreased cerebral perfusion and oxygenation
- cool, clammy skin and cold peripheries due to vasoconstriction and sympathetic stimulation of sweat glands
- decreased urinary output, due to renal artery vasoconstriction and endocrine compensatory mechanisms
- lowered body temperature, which may be related to altered metabolism, perfusion and oxygenation and, possibly, heat loss from evaporation of sweat from the skin
- thirst and a dry mouth related to fluid depletion and possibly to sympathetic nervous system stimulation
- fatigue, probably related to inadequate perfusion and oxygenation of the tissues and vital organs.

As stated earlier, it is relatively easy to diagnose hypovolaemic shock when a patient is bleeding externally. Diagnosis is more difficult when hypovolaemia is developing as a consequence of an internal crisis. Nurses must be alert to recognise the above signs and context of the crisis and to ensure that prompt action is taken and/or help is sought.

Cardiogenic shock

The clinical definition of cardiogenic shock is hypotension with evidence of impaired perfusion, in the setting of acute myocardial infarction. A variety of other causes, such as myocardial contusion, myocarditis and cardiomyopathy can produce cardiogenic shock, but the majority of cases result from atherosclerosis and resulting myocardial necrosis (Tiffany & Jorden 2001).

STOP THINK

18.1 Refresh your knowledge of cardiac function by reviewing Chapter 2.

18.2 Review the terms listed in Box 18.1 to ensure that you understand how they would be applied in the course of treatment and monitoring for cardiogenic shock.

Ischaemic muscle is deprived of adequate oxygen and substrates for effective contraction, and infarcted muscle or scar tissue is unable to contract. When more than approximately 40% of the left ventricle is infarcted the ability to maintain the systemic circulation is significantly impaired.

The compensatory mechanisms that normally act to prevent hypotension can worsen the situation. The catecholamine release produces tachycardia, vasoconstriction and increased cardiac contractility, all of which increases the workload of the left ventricle and increased myocardial oxygen demand, potentially causing extension of the infarct and further compromising left ventricle function (Jowett & Thompson 2002).

In addition, since the left ventricle is not being emptied effectively, pressure will rise in the left atrium, the pulmonary circulation and the right side of the heart. As the pressure rises, pulmonary oedema will eventually ensue, reducing oxygenation. Thus, not only will the tissues be poorly perfused, but also the blood which does reach the tissues will carry less oxygen. As shock progresses, without effective intervention the vicious circle of effects shown in Figure 18.3 will occur.

Signs of cardiogenic shock

The signs of cardiogenic shock include:

- systolic pressure <80 mmHg
- tachycardia and a weak, thready pulse
- cold, clammy skin
- oliguria — urine output <20 mL/h
- confusion
- mottling of the extremities, particularly the legs
- if measured, pulmonary artery wedge pressure is >18 mmHg, cardiac index is <1.8 L/min per m^2 (see Box 18.1).

Box 18.1

Key terms relating to cardiac status

Cardiac output
This is the product of the heart rate multiplied by the stroke volume and represents the amount of blood ejected from the heart each minute. In the adult, cardiac output is normally 5–8 L/min.

Cardiac index
This is the patient's cardiac output divided by the body surface area. It indicates how many litres per min per square metre of body surface the heart ejects. The normal range for an adult is 2.7–4.3 L/min per m^2.

Stroke volume
This is the amount of blood delivered to the aorta during a left ventricular contraction (normally 80–120 mL in an adult). Three factors influence stroke volume: preload, afterload and contractility.

Preload
Indicators are central venous pressure (CVP) and pulmonary artery wedge pressure (PAWP). By means of a CVP transducer, right atrial pressure can be measured. CVP reflects the pressure in the right atrium and systemic veins but does not reliably reflect left ventricular pressures. PAWP gives an indication of the compliance of the left ventricular myocardium during diastole and the left atrial filling pressure necessary to fill the left ventricle with blood prior to systole.

Afterload
This is the resistance to systolic ejection of blood from the ventricle and can be assessed by measuring pulmonary vascular resistance and systemic vascular resistance. The pulmonary vascular resistance is the ratio of the pressure drop across the pulmonary vascular system to the total flow passing through the pulmonary circulation. Systemic or peripheral vascular resistance is a measurement of the vascular resistance to blood flow.

Contractility
This refers to the ability of the myocardium to contract effectively and act as a pump to maintain the circulation of blood.

Tiffany and Jorden (2001) state that signs and symptoms can vary from patient to patient and can also rapidly deteriorate in any given patient. Therefore close observation and assessment are required by the health care team.

Obstructive shock

This type of shock is caused by obstruction to blood flow in the circulation (Haslett et al 2002). Examples of obstructive shock include pulmonary embolism, cardiac tamponade or tension pneumothorax. Clinical signs of shock are similar to hypovolaemic and cardiogenic shock, producing cold peripheries, weak central pulses and low cardiac output.

Distributive shock

Distributive shock can be divided into three different types: septic, neurogenic and anaphylactic. All are characterised by a loss of blood vessel tone, enlargement of the vascular component and displacement of the vascular volume away from the heart (Hand 2001). Although the blood volume remains the same, due to vasodilatation the vascular compartment has expanded, resulting in a reduction in cardiac output. This is described by Dipenbrock (1999) as the 'tank being too large'.

Septic shock

Septic shock is a medical emergency and is the most common type of shock that develops as a result of widespread infection (Smelzer & Bone 2000). Full assessment of the patient may need to wait until resuscitation and antimicrobial drugs have commenced (Green & Lynn 2000).

Sepsis and septic shock encompass a spectrum of clinical conditions caused by the systemic response to infection (see Box 18.2). Patients with sepsis usually present with a localised infection, which progresses into an uncontrolled systemic reaction. Patients can then develop acute organ failure at locations distant from the initial infective site, ultimately leading to death. The incidence of sepsis is thought to be rising (Bone et al 1997). Factors that can contribute to this include:

- an increased use of invasive surgery
- an increased incidence of bacterial resistance
- a greater number of immunocompromised patients.

Box 18.2

Working definitions for conditions related to sepsis

- *Infection* — invasion of microorganisms into a normally sterile site, often associated with an inflammatory host response
- *Bacteraemia* — viable bacteria in bloodstream
- *Septicaemia* — no uniform definition, often interpreted as bacteraemia plus severe illness
- *Sepsis* — clinical evidence of infection plus systemic response indicated by two or more of:
  - — hyper- or hypothermia: core temperature >38°C or <36°C
  - — tachycardia: heart rate >90 bpm
  - — tachypnoea: respiratory rate >20 resps/min
  - — white blood count $>12 \times 10^9$
- *Severe sepsis* — sepsis associated with organ dysfunction:
  - — hypotension
  - — oliguria
  - — hypoxia
  - — confusion
  - — metabolic acidosis
  - — disseminated intravascular coagulation
- *Septic shock* — severe sepsis with hypotension unresponsive to intravascular volume replacement
- *Refractory shock* — hypotension not responding to vasoactive agents
- *Systemic inflammatory response syndrome (SIRS)* — similar physiological response to sepsis but unrelated to infection. May be caused by a variety of acute insults, e.g. pancreatitis

Adapted from Bone et al (1992).

Septic shock is commonly seen as a complication of bacterial infection and is characterised by a wide range of metabolic and haemodynamic abnormalities (Bone et al 1992).

Bacteraemia Bacteraemia is a serious condition with potentially fatal consequences. Recognition and prompt use of empiric antibiotic therapy will reduce the risk of severe sepsis and may be life saving (Green & Lynn 2000). Septic shock may be caused by any invading microorganism. However, this condition is commonly associated with Gram-negative bacteria such as *Escherichia coli, Meningococcus, Klebsiella, Pseudomonas, Bacteroides* and *Proteus*.

For further reading, see British Infection Society (2003).

Gram-negative bacteria contain a lipopolysaccharide in their cell walls called endotoxin. When released into the bloodstream, endotoxin produces a variety of adverse biochemical changes and activates immune and other biological mediators that contribute to the development of septic shock (Hudak & Gallo 1998).

Gram-positive organisms such as *Staphylococcus, Streptococcus* and *Pneumococcus* are also implicated in the development of sepsis. Necrotising fasciitis is a soft tissue infection often caused by two or more bacteria, most commonly Group A streptococcus bacteria.

For further reading, see Gully (2002).

Phases of septic shock The clinical effects of septic shock occur in two distinct phases: the warm hyperdynamic stage and the cold hypodynamic stage (Hudak & Gallo 1998).

The hyperdynamic phase This first stage is characterised by:

- high cardiac output
- low systemic vascular resistance
- vasodilatation
- volume depletion and hypotension
- fever and chills
- low urine output
- tachycardia
- tachypnoea
- restlessness, agitation and confusion.

Unlike the other types of shock, which are characterised by a compensatory increase in systemic vascular resistance, septic shock often presents with a relative hypovolaemia due to massive vasodilatation and leakage of fluid into the interstitial space (Hand 2001).

The hypodynamic phase Following the hyperdynamic phase, the hypodynamic stage occurs. This is characterised by:

- high systemic vascular resistance
- vasoconstriction
- hypotension
- hypoperfusion
- cold, clammy skin
- subnormal or elevated temperature
- depressed conscious level.

At this stage, clinical findings begin to resemble more closely those typically associated with shock. Catecholamine release results in vasoconstriction and the patient's skin becomes cold, moist and possibly mottled at the peripheries. The pulse becomes rapid, thready and weak, and ECG changes suggest an inadequate coronary blood flow. Patients who reach this clinical state are particularly at risk of developing multisystem failure.

During this phase it is common for haematological problems to become evident. The released endotoxins damage the endothelium and cause adhesion of platelets and subsequent destruction of the microcirculation. These effects, together with the activation of the coagulation and fibrinolytic systems, may give rise to DIC (see p. 732). Hyperventilation persists but fails to overcome hypoxia. Lactic acid builds up and there is increasing metabolic acidosis, further compromising cell function.

All the body systems will become affected. As blood flow to the brain is reduced, conscious level falls and the patient is unable to respond to verbal stimuli. In the gastrointestinal tract, ischaemia may cause stress ulceration, leading to potential bleeding. The liver loses its ability to remove bilirubin, resulting in jaundice (Hand 2001) (see Case History 18.1 and Nursing Care Plan 18.1).

STOP THINK **18.3** Which stage of shock do the clinical findings in Case History 18.1 represent: hyperdynamic or hypodynamic?

Neurogenic shock

This type of distributive shock is associated with the central nervous system. It can occur when a disease process, drug or traumatic injury blocks sympathetic nerve impulses from the brain's vasomotor centre and thus increases parasympathetic activity. Neurogenic shock produces a picture of vasodilatation with loss of vascular tone. Venous return is reduced, cardiac output falls and hypotension rapidly follows.

There are a number of preconditions which may, over the course of several hours, or even a few weeks or months,

CASE HISTORY 18.1

Mr R (see also Nursing Care Plan 18.1)

Mr R, a 50-year-old bank manager, was admitted to the surgical unit for a hemicolectomy for diverticular disease. The surgery went according to plan and Mr R appeared to be progressing well. On the fifth postoperative day, however, the staff nurse noticed that he looked ill, and Mr R admitted that he was 'not so well today'.

Physical findings included:

- tachycardia
- tachypnoea
- warm, pink skin
- restlessness
- pyrexia
- polyuria.

The doctor concluded that Mr R was in the early stages of septic shock. Nursing staff then implemented the interventions summarised in Nursing Care Plan 18.1.

Nursing Care Plan 18.1 Mr R — care of a patient with septic shock (see Case History 18.1)

Nursing considerations	Goal	Action	Rationale
1. Potential risk of fluid volume depletion due to peripheral vasodilatation and capillary leakage	To restore and maintain circulating blood volume	• Assess vital signs, skin colour and capillary refill time	Depending on the shock phase, Mr R may present with an increased cardiac output, which causes a flushed, pink appearance. As the hypodynamic phase develops, the cardinal signs of shock become evident (see p. 719)
		• Ensure i.v. access with a minimum of two large-bore catheters	Fluid volume loss due to redistribution requires blood, colloid and crystalloid replacement
		• Monitor and record vital signs and core body temperature	Alterations in vital signs determine stability, improvement or deterioration and indicate whether changes need to be made to therapy
		• Insert a urinary catheter	Renal function is a good indicator of overall tissue perfusion. A urine output of 0.5–1.0 mL/kg per h is desirable. In the early stages of septic shock, an inappropriately large volume of urine may be passed due to renal vasodilatation caused by bacterial toxins. In such circumstances, urine output can be more than 100 mL/h
		• Assist with the insertion of a pulmonary artery catheter	Ideally the left ventricular function should be monitored by means of a PA catheter. If this is not possible then a central line will monitor the CVP and serve as a guide to fluid replacement
		• Administer and evaluate the effectiveness of inotropic agents: – dobutamine – dopamine – dopexamine	Inotropic agents increase cardiac output and therefore improve renal, coronary, mesenteric and cerebral blood flow
2. Potential for impaired gas exchange due to interstitial fluid overload	Restore and maintain optimal pulmonary function	• Assess Mr R's respiratory status, rate and rhythm: – Is he distressed? – Does he have any bronchospasm? – Monitor arterial blood gases – Monitor O_2 saturation via pulse oximetry	Escalating demands on the cardiovascular system increase oxygen consumption. In the early hyperdynamic stage, the ABGs may be relatively normal and it is not until the hypodynamic stage that they reflect hypoxia or metabolic acidosis
		• Encourage Mr R's cooperation in optimising respiratory function by means of: – breathing exercises – chest physiotherapy – incentive spirometry (see Ch. 3) – progressive O_2 therapy	Mr R may eventually need intubation and ventilation to maintain acceptable ABGs. To try to avoid this the nurse can employ these interventions

Nursing Care Plan 18.1 Mr R — care of a patient with septic shock (see Case History 18.1) *(Continued)*

Nursing considerations	Goal	Action	Rationale
2. Potential for impaired gas exchange due to interstitial fluid overload *(Continued)*		• Administer bronchodilators as prescribed by the physician	Bronchodilators cause airway dilatation by acting directly on β_2 receptors
3. Potential for further systemic infection	Reduce or eliminate the systemic risk of further infection	• Administer appropriate antibiotic therapy via i.v. route	Antibiotics are given i.v. to ensure a high level of the drug in the blood, body cavity fluids and tissues
		• Minimise the introduction of further infection by: – careful and frequent hand washing – maintaining aseptic techniques for all invasive procedures	Shock states alter the immune response and these patients are even more susceptible to infection. The increased use of invasive monitoring techniques offers more opportunities for invading pathogens
		• Perform frequent bacteriological screening	The use of antibiotic 'cocktails' to treat one organism may allow others to proliferate

lead to the development of neurogenic shock. One of the most common causes is spinal anaesthesia, especially that which extends up the length of the spinal cord and results in a blockage of sympathetic impulses. Cerebral trauma such as contusions or concussion, particularly to the brain stem or medulla oblongata, may also produce severe neurogenic shock. Another potential cause is spinal cord trauma in which all reflex activity below the level of the lesion is lost.

Spinal shock

Trauma to the head, neck, back or shoulders resulting from an accident may cause injury to the vertebral column and/or spinal cord. Spinal injuries are most prevalent among young men who have been previously healthy and for whom the injury is a catastrophic event necessitating major changes in lifestyle.

The degree and type of force exerted on the spine at the time of injury will determine the nature and severity of the injury. The most frequently seen and, unfortunately, the most damaging type of spinal injury as a result of a road traffic accident is a sudden hyperflexion and rotation with fracture–dislocation of the vertebral column at C5 and C6, and T12 to L1. Within 30–60 min of the trauma, autonomic and motor reflexes below the level of the injury are suppressed. This state is known as spinal shock and it may last hours or even weeks.

For further reading on spinal shock, see Fahey (2001).

Anaphylactic shock

If it is not dealt with immediately, this type of shock is life threatening. It arises when the individual develops a hypersensitivity response to an antigen, drug or foreign protein in which the release of histamine causes widespread vasodilatation resulting in hypotension and increased capillary permeability with loss of fluid into the interstitium.

The main causes of systemic anaphylaxis are insect bites and stings, particularly from bees and wasps, drugs, notably penicillin, and food such as peanuts, eggs or shellfish. Occasionally, diagnostic contrast media, e.g. iodine based, may also precipitate anaphylactic reactions.

STOP THINK **18.4** What precautions might be observed before a patient undergoes a diagnostic test involving a contrast medium?

The individual developing anaphylactic shock presents with a combination of the following symptoms:

- laryngeal stridor, dyspnoea, cough and, occasionally, cyanosis
- local oedema, particularly around the face
- a weak and rapid pulse
- skin eruptions, large weals.

Treatment will be needed urgently because of the respiratory problems caused by local tissue swelling, laryngeal oedema and/or bronchospasm in addition to circulatory insufficiency (see Ch. 16, p. 682).

Box 18.3 provides a summary of interventions used in the treatment of shock.

FIRST AID TREATMENT FOR SHOCK

Nurses may be called upon occasionally to help people on the street or in other public places who have gone into

Box 18.3

Definitive and supportive therapy in clinical shock

Definitive therapy

Hypovolaemic shock
- Maintain or increase intravascular volume
- Decrease any future fluid/blood loss via i.v. fluid regimen
- Give supplementary O_2 therapy

Cardiogenic shock
- Reduce cardiac muscle damage by O_2 supply and reduce cardiac demand by O_2 therapy and cardiac medication to dilate the coronary vessels and by decreasing pain and activity
- Increase effectiveness of heart as a pump via inotropic medication

Septic shock
- Restore adequate intravascular volume via i.v. fluids
- Give supplemental O_2 therapy
- Identify and control source of infection via bacterial screening
- Administer appropriate antibiotics
- Remove nidus of infection if possible

Anaphylactic shock
- Identify and remove causative antigen
- Reduce effects of mediator substances that have caused massive vasodilatation, e.g. give adrenaline to restore vascular tone, antihistamines to reverse histamine effects, bronchodilators to oppose bronchial constriction
- Give O_2 therapy and i.v. fluid replacement

Supportive therapy
- Give adequate ventilation and oxygenation via optimal airway maintenance, optimal breathing technique and supplemental O_2
- Maintain or restore adequate perfusion of tissues to ensure oxygen delivery, via maintenance of cardiac pump to effectively circulate the blood and medication to improve contractility and reduce cardiac workload
- Maintain or restore metabolic equilibrium
- Reverse metabolic acidosis via hyperventilation and, if severe, by i.v. sodium bicarbonate administration

Adapted from Rice (1991).

shock as the result of an accident, heart attack or severe allergic reaction, and so should be aware of the appropriate first aid to give in the absence of clinical facilities.

The main objectives of intervention in such an emergency should follow the chain of survival used in basic life support (Colquhoun et al 2003):

- Maintain an adequate supply of blood to the heart, lungs and brain
- Limit haemorrhaging and prevent further injury
- Ascertain the cause of the shock
- Arrange for transfer to hospital.

Box 18.4 lists the steps to take in the event of an emergency, especially where hypovolaemic shock is suspected or imminent.

For further reading, see Resuscitation Council (UK) (2000).

Box 18.4

Emergency interventions at the scene of an accident

1. Immediately reassure and comfort the person.
2. Check the airway for patency. If breathing is laboured or difficult, lie the individual in the recovery position if it is safe to do so. This will reduce the risk of aspiration of stomach contents. The jaw may need to be lifted, without hyperextension of the neck, to aid in the maintenance of the airway. Loosen any tight clothing, especially around the neck. NB: do not attempt to move the person if there is any likelihood of cervical or other spinal injury.
3. If haemorrhaging is obvious, try to control it by applying pressure.
4. Call 999. Give clear instructions, i.e. what kind of help is needed and the correct location of the accident. People tend to panic when a crisis occurs and someone needs to assume the position of leader and maintain an air of calm efficiency. Discourage onlookers from gathering as this only distresses the individual even further.
5. If relatives or friends are at the scene, ask them for a brief history. This may help to ascertain the cause of the shock.
6. Someone may be able to provide a blanket or coat to cover the person. However, do not accept the offer of a hot water bottle, as the application of heat would only increase peripheral vasodilatation and draw some of the blood supply away from the vital organs.
7. If the person complains of thirst, moisten the lips with water but do not allow drinking.
8. If a cardiac or respiratory arrest develops, commence artificial resuscitation immediately.
9. Transfer the person to hospital as soon as possible.
10. Try to ensure safety, considering the cause of the problem. For example, in the case of a road traffic collision, ask someone to warn and divert traffic, whilst maintaining personal safety.

GENERAL PRINCIPLES OF THE MANAGEMENT AND TREATMENT OF SHOCK

As well as being able to recognise the warning signs of shock (see p. 715), the nurse should be able to identify those patients who are most at risk of developing shock. Increasingly, hospitals are implementing early warning teams who can be called upon for advice and, if required, to treat patients in the early stages of shock. Examples of this initiative include ALERT – Acute Life Threatening Events Recognition and Treatment, and MEWS – Medical Early Warning Systems.

For further reading, see http://web.port.ac.uk/alert/intro.htm and McArthur-Rouse (2001).

In its early stages, shock demands immediate intervention. The initial treatment priority is the control of life-threatening abnormalities through assessment of airway, breathing and circulation (Sepsis Care Initiative 2002). When obtaining a patient's initial history the nurse should take note of the risk factors listed in Box 18.5. Thereafter, the

Box 18.5

Identifying patients at risk of experiencing shock

- Has the patient experienced multiple trauma?
- Has the patient had surgery recently?
- Has the patient suffered severe burns?
- Is the patient postpartum?
- Does the patient have a history of oesophageal varices or peptic ulceration?
- Is the patient taking anticoagulant therapy?

The above factors put the patient at risk of *hypovolaemic* shock.

- Has the patient experienced chest pain recently or suffered a myocardial infarction — especially in vessels supplying the anterior wall of the left ventricle?
- Does the patient have a history of cardiac failure or cardiac dysrhythmias?

The above factors put the patient at risk of *cardiogenic* shock.

- Does the patient have impaired immunity, e.g. are they suffering from AIDS or cancer, or undergoing chemotherapy?
- Does the patient have a resistant deep-seated infection?
- Is the patient seriously ill and requiring multiple invasive catheters and devices?

The above factors put the patient at risk of *septic* shock.

- Does the patient suffer from any disordered state resulting in impaired nervous stimuli to vascular smooth muscle?
- Has the patient experienced recent spinal anaesthesia?
- Has the patient experienced trauma to the brain and/or spinal cord?

The above factors put the patient at risk of experiencing *neurogenic* or *spinal* shock.

- Does the patient have significant allergies or sensitivities?
- Is the patient undergoing tests requiring contrast media?

The above factors put the patient at risk of experiencing *anaphylactic* shock.

management of shock includes treatment of the underlying cause, restoration of tissue perfusion and patient support (see Fig. 18.4). The purpose of oxygen support is to restore and help maintain adequate tissue oxygenation. The goals of haemodynamic support are to restore an effective blood pressure, to ensure tissue perfusion and to normalise cellular metabolism.

STOP THINK **18.5**

(a) Read Case History 18.2. In your opinion, is Mr A suffering from shock? If so, which type?
(b) Why might his abdomen be rigid?
(c) What initial steps should medical and nursing staff take?

Management and treatment of hypovolaemic shock

Regardless of what may have triggered the patient's hypovolaemia, the restoration of circulating fluid volume is the key to management. As soon as the patient's airway has been secured and oxygen therapy instituted, the next priority is to assess circulatory status and commence replacement i.v. fluids via two large-bore cannulae. Fluid therapy remains the cornerstone for almost every form of shock, although the original insult must also be identified and resolved where possible.

The nurse must ask:

- What kind of fluid is required?
- How much fluid does the patient need?

Fluid replacement must be accurately recorded and observations taken regularly to assess the patient's response.

Crystalloids

Normal saline solution (sodium chloride 0.9%) is often the first replacement fluid administered to the shocked patient, although its large concentration of chloride ions could be disadvantageous to the patient whose renal function is

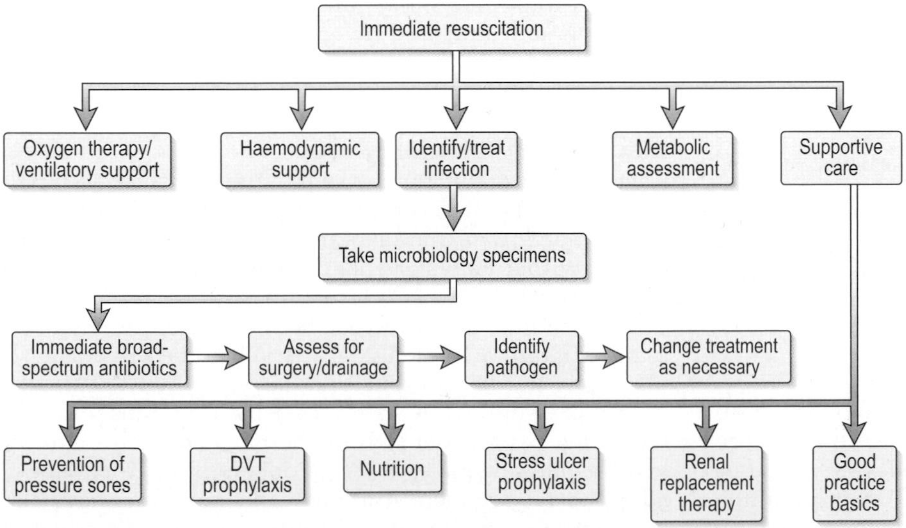

Fig. 18.4 Treatment: general approach to septic shock. (Reproduced with kind permission from Eli Lilly & Co. Ltd.)

CASE HISTORY 18.2

Mr A

Mr A, aged 35, is married and has two young children. While travelling to work one morning he was involved in an RTA. Within 30 min he was admitted to the nearest emergency department, where initial assessment showed the following:

Vital signs

- Blood pressure — systolic = 70 mmHg but diastolic difficult to hear
- Heart rate — 150/min; pulse weak, thready and rapid
- Respirations — 40/min; breathing shallow
- Temperature — 35.5°C

Neurological signs

- Little response to painful stimuli
- Poor gag and cough reflex
- Right pupil unresponsive to light
- Left pupil reacting sluggishly
- Glasgow Coma Scale score = 4

General examination

- Large swelling in right occiput
- Rigid abdomen; bowel sounds absent
- Obvious fracture to right femur with large gaping wound
- Possible fractured pelvis
- Skin moist and clammy; mouth dry

already impaired. It may also cause hypernatraemia, hypokalaemia or a hyperchloraemic metabolic acidosis.

Dextrose 5% is not considered a suitable fluid for the patient in shock, although it may maintain water balance and supply the calories necessary for cell metabolism.

Hartmann's solution, an electrolyte solution consisting of sodium chloride, potassium chloride, calcium chloride and sodium lactate in water, is one of the most common resuscitative fluids used in haemorrhagic shock. As it closely resembles blood plasma, but without the formed elements, it can be used as an emergency plasma expander until the patient's blood has been grouped and cross-matched. It rarely causes any adverse reaction, is inexpensive and readily available.

Colloids

A colloid is a solution containing large particles, such as protein, which help to restore the interstitial osmotic pressure. Examples of colloids are albumin and fresh frozen plasma. However, synthetic solutions, such as succinylated gelatin (Gelofusine) or dextran, are being used increasingly, due to the expense of human products.

Combined solutions

Mayor (2004) in a recent research study involving 7000 critically ill patients, suggested that there was no difference in outcomes for those patients resuscitated with saline or albumin. Intravenous therapy needs to replace fluid in the cells as well as the vascular compartment, therefore the use of both crystalloid and colloid is indicated.

Blood

The rapid replacement of blood and blood products is essential in the haemorrhagically shocked patient. Blood replaces volume in the intra- and extracellular spaces and, in addition, has oxygen-carrying capacity as well as clotting factors. It is often necessary to use a pressure infuser to increase the rate of delivery and a blood warmer to bring the blood up to body temperature in order to avoid excessive cooling of the patient (see Ch. 27).

Autotransfusion This procedure, normally carried out in the operating theatre, involves collecting the lost blood from the patient, filtering the blood, treating the blood with an anticoagulant and reinfusing the patient. Autotransfusion is a popular practice in large trauma centres.

For further reading, see Vanderlinde et al (2002).

Management and treatment of cardiogenic shock

The main goals of therapy in cardiogenic shock are:

- to re-establish circulation to the myocardium
- to minimise heart muscle damage
- to improve the effectiveness of the heart as a pump.

Damage to cardiac muscle can be minimised by improving the heart's oxygen supply and, at the same time, reducing its own oxygen demand. Oxygen supply can be increased by the administration of a high percentage of O_2 via a non-rebreathing face mask. Monitoring via pulse oximetry and blood gas analysis should guide administration (Hand 2001).

An essential part of management is the control of pain, including the administration of intravenous morphine. Morphine also dilates the blood vessels and reduces peripheral resistance, which in turn will further reduce oxygen demand. Tiffany and Jorden (2001) describe the challenges of maintaining an adequate blood pressure by careful fluid management and the use of vasopressor drugs.

The catecholamines, such as adrenaline and noradrenaline, are commonly used to improve contractility and correct hypotension, and since the patient with myocardial ischaemia and impaired myocardial contractility will also be at risk of arrhythmias, anti-arrhythmic agents may also be administered.

Medications commonly used

Catecholamines function by stimulating the smooth muscle receptors of the myocardium. This leads to an increase in the contractility of the myocardium and thereby increases cardiac output, raises arterial pressure and improves tissue perfusion.

Dobutamine is considered the medication of choice by many (Tiffany & Jorden 2001) as it has the advantage of increasing cardiac output and lowering left ventricular filling pressure while not increasing the pulse rate or increasing oxygen demand. If the blood pressure remains low despite adequate doses of dobutamine, dopamine is added to the regimen. Amrinone and milrinone have also been effective in improving cardiac output. Vasodilators such as intravenous nitroglycerin and nitroprusside can be added to decrease afterload and therefore reduce left ventricular work and oxygen consumption. Extreme caution must be used when using these potent medications because of their hypotensive effects.

The intra-aortic balloon pump (IABP)

The IABP is often used in conjunction with medication to improve afterload. It assists a weakened or damaged left ventricle by aiding left ventricle ejection and thus improving coronary artery and peripheral tissue perfusion.

There are various types of IABP, all of which work on the same principle. A balloon-tipped catheter is inserted via the femoral artery and is advanced into the aorta until the balloon is just distal to the left subclavian junction. The cardiac cycle triggers the inflation and deflation of the balloon with carbon dioxide or helium. Inflation during diastole increases intra-aortic blood pressure, thereby improving coronary artery perfusion.

Ventricular assist device

For some patients, the above therapies are not sufficient and ventricular assist may be needed. This device is basically a pump which bypasses a failing ventricle and physically removes blood from the circulation, allowing the ventricle to rest and recover. A large-bore cannula is inserted from the atria to drain blood to the pump and back via another inflow cannula from the pulmonary artery or aorta. The decision to use a ventricular assist device should not be taken lightly, due to the possibility of life-threatening complications such as haemorrhage, arterial occlusion or pulmonary embolism. There is increasing interest in applying this technology to provide implantable assist devices to patients with refractory heart failure until recovery or consideration for heart transplant (Westaby 2000). Both therapies require highly skilled nursing.

Management and treatment of septic shock

Treatment of septic shock is summarised in Figure 18.4. The initial priority is assessing airway, breathing and circulation (Green & Lynn 2000).

Blood gases

Blood gases should be monitored regularly. Access can be gained by arterial cannulation and increasingly nurses are taking responsibility for arterial line sampling in the light of the *Code of Professional Conduct* (Nursing and Midwifery Council 2004). Many patients with septic shock present with a mixed acidosis due to respiratory and metabolic elements. Treating the cause is obviously vital and most patients will require artificial ventilation in a critical care unit.

Nitric oxide and nitric oxide inhibitors

The action of nitric oxide was first identified by Furchgott as early as 1980. Many studies have been carried out to determine the benefits of treatment and successful applications have been made in North America, Europe and Australia (Cuthbertson & Webster 1995).

Vasoactive substances essential in the physiological regulation of blood vessel tone are produced within the endothelial layer of the pulmonary vasculature. One of these substances is endothelium-derived relaxing factor (EDRF). Nitric oxide is the gaseous form of this potent vasodilator.

The physiological effects of nitric oxide The release of nitric oxide is responsible for many physiological effects, including control of vessel tone and tissue perfusion, platelet aggregation, white cell function and neuronal activity. Nitric oxide is produced by the enzyme nitric oxide synthase from the substrate amino acid L-arginine. The nitric oxide produced then diffuses to the vascular smooth muscle layer, stimulating the enzyme guanylate cyclase. Guanosine triphosphate is formed, which then catalyses the production of guanosine monophosphate. This chemical cascade is responsible for smooth muscle relaxation and vasodilatation.

In septic shock, endotoxin stimulates the formation of excessive amounts of endogenous nitric oxide, resulting in profound vasodilatation and hypotension.

Inhalational nitric oxide In many critical care units, nitric oxide in the form of inhalation therapy is currently being used successfully for the treatment of adult respiratory distress syndrome (ARDS; see p. 732) and pulmonary hypertension. Inhalational nitric oxide (INO) improves ventilation–perfusion matching by selectively dilating blood vessels adjacent to ventilated alveoli, without affecting systemic circulation. Although a number of studies have noted an improvement in oxygenation, a multicentre trial failed to show any demonstrable effect on outcomes (Dellinger et al 1998).

Microcirculatory changes

The patient suffering from septic shock needs particular nursing attention to the condition of their skin. The administration of inotropic agents increases peripheral vasoconstriction and the resulting decrease in tissue perfusion puts the patient at risk of pressure ulcers. Moreover, the patient may not be sufficiently haemodynamically stable to allow frequent repositioning or assessment of pressure areas. Such critically ill patients often require the expertise of a tissue viability nurse or specialist nurse to assess and implement a strategy for the prevention of pressure ulcers (see Ch. 29). A number of therapeutic beds are now available for purchase or rent which will provide appropriate therapy; in addition some beds rotate the patient, providing a useful adjunct to postural drainage and physiotherapy (James 1997).

Management and treatment of anaphylactic shock

Swift recognition of anaphylactic shock, which results from a severe allergic reaction to a specific antigen, is vital to the individual's survival. Intervention should aim first at identifying and removing the cause. If this is not possible, the effects of the reaction must be reversed.

In extreme circumstances, intubation and artificial ventilation may be needed to overcome respiratory complications. The medication of choice is i.v. adrenaline to restore vascular tone. Aminophylline may be given to counteract bronchoconstriction and antihistamines may be administered to reverse the adverse effect of the mediator histamine involved in the reaction. As with other forms of shock, oxygen therapy and i.v. fluid replacement will usually be required (see also Ch. 16, p. 682).

Definitive and supportive therapy

From the above, it can be seen that the interventions used in the management and treatment of shock may be described as either 'definitive' or 'supportive' (Rice 1991). The goal of definitive therapy is to locate and correct the cause of the shock and to restore and maintain adequate perfusion and oxygenation of the tissues, whereas the goal of supportive therapy is to improve oxygen delivery to the tissues, to restore and maintain tissue perfusion, and to restore cellular function.

For further reading on the management of shock occurring as a result of fractures and burns, see Chapters 10 and 30, respectively.

MONITORING THE PATIENT IN SHOCK

Monitoring and observation of the patient's ever-changing condition will allow for the prompt correction of deficits. The following are the most important indicators of tissue perfusion and will be discussed in the following sections:

- cardiac status
- respiratory status
- haemodynamic status
- level of consciousness
- renal function
- body temperature
- skin condition.

Monitoring cardiac status

Electrocardiography

An electrocardiogram (ECG) is a recording of the electrical activity of the myocardium and indicates the changes which occur as a result of contraction. The contraction of any heart muscle is associated with electrical changes called depolarisation and these can be detected by electrodes attached to the surface of the body (see Ch. 2). An ECG can be obtained quickly in an emergency department or with a portable electrocardiograph at the site of an accident and can give useful information about the rate and rhythm of the heart. Thus, if arrhythmias arise, they can be detected and treated immediately. All patients who are likely to be suffering from shock should be monitored by electrocardiograph. In addition, heart sounds should be assessed, as should major arterial pulses, for rate, rhythm and pressure.

STOP THINK **18.6** What might cause a shocked patient to experience:

(a) tachycardia — heart rate >100 beats/min
(b) bradycardia — heart rate <60 beats/min?

Monitoring respiratory status

The shocked patient's respiratory status may change rapidly and therefore should be monitored at frequent intervals, allowing for the early detection of potential deterioration. In the early stages, the nurse should be alert to hyperventilation, resulting in respiratory alkalosis followed by fatigue of the respiratory muscles. This may lead to shallow breathing and the risk of respiratory distress, necessitating mechanical ventilation.

Monitoring oxygen saturation

The level of O_2 saturation in the patient's blood (S_aO_2) will give some indication of respiratory status. Continuous monitoring will give valuable information on the individual's response to interventions and can provide early warning of hypoxaemia. Both invasive and non-invasive techniques are available for S_aO_2 measurement.

Pulse oximetry Arterial O_2 saturation along with pulse rate can be monitored continuously by means of a non-invasive electronic device called a pulse oximeter. This functions by measuring the absorption of red and infrared light passed through living tissue, usually a finger, toe or ear lobe. Since results correspond closely to arterial blood gas values, this instrument reduces the need for blood samples. Readings are not affected by skin colour but can be distorted by high blood bilirubin levels, as in jaundice, and in cases of carbon monoxide poisoning and smoke inhalation. Results for very heavy smokers may also be difficult to interpret.

For further reading, see Woodrow (1999) and Casey (2001).

The fibreoptic catheter The fibreoptic catheter can be used to measure the patient's venous oxygen saturation. This pulmonary artery catheter contains two optical fibres: one transmits light from the optical module to the catheter tip; the other collects reflected light at the catheter tip and transmits it back to the optical module. These signals are transmitted to a computer which calculates oxygen saturation percentage values. These values are continuously displayed in numerical form and recorded as a graph. Acceptable oxygen saturation levels are considered to be above 90%, although observing for changes in trends should be the nursing priority.

Monitoring haemodynamic status

In the shocked patient, blood pressure may initially be kept within normal limits by the compensatory mechanisms described earlier (see p. 716). However, as shock progresses and cardiac output decreases, blood pressure will fall. In progressive decompensating shock, the use of a sphygmomanometer to estimate blood pressure is inaccurate and inadequate, and more sophisticated investigation will be required.

Central venous pressure (CVP) monitoring

CVP is the blood pressure within the right atrium and vena cava. Its measurement can give information about blood volume or venous system capacity. It can also give an indication of vascular tone and pulmonary vascular resistance, as well as of the effectiveness of the right heart pump. However, it does not measure left ventricular function and it can be unreliable in the critically ill patient with chronic lung disease, right and left heart failure and valve disease.

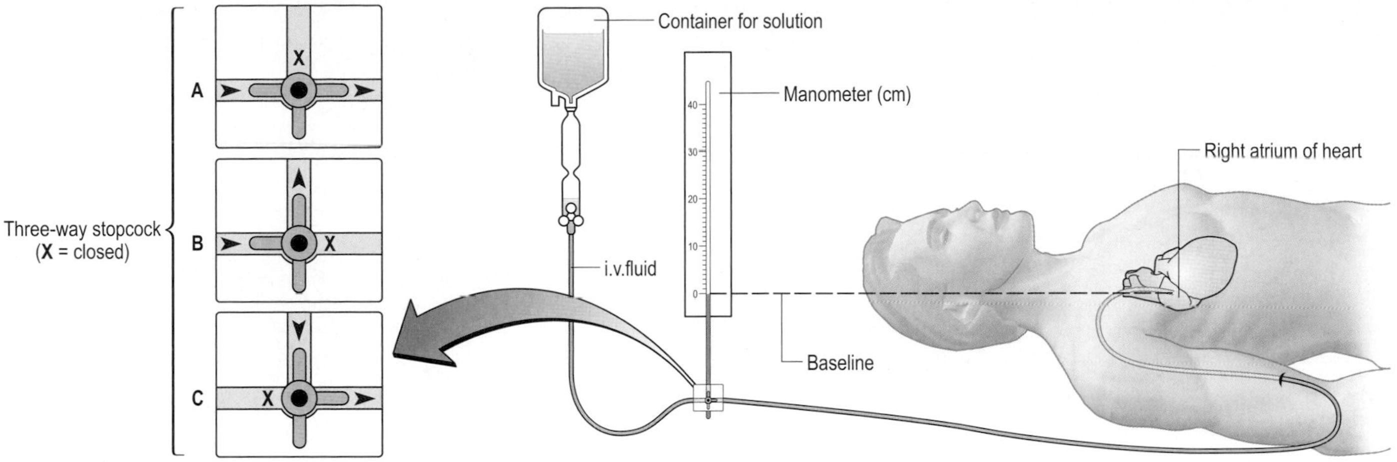

Fig. 18.5 Diagram of a CVP water manometer. A: Before measuring central venous pressure (CVP), the infusion flow is to the patient and the three-way stopcock is closed to the manometer. B: To measure CVP, the stopcock is turned so that it is closed to the patient. This allows the manometer to be refilled with fluid. C: The stopcock is turned so that it is closed to the infusion fluid. This allows a free flow of fluid from the manometer to the intravenous catheter. The fluid level will fall until the level corresponds with the pressure in the right atrium or superior vena cava. (Adapted from Jamieson et al 2003.)

CVP monitoring reflects the rate of blood return to the right side of the heart and can be an accurate guide for fluid replacement. A CVP of approximately 0.5 cm H_2O in the presence of a low arterial blood pressure usually indicates hypovolaemia, whereas a CVP above 14 cm H_2O in the presence of a low arterial blood pressure indicates cardiac failure (see Fig. 18.5).

Technique A large-bore catheter should be inserted under aseptic conditions into the internal or external jugular, subclavian or femoral vein, either using the percutaneous technique via a large-bore needle or by means of a venous cutdown by a member of the medical staff. The site of the central line is checked radiologically prior to the commencement of fluid therapy.

In the intensive therapy or high-dependency unit, a transducer can be attached to the central line in order to obtain a waveform and digital display of the CVP reading in mmHg. Continuous monitoring will indicate the effectiveness of treatment.

Central venous lines, although extremely important for a critically ill patient, present a danger of bacterial infection. Nurses can make an important contribution to care by ensuring that aseptic techniques are adhered to when the line is inserted initially and that the insertion site is kept clean and dry. Once it is no longer needed, the line should be removed as quickly as possible to reduce the risk of infection.

Arterial pressure monitoring

An accurate assessment of blood pressure can be made by measuring the arterial pressure directly. This is performed by medical staff by the insertion of a flexible catheter into an easily accessible artery. The most commonly used site is the radial artery, as the line can be readily secured and observed at this point, and the hand has a good collateral circulation. Other frequently used sites include the brachial, femoral and dorsal arteries.

Once the catheter is inserted, it is attached to a bag of normal saline, which is normally pressurised to around 300 mmHg (see Fig. 18.6). Approximately 2–3 mL/h of the solution is delivered into the artery to maintain patency. By means of a transducer the arterial waveform is displayed on a monitor along with arterial pressure readings.

Patients with an arterial catheter in place require constant nursing supervision in order to ensure that the catheter does not become disconnected — should this happen, the patient could exsanguinate in a matter of minutes. The nurse should ensure that the catheter is securely positioned and covered with a sterile dressing. In addition, the catheter should be clearly labelled to prevent the line being used as an injection port.

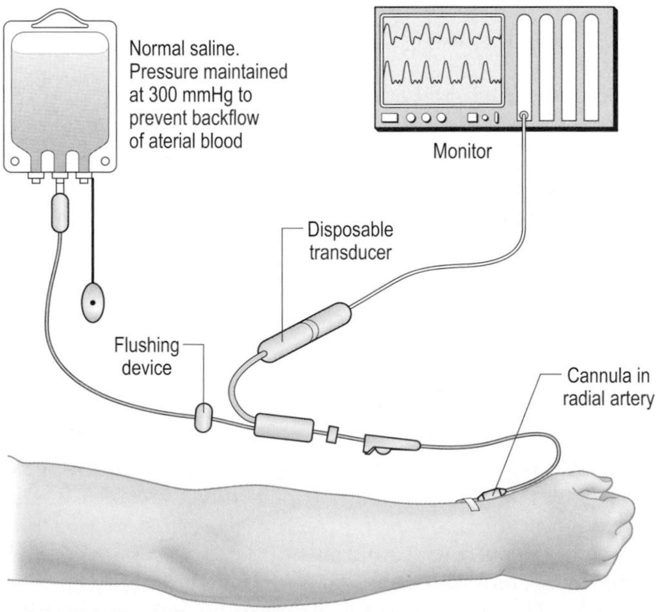

Fig. 18.6 Arterial pressure monitoring equipment.

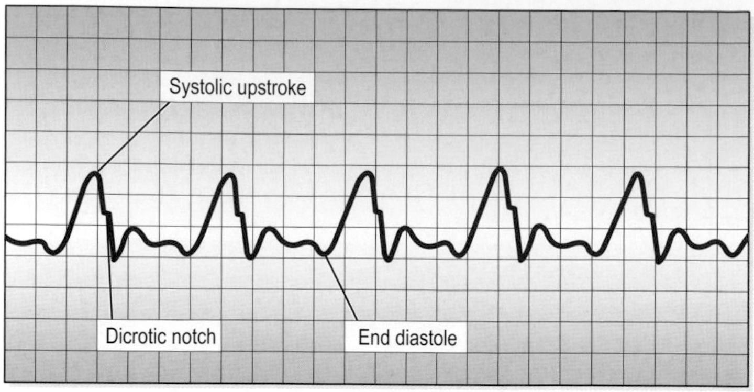

Fig. 18.7 Normal arterial waveform.

The normal waveform will indicate that the arterial catheter is functioning and that the digital blood pressure display is accurate. The nurse must be able to recognise its distinct pattern, which is composed of a systolic upstroke and a dicrotic notch on the downstroke (see Fig. 18.7). The dicrotic notch occurs as a result of the aortic valve closing and a simultaneous increase in aortic pressure. If this pattern becomes dampened, the nurse must be aware that it may indicate a clot in the catheter, air in the line or pressure from the tip of the catheter against the vessel wall itself.

STOP THINK **18.7** If the patient has a pulmonary artery wedge pressure (PAWP) of <8 mmHg, what does that indicate?

18.8 If the PAWP is >25 mmHg, what might be the medical diagnosis?

Cardiac output monitoring

The critically ill patient (see Ch. 29) may require invasive monitoring to allow measurement of cardiac output and oxygen content of both arterial and mixed venous blood.

Cardiac output, and right and left ventricular pressures can be measured by inserting a pulmonary artery catheter into the internal jugular, subclavian, basilic or cephalic veins (see Fig. 18.8). The readings obtained allow the clinician to determine the intervention and therapies required (see Fig. 18.9).

There is much debate in the literature regarding the usefulness and safety of invasive haemodynamic monitoring (Vincent & De Backer 2002). Complications in the use of pulmonary artery catheters have led to ongoing interest in non-invasive or minimally invasive monitoring including Doppler technology, thoracic electrical bioimpedance and pulse contour devices.

For further reading, see Chaney & Derdak (2002).

Monitoring level of consciousness

In the early stages of shock, the patient may still be quite alert and anxious. They may complain of pain and may be able to give a history which will help the clinician to establish a diagnosis. However, if cerebral perfusion pressure falls, with resulting cerebral hypoxia, the patient will gradually become less coherent and may eventually become comatose. The nurse should observe the patient carefully at this stage and ensure the airway is maintained. It may be

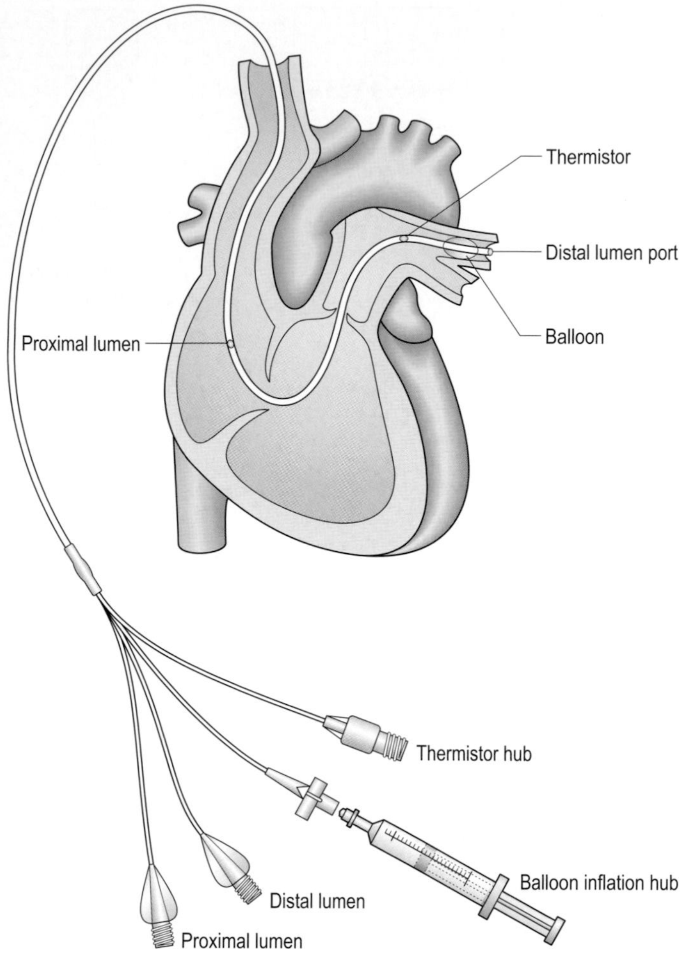

Fig. 18.8 A pulmonary artery catheter. *Distal lumen*: located at the tip of the catheter in the pulmonary artery. Pulmonary artery pressure (PAP), pulmonary artery wedge pressure (PAWP) and mixed venous gas pressures are obtained at this port. *Proximal lumen*: used for central venous pressure (CVP) monitoring or main fluid infusion lumen. It is situated in the right atrium and can also be utilised to measure the right atrial pressure. *Balloon inflation valve*: the balloon situated at the end of the catheter may be inflated to read the PAWP. *Thermistor hub*: situated 4 cm from the tip of the catheter and used to measure cardiac output by thermodilution methods (see Fig. 18.10).

advisable to place the patient in the lateral position. In a clinical setting, medical staff may elect to intubate and artificially ventilate the patient. The Glasgow Coma Scale (see Fig. 28.4, p. 971) is a useful tool with which to assess the patient's cerebral function.

For a detailed discussion of consciousness levels, see Chapter 28, page 967.

Monitoring renal function

Renal function is a very good indicator of tissue perfusion and should therefore be monitored carefully in patients suffering from shock. Since the kidneys are dependent on adequate tissue perfusion, a drop in urinary output will indicate poor perfusion. Unless the patient is dehydrated, urinary output should be 0.5–1.0 mL/kg per h.

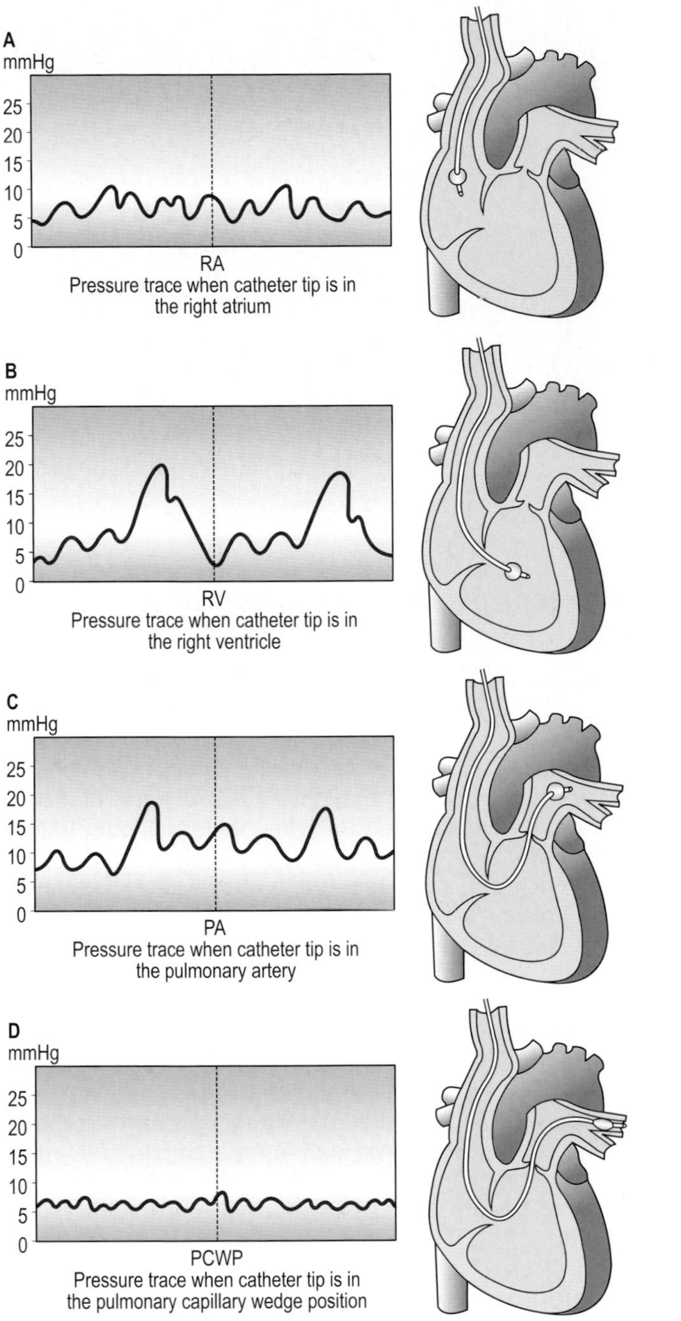

Fig. 18.9 Waveform changes during monitoring by pulmonary artery catheter. A: The catheter is advanced by the doctor until it is in the right atrium. The balloon is then inflated. B: The balloon carries the catheter through the tricuspid valve and into the right ventricle. C: The pressure of blood flow carries the catheter through the pulmonary valve into the pulmonary artery. D: When the catheter has become wedged in a branch of the pulmonary artery, the balloon is deflated and falls back into the pulmonary artery, where it can be used to monitor continuously the pulmonary artery pressure.

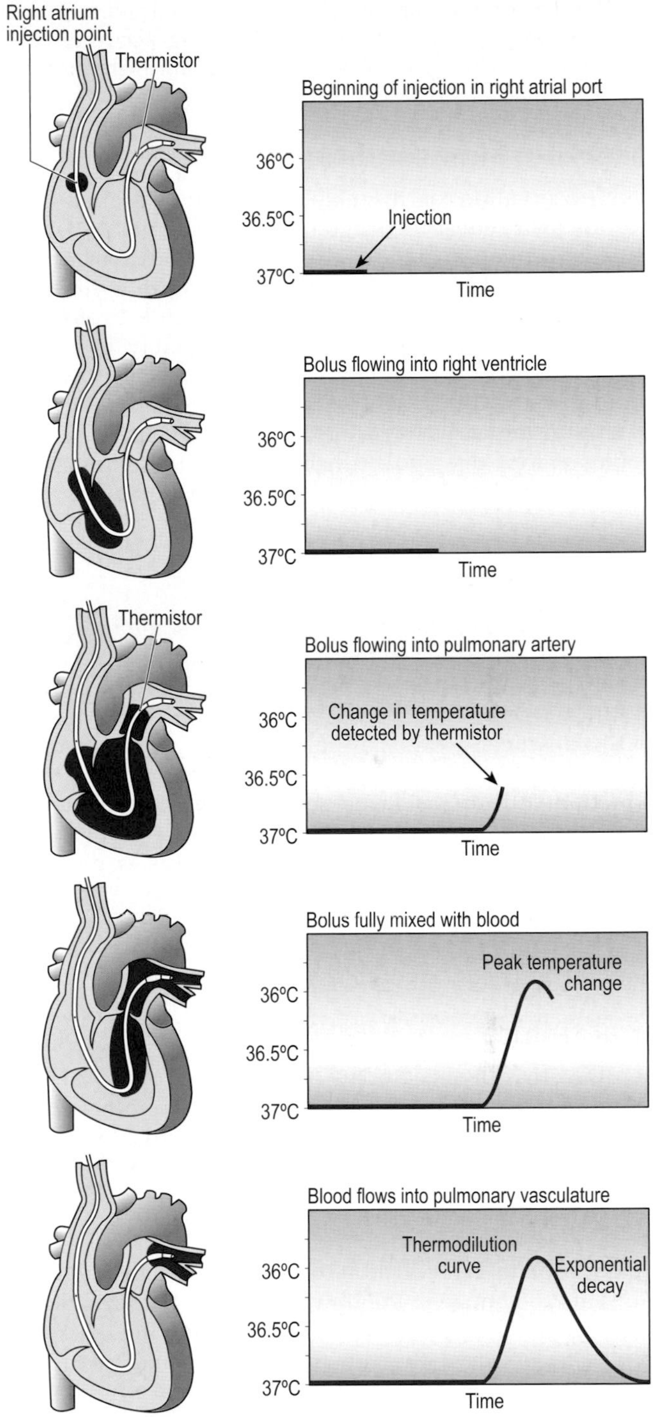

Fig. 18.10 The thermodilution technique for assessing cardiac output.

Urinary catheterisation and hourly urine volumes can assist in early detection of decreasing renal perfusion.

Measurement of specific gravity and osmolality will reflect the concentration of the urine. In the early stages of shock, when urine volume falls, the concentration of excreted waste products rises. However, if the shocked state progresses, urine volumes remain low but the ability to concentrate the urine and blood and the osmolality are fixed or low (Hand 2001).

Monitoring body temperature

The importance of obtaining accurate body temperature measurements should not be underestimated, as many clinical interventions are based on these readings. These factors, as well as procedures for obtaining accurate core temperature readings, are described in detail in Chapter 22.

Observing skin condition

Direct observation of the skin colour, temperature and condition will reflect the stage of shock that the patient is in. Intense activation of the sympathetic nervous system will result in pale, clammy skin and a dry mouth. Failure of capillary refill will indicate sustained and prolonged vasoconstriction. If oxygen delivery is severely impaired, the skin will become cold, mottled and cyanosed. However, it should be noted that the clinical picture in septic shock is different. In the early stages of this type of shock, the skin becomes warm, dry and flushed as bacterial toxins cause vasodilatation.

Laboratory and diagnostic tests

Arterial blood gas (ABG) analysis can give some indication of circulatory efficiency. In the early stages of shock, it is not uncommon to find a fall in the partial pressure of oxygen (PO_2) and a rise in the partial pressure of carbon dioxide (PCO_2). However, PCO_2 may fall due to hyperventilation. With an increase in anaerobic metabolism and in the production of lactic acid, metabolic acidosis is frequently seen in the severely shocked patient.

Information on a range of diagnostic tests is given in Appendix 1.

COMPLICATIONS OF SHOCK

Renal failure

When the crisis of shock occurs, blood flow to the kidneys is reduced both by the original hypovolaemic or other circulatory problem and by the vasoconstriction which occurs as part of the body's compensatory mechanisms (see p. 716).

STOP THINK **18.9** What are the functions of noradrenaline?

In addition to the reduction of blood flow to the kidneys, there is also a change in the flow within the kidneys. Blood flow is directed away from the renal cortex to the renal medulla to preserve the function of the juxtamedullary nephrons. This is essential if the countercurrent system of concentrating the urine is to function (see Ch. 8). If, however, the shock persists without prompt treatment, then the countercurrent mechanism will fail and the urine will become dilute, leading to the early stages of acute renal failure.

Haemofiltration

Many patients with acute renal failure will require renal replacement therapy as part of their treatment. Haemofiltration is the removal of excess fluid and waste products from the blood by a filter in conjunction with fluid replacement. Increasingly, haemofiltration is being used in the critical care area and offers a number of advantages to dialysis (see Fig. 18.11).

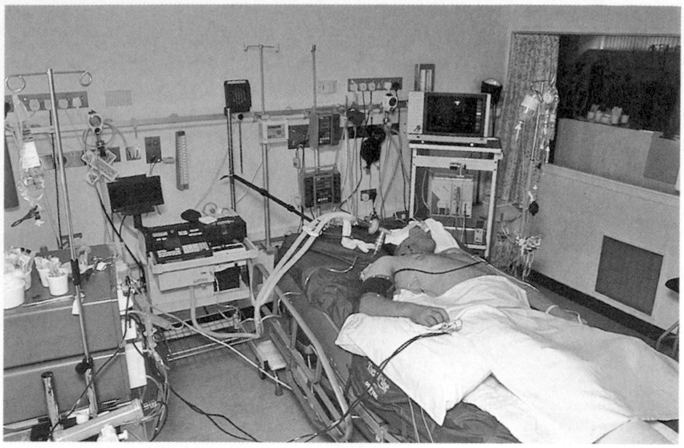

Fig. 18.11 Patient on haemofiltration therapy. (Reproduced with kind permission from NHS Lothian.)

Adult respiratory distress syndrome (ARDS) or acute lung injury

ARDS, now referred to more commonly as acute lung injury (ALI), is characterised by acute, severe and progressive respiratory distress, increased stiffness of the lungs and diffuse lung opacification. At cellular level, a number of substances are activated, including macrophages, platelets, proteases, lysosomes, endotoxins, polymorphonuclear lysosomes and free oxygen radicals, which cause damage to the alveolar capillary membrane and lead to the classic signs of pulmonary oedema. In addition, surfactant production is decreased, secondary to atelectasis, resulting in dyspnoea.

Although treatment has become sophisticated, there is still no medication or procedure which will cure ARDS/ALI. The mortality rate remains approximately 60% and has shown little reduction despite increased technology and intervention (Brower et al 2001). Standard supportive care for patients with ARDS/ALI will involve therapeutic intervention in an intensive care unit. Increasingly, novel modes of mechanical ventilation are being used to treat this group of patients.

Positioning of patients

The body position of critically ill patients may have a profound effect on arterial oxygenation. The prone position is used primarily for the treatment of ARDS/ALI and can significantly improve oxygenation in this group of patients (Marion 2001).

For further reading, see MacDonald & Armstrong (2000).

Disseminated intravascular coagulation (DIC)

DIC is a serious disorder of coagulation that may cause severe organ damage or failure. Some of the pathophysiological processes leading to DIC have already been described in relation to septic shock (see p. 720). In DIC the patient's normal clotting mechanisms do not function correctly. Clots may be produced in capillaries where they are not

Table 18.1 Signs of disseminated intravascular coagulation (DIC)

System	Haemorrhagic signs	Microemboli signs
Integumentary	Oozing/bleeding from i.v. sites, arterial lines, previous surgical sites and mucous membranes	Patchy cyanosis, gangrene
Neurological	Altered level of consciousness, subarachnoid bleeding	Altered level of consciousness, cerebral vascular accident
Pulmonary	Haemoptysis	Pulmonary embolus, adult respiratory distress syndrome
Gastrointestinal	Gastrointestinal bleed, abdominal distension	Bowel infarction, constipation, diarrhoea
Renal	Haematuria	Haematuria, oliguria, renal insufficiency/failure

required, and sites where clotting factors could be utilised are deprived of them. Fibrinolytic (clot-dissolving) factors then go into action where they are not needed, and the end result is uncontrolled haemorrhage. The nurse plays an essential role in early recognition of DIC and Table 18.1 lists the signs of DIC (Geiter 2003). Treatment is aimed at replacing the clotting factors by administering blood and blood components, platelets, fresh frozen plasma and possibly cryoprecipitates.

CONCLUSION

Although there have been important advances in the resuscitation and treatment of patients in shock, survival can be further improved by early recognition and supportive therapy.

Assisting individuals suffering from shock, whether in a hospital or a community setting, presents the nurse with a major challenge. Intervention will require not only a sound understanding of the pathophysiological processes of shock, but also the ability to act swiftly on the basis of that understanding and to assist with a range of resuscitative and investigative procedures. Above all, the nurse is in a unique position to ensure that patients and their loved ones are supported and informed throughout this life-threatening experience.

REFERENCES

ALERT — Acute Life-Threatening Events Recognition and Treatment. Home page http://web.port.ac.uk/alert/intro.htm

Bone R C, Balk R A, Cerra F B et al 1992 Definitions for sepsis and organ failure and guidelines for the use of innovative therapies in sepsis. Chest 101: 1644–1655

Bone R C, Grodzin C J, Balk B A 1997 Sepsis: a new hypothesis for pathogenesis of the disease process. Chest 112: 235–243

Brower R G, Ware L B, Berthiaume Y, Mattay M A 2001 Treatment of ARDS. Chest 120(4): 1347–1367

Colquhoun M C, Handley A J, Evans T 2003 ABC of resuscitation. BMJ Publications, London

Cuthbertson B H, Webster N R 1995 Nitric oxide in critical care medicine. British Journal of Hospital Medicine 54(11): 579–582

Dellinger R P, Zimmerman J L, Taylor R W 1998 Effects of inhaled nitric oxide in patients with acute respiratory distress syndrome: results of a randomized phase II trial. Critical Care Medicine 26: 15–23

Dipenbrock N 1999 Quick reference guide to intensive care. Lippincott, Philadelphia

Geiter H 2003 Disseminated intravascular coagulopathy. Dimensions of Critical Care Nursing 22(3): 108–114

Green J, Lynn W A 2000 Presentation and clinical features of severe sepsis. Journal of the Royal College of Physicians of London 34(5): 418–423

Guyton A C, Hall J E 2000 Textbook of medical physiology, 10th edn. W B Saunders, Philadelphia

Hand H 2001 Shock. Nursing Standard 15(48): 45–52

Haslett C, Chilvers E R, Burn N A, Colledge N R 2002 Davidson's principles and practice of medicine, 19th edn. Churchill Livingstone, Edinburgh

Hudak C M, Gallo B M 1998 Critical care nursing: a holistic approach. Lippincott, Philadelphia

James H 1997 Pressure sore prevention in acutely ill patients. Professional Nurse 12(Suppl 6): S8–10

Jamieson E M, McCall J M, Blythe R, White L A 2003 Guidelines for clinical nursing practices, 4th edn. Churchill Livingstone, Edinburgh

Jowett N I, Thompson D R 2002 Comprehensive coronary care. Scutari, Harrow

Marion B 2001 A turn for the better: prone positioning of patients with ARDS. A guide to the physiology and management of this effective, underused intervention. American Journal of Nursing 101(5): 26–35

Mayor S 2004 Saline has a similar effect to albumin in critically ill patients. British Journal of Medicine 328: 852

Nursing and Midwifery Council (NMC) 2004 Code of professional conduct: standards for conduct, performance and ethics. NMC, London

Rice V 1991 Shock: a clinical syndrome. Parts 1–4. Critical Care Nurse 11(4–7): 20–27; 74–82; 34–39; 28–39

Sepsis Care Initiative 2002 Slide kit and bibliography – CD-ROM. Eli Lilly & Co. Ltd, Basingstoke

Smelzer S, Bone B 2000 Brunner and Suddart's textbook of medical–surgical nursing. Lippincott, Philadelphia

Tiffany B R, Jorden R C 2001 Cardiogenic shock. In: Harwood-Nuss A, Wolfson A B, Linden C H, Shepherd S M, Stenk P H (eds) The clinical practice of emergency medicine, 3rd edn. Lippincott, Williams and Wilkins, Baltimore

Vincent J, De Backer D 2002 Cardiac output measurement: is least invasive always best? Critical Care Medicine 30(10): 2380–2382

Westaby S 2000 New implantable blood pumps for medium and long term circulatory support. Perfusion 15(4): 319–325

FURTHER READING

ALERT – Acute Life-Threatening Events Recognition and Treatment. Home page http://web.port.ac.uk/alert/intro.htm

British Infection Society 2003 Early management of suspected bacterial meningitis and meningococcal septicaemia in adults. Online. Available: www.britishinfectionsociety.org

Casey G 2001 Oxygen transport and the use of pulse oximetry. Nursing Standard 15(47): 46–53

Chaney J C, Derdak S 2002 Minimally invasive haemodynamic monitoring for the intensivist. Critical Care Medicine 30(10): 2338–2345

Fahey M 2001 Spinal shock: a nurse's perspective. Journal of Orthopaedic Nursing 6(1): 18–22

Gully S 2002 Nursing management of necrotising fasciitis. Nursing Standard 16(52): 39–42

MacDonald C, Armstrong D 2000 The prone position – a nursing perspective. Nursing in Critical Care 5(5): 215–219

McArthur-Rouse F 2001 Critical care outreach services and early warning scoring systems: a review of the literature. Journal of Advanced Nursing 36(5): 696–704

Resuscitation Council (UK) 2000 ABC – airway, breathing, circulation. Online. Available: www.resus.org.uk/pages/bls.htm

Tortora G J, Grabowski S R 2003 Principles of anatomy and physiology, 10th edn. HarperCollins, New York

Vanderlinde E S, Heal J, Blumberg N 2002 Autologous transfusion. British Medical Journal 324(7340): 772–775

Woodrow P 1999 Pulse oximetry. Nursing Standard 13(42): 42–46

Woodrow P 2002 Central venous catheters and central venous pressure. Nursing Standard 16(26): 45–52

PAIN

19

Sue Duke

INTRODUCTION

Although pain is a common experience, it is a complex one, unique for each individual every time it is experienced. The experience of pain is influenced by an interaction between physiological, psychological and sociocultural factors and encompasses sensory, emotional, cognitive and behavioural components (Melzack & Wall 1996). This means that it is difficult to understand what pain is like for another person. Much is known about the pathophysiology of pain and treatment modalities but less about the lived experience of pain. Research is beginning to address this deficit, through studies that vividly portray the individual's personal description of their pain experience, and also those which focus on clinical decision making about pain management. This chapter will commence with two such personal descriptions, followed by a discussion of various definitions of pain. The many and complex factors which influence the experience of pain will then precede discussion of the mechanisms of pain and the implications for nursing care.

THE EXPERIENCE OF PAIN AND THE ADEQUACY OF DEFINITIONS OF PAIN

STOP THINK **19.1** Think about a time when you were in pain. Write down your description of this experience. Compare your description with the discussion below.

Here is how one person described the pain she experienced: 'Bodily feelings were shrieking agony at the top of their voices, mental feelings were fury and total frustration' (Seers & Friedli 1996).

Another quotation from the same study describes the overwhelming nature of pain:

> *Pain is now beyond coping with … it has stopped me leading my whole life. I'm petrified they'll say I have to learn to live with this level of pain … I would rather die. I'd like to be unconscious. Deep inside I feel suicidal … Can't see through the pain when there is so much and I know I do not want to live with it.*

These quotations give vivid insight into the impact that pain has on an individual's life. In contrast, many definitions of pain emphasise the physiological sensation of pain. For example, the International Association for the Study of Pain (1994) defined pain as 'an unpleasant sensory and emotional experience associated with actual or potential tissue damage, or described in terms of such damage'. This definition has been criticised for not accounting for other peripheral stimuli, for central nervous system (CNS) activity and the variable way in which the nervous system responds to stimuli, especially after injury (Melzack & Wall 1996).

The concept of pain as a sensation is criticised by Bendelow and Williams (1995) from a sociological perspective. They argued that this emphasis elevates sensation over emotion and ignores social and cultural perspectives. They draw on Morris (1991) who suggested that pain emerges at the intersection of bodies, minds and cultures. Some definitions have tried to encompass this interaction, e.g. National Institutes of Health (1987):

> *Pain is a subjective experience that can be perceived directly only by the sufferer. It is a multidimensional phenomenon that can be described by pain location, intensity, temporal aspects, quality, impact and meaning. Pain does not occur in isolation but in a specific human being in psychosocial, economic, and cultural contexts that influence the meaning, experience and verbal and non-verbal expression of pain.*

Some definitions emphasise the invisibility of pain and its inexplicability, qualities that Scarry (1985) first proposed as being intrinsic to the experience of pain. These qualities make it possible to be physically near someone in pain yet to be unaware of their pain (Whelan 2003). McCaffery (1972) referred to the invisibility of pain in her seminal definition: 'Pain is whatever the experiencing person says it is, existing whenever he says it does'. This definition has encouraged nurses to value a patient's self-report of pain, although in clinical practice this is often balanced against other information, such as the nurse's expectations of how much pain a patient should be in (Carr & Mann 2000). As Scarry (1985) argued, health professionals can 'perceive the voice of the patient as an "unreliable narrator" of bodily events and discount patient report in favour of what the body reveals'. On the other hand, if nurses believe the patient's self-report of pain at face value, they may not take into account personal and contextual issues that can influence an individual's self-report (Price & Cheek 1996). For example, surgical patients have been reported to underplay their pain if they see nurses are busy (Carr & Mann 2000), older people may minimise their pain for fear of being 'taken over' by medicine (Frampton 2003), and Thomas (2000) stated that people with persistent pain do not talk about their pain for fear of adverse reactions from others. Thus, accepting the patient's report at face value may not enable the practitioner to explore the person's experience of pain in order that it can be understood in terms of the impact of pain on their self-concept and their quality of life. To achieve this, a patient's report of pain must be framed within the context of their experience and the depth of interaction between practitioner and patient (Price & Cheek 1996).

McCaffery's (1972) definition depends on an individual being able to say that they are in pain and to describe this experience. As Whelan (2003) states: 'Pain is ineffable and elusive: it confounds the grasp of language'. This perhaps explains why, as yet, no definition adequately describes the all-encompassing experience of pain.

Despite the lack of an adequate definition of pain, research over the last decade or more has expanded understanding of the experience of pain. Using the philosophical concept of embodiment, Bendelow and Williams (1995) presented a sociological response to their criticism of the dominance of the sensation of pain over the emotional experience.

- *Embodiment* describes the usual state in which the body is experienced in health. On the whole, people are unaware of their body. In illness or pain the body can become the focus of experience; it is monitored for changes and life is lived in relation to this. People in persistent pain describe the body as an obstacle to daily living (Thomas 2000, Paulson et al 2002) and wait to feel 'themselves' again — paradoxically meaning that they will no longer be aware of their body.
- In severe or persistent pain, people begin to define themselves in terms of pain. This is called *disembodiment*. The participants in Paulson et al's (2002) study described how pain altered their perception of themselves, so that each became a different person to the one before they had pain. Madjar (1998) and Thomas (2000) described how pain blocked all other sensations and thoughts. Participants in Thomas's (2000) study felt continually tied to their internal pain, which was described as 'tormentor', 'opponent' or 'monster'.

Pain also took over lived space and time. Space became reduced to the immediate environment and people felt isolated as a consequence (Paulson et al 2002). Time became defined in terms of the 'moment' (Thomas 2000), the moment in which pain is experienced and the thought of future suffering. When pain was at its worst, people experienced a stopping of time, as if the moment would never end. Madjar (1998) quoted one participant who said:

> *... everything just slowed down because that was hurting so much and relief was not coming soon enough. So I think a second turns into a minute and a minute into an hour.*

Madjar (1998) and Paulson et al (2002) also pointed to the exhaustion that accompanies being in, and enduring pain. They described how participants were exhausted by the intensity of pain, the tension and vigilance needed to face and endure it, and, in Madjar's study, by the energy expended to cope with nursing procedures that accompanied their condition. One participant explained:

> *I've got no choice but to sit in here and face this pain. All my energy is going in [to] this pain and that's getting it away from me.*

FACTORS INFLUENCING THE EXPERIENCE OF PAIN

STOP THINK **19.2** Think back to the experience of pain that you described in stop-think 19.1 and to your experiences of caring for people in pain. From these experiences, make a list of factors that might influence someone's pain. Organise your thoughts under the following headings: factors related to individual differences; factors related to small systems such as families and care teams; factors related to organisations, society and cultures. Compare your thoughts with the following discussion.

How pain is experienced is influenced by a number of factors.

Individual influences

Past learning

Learning about pain takes place throughout life, through the process of socialisation. If a child falls over and hurts their knee, they learn that this feeling is called pain. They also learn how they are expected to react by the response that they elicit, e.g. sympathy and a cuddle may reinforce crying when in pain, whereas ignoring the complaint and subsequent praise may reinforce the minimisation of pain.

Gender

It has been suggested that men are better able to tolerate pain than women, but the evidence for this is inconclusive and mostly taken from data reporting the incidence of pain. A population prevalence study (*n* = 10 000) in Sweden, found women reported significantly more incidence of pain than men (Müllersdorf & Söderback 2000). Similar findings were reported from an epidemiological study of pain in the Grampian region of Scotland (*n* = 3605) (Elliott et al 1999) and from a population-based telephone survey by Portenoy et al (2004). These findings may be explained by the different ways in which men and women are socialised (Bendelow 1993). In some societies men are expected to be 'brave', and tend not to report pain, whereas women are expected to be expressive or 'emotional', and tend to report pain. Another possibility is that gender differences can be explained in terms of coping style. Rollnik et al (2003) found that women were more likely to adopt passive coping strategies, whereas men were more likely to adopt active coping strategies. Passive coping strategies are more likely to result in disability as a consequence of pain.

Coping is also influenced by socioeconomic factors. Portenoy et al (2004) argue that women are more likely to have poorer socioeconomic conditions than men, which may provide an alternative explanation for gender differences in the pain experience and behavioural response.

Age

The evidence with respect to the influence of age on the experience of pain is conflicting. It has been suggested that age diminishes the experience of pain. In a study examining the influence of age on women with fibromyalgia, Burckhardt et al (2001) found that younger women perceived pain severity to be higher than older women. This is in contrast to evidence that pain is more common and more severe in older people (Elliott et al 1999) and that older people do not seek help because they feel their pain is to be expected and tolerated (Yates et al 1995, Lansbury 2000). In Yates et al's (1995) study, one participant stated:

> *Well, I just realised that I've got to live with it you know ... it's always there ... it's no good. I've just got to learn to live with it, I know fully well that nothing will help me now.*

The underplaying of pain in older people is likely to be reinforced by a lack of recognition and assessment of pain in this group by health and social care professionals (Blomqvist & Edberg 2002, Blomqvist 2003, Frampton 2003), and by a desire to remain independent on the part of the older person (Frampton 2003):

> *I'm concerned of others' reactions. I don't like to tell others about my pain for fear of worrying them. I am concerned that they will try and take me over and I will lose control.*

Personality

An individual's personality will influence the way in which they express and cope with pain. For example, drawing on Eysenck's theory of the personality, several studies have demonstrated that an internal locus of control, in combination with active coping strategies leads, to less depression and pain compared with an external locus of control and passive coping strategies (Arraras et al 2002, Smith et al 2002, Bishop & Warr 2003).

The ability to cope

Several studies suggest that a person's ability to cope with pain influences perceptions of disability and quality of life (Walker et al 1990, Melanson & Downe-Wamboldt 2003, Tsai et al 2003). These studies adopt the definition of coping given by Lazarus (1993):

> *What a person does to cope depends on the context in which the disease occurs, and this will change over time because of what is attended to, and the threats themselves also change.*

Walker et al (1990) found that older people were less likely to cope if they were lonely, or coping with other problems such as financial difficulties or the illness or death of a friend. From a descriptive longitudinal study (*n* = 39; 75 years+), Melanson and Downe-Wamboldt (2003) suggested that the ability of older people to cope with the pain resulting from rheumatoid arthritis influenced their ability to be independent and have a sense of control in their lives. The majority of participants perceived pain as signifying harm and coped through problem-solving strategies.

From a study examining the relationship between pain and other influences on daily stresses and between stress and depression in a group of older people with arthritis (*n* = 71; mean age 71.6, range not given), Tsai et al (2003) suggested that people's ability to cope was influenced by the degree to which they felt supported by others. Their results demonstrated that pain, disability and social support were predictors for daily stress and that daily stress *per se* was predictive of depression.

The meaning of pain

Pain will have different meanings for different people. Some patients may view pain as a punishment, while others may see it as having some value for self-testing or personal growth; yet others may see it as something that must be eradicated. Pain from a recurrence of cancer, for example, is likely to have a different significance for the patient compared to pain following elective surgery. People with cancer often fear that pain means that their disease is progressing, or that pain will increase as death approaches (Oldham & Kristjanson 2004). Pain following surgery is expected, although people often underestimate the intensity of the pain to be experienced (Carr & Thomas 1997), causing them to fear that the pain signifies complications. Persistent pain may also have implications for the individual's self-image by necessitating a change in or loss of role. The meaning of pain will also be influenced by individual pain beliefs (Williams & Thorn 1989). In an influential analysis, Williams and Thorn (1989) described three beliefs that negatively influence the experience and severity of pain — whether the individual blames themselves for the pain, sees the pain as mysterious and/or sees pain as something that has to be endured. They argued that any of these beliefs could negatively affect self-esteem, and predispose to psychological distress and a feeling of loss of control.

Body part affected

The part of the body involved may influence the expression of pain (McCaffery & Pasero 1999). Some areas of the body, such as the rectum or genitals, may be difficult for some people to talk about, and thus pain in these areas may go unreported and potentially have a negative effect on an individual's sexuality and self-concept. The assessment and relief of pain in these areas therefore needs skilled management and the patient may benefit from referral to a nurse specialist in pain management.

Factors related to families and the care teams

Interaction between the person in pain and their partner

Pain rarely has an isolated influence. The influence of pain in relationships has been long recognised. Witnessing pain is distressing (Coyle 2004) and can affect the physical and psychological health of a partner (Turk et al 1987, Taylor et al 1990). In Ferrell et al's (1991a) study, family carers described their feelings of fear, suffering, helplessness, heartbreak and denial. They quote one spouse who said: 'It is the saddest thing in the world. I share her pain. If she hurts, I hurt. What else can I say?'. Sometimes, such feelings can influence the way in which couples communicate and cope with the experience of pain. In a phenomenological study describing seven people's experience of cancer pain, Coyle (2004) reported that severe pain can influence an individual's desire for death and this can cause conflict with family members' wish for that person to live.

The impact of pain on styles of interaction between couples has been studied more comprehensively in persistent pain, some research suggesting that particular styles of communication can reinforce an individual's disability. Romano et al (1995) and Schwartz et al (1996) found that physical and psychosocial disabilities were more likely in spouses responding in a concerned way, who were solicitous, and less likely in those whose spouses responded in a negative way. A review of 27 studies examining patient–spouse interactions confirmed these findings (Newton-John 2002) but warned that interactions are more complex than suggested by the research on which these findings are based.

Some of the complexity of spousal experience of pain is elicited in a narrative study of five men married to women with fibromyalgia, undertaken by Söderberg et al (2003). The analysis highlighted how pain influenced many aspects of the spouses' lives, in addition to their relationship with their wife. This included changing relationships with friends and relatives, i.e. less frequent contact, and deepening relationship with their children, as well as taking responsibility for work within the home and acting as an advocate for their wife.

Family dynamics

Families play an important role in the health of individuals and in their care (Oldham & Kristjanson 2004). Thus the experience of pain will be influenced by how family members cope. Families who have effective coping strategies can positively influence an individual's experience of pain through support. On the other hand, families who have ineffective coping responses may aggravate an individual's pain and, in turn, the family dynamics (Schwartz et al 1996). Dura and Beck (1988) observed that families with ineffective coping strategies are typically characterised by:

- enmeshed relationships where interactions are polarised — either overprotective or detached
- lack of cohesion within the family group
- controlling and manipulative behaviour
- conflict and a lack of expression of their feelings.

Team dynamics

A patient's experience of pain can be influenced by the response of health care professionals (Carr & Mann 2000). If a nurse can be with someone in pain without becoming unduly distressed or without judging that person's response, then nurse and patient are likely to interact in a way that encourages discussion and optimal pain management. Conversely, a nurse who feels overwhelmed by such situations is likely to use distancing strategies such as depersonalising the pain and playing down its severity (Madjar 1998). Such strategies result in poor assessment of pain and the exacerbation of patient and nurse distress. An individual's experience of pain will also be influenced by the way in which the health care team functions. Nursing is predominantly a team endeavour, irrespective of where it is taking place. For example, effective pain relief postoperatively is dependent on a congruent plan between anaesthetists, ward-based nursing and medical personnel, general practitioners and district nurses. Where there is disagreement about a care plan, tension may arise and this can negatively affect the patient's experience of pain (Carr & Mann 2000).

Social and environmental factors

Cultural influences on the experience of pain

The relationship between culture and pain has been researched by what Lasch (2002) describes as two genres of studies. The first — culture *of* pain — refers to research investigating the way in which society shapes the meaning and treatment of pain. The second — culture *in* pain — refers to research addressing the ways in which pain is moulded by an individual's perception and expression of pain. Few studies have been undertaken to understand the way in which society shapes the meaning and treatment of pain (Lasch 2002), although Carr and Mann (2000) and Portenoy et al (2004) suggest that people from minority cultural groups are more likely to experience poor pain management. However, more research has been undertaken about cultural perception and expression of pain. Each cultural group has its own behaviours, beliefs, values and meaning 'scripts' that shape responses to pain, as well as help-seeking activities and receptivity to health care interventions. For example, most British people traditionally value control over the display of emotions — maintaining a 'stiff upper lip' — which has the effect of discouraging people from reporting pain.

A classic study by Zborowski (1952) illustrates the link between culture and pain. Men from three groups were compared: 'old Americans', i.e. their grandparents or earlier forebears were born in America and they did not identify with a particular cultural group, Italian Americans and Jewish Americans. The 'old Americans' attempted to avoid showing any pain, tended to withdraw and preferred to be alone when in severe pain. The Italian and Jewish Americans, however, openly expressed their pain and did not want to be alone. The Italian Americans were concerned with relief of their pain, while the Jewish Americans were concerned about the implications of their pain for the future. This study has been criticised for selecting people whose culture, and consequently their responses, may have been 'diluted' by their residence in America; nevertheless, the study points to the influence of culture on expression and experience.

The influence of culture on the experience and expression of pain has more recently been explored through narrative research. This approach to understanding the influence of culture on the experience of pain enables the beliefs and values that shape this experience to be understood. Lasch (2002) gives an overview of this work on the International Association for the Study of Pain website (see 'Useful websites and addresses').

Socioeconomic factors

Several studies have demonstrated that socioeconomic factors influence pain experience. In their epidemiological study of pain, Elliott et al (1999) found that persistent pain was associated with living in rented council accommodation, being retired and being unable to work. Portenoy et al (2004) found a similar relationship between persistent pain and low income. Richards et al (2002) found that people from a socioeconomically deprived area were less likely to report chest pain than people from more affluent areas. In a qualitative study examining variations in perception and behavioural response to pain, they found that people from deprived areas were less likely to present to medical services following chest pain because they were concerned that they would be chastised for their risk behaviours, e.g. smoking. The authors suggested that this affects their access to health services.

Organisational factors

Organisational culture can influence pain experience; for example, patients may respond to their pain in hospital according to how they feel they should respond, rather than according to the pain experienced. Davidson (1988) suggested that organisations utilise a variety of strategies to manage difficult situations such as pain. He describes these strategies as the 'institutional denial of pain'. The most powerful of these strategies is to render the patient a passive receiver of care. Carr and Thomas (1997) described how patients may be reluctant to tell nurses that they are in pain because they feel dehumanised and helpless while in hospital. In an extensive phenomenological study, Madjar (1998) illustrates how the clinical environment encourages patients to behave with composure and cooperation, despite being in considerable pain. In this study, patients with severe burns described how they controlled their expression of pain during dressing changes, in order not to impede the work of nurses, so as to have the best possible chance of recovery.

Organisational issues also influence how nurses respond to pain. Madjar (1998) described several instances where nurses expect patients to cope with pain through their ability to endure pain rather than through having adequate analgesics, as the following excerpt from the study illustrates:

> *His requests for pain relief, his obvious distress, obvious physical distress, and just his communication, his whole attitude ... I think he is at the stage now where we have to be firm with him, talk to him, try and talk him through [painful procedures without the use of opioids], to make him more comfortable in other ways.*

In addition to environmental influences, several structural organisational issues influence pain, such as the availability of medications. In some countries, common analgesics such as morphine are unavailable and, in the UK, these medications may be unavailable or restricted out of hours and at weekends. Similarly, prescription practices may influence the availability of medications (Schafheutle et al 2001).

MECHANISMS OF PAIN

In addition to individual, group and contextual influences on pain, physiological mechanisms mediate how individuals experience pain. Emotional, cognitive and behavioural influences interact with sensory mechanisms of pain, sometimes exacerbating the sensory perception of pain and sometimes modulating it (Frischenschlarger & Pucher 2002). Understanding this interaction is key to understanding how to manage pain from a pharmacological, a medical and a nursing perspective.

ANATOMY AND PHYSIOLOGY

STOP THINK **19.3** Before reading the next section, try to describe the physiological 'pathway' of pain from an injury to your leg to your cognitive awareness of pain.

Nociceptors

As in all sensations, pain is recognised by specific receptors. These are nociceptors — free sensory nerve endings that detect physical and chemical damage to the tissues and form a widespread and overlapping network in almost all tissues of the body. Like other neurones, nociceptors are classified according to their speed of conduction and their diameter. Most nociceptors fall into the A and C groups of sensory neurones. Nociceptors are structurally similar to other sensory neurones but differ in respect of their thresholds, i.e. the minimum stimulus that activates them, and their specificity (Carpenter 2003). Some nociceptors, such as the fast conducting myelinated A-delta (A-δ) neurones, are unimodal and respond to high threshold mechanical stimulus. Other A-δ neurones are bimodal, responding to both chemical and mechanical or thermal stimuli. Most of the slower conducting non-myelinated C fibres are polymodal and respond to chemical, thermal, mechanical and touch stimuli. The differentiation between A and C nociceptors is a fundamental principle of the gate control theory of pain, discussed below. However, it is important to appreciate that this differentiation is simplistic, since there is a dynamic interaction between all nociceptors.

Chemical stimulation is usually a result of tissue damage and the subsequent release of chemicals around the free nerve endings. These chemicals are released by damaged cells and by the action of neurotransmitters released by nociceptors. For example, damaged cells synthesise prostaglandins and leukotrienes from membrane phospholipids. The neurotransmitter, substance P, and other peptides are released from C fibres, causing sensitisation, vasodilatation and leakage from blood vessels. In addition, substance P induces histamine release from mast cells and 5-hydroxytryptamine — 5-HT, serotonin — from platelets. Chemicals are also released from the sympathetic fibres and contribute to pain and aspects of the inflammatory process (Stannard & Booth 2004; see also Ch. 23, p. 835). Such chemicals either directly initiate a response in the nociceptor or sensitise it to further stimulation, i.e. lower the threshold.

Peripheral nerve pathways

Once a nociceptor has been activated, an electrical impulse is conducted along afferent, i.e. sensory, neurones to the CNS. This is achieved through the exchange of sodium and potassium across the neurone membrane through the sodium pump, a specialised membrane-bound protein.

Spinal cord pathways

Nociceptors communicate with the CNS at the dorsal horn of the spinal cord (see Fig. 19.1). The dorsal horn is the posterior part of the grey, butterfly-shaped area seen on cross-section of the spinal cord. This is surrounded by white matter — myelinated axons stretching the length of the spinal cord. These fibres are either ascending or descending pathways connecting the brain with the dorsal horn.

The grey matter comprises the cell bodies of interneurones, small neurones that link the peripheral nervous system with the CNS via specialised nerve pathways. A cross-section of the spinal cord shows a loose structural organisation of these cells in 10 layers called lamina. Six of these laminae are in the dorsal horn and roughly correspond to the cells responsible for nociception. The outer two, laminae I and II, comprise the substantia gelatinosa, identified by Melzack and Wall (1996) as a key area in nociception, central to the gate control theory. However, research has shown that most noxious stimuli are assessed by nociceptive-specific (NS) cells in lamina I (Lima 1997). Other stimuli, such as those caused by heat, pressure and touch, are assessed by wide dynamic range (WDR) neurones predominately found in laminae IV, V and VI (Lima 1997). Thus peripheral fibres interact with NS and WDR fibres depending on the stimulus they are conveying. The role of the NS and WDR neurones in assessing impulses from the peripheral nervous system is an important one and determines whether the impulse will be transmitted to the brain (Carpenter 2003). For example,

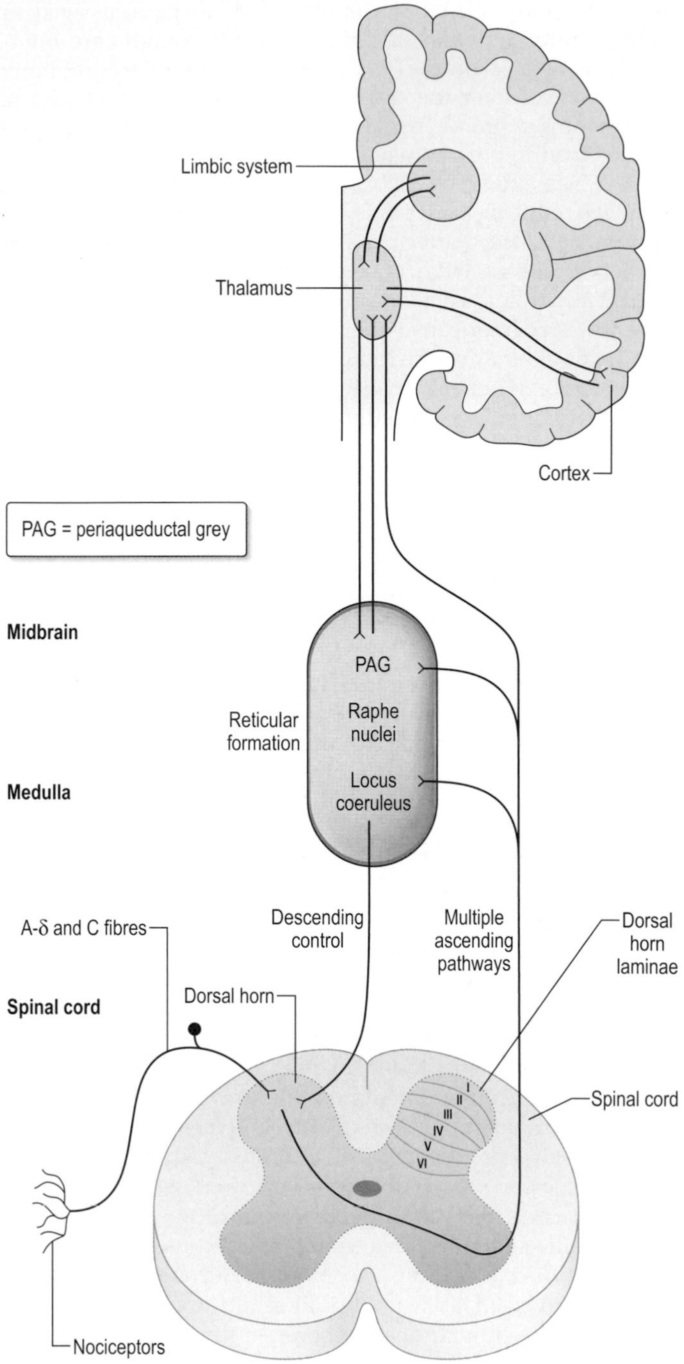

Fig. 19.1 Diagrammatic representation of some neural pathways involved in pain transmission.

research has shown that brief stimuli are sufficient to activate NS neurones, whereas prolonged stimulation is required to activate WDR neurones (Lima 1997). Carpenter (2003) suggests that the evidence now available points to NS and WDR neurones being part of two distinct but complementary nociceptive systems.

Ascending pathways

Ascending pathways consist of neurones that link the dorsal horn with centres in the brain. There has been significant growth in knowledge about these pathways. Perhaps the most important information to come to light is the number of pathways identified in nociception and their role in a compound processing system activated by any kind of sensory input (Lima 1997).

From a review of research using chemical and electrophysiological tracing techniques, Lima (1997) has identified the following ascending tracts as nociceptive pathways: lateral spinothalamic, medial spinothalamic, spinomesencephalic, spinoreticular medial, spinocaudal ventrolateral medullary reticular, spinodorsomedullary reticular, spinosolitary, spinohypothalamic, spinoamygdalian and spino-orbital cortex. However, although all of these pathways are capable of transmitting pain, they are not, in most cases, pain specific. Each of these tracts connects a particular area of the dorsal horn with a specific area in the brain. While much remains to be discovered about the operation of these tracts, their apparently overlapping functions may include (Carpenter 2003):

- signalling the 'sensory–discriminative' aspects of pain, e.g. location, identification
- signalling its 'motivational–affective' aspects, e.g. unpleasantness of the sensation, desire to escape, anxiety
- triggering motor and autonomic responses
- activating descending analgesia systems.

Brain mechanisms

From the number of ascending tracts described above, it can be seen that many areas of the brain are involved in pain transmission. Each of these centres receives and integrates sensory inputs, relates them to past experiences and thus brings about behaviour to promote survival. Central to these centres is the reticular formation in the central core of the medulla, pons and midbrain (see Ch. 9). The reticular formation contains the periaqueductal grey (PAG), the locus coeruleus and the raphe nuclei. Of these, the PAG has particular importance for receiving inputs from the frontal cortex, the limbic system, particularly the thalamus and hypothalamus, as well as some ascending tracts. In turn, the PAG relays information to the nuclei of the rostral ventral medulla (RVM), such as the nucleus raphe magnus (NRM), the nucleus reticularis magnocellularis (Rmc), the reticularis paragigantocellularis (Rpgl) and the medullary adrenergic cellular groups (MA). The neurotransmitters involved in this relaying of information appear primarily to be serotonin and neurotensin (NT). Through these connections the PAG has a monitoring as well as a response role in pain sensation and perception, coordinating a negative feedback loop between the ascending tracts and the cortex, and the descending tracts and the dorsal horn. It is proposed that this feedback loop modulates the responses of convergent, i.e. multireceptive neurones (Carpenter 2003).

Descending pathways

Descending pathways connect the brain centres described above with the dorsal horn. They have a key role in the modulation of pain, primarily through the release of specialised neurotransmitters at the dorsal horn. The principal neurotransmitters associated with these pathways are noradrenaline (NA) and serotonin (5-HT). They coexist with other neuropeptides such as the endogenous opiates, endorphins and encephalins.

Throughout the central nervous system pain is further influenced by excitatory and inhibitory receptor mechanisms. These can be broadly divided into two groups: excitatory mechanisms are managed by glutamate synapses, particularly N-methyl-D-aspartate (NMDA) receptors; inhibitory mechanisms are managed by gamma-aminobutyric acid (GABA)-ergic synapses.

The primary excitatory mechanism in the CNS is glutamate synapses, in which the key neurotransmitters are L-glutamate acid and L-aspartic acid. These amino acids open sodium channels and so increase sodium concentration. This leads to depolarisation and increased neuronal firing (Carpenter 2003). These neurotransmitters bind with two main types of receptor that have been distinguished pharmacologically: AMPA receptors and NMDA receptors. Both receptors are elements of a complex protein molecule that forms part of a postsynaptic ionic channel.

The NMDA channel has several critical properties:

- it is voltage dependent, due to the ability of magnesium to block the channel
- it has several binding sites, including a phencyclidine site that binds with some opioids and dissociate anaesthetics such as ketamine that then prevent ion transfer
- it has a high permeability for calcium.

These properties are thought to be key to the mechanisms involved in persistent pain.

The primary inhibitory mechanisms in the CNS are GABA-ergic. The key neurotransmitters in these synapses are amino acids such as gamma-aminobutyric acid (GABA), glycine, aurine and proline. These inhibitory amino acids open chloride channels and so increase conductance of postsynaptic membranes, leading to hyperpolarisation and decreased neuronal firing (Carpenter 2003). These amino acids bind with GABA receptors.

The GABA receptor is found in neuronal membranes throughout the CNS, particularly in the thalamus, hypothalamus, hippocampus and basal ganglia of the brain and the substantia gelatinosa of the dorsal horn of the spinal cord. This receptor is a complex protein that can be classified into two types – $GABA_A$, selective for chloride as described above, and $GABA_B$, selective for potassium.

$GABA_A$ receptors are complex proteins consisting of five different subunits arranged around a central core. Each subunit has an affinity for different neurotransmitters and thus the binding of different substances to different subunits brings about a large number of possible actions.

RELATING THE PHYSIOLOGY OF PAIN TO ANALGESICS

Peripheral mechanisms and non-steroidal anti-inflammatory drugs

Pain is stimulated by the release of noxious substances such as prostaglandins, histamines and kinins within the tissues, 'released' in response to tissue damage such as that caused by injury, tumour infiltration or inflammation. Of these chemicals, the synthesis of prostaglandins is of interest, since preventing its synthesis, and therefore preventing pain stimulation, is possible through administration of glucocorticoids and non-steroidal anti-inflammatory drugs (NSAIDs).

Prostaglandins

Prostaglandins are synthesised in response to tissue damage from arachidonic acid (AA). AA is an important constituent of the lipid component of phospholipids that constitute cell membranes. AA is obtained from dietary animal fats or converted from dietary linoleic acid found in animal and plant fats, especially seed oils. The amount of AA that is 'free' and not incorporated within cells is very small and this is one of the main factors limiting the production of prostaglandins. AA is freed from cell membranes by the enzyme phospholipase A_2 (PLA_2). This enzyme is found in cell lysosomes. PLA_2 separates the phosphate from the lipid element of the phospholipid. The AA liberated may be synthesised by two pathways to form potent biological mediators that include prostaglandins. Collectively these mediators are called eicosanoids. Two different enzymes initiate the two pathways of AA metabolism: cyclo-oxygenase (Cox), an enzyme bound to the reticulum of the cell, and lipo-oxygenase (Lox), an enzyme found in cytosol. Cox synthesises AA into endoperoxides, short-living intermediates. These are further synthesised into prostaglandins and thromboxanes (collectively called prostanoids) by the enzyme synthetase. Two types of Cox are now recognised: Cox I is involved in gastric cytoprotection and renal function; Cox II is involved in inflamed tissue (Pace 1995). Lox converts AA into non-cyclised hydroxy acids. These are further synthesised into leukotrienes.

Non-steroidal anti-inflammatory drugs (NSAIDs)

NSAIDs are a group of compounds that share common pharmacological properties but are not necessarily chemically related. NSAIDs all possess anti-inflammatory, analgesic and antipyretic actions. With respect to pain, NSAIDs have an analgesic effect by:

- inhibiting prostaglandin (PG) synthesis through inhibiting the enzyme Cox and thereby reducing peripheral nociceptor stimulation. Cox also inhibits the role of PG in sensitising the CNS to noxious stimulus
- inhibiting superoxide anion formation — superoxide anion is formed by polymorphonuclear cells in response to inflammation and is one of the chemicals that can stimulate nociceptors peripherally. NSAIDs block the action of the enzyme produced by polymorphonuclear cells to initiate the production of superoxide anion and thereby reduce peripheral nociceptor stimulation. Diclofenac is an example of a NSAID that has been found to have this effect
- increasing beta-endorphins and therefore inhibiting the action of nociceptive neurotransmitters
- stimulating serotonin (5-HT) synthesis in the CNS and so inhibiting nociceptor transmission by blocking the action of neuromodulators.

The way in which these effects are brought about varies with different groups of NSAIDs because the chemical effects and potency of NSAIDs vary. NSAIDs have a range of side-effects, the most serious being adverse gastrointestinal events such as ulceration, bleeding and perforation. Patients at high risk of these side-effects include those who are 65 years or older, those with a previous history of such events, concomitant use of medications, e.g. steroids or anticoagulants, the presence of co-morbidity such as cardiovascular disease, renal or hepatic impairment, diabetes and hypertension (National Institute for Clinical Excellence 2001). Some of these side-effects, it is argued, are minimised by a new group of NSAIDs – the Cox II selective inhibitors. The enzyme Cox II is thought to be specific to prostaglandins synthesised as a result of inflammation. The NSAIDs such as celecoxib have been developed to act specifically to prevent the synthesis of this form of the Cox enzyme. They are more expensive than other NSAIDs and evidence about the claims that they minimise side-effects is limited. However, the National Institute for Clinical Excellence (2001) stated that there is 'pragmatic evidence of a reduced incidence of serious gastrointestinal events compared to standard NSAIDs'. The complete version of the evidence and guidance is available on the NICE website (see 'Useful websites and addresses'). This evidence is under review following withdrawal of the Cox II drug, rofecoxib, by the manufacturers because of recent controlled trial evidence suggesting similar side-effect dangers to a Cox I comparative NSAID (naproxen). An overview of the pharmacology, effectiveness and clinical use of NSAIDs is given on the Bandolier website (see 'Useful websites and addresses').

Central mechanisms and opioids

Analgesic opioids, e.g. morphine, mimic the effect of endogenous opiates and bind to opioid receptors found throughout the CNS. Naturally occurring endogenous opiates are neuropeptides, neurotransmitters synthesised and released by descending fibres in the CNS. When bound with an opioid receptor they have a modulating effect on pain. Their effect is determined by a complex multiple messenger system, sometimes referred to as co-transmission, meaning that other substances, e.g. serotonin and substance P, are involved in the effect that endogenous opiates have when bound to a receptor. Co-transmission enables an increased level of control at the synapse, compared with simple synapse mechanisms.

Neuropeptides are found in the gut, hypothalamus, anterior pituitary and posterior pituitary gland.

At least 10 opioid neuropeptides have been identified. They arise from three major groups of endogenous opiates: encephalins, endorphins and dynorphins.

The release of neuropeptides from a descending fibre is dependent on calcium activation. Termination of the activity of neuropeptides is believed to be initiated by enzymes, which release the neuropeptide from the receptor binding site.

Opioid receptors

A number of key opioid receptors have been identified:

- Mu (μ) receptors preferentially bind with opioids such as morphine and fentanyl, i.e. as an agonist to these drugs. When an opioid binds with a mu receptor it activates the cyclic adenosine monophosphate (AMP) secondary messenger system within the nerve cell, and this causes the opening of potassium channels. This reduces the excitability of the cell and consequently reduces the firing rate of the nerve. Mu receptors are distributed in the peripheral and central nervous system, with high densities in the brain stem, trigeminal nuclei, spinal cord, periaqueductal grey region, amygdala and cerebral cortex. Naloxone, an antagonist to morphine, also binds to mu receptors, so preventing morphine from binding at this site.

- Delta (δ) receptors are located throughout the peripheral and central nervous system and preferentially bind with the neuropeptide, leucine–encephalin. When bound with an opioid, delta receptors mediate hyperpolarisation and inhibit the release of noradrenaline. This reduces nociception by decreasing firing and reducing neurotransmission at the dorsal horn synapse. Delta receptors are partially agonistic to naloxone whereby there is a small attraction between naloxone and these receptors.
- Kappa (κ) receptors have a different spectrum of action to mu and delta receptors. They are agonistic to pentazocine and endogenous dynorphin and are predominant at spinal sites. Binding with an opioid causes less respiratory depressive effect but more hallucinogenic effects.

Therapeutic use of opioids

Morphine is the standard, first choice, 'strong' opioid for nociceptive pain. When titrated against an individual's pain, it provides effective and safe analgesia. Other opioids in clinical use include diamorphine, tramadol, fentanyl, oxycodone, buprenorphine and methadone.

The side-effect profile for each of these opioids varies in the degree to which they are experienced. In persistent and cancer pain, rotation between opioids may be necessary to find the opioid that gives the best therapeutic effect with the minimum side-effects. Typical opioid side-effects include the following (Stannard & Booth 2004):

- Respiratory depression and sedation due to binding with mu receptors in the pons and medulla. Respiratory rate, depth and rhythm can be altered, leading to carbon dioxide retention. Respiratory depression is rarely a problem in long-term opioid therapy but is more common postoperatively because of the compounding influence of anaesthetic agents. Sedation usually declines within a few days.
- Nausea and vomiting due to stimulation of the chemoreceptor trigger zone in the CNS and gastric stasis due to binding with mu receptors in the gut. This tends to be a transient side-effect that will pass within a few days.
- Constipation due to direct effect on the smooth muscle of the gut. This is a persistent side-effect that is likely to require treatment with laxatives.
- Hallucinations and agitation, thought to be due to the action at kappa and sigma (σ) receptors.
- Myoclonus, i.e. jerking or twitching of muscle groups.
- Itching, due to histamine release in the skin.
- Urinary retention, due to increased smooth muscle tone in the urinary tract.

Morphine is contraindicated in patients with raised intracranial pressure because the respiratory depressant effect may cause an increase in arterial PCO_2, resulting in a further rise in intracranial pressure. Care also needs to be taken in patients with renal impairment since the excretion of morphine and its metabolites will be impaired and the likelihood of side-effects therefore increased. Careful titration and increasing the time interval between doses is often necessary for these patients.

THEORIES OF PAIN

STOP THINK **19.4** Before reading the following section, make a note about how theories might help you to understand pain. As you read the section, judge the contribution of each theory to your understanding of pain.

Several theories have been developed to explain pain. The philosopher Aristotle drew on Plato's theory about extremes and opposites, arguing that pain was the opposite of pleasure and that both pain and pleasure were 'quales' — emotional qualities of the soul. An important part of Aristotle's differentiation between pleasure and pain was the belief that pleasure is good whereas pain is bad. Thus Aristotle viewed both pain and pleasure as having moral value and, indeed, he argued that these quales were fundamental moral drives directing human action. Furthermore, he suggested that pain could be overcome by reason.

The specificity theory

Descartes (1596–1650) proposed a direct channel for pain from the periphery of the body to the brain, proposing that when the body was exposed to a painful stimulus, this was relayed to the brain by a specific pain pathway. This is known as the specificity theory and is challenged by Melzack and Wall (1996), who point to clinical evidence such as phantom limb pain that contradicts the existence of specific pain pathways.

The pattern theory

This theory develops the concept that any stimulus is capable of producing pain if it reaches sufficient intensity. Pattern theory differs from the specificity theory in that it proposes that all fibre endings are alike (except innervate hair cells) and that the pattern for pain is produced by intense stimulation of non-specific receptors (Melzack & Wall 1996). The pattern theory also introduced the concept of summation – that successive impulses collectively 'summate' to reach a critical firing level. Pattern theory suggests that summation can be prevented by specialised rapidly conducting fibres. Melzack and Wall (1996) later developed the concept of summation in the gate control theory.

The gate control theory

The gate control theory of pain, developed by Melzack and Wall (1965), combines pertinent aspects of older theories with an account of what happens in clinical practice. According to this theory, the transmission of information from a potentially painful stimulus can be modified by a gating mechanism situated in the substantia gelatinosa in the dorsal horn of the spinal cord. This mechanism can increase or decrease the flow of nerve impulses from the periphery to the CNS. If the gate is open, impulses pass through; if it is partially open some pass through; and if shut, no impulses get through and pain is not experienced.

Melzack and Wall (1965), in their seminal text, argued that whether the gate is open or closed is determined by:

- activity in small diameter fibres (A-δ and C fibres, which transmit pain)
- activity in large diameter fibres (A-β fibres, which transmit touch)
- descending influences from higher centres, including those concerned with motivational and cognitive processes.

Melzack and Wall (1965) proposed that the substantia gelatinosa is activated by large A-β fibres that shut the gate and inhibited by small A-δ and C fibres that open the gate. This activity then influences the information sent to the brain, which in turn initiates descending inhibitory controls depending on the information from other areas such as the cortex.

Implications of the gate control theory

The physiology of pain has developed since the gate control theory was first proposed. However, the inherent fundamental principles have stood the test of time and influenced pain management. Clinically, the gate control theory has been applied to nursing care (Carr & Mann 2000) through measures such as massage and the application of heat. The use of touch and massage can stimulate the skin, increasing large fibre (A-β) activity and thereby closing the gate at the spinal cord level and relieving pain. This rationale also explains the benefit of the advice: 'rub it better'.

Closing the gate at the brain stem level can sometimes be achieved by ensuring sufficient sensory input, e.g. by using distraction and imagery (see p. 754). Similarly, at the level of the cortex/thalamus, the gate can be closed by reducing anxiety, e.g. by providing accurate information about the cause, likely course and relief of pain and thereby increasing the patient's confidence and sense of control.

Developments since the gate control theory

The pain control system described by the gate control theory is one that acts rapidly. Research has demonstrated the existence of 'plasticity' or adaptability in the nervous system, which allows for both rapidly transmitted impulses and slow-onset, long-duration changes. It is thought that C fibres, especially those originating in deep tissues, trigger these slower messages (Price 2002). This prolonged mechanism, referred to as 'wind up', results in a sustained experience of pain, which may account for some cases of neuropathic pain (Price 2002). In addition, there is some evidence that this kind of pain can be explained by changes in central neural function (Coderre et al 1993).

More recently, spinal cord glial cells have been implicated in persistent pain. Glia regulate extracellular ions and neurotransmitters, and clear debris such as dead cells. It has been suggested that these cells are responsible for amplifying pain by releasing proinflammatory cytokines, which stimulate the CNS pain response (DeLeo & Yezierski 2001, Watkins & Maier 2003, Wiesler-Frank et al 2003).

KEY CONCEPTS IN PAIN

STOP THINK **19.5** When reading the following section, think about the meaning of the words acute and chronic. How might this influence someone's pain experience and management?

Pain threshold

Pain threshold is 'the least experience of pain which a subject can recognise' (International Association for the Study of Pain 1994). Laboratory studies of pain have demonstrated that pain thresholds are fairly constant across the population. In other words, the vast majority of people agree on the point at which a sensation becomes painful.

Pain tolerance

Pain tolerance is 'the greatest level of pain which a subject is prepared to tolerate' (International Association for the Study of Pain 1994). Pain tolerance needs to be distinguished from drug tolerance.

Acute and chronic pain

Pain was traditionally classified as either acute or chronic. Acute pain distinguished pain that was short lived and related to injury, e.g. following surgery or trauma. Chronic pain described pain that was long lived, most definitions suggesting 3 months or more (Royal College of Anaesthetists and The Pain Society 2003), and that was typically harder to control. Chronic pain was further divided into chronic malignant pain, due to cancer or other similar progressive illnesses, and chronic non-malignant pain, due to injury, such as prolapsed intervertebral disc, but persisting beyond the healing of the injury. The physiological mechanisms present in pain due to trauma reinforce this view — there is usually an associated sympathetic nervous system response which results in observable changes: nausea and vomiting, increased oxygen consumption, raised blood pressure and pulse rate and vasoconstriction or, less commonly, a parasympathetic stimulation resulting in decreased pulse rate and blood pressure. In chronic pain these signs are not present and can lead to assumptions that someone is not in pain.

More detailed knowledge of the physiology of conditions that were associated with chronic pain makes the classification of chronic pain by time frame redundant (International Association for the Study of Pain 1994). There is therefore a growing use of the term persistent pain to describe chronic pain and to classify pain by its physiological mechanism, 'nociceptive' describing pain caused by tissue damage and 'neuropathic' describing pain that persists beyond the original cause as a result of disruption to the normal transmission of pain, e.g. through nerve injury, nerve infection and nerve compression. Classifying pain by the physiological mechanism in this way has the advantage of informing decision making about how best to manage the pain (Arnér 2000, Dann et al 2000, Caraceni 2001).

Nociceptive and neuropathic pain

Nociceptive pain is typically experienced as sharp or aching and it may be intermittent or continuous. Neuropathic pain is characterised by continual severe unremitting pain, often associated with burning or shooting or stabbing sensations and with allodynia – where light touch normally not painful is excruciating. In practice, people use phrases such as: 'It feels as though a knife is digging into me'; 'I can't bear to put my pyjamas on because they hurt so much'. One patient said: 'It feels as though my knee cap is going to explode'.

The cause of neuropathic pain will determine some of the symptoms that people experience as a consequence. For example, nerve root compression can cause pain along the distribution of the nerve being compressed, the compression preventing the action potential moving smoothly along the neuronal membrane. The notion of a 'short circuit' in the nerve is helpful to explain this. The resultant excessive firing exacerbates the strength of the sensation being interpreted at the dorsal horn and is responsible for the sensation of severe pain. Where pain is persistent, such as in nerve damage, the CNS can undergo particular changes that make it very responsive to any received sensory information, causing it to fire in circumstances when the strength of this sensation would not normally cause this reaction. This is called 'wind up', a term used to describe the enhanced responsiveness of the CNS to sensory stimuli.

Referred pain

Normally, if one stubs a toe or cuts a finger, it is apparent exactly where the injury has occurred. However, this localisation of pain is limited to the skin. Pain from the viscera and from deep somatic tissue can be felt in apparently unrelated but predictable locations. For example, the pain of a heart attack is often referred to the left arm, and pain in the early stages of appendicitis may appear to originate from above the umbilicus. Pain is usually referred to a structure developed from the same embryonic structure or sclerotome.

Another type of referred pain is associated with trigger points. These are small hypersensitive regions in muscle or connective tissue that may be located in the area of pain or at some distance from it. This referred pain does not follow any known dermatomes, but stimulation produces pain in a relatively constant and predictable location (Stannard & Booth 2004).

PAIN MANAGEMENT

Nursing assessment

STOP THINK **19.6** Think back to the last time that you assessed a person in pain. How did you go about this? What influenced this process?

Assessment is fundamental to pain management. It is a crucial nursing activity that must be carried out as part of the initial nursing assessment and at regular intervals thereafter in order to obtain a complete and evolving picture of the patient's pain. Sjöström et al (2000) emphasise the importance of this individual assessment rather than relying on typologies of patients (such as 'major' or 'minor' surgery) as this leads to underestimation of pain.

Pain assessment is complex and dependent upon the interaction between patient, nurse and clinical context (Manias 2003). It includes observing the patient's behaviours, taking account of relevant physiological measurements, interviewing the patient, understanding their concerns and responding to cues appropriately. Assessment may incorporate a framework such as a pain assessment tool, but it should be remembered that a pain tool is only one facet of an adequate assessment.

Observation

Observation of pain is difficult and unreliable, but is usually based on verbal clues such as direct statements, as well as moaning, crying, sighing and grimacing, and non-verbal clues such as guarding, bracing and lying perfectly still. However, these clues do not have to be present for someone to be in pain. Indeed, such clues are frequently absent. Thus, caution should be exercised in the interpretation of non-verbal signals. However, they remain an important source of assessment for people who cannot respond verbally, such as those who are unconscious or disorientated and confused. Where this is the case, observational assessment needs to be systematic and may be enhanced by the use of an observational tool such as that reported by Simons and Malabar (1995).

Asking the patient

Observation must be combined with discussion with the patient wherever possible, in order to assess whether someone is in pain and, if so, to understand the nature of the pain and the degree to which it is influencing that individual's experience of life. On the whole, this aspect of pain assessment is undervalued, with some studies demonstrating that few patients are asked about their pain (Carr & Thomas 1997) and as a consequence experience pain unnecessarily. Results of studies in which patients and carers were asked how nurses could help to relieve pain reinforce the importance of nurses listening and being sensitive to their concerns and experience in order to understand and anticipate these, and guide the patient and carer to information that may be helpful (Walker et al 1990, Ferrell et al 1991a,b, Madjar 1998, Manias et al 2002, White 2003). Box 19.1 gives an example of how assessment can be shaped to gain an understanding of a person's experience of pain.

Pain assessment tools

Assessment is often complemented by a pain assessment tool, and there are many different tools available for this purpose. The characteristic of a tool is shaped by the underpinning interpretation of pain (Coll et al 2004a). Pain scales, such as the visual analogue scale or numerical rating scale, assess pain sensation and intensity (see Figs 19.2–19.4). Tools such as the McGill Pain Questionnaire (MPQ) assess multidimensional aspects of pain such as sensation, intensity, quality, physical function and the effectiveness of pain-relieving strategies. Tools such as pain diaries are designed to assess the impact of pain on the quality of a person's life.

Box 19.1

One nurse's process of pain assessment

Setting the scene

I explain who I am and what I am doing. I might say something like: 'I am one of the nurses in the unit and have a responsibility to make sure that you are comfortable. Is it alright if I talk to you for a few minutes about this?'. If this is acceptable, then I proceed with a question such as: 'Can you tell me if you have any pain or discomfort?'. If it is not acceptable, then I negotiate another time when it is convenient. The question about pain is quite a closed one and has the disadvantage that it focuses attention on one facet of the patient's illness but I find that this means we have a place to start. If I feel someone will be comfortable with an open question I will say something like: 'Tell me what's been happening to you'. Within the conversation that follows I will include the following pain themes: location, severity, quality, pattern and effect on other aspects of life.

The location of pain

I ask where the pain is and check the location, and also ask whether the patient has more than one pain. A question such as 'Can you tell me where you get the pain' will often prompt people to point to the pain. If this is easily reachable, important information can be gained by watching how the affected part is touched. For example, if someone has nerve pain they often show the location along the sensory distribution of a nerve and this can give a clue as to which nerve is affected. If the place is difficult to reach, I ask the patient just to describe where the pain is so that their discomfort is not increased.

The severity of pain

In assessing the degree to which pain is affecting a person's ability to be independent and what coping strategies are used, a question I often ask is: 'Can you divert your attention away from the pain?'. If pain is all-embracing, in the way that Bendelow and Williams (1995) suggest, then it is difficult for someone to forget the pain because 'they become the pain'. If a patient tells me that this is really difficult to do, I suggest that their pain is really severe; this is typically followed with relief that someone has recognised how awful their experience is.

The quality of pain

How pain is described provides information about the mechanisms of the pain. Common words include throbbing, shooting, stabbing, sharp, cramping, gnawing, hot/burning, aching, heavy, tender, splitting, tiring/exhausting, sickening, fearful and punishing/cruel. It is important to be aware that some people may not actually use the word 'pain' when asked about their discomfort and may even deny having pain. In these cases it can be helpful to incorporate words such as 'ache', 'hurt', 'sore' and 'discomfort' into an assessment.

The pattern of pain

Pain often follows a pattern that gives a clue about its nature and what can be done to relieve it. For example, pain in arthritis is often worse in the morning and knowing this can influence the medication that is given at night in an attempt to alleviate it. Similarly, persistent pain is sometimes worse when the individual is tired; knowing this can help the individual to plan their day. Questions that enable such patterns to be identified include:

- When did the pain start?
- How long does it last?
- Does it come and go or is it there all the time?
- Does anything relieve it?
- Does anything make it worse?

The effect of pain on other aspects of life

Pain often influences whether someone can sleep or socialise and so a question about how pain is influencing the quality of life is important as there may be ways to help with this. I sometimes ask: 'How are you coping?', both to elicit this information and to find out how the person is feeling in themselves. This sort of question not only gives people an opportunity to explain how pain is influencing their life but also to raise other related concerns, such as finances or care needs, or fears about medications or their illness. This gives me an opening to ask questions about the sense that they might be making of the pain, which in turn helps me to understand the meaning they are attributing to their experience.

Anything else?

This last question makes sure that I have not missed any cues given to me earlier. I ask something like: 'What else do you think I should know?' or 'Is there anything else you would like to tell me?'.

Summary

After this assessment I summarise what I have been told by affirming that someone has pain and by explaining what is possible to help this pain. A typical comment would be: 'From what you have told me the pain in your [place of the body] has been really difficult to cope with. I think we can do something to relieve this pain'. I then go on to discuss what this might be. In the case of complex pain I explain that easing the pain might take a little time ('to get the recipe right') but that there is much that can be done ('there is a lot left in the tool kit yet'). If it is clear what can be tried straight away, I go on to discuss this. If I am not sure, I explain that I need to take some advice and will come back to explain what the possibilities might be. However, for the majority of people in pain there are simple strategies which can be implemented immediately that will make a significant and positive difference to their experience of pain.

STOP THINK

19.7 Compare the following discussion with the pain tool that you use, or that is available, in your ward, team or organisation. What sort of tool is used? How applicable is it to the patient group that you care for?

Pain scales

Typically, intensity of pain is determined using a scale designed to enable the patient to rate the degree of pain felt. These scales can also be used to note any change in pain levels following an intervention or to indicate when the 'worst pain' or 'least pain' was felt, thus giving a profile of the pain experience over time. Scales can also be used to help the patient quantify the distress caused by the pain or to determine at what level of intensity the patient would like to be given analgesics. It should be remembered, however, that this level is not necessarily constant and that the patient's pain tolerance may fluctuate from day to day or within a 24-h period. Scales also have a place in minimising the discrepancy between a patient's experience of pain and the nurse's judgement of it, as observed by authors such as Whelan (2003).

Three pain scales in current use that have been demonstrated to be both reliable and valid in people with cognitive function (Lundeberg et al 2001, Coll et al 2004a) are the visual analogue scale, the numerical rating scale and the verbal rating scale. Details of the research underpinning the reliability and validity of these tools is given in McCaffery and Pasero (1999). Closs et al (2004) found that the verbal rating scale provided a more reliable guide to the intensity of an individual's pain compared to the other scales, but that this was possible only in people with a small degree of cognitive impairment, the scales being inadequate to assess pain in people with severe cognitive impairment.

Visual analogue scale (VAS) This consists of a 10 cm line with the words 'no pain at all' at one end and a phrase such as 'agonising pain' or 'worst pain possible' at the other end (see Fig. 19.2). The line is usually horizontal but can be vertical. The patient is asked to mark this line at whatever point corresponds to the degree of pain being experienced at that moment. The assessor then measures in centimetres from the left-hand side of the pain scale (or the foot if a vertical line is used) to the mark in order to obtain the pain 'score'.

The advantages of this scale include the absence of numbers or words; the person in pain is not required to assign a precise numerical value to the pain or to choose a word that may not exactly represent their pain.

Numerical rating scale (NRS) This scale is like the VAS but is calibrated with the numbers 0–10 (see Fig. 19.3). The patient is asked to make a mark at a point that indicates the intensity of their pain. McCaffery and Pasero (1999) provide translation of the numerical rating scale into several languages that can be copied for clinical use.

Verbal rating scale (VRS) This scale provides graded categories, e.g. 'no pain at all', 'slight pain', 'moderate pain', 'very bad pain' and 'agonising pain' (see Fig. 19.4). The patient marks whichever category is most like their pain and this is assigned a score from 0 to 4. Many patients find this scale easy to use although it has the disadvantage of fewer assessment points compared to a 0–10 scale and therefore is not as sensitive.

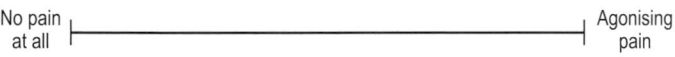

Fig. 19.2 The visual analogue scale.

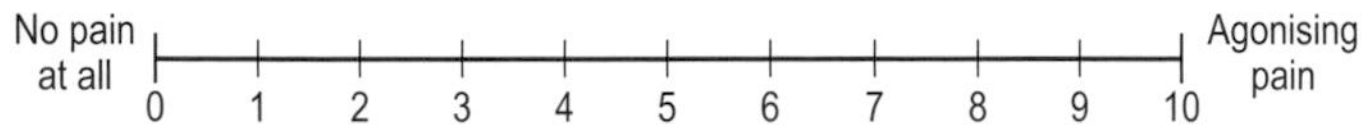

Fig. 19.3 The numerical rating scale.

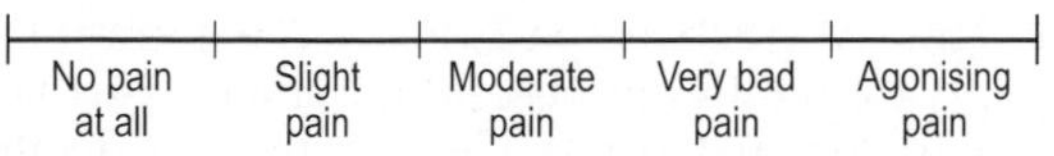

Fig. 19.4 The verbal rating scale.

The visual, numerical and verbal pain scales rate pain intensity, which is only one aspect of pain experience. These tools also encourage a linear assessment of pain intensity. Turk (1989) was one of the first authors to note that pain intensity may not be perceived in a linear fashion, and that linear scales may constrain and distort patient experience. This was borne out by a participant in Whelan's (2003) study who commented on the difficulty of expressing the meaning of the pain when using a numerical scale:

> *I wanted to put a meaning next to those numbers, so that if I said to my doctor 'I'm having pain that's about a seven' what I mean is, it's really bad, it's incapacitating enough that I'm not able to do my daily duties, but it's not so bad that I'm not able to get out of bed.*

Furthermore, the effectiveness of any of the above assessment tools may be distorted by the patient's inadvertent and deliberate denial or minimisation of pain (McCaffery & Pasero 1999).

Multidimensional pain tools

The scales described above are relatively simple forms of pain assessment tools. Many tools are more comprehensive and incorporate a body outline on which the site(s) of pain can be noted, scales to rate the intensity and quality of the pain and words that can be used to describe the pain, e.g. the McGill Pain Questionnaire (MPQ) and Brief Pain Inventory. McCaffery and Pasero (1999) provide examples of multidimensional assessment tools that can be copied for clinical use.

Pain tools to assess the impact of pain on a person's quality of life

There are several ways in which the impact of pain on an individual's life can be assessed. Pain diaries are useful assessment tools for this purpose. These are kept by the patient to record intensity of pain, effect of medication, other pain-relieving measures used and major activities, e.g. lying, sitting, walking. General impact of health questionnaires, such as the Sickness Impact Profile and the Nottingham Health Index, reviewed by Bowling (2004), are used by some pain clinics and in pain research to elicit disruption in daily activities and family relationships.

Selecting an appropriate tool

Coll et al (2004a) advocate using the framework developed by Fitzpatrick et al (1998) to select the most appropriate tool to complement pain assessment. The framework was developed from a review of 5621 abstracts and articles that focused on methodological aspects of patient-based outcome measures and consists of the following eight criteria, which state that the tool must be:

- appropriate — for the purpose intended and the setting in which it will be used
- reliable — in terms of reproducibility and internal consistency
- valid — in that it measures patients' perceptions of pain

- responsive — to changes of importance to patients
- precise — accurate and discriminating
- interpretable — in that meaningful information is produced
- acceptable — to those completing it
- feasible — in that the degree of burden and effort involved in using it is acceptable.

Nursing care

STOP THINK **19.8** Before reading this section, consider your own feelings about pain and pain relief. If you were in pain, what sorts of things would be important to you to help you cope? Would this be different if you were at home rather than in hospital? Would different things be important for different types/causes of pain?

Nurses have a very significant role to play in pain management. Effective pain management depends upon the relationship developed between the nurse and the patient and, in part, this is why pain assessment is so important, as it sets the 'spirit' of that relationship, whether the patient's concerns will be taken seriously and how they will be responded to. The importance of this kind of nursing relationship, and of the nature of the characteristics required to achieve it, can be drawn from several studies that represent the patient view. A respondent in Carr and Thomas's (1997) study emphasised the importance of this relationship:

> *If she [the acute pain nurse] had just walked away I don't know what I would have done. Her being with me enabled her to understand what I was going through. I didn't feel alone. I felt that I had someone who was helping ... you know. She was sort of experiencing it with me. Really, it was a wonderful feeling in that way ... that she was with me.*

The patient respondents in Madjar's (1998) research identified particular qualities that they valued in the ways that nurses responded to their pain. These included:

- *gentleness* — a softness and tenderness in the way a nurse saw to their comfort
- *trustworthiness* — a combination of characteristics such as calmness and ability to inspire confidence
- *sensitivity* — responding through appropriate use of talk and silence and pacing nursing care according to the person's ability to tolerate it
- *technical competence* — being organised and efficient and able to perform technical tasks with skill and agility
- *knowledge and skilful communication* — being able to judge what information would be important at a particular time and the ability to communicate it in a way that fostered reassurance and encouragement.

Manias et al (2002) point to another nursing skill in pain management. This study highlighted that nurses are regularly interrupted in their work and needed skill in managing frequent interruptions and the competing demands placed on their time, since these qualities influenced pain management, e.g. how long a patient waits for analgesics.

Information and explanation are important aspects of support and therefore crucial to the nurse's role. The purpose of these activities is to ensure the patient has realistic expectations and that the nurse works towards achieving these. The aim is to achieve congruence between patients' expectations and their experience, since this has been shown by studies to reduce distress (Carr & Thomas 1997, Boström et al 2004).

Congruence between expectation and experience will also depend on the type of pain. In neuropathic pain it may take time to achieve a reduction in pain, although much can be done to help people cope. On the other hand, nociceptive pain can be relieved in nearly everyone and it is realistic to work towards considerable pain relief. However, despite advances in pain management, some doctors and nurses still believe that pain is an inevitable consequence of treatment and care (McCaffery & Pasero 1999, Carr & Mann 2000) and overestimate patients' ability to cope with pain (Madjar 1998). This is compounded by patients not realising that they can ask for pain relief (Carr & Thomas 1997, McCaffery & Pasero 1999) or waiting until they are in severe pain before requesting an analgesic (Carr & Mann 2000). Carr and Thomas (1997) suggest that this is due both to the lack of information and to the fact that patients can see that nurses are busy: 'Well, you could see the bells ringing here, there and everywhere and I wasn't that bad, so why worry them'.

The nurse's role in pain management extends to the family. Part of the nurse–family relationship is to recognise that family members have information needs of their own, particularly if they are the key carers. The carers in Oldham and Kristjanson's (2004) study of cancer pain identified the need to have the following concerns addressed: the nature of pain, concerns about medication and how to provide comfort.

The principles of the nursing management and the issues that challenge this are summarised in Table 19.1.

The role of the person in pain

The role of patients in the management of their own pain has been largely ignored. In part, this can be explained by the way in which health care professionals have encouraged a passive patient role. In addition, patients have not been given sufficient information about pain relief (Carr & Mann 2000), with the result that they have low expectations about what level of relief can be achieved.

Health care professionals can encourage patients to play a role in their pain management by adopting a partnership approach to care, involving patients in the assessment of their pain and its relief. This approach can foster a sense of control and reduce reliance on health care professionals. Control can be enhanced by giving adequate information about pain and pain relief prior to surgery (Carr & Thomas 1997) and by the self-administration of medications, e.g. by the use of patient controlled analgesia (PCA), postoperatively. In addition, with appropriate instruction and support, patients may contribute to their pain management by using complementary methods of pain relief (see p. 754).

Patients can also be helped to have a sense of control in their pain management if their coping strategies are built on, rather than ignored (Richardson & Poole 2001); finding out how people cope with pain becomes a crucial part of assessment. Richardson and Poole (2001) advocate using Turk et al's (1987) taxonomy of coping with pain to achieve

Table 19.1 Principles of pain management

Principles	Issues in practice
Base your management on a thorough assessment	Nurses often rely on their ability to judge a patient's pain rather than asking the patient about it (McCaffery & Pasero 1999). Many nurses assume that a patient who does not appear to be in pain is in no discomfort when the opposite might be true. Moreover, they assume that analgesics have been effective because the patient does not say anything to the contrary (Carr & Mann 2000)
Believe that it is possible and desirable for people to be pain free	Both nurse and patient may view pain as something to be tolerated. Research has shown that both patients and nurses often have low expectations of analgesics, and accordingly are satisfied with pain 'relief' that allows significant levels of pain to remain (Carr & Thomas 1997, Schafheutle et al 2001)
Provide analgesics until the person is pain free or experiences side-effects	PRN is sometimes wrongly interpreted as 'as little as possible' rather than 'as needed' until pain free. PRN prescriptions can be given in addition to regularly prescribed medication
Provide regular analgesics throughout the 24-h period to maintain pain-free state	Giving analgesics 'around the clock' at set times has been shown to maintain constant plasma blood levels of the drug (see Fig. 19.5) and thus prevent the peaks and troughs associated with PRN prescription (WHO 2004). This method of administration breaks the pain–anxiety cycle and decreases the patient's anticipation of pain worsening or returning
Use the analgesics prescribed to their full prescription to achieve the pain-free state	Very often nurses give the minimum dose prescribed and give analgesics less frequently than prescribed. As a consequence, many people experience pain unnecessarily. Sometimes prescribing is inadequate to provide pain relief (Schafheutle et al 2001)
Do not rely on the patient to tell you they are in pain or to remind you to provide analgesics — base your management on regular review	Few nurses accurately document their pain assessment or their evaluation of the effectiveness of any drug or comfort measure given to relieve pain (Carr & Mann 2000). Nurses may not trust the pain assessment and instead rely on their own judgement (Schafheutle et al 2001). Nurses may not ask patients if they have pain if they have recently had analgesics, if they have a PCA device or epidural in place or if they have been asleep (Schafheutle et al 2001)
Address fears of medication so that patients can make an informed choice about the analgesics you are offering	Many patients and family members have fears associated with the prescription of opioids, such as fear of becoming addicted, and fear that tolerance will prevent adequate analgesia later in their illness (McCaffery 2001). These fears are not always recognised or addressed by health professionals
Remember the importance of the environment on an individual's ability to cope and their spiritual well-being	Carr and Thomas (1997) suggest that depersonalisation, helplessness and passiveness are inherent in being a patient and influence people's ability to have a sense of control over their pain management (Arraras et al 2002, Smith et al 2002, Bishop & Warr 2003)

PCA, patient controlled analgesia; PRN, as required (*pro re nata*).

this. This taxonomy consists of three classifications of coping:

- *dysfunctional coping* — coping that does not influence the impact of pain on daily life, with the consequence that pain interferes with daily activities of living and results in psychological distress
- *interpersonally distressed* — where a perceived lack of support makes coping difficult
- *adaptive coping* — where coping is successful in managing pain.

Richardson and Poole (2001) suggested that these taxonomies can be identified from nursing assessment of activities of daily living.

The role of family members and carers

Family members have a key role in pain management. Ferrell et al (1991a) noted that family carers contribute to pain assessment by identifying the nature of pain through descriptors such as those used by patients — e.g. 'aching', 'horrendous', 'excruciating' — and by referring to anatomical locations of pain. Carers are also perceptive as to the degree to which pain is hidden by patients or minimised: 'A lot of the time I can sense what she is going through, but she doesn't want to burden others, so she minimises' (Ferrell et al 1991a). However, the degree to which family carers' assessment of pain is congruent with that of the patient is dependent on the severity of the pain. McMillan (1996) found that congruence was more likely when pain was at its least, rather than when it was at its worst, which is likely to be due to the distress experienced by family members when the patient's pain is severe.

Family members also play a very significant role in pain relief at home. With respect to people with cancer pain, Ferrell et al (1991b) found that carers often had a 24-h responsibility for deciding which analgesic to give and when. In addition, they were involved in reminding and encouraging the patient to take the analgesic and in keeping a record of what was taken and when. They were also involved in non-pharmacological pain management such as positioning, massage, the use of heat, cold and touch, and the use of talk and other distraction techniques.

Pharmacological management

Pain can be relieved pharmacologically through the use of analgesics to provide analgesia — the 'absence of pain in response to stimulation which would normally be painful' (International Association for the Study of Pain 1994). Analgesics are commonly divided into the following groups:

- NSAIDs/non-opioids, e.g. paracetamol, ibuprofen
- weak opioids, e.g. codeine
- strong opioids, e.g. morphine.

Frameworks for the use of analgesics

Two frameworks can guide the use of analgesics: the World Health Organization pain ladder (WHO 2004) and systematic reviews of analgesic effectiveness. These frameworks have in common the principle that safe and effective analgesia can be provided by titrating the dose of analgesics to gain a balance between therapeutic effect and side-effect.

The World Health Organization pain ladder

The World Health Organization pain ladder (WHO 2004) is a three-step ladder that guides analgesic decision making. In clinical studies assessing the effectiveness of this framework, pain relief was attained in 80–90% of cases (WHO 2004). The underpinning principle of this framework is that the right drug should be given, at the right dose, at the right time. In persistent pain, titration should be done by moving from non-opioids, e.g. paracetamol, and NSAIDs through to weak opioids, e.g. codeine, and through to strong opioids, e.g. morphine, i.e. moving up the ladder. In surgical or trauma pain, titration will move in reverse order, from strong opioids to weak opioids to non-opioids and NSAIDs. In both cases analgesics should be given regularly to maintain a constant analgesic plasma concentration (see Fig. 19.5). For example, if a patient needs morphine, this will require to be given 4-hourly unless given in a sustained release preparation such as Zomorph, which enables a twice a day dose.

The right dose of analgesic is that which provides pain relief with the lowest side-effect profile. When moving from strong opioids to weak opioids, or vice versa, it is important to take into account the equipotency of the drugs involved. If a patient has been having 60 mg oral codeine 6-hourly and still has pain, the starting dose of oral morphine needs to be equivalent to more than this dose, in order to increase analgesia. For example, 60 mg oral codeine 6-hourly is approximately equivalent to 4 mg oral morphine 4-hourly. The starting dose of oral morphine therefore needs to be in the order of 7.5 mg 4-hourly rather than the typical oral starting dose of 5 mg 4-hourly.

Calculating an appropriate dose is equally important when changing routes of analgesic delivery. For example, patient controlled analgesia (PCA) and epidurals have significantly diminished people's experience of pain in the immediate postoperative period (Buggy & Smith 1999, Chang et al 2004) but, when discontinued, pain escalates

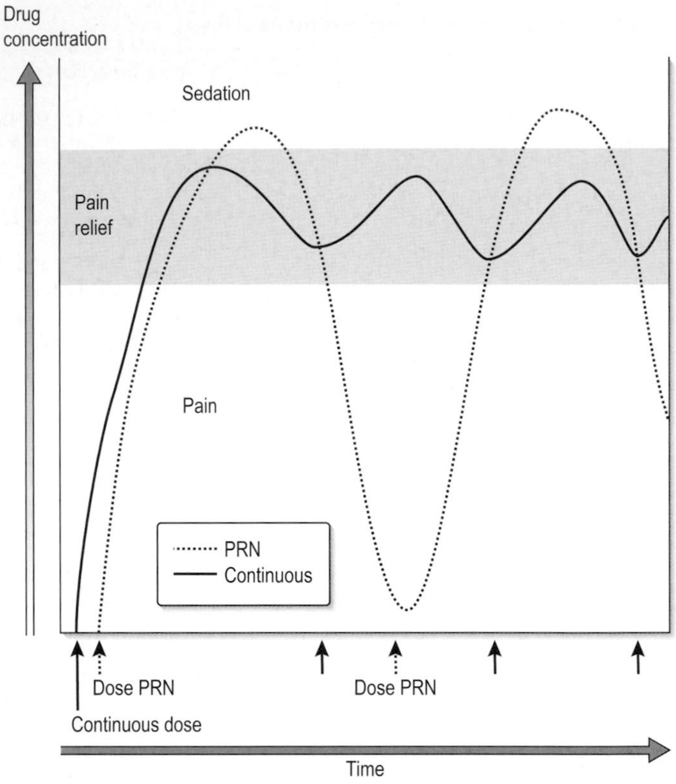

Fig. 19.5 PRN versus around-the-clock administration of analgesics.

because insufficient analgesics are given in their place (Carr & Thomas 1997). For example, if someone has had PCA and used 20 mg morphine over the course of 24 h, 5 mg oral morphine would be needed, 4-hourly, to achieve a similar level of pain control.

The principles of using the WHO framework discussed here are summarised on the WHO website (see 'Useful websites and addresses', p. 761). Equipotent doses for morphine are given in Table 19.2 for commonly prescribed weak and strong opioids.

Number needed to treat (NNT)

In systematic reviews, the effectiveness of analgesics is expressed as 'number-needed-to-treat' (NNT). NNT means the number of people needed to receive the medication to achieve at least a 50% reduction of pain compared with a placebo over a 6-h treatment period. The most effective drugs have a low NNT of around 2 (McQuay & Moore 1998). Systematic reviews of surgical pain suggest that oral diclofenac 25–50 mg, oral ibuprofen 400 mg (both NSAIDs) and morphine 10 mg i.m. have low NNTs of between 2.3 and 2.9 over the 6-h test period, and tramadol 100 mg has a NNT of 4.8.

Comparisons between opioids show 'no compelling evidence' that any opioid is better than another, although pethidine 'has a specific disadvantage and no specific advantage' (McQuay & Moore 1998). The disadvantage referred to is the irritation caused to the CNS by one of the drug's metabolites, norpethidine, which can cause convulsions, especially in patients who have renal dysfunction

Table 19.2 Equipotent doses of commonly used analgesics

Analgesic	Equipotent dose	Example
Oral morphine: subcutaneous morphine	Two-thirds of the oral dose = s.c. dose	Morphine 10 mg orally is roughly equivalent to 6.5 mg s.c./i.m.
Oral morphine to subcutaneous diamorphine	One-third to one-half of oral dose	Morphine 10 mg orally is roughly equivalent to diamorphine 3–5 mg s.c.
Oral codeine to oral morphine	One-tenth of the dose	Codeine 60 mg orally is roughly equivalent to 6 mg oral morphine
Oral tramadol to oral morphine	One-fifth of the dose	Tramadol 100 mg is roughly equivalent to 20 mg oral morphine
Oral morphine to oral oxycodone	One-half of the dose	Morphine 10 mg orally is roughly equivalent to oxycodone 5 mg orally

where the metabolites are likely to accumulate in the blood, rather than be excreted. NNTs for commonly prescribed analgesics are given on the Bandolier website (see 'Useful websites and addresses').

Neuropathic pain and adjuvant drugs

Most neuropathic pain can be relieved using the principles discussed above. Until the late 1990s it was believed that neuropathic pain was not responsive, or only partially responsive, to opioids. However, reviews by Arnér (2000) and on the Bandolier website (see 'Useful websites and addresses') have shown that many people with neuropathic pain gain effective pain relief from opioids, provided the principle of balancing therapeutic effect with side-effects is followed, i.e. it is important to give a dose large enough to gain maximum analgesic benefit with minimal side-effects. Nevertheless, for a small number of people with neuropathic pain it is likely that adjuvant drugs will also be needed. These include the following:

Anticonvulsants, e.g. sodium valproate, are membrane stabilisers and work by blocking the channels through which sodium and potassium are exchanged across the membrane. As a consequence, an action potential is not produced and thus the pain is prevented. Local anaesthetics work in a similar way (Colvin & McClure 1997). Anticonvulsants also enhance the activity of GABA-ergic synapses (Stannard & Booth 2004). As described above, this receptor complex inhibits pain transmission, so an enhancement of its function will reduce pain transmission.

Gabapentin is a new anticonvulsant, licensed for the treatment of neuropathic pain, that has a slightly different action from other drugs in this group. The precise mode of action of gabapentin is unknown but it is thought that it binds with a specific protein in the CNS, involved in the amino acid cell transport system and in this way influences a cell's responsiveness (Stannard & Booth 2004). A Cochrane Review of pain relief using anticonvulsant drugs concluded that, although gabapentin was increasingly being used to treat neuropathic pain, there is no evidence that it is superior to other anticonvulsants (Wiffen et al 2004).

Antidepressants, e.g. amitriptyline, work by preventing the reuptake of noradrenaline from the synaptic cleft after it has been released by the neurone to transfer chemically an action potential. This depletes the available neurotransmitter and therefore diminishes pain (McQuay et al 1996).

Glucocorticoids, e.g. dexamethasone, are helpful in reducing nerve compression, e.g. as a consequence of tumour. Swelling often occurs around a tumour and these drugs reduce the swelling, so relieving the degree of pain experienced.

Routes of administration

Analgesics are administered via a number of routes — oral, intramuscular, intravenous, rectal, sublingual, buccal, transdermal, subcutaneous, by inhalation, intrapleural, respiratory and spinal — depending on such factors as efficacy, convenience, desired onset of analgesia, acceptability to the patient, side-effects and cost. The choice of route should be made after careful consideration of the comparative risks and benefits of the various routes possible for a given drug. The following discussion provides only a brief introduction to the routes of analgesic administration in common use.

Oral Tablets or liquids are usually easy to administer and place no restrictions on patient mobility. However, their effectiveness is dependent on patient adherence. Sustained-release preparations can enhance adherence by limiting the number of tablets needed each day and have the advantage of attaining consistent blood plasma levels. However, absorption of drugs given by the oral route will be compromised if the patient has nausea and vomiting. In addition, this route has the disadvantage that it is susceptible to the 'first-pass effect' in the liver and intestine, by which some of the drug is metabolised and thus inactivated before it enters the circulation. The oral route is often thought to be appropriate only for mild to moderate pain, but there is much research to show that oral opioids such as morphine and oxycodone can be effective against severe pain if they are given regularly and the dose is titrated to the pain (Hanks 2001).

Intramuscular This route is often used in the treatment of postoperative pain. It has the advantage that it enables the rapid absorption of drugs, although morphine, because of its particular molecular structure, may be more slowly and erratically absorbed than water-based drugs, such as diamorphine. Intramuscular injections can be painful as the needle passes through subcutaneous tissue densely packed with pain receptors. In addition, the injection of the solution can be painful at the site of injection, particularly if the volume of drug exceeds 4 mL. Patients may have to move to expose an injection site and this may cause additional pain. This route also has the disadvantage that it takes time to prepare the injection and have it checked, which can delay analgesia for the patient.

Intravenous The action of analgesics administered by this route is rapid in onset but of short duration, and therefore a continuous infusion rather than bolus injection may be more effective in maintaining the level of analgesic in the bloodstream.

Rectal Medications given by the rectal route are absorbed across the mucous membrane and generally the bioavailability of opioids given via this route is similar to that obtained via the oral route (Hanks et al 1996). Indeed, there is some indication that this route may be better, because the first-pass effect might be avoided as a result of venous drainage (McQuay 1990). However, absorption can be incomplete or erratic, particularly if the patient is constipated. This is a useful route for people unable to take drugs by the oral route, e.g. if they have nausea and vomiting or difficulty in swallowing. Rectal preparations may not be suitable for people who are neutropenic or in danger of being so. Minor trauma on inserting the drug may allow entry of gastric intestinal tract commensals into the systemic circulation and result in septicaemia. Examples of analgesic drugs given rectally include the NSAID diclofenac (Voltarol) and paracetamol suppositories. Most drugs come as a suppository preparation. These preparations have the advantage that they can be given at home and are useful in the management of terminally ill people. However, some people find drug administration by this route unacceptable (Stannard & Booth 2004).

Sublingual and buccal In sublingual administration, the medication is placed under the tongue; in buccal administration it is placed between the upper lip and gum or between the cheek and gum. These routes may avoid the first-pass effect and are rapid in onset of action. However, there is the disadvantage that the patient may inadvertently swallow the drug, and buccal administration may be difficult if the patient has upper dentures. The Expert Working Group of the European Association of Palliative Care (EAPC) (Hanks 2001) has recommended that this route be avoided in cancer pain therapy as it has no clinical advantage over other routes and drug absorption is unpredictable. An example of an analgesic drug available for administration via this route is the opioid buprenorphine.

Transdermal This method of pain relief involves placing a drug-containing patch directly onto the skin, where absorption occurs. The opioid fentanyl has been shown to give effective pain relief by this route and is currently licensed for people with cancer pain and non-cancer pain. Patches need to be changed, usually every 3 days, and have the advantage of continuous pain relief without the need to remember to take tablets throughout the day and night. Research has shown that once the correct dose to manage the pain is achieved, this route of providing analgesia is effective and improves the person's quality of life (Ahmedzai & Brooks 1997). Successful management of pain by this route is dependent on the patch being in contact with the skin and on the availability of oral morphine to control 'breakthrough' pain. Absorption can be speeded up by warmth, so care is needed when bathing or sunbathing.

Subcutaneous infusion is the recommended preferred route for administration of opioids and NSAIDs for people with chronic illness who are unable to take oral medications (Hanks 2001). This route offers a simple, safe and effective alternative to i.v. or i.m. injections and can be used safely in the patient's home.

Inhalation This route enables rapid absorption of gaseous, volatile and atomised substances. For example, nitrous oxide (Entonox) administered with a mask or inhaler can help the patient to deal with bursts of pain, as in childbirth, or during dressing changes or other painful minor procedures. However, this route has the disadvantage that it can be difficult to administer an exact dose and the drug may cause airway irritation.

Spinal This route enables medications to be given directly into the epidural or subarachnoid space of the spinal column. This has a rapid onset of effect and can offer effective pain relief for a wide variety of pain (Stannard & Booth 2004). Medications typically given by this route are opioids and anaesthetic agents which, if given together, can have a synergistic effect. Because of the direct access to the CNS afforded by this route, much smaller doses are required. Whilst this route has many advantages — including a reduction in postoperative complications (Buggy & Smith 1999) and neuromodulation of persistent pain, using opioids to reduce wind-up in neuropathic pain — it has important and potentially serious complications such as respiratory depression and sudden dramatic lowering of blood pressure. Giving analgesics by this route is an extended role for the nurse and subject to the same requirements as discussed under the i.v. route. Despite the need for caution, many people with persistent pain are managed at home for long periods of time, with spinal analgesics administered via a small portable syringe pump or through a medication pump implanted under the skin. Although this treatment has high initial costs, it significantly reduces long-term costs (Winkelmüller 1999).

Patient controlled analgesia (PCA)

PCA refers to the administration of analgesics by any appropriate and safe route over which the patient has control. It usually refers to the self-administration of i.v. boluses of an opioid analgesic, usually morphine, via a specifically designed pump. The pump is set with 'lock-out' intervals and doses to regulate the dose of medication received. This method is typically used postoperatively, but can be used for people with incident-related pain. PCA is dependent on the patient being able and willing to use it and therefore attention to patient information needs is important. From focus group discussions with patients who had experience of using PCA, Chumbley et al (2002) identified that information should include detail about side-effects, but give reassurance that it was safe, and that overdose and addiction was not possible. Information was also sought on how to use PCA and the support available from staff. Despite these concerns, satisfaction with PCA is generally high (Shiloh et al 2003, Chang et al 2004).

PCA has been found to be a safe method of analgesic administration although, depending on the opioids used, side-effects such as nausea and sedation have been reported (Sidebotham et al 1997, Chang et al 2004). There is evidence that PCA offers improved pain relief and quicker recovery following surgery, resulting in earlier discharge (Chang et al 2004). However, results from randomised controlled trials comparing PCA and i.m. injection of morphine are mixed. Snell et al (1997) found no significant difference, whereas Chang et al (2004) found significantly lower levels of pain in the PCA group compared to the i.m. injection group. Thomas and Rose (1993) pointed out that the efficacy of PCA is influenced by the opioid chosen, the demand dose and the lock-out interval set on the PCA pump, as well as by patient psychological variables.

The most frequently purported psychological benefit of PCA is the patient's specific control over pain, PCA eliminating the need for a patient to wait for a nurse to administer pain relief. To test the influence of this on pain experience, Shiloh et al (2003) undertook a randomised quasi-experimental design trial in which postoperative patients (n = 120) were assigned to one of three groups, each receiving different pain management regimens. These were PCA; perceived PCA (PPCA), i.e. a continuous intravenous infusion of analgesics, but without actual control; and continuous intravenous infusion of analgesics (CII). The PPCA and the CII groups received the same dose of morphine over a 24-h period. The PCA group received a background dose equivalent to 50% of the dose received by the other two groups and they could demand bolus doses of morphine up to a total of one and a half times the total dose of morphine received by the other two groups. The groups were compared on reported pain, morphine consumption and satisfaction with pain relief, and individual differences in preferences for control and in state trait anxiety were measured. The study found that the PCA group consumed less morphine than the PPCA and CII groups, reported more pain, but had slightly higher satisfaction with pain relief. The PPCA group were intermediate in relation to both other groups in their reports of pain and morphine consumption, but had the lowest satisfaction with pain relief. Individual differences did not alter the effects of PCA. The authors suggest that the main effect of PCA is increased pain tolerance and that this may be due to the patient's control over their pain and thus a decrease in uncertainty about the availability and effectiveness of pain relief. This may in turn lead to an increase in the use of strategies such as diversion to help the pain.

In a cost-effective analysis, Chang et al (2004) found PCA to be more costly, but this might be explained by the amount of opioid used — being sufficient to control pain in the PCA group but insufficient to control pain in the i.m. injection group.

Other medical interventions

Local anaesthesia and regional nerve blocks These interventions work by injecting local anaesthetic, sometimes together with a steroid, near to or in a peripheral nerve or major nerve plexus or into the spine. Although there can be adverse reactions and complications, the pain-relieving effects often outlast the duration of the local anaesthetic. A review of the efficacy of nerve blocks by Raj and Schwiers (1999) concluded that they are important in the management of pain, particularly for intractable cancer pain and for some people with persistent pain. McCaffery and Pasero (1999) provide an overview of this method and the nursing implications.

Surgery Nerves can be transected in an attempt to reduce or eliminate intractable pain. Examples of surgical methods of pain relief include sympathectomy and cordotomy. Although this measure may work initially, pain often returns and may be worse than it was pre-surgery (Stannard & Booth 2004). For this reason, other techniques, such as spinal cord stimulation, are more common.

Spinal cord stimulation involves the implanting of epidural electrodes, which are controlled either via an external radio frequency transmitter or an implanted pulse generator. Spinal cord stimulation is used for the management of neuropathic pain which has not been relieved by less invasive techniques. Evidence for this technique is limited and predominantly retrospective in design but suggests lasting pain relief in about 50% of patients (Winkelmüller 1999).

Radiotherapy, chemotherapy and hormone therapy may relieve pain by reducing invasive tumours (Stannard & Booth 2004). The effectiveness of radiotherapy in pain relief has been subjected to Cochrane systematic reviews (McQuay et al 2004, Sze et al 2004). These concluded that radiotherapy provided pain relief for three-quarters of patients treated at 1 month after treatment, although the degree to which pain was relieved varied. A single fraction of radiotherapy was found to be as effective as a course of radiotherapy. Radiopharmaceuticals such as strontium chloride-89 have also been shown to be effective in pain due to bone metastases (Robinson et al 1995). There is also growing evidence that bisphosphonates such as pamidronate are effective in relieving bone pain (Wong & Wiffen 2004) (see also Ch. 31).

Specialised pain services

Acute pain services

In response to continuing documentation of inadequate postoperative pain relief, adoption of multiprofessional acute pain services in hospitals is recommended by the Royal College of Anaesthetists and The Pain Society (2003). They recommend that the objectives of a service should include:

- establishment of a system for regular assessment and individual treatment of acute pain
- provision of specialist care and advice for difficult acute pain problems such as occur in patients already taking strong analgesics for persistent pain, and who are drug users

- seamless liaison with other health care teams responsible for the shared care of patients with acute pain
- provision of back-up arrangements, education programmes and appropriate guidelines or protocols to ensure that there is continuous cover for acute pain management around the clock, 7 days a week
- information, education and reassurance for patients, presented in a way that they can understand
- education for nurses, medical staff and allied health care professionals leading to increased awareness of the consequences of unrelieved acute pain and of the techniques available to relieve pain
- continuing audit and evaluation of the service and the needs of patients.

Evidence of the effectiveness of such services is sparse. A systematic review and meta-analysis undertaken by McDonnell et al (2003) concluded that there is insufficient robust research to assess the impact of acute pain teams on adult patients or on the process of postoperative pain relief. There is a little evidence of the cost utility and cost-effectiveness of acute pain services. An analysis by Stadler et al (2004) showed minor reductions in postoperative complication rates in some surgery but no change in duration of hospital stay and postoperative mortality.

Although these studies show a modest influence of acute pain services on patient care, there is emerging evidence of the impact of specialist acute pain teams on nurses' knowledge and attitudes towards pain management. Mackintosh et al (2000) found a consistent positive trend in improved knowledge and attitudes in pain management following the development of a pain service. Similar findings were demonstrated from a survey study (n = 286) by Barton et al (2004), who found that nurses who were unaware of an acute pain service in their organisation had less knowledge about pain than nurses who were aware of the service.

Hospice/palliative care teams have a wealth of expertise in pain and symptom control and can be a valuable resource (see Ch. 33). Such teams are usually multidisciplinary and situated in a variety of care settings. The key functions of such teams are to provide support to other professionals in caring for people with life-threatening illness. Pain is a typical reason for referral to these services, accounting for approximately 64% of referrals (Potter et al 2003). To meet this level of need, palliative care services provide pain control for 2800 patients per million population (Franks et al 2000). A large and thorough review of the research, *Improving Supportive and Palliative Care for Adults with Cancer* (Gysels & Higginson 2004), demonstrated that palliative care teams positively influence patients' experience of pain (see Ch. 33).

Chronic or 'persistent' pain services

These offer a service to people with persistent pain. Clinics are usually multidisciplinary and may be staffed by anaesthetists, nurses, psychologists, physiotherapists, occupational therapists and pharmacists with the aim of increasing the person's ability to function and lead a more fulfilled life. This aim incorporates the belief that persistent pain is the result of multiple interrelating physical, psychological and social or occupational factors.

For detailed objectives of such a service, see the Royal College of Anaesthetists and The Pain Society (2003); for a systematic review of the effectiveness of these services in the care of people with back pain, see Guzmán et al (2001).

Complementary methods of pain relief

'Complementary' methods of pain relief have gained in popularity and include distraction, relaxation, imagery, transcutaneous electrical nerve stimulation (TENS), massage, the application of heat or cold, hypnosis, biofeedback and acupuncture. There is some overlap between certain of these techniques; for example, imagery contains elements of distraction and relaxation.

As with all aspects of pain management, the success of the therapy is dependent on the quality of the relationship between the therapist and the patient. Many nurses have incorporated complementary therapies into nursing practice in order to develop their caring relationship with patients (Royal College of Nursing 2003). Integration of such complementary therapies into nursing practice must be undertaken within the context of the Nursing and Midwifery Council's *Code of Professional Conduct* (2004) and the principles of clinical governance, with the aim to enhance safe, effective and appropriate patient care (Royal College of Nursing 2003).

For guidance on issues which must be taken into account when introducing complementary therapies, see Royal College of Nursing (2003).

Many nurses may use such complementary techniques without realising that they are using them, or explicitly recognising their value. For example, a nurse may distract a patient during a dressing change by asking about holidays or their family. Equally, many patients incorporate complementary techniques into their lives without realising it — they might, for example, use distraction such as watching television, listening to music, or thinking about pleasant times and memories to help them relieve their pain.

Nevertheless, whilst many people find specific complementary therapies helpful, some are sceptical. In part, this is due to the lack of sound research demonstrating their effectiveness, but it may be that pharmacological methods are seen as the only legitimate treatment for pain. In addition, some people, when offered complementary therapies, might feel there is a suggestion that their pain is 'all in the mind'. Some people may refuse complementary therapies because they believe that their pain is too bad. If complementary therapies are offered, explanation about them is best given when pain is either not present, i.e. before surgery, or not at its worst.

Distraction

Distraction involves diverting attention away from the distressing stimulus so that it is no longer the main focus. This can be achieved, as noted above, by encouraging patients to participate in activities that they find absorbing, e.g. conversation, listening to music or focusing on everyday stimuli in the immediate environment. Distraction can give patients a sense of control over their pain and can improve mood (McCaffery & Pasero 1999). However, it also has the following potential disadvantages:

- the validity of the individual's pain may be doubted if distraction is successful
- distraction may not reduce the need for analgesics
- no lasting effect follows a period of distraction; indeed, an individual may be more aware of the pain afterwards
- distraction needs energy and therefore a person might feel fatigued and irritable afterwards.

Relaxation

McCaffery and Pasero (1999) define relaxation as 'a state of relative freedom from both anxiety and skeletal muscle tension'. Relaxation may help to reduce the distress associated with having pain. Relaxation needs to be taught; face-to-face teaching has been found to be more effective than using taped instructions (Seers & Friedli 1996), although once the patient has been given personal instruction, a tape could be given to refresh their memory.

Various methods may be used to promote relaxation; some of these highlight breathing techniques and others attempt to focus the attention sequentially on various parts of the body and then 'letting go' of the tension in those areas. Relaxation can be used to help people cope with specific painful procedures or events or to help people live with persistent pain. Systematic reviews of relaxation in acute and persistent pain are inconclusive overall (Carroll & Seers 1998, Seers & Carroll 1998).

Guided imagery

This technique involves using the imagination to help control pain. Typically, it involves a variety of senses in conjuring up an image. For example, an image about the seaside might include 'seeing' the sand and waves at a beach, 'hearing' the waves and the wind, 'feeling' the sand and the warmth of the sun, 'smelling' the sea air and 'tasting' the salty sea spray.

Evidence for the effectiveness of imagery is weak. In a review, Wallace (1997) found few controlled studies, lack of control groups, small sample sizes, weak theoretical frameworks and few complete descriptions of the nature of the pain being treated. However, notwithstanding methodological problems, some studies suggest benefit, particularly when a person chooses their own image and controls when to use it. Imagery is not advised for people who are psychotic because of the risk that it might exacerbate their psychosis by making it more difficult for them to differentiate between what is real and what is imagined.

Cutaneous stimulation

Transcutaneous electrical nerve stimulation (TENS) In this intervention, low-voltage electrical stimulation is delivered via electrodes placed on the skin near to or on the site of pain. This usually causes a sensation of vibration or tingling and can be used in an intermittent or continuous mode. The device is powered by a battery pack and can be operated by the patient. Care needs to be taken to discriminate the standard TENS device from a variety of commercial devices being marketed, such as microcurrent electrical therapy devices, TENS-pens. In a thorough review of the available devices and the effectiveness of TENS, Johnson (2001) concluded that TENS is not effective for labour pain and postoperative pain and that evidence is inconclusive for persistent pain. However, the studies on which these conclusions are based have methodological problems, therefore health professionals are advised not to dismiss the use of TENS until the methodological issues have been resolved. TENS is not suitable for people with cardiac pacemakers or people suffering from cognitive impairment and should not be placed over a pregnant uterus or the carotid sinus (McCaffery & Pasero 1999).

Massage Throughout history, massage has been used to alleviate pain and suffering (Ernst 2003). Evidence for the effectiveness of massage in relieving pain is sparse. The exception is a Cochrane Review of massage treatment for back pain. This concluded that massage was superior to placebo, relaxation treatment, acupuncture or self-care education; inferior to manipulation, shiatsu or TENS; and no different from treatment with corsets or exercise. The benefit lasted 1 year (Furlan et al 2000). There are several reasons for the scarcity of research, including methodological difficulties, such as the variety of massage techniques practised and the difficulty of designing a placebo with which to compare massage intervention, and a lack of research culture amongst massage therapists (Ernst 2003). Massage should not be confused with therapeutic touch, a technique designed to realign energy fields through the transfer of energy from a healer or therapist.

Heat and cold The application of heat or cold may relieve pain through a 'counter-irritant' effect as well as by direct effects on peripheral and free nerve endings (McCaffery & Pasero 1999). Care should be taken when using this method with patients who have impaired sensation or a reduced level of consciousness as their skin could be inadvertently damaged.

Hypnosis

The nature of hypnosis and the mechanism of its effects are unclear. However, it seems to be an altered state of consciousness in which concentration is focused and distractions are minimised. Success appears to be determined by the individual's ability to respond to suggestion (McCaffery & Pasero 1999), although the person may choose to inhibit this responsiveness. In addition, it seems to be dependent on the type of pain being treated, the context and goals of treatment, the skill of the therapist and the expectations and motivations of the patient. A systematic review of hypnosis concluded that it increased pain relief (Hawkins 2001). However, this technique is not one that should be attempted without special education and training.

Biofeedback

Biofeedback is a method used to encourage and develop relaxation skills. An individual is encouraged to use relaxation to alter specific body functions, such as muscle tension, blood pressure, pulse and/or temperature. Information about these functions is fed back to the individual as they relax, enabling them to learn how to influence positively tension and anxiety.

Acupuncture

Acupuncture originated in China thousands of years ago. It involves inserting needles into the skin at specific acupuncture or Hoku points that are located in a series of channels or meridians. These needles may be manipulated to maximise the effect. The mechanism of action has been the subject of many debates, and activation of endorphins has been implicated.

Studies examining the effectiveness of acupuncture show varying results. A randomised trial comparing acupuncture for the treatment of headache with the accepted management in primary health care (n = 401) found that acupuncture led to significant lasting benefits for patients, including a reduction in pain, medication and sick leave (Vickers et al 2004). Reduction in pain and improvement of movement was demonstrated by Irnich et al (2001) in a randomised trial of acupuncture compared with conventional massage and 'sham' laser acupuncture for neck pain (n = 177). In this trial, benefits were significantly greater for people who had had pain for more than 5 years and in patients with myofascial pain syndrome. Little detail is given about differences between assessment time points in this study so it is difficult to comment on the lasting effects of acupuncture. A Cochrane Review examining the effectiveness of acupuncture for the relief of low back pain found little evidence for its effectiveness and commented on the poor quality of the majority of the studies reviewed (van Tulder et al 2004).

In acupressure, the acupuncture points are stimulated by pressing and/or rubbing rather than by the insertion of needles.

Behaviour therapy

The development of behaviour therapy programmes for pain management owes much to Fordyce (1978), who first drew attention to the rewards a person in persistent pain may receive for 'pain behaviour', such as sympathy, attention and exemption from certain tasks. Since behavioural psychologists believe that all behaviour is governed by its consequences, it is felt that discouraging pain behaviours, such as moaning or grimacing, and encouraging 'well behaviours', the person may adopt a more normal pattern of behaviour. This has been described as operant conditioning. A cognitive–behavioural approach includes the modification of the patient's thoughts and feelings as well as behaviours; it also includes a commitment on the patient's part to behaviour therapy procedures in promoting change, such as graded practice and homework assignments. A systematic review and meta-analysis of cognitive and behavioural therapy for chronic pain found evidence that these therapies were effective in reducing pain experience, and in improving appraisal and coping (Morley et al 1999). Pain clinic programmes usually contain some element of behaviour therapy.

Chiropractic and osteopathy

There is much overlap between the methods and techniques of chiropractic and osteopathy, with what Tanner (1987) describes as 'subtle' differences. He argues that chiropractors are more likely to emphasise the structure of the spine, whereas osteopaths emphasise abnormal movement of the spine. Research supporting these practices is sparse.

Other therapies

Discussion of other therapies such as faith healing, herbal remedies, music therapy, art therapy, aromatherapy and reflexology are not addressed here. However, much of what has already been said above is equally applicable to these therapies, in that they promote well-being and relaxation and may decrease anxiety and thus pain. Art and music therapy may also enable active expression of feelings, which can contribute towards pain relief.

Support and self-help groups

People suffering from pain often seek help from relatives and friends before approaching a professional, such as their GP, within the health care system. Examining the 'trigger' that converts a 'person' into a 'patient' can help to determine how best to help those who do seek help. Examining this in people with persistent pain, Reitsma and Meijler (1997) found that those employing effective coping strategies were less likely to be consumers of health care. In contrast, those people without effective coping strategies were more likely to see themselves as patients and have a greater degree of disability. This suggests that if individual coping skills are developed then disability and distress might be reduced. Emotional coping skills may be developed through self-help groups and organisations such as the National Back Pain Association and the Migraine Action Association (formerly the British Migraine Association) (see 'Useful websites and addresses').

BARRIERS TO PAIN MANAGEMENT

The theory–practice gap

STOP THINK **19.9** Why do you think that the gap between theory and practice exists in respect of pain management? What would influence your ability to provide adequate pain relief for someone you were looking after?

There is arguably a gap between theory and practice in current pain management. Despite significant developments in research-based knowledge, people still experience pain that could be adequately relieved. Surveys of the incidence of postoperative pain demonstrate that moderate to severe pain is common (Royal College of Anaesthetists and The Pain Society 2003). In a critical literature review of pain after day surgery, Coll et al (2004b) found that pain management strategies had been overlooked, resulting in people experiencing pain unnecessarily. These results suggest very little improvement in pain management in the past 10–15 years since the results are very similar to those reported by Seers (1989), Carr and Thomas (1997) and McQuay et al (1997).

The picture is no better with respect to persistent pain. In a large (n = 3605) epidemiological study in the Grampian region of Scotland, 50% of the sample reported having persistent pain (Elliott et al 1999). One-quarter of the people reporting pain had pain that was disabling and limited their daily activities. There are indications from the study that much of the reported pain was poorly treated (for a review and commentary of this paper, see www.jr2.ox.ac.uk bandolier/band70/b70-3.html).

The World Health Organization (WHO) guidelines for analgesia are frequently not utilised in practice (Kuuppelomäki 2002) despite evidence that they are effective (WHO 2004).

Fears associated with opioids

Pain management is influenced by fears about opioids (Carr & Mann 2000) and these fears tend to be common to nurses, patients and their family members/carers. They include fear of addiction and dependence, fear of tolerance and fear of side-effects. Most of these fears are propagated by reports of addiction in people using opioids for recreational use, the dangers to which this use exposes them and the difficult symptoms that they experience when trying to withdraw from this use. In order to examine these fears, it is important to clarify the terms 'addiction', 'tolerance' and 'dependence' (see Ch. 36 for a discussion of these terms).

Addiction to opioids when used specifically in pain management is rare. Two seminal studies found the following incidence of addiction in patients receiving opioid analgesics was virtually non-existent:

- Porter and Jick (1980), n = 12 000; four cases of addiction reported, only one of which required treatment
- Perry and Heidrich (1982), n = 10 000; no cases of addiction reported.

Dependence on opioids occurs in prolonged use and therefore care is needed when reducing the dose. If the dose is reduced gradually, withdrawal symptoms will not occur.

Tolerance to opioids is varied. It is not usually necessary to increase the dose of an opioid to maintain a similar therapeutic effect. In other words, more of the drug is not needed as someone 'gets used to it'; in cancer pain, an increase in dose is normally only needed with disease progression. Therefore, concerns that if morphine is started too soon it will not be possible to control the pain later are unfounded. On the other hand, tolerance does develop to some of the side-effects of opioids. For example, it is common for people to experience nausea and vomiting and drowsiness in the first few days of taking an opioid, but this then passes and is rarely a continuing problem. It is important to note that constipation is a continuing side-effect of opioid use.

Issues in professional education and training

A number of researchers have demonstrated that there is insufficient education in pain management throughout the world (Brunier et al 1995, McCaffery & Ferrell 1995, Clarke et al 1996, Kubecka et al 1996). This can lead to attitudinal barriers and inappropriate behaviours in pain management (McCaffery & Pasero 1999). For example, most nurses in these studies did not understand the fundamental principles of pain relief or take responsibility for pain assessment, and they misunderstood the extent to which opioids induce respiratory depression and addiction. However, such attitudes have been shown to respond positively to education when this is provided (Brunier et al 1995, Dalton et al 1996, McCaffery & Ferrell 1997).

Professional and cultural biases in inferences of pain

At the beginning of this chapter, it was argued that it is very difficult to know what anyone's experience of pain is like. However, many studies have shown that nurses make assumptions and judgements about the amount or type of pain their patients are suffering, which significantly influence the quality of care provided (McCaffery & Pasero 1999).

There is a significant body of evidence that supports the view that nurses and other health care professionals view pain as 'normal' or to be expected and thus underestimate the severity of the patient's experience (Carr & Mann 2000). Underestimation of pain may also be due to nurses adopting a detached, rather than an involved, stance towards someone in pain. For example, Madjar (1998) noted that some nurses distanced themselves from the pain that patients were experiencing as a way of protecting themselves from the emotional experience of caring for someone in pain. In this way, these nurses became desensitised to patients' distress.

Evidence suggests that factors influencing the patient's experience of pain also influence a nurse's judgement of pain. For example, McCaffery and Pasero (1999) draw attention to societal prejudices that can influence nurses' inferences of pain and psychological distress, such as patients' socioeconomic, religious or ethnic backgrounds.

Furthermore, there is evidence that nurses make judgements about pain based on whether or not they believe it has a cause. In a study examining nurses' discourse of pain, Wakefield (1995) found that nurses believe that pain can, and should, only be manifest in the presence of an identifiable cause and that, if no cause was identified, nurses were likely to believe that patients were trying to get analgesics by immoral means. This 'acute pain model' is noted by McCaffery and Pasero (1999) as being a major obstacle to effective pain management and has a profound effect on patients, as illustrated by another example from the study by Seers and Friedli (1996):

> *I had something that was medically unacceptable. The GPs labelled me as neurotic because they couldn't find anything wrong. Their dismissive 'unlistening' attitude to my mysterious pain almost amounts, in my opinion, to mental cruelty.*

Madjar (1998) found that nurses were more likely to label patients as complainers if they felt that they were exaggerating their report of pain or that they were not coping adequately with their pain. McCaffery and Pasero (1999) also suggest that unpopular or difficult patients are often labelled as not having 'real' pain.

The research referred to in this chapter has begun to explain why it is so difficult to put knowledge about pain management into practice. The complexity of practice cannot be underestimated. Competing demands and resource limitations challenge the ability to care for people in pain but the distress of pain makes it imperative that these challenges are conquered.

CONCLUSION

STOP THINK **19.10** Now that you have read this chapter, make an action plan of how you are going to improve the care that you provide to people in pain. Share this action plan with your mentor or a colleague to help you implement it.

Pain and its relief form a central part of nursing in almost all care settings. Ongoing education for health professionals and an understanding of the complexities of pain and its management are crucial in forming a sound basis for practice (Royal College of Anaesthetists and The Pain Society 2003). The person in pain should be believed, their pain should be systematically assessed, treated and reassessed, and they should be involved in pain management whenever possible. Pain and its relief must be given a high priority in care, and health professionals should be accountable for the pain relief of people in their care. Indeed, failure to do so contravenes the Nursing and Midwifery Council *Code of Professional Conduct* (2004). Nurses are in the fortunate position of being able to make an important contribution towards the comfort and well-being of people in pain and to rise to the challenges of influencing the contextual factors that shape this care.

REFERENCES

Ahmedzai S, Brooks D 1997 Transdermal fentanyl versus sustained release morphine in cancer pain: preference, efficacy and quality of life. Journal of Pain and Symptom Management 13(5): 254–261

Arnér S 2000 Opioids and long-lasting pain conditions: 25-year perspective on mechanism-based treatment strategies. Pain Reviews 7: 81–96

Arraras J I, Wright S J, Jusue G et al 2002 Coping style, locus of control, psychological distress and pain-related behaviours in cancer and other diseases. Psychology, Health and Medicine 7(2): 181–188

Barton J, Don M, Foureur M 2004 Nurses' and midwives' pain knowledge improves under the influence of an acute pain service. Acute Pain 6(2): 47–51

Bendelow G A 1993 Pain perceptions, emotions and gender. Sociology of Health and Illness 15(3): 273–294

Bendelow G A, Williams S J 1995 Sociological approaches to pain. Progress in Palliative Care 3(5): 169–174

Bishop S R, Warr D 2003 Coping, catastrophizing and chronic pain in breast cancer. Journal of Behavioural Medicine 26(3): 265–282

Blomqvist K 2003 Older people in persistent pain: nursing and paramedic staff perceptions and pain management. Journal of Advanced Nursing 41(6): 575–584

Blomqvist K, Edberg A-K 2002 Living with persistent pain: experiences of older people receiving home care. Journal of Advanced Nursing 40(3): 297–306

Boström B, Sandh M, Lundberg D, Fridlund B 2004 Cancer-related pain in palliative care: patients' perceptions of pain management. Journal of Advanced Nursing 45(4): 410–419

Bowling A 2004 Measuring health: a review of quality of life measurement scales, 2nd edn. Open University Press, Milton Keynes

Brunier G, Carson M G, Harrison D E 1995 What do nurses know and believe about patients' pain? Results of a hospital survey. Journal of Pain and Symptom Management 10(6): 436–445

Buggy D J, Smith G 1999 Epidural anaesthesia and analgesia: better outcome after major surgery? British Journal of Medicine 319: 530–531

Burckhardt C S, Clark S R, Bennett R M 2001 Pain coping strategies and quality of life in women with fibromyalgia: does age make a difference? Journal of Musculoskeletal Pain 9(2): 5–8

Caraceni A 2001 Evaluation and assessment of cancer pain and cancer pain treatment. Acta Anaesthesiologica Scandinavica 45: 1067–1075

Carpenter R H S 2003 Neurophysiology, 4th edn. Oxford University Press, Oxford

Carr E C J, Mann E 2000 Pain: creative approaches to effective pain management. Palgrave, Basingstoke

Carr E C J, Thomas V J 1997 Anticipating and experiencing post-operative pain: the patient's perspective. Journal of Clinical Nursing 6(3): 191–201

Carroll D, Seers K 1998 Relaxation for the relief of chronic pain: a systematic review. Journal of Advanced Nursing 27: 476–487

Chang A M, Ip W Y, Cheung T H 2004 Patient controlled analgesia versus conventional intramuscular injection: a cost effectiveness analysis. Journal of Advanced Nursing 46(5): 531–541

Chumbley G M, Hall G M, Salman P 2002 Patient-controlled analgesia: what information does the patient want? Journal of Advanced Nursing 39(5): 459–471

Clarke E B, French B, Bilodeau M L et al 1996 Pain management knowledge, attitudes and clinical practice: the impact of nurses' characteristics and education. Journal of Pain and Symptom Management 11(1): 18–31

Closs S J, Barr B, Briggs M 2004 Cognitive status and analgesic provision in nursing home residents. British Journal of General Practice 54(509): 919–921

Coderre T J, Katz J, Vaccarino A L, Melzack R 1993 Contribution of central neuroplasticity to pathological pain: review of clinical and experimental evidence. Pain 52(3): 259–285

Coll A M, Ameen J R M, Mead D 2004a Postoperative pain assessment tools in day surgery: literature review. Journal of Advanced Nursing 46(2): 124–133

Coll A M, Ameen J R M, Moseley L G 2004b Reported pain after day surgery: a critical literature review. Journal of Advanced Nursing 46(1): 53–65

Colvin L A, McClure J H 1997 Local anaesthetics: structure–activity relationships and their role in pain treatment. Pain Reviews 4: 59–77

Coyle N 2004 In their own words: seven advanced cancer patients describe their experience with pain and the use of opioid drugs. Journal of Pain and Symptom Management 27(4): 300–310

Dalton J A, Blau W, Carson J et al 1996 Changing the relationship among nurses' knowledge, self-reported behaviour and documented behaviour in pain management: does education make a difference? Journal of Pain and Symptom Management 12(5): 308–319

Dann K, Yokota T, Koyama N et al 2000 Mechanism-based treatment of zoster-associated pain. Pain Reviews 7: 157–180

Davidson P 1988 Facilitating coping with cancer pain. Palliative Medicine 2: 107–114

DeLeo J A, Yezierski R P 2001 The role of neuroinflammation and neuroimmune activation in persistent pain. Pain 90: 1–6

Dura J R, Beck S J 1988 A comparison of family functioning when mothers have chronic pain. Pain 35(1): 79–89

Elliot A M, Smith B H, Penny K I, Smith W C, Chambers W A 1999 The epidemiology of chronic pain in the community. Lancet 354: 1248–1452

Ernst E 2003 Massage treatment for back pain. British Medical Journal 326: 562–563

Ferrell B, Rhiner M, Cohen M Z, Grant M 1991a Pain as a metaphor for illness. Part 1: impact of cancer pain on family caregivers. Oncology Nurse Forum 18(8): 1303–1308

Ferrell B, Cohne M Z, Rhiner M, Rozek A 1991b Pain as a metaphor for illness. Part 2: family and caregivers' management of pain. Oncology Nurse Forum 18(8): 1313–1322

Fitzpatrick R, Davey C, Buxton M J, Jones D R 1998 Evaluating patient-based outcome measures for use in clinical trials. Health Technology Assessment 2: 1–4

Fordyce W E 1978 Learning processes in pain. In: Sternbach R A (ed) The psychology of pain. Raven Press, New York, p 49–72

Frampton M 2003 Experience assessment and management of pain in people with dementia. Age and Aging 32: 248–251

Franks P J, Salisbury C, Bosanquet N et al 2000 The level of need for palliative care: a systematic review of the literature. Palliative Medicine 14: 93–104

Frischenschlarger O, Pucher I 2002 Psychological management of pain. Disability and Rehabilitation 24(8): 416–422

Furlan A D, Brosseau L, Welch V et al 2000 Massage for low back pain. Cochrane Database Systematic Review (4): CD001929

Guzmán J, Esmail R, Karjalainen K et al 2001 Multidisciplinary rehabilitation for chronic low back pain: systematic review. British Journal of Medicine 322: 1511–1516

Gysels M, Higginson I J 2004 Improving supportive and palliative care for adults

with cancer: research evidence manual. National Institute for Clinical Excellence, London
Hanks G 2001 Morphine and alternative opioids in cancer pain: the EAPC recommendations. British Journal of Cancer 84(5): 587–593
Hanks G, de Conno F, Ripamonti C et al 1996 Morphine in cancer pain: modes of administration. British Medical Journal 312: 823–826
Hawkins R M F 2001 A systematic meta-review of hypnosis as an empirically supported treatment for pain. Pain Reviews 8: 47–73
International Association for the Study of Pain (IASP) Task Force on Taxonomy 1994 IASP pain terminology. In: Merksey H, Bogduk N (eds) Classification of chronic pain, 2nd edn. IASP Press, Seattle, p 209–214
Irnich D, Bechrens N, Molzen H et al 2001 Randomised trial of acupuncture compared with conventional massage and 'sham' laser acupuncture for treatment of chronic neck pain. British Journal of Medicine 322: 1574–1578
Johnson M I 2001 Transcutaneous electrical nerve stimulation (TENS) and TENS-like devices: do they provide pain relief? Pain Reviews 8: 121–158
Kubecka K E, Simon J M, Boettcher J H 1996 Pain management of hospital-based nurses in rural Appalachian area. Journal of Advanced Nursing 23(5): 861–867
Kuuppelomäki M 2002 Pain management problems in patients' terminal phase as assessed by nurses in Finland. Journal of Advanced Nursing 40(6): 701–709
Lansbury G 2000 Chronic pain management: a qualitative study of elderly people's preferred coping strategies and barriers to management. Disability and Rehabilitation 22(1/2): 2–14
Lasch K E 2002 Culture and pain. Pain Clinical Updates X(5): 1–10
Lazarus R 1993 Coping theory and research: past, present and future. Psychosomatic Medicine 55: 234–247
Lima D 1997 Functional anatomy of spinofugal nociceptive pathways. Pain Reviews 4: 1–19
Lundeberg T, Lund I, Dahlin D 2001 Reliability and responsiveness of three different pain assessments. Journal of Rehabilitation Medicine 33(6): 279–283
Mackintosh C, Bowles S, Mackintosh S 2000 The effect of an acute pain service on nurses' knowledge and beliefs about post-operative pain. Journal of Clinical Nursing 9(1): 119–126
Madjar I 1998 Giving comfort and inflicting pain. Qualitative Institute Press, Edmonton
Manias E 2003 Pain and anxiety management in the postoperative gastro-surgical setting. Journal of Advanced Nursing 41(6): 585–594
Manias E, Botti M, Bucknell T 2002 Observation of pain assessment and management – the complexities of clinical practice. Journal of Clinical Nursing 11: 724–733
McCaffery M 1972 Nursing management of the patient in pain. Lippincott, Philadelphia
McCaffery M 2001 Controlling pain: overcoming barriers to pain management. Nursing 31(4): 18
McCaffery M, Ferrell B R 1995 Nurses' knowledge about cancer pain: a survey of five countries. Journal of Pain and Symptom Management 10(5): 356–369
McCaffery M, Ferrell B R 1997 Nurses' knowledge of pain assessment and management: how much progress have we made? Journal of Pain and Symptom Management 14(3): 175–188
McCaffery M, Pasero C 1999 Pain: clinical manual for nursing practice, 2nd edn. Mosby, Aylesbury
McDonnell A, Nicholl J, Read S M 2003 Acute pain teams and the management of postoperative pain: a systematic review and meta-analysis. Journal of Advanced Nursing 41(3): 261–273
McMillan S C 1996 Pain and pain relief experienced by hospice patients with cancer. Cancer Nursing 19(4): 289–307
McQuay H 1990 The logic of alternative routes. Pain and Symptom Management 5(2): 75–77
McQuay H, Moore A 1998 An evidence-based resource for pain relief. Oxford University Press, Oxford
McQuay H, Tramer M, Nye B A et al 1996 A systematic review of antidepressants in neuropathic pain. Pain 68(2): 217–227
McQuay H, Moore A, Justins D 1997 Treating acute pain in hospital. British Medical Journal 314: 1431–1535
McQuay H, Collins S L, Carroll D, Moore R A 2004 Radiotherapy for the palliation of painful bone metastases (Cochrane Review). In: The Cochrane Library, Issue 3. Wiley, Chichester
Melanson P M, Downe-Wamboldt B 2003 Confronting life with rheumatoid arthritis. Journal of Advanced Nursing 42(2): 125–133
Melzack R, Wall P D 1965 Pain mechanisms: a new theory. Science 150: 971–979
Melzack R, Wall P D 1996 The challenge of pain. Penguin, Harmondsworth
Morley S, Eccleston C, Williams A 1999 Systematic review and meta-analysis of randomised controlled trials of cognitive behaviour therapy for chronic pain in adults, excluding headache. Pain 80: 1–13
Morris D 1991 The culture of pain. University of California Press, Berkeley
Müllersdorf M, Söderback I 2000 The actual state of the effects, treatment and incidence of disabling pain in a gender perspective – a Swedish study. Disability and Rehabilitation 22(18): 840–854
National Institute for Clinical Excellence (NICE) 2001 Guidance on the use of cyclo-oxygenase (Cox) II selective inhibitors, celecoxib, rofeecoxib, meloxicam and etodolac for osteoarthritis and rheumatoid arthritis. NICE, London
National Institutes of Health Consensus Development Conference 1987 The integrated approach to the management of pain. Journal of Pain and Symptom Management 2(1): 35–44
Newton-John T R O 2002 Solicitousness and chronic pain: a critical review. Pain Reviews 9(1): 7–21
Nursing and Midwifery Council (NMC) 2004 The NMC code of professional conduct: standards for conduct, performance and ethics. NMC, London
Oldham L, Kristjanson L J 2004 Development of a pain management programme for family carers of advanced cancer patients. International Journal of Palliative Care 10(2): 91–98
Pace V 1995 Use of non-steroidal anti-inflammatory drugs in cancer. Palliative Medicine 9: 273–286
Paulson M, Danielson E, Söd S 2002 Struggling for a tolerable existence: the meaning of men's lived experience of living with pain of fibromyalgia type. Qualitative Health Research 12(2): 238–249
Perry S, Heidrich G 1982 Management of pain during debridement: a survey of US burn units. Pain 13(3): 267–280
Portenoy R K, Ugarte C, Fuller I, Haas G 2004 Population-based survey of pain in the United States: differences amongst White, African, American and Hispanic subjects. Journal of Pain 5(6): 317–328
Porter J, Jick H 1980 Addiction rare in patients treated with opioids. New England Journal of Medicine 302(2): 123
Potter J, Hami F, Bryan T et al 2003 Symptoms of 4000 patients referred to palliative care services: prevalence and patterns. Palliative Medicine 17: 310–314
Price D 2002 Brain mechanisms of persistent pain states. Journal of Musculoskeletal Pain 10(1–2): 73–83
Price K, Cheek J 1996 Exploring the nursing role in pain management from a post-structuralist perspective. Journal of Advanced Nursing 24(5): 899–904
Raj P P, Schwiers R J 1999 Nerve blocks: are they useful and significant in the management of pain patients? Pain Reviews 6: 193–201
Reitsma B, Meijler W J 1997 Pain and patienthood. Clinical Journal of Pain 13: 9–21
Richards H M, Reid M E, Murray G C et al 2002 Socioeconomic variations in responses to chest pain: qualitative study. British Journal of Medicine 324(7349): 1308–1318
Richardson C, Poole H 2001 Chronic pain and coping: a proposed role for nurses and nursing models. Journal of Advanced Nursing 34(5): 659–667
Robinson R G, Preston D F, Schiefelbein M, Baxter K G 1995 Strontium 89 therapy for the palliation of pain due to osseous metastases. Journal of the American Medical Association 4(5): 420–424
Rollnick J D, Karst M, Pieoenbrock S et al 2003 Gender differences in coping with tension-type headaches. European Neurology 50(2): 73–78
Romano J M, Turner J A, Jenson M P et al 1995 Chronic pain patient–spouse behavioural interactions predict patient disability. Pain 63(3): 353–360
Royal College of Anaesthetists and The Pain Society 2003 Pain management services: good practice. Royal College of Anaesthetists and The Pain Society, London
Royal College of Nursing 2003 Complementary therapies in nursing, midwifery and health visiting practice. Royal College of Nursing, London
Scarry E 1985 The body in pain. Oxford University Press, New York
Schafheutle E I, Cantrill J A, Noyce P R 2001 Why is pain management suboptimal on

surgical wards? Journal of Advanced Nursing 33(6): 728–737
Schwartz L, Slater M A, Birchler G R 1996 The role of pain behaviours in the modulation of marital conflict in chronic pain couples. Pain 65(2/3): 227–233
Seers K 1989 Patients' perceptions of acute pain. In: Wilson-Barnett J, Robinson S (eds) Directions in nursing research: ten years of progress at London University. Scutari, London, p 107–116
Seers K, Carroll D 1998 Relaxation techniques for acute pain management: a systematic review. Journal of Advanced Nursing 27: 466–475
Seers K, Friedli K 1996 The patients' experience of their chronic non-malignant pain. Journal of Advanced Nursing 24(6): 1160–1168
Shiloh S, Zukerman G, Butin B et al 2003 Postoperative patient-controlled analgesia (PCA): how much control and how much analgesia? Psychology and Health 18(6): 753–770
Sidebotham D, Dijkhuizen M R J, Schug S A 1997 The safety and utilization of patient controlled analgesia. Journal of Pain and Symptom Management 14(4): 202–209
Simons W, Malabar R 1995 Assessing pain in elderly patients who cannot respond verbally. Journal of Advanced Nursing 22(1): 663–669
Sjöström B, Dahlgren L O, Heljamäe H 2000 Strategies used in post-operative pain assessment and their clinical accuracy. Journal of Clinical Nursing 9: 111–118
Smith J A, Lumley M A, Longo D J 2002 Contrasting emotional approach coping with passive coping for chronic myofascial pain. Annals of Behavioural Medicine 24(4): 326–346
Snell C C, Fothergill-Bourbonnais F, Durocher-Hendrikis S 1997 Patient controlled analgesia and intramuscular injections: a comparison of patient pain experiences and post operative outcomes. Journal of Advanced Nursing 25(4): 681–690
Söderberg S, Strand M, Haapala M, Lundman B 2003 Living with a woman with fibromyalgia from the perspective of the husband. Journal of Advanced Nursing 42(2): 143–150
Stadler M, Schlander M, Braeckman M et al 2004 A cost-utility and cost-effectiveness analysis of an acute pain service. Journal of Clinical Anaesthesia 16(3): 159–167
Stannard C, Booth S 2004 Pain, 2nd edn. Churchill Livingstone, Edinburgh
Sze W M, Shelly M, Held I, Mason M 2004 Palliation of metastatic bone pain: single fraction versus multifraction radiotherapy (Cochrane Review). In: The Cochrane Library, Issue 3. Wiley, Chichester
Tanner J 1987 Beating back pain: a practical self-help guide to prevention and treatment. Dorling Kindersley, London
Taylor A G, Lorentzen L J, Blank M B 1990 Psychological distress of chronic pain sufferers and their spouses. Journal of Pain and Symptom Management 5(1): 6–10
Thomas S P 2000 A phenomenological study of chronic pain. Western Journal of Nursing Research 22: 683–699
Thomas V, Rose F D 1993 Patient controlled analgesia: a new method for old. Journal of Advanced Nursing 11(1): 1719–1726
Tsai P-F, Tak S, Moore C, Palencia I 2003 Testing a theory of chronic pain. Journal of Advanced Nursing 43(2): 158–169
Turk D C 1989 Assessment of pain: the elusiveness of latent constructs. In: Chapman C R, Loeser J D (eds) Issues in pain measurement. Advances in pain research and therapy, Vol 12. Raven Press, New York, p 267–279
Turk D C, Flor H, Rudy T E 1987 Pain and families I: etiology, maintenance and psychological impact. Pain 30(1): 2–27
Van Tulder M W, Cherkin D C, Berman B et al 2004 Acupuncture for low back pain (Cochrane Review). In: The Cochrane Library, Issue 3. Wiley, Chichester
Vickers A J, Rees R W, Zollman C E et al 2004 Acupuncture for chronic headache in primary care: large, pragmatic, randomised trial. British Journal of Medicine 328: 744–747
Wakefield A B 1995 Pain: an account of nurses' talk. Journal of Advanced Nursing 21(5): 905–910
Walker J M, Akinsanya J A, Davies B D, Marcer D 1990 The nursing management of elderly patients with pain in the community: study and recommendations. Journal of Advanced Nursing 15(4): 1154–1161
Wallace K G 1997 Analysis of recent literature concerning relaxation and imagery interventions for cancer pain. Cancer Nursing 20(2): 79–87
Watkins L R, Maier S F 2003 When good pain turns bad. Current Directions in Psychological Science 12(6): 232–236
Whelan E 2003 Putting pain to paper: endometriosis and the documentation of suffering. Health 7(4): 463–482
White A K 2003 Interactions between nurses and men admitted with cardiac pain. European Journal of Cardiovascular Nursing 2(1): 47–55
Wiesler-Frank J, Maier S F, Watkins L R 2003 Glial activation and pathological pain. Neurochemistry International 45: 389–395
Wiffen P, Collins S, McQuay H et al 2004 Anticonvulsants for acute and chronic pain (Cochrane Review). In: The Cochrane Library, Issue 3. Wiley, Chichester
Williams D A, Thorn B E 1989 An empirical assessment of pain beliefs. Pain 36(3): 351–358
Winkelmüller W 1999 Neuromodulation techniques in the treatment of chronic painful diseases. Pain Reviews 6: 203–209
Wong R, Wiffen P J 2004 Bisphosphonates for the relief of pain secondary to bone metastases (Cochrane Review). In: The Cochrane Library, Issue 3. Wiley, Chichester
World Health Organization 2004 WHO analgesic ladder. Online. Available: www.who.org
Yates P, Dewar A, Fentiman B 1995 Pain: the views of elderly people living in long term residential care settings. Journal of Advanced Nursing 21(4): 667–674
Zborowski M 1952 Cultural components in response to pain. Journal of Social Issues 8(4): 16–30

FURTHER READING

Carpenter R H S 2003 Neurophysiology, 4th edn. Arnold, London
Carr E C J, Mann E 2000 Pain: creative approaches to effective pain management. Palgrave, Basingstoke
Guzmán J, Esmail R, Karjalainen K et al 2001 Multidisciplinary rehabilitation for chronic low back pain: systematic review. British Journal of Medicine 322: 1511–1516
Kearney M 2000 A place of healing. Working with suffering in living and dying. Oxford University Press, Oxford
Madjar I 1998 Giving comfort and inflicting pain. Qualitative Institute Press, Edmonton
McCaffery M, Pasero C 1999 Pain: clinical manual for nursing practice, 2nd edn. Mosby, Aylesbury
Melzack R, Wall P D 1996 The challenge of pain. Penguin, Harmondsworth
Royal College of Anaesthetists and The Pain Society 2003 Pain management services: good practice. Royal College of Anaesthetists and The Pain Society, London
Royal College of Nursing 2003 Complementary therapies in nursing, midwifery and health visiting practice. Royal College of Nursing, London
Salmon P, Manyande A 1996 Good patients cope with their pain: postoperative analgesia and nurses' perceptions of their patients' pain. Pain 68(1): 63–68

USEFUL WEBSITES AND ADDRESSES

Bandolier – evidence-based thinking about health care
www.jr2.ox.ac.uk/bandolier

International Association for the Study of Pain
www.iasp-pain.org

Migraine Action Association (formerly British Migraine Association)
www.migraine.org.uk

Migraine Sufferers Support Group
www.migraine.co.nz

National Back Pain Association
www.backpain.org.uk

National Institute for Clinical Excellence
www.nice.org.uk

Pain Wise UK (formerly Self-help in Pain, SHIP)
33 Kingsdown Park
Tankerton
Kent CT5 2DT
(No website)

Palliative care formulary
www.palliativedrugs.com

World Health Organization
www.who.org

FLUID AND ELECTROLYTE BALANCE

20

Mary Gobbi
Michelle Cowen
Debra Ugboma

INTRODUCTION

Monitoring and manipulating body fluid and electrolytes form a crucial aspect of nursing care. For the average male, only about 18% of the body weight is protein with 15% fat and 7% minerals; 60% is water. For health, body water and electrolytes must be maintained within a limited range of tolerances. Homeostatic mechanisms regulate parameters such as body fluid volume, acid–base balance (pH) and electrolyte concentrations, maintaining a delicate, dynamic balance which can be destabilised during illness. In extreme cases, the fluid or electrolyte deficit can lead to death. Consequently, nurses must have a clear understanding of fluid and electrolyte homeostasis so that they can assess fluid and electrolyte status, anticipate/recognise deterioration and implement corrective interventions.

Nursing interventions in relation to fluid therapy may range from encouraging the patient to drink an afternoon cup of tea to managing a complicated intravenous fluid regimen. Ill-defined terms, such as 'restrict fluids' or 'push fluids', and instructions to record fluid intake/output or daily weight, are commonly encountered. However, without a knowledgeable appreciation of the physiology and pathophysiology of fluid and electrolyte balance there is a real risk that these tasks will be performed in a somewhat mechanistic fashion, without sufficient thought or understanding.

This chapter reviews the normal mechanisms which regulate body fluid and outlines some of the basic adaptive responses to stress. The regulation of acid–base balance is also considered, along with basic principles in the management of fluid and electrolyte disorders. Throughout the chapter, typical clinical situations where fluid and electrolyte control may be compromised are reviewed. Reference is made to the ethical dilemmas which may be associated with the administration/withdrawal of hydration measures.

Students who are unfamiliar with the physiology of fluid, electrolyte and acid–base balance are advised to read this chapter in conjunction with their physiology and pathophysiology textbooks. It is important for the reader to be familiar with units and terms such as 'moles', 'molality', 'equivalents', 'diffusion', 'osmosis', 'osmoles', 'osmolality', 'tonicity' and 'filtration'.

For more detailed information, see Smith & Kinsey (1991), Porth (2002) and Marieb (2004).

Nursing goals in the care of patients with existing or potential fluid and electrolyte problems include:

- the promotion and maintenance of a healthy pattern of fluid intake/output appropriate to the patient's lifestyle and wishes

- the detection of existing or potential fluid and electrolyte imbalances
- the re-establishment of fluid and electrolyte balance when homeostasis is disturbed
- the development of educational programmes on the maintenance of fluid and electrolyte balance.

It is hoped that this chapter will provide some of the essential background knowledge necessary to achieving these aims.

BODY WATER

Water has a range of functions within the body which are essential to sustaining life and maintaining health. These include:

- giving form to body structures and cushioning the body from shock
- acting as a transport medium for nutrients, electrolytes, blood gases, metabolic wastes, heat and electrical currents
- providing insulation
- aiding in the hydrolysis of food
- acting as a medium and reactant in chemical processes
- acting as a lubricant.

Body tissues contain varying proportions of water, ranging from 10% for fat to 83% for blood. A young 70 kg man of average build has a total body water (TBW) of about 60% of body weight, or 40 L. The percentage of body weight represented by the TBW varies from one individual to another, depending on factors such as age, gender and build. Fat contributes little towards TBW and is the main source of this variation. A 70 kg woman of average build would have a TBW of about 52% (36 L) due to the greater proportion of adipose tissue. In both genders, the percentage of body water tends to decrease with age. Lean tissue has a fairly constant water content of 71–72 mL/100 g, and if adipose tissue is disregarded as a non-functional storage tissue, then the TBW of the lean body mass is about 73%. As water makes up nearly three-quarters of the body's active tissues, homeostatic regulation of body fluids is essential to normal function and health.

Fluid compartments

Body water is distributed between two major compartments: the intracellular fluid (ICF) and the extracellular fluid (ECF). The distinction between the two compartments is maintained by the selective permeability of cell membranes. The intracellular environment is not homogeneous but varies greatly between cell types. However, all cells can tolerate only a limited variation in the volume and composition of their ICF before function is disrupted.

Large proteins which are synthesised by the cell remain inside as they are too big to pass through the membrane. However, the membrane is freely permeable to water. Selective membrane transport processes regulate the distribution of electrolytes, and hence water, across the cell membrane. The ICF has been estimated to be approximately 40% of TBW, or about 28 L in a 70 kg male.

The ECF bathes and surrounds the cells, forming a relatively constant environment. It has a smaller volume than the ICF, accounting for about 20% of TBW (or 14 L), and can be divided into four subcompartments:

- the extravascular fluid (interstitial or tissue fluid)
- inaccessible bone water (skeletal water)
- the intravascular fluid compartment (blood plasma)
- transcellular fluids.

Interstitial fluid includes lymph and accounts for about 15% (10.5 L) of TBW. Interstitial fluid is defined by two membranes: the cell membrane which separates the lymph from the ICF, and the capillary endothelium which separates it from plasma. Interstitial fluid forms the interface and exchange route between the ICF and plasma. Plasma represents about 4% of body weight (3 L).

Transcellular fluids are specialised fluids which are separated from the ECF by an additional epithelial cell layer. They include:

- cerebrospinal fluid (CSF)
- aqueous and vitreous humor of the eye
- glandular secretions
- synovial fluid
- pleural fluid
- peritoneal fluid
- glandular secretions
- saliva and other gastrointestinal secretions
- respiratory tract fluid
- fluid within the urinary system.

Transcellular fluid volume is highly variable, and some transcellular fluids have a very high turnover; in the gastrointestinal tract alone it can be greater than 20 L/day. Some water is trapped in the deeper layers of bone; this is inaccessible and, because it does not readily exchange with the rest of the ECF, is difficult to measure. The relative contribution of each compartment is summarised in Box 20.1. In infants and children, although the actual ECF volume is much smaller than in adults, the ECF:ICF ratio is larger, i.e. the ECF represents a greater percentage of the TBW, and fluid loss can rapidly lead to dehydration. The consequences of ECF losses from, for example, vomiting, sweating or diarrhoea are potentially more serious in the infant than in the adult.

For further details, see Porth (2002) and Marieb (2004).

Box 20.1

The major fluid compartments of the body in the average young male weighing 70 kg and containing 40 L of body water

- Intracellular fluid: 40% body weight and 25 L
- Extracellular fluid: 20% body weight and 15 L, of which:
  - 80% (12 L) is interstitial/tissue fluid
  - 20% (3 L) is plasma

These figures include water found in serous fluid, cerebrospinal fluid and bones.

Solutes and electrolytes

Body fluids cannot be equated simply with water, as they also contain dissolved substances or solutes as well as larger particles in suspension (colloids). Solutes may be complete molecules (non-electrolytes) or parts of molecules (electrolytes). Measures of body fluid volume, such as the litre, refer to the volume of water and its dissolved solutes. Glucose is a good example of a non-electrolyte. It dissolves in body water but does not dissociate into component parts. An electrolyte, however, will dissociate in solution into its constituent ions. Sodium chloride (Na^+Cl^-) is the most important example of this. In solution, a molecule of sodium chloride dissociates into a positively charged sodium ion (cation) and a negatively charged chloride ion (anion). Sodium is the dominant cation in the ECF but smaller concentrations of potassium (K^+), magnesium and calcium ions are present. Chloride and bicarbonate are the major extracellular anions.

Inside the cell, potassium is the dominant cation. Lower concentrations of magnesium, calcium and sodium are also present. Intracellular anions include phosphate, sulphate and intracellular proteins which also behave as anions. The cell regulates the movement of ions across its membrane, and maintenance of an appropriate distribution of ions between the ECF and ICF is essential for cell function, particularly in excitable tissues such as nerve and muscle.

Fluid exchange

Fluid exchange between ICF and ECF

The movement of body fluids and their constituents between the different compartments involves both active and passive transport processes (Porth 2002). The main mechanisms which enable body fluids to enter the cell membrane are:

- diffusion
- facilitated diffusion
- voltage-gated channels
- ligand-gated channels
- mechanically gated channels
- active and co-transport.

For further reading, see Marieb (2004).

Lipid-soluble substances diffuse directly through the cell membrane, while water and electrolytes utilise channels formed by membrane proteins. The membrane is freely permeable to water but is only selectively permeable to electrolytes. Permeability is affected by the size and charge of the hydrated ion; for example, the membrane is 50–100 times more permeable to K^+ than to Na^+. Movement into the cell via membrane proteins may be by simple diffusion, facilitated diffusion (carrier-mediated transport) and active transport. Glucose, for example, enters the muscle cell by facilitated diffusion under the influence of insulin. The most important example of active transport is the sodium–potassium pump. This pump is a membrane protein that couples the active transport of Na^+ out of the cell with the active transport of K^+ inwards. It requires energy derived from the hydrolysis of adenosine 5-triphosphate (ATP) to function.

Tissue–capillary fluid exchange

Just as the cell membrane separates the ICF from the ECF, the capillary wall represents the boundary between the intravascular and interstitial compartments of the ECF. The capillary wall is selectively permeable to substances of a molecular weight less than 69 000 Daltons (67.0 kDa) and to lipid-soluble molecules. The exchange of water, electrolytes, metabolites and waste products between the plasma and interstitial fluid occurs in the capillary bed. Fluid movement is determined by three forces: diffusion, osmosis and filtration. The capillary endothelium is freely permeable to water and solutes but the larger plasma proteins are retained. At the arterial end, fluid is forced out of the capillary by hydrostatic pressure. As water is lost from the capillary, the plasma proteins become more concentrated and the colloid osmotic or oncotic pressure exerted by the plasma proteins increases. Oncotic pressure reflects osmotic pressure caused by the presence of colloids, i.e. colloid osmotic pressure. At the venous end, the hydrostatic pressure, lower than the osmotic pressure, draws fluid back into the capillary.

Because the capillary endothelium is a very imperfect barrier, plasma proteins may leak into the interstitial fluid, complicating the situation described above. If these proteins were not removed, the oncotic pressure of the interstitial fluid would rise, disrupting capillary fluid exchange and favouring retention of water in the interstitial spaces. The lymphatic system is central to maintaining interstitial fluid volume. Blind-ended lymphatic capillaries in the interstitium are more permeable than the capillaries and easily take up and remove plasma proteins and fluid from the interstitial space. The fluid formed in these vessels — lymph — is carried through the lymphatic system, eventually returning to the circulation via the central lymphatic and the thoracic duct.

As approximately 20% of body fluid is found in the interstitial or tissue spaces, the maintenance of fluid volume in this compartment plays a key role in homeostasis. Normally, a dynamic equilibrium exists which maintains the extracellular fluid content of both the plasma and the tissue spaces. However, this delicate balance can easily be disturbed by the following factors:

- *Alterations in capillary pressure* — changes in pressure at either end of the capillary bed will alter net movement of fluid. Increased arterial pressure or venous congestion both tend to favour the loss of fluid to the interstitial space. Examples include hypertension, hypotension, heart failure, and arterial or venous obstruction.
- *Alterations in the plasma proteins* — a reduction in plasma proteins due to malnutrition, liver or renal disease, loss of circulating plasma or leakage of proteins into the tissue fluids will alter the osmotic pressure gradient and prevent fluid being reclaimed from the tissue spaces. Failure of the lymphatics to remove this fluid will increase the osmotic pressure of the interstitial fluid and favour fluid retention.
- *Changes in the integrity of the capillary membranes* — factors which alter the normal mechanisms regulating the permeability/pore size of the capillary membranes also change the osmotic or hydrostatic pressures. These

effects may be local or systemic. Examples include membrane damage from burns, anoxia, pressure, septicaemia and the presence of inflammatory mediators such as bradykinin or histamine.
- *Accumulation of metabolites* — an accumulation of metabolites within the tissue fluid can alter the hydrostatic and colloidal osmotic pressures with consequent changes in fluid movement. For example, in some states of shock or tissue hypoxia, the cumulative effects of lactic acid and carbon dioxide when combined with vasoactive substances may result in oedema.

Oedema

Oedema is an accumulation of fluid in the interstitial spaces or other sites, such as the pericardial sac, between the pleura, in the peritoneal cavity or within the joint capsule. Oedema alters the natural turgor of the tissue spaces and may be noticed by swelling or distension. If the swollen tissue is indented by slight pressure, it is called pitting oedema. In the case of blocked lymphatics for example, protein leakage from the capillaries is not reclaimed from the tissue fluid and the oedema so caused is firm due to the presence of the proteins and does not tend to pit — a characteristic sign of lymphoedema. Oedema may be localised, as in the case of inflammation and tissue damage, or generalised, as seen in heart failure.

General features

Oedema presents several problems to the patient. Its characteristic features may be described as follows:

- it accumulates in dependent areas, especially soft tissues
- it presents as swelling and distension which sometimes 'pits' under pressure
- it hinders the diffusion of gases and transport of nutrients and waste products
- the oedematous tissues lose integrity and are easily traumatised
- tissues adjacent to the oedema may be damaged by the pressure.

STOP THINK

20.1 Oedema can occur for the following reasons:

(a) cardiac failure
(b) protein loss
(c) renal dysfunction
(d) soft tissue injury
(e) deep vein thrombosis
(f) arterial insufficiency and the accumulation of metabolites liberated from hypoxic cells.

20.2 Why should one try to avoid giving injections in oedematous areas?

Management

It is important to ascertain the cause(s) of the oedema before initiating any nursing actions.

Consideration of the points listed below may enable a safe, effective plan of care to be initiated which is specific to the person concerned.

- Identify the cause of the oedema and ascertain the appropriate management by liaising with medical staff and other health professionals, e.g. physiotherapists or podiatrists may advise in the case of sports or orthopaedic problems and dietitians where there is protein loss.
- Consider the use and effects of gravity, which may alter fluid drainage or blood flow.
- Monitor and record the extent and nature of the oedema. Communication between day and night staff may identify oedema due to the effects of gravity/position. For example, oedematous feet in the evening may appear to be resolved by a night in bed, only to be replaced in the morning by sacral or orbital oedema, the latter recognised by puffy eyes.
- Assess the effects of the oedema on local tissues and take appropriate action. For example, sacral oedema increases the risk of a pressure ulcer, and severe oedema of the fascia may restrict blood flow and lead to tissue hypoxia.
- Implement medical therapies with appropriate interventions, e.g. administration of diuretics.
- Consider the potential implications and complications of specific types of oedema, e.g. pulmonary or cerebral, and initiate appropriate nursing assessment.
- Consider how oedema may restrict movement, alter a person's self-image and cause practical difficulties in daily life. Ankle oedema may be exacerbated by tight-fitting shoes, whilst ascites may cause respiratory embarrassment and affect the body image. Attention to small details may greatly enhance the comfort of a person with oedema.

STOP THINK

20.3 What advice would you give to an older person who suffers from persistent ankle oedema and who wishes to buy a new pair of shoes?

WATER AND ELECTROLYTE HOMEOSTASIS

Constancy of the internal environment is essential for efficient cell function. In health, the volume and composition of the different fluid compartments is finely regulated, with daily fluctuations in TBW of less than 0.2%. Water and electrolytes are ingested and absorbed through the gastrointestinal (GI) tract, although a small volume of water is produced through the oxidation of hydrogen in food. Excess water, electrolytes and waste products are excreted via the kidneys and in faeces. Additional water and salt loss occurs via the skin and respiratory tract.

Since losses from the GI and respiratory tracts are not subject to fine regulation, the kidney is the main regulator of fluid and electrolyte balance. Plasma represents about 4% of the body weight, or only 3 L, but the glomerular filtration rate is 125 mL/min, or about 180 L/day (Marieb 2004). This means that the 3 L of plasma contained within the body is filtered and reabsorbed about 60 times a day! With such a large turnover, the kidney can exert a major influence on plasma composition and, through plasma, on the composition of interstitial and, ultimately, intracellular fluid. Basal urine production in the absence of fluid ingestion is about 300 mL/day. The maximum rate seen in some disease states is 23 L/day, and a normal volume is approximately 2–2.5 L/day. The kidney regulates not only fluid volume, but also electrolyte composition, pH and osmolality. (Osmolality is the concentration of a solution defined in terms of the number of osmoles per kg of solvent; this is a measure of a solution's osmotic property.) Central to the renal regulation of body fluid, osmolality and volume is the kidney's role in the handling of sodium and water.

STOP THINK **20.4** How much daily water is required by a 26-year-old woman who weighs 62 kg? How much extra water might she need if she had a pyrexia of 39°C?

Regulation of ECF volume, osmolality and sodium

Volume and osmolality regulation involves a series of homeostatic mechanisms which regulate the constancy of the ECF. Although the plasma compartment is small, it is dynamic, with shifts in volume and pressure occurring in response to internal and external stimuli. The rapid turnover of the plasma makes it the ideal target for regulatory mechanisms. Although plasma volume and osmolality are monitored, sodium is also a major factor in the regulation of ECF. Changes will also occur in the interstitial and intracellular fluid volumes, but these are usually slower than changes in plasma volume and the body can adapt to them with less functional disruption. The kidney regulates sodium and water ingestion/excretion under the influence of two hormones, aldosterone and vasopressin, also known as antidiuretic hormone, ADH, with additional input from the renin–angiotensin system.

Osmolality and ADH

Within the hypothalamus are specialised cells called osmoreceptors which monitor and respond to changes in plasma osmolality. They are very sensitive and respond to changes of as little as ±3 milliosmoles (mOsml). Plasma osmolality is normally in the range of 280–290 mOsml/kg water. The osmoreceptors respond to variations in plasma osmolality by stimulating two mechanisms: ADH release and thirst.

ADH acts on the epithelial cells of the nephron collecting ducts to increase tubular permeability to water and therefore water reabsorption. If a large volume of water is ingested, the plasma sodium is diluted, causing a fall in the plasma osmolality. This fall is registered by the osmoreceptors, with a resultant decrease in ADH release. Lowered plasma ADH then results in decreased tubular permeability, less water is reabsorbed and water is excreted in the form of a more dilute urine. Conversely, if plasma osmolality is increased, e.g. after fluid loss or after the ingestion of excess salt, a higher plasma ADH results, with an increased permeability of the collecting ducts, and water is absorbed to dilute the hypertonic plasma.

The presence of a non-absorbable solute in the tubular lumen will increase water loss. For example, when plasma glucose levels are raised, as in diabetes mellitus, and filtered glucose exceeds the ability of the nephrons to reabsorb it, urine production is increased. The glucose exerts an osmotic force, keeping water in the tubule. Osmotic diuresis can also be induced therapeutically by the i.v. administration of a non-absorbable molecule such as mannitol.

Other factors affecting ADH regulation of osmolality

ADH release may be altered by some drugs, including nicotine and alcohol. Alcohol inhibits the release of ADH, with a resulting diuresis. Nicotine, morphine and barbiturates are drugs which increase ADH release. Adrenal insufficiency alters the renal response to water loading. Deficiency in adrenal glucocorticoids causes an increase in distal tubular permeability to water. Water reabsorption is increased and dilute urine cannot be produced. Tubular response to ADH is decreased and, even in the absence of ADH, permeability to water remains high.

Regulation of ECF volume and sodium

ECF volume is principally determined by sodium, and body sodium is regulated by the kidney, mainly under the influence of aldosterone. Aldosterone is a mineralocorticoid essential for sodium (with associated water) reabsorption. It has a complex effect: it stimulates Na^+ reabsorption but is not the main regulator of this process, i.e. excess aldosterone production does not usually lead to excess sodium retention. When aldosterone is lacking, Na^+ reabsorption does not occur; this can rapidly lead to death from sodium and water depletion. Aldosterone is also important in hydrogen/potassium ion exchange in the kidney, and in the reabsorption of sodium in the gut and from sweat and the salivary glands. Aldosterone release is stimulated by plasma potassium concentration, plasma sodium concentration and changes in ECF volume. Increases in serum potassium levels of as little as 0.1 mmol can cause a marked increase in aldosterone release.

However, hypovolaemia, which reflects a fall in sodium content (as opposed to concentration), will increase aldosterone secretion via the renin–angiotensin system. Changes in the effective circulating volume, i.e. the blood volume actually perfusing the tissues, which may be less than the total blood volume, stimulate renin release.

Renin is a proteolytic enzyme released from the juxtaglomerular apparatus when sodium loss causes a drop in the effective circulating volume. Renin acts on a plasma protein called angiotensinogen, causing it to release angiotensin I. Angiotensin I is in turn split by a converting enzyme into angiotensin II. Angiotensin II has several actions:

- it is a potent vasoconstrictor
- it stimulates the release of aldosterone
- it increases the reabsorption of sodium by the proximal convoluted tubule
- it acts on the hypothalamus, which then stimulates the thirst centre and increases ADH secretion.

For further information, see Marieb (2004).

DISORDERS OF WATER AND SODIUM BALANCE

Water volume and sodium imbalances frequently occur in combination with other electrolyte problems, although occasionally they occur alone. Principal causes of disturbance can be related to:

- insufficient or excessive intake or output
- problems in the regulation of intake and output which may be associated with disease states, e.g. heart failure or renal failure
- problems related to fluid shifts within the body.

It merits beginning by considering the effects of water deprivation (dehydration) and excessive intake (water overload).

Fluid volume deficit (see Boxes 20.2 and 20.3)

An ECF volume deficit will arise when water loss exceeds water intake. Insufficiency of intake may be related to a number of factors. For example, a patient may be reluctant to swallow because of oral or pharyngeal pain and so may take in less fluid and food. Depressed, anorexic, nauseated or fatigued patients may also fail to take in adequate fluid. Patients suffering from neuromuscular impairment or who are unconscious will have an impaired ability to swallow and thus will also be prone to fluid volume deficit.

Dehydration

Strictly speaking, dehydration refers only to water losses from the body which exceed intake, leaving the person with a corresponding accumulation of sodium (hypernatraemic dehydration). However, 'free water' losses are unusual and it is more common for water to be lost in conjunction with sodium and/or in its role as the biological solvent. Dehydration may thus be isotonic, hypernatraemic or hyponatraemic with respect to the ECF. Isotonic dehydration occurs when the fluid lost is isotonic with the ECF in relation to water and sodium content, whereas in hyponatraemic dehydration the sodium losses exceed the water losses.

Water-only depletion causes a volume deficit in the ECF. Sodium concentration is increased, hypernatraemic dehydration, with a consequent rise in osmolality and haematocrit (packed cell volume, PCV; see Appendix 2). If the dehydration is not resolved, the cells will ultimately become dehydrated. Compensatory mechanisms initially maintain blood pressure, heart rate and haematocrit, but as the dehydration continues, blood pressure falls, pulse volume weakens, and heart rate and haematocrit rise. Haemoconcentration also causes apparent rises in haemoglobin and albumin levels. Eventually the person will be unable to meet the obligatory volume necessary to excrete waste products in the urine. The sequelae of this — metabolite accumulation, acidosis, renal failure and toxaemia — may lead to death.

Dehydration can be assessed according to the approximate percentage of body water that is lost; in the adult this may be defined as follows:

- mild: 4% (3 L)
- moderate: 5–8% (4–6 L)
- severe: 8–10% (7 L).

The management of dehydration is often complex, especially in severe states where there is gross derangement of body chemistry. In mild to moderate dehydration, fluid losses should be replaced slowly to prevent sudden shifts of water and/or electrolytes between fluid compartments, which would aggravate ionic balance. However, as severe dehydration, as seen in diabetes insipidus, heat illness or

Box 20.2

Causes of fluid volume deficit and excess

Complete this box with reference to your textbooks and discussion with your practice mentors.

Fluid deficit

Reasons for inadequate fluid intake: give at least seven reasons

—

Reasons for excessive fluid losses

- Gastrointestinal losses: give at least six reasons
  —
- Urine losses: give at least five reasons
  —
- Skin losses: give at least three reasons
  —

Third space losses (Na^+ and H_2O): give at least four reasons

—

Fluid excess

Reasons for excessive sodium and water intake: give at least three reasons

—

Reasons for inadequate renal losses: give at least three reasons

—

Reasons for increased corticosteroid levels: give at least two reasons

—

For further information, see Porth (2002) and Marieb (2004).

Box 20.3

Signs and symptoms of fluid volume deficit and excess

Complete this box with reference to your textbooks and discussion with your practice mentors.

Fluid deficit

- Thirst
- Acute weight loss: how might this be noticed?
  —
- Alteration in renal function: how might this be noticed?
  —
- Alteration in cardiovascular function: how might this be noticed?
  —
- List six other signs or symptoms of fluid deficit
  —

Fluid excess

- Acute weight gain (in excess of 5% body weight)
- Alteration in cardiovascular function: list five signs or symptoms and give a reason why this has occurred, e.g.
  — pitting oedema (cardiac failure)
- Alteration in respiratory function: list five signs and symptoms and give a reason why this has occurred, e.g.
  — frothy white sputum (pulmonary oedema)

For further information, see Porth (2002) and Marieb (2004).

severe heat exhaustion, may lead to fatal hypovolaemia, aggressive therapy is required (see Ch. 22). The effects of hyponatraemia and hypernatraemia which may accompany dehydration will be discussed later (see p. 770).

Gastrointestinal losses

Within the GI tract there is a continuous exchange of fluids, with most of the fluid produced being absorbed. Illnesses which present with diarrhoea or vomiting, or conditions in which fistulae, drainage tubes or GI suction are involved, can result in excessive fluid volume losses, potentially up to about 8–9 L/day. Continuous GI or fistula drainage will have the same consequences for a patient as severe diarrhoea and vomiting.

Urinary loss

Patients who have incurred head injury, have undergone hypophysectomy, or who have a primary diagnosis of diabetes insipidus, may excrete excessive volumes of water and electrolytes due to a disruption in the hypothalamo-pituitary release of ADH. Diabetes insipidus occurs when there is either a deficiency in the manufacture and release of ADH, or an inability of the kidney to respond to ADH. ADH deficiency and its consequences are discussed in Chapter 5.

Osmotic diuresis

In osmotic diuresis, polyuria results from the presence of large quantities of solutes in the blood which enter the glomerular filtrate and are not reabsorbed. The high osmolality produced in the renal tubules inhibits the action of ADH and prevents reabsorption of water. This principle can be used to produce an osmotic diuresis therapeutically, e.g. mannitol can be administered to reduce intracranial pressure.

Osmotic diuresis will occur in the following circumstances:

- when the production of large particles exceeds the body's ability to reabsorb or excrete them — classic examples are glucose excess in diabetes mellitus and urea excess in renal failure
- when solutes which can be filtered by the kidney are not reabsorbed, e.g. when mannitol and polysaccharides are administered
- when substances are infused beyond the capacity of the nephron to reabsorb them, e.g. sodium chloride and urea.

Skin losses

The loss of sodium and water from the skin increases dramatically during excessive sweating or if large areas of the skin have been damaged. For example, in extreme hot weather as much as 1.5–2.0 L/h can be lost through sweat. In the patient with fever, water loss may be up to 3 L/24 h. Burns patients suffer excessive fluid losses; evaporation losses can increase ten times with severe burns (Porth 2002; see also Ch. 30). Total loss from burns can be as much as 6–8 L/24 h.

Third space losses

The concept of the 'third space' is used to describe the presence of fluids in areas of the body where they are usually absent, or present only in small quantities, e.g. the peritoneal cavity. Although not lost from the body, the fluid is physiologically unavailable and thus many of the effects of fluid loss may be produced. Whilst the total body weight may remain constant with no net change in body water, the distribution of fluid within the body may be altered. The difficulty in ascertaining the actual problem experienced by a patient is illustrated in 'Stop-think' 20.5.

STOP THINK **20.5** Mrs Jones, aged 26, is receiving a continuous infusion of opiates to relieve postoperative pain, and she has a urinary catheter in situ. Mrs Jones's urinary output has been measured at <25 mL/h for the past 3 h.

(a) Identify at least five potential causes of this reduced urinary output.
(b) How might you ascertain which was the most likely cause?

While diagnosis may be the physician's role, astute nursing assessment and implementation of a sound plan of care for such a patient may prevent or anticipate likely problems in relation to the patient's fluid and electrolyte balance.

STOP THINK **20.6** What might be the significance of a patient complaining of being very thirsty?

Fluid volume excess (see Boxes 20.2 and 20.3)

The retention of fluid results in a fluid volume excess. Such an imbalance can be caused by overloading with fluids or by reduced functioning of the body's homeostatic mechanisms responsible for maintaining fluid and electrolyte balance. Circulatory overload is a condition associated with an increase in the intravascular blood volume. It is most often observed during the administration of i.v. fluids or in blood transfusion, especially if the amount or rate of the administration is excessive. Isotonic fluids such as 0.9% sodium chloride (normal saline) or Ringer's lactate contain large amounts of sodium. With some patients, e.g. older people or those who have a history of heart disease, careful attention must be given to i.v. fluid therapy. Other sources of sodium gain include some proprietary drugs, e.g. Alka-Seltzer.

Effects of drinking large amounts of hypotonic fluid, e.g. water When a large volume of water is ingested, it begins to be absorbed within about 15 min, in consequence of which the osmolality of the blood decreases. This causes an inhibition of the production and secretion of ADH. Absence of ADH makes the distal convoluted tubule and collecting duct impermeable to water and so more urine is excreted by the kidney, thus producing a more dilute urine and a water diuresis. Following a single large intake of oral fluid, the maximum effect upon diuresis will be noticed about 40 min later. A similar effect is achieved if a bolus or fluid challenge of i.v. fluid is administered.

Water intoxication The kidney has a maximum rate at which it can excrete fluid. If water ingestion, or a hypotonic i.v. fluid administration, exceeds this capacity, then the ECF remains hypotonic. The hypotonic ECF results in fluid moving into the ICF, with a subsequent swelling and bursting of cells. This is most serious in the brain, causing raised intracranial pressure, convulsions and death. Another significant cause of death from water intoxication occurs as a consequence of the use of recreational drugs like ecstasy. Ecstasy reduces or suppresses the thirst sensation with a resultant risk of dehydration. To prevent the likelihood of dehydration, ecstasy users are advised to drink approximately a litre of water an hour if they become hot and/or expend energy, e.g. while dancing. The particular danger is that the user misjudges how they should compensate their fluid intake while taking ecstasy (see Ch. 36).

Fluid volume adjustments

Chapter 2 describes how the circulatory system comprises the arterial system of high pressure and low volume and the venous system which operates with a lower pressure and higher volume. Approximately 55% of the plasma volume is in the venous system, 10% in the arterial system and the remaining 35% distributed in the heart, lungs and capillaries. Thus changes in volume are usually accommodated by the venous system. The effect of gravity upon fluid in the circulatory system is marked, causing pooling of blood in the venous system with a consequent reduction in the arterial blood volume. If an individual stands for a prolonged period, particularly in a warm environment, there is a reduction in arterial flow to the cells; inadequate venous return then leads to a fall in end-diastolic volume and hence cardiac output. Inadequate perfusion of the brain can then lead to fainting.

The tissue spaces can accommodate large volumes of fluid, but the process is slow and causes fewer disturbances to the ICF or plasma. Adults can usually tolerate changes of about 2 L in the tissue spaces before there are noticeable signs of a volume shift. This 'hidden' accumulation of fluid may, however, be noticed by changes in body weight, 1 L of water being equivalent to 1 kg.

THE ELECTROLYTES

Sodium

Sodium is a major cation found in the ECF, and its concentration is maintained within the range 135–145 mmol/L. Its importance for a number of body functions is related to its role in maintaining the osmolality of extracellular fluids, normal muscular functioning, acid–base balance and a number of other chemical reactions. While hyper- or hyponatraemia usually indicates changes in body water content rather than in the intake of sodium, it is not unknown for individuals to have bizarre eating habits and thus become hypernatraemic, e.g. eating excessive amounts of peanuts or crisps. Furthermore, as sodium is the main extracellular cation, addition of substances to the plasma may cause a dilution effect rather than an actual loss of sodium. For example, serum sodium may appear to have fallen when glucose levels suddenly rise, either due to parenteral nutrition or in diabetes mellitus. Sodium losses may occur from the GI tract, kidney, skin or traumatised limbs.

Normally, the kidneys are extremely efficient in controlling sodium when the intake is reduced. Hyponatraemia, i.e. sodium depletion in the extracellular fluids, is defined as a sodium concentration in the blood of less than 135 mmol/L. The loss of sodium from the ECF is usually a result of excessive fluid loss and not a deficit in intake (see Boxes 20.4 and 20.5).

Box 20.4

Key signs, symptoms and reasons for hyponatraemia (serum sodium <135 mmol/L)

Reasons	Clinical examples
Excess sodium loss	Gastrointestinal loss Exercise
Sodium dilution	Excessive fluid intake
Hormone-induced water gains	Renal tubule dysfunction Increased ADH

Typical signs and symptoms of hyponatraemia
- Muscle cramps
- Weakness
- Headache
- Hypotension
- Oedema
- Mood changes
- Depression
- Lethargy
- Coma

Box 20.5

Key signs, symptoms and reasons for hypernatraemia (serum sodium >148 mmol/L)

Reasons	Clinical examples
Excess sodium intake	Diet Near drowning Excessive i.v. administration of Na^+-containing solutions
Decreased extracellular water	Dehydration
Water deprivation and decreased water intake	Confusion Impaired thirst sensation Communication difficulties
Hormone related	Diabetes insipidus

Typical signs and symptoms of hypernatraemia
- Confusion
- Lethargy
- Twitching
- Convulsions
- Polydipsia (diabetes insipidus)

Chloride

Chloride is ingested either with sodium or as potassium chloride. Normal daily intake is approximately 70–120 mmol, and the minimum requirement is 75 mmol. Chloride output is via sweat (15 mmol/L), gastric juice (90–150 mmol/L) and other intestinal secretions (50–100 mmol/L). Renal excretion is in conjunction with ammonia (NH_4Cl) and occurs mainly in the proximal tubule. Reabsorption occurs in the ascending limb of the tubule and is passively linked with Na^+ reabsorption. Cl^- reabsorption is inversely linked to bicarbonate. As Cl^- is linked to Na^+ reabsorption, aldosterone is an indirect regulator.

Potassium

Potassium (K) is the major intracellular cation. The body contains 2900–3500 mmol of potassium, of which 98% is intracellular and 2% is in the ECF. The intracellular potassium level is approximately 150 mmol/L, as compared with a plasma concentration of 3.5–4.8 mmol/L. Of the body's potassium, 90% is exchangeable while the remaining 10% is bound, mainly in the red blood cells. Men have approximately 45 mmol/kg body weight and women 37 mmol/kg body weight of exchangeable K. The total body K declines significantly with increasing age in both genders. Potassium continually leaks out of the cells, but a high intracellular level is maintained by the sodium–potassium pump. Although extracellular K is low, both intracellular and extracellular K^+ are essential for normal physiological function.

As the muscle cell membrane potential is largely a function of the ratio of intracellular K^+ to extracellular K^+, any alteration of this ratio can adversely affect neuromuscular function. The low ECF potassium means that large changes can occur in total body potassium without a significant effect on plasma K^+.

Potassium is acquired through the diet. Although the potassium content of food varies widely, any diet providing sufficient energy will invariably supply more than enough K, and a normal intake would be 40–200 mmol/day. Potassium is not as well conserved by the kidney as sodium and the minimum daily K loss is approximately 40 mmol: obligatory losses are approximately 15–20 mmol from the gastrointestinal tract and skin, and 10–20 mmol in urine. As noted above, dietary K is usually sufficient to cover the individual's needs, but additional potassium may be required during trauma and stress. Potassium excretion is regulated mainly by the kidney, and plasma K^+ levels are regulated by both renal mechanisms and shifts between the intracellular and extracellular compartments. Although only small amounts are normally lost through the GI tract, diarrhoea and vomiting can quickly lead to potassium imbalances (see Boxes 20.6 and 20.7).

Potassium cannot be conserved by the body, and so a daily intake is required. In the proximal tubule, 80–90% of filtered potassium is reabsorbed; this is essentially an obligatory process little influenced by regulatory factors. Renal regulation of potassium excretion occurs in the distal tubule and collecting duct. Aldosterone is the regulatory hormone for potassium ions. A rise in plasma K^+ concentration increases aldosterone secretion, resulting in increased potassium excretion; a fall in plasma K^+ decreases aldosterone secretion. It is important to recognise that some medications may influence potassium levels, particularly the use of diuretics and angiotensin-converting enzyme (ACE) inhibitors.

Box 20.6

Key signs, symptoms and reasons for hypokalaemia (serum potassium <3.5 mmol/L)

Reasons	Clinical examples
Inadequate intake	Starvation Anorexia
Excessive gastrointestinal losses	Diarrhoea Vomiting Excessive nasogastric tube aspirate
Excessive renal losses	Diuretic therapy Hyperaldosteronism
Intercellular movement	Side-effect of some beta-blockers Insulin therapy, e.g. diabetic ketoacidosis

Typical signs and symptoms of hypokalaemia

- Muscular weakness
- Cardiac dysrhythmias
- Cardiac arrest
- Hypoventilation
- Alkalosis
- Mental confusion

Box 20.7

Typical signs, symptoms and reasons for hyperkalaemia (serum potassium >5.5 mmol/L)

Reasons	Clinical examples
Excessive intake or gain	Oral or i.v. potassium
Inadequate renal losses	Renal failure Renal tubule dysfunction Side-effects of ACE inhibitors
Release from intracellular compartment	Tissue trauma Burns Crush injuries

Typical signs and symptoms of hyperkalaemia

- Cardiac dysrhythmias
- Cardiac arrest
- Twitching
- Skeletal muscle weakness
- Nausea, vomiting and gastrointestinal disturbances

Hyperkalaemia

Body regulation of potassium is geared mainly towards management of hyperkalaemic states, with general excretion occurring via the colon and kidney, whilst serum levels are also influenced by the catecholamines, the pancreatic hormones (insulin and glucagon) and by acid–base states. Due to the cation exchange mechanism which operates in the regulation of acid–base balance, potassium secretion is increased by the nephron in alkalotic states and decreased in acidosis. For example, in metabolic alkalosis the potassium levels rise in the ICF to compensate for hydrogen ion loss. Potassium levels are thus high in the nephron and so excretion takes place with a resultant total body loss of potassium. Hyperkalaemia may be associated with acidosis when there are shifts in the potassium and hydrogen ion concentrations. This may be aggravated by medications such as ACE inhibitors, and require dietary restriction of potassium.

Changes in serum potassium levels tend to reflect either total body changes of potassium or movement of potassium from one fluid compartment to another. Potassium levels are interrelated with sodium and body water levels. This relationship is disturbed by illness, especially if cell membrane function is disrupted. Cell membrane function is itself very susceptible to changes in potassium concentrations; even small alterations affect membrane excitation, with potentially dire consequences for cardiac tissue. In diabetes mellitus, the administration of insulin causes potassium to enter the cells with glucose in a co-transporter system, leading to a fall in serum potassium. Thus potassium depletion decreases insulin secretion, with the cells having a lower tolerance to glucose. This action of insulin can be utilised in the management of patients with hyperkalaemia: insulin and glucose can be administered to reduce serum potassium.

Hyperkalaemia may also be managed by creating GI losses through the induction of diarrhoea or by using an ion exchange, i.e. a sodium or calcium resin which exchanges with the potassium (Porth 2002). Intravenous calcium gluconate or chloride may temporarily reverse the toxic effect of potassium upon cardiac tissue.

Hypokalaemia

Management of hypokalaemia involves the treatment of any accompanying alkalosis or potassium losses. Potassium supplements may be given orally or intravenously. However, i.v. potassium can cause peripheral vein phlebitis and overly rapid infusion may cause cardiac dysrhythmias and death. Intravenous potassium should not be added to blood products, where it may cause erythrocyte lysis, nor should it be added to solutions of mannitol, amino acids or lipids, as precipitation may occur. Nursing considerations in the administration of potassium are summarised in Boxes 20.8 and 20.9.

Calcium

Calcium is the fifth most abundant element in the body, constituting 2% of body weight. Of the total body calcium, 99% is found in bone, 0.5% in teeth and the remaining 0.5% in soft tissues. Total plasma content is low (8 mmol) and over half of this is bound to albumin. Binding to plasma proteins is pH sensitive, so that acidosis can cause an increase in plasma Ca^{2+} without changes in the total Ca^{2+}. Spuriously high Ca^{2+} levels will be measured if a tourniquet is used to obtain blood for calcium levels. This is due to venous constriction increasing fluid loss with an apparent concentration of the Ca-binding plasma proteins. Normal plasma levels are 2.2–2.6 mmol/L and urinary excretion is 2.5–7.5 mmol/day.

Calcium is required for a range of physiological functions, including:

- calcification of bones and teeth
- regulation of cell metabolism

Box 20.8

Critical factors to observe when administering i.v. potassium

- Never give a rapid bolus of potassium, as this may cause cardiac arrest
- 10 mmol/h via a peripheral line and 20 mmol/h via a central line are maximum recommended infusion rates
- Maximum adult dose is 100–200 mmol/24 h
- Avoid giving higher concentrations of i.v. potassium via a peripheral vein, as this causes venous pain and sclerosis
- Use an infusion pump to control rate when giving higher concentrations intravenously. Observe closely for signs of extravasation
- Observe for signs of thrombophlebitis
- Use ready-prepared solutions when possible
- Ensure thorough mixing of the infusate when potassium is added to infusion solutions. Never add potassium to an infusion bag which is hanging in the upright position because the patient may receive a bolus of undiluted potassium due to inadequate mixing
- Avoid i.v. potassium if the patient is dehydrated or has seriously impaired renal function. Adequate urine flow is required before i.v. potassium can be administered
- Always dilute potassium ampoules before administration. Usual concentration is 40 mmol/L (range 40–60 mmol/L); do not exceed 80 mmol/L
- Monitor the patient carefully, noting excretion of urine, cardiovascular parameters, infusion rate and infusion site. Potassium is highly irritating if it leaks into subcutaneous tissues and may lead to serious tissue damage

Adapted from Metheny (2000).

Box 20.9

Oral potassium supplements: nursing implications

Common side-effects of the administration of oral potassium are nausea, vomiting, gastrointestinal discomfort and diarrhoea. These are due to gastrointestinal irritation and can be reduced by the steps listed below. Because of these side-effects, oral potassium supplements are used with caution in patients who have gastrointestinal problems and patient adherence may be poor, limiting the effectiveness of the supplements. Liquid preparations are preferred to slow-release tablets. Potassium-sparing diuretics are used where possible as they do not require potassium to be supplemented, unlike other diuretics. Potassium supplements can be a cause of hyperkalaemia.

Prevention of gastrointestinal irritation/ulceration

- Always dilute potassium preparations according to the manufacturer's instructions
- Advise patients to sip the diluted solution slowly, over a 5–10 min period
- Effervescent products must be fully dissolved and should not be swallowed until they have stopped fizzing
- Advise the patient to drink a full glass of water with slow-release tablets to help them dissolve in the gastrointestinal tract
- Give potassium supplements after meals
- Observe patients on slow-release potassium tablets for signs of gastrointestinal bleeding
- Check manufacturer's information before crushing potassium tablets — some types must not be crushed

Adapted from Metheny (2000).

- excitability of nerve and muscle, synaptic neurotransmitter release, muscle contraction
- cardiac conduction
- haemostasis
- complement activation.

Calcium is an important intracellular cation, with free calcium ion levels of 10^{-7} mol/L. Within the cell, calcium may be contained within organelles or bound to proteins. A calcium/magnesium ATPase may maintain the concentration gradient of calcium across the cell membrane.

Bone calcium, found in the hydroxyapatite form, provides a large reserve of calcium. The continual formation and destruction of bone, together with soft tissue calcium and calcium in the ECF, provides a small, exchangeable pool which can compensate for decreases in plasma Ca.

Calcium is ingested through the diet. Its absorption from the gut varies according to the presence of vitamin D, parathyroid hormone, growth hormone, corticosteroids and lactose (see Ch. 5). Calcium exists in two major forms within the ECF: as plasma, namely as freely ionised calcium ions, and as a complex bound to proteins (usually albumin). It is the freely ionised calcium which is important for nerve and muscle function. In the plasma, the ratio of the two forms of calcium is usually 50:50, although in the tissue fluid there is only freely ionised calcium.

The location of plasma calcium varies according to pH. The more acidic the plasma, the less protein is available for binding with calcium, and thus the free calcium ion level rises. In a patient with alkalosis there may be signs of hypocalcaemia because the free ions are reduced, yet total plasma levels remain unchanged. Any sudden change in pH will change the free calcium levels and cause clinical effects. This is one reason why, in the treatment of metabolic acidosis, e.g. after a cardiac arrest, any infused sodium bicarbonate should be given slowly and with caution. Where there is a low serum albumin, the free calcium ion level will be normal, although the total plasma calcium will be low. A total serum calcium that is corrected for albumin is the result routinely used in clinical practice. It should be noted that calcium should not be added to blood, lipid, bicarbonate or amino acid preparations, as precipitation may occur.

It is known that cardiac muscle contraction is dependent not only upon the concentration of calcium ions, but also upon the acidity of the extracellular environment. Myocardial depression may occur when there is a rapid drop in calcium levels, as for example following massive blood transfusion when the calcium may have been chelated by the citrates and the bone reservoir cannot release calcium quickly enough to compensate.

The myocardial depression will be aggravated in states of shock where there is poor coronary perfusion. The normal ionic regulation of the cardiac cells is disturbed when there is myocardial necrosis; in this circumstance calcium ions can pour into the cells and overactivate the ATPases, which in turn aggravate and worsen the cardiac necrosis. Thus, where the cell becomes overloaded with calcium ions, uncoordinated and disturbed waves of contraction spread through the muscle, inhibiting effective contraction. Unfortunately, following myocardial ischaemia, immediate reperfusion of the cells with oxygen and nutrients does not necessarily reverse the problem.

Box 20.10

Key signs, symptoms and reasons for hypocalcaemia (serum calcium <2.12 mmol/L)

Reasons	Clinical examples
Impaired ability to mobilise calcium from bone	Hypothyroidism
Abnormal calcium binding	Raised pH Rapid transfusion of citrated blood
Abnormal losses	Pancreatitis
Renal failure, liver disease	Reduced absorption or intake

Typical signs and symptoms of hypocalcaemia

- Paraesthesia
- Spasms
- Cramps
- Tetany
- Hypotension
- Cardiac dysrhythmias
- Bone pain
- Osteomalacia
- Deformity
- Fracture

Calcium-blocking drugs such as verapamil, nifedipine and beta-blockers can slow the entry of calcium into the cells, thus reducing the effects of the necrosis. Calcium blockers may be used for their two major effects, namely to relax muscle and cause vasodilatation, and to alter cardiac rhythm.

Digoxin is known to ultimately change intracellular calcium levels through its action on the sodium–potassium pump. It is this action which enables digoxin to improve the contractility of cardiac muscle.

Signs, symptoms and reasons for calcium deficit and excess are listed in Boxes 20.10 and 20.11.

Box 20.11

Key signs, symptoms and reasons for hypercalcaemia (serum calcium >2.62 mmol/L)

Reasons	Clinical examples
Excessive gains	Increased vitamin D or calcium in diet
Increased bone resorption	Malignant neoplasms
Increased levels of parathyroid hormone	Hyperparathyroidism
Inadequate losses	Thiazide diuretics Lithium therapy
Renal insufficiency	Altered calcium and phosphate absorption or binding

Typical signs and symptoms of hypercalcaemia

- Polyuria
- Polydipsia
- Anorexia
- Nausea and vomiting
- Constipation
- Muscle weakness
- Lethargy
- Cardiac disturbances

Tetany

If there is a decrease in extracellular freely ionised calcium ions, then a condition known as hypocalcaemic tetany may be observed. In the absence of sufficient calcium ions in the ECF, neurotransmission is inhibited, but the deficit of calcium ions in the cell leads to an excitatory effect on nerve and muscle cells, giving rise to increased motor activity. The outcome of this neuromuscular activity is marked spasms of skeletal muscle, particularly affecting the larynx and extremities. If laryngospasm becomes severe, then the person may suffer respiratory obstruction and arrest.

ACID–BASE BALANCE

Body fluids are normally slightly alkaline, within a pH range of 7.36–7.44 (hydrogen ion concentration ($[H^+]$) 35–45 nmol/L). Blood has a H^+ concentration of 40 nmol/L, or a pH of 7.4. Acidaemia occurs when the arterial blood pH is less than 7.36 (greater than 44 nmol/L H^+). An arterial pH greater than 7.44 (or less than 36 nmol/L H+) is alkalaemia. The body enzymes which control most physiological processes are optimally active within the normal pH range, and variations from this range can rapidly result in severe disability or death. It is therefore essential to understand the basis of acid–base balance in health and the effects of disease on this balance. A pH outside the range 6.9–7.7 is incompatible with life and variations outside 7.36–7.44 are serious and may be difficult to rectify. Whilst the blood pH is maintained at a slightly alkaline level, the pH of urine is frequently acidic as the body seeks to excrete surplus acids which have been produced by both metabolic and respiratory processes.

The long-term regulation of pH occurs through the lungs and kidneys, whilst buffers in the blood provide an immediate response to changes in pH. With adjustments in respiratory rate, carbon dioxide levels, and hence pH, can also change. The response, involving the kidney, is slower and sometimes referred to as the 'renal lag'. The kidney's ability to regenerate bicarbonate ions whilst excreting hydrogen ions enables it to aid the regulation of pH. Crucial to the management of these problems is the reversal or removal of the causative factor (Porth 2002, Marieb 2004).

Acidosis and alkalosis

The terms acidosis and alkalosis refer to abnormal situations which lead to acidaemia and alkalaemia, respectively, if there are no secondary compensatory mechanisms to reverse the situation. Both situations can be equally disruptive.

Acidosis occurs when there is a high hydrogen ion concentration and thus a low pH of <7.36. It can arise through:

- metabolism of proteins producing sulphuric and phosphoric acids
- anaerobic metabolism producing lactic acid
- metabolism of fats producing acetoacetic acid and ketone bodies
- excessive intake of acidic products orally or intravenously
- excessive loss of bicarbonate from the body
- hypoventilation with resulting retention of carbon dioxide.

Alkalosis occurs when there is a loss of hydrogen ions or a gain in bicarbonate ions and hence a correspondingly high pH >7.44. Alkalosis can occur through:

- excessive loss of gastric juices, e.g. vomiting, gastric aspiration
- excessive intake of alkaline products, e.g. overdose of antacids
- hyperventilation with resulting removal of carbon dioxide.

Changes in carbon dioxide tension which have a respiratory origin result in respiratory acidosis or alkalosis. Changes in bicarbonate levels reflect metabolic causes: metabolic acidosis or alkalosis. Whilst the primary causes may be metabolic or respiratory, the adaptive responses involve both systems and lead to compensatory states. Occasionally both metabolic and respiratory problems occur simultaneously and a confused picture presents, as in respiratory failure in a patient with renal failure.

Buffers

STOP THINK **20.7** Refer to your physiology textbook to review the Henderson–Hasselbalch equation.

Regulation of blood pH involves complex chemical reactions in which buffers play a critical role. Buffers are substances which prevent major changes in the pH of a solution by removing or releasing hydrogen ions. In humans there are three main buffer systems:

- carbonic acid bicarbonate
- phosphate and sulphate compounds
- proteins and haemoglobin (main ICF system) (see Porth 2002).

Buffers are found in both the ICF and the ECF and enable products to be safely transported to the site of excretion.

For further reading on buffers and pH regulation, see Porth (2002) or Marieb (2004).

Carbonic acid bicarbonate

This is the main buffer in humans and will serve as an illustration of the role of buffers in the body. This mechanism operates through the following reversible reaction:

$$H_2O + CO_2 \rightleftharpoons H_2CO_3 \rightleftharpoons H^+ + HCO_3^- \text{ (bicarbonate ion)}$$

In situations where hydrogen ions are added to body fluids, they combine with the bicarbonate ion:

$$H^+ + HCO_3^- \rightleftharpoons H_2CO_3$$

In situations where the hydrogen ion levels become low or there is an excess of hydroxyl ions, carbonic acid dissociates, releasing hydrogen ions into solution:

$$H_2CO_3 \rightleftharpoons H^+ + HCO_3^-$$

In alkalotic states, the level of bicarbonate ions rises (metabolic alkalosis) or the amount of carbon dioxide in solution falls (respiratory alkalosis). In acidic states, the level of bicarbonate decreases (metabolic acidosis) or the amount of carbon dioxide in solution rises (respiratory acidosis). There is thus a reciprocal relationship between the levels of carbon dioxide and the bicarbonate ions. This dynamic relationship, which enables pH to be regulated, is utilised in several ways within the respiratory system and the renal tubule. The enzyme carbonic anhydrase catalyses the formation of carbonic acid from water and carbon dioxide. Acetazolamide is an example of a drug which blocks carbonic anhydrase and thus inhibits both the regeneration of bicarbonate ions and the production of hydrogen ions in the renal tubule.

Alterations in the pH of the body may be indicated by clinical signs and laboratory results. The acidity of plasma is determined using arterial blood gas samples, but changes in other body fluids may be detected by testing urine, intestinal fluids, CSF and other exudates.

Handling blood gases

Obtaining a sample for the analysis of blood gases can be effected by direct arterial puncture or the withdrawal of blood from an arterial line. The nurse responsible for the patient will need to ensure that several precautions are taken to prevent a false result. The specimen form should include such details as:

- the patient's temperature
- respiratory pattern
- concentration of oxygen in the inspired gases
- any relevant recent therapies, e.g. physiotherapy, administration of bicarbonate or blood
- time the sample was taken.

The sample is collected in a small prepared heparinised syringe (1 or 2 mL). Should this be unavailable, add a small quantity of dilute heparin (100 units/mL) to a syringe to prevent coagulation. The amount of heparinised saline added should be just enough to fill the dead space of the syringe. In the case of collecting a blood sample from an arterial line, it will be necessary first to withdraw and discard the heparinised saline in the arterial line tubing (excess heparin itself reduces the measured pH). A second syringe may then be used to withdraw the arterial blood itself. As soon as the sample has been collected, a bung or stopper is attached to the end to prevent air contamination. The syringe should be labelled and sent to the laboratory as soon as possible. If the ambient temperature is warm then the sample can be transported in ice. The arterial line will need to be flushed and reset in order to remove the blood which has been drawn back into the line. With direct puncture, firm digital pressure will be required over the puncture site for at least 5 min to prevent arterial haemorrhage or subsequent aneurysm formation. The circulation of the limb distal to the puncture should be checked later. Normal blood gas results are listed in Box 20.12.

Box 20.12

Normal blood gas results (slight variations according to local laboratory)

pH	7.36–7.44
$[H^+]$	35–45 nmol/L
P_aCO_2	4.6–5.6 kPa (35–42 mmHg)
P_aO_2	11.3–14 kPa (90–105 mmHg)
HCO_3	23–31 mmol/L
Standard HCO_3^-	22–26 mmol/L
Base excess	–2 to 2 mmol/L
Saturation O_2	97%

The acidotic/alkalotic states

STOP THINK **20.8** Disorders of acid–base balance are primarily respiratory or metabolic in origin. From the information given so far, draw up a chart to indicate how the respective acid/base states may influence the pH, the bicarbonate ion levels (HCO_3^-) and the partial pressure of carbon dioxide in the plasma (PCO_2) in:

(a) metabolic acidosis
(b) respiratory acidosis
(c) metabolic alkalosis
(d) respiratory alkalosis.

Recognition and management of metabolic alkalosis

Metabolic alkalosis is caused by a loss of hydrogen ions, e.g. through vomiting, or a gain of alkali, as seen in the excess intake of sodium bicarbonate. It is characterised by high pH and a high concentration of bicarbonate ions. This rise in pH decreases the ionisation of calcium, thus giving signs of hypocalcaemia. Indicators of hypokalaemia may also arise. The respiratory response seeks to compensate for the alkalosis by raising the PCO_2 through a decreased respiratory effort: thus a respiratory acidosis may accompany the metabolic alkalosis. The increasing numbers of bicarbonate ions utilise free sodium ions, thus decreasing the ratio of free sodium ions to chloride ions. There is a slight renal compensation which attempts to conserve hydrogen ions. Usually, a metabolic alkalosis is successfully treated by management of the cause with appropriate monitoring of any hypokalaemia and/or by restoration of fluid volume. Occasionally, acidification of the plasma may be required, or the administration of acetazolamide to inhibit carbonic anhydrase.

Antacid use Antacids are bases used to neutralise the acidity of gastric juices. Injudicious use can lead to metabolic alkalosis and problems associated with other side-effects of the substances used. Most antacids comprise a combination of aluminium or magnesium hydroxides, or derivatives of carbonates. It is important that patients who take antacids are aware of the necessity to keep within the prescribed doses and to report side-effects or failure of the therapy to their physician or community pharmacist; some antacids, for example, are contraindicated in patients with peptic ulcers (see *British National Formulary*, www.bnf.org).

Recognition and management of metabolic acidosis

Metabolic acidosis is characterised by a low pH and low levels of bicarbonate ions. The lowered pH leads to a compensatory respiratory drive to hyperventilate, thus causing a transitory fall in the PCO_2. If this is successful, the pH will return towards normal. However, if the acidosis is severe, cardiac output may drop with accompanying bradycardia, because acidosis impairs cardiac contractility. Renal compensation is made through the excretion of extra hydrogen ions. Hyperkalaemia may also be present, depending upon the cause of the acidosis. The features of the underlying acidotic state, e.g. peripheral vasodilatation, will also be present. The main aim of treatment is to reverse the cause. This may involve the administration of bicarbonates, but it is important to recall that each mmol of sodium bicarbonate given contains 1 mmol of sodium ions. The three most common causes of metabolic acidosis are renal failure, diabetic ketoacidosis and hypoxia.

Recognition and management of respiratory alkalosis

The most common cause of respiratory alkalosis is an anxiety attack which has led to the person noticeably hyperventilating. The subsequent removal of carbon dioxide leads to a raised pH and eventually a fall in the bicarbonate level when renal compensation has occurred. The aim in managing the anxiety attack is to enable the person to breathe more slowly, to calm them, with a sedative if necessary, and, if it is safe, to enable them to rebreathe expired air, thus raising the carbon dioxide level. This can be achieved by having the person breathe in and out of a paper bag. While this technique is effective, it must be supervised to ensure that the person does not suffocate or do it to excess. Other instances of alkalosis will require management of their specific causes.

Recognition and management of respiratory acidosis

Respiratory acidosis is caused by an excess of carbon dioxide. It is most frequently caused by primary disorders of the respiratory tract, or by conditions which affect the respiratory centre, e.g. drug overdose and central nervous system problems. Faults in the management of mechanical ventilation may also lead to respiratory acidosis.

Respiratory acidosis may be detected when the underlying respiratory problem is recognised, e.g. asthma or bronchitis, and/or when the signs of acidosis become apparent. People with chronic respiratory problems may already have well-established compensatory mechanisms; for example, in chronic obstructive pulmonary disease (COPD) there may be a renal compensation which retains bicarbonate ions to counter the respiratory acidosis generated by a chronic high level of PCO_2 (see Ch. 3). In these situations, biochemical results may have a different significance from those associated with acute respiratory acidosis.

NURSING CONSIDERATIONS IN MAINTAINING FLUID AND ELECTROLYTE BALANCE

Assessment

Assessing fluid and electrolyte status

The effects of a fluid/electrolyte loss or gain depend to a large extent on the volume of the loss or gain and the rate at which it occurs. Effects are more acute when they develop rapidly, when the person is older and when the person is debilitated. Signs and symptoms observed by the nurse will depend upon the effects of the fluid loss or gain on the serum osmolality. A major problem in the assessment of fluid and electrolyte imbalance is that significant changes occur before they can be detected by clinical measurements such as blood pressure or central venous pressure. The nurse therefore needs to be able to use a wide range of skills to detect early changes. These include the following:

- *Knowing what to look for* — using a sound knowledge of physiology, the nurse will know what early and late clinical signs may be present, including signs of compensation by the body in its attempt to maintain homeostasis.
- *Knowing how often to look* — the nurse will be able to assess the severity of the situation and assess/monitor the patient accordingly.
- *Knowing what the anticipated effects of a variety of medical interventions are* — in order to assess effectiveness of treatment and plan further care.

Changes in tissue fluid volume are noticed mainly through observation of mucous membranes and skin elasticity, the latter being more easily observed over bony prominences. With an infant, the anterior fontanelle provides a good indication of hydration status.

The nurse's frequent contact with the patient should enable detection of any disturbances of features which may be related to fluid and electrolyte status. Unfortunately, nursing management of patients' needs for food and fluid is often neglected and notoriously full of errors and confusion (see Research Abstract 20.1). In illness, certain groups of patients, such as older people, children and pregnant women, are particularly susceptible to fluid and electrolyte problems. Others are at risk by virtue of an underlying pathological problem and/or as a result of nursing or medical interventions.

RESEARCH ABSTRACT 20.1

Nutritional care of the unconscious patient

Jones (1975) published the results of a study into the nutritional care of unconscious patients being fed by a nasogastric tube. Amongst the many findings of this study were several points pertinent to the fluid status of the patient. We suggest that you consult this seminal study which discusses some of the errors commonly made in fluid measurement and administration, problems which are still valid today. Metheny (2000) identifies other potential sources of error when recording fluid input and output.

Jones D C 1975 Food for thought. Royal College of Nursing, London

Metheny N 2000 Fluid and electrolyte balance: nursing considerations, 4th edn. Lippincott, Philadelphia

STOP THINK **20.9** Carry out the activities listed below. What are the implications of your findings with regard to a patient's hydration status?

(a) Measure out 100 mL quantities of liquid using a syringe or i.v. burette and inject them into the following utensils, observing the water levels:
- urinal
- catheter bag

- measuring jugs
- standard hospital glass, cup and cereal bowl.

(b) Determine how much liquid is contained in the standard hospital glass, cup and bowl when:
- full to the brim
- half full
- filled to the level usually served by the catering staff.

20.10 Select a suitable person on your next clinical allocation and make an assessment.

(a) What is the state of the person's hydration?
(b) What is the person's ability to regulate fluid and electrolyte intake and to excrete necessary fluids?
(c) Give reasons for your conclusions.

A number of parameters may indicate changes in fluid or electrolyte status, but minor changes are often recognised only by those familiar with the person. Thus effective communication is crucial between nurses, e.g. at handover reports, and with relatives and carers who may notice changes. The rapid detection of patterns and trends can be important in identifying deterioration or improvement in the patient's condition.

A structured approach to nursing assessment should facilitate the identification of actual and potential patient problems. Indeed, the initial assessment may not be completed until a 24-h observation of the patient has been undertaken. Assessment of the patient's fluid and electrolyte status involves a four-stage process, some of which may run concurrently.

Stage 1: Consider observable and reported parameters
Stage 2: Consider measurable parameters
Stage 3: Consider the underlying pathophysiology
Stage 4: Consider the effects of medications.

Observable and reported information

Many changes in tissue volume can be noticed through sensory observation or by the patient reporting symptoms. When this information is combined with the measurable data, it can give a reliable indicator of the patient's fluid status.

For further details of the physiological processes which influence fluid and electrolyte status, see Porth (2002), Marieb (2004) and Tables 20.1 and 20.2.

Effects of underlying pathophysiology and/or medications

Underlying pathological processes and the effect of medications frequently distort clinical signs. The examples in Table 20.1 indicate their possible effect when assessing a patient's fluid and electrolyte status.

Monitoring fluid balance

The two most important components of monitoring a patient's fluid balance are measurements or estimations of fluid intake/output and weight. Insensible fluid losses are estimated according to standard norms and often account for a much larger volume than is usually estimated in clinical practice (Marieb 2004). It is therefore important to make adjustments for the following factors:

- body temperature
- ambient temperature
- basal metabolic rate
- respiratory rate
- respiratory assistance, e.g. use of oxygen, humidification
- other pathologies
- fluid content in stools
- internal losses due to fluid movement
- losses through skin trauma.

Whilst some losses and gains have to be estimated, in appropriate circumstances others can be measured, for example:

- volume of oral fluid intake and fluid in foods
- i.v. fluids
- GI gains through enteral sources
- GI losses
- losses from fistulae and drains
- urine: volume and concentration, i.e. an output <0.5 ml/kg body weight per h
- fluid pressures through observing the jugular venous pressure or measuring central venous pressure.

Unfortunately, the volume of oral fluid intake or fluid in food is usually estimated rather than measured. Indeed, some 'fluid foods' such as soups and custards are not necessarily included in fluid recording. This is particularly important in patients who are restricted to a liquefied diet or whose fluid intake is restricted, as in renal failure.

Fluid balance charting: possible sources of error

Nurses should be aware of the many ways in which the accuracy of fluid intake/output calculations may be compromised. Examples include:

- duplication or omission of items
- use of estimations rather than measurements
- arithmetical errors
- i.v. fluids administered in theatre and not correctly accounted for
- shift change errors, i.e. in carrying forward from the previous shift
- not specifying whether fluid is colloid or crystalloid in calculations
- recording wrong i.v. bag — confusion between treatment chart and fluid chart
- failure to observe patterns in consecutive daily balance
- the patient is unable to accurately recall events and forgets their fluid or food intake.

Measurement errors also arise when inappropriate utensils are used. To reduce the margin of error, low volumes of urine should be measured in containers with graduations designed for low volumes. Large volumes measured from catheter bags may prove to be different if the bag is emptied and then measured from a rigid jug. Similarly, i.v. fluid bags may contain more than the actual amount specified. Understanding the relative acceptable margins of error is an essential but neglected aspect of fluid monitoring. In a fit, healthy person, small errors may not be significant, but in a vulnerable person they can lead to inappropriate treatment

Table 20.1 Observable/reportable signs of fluid and electrolyte disturbance and their possible significance

Clinical signs/symptoms	Clinical significance	Cautions in interpretation
Mucous membranes will appear dry and the patient will complain of thirst	Decreased saliva production will result in a dry mouth and sensation of thirst Osmoreceptors detecting hypovolaemia will also trigger a feeling of thirst. This acts as a useful backup, as good mouth care often disguises the decreased saliva production	Mouth breathing Oxygen administration Anticholinergic drugs
Tongue furrows	A normal tongue has one long longitudinal furrow, but in dehydration additional furrows will be present and the tongue will appear smaller due to fluid loss (Lapides et al 1965)	—
Sunken eyes	As a result of decreased intraocular pressure	—
Increased jugular venous pressure (JVP) With a patient at 45°, venous distension should not exceed 2 cm above the sternal angle	Distended veins indicate fluid overload; flat veins indicate decreased plasma volume	Assessing the right internal jugular vein gives a more reliable reading than on the left as it is the most anatomically direct route to the right atrium
Reduced capillary refill time	Capillary refill taking 2–3 s indicates a mild fluid deficit Refill times in excess of 3 s signify severe fluid deficits	Peripheral shutdown due to cold will slow capillary refill irrespective of fluid status
Reduced skin turgor	Reduction in interstitial and intracellular fluid will reduce skin elasticity	In an older person it is difficult to detect changes in skin turgor due to the gradual loss of skin elasticity with age
Cool peripheral temperature and pale skin colour	As a result of the renin–angiotensin cycle, hypovolaemia will result in peripheral vasoconstriction and therefore reduced temperature and colour	Patients with poor circulation, e.g. peripheral vascular disease/Raynaud's disease, will normally have cool peripheries Certain antihypertensives including vasodilators and ACE inhibitors will disguise the body's normal compensatory mechanism
Dark urine	Hypovolaemia will trigger release of ADH, leading to more concentrated urine	Patients with liver disease may have bilirubin present in their urine giving it a very dark colour Administration of diuretics will override the body's production of ADH
Peripheral oedema	Oedema occurs as a result of movement of fluid into interstitial spaces as a result of fluid excess and/or reduced levels of plasma proteins A consequent decrease in intravascular fluid may lead to a drop in blood pressure	—
Pulmonary oedema, observable through frothy sputum and/or shortness of breath	Pulmonary oedema will result in decreased gaseous exchange, with a reduction in oxygen saturations and arterial oxygen levels	—

regimens with consequent problems. Due to the problems associated with estimating and measuring fluid intake and output volumes, many view the use of daily weight recordings as a more reliable indicator of fluid status. However, for these measurements to be accurate and meaningful, the weight should be taken at the same time each day and with the patient wearing the same clothes and shoes. Lean body mass changes do not occur quickly and the measurement of daily weight is particularly useful when assessing the older person and those with renal or cardiac impairment. Finally, measurement of bioimpedance may be a way forward in the assessment of fluid volumes within the body. Bioimpedance measures the extent to which the body conducts electricity. However, interpretation of measurements is complex and it is unlikely that this will become a widely used technique.

Table 20.2 Measurable parameters and their possible significance in fluid and electrolyte imbalance

Clinical measurements	Clinical significance	Cautions in interpretation
Pulse	If there is a reduction in circulating volume and therefore stroke volume, the heart rate will increase to compensate and maintain cardiac output Initial assessment of rhythm, based on the regularity of the pulse, may be useful and indicate a need for an ECG recording	Cardiac drugs, e.g. beta-blockers, will inhibit the body's compensatory mechanism and therefore block an increase in heart rate
Blood pressure	Measurement of blood pressure will give an indication of circulating volume Pulse pressure, the difference between systolic and diastolic pressure, will give an indication of vasoconstriction, i.e. compensation by the body	As a result of numerous compensatory mechanisms, blood pressure is maintained by the body for as long as possible. A 'normal' blood pressure in the presence of compensation must be acted upon immediately
Central venous pressure (CVP)	Will be reduced as a result of hypovolaemia and/or vasodilatation An increase in CVP does not necessarily indicate fluid overload as CVP is influenced by numerous other factors including cardiac competence, systemic vascular resistance, intrathoracic and intra-abdominal pressure. For further information, see Chapter 18	—
Urine volume	In health, the body produces 1 mL urine/kg of body weight per h Acceptable urine output in the critically ill patient is equal to 0.5 mL urine/kg per h	A knowledge of the patient's weight and calculation of desired urine output based upon that is essential Administration of diuretics will override normal physiological processes. Their use must be noted when assessing volume of urine produced
Specific gravity of urine	Demonstrates the body's ability to concentrate urine as an indicator of kidney function and/or response to ADH production	Administration of diuretics will override normal physiological processes. Their use must be noted when assessing urinary specific gravity

Managing fluid and electrolyte therapy

Aims

The aims of all fluid and electrolyte therapy are:

- to regulate, where possible, the patient's fluid and electrolyte balance by controlling the content and volume of the oral/enteral route; when oral/enteral routes are inadequate, venous access is used
- to control excessive losses and gains, e.g. by means of surgical intervention to prevent blood loss or by the use of diuretics to regulate fluid balance.

Both the medical and nursing management of the patient's fluid and electrolyte status will be derived from the initial assessment. The patient may require one or more of the following interventions:

- Assistance with the maintenance of normal fluid and electrolyte requirements; this usually occurs for a short period of time in a previously well-nourished person, e.g. following surgery or during a brief period of coma
- Correction of fluid/electrolyte imbalances
- Parenteral nutrition (PN) (see Chs 4 and 21).

Occasionally, a person will require all three measures simultaneously; for example, someone with a major injury to the abdomen may need immediate correction of blood losses and electrolyte disturbances. There would then be a need to ensure that normal fluid and electrolyte requirements are met, with consideration being given to changes in demand due to the injury.

If oral/enteral feeding is unlikely to be resumed within 2–3 days, then immediate plans should be made to commence parenteral feeding.

In deciding on the most appropriate plan for a patient, consideration is given not only to the content of the therapy, but also to the resources available, the patient's coexisting problems, e.g. cardiac failure or diabetes mellitus, and the particular hazards associated with the respective methods of administration. The timing, rate and duration of the therapy can also determine which route will be most effective.

Determining the volume and content of the therapy

The regimen prescribed for the patient will be based on the following essential considerations:

- What needs to be replaced — measured and insensible or hidden losses from the body
- What needs to be removed — where there is excess production or excretory failure

- What needs to be adjusted — where there is translocation of fluids or electrolytes
- What needs to be resolved — the cause of the problem, e.g. vomiting, haemorrhage.

The identification of these requirements will be based on nursing observation, medical assessment and laboratory analysis of specimens. However, the method of administration will influence the nature of the fluid regimen.

Routes for fluid and electrolyte therapy

The oral route

Replacing fluids via the oral route is without doubt the safest method. In a healthy adult who has no circulatory or renal insufficiency, the need for fluid is 1500–3000 mL/24 h. Replacing fluids orally will involve identifying the person's preferred drinks and then making these available, where reasonable, in the desirable quantity.

In some situations the patient may be prescribed 'restricted fluids', the amount usually being stated. For example, a person with renal failure may have a restricted fluid intake of 1000 mL/24 h. In other circumstances the nurse may be instructed to 'encourage fluids', especially when the goal is to prevent urinary stasis in the catheterised patient.

Two key points for the nurse to bear in mind when caring for patients requiring replacement of fluid and electrolytes by the oral route are as follows:

- Always ascertain the exact meaning of any rather vague verbal or written orders concerning fluid replacement, e.g. 'push fluids', 'encourage fluids', 'taking sips'. Remember that fluid and electrolyte balance is important and that the nurse has a key role to play in preventing further problems.
- If at all possible, know exactly how much fluid a person is required to have over a 24-h period. Medical orders can easily be written to identify appropriate daily fluid intake targets, e.g. 2000–2500 mL/24 h.

Sometimes patients on fluid replacement therapy still complain of thirst. Whilst the thirst reflex will be permanently relieved if the thirst sensors in the hypothalamus are no longer stimulated, a temporary depression of the thirst mechanism has been associated with interventions related to the oropharyngeal region (Anderson & Rundgren 1982). The patient troubled by thirst may be comforted by the following nursing actions:

- Carrying out frequent oral hygiene
- Applying lubricant to lips
- Giving mouth rinses with fresh water
- Choosing carefully the type and temperature of fluids
- Offering ice chips for the patient to suck.

The parenteral route

For a number of patients, fluid and electrolyte therapy must be administered via the parenteral (i.v.) route. Parenteral fluid administration enables solutions to enter into the extracellular compartment directly, enabling a rapid and controlled method of delivery. Managing an i.v. therapy regimen has become a common nursing responsibility, with some practitioners being qualified to initiate specified therapies under specified authority. Before commencing an i.v. therapy regimen, assessment should consider the adequacy of the patient's renal/cardiac function and current fluid/electrolyte status, referring to such objective measures as laboratory results, body surface area and intake/output.

The subcutaneous route

In older patients who have impaired venous access, in those who are confused or find it difficult to tolerate an alternative route, or in the terminally ill patient, the use of subcutaneous fluid administration (SFA) can be both appropriate and preferred (Mansfield & Monaghan Hall 1998). The sites of choice include the anterior or lateral aspects of the chest wall, the abdominal wall, the anterolateral aspects of the thigh and the scapula. The site of the subcutaneous administration should be regularly inspected and changed every 24 h.

Other routes

Fluids can be administered through the rectum and through ostomies, although these routes are not always effective. A feeding tube may be inserted into the stomach, e.g. via a percutaneous endoscopic gastrostomy (PEG), or into the jejunum and used to administer fluids (see Ch. 4). When the oral route is inadequate, arteriovenous (AV) access may be used for i.v. therapy. In renal failure, fluid and electrolyte regulation may also involve the use of human or artificial membranes in the case of peritoneal dialysis or haemodialysis.

Major complications of i.v. therapy

Due to advances in technology, i.v. therapy is now relatively safe; however, it is still possible for serious complications to arise. Unfortunately, as noted by Speechley and Toovey (1987), complications are sometimes regarded as routine occurrences or a mere 'nuisance', but to overlook or underestimate the potential risks of i.v. therapy is to lose sight of the aim of therapy, which is to effectively replace fluid and electrolytes without causing the patient discomfort or further injury. The most common complications are:

- occlusion
- infiltration, i.e. leakage of non-irritant or vesicant fluid into the tissues surrounding the vein
- extravasation, i.e. infiltration of irritants or vesicants that cause tissue damage
- phlebitis.

Factors associated with an increased incidence of phlebitis include:

- cannula location — insertion in the lower extremities or movable joints presents an increased risk
- duration of therapy — increasing length of time raises the incidence, especially over 24 h
- blood flow problems in the region of the cannula site
- inadequate sterilisation of the cannula site
- pre-existent infection
- pH and osmolality of the fluid — acidic infusates in particular

- particulate matter which may contaminate the delivery system.

Selecting the site

Patients who are particularly vulnerable to complications are those with existing infections or immune suppression and those whose restlessness or mental state may lead them to traumatise the cannula site. In their seminal work, Maki et al (1973) pointed out that the cannula site is similar to an open surgical wound containing a foreign body and should be treated as such.

For a summary of the potential complications associated with i.v. devices, see Dougherty & Lamb (1999) or Finlay (2004).

Some practical considerations are involved in site selection, namely:

- the nature and anticipated duration of the therapy
- situational and environmental factors
- patient and safety factors
- availability of products
- staff expertise.

Insertion of the i.v. cannula, although often considered to be an expanded role of the nurse, is usually undertaken by medical staff or specially trained nurses. Some suggested competencies for i.v. drug administration are outlined by Finlay (2004) and are the subject of ongoing development by the Royal College of Nursing IV Therapy Forum. Effective communication between patient, nurse and doctor may enable a more effective and safe selection of site, materials and insertion technique. In life-threatening circumstances, the selection of the i.v. site is largely dependent upon the expertise of the staff available, the products to hand and the purpose of the line. Whilst infection control measures are important, at the scene of a disaster or accident, environmental contaminants may be inevitable and speed may take priority. The more invasive the procedure, the greater is the importance of environmental control. Where possible, central vein devices, especially those involving a cutdown procedure, should be inserted in an operating theatre environment. Local factors which may be controlled during the time of insertion include the elimination of airborne contaminants and the avoidance of debris or bacteria entering via the insertion site.

Patient factors Patient mobility and comfort may be enhanced or hindered by site selection. It is wiser, and causes less discomfort, to site the i.v. cannula away from movable joints or sites where clothes may rub. Skin areas which are vulnerable to breakdown should also be avoided, including areas which are burned, oedematous, traumatised, inflamed or affected by dermatological conditions such as eczema or psoriasis. The integrity and state of the veins themselves should also influence selection.

The safety of lines in patients who are restless often poses a practical problem for nursing staff. Stability of the line may be enhanced by the method of attachment to the patient, and applying principles of countertraction, through the use of loops, may prevent unnecessary trauma. Personal and environmental hygiene factors may necessitate that the insertion site be covered.

Central lines

Chapter 18 discusses the management of central lines used for the measurement of central venous pressure (CVP) and summarises the potential problems associated with the insertion, maintenance and removal of CVP lines. Similar principles apply when the central line is used for the long-term administration of infusates, e.g. patients requiring PN, cytotoxic and antibiotic therapy. However, the greatly increased incidence of complications associated with the use of central lines necessitates a very cautious and competent approach to their management. Finlay (2004) reminds us of the dangers associated with central line insertion and maintenance, namely pneumo- or haemothorax, arterial puncture, atrial fibrillation, venous embolism on insertion, during maintenance or upon withdrawal, infection and thrombosis.

STOP THINK

20.11 This résumé of the numerous issues involved in the safe management of a person with an i.v. device illustrates the complexity and importance of skilful and knowledgeable nursing practice. The professional accountability of the nurse practitioner is outlined by the Nursing and Midwifery Council in their standards and guidance regarding *Professional Conduct, the Administration of Medicines, Records and Record Keeping* (NMC 2004). In the light of these standards, review your local Trust or Unit protocols and evaluate the 'customs and practices' in your own clinical areas. It would be a useful management exercise to attempt to devise some criteria/standards and actions which could be employed to evaluate the effectiveness of local policies.

20.12 Identify the observations you should make when a patient has (a) a peripheral device and (b) a central device. How might you recognise signs of a problem associated with the maintenance of these i.v. devices?

20.13 What specific problems may be encountered in a person with an infusion device who is being cared for at home?

Types of parenteral fluids

The nature of the products to be infused determines both the number and location of the lines. Some infusates cannot be mixed, and if concurrent administration is required, two or more lines may be needed. Infusates which increase the likelihood of microbial contamination include those used in PN, especially those containing high concentrations of glucose. Each infusate carries with it particular risks, and nurses should familiarise themselves with the specific potential side-effects associated with different infusates.

Broadly speaking, the infusates commonly used in i.v. therapy, as opposed to PN, may be categorised as follows:

- colloidal solutions:
  — blood and blood products
  — plasma and plasma substitutes
- crystalloids — water, electrolytes and isotonic solutions.

There is ongoing clinical debate as to which type of i.v. fluid is preferable. Research has provided mixed evidence, and several Cochrane Reviews have added to the debate but have not drawn firm conclusions (Alderson et al 2003, Bunn et al 2003).

Infusates can also be categorised with respect to their tonicity.

Isotonic solutions have the same osmolarity (tonicity) as serum or other body fluids and expand the intravascular compartment without affecting the intracellular and interstitial compartments; 0.9% saline is an isotonic fluid with respect to plasma.

Hypotonic solutions have a lower serum osmolarity and cause body fluids to shift away from the blood vessels and into the intracellular and interstitial spaces to areas of higher osmolarity. Hypotonic solutions may be used in the case of cellular dehydration due to diabetic ketoacidosis.

Hypertonic solutions cause fluid to move from the interstitial and intracellular compartments towards the intravascular compartments. For example, hypertonic saline will increase plasma and interstitial fluid osmolality.

For further information, see Finlay (2004).

Dehydration and hydration in the terminally ill individual The ethical and clinical debates continue as to whether, and when, to withhold or withdraw intravenous, subcutaneous or nasogastric hydration in the terminally ill patient (see Ch. 33). Nurses may well be presented with situations where a decision regarding hydration of their patients must be made. Nurses need to be knowledgeable of the benefits and disadvantages of both terminal dehydration and the rationale for hydration (Jackonen 1997). Decisions made must be individualised and based on careful assessment that considers the clinical and ethical problems related to dehydration, the potential risks and benefits of fluid replacement and the patient's and family's wishes. Guidance is forthcoming associated with the outcomes of the current Draft Mental Capacity Bill and the Glass family case in the European Courts. There is also ongoing guidance from the General Medical Council (www.gmc-uk.org).

PROBLEMS ASSOCIATED WITH DISORDERS OF FLUID AND ELECTROLYTE BALANCE

This section outlines some areas in which patients commonly experience difficulties with fluid and electrolyte control. Nurses in many areas of practice will encounter patients whose fluid and electrolyte balance has been challenged, with potentially dire consequences, e.g. patients with burns, cardiac failure or respiratory problems. The reader is referred to the relevant chapter of this book for information on fluid and electrolyte management in these more specialised contexts.

Gastrointestinal disorders

Disorders of the GI system are very likely to lead to derangements in the normal balance of fluid and electrolytes, with subsequent problems in acid–base control (British National Formulary 2005). Fundamental problems can arise in circumstances such as the following:

- fluids are lost from the body by vomiting, diarrhoea or from a stoma
- the body is unable to absorb ingested fluids and foods
- the usual GI fluids are produced either normally or in excess but the body is unable to reabsorb them; thus the gut acts as a third space, as seen in paralytic ileus
- body fluids leak into the gut or GI fluids leak into adjacent organs or cavities (which again act as a third space) — examples include GI bleeding from oesophageal varices or GI ulcers, fistulae and peritonitis.

It is possible for several of these conditions to occur simultaneously, e.g. in a person with intestinal obstruction who is vomiting, has abdominal distension from the obstruction and may develop paralytic ileus. Two common problems of the GI tract which can be fatal if left untreated are vomiting and diarrhoea.

Vomiting

Loss of fluid through vomiting can rapidly cause dehydration and, if prolonged or severe, may lead to metabolic alkalosis and malnutrition. Following surgery to the thoracic and abdominal regions, vomiting can exacerbate the pain experience and delay healing, due to the strain imposed upon the abdominal muscles. In the case of a person's inability to protect their airway, e.g. through coma, inhalation of vomitus may lead to inhalation pneumonia and possibly death.

Vomiting causes fluid loss through the ejection of recently ingested foods and fluids, the loss of gastric or upper intestinal juices, the loss of blood from GI lesions and the prevention of oral fluid and nutritional replacement. Thus prolonged or severe vomiting requires not only the prevention and/or control of the vomiting itself, but also adequate fluid replacement.

The loss of gastric juices, which contain hydrochloric acid and potassium ions, initially leads to metabolic alkalosis due to a surplus of bicarbonate ions. In severe, prolonged vomiting without adequate nutritional replacement, the body begins to metabolise fats as an energy source, producing ketone bodies and further exacerbating the metabolic acidosis.

Thus fluid and electrolyte losses caused by vomiting may be summarised as follows:

- depletion of the ECF volume
- hypochloraemia (Cl^- loss)
- alkalosis
- hypokalaemia
- possible acidosis
- anaemia due to any blood losses.

Nursing management The actual control and the prevention of further episodes of vomiting will depend upon the cause of the vomiting and on available resources. However, whilst the patient is vomiting, some practical measures can help to alleviate some of the distress. These include providing a receptacle to vomit into, ensuring privacy if possible, and providing something to wipe away the vomit and mucus. The controlled use of breathing and swallowing techniques can sometimes enable the patient to regain control of the waves of contraction that accompany the vomiting episode.

The ability to enable a patient to adopt such techniques often rests on the nurse's interpersonal skills and confidence.

The use of touch can also help the patient to relax and thus avoid unnecessary muscular contractions which may aggravate any wound pains. In the presence of a wound, it is important for the patient or nurse to support the wound. When the immediate episode is over, a method of refreshing the mouth is essential. Judicious use of pharmacological agents, e.g. antiemetics, may prevent vomiting episodes, especially if their timing is sequenced for maximum benefit, e.g. taken before anticipated vomiting triggers. With very severe vomiting episodes there is a risk that inhalation may occur; in such cases observation of the patient's breathing pattern is essential. Indeed, occasionally gastric contents may be emitted via the nose. If a patient vomits whilst a nasogastric tube is in place, the nurse should investigate the following possibilities:

- Is the tube blocked, kinked, in the wrong place or spigoted?
- Is the tube too fine for the aspirate?
- Does the frequency of gastric aspiration need to be altered?
- Is there a deterioration in the patient's condition, e.g. haemorrhage?
- Should the tube be removed?

The best action is to leave the tube on free drainage and aspirate intermittently, unless this is contraindicated. At a suitable point, the effectiveness of the tube should be re-evaluated.

STOP THINK

20.14 What actions could be taken when the following patients seem likely to vomit?

(a) A patient with a spinal injury.
(b) A patient with a wired jaw.

20.15 What is the significance of the information that may be obtained through observation of vomitus and the accompanying episodes of vomiting?

Diarrhoea

Worldwide, diarrhoea is a serious problem and the most important indication for fluid and electrolyte replacement. It occurs when the body is unable to reclaim/absorb the fluids in the intestinal tract and the peristaltic contractions of the gut expel the intestinal contents. Generally, intestinal fluids are isotonic with the ECF until the colon is reached, at which point the contents gradually become hypotonic due to the colon's role in water reabsorption. Severe and prolonged diarrhoea, as seen in cholera or in some forms of infant enteritis, can lead to severe electrolyte imbalance, dehydration and, ultimately, death if treatment is unsuccessful or delayed. The fluid losses may cause:

- depletion of ECF volume
- hyponatraemia
- hypokalaemia
- metabolic acidosis due to loss of bicarbonates in the digestive juices
- severe water dehydration (if the problem is located in the colon).

The causes of diarrhoea are identified and its nursing and medical management discussed in Chapter 4. Fluid and electrolyte replacement is an essential component in the management of the effects of diarrhoea, with accompanying management of the causative agent. Oral rehydration therapy is frequently employed in cases of enteritis and dehydration, providing the gut is able to absorb ingested fluids (see Box 20.13).

Box 20.13

Contents of a solution to use in oral rehydration therapy (to be reconstituted with water to make a total volume of 1 L)

Substance	WHO formulation
Sodium chloride	3.5 g
Potassium chloride	1.5 g
Sodium citrate	2.9 g
Anhydrous glucose	20.0 g

This combination gives (mmol/L):

- sodium: 90
- potassium: 20
- chloride: 80
- citrate: 10
- glucose: 111.

In UK practice, where less severe forms of dehydration are found than in developing countries, the sodium content is slightly less and the glucose higher. It is important to ensure that the water additive is safe and free from contaminants.

Adapted from British National Formulary (2005).

STOP THINK

20.16 Why do oral preparations to rehydrate a person suffering from diarrhoea/dehydration contain salts and glucose? (See British National Formulary 2005, section 9.2.)

Special needs of the person undergoing surgery

The person undergoing surgery, whether elective or emergency, is particularly vulnerable to several disturbances of fluid and electrolyte balance. Disturbances in the composition and placement of the body fluids and electrolytes accompany many procedures and include blood loss, dehydration from preoperative fasting, bowel preparation and surgical exposure (see Ch. 26). Problems due to the underlying pathology and the patient's general health status can exacerbate the situation. Surgery/trauma causes a defensive metabolic response which conserves water and sodium and changes the plasma levels of sodium, potassium, nitrogen and albumin. The basis of the response is vasoconstriction of the renal artery, stimulation of osmoreceptors and the release of antidiuretic hormone (ADH), whilst any changes in blood pressure which affect the juxtaglomerular apparatus will stimulate the renin/aldosterone systems. This response enables conservation of plasma volume and the retention of sodium, whilst an increase in catecholamines raises the cardiac output and heart rate.

The renal response to trauma usually takes 24–72 h to recover and during this time the patient is unable to cope normally with electrolyte control and cannot produce hypotonic urine. The risks of fluid overload and water intoxication are thus high; yet, conversely, inadequate replacement therapy may lead to dehydration and shock. Thus, in a vulnerable patient, it is important not only to measure daily fluid balance but also to keep a record of the consecutive daily balances over the first 72 h. Oedema may occur due to changes in vascular permeability, with translocation of fluids into the third space. The fundamental nursing activities of patient assessment and effective implementation of treatment regimens are often critical to the patient's recovery.

By convention, it is normally assumed that intraoperative fluid losses are replaced in theatre and that fluid balance recording commences postoperatively from a state of 'zero' balance. It is important to note the losses during surgery in order to anticipate any potential problems, which should be indicated in the theatre notes and postoperative guidelines from the anaesthetist. However, the picture is occasionally confused by poor record keeping and inadequate communication between staff in theatre and the ward. This may cause the postoperative fluid balance data to be misleading. Insensible losses may also pass unnoticed, e.g. loss from sweating, as in shock or pyrexia.

STOP THINK **20.17** Select a person who is to undergo surgery and you can follow up postoperatively. Assess your chosen patient and identify actual and potential needs with particular reference to:

(a) comfort needs in respect of hydration and elimination
(b) potential fluid and electrolyte losses or gains
(c) other factors influencing fluid and electrolyte balance
(d) the changing needs of the patient from the preoperative assessment through surgery to the postoperative phase.

Critically evaluate the planned and implemented nursing care of your selected patient in respect of the identified problems derived from items (a)–(d).

CONCLUSION

This chapter has demonstrated the key skills required by the nurse when assisting patients with their fluid and electrolyte needs. These essential skills include:

- effective observation and assessment
- good communication
- detailed attention to the accuracy and frequency of taking measurements and recording
- proficient use of interventions
- a sound knowledge base of the patient as a unique individual coping with particular health and social problems
- ethical and professional commitment.

REFERENCES

Alderson P, Schierhout G, Roberts I, Bunn F 2003 Colloids versus crystalloids for fluid resuscitation in critically ill patients (Cochrane Review). In: The Cochrane Library, Issue 4. Wiley, Chichester

Anderson B, Rundgren M 1982 Thirst and its disorders. Annual Review of Medicine 33: 231–239

British National Formulary 2005 No. 49 (March). Pharmaceutical Press, London. Online. Available: www.bnf.org

Bunn F, Roberts I, Tasker R, Akpa E 2003 Hypertonic versus crystalloids for fluid resuscitation in critically ill patients (Cochrane Review). In: The Cochrane Library, Issue 4. Wiley, Chichester

Finlay T 2004 Intravenous therapy. Blackwell Science, Oxford

Jackonen S 1997 Dehydration and hydration in the terminally ill: care considerations. Nursing Forum 32(3): 5–13

Jones D C 1975 Food for thought. Royal College of Nursing, London

Lapides J, Bourne R, Maclean L 1965 Clinical signs of dehydration and extracellular fluid loss. Journal of the American Medical Association 191: 413

Maki D G, Goldman D, Rhame S 1973 Infection control in IV therapy. Annals of Internal Medicine 79(6): 867–887

Mansfield S, Monaghan Hall J 1998 Subcutaneous administration and site maintenance. Nursing Standard 13(12): 56–62

Marieb E N 2004 Essentials of human anatomy and physiology, 7th edn. Benjamin Cummings, San Francisco

Metheny N 2000 Fluid and electrolyte balance: nursing considerations, 4th edn. Lippincott, Philadelphia

Nursing and Midwifery Council (NMC) 2004 The NMC code of professional conduct: standards for conduct, performance and ethics. NMC, London. Online. Available: www.nmc-uk.org/nmc/main/publications/$publicationsMain

Porth C M 2002 Pathophysiology: concepts of altered health state, 6th edn. Lippincott, Philadelphia

Speechley V, Toovey J 1987 Problems in i.v. therapy. Professional Nurse 2(8): 240–242

FURTHER READING

Dougherty L, Lamb J (eds) 1999 Intravenous therapy in nursing practice. Churchill Livingstone, Edinburgh

Fan S T, Teoh-Chan C H, Lau K F et al 1988 Predictive value of surveillance skin and hub cultures in central venous catheters sepsis. Journal of Hospital Infection 12(3): 191–198

Ganong W F 2001 Review of medical physiology, 20th edn. Lange Medical, New York

Guyton A C, Hall J E 2000 Textbook of medical physiology, 10th edn. W B Saunders, Philadelphia

McVicar A, Clancy J 1992 Which infusate do I need? Professional Nurse 7(9): 586–591

Maki D G 1977 Preventing infection in IV therapy. Current Researches in Anesthesia and Analgesia 56(1): 141–153

Maki D G, Ringer M 1987 Evaluation of dressing regimens for prevention of infection with peripheral IV catheters. Journal of American Nursing 258(17): 2396–2403

Maki D G, Goldmann D, Rhame S 1993 Infection control in IV therapy. Annals of Internal Medicine 79(6): 867–887

Mallett J, Dougherty L 2003 The Royal Marsden Hospital manual of clinical nursing procedures, 6th edn. Blackwell Science, Oxford

Manley K M 1992 Flow control devices in intravenous therapy. Surgical Nurse 5(3): 11–15

Marieb E N 2004 Essentials of human anatomy and physiology, 6th edn. Benjamin Cummings, San Francisco

Neeser M, Ruedin P, Restellini J P 1992 Thirst strike: hypernatraemia and acute prerenal failure in a prisoner who refused to drink. British Medical Journal 304(6838): 1352

Porth C M 2002 Pathophysiology: concepts of altered health state, 6th edn. Lippincott, Philadelphia
Rochon P A, Gill S S, Litner J et al 1997 A systematic review of the evidence for hypodermoclysis to treat dehydration in older people. Journal of Gerontology: Medical Sciences 52A(3): M169–176
Smith E, Kinsey M 1991 Fluids and electrolytes: a conceptual approach, 2nd edn. Churchill Livingstone, Edinburgh
Smith S A 1997 Controversies in hydrating the terminally ill patient. Journal of Intravenous Nursing 20(4): 193–200
Weinstein S 2005 Plumer's principles and practice of intravenous therapy, 8th edn. Lippincott, Williams and Wilkins, Philadelphia

NUTRITION

Sue Green
Pam Jackson

21

INTRODUCTION

Eating and drinking are integral parts of human existence. An adequate intake of nutrients and water is required to maintain physiological function, to allow for growth and maintenance of tissues, and to provide energy to meet the demands of daily living. Although a biological necessity, eating and drinking have significance beyond the merely physiological, forming an important part of social and psychological well-being. In any society, food production and preparation are central activities; the preparation and consumption of food may take up several hours a day. Meals are used as a time for people to come together, food or drink may be offered to make a guest feel welcome, and formal meals may be a feature of family, religious or national ceremonies.

The importance of the role of the nurse in ensuring nutritional needs are met is well recognised. Indeed, food and nutrition is one of the eight aspects of fundamental and essential care highlighted in *Essence of Care* (DH 2003a). The responsibilities of the nurse concerning nutritional care are extremely varied and range from preventing malnutrition to caring for the malnourished. For example, nurses may be involved in aspects of nutritional care relating to health education, particularly activities related to the rise in the incidence of obesity and type 2 diabetes mellitus. Nurses may also be involved with the care of the individual receiving enteral or parenteral nutrition. Nurses now play a more minor role in the preparation and serving of food to individuals in their care than in previous years. Changes in food delivery and serving methods have acted to reduce the nursing input required at mealtimes. In many areas there is a necessary delegation of responsibility concerning mealtime care to qualified health care assistants or unqualified staff. However, it must be remembered it is the qualified nurse who is responsible for ensuring food is provided, as appropriate, to the patient in their care; 'Nurses have a clear responsibility for ensuring that the nutritional needs of patients are met' (United Kingdom Central Council for Nursing, Midwifery and Health Visiting 1997).

STOP THINK **21.1** One of the factors considered to be an *Essence of Care* (DH 2003a) is Food and Nutrition. Access the document outlining the Essence of Care Programme on the website of the Clinical Governance Support Team of the NHS Modernisation Agency (www.cgsupport.nhs.uk/Programmes/Essence_of_Care_Programme/default.asp).

Consider the 10 factors identified under Food and Nutrition. To what extent are the benchmarks being achieved in your current practice area?

This chapter will consider the principles of nutritional science, public health nutrition and the nutritional care of individuals by nurses.

PRINCIPLES OF NUTRITIONAL SCIENCE

To maintain health, an adequate supply of nutrients is required. The foods that make up the diet can vary considerably but the basic nutritive constituents of the diet fall into two main groups: macronutrients and micronutrients. The macronutrients are carbohydrate, protein and fat and the micronutrients are vitamins and minerals. Alcohol, usually in the form of ethanol, may also be considered a form of macronutrient in that it does provide the body with energy. Water is an essential component of the diet but is not usually classed as a nutrient. Water intake is discussed in Chapter 20. Some compounds present in the diet, such as food colourings and preservatives, are also important components of food.

Nutrients have a complex role in physiological function and most nutrients are involved in several processes. Nutrients are required to form the structural components of the body; for example, protein is the major constituent of muscles. Nutrients are also important in metabolic pathways and enzyme systems that enable the body to function appropriately. They can either form a part of the pathway or assist in the enzymatic reactions in that pathway (a co-factor). For example, vitamin C is required in the pathway that forms collagen; inadequate intake of vitamin C will result in collagen not forming properly.

Nutrients also provide energy for metabolism. Metabolic demand for energy comes from three essential physiological tasks: transport, turnover and work:

- Transport of nutrients and electrolytes across cell membranes can be an active process, which requires energy.
- Turnover of substrates includes activities such as converting amino acids into body protein and fatty acids into triglycerides, and vice versa.
- Mechanical work, such as maintaining cardiac output or respiration.

Metabolic demand needs to be met by an effective supply of nutrients. These come primarily from two sources: the food we eat and the breakdown of tissues in the body. There is a dynamic process between food eaten, body tissues and metabolism. Carbohydrate and fat are the body's predominant energy sources but protein may be used if these are not readily available. If the supply of nutrients from food intake is inadequate, body tissues such as adipose or muscle will be used to supply the energy needed for metabolic demand. Whilst only the macronutrients and not the micronutrients can act as sources of energy, both can form the structural components of the body and participate in metabolic pathways and enzymatic processes. Non-nutrients, such as non-starch polysaccharides, may be important for physiological function, and others such as caffeine may fulfil other lifestyle functions. Alcohol is energy rich and has a complex role in many societies but taken in excess can be damaging to health. The macro- and micronutrients are described briefly below although their digestion and metabolism are not considered.

For a more comprehensive description, refer to a physiology or nutrition textbook such as Garrow et al (2000) or Barasi (2003).

Macronutrients

Carbohydrate

Carbohydrates are classified into three major groups according to the number of 'saccharides' that make up their structure: monosaccharides, oligosaccharides, which include disaccharides, and polysaccharides.

- The monosaccharides — also known as simple sugars — include glucose and fructose. The body absorbs carbohydrate across the intestine wall in the form of monosaccharides.
- Disaccharides include sucrose (table sugar), lactose (milk sugar) and maltose.
- The polysaccharides — also known as complex carbohydrates — include starch and non-starch polysaccharides ('fibre').

Carbohydrate is the main energy source for the body and, as glucose, it is the preferred fuel for the brain. Each gram of carbohydrate yields about 17 kJ/g (4 kcal/g) (see Box 21.1). Carbohydrate is stored in the body in the form of glycogen in the liver and muscles.

Foods which are rich in complex carbohydrates, such as bread, cereal, rice and pasta, are recommended as the main energy source of a healthy diet. Generally speaking, the more refined the food the less non-starch polysaccharide ('fibre') it contains; for example white rice contains less 'fibre' than brown rice and white bread less than brown bread. Vegetables such as potatoes, peas and corn are also rich sources of polysaccharides. Fruit contains carbohydrates in the form of monosaccharides and disaccharides as well as polysaccharides. Foods such as cakes, biscuits and chocolates contain high levels of carbohydrate, particularly in the form of monosaccharides and disaccharides.

Non-starch polysaccharides ('fibre')

Non-starch polysaccharides are a very important component of the diet. They give bulk to food passing through the gastrointestinal (GI) tract, thus reducing the amount of time it takes for food to pass through the gut (bowel transit time) and increasing feelings of satiety. Non-starch polysaccharides may be classed as soluble or insoluble fibre. Soluble fibre forms a gel when mixed with water and is

Box 21.1

Energy value of macronutrients

Carbohydrate	17 kJ/g (4 kcal/g)
Protein	17 kJ/g (4 kcal/g)
Fat	38 kJ/g (9 kcal/g)
Alcohol	29 kJ/g (7 kcal/g)

found in oats, fruit and vegetables. Insoluble fibre does not mix well with water and is found in the bran layers of cereal grains and some vegetables. Soluble fibre can slow the absorption of monosaccharides into the bloodstream, enabling a slower and more sustained rise in blood glucose levels. It may also lower blood cholesterol levels by reducing absorption of dietary cholesterol and bile acids in the large intestine (Webb 2002). Some types of non-starch polysaccharide, in particular unprocessed bran, may reduce the absorption of some micronutrients, such as calcium, in the intestine (Sullivan 2000).

Protein

The smallest component of protein is an amino acid; amino acids bond together to form a protein. Some amino acids are synthesised by the body; others, the essential amino acids, cannot be synthesised by the body and must be obtained from food. There are approximately 20 different types of amino acid, of which about eight are considered to be essential. Protein is required to build new tissue as a result of growth, to replace tissue lost through injury or as a result of normal body function. Nearly all cells need to be replaced on a regular basis and, in addition, cell proteins are regularly replaced and renewed. Many enzymes and hormones are proteins. If there is no other nutrient available, the body will use protein as an energy supply. Each gram of protein yields about 17 kJ/g (4 kcal/g) (see Box 21.1). Proteins are present in most foods, including meat, fish, cereals, legumes and vegetables, but the amount and quality varies. Foods that contain all the essential amino acids required by the body are often termed 'high-quality protein foods'. Meat, milk, cheese, egg and soy are usually considered to be high-quality protein foods. If plant foods are to provide the major source of protein, a wider mix of food types is required to ensure all the essential amino acids are consumed. Foods that are traditionally eaten together often contain most if not all of the essential amino acids when combined, e.g. rice and beans. Vegetarians and vegans need to plan their dietary intake to ensure the foods they eat complement each other in that the essential amino acids absent in one food are present in another, e.g. baked beans on toast.

Fat

There are three main types of fat: triglycerides, phospholipids and sterols. Most of the fat in foods is in the form of triglycerides. Triglycerides are made up of fatty acids and glycerol. Fatty acids are classified according to their chemical structure, more specifically the number of hydrogen atoms bonded to carbon atoms in the fatty acid. Fatty acids can therefore be saturated, i.e. all the carbon atoms are fully saturated with hydrogen atoms, or unsaturated, i.e. some of the hydrogen atoms are absent and the usual single bond between carbon atoms has been replaced by a double bond. Unsaturated fatty acids may be monounsaturated, i.e. one double bond between carbon atoms, or polyunsaturated, i.e. more than one double bond between carbon atoms. Polyunsaturated fatty acids are often termed 'essential fatty acids' as the body is unable to make this type of fatty acid. These include alpha-linolenic and linoleic fatty acids, often called omega 3 and omega 6 fatty acids. *Trans* fatty acids are a type of polyunsaturated fatty acid which may occur naturally, but most that we consume are produced as a result of food processing. A high intake of saturated and *trans* fatty acids is associated with the development of some diseases, particularly cardiovascular disease.

Fat is a good energy source as it is easily stored by the body and provides a large energy store. Each gram of fat yields approximately 38 kJ/g (9 kcal/g) (see Box 21.1). Fat also provides an important insulating layer beneath the skin and surrounds some body organs, giving support and cushioning the organs from mechanical trauma. In addition, fat is a structural element forming the major component of the cell membrane. Fat is used in the formation of substances such as lipoproteins, cholesterol and phospholipids and the steroid hormones. Adequate dietary fat is important, as the essential fatty acids (polyunsaturated fats) and fat-soluble vitamins are found mainly in high fat foods. Fat also enhances the palatability of food.

Most foods contain a proportion of each of these basic types of fatty acid but are usually described according to which type predominates. It is generally quite easy to identify a saturated fat because it is usually solid at room temperature. Saturated fats originate from animals with the exception of fish and shellfish. Unsaturated fats derive from plant and seafood oils. *Trans* fats are contained in significant amounts in commercially prepared foods such as biscuits and hard margarine.

Micronutrients

Vitamins

Apart from vitamin D, which can be synthesised through the action of sunlight on the skin, and vitamin K, which can be synthesised by intestinal bacteria, all the vitamins must be obtained from the diet. Only small amounts are needed and a varied diet will normally supply all the vitamins required. Vitamins are important in many metabolic pathways in the body and also act as antioxidants. The two main groupings are the fat-soluble and the water-soluble vitamins.

- The fat-soluble vitamins (A, D, E and K) are absorbed from the small intestine along with dietary fat. They are found in foods such as fish, meat, butter, milk and plant oils. Fat-soluble vitamins can be stored in the body and excessive intake may lead to toxic levels.
- The water-soluble vitamins include B_2 (thiamine), B_1 (niacin), B_3 (riboflavin), B_6 (pyridoxine), B_{12} (cobalamin), C (ascorbic acid), folic acid, pantothenic acid and biotin. Water-soluble vitamins are easily lost from foods and from the body and little storage occurs within the body.

Vitamin deficiency is a common feature in some countries but is generally rare in the UK unless it is associated with protein-energy malnutrition. Table 21.1 outlines the vitamins required by the body, and gives details of rich food sources, at-risk groups and symptoms of deficiency.

Minerals

Some minerals play an essential role in human nutrition. Minerals are important in metabolic pathways and also form structural components of the body. A balanced diet

Table 21.1 **Vitamins: rich food sources, at risk groups and symptoms of deficiency***

Nutrient	Rich food sources	Groups at risk of deficiency or excessive intake affecting health	Symptoms of deficiency
Vitamin A (retinol)	Liver, fish oils, dairy products, fortified margarine, some green, yellow and orange fruits and vegetables	*Deficiency associated with*: fat malabsorption *Excessive intake affecting health*: pregnant women should avoid supplements containing vitamin A (unless advised otherwise at antenatal clinic) and liver and liver products	Dryness of the conjunctiva and cornea, impaired adaptation to dim light (night blindness), skin changes, impaired immune function, growth retardation
Vitamin B_1 (thiamine)	Found in most foods, particularly unrefined cereal grains, fortified flour, some breakfast cereals, meat, dairy products and legumes	*Deficiency associated with*: alcoholism	Headaches, tiredness, anorexia, muscle wasting. Deficiency disease (beriberi) affects the cardiovascular and nervous systems. Wernicke–Korsakoff syndrome can develop in alcoholism
Vitamin B_2 (riboflavin)	Found in many foods, particularly dairy products, eggs, fortified cereals, ice cream, liver	*Deficiency associated with*: intestinal malabsorption, biliary atresia, older people with poor dietary intake, regular use of fibre-based laxatives, women who exercise excessively, alcoholism	Lesions of the mucocutaneous surfaces of the mouth, seborrhoeic skin lesions, vascularisation of the cornea, anaemia, retarded growth in childhood
Vitamin B_3 Niacin (nicotinic acid and nicotinamide)	Red meat, wheat flour, maize, eggs, milk	*Deficiency associated with*: alcoholism, long-term use of isoniazid medication	Changes in skin, mucosa of the mouth, GI tract and nervous system Deficiency disease (pellagra) is characterized by skin lesions in areas exposed to sun and pressure, and by diarrhoea and dementia
Vitamin B_6 (pyridoxine)	Meat, fish, eggs, milk, wheatgerm, brewers' yeast, brown rice, soybeans, unrefined wheat grains, some nuts	*Deficiency associated with*: use of drugs which cause depletion (e.g. isoniazid), intestinal malabsorption, renal dialysis, alcoholism *Excessive intake affecting health*: women may take large amounts (without medical advice) to relieve premenstrual syndrome symptoms. The Food Standards Agency (2003) advises against taking more than 10 mg/day to avoid the development of neuropathy. Supplements may reduce therapeutic effects of levodopa. Pyridoxine interacts with some drugs, e.g. phenytoin, theophylline and phenobarbital	Severe deficiency rare Inflammation and skin changes around the mouth, weakness, irritability
Vitamin B_{12} (cobalamin)	Made by microorganisms and incorporated into the food chain by animals Appears in meats or foods of animal origin	*Deficiency associated with*: lack of intrinsic factor, strict vegetarians and vegans, malabsoprtion syndrome, older people in institutional environments	Neuropathy (subacute combined degeneration), megaloblastic anaemia
Folate (folic acid)	Widely distributed in foods, particularly liver, yeast extract, leafy green vegetables, fortified grains and breakfast cereals	*Deficiency associated with*: malabsorption, alcoholism, some anticonvulsant drugs, older people on restricted diets Women in the first trimester of pregnancy or those thinking of becoming pregnant should take a daily supplement of 400 mcg (Food Standards Agency 2003). A higher dose may be recommended by the doctor or midwife if there is a history of neural tube defect	Effect on cell division leading to megaloblastic and macrocytic anaemia, elevation of plasma homocysteine, association with neural tube defect in pregnancy
Pantothenic acid	Widely distributed in foods, particularly animal products, whole grains, potatoes and tomato products	—	Rare and only demonstrated in those eating a very restricted diet

Table 21.1 Vitamins: rich food sources, at risk groups and symptoms of deficiency* *(Continued)*

Nutrient	Rich food sources	Groups at risk of deficiency or excessive intake affecting health	Symptoms of deficiency
Biotin	Widely distributed in foods, particularly liver, egg yolk, soy flour, cereals and yeast	—	Rare and only demonstrated in those receiving parenteral nutrition or eating a very restricted diet
Vitamin C	Fresh vegetables and fruit, particularly spinach, tomatoes, broccoli, strawberries and citrus fruits	*Deficiency associated with*: smokers, an absence of fruit and vegetables in the diet	Hair follicle eruption, petechial haemorrhage on limbs, bleeding gums, impairment of connective tissue formation in wound repair, joint pains, fatigue Symptoms of deficiency disease (scurvy) result from the failure of the body to synthesise collagen
Vitamin D (calciferols)	Major source is exposure to sunlight Found in fatty fish, liver, milk, eggs, fortified food such as margarine, breakfast cereals	*Deficiency associated with*: inadequate exposure to sunlight (e.g. nursing home residents, dark skinned people who habitually cover their skin), malabsorption *Excessive intake affecting health*: people with sarcoidosis should not take vitamin D supplements	Rickets in children, osteomalacia, muscle weakness, bone tenderness
Vitamin E (tocopherols)	Synthesised by plants Plant oils, nuts and seeds are a rich source	—	Deficiency only demonstrated in premature infants and those unable to absorb or utilise vitamin E Deficiency results in cell membrane dysfunction
Vitamin K (phylloquinone and menaquinones)	Green leafy vegetables and vegetable oils Also produced by bacteria in intestine	*Deficiency associated with*: malabsorption or impaired gut synthesis Vitamin K supplement given prophylactically to prevent haemorrhagic disease of the newborn in many countries due to vitamin K deficiency in the newborn	Deficiency very rare in adults and results in bleeding disorder

*For further details, see Garrow et al (2000) and Food Standards Agency (2003).

featuring a range of different foods is likely to meet daily requirements but deficiency of some minerals is very common, e.g. iron and iodine. Iron deficiency affects many people in the developed as well as the developing world. One of the major functions of iron in the body is as a component of haemoglobin. It is also important in some metabolic pathways and in the immune response. Women are particularly at risk of iron-deficiency anaemia due to loss from menstruation.

Iron is found in the haem form in meats, and in the non-haem form in plants (see Ch. 11). Non-haem iron is not absorbed by the body as well as haem iron. Other factors may also affect the absorption of iron in the digestive system, e.g. the presence of vitamin C.

Iodine deficiency is a devastating problem in some regions of the world. People living in areas where the soil, and consequently food grown in the soil, is deficient in iodine can develop signs and symptoms of iodine deficiency. These include an enlarged thyroid gland (goitre), lethargy, mental impairment and congenital abnormalities. Programmes which provide iodine supplementation by iodising salt have proved very successful in reducing the incidence of iodine deficiency (WHO 2003a). Table 21.2 shows some of the minerals required by the body, and gives details of rich food sources, at-risk groups and symptoms of deficiency.

Some nutrients are termed essential nutrients because they cannot be made by the human body and have to be obtained from the diet. If an essential nutrient, or enough of a non-essential nutrient, is unavailable to the body, then the body will be unable to function as it should. The physiological processes in which the nutrient takes part will be affected. For example, growth will be stunted if protein intake is below that which is required for the normal growth of body tissues, and if iron intake is less than required, the formation of haemoglobin will be reduced.

If intake of a particular nutrient or range of nutrients affects physiological function adversely, then the person can be said to be malnourished. Malnutrition can refer to both overnutrition, i.e. intake of energy and nutrients in excess of requirements, and undernutrition, i.e. intake of insufficient energy and nutrients to meet requirements. Malnutrition may jeopardise health status in general and can affect morbidity and mortality. The body can adapt to a low intake of some nutrients but this will affect body composition and function (see p. 800).

The amount of nutrient a person requires is influenced by their basal metabolic rate (BMR), activity level and

Table 21.2 Minerals: rich food sources, at risk groups and symptoms of deficiency*

Nutrient	Rich food sources	Groups at risk of deficiency or excessive intake affecting health	Symptoms of deficiency
Calcium	Milk, cheese, small fish, e.g. sardines, some green leafy vegetables, soybean products, fortified wheat flour and breakfast cereals, some nuts	*Deficiency associated with*: fat malabsorption, consumption of large amounts of phytates *Excessive intake affecting health*: excessive intake of calcium (e.g. antacids) and those with renal failure may be susceptible	Widespread effects of deficiency. Stunted growth and bone malformation in children, skeletal and tooth changes in adults
Magnesium	Found widely in foods, particularly green leafy vegetables, grains, nuts	*Deficiency associated with*: malabsorption, excessive renal loss (e.g. diuretic use) *Excessive intake affecting health*: those with renal glomerular failure susceptible	Widespread effects including cardiovascular and skeletal system disorders, hypocalcaemia
Phosphorous	Found widely in foods, particularly fish, poultry, red meat, dairy products, cereal grains	*Deficiency associated with*: some forms of rickets, excessive intakes of aluminium-containing antacids, vitamin D deficiency, alcoholism, diabetic ketoacidosis *Excessive intake affecting health*: those with renal glomerular failure susceptible	Widespread effects including osteomalacia, myopathy, growth failure
Sodium chloride	Salt and salty foods	*Excessive intake affecting health*: young infants should not have salt added to food as renal excretion is limited. In adults intake of no more than 6 g/day recommended to promote health	Rare except following excessive loss of body fluids, e.g. sweating Low blood pressure, dehydration and muscle cramps
Potassium	Milk, fruit, e.g. bananas, and vegetables, shellfish, red meat, white meat, liver	*Deficiency associated with*: use of some diuretics, very low energy diets *Excessive intake affecting health*: those taking potassium-sparing diuretics and some other types of drug Those with renal disease, adrenal insufficiency and insulin deficiency susceptible	Rare except following excessive loss of body fluids, e.g. diarrhoea Muscle weakness, arrhythmias, irritability, cardiac arrest
Iron (haem and non-haem form)	Liver, meat, beans, nuts, dried fruit, fish, enriched cereals, soybean flour, dark leafy green vegetables Dietary factors influencing uptake include: form of iron ingested; presence of vitamin C, phytates, calcium, soy protein	*Deficiency associated with*: infants over 6 months, toddlers, adolescents, pregnant women, menstruating women, older people, people with parasitic infestations, high intake of inhibitors of absorption, e.g. tea *Excessive intake affecting health*: frequent blood transfusion recipients susceptible	Normocytic anaemia, microcytic anaemia, reduced work capacity, reduced intellectual performance, impaired resistance to infection, impaired thermoregulation
Zinc	Meat, unrefined cereals, fortified cereal products	—	Growth retardation, defects of rapidly dividing tissues, e.g. skin, intestinal mucosa, immune system
Selenium	Fish, offal, brazil nuts, cereals	Dietary deficiency endemic in some areas of the world, e.g. China	Deficiency associated with Keshan disease, a form of cardiomyopathy; inflammatory joint disease
Iodine	Marine fish, shellfish, sea salt, supplemented salt	Dietary deficiency endemic in some areas of the world	Goitre, hypothyroidism, cretinism if fetal growth affected
Fluoride	Generally obtained from drinking water and dental products Rich food sources include tea and fish	—	Fluoride is implicated in the development of tooth health

Molybdenum, manganese, copper, chromium also required but these are widespread in foods and deficiency is only demonstrated in very restricted diets or certain medical conditions.

*For further details, see Garrow et al (2000) and Food Standards Agency (2003).

response to certain factors such as cold exposure and ingestion of food. BMR is the metabolic rate at rest and is influenced by several factors, including genetic makeup and body mass. The amount of energy required by a person can be worked out using an equation which considers BMR and activity level (DH 1991). Illness can increase BMR, but the consequent rise in energy required by the body may be counteracted by a reduction in physical activity level. If an individual has an inadequate intake of energy for a period of time, the body can adapt by reducing BMR.

Although foods containing all known nutrients can be formulated, no single naturally occurring food can meet all the daily nutritional demands. Different types of food contain different proportions of macro- and micronutrients and therefore a range of foods is necessary to provide the daily requirement of individual nutrients. In general, plant products are richer in carbohydrate but lower in protein and fats than animal products. Plants are the major source of fibre. Some foods are particularly rich in a single nutrient, although they may contain other nutrients; thus, meat should be classed as protein-rich rather than as a protein, as it also contains fat and other nutrients. Cereals are rich in carbohydrate; for example, of 100 g of wheat flour, over 70% is carbohydrate, but approximately 10% is protein and 1% is fat. Very few foods, such as sugar, almost pure carbohydrate, or cooking oils, almost pure fat, fall predominantly into one macronutrient group. Some nutrients are better absorbed by the body, i.e. they are more 'bioavailable', in certain forms and under certain conditions, e.g. iron (see above). The bioavailability of some medications can also be changed by particular foods (see p. 795).

PUBLIC HEALTH NUTRITION

The diet consists of the foods we eat from day to day. The diet we eat must supply the essential nutrients, i.e. those which are necessary for survival but cannot be synthesised by the body from other sources. It should supply all the necessary components in the correct quantities and proportions, whilst avoiding excessive intake. For optimal health, nutrient intake must balance nutrient usage; an excess intake may be damaging. There is considerable debate about the safety of some vitamin and mineral supplements that are not medically prescribed, as a result of which the UK Food Standards Agency has published a comprehensive review of the safety of vitamin and mineral supplements (Food Standards Agency 2003).

Nutritional requirements will vary depending on a person's size, gender, activity level and state of health. Nutritional requirements also vary across the life span. Infants and children require sufficient nutrients to grow and develop. Requirements for some nutrients are increased pre-conception, during pregnancy and whilst breast feeding, and also change with ageing (Barasi 2003). In the UK, estimated nutritional requirements for different groups of people within the population have been established and are published by the Department of Health (1991). These are termed dietary reference values. It is important to recognise that these are not recommendations for intake by individuals but are estimates for healthy populations only; within a clinical setting the advice of a dietitian must be sought.

STOP THINK **21.2** Apart from pregnancy and lactation, when else during their life span may a person have sudden changes in their nutrient demand?

The diet in the UK has changed quite drastically in the last 50 years. Access to an extensive range of foods has never been greater. Nutrient intake has changed as a result of the changes in the type and amount of food eaten and few people now suffer from undernutrition. Current government guidelines on dietary intake recommend an intake thought to promote maximum health for the population. These recommendations include a fat intake of less than 35% of dietary energy intake, of which no more than one-third should be in the form of saturated fats, and a carbohydrate intake of approximately 50% of dietary energy intake (DH 1994). A salt intake of less than 6 g/day is also recommended (Scientific Advisory Committee on Nutrition 2003). How this relates to food is discussed below. The amount of fat consumed in the UK is less than in recent years but saturated fat intake is still higher than recommended (Henderson et al 2003).

The type of diet an individual eats is determined by many factors. At a global level, government policies influence food supply and legislation. Fortification of foods or water with particular nutrients is a feature in many countries and is usually managed at a central government level, e.g. the fluoridation of water supplies. The policy for food labelling is also determined centrally.

Within a country, there are regional and socioeconomic differences in dietary intake; for example, intake of fruit and vegetables in Scotland is lower than in the rest of UK and lower income households tend to eat less fresh fruit and vegetables but more canned and frozen vegetables (Buttriss 2002).

At an individual level, a person chooses to eat a particular type of diet for a variety of reasons which include sociological, psychological, economic and behavioural issues. Some of these factors are shown in Figure 21.1.

- Sociological issues include age, culture, religion, income, food availability and cooking facilities.
- Psychological issues encompass a variety of factors ranging from aversions to particular foods, to a fear of food in general.
- Economic factors are important and influence both the quality and quantity of dietary intake. If a type of food, such as fruit, is not available to buy or if there is insufficient money to buy a range of foods in appropriate amounts, dietary intake will be reduced in quality and quantity.
- Behavioural elements of food choice can also influence dietary intake. For example, toddlers can be very particular about the type of food that they will eat.

When food is available, the amount eaten is determined by appetite. Appetite is controlled by many factors, including the presence of nutrients in the GI tract, levels of GI hormones, levels of nutrients in the blood and the response of the central nervous system to hunger signals from the rest of the body. Emotional factors may also influence what is eaten; for example, some people eat particular foods to 'cheer themselves up' or a celebratory meal may be eaten. The environment to which we are exposed also affects

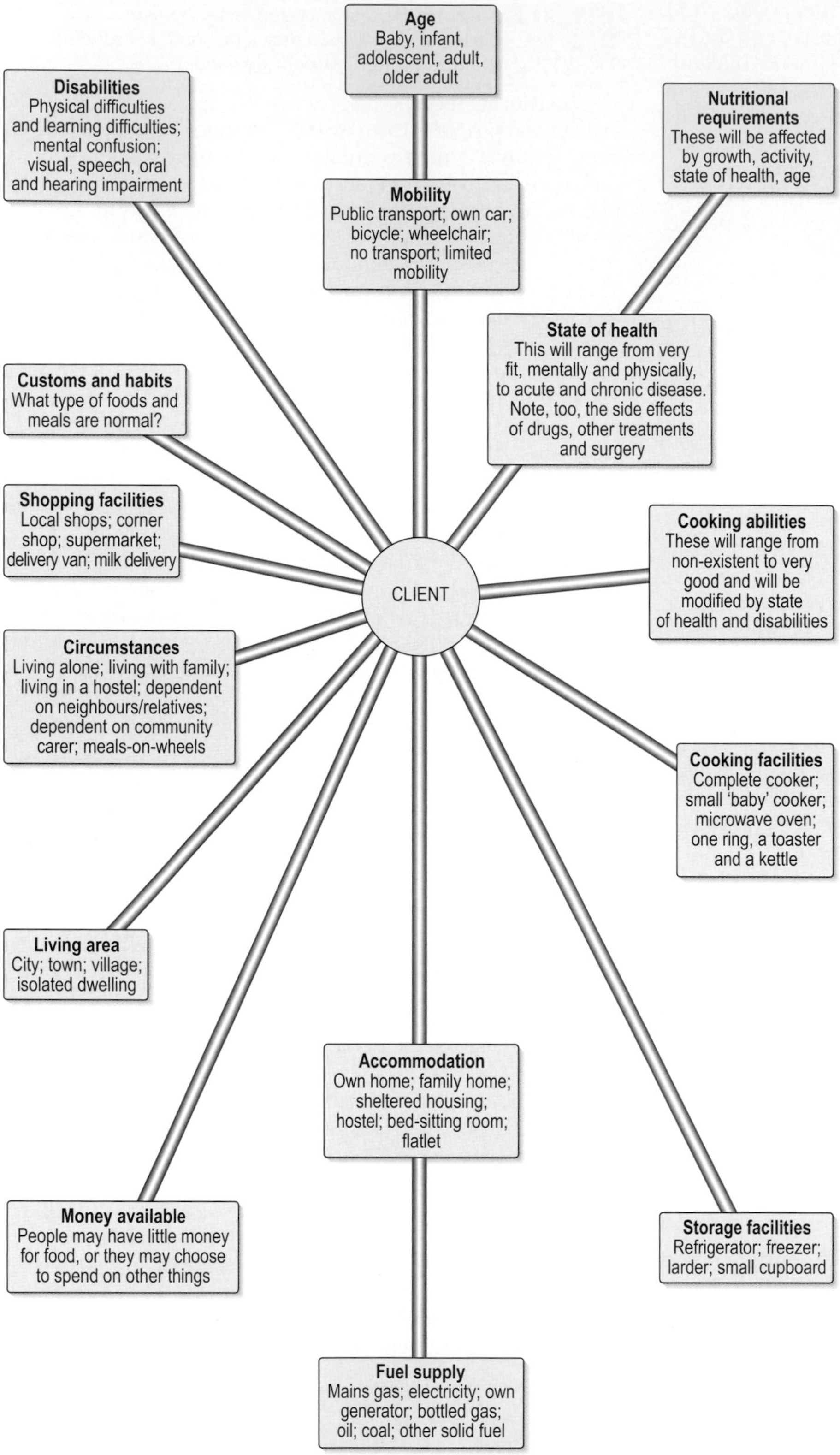

Fig. 21.1 Factors to consider when screening, assessing and planning nutritional needs. (Reproduced with permission from Sandy 1997.)

appetite; for example, the smell of freshly baked bread when passing a bakery may instigate feelings of hunger. Conversely, smelling a very unpleasant odour when eating tends to diminish appetite. People tend to eat more when eating with other people in a social setting, although this is not always the case (see p. 802).

Nurses should ascertain the dietary intake of individuals on admission to care and it is important not only to think of dietary intake in terms of nutritional content but also to consider the reasons why a particular type of diet is consumed. It is the role of the nurse to ensure that patients are provided with a diet that is acceptable to them, unless

Table 21.3 Common food-borne infections

Microorganism	Common source	Symptoms
Bacillus spp.	Cereals, dried foods, dairy products	Vomiting, 1–5 h after ingestion; diarrhoea few hours after ingestion
Campylobacter spp.	Raw or undercooked meat, poultry, untreated water, unpasteurised milk	Profuse diarrhoea, severe abdominal pain; incubation 2–5 days; prodromal phase of headache and photophobia
Clostridium perfringens	Cooked meats, gravy, fish, dried foods, vegetables	Diarrhoea, abdominal pain 8–12 h after ingestion
Escherichia coli (toxogenic strains)	Raw or undercooked beef, milk, vegetables, infected animals	Diarrhoea (can progress to haemolytic uraemic syndrome). Incubation period 1–6 days
Salmonella *typhi/paratyphi* Other salmonellas	Food in contact with an infected human carrier or contaminated by sewage Meat, especially poultry, eggs, milk, dairy products	Fever, malaise, constipation followed by diarrhoea. Incubation 1–3 weeks Diarrhoea, vomiting, fever, 12–72 h after ingestion
Shigella spp.	Faecally contaminated water and food, e.g. salads	Diarrhoea, fever, abdominal pain, 1–7 days after ingestion
Staphylococcus aureus	Cold food handled during preparation, dairy products	Vomiting, abdominal pain 1–7 h after ingestion
Gastrointestinal viruses, e.g. SRSV, Norwalk agent, rotavirus	Contaminated water, shellfish, cold foods handled during preparation	Vomiting, diarrhoea, fever, abdominal pain 24–48 h after ingestion

Source: PHLS Salmonella Committee (1995).

contraindicated by their medical condition. The quality of foods consumed in the diet is also an important factor and issues of food safety need to be considered.

Food safety

Food safety is a topic encompassing a wide range of factors which influence the quality of the foods that we eat. These include the use of aluminium foil and plastic to wrap food, pesticide residues in foods, natural toxins in foods and food-borne illness. Food-borne illnesses are a particular topic of nursing concern due to their impact on the health of individuals. Food-borne illnesses can be caused by improperly prepared or stored food. Older people and children are particularly susceptible as they are less able to withstand the consequences of food-borne illness, such as prolonged nausea and vomiting. Table 21.3 lists some common food-borne infections. Nurses must ensure that Food Safety Regulations are adhered to in clinical practice areas (see Ch. 16).

STOP THINK **21.3** What regulations are in place to help to prevent food poisoning in the hospital environment?

Functional foods

In recent years the concept of consuming a food with the aim of promoting health has developed. Foods which promote health can be termed functional foods. A functional food is defined as one which has health-promoting benefits and/or disease-preventing properties, in addition to the usual nutritional value (Barasi 2003). Included in this category are fortified foods, foods containing components that do not occur generally in the normal diet and foods containing bacteria thought to promote GI function, e.g. omega-enriched eggs and probiotic-enriched yoghurts. This is a rapidly expanding area of nutrition and one about which nurses need to be informed, as patients may seek advice on the use of functional foods.

Drug–nutrient interactions

Some medications may influence food intake, absorption and metabolism. In addition, some nutrients may influence medication absorption and metabolism. The interaction may potentiate or inhibit the activity of the medication or result in side-effects. The type of interaction will vary depending on the medication and the nutrient. This is an important issue in the administration of medications and the nurse should be aware of the potential of commonly prescribed medications to interact with food. The hospital or community pharmacist can provide advice on this issue in a clinical setting.

For further reading on this topic, see Barasi (2003) and Jordan et al (2003).

NUTRITIONAL CARE

Nutritional care by nurses involves screening, assessment, planning, intervention and evaluation. This process is illustrated in Figure 21.2 (McLaren & Green 1998).

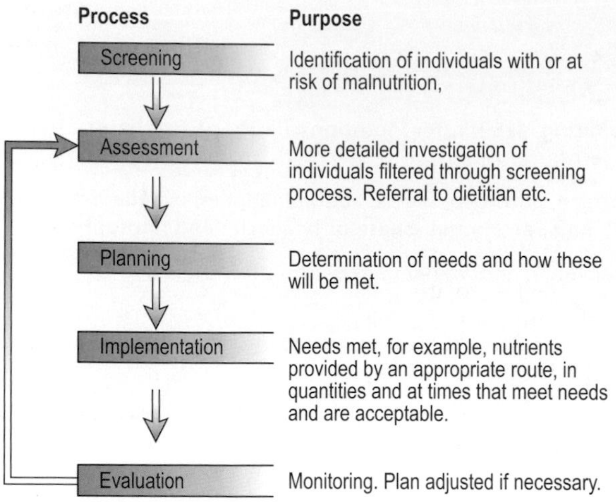
Process
Purpose
Screening
Identification of individuals with or at risk of malnutrition,
Assessment
More detailed investigation of individuals filtered through screening process. Referral to dietitian etc.
Planning
Determination of needs and how these will be met.
Implementation
Needs met, for example, nutrients provided by an appropriate route, in quantities and at times that meet needs and are acceptable.
Evaluation
Monitoring. Plan adjusted if necessary.

Fig. 21.2 Process of nutritional care of individuals by nurses. (Adapted from McLaren & Green 1998, with permission.)

NUTRITIONAL SCREENING AND ASSESSMENT

Nutritional screening aims to identify those with, or at risk of, malnutrition and can highlight potential causes. If an individual is considered to be at risk of or to have malnutrition, then a more detailed assessment must be undertaken. A variety of health care professionals may undertake this assessment depending on the type of problem identified at screening. The majority of patients will be referred to the dietitian if malnutrition is suspected. However, referral to another health care professional may also be appropriate; for example, referral to the speech and language therapist (SALT) if a swallowing deficit is identified, or to the occupational therapist if difficulty with manipulation of cutlery is an issue. Screening and assessment will allow identification of needs, planning of interventions and setting of goals (McLaren & Green 1998). Following this, interventions can be implemented. As always, interventions should be recorded and regularly evaluated and modified by assessment. Screening and assessment can also establish a baseline from which to monitor changes in status.

There are five principal methods of screening or assessing for nutritional status:

- Dietary history and intake
- Clinical examination
- Functional tests
- Anthropometric measures
- Biochemical tests.

Dietary history and intake

Elementary assessment by nurses of dietary history and intake is essential to determine the risk of malnutrition as well as to examine other factors, such as dietary habits, food preferences and economic factors affecting food intake. Changes in appetite, reduced food intake and absorption, the use of supplements and other issues, e.g. dietary adherence, can also be considered. The type of diet a person consumes is influenced by many factors, particularly in a home environment (see Fig. 21.1). In care environments, food charts can be used to record food intake over a period of time to assess whether dietary needs are being met. Asking a person to recall what they have eaten over the previous day, or to describe what they generally eat, are also useful ways of assessing dietary intake. These methods can also be used to identify food that may have caused a reaction. Assessment of food intake over a longer period of time, e.g. 7 days, by the use of a food diary can be useful in some circumstances, for example when working to promote dietary change in a person with obesity. Assessment of habitual intake will increase a person's awareness of their dietary intake and can highlight aspects that can be modified to help achieve an intake that follows the 'healthy eating guidelines'. The nurse is able to carry out an elementary assessment of food intake but more comprehensive dietary analyses should be undertaken by a dietitian; assessment of any individual's specific intake is a complex process.

STOP THINK **21.4** What provision is there in your current clinical practice to meet the nutritional needs of people who eat the following:

(a) Halal food
(b) A vegan diet
(c) A gluten free diet?

Clinical examination

A clinical examination can identify medical conditions and treatment that may influence intake, digestion and absorption of nutrients. Drug and alcohol use can adversely affect nutritional status and should be considered in assessment. Changes in appetite, taste or smell, dental problems or ill-fitting dentures should be investigated. The person's usual activity level should also be considered, as well as general appearance and fit of clothes, condition of the hair, skin, eyes and mouth, and neurological and musculoskeletal systems. It is also important to assess a person's functional ability to eat; for example, are there physical or mental factors that might impair the process of eating? In addition, assessment of whether a person is able to read the language in which any dietary advice is written is essential. Issues such as literacy and visual impairment need to be considered if written dietary advice is to be given.

Functional tests

Functional tests of nutritional status are usually performed by the doctor or dietitian and include tests such as handgrip strength, using a dynamometer, and respiratory muscle strength.

Anthropometric measures

Simple anthropometric measures can be used by nurses to screen and assess nutritional status. Anthropometry refers to the measurement of the human body. It is important to weigh individuals on admission to care and periodically thereafter to identify any subsequent losses or gains. To ensure accuracy, the person should, if possible, be weighed on the same scales at the same time each day, preferably in the same clothes, and after emptying their bladder and bowel. Single measurements of weight are of limited value, but serial measurements permit trends in weight loss or gain to be identified.

Percentage weight change can be calculated using the equation:

$$\% \text{ weight loss/gain} = \frac{\text{usual weight} - \text{current weight (kg)} \times 100}{\text{usual weight (kg)}}$$

A loss of 10% in the previous 3 months is suggestive of malnutrition. However, caution is required when interpreting weight changes as factors such as dehydration, oedema or tumour growth can complicate the picture.

Weight considered in relation to height gives a more accurate assessment of the degree to which a person is under- or overweight. Body mass index (BMI) is commonly used to assess weight in relation to height. This is simply the body weight in kilograms (kg) divided by the height in metres squared (m^2). For example, someone with a body weight of 57 kg and a height of 1.62 m has a BMI of $57/1.62^2 = 21.7\ kg/m^2$. Height can be difficult to determine, due to factors such as spine curvature and inability to stand. An estimation of height can be made using demi-span, i.e. distance from web between middle and ring finger along outstretched arm to sternal notch (Webb & Copeman 1996) or ulna length (Elia 2003). In the clinical setting, further information on these measures can be obtained from the dietitian.

The International Obesity Task Force (2000) has outlined the following categories associated with BMI: <18.5 as underweight, 18.5–24.9 as normal range, 25.0–29.9 as overweight, 30.0–34.9 obese (class 1), 35.0–39.9 obese (class 2) and >40.0 obese (class 3). When using BMI with older people the resulting plan and intervention need to be carefully considered as the usefulness of BMI as a predictor of risk of morbidity and mortality in the very old has been questioned (British Dietetic Association 2003).

Waist circumference can be used to assess the amount of fat carried in the abdominal region. This measure is increasingly being used to screen for cardiovascular risk in primary care. Men with a waist circumference >102 cm and women with a waist circumference >88 cm should be advised that weight reduction would be beneficial (Lean 2000).

Anthropometric measures that assess fat levels or muscle mass of the body can be used by dietitians or doctors in clinical environments. Nurses may use these measures in specialist units following education in their use. These measures include skinfold measures to estimate body fat, and mid-arm muscle circumference to estimate skeletal muscle mass. Electrical bioimpedance is a method of assessing the fat mass of the body, which is being used increasingly in some environments such as health clubs.

Regular checks of accuracy and, if necessary, recalibration are essential for all equipment used to measure individuals, including weighing scales.

Biochemical tests

Biochemical measures to assess nutritional status include a number of parameters, obtained from investigation of plasma, urine and tissues.

Measurement of proteins present in the blood, such as albumin and retinol-binding protein, can be useful in some clinical situations but the interpretation of what the level means needs to be considered carefully. Serum protein levels are usually more an indicator of clinical state than nutritional status in the acutely ill, as protein levels in the blood change in response to the trauma the body is experiencing. In addition, treatments such as administration of blood products will change serum protein levels. The clinical biochemist, doctor and dietitian are key members of the multidisciplinary team when considering the relationship between a patient's nutritional status and serum protein level.

Biochemical investigations can also assess circulating lipoprotein levels to give an indication of cardiovascular risk. In addition, specific vitamin, e.g. vitamin C, or mineral, e.g. iron and selenium, levels can be evaluated.

Nitrogen balance studies provide an index of protein status. Nitrogen balance is determined by estimating protein intake and subtracting urinary nitrogen excretion with an allowance for nitrogen loss via hair, skin and faeces. Additionally, losses from wound drainage or GI fistulae must be considered. A positive nitrogen balance indicates that the patient is in an anabolic state, whereas a negative balance indicates catabolism.

Accurate nutritional assessment relies on utilisation of data from a number of sources. Data from only one source can be open to misinterpretation due to the many factors, such as disease processes, that can influence individual parameters. A combination of two or more measures obtained from dietary history and intake, clinical examination, functional tests, anthropometric measures and biochemical tests is required to gain an accurate picture of an individual's nutritional status. The methods described above may be used by nurses in the context of a busy clinical environment. Other methods can be employed by dietitians and other health care professionals in the clinical environment and research settings (Garrow et al 2000).

Nutritional screening tools

Recently there has been an increase in the number of nutritional screening tools which are for use by nurses. These tools use risk factors that may lead to or be associated with malnourishment and are similar in format to a pressure ulcer risk assessment tool (see Ch. 23). They are typically in questionnaire format and are useful as an aide-mémoire for screening and as a record of information. An appropriate plan of action is identified by some. Of the many screening tools published, only a few have undergone rigorous testing of reliability and validity (Jones 2002, Green & Watson 2005). The British Association of Parenteral and Enteral Nutrition has introduced a screening tool for malnutrition for use by nurses in all areas of clinical practice (Elia 2003). This tool has undergone testing to ensure it is a valid and reliable tool with which to screen for malnutrition (Elia 2003).

A number of recent national publications (Nursing and Midwifery Practice Development Unit 2002, DH 2003a) have highlighted the need for nutritional screening and assessment, and local guidelines for nursing practice have been developed from these.

NUTRITIONAL INTERVENTION

Following screening and assessment of an individual, the nurse will plan appropriate interventions. The following sections outline interventions that may be planned by the nurse, usually in association with other health care professionals such as the dietitian. These include advising on a 'healthy diet', promoting oral intake and enteral and parenteral nutrition. Obesity and undernutrition are also discussed. In many situations referral to the dietitian is a necessary part of the nutritional plan of care. However, in some circumstances — for example, giving advice concerning healthy eating to an individual who is overweight — this can be given by the nurse. Local guidelines should outline when referral to a dietitian is appropriate. Individuals who require therapeutic diets, e.g. those with diabetes mellitus, renal disease, coeliac disease, hyperlipidaemia and food allergy, should always be referred to the dietitian. Nurses may then follow through a plan of care prescribed by the dietitian. The dietitian is the expert on nutritional care in the health care environment.

A healthy diet

The diet which is currently recommended to promote the health of the general population in the UK is shown in Figure 21.3. This pictorial representation is termed the 'Plate model'. It illustrates five food groups and the proportion in which each group should be consumed. The model is based on guidelines for a healthy diet approved by the Department of Health (British Nutrition Foundation 2004) (Box 21.2) and is a useful health promotion tool. Such a diet is sometimes termed a 'balanced diet', i.e. it provides the appropriate amounts of all nutrients in the correct proportions to meet the requirements of the body. This diet consists of 33% vegetables and fruit, 33% complex carbohydrate, 12% protein-containing foods, 15% dairy products or similar foods and 8% fat- and sugar-containing foods. Current recommendations from the Department of Health suggest that each individual should eat five or more portions of a variety of fruit and vegetables a day (DH 2003b). The type of diet outlined above is not suitable for those under 5 years of age or those following a diet prescribed by the dietitian.

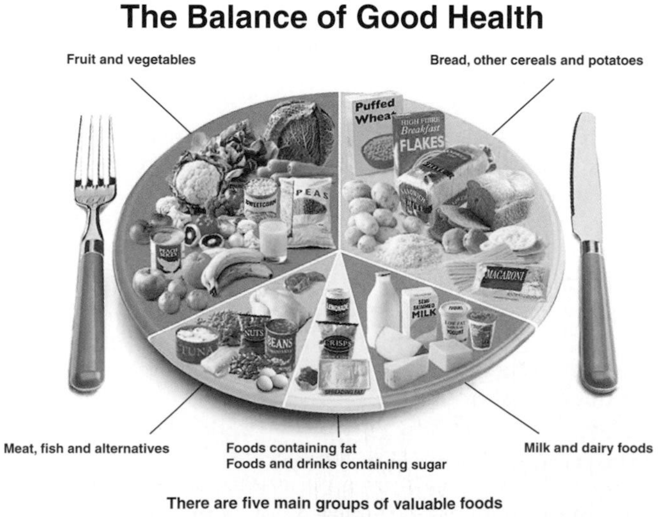

Fig. 21.3 'Balance of Good Health' plate model. (Reproduced with kind permission of the Food Standards Agency.)

Box 21.2

Guidelines for a healthy diet

- Enjoy your food
- Eat a variety of different foods
- Eat the right amount to be a healthy weight
- Eat plenty of foods rich in starch and fibre
- Eat plenty of fruit and vegetables
- Don't eat too many foods that contain a lot of fat
- Don't have sugary foods and drinks too often
- If you drink alcohol, drink sensibly

Reproduced with kind permission from the Food Standards Agency (2003).

Obesity

Obesity is the condition of excessive accumulation of fat in the body, leading to an increase in weight beyond that considered desirable. Obesity quite simply results when intake of energy is greater than energy usage. However, the reasons why this happens are complex. Many people have the genetic propensity to develop obesity. However, the propensity does not mean the person will become obese; customary diet and lifestyle play a major role (British Nutrition Foundation Task Force 1999). A high dietary fat intake (Golay & Bobbioni 1997) and low levels of activity are strongly implicated (Prentice & Jebb 1995). Emotional factors may trigger overeating in some but it is generally thought that personality and emotional factors play only a minor role in the development of obesity, although they may be important in terms of response to treatment (British Nutrition Foundation Task Force 1999). Rarely, obesity may result from a medical condition, such as hypothyroidism.

Obesity is considered a major world health problem as the number of people who are obese is rapidly escalating (WHO 2003b). Obesity is associated with many common disorders such as cardiovascular disease, hypertension, stroke, type 2 diabetes mellitus and certain forms of cancer (WHO 2003c). The extra strain placed on the musculoskeletal system may contribute to arthritic disease, particularly of the hips and knees, and excess fat in the thoracic cavity may lead to sleep apnoea (British Nutrition Foundation Task Force 1999) (see Ch. 25). Individuals with obesity, particularly morbid obesity, may also be subject to psychological distress and social penalties. The economic costs of obesity may also be high. The National Audit Office (2001) estimated that obesity accounted for 18 million days of sickness absence and 30 000 premature deaths in 1998, and costs the NHS at least £0.5 billion a year.

Treatment of obesity

There are a number of approaches to the treatment of obesity. Currently few specialist obesity clinics exist and most people with obesity who seek help from health care professionals are assessed and managed by the primary care team. Interventions to reduce weight instigated or maintained by nurses include strategies to promote 'healthy eating' and lifestyle change. Treatment programmes within the primary care setting should be individualised and involve assessment and goal setting.

As outlined by Green and O'Kane (2002), advice given by nurses on weight management can be considered within four identified stages of health promotion:

1. Eliciting the person's views, beliefs and readiness to change
2. Explaining the nature of and reasons for advice
3. Negotiating and agreeing goals
4. Supporting the achievement of goals and maintenance of change.

Readiness to change, and the aspects of behaviour the person is willing and able to change, must be assessed. The 'stages of change' model may be used to facilitate this process (Hunt & Hillsdon 1996) (see Ch. 36). Nurses must have an understanding of the causes and effects of obesity in order to explain why weight loss is desirable. With most people the first goal should be to stabilise weight and therefore prevent further weight gain. If this is successful, moderate weight loss can then be attempted; a weight loss of just 10% can reduce the health risks associated with obesity (British Nutrition Foundation Task Force 1999). Weight loss beyond this may be attempted if the individual wishes.

Dietary change Dietary advice given by nurses to obese or overweight individuals should follow the guidelines for a healthy diet shown above. Adhering to healthy eating guidelines should lead to the consumption of a low-fat diet. The concept of healthy eating, rather than a prescriptive short-term reducing diet, is useful as it may encourage long-term or permanent changes to the individual's diet. Restriction of energy intake may be considered appropriate for some individuals, e.g. those with reduced mobility. Whilst some research has suggested weight loss has been more strongly associated with a change in the percentage of energy derived from fat, rather than with change in total energy intake (Toubro & Astrup 1997), a recent systematic review has suggested energy-restricted diets are as effective as fat-restricted diets in achieving long-term weight loss (Pirozzo et al 2003). A further review, however, suggests that whilst both low-fat diets, i.e. with 30% or less of total daily energy derived from fat, and low-fat, energy-restricted diets can promote weight loss (Mulvihill & Quigley 2003), their relative effectiveness is not clear.

There are many types of diet published, advocating various types and combinations of foods. The long-term efficacy of many of these has not been ascertained and some may be very low in energy and result in a deficiency of some nutrients. Many of these diets encourage a short-term drastic change in dietary habit, which is difficult to maintain, and most people find themselves reverting to their old eating habits.

Physical activity Increased physical activity can facilitate weight management (Mulvihill & Quigley 2003) and maintenance of a new eating pattern (Hunt & Hillsdon 1996). Some individuals may be unable to increase their physical activity levels due to their medical condition, and the advice of the doctor should be sought. The British Nutrition Foundation Task Force (1999) recommends building up slowly to walking at a pace that achieves mild breathlessness for 30 min/day at least 5 days per week. Eventually the person may consider extending some sessions to 40 min or more to encourage fat burning. Activity within the daily routine, e.g. walking rather than driving, should be encouraged. Resistance training can also help, as it will conserve muscle mass and maintain resting metabolic rate as weight is lost. Exercise on prescription may also be a useful way of promoting activity level (British Nutrition Foundation Task Force 1999).

Behaviour Strategies to promote behavioural change and modification may help individuals to avoid or cope with situations that promote overeating, and encourage the adoption of a healthier lifestyle (Hunt & Hillsdon 1996). Some individuals may find that they benefit from the support they gain from attending a reputable 'slimming club'.

Medication Drug therapy may be indicated when an obese or overweight individual with co-morbidities has been unable to lose weight by dietary change (National Institute for Clinical Excellence 2001a). In the UK there are currently two main types of medication that may be prescribed by the doctor for the treatment of obesity: one type inhibits the actions of lipases in the GI tract, thus limiting the absorption of fat, which is consequently excreted in the stools; the other type is a re-uptake inhibitor of noradrenaline and serotonin that works to reduce energy intake by increasing satiety and reducing hunger (National Institute for Clinical Excellence 2001b). Both these types of medication have been shown to be useful in promoting weight loss but there are side-effects associated with their use.

Surgery Obesity can be treated by surgical means if other methods of obesity management have failed (National Institute for Clinical Excellence 2002), although currently in the UK only a few hospitals offer this kind of surgery. The decision to undertake surgical treatment is not taken lightly as there are risks involved and eating patterns following surgery are vastly different from those before. Surgical treatments involve reducing the size of the stomach ('stomach stapling' or gastric banding) or bypassing sections of the upper GI tract. Reducing the size of the stomach restricts the amount of food a person can eat; bypassing sections of the GI tract results in less food being absorbed by the body. Care of the patient pre- and post-surgery is discussed in Chapter 26. It is important that anyone undergoing surgical treatment for obesity is referred to the dietitian. Surgical treatment for obesity will not automatically result in the consumption of a healthier diet, and may actually lead to a poorer quality of diet being consumed. The nurse must be aware that, following surgery, whilst the patient may be pleased with a very fast weight loss, a poor diet may be the cause, which can lead to a risk of malnutrition. As with any method of weight loss, weight loss maintenance is important and diet and lifestyle changes are essential factors in this.

Prevention of obesity is an important issue, as obesity levels, particularly in children, continue to escalate. Where appropriate, health promotion and education strategies by nurses should promote adherence to healthy eating guidelines and increased activity levels, not only for individuals but also for their families.

Undernutrition

Undernutrition is an endemic problem; protein-energy malnutrition (PEM) affects large numbers of the world's population and contributes significantly to human mortality and morbidity. However, in developed countries, while outright starvation might be thought to be unlikely, levels of undernutrition do exist and can result in significant morbidity and mortality. Certain groups may be at particular risk, including older adults, homeless people, substance abusers, those with eating disorders such as anorexia nervosa, those suffering from dementia and those who are hospitalised (Holmes 1999a). Undernutrition can occur as a result of:

- reduced food intake
- increased nutritional requirements
- impaired ability to digest, absorb or metabolise nutrients.

Metabolically active disease can alter or increase the need for nutrients. Disease processes may cause a reduction in food intake or absorption of nutrients; pyrexia and infection may increase metabolic rate and nutritional demands; surgery and trauma have a profound impact on metabolism, initiating a complex neuroendocrine response, resulting in an increased metabolic demand. The effects are cumulative, so that two or more of these factors occurring together will result in an even higher metabolic demand. However, the level of physical activity may be reduced, so the overall energy demand may not be raised.

Undernutrition is often associated with chronic disease and is a risk whether the person is nursed at home or in hospital, but there is also evidence of significant undernutrition in acute hospital wards. Holmes (1999a) has reviewed the literature on malnutrition in hospital patients. Surveys suggest that up to 50% of patients hospitalised for 2 weeks or longer could suffer from malnutrition. McWhirter and Pennington (1994) found that PEM was common in both surgical and medical patients. On admission, 38% of patients were undernourished and 66% suffered further weight loss whilst in hospital. A review of case notes of the 200 undernourished patients in this study revealed that only 96 had any nutritional information documented. Elmstahl et al (1997) found that, of 61 older patients in a Swedish long-stay unit, those with a low energy intake were at increased risk of morbidity or mortality.

In people undergoing surgery, undernutrition is associated with increased postoperative morbidity and mortality and studies have demonstrated that preoperative nutritional support can reduce these rates (Delmi et al 1990). Postoperative infection is particularly linked to undernutrition. Infection can induce a stress-related, catabolic response similar to that seen in surgical trauma and it is also often associated with anorexia. The links between nutrition and depression of the immune system are complex, but it is clear that a wide range of immunological functions may be affected.

Hospitalisation may predispose to undernutrition due to a number of factors:

- The patient or client may find that the anxiety and unfamiliarity of the environment reduce appetite.
- Food may not be to their taste and the presentation of meals and environment for eating may be less than ideal.
- Pain, fatigue, respiratory distress or other symptoms may affect appetite or ability to eat.
- Treatment, such as chemotherapy, may alter taste sensation (Holmes 1999b).

In addition, investigations may require periods of fasting and missed meals may not be replaced. Recommended practice is to fast patients from food for 4 h and fluids for 2–4 h prior to surgery (Maltby 1993) in order to empty the stomach and avoid perioperative or postoperative vomiting and the risk of aspiration into the lungs. However, actual fasting times for elective surgery ranging from 5 to 22 h have been reported and, in one study cited in Chapman (1996), only 16% of patients on an afternoon list were fasted for 6 h or less (Hamilton-Smith 1972, Chapman 1996); 33% had been deprived of food for more than 13 h. The theoretical 4–6 h preoperative fast appears to result, in practice, in periods of abstinence that might be better termed preoperative starvation, which could lead to a state of catabolism possibly detrimental to a patient undergoing major surgery. Smith et al (1997) found that shortening the preoperative fast time actually reduced postoperative nausea and vomiting.

For a discussion of strategies to reduce unnecessary preoperative fasting, see Jester & Williams (1999).

ENCOURAGING DIETARY INTAKE

Nurses are ideally placed to help individuals, whether at home or in hospital, to manage their nutritional needs. It is important to acknowledge that food has a number of non-nutritional roles, fulfilling a range of psychosocial and cultural needs. Eating will have very different expectations and associations for different people. Loss of menu choice, unfamiliar foods, food presentation, ethnic or cultural preferences, eating alone, eating in company, timing of meals, and even the eating utensils can all influence the motivation to eat. In addition, the patient's psychological state, e.g. stress due to the hospital environment, illness or bereavement, may modify eating behaviour. Physical factors such as ability to manipulate cutlery, ability to keep the lips together, chew and swallow, to taste food and even to reach food independently are all important. Box 21.3 outlines ways in which appetite can be promoted.

Oral intake

Individual physical and psychological factors, together with environmental or organisational factors, will influence a person's ability or willingness to eat an adequate diet. For an individual to successfully ingest an adequate oral diet at home, a number of activities are required and have to be assessed:

- Is the person able to go shopping and to choose and purchase appropriate foods?
- Is the person's nutritional knowledge adequate for informed choice and have they the financial resources to purchase the required foods?

Box 21.3

Promoting appetite

- *Presentation of food* — is the portion size appropriate? Does the food look attractive? Is it served at the correct temperature? Are mealtimes convenient?
- *Variety and choice of food* — are familiar foods served? Are they an appropriate type and consistency? Have individual food preferences and the needs of minority groups been acknowledged?
- *Frequency* — is there an option to have smaller, more regular meals? Are mealtimes spaced evenly through the day?
- *Duration* — are meals rushed?
- *Assistance* — is help with eating available, if required? Are there feeding aids to assist independence?
- *Oral hygiene* — are mouthwashes/mouth care offered after a meal? Are dentures well fitting? Is the mouth clean, fresh and without infection?
- *Toileting* — are individuals offered toilet and hand washing facilities prior to meals?
- *Positioning* — are individuals positioned comfortably and supported, if necessary, to allow them to manage their meal as independently as possible?
- *Exercise* — is activity or exercise encouraged during the day, to help improve appetite?
- *Social event* — do individuals eat alone or do they have company during meals?
- *Distractions* — are there other activities taking place at mealtimes? Are there unwanted smells/sounds/sights that may be off-putting?

Adapted from Jackson (2003).

- Once purchased, can food be transported home or is a delivery service available?
- Are there adequate facilities for storing food at home, e.g. refrigerator/freezer?
- Are adequate cooking facilities available and can the person use them safely?
- Can the person eat independently or do they need help?

If a deficit occurs in any of these areas, the nurse may need to look at alternative strategies and the occupational therapist may have a major role in assessing the home environment.

Shopping for food can be difficult for people with disabilities, the ill older adult and some people with behavioural disturbances. Ordering shopping over the internet, mobile shops and delivery services may help overcome these problems, if they are available and the individual can cope with ordering the food. However, these services may not be available or appropriate, and then the person will require outside assistance. The family or informal carers may be involved, as can social services, e.g. home helps, or voluntary agencies.

Food preparation can also be a problem. The home environment should be assessed for access to the kitchen, and access to worktops, cupboards, fridge and cooker. For example, a person who is dependent on a wheelchair may need substantial alteration to the kitchen to enable independent food preparation. People with chronic illness such as multiple sclerosis or rheumatoid arthritis may have limited mobility or may find food preparation tiring and need adapted equipment and lightweight cooking utensils. Perceptual problems and confusion may also interfere with independent food preparation. Again, if the person cannot cope, or can cope only with assistance, family or community services may need to be involved.

Physical factors influencing eating

To eat and drink normally requires the ability to transfer food to the mouth, the ability to retain food in the mouth, to chew and to swallow. Sensory function is also important; appetite is improved and eating is easier if the individual can see, smell and taste the food. Digestion and the absorption of nutrients are dependent on effective GI function, and utilisation is dependent on metabolism. The state of the teeth and mouth is important. Cleft lip and cleft palate are examples of congenital abnormalities that can reduce a baby's ability to suck. Teeth are needed for effective chewing; edentulous people may require food of a softer texture or food cut into smaller pieces, but seldom a diet of only mashed or minced foods. Such people are likely to eat fewer vegetables, less dietary fibre and be deficient in vitamins such as D (Finch et al 1998).

If the oral tissues are dry, inflamed or painful, a person may be reluctant to eat (see Ch. 15). In xerostomia, artificial saliva can be used to help lubricate food. Oral health may also contribute to improving the taste and enjoyment of a meal; poor oral hygiene can mask taste and reduce appetite. The number of taste buds per papilla of the tongue decreases with age and taste changes can occur in some conditions such as cancer. In the older adult, the perception of sweetness and saltiness may change and more highly seasoned food may be preferred.

STOP THINK **21.5** What are the particular nutritional needs of older people? Discuss this with your mentor and lecturer.

Odour, visual appearance and texture of food

The odour of food is an important aspect of taste and enjoyment. Conditions such as upper respiratory tract infections can cause a temporary reduction in the sense of smell. Ageing may also be associated with alterations in the sensation of smell. Reduced oral sensitivity or confusion may cause the temperature of food to be misjudged, resulting in a greater risk of scalds and burns.

The visual appearance of food is also important; meals that look unappetising or are poorly presented may reduce interest in eating. The visually impaired will appreciate knowing where different foods are positioned on the plate, and some individuals who have experienced a stroke may only perceive half the plate and therefore need to be reminded about the remainder (see Chs 2 and 13).

The texture of food and the person's perception of their ability to chew it are also important. Problems with mastication appear to increase with age and may often be related to poorly fitting dentures. In some conditions there may be difficulty in coordinating chewing, and the movements of the mouth may be uneven, with a tendency for food to dribble out of one side.

Difficulty in swallowing

Difficulty in swallowing — dysphagia – has a number of causes. It may be due to neurological injury, as in stroke, mechanical or motor obstruction of the oesophagus, oesophagitis and oesophageal cancer. The degree of dysphagia must be assessed by the SALT and local guidelines for the management of patients with swallowing difficulties should be followed. It may be that no oral intake or only soft foods or thickened fluids can be tolerated. If oral intake is problematic or impossible, then enteral feeding must be considered. McLaren (1996), in a study of nutrition in patients with a stroke, found that the responsibility for assisting patients to eat was principally devolved to student nurses and care assistants. Although attention was paid to activities related to positioning of the body, arm movement, communication and attention deficits, little interest was shown in nursing activities relating to impaired lip closure, chewing, swallowing or perception.

Food access

Reduced mobility may cause problems in access to food, choice of place for eating and attaining a comfortable eating position. Care and perhaps some dietary alterations may be required if supine or prone positions have to be adopted for eating. Any difficulty of arm or hand movement or hand–eye coordination may diminish the ability to eat. The person may need assessment for eating aids such as cutlery with special grips or shapes. If the person has to eat one-handed, stabilisation of plates, using a mat, the use of deeper plates or the provision of plate guards may help. Drinking may also be a problem and special cups and glasses are available. If the patient or client suffers from muscle weakness, special lightweight utensils can be ordered. A number of problems may result in difficulties with eating and drinking, but stroke is just one example that can markedly alter many aspects of eating and drinking behaviour (McLaren 1996).

Organising effective mealtimes

Ensuring a supply of nutritious food, at the right temperature and in an attractive and hygienic manner is the responsibility of both nursing and catering services. Although nurses remain responsible for ensuring adequate nutrition (Royal College of Nursing 1996), their role in the preparation and distribution of food has tended to be reduced. Food preparation is not usually a nursing task, but the nurse is responsible for ensuring that food is ordered and should act as advocate between the patient and the centralised catering services. Meals are often delivered to the wards pre-plated in heated trolleys at times dictated by catering service needs. However, some people may need or prefer more frequent, smaller meals. Patients may miss meals due to investigations or treatments and obtaining meals in these cases will require effective liaison with catering services. In the *Guide to the NHS* (DH 2001), the promise is given that people will be provided with good food and given any help needed to order or eat meals. The Guide also states that there should be a 24-h catering service.

Mealtimes

Mealtimes should be a planned part of nutritional care; used appropriately they can be an effective therapeutic event. Meals are often the focal point of the day, providing landmarks that break up the day and lend a familiar pattern to the ward routine. For the older person at home, the arrival of a midday meal may be an important social event; in a busy ward sharing a table may help patients to improve appetite. Mealtimes must not be considered as an inconvenience, disrupting ward activities three times a day. Rather they should be organised to be, where possible, a pleasurable social activity. Properly managed, they can provide a useful focus for social activities in continuing care environments.

To make the most of meals, they should be planned in relation to timing, environment, menu and nutritional value. Allowing individual patients to continue with their normal pattern of mealtimes is good practice; however, the necessities of catering for large numbers may preclude this.

Timing Mealtimes should, ideally, not coincide with other structured ward activities such as medication administration, shift handovers or staff breaks, since there is a risk that they will then be hurried and unsatisfactory for both nurse and patient. Some patients or clients may like to take their time over meals and others will require assistance in eating. Hovering staff, in a hurry to clear away dishes, will not encourage appetite. Even when meals are pre-plated and the trays distributed by domestic staff, it is essential for the nurse to be involved. Timing of meals may have to be a compromise, reflecting the needs of the patient, the ward and the catering service. In continuing care environments, for example, breakfast time could be flexible, especially if cold cereals or a continental style breakfast have been chosen. If the evening meal is served early, a snack and hot drink later in the evening is a useful way of increasing nutrient intake. Some flexibility over mealtimes is preferable in the acute setting but it is essential that an effort is made to meet residents' needs and norms in long-term care. It may be possible for residents to take an active role in choosing menus and deciding on mealtimes.

Environment Ideally the patient will have a choice of where to eat, particularly for individuals in long-stay units. While some may prefer to eat by their bed or in their own room, a separate dining area, distinct from the bed spaces and treatment area of the unit, is ideal. The nature of the open ward, with inevitable sights, sounds and smells of illness, is not conducive to appetite.

The dining area should be decorated to provide a social atmosphere and provided with small tables to allow people to eat in their natural groupings. Provision for those who wish to eat alone or who need assistance is also necessary. Forcing relative strangers to eat together or to have to watch a person with eating difficulties may not aid appetite. Although the eating area may also function as the day room, it can be specifically set up at mealtimes. If a person has visitors during meals, this can be helpful, as relatives can be involved in assisting with eating or enjoy a meal with them. Some Trusts have employed hostesses or volunteers at mealtimes to assist patients with eating (Hobday 1997).

Food selection and presentation

Although nurses do not always serve meals, it is important for them to make sure that each patient receives the right food in sufficient quantities. Patients need to be active in food selection where possible. In a care setting, helping a person to fill in a menu card or offering a choice from a bulk trolley is an important nursing function. Foods should be attractively served, with small inviting portions placed separately on the plate. Presenting a heaped plate of food to a patient with a poor appetite will be counterproductive. For some, large portions of food can be daunting. For those requiring a soft diet, food moulds can enhance the presentation of a meal.

The temperature of food is another factor that affects appetite; care should taken to ensure hot foods are served hot and cold foods are served cold (Ellis 2002). It is also important that food is served using a no-touch technique. Chipped or cracked crockery should not be used as it will not clean properly and can become a source of cross-infection.

Assisting people to eat

When someone has difficulty eating, it becomes the nurse's responsibility to help with this basic activity of living. Assisting a person to eat requires considerable skill. Having to be fed by someone can be a threat to the individual's integrity and self-esteem. This should be recognised and every effort made to minimise the negative aspects. Before preparing for the meal, the dependent person should be offered toilet facilities, followed by the opportunity to wash their hands. Eating is easier and more natural sitting out of bed, but the person on bed rest can be assisted to sit upright and be made comfortable, if this is not contraindicated. An appropriate table is required so that the food can be set out, allowing the person to see the food and indicate preferences. The nurse should sit level with the person and encourage a relaxed social atmosphere.

Food habits The person's food habits must be identified and the rate and manner of assistance with eating and drinking should be at the person's normal pace and pattern. The pace of eating can be controlled by the person if their hand is placed on the nurse's forearm during assistance with feeding and drinking. Plenty of time is essential to allow the person to chew, to pause between mouthfuls and to have a drink when desired. If protection for clothing is required, a normal serviette can be used. The use of plastic bibs or rolls of paper towel may damage self-esteem. Normal crockery should be used if the nurse is assisting the person to eat and drink; if the person is able to participate, then feeding aids may improve independence. Spoons have their place, but knife and fork should be used if possible. The nurse should check that plates and food are at an appropriate temperature and ensure that any bones or fruit pips are removed. The person should be offered mouth care after the meal.

Patient participation A study by ACHCEW (1997) suggested that staff shortages, combined with pressure to undertake other duties, prevented nurses from offering assistance at mealtimes to those who needed it. What the patient can do for themselves they must be given the time and encouragement to attempt. Food and drink can be positioned on the dominant side, well within reach. If a person cannot manage to pour a drink, a glass can be left ready filled. Some individuals are unable to cut up food and require assistance with this. By giving individuals your full attention and allowing them to control the process of eating and drinking as much as possible, the negative effects of having to be assisted to eat and drink can be minimised.

Food supplements People with a poor appetite or dysphagia may not be able to ingest enough food to meet nutritional needs, and supplements of liquid foods between meals may be required. These may be powdered supplements, which are added to milk, or complete formulae supplied ready packaged. Although providing a range of nutrients, these are particularly useful for providing a supplementary energy intake.

Some individuals may need some encouragement to take supplement drinks. Supplements can be presented in a range of ways: frozen to the consistency of a mousse or ice cream or warmed to resemble soup. If an individual's intake is poor, it is important to 'make every mouthful count'. This can be achieved through strategies such as the addition of butter or cheese to vegetables, ice cream to puddings and milk drinks, vanilla or neutral flavour supplements in place of milk on cereals. If a person has a poor intake or requires assistance with eating and drinking, it is important to chart daily intakes of food and fluid and to note in the nursing records which assistance strategies were effective.

For further information, see 'Small is beautiful', in *Eating Matters* (Bond 1997).

ENTERAL FEEDING

Enteral feeding in the context of this chapter refers to the delivery of nutrients directly to the patient's stomach or small intestine via a tube. If a patient is not able to eat or drink sufficiently adequately to maintain nutritional status, enteral feeding should be considered and can be used as the sole form of nutrition or as a supplement to oral intake. Indications for enteral feeding are shown in Box 21.4.

If a person has a functioning gut, enteral nutrition should always be considered before parenteral nutrition (BAPEN 1999). Enteral nutrition is less costly, safer, easier to manage and has fewer side-effects than parenteral nutrition. Compared to parenteral nutrition it is thought to preserve intestinal mucosal structure and function and allow for the absorption and utilisation of nutrients in a more physiologically normal way (BAPEN 1999).

Enteral nutrition is contraindicated in some conditions, e.g. obstruction or incompleteness of the GI tract. The decision as to whether a person is enterally or parenterally fed should be informed by the Nutrition Support Team if present in the clinical setting, or with the input of a dietitian and pharmacist if not. When deciding whether enteral nutrition is appropriate for an individual, ethical and legal issues need to be considered.

For further information on this complex and important area of clinical practice, see Lennard-Jones (1999).

Box 21.4

Indications for enteral feeding

Increased nutritional needs

- Hypercatabolic states, e.g. following extensive burns, major sepsis or severe trauma
- Major surgery. Enteral feeding may be commenced prior to surgery to improve nutritional status

Compromised access to GI tract

- Head and neck surgery
- Obstruction due to tumour, e.g. carcinoma of the mouth or oesophagus
- Oesophageal stricture
- Oesophageal fistula

Inability to eat

- Unconscious
- Confused
- Unwilling to eat, e.g. persistent anorexia due to chemotherapy
- Persistent nausea and vomiting
- Dysphagia, e.g. following stroke

Gastrointestinal disorders

- Fistula
- Reduced absorption in GI tract, e.g. short bowel syndrome, inflammatory bowel disease, gastrectomy

It is essential that a patient receiving enteral feeding has a written plan of care so that all involved with the care of that person are aware of the goals of care, interventions planned and the evaluation strategies. It is also important that the plan of care is made in partnership with the patient or client where possible and that carers are informed where appropriate. Often it seems there is a lack of clarity in care settings as to what the overall plan of care is for an individual, for example why a particular type of tube is used, when it has been placed and the duration of any side-effects.

For examples of plans of care, see Scott et al (1998) and Dougherty & Lister (2004).

The major enteral route via the nose is to the stomach (nasogastric tube), although a tube may also be inserted from the nose to the duodenum (nasoduodenal tube) or jejunum (nasojejunal tube). Post-pyloric placement is indicated when the risk of aspiration is considered high or when the patient's medical condition, e.g. obstruction by tumour, or treatment, e.g. oesophageal surgery, indicates this. Less commonly a tube may be passed via the mouth to the stomach (orogastric tube). Tubes may also be inserted through the body wall into the stomach (gastrostomy) or jejunum (jejunostomy). For short-term feeding, enteral feeding tubes are usually inserted via the nose, but if a tube is required in the longer term, a gastrostomy is the preferred route of choice. As nasogastric and gastrostomy tubes represent the most common approaches to tube feeding, they will be the focus of the rest of this section.

Nasogastric tube insertion and care

Nasogastric tube feeding is indicated when short-term nutritional support is required. As the nasogastric route interferes minimally with oral function, it can be used to supplement oral intake. The tube used should be narrow in diameter and flexible. Tubes that have a wide diameter are poorly tolerated as they are uncomfortable, can cause pressure necrosis in the nose and oropharynx and may encourage cardiac sphincter incompetence, thus increasing the risk of gastric reflux and aspiration. As fine-bore tubes are flexible, a wire introducer may be required when the nurse is inserting the tube. Fine-bore (6–8 FG) feeding tubes of PVC, silicone or polyurethane are available. PVC tubes degrade quite quickly and are less flexible but can be useful for feeding in the short term as they are less expensive. Polyurethane or silicone tubes are for longer term use and can be left in position for up to a month. The exact length of time is detailed in the manufacturer's guidelines. Some of those with a guide wire (single-patient use) may also be reused on the same patient if they are displaced, although the guide wire must only be reinserted into the tube if the tube has been removed from the patient (Bowling 2004).

Insertion of the tube must follow guidelines approved by the clinical setting. Procedures on how to insert tubes with and without guide wires are described in Dougherty and Lister (2004). Nurses may insert tubes safely and effectively in most individuals; however, the insertion of fine-bore tubes following maxillofacial surgery and laryngectomy, or in those individuals with maxillofacial or oesophageal disorders, is not straightforward and in these situations either a doctor (BAPEN 1996) or a nurse with advanced clinical skills in this procedure should place the tube.

Once the tube is in place, then its position may be checked by pH testing of aspirate using pH indicator strips or X-ray (Colagiovanni 1999, Burnham 2000). Air auscultation — the 'whoosh' test — involving the rapid injection of 20–30 mL of air down the tube while listening over the stomach with a stethoscope, is no longer recommended (National Patient Safety Agency 2005). However, no method is foolproof; gastric aspirate may be obtained from the trachea if the person has aspirated, and an X-ray is only accurate at the time it was taken. Guidelines approved by the clinical setting must be followed when ascertaining the placement of a tube and the patient carefully observed for signs of respiratory distress or general discomfort once feeding has commenced.

Following insertion, the position of the tube should be checked before administration of any solution or medication, if the patient complains that the tube feels uncomfortable, if feed is seen in the mouth and following episodes of vomiting, coughing or suctioning. Regular flushing of the tube with water is essential to reduce the chance of blockage (Colagiovanni 2000). A 50 mL syringe is considered to be the most appropriate size of syringe to use for flushing or aspirating, as use of a smaller syringe is thought to generate a higher pressure within the tube (Cannaby et al 2002). Excessive pressure should not be used to force fluids down the tube as this may split the tube wall. It has been suggested that the tube should be flushed with 30 mL of water using a 50 mL syringe at the beginning and end of each feed and before and after giving medication (BAPEN 1999). For some patients, fluid intake may be limited due to their medical condition and therefore smaller amounts of water should be used to flush the tube. Recent guidelines from the Infection Control Nurses Association (Skipper et al 2003) suggest that sterile water should be used to flush tubes in acute health care settings and all tubes which terminate in the jejunum. In the community setting, guidelines suggest cooled, freshly boiled water or sterile water from a newly opened container should be used if the patient is immunosuppressed (National Institute for Clinical Excellence 2003). A 50 mL catheter-tipped syringe should be used to administer fluids. Syringes intended for i.v. use should not be used due to the risk of accidental parenteral administration (BAPEN 2004). Syringes used for the administration of medication or flushing should be discarded after use (Skipper et al 2003).

Premature removal of nasogastric tubes by patients is common (Pancorbo-Hidalgo et al 2001). A nasogastric tube should be secured to the nose and side of the face to prevent the tube from being displaced (Burnham 2000).

The act of eating and drinking cleanses and hydrates the mucosa of the mouth. In patients who are tube fed, frequent mouth care is a priority to keep the mouth in a clean and comfortable condition.

Gastrostomy tube insertion and care

Gastrostomy feeding is used if enteral feeding is likely to continue for longer than a month (Garrow et al 2000) or in some situations where a nasogastric tube is poorly tolerated. This has become a relatively common nutritional intervention. The procedure most commonly used to place a gastrostomy is termed a percutaneous endoscopic gastrostomy (PEG) although tubes may also be inserted radiologically or surgically (radiologically inserted gastrostomy or percutaneous fluoroscopic gastrostomy). Prior to the procedure the patient will require preoperative preparation (see Ch. 26). Gastrostomy placement is contraindicated in a number of medical conditions such as ascites, liver disease and morbid obesity (BAPEN 1996). The doctor in charge of the patient's medical care will assess their suitability for gastrostomy placement prior to the procedure and obtain the patient's written consent. A gastrostomy is normally performed after the patient has received a sedative medication, therefore postoperative care should follow the general guidelines following an operative procedure under sedation outlined in Chapter 26. Complications of gastrostomy insertion can occur, such as bleeding and pneumoperitoneum (BAPEN 1999) and the nurse should observe the patient's condition in the postoperative period carefully.

Following the procedure, tube feeding can usually commence within 6 h but local clinical setting guidelines must be followed because opinion as to when it is safe to proceed with feeding varies (Srinivasan & Fisher 2000). Usually a dressing is not required over the gastrostomy site. Once the site has healed and the stoma formed, the site should be washed daily with water and dried thoroughly (National Institute for Clinical Excellence 2003). Some types of gastrostomy tube need to be rotated regularly once the tract is healed to prevent skin from growing around the tube. The frequency with which this should be carried out is variable, therefore local clinical guidelines must be followed. It is suggested that the tube should be gently pushed in by 1 cm and then returned to its original position whilst rotating it through 360°. The fixation plate should be approximately 5 mm distance from the abdomen and should be undone and pulled back to facilitate cleaning. The patient with a gastrostomy tube should not swim or bathe until the tract has healed.

If the gastrostomy tube is removed accidentally, then immediate action must be taken as the tract will close over within a matter of hours. If the tube cannot be reinserted by the Nutrition Nurse Specialist or doctor within a short period of time, then a replacement may be inserted to keep the stoma patent; fluid should never be infused until the position of the tube has been confirmed by a health care professional experienced in the care of gastrostomy tubes.

Complications as a result of gastrostomy formation are not uncommon and may include infection and leakage (Platt & Roe 2000). Overgranulation of the stoma may also occur; advice on this may be sought from the Nutrition Nurse Specialist or in some situations from the Tissue Viability Nurse. Local guidelines on how to prepare and care for individuals post procedure must be adhered to.

The procedure for the removal of a gastrostomy tube varies according to the type of tube placed. Some tubes can be withdrawn through the stoma, following deflation of the retainer in the stomach; some tubes may be cut and the portion remaining in the stomach removed endoscopically or allowed to pass through the GI tract. If a tube is to be removed, local clinical area guidelines should be followed or the advice of the Nutrition Nurse Specialist or Unit personnel who have placed the tube should be obtained.

Administration of medications via enteral tube

The pharmacist should be consulted if medication is to be given via an enteral tube as there are risks associated with this route of administration such as tube blockage, drug toxicity and a reduction in drug efficacy. The pharmacist is able to advise on the appropriate route, formulation, timing and monitoring. Nurses must be aware that administration of a licensed medicine via an enteral tube is an unlicensed use and that they are professionally accountable for any adverse effects experienced as a result of using this route (Bowling 2004).

The location of the enteral tube needs to be considered before medication is given as some drugs are not absorbed effectively when delivered directly into the small intestine rather than to the stomach. Medications in the form of oral liquid and dispersible tablets are most easily administered via an enteral tube. However, some liquids may be hyperosmolar and cause diarrhoea, especially if directly administered further down the small intestine. Some viscous oral liquids may be diluted with water to ease administration. Tablets may be crushed, but the advice of the pharmacist must be sought. Medication which is coated (film or enteric) is rarely suitable for administration via an enteral tube. Tablets or capsules of cytotoxic, hormonal, steroidal or antibiotic medications should not be crushed or opened because of the potential risk of exposure to staff and others.

The pharmacist is also able to advise on the potential for drug–nutrient interactions; for example, the drugs phenytoin, carbamazepine and tetracycline should not be administered with feed as this can affect the amount of drug absorbed from the GI tract. If several medications are to be given at one time, the tube should be flushed with at least 10 mL of water between each medication (BAPEN 2004) or advice on the suitability of mixing medications sought from the pharmacist. Two drugs may interact with each other and their effects may change as a result.

Selection of enteral solution

There is a wide range of commercially prepared enteral solutions ('feeds') that may be prescribed. Commercially prepared feeds are of a known nutritional content, are sterile and are designed for ease of administration. The dietitian will choose the most appropriate feeding regimen for the patient, basing such choice on assessment of the patient's needs and medical condition. Generally, the dietitian will also order the feed and ensure it is available for the nurses to administer. Feeds may cause GI disturbances when feeding is being initiated or if they are infused too rapidly. Enteral solutions should be administered at room temperature, as administration of a cold feed can cause the patient to experience abdominal discomfort. Enteral solution should be stored according to the manufacturer's instructions and usually requires shaking prior to administration to disperse any sediment formed. 'Use by' dates should always be checked prior to administration.

Method of administration of enteral solution

The equipment for feeding consists of a reservoir, the nasogastric tube, and usually a giving set that connects to the reservoir and a pump. The reservoir may be a bottle or soft pack and may require filling or may be filled with feed at the manufacturing stage. Nasogastric feeds can be delivered intermittently or continuously. Intermittent feeding is the administration of a 'bolus' of feed periodically. Continuous feeding involves the delivery of a feed over a period of many hours. In clinical settings, enteral feeding pumps are commonly used to deliver a steady flow of solution over a period of time. Feeding intermittently reflects more closely the normal eating pattern and permits free movement between feeds; however, it may be more likely to result in feelings of nausea, intestinal distension, cramps and diarrhoea. There may also be an increased risk of reflux and aspiration. The dietitian will prescribe the rate at which a solution should be administered following assessment of the individual. During feeding and for 1 h after, unless contraindicated, the patient should sit up at 30° or higher to reduce the risk of aspiration (BAPEN 1999). The amount of feed remaining in the stomach (gastric residue) can be checked if the individual complains of nausea or gastric distension. In some clinical settings, e.g. intensive care units, checking the amount of feed in the stomach should be carried out periodically; local guidelines should be consulted on this issue.

Monitoring and complications of enteral feeding

Monitoring of a patient on enteral feeding is essential to observe for signs of complications and to ensure nutritional goals are being met:

- Food and fluid intake and urine output should be recorded to identify any changes in fluid balance.
- Temperature, pulse and respiration should be recorded at least twice weekly.
- The patient should be observed for any signs of respiratory distress and their general clinical condition monitored.
- If a gastrostomy is present, the site should be observed daily for signs of infection, skin irritation, leakage, stoma overgrowth or excessive movement of the tube.
- Stool frequency should be recorded.
- Biochemical monitoring should be carried out as directed (BAPEN 1999).
- The patient should be weighed weekly.

Complications of enteral feeding can be categorised into three broad groups: mechanical, biochemical and gastrointestinal/infectious (see Box 21.5). The psychological effects of tube feeding should also be considered, since food has a profound influence on psychosocial well-being. One study highlighted that the placement of a gastrostomy has a major impact on the lifestyle of patients and their carers which can lead to feelings of frustration, loss of freedom, embarrassment and anxiety (Rickman 1998). Those who felt they coped best were those who felt supported by professionals. The enteral tube may affect self-image and impose feelings of loss of control. The nurse should ensure that the nursing care recognises and meets the patient's and carer's needs.

If a patient is likely to be discharged from hospital with an enteral feeding tube in situ, then it is essential that appropriate discharge arrangements are made for the continuation of nutritional care (BAPEN 1994). Russell and Rollins (2002) highlight that there are more people receiving enteral tube feeding in a community setting than in the hospital setting.

PARENTERAL NUTRITION

In parenteral feeding, nutrients in solution are infused directly into the venous system (Finlay 1997). Parenteral nutrition (PN) may be used as a supplement to oral or enteral feeding or it can be the sole form of feeding. The term TPN (total parenteral nutrition) is commonly used, but PN is preferred. This invasive technique is associated with several hazards and problems and should be used only when other methods have been excluded. Appropriate early intervention by PN can prevent or reduce the likelihood of malnutrition developing.

Indications for PN

The risks and expense associated with PN are significant and the key factor to consider when deciding to use this form of feeding is the availability of the GI system. PN will be the method of choice if the GI system is unavailable,

Box 21.5

Complications associated with enteral feeding

Mechanical complications of enteral feeding

Potential complication	Prevention/management
Tube blockage	Flush tube with water regularly (Cannaby et al 2002) Maintain continuous flow of feed Replace tube as required Consult pharmacist concerning appropriate medications Clear tube blockage using solution detailed in local guidelines; these may include carbonated drinks or enzymes
Knotted tubes	Note any pain on tube withdrawal Consult Nutrition Nurse Specialist or doctor if pain is present
Tube displacement	Use correct procedure to insert tube Use appropriate type and length of tube Secure tube firmly Explain need for tube to patient
Aspiration of feed	Elevate head and shoulders by 30° or more whilst feeding and for 1 h after Confirm position of tube prior to use Check gastric residual volume as indicated
Discomfort	Give mouthcare regularly Lubricate lips Use smallest appropriate bore of tube Use alternate nostril for tube insertion
Excessive or inadequate feed flow	Use appropriate procedure to administer feeds Use an enteral feeding pump to administer feeds or follow dietitian's instruction concerning bolus feed administration

Biochemical complications of enteral feeding

Potential complication	Prevention/management
Changes in electrolyte levels	Monitor electrolyte levels in blood as required and act promptly if changes detected
Changes in hydration status	Record fluid input and output Weigh the patient weekly
Refeeding syndrome	Follow dietitian's instructions concerning rate and type of feed Monitor electrolyte levels in blood (see Bowling 2004) Record temperature, blood pressure, pulse and respiration frequently initially Record fluid input and output

Gastrointestinal and infectious complications of enteral feeding

Potential complication	Prevention/management
Nausea and vomiting	Avoid administering high osmolality fluids Avoid rapid infusion rates Administer fluids at room temperature Consult dietitian if nausea is experienced Check residual gastric volume if nausea is experienced Stop feed if vomiting is experienced and consult dietitian Consider antiemetic administration Review procedures used to administer feeds and ensure giving set changed according to clinical setting guidelines
Diarrhoea	Establish cause of diarrhoea: consider medications used, e.g. antibiotic therapy, laxatives and high osmolality fluids, and medical diagnosis Consult dietitian as feed type and rate may need reviewing Administer feed at room temperature If diarrhoea persists, send a stool sample for culture Review procedures used to administer feeds and ensure giving set changed according to clinical setting guidelines
Constipation	Monitor frequency and consistency of stool Contact dietitian, as feed type may need reviewing Encourage mobility Give laxatives as prescribed Ensure adequate water intake
Distension/cramps	Check gastric residual volume of feed Follow dietitian's instructions concerning rate and type of feed Consider antiemetic or antispasmodic use
Stoma site inflammation	Clean site daily Ensure fixation device is in the appropriate position to avoid external pressure at stoma site Avoid the use of a dressing around the site Rotate tube according to clinical setting guidelines Consult Nutrition Nurse Specialist or Tissue Viability Nurse Specialist for advice Send swab from site for microbiological analysis Observe for signs of systemic infection

i.e. cannot be accessed or there is GI failure. Severely malnourished patients may not be able to tolerate the oral or enteral intake required to rectify their nutrition deficits, and supplementary parenteral feeding may be considered. Severe trauma, including extensive surgery, some malignancies and major sepsis can induce a state of hypercatabolism that imposes an enormous demand on nutritional resources. If exogenous nutrients are not available, the catabolic demands can result in a marked loss of body tissues. PN should be considered if a person is likely to be starved for 7 days or more, or, if severely malnourished, after 3 days (BAPEN 1996). Indications for PN include:

- trauma to the GI system which may result in an inability to ingest or absorb foods, e.g. fistulae, perforated bowel
- preoperative malnutrition, e.g. BMI <18 or 20% weight loss
- postoperative complications delaying enteral feeding, e.g. paralytic ileus, obstruction, short bowel syndrome, fistulae, peritoneal sepsis
- acute or chronic GI inflammation which is not responding to treatment, e.g. Crohn's disease, ulcerative colitis, severe gastroenteritis
- malabsorption, e.g. in cancer and cancer chemotherapy or radiotherapy, where there is inflammation of the mucosa
- severe trauma, burns, sepsis and other conditions resulting in a hypermetabolic state
- some cases of pancreatitis
- nausea and vomiting secondary to disease of the central nervous system.

Many people will require only short-term PN, for less than 2 weeks, until GI function has improved sufficiently. Some, however, with prolonged GI failure, will need long-term PN, either at home or in hospital. Whilst there may be 'typical' indications for PN, each patient will have individual needs. In order to support and maintain a patient with PN successfully, a team approach is needed, involving not only the nursing and medical staff, but also the biochemist, pharmacist and dietitian, and the primary care team if the patient is to receive PN at home. Specialist nutrition teams assist patients and their carers to manage PN successfully at home, giving advice on such things as storage of PN bags, management of the regimen and equipment use.

Venous access for PN

PN can be administered through a peripheral or central vein. Central venous catheterisation is currently the route of choice for long-term PN and for those with inaccessible peripheral veins. Infusion into the superior vena cava promotes rapid dilution of the hyperosmolar fluids. The vena cava can be accessed by direct cannulation via the subclavian, external jugular, internal jugular or brachiocephalic veins. Catheters can be inserted by percutaneous puncture or a cutdown procedure. For long-term feeding, i.e. >1 month, then this may be tunnelled. With tunnelling, there is some distance between where the catheter enters the skin and the point at which it enters the vein, which may facilitate better positioning of the catheter and reduce the risk of infection. Increasingly, central venous catheterisation is being carried out through a peripheral vein in the antecubital fossa, using a long catheter that is threaded up to the vena cava (peripherally inserted central catheter, or PICC line). PICC lines are suitable for medium- to long-term PN.

Peripheral lines are often referred to as PIC lines (peripherally inserted catheters) and include both peripheral cannulae and midline catheters. Peripheral cannulation is not suitable for long-term parenteral feeding as the solutions infused are often hypertonic and chemical irritation will result in thrombophlebitis (Kingsbury 1999), but Colagiovanni (1997) advocates peripheral vein access for short-term use, if there is no alternative. The cannula should only be in place for 24–48 h before re-siting it in the opposite arm. The leg veins should not be used for PN because of the risk of deep vein thrombosis and phlebitis. Peripheral midline catheters are typically 20 cm, 22 FG catheters, which are sited in the antecubital fossa and stretch along the vein toward the superior vena cava. These catheters are suitable for short- to medium-term use.

Regardless of the approach adopted, an aseptic insertion technique and careful insertion site management are essential (see Ch. 20). The central venous line should be inserted either in the operating theatre, where maximum control of the environment is possible, or on the ward, using barrier or expanded infection control measures (see Ch. 16). After insertion of a central catheter, an X-ray should be performed to ensure that the line is in the correct position and complications have not occurred.

Administration equipment

All nutrient solutions should be administered through a dedicated feeding line, using a volumetric pump as flow control is important (BAPEN 1996). A large variety of i.v. catheters is available for parenteral feeding. A rigid catheter is more likely to damage the internal lining of the vein and cause phlebitis. A flexible, strong catheter made from an inert, soft material is ideal. It should also be detectable by X-ray, so that the tip position can be checked prior to PN commencing. Silicone or polyurethane catheters are often used, as they appear to be less thrombogenic, although other materials are also common. For peripheral PN, fine-bore catheters (22–23 FG) are being increasingly used. Infusion sets with Luer locks should be used, to allow access to the catheter whilst maintaining a closed system. In-line filters can be used to reduce particulate matter and may help to reduce bacterial contamination, depending on the type of filter employed.

Solutions for PN

Parenteral nutrition, if used exclusively, must meet, as closely as possible, all of a patient's requirements for water, energy, macro- and micronutrients. The fluid and electrolyte intake should cover loss via urine, faeces (especially if diarrhoea occurs), respiration, perspiration and any abnormal losses via wounds or drains. Energy is most commonly provided by glucose and lipid solutions, compounded with other nutrients in a single bag. Lipid solutions provide essential fatty acids and supply 40–50% of the energy. A mixture is better tolerated than glucose alone, as fat reduces the overall concentration of the infusate, relative to glucose, which will reduce the risk of thrombophlebitis.

Nitrogen is generally supplied by amino acid solutions with varying proportions of essential and non-essential amino acids. Micronutrients can be provided by a number of additive preparations that should be added to the bag in pharmacy, as close in time to administration as possible. All nutrient solutions should be compounded, under aseptic conditions, by the pharmacy department or a licensed manufacturer. This will ensure stability of solutions and minimise the risk of microbial contamination.

Complications of PN

General complications associated with PN can be classed as:

- catheter-related complications
- complications associated with the feeding regimen
- difficulties arising from coexisting medical problems
- the psychosocial impact of parenteral nutrition.

Catheter-related complications

Chapter 20 considers the general problems of i.v. therapy. In PN, the particular risks are those related to the long-term use of a central venous catheter and the administration of large quantities of viscous and hypertonic fluid. Chapter 26 discusses the complications which may arise from the insertion of a central venous catheter. Displacement of a peripheral PN catheter can result in damaging extravasation and tissue necrosis. Catheters should be well secured when initially inserted. Catheter fracture can occur from frequent clamping and unclamping of the catheter and can result in air or bacteria entering the system. Air embolism can result from detachment of the catheter from the tubing and is potentially fatal. However, it is quite rare with modern equipment.

Catheter blockage can occur due to blood clots, lipid deposits or precipitation of drugs within the lumen of the catheter, or to equipment failure. The need to change PN bags should be foreseen and changeover accomplished with minimum delay. There is insufficient evidence to support or reject the use of heparin to reduce the incidence of catheter-related thrombosis. Catheters should be irrigated with caution and never if there is no blood return. As with all i.v. therapy, local and systemic infections are a serious risk. It is a particular risk for the patient with a long-term cannula who may be immunocompromised and is receiving PN, as this forms an ideal growth medium if there is any breach of sterility. The sources of infection in PN are essentially the same as those discussed in Chapter 20 for i.v. lines. Thrombophlebitis is often cited as the most common complication associated with peripheral PN (Kingsbury 1999). It is also important to reduce the number of 'breaks' in the infusion system. Feeding lines should not be used for the administration of medications or the withdrawal of blood.

These complications can be avoided or reduced if attention is paid to the management of the line. The emphasis should be on prevention of catheter-related complications. Scrupulous attention to the care of the insertion site, infusion lines and bag changes is essential, and hospital protocols should be observed. Management by Nutrition Support Teams or Nutrition Nurse Specialists has significantly reduced the problem (Lennard-Jones 1992). Usually, changing of PN infusion bags is considered an extended role for the nurse.

Complications associated with the feeding regimen

An understanding of the processes involved in the absorption and metabolism of the nutrients used in PN enables the nurse to appreciate the potential complications that may arise during therapy. On the whole, these complications are metabolic or are associated with the nature of the fluid being administered or the speed of administration, i.e. over- or underinfusion. All feeds should be commenced at the prescribed rate, to reduce the risk of metabolic complications. As with enteral feeding, if the patient has been starved for a long period, problems can arise from sudden feeding, known as re-feeding syndrome. This is caused by a rapid shift of electrolytes, glucose and water, from extracellular to intracellular compartments, and can cause deficits in the extracellular fluid. In severely malnourished patients, feeding should always be commenced very slowly, to avoid this complication, and liaison with the Nutrition Support Team is essential (Riley 2002). The biochemical problems arise because the body's attempts to utilise different energy sources have metabolic effects and the body may not be able to cope with them. For example, high-carbohydrate infusions produce raised levels of carbon dioxide, which in turn influence the respiratory pattern, particularly of patients with concurrent respiratory problems.

Monitoring of PN

Patients need careful monitoring of clinical, laboratory and nutritional indices. These are defined in the BAPEN standards (BAPEN 1996). Baseline measurements of weight, height, temperature, pulse, respiration, blood pressure, full blood count, urea and electrolytes and liver function tests must be established. Monitoring of vital signs, weight, blood glucose and lipidaemia is critical during the immediate period following initiation of PN and regular checks are still required, daily, once PN has been established (Hamilton 2000). For those patients with diabetes, controlled with insulin, use of sliding scale prior to PN is recommended (see Ch. 5, Part 2). Those not controlled with insulin should have blood glucose monitored closely and, if it is regularly above 11 mmol/L, it is recommended that sliding scale insulin is commenced. Local protocols for monitoring the progress of PN should be consulted.

Difficulties arising from coexisting medical problems

The complexity of managing the patient receiving PN is often related to underlying medical problems, e.g. patients with hypertension, arthritis, diabetes, and renal, hepatic or respiratory diseases. Whatever the coexisting medical problems, they will influence the patient's need for, or response to, nutritional support and must be considered in the patient's nursing and medical management.

The psychosocial impact of PN

Many patients receiving PN take nothing by mouth and may have altered sensations and drives associated with both the physical and social aspects of eating. For instance, some individuals experience taste disturbances. A number may be affected by alterations to body image (McDermott 1995). Social and leisure activities may be disrupted and dress code affected by the presence of the line. It is important to support the patient and family and involve them, helping them to explore ways of adjusting or coping with the restrictions. They may require appropriate counselling. Patients on Intravenous and Naso-gastric Nutrition Therapy (PINNT) is a self-help group set up to provide support and network between patients receiving long-term PN and enteral nutrition by tube (see 'Useful websites', p. 812).

THE ROLE OF THE NUTRITION SUPPORT TEAM AND THE CLINICAL NURSE SPECIALIST IN NUTRITION

The establishment of an expert, multidisciplinary nutrition team within care settings to coordinate nutritional care has been recommended by a number of authorities (Silk 1994). Such a team is usually termed a Nutrition Support Team. In a recent UK survey, 41% of hospitals who responded reported they had a Nutrition Support Team (Elia 2002). Membership of a Nutrition Support Team varies between practice settings, but at a minimum usually includes a senior medical doctor, a Nutrition Nurse Specialist, a dietitian and a pharmacist. The team may also include a chemical pathologist and a microbiologist. The responsibilities of a team vary according to the practice setting but usually include ensuring enteral and parenteral nutrition is administered appropriately, providing nutritional education and training, conducting audit and setting standards of clinical practice in nutritional support through the development of policies and procedures. It has been suggested that the presence of a coordinated team approach leads to a reduction in complications associated with enteral and parenteral feeding (Silk 1994, BAPEN 2003). The team can also ensure that the nutritional care of patients within each care setting is standard and follows local and national policy and guidelines.

The Nutrition Nurse Specialist (NNS) is a clinical nurse specialist who works with the Nutrition Support Team. The NNS acts to ensure nursing practice concerning nutritional care is appropriate, follows policy and guidelines and is patient centred. The role of the NNS varies according to the practice setting but generally includes clinical practice, education and training, management, audit and provision of advice and guidance. Research activity may also form part of the role of the NNS.

FUTURE DIRECTIONS

Currently the nutritional care of patients in care settings does vary, both at a regional and a national level. The Council of Europe has recently published national guidelines for hospital food provision, nutritional care and support in response to concerns about levels of malnutrition in hospitals (Council of Europe 2002). In the UK, the advent of national guidelines is a big step forward in ensuring that the practice of health care professionals in the UK is guided by appropriate evidence. Within Scotland, the Nursing and Midwifery Practice Development Unit of NHS Scotland has developed several 'Best Practice Statements' which address nutritional aspects of care (see 'Useful websites', p. 812). The Clinical Resource Efficiency Support Team in Northern Ireland is developing guidelines concerning nutritional care, including home enteral tube feeding, and obesity (see 'Useful websites', p. 812). In England and Wales, the National Institute for Clinical Excellence (NICE) is currently developing guidelines focusing on nutritional support (see 'Useful websites', p. 812).

CONCLUSION

Nutritional care of patients is fundamental to good nursing practice. The importance of the role of the nurse in ensuring nutritional care is carried out appropriately and in accordance with the patient's wishes cannot be underestimated. However, the nurse does not act independently to ensure nutritional needs are met — the involvement of the whole health care team is crucial. The dietitian is central to the nutritional care of the patient and other members of the team make important contributions.

REFERENCES

ACHCEW 1997 Hungry in hospital? Association of Community Health Councils for England and Wales, London

BAPEN 1994 Enteral and parenteral nutrition in the community. British Association for Parenteral and Enteral Nutrition, Maidenhead

BAPEN 1996 Standards and guidelines for nutritional support of patients in hospitals. British Association for Parenteral and Enteral Nutrition, Maidenhead

BAPEN 1999 Current perspectives on enteral nutrition in adults. British Association for Parenteral and Enteral Nutrition, Maidenhead

BAPEN 2003 Nutrition support teams dramatically improve patient care. British Association for Parenteral and Enteral Nutrition, Redditch. Online. Available: www.bapen.org.uk/pressrelease14.htm

BAPEN 2004 Drug administration via enteral feeding tubes. BAPEN, Redditch. Online. Available: www.bapen.org.uk/drugs-enteral.htm

Barasi M E 2003 Human nutrition. A health perspective. Arnold, London

Bond S 1997 Eating matters. Centre for Health Services Research, University of Newcastle, Newcastle-upon-Tyne

Bowling T 2004 Nutritional support for adults and children. Radcliffe Medical Press, Abingdon

British Dietetic Association 2003 Effective Practice Bulletin, issue 32: Challenging the use of body mass index (BMI) to assess under-nutrition in older people. Dietetics Today 38(3): 15–19

British Nutrition Foundation (BNF) 2003 Healthy eating: a whole diet approach. BNF, London

British Nutrition Foundation (BNF) 2004 Welcome to the British Nutrition Foundation. BNF, London. Online. Available: www.nutrition.org.uk

British Nutrition Foundation Task Force 1999 Obesity. Blackwell Science, Oxford

Burnham P 2000 A guide to nasogastric tube insertion. Nursing Times 96(8): 6–7

Buttriss J 2002 Findings of the National Food Survey for 2000. British Nutrition Foundation Nutrition Bulletin 27: 37–40
Cannaby A M, Evans L, Freeman A 2002 Nursing care of patients with nasogastric feeding tubes. British Journal of Nursing 11(6): 366–372
Chapman A 1996 Current theory and practice: a study of pre-operative fasting. Nursing Standard 10(18): 33–36
Colagiovanni L 1997 Parenteral nutrition. Nursing Standard 12(9): 39–43
Colagiovanni L 1999 Taking the tube. Nursing Times 95(21): supplement
Colagiovanni L 2000 Preventing and clearing blocked feeding tubes. Nursing Times 96(17): 3–4
Council of Europe 2002 Practices in relation to nutritional care and support – report from the Council of Europe. Clinical Nutrition 4: 351–354
Delmi M, Rapin C H, Bengoa J M et al 1990 Dietary supplementation in elderly patients with fracture of neck of femur. Lancet 335(8696): 1013–1016
Department of Health 1991 Dietary reference values for food energy and nutrients for the United Kingdom. HMSO, London
Department of Health 1994 Nutritional aspects of cardiovascular disease. Report on health and social subjects, No. 46. HMSO, London
Department of Health 2001 Your guide to the NHS. Department of Health, London
Department of Health 2003a The essence of care: patient-focused benchmarks for clinical governance. TSO, London
Department of Health 2003b Five a day, UK. DH, Leeds
Dougherty L, Lister S 2004 The Royal Marsden Hospital manual of clinical nursing procedures. Blackwell Science, Oxford
Elia M 2002 BANS Report: current aspects of artificial nutrition support in the UK. BAPEN, Redditch
Elia M 2003 The 'MUST' report. BAPEN, Redditch
Ellis J 2002 How benchmarking can improve patient nutrition. Nursing Times 98(44): 30–34
Elmstahl S, Persson M, Andren M et al 1997 Malnutrition in geriatric patients: a neglected problem? Journal of Advanced Nursing 26(5): 851–855
Finch S, Doyle W, Lowe C et al 1998 National diet and nutrition survey: people aged 65 years and older. Volume 1: Report of the diet and nutrition survey. TSO, London
Finlay T 1997 Making sense of parenteral nutrition in adult patients. Nursing Times 93(2): 35–36
Food Standards Agency 2003 Safe upper levels for vitamins and minerals. Food Standards Agency Publications, London
Garrow J S, James W P T, Ralph A 2000 Human nutrition and dietetics. Churchill Livingstone, Edinburgh
Golay A, Bobbioni E 1997 The role of dietary fat in obesity. International Journal of Obesity 21(3): S2–S11
Green S, O'Kane M 2002 Learning to support practice: management of obesity in adults. Practice Nurse 23(2): 36, 38, 40, 42–46
Green S M, Watson R 2005 Nutritional screening and assessment tools for use by nurses: literature review. Journal of Advanced Nursing 50(1): 69–83
Hamilton H 2000 Total parenteral nutrition: a practical guide for nurses. Churchill Livingstone, Edinburgh
Hamilton-Smith S H 1972 Nil by mouth? Royal College of Nursing, London
Henderson L, Gregory J, Irving K 2003 The National Diet and Nutrition Survey: adults aged 19 to 64 years. Volume 2. TSO, London
Hobday S 1997 Helpers at mealtimes. In: Bond S (ed) Eating matters. Centre for Health Services Research, University of Newcastle, Newcastle-upon-Tyne, p 156
Holmes S 1999a Hospital-related malnutrition. Nursing Times Books, London
Holmes S 1999b Nutrition and chemotherapy. Nursing Times Books, London
Hunt P, Hillsdon M 1996 Changing eating and exercise behaviour. Blackwell Science, Oxford
International Obesity Task Force 2000 About obesity. International Obesity Taskforce, Quebec. Online. Available: www.iotf.org
Jackson P 2003 Insights into meeting nutritional needs. In: Grandis S, Long G, Glasper A, Jackson P (eds) Foundation studies for nursing, using enquiry-based learning. Palgrave Macmillan, Basingstoke
Jones J M 2002 The methodology of nutritional screening and assessment tools. Journal of Human Nutrition and Dietetics 15: 59–71
Kingsbury S D 1999 The development of a policy for the administration of peripheral parenteral nutrition. The Pharmaceutical Journal 263(7063): 46–47
Lean M E J 2000 Pathophysiology of obesity. Proceedings of the Nutrition Society 59: 331–336
Lennard-Jones J E 1992 A positive approach to nutrition as treatment. Report of a working party on the role of enteral and parenteral feeding in hospital and at home. King's Fund, London
Maltby J R 1993 New guidelines for preoperative fasting. Canadian Journal of Anaesthesia 40(5 II Suppl): R113–R117
McDermott M K 1995 Patient education and compliance issues associated with access devices. Seminars in Oncology Nursing 11(3): 221–226
McLaren S 1996 Nutrition risks after a stroke. Nursing Times (Nutrition Supplement) 16(42): 64–70
McLaren S, Green S 1998 Nutritional screening and assessment. Professional Nurse (Nutrition Study Guide: Supplement for Self-Assessed Learning) 13(6): S9–S14
McWhirter J P, Pennington C R 1994 Incidence and recognition of malnutrition in hospital. British Medical Journal 308(6934): 945–948
Mulvihill C, Quigley R 2003 The management of obesity and overweight: an analysis of reviews of diet, physical activity and behavioural approaches. Evidence briefing. Health Development Agency, London
National Audit Office 2001 Tackling obesity in England. TSO, London
National Patient Safety Agency (NPSA) 2005 Advice to the NHS on reducing harm caused by the misplacement of nasogastric feeding tubes. NPSA, London. Online. Available: www.npsa.nhs.uk/health/alerts
National Institute for Clinical Excellence (NICE) 2001a Technology Appraisal Guidance No. 22. Guidance on the use of orlistat for the treatment of obesity in adults. NICE, London
National Institute for Clinical Excellence (NICE) 2001b Technology Appraisal Guidance No. 22. Guidance on the use of sibutramine for the treatment of obesity in adults. NICE, London
National Institute for Clinical Excellence (NICE) 2002 Technology Appraisal Guidance No. 46. Guidance on the use of surgery to aid weight reduction for people with morbid obesity. NICE, London
National Institute for Clinical Excellence (NICE) 2003 Prevention of healthcare-associated infections in primary and community care. NICE, London
Nursing and Midwifery Practice Development Unit 2002 Best practice statement: nutrition assessment and referral in the care of adults in hospital. Nursing and Midwifery Practice Development Unit, Edinburgh
Pancorbo-Hidalgo P L, Garcia-Fernandez F P, Ramirez-Pérez C 2001 Complications associated with enteral nutrition by nasogastric tube in an internal medicine unit. Journal of Clinical Nursing 10: 482–490
PHLS Salmonella Committee 1995 The prevention of human transmission of gastrointestinal infections, infestations, and bacterial intoxications. Communicable Disease Report 5: Review No. 11, R158–R172
Pirozzo S, Summerbell C, Cameron C, Glasziou P 2003 Advice on low-fat diets for obesity (Cochrane Review). In: The Cochrane Library, Issue 1. Wiley, Chichester
Platt M S, Roe D C 2000 Complications following insertion and replacement of percutaneous endoscopic gastrostomy (PEG) tubes. Journal of Forensic Science 45(4): 833–835
Prentice A M, Jebb S A 1995 Obesity in Britain: gluttony or sloth? British Medical Journal 311(7002): 437–439
Rickman J 1998 Percutaneous endoscopic gastrostomy: psychological effects. British Journal of Community Nursing 7(12): 723–729
Riley M E 2002 Establishing nutritional guidelines for critically ill patients. Part 1: Professional Nurse 17(10): 580–583; Part 2: Professional Nurse 17(11): 655–658
Royal College of Nursing 1996 Statement on feeding and nutrition in hospitals. RCN, London
Russell C A, Rollins H 2002 The needs of patients requiring home enteral tube feeding. Professional Nurse 17(8): 500–502
Sandy D 1997 Food in care. Macmillan, London.
Scientific Advisory Committee on Nutrition 2003 Salt and health. TSO, London
Silk D B A (ed) 1994 Organisation of nutritional support in hospitals. BAPEN, Maidenhead
Skipper L, Cuffling J, Pratelli N 2003 Enteral feeding infection control guidelines. Infection Control Nurses Association, Bathgate
Smith A F, Vallance H, Slater R M 1997 Shorter preoperative fluid fasts reduce postoperative emesis. British Medical Journal 314: 1486
Srinivasan R, Fisher R S 2000 Early initiation of post-PEG feeding: do published recommendations affect clinical practice?

Digestive Diseases and Sciences 45(10): 2065–2068
Sullivan A 2000 Healthy eating: something to chew over? Nursing Standard 14(21): 43–46
Toubro S, Astrup A 1997 Randomised comparison of diets for maintaining obese subjects' weight after major weight loss: ad lib, low fat, high carbohydrate diet vs. fixed energy intake. British Medical Journal 314: 29–34
United Kingdom Central Council for Nursing, Midwifery and Health Visiting 1997 Nurses are responsible for feeding patients. Register 20: 5
Webb G P 2002 Nutrition. A health promotion approach. Arnold, London
Webb G P, Copeman J 1996 The nutrition of older adults. Arnold, London
World Health Organization 2003a Nutrition. Micronutrient deficiencies. WHO, Geneva. Online. Available: www.who.int/nut/idd.htm
World Health Organization 2003b Nutrition. Controlling the global obesity epidemic. WHO, Geneva. Online. Available: www.who.int/nut/obs.htm
World Health Organization 2003c Diet, nutrition and the prevention of chronic diseases. WHO Technical Report Series 916. WHO, Geneva

FURTHER READING

Barasi M E 2003 Human nutrition. A health perspective. Arnold, London
Bond S 1997 Eating matters. Centre for Health Services Research, University of Newcastle, Newcastle-upon-Tyne
Bowling T 2004 Nutritional support for adults and children. Radcliffe Medical Press, Abingdon
British Association for Parenteral and Enteral Nutrition 2004 Welcome to BAPEN. BAPEN, Redditch. Online. Available: www.bapen.org.uk
British Nutrition Foundation 2004 Welcome to the British Nutrition Foundation. BNF, London. Online. Available: www.nutrition.org.uk
Department of Health 2003 The essence of care: patient-focused benchmarks for clinical governance. TSO, London
Dougherty L, Lister S 2004 The Royal Marsden Hospital manual of clinical nursing procedures. Blackwell Science, Oxford
Food Standards Agency 2003 Safe upper levels for vitamins and minerals. Food Standards Agency Publications, London
Garrow J S, James W P T, Ralph A 2000 Human nutrition and dietetics. Churchill Livingstone, Edinburgh
Jester R, Williams S 1999 Pre-operative fasting: putting research into practice. Nursing Standard 13(3): 33–35
Jordan S, Griffiths H, Griffith R 2003 Administration of medicines part 2: pharmacology. Nursing Standard 18(3): 45–54
Lennard-Jones J 1999 Ethical and legal aspects of fluid and nutrients in clinical practice. Nursing Times Books, London
McLaren S, Crawley H 2000 Promoting nutritional health in older adults. Nursing Times Books, London
Scott A, Skerratt S, Adam S 1998 Nutrition and the critically ill. A practical handbook. Arnold, London

USEFUL WEBSITES

Best Practice Statements (NHS Scotland)
www.nhshealthquality.org/nhsqis/files/20387_Report.pdf

British Association for Parenteral and Enteral Nutrition (BAPEN)
www.bapen.org.uk

British Nutrition Foundation (BNF)
www.nutrition.org.uk

Clinical Resource Efficiency Support Team (CREST)
www.crestni.org.uk/index.html

International Obesity Task Force
www.iotf.org

National Institute for Clinical Excellence (NICE)
www.nice.org.uk

National Patient Safety Agency (NPSA)
www.npsa.nhs.uk

Patients on Intravenous and Naso-gastric Nutrition Therapy (PINNT)
www.pinnt.co.uk

World Health Organization
www.who.int

TEMPERATURE CONTROL

22

Charmaine Childs

INTRODUCTION

The aim of this chapter is to provide an understanding of the factors and processes involved in thermoregulation, i.e. the maintenance of body temperature at a near-constant level. An understanding of the physical, physiological and biological mechanisms will facilitate provision of rational treatment for patients whose thermoregulatory system is disturbed (Edwards 1998). There are a number of reasons why body temperature might rise or fall from the 'normal' range, but before any decisions are made about treatment, the first step is to ensure that measurement is accurate.

Taking a person's temperature is one of the most commonly used methods for detecting disturbances in health, e.g. fever. It is therefore an extremely important clinical measurement but one which is often based on ritual rather than on rational decision making (Edwards et al 2003). The responsibility of the nurse, whether practising in the home or in hospital, is to:

- understand the mechanisms for 'normal' control of body temperature at approximately 37°C
- ensure that temperature measurements are accurate and that the body site used for temperature measurement is appropriate
- monitor and evaluate the impact of any treatments used to regulate body temperature.

It is for the above reasons that patients should have their temperature measured and assessed by a qualified nurse or nursing student under supervision.

NORMAL BODY TEMPERATURE

'Body temperature' is a rather imprecise term, because the body is not at a uniform temperature. For example, skin temperature varies considerably. The skin has been described as a mosaic of temperatures and even 'core' (deep body) temperature can vary slightly. For this reason it is good practice to use the same body site for each temperature measurement and to report the temperature of the site used, e.g. 'Axilla temperature of Mr A on admission to hospital was 36.9°C' or 'Oral temperature of Mrs B was 37.1°C'.

The temperature of the tissues of the body

Surface temperature

Under most circumstances, the skin surface or 'body shell' is the coolest part of the body. The organs, blood and deeper tissues are described as the body 'core' (Tortora & Derrickson 2006). Because the temperature of the skin is influenced greatly by the temperature and humidity of the air (ambient conditions) (see Fig. 22.1), thermometers which measure skin temperature (see 'Infrared radiation thermometers', p. 820) are not sufficiently accurate for precise monitoring of temperature in sick patients where deep body temperature measurements are more reliable. In most circumstances the skin temperature will be lower than the temperature of the axilla, ear, mouth or rectum.

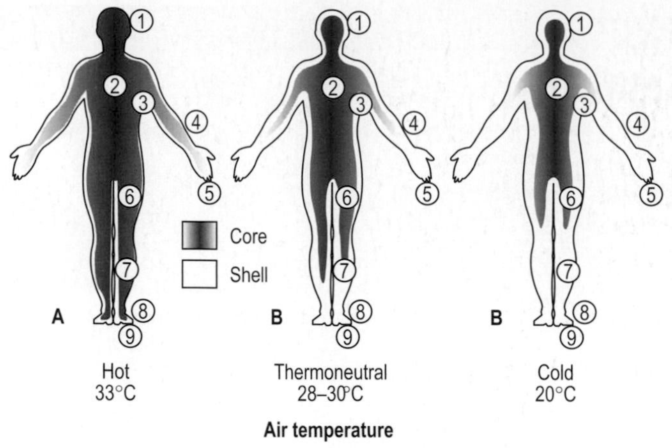

	Site	A (°C)	B (°C)	C (°C)
1	Scalp	36.0	34.8	32.8
2	Chest	35.8	34.5	31.3
3	Axilla	36.5	36.4	36.4
4	Arm	35.9	33.5	27.6
5	Finger	35.9	33.2	21.0
6	Thigh	35.2	33.4	27.8
7	Leg	35.3	30.1	25.2
8	Foot	35.5	29.7	22.7
9	Toe	36.2	29.1	21.4

Fig. 22.1 Core temperature and temperature of the skin surface at various sites in a hot, a thermoneutral and a cold environment. (Based on an original figure by Aschoff & Wever, cited in Stainer et al 1984, with additional data from Childs C.)

STOP THINK

22.1 After examining the temperature data given in Figure 22.1, answer the following questions:

(a) What is the reason for the change in the size of the shell between A and C?

(b) What is the explanation for the higher skin temperatures at the extremities in A compared with C?

(c) What do you notice about the skin temperatures measured over the thigh, leg, foot and toe in A? Why is the pattern of skin temperature in A different from the patterns in B and C?

Deep body (core) temperature

The organs, e.g. heart, liver and brain, and blood (i.e. body core tissues) are 'insulated' from environmental conditions by body fat and skin. The temperature of the body core is generally higher than skin temperature. The liver, kidneys, brain and myocardium have a high metabolic rate and consequently a higher temperature than tissues with a lower rate of metabolic activity such as smooth muscle (Houdas & Ring 1982). Just how much the different core temperatures vary has been the subject of a study by LeFrant et al (2003). This study supports earlier work demonstrating that whilst differences exist between body core sites such as rectum and urinary bladder, any differences are small (Childs et al 1999). This goes some way to dispel the notion that rectal temperature 'lags behind' other core sites.

REGULATION OF BODY TEMPERATURE

Current understanding is that mammalian thermoregulation is controlled by the brain. Observations made in the early 19th century revealed that the body cooled down after severe damage to the spinal cord. Over a century later, the importance of the hypothalamus in the control of body temperature, specifically the pre-optic region within the anterior portion of the hypothalamus (POAH), became recognised as the integrating centre for temperature regulation in the mammalian brain (Berner & Heller 1998). Sensory signals (afferents) from thermoreceptors in the skin and organs are transmitted to and integrated within the POAH, which then responds appropriately by transmitting outgoing (efferent) signals to effector organs. If incoming signals indicate that the body is above the 'normal' thermostat temperature, i.e. >37°C, often referred to as the temperature 'set-point', an 'error signal' is received. The error signal is a useful concept borrowed from engineering theory to describe incoming sensory signals which differ from the brain's thermostat reference temperature. When an error signal is received, the nervous system stimulates activities which protect the person from overheating or from becoming too cold.

For example, if the temperature of the blood bathing the cells of the hypothalamus starts to rise above 'normal' (37°C), as in a fever, the outgoing, or efferent, signals stimulate 'effector' mechanisms so that heat is lost from the body. Conversely, if the incoming blood is at a lower temperature than the reference (set-point) temperature (i.e. <37°C), mechanisms to conserve or produce heat will be activated. In this way, deep body temperature is prevented from fluctuating greatly from its biological set-point of 37°C. The pathways which help maintain body temperature at a constant level are discussed below (see also Fig. 22.2A).

Mechanisms of heat conservation and heat production

Heat conservation

If skin or blood temperature falls, signals from peripheral thermoreceptors, e.g. in skin, are interpreted at the POAH and the heat-promoting centre stimulates mechanisms to retain heat as well as to increase the amount of heat produced within the body (endogenous heat production).

Behavioural thermoregulation The ability of humans to conserve heat by putting on more clothes or seeking shelter from a 'hostile' environment is often overlooked or forgotten, but such behaviours are the most fundamental of the protective thermoregulatory activities and are the 'first line' of defence against extreme heat or cold. Very young and very old people, as well as those who are immobile due to illness or sedation, are unable to protect themselves from heat or cold in this way and are therefore more vulnerable to changes in environmental temperature. It then becomes the responsibility of the nurse to place the patient in a warm and comfortable environment to ensure that thermal homeostasis is achieved.

Peripheral vasoconstriction At about the same time that a person begins to feel cold, changes in the flow of blood to the skin also occur. Nerve impulses from the POAH which are concerned with heat conservation cause blood vessels, particularly in the hands, feet, ears and nose, to constrict. Sympathetic stimulation to nerves supplying the blood vessels in these acral regions results in both peripheral vasoconstriction and a reduction in the flow of warm blood from internal organs to the skin. The result is that heat is retained or stored within the body, where it helps maintain the core tissues at or close to 37°C.

In situations where body temperature continues to fall, despite the above measures, additional mechanisms that involve endogenous metabolic heat production come into play in order to restore body temperature to normal (see non-shivering and shivering thermogenesis below).

STOP THINK **22.2** What steps should be taken by a nurse to help a patient with a low core temperature to retain body heat? What are the harmful or adverse effects of allowing a patient to shiver continuously?

Heat production

In a healthy young adult, the metabolic rate is between 35 and 39 kcal/m^2 body surface/h. In an infant, metabolic rate is 53 kcal/m^2 body surface/h. This difference can be explained by the fact that the rapid synthesis of cells in the growing body of a child contributes to an increased metabolic heat production. Metabolic rate may rise well above the normal limit for a given age in sick or injured patients, particularly those who are febrile and/or have an infection (Childs & Little 1994, Jenney et al 1995).

In early studies (Wilmore 1977), patients suffering from serious burns (see Ch. 30) were found to have a very high metabolic rate; consequently endogenous heat production was almost double that of a healthy person of the same age. The high metabolic rate and heat production were thought to contribute to the very high fever which developed after a major burn. More recent studies suggest, however, that improvements in surgical management, wound care and analgesia have ameliorated the enormous increases in metabolic rate and demand for energy (Childs 1994). As a consequence, the metabolic response to major burn injury is lower than shown in earlier studies; however, fever persists as a common symptom of burn injury (Childs 1994).

Any activity or event which increases the rate of chemical reactions in cells and rate of oxygen uptake by the cell increases metabolic rate and thus the amount of metabolically produced heat (Frayn 1997). Body heat is produced in two ways: chemically by non-shivering thermogenesis and physically by the rhythmical contraction of skeletal muscle, i.e. shivering thermogenesis.

Non-shivering thermogenesis Although peripheral vasoconstriction is very effective in helping to conserve heat, additional heat may be needed to restore body temperature to 'normal'. Initially, this is achieved by non-shivering thermogenesis (NST). As its name implies, NST does not involve muscular contraction to stimulate endogenous heat production, but relies upon release of the thermogenic hormone noradrenaline under the control of the sympathetic nervous system. Although muscle tissue is the most important source of chemically produced heat, other important heat-producing organs are the brain and liver.

Shivering thermogenesis People who are cold shiver, but it should be remembered that shivering does not continue indefinitely (see 'Hypothermia', p. 827). The heat conservation area of the brain stimulates an increase in muscle tone, i.e. shivering, which can increase heat production to five times the basal rate. Shivering occurs in most skeletal muscles but the greatest intensity of shivering thermogenesis is in the jaw and neck and is least in the legs. The repetitive contraction of muscle is not, however, a very economical process, as only 40% of the heat generated in shivering is retained by the body.

Mechanisms of heat loss (see Fig. 22.2B)

High air temperatures and strenuous exercise will raise the temperature of the blood. If the heat gained during the exercise is not matched by an equivalent rate of heat loss, heat-losing mechanisms are initiated and heat-conserving mechanisms are inhibited. The series of events which protect the brain and core tissues from reaching dangerously high temperatures are as follows:

- A high air temperature warms the skin. The rise in skin temperature is detected by skin thermoreceptors which send afferent signals to the thermoregulatory centre in the POAH.
- The first reaction of the person is to reduce body insulation by removing some clothing.
- At the same time, blood vessels in acral regions (hands, feet, ear lobes and nose) dilate so that more blood is brought to the surface of the skin. Areas of the body, such as the face and ears, will then appear 'flushed', pink and warm.
- Providing the air temperature is lower than the skin temperature, heat will be lost by radiation and convection (see Table 22.1). If, however, the air temperature is higher than skin temperature, the person will gain heat from the environment. This is why evaporative heat loss becomes so important when the temperature gradient between skin and air is narrow, i.e. when skin temperature is close to air temperature.
- Stimulation of sweat glands in hot conditions is controlled by the sympathetic nervous system. Production of a fluid consisting mostly of water, but also containing salt, urea, lactic acid and potassium ions, onto the skin causes cooling when the thermal energy needed to transfer the fluid to a gas is removed from the body, i.e. from the skin surface to the air. This transfer of energy from a fluid to a gaseous state is called vaporisational heat loss and occurs during heat loss by sweating.

STOP THINK **22.3** What is the most important route for heat loss in a warm environment?

22.4 What is the collective term used to describe heat loss by radiation and convection?

22.5 Find out which areas of the body are described as 'acral regions'. What is their specific function in thermoregulation?

22.6 After a bath, patients often feel cold and uncomfortable if the nurse is slow in helping them to dry themselves. What is the cause of this feeling of

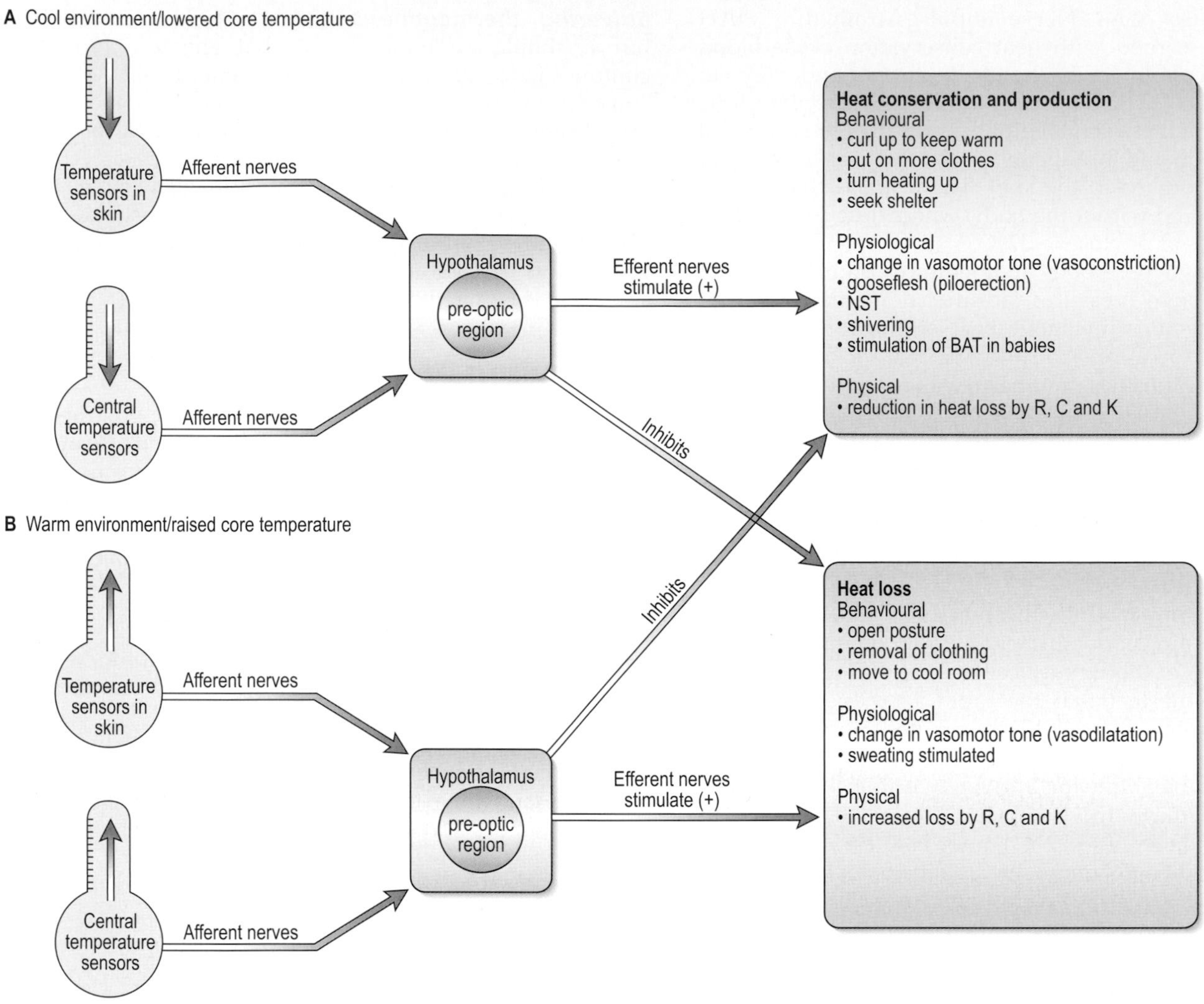

Fig. 22.2 Control of body temperature. A: Responses to a cool environment or lowered core temperature. B: Responses to a warm environment or raised core temperature.

discomfort when the body is wet and the room temperature low? Why would leaving the door of the bathroom open make the patient feel cold? How can the nurse improve the patient's comfort when preparing them for a bath?

FLUCTUATIONS IN A HEALTHY PERSON'S TEMPERATURE

Humans are able to make both physiological and behavioural adjustments to maintain deep body temperature close to 37°C. Like many mammals, humans have the ability to increase the amount of heat in the body as air temperature falls, or to increase heat loss when conditions become uncomfortably hot. It is for this reason that humans are able to survive in most climates on Earth.

Normal temperature range

Although central or hypothalamic temperature is 'set' at a relatively constant level, fluctuations do occur in healthy people, e.g. following exercise. No harm is done to the cells of the body by a change in temperature, providing core temperature does not rise above or fall below certain limits. Indeed, the ability of the thermoregulatory system to stimulate changes in heat production or heat loss indicates that the system is operating efficiently.

In his classic monograph, DuBois (1948) illustrates the range of 'normal' temperature in health. In the early morning or during cold weather, body temperature may fall to 35–36°C. After moderate exercise, and also, for example, in crying babies, core temperature may rise to approximately 38°C; after hard exercise, body temperature can reach 40°C without causing harm. However, an increase of approximately 5°C above 37°C indicates a serious disruption of thermoregulation and a person's life may be at risk if deep body temperature rises above 43°C or falls below 24°C.

STOP THINK **22.7** During one shift of duty, find out how many patients have a high temperature and then answer the following questions:

(a) Give the highest and lowest measured temperatures for each of the patients you have identified as having a pyrexia.
(b) State the site used to measure deep body temperature for each patient.
(c) Has the pyrexia been reported?

Table 22.1 Principles of heat transfer

Route for heat loss	Principle	Relevance to clinical practice
Radiation (R)	Transfer of energy in the form of electromagnetic waves. The human body emits heat as infrared radiation. At the same time all dense objects (furniture, buildings, other people) are also radiating heat. The rate at which heat is emitted from the human body is dependent upon the temperature difference (gradient) between the skin and other objects and surfaces in the room. If the skin is hotter than the average temperature of objects in the room, heat will be lost. If the objects in the room are hotter, the body will gain heat	A person, naked, sitting quietly in a room at 25°C loses between 50 and 70% of heat by R, the major route for heat loss under such conditions. As air temperature increases, the temperature gradient between skin and air falls such that less heat is lost by this route. As air temperature rises towards skin temperature (35°C), the gradient will be so small that very little heat loss can take place by this route. Evaporative heat loss then becomes an important route for heat loss
Convection (C)	Air (or water) next to the body warms and moves slowly away because warm air is less dense and rises. As it moves away from the body, cooler air replaces it. This process can be speeded up if a strong draught (e.g. electric fan) is used to force the air away and cause a rapid replacement of warmed air with cool air	Nurses frequently increase the rate of heat loss by convection by placing electric fans close to their patients. This can be a very efficient way to lower skin temperature, but frequently the cool stimulus results in an inappropriate response, i.e. peripheral vasoconstriction. Heat retention within core tissues then causes core temperature to rise rather than fall. In febrile patients who have an elevated set-point, the use of electric fans is likely to exacerbate the problem of pyrexia
Conduction (K)	Heat loss by K involves transfer of thermal energy from atom to atom. The skin must be in contact with cooler or hotter objects for heat exchange to take place by K	Critically ill patients are often nursed on special beds designed to reduce the incidence of pressure ulcers. These beds are often maintained at a constant temperature to help prevent heat loss from the body. Sometimes the thermostat can fail and patients have been known to overheat or to cool because the temperature of the bed is too high or too low. Patients must be protected from body temperature disturbances of such an iatrogenic nature
Evaporation (E)	Evaporation of water from the skin and respiratory passages is the most important route for heat loss in hot conditions. The evaporation of water occurs when energy transforms water and sweat droplets to a gas. The heat (or thermal energy) needed to drive this process is taken from the body. Thus the more water there is on the skin, the more heat is taken from the body to turn it into a gas (vaporisation). The more heat removed from the body in the process of E, the more the body cools. The function of sweat (produced under the control of the sympathetic nervous system) as an agent for vaporisational heat loss can be enhanced by spraying the body with a fine mist of warm water	Patients with a high core temperature may not always sweat. During a rise in rectal temperature the body responds as though it were too cold and if patients are observed carefully it will be seen that their skin is dry. At this stage the hypothalamic set-point is above normal but the body continues to activate heat-conserving mechanisms to achieve the new set-point temperature. Only when the patient has reached the new central temperature set-point will heat loss by all routes (E included) be activated. Thus when nurses notice that patients with a high core temperature are sweating, it is more likely to indicate that core temperature has reached the new set-point. A fall in body temperature may then follow

(d) What are the possible reasons for the pyrexia?
(e) Has the cause been identified and treated?
(f) How frequently is the temperature being monitored?

Circadian rhythm

Body temperature fluctuates in a characteristic pattern over a 24-h period. It is thought that this pattern is a result of regular, but normal, deviations of the body's own thermostat or hypothalamic set-point temperature. As with many other physiological functions, thermoregulation displays a circadian rhythm or diurnal variation. This rhythm persists during short periods of night work. Eventually, however, regular night work will reverse the normal pattern so that lower temperatures occur during the day and higher temperatures at night.

In general, the lowest temperatures recorded over a 24-h cycle will be approximately 0.5°C lower than the afternoon temperature. By the evening, body temperature may be as much as 1.0°C above the early morning temperature. In the newborn, a circadian rhythm of core temperature is not fully developed (Waterhouse et al 2000).

An awareness of the normal changes in deep body temperature in health is necessary if nurses are to interpret temperature measurements correctly. For example, a moderately elevated axilla temperature recorded during the afternoon should be monitored closely before any action is taken because of the cyclical nature of body temperature, otherwise treatment for pyrexia could be instigated unnecessarily.

STOP THINK **22.8** For this project you will need to measure the temperature of a healthy person every 2–4 h. You will need to ask for help from your partner, parents, siblings or friends — someone who will not mind being woken at night for the sake of this exercise. Plot your subject's oral temperature every 2–4 h for 24 h onto graph paper. From the data you collect, try to identify a circadian rhythm in your subject. State the highest and lowest temperatures recorded over the 24-h period. You should now be able to state the overall variation in body temperature of a healthy subject.

Other factors affecting a healthy person's temperature

Age The age of a patient must be taken into account in the interpretation of body temperature.

Babies and young children As long ago as 1937, Bayley and Stolz showed that rectal temperature begins to rise during the first 7 months of life, remaining fairly constant until the age of 2 years, after which it begins to fall. Average rectal temperature at age 1 month was reported to be 37.1–37.2°C, at 8 months 37.6–37.7°C, and at 18 months 37.7°C. By the time the children in the Bayley and Stolz study approached their third birthday, rectal temperature had settled to 37.1°C.

Healthy children tend to have a higher deep body temperature than adults and therefore their 'normal' range differs slightly. Higher temperatures in early childhood are thought to be a result of increased cellular and metabolic activity. The young of most mammals have a large body surface area relative to their body weight. As a result, babies have a higher risk of hypothermia because they cannot shiver and cannot increase their body insulation, as can adults, by putting on more clothes. This means that the naked baby will lose relatively more heat than the adult for every square metre of their body surface. Babies are therefore reliant on parents and carers to protect them from extremes of environmental temperature.

To counteract their vulnerability to increased heat loss, babies have an important source of body heat in the form of brown adipose tissue (BAT), a specialised type of fat cell (Cannon & Nedergaard 2004). BAT is a unique type of adipose tissue, shown by Hull (1976) to be an important source for heat production in small hibernating mammals and has been described as the 'hibernating gland'. BAT is also stimulated in the human newborn infant. Under the control of the sympathetic nervous system, the function of BAT is to transfer energy from food into heat (Cannon & Nedergaard 2004). BAT is activated after birth. In babies, BAT has probably played a role in the evolutionary success of mammals. BAT can be found around the kidneys, between the shoulder blades, around the great vessels and deep within the axillae (Frayn 1997). BAT is richly supplied with blood and oxygen and this dense blood supply is responsible for its brown colour. It becomes much less important in maintaining the temperature of the body as a baby gets older. In adults, BAT is scarce and probably not functional (Klaus 2004).

Adults and older people Unlike small infants, who rely principally on 'switching on' heat production to maintain a stable deep body temperature, adults are more efficient at conserving body heat. In other words, they rely on preventing body heat from being lost, either by putting on more clothes (behavioural thermoregulation) or by vasoconstriction at the extremities (physiological thermoregulation).

Older people, however, often have a lower body temperature than children or younger adults, for which there are a number of reasons:

- After the age of about 50 years, the metabolic rate starts to decline and, correspondingly, metabolic heat production also falls. Consequently, deep body temperature tends to be lower.
- Social and economic factors contribute to the inability of some older people to keep warm, particularly in winter, because, as people grow older, it is more difficult for them to detect extremes in temperature (see Ch. 35). This puts them at risk of hypothermia (see Box 22.1).
- In warm conditions, deep body temperature in older people may rise slightly because the ability to sweat is reduced. Evaporative heat loss is therefore less efficient at a time when increased heat loss is needed to keep the temperature within the normal range.

STOP THINK **22.9** When you have the opportunity, either at work or at home, record the temperatures of three or four people before and after they take a hot drink and before and after they smoke a cigarette. What differences do you observe?

Exercise Vigorous exercise can raise both oral and rectal temperature by several degrees. Temperatures above 40°C have been recorded in marathon runners and, after a game of rugby, rectal temperatures over 39°C can occur. This rise in temperature can persist for many hours and represents an imbalance between heat production and heat loss (see pp. 814–816).

The menstrual cycle It is now well recognised that 80% of healthy women have higher oral temperatures at the time of ovulation and a record of early morning oral temperature is used to reflect this.

On waking, oral temperature should be recorded before getting out of bed. This provides a resting, baseline temperature. Body temperature should then be recorded at the same time every day throughout the cycle. A slight drop in temperature occurs 24–36 h after ovulation. Temperature then rises abruptly by 0.3–0.4°C and continues at this slightly higher level for the rest of the cycle. Three days after the onset of the higher temperature is generally thought to coincide with the end of the fertile phase. The 'hot flushes' associated with the menopause are discussed in Box 22.2.

Eating a meal Mastication, digestion, absorption and assimilation of nutrients produce body heat. This metabolic heat production was originally described as the specific

Box 22.1

Helping older people to keep warm in winter

There will always be cold spells during the winter months and some will be much worse than others. Weathermen frequently refer to the more extreme conditions as a 'cold snap' and their advice, particularly to older people who are watching their forecast on television, is to make sure that they keep warm. The problem is that keeping warm usually means keeping the heating on for longer than usual, with a consequent rise in heating bills. In recognition of this, the government provides a small annual winter fuel payment to all pensioners. However, older people become cold for many reasons and not only during extremely cold spells.

The housing stock in which many older people live becomes damp and cold if maintenance and repairs are not kept up to date. It is expensive to keep old houses warm at any time of year, but especially in winter. If older people cannot be persuaded to keep their heating on during the winter, it can be helpful for family, friends and neighbours to offer good advice about keeping warm.

The obvious suggestion for someone on a low income would be to heat just one room, i.e. the room in which most time is spent. An alternative is to conserve body heat by wearing extra layers of clothes. These should be comfortable but effective in retaining body heat. The most important principle to remember is that there is no particular merit in one kind of material compared to another, except in its capacity to trap air. Clothes made of cotton are as good as down feathers in this respect. The problem is that feathers can be easily compressed, and when this happens the insulating properties are reduced. It is worth advising people who use a down quilt to keep it 'fluffed' for maximum insulation.

Covering parts of the body exposed to draughts, i.e. hands, feet and head, should be done in much the same way as for a person in a cold climate. Although the head is generally heated by a plume of warm air rising upwards from the body, this band of warm air can be blown away if the person is sitting in a draught. People who spend a lot of time relatively immobile in a draughty house should be advised to wear something on their head like a hat, cap or even a Balaclava. The reasons for taking so much care to keep warm are obvious: lives can be saved by these simple yet effective actions.

In December 2003, the discovery of two pensioners who had died weeks after their gas supply was cut off, because of an unpaid bill, sparked huge media coverage and general concern about the plight of older people dying as a result of fuel debt. Age Concern has published data on their website (see 'Useful websites'), stating that in 2001 there were 10.8 million older people in the UK. In the year 2000, 165 people aged 65 years or over died as a direct result of hypothermia. These data were obtained from the information given on the death certificate. However, many more deaths may be indirectly related to accidental hypothermia in our older population.

The UK remains one of the worst countries in the world at coping with unseasonal low temperatures and everyone needs to be vigilant about looking after older family members and neighbours during a 'cold snap'.

Box 22.2

Hot flushes

The exact cause of 'hot flushes' in menopausal women is not known, but there is evidence that a defect in thermoregulatory function may be responsible for the discomfort and distress associated with the hot flush. The two physiological changes which characterise hot flushes are sweating and cutaneous vasodilatation. During a hot flush, central temperature falls in response to heat lost from the skin surface after peripheral vasodilatation and sweating. Sufferers feel very warm and uncomfortable and want to cool themselves. Since the flushes frequently occur at night (night sweats), they can cause great distress and make it difficult to get a good night's sleep.

It is thought that hot flushes are the result of a sudden fall in the central hypothalamic thermostat. This would result in the body being too hot and stimulating heat loss mechanisms such as sweating and vasodilatation. Over 25% of women who had between 3 and 12 months' amenorrhoea, and 37% who were menopausal, experienced hot flushes several times a day (Guthrie et al 1996). Because hot flushes occur during the climacteric and are associated with cessation of ovarian function, their underlying cause is thought to lie in changes in the endocrine system.

Reporting of hot flushes is greatest 3 months or more after the final menstrual period. The frequency of hot flushes is associated with increasing follicle-stimulating hormone (FSH), a reduction in estradiol and a history of menstrual complaints. Since oral oestrogen replacement therapy is highly effective in alleviating hot flushes and night sweats, a hormonal cause for the symptoms seems evident (MacLennan et al 2001).

dynamic action (SDA) of food. Metabolism of protein has a greater effect in generating heat than the metabolism of carbohydrate or fat. Today, the term 'diet-induced thermogenesis' (DIT) is more often used (Frayn 1997).

The source of body heat — chemical thermogenesis

Heat is expressed in 'energy units' called calories (cal), or more usually in larger units, kilocalories (1 kcal = 1000 cal). The SI unit for energy is the kilojoule (1 kJ = 4.18 kcal).

Since nurses are involved in measuring body temperature, it is important for them to understand how body heat is generated. Most of the energy needed for growth and repair of tissues, for work and for body warmth comes from the food we eat. Most packaged foods have a label which gives the amount of energy (in kcal or kJ) contained in an average serving (or per 100 g) when oxidised or burned by the body. Heat is a by-product of oxidation and the process by which it is produced is called chemical thermogenesis. The rate at which heat is produced in the body is referred to as the metabolic rate.

Metabolic rate

If an awake, resting, lightly clothed man fasts overnight for 12 h in a warm (28–30°C) room, his metabolic rate, and thus his energy expenditure, will be at a minimum or basal level (basal metabolic rate, BMR). If the man increases his activity, by walking, exercising or even shivering, metabolic rate will rise because more oxygen is being utilised. When this happens, some of the additional energy will be used in order to perform the exercise, i.e. to move from sitting to walking (between 2 and 25%, depending on the activity), but most will be lost as heat.

A business man or woman spending most of the day at the office and taking little exercise has a relatively sedentary lifestyle. They can expect to increase their energy requirements by 25–40% above the basal rate during the course of a day. Assuming that all their energy requirements were provided from the food they ate on that day (100%) and no energy was stored, approximately 10% would be lost as heat, as a by-product of the work involved in processing their food, 50% would be lost as heat in the conversion of potential energy in food to high-energy biochemical bonds, and 20% would be lost as heat as a result of internal work, e.g. respiration, cell pumps, glandular activity. In this example, only 20% of the individual's energy intake would be used for external work, e.g. muscular contraction for walking, and the remaining 80% is lost as heat (Wilmore 1977). It is clear that utilisation of food energy is a very inefficient process because most of our energy intake is lost as heat. However, the rate at which heat is produced does not necessarily reflect the rate at which it is lost from the body, because heat can be retained and stored. One of the most important stimuli for body heat storage is a slight fall in core temperature, particularly if the person is in a cool environment. Although a large amount of the energy from food is lost from the body as heat, it is known that many people eat more than is required. Thus, if the amount of calories ingested in food is in excess of the amount of calories used, then energy is stored and the person gains weight. If this is the case, the person is said to be in positive energy balance (see Ch. 21).

THE MEASUREMENT OF BODY TEMPERATURE

Thermometers

The clinical thermometer

The development of a reliable thermometer was made possible only after scientists came to an agreement about the meaning of temperature and devised a scale to measure it. The scale with which most nurses will be familiar in clinical practice is the Celsius or centigrade scale determined by Anders Celsius (1701–1744). The mercury-in-glass thermometer has been the standard temperature-taking instrument for the last century. For many years it was the most practical way of measuring oral, axilla and even rectal temperature, but with modern instruments and techniques the mercury-in-glass thermometer is now rarely used.

Infrared radiation thermometers

Radiation from the sun travels through space mostly in the form of visible light and infrared rays. On striking a body, these waves are partly reflected and partly absorbed and can cause a rise in temperature. The skin absorbs as well as radiates infrared waves (infrared radiation). These waves are part of a 'family' of waves called the electromagnetic spectrum and can be detected with the aid of a special lens (detector) incorporated into a hand-held thermometer.

The tympanic thermometer

This is the basic principle behind the tympanic (ear) thermometer which detects radiant heat emitted from the tympanic membrane. Since the tympanum (ear drum) shares a blood supply with deep parts of the brain, tympanic temperature is considered to be a very good substitute for deep body, even brain temperature.

The key point in this measurement technique is to ensure that the 'lens' is inserted correctly so that it can 'see' the tympanum. If the lens is focused towards the skin of the ear canal, the measurement is likely to be inaccurate. Tympanic thermometers are safe for use even in babies, do not present any risk of perforation to the ear drum and a recording is available in 1–2 s. The problem is that the accuracy of tympanic thermometers has been questioned. When comparisons were made of results from three different brands of tympanic thermometer with results from rectal thermometers, the data suggested that the tympanic thermometers had an unacceptable sensitivity (Hoffman et al 1999). In the Emergency Department where the thermometers were tested, differences between tympanic and rectal temperature were as much as 2°C. These data support the results of earlier studies (Talo et al 1991, Brogan et al 1993, Childs et al 1999) and a more recent meta-analysis (Craig et al 2002) confirmed that tympanic thermometers are frequently unreliable as a surrogate for 'true' core temperature.

Skin surface thermometers

Small infrared thermometers have also been developed to measure the skin surface temperature. The great benefit of these instruments is that they can be held in the nurse's hand just a few centimetres from the skin surface and a measurement can be made in a few seconds. The thermometer does not need to touch the skin. This is a useful way to measure skin temperature, e.g. after trauma or vascular surgery, since the temperature of the skin surface gives a reasonable indication of skin blood flow (Stoner et al 1991).

In plastic surgery, surface temperature measurements are a useful and often important way of diagnosing burn depth (Cole et al 1991, Wyllie & Sutherland 1991), the deeper burn being colder than surrounding tissue (see Ch. 30). After transplantation of skin flaps, a change in temperature of a flap could indicate poor vascular supply, if lowered, or infection, if raised.

Electronic thermometers

Although the mercury-in-glass thermometer is a reliable method for body temperature measurement, electronic thermometers have improved both safety and speed of measurement and revolutionised temperature monitoring for nurses in the UK over the last 20 years. Thermometers such as the IVAC reduce the time taken to obtain an accurate measurement using the traditional clinical (mercury-in-glass) thermometer from approximately 9 min to 1 min. For a single 'spot' measurement, electronic thermometers are quick and simple to use.

Tempa-Dot thermometers

In 1999 a new 'generation' of single-use clinical thermometers became available. The 3M company introduced a single-use (disposable) clinical thermometer which was considered to be a more convenient and hygienic alternative to mercury-in-glass and electronic thermometers. This thermometer is also useful in frail older patients, as well as those patients with stroke, where keeping the electronic thermometer in the mouth can be difficult and uncomfortable. Each thermometer has a series, or matrix, of temperature-indicating dots at the tip. Within each dot, a different combination of chemicals melts, changing colour from beige to blue at intervals of 0.1°C. The temperature is read from the number of dots that have changed colour. The range of temperature which can be measured with the Tempa-Dot thermometer is 35.5–40.4°C.

Whilst Tempa-Dot thermometers have some advantages over other methods, nurses should be aware that temperatures below 35.5°C or above 40.4°C will not be detected. These thermometers are therefore not suitable for temperature measurement when hypo- or hyperthermia is suspected but are considered useful in paediatrics (Macqueen 2001), correctly identifying fever in children with a sensitivity of 92% (Morley et al 1998).

Taking temperatures

Recording an accurate body temperature depends not only on the reliability of the instrument, but also on the clinical skill of the nurse. Even the most accurate of instruments will give an incorrect reading if the nurse has a poor temperature-taking technique. Table 22.2 gives some useful tips to help nurses improve clinical practice.

Table 22.2 Sites for body temperature measurement: advantages and disadvantages

Site	Nursing practice	Advantages	Disadvantages
Axilla	Place in centre of armpit, hold arm against chest. Leave in position for 9 min	Ideal for temperature measurement in babies and toddlers	Less accurate than oral or rectal measurements but can be a reasonable indicator of core temperature if thermometer is left in situ for the required length of time. Since measurement is not taken in a body cavity, there is more chance of external influences affecting the result
Rectum	Insert rectal thermometer 4 cm into the anus (adults) or 2–3 cm in an infant. Leave in situ for 4 min	Suitable site for babies or for unconscious patients who need continuous temperature monitoring	Unacceptable for routine monitoring in some conscious patients, although seriously ill patients with fluctuating conscious levels may require rectal temperature monitoring. Rectal temperature may be higher than at other sites.
Ear (auditory canal) (e.g. using the Core Check thermometer, Ivac, Basingstoke, UK)	Ensure the 'lens' of the thermometer is clean (free from cerumen or ear wax). Apply lens cover. Gently hold the pinna and insert probe into the auditory canal. In small children it is important to pull the pinna gently backwards to straighten the ear canal (refer to manufacturer's instructions). Ensure lens is directed towards the tympanum and not to the skin inside the ear canal. After pressing the thermometer 'start' button, a bleep will be heard. It is advisable to repeat the measurement in the opposite ear to ensure parity of measurements in both ears. However, there is sometimes a difference between the temperature of the ears. This is particularly true in hospital where measurements are made on patients who have recently been lying on their side, with their ear on a pillow	Quick and easy to use, with little danger of ear perforation, even in babies. Always remember that thermometers must be calibrated regularly (6-monthly) by the hospital technical department	Unreliable measurements can occur if the ear is inadvertently cooled or warmed, either naturally or by recent local heating/cooling; e.g. if a tympanic temperature measurement is taken in patients who have recently been in a cold environment, or if patients are receiving body cooling treatment for a high temperature, especially where the scalp is involved. Where repeat measurements are made in the same ear, repeated placement of the thermometer in the same ear may cause the measurement to be lower each time it is made, because the instrument casing may slightly lower the temperature inside the ear canal

In the conscious patient, the options for deep body temperature measurement are limited to conventional sites such as the axillae, mouth and tympanum (auditory canal). However, when patients are critically ill, accurate temperature measurement becomes a priority. The patient's temperature may need to be measured at a site which allows the thermometer to remain in situ for many hours, i.e. for continuous monitoring. This is common in the intensive care unit. In such cases, body core temperature can be measured using indwelling thermometers (thermistors) placed in the rectum, oesophagus, nasopharynx or urinary bladder. Continuous temperature measurements are provided from bedside monitoring systems.

Special cases

In the brain-injured patient, a rise in temperature of 1–2°C above normal is linked to a poor neurological outcome (Natale et al 2000). Accurate measurement of brain temperature is therefore desirable. For many years this was not possible outside the laboratory but today, brain temperature monitoring can be performed at the bedside. Brain temperature can be measured within brain tissue (parenchyma) as well as in the ventricles and is usually undertaken in conjunction with routine monitoring of intracranial pressure (Childs et al 2005).

STOP THINK

22.10 Ask a qualified nurse to help you with this exercise. With a patient's consent and cooperation, measure oral and axilla temperature at intervals of 1, 3, 5 and 9 min. Compare the results. Are there differences in the values recorded at the two sites?

22.11 If you have some experience of using an electronic thermometer, comment on the advantages (if any) of this technique of measuring deep body temperature compared with the mercury-in-glass thermometer.

22.12 Ask your mentor or the charge nurse on the ward where you are working to tell you about the cost of temperature taking and how much of the ward/unit budget is allocated to temperature measurement.

DISTURBANCES IN TEMPERATURE REGULATION

The aim of this section is to supplement the nurse's understanding of thermal physiology with examples of abnormal or disturbed thermoregulation.

Table 22.3 gives examples of clinical conditions associated with a rise in body temperature. The causes of increased body temperature can be divided into two categories:

- a rise due to fever
- an increase as a result of heat illness.

Table 22.3 Changes in body temperature

	Cause	Clinical examples	Appropriate treatment
Fever	Elevation of hypothalamic set-point by endogenous pyrogens such as cytokines, interleukin-1 and interleukin-6. Both are released from the patient's own white cells in response to bacterial or viral infection or to damage to skin and tissues	Infection: bronchitis, malaria, sepsis, meningitis Trauma: burn injury, minor and major surgery, myocardial infarction, thrombophlebitis	Antipyretic medications such as aspirin or paracetamol return altered set-point temperature to a lower level. Avoid external cooling as this may exacerbate the rising core temperature
Heat illness	Increased metabolic heat production, *or* Reduction in the rate of heat loss (by R, C and E) from the body surface (see Table 22.1)	Heat stroke resulting from high air temperature, overwrapping (children/older people) and excessive clothing, or due to increased exercise or work in hot conditions where dehydration and reduced sweating are common associated factors	External cooling: 1. Increase radiant and convective heat loss by removing clothing and helping 'stir' the air around the subject. Avoid cold draughts. Do not use ice packs, as these can increase vasoconstriction 2. Increase evaporative heat loss by applying a fine mist of warm water (40°C) over the body and exposing as much of the skin surface as possible to the air
Malignant hyperpyrexia	Largely unknown. Patients found to have an underlying inborn error of muscle metabolism, usually triggered by general anaesthesia	Hyperthermia occurs shortly, or immediately, after general anaesthetic, in apparently normal patients. Once body temperature starts to go up, it does so very rapidly, by as much as 1°C every 5 min. Temperatures as high as 46°C may be reached, with tachycardia, cyanosis and loss of consciousness	Active cooling, maintenance of cardiac output, correction of metabolic disturbances, e.g. hyperkalaemia, acidosis. Administration of dantrolene sodium

It is important to recognise the fundamental differences between these two main causes of raised body temperature as well as to appreciate their implications for treatment.

Fever

The high 'core' or deep body temperature associated with fever is due to an upward re-set in the central hypothalamic set-point temperature (see p. 814). If the set-point is shifted, for example from 37° to 39°C, thermoreceptors in the brain detect a discrepancy between the set-point temperature and the temperature of the blood circulating (37°C) through the hypothalamus. This is the error signal described on page 814. Since blood temperature is lower than the new, raised set-point temperature, heat gain mechanisms will be stimulated to achieve an increase in the temperature of the 'core'. This can be observed when the febrile patient complains of being cold and pulls on more bedclothes or turns the heating up. Patients do this even when their core temperature has started to rise. They complain that their hands and feet feel cold and this is due to the blood in the skin being diverted away from the 'shell' to the central 'core'. The patient may also start to shiver. Very vigorous shivering is called a rigor. The occurrence of febrile convulsions in young children and the related nursing care is discussed in Box 22.3.

As body temperature rises, heat loss mechanisms are inhibited or 'switched off'. These thermoregulatory changes help the temperature to reach the new set-point level. At this stage, the nurse should not try to lower the patient's temperature by cooling, either by tepid sponging or with electric fans, because by doing so the stimulated heat conservation mechanisms already in operation will be counteracted. However, once the temperature of the blood and core tissues are at the new 'set-point' level and sufficient heat has been stored within the body to sustain the new set-point temperature, the patient will become more comfortable despite the higher (febrile) temperature.

The set-point will not remain at the higher level. Eventually, the biological effects of the pyrogen (see below) will wear off and the thermoregulatory 'set-point' will abruptly return to normal. When this happens, the patient will feel uncomfortable and hot. Hands, face and feet will become red as peripheral vasodilatation replaces vasoconstriction. Vasodilatation allows skin blood flow to reach the most superficial layers of skin so that heat exchange from core tissues to the skin surface and from the skin to the air can take place. At this stage the patient should be put in the best position to allow dissipation of body heat naturally. Forcing heat loss by causing excessive draughts or allowing the temperature of the room to fall so low that the patient quickly becomes cold will make them uncomfortable and possibly induce peripheral vasoconstriction again. If this happens, heat loss by radiation and convection will be reduced. Patients often have a drenching sweat when their set-point returns to normal. It is, however, possible to encourage heat loss by evaporation by spraying the patient with a fine mist of warm water. The use of non-steroidal anti-inflammatory drugs (NSAIDs) in the treatment of fever is discussed in Box 22.4.

Box 22.3

What to do in the event of a febrile convulsion

Febrile convulsions occur in 40 out of 1000 children and it has been estimated that 30% of all convulsions in children occur during a febrile episode. Approximately 2–5% of all children have at least one convulsion in association with fever by the time they are 5–7 years of age.

Febrile convulsions generally occur in normal children between the ages of 6 months and 5 years. Simple febrile convulsions are probably not harmful. They are brief, lasting only seconds or a few minutes. They occur soon after the onset of fever and it is the height of the fever rather than the speed of the rise in temperature that is thought to be an important contributing factor. However, there are some situations in which a rapidly developing high fever (of 39–40°C) in infants and young children is not associated with convulsions (Childs 1988) and this raises questions about the precise contribution of level of fever and rapidity of onset to the development of a convulsion.

Certain infections, particularly those of the central nervous system, have a high incidence of associated seizures. Bacterial and viral meningitis have been associated with a high incidence of convulsions, but these conditions may well precipitate convulsions by virtue of the nature of the underlying disease rather than because of the fever *per se*.

Nurses play an important role in the acute management of the child with a febrile convulsion. Convulsions can cause fear and misunderstanding and, since they generally occur in very young children, the parents may feel particularly helpless. Nurses are often in a good position to explore these fears and misconceptions with parents and to provide them with information about what to do if their child experiences a febrile convulsion; this information will help to reduce anxiety and feelings of helplessness.

When a convulsion starts, the child needs to be protected from falling on to the floor or against furniture. If they are in a cot or bed, care should be taken to prevent them from falling out or hitting themselves against sharp corners which may be within reach. The airway should be cleared but nothing should be inserted into the mouth. A common misconception is that the use of spoons or gags is necessary to prevent the tongue from blocking the airway. This practice is dangerous and can harm the child. As long as the nurse puts the child in the recovery position (see Ch. 26), observes the airway and takes the necessary actions to maintain a clear airway by, for example, wiping away accumulated secretions, little more can be done. However, if the convulsion does not resolve after a period of 10–20 min, medications may be needed to control it. In such a case, medical help will be needed.

In addition to protecting the child from injury during the convulsion, the nurse should document its characteristics. Notes should be made relating to the child's temperature at the time of the convulsion or the last measurement made before it started, the type of movements made during the convulsion, where they started, how they developed and for how long they lasted. The clinical condition of the child should also be described.

Box 22.4

Non-steroidal anti-inflammatory drugs (NSAIDs)

In addition to their anti-inflammatory effects, NSAIDs are antipyretics. They act by inhibiting the production of prostaglandins from arachidonic acid in the cyclo-oxygenase pathway.

Since 1986, the NSAID aspirin (acetylsalicylic acid) has been withdrawn from general use in children under the age of 12 years because of the association between this drug and a serious condition called Reye's syndrome.* Paracetamol (acetaminophen) is now the most commonly used antipyretic in children. Although not an NSAID, its antipyretic properties are thought to lie in its ability to prevent the synthesis of prostaglandins, which are thought to affect the temperature set-point when released into the brain (see p. 814).

Antipyretic drugs are not effective in conditions where high core temperatures are caused by heat illness; neither are they effective in lowering normal body temperature.

*Reye's syndrome is a rare illness that occurs typically in children and teenagers. The onset is usually during a viral illness such as influenza or chickenpox. This is then followed by protracted vomiting and neurological changes at just about the time when the child is beginning to recover from the original illness (Ward 1997). The use of aspirin during the illness has been identified as a factor contributing to the very serious metabolic disorders associated with it, i.e. encephalopathy and fatty degeneration of organs. Unexpected vomiting and disturbed brain function after a viral illness are symptoms of Reye's syndrome in children and teenagers, but in infants the symptoms may be slightly different and include diarrhoea, breathing difficulties and fits. The number of cases reported has fallen in countries where aspirin has been withdrawn from use in children (Larsen 1997).

How fever develops

Fever is caused by the action of proinflammatory cytokines acting within the brain. Cytokines are peptide molecules released from a variety of cells, including those of the immune system (see Ch. 16). In health, cytokines are essential for cell–cell communication. During episodes of disease, such as inflammation and injury, they are responsible for many of the exaggerated inflammatory changes which can lead to sepsis and multiple organ failure. However, cytokines are not always harmful in disease, because these molecules also have beneficial effects for the host. The anti-inflammatory cytokines, such as interleukin-10 (IL-10) and transforming growth factor beta (TGFβ) for example, are important for healing and repair. Cytokines therefore have harmful as well as beneficial effects upon the patient.

For many years, the substances thought to be responsible for the fever associated with infection, tissue breakdown and necrosis, e.g. after traumatic injury or myocardial infarction, were a group of peptides called endogenous pyrogens (EPs). The endogenous pyrogens have now been shown to include specific molecules and are collectively called interleukins. Interleukin-1 (IL-1) is generally believed to be the pyrogen which acts in the brain to raise the set-point temperature to a higher level. IL-1 can be detected in the circulation in some but not all diseases. For example, after severe acute respiratory syndrome in children, patients have markedly elevated levels of IL-1 (Ng et al 2004). High levels of circulating IL-1 are also reported after acute myocardial infarction (Francis et al 2004).

Release of IL-1 into the circulation is probably stimulated by other interleukins produced outside the brain. Interleukin-6 (IL-6), for example, is a cytokine produced by a number of different cells such as activated macrophages, monocytes, keratinocytes, fibroblasts and others. It is thought that IL-6 released at the site of inflammation or injury triggers the production of IL-1 in the brain. In the brain, IL-1 probably stimulates production of a group of substances called prostaglandins. These substances are thought ultimately to be responsible for elevating the thermoregulatory set-point (Ranels & Griffin 2003).

Chills and rigors

A sudden onset of fever with a 'chill' or 'rigor' is characteristic of some diseases. For example, the rigors associated with malaria are diagnostic of the disease and are often portrayed in novels and films as a serious symptom of tropical disease. Repeated rigors are typical not only of pyrogenic infections and bacteraemia but are now also recognised as a symptom of viral as well as bacterial infections. Rigors and chills also occur in other febrile illnesses and can be demonstrated experimentally. For example, fever can be induced in human volunteers by safe, intravenous administration of a pyrogen called endotoxin. Endotoxin is a lipopolysaccharide molecule produced from Gram-negative bacteria. In human volunteer studies of thermoregulation and metabolism, endotoxin administration produces a 1–1.5°C rise in body temperature, accompanied by chills, shivering, myalgia and flu-like symptoms. These symptoms begin approximately 90 min after the endotoxin is administered. All the symptoms disappear after 5–6 h (Soop et al 2002).

A chill or rigor is accompanied by intense feelings of cold. The patient's skin will be white and cold and they will probably pull their bedclothes tightly around their body and curl up into a ball. Their teeth may chatter and they will feel very uncomfortable. Intense shivering and violent jerking movements will be uncontrollable.

Fever in myocardial infarction

Myocardial infarction is an example of a condition in which there is an acute rise in deep body temperature, probably due to release of proinflammatory cytokines from the injured myocardium (Francis et al 2004). Typically, body temperature rises after the first 24 h to 37.8–39.9°C and remains elevated for 2–3 days. Temperatures may be even higher. By day 5, however, deep body temperature returns to normal. It is thought that the pattern of elevated body temperature reflects necrosis of myocardial tissue (see Ch. 2). If fever persists after the fifth day, the nurse should consider infection, e.g. pneumonia, thrombophlebitis or a systemic infection, as a possible cause.

STOP THINK **22.13** Each of the following illnesses and conditions may result in fever:

- otitis media
- meningitis
- blood transfusion
- acquired immune deficiency syndrome (AIDS).

Construct a table to give the cause of the fever and its appropriate nursing care. You will need to refer to Nursing Care Plan 22.1 as well as to other chapters in this book to complete the table. When you have done so, answer the following questions:

(a) What is the common cause of the raised deep body temperature in the above examples?
(b) Why would you expect your chosen methods of treatment to be effective in lowering deep body temperature in each case?

Fever or heat illness?

Confusion sometimes surrounds the use of the word 'fever' to describe an elevated body temperature. 'Fever' is often used to describe a 'generic' increase in temperature, but in fact it has specific characteristics. To add to the confusion, the words 'hyperthermia' (wrongly) and 'hyperpyrexia' (correctly) are also used to describe febrile illness. In caring for patients with an elevated deep body temperature, it is important to appreciate the distinction between the mechanisms of fever on the one hand, and of heat illness on the other. When planning to treat the patient, the nurse should consider: 'Does this patient have a high temperature because of an altered set-point or because of a problem with dissipating their body heat loss?'. If the former is the case, the patient is febrile; if the latter seems more likely, then hyperthermia and heat illness should be suspected. The problem is that, in many cases, it is difficult to be sure of the cause of high body temperature.

How heat illness develops Heat illness is a term which includes the following three clinical conditions:

- heat cramps
- heat exhaustion
- heat stroke.

An elevated body temperature is not a diagnostic criterion for heat illness, but it may occur in association with clinical symptoms secondary to environmental heat stress or to a disturbance in the body's ability to dissipate body heat.

The cause of heat illness is quite different from that of fever. Fever and the concept of an upward re-setting of the hypothalamic set-point have already been discussed. Heat illness can be a minor medical problem or so severe that it poses a threat to life. Its primary cause is not the production of pyrogenic cytokines (IL-1, IL-6) but a variety of other factors, e.g. drugs, extremely hot and humid conditions, excessive overwrapping and body insulation, and very intense work in a hot environment, which causes heat to be stored in the body and which cannot be dissipated quickly enough from the body surface. A mild form of heat illness leads to heat cramp, and the most severe leads to heat stroke (see Case History 22.1).

Table 22.4 presents some of the signs which may alert the nurse to the fact that a patient is becoming overheated.

CASE HISTORY 22.1
Mr G

While making the weekly call to the home of Mr G, an 81-year-old widower, the community nurse finds him in the garden sitting in his wheelchair in a state of collapse. A relative arrives shortly afterwards and explains that since it was a nice day she thought Mr G would benefit from some fresh air and sunshine whilst she did his shopping.

Mr G feels hot and his hands and feet are red and sunburned. His skin is dry (he is not sweating) and his lips are slightly cracked. His axilla temperature (measured when taken indoors) is 39.2°C.

After being taken indoors, Mr G is sponged with warm water and his clothing removed or loosened. Cool drinks are given and his temperature gradually returns to normal over the next 4 h.

Nursing care of a febrile patient

Fever may start abruptly with a shaking chill, or it can develop without the patient even being aware that their

Table 22.4 Clinical appearance and observations of an apyrexial patient who complains of feeling hot: evidence for behavioural and physiological thermoregulation

Observation	Response
The bedclothes have been pushed to the bottom of the bed by the patient	This is a behavioural response to the sensation of feeling too warm. Removal of bedclothes/clothing exposes a larger area of the body surface for heat exchange by radiation and convection. If bedclothes/clothing are removed then sweat can freely evaporate to the room and so facilitate evaporative heat loss
Close inspection of the patient shows that the skin of the hands and feet is red and the veins in these areas dilated	Under control of the sympathetic nervous system, veins of the feet and hands vasodilate due to a reduction in vasomotor tone. Blood is therefore directed to the skin surface, resulting in the core tissues extending to the shell (see p. 814) and the skin appearing flushed. The skin is now at a higher temperature, thus creating a wider temperature gradient between the body and the environment. The greater the temperature difference between the body surface and its surroundings, the greater the heat loss by dry routes
Small droplets of sweat appear on the forehead and trunk	Sweating is stimulated in response to either an increase in skin temperature or a rise in core temperature (note the exception to this described in Table 22.1). Sweating occurs first on the forehead, followed by the upper arms, hands, thighs, feet and, finally, the abdomen. Sweating has been shown to start when the average skin temperature is 34°C; as skin temperature increases so does the sweat rate

Nursing Care Plan 22.1 Care of a febrile patient

Time scale	Problem	Action	Rationale
08.00	When measured, the patient's oral temperature has risen to 37.5°C	• Measure patient's temperature every 10 min	During a chill, frequent measurements should be made to determine the pattern of temperature and the maximum values reached
09.00	Oral temperature continues to rise, and now does so rapidly and is accompanied by shivering. The trunk is hot but the limbs are cold	• Cover the patient's body with blankets and raise the air temperature slightly. Avoid exposing the patient to cold draughts	At this stage the temperature regulating system is disturbed. Mechanisms are initiated to raise body heat to meet the new, raised set-point temperature. Any attempt at this stage to cool the patient will worsen their chill and delay the time in which the new set-point temperature is reached
11.00	Oral temperature has reached a plateau of 39.5°C	• Once deep body temperature has settled and is no longer rising, temperature measurements can be made every 30 min	A patient's temperature can be considered to be stable when there are at least two consecutive readings of the same value over a period of 1 h. Once the temperature is stable, measurements can be made every 2–4 h but observations of the patient's general condition should continue
11.30	Pulse rate has increased to 100 beats/min and respiratory rate to 20/min	• Frequent observations of pulse and respiratory rate should be part of the overall assessment of the febrile patient	As body temperature goes up so does cellular activity, i.e. there is a rise in metabolic activity. There are direct effects upon the cardiovascular and pulmonary systems as a consequence of a rise in temperature and metabolic activity. Metabolic activity increases by 13% for every 1°C rise in core temperature. Because of the increased energy demands brought about by fever, persistent pyrexia represents a drain on energy stores. In addition, febrile patients become anorexic and are reluctant to eat and so their energy intake falls. A poor energy intake in conjunction with increased energy expenditure results in negative energy balance or weight loss
11.45	An antipyretic has been prescribed to lower core temperature	• Administer aspirin/paracetamol as indicated. Note the patient's temperature at the time of giving the medication. Monitor the patient's temperature regularly (every 15 min) and record the changes on the patient's temperature chart to determine the efficacy of the treatment given	Antipyretics such as aspirin return the upwardly reset temperature to the original set-point level of approximately 37°C. Once this happens, the excess heat stored within the body represents an excessive heat load which must be dissipated. In addition to heat loss by the dry routes, radiation, convection and evaporative heat losses are switched on and patients may sweat profusely. Body temperature subsequently falls
		• Remove blankets and switch off any form of external heating	During the phase of heat dissipation the surface of the body needs to be exposed so that heat loss by all routes can be encouraged
13.00	The patient's mouth is dry. Patient is drenched in sweat and feels uncomfortable	• Frequent mouth care should be given if the patient cannot eat or drink, but whenever possible clear fluids should be encouraged. These can be refreshing and will provide glucose for energy	Some authors claim that as much as 3 L water can be lost each day in a febrile sweating person. An inadequate fluid intake is accompanied by excretion of a small amount of concentrated urine. An inadequate urine output indicates poor hydration and this is often accompanied by the development of sordes. Drenching sweats are uncomfortable, particularly if nightwear and sheets are wet. The patient can be made more comfortable by giving a bedbath and by sponging with warm water. Cold water should be avoided as this causes external cooling and worsens the feeling of discomfort

temperature has risen. When measured, core temperature may remain high or it may fluctuate (Edwards 1998). A fluctuating temperature with peaks and troughs can occur naturally, as discussed on page 816, but in hospital, a peak followed by a trough is more likely to be due to the effects of administration of an antipyretic, such as aspirin or paracetamol, or to vigorous use of surface cooling.

Nursing the patient with fever is a skill. It demands knowledge of the mechanisms of thermoregulatory disturbance as well as good clinical practice. The care that might be given to a febrile patient in the course of a few hours is described in Nursing Care Plan 22.1.

It is important for the nurse to appreciate the differences between managing the patient with fever compared to hyperthermia caused by heat stroke. In heat stress or heat stroke the primary problem is one of heat imbalance: too much heat stored, not enough body heat lost. This can occur after a marathon or after too much sunbathing. In both situations the problem for the person is the same. Antipyretics are ineffective because the set-point remains unchanged. The first line of treatment is to aid the dissipation of heat from the body and to rehydrate the person. Mild cases of 'sunstroke' can be corrected by moving out of the sun and to a cool environment so that heat can be lost from the body by radiation and convection: the dry heat loss routes. Cold drinks will also be helpful and comforting. In extreme situations, heat exhaustion may occur. The person is unable to lose heat by sweating because the sweat glands fail to produce sweat. The most effective treatment is to expose the body and spray the skin with warm (not cold) water to promote vaporisational heat loss, whilst taking care not to cause peripheral vasoconstriction. Heat exhaustion is a major risk for soldiers during combat in a hot climate.

Hypothermia

Hypothermia is a state in which the temperature of the body is lower than the thermoregulatory set-point. This situation can occur accidentally, i.e. spontaneous or accidental hypothermia, or it can be induced deliberately, i.e. therapeutic hypothermia. Nurses may encounter patients who have had a prolonged period of cold exposure due to an accident either inside or outside the home. In hospital, a subnormal temperature may occur in a patient who has undergone a prolonged surgical procedure. Nurses also now encounter therapy designed deliberately to lower the temperature of the body for therapeutic reasons (see Box 22.5).

The physiological mechanisms that lead to the development of hypothermia can be explained with reference to the hillwalker described in Case History 22.2. With nightfall, a drop in air temperature will stimulate a number of physiological responses to limit the rate of heat loss from the surface of Mr E's body. First of all, a fall in skin temperature, detected by skin thermoreceptors, will cause a reduction in blood flow to the skin at the extremities, i.e. nose, fingertips, toes and ears. Whilst peripheral vasoconstriction is extremely effective in maintaining body temperature with a moderate fall in air temperature, the conditions on the hillside will be more severe and eventually peripheral vasoconstriction will become maximal. When the vessels cannot constrict further, other mechanisms will be stimulated to prevent a further fall in deep body temperature. This will involve activation of the thermoregulatory mechanisms of heat production.

The first response to a modest reduction in air temperature which causes mild sensations of discomfort is an increase in non-shivering thermogenesis (NST; see p. 815). Shivering quickly follows NST as the major thermoregulatory mechanism to raise heat production. The main stimulus to shivering thermogenesis is a fall in skin temperature, but the intensity of shivering increases when core temperature falls as well. Shivering starts first in the muscles of the jaw and neck and progresses to all skeletal muscles. Although shivering increases heat production by approximately five times the basal rate, only about 40% of the heat produced is retained within the body. The rest is lost from the body

Box 22.5

Deliberate cooling — new treatments using therapeutic hypothermia

Although accidental hypothermia is undoubtedly harmful and can lead to death, deliberate cooling of the body may have beneficial effects in specific conditions. Refrigeration of human tissue has a long history (Fay & Smith 1941). In patients with neurological conditions, such as brain tumours, or in patients with cancer, early research undertaken in the middle of the last century claimed positive benefits in reducing the size of the brain tumour as well as helping patients with intractable pain.

In the last few years, interest in therapeutic hypothermia has grown. Cooling is reported to be helpful in limiting the size of brain lesions, for example after stroke (Reith et al 1996) and after severe head injury. However, the results of therapeutic hypothermia in patients with severe head injury were not as encouraging as expected. A multicentre randomised trial in the USA of patients with severe head injury (Clifton et al 2001) failed to show that mild body hypothermia (bladder temperature 32–33°C) had any benefit. Nevertheless, there is new evidence that whole body cooling, to a core temperature of 33°C, provides neurological benefit for those patients who survive a cardiac arrest out of hospital (Bernard et al 2002).

CASE HISTORY 22.2

Mr E

Mr E, a novice hillwalker, becomes separated from his fellow hikers and is lost for many hours in the mountains of the Lake District. As evening approaches, the air temperature falls and Mr E begins to feel tired, hungry and cold. After putting on an extra woollen jumper he sets off to find shelter. He is found early the next morning huddled under an outcropping of rock. The rescue team recognise that he is suffering from hypothermia and take him to hospital.

On his admission to hospital, his rectal temperature is found to be 33.8°C. Although mortality accompanying this degree of cold exposure is approximately 50% (Houdas & Ring 1982) and Mr E is confused and unable to speak clearly when found, he does in fact recover after successful rewarming and emergency treatment.

surface. Although shivering is not a very economical process, it is very important in humans to increase heat production and so prevent hypothermia.

Shivering is maximal when core temperature is approximately 35°C. It does not go on indefinitely in response to continued cold exposure but stops when deep body temperature falls to approximately 32°C. At this point, energy stores in skeletal muscle will be exhausted; the muscular contractions of shivering rapidly utilise these stores. The cold also prevents optimum contraction of muscle tissue. As the protective thermoregulatory mechanisms fail, core temperature falls further and body systems begin to fail. Although the hillwalker in Case History 22.2 initially took sensible steps to protect himself from the cold and exposure to the weather, he continued to lose body heat. Under less severe conditions, his normal thermoregulatory mechanisms would have been adequate to prevent a serious fall in deep body temperature but the prolonged exposure in Mr E's case was obviously of major importance in the development of hypothermia.

STOP THINK **22.14** Why is it so important for Mr E (Case History 22.2) to find shelter on the hillside? Why would rain have made the hillwalker's problem of becoming cold worse?

Causes of accidental hypothermia

Although accidental hypothermia does occur in fit young people, it is more often seen in neonates shortly after birth or in older people living at home. The young and the old are the most vulnerable to the effects of cold, particularly during the winter months. Resistance to cold in the fit and healthy person depends upon an efficient thermoregulatory system (see Fig. 22.2). Some impairment of thermoregulation may play a role in the predisposition of older people to the adverse effects of cold. Perception of cold, for example, may be impaired and the individual may therefore not respond to falling temperatures appropriately, for example by putting on extra clothing. Many older people become confined to a chair or their bed, so it is difficult for them to get up for extra clothes even when they do begin to feel the cold. Those caring for older people at home can help by leaving extra warm clothing close at hand to be used when needed; even wearing a hat at home may be useful to reduce heat loss from the head. Ensuring they have warm drinks close by, perhaps in a flask, and encouraging them to take these, will help to warm the body (see Box 22.1, p. 819).

Older people do not have the same ability as young adults to generate heat within the body, and therefore NST and shivering thermogenesis may not be as efficient. Other factors which, if present, may reduce the ability of the body to produce heat when needed (see Box 22.6) include:

- malnutrition
- hypothyroidism
- hypoglycaemia, which may be a particular problem in the older diabetic patient, as it lowers the threshold for the onset of shivering (Passias et al 1996); this means that a much greater fall in body temperature can occur before a hypoglycaemic patient starts to shiver
- intoxication with alcohol, because it limits the availability of glucose; the resulting hypoglycaemia inhibits shivering thermogenesis.

Box 22.6

Hypothermia in malnourished older people

During the winter months we often hear of older people becoming hypothermic after an injury, usually a fall. Why do some injured older people have such a problem in maintaining their body temperature at or around 37°C? Do older people become hypothermic because they get cold as a result of the fall, e.g. outside in the snow, or is there another reason? Studies have shown that very thin older women are more prone to fracture of the femur. They do not, as popularly believed, fall outside the home — 80% of falls in one study occurred indoors (Allison 1997).

It seems that in thin, underweight patients the central thermoregulatory 'thermostat' does not respond in the usual way to the cold, and if the patient is injured the problem is worsened. Injury *per se* has its own effects on thermoregulation, resulting in an inability to produce heat by shivering when body temperature falls. Body temperature of injured patients can fall well below 35°C, at which shivering is maximal in healthy subjects exposed to cold, before shivering heat production begins.

In summary, very thin, undernourished older people have a problem maintaining their body temperature because they do not produce heat when they need it most, i.e. when core temperature falls. When people get cold, they become confused and muscles get stiff, so it is not surprising that frail and older people are most at risk of a fall, especially in winter. Whether in the community or in hospital, nursing care should be directed towards ensuring that older people maintain their body weight and are protected from the cold. By doing this, injury and hypothermia may be prevented.

In the UK, accidental hypothermia in older people is a real hazard (Ranhoff 2000). Sadly, each winter, there are newspaper reports of older people who have died of hypothermia — deaths which are preventable. The British media (BBC News Online 2001) report that the British government is being urged to end the health risks for millions of older people who live in a cold home and who cannot afford to pay their fuel bills. With an estimated 30 000 deaths each year in cold weather, schemes to improve home insulation could make a positive impact in reducing accidental hypothermia in the older population. Mortality rate from hypothermia is considered to be approximately 40% (Stoner & Randall 1990).

Donaldson et al (1998) have shown that even in the coldest regions of the earth, such as Eastern Siberia, mortality from hypothermia is not as high as it is during winter in regions where the climate is more temperate. This is thought to be because the population in extremely cold regions takes what are quite simple precautions to prevent themselves becoming cold. For example, they wear very warm clothing in several layers and stay indoors as much as possible in their houses, which they keep warm.

The importance of temperature measurements in older people at home

When the community nurse visits older people during the winter months, some assessment of their environment and of their thermoregulatory system should be made. If the nurse thinks that the patient's house is too cold, assessment of the risk of hypothermia should be carried out. The nurse should ensure that the thermometer selected, e.g. tympanic thermometer or Tempa-Dot thermometer, is adequate for use with patients who may have a temperature well below normal, i.e. 33–34°C.

Rewarming the hypothermic patient

Safe rewarming of a person who has developed hypothermia must be undertaken with care because patients may die several hours after arriving in the Emergency Department, even following an apparently successful rescue. This phenomenon, which has become known as 'after-drop', first came to prominence during the First World War during sea rescues of servicemen and women. After prolonged immersion in cold water, victims, alive when rescued and taken on board ship, died shortly afterwards despite receiving emergency rewarming treatment. These 'late' deaths after apparently successful rescue were a real tragedy and for many years were unexplained. It is now known, however, that 'after–drop' is a consequence of inappropriate rewarming. As the patient is warmed, blood vessels at the extremities dilate and a large volume of very cold blood flows from the extremities to the heart. This results in severe cardiac complications, e.g. ventricular fibrillation, and death follows.

The most appropriate way to rewarm a hypothermic patient after immersion in cold water also applies to the person subjected to cold exposure. The first step is to stop any further heat loss from the body. Next, a shock blanket is used to retain body heat. This is called 'passive' rewarming and it allows core temperature to rise slowly by the gradual build-up of body heat resulting from natural heat production. Providing that all endogenously produced body heat is retained within the body, organ temperature will rise gradually. If core temperature is above 32°C, passive rewarming is the method of choice. If core temperature is below 32°C and the patient is a young adult who has become hypothermic as a result of immersion in cold water or from exposure, 'active' rewarming of core tissues is required. There are a number of methods available, including:

- gastric lavage with warmed saline
- the introduction of warmed humidified oxygen in air via a ventilator
- the administration of warmed intravenous fluids
- warm peritoneal lavage.

It remains to be determined whether active or passive rewarming procedures are better in the treatment of accidental hypothermia in patients receiving intensive care (Vassal et al 2001).

In older patients, careful active rewarming is recommended (Ranhoff 2000)

In all patients it is important to remember that if the skin surface is warmed first, blood flow to the extremities will be increased. For older people with pre-existing cardiovascular disease, this could precipitate a fall in blood pressure. With active rewarming, core temperature can rise from 0.6 to 1.9°C/h (Stoner & Randall 1990). As core temperature rises, shivering may start and will become maximal at about 35°C.

Box 22.7

The metabolic 'cost' of a polar expedition

In 1992, two explorers, Mike Stroud and Sir Ranulph Fiennes, completed the first unaided crossing of Antarctica. The 1700 km journey took 95 days. Throughout the journey the men conducted a series of medical experiments to assess the effect of the extreme climate and hard work on their bodies. In air temperatures of between –10 and –50°C and strong winds, the men dragged their sleighs for 10–12 h each day. The journey took these men to the limits of human endurance. Despite a high food intake, each man lost an extreme amount of weight (26% and 29%), all of their body fat as well as a proportion of lean tissue (muscle). As body fat, and therefore insulation was lost, the men felt even colder and weaker and they became extremely malnourished. The hard work, the extreme cold over such a long time, together with a number of injuries, resulted in an enormous demand for energy. The food they ate was not enough to stop them from breaking down their energy stores of fat, and as time went on they also began to break down their muscle to provide a source of energy. The results of the tests and measurements on their body composition illustrate how the human body adapts to the most extreme conditions and climate (see Stroud 1997, 1998).

Local cold injuries (see also Box 22.7)

Frostbite

When tissue freezes, ice crystals form and the substances in tissue fluid become concentrated. The ice crystals can be many times the size of the cell itself. The degree of cell death after freezing depends on the concentration of the solute. Tissue damage resulting from freezing very much resembles a burn injury.

The milder form of freezing injury is called 'frost nip'. The extremities, i.e. nose, ear lobes, cheeks, fingertips, hands and feet, can be affected, but treatment is by simple rewarming of the affected area. A more serious form of cold injury is frostbite. In this condition, blood vessels are damaged and blood circulation to the affected part stops. The congested blood causes agglutination of cells, resulting in thrombus formation. The severe conditions which result in frostbite can mean that the person is so cold that they neglect to care for the frostbitten tissues and that, if rewarming does occur because of improvements in weather conditions, the frostbitten areas become macerated.

Treatment for frostbitten limbs should aim to warm the core tissues first before treating the local damage. The affected limb can then be immersed in water at 10–15°C. The water temperature should then be raised every 5 min by 5°C to a maximum of 40°C.

Once the core and the affected extremities have been rewarmed, the patient should remain on bed rest. The affected limbs should be elevated and tetanus toxoid administered. Antibiotics may be necessary if there is any evidence of infection. Local treatment should consist of care of the wound together with early physiotherapy.

Raynaud's phenomenon

Raynaud's phenomenon develops most often in young women and is due to abnormal stimulation of vasoconstrictor nerves (see Ch. 2). The cause of this abnormal vasoconstriction is thought to be more complex than simply increased vasoconstriction on exposure to a change in air temperature and may involve microvascular changes in the endothelium (Gardner-Medwin et al 2001). Mainly affected are the fingers; spasm of the digital arteries causes sluggish circulation in the fingers, which then become cyanosed. The intense vasoconstriction causes the arteries to empty of blood and this leads to the typical 'dead' white appearance of the fingers. When the vasoconstrictor spasm has passed the circulation starts to flow again. At this stage the individual experiences tingling and throbbing followed by intense pain. In some individuals, vasoconstriction can be so severe and prolonged that the skin of the fingertips becomes ulcerated and necrosed, a condition known as 'Raynaud's disease'. Raynaud's phenomenon generally worsens in winter.

Nursing care of individuals with Raynaud's phenomenon should be directed towards helping them to avoid the stimuli which they know cause their fingers, and toes, to go 'dead'. For some people, simply wearing gloves may be sufficient precaution. Pocket handwarmers, often used by people involved in outdoor sports and pursuits, e.g. golfers and hillwalkers, are very useful in preventing attacks but they should be used before the person goes out into the cold, as once the hands have become cold a pocket handwarmer is unlikely to be sufficient to prevent vasoconstriction. In severe cases, vasodilator drugs or sympathectomy may be necessary.

STOP THINK **22.15** Now try to apply the knowledge you have gained in reading this chapter to the following situations. In formulating your answers, refer to the relevant sections of this chapter as well as to the books and articles listed in the references and further reading.

STOP THINK **22.16** 85-year-old Mrs K was being cared for by her husband until his recent death. Now alone, Mrs K is visited daily by her daughter and the community nurse. Mrs K has become very depressed, her appetite is poor and she has lost weight. On one of your morning visits, you find Mrs K collapsed in the cold hallway of her home. You suspect she may have been on the floor for some hours. You notice that her skin is very cold. Her axilla temperature is 34°C.

(a) What is the rationale for the immediate management of this patient?
(b) What steps would you take to rewarm the patient at home and once admitted to hospital?
(c) What method of temperature measurement would be needed to record deep body temperature?
(d) What would you expect the method of rewarming to be in the Emergency Department?
(e) What advice would you give to the patient's family so that further episodes of hypothermia could be avoided?

22.17 In the following situations, what decisions would you consider appropriate in the management of a patient with a disturbance in body temperature? (Note: you may decide that no action is necessary in some cases; if so, give your reasons.)

(a) A patient admitted to hospital with abdominal pain has had a fluctuating oral temperature (between 36.5 and 37.5°C) for 2 days. When you last took her temperature it was 39°C and she was complaining of feeling cold. Her hands and feet were cold and she looked 'mottled' blue. The patient then started to shiver.
(b) A patient on his second postoperative day has had a raised axilla temperature for 6 h. Treatment with aspirin was given 30 min previously. The patient is flushed and droplets of sweat are present on his forehead.

REFERENCES

Allison S P 1997 Impaired thermoregulation in malnutrition. In: Kinney J M, Tucker H N (eds) Physiology, stress, and malnutrition – functional correlates, nutritional intervention. Lippincott-Raven, Philadelphia, p 571–593

Aschoff J, Wever R 1958 cited in Stainer M W, Mount L E, Bligh J 1984 Energy balance and temperature regulation. Cambridge University Press, Cambridge

Bayley N, Stolz H R 1937 Maturational changes in rectal temperature of 61 infants from 1–36 months. Child Development 8(3): 195–206

BBC News Online 2001 Plan to cut deaths in cold homes. Online. Available: news.bbc.co.uk

Bernard S A, Gray T W, Buist M D et al 2002 Treatment of comatose survivors of out-of-hospital cardiac arrest with induced hypothermia. New England Journal of Medicine 346: 557–563

Berner N J, Heller H V 1998 Does the preoptic anterior hypothalamus receive thermoafferent information? American Journal of Physiology 274: R9–18

Brogan P, Childs C, Phillips B M et al 1993 Evaluation of a tympanic thermometer in children. Lancet 342: 1364–1365

Cannon B, Nedergaard J 2004 Brown adipose tissue: function and physiological significance. Physiological Review 84(1): 277–359

Childs C 1988 Fever in burned children. Burns 14(1): 1–6

Childs C 1994 Studies in children provide a model to re-examine the metabolic response to burn injury in children treated by contemporary burn protocols. Burns 20: 291–300

Childs C, Little R A 1994 Acute changes in oxygen consumption and body temperature after burn injury. Archives of Disease in Childhood 71: 31–34

Childs C, Harrison R, Hodkinson C 1999 Tympanic membrane temperature as a measure of core temperature. Archives of Disease in Childhood 80(3): 262–266

Childs C, Vail A, Protheroe R at al 2005 Differences between brain and rectal temperatures during routine critical care of patients with severe traumatic brain injury. Anaesthesia 60: 1–7

Clifton G L, Miller E R, Choi S C et al 2001 Lack of effect of induction of hypothermia after acute brain injury. New England Journal of Medicine 344: 556–562

Cole R P, Shakespeare P G, Chissell H G et al 1991 Thermographic assessment of burns using a non permeable wound covering. Burns 17: 117–122

Craig J V, Lancaster G A, Taylor S et al 2002 Infrared ear thermometry compared with rectal thermometry in children: a systematic review. Lancet 360: 603–609

Donaldson G C, Ermakov S P, Komarov Y M et al 1998 Cold related mortalities and protection against cold in Yukutsk, Eastern Siberia: observation and interview study. British Medical Journal 317: 978

DuBois E F 1948 Fever and the regulation of body temperature. Thomas, Springfield, IL

Edwards H E, Courtney M D, Wilson J E et al 2003 Fever management audit: Australian nurses' antipyretic usage. Pediatric Nurse 29(1): 31–37
Edwards S L 1998 High temperature. Professional Nurse 13(8): 521–526
Fay T, Smith G W 1941 Observations on reflex responses during prolonged periods of human refrigeration. Archives of Neurology and Psychiatry 45: 215–222
Francis J, Zhang Z H, Weiss R M et al 2004 Neural regulation of the pro-inflammatory cytokine response to acute myocardial infarction. American Journal of Physiology – Heart and Circulatory Physiology 287(2): H791–797
Frayn K N 1997 Metabolic regulation – a human perspective. Portland Press, Oxford
Gardner-Medwin J M, Macdonald I A, Taylor J Y et al 2001 Seasonal differences in finger skin temperature and microvascular blood flow in healthy men and women are exaggerated in women with Raynaud's phenomenon. British Journal of Clinical Pharmacology 52(1): 17–23
Guthrie J R, Dennerstein L, Hopper J L et al 1996 Hot flushes, menstrual status, and hormone levels in a population-based sample of midlife women. Obstetrics and Gynecology 88: 437–442
Hoffman C, Boyd M, Briere B et al 1999 Evaluation of three brands of tympanic thermometer. Canadian Journal of Nursing Research 31(1): 117–130
Houdas Y, Ring E F J 1982 Human body temperature. Plenum Press, New York
Hull D 1976 Temperature regulation and disturbance in the newborn infant. Clinics in Endocrinology and Metabolism 5: 39–54
Jenney M E M, Childs C, Mabin D et al 1995 Oxygen consumption during sleep in atopic dermatitis. Archives of Disease in Childhood 72: 144–146
Klaus S 2004 Adipose tissue as a regulator of energy balance. Current Drug Targets 5(3): 241–250
Larsen S U 1997 Reye's syndrome. Medicine, Science and the Law 37: 235–241
LeFrant J-Y, Muller L, Emmanuel Coussaye J et al 2003 Temperature measurement in intensive care patients: comparison of urinary bladder, oesophageal, rectal, axillary and inguinal methods versus pulmonary artery core method. Intensive Care Medicine 29: 414–418
MacLennan A, Lester S, Moore V 2001 Oral oestrogen replacement therapy versus placebo for hot flushes. Cochrane Database Systematic Reviews (1) CD002978
Macqueen S 2001 Clinical benefits of 3M Tempa-Dot thermometer in the paediatric setting. British Journal of Nursing 10(1): 55–58
Morley C, Murray M, Whybrew K 1998 The relative accuracy of mercury, Tempa-Dot and Fever Scan thermometers. Early Human Development 53: 171–178
Natale J, Joseph J G, Helfaer M et al 2000 Early hyperthermia after traumatic brain injury in children: risk factors, influence on length of stay and effect on short-term neurological status. Critical Care Medicine 28: 2608–2615
Ng P C, Lam C W, Li A M et al 2004 Inflammatory cytokine profile in children with severe acute respiratory distress syndrome. Pediatrics 113(1): e7–14
Passias T C, Meneilly G S, Mekjavic I B 1996 Effect of hypoglycaemia on thermoregulatory responses. Journal of Applied Physiology 80(3): 1021–1032
Ranels H J, Griffin J D 2003 The effects of prostaglandin E2 on the firing rate activity of thermosensitive and temperature insensitive neurons in the ventromedial preoptic area of the rat hypothalamus. Brain Research 964(1): 42–50
Ranhoff A H 2000 Accidental hypothermia in the elderly. International Journal of Circumpolar Health 59: 255–259
Reith J, Jorgensen H S, Pederson P M et al 1996 Body temperature in acute stroke: relation to stroke severity, infarct size, mortality and outcome. Lancet 347: 422–425
Soop M, Duxbury H, Agwunobe A O et al 2002 Euglycaemic hyperinsulinaemia augments the cytokine and endocrine responses to endotoxin in humans. American Journal of Physiology, Endocrinology and Metabolism 282: E1276–E1285
Stainer M W, Mount L E, Bligh J 1984 Energy balance and temperature regulation. Cambridge University Press, Cambridge
Stoner H B, Randall P E 1990 The metabolic aspects of hypothermia. In: Cohen R D, Lewis B, Alberti K G M M, Denman A M (eds) The metabolic and molecular basis of acquired disease. Baillière Tindall, London
Stoner H B, Barker P, Riding G S G et al 1991 Relationships between skin temperature and perfusion in the arm and leg. Clinical Physiology 11: 27–40
Stroud M A 1997 Thermoregulation, exercise and nutrition in the cold: investigations on a polar expedition. In: Kinney J M, Tucker H N (eds) Physiology, stress and malnutrition: functional correlates, nutritional intervention. Lippincott-Raven, Philadelphia, p 531–548
Stroud M A 1998 Survival of the fittest? Jonathan Cape, London
Talo H, Macknin M L, Medendorp S V 1991 Tympanic membrane temperatures compared to rectal and oral temperatures. Clinical Pediatrics (Suppl.): 30–35
Tortora G J, Derrickson B 2006 Principles of anatomy and physiology, 11th edn. John Wiley & Sons Inc., N.Y.
Vassal T, Benoit-Gonin B, Carrat F et al 2001 Severe accidental hypothermia treated in an ICU: prognosis and outcome. Chest 120(6): 1998–2003
Ward M R 1997 Reye's syndrome: an update. Nurse Practitioner 12: 45–53
Waterhouse J, Weinert D, Nevill A et al 2000 Some factors influencing the sensitivity of body temperature activity in neonates. Chronobiology International 17(5): 679–692
Wilmore D W 1977 The metabolic management of the critically ill. Plenum, London
Wyllie F J, Sutherland A B 1991 Measurement of surface temperature as an aid to the diagnosis of burn depth. Burns 17: 123–128

FURTHER READING

Childs C 1994 Temperature regulation in the burned patient. British Journal of Intensive Care 4: 129–134
Stroud M A 1993 Shadows on the wasteland. Jonathan Cape, London
Stroud M A 1997 Thermoregulation, exercise and nutrition in the cold: investigations on a polar expedition. In: Kinney J M, Tucker H N (eds) Physiology, stress and malnutrition: functional correlates, nutritional intervention. Lippincott-Raven, Philadelphia, p 531–548
Stroud M A 1998 Survival of the fittest? Jonathan Cape, London

USEFUL WEBSITE

Age Concern
www.ageconcern.org.uk

WOUND HEALING

Sue Bale

23

INTRODUCTION

For most healthy individuals, the term 'wound' conjures up thoughts of a cut, a graze or even a surgical incision that heals rapidly without difficulty. For nurses, however, the management of wounds is a complex aspect of patient care, requiring much skill and expertise. A nurse may care for a patient with a wound in a variety of settings, ranging, for example, from patients with surgical incisions nursed in hospital, to patients with chronic leg ulcers nursed in their own homes, to patients with industrial injury or trauma treated in their workplace.

The impact of a wound on an individual can be considerable. Pain, fear and scarring are the most obvious, but individuals vary in their response to having a wound (see Ch. 26). For some, restriction in social activity, or the financial implications of not being able to work, should also be considered alongside the psychological effects of altered body image (Wilson 2000).

Tissue injury and the resulting wound problems have existed for as long as humans have walked the earth (Leaper 1998). For many centuries, trauma and war injury caused most wounds. A variety of readily available materials were used as wound coverings, the forefathers of today's dressing materials. Prehistoric humans had a wide range of salves, which were used to achieve haemostasis, and plant extracts, herbs, cold water, snow and clay were used to ease pain. Surprisingly, throughout human history, wound management has been well documented. One of the first records of wounds was found in cave paintings. Archaeologists have found skulls dating back to the New Stone Age that show evidence of healing following skull trephining. This demonstrates not only that this surgical procedure was performed then, but also that people survived it long enough to heal. Injuries that did not result in death were likely to have been lacerations, contusions (bruises) and fractures. First-aid priorities in these situations would have been to arrest bleeding, bring the tissue edges together, hold them in place and protect the damaged tissues with a covering.

Scandinavian folklore suggests that for thousands of years plant extracts have been applied to wounds for a variety of reasons (Leaper 1998). Of these 2500 agents, some were antimicrobial, others astringent and others used to effect healing. Towards the end of the Roman era, Galen, the famous Greek physician and anatomist, AD 129–200, developed his theory of laudable pus — pus bonum et laudabile. The basis of this theory was that, should a wound become infected, its temperature would increase and this localisation of infection should be allowed to continue. Galen wrote that, when infection localised and then discharged itself, the wound would go on to heal without problems. In the years that followed, medical practitioners became so keen on this idea that they believed not only that pus was acceptable, but also that it was essential and desirable for good wound healing. Clean, uninfected wounds were inoculated with various noxious substances in order to stimulate pus formation. These practices continued from the 7th to the 14th century. It was not until the 19th century that Pasteur and Lister managed to persuade their medical colleagues that mortality rates could be reduced by using antiseptics and aseptic principles.

Throughout time, individual species have varied in the way in which their tissues are renewed. Primitive vertebrates such as reptiles and amphibians have retained the ability to regenerate lost tissue. However, in humans, only liver and epidermal tissue can regenerate. Where tissue loss in humans occurs, healing is achieved by tissue repair, and the body's ability to deal with injury quickly and effectively has been important throughout human evolution for survival of the species.

The healing process comprises a complex series of events that depends on a number of factors, and in order for it to proceed at its optimal rate the individual concerned should be in good health. In caring for patients with wounds nurses have an important role in promoting health. Their skills as health promoters and health educators are called upon to optimise the healing time.

As in other aspects of nursing, the issues of clinical effectiveness and the delivery of evidence-based care are key to wound management. As wound healing is a relatively new specialty, the evidence base and research strategies are still being developed (Cullum & Roe 1995, Harding 1998, Bale 2004).

Definition of a wound

A wound can be defined as a defect or breach in the continuity of the skin. This is an injury to the skin or underlying tissues/organs caused by surgery, a blow, a cut, chemicals, heat/cold, friction/shear force, pressure or as a result of disease, such as in leg ulcers and carcinomas.

Box 23.1 lists the terms that are used in wound healing.

Box 23.1

Terms used in wound healing

Aseptic technique. A precautionary method, using sterile equipment and a 'no-touch' technique to prevent infection.

Autolysis. The disintegration or breakdown of cells or tissues by endogenous enzymes.

Autolytic debridement. The natural process by which the body's own enzymes degrade devitalised tissue on a wound bed.

Chemotaxis. The process by which chemical attractants (kinins) stimulate polymorphs to move towards damaged cells.

Collagen. Fibrous protein strands which provide the strength and structure of granulation tissue.

Collagenase. An enzyme which breaks down collagen during remodelling.

Debridement. The removal of devitalised tissues from a wound.

Dehiscence. Bursting open of a wound.

Elastin. Fibres in connective tissue which provide elasticity.

Epithelium. The cells which form the epidermis.

Exudate. The extracellular fluid which bathes a wound and is rich in nutrients, phagocytes and antibodies.

Fibronectin. An adhesive protein that is a component of extracellular matrix.

Glycosaminoglycans. A polysaccharide that is a component of extracellular matrix.

Granulation. The process of healing by secondary intention.

Ground substance. A gel-like material in which connective tissue cells and fibres are embedded.

Necrotic tissue. Dead tissue, often black in colour.

Proteoglycans. A polysaccharide that is a component of extracellular matrix.

Pus. A protein-rich liquid consisting of exudate, dead macrophages and bacteria.

Slough. Devitalised white/yellow tissue — dead tissue that separates (and is 'sloughed' off) from healthy tissue after inflammation and infection.

Tensile. The ability to be stretched.

Wound abscess. A localised collection of pus, caused by invading microorganisms, which forms as a result of liquefaction of disintegrated tissue and an accumulation of polymorphs — the process of abscess development is in response to the defences of the body attempting to 'wall off' the damage.

Wound types and the classification of wounds

There is no clear-cut method of classifying wounds. Some practitioners refer to wounds by anatomical site, e.g. abdominal wall wounds, axillary wounds. Others classify wounds by their depth, e.g. epidermal loss, subcutaneous wounds. Another possible classification is by degree of tissue loss (Dealey 1999). In the first group, there are wounds with little or no tissue loss where the skin edges can be brought together and sutured. In the second, there has been substantial tissue loss and the skin edges cannot be brought together.

Epidemiology

The epidemiology of wounds is not clearly documented. Because patients with wounds can be found in almost every specialty, information relating specifically to wounds is not collected. However, although there are currently no centrally collected data on wounds, information is available for some wound types, for example leg ulcers.

Leg ulcers

Leg ulcers have been described as 'loss of skin below the knee on the leg or foot which takes more than 6 weeks to heal' (Morison & Moffatt 1997). Leg ulceration has affected humans over the centuries and is associated with venous disease of the lower limb in approximately 80% of cases (Cullum et al 1997). It is estimated that between 1 and 22% of those over 60 years of age have a lower limb ulcer (Sieggreen & Kline 2003). The largest survey of patients with leg ulcers, carried out in Scotland in 1985 (Callam et al 1987), found that the prevalence of ulceration increased with age and that by 85 years, more than ten times more women than men experienced ulceration.

The social and economic burden of managing these patients is considerable. Estimates vary, but Cullum et al (1997) estimated the costs to be between £230 and £400m annually for the UK alone. The cost of home care has been estimated at a minimum of £400m and this figure is likely to increase with the rising numbers of older people in the population (Moffatt 1995). For the most part these patients are cared for by their GP and by nurses within the community setting. However, there is an increasing trend towards referral to a specialist leg ulcer service or centre.

The individual's lifestyle can be greatly affected by the presence of a leg ulcer. These wounds are difficult to manage, traditionally slow to heal and, even once healed, likely to recur (Dale & Gibson 1986).

Pressure ulcers

Throughout the history of nursing, the issue of patients developing pressure ulcers has been associated with guilt and failure (Dealey 1997). Indeed, it has been suggested that many if not all pressure ulcers are preventable (Dealey 1999). In long-term care facilities as well as in the acute hospital setting, incidence and/or prevalence of pressure ulcers are used as the key quality indicators in patient care (DH 1993a). There is a growing awareness that the problem of pressure ulcers in patient care is not only a nursing issue but also involves medical staff, management and government (Sussman & Bates-Jensen 1998, Pieper 2000, European Pressure Ulcer Advisory Panel 2003). Improvement in patient care needs a number of approaches, including the development of local prevention strategies and educational programmes for all health care professionals (Dealey 1997).

Pressure ulcers are among the most difficult wounds to manage. UK surveys have documented the prevalence rate as being between 10.3 and 18.6% (Clark & Cullum 1992, O'Dea 1993, Pieper 2000). Across Europe this figure is similar, reported to be 18.1% (Clark et al 2004).

The incidence of pressure ulcers within hospital ranges from 4.3 to 43% (Gebhardt 1992, Clark & Watts 1994) and within nursing homes ranges from 5 to 23% (Pieper 2000). However, in the most acute settings the incidence is reported to be as low as between 1.1 and 2.7% (Williams et al 2004). The variation in rates depends on the specialty in which the patients are being nursed; orthopaedic units and wards where patients are older, immobile, chronically ill and disabled have the higher rates.

The cost implications of a patient developing a pressure ulcer are high. Such patients need to spend longer in hospital and, even when discharged home, frequently require a district nurse to continue treatment. This financial cost is thought to be rising. In 1982 the estimate was £150m (Scales et al 1982), and it subsequently increased to £300m in 1988 (Waterlow 1988) and £755m in 1993 (DH 1993b). Given the rising numbers of older and debilitated people, the figure could be much higher today; the costs have been estimated to be a minimum of £250 000 a year in one community unit (Dealey 1999).

The personal costs to the individual of developing a pressure ulcer also need to be taken into account. Apart from the disappointment of having discharge from hospital postponed and return to normal function delayed, there is the pain and distress, all of which are difficult to measure (Dealey 1997).

Given the suggestion that many if not all pressure ulcers can be prevented (Dealey 1999), the extent of the challenge for practising nurses is clear (p. 849).

Table 23.1 Important cells in wound healing

Cell	Function
Endothelial cells	Help to achieve haemostasis
Polymorphs	Take part in the initial inflammatory response
Macrophages	Digest debris and stimulate other cells to function; orchestrate wound healing processes
Fibroblasts	Produce collagen
Myofibroblasts	Aid wound contraction by producing mature collagen

STOP THINK **23.1** What are the mechanisms in your organisation for measuring the prevalence and incidence of pressure ulcers? How does this compare with national figures?

THE PHYSIOLOGY OF WOUND HEALING

A number of cell types are involved in the process of healing (see Table 23.1).

Tissue repair

The wound healing process comprises a complex series of events, whereby the continuity and strength of damaged tissues are restored by the formation of connective tissue and regrowth of epithelium. The process can be divided into four phases (see Fig. 23.1) but, since wound healing is a continuous biological process, there is some overlap between them (see Table 23.2).

Phase I — haemostasis

As soon as a wound occurs, it bleeds and blood initially fills the wound defect. Platelets aggregate and degranulate, resulting in clot formation and haemostasis (Witte & Barbul 1997). Haemostasis is the arrest of bleeding at the site of blood vessel damage, and is essential to preserve the integrity of the closed and high-pressure circulatory system in order to limit blood loss. A fibrinous clot forms as the blood coagulates, which now acts as a preliminary matrix or scaffold within the wound space into which cells can migrate.

Phase II — inflammation

The fibrin clot begins to degrade and the surrounding capillaries dilate and become permeable, allowing fluid into the wound site. This activates the complement system, which is composed of a series of interacting soluble proteins found in serum and extracellular fluid that induces lysis and destruction of target cells, such as bacteria. Cytokines and proteolytic fragments are also found in the wound space (Steed 1997), their accumulation initiating a massive

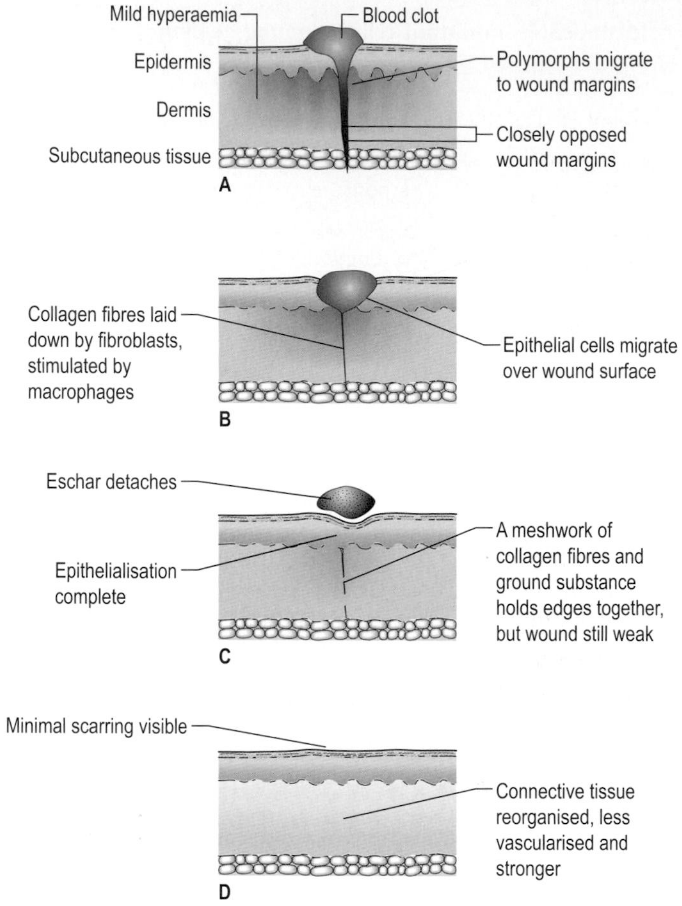

Fig. 23.1 Wound healing by primary intention. A: Haemostasis. B: Inflammation. C: Proliferation/reconstruction phase. D: Maturation phase.

Table 23.2 Phases of wound healing

Phase	Time after sustaining wound
Haemostasis	0–3 days
Inflammation	2–5 days
Proliferation	4–28 days or until defect is filled
Maturation	15 days–1 year

influx of other cells. The two main inflammatory cells are neutrophils and macrophages (Martin 1997).

- Neutrophils flood into the wound shortly after injury and reach their peak number within 24–48 h, their main function being to destroy bacteria through the process of phagocytosis. Neutrophils have a very short life span and their numbers reduce rapidly 3 days post injury, provided there is no infection.
- Tissue macrophages, like neutrophils, destroy bacteria and debris through phagocytosis. However, the macrophage is also a rich source of biological regulators, including cytokines and growth factors, bioactive lipid products, and proteolytic enzymes, elements essential for the normal healing process (Steed 1997, Slavin 1999).

This phase can be looked on as one of biological cleansing. It does, however, make a considerable metabolic demand on the body. Much heat and fluid can also be lost where a cavity wound exists. The shorter the duration of this phase, the better, because as it nears completion, proliferation or formation of new tissue can begin. Following the inflammation phase, the wound site is prepared for the repair process to begin.

Phase III — proliferation/reconstruction

Tissue repair takes place during this phase. It usually begins at around day three and lasts for some weeks. Proliferation is characterised by the formation of granulation tissue in the wound space. This new tissue consists of a matrix of fibrin, fibronectin, collagens, proteoglycans and glycosaminoglycans, and other glycoproteins (Hart 2002). Fibroblast cells move into the wound space and proliferate. Their function is to synthesise and deposit extracellular proteins, producing growth factors and angiogenic factors that regulate cell proliferation and angiogenesis (Stephens & Thomas 2002). Fibroblasts will multiply rapidly in the well-nourished individual and, to be most effective, need adequate amounts of vitamin C, iron, oxygen and nutrients. Accounting for 70–80% of the dry weight of dermis, collagen is the most abundant protein in human tissue (Wysocki 2000). Collagen is usually produced by fibroblasts and at least 19 genetically distinct collagens have been identified. Granulation tissue also contains elastin, providing the wound with elasticity and resilience (Wysocki 2000).

Angiogenesis is the formation of new blood vessels in the wound space and such vessels are essential for the delivery of oxygen and other nutrients. The key cells involved in angiogenesis are the vascular endothelial cells, which arise from the damaged end of vessels and capillaries (Neal 2001). New vessels sprout from existing small vessels at the wound edge, endothelial cells detaching from these small vessels and penetrating the wound space. These sprouts are then extended in length until they meet other capillaries, connecting together to form new vascular loops and networks.

Re-epithelialisation begins a few hours after injury and continues as the wound begins to fill with granulation tissue. At the wound edges, epithelial cells divide and, gradually, epithelium migrates from the edges towards the middle of the wound. Epithelialisation of larger areas is achieved not only by migration, but also by rapid division of epithelial cells near hair follicles, which might be present deep in the dermis. Islands of epithelium appear wherever a follicle is present. Cells migrate from these islands to meet each other, while cells from the edges of the wound grow inwards to cover the raw surface.

The final feature of proliferation is wound contraction, beginning around day five. Wound contraction is a dynamic process where cells reorganise the surrounding connective tissue, reducing the amount of granulation tissue. This effect is mostly due to the activity of fibroblasts and myofibroblasts which, under the influence of cytokines, contract to pull the wound edges together.

Phase IV — maturation

This phase usually begins around 7 days post injury and continues for many months or years, long after the wound appears to the naked eye to be closed or healed. The immature collagen laid down in phase II is gradually replaced by a mature collagen. The formation of new collagen and the lysis of immature collagen are balanced so that the amount of collagen present at any one time remains constant. The immature collagen is laid down in a random, haphazard fashion, its function being to fill the wound defect as quickly as possible. The remodelling process involves the balance between synthesis and degradation of collagen, where the cells producing the different types of collagen are subjected to apoptosis (programmed cell death) (Tjero-Trujeque 2001). Mature collagen is laid down following lines of tension within the wound, and at the same time it is cross-linked to give strength. Tensile strength at 14 days in sutured wounds is approximately 10% of the original strength of the skin. Within 3 weeks this increases to 20%, gradually reaching a maximum of 70–80% about 1 year later.

Healing by primary/first intention

When injury occurs, whether through accident or as a surgical necessity, the aim of treatment is to effect complete healing as quickly as possible with minimal scarring. To achieve this, the method of choice is healing by primary intention, which occurs when wound edges are in apposition (see Fig. 23.1). There is minimal formation of granulation tissue and once the wound has healed, only a thin seam remains. Healing by primary intention is only possible where there is adequate, mobile tissue and no complicating bacterial contamination. In situations where contamination is suspected, closure of the wound is accompanied by the use of prophylactic systemic antibiotics. For healing to take place by primary intention, the wound edges need to be closely approximated and held together until the wound has healed sufficiently. The skin may be closed by using tapes, clips, continuous or interrupted sutures, or glue. However, a Cochrane systematic review of tissue adhesives reports that it is unclear whether these are more or less effective than sutures or tapes (Coulthard et al 2004). The skill of the surgeon ensures that the sutures are not inserted too tightly and that the skin edges are closely apposed. The choice of suture material depends on the type of tissue being closed and on the particular function of the tissue (Leaper & Gottrup 1998).

Healing by secondary intention

Where there is significant tissue loss and/or bacterial contamination, wounds are usually left open to heal by secondary intention through the formation of granulation tissue and, later, wound contraction (see Fig. 23.2). Due to the amount of tissue excised or lost during injury, wound healing by secondary intention is a longer process, taking weeks or even months to complete. The healing process itself proceeds in much the same way as for healing by primary intention. The proliferative phase is much extended, as this is when granulation tissue forms and fills the wound defect. It was established many years ago (Marks et al 1983) that, for some wounds, the length of time taken to heal depends on the original size, i.e. small wounds heal more quickly than larger ones, and it is therefore possible in some wound types (pilonidal sinus, abdominal and axillary wounds) to predict when wounds of a given size that are free from infection will heal.

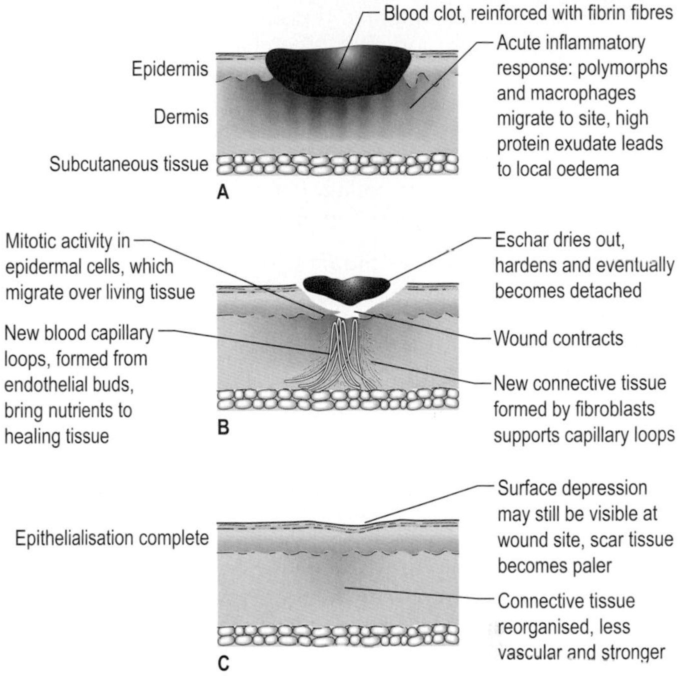

Fig. 23.2 Wound healing by secondary intention. A: Haemostasis/inflammation. B: Proliferation phase. C: Maturation phase.

For methods of wound closure and types of suture material, see Leaper & Gottrup (1998) and Coulthard et al (2004).

Scar tissue

A scar is the mark that may remain after a wound has healed. A scar consists of relatively avascular collagen fibres covered by a thin layer of epithelium.

Most scars fade with time (see Table 23.3) and the resultant cosmetic effect is generally acceptable, but abnormal scarring can lead to problems, as follows:

- *Stretching of scar tissue* — this can occur where sutures have been removed prematurely, especially over areas

Table 23.3 The maturation of scar tissue

Time after sustaining wound	Characteristics of scar
0–28 days	The scar is fragile and soft
28 days–3 months	The scar becomes denser, stronger and is red or purplish in colour
3 months onwards	Over time the colour fades to white and the tissues become softer and more elastic

that are under tension, e.g. the skin over the scapula and back are common sites where stretching occurs
- *Hypertrophic scar tissue* — here collagen lysis and collagen production are out of synchrony and excessive tissue lies within the boundaries of the scar
- *Keloid* — this is a protuberant, prominent scar that results from excessive collagen formation in the dermis during connective tissue repair.

Hypertrophic and keloidal scarring are examples of excessive scar formation. Such scarring is more common in young people, especially during pregnancy and puberty, and also in deeply pigmented skins, the peristernal area being particularly susceptible.

A number of factors influence scarring (see Table 23.4).

Why some wounds are sutured and others are left open

Wound closure, enabling wounds to heal by primary intention, is considered to be the method of choice whenever possible, as healing by primary intention is much quicker than healing by secondary intention.

Wound closure is undertaken where:

- the procedure will result in cosmetically acceptable scars; adhesive tapes and clips can be used to avoid undesirable suture marks
- sufficient mobile tissue exists to allow the edges of the wound to be brought together easily without tension or without causing trauma which could lead to subsequent wound breakdown
- the wound site is clean, e.g. when an operation is considered to be a clean procedure as in excision of lipoma, a benign tumour containing fatty tissue.

Secondary intention is chosen as the method of healing where:

- the final cosmetic effect is likely to be an improvement over either suturing or skin grafting
- there is insufficient tissue to allow the wound edges to be approximated, e.g. in some chronic open wounds such as leg ulcers (see p. 852) and pressure ulcers (see p. 849)
- the wound area is heavily contaminated or infected, e.g. in a contaminated injury or surgical procedure such as excision of an infected pilonidal sinus.

FACTORS THAT ADVERSELY AFFECT HEALING

STOP THINK **23.2** Before considering factors that adversely affect wound healing, identify the requirements for optimal wound healing.

A number of factors can adversely affect the normal rate of healing, slowing it down and, in severe cases, impairing it altogether. These factors can be intrinsic or extrinsic.

Intrinsic factors

Advanced age (see Ch. 35). With advancing years the dermis gradually becomes thinner and the underlying structural support, collagen, diminishes at a rate of 1% per year (Hunter 1995). In addition, as fewer fibroblasts produce less collagen, skin loses its elasticity and its ability for elastic recoil, leading to creases and wrinkles. At the same time the amount of subcutaneous fat reduces, and there is less of a cushion for underlying bone. As individuals age, the natural moisture from sebum secretions lessens as sweat glands become smaller, leading to increasing dryness of the skin. The consequence of ageing is dry, thin, inelastic skin that is susceptible to damage, with a reduced metabolic rate and a prolonged healing period. These factors together with poor circulation associated with old age affect the tensile wound strength.

Malnutrition Malnutrition may result in delayed wound healing and the production of weak, poor quality scars (Pinchcofsky-Devin 1994). McLaren (1997) describes two types of malnutrition that affect healing: protein-energy malnutrition and nutrient deficiencies.

Protein-energy malnutrition (PEM) is caused by an absolute or relative deficiency of energy and protein that affects between 19 and 50% of hospitalised patients (McLaren 1997). Several factors contribute to PEM including a reduced intake of nutrients, reduced absorption and digestion of nutrients, and increased metabolic use. McWhirter and Pennington (1994) reported that 200 out of 500 patients admitted to hospital were undernourished, and just over 100 lost weight during their admission. Other research supports these findings. McLaren (1997) estimates that although 70% of patients admitted to hospital are malnourished prior to admission, the remaining 30% develop PEM during their hospital stay.

For a review of the literature related to complications experienced by patients admitted to hospital when they

Table 23.4 Factors influencing scarring

Cause of injury: Burn/trauma	Cause of injury: Surgery	Race	Age	Wound site
1. Over joints contractures can occur 2. Dirty injuries caused by gravel can cause pigmentation	1. The skill of the surgeon 2. The type of suture material used, i.e. non-absorbable sutures, alongside the wound	1. Extreme hypertrophic scarring is common in deeply pigmented races and rare in Caucasian races	1. In infancy and childhood, scars resolve quickly 2. In pregnant women, hypertrophic scarring is more common	1. Scars which follow the body's natural lines of skin tension do best 2. Scars which cross skin folds do less well 3. Scars on the shoulders, sternum and back produce unsightly scarring

are undernourished and starved during their stay, see Stotts (2000).

Malnutrition can adversely affect wound healing by reducing tensile strength, increasing wound dehiscence and increasing susceptibility to infections (Dickerson 1995) and to developing pressure ulcers (Meaume et al 1994).

Nutrient deficiency The European Pressure Ulcer Advisory Panel (2003) has produced nutrition guidelines that recommend a minimum daily intake of 30–35 g/kg body weight, with 1–1.5 g/kg/day of protein and 1 mL/kcal/day of fluid intake. These guidelines also recommend that nurses consider the quality of the food that patients are offered, along with removing the physical or social barriers to its consumption. For some patients it is not always easy to maintain adequate nutrition, e.g. an older person living alone may lose interest in cooking or a terminally ill patient may be unable to eat due to nausea. The importance of diet cannot be overemphasised, and wherever possible the nurse should ensure that the patient receives all the nutrients required for healing. The advice of a dietitian may be sought in an attempt to improve or supplement the nutritional status of vulnerable individuals (see Ch. 21).

Dehydration The normal metabolic processes of an individual require approximately 2500 mL of water every 24 h (see Ch. 20). A dehydrated individual will not be able to metabolise efficiently and this will adversely affect the healing process.

Disease processes The metabolic effects of a number of disease processes can delay healing. Anaemia, arteriosclerosis, cardiovascular disorders, diabetes mellitus, cancer, inflammatory disease, immune disease, rheumatoid arthritis and jaundice are included in this group, as is any other disease that impairs the body's immune response. It is important to remember that in some patients, particularly older people, several disease processes may be present at the same time.

Impaired blood supply to the area Where the blood supply to the wounded area is impaired, insufficient nutrients and oxygen are supplied and the healing period is prolonged. This happens, for example, in patients with peripheral vascular disease and lower limb ulcers.

Smoking adversely affects the healing process in a number of ways. Smoking and the absorption of nicotine has a vasoconstricting effect. After smoking one cigarette, peripheral blood flow has been shown to be reduced by 50% and to remain so for more than an hour (Siana et al 1992). The main influences of nicotine and carbon dioxide relate to the effects on peripheral tissues, with a reduction in oxygen tension in these tissues and the formation of thrombi. Nicotine has been demonstrated to inhibit epithelialisation (Waldrop & Doughty 2000) and the healing of abdominal wounds, the overall cosmetic effect of a scar being poorer in patients who were smokers (Siana et al 1992).

Extrinsic factors

Poor surgical technique Tissues handled excessively during surgery can be damaged, resulting in haematoma formation. This can lead to the development of infection as the haematoma is broken down. A dead space may also occur if tissues are not correctly approximated during surgery, again encouraging the development of infection. In addition, where sutures are inserted too tightly, the tissue becomes damaged and tissue death can occur.

Medication A whole range of medications can affect healing. Cytotoxic medication given during chemotherapy can destroy healthy as well as malignant cells. Ideally, their use is withheld until any wound healing is complete, usually a period of 4 weeks. Steroids also slow down, or prevent, healing taking place and their use is closely monitored in individuals with wounds.

Inappropriate wound management The healing process may be adversely affected by the use of poor dressing technique, the wrong dressing material or antiseptics where they are not needed (see p. 844). It is essential that the nurse is aware of what is required from a dressing material in order to ensure that each product is used cost-effectively.

Psychosocial factors There is a close association between psychological and physical well-being. Stress and anxiety can affect the immune system (Waldrop & Doughty 2000) through elevation of serum levels of corticosteroid, which impairs immune function (Kiecolt-Glaser 1995). Researchers have also studied the effects of stress on the sympathetic nervous system, where vasoactive substances (catecholamines) impair blood perfusion to the wound bed (Stotts & Wipke-Tevis 1996, Padgett et al 1998). Sleep disturbances are linked to being stressed and sleep is thought to be essential for healing and tissue repair (Dealey 1999).

Infection Of all the factors that can delay or prevent healing, infection is the most important (see Ch. 16).

WOUND INFECTION

All wounds are likely to be colonised by bacteria, though many of these do not delay or affect healing. It is pathogenic organisms, growing in large numbers, which usually produce wound infection (Leaper & Harding 2000). Established infection in a healing wound often delays healing and may even cause wound breakdown, herniation of the wound or complete wound dehiscence. The clinical signs and symptoms of a wound infection are summarised in Box 23.2. Despite all the technological advances that have been made in surgery and wound management, the problem of wound infection persists. This happens because the causes of wound infection are so varied and are often linked to the individual's general condition; both nutritional status and immune status are important factors in resistance to infection (Bale & Jones 1997, Williams & Leaper 1998).

The wound environment itself can encourage bacterial growth. Anaerobic organisms, for example, thrive in wounds with a poor oxygen supply. A wound bed or area that is free from haematoma and dead tissue and is clean reduces the risk of infection.

The way in which the wound is managed can also affect infection. Contamination by bacteria, through poor

Box 23.2

Clinical signs and symptoms of wound infection

The local effects of wound infection are:

- Pain — throbbing
- Redness — erythema
- Swelling — of the area surrounding the wound
- Discharge — haemoserous and/or purulent
- Loss of function — to protect the area
- Unhealthy appearance of the wound bed (p. 842).

Wound infection prolongs the inflammatory healing phase and delays healing by secondary intention. Systemic effects on the patient are:

- Raised temperature
- Increased metabolic rate
- General malaise
- Anorexia.

technique on the part of the nurse, poor hygiene or incontinence on the part of the patient, can all increase the risk of wound infection. The consequences of wound infection vary depending upon the condition of the patient and the environment in which they are being nursed: in hospital, a patient with a surgical wound infection poses a considerable risk to other patients with wounds on that ward; at home, that patient is less of a risk to the family and community, who are unlikely to be vulnerable.

Factors that predispose to wound infection

Factors associated with the patient

There are several factors that, in addition to delaying the healing process, can predispose a patient to wound infection. These can be identified on first assessment:

- Poor nutritional status — McLaren (1997) has described in detail the effects of deficiencies in nutrition on wound healing. Protein-energy malnutrition (PEM) has been linked to hospitalisation and impacts on all aspects of patient care, including developing pressure ulcers and influencing postoperative wound infection.
- Immunosuppression — suppression of the immune system, e.g. in diabetes mellitus or after steroid therapy, can lead to an increased rate of infection (Kindlen & Morison 1997).
- Excessive body weight.
- Advanced age.

Factors specifically related to the hospital environment

- Adverse spatial arrangements — when too many patients are nursed in close proximity to each other, especially in an open ward, the wound infection rate increases. An increase occurs when more than 25 patients are being nursed in an open ward (NHS Estates 2002).
- Length of preoperative stay — the wound infection rate is linked to the length of time a patient spends in hospital prior to operation. The longer this period, the more likelihood there is of the individual being colonised by the pathogenic bacteria found in hospitals.
- Inappropriate preoperative care — it is not usually necessary to shave the site preoperatively (Williams & Leaper 1998). Where shaving is required, it should occur immediately prior to surgery to reduce the risk of bacterial growth on newly shaved skin (see Ch. 26). These precautions should result in a wound infection rate of less than 1%.
- Prolonged operative procedure — since 1980, research has suggested that the longer the operation, the greater is the risk of infection in clean wounds (Cruse & Foord 1980, Williams & Leaper 1998).
- Surgical contamination — in elective surgery, e.g. excision of a benign breast lump, the rate of infection should be less than 5%, and with effective surveillance and control this can be reduced to less than 2% (Leaper & Harding 2000). In emergency operations where the area is contaminated, e.g. for perforated bowel, the rate soars to between 20 and 40% (Leaper & Harding 2000).
- Use of drains — these are used to close or minimise dead space in a wound or to evacuate haematomas or body fluids, with the intention of reducing the risk of infection (Bale & Leaper 2000). They should be used with caution, as all drains are foreign bodies and may cause tissue reactions.

As a wound infection develops, localisation of the infection leads to the formation of a wound abscess. This may drain through the suture line or into the wound in the case of cavities. Occasionally, if deep-seated, the abscess will need a surgical incision to drain it properly. Where partial wound breakdown occurs, extra caution is needed to explore and assess the wound as being suitable for healing by secondary intention (Bale & Jones 1997).

Sources of wound infection

Endogenous Organisms found on the patient's own skin are endogenous sources of wound infection. These organisms, usually *Staphylococcus aureus* or gut commensals, are either present under normal circumstances or are hospital pathogens that colonise the body after the patient is admitted to hospital. Shortening the time between admission and surgery reduces the possibility of skin contamination by hospital acquired bacteria (Williams & Leaper 1998, Dealey 1999).

S. aureus is found on the skin and sometimes in the upper respiratory tract. This organism does not normally affect the patient adversely, but when a wound has been created, *S. aureus* can invade the wound from adjacent skin or be breathed into the wound from the nose.

Exogenous Infections from exogenous sources are those that occur following contamination of the wound from a source external to the patient. This may happen in theatre or later in the ward when pathogens are allowed to fall onto the wound and penetrate it. Bacteria such as *Pseudomonas aeruginosa* can be found in wet areas or where moisture is present, i.e. in water, other fluids or ventilators. *P. aeruginosa* is also found in flower vases, sinks and drains.

Accidental injuries are highly likely to have been contaminated by bacteria. *Clostridium tetani* and *Clostridium welchii* are present in the soil and can be hazardous. People who receive minor injuries whilst gardening are at risk and, if they have not already had antitetanus immunoglobulin, should be immunised.

Bacteria

Bacteria consist of a variety of single-celled organisms that have a primitive nucleus with no nuclear membrane. Bacteria vary in size, but are larger than viruses and can be seen under a light microscope. They reproduce by simple binary fission, i.e. each bacterial cell divides into two, both of which can divide again. The rate of division of bacteria, and so multiplication, depends on their environment, and in suitable conditions they divide rapidly.

Many of the harmful effects of bacteria on humans are caused by products of the bacteria, namely toxins, when these are released into the bloodstream. Endotoxins are released when a bacterial cell dies and breaks up, whereas exotoxins are released continually by thriving bacteria.

Bacterial cell walls The cell wall of a bacterium can have a number of characteristics. These ultimately influence how capable a host will be at destroying that bacterium (see Box 23.3). It is the cell wall that the body's immune system penetrates in order to destroy it.

STOP THINK **23.3** Identify the major microorganisms that cause wound infection. Can you identify their sources?

WOUND MANAGEMENT — A HOLISTIC APPROACH

Ideally, assessment and management of a patient with a wound utilises a systematic approach (Bale 2000). This begins with an initial assessment (see Box 23.4) of both the patient and the wound so that management can be planned. Following implementation, evaluation of that management is required to ensure that the needs of the patient have been met.

Box 23.3

Gram-positive versus Gram-negative bacteria

The differing characteristics of the bacterial cell wall can be determined by the staining reaction first used by Professor Hans Gram in the late 19th century. Gram, who developed the procedure quite accidentally, found that due to the properties of the cell wall, certain bacteria retain staining with crystal violet and resist any attempt to decolorise with ethanol. Other bacteria lose the stain, or respond to decolorisation and then respond to a pink counterstain: the former are described as Gram-positive bacteria and include such organisms as the cocci and clostridia; the latter are described as Gram-negative and include such organisms as *Escherichia coli* and *Pseudomonas aeruginosa*. This staining reaction is now considered a major classification distinction between bacteria.

Box 23.4

Assessment in wound care

1. Assess the patient:
   - Identify factors that might impede healing, such as intercurrent disease processes or certain medications (see p. 838)
   - Where disease processes are identified, attempt to ensure that they are corrected
   - Where they cannot be corrected, build an expected delay in healing into the nursing care plan.
2. Assess the wound:
   - Consider whether the wound is healthy for the stage of healing and free from infection
   - Assess the wound's physical characteristics
   - Where appropriate, measure and record wound size and shape.
3. Assess the environment in which the patient is being nursed.
4. Assess the appropriateness of wound agents and wound dressing materials.

This approach can be adapted to suit the environment in which the patient is being cared for, whether this is in the patient's own home or in the hospital setting.

Wound management is an aspect of nursing that is undergoing rapid change and expansion. Research has been undertaken using different study designs to answer a diverse range of clinical questions, and to explore the lived experiences of patients. Best available evidence is used not only to inform practice but also to develop clinical guidelines (National Institute for Clinical Excellence 2001, European Pressure Ulcer Advisory Panel 2003). Journals (paper and electronic), the internet, study days and conferences provide access to much of the research data. A wide range of educational opportunities at undergraduate and postgraduate levels is available for those wishing to further their knowledge regarding wound care.

Patient assessment

This should be patient-centred, comprehensive and should consider the physical and social environment.

Whether the patient is being cared for in hospital or in the home, or is young or old, assessment of the patient's general condition should be undertaken. This is done to identify any of the factors that might impair the wound-healing process (p. 838): for those factors seen as reversible, treatment should be sought; for those factors uncovered for which no treatment is possible, some degree of delay in healing should be anticipated and allowed for in the care plan.

The patient's social environment can affect the treatment options. For example, when caring for a frail older person living alone, the nurse may need to select a dressing that is waterproof, in order that carers who come in to bathe the person on days when the district nurse does not visit need not disturb the wound unnecessarily.

For further reading, see Bannon (1993). In this article, the author explains the importance of the holistic approach to wound care in the setting of an intensive care unit.

Assessment of the wound

In the assessment of the wound and surrounding skin, a range of wound criteria are considered which can help ensure that the patient receives the most appropriate care to suit their needs (Bale & Jones 1997).

Assessment of wounds that are healing by primary intention

Three questions should be addressed:

1. *What has caused this wound?* The answer may be surgical incision to perform an operation, or surgical excision of an abscess. Once the cause of the wound has been established, the expected prognosis for complete healing can be estimated. For example, a surgical incision in a fit, 20-year-old woman to remove a benign breast lump should result in a wound that will heal quickly and without complications. The expected healing potential in an older person who has had emergency bowel surgery for removal of colonic cancer is less good.
2. *Is the wound healthy for the stage of healing?* During the first 3 days of healing by primary intention, the area surrounding the wound will be red, swollen, indurated and often painful. This is normal during the inflammatory phase of healing. It would not be considered normal if the patient presented with the same symptoms 7–10 days postoperatively, and would indicate the presence of infection. Recognising what is normal throughout the healing process is essential. Only when this has been achieved can the abnormal be identified.
3. *What needs to be done in the days before the sutures or clips are removed?* Nothing; if the wound remains healthy during the early days, the original dressing, if unstained and intact, can be left in place until the wound closure material is removed.

Assessment of cavity wounds

If wound management materials are to be used effectively, the appropriate product must be applied to the wound throughout the stages of healing. During the assessment the following factors should be taken into consideration (Bale 2000).

Appearance of the wound bed In the pregranulation stage, cavity wounds often appear red and raw, and have the very uneven surface of adipose tissue. It is important to recognise that this is normal for this early stage of healing. Within 10–13 days the appearance of the wound will change as granulation tissue is formed. A healthy wound should be pale pink in colour, sometimes covered with a pale yellow membrane, pain-free and should not bleed easily if touched. If infection is present, the appearance of the wound will alter. The colour of the tissue may change to a dark red and the wound will show a tendency to bleed easily on light contact and become uncomfortable or painful. Superficial bridging of tissue can also be seen within the cavity (Bale 2000). As the presence of infection can delay healing, prompt treatment is needed in these situations. For deep-seated infection, a wound swab (see Box 23.5) followed by the appropriate course of antibiotics is generally indicated, but more superficial infections can sometimes be treated topically. Until the infection is cleared, no dressing material will be fully effective.

> **Box 23.5**
>
> **Taking a wound swab**
>
> Points to remember:
>
> - Use an aseptic technique
> - Use a sterile, microbiological cotton wool swab
> - This swab should be moistened in a transport medium before use
> - If the wound is flat or shallow, gently rotate the swab across the middle of the wound bed. Care needs to be taken not to contaminate the swab with skin flora from the edges of the wound
> - If the wound is deep, or has a recess, insert the swab into the depths of the wound. Bacteria present in the depths of a wound are different from and more likely to be pathogenic than bacteria on the surface of a wound
> - Carefully replace the swab directly into its storage tube containing culture medium
> - Deliver to the laboratory as soon as possible, but at the latest within 24 h
> - Record antibiotic drugs being given, the site of the wound, together with any other information likely to be of help to the laboratory.

Wound size In general, the larger a wound, the longer it will take to heal; therefore the size of a wound provides a useful indication of the probable healing time. The healing rates of some wound types, such as pilonidal sinus excisions, axillary wounds and abdominal wall wounds, have been carefully measured, and so it is possible with these wound types to predict with some accuracy how long they will take to heal (Leaper & Gottrup 1998, Wilson 2000).

The size of a wound may also influence the choice of dressing. Whilst small cavities may be dressed with one of a number of products, it may not be practical to use some products on larger wounds where multiple pieces or packs would be required. In these situations, the choice of dressing material may be limited to products that provide the bulk with just one or two packs. This is an especially important consideration in the community where the available size range of modern dressing materials may be limited.

Wound measurement In order to assess the effectiveness of a particular treatment, it is necessary to monitor changes in the size of the wound. For the majority of wound situations this should be the way a wound progresses towards complete healing. Surgically created cavities are usually of even contour and depth; the length and breadth of such a wound can generally be determined fairly easily (Bale 2000). Weekly measurement is often sufficient and steady progress should be evident.

Wound volume is more difficult to assess and does not really offer any advantages over the measurement of linear dimensions.

Chronic wounds, such as pressure ulcers, are often more difficult to measure as these wounds can extend under the skin edge. The simplest way of assessing the extent of these wounds is to measure by using a cotton wool bud or probe gently inserted into the wound, under the edge of the cavity, marking the boundary on the skin with an ink marker. This outline of the extent of the wound can then be traced onto paper and stored as a permanent record of wound progress.

For leg ulcers, the circumference of the wound can be traced onto clean acetate or plastic sheets and, again, can be stored as a permanent record.

Re-measurement of chronic wounds may only be necessary every 2–3 weeks, as healing is generally slower in these situations. Accurate measurement and record keeping avoids the need to depend upon clinical impression. More sophisticated and expensive methods of wound measurement are available, including structured light and computer imagery, which assess wound area and volume (Bale 2000). Photography, using instant Polaroid or a digital camera, is valuable in providing a permanent record of the appearance of the wound.

STOP THINK **23.4** How are wounds measured in the areas in which you have worked? Devise a way of recording the wound dimensions in the care plan of one of your patients.

Wound shape and depth When managing cavity wounds, it is necessary to recognise the importance of wound shape. Ideally, cavities created surgically should be boat- or saucer-shaped, with evenly sloping sides. Where pockets, tracts or sinuses occur within a cavity, drainage of exudate may be inadequate, and this in turn may greatly delay healing. Poor wound shape also restricts the range of dressing materials that can be used. For example, a long narrow cavity will require a dressing material that is conformable enough to be inserted into the restricted space but which can be easily removed from the depth of the wound without leaving behind fibres and particles which could then become a focus for infection.

In a wound where the shape is so poor that progress towards healing is unacceptably slow, surgical revision may be required in order to create a wound with more regular contours. This is occasionally necessary when wounds that have undergone primary closure subsequently break down. Pressure ulcers are particularly prone to develop into poorly shaped wounds and, as surgical revision here is not always possible or advisable due to the poor health of the individual, careful choice of an appropriate dressing material is essential (Bale 2000).

Exudate production Cavities vary enormously in the amount of exudate they produce. New, surgically created wounds can exude heavily, whereas some deep pressure ulcers produce very little exudate. This variation will affect management, especially the choice of dressing material. Some products are highly absorbent and are able to deal with copious discharges, whereas others have a limited capacity for absorption. The inappropriate use of a dressing material can sometimes have serious consequences. If, for example, a dressing material is chosen that is unable to cope with heavy exudate production, the surrounding skin can quickly become macerated. Alternatively, a very hydrophilic dressing material applied to a lightly exuding wound may cause excessive drying of the wound surface, delaying healing and sometimes even causing pain.

Presence of slough or necrotic tissue When slough or necrotic tissue is present on the wound surface, healing will be delayed or, in some cases, prevented altogether. This material needs to be loosened and removed to allow wound healing to progress. This procedure is known as debridement and is a difficult task that requires intensive and skilled nursing intervention (see p. 845) (Bale 1996).

The location of care

This can affect patients' progress. Those nursed in hospital are in an environment where their dietary intake and fluid balance can be monitored and their general well-being assured. Nursing care is available continuously and, to a certain extent, the nurse 'controls' the environment in which the patient is being nursed. In the community, when patients are being cared for in their own homes, the nurse has far less influence over a patient's environment. As a guest, the district nurse is able to advise and recommend an adequate food and fluid intake but is unable to monitor this accurately, as each visit may only be for a comparatively short period once or twice a day.

Creating an environment for healing

Principles of moist wound healing

Healing proceeds at its optimal rate when the wound is enclosed in a warm, moist environment (see Fig. 23.3). Under these conditions, cellular activity is maximised; the benefits of such an environment have been recognised since the early 1960s (Winter 1962). This is true for the whole spectrum of wounds encountered, from superficial cuts and grazes to large, extensive granulating wounds. Exposure of a wound to the air precipitates drying out of the wound surface and scab formation. Nurses should consider the importance of providing a suitable environment for wound healing when choosing a wound management material. The term 'dressing' traditionally depicted some form of absorbent cotton/gauze-type material that was used to soak up excess wound secretions and protect the wound from trauma. By the 1990s a wide range of sophisticated materials had been developed to cater for the diversity of individual wound situations. Many of these materials interact with the wound surface (so-called interactive materials) and are designed to optimise the local conditions for wound healing (Bale 2000). Box 23.6 summarises the characteristics of an ideal wound dressing material.

As therapies continue to be developed, the use of growth factors, cultured human skin and synthetic substitutes are being introduced into patient care (Gentzknow et al 1996). Although such therapies are not appropriate for many patients whose wounds are healing rapidly, their use can be invaluable for wounds in life-threatening and other difficult situations such as burns and chronic and indolent ulcers.

Principles of cleansing

Why cleanse a wound? Sutured wounds rarely need cleansing unless leakage has occurred. In this situation

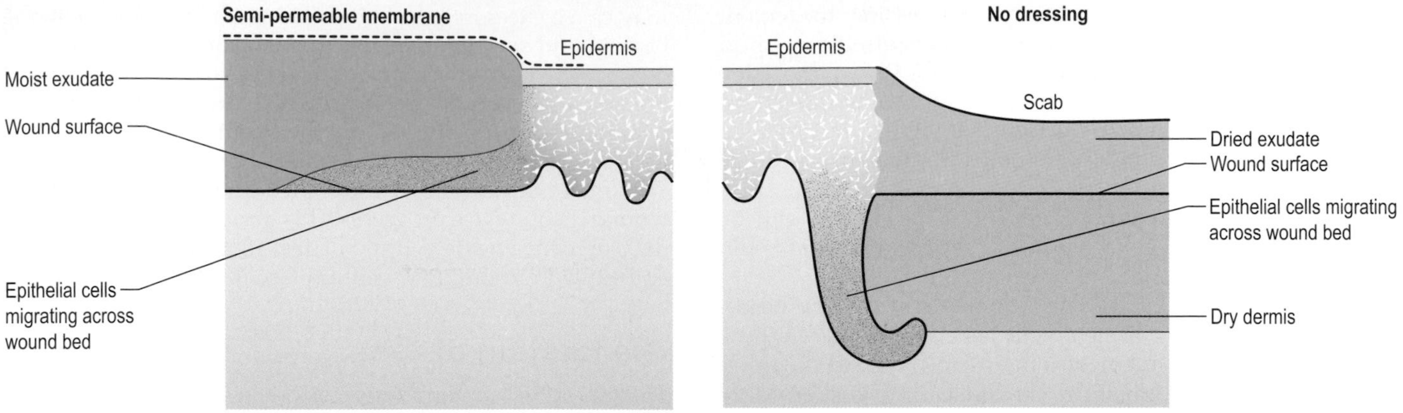

Fig. 23.3 Healing of skin wounds with and without a semi-permeable membrane dressing (Adapted from Winter 1962).

Box 23.6

Characteristics of an ideal dressing

- Non-adherent
- Impermeable to bacteria
- Capable of maintaining a high humidity at the wound site while removing excess exudate
- Thermally insulating
- Non-toxic and non-allergenic
- Comfortable and conformable
- Capable of protecting the wound from further trauma
- Requires infrequent dressing changes
- Cost-effective
- Long shelf-life
- Available both in hospital and in the community

Reproduced with permission from Morison et al (1997).

the suture line can be gently, aseptically cleansed with sterile normal saline. With open wounds, strict asepsis is not always required. The patient can use the bath or preferably the shower to irrigate the wound with warm water (Bale & Jones 1997). For patient comfort, fluids used for wound cleansing should be warmed to body temperature. The main reason for cleansing open cavity wounds is to remove any loose debris and excess wound secretions. A shower is particularly useful in achieving this. The gently flushing action of the spray will remove any particles that are loose, and flushing for 10–15 s is usually sufficient. If bathing, the wound should be flushed by splashing water into it. Wounds of the lower limb can be bathed in a bucket or bowl, gently splashing the wound to remove loose debris. A bucket can be lined with a commercial bin liner. This protects the bucket from contamination and makes cleaning of the bucket much easier and so reduces the potential risk of cross-infection.

For further reading on wound irrigation, see Cunliffe & Fawcett (2002).

The role of antiseptics and topical agents (see Table 23.5). The actions of the whole range of antiseptics and cleansing agents are generally poorly understood, though researchers have attempted to investigate their effects on healing tissue. Some antiseptics are reported to have adverse effects on healing (Williams & Leaper 1998), whilst others have a positive effect (Gilchrist 1997). The challenge for nurses is to match these results with the clinical situations they

Table 23.5 Topical cleansing agents

Agent	Action
Cetrimide	A detergent that cleanses the wound bed, useful for traumatic injuries that are contaminated or require debridement. Bacteriostatic against Gram-negative bacteria though rapidly deactivated on contact with organic material
Chlorhexidine	Aqueous version used for wound cleansing. Bacteriostatic against both Gram-positive and Gram-negative bacteria though rapidly deactivated on contact with organic material
Iodine preparations: povidone and cadexomer products	Have a broad action against both Gram-positive and Gram-negative bacteria
Isotonic saline 0.9% sodium chloride	Physiologically compatible with body fluids. Suitable for mechanical cleansing of excess or stale wound exudate and loose debris
Drinking and boiled water	Suitable for mechanical cleansing of excess or stale wound exudate and loose debris

encounter. All wounds become colonised from the surrounding skin by bacteria, which are particular to that individual and their presence rarely delays healing (Williams & Leaper 1998).

Bacterial studies on pilonidal sinus excisions, axillary wounds and abdominal wall wounds have shown that the vast majority of bacteria present in these wound types do not cause problems to the patient or, in fact, delay healing. Similarly, in a study of the bacteriology of leg ulcers, the presence of bacteria on the wound surface again did not delay healing (Gilchrist 1999). Patients with leg ulcers appeared to keep their initial bacterial flora irrespective of the type of treatment and its eventual outcome. The organisms here included *Staphylococcus aureus*, *Escherichia coli* and *Pseudomonas aeruginosa*.

Wound cleansing The purpose of cleansing a wound is to gently remove loose debris and other surface contaminants, so providing an optimal healing environment prior to applying a dressing. However, wound exudate bathes the surface of wounds and provides nutrients and cytokines essential for healing. Cleansing the surface of a wound removes exudate and in some cases this inhibits the healing process (Barone et al 1998). Nurses need to consider carefully why they are cleansing a wound and to balance the need to remove exudate because of harmful effects, against leaving it in place to enhance healing. Exudate needs to be removed if:

- it is causing maceration to the wound bed and/or surrounding tissues
- there are signs of infection
- foreign bodies are present
- devitalised tissue is present
- it has an unpleasant odour and is embarrassing and nauseating for the patient
- it is excessive and is oozing through dressings and onto clothing/bedding/furniture.

Where the wound is healthy with minimal amounts of exudate, routine wound cleansing is of little benefit (Davies 1999). Nurses should use a realistic approach when cleansing wounds. Many antiseptics have a short-lived action and so bacteria will quickly re-colonise the wound surface. If these organisms are not harmful, why seek to eradicate them?

Removal of devitalised tissue

Chemical debridement Before the advent of modern dressing materials, a range of chemicals was applied to sloughy and necrotic tissue in an attempt to soften and remove it (Bale 1996), but with varying degrees of success. These agents have difficulty penetrating the surface of leathery and hard necrotic tissue, so rendering them ineffective. Where healthy granulation tissue is present, damage can occur due to the toxicity of the chemicals.

Surgical or sharp debridement is the removal of devitalised tissue using a scalpel and scissors. It is sometimes possible for a surgeon to excise devitalised tissue with or without anaesthesia depending on the site and depth of the problem. Alternatively, experienced and specialist nurses can also perform this procedure. If general anaesthesia is not indicated then careful consideration is needed to ensure that the patient does not feel pain or discomfort, and that the area is not painful. The advantages of this method are that debridement is instant and a healthy cavity results. Where patients are being cared for in the community, access to a surgeon or specialist nurse may be limited and this is not always a practical alternative for many patients.

Autolytic debridement Autolysis is the lysis of devitalised tissue from the wound bed by white blood cells and proteolytic, fibrinolytic and collagenolytic enzymes (Ramundo & Wells 2000), which work best under moist conditions. Several types of wound dressing provide this moist environment that facilitates cleaving of the devitalised tissue from the wound bed. These dressings can effectively remove devitalised and necrotic tissue without damaging either the skin surrounding the wound or healthy tissue within the wound. Included in these are the hydrogels and hydrocolloids (see Table 23.6).

Excessive granulation

From time to time, re-epithelialisation fails to take place due to the presence of excessive granulation tissue or 'proud flesh'. Treatment is needed to flatten the granulation tissue so that it is level with the epithelial edge, as new epithelium cannot migrate up over this 'proud flesh'. An application of 75% silver nitrate stick will cauterise the tissue, but a less traumatic method is the use of a cream containing a corticosteroid, although this should be used under medical supervision. The need for careful assessment is paramount in the successful treatment of cavity wounds. When planning a wound care programme, consideration of these factors should provide the nurse with an accurate picture of the needs of each patient and also provide some assistance with the dressing selection process.

New wound healing therapies

The drive to develop therapies that accelerate wound healing continues. Such therapies are designed to interact with the wound and enhance the wound environment. These include growth factors, skin substitutes, antimicrobials, vacuum-assisted closure and wound warming.

Growth factors aim to regulate cellular activity, including:

- the movement of cells into a wound
- replacement of damaged epidermal and dermal cells
- formation of scar tissue
- remodelling of scar tissue (Schulz 2000).

One example of a product available for such use is recombinant growth factor, platelet derived growth factor (PDGF), which is used to stimulate the formation of extracellular matrix and granulation tissue. Other examples include basic fibroblast growth factor (bFGF), transforming growth factor, b family (TGFb), and the interleukin family of proteins. Research continues to determine which wounds are likely to benefit most from the application of such agents.

Tissue engineering A range of artificial skin, cultured skin and living skin equivalents has been developed, though

Table 23.6 Dressings and topical wound products

Material	Presentation	Action	Indications for use	Special considerations
Alginates (fibres of calcium or sodium alginate derived from seaweed)	Flat sheets, ropes and packing	Absorbent; gels in contact with exudate Non-adhesive, non-occlusive	Partial and full thickness wounds Moderate to heavily exuding wounds	Can be packed into cavities and sinuses Can be rinsed from wound bed, cavity or sinus Usually require a secondary dressing
Antimicrobial dressings (impregnated with iodines, silvers)	Flat sheets and packing	Have an antimicrobial effect on the wound bed	Heavily contaminated or infected partial and full thickness wounds Moderate to heavily exuding wounds as these products usually need exudate to activate the antimicrobial effect	Usually require a secondary dressing Silver products can cause staining of surrounding skin and clothing if not contained
Foams (hydrophilic polyurethane/ polymer)	Flat sheets and cavity dressings Some are adhesive, some are semi-occlusive	Absorbent; some can retain exudate in foam	Partial and full thickness wounds Moderate to heavily exuding wounds	Removed in one piece Some are reusable and can be disinfected
Films (polyurethane or co-polymers)	Adhesive sheets	Transparent dressing Maintain a moist environment Impermeable to fluids and microorganisms	Partial and full thickness wounds Moderate to heavily exuding wounds	Removed in one piece Can be used as a primary wound contact dressing or to hold other dressings in place (e.g. hydrogels)
Hydrocolloids (hydrophilic colloid particles derived from cellulose, gelatins and pectins bound to a polyurethane foam backing)	Adhesive flat sheets in different thicknesses Gels Powders	Maintain a moist environment Provide an environment for autolysis Impermeable to fluids and microorganisms	Partial and full thickness wounds Dry to moderately exuding wounds Often not recommended for heavily exuding wounds, tracts and sinuses	Usually leave a residue that can be malodorous
Hydrofibres (fibres of carboxymethyl-cellulose)	Flat sheets and packing	Absorbent product that gels on contact with exudate	Partial and full thickness wounds Moderately to heavily exuding wounds	Require a secondary dressing
Hydrogels (water- and glycerin-based crossed-linked hydrophilic polymers)	Sachets of gel Sheets available Packing available Some are a carrier for antibiotics	Maintain a moist environment Provide an environment for autolysis	Partial and full thickness wounds Dry to moderately exuding wounds Provide an environment for autolysis	Usually require a secondary dressing to hold gel in contact with wound bed May cause maceration of skin surrounding wound and so often not recommended for heavily exuding wounds
Hydropolymers (multilayered)	Adhesive sheets of different thicknesses	Absorbent, some can retain exudate in the layers of dressing	Partial and full thickness wounds Minimal to heavily exuding wounds	Adhesive dressing that has the ability to be peeled away and reapplied
Low adherent dressings (woven mesh or net of polyamide)	Sheets Often silicone coated	Wound contact layers that wick exudate onto a retention dressing	Partial and full thickness wounds Moderately to heavily exuding wounds	Used under compression bandaging systems and in situations where a secondary dressing absorbs exudate

Table 23.6 Dressings and topical wound products *(Continued)*

Material	Presentation	Action	Indications for use	Special considerations
Skin substitutes or equivalents (bioabsorbable matrix containing fibroblasts and/or keratinocytes)	Single or multilayers of living cells, transported on a mesh or medium	Replaces skin and provides wound coverage with cellular activity	Partial and full thickness wounds Usually indicated for chronic and slow or non-healing wounds such as diabetic foot ulcers and venous leg ulcers Have been used extensively in burns patients	Usually require specialist skills and facilities Require special transportation and storage as some products are provided frozen and others are incubated Some wound bed preparation is needed prior to application

NB: This table provides examples of the main groups of dressings and topical wound products. However, it is not an exhaustive list and other products are available as combinations or variations of these main groups.

these are expensive to produce. They are recommended for indolent wounds, burns and diabetic foot ulceration (Gentzknow et al 1996) and usually comprise a bioabsorbable matrix of collagen that has been inoculated with living fibroblasts or keratinocytes. This technology is unlikely to be widely available but could enhance the care of and improve outcomes for patients with the most difficult wound healing problems.

Dressing change techniques

Throughout the UK there are many different policies, procedures and protocols for dressing changes. However, there are fundamental principles that need to be adhered to when undertaking wound care procedures (Rolstad et al 2000), namely standard infection control precautions where clean, non-sterile gloves are used to remove a soiled dressing and these discarded and a new pair of gloves used for any further procedures (Stotts 1997). A dressing needs changed when:

- there is a specific purpose, e.g. to remove sutures
- clinical signs of infection are present
- wound discharge has leaked through the dressing
- cleansing of an open wound is necessary — this may be as frequently as twice a day or as infrequently as once a week (see Table 23.6 for different dressings)
- special treatments are needed, e.g. burns dressings.

Aseptic technique

In hospital When dressing changes are being performed within a hospital, the nurse must always take into consideration the possibility of transferring bacteria from one patient to another, due to the close proximity in which patients are cared for. This is more of a risk when several patients with wounds are being nursed in the same ward and by the same nurses. Once a wound has become contaminated, clinical infection can quickly develop (see Ch. 16). Aseptic technique aims to prevent pathogenic organisms from contaminating a wound (see Box 23.7). In hospital, dressings are generally changed using an aseptic technique. There may, however, be occasions when dressing changes require a technique that is socially clean without being fully aseptic. It is an individual nurse's responsibility to understand the principles of asepsis and standard infection control precautions and adapt knowledge to the situation being managed.

In the community In the hospital, equipment is provided which allows the nurse to manage safely all the wound management situations encountered. Maintaining asepsis may pose different problems in the patient's own home. The district nurse may have little control over the cleanliness of the area and needs to take extra care when changing dressings. It is just as important in the community to avoid cross-infection between households and contamination of

Box 23.7

Principles of aseptic technique

- Perform the procedure in an area which is closed, clean and well ventilated at least 1 h after periods of activity — bed making and ward cleaning, for example, increase the circulation of dust particles and airborne bacteria
- Use a clean trolley — this should be thoroughly cleaned daily and wiped with an alcoholic solution before and after use
- Wash hands (p. 666) before, after and at any point during the procedure should they become contaminated. The use of an alcoholic hand-rub can sometimes be substituted
- Wear a clean plastic apron to protect the patient from bacteria on the nurse's uniform
- Use sterile equipment for the procedure — be aware of how your health authority/board identifies equipment which is sterile and therefore safe to use
- Discard equipment which has broken or damaged packaging
- Use sterile fluids and dressing materials
- Prepare equipment before dressings are removed
- Use gloves to remove any dressings and dispose of both immediately
- Carry out the procedure using forceps or sterile gloves, discarding equipment as it becomes contaminated
- Dispose of used equipment in the appropriate bin

wounds. The district nurse in these situations has many opportunities for health education.

The use of a clean technique

For many dressing changes, the use of a clean technique (see Table 23.7) is safe and acceptable (Flanagan 1997). The types of wound suitable for this method include the majority of granulating wounds.

Involving the patient in wound care

Whether patients are being cared for at home or in hospital, there are many opportunities for the nurse to involve patients in wound management. This is important in giving the patient a sense of independence and will help promote return to normality. Patients with sutured wounds can be taught to monitor themselves for clinical signs of infection and to give good self-care in terms of nutrition, fluid intake, rest and avoidance of excessive movement of the affected area. Patients with open wounds can become much more involved. In addition to the self-care elements outlined above, they can be taught about the appearance of the wound surface and what can be expected to happen during the healing phase. In the community, patients and their relatives can be taught the basic dressing-change technique where asepsis is not necessary and the district nurse can assume a supervisory role. This obviously depends on individual circumstances and the patient's level of understanding, but certainly many patients with open wounds are able to play a major role in wound management. This is important as the patient begins to resume a more normal lifestyle and it also avoids the need for routine daily visits by the district nurse.

Patients with chronic wounds, such as leg ulcers and pressure ulcers, need special help, but it is very important to gain their cooperation. Patients with venous leg ulcers (see p. 852) require advice on leg elevation techniques and calf pump muscle exercises, which stimulate the circulation and aid drainage of the lower limb. Carers of patients with pressure ulcers (see p. 849) need advice and training on manual handling, i.e. turning and repositioning the patient. Carers also need to know how the pressure-relieving aids work, so that these are used correctly at all times and not just when the district nurse is in the home.

Nurse prescribing

In 1999 a *Review of Prescribing, Supply and Administration of Medicines* recommended that new forms of prescribing — 'supplementary prescribing' and 'independent prescribing' — be carried out by nurses and pharmacists as non-medical professionals (DH 2004). Since then programmes for the education, training and regulation of nurses and pharmacists have been developed. There are plans to extend some aspects of this patient service to include physiotherapists, radiographers, podiatrists, chiropodists and optometrists. In addition, patient group directives (PGDs) enable nurses to supply and administer prescription only medicines to patients under the direction of a doctor. It is envisaged that these PGDs will be on an individual, patient-specific basis.

STOP THINK **23.5** Discuss with a community nurse some examples of nurse prescribing in relation to wound care.

Wound management policies and guidelines

Most health care providers in the UK have developed wound treatment and prevention policies to help guide their staff towards safe and standardised nursing care. Ideally, these are based on the best available evidence sourced from systematic reviews of the literature covering randomised, controlled trials (Cullum et al 1997). Given the rapid development of wound dressings and associated devices such as bandages and pressure-relieving equipment, and the wide range of therapies available to patients, such protocols and guidelines can enhance quality of care for patients by ensuring they receive treatment that is evidence based.

The transition from hospital to home

The transition from hospital to home for patients with wounds usually takes place without any problems. Liaison nurses are available to organise the discharge home and to arrange for any visits needed by the district nurse for the newly discharged patient. In emergency departments, a liaison service may also be available. It is important, however, that wherever patients receive treatment they have a point of contact so that they are well supported when discharged home (Bale & Jones 1997).

Table 23.7 Clean technique

Procedure	Rationale
1. Use non-sterile gloves to remove dressing. Change gloves	Protects both nurse and patient from cross-infection
2. Shower or bathe patient's wound	Mechanically removes loose wound debris (NB: ensure thorough cleansing of shower/bath whether at home or in hospital)
3. Use clean bowl/bucket with bin liner for patients with small wounds or foot/leg wounds in the home	Prevents contamination of equipment
4. Use clean paper or a clean towel to dry area surrounding wound	Prior to application of dressing, area needs to be dry
5. Encourage patient involvement in treatment	Increases patient compliance and encourages return to normal activity

Provision of materials in hospitals and in the community

Nurses may be unaware of the vast differences which exist in the provision of wound management materials to patients cared for in hospital compared with those cared for in the community. Although most hospitals impose some form of restriction on which materials are provided, generally all the main groups of manufactured materials are available. These are supplied not only to inpatients but also to outpatients who are under the care of a hospital consultant. All materials needed for inpatient treatment are provided without direct cost to the individual patient. It is the norm, then, for patients treated in hospital to have access to a comprehensive range of wound management materials for their wound care, and supplies of these continue as long as the patient remains in hospital.

Patients managed in the community are in a different position. Materials needed for their treatment are generally obtained from the general practitioner (GP), practice nurse or district nurse who writes a prescription for those items required. Unless the patient is exempt from paying, a charge is made for each item dispensed, though provision is made to enable patients to purchase a 'season ticket' lasting 4 months or 1 year. The products that can be prescribed are listed in the Drug Tariff that is controlled by the Department of Health. This list defines those dressing products that can be prescribed for use in the community and can be accessed on www.drugtariff.com.

STOP THINK **23.6** Ask the pharmacist what products are available on FP10 and GP10 (NHS Scotland) to patients in the community. Look also at the sizes of prescribable products.

Expectations of outcome and effectiveness of treatment

Following individual patient and wound assessment, the nurse should have reasonable expectations regarding the prospects of achieving complete healing. In some wounds, complete healing is expected rapidly, as in primary wound closure following excision of a lipoma in a healthy young person. For others, the prognosis for healing is less good, e.g. an older woman with arthritis and a venous leg ulcer. The expected outcome affects the choice of treatment for individual patients. For patients with a poor prognosis for healing, treatment is often directed towards minimising symptoms and preventing further wound breakdown. This situation can arise in terminally ill patients with superficial pressure ulcers where the aim is to prevent penetration of the ulcer into deeper tissues. Patient comfort and convenience become the priorities and provide some measure of the effectiveness of the treatment. Where healing is expected, effectiveness means complete healing is achieved in the minimum number of days.

Cost-effectiveness

Efficacy is also measured in terms of the cost of treatments. Hospital doctors, GPs, practice nurses or district nurses and the pharmacists who supply materials for wound management can be misled into believing that, because the initial cost of a material is high then it follows that the total treatment costs will also be high. Modern wound dressing materials can be very expensive to buy per unit. However, these dressings can often be left on the wound for several days and, in some cases, for a full week.

It is important, when comparing the costs of dressing materials, to consider:

- how long the product can be left on the wound
- how much nursing time is needed to change and apply dressings
- the benefits of using a material which is interactive and so stimulates tissue growth to achieve rapid healing or stimulate healing in a chronic wound.

Clinical evidence for improvement in healing or other outcome measures

It is in the area of materials that there has been most benefit, especially in the community, where much of the chronic wound care is undertaken. Modern wound treatments are helping to control wound symptoms and to achieve healing in chronic wounds, thus enabling more efficient use of nurses' time. Discharging such patients after many months, if not years, of treatment also improves their quality of life.

SPECIFIC WOUND TYPES

Pressure ulcers

Definition A pressure ulcer is an area of localised damage to the skin caused by disruption of the blood supply to the area, usually caused by pressure, shear or friction, or a combination of any of these (Dealey 1999). Tissue damage can be restricted to superficial epidermal loss or may involve underlying structures, extending to involve muscle and bone (European Pressure Ulcer Advisory Panel 1998).

The prevention and management of pressure ulcers present major challenges for nurses. The pressure ulcer problem is widespread and persistent, affecting patients from all walks of life and with a range of illnesses. It causes diminished quality of life and distress to patients and carers and makes major financial demands on the health service. As a result, in many hospital and community trusts, nurses are now supported by a 'tissue viability service' (Dealey 1997). Particular difficulties arise in trying to identify patients who might develop a pressure ulcer, and when they are at risk of doing so.

It is a basic responsibility of nurses to:

- assess accurately the patients in their care for being 'at risk' of developing a pressure ulcer
- ensure that any predisposing factors are reduced
- ensure that patients are nursed on the most suitable surface, depending on their individual needs
- ensure that established pressure ulcers are efficiently managed
- undertake regular and ongoing reassessments of individual patients; a patient's needs vary from one day to the next, and in the very ill from one hour to the next.

Aetiology

Pressure ulcers result from areas of previously healthy tissue becoming devitalised, resulting in localised tissue death. Pressure ulcers develop in a number of ways:

- as a result of direct, unrelieved pressure of soft tissues against bone
- where friction occurs between the patient and the surface of a bed or chair; this can happen if the patient is moved and the skin is dragged over a sheet
- as a result of the shear forces that frequently accompany both direct pressure and friction; shear forces develop in tissues that are distorted and pulled, so that the blood supply is disrupted.

Classification

In order to assess the extent or degree of damage, grading systems have been developed (European Pressure Ulcer Advisory Panel 1998). The EPUAP system has four grades of tissue damage:

- *Grade 1* — non-blanchable erythema of intact skin. Discoloration of the skin, warmth, oedema, induration or hardness may also be used as indicators, particularly on individuals with darker skin.
- *Grade 2* — partial-thickness skin loss involving epidermis, dermis or both. The ulcer is superficial and presents clinically as an abrasion or blister.
- *Grade 3* — full-thickness skin loss involving damage to or necrosis of subcutaneous tissue that may extend down to, but not through, underlying fascia.
- *Grade 4* — extensive destruction, tissue necrosis or damage to muscle, bone or supporting structures with or without full thickness skin loss.

Assessment of risk

In an acute illness, even the most unlikely individual may become 'at risk' of developing a pressure ulcer; therefore, all patients should be assessed on admission either to a hospital ward or unit or onto a district nurse's caseload — 'The importance of assessing all patients (except perhaps some short-stay cases) cannot be overemphasised' (Dealey 1999). A combination of disease processes and/or drug therapies or surgery, for example, can quite suddenly put an individual into an 'at risk' category.

The following patients are at risk of developing pressure ulcers:

- older people
- the immobile, e.g. paraplegic or following certain types of orthopaedic surgery
- those with sensory loss, e.g. in a coma, or in the diabetic
- those with a range of systemic diseases, e.g. anaemia, peripheral vascular disease, carcinoma
- those having a range of medication, e.g. anti-inflammatory, cytotoxic or steroid medication
- those with impaired continence
- poorly nourished individuals
- the obese and those with below-average body weight.

Several scales and scoring systems have been devised for assessing risk; the most widely used in the UK is probably the Waterlow score (see Fig. 23.4). There are other risk assessment scores available, though only some — the Norton Scale, the Braden Scale and the Central Begeleidings Orgaan (CBO) — have undergone validity testing (Braden 1997, Schoonhaven et al 2002). National (National Institute for Clinical Excellence 2001) and international (European Pressure Ulcer Advisory Panel 1998) guidelines have been produced to guide nurses towards adopting an evidence-based approach to caring for patients. Many health care providers have adapted guidelines for local use to suit their own patients' needs and as part of a pressure ulcer prevention policy. Guidelines are designed to rationalise and standardise patient care so that all patients receive a reasonable level of care. Guidelines also help to ensure that the available pressure-relieving equipment is used most efficiently. However, all health care professionals have a responsibility for taking action once risk is identified (Dealey 1997).

As part of guideline recommendations, risk assessment tools are designed to support nurses' clinical judgement and not to replace it (Bates-Jensen 1997, Braden 1997, National Institute for Clinical Excellence 2001). They are useful only if used regularly — on admission and again each time the patient's condition changes. The scores need to be accurately documented and then used to determine the most appropriate pressure-relieving devices on which to nurse the patient.

23.7 What scoring system does your ward/area use? Where is the score documented and how often are patients reassessed?

For further information, see Dealey (1997).

Prevention of pressure ulcers

Once patients have been identified as being 'at risk', they should be nursed on the most appropriate surface. This includes not only the mattress on the bed but also any chairs in which they may sit during the day (Dealey 1999). Other areas worth considering are theatre operating tables and trolleys on which patients are transported around the hospital. Liaison with other professionals may be indicated, for example with the physiotherapist to assess the degree of mobility an individual has and where help and treatment can be given.

Attempts to reduce friction and shearing when nursing patients are essential. At home this is easier than in hospital where sheets may become hard when washed in very hot water and dried in very hot dryers. Where possible, patients should be nursed on soft sheets and covered with a duvet or soft blankets, as hard rigid surfaces increase friction.

Friction also increases with moisture. As increased skin moisture can result from incontinence and sweating, these should be avoided where possible. Nutrition and fluid balance also need attention. It has been estimated that dehydrated patients and patients in a negative nitrogen balance are more likely to experience tissue breakdown.

For further information, see the European Pressure Ulcer Advisory Panel website, www.epuap.org.

Management of patients with established pressure ulcers

In addition to providing a suitable surface on which to nurse the patient, and ensuring adequate nutrition and using

A

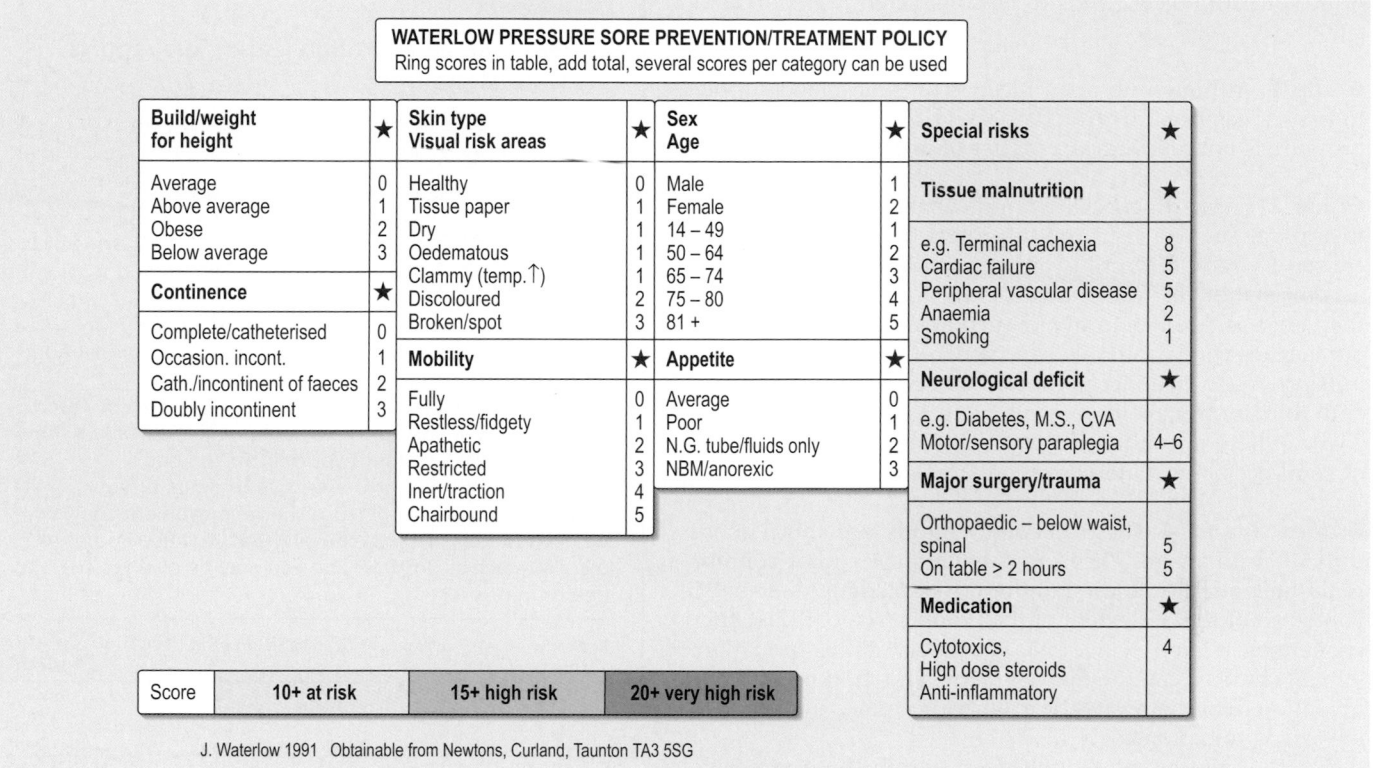

WATERLOW PRESSURE SORE PREVENTION/TREATMENT POLICY
Ring scores in table, add total, several scores per category can be used

Build/weight for height	★
Average	0
Above average	1
Obese	2
Below average	3

Continence	★
Complete/catheterised	0
Occasion. incont.	1
Cath./incontinent of faeces	2
Doubly incontinent	3

Skin type Visual risk areas	★
Healthy	0
Tissue paper	1
Dry	1
Oedematous	1
Clammy (temp.↑)	1
Discoloured	2
Broken/spot	3

Mobility	★
Fully	0
Restless/fidgety	1
Apathetic	2
Restricted	3
Inert/traction	4
Chairbound	5

Sex Age	★
Male	1
Female	2
14 – 49	1
50 – 64	2
65 – 74	3
75 – 80	4
81 +	5

Appetite	★
Average	0
Poor	1
N.G. tube/fluids only	2
NBM/anorexic	3

Special risks	★
Tissue malnutrition	★
e.g. Terminal cachexia	8
Cardiac failure	5
Peripheral vascular disease	5
Anaemia	2
Smoking	1
Neurological deficit	★
e.g. Diabetes, M.S., CVA	
Motor/sensory paraplegia	4–6
Major surgery/trauma	★
Orthopaedic – below waist, spinal	5
On table > 2 hours	5
Medication	★
Cytotoxics, High dose steroids Anti-inflammatory	4

Score	10+ at risk	15+ high risk	20+ very high risk

J. Waterlow 1991 Obtainable from Newtons, Curland, Taunton TA3 5SG

B

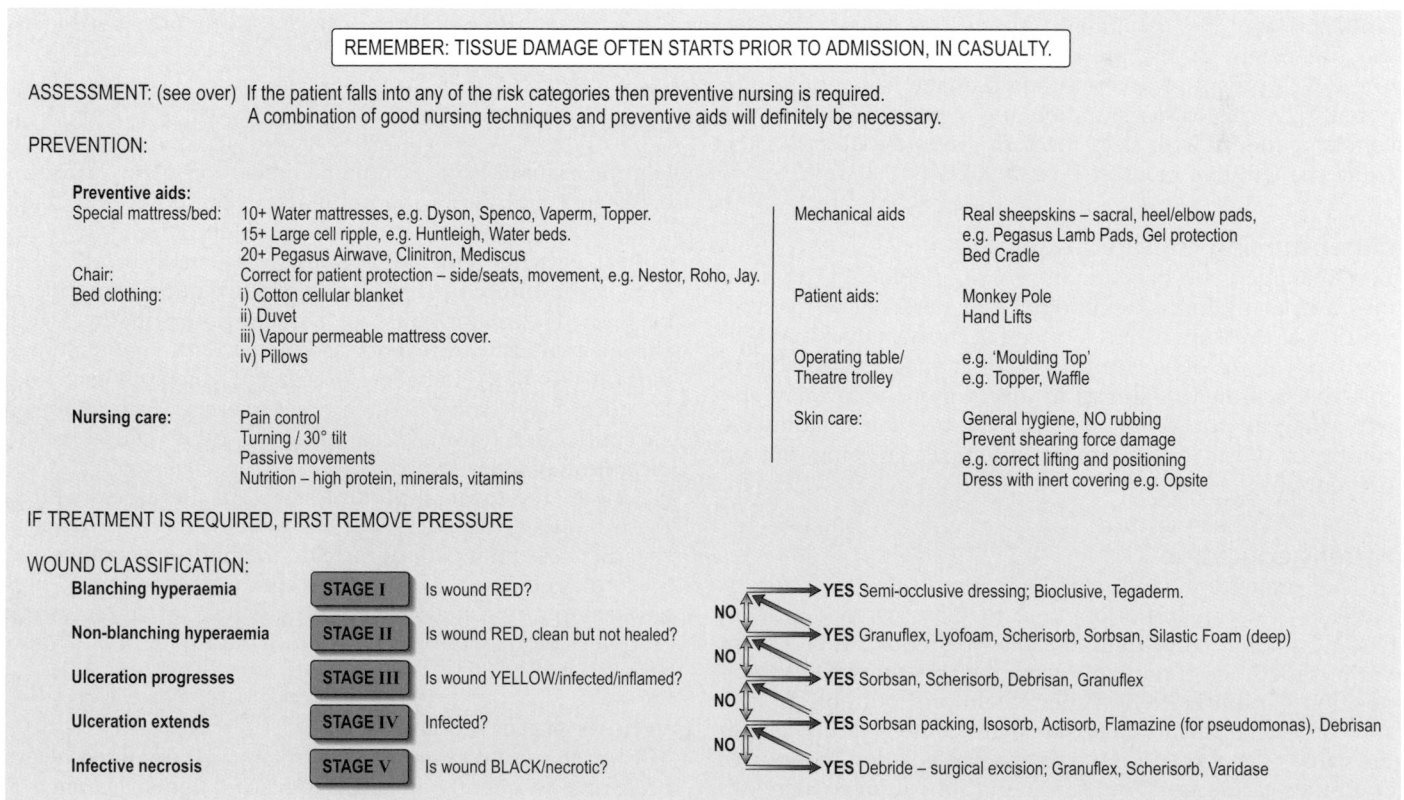

REMEMBER: TISSUE DAMAGE OFTEN STARTS PRIOR TO ADMISSION, IN CASUALTY.

ASSESSMENT: (see over) If the patient falls into any of the risk categories then preventive nursing is required.
A combination of good nursing techniques and preventive aids will definitely be necessary.

PREVENTION:

Preventive aids:

Special mattress/bed: 10+ Water mattresses, e.g. Dyson, Spenco, Vaperm, Topper.
15+ Large cell ripple, e.g. Huntleigh, Water beds.
20+ Pegasus Airwave, Clinitron, Mediscus

Chair: Correct for patient protection – side/seats, movement, e.g. Nestor, Roho, Jay.

Bed clothing: i) Cotton cellular blanket
ii) Duvet
iii) Vapour permeable mattress cover.
iv) Pillows

Nursing care: Pain control
Turning / 30° tilt
Passive movements
Nutrition – high protein, minerals, vitamins

Mechanical aids: Real sheepskins – sacral, heel/elbow pads,
e.g. Pegasus Lamb Pads, Gel protection
Bed Cradle

Patient aids: Monkey Pole
Hand Lifts

Operating table/ Theatre trolley: e.g. 'Moulding Top'
e.g. Topper, Waffle

Skin care: General hygiene, NO rubbing
Prevent shearing force damage
e.g. correct lifting and positioning
Dress with inert covering e.g. Opsite

IF TREATMENT IS REQUIRED, FIRST REMOVE PRESSURE

WOUND CLASSIFICATION:

Blanching hyperaemia	STAGE I	Is wound RED?	**YES** Semi-occlusive dressing; Bioclusive, Tegaderm.
Non-blanching hyperaemia	STAGE II	Is wound RED, clean but not healed?	**YES** Granuflex, Lyofoam, Scherisorb, Sorbsan, Silastic Foam (deep)
Ulceration progresses	STAGE III	Is wound YELLOW/infected/inflamed?	**YES** Sorbsan, Scherisorb, Debrisan, Granuflex
Ulceration extends	STAGE IV	Infected?	**YES** Sorbsan packing, Isosorb, Actisorb, Flamazine (for pseudomonas), Debrisan
Infective necrosis	STAGE V	Is wound BLACK/necrotic?	**YES** Debride – surgical excision; Granuflex, Scherisorb, Varidase

(NO → next question)

Fig. 23.4 The Waterlow pressure ulcer prevention/treatment policy. (Reproduced with permission from Waterlow 1991.)

good handling techniques when moving a patient, local care of the pressure ulcer needs to be considered (Morison et al 1997).

Grade 1 Although no open ulcer is present, blood supply to tissues has been disrupted and will rapidly deteriorate if pressure is not relieved as a matter of urgency.

Grade 2 These superficial wounds usually need a dressing to assist tissue recovery and to protect the area. A common cause of Grade 2 ulcers is either friction or, more usually, a combination of friction and shear force. Elimination of the cause is needed to avoid further and more extensive damage. Several materials can be chosen as dressings that will provide a healing environment: semi-permeable films and thin hydrocolloids are all good examples (see Table 23.6). Where incontinence is a problem, these occlusive or semi-occlusive materials are invaluable.

Grades 3 and 4 These deeper wounds are much more difficult to manage. They often have an irregular contour with the wound extending under the skin edge. Assessment is needed of the full extent of the wound (see p. 842). Other challenges related to wound shape are sinus formation, which requires careful management, and packing and/or irrigation. This is a situation where surgical intervention may need to be considered.

Necrotic tissue and slough deep within these extensive wounds must be removed if healing is to proceed, and there are several ways of achieving this (Bale 1996) (see p. 845). Until most of the devitalised tissue has been removed, the full extent of the pressure ulcer cannot be assessed. The development of severe tissue damage is a serious and potentially hazardous situation for a patient. Ninety per cent of patients with deep necrotic pressure ulcers of the trunk die within 4 months (Bliss 1990).

Other nursing considerations

The management of patients with established pressure ulcers is costly in both economic and personal terms. Prevention of pressure ulcers is often far cheaper than management (Dealey 1997). Health service managers are able to cost the treatment of pressure ulcers more accurately and with the call for pressure ulcers to become a notifiable condition (Dealey 1997) more emphasis is being put on prevention.

Patient education

In the prevention and management of pressure ulcers, patients have an important role to play. All patients, including young, chronically disabled patients can be taught various methods of regularly relieving pressure by changing position (Colburn 1997). Patients who are not able to take such an active part in their own management can be taught the value of and need for the changes of position that nurses and other carers carry out for them. Concordance increases when patients understand why intervention is necessary.

Education leaflets can also be useful. An extract from a typical patient information leaflet demonstrates how the nurse and the patient share in the prevention of pressure ulcers (see Box 23.8).

Box 23.8

Extract from an education leaflet: preventing pressure ulcers

As most pressure ulcers are the result of staying in one position for too long, the answer is to:

Relieve the pressure by changing position
Ideally, you should get up out of bed or your chair at least once every 2 hours during the day and take a short walk. This activity also helps your blood circulation and stops your muscles getting lax.

If you are confined to a chair, you should lift your bottom off the seat for a few moments every half an hour by pushing up on the arms of the chair.

If you have to stay in bed, then your bed may be fitted with a 'monkey pole' or rope ladder — the nurse will show you how to use this to lift yourself off the bed.

If your pressure ulcer is extensive or deep, or your movement is very restricted, a special movement chart will be devised for you by the nursing staff to keep you off the ulcer as much as possible, and you may be given a special bed or mattress.

Reproduced with permission from Morison et al (1997).

Throughout the UK and mainland Europe guidelines for the prevention and treatment of pressure ulcers have been produced in different languages for professionals, carers and patients (European Pressure Ulcer Advisory Panel 1998).

Leg ulcers

Leg ulceration is a common clinical problem, affecting between 1 and 2% of the population (Doughty et al 2000). Essentially a community-based problem, the day-to-day care of patients with these wounds is usually undertaken in the community by district and practice nurses, supported by GPs. The major cause of leg ulceration in the UK is chronic venous insufficiency associated with venous hypertension (70–75%). Between 20 and 30% of patients with a leg ulcer have some degree of ischaemia, with diabetes, vasculitis and trauma accounting for other causes of leg ulceration (Collier 1999).

One of the most important stages in the assessment of these patients is to diagnose the aetiology of the ulcer, as this dictates the most appropriate method of management. Such diagnosis is achieved by conducting a lower limb assessment in conjunction with the use of a hand-held Doppler (Morison & Moffatt 1997, Doughty et al 2000) (see Box 23.9 and p. 853).

Venous stasis leg ulcers

This is the most commonly encountered group of leg ulcers, occurring frequently in older female patients. Damage to the veins deep in the calf causes incompetence of the perforators, the veins which link the deep and superficial veins in the calf (see Fig. 23.5).

Drainage of the skin in the lower leg is affected, leading to oedema, induration and pigmentation. Fibrin is laid

Box 23.9

How to take the ankle pressure index

- Lay the patient flat and allow the patient to rest quietly for 20 min. This is necessary to eliminate the effects of gravity on the legs
- Place the sphygmomanometer cuff on the upper arm, and apply gel over the brachial artery. Hold the Doppler probe at a 45° angle and measure the systolic pressure
- Place the sphygmomanometer cuff around the malleolus (should the ulcer be sited here, place the cuff above the ulcer). Apply gel around either the dorsalis pedis or posterior tibial pulse
- Locate the pulse and inflate the cuff until Doppler sound disappears. Gradually deflate the cuff and, when sound returns, record this as the ankle systolic pressure. The ankle pressure index is calculated by dividing the ankle pressure reading by the brachial pressure reading

Normal ankle pressure index ≥1
Abnormal ankle pressure index ≤1
If ankle pressure index is ≤0.8, the arterial impairment is likely to be significant

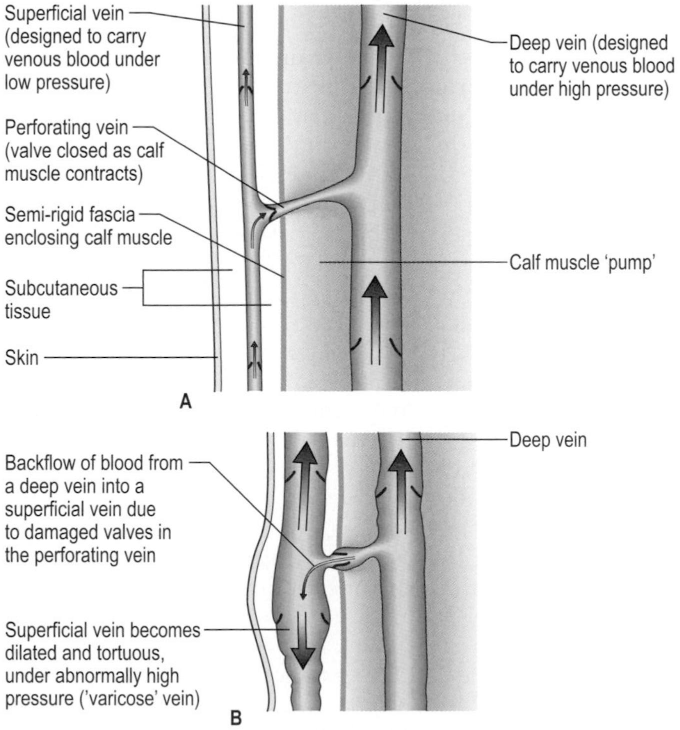

Fig. 23.5 A: Healthy, intact valves prevent backflow of blood from the deep to the superficial veins. B: An incompetent valve in a perforating vein allows backflow of blood from the deep to the superficial venous system.

down around the capillaries in this area, which interferes with oxygen diffusion into the tissues. Following this, any knock or minor injury to the lower leg leads rapidly to breakdown of the skin and ulceration. Most commonly, ulceration occurs around the medial malleolus; the ulcers are shallow and pain is not usually a factor. A typical past history reveals previous phlebitis, deep vein thrombosis (DVT), leg fracture or severe leg injury, or varicose veins.

It can take many months for venous ulcers to heal. Due to the poor condition of the tissues, ulceration can recur and these patients need to wear compression stockings, even after healing, to help maintain drainage of the affected limb.

For further reading, see the European Wound Management Association position document on understanding compression therapy (2003).

Assessment One of the primary aims of assessment in a patient with a leg ulcer is to determine the cause. This is frequently undertaken by both the nurse and doctor working together as part of the primary health care team. Assessment includes:

- taking a comprehensive medical history which might indicate the presence of venous disease, e.g. history of previous DVT, venous claudication, previous vein surgery or pelvic trauma
- undertaking a thorough clinical examination to support the medical history
- undertaking the appropriate investigations: a Doppler assessment will give the ankle pressure index (see Box 23.9) but other investigations may include haemoglobin to exclude anaemia, ESR to indicate the presence of infection, glucose levels to exclude diabetes mellitus, and wound swab where infection is suspected.

Management

Bandaging The most important component in the treatment of venous stasis ulcers is the control of oedema by compression bandages or support stockings (Morison & Moffatt 1997). Compression bandages are designed to give a graduated compression that provides more support at the ankle and less at the knee, to compensate for the failure of the perforators in the leg. The bandages need to be worn constantly during the day when the patient is walking and upright, to reduce oedema. It may be necessary to prescribe diuretics to assist drainage of oedema.

The principles of compression bandaging are to:

- bandage from toes to below the knee (see Fig. 23.6)
- apply graduated compression by applying even tension to a compression bandage; more pressure is applied to the ankle and less as the circumference of the leg increases to the knee — 30–40 mmHg of pressure may be required at the ankle, graduating to 15–20 mmHg below the knee (Morison & Moffatt 1997)
- maintain the level of compression
- ensure that the bandage/stocking does not slip, causing constriction of the limb (Morison & Moffatt 1997, European Wound Management Association 2003).

The pressure exerted by a bandaging system can be calculated using Laplace's law (see Box 23.10).

Selection of a bandage depends on the amount of compression required. Three grades of compression bandage are available:

- grade I provides very light compression or support for mild oedema

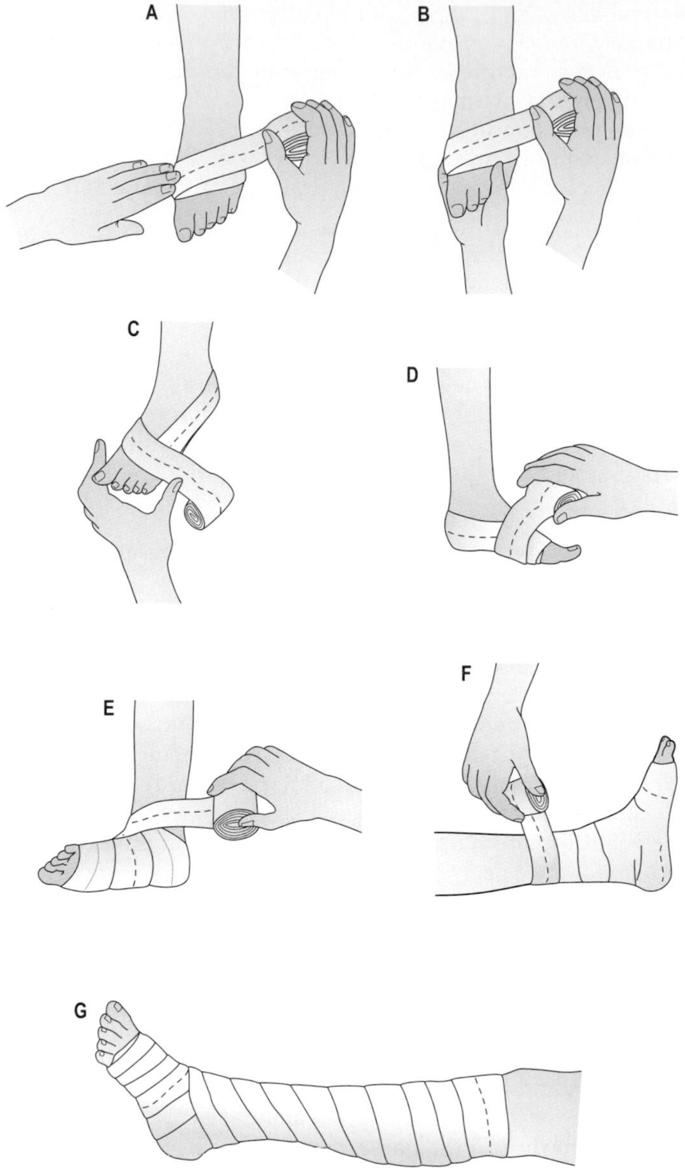

Fig. 23.6 Elastic web bandage. A: Start bandage on the inner side of the sole of the foot, with the lower edge of bandage at the root of the toes. Turn 1½ times round the foot. B: The thumb fixes the bandage for the start of the turn around the heel. C: View from the outer side of the foot. Thumb and finger hold bandage in place prior to completing turn around base of toes. D: View from the inner side of the foot. E: View from the outer side of the foot. Continuation of the bandaging, keeping lower edge of the bandage along red or blue line of the previous turn. F: View from the outer side of the foot. Tension used is about half the full stretch of the bandage. G: View from the outer side of the leg. Note the position of the final turn of bandage immediately below the knee. (Reproduced with permission from Ryan 1991.)

- grade II provides moderate compression at the ankle of between 18 and 24 mmHg
- grade III provides strong compression, giving between 25 and 35 mmHg at the ankle.

Control of infection Where pain, cellulitis, erythema, enlarging of the ulcer and purulent discharge occur,

Box 23.10

Formula for calculating the pressure exerted by a bandaging system

$$P = \frac{T \times N \times \text{constant}}{C \times W}$$

P = sub-bandage pressure
T = tension
N = number of layers
C = limb circumference
W = width of bandage

Reproduced with permission from Morison & Moffatt (1997).

antibiotics may be necessary to control the infection. These should be administered systemically. Superficial infection can sometimes be controlled by the topical application of an antiseptic.

Physiotherapy Exercises to stimulate the calf muscle pump, which assists venous return, can be taught to each patient, and these are encouraged regularly throughout the day to stimulate circulation and aid drainage of the lower legs. Some period of leg elevation should also be encouraged around the middle of the day, again to allow drainage of the lower legs.

Dressings Dressing management should be carefully considered once the factors outlined above have been successfully tackled. The ulcer should be assessed as for wounds (p. 842) and the appropriate material then selected (p. 846). Caution should be exercised with dressings and lotions as these patients quickly develop sensitivities to many of the commonly used products. The simplest treatments should be used first: non- or low adherent textile dressings, with hydrocolloid, alginate, impregnated textile dressings and foam dressings having a useful role when used in combination with an appropriate compression bandage.

A comprehensive patient assessment should aim to result in a complete treatment package. A suitable wound contact dressing and skin care combined with adequate compression therapy, physiotherapy and education are likely to produce the best patient outcomes.

Arterial ulcers

These are often the result of arteriosclerosis (Doughty et al 2000) of the lower leg and the underlying disease processes are different from venous disease (see Table 23.8). Arteriosclerosis may occur anywhere throughout the arterial circulation, causing narrowing and occlusion due to calcification of the artery wall. Damage to the arteries supplying the leg can be caused by vascular disease and this gradually occludes and blocks them. Additionally, infarction of smaller arteries is caused by embolus formation, which causes ischaemia in the area of skin normally supplied by that artery. What follows is a very rapid breakdown of the skin.

The characteristics of these ulcers are a history of intermittent claudication and rapid onset of a deep ulcer that is often extremely painful. Relief is gained by lowering the

Table 23.8 Characteristics of venous and arterial disease of the lower limb

Characteristic	Venous disease	Arterial disease
Site of ulcer	Around the 'garter' area, commonly above the medial malleolus	Anywhere on the lower limb including the foot, but commonly affecting the toes
Depth of ulcer	Shallow and spreading	Deep, with a punched-out appearance
Presence of oedema	Common, due to poor venous return	Often not detected
Onset	Gradual, unless precipitated by trauma	Rapid
Pain	Often uncomfortable, nagging in character	Pain on elevation of limb relieved by lowering it (the blood flow is increased when the limb is in the dependent position). The pain of ischaemia can be unremitting
Temperature of foot	Warm and well perfused	Cool or cold and poorly perfused
Condition of the skin surrounding the ulcer	Lipodermatosclerosis present Varicose eczema	
Ankle pressure index	>0.8	<0.8

affected limb and hanging it over the edge of the bed or chair. These patients rarely go to bed to sleep, or if they do, they have to get up in the night because of the pain. They tend to sleep in a chair, which allows the affected limb to hang down, thus optimising the blood supply.

These ulcers can occur anywhere on the lower leg, but usually present on the foot and lateral aspect of the lower leg. Foot pulses are often absent or very difficult to palpate. Doppler assessment reveals a pressure index of below 0.8. The patient may also have a history of cardiovascular disease, typically hypertension, myocardial infarction, strokes or transient ischaemic attacks.

Management Surgical intervention may be necessary to improve the circulation through reconstruction of vessels or to debride dead tissue within the ulcer, and skin grafting may be considered. Light bandaging only is applied to keep a dressing in place; compression is to be avoided at all costs as this would further impede an already poor blood supply to the area.

Healing of these wounds is slow and the prognosis for eventual healing often poor. Treatment aims to keep the patient as comfortable as possible and to achieve debridement and cleansing where necessary. Useful dressings include alginate sheets, medicated dressings and hydrogel sheets.

Mixed aetiology ulcers

Around 20% of venous ulcers also have a significant arterial blood supply deficiency (Morison & Moffatt 1997). This further complicates management, as control of oedema is needed but without restricting the already poor blood supply.

Diagnosis Accurate diagnosis is fundamental to successful treatment. Those giving care should be absolutely certain of exactly what the aetiology of the ulcer is before any type of treatment begins. Lower limb assessment together with Doppler assessment (p. 853) will assist diagnosis (Doughty et al 2000). Clearly, if arterial problems are allowed to go unrecognised and strong compression bandaging applied, treatment will not only be ineffective but could also cause the patient harm. Information on other types of leg ulcer is summarised in Box 23.11.

Patient education

Individual education regarding wound management can have a dramatic effect on progress. This aspect of care is particularly appropriate in patients with leg ulcers, especially venous leg ulcers, as unless these patients know the cause of their ulcer, they may not comply with treatment. Leg exercises, leg elevation and the need for adequate

Box 23.11

Other types of leg ulcer accounting for between 2 and 5% of lower limb ulcers

- *Vasculitic ulcers* — these are due to connective tissue disease, e.g. rheumatoid arthritis, scleroderma, and also occur on the lower leg. They are unusual and extremely difficult to manage due to the underlying disease process and the medication that these patients require.
- *Diabetic ulcers* — these occur most commonly on the foot. Again, due to the general condition of the patient, they heal slowly. It is worth noting that people with diabetes mellitus may give a falsely high reading on Doppler assessment due to peripheral hypertension. The management of rheumatoid and diabetic ulcers is generally under specialist care and treatment is prescribed by the individual consultant.
- *Traumatic ulcers*
- *Miscellaneous causes* — neoplastic and tropical ulcers are examples in this category.

Based on data from Morison & Moffatt (1997) and Doughty et al (2000).

compression are the key factors to success. Without this education the patient is not fully equipped to participate in management of the ulcer. Patient education can be helped by providing patients with leaflets that can be read at home (see Box 23.12).

Box 23.12

An education leaflet for patients with venous ulcers and their carers: how to care for your legs

How long must I keep the dressing and bandage (or stocking) in place?
Wear the support bandages or elastic support stockings as advised by the doctor and nurse. They will make arrangements for your next dressing change.

Do not be tempted to look under the bandage or disturb the dressing in the meantime, as this may delay healing. It is particularly important not to scratch the skin around the ulcer as this skin is easily damaged.

Ask for help AT ONCE if:

- your leg itches excessively, is hot, or more painful than usual
- you feel that the bandage is too tight anywhere
- you lose sensation in your toes, or they turn cold or blue
- you need any other advice.

Contact person:
Contact telephone number:

Can I exercise?
Yes. Exercise is good for your circulation and your general health. If possible, take a gentle walk every day. Even indoors, you can bend and stretch your toes while sitting, and bend, flex and circle your ankles to prevent them from becoming stiff. It is important not to stand still for too long. It is a good idea to do the dishes and the ironing sitting down, if you can obtain a chair of the correct height.

Should I sit with my legs up?
Yes. Sitting with your legs hanging down is almost as bad as standing in one place for too long. You should sit with your legs supported on a stool, on a cushion or pillow, i.e. above the level of your hips. It is also helpful to raise the foot of your bed 9 inches (23 cm) as this aids return of blood from the legs to the heart overnight.

Do I need a special diet?
You do not need a special diet, but try to eat a balanced one that includes protein (meat, fish, eggs), fresh fruit and vegetables. Being overweight does not help the circulation in your legs. Ask the doctor for advice on weight loss if this is a problem for you.

Are there any other ways I can help my legs?
Yes.

- Avoid knocks to your legs, as this could lead to another ulcer.
- Keep your legs warm, but do not sit too close to the fire as this can damage the skin.
- Do not wear anything tight around the tops of your legs, such as garters or girdles, as your circulation will be hindered.
- Stop smoking.

Reproduced with permission from Morison & Moffatt (1997).

Sutured wounds

Although the vast majority of sutured wounds heal without complication, there is a need for careful observation of both the patient and the wound site:

- Observe the patient for changes in vital signs, pulse, temperature, or malaise that could indicate the presence of infection, especially wound infection. Surgical wound infection accounts for 10.7% of all hospital acquired infections (Emmerson et al 1996) and is a major cause of postoperative morbidity.
- Observe the wound area for signs of infection after the initial inflammatory response has passed, i.e. redness, swelling, pain, discharge, heat.

When are the sutures removed? The best time for removal of suture material depends upon a number of factors:

- *The site of the wound* — wounds on the head and neck usually heal within 2 days due to the rich blood supply to the area, whereas wounds on the back may take 10–14 days to heal. The skin here is thicker and less well supplied with blood.
- *Patient variation* — if, during suture removal, the wound begins to gape then the nurse should stop and refer to the surgeon or a nurse specialist for advice. The skin edges can be pulled back together and held for a few more days with paper sutures.
- *Cosmetic considerations* — it should also be noted that leaving sutures in for too long can cause excessive scarring.

In general, the principles for managing sutured wounds are to leave the wound undisturbed and the theatre dressing intact unless either the patient or the wound area begins to develop signs which indicate the presence of infection (Bale & Jones 1997). Disturbing dressings unnecessarily can lead to the entry of bacteria into the wound itself or disturb the newly forming epithelium. Local wound infection can slow down the rate of healing and also increase the amount of scar tissue produced. Careful postoperative observation is important. Ultimately a severe wound infection can spread into the tissues and also the bloodstream, causing septicaemia which could be life threatening (Williams & Leaper 1998).

Traumatic wounds

Patients who present to the emergency department with traumatic wounds need special consideration. These patients may be shocked or have other injuries and their wounds are often contaminated due to the nature of the trauma (see Ch. 27).

These wounds are frequently an irregular shape, with varying degrees of tissue loss (Whiteside & Moorehead 1999). Due to contamination, wound closure is often not attempted (Bale & Leaper 2000). Mechanical cleansing of the wound is undertaken to remove debris such as glass, wood or tarmac. Where wound closure is attempted, antibiotic cover is given to prevent infection, and the patient also needs to be given prophylactic tetanus protection if they are not already covered (Whiteside & Moorehead 1999).

Patients with extensive injuries are admitted for inpatient treatment. However, the majority of patients with wounds are discharged home to be cared for in the community. They may be instructed to care for the wound themselves or asked to return to the emergency department for any dressing changes, or the community nurse may be asked to take over the wound management.

For further information, see Bale & Jones (1997), part 2: intervention.

Malignant wounds

This is one group of wounds where healing is not always the expected outcome of wound management. Carcinomas and sarcomas are most likely to result in ulceration and fungation in the latter stages of the disease (Bale & Harding 2000, Goldberg & McGinn-Byer 2000). Such lesions include fungating carcinoma of the breast, fungating lesions of malignant melanoma and a variety of other non-healing, extending or fungating wounds. Mortimer (1993) has defined the term 'fungating' as describing a malignancy that has ulcerated and infiltrated through the epithelium. Fungating wounds can result either in a protruding growth or in an ulcerating cavity (Carville 1994). These patients are generally managed by a combination of hospital and home care and over a period of time become well known to both agencies.

The growth of tumours is a complex process that controls blood flow and tissue oxygenation (Grocott 1995). Bridel-Nixon (1997) describes the process of fungation as a mixture of concurrent and progressive disease that affects haemostasis, lymph, interstitial and cellular environments. Hypoxia of the tissues causes tissue breakdown and encourages anaerobic and aerobic bacterial growth, producing malodour.

Problems encountered with malignant wounds (see Ch. 31) are as follows:

- *Wound site* — often these wounds are present in an area which is extremely difficult to dress in terms of keeping the dressing in place, e.g. on the chest wall, in the groin and on the lower limb.
- *Exudate production* — the exudate tends to be thick and sticky. Many dressings that do not adhere to other wound types will do so in the presence of this particularly viscous exudate. Hydrogel sheets and gel are very useful dressings for these wounds.
- *Pain* — where nerve endings are exposed, changing dressings and rubbing of dressings can be painful. Keeping the wound covered reduces the irritation to the nerve endings, and using gel dressings reduces pain at dressing changes.

Where healing is not the ultimate aim, wound management should maximise convenience and minimise distress.

For further reading, see Morison et al (1997), Chapter 11.

Burns

The management of burns is a specialised area (see Ch. 30). The treatment given depends on the individual burns unit. However, all follow the same basic principles for management. Treatment will depend on the physical well-being and age of the individual, the area burnt and the depth and extent of the burn.

Psychosocial factors

The presence of a wound will inevitably have some effect on well-being. There may be no difficulty when a wound is small and heals rapidly, but for many patients some degree of anxiety is felt relating to the wound. This can disrupt sleep patterns, increase the perception of pain and even suppress the immune system. In more serious wounds, a disturbance of body image may also cause lasting distress, particularly if the patient is unprepared for this (Wilson 2000).

STOP THINK **23.8** How would you help the following patients to overcome their fears and worries?

- An older lady living alone has a chronic venous ulcer requiring frequent dressing by the community nurse. She is increasingly confined to the house.
- A small girl recovering from a hernia repair fears that when the sutures are removed her wound will break open.
- A young woman has been mugged on her way home from work. The knife wound to her face required suturing in the Emergency Department. She has had no opportunity to see the wound and is fearing the worst.

CONCLUSION

The effective management of patients with wounds requires an understanding of the healing process in conjunction with a systematic approach to both assessment and management, and includes:

- assessment of the individual's overall health, taking into account factors which might impair healing
- assessment of the wound
- planning the management of the individual and the wound, taking into account the social and physical environment, and using the most appropriate dressing materials available
- involving the patient, where possible, in wound care
- evaluation and reassessment of the individual until the wound heals or the needs of the patient change.

STOP THINK **23.9** Which types of dressing material are available in your hospital/community?

Estimate the cost of dressings needed to manage four different patients for 1 week. Include dressing packs, surgical tapes and lotions as well as the dressing materials themselves.

How much variation is there between the four? Which patient is the most expensive to manage?

23.10 Go to the operating theatre and find out how pressure ulcers are prevented in theatre.

23.11 Go to the hospital pharmacy/chemist's shop to find out how dressing materials are ordered and dispensed. Who decides which products are made available in the hospital?

REFERENCES

Bale S 1996 A guide to wound debridement. Journal of Wound Care 6(4): 179–182

Bale S 2000 Principles and practices of wound assessment and management. In: Bale S, Harding K, Leaper D (eds) An introduction to wounds. Emap Healthcare, London

Bale S 2004 Using different designs in wound healing research. Nurse Researcher 11(4): 42–53

Bale S, Harding K 2000 Chronic wounds 2: diabetic foot ulcers and malignant wounds. In: Bale S, Harding K, Leaper D (eds) An introduction to wounds. Emap Healthcare, London

Bale S, Jones V 1997 Wound care nursing: a patient centred approach. Baillière Tindall, London

Bale S, Leaper D 2000 Acute wounds. In: Bale S, Harding K, Leaper D (eds) An introduction to wounds. Emap Healthcare, London

Barone E J, Yager D R, Pozez A L 1998 Interleukin-1 alpha and collagenase activity are elevated in chronic wounds. Plastic and Reconstructive Surgery 102: 1023–1027

Bates-Jensen B M 1997 Pressure ulcer assessment and documentation: the pressure sore status tool. In: Krasner D, Kane D (eds) Chronic wound care. Health Management Publications, Wayne, PA

Bliss M 1990 Geriatric medicine. In: Bader D L (ed) Pressure sores. Clinical practice and scientific approach. Macmillan, London

Braden B J 1997 Risk assessment in pressure ulcer prevention. In: Krasner D, Kane D (eds) Chronic wound care. Health Management Publications, Wayne, PA

Bridel-Nixon J 1997 Other chronic wounds. In: Morison M, Moffatt C, Bridel-Nixon J, Bale S (eds) Chronic wounds. Mosby, London

Callam M J, Harper D R, Dale J J, Ruckley C V 1987 Chronic ulceration of the leg: clinical history. Lothian and Forth Valley Leg Ulcer Study. British Medical Journal Clinical Research 294(6577): 929–931

Carville K 1994 Assessment and management of cancerous wounds. Primary Intention 2(1): 20–26

Clark M, Cullum N 1992 Matching patients' needs to pressure sore prevention with the supply of pressure redistributing mattresses. Journal of Advanced Nursing 17: 310–316

Clark M, Watts S 1994 The incidence of pressure sores within a National Health Service trust hospital during 1991. Journal of Advanced Nursing 20: 30–36

Clark M, Defloor T, Bours G 2004 A pilot study of the prevalence of pressure ulcers in European hospitals. In: Clark M (ed) Pressure ulcers: recent advances in tissue viability. Quay Books, Salisbury

Colburn L 1997 Prevention of chronic wounds. In: Krasner D, Kane D (eds) Chronic wound care. Health Management Publications, Wayne, PA

Collier M 1999 Venous leg ulceration. In: Miller M, Glover D (eds) Wound management: theory and practice. NT Books, London

Coulthard P, Worthington H, Esposito M et al 2004 Tissue adhesives for closure of surgical incisions (Cochrane Review). In: The Cochrane Library, Issue 2. Wiley, Chichester

Cruse P J E, Foord R 1980 The epidemiology of wound infection: a 10 year prospective study of 62,939 wounds. Surgical Clinics of North America 60(1): 27–40

Cullum N, Roe B (eds) 1995 Leg ulcer research and practice: the way forward. In: Leg ulcers: nursing management. A research-based guide. Scutari Press, London

Cullum N, Sheldon T A, Fletcher A et al 1997 Compression therapy for venous leg ulcers. Effective Health Care 3(4): 1–12

Dale J, Gibson B 1986 The epidemiology of leg ulcers. Professional Nurse 1(8): 215–216

Davies C 1999 Cleansing rites and wrongs. Nursing Times 95: 43

Dealey C 1997 The politicisation of pressure sores. In: Managing pressure sore prevention. Mark Allen, Guildford

Dealey C 1999 The management of patients with chronic wounds. In: The care of wounds. Blackwell Science, Oxford.

Department of Health 1993a Pressure sores: a key quality indicator. DH, London

Department of Health 1993b The costs of pressure sores. DH, London

Department of Health 2004 Review of prescribing, supply and administration of medicines. DH, London

Dickerson J W T 1995 The problem of hospital induced malnutrition. Nursing Times 91(4): 44–45

Doughty D B, Waldrop J, Ramundo J 2000 Lower-extremity ulcers of vascular etiology. In: Bryant R A (ed) Acute and chronic wounds: nursing management, 2nd edn. Mosby, St Louis

Emmerson A M, Enstone J E, Griffin M et al 1996 The second national prevalence survey of infection in hospitals – overview of the results. Journal of Hospital Infection 32: 175–190

European Pressure Ulcer Advisory Panel (EPUAP) 1998 A policy statement on the prevention of pressure ulcers from the European Pressure Ulcer Advisory Panel. British Journal of Nursing 7(15): 888–890

European Pressure Ulcer Advisory Panel (EPUAP) 2003 EPUAP guidelines on the role of nutrition in pressure ulcer prevention and management. EPUAP Review 5(2): 50–53

European Wound Management Association (EWMA) 2003 Position document: understanding compression therapy. Medical Education Partnership, London

Flanagan M 1997 Wound cleansing. In: Morison M, Moffatt C, Bridel-Nixon J, Bale S (eds) A colour guide to the nursing management of chronic wounds. Mosby, London

Gebhardt K 1992 Preventing pressure sores in orthopaedics. Nursing Standard 6(23): 3–5

Gentzknow G D, Iwasaki S D, Hershon S 1996 Use of dermagraft, a cultured dermis, to treat diabetic foot ulceration. Diabetes Care 19(4): 350–354

Gilchrist B 1997 Should iodine be reconsidered in wound management? Journal of Wound Care 6(3): 148–150

Gilchrist B 1999 Wound infection. In: Miller M, Glover D (eds) Wound management: theory and practice. NT Books, London

Goldberg M T, McGinn-Byer P 2000 Oncology-related skin damage. In: Bryant R A (ed) Acute and chronic wounds: nursing management, 2nd edn. Mosby, St Louis

Grocott P 1995 The palliative management of fungating malignant wounds. Journal of Wound Care 4(5): 240–242

Harding K G 1998 The future of wound healing. In: Leaper D J, Harding K G (eds) Wounds: biology and management. Oxford University Press, Oxford

Hart J 2002 Inflammation 2: its role in the healing of chronic wounds. Journal of Wound Care 11: 245–249

Hunter J A A 1995 Clinical dermatology, 2nd edn. Blackwell Science, Oxford

Kiecolt-Glaser J 1995 Slowing of wound healing by psychological stress. Lancet 346(8984): 1194–1195

Kindlen S, Morison M 1997 The physiology of wound healing. In: Morison M, Moffatt C, Bridel-Nixon J, Bale S (eds) A colour guide to the nursing management of chronic wounds, 2nd edn. Mosby, London

Leaper D J 1998 History of wound healing. In: Leaper D J, Harding K G (eds) Wounds: biology and management. Oxford University Press, Oxford

Leaper D J, Gottrup F 1998 Surgical wounds. In: Leaper D J, Harding K G (eds) Wounds: biology and management. Oxford University Press, Oxford

Leaper D, Harding K 2000 The problems of wound infection. In: Bale S, Harding K, Leaper D (eds) An introduction to wounds. Emap Healthcare, London

Marks J, Hughes L E, Harding K G et al 1983 Prediction of healing time as an aid to the management of open granulating wounds. World Journal of Surgery 7: 641–645

Martin P 1997 Wound healing: aiming for perfect skin regeneration. Science 276: 75

McLaren S 1997 Nutritional factors in wound healing In: Morison M, Moffatt C, Bridel-Nixon J, Bale S (eds) A colour guide to the nursing management of chronic wounds, 2nd edn. Mosby, London

McWhirter J P, Pennington C 1994 Incidence and recognition of malnutrition in hospital. British Medical Journal 308: 945–948

Meaume S, Merlin L, Ramamonjisoa M 1994 Major risk factors associated with pressure sores in geriatric patients. A study of 87 hospitalised elderly people with decubitus ulcers. In: Cherry G N, Leaper D J, Lawerence J C, Milward P (eds) Proceedings of 4th European Conference on Wound Management. Macmillan, London

Moffatt C 1995 The organisation and delivery of leg ulcer care. In: Cullum N, Roe B (eds) Leg ulcers: nursing management. A research-based guide. Scutari Press, London

Morison M, Moffatt C J 1997 Leg ulcers. In: Morison M, Moffatt C, Bridel-Nixon J, Bale S (eds) A colour guide to the nursing management of chronic wounds, 2nd edn. Mosby, London

Morison M, Moffatt C, Bridel-Nixon J, Bale S

1997 A colour guide to the nursing management of chronic wounds, 2nd edn. Mosby, London
Mortimer P 1993 Skin problems in palliative care: medical aspects. In: Doyle D, Hanks G, MacDonald N (eds) Oxford textbook of palliative medicine. Oxford Medical Publications, Oxford
National Institute for Clinical Excellence (NICE) 2001 Inherited clinical guideline B: pressure ulcer risk assessment and prevention. NICE, London
Neal M 2001 Angiogenesis: is it the key to controlling the healing process? Journal of Wound Care 10: 281–287
NHS Estates 2002 Infection control in the built environment. TSO, Norwich
O'Dea K 1993 Prevalence of pressure damage in hospital patients in the UK. Journal of Wound Care 2(4): 221–225
Padgett D, Marucha P, Sheridan J 1998 Restraint stress slows cutaneous wound healing in mice. Brain Behavior and Immunity 12: 64
Pieper B 2000 Mechanical forces: pressure, shear and friction. In: Bryant R A (ed) Acute and chronic wounds: nursing management, 2nd edn. Mosby, St Louis
Pinchcofsky-Devin G 1994 Nutritional wound healing. Journal of Wound Care 3(5): 231–234
Ramundo J, Wells J 2000 Wound debridement. In: Bryant R A (ed) Acute and chronic wounds: nursing management, 2nd edn. Mosby, St Louis
Rolstad B S, Ovington L, Harris A 2000 Principles of wound management. In: Bryant R A (ed) Acute and chronic wounds: nursing management, 2nd edn. Mosby, St Louis
Ryan T 1991 The management of leg ulcers. Oxford University Press, Oxford
Scales J T, Lowthian P T, Poole A G et al 1982 'Vaperm' patient support system: a new general purpose hospital mattress. Lancet 2: 1150–1152
Schoonhaven L, Haalboom J R E, Buskens E et al 2002 Prognostic ability of risk assessment scales. EPUAP Review 4(1): 17–18
Schultz G 2000 Molecular regulation of wound healing. In: Bryant R A (ed) Acute and chronic wounds: nursing management, 2nd edn. Mosby, St Louis
Siana J E, Frankild S, Gottrup F 1992 The effect of smoking on tissue function. Journal of Wound Care 1(2): 37–41
Sieggreen M Y, Kline R A 2003 Vascular ulcers. In: Baranoski S, Ayello E A (eds) Wound care essentials: practice principles. Lippincott, Williams and Wilkins, Springhouse, PA
Slavin J 1999 Wound healing: pathophysiology. Surgery 17(4): I–V
Steed D 1997 The role of growth factors in wound healing. Surgical Clinics of North America 77: 575
Stephens P, Thomas D W 2002 The cellular proliferative phase of the wound repair process. Journal of Wound Care 11: 253–261
Stotts N A 1997 Sterile versus clean technique in postoperative wound care of patients with open surgical wounds: a pilot study. Journal of Ostomy Continence Nursing 24: 10
Stotts N 2000 Nutritional assessment and support. In: Bryant R A (ed) Acute and chronic wounds: nursing management, 2nd edn. Mosby, St Louis
Stotts N, Wipke-Tevis D 1996 Co-factors in impaired wound healing. Ostomy Wound Management 42(2): 44
Sussman C, Bates-Jensen B M 1998 Introduction: the need for collaborative practice. In: Wound care: a collaborative practice manual for physical therapists and nurses. Aspen, Gaithersburg, MD
Tjero-Trujeque R 2001 Understanding the final stages of wound contraction. Journal of Wound Care 10: 259–263
Waldrop J, Doughty D 2000 Wound-healing physiology. In: Bryant R A (ed) Acute and chronic wounds: nursing management, 2nd edn. Mosby, St Louis
Waterlow J 1988 Prevention is cheaper than cure. Nursing Times 84(25): 69–70
Waterlow J 1991 A policy that protects: the Waterlow pressure sore prevention/ treatment policy. In: Horne E M, Cowan T (eds) Staff nurse's survival guide, 2nd edn. Wolfe, London
Whiteside M C R, Moorehead J R 1999 Traumatic wounds: principles of management. In: Miller M, Glover D (eds) Wound management. NT Books, London
Williams N A, Leaper D J 1998 Infection. In: Leaper D J, Harding K G (eds) Wounds: biology and management. Oxford Medical Publications, Oxford
Williams S, Watret L, Pell J 2004 Case-mix adjusted incidence of pressure ulcers in acute medical and surgical wards. In: Clark M (ed) Pressure ulcers: recent advances in tissue viability. Quay Books, Salisbury
Wilson R 2000 Massive tissue loss: burns. In: Bryant R A (ed) Acute and chronic wounds: nursing management, 2nd edn. Mosby, St Louis
Winter G D 1962 Formation of the scab and rate of epithelialization of superficial wounds in the skin of the young domestic pig. Nature 193: 293–294
Witte M, Barbul A 1997 General principles of wound healing. Surgical Clinics of North America 77: 509
Wysocki A B 2000 Anatomy and physiology of skin and soft tissue. In: Bryant R A (ed) Acute and chronic wounds: nursing management, 2nd edn. Mosby, St Louis

FURTHER READING

Bale S, Jones V 1997 Wound care nursing: a patient centred approach. Baillière Tindall, London
Bale S, Harding K, Leaper D (eds) 2000 An introduction to wounds. Emap Healthcare, London
Bannon M 1993 Healing the whole person. Nursing Times 89(13) (Wound Care Supplement): 62–68
Bryant R A 2000 Acute and chronic wounds: nursing management, 2nd edn. Mosby, St Louis
Cameron J 1997 Dermatological aspects of wound healing. In: Morison M, Moffatt C, Bridel-Nixon J, Bale S (eds) Chronic wounds. Mosby, London
Coulthard P, Worthington H, Esposito M et al 2004 Tissue adhesives for closure of surgical incisions (Cochrane Review). In: The Cochrane Library, Issue 2. Wiley, Chichester
Cullum N 1994 The nursing management of leg ulcers in the community: a critical review of the research. HMSO, London
Cullum N, Roe B 1995 Leg ulcers: nursing management. A research-based guide. Scutari Press, London
Cunliffe P J, Fawcett T N 2002 Wound cleansing: the evidence for the techniques and solutions used. Professional Nurse 18(2): 95–99
Dealey C 1997 Managing pressure sore prevention. Mark Allen, Guildford
Dealey C 1999 The care of wounds: a guide for nurses. Blackwell Science, Oxford
European Wound Management Association (EWMA) 2003 Position document: understanding compression therapy. Medical Education Partnership, London
Jones V, Bale S 2000 Wound management: the module. Emap Healthcare, London
Krasner D, Kane D 1997 Chronic wound care: a clinical source book for healthcare professionals, 2nd edn. Health Management Publications, Wayne, PA
Leaper D J, Gottrup F 1998 Surgical wounds. In: Leaper D J, Harding K G (eds) Wounds: biology and management. Oxford University Press, Oxford
Leaper D J, Harding K G (eds) 1998 Wounds: biology and management. Oxford University Press, Oxford
Morison M, Moffatt C J, Bridel-Nixon J, Bale S 1997 A colour guide to the nursing management of chronic wounds, 2nd edn. Mosby, London
Sussman C, Bates-Jensen B M 1998 Wound care: a collaborative practice manual for physical therapists and nurses. Aspen, Gaithersburg, MD

USEFUL WEBSITES

Diabetic Foot Study Group
www.dfsg.org

European Pressure Ulcer Advisory Panel
www.epuap.org

European Wound Management Association
www.ewma.org

Leg Ulcer Forum
www.legulcerforum.org

Tissue Viability Society
www.tvs.org.uk

The Wound Care Society
www.woundcaresociety.org

CONTINENCE

24

Linda Morrow

INTRODUCTION

Having control over urinary and faecal elimination is an expected norm within every society. In all but the very young, incontinence is generally not viewed with sympathy, and the real suffering it causes to individuals and their carers has not received the attention it deserves. Epidemiological research has shown that the number of people suffering from incontinence in some form or other far exceeds the number of cases reported to health professionals. An underlying theme of this chapter is the need to acknowledge the extent of the problem and to promote continence by improving screening practices and raising public and professional awareness of preventive measures against incontinence and of the range of treatments available.

Incontinence is a symptom that is often wrongly labelled as a disease. This chapter describes the underlying conditions that can prevent the acquisition of continence or provoke its loss. It is argued that a sound understanding of the causes and types of incontinence is essential for its proper investigation, treatment and management and that diagnostic assessment must recognise the individuality of each patient. Similarly, where incontinence is intractable, assessment for aids and equipment must be sensitive to the values, needs and priorities of each patient in order to ensure that an optimum quality of life is achieved.

Throughout the chapter the nurse is encouraged to take a positive, problem-solving approach towards this often hidden problem, to assess personal attitudes towards the subject of incontinence, and to base nursing decisions and actions on up-to-date, research-based knowledge.

URINARY CONTINENCE

The acquisition of continence in early childhood is a much valued developmental milestone. In the adult, the ability to control urinary and faecal elimination is largely taken for granted, and a loss of continence will have profound implications for the individual's ability to participate fully within society. While it may be deemed acceptable for a child to have an occasional 'accident', this is not generally the case for adults. The subject of incontinence is one which many people find difficult to discuss openly, and one which is poorly understood.

The onus is on health professionals to foster a change in social attitudes by acquiring a clear understanding of how continence is attained and how incontinence can develop. Nurses can make an important contribution to the promotion of continence among particularly vulnerable groups.

Defining continence

Continence may be defined in terms of the actions and abilities necessary for the appropriate management of urinary and faecal elimination. These include:

- recognising the need to pass urine or faeces
- identifying the correct place to pass urine or faeces
- delaying elimination until the appropriate place is reached
- reaching the correct place
- passing urine or faeces appropriately once a suitable place is reached.

Acquiring continence

Urinary continence cannot be acquired until the physiological systems necessary for micturition have matured. Once the prerequisite physical development has taken place, becoming continent is a matter of imitation, skill attainment and social conditioning.

The anatomy of the bladder is detailed in Chapter 8. The bladder is a simple organ which has a dual function: it acts as a reservoir for urine and it expels urine at the volition of the individual. Urine remains in the bladder as long as the intravesical pressure does not exceed the urethral resistance.

In normal micturition, the contraction of the detrusor muscle of the bladder induces the bladder neck to open while the pelvic floor muscles and the external sphincter relax. For a child to obtain continence they must acquire control of the mechanisms which prevent the bladder from automatically emptying when it is full; this is usually achieved by the age of 3 years.

The neurological control of the bladder at birth involves a simple sacral reflex arc whereby automatic filling and emptying of the bladder are under the control of sacral segments 3 and 4 of the spinal cord. Nerve endings in the bladder wall are activated by urine accumulation. These relay impulses with increasing frequency through the parasympathetic nerves to the spinal cord until the motor parasympathetic nerves react by causing the bladder muscles to contract and the urethral sphincter to open, whereupon reflex emptying occurs.

In order to achieve continence, a child needs to become aware of the sensation of the bladder becoming full and through trial and error attempt to overcome the reflex emptying mechanism by using the pelvic floor to keep the urethral sphincter closed. The sensory tracts of the spinal cord involve the cerebral cortex in the brain to overcome or inhibit the contractions; this requires practice as well as maturation of the central nervous system (see Fig. 24.1).

Continence thus involves the active inhibition of nerve impulses. When micturition is initiated, the brain ceases to send out inhibitory impulses, allowing the spinal reflex arc to be completed. Figure 24.2 illustrates the innervation of the bladder.

'Normal' patterns of micturition can vary markedly from one individual to another. Most people empty their bladder four to six times a day and have a bladder capacity of up to 600 mL; this may be altered, however, by age, fluid intake, medication, perspiration, body temperature, activity and stress. People in a state of anxiety generally feel the need to empty their bladders more often; in the event of acute emotional distress or sudden shock, it is possible for incontinence to occur.

ATTITUDES TOWARDS INCONTINENCE

In modern British society, attitudes towards many previously taboo subjects are rapidly changing. This is particularly evident in the topics that are now permissible within 'polite' conversation, e.g. intercourse, AIDS and homosexuality. Incontinence is also gradually becoming an acceptable subject for open discussion and began to be addressed openly in newspaper and magazine articles, and radio and television programmes from 1985 onwards (Glew 1985, Horsfield 1986, Walker 1987). Indeed today, advertisements for absorbent products fill many magazine pages and television commercials. Nevertheless, certain myths still persist, such as the notion that incontinence is an inevitable consequence of old age, or that wearing pads is the only solution. Such mistaken ideas must be dispelled in favour of seeking the underlying cause of incontinence in each individual case.

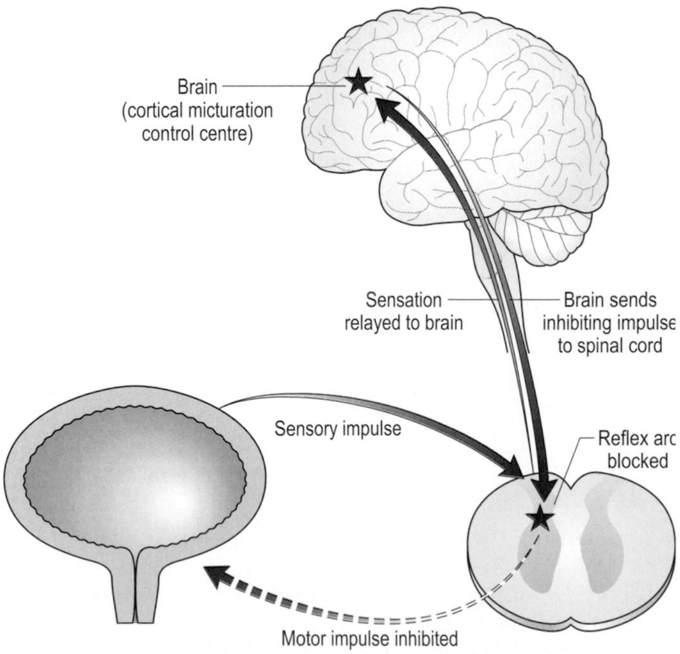

Fig. 24.1 Bladder-filling phase. The brain inhibits the spinal reflex arc. (Reproduced with kind permission from Coloplast.)

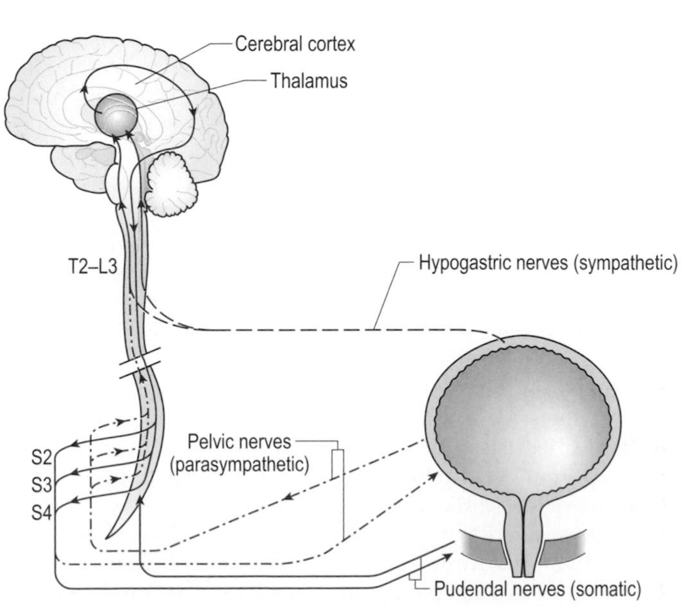

Fig. 24.2 Nerve pathways between the bladder, spine and micturition control centre. NB: nerves supplying the urethra have been omitted for clarity. (Reproduced with kind permission from Coloplast.)

For the nurse, perhaps the best starting point in this process of re-education is an examination of personal attitude to patients' toilet requirements, and what they can do to prevent the onset of incontinence. It has been found that some nurses consider routine or service requirements to be more important than assisting patients to use the toilet (Willis 2000, Morrow 2002, Nazarko 2003a).

Types of incontinence

The International Continence Society (ICS), which has coordinated the publication of a consensus document defining the terminology associated with the lower urinary tract, defines urinary incontinence as 'a condition in which involuntary loss of urine is a social or hygienic problem' (ICS 2002).

Urinary incontinence may take a variety of forms:

- stress incontinence
- urge incontinence
- overflow incontinence
- reflex incontinence
- nocturnal enuresis
- functional incontinence.

It is only when the specific type and cause of an individual's incontinence are known that appropriate treatment can be offered.

Stress incontinence results from a failure of the urethral sphincter to remain closed when a sudden increase in abdominal pressure on the bladder occurs, e.g. during coughing, sneezing or laughing. The weak pelvic floor allows the urethra to descend and the sphincter to open, releasing urine.

Urge incontinence results from the contraction of the detrusor muscle of the bladder as if to void, although the bladder may not be full. This may be caused by overactive detrusor function (motor urgency) or by hypersensitivity (sensory urgency).

Overflow incontinence occurs as a consequence of urinary retention, which may in turn result from:

- an obstruction, e.g. that caused by a tumour, faecal impaction or an enlarged prostate gland
- an underactive detrusor muscle, resulting in a flaccid bladder and thus failure to generate enough pressure to open the urethra
- failure of the urethra to open.

Reflex incontinence may occur as a result of damage to the spinal cord and loss of sensation associated with the desire to micturate, leading to failure to inhibit the simple reflex arc.

Enuresis refers to any involuntary loss of urine. Nocturnal enuresis is the term for urinary incontinence which occurs during sleep, in the absence of any organic disease or infection. Nocturia refers to being woken at night by the urge to pass urine.

Functional incontinence The individual with this type of incontinence would, in favourable circumstances, be able to remain continent but is prevented by pre-existing disease or disability from gaining access to an appropriate place at an appropriate time to pass urine. Diseases which may affect mobility and dexterity, and therefore continence, include multiple sclerosis, spina bifida, arthritis and spinal cord injury. In addition, conditions associated with ageing, such as slowness of movement, pain, joint stiffness, inability to climb stairs or difficulty in manipulating fastenings, may all contribute to incontinence.

EPIDEMIOLOGY

In conducting their seminal research into the prevalence of incontinence, Thomas et al (1980) used the following definition to identify all those in two London health districts over the age of 5 years who were incontinent: 'involuntary excretion or leakage of urine and/or faeces in inappropriate places or at inappropriate times, and production of two or more "accidents" a month or continuous leakage of urine'. This categorisation included individuals with 'long term catheters and urinary diversions'.

In the early stages of the study, this definition was applied to known patients who were already in touch with health and social services agencies. These individuals were monitored over a 1-year period, and the following information was obtained:

Age (years)	*Percentage of incontinence in this sample*
15–64	0.2% in women
	0.1% in men
65+	2.5% in women
	1.3% in men

In an extension of the study, a postal questionnaire was sent to all individuals over the age of 15 on the lists of 12 general practitioners (n = 22 430 patients) and an 89% return was obtained. The results, when compared with those of the first stage of the study, were illuminating, as they revealed a markedly higher incidence of incontinence, as follows:

Age (years)	*Percentage of incontinence in this sample*
15–64	8.5% in women
	1.6% in men
65+	11.6% in women
	6.9% in men

While incontinence was most prevalent among older women, its occurrence was significant across all age groups. Stress incontinence was reported less often by nulliparous than by parous women of all ages, and was especially prevalent among those who had borne four or more children. Urge incontinence also occurred more commonly among parous than nulliparous women. No significant class differences were found among men or women, but individuals of Afro-Caribbean or part Afro-Caribbean descent were more likely to have some form of incontinence than those with an Asian background. Differences have also been found within groups of Asiatic women working in the east end of London (Haggar 1995).

The most important finding of the study, however, was the 1:10 ratio of known to unknown cases of incontinence. This suggests that for every incontinent person who is known to health or social services professionals, there are 10 others who are unidentified. As further in-depth interviews revealed, many people try to 'cope' with moderate to severe problems of incontinence without professional support. These findings identify the need for health care workers to take advantage of all appropriate opportunities in hospital or community care settings to identify those who require assessment and treatment for incontinence.

Brocklehurst (1993), in an analysis of a MORI poll, suggested that there has been some improvement in the number of people coming forward for help. Annual national awareness campaigns coordinated by the Department of Health and the Continence Foundation since 1994, the Continence Foundation helpline in London and the Continence Resource Centre in Glasgow all help to direct people to the professional services that they need by helping to remove the stigma in talking about the problem (Association for Continence Advice 2000).

Data presented by the Royal College of Physicians (1995) showed an increase in the number of people with incontinence, but this may be evidence of more people coming forward for help or admitting to the problem.

Surveys of health care institutions and social services homes between 1964 and 1986 showed a high prevalence of incontinence; however, it has been suggested that this was to some extent a consequence of the quality of care given. A high failure rate in addressing the problems of incontinence was apparent and this was attributed to insufficient knowledge (Townsend 1964, Egan et al 1983, Edginton et al 1986). In 1995, Peet et al found that 44% of residents in long-term care were incontinent, which suggests that despite the evidence gathered over several decades there had been little improvement in practice. The Audit Commission (1999), when auditing first assessments by community nurses, found that district nurses were primarily assessing incontinent patients for absorbent products rather than assessing their incontinence with a view to improved management or regaining continence.

The implication of these research findings is that there is a need not only to identify patients who are incontinent, but also to improve public and professional understanding of incontinence, to evaluate services available for those requiring assessment and to improve methods of treatment and management (Scottish Intercollegiate Guidelines Network (SIGN) 2004).

Continence care is an area which lends itself to nursing initiatives and there are some excellent nurse-led projects being established throughout the country. In 2002, the *Nursing Times* award in the privacy and dignity category was awarded to a nurse-led, community continence assessment clinic (Armstrong 2003).

STOP THINK

24.1 Determine how many patients in your ward or on your community caseload are incontinent.

24.2 What percentage of your caseload does this represent?

24.3 To the best of your knowledge, how many of those who are incontinent have been fully investigated?

24.4 From what you have been told, try to identify the type of incontinence suffered by each person.

24.5 Compare your findings with the prevalence figures quoted in Peet et al (1995) or the Royal College of Physicians (1995).

24.6 Discuss your findings with a senior member of staff in your working area.

Sociological factors in underreporting of incontinence

The fact that incontinence remains to such a large extent a hidden problem among the general population can be attributed in part to the embarrassment felt by many people, leading to reluctance to admit to their incontinence and seek treatment (Mason et al 2001). Several authors agree that the more severe the incontinence, the more likely a patient is to seek medical help (Roe et al 1999, Shaw 2001). However the severity of the symptoms is only one factor which influences the patient in their choice to seek help or to hide their condition. Shaw (2001) identifies other factors which influence this decision:

- Lack of knowledge of causes, not considering incontinence to be a medical problem.
- Lack of knowledge of treatment options, not aware that the condition is amenable to cure.
- Belief that incontinence is a long-term condition related to age and parity.
- Previous experience or experience of friends/family.
- Variation of approach due to ethnic background and different attitudes to discussing such intimate problems.
- Personality of the individual and their relationship with individuals in their health care team.

The fact that it is 'comparatively rare for someone to decide in favour of or against a visit to the surgery without discussing his or her symptoms with others' — Freidson (1970) refers to this as 'a lay referral system' — may go some way towards explaining why incontinence is underreported. Many people prefer not to mention their incontinence to others; indeed Roe et al (1999) found that only 25% of one sample had discussed their incontinence with a friend, and so the opportunity for friends to encourage them to seek advice did not arise. Moreover, it may also be true that, in the case of women, the private and, to some degree, secretive management of menstruation gives an easily transferable model of management to follow should incontinence develop. Many women conceal the leakage of urine as they have concealed menstruation previously.

For many people, incontinence is a source of embarrassment or shame rather than a signal to them that they should seek medical help. The dysfunction is seen mainly in terms of its social consequences rather than as a symptom of a possible underlying illness or disease process.

Personal and social attitudes towards incontinence are not, however, the only factors that account for the underreporting of this widespread health problem. The way that particular health services are marketed or presented can also influence an individual's decision whether to seek help or cope on their own. In the words of one patient, 'I would find it too embarrassing to go to a special clinic ... perhaps a home visitor would be more helpful' (Association for Continence Advice 2000).

It is therefore important that available services reflect positive approaches to the promotion of continence, and progress on this is demonstrated in the setting of standards by nurses and monitoring of services and treatment.

In England and Wales, the Department of Health issued guidance to the NHS called *Good Practice in Continence Services* (DH 2000). This guidance included targets for health authorities for both inpatient and community care. The guidance has also influenced the content of the National Service Frameworks for Older People (see Ch. 35).

In Scotland, NHS Quality Improvement Scotland (NHSQIS) took a different approach in developing *Best Practice Statements for Adults with Urinary Dysfunction* (Nursing and Midwifery Practice Development Unit (NMPDU) 2002) and *Urinary Catheterization and Catheter Care* (NHSQIS 2004). NHSQIS has also published an evidence-based guideline on the *Management of Urinary Incontinence in Primary Care* (SIGN 2004). These publications have been widely disseminated through practice development initiatives to the NHS, general practice and the private care home sector. All these publications are available on the NHSQIS website (see 'Useful websites and addresses', p. 882).

In line with patient charter initiatives, a *Charter for Continence* was developed by a group of professional organisations in 1995 (see Box 24.1). This approach to involving patients has been strengthened by including patients on all the working parties for national continence publications, and including sections on patient information in those publications.

Box 24.1

Charter for Continence*

The Charter for Continence presents the specific needs and rights of people with bladder or bowel problems. It outlines the resources available and the standards of care that can be expected.

As a person with bladder or bowel problems you have the right to:

- Be treated with sensitivity and understanding
- Become continent if achievable
- Receive a thorough individual assessment of your condition by a doctor or nurse knowledgeable in this aspect of care
- Request specialist advice about continence care
- Be provided with a clear explanation of your diagnosis
- Participate in a full discussion of treatment options, their advantages and disadvantages
- Be provided with full, impartial information on the range of products which are available and how to obtain them
- Expect products to have clear instructions for use
- Receive regular reviews of treatment and be given the opportunity to change treatments if your condition has changed
- Be made aware of any treatments or products as they become available
- Be provided with a personal contact point able to give you ongoing advice and support.

*Developed by The Continence Foundation, InconTact, Association for Continence Advice (ACA), the RCN Continence Care Forum, Education and Resources for Improving Childhood Continence (ERIC), the Spinal Injuries Association and the Multiple Sclerosis Society. (Produced by an educational grant from Bard Ltd, March 1995.)

The Cochrane Urinary and Faecal Incontinence Review Group (CURE), based at the University of Aberdeen, maintains and disseminates systematic reviews of the effectiveness of the interventions for incontinence, including prevention, treatment and rehabilitation, concentrating on randomised controlled trials. Publications developed by this group can be accessed via the NHS Scotland e-library (see 'Useful websites and addresses', p. 882).

Care pathways, a process approach to managing integrated patient-focused care, have been designed to improve quality and standards of care for all incontinent people (Bayliss et al 1998, Cherry 2000).

An audit package, *Promoting Continence*, has been developed by the Royal College of Physicians (1998) which can be used for assessing continence care in relation to a single patient, multiple patients or for a facility audit. It covers urinary incontinence, faecal incontinence and urethral catheter management, and is intended to encourage staff to reflect on their management of incontinence and to consider areas where standards of care could be improved.

Identifying patients

Most people who are incontinent do not regard themselves as ill. It is therefore incumbent upon nurses and other professionals working in hospitals and the community to take advantage of every opportunity to identify those who are suffering in silence. Table 24.1 outlines potential opportunities for professionals to identify patients with continence problems and demonstrates that it is not always medical professionals who have the greatest opportunity to help these individuals. This supports the view that non-medical professionals and others should become better informed about this aspect of health. Pharmacists and home carers, to choose two very different examples, are well placed to provide information and foster positive attitudes towards treatment and should therefore be included in educational initiatives to promote continence.

PRIMARY REASONS FOR INCONTINENCE

Delay in achieving continence

In childhood, the acquisition of the skills necessary to achieve continence may be delayed. Nocturnal enuresis may present as a primary or secondary feature; its cause is not known. Although for many sufferers it often spontaneously resolves, it is sometimes not resolved during childhood. In such cases, if it remains untreated, it may be a problem throughout life (Butler 1994, Hjalmas et al 2004). The NHS Centre for Reviews and Dissemination (1997) published a systematic review of the effectiveness of interventions for managing childhood enuresis. Its impact on both individual and family has been researched by Morrison et al (2000).

Sometimes learning difficulties will prevent a person from attaining continence. Professionals working with individuals with learning difficulties, however, should base their interventions on the assumption that, although the process of toilet training may be slow, continence will eventually be achieved provided interventions are tailored to the individual and their family's requirements (Rogers 1998). Physical difficulties can also hinder the acquisition

Table 24.1 Lifespan opportunities for helping people who are incontinent

Lifespan stage	Potential problem areas	Sources of help	
		Nurses	Others
Childhood	Toilet training Enuresis Urinary control Learning disability Ureteric reflux	Health visitor, practice nurse, school nurse, community learning disability nurse, nursery nurse, community paediatric nurse	Doctor, consultant, dietitian, social worker, teachers
Teenager	Enuresis Sex education Cystitis	Health visitor, school nurse/matron, family planning nurse	Teachers, health educator
Pregnancy, childbirth	Antenatal frequency Difficult birth — tissue/nerve injuries, postnatal stress incontinence	Health visitor, midwife, district nurse	GP, physiotherapist, gynaecologist, obstetrician, self-help groups, pharmacist
Adulthood and hormone changes	Symptoms of incontinence from urological, gynaecological, neurological, psychological conditions	Continence advisor, practice nurse, clinic nurse, district nurse, health visitor, outpatients/occupational health nurse, specialist ward or urodynamics nurse	Urologist, neurologist, psychologist, physiotherapist, occupational therapist, dietitian, GP
Old age	As above, combined with the ageing process, prostatic enlargement and disability	District nurse, health visitor, practice nurse, day/ward nurse, older people's nurse	Home help, home carers, social workers and aides, GP, senior citizens advisors, consultant in medicine for older people

Reproduced with kind permission from the Continence Foundation.

of continence. Some children are incapable of acquiring continence, without medical intervention, because of spinal lesions, as in spina bifida, or other congenital conditions. A baby who is continuously wet should always be investigated for either congenital fistula or failure to empty the bladder. Such symptoms should be taken seriously. Ureteric reflux caused by failure of the bladder to empty will put pressure on the kidneys and may ultimately lead to renal failure.

Problems in maintaining continence

Childbirth Giving birth can cause damage to the mother's pudendal nerve, preventing the tone of the pelvic floor muscles from returning to normal. Van Kessel et al (2001) suggest that prolonged second-stage labour and the use of forceps put mothers at particular risk of incontinence.

Chronic disorders Cerebral, nerve or muscle damage can have varying effects on continence, as can trauma and damage resulting from injury or accident (see Fig. 24.3). Tumours or growths in the area of the bladder or cauda equina are also contributory factors, as is constipation.

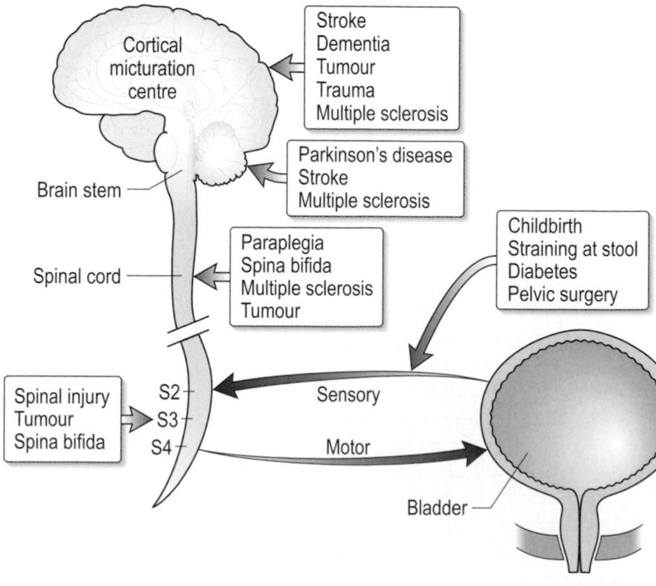

Fig. 24.3 Possible neurogenic causes of incontinence. (Reproduced with kind permission from Coloplast.)

Medications Many medications, especially diuretics, can have an effect on the bladder and its function. They may cause incontinence because of the sheer volume of output that they induce, and because of the demands they place on individuals with limited mobility in reaching an appropriate place where they can pass urine in time.

The sedative and diuretic effects of alcohol can contribute to incontinence. Sedatives and hypnotics make people less responsive to signals from the bladder. Antimuscarinic medications and others with some antimuscarinic action, such as phenothiazines and antidepressants, can cause retention in people with previously normal bladder function. Beta-blockers generate a variety of urinary dysfunctions.

For further information, see Greenstein & Gould (2004).

The effects of ageing Age can affect an individual's ability to maintain continence. It should be emphasised, however, that while incontinence is more prevalent among older people (especially women), it is not an inevitable consequence of ageing (Heath & Schofield 1999). The prevalence rates previously discussed cite the prevalence of incontinence in care home residents as 44% (Peet at al 1995) so even in this frail older population more than 50% remain continent. With age comes an increasing degeneration of the glomeruli in the kidneys; their function is reduced by up to 50% by the age of 80, thus impairing the ability of the kidney to concentrate urine. This consequence of ageing occurs alongside a decrease in the bladder's urine-storing capacity (Hald & Horn 1998).

The failure of ageing kidneys to eliminate sufficient waste products from the body during the day means that at night they remain very active. This results in an increased nocturnal output of urine leading to a change in the individual's pattern of micturition.

Ageing may also have some effect on the cerebral control of micturition, through the diminishing of cell function.

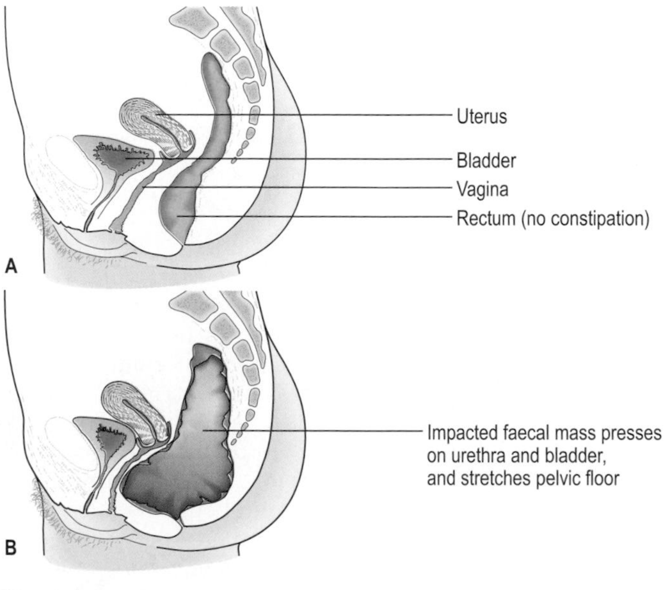

Fig. 24.4 How constipation can cause incontinence. Female, side view. (A): Normal. (B): Impacted. (Reproduced with kind permission from Coloplast.)

Ageing of the cerebral cortical neurones can reduce their effectiveness in inhibiting the sacral reflex arc, so that involuntary emptying of the bladder occurs.

In older women, vaginal dryness, soreness and atrophic changes may give a number of clues as to why incontinence has developed. Glycosuria or atrophic changes in the vulva may lead to vaginitis and urethritis (note that the lining of the vagina is continuous with that of the urethra). After the menopause, hormonal changes resulting in a decrease of oestrogen can cause dryness in the vagina and urethra. This may interfere with functioning of the moist seal of the urethral sphincter, thus allowing urine to leak through (International Continence Society 2002).

Constipation can also lead to urinary incontinence. Because of the anatomical proximity of the rectum and the urethra, it is possible for the urethra to be closed off by a faecal mass (see Fig. 24.4). This can result in incomplete voiding and thus stasis of urine, which in turn can encourage growth of bacteria in the bladder. A full rectum and patulous anus are signs of constipation.

PROMOTING CONTINENCE: A PROBLEM-SOLVING APPROACH

The problem-solving approach to nursing intervention consists of four stages:

1. Identifying the problem through assessment
2. Setting goals
3. Implementing care or treatment
4. Evaluating outcomes to ascertain that the goals have been achieved.

Involvement of the patient in all aspects of the nursing process will help to improve motivation and willingness to agree to treatment and will enhance the patient's feeling of independence and self-esteem.

Assessment

Assessment should be carried out in a manner which respects the patient's privacy and dignity (Armstrong 2003) with reference to a professionally agreed protocol and be tailored to the individual (SIGN 2004). It is vital that this assessment is conducted with a view to ascertaining the cause of any incontinence, for only then can the correct type of treatment be instigated (NMPDU 2002). In collecting information from patients, the nurse must have a clear understanding of the rationale behind the questions asked and of the implications for diagnosis and treatment of the patient's responses (see Table 24.2).

A full assessment should include:

- the patient's own account of the problem
- a detailed history, using closed and open-ended questions
- recording of micturition and incontinence over a few days
- physical examination by a competent professional
- urine testing
- further investigations as required.

Assessment should take place in a private setting and allow adequate time for the patient to air concerns and ask questions.

Table 24.2 Incontinence assessment questions

Question	Rationale
How long have these symptoms been present?	The symptoms may have begun at a life crisis or on taking a new medication, or they may have been a long-standing problem, but some new development has prompted the patient to ask for help
Are you wet every time?	It is important to establish the degree and frequency of wetting
How many times do you pass water each day?	A baseline needs to be established in order for progress to be charted
Are you wet at night as well as by day?	This gives an indication of the degree of the problem as well as the type of incontinence
Are you aware of the need to go to the toilet before you are wet?	This will determine whether signals are normal or absent
Do you have feelings of urgency to go to the toilet?	This indicates whether signals are present and their degree of urgency
Do you lose urine if you laugh, cough, jump or run?	A positive response often indicates genuine stress incontinence
Do you pass small amounts of urine?	Passing small amounts of urine may be due to urge, stress or overflow incontinence. It may also be indicative of reduced fluid intake
Do you pass a full stream?	Passing a full stream suggests the bladder capacity is normal
Is the stream of urine poor?	The flow rate may indicate a degree of obstruction or the bladder's inability to contract
Does passing urine sting?	Stinging urine usually indicates infection or a sore or broken area
Does the urine have a strong smell?	Urine invaded with bacteria or concentrated often has a strong smell
Do you have difficulty in starting to pass urine?	Hesitancy may be caused by an obstruction, e.g. prostatic enlargement
Do you dribble urine before or after going to the toilet?	Dribbling before suggests overflow; dribbling after suggests a failure to completely empty the bladder or an incompetent sphincter
Do you need to use pads or other aids, and if so how many and how often?	The answer may indicate the degree of urine loss
Are you constipated?	Constipation is the most common cause of urinary incontinence
Have you had any operations 'down below' (lower abdomen)?	Surgical trauma may be significant
Have you difficulty in getting to the toilet, problems with undoing clothes or any sight problems?	If the patient has problems with mobility or dexterity, clothes may need to be adapted and toilet seats raised. Supports to steady patients and aids to help them locate the toilet may be required
Are you taking any medication?	Many medications can affect the functioning of the urinary tract
Is the patient mentally aware?	Dementia may be the cause of incontinence due to a failure to remember the routines of the day

Questioning the patient

In order to establish a good rapport with patients, it is important to meet their own agenda when discussing the potentially embarrassing topic of incontinence. Open-ended questions such as 'Tell me about the problems with wetting that you have been having' or 'Could you describe what happens when wetting occurs' will give the patient a greater opportunity to relate the problem in detail than will questions that require a simple 'yes' or 'no' response. Open-ended questions will allow them to set out their own agenda for the interview. However, yes/no questions are useful with patients who are acutely embarrassed and have trouble finding a comfortable vocabulary to describe their problems.

The nurse's choice of language and sensitivity to the patient's preferred terminology will be important to the patient's comfort during the assessment interview. Patients generally use terms such as 'passing water', 'peeing' or 'making water' rather than medical terms such as 'micturition' or 'voiding' and many find words such as 'accidents', 'wetting' or 'leaking' more acceptable than the term 'incontinence'. Where the patient uses a euphemism or is vague, the nurse should seek clarification if there is any danger of misunderstanding, e.g. by asking 'When you said "at it" did you mean "having sex"?' or 'What do you mean by "a little"?'.

More specific questions may be indicated when the patient has a pre-existing illness, e.g. multiple sclerosis, or where bleeding, pain or discharge has occurred. Obviously, some questions, such as those concerning childbirth or prostate problems, will be gender-specific. Supplementary questions can be asked by means of a written assessment form.

Table 24.2 provides a checklist of questions that can be used during the assessment interview, together with a rationale for each item of information requested. These questions should be posed only after the patient has described their symptoms and has been given the opportunity to articulate their own agenda of concerns.

Charting information

The patient's history may yield enough information to determine the probable type and cause of the incontinence. A baseline chart, recorded over a few days, can confirm the accuracy of the history by supplying information indicating frequency of micturition and incontinence and, where required, the volume of urine passed. Charting such information again at intervals of a few weeks or at the end of treatment will produce a means of evaluating the treatment implemented. Any chart provided should be straightforward and easily understood so that patients are encouraged to use it, as the success of any future treatment will depend upon the patient's motivation. A sample chart which can be photocopied for use is available in the SIGN guideline (2004).

After careful explanation, the patient should be given the chart to fill in for a few days. Discussion concerning keeping the chart easily accessible to the bathroom, but bearing in mind the need for discretion, will help the patient to identify what will work best for them. The times of voiding and times of wetting are the most important pieces of information. Ticking or a range of ++++ may be sufficient to quantify volumes of urine lost. Although cumbersome, before and after weighing of pads is possible if objective testing is required (Groutz et al 2000). The amount of detail requested should be tailored to each patient, to balance the need for as detailed a clinical picture as possible with the patient's ability to understand and complete the chart.

The above approach is advocated for most patients, whether in the hospital or the community. Many specialists in the field of continence care suggest that admission to hospital for a barrage of invasive tests to diagnose the type of incontinence is not required for the majority of patients (SIGN 2004). For many patients, thorough assessment will indicate the likely type, or cause, of the incontinence and a care/treatment plan can be devised.

Physical examination

Women In women, a physical examination can determine whether atrophic vaginal changes, vaginitis or painful excoriation are features, and whether prolapse(s) or constipation is present. In the case of genuine stress incontinence, provocative testing such as asking the patient to cough while they are in a semi-recumbent position may demonstrate leakage. Assessing the ability of the pelvic floor to contract should be undertaken before initiating a pelvic floor muscle re-education programme. Such an assessment should be performed by professionals who have developed the appropriate knowledge and expertise (SIGN 2004).

Men
should be examined for prostate enlargement and to determine whether the bladder is palpable. If the bladder is palpable or the history suggests inability to empty the bladder completely, it may be necessary to ask the patient to pass urine, after which an intermittent catheter can be introduced, or a portable bladder scanner used to assess the residual volume of urine.

Urine testing

A cloudy appearance of the urine and a strong odour are indications of a urinary tract infection. A urine sample should be obtained and tested for further indications of infection, proteinuria, leucocytes or blood. If indicated, a midstream sample should be sent for culture and sensitivity analysis. Routine testing of urine can identify problems which may contribute to incontinence; haematuria, for example, may be an indication of infection, stones in the bladder or tumour. Poorly controlled diabetes mellitus, evidenced by glycosuria, is associated with continence difficulties for a number of reasons:

- Glycosuria itself can irritate the bladder causing bladder spasm.
- The intense thirst which leads diabetic patients to drink excessive amounts of fluid results in the production of large volumes of urine which can overwhelm the bladder's storage ability.
- In the longer term, peripheral neuropathy may result in damage to the nerve endings in the bladder, leading to reduced sensation of bladder filling and reduced ability to block reflex emptying.

Further investigations

Once the type of incontinence has been diagnosed, goals can be set for the patient's achievement or recovery of continence. If the incontinence is of an intractable nature, requiring long-term management rather than cure, further assessment for toileting programmes, aids or equipment will be required. It may be the case that further investigation into the cause of the incontinence is needed and that referral is indicated.

Urodynamics Where the probable cause of incontinence is difficult to establish, or where surgery is being considered, patients are often referred for urodynamic testing. Depending on local protocols, this may be undertaken by a clinical nurse specialist, a urologist or a urogynaecologist.

Urodynamic tests measure the pressure and flow relationships in the bladder and urethra. They can aid diagnosis of the type of incontinence by showing sphincter incompetence, detrusor instability, urethral instability and problems with voiding due to obstruction or an underactive detrusor. The procedures are invasive, unpleasant, potentially very embarrassing, but generally not painful. Clear explanations and psychological support must be given to the patient throughout. Table 24.3 outlines the most common urodynamic investigations; further details can be found on the International Continence Society website (see 'Useful websites and addresses', p. 882).

Radiography Radiographs can reveal signs of stones or large tumours in the bladder and may be required to assess

Table 24.3 Urodynamic investigations

Test	To establish:	Indications
Post void residual urine (PVR)	the volume of urine remaining in the bladder after voiding	Should be done in all patients to exclude incomplete emptying and consequent recurrent infections, or damage to the upper urinary tract
Uroflowmetry	the rate of urine flow via the urethra	Advised for all patients to exclude voiding difficulties
Pressure/flow studies	voiding pressures (related to voiding, not incontinence)	Follow-up from abnormal PVR or uroflowmetry, to distinguish between possible causes, e.g. poor bladder contraction or urethral obstruction
Cystometry	the pressure/volume relationship within the bladder, detrusor activity, bladder capacity and bladder compliance	Basic urodynamic evaluation for patients experiencing incontinence to assess bladder function, especially prior to considering surgery
Urethral pressure profile	the closure pressure within the urethra available to counteract increase in bladder pressure	Suggested, though not proven, for individuals in whom urethral dysfunction is suspected
Leak point pressure	the bladder pressure at which involuntary leakage of urine from the urethra is observed (the rise in bladder pressure may be from detrusor contraction or increased abdominal pressure)	Detrusor leak point pressure estimations allow assessment of risk to the upper urinary tract Abdominal leak point pressure assesses the increase in abdominal pressure which causes stress incontinence, and thus assesses the urethral contribution to continence
Surface electromyography	the efficiency of the pelvic floor muscles during the filling and voiding phases	Limited value in routine urodynamics
Videourodynamics	the simultaneous measurement of pressure and visualisation of anatomy	Useful in patients with a complex history, for example individuals with neurological disease
Ambulatory urodynamic monitoring	leakage, flow rates and bladder and abdominal pressure while the individual is ambulant	Useful to assess therapeutic effects of medication or to establish patterns which can not be exhibited in a clinic

the extent of faecal impaction in the colon and to show any narrowing or obstruction.

Cystoscopy A cystoscope is an instrument fitted with a fine telescope which is introduced via the urethra into the bladder. Modern types of cystoscope are quite flexible and allow the procedure to be carried out with only a local anaesthetic. Cystoscopy allows the urologist the opportunity to inspect the bladder and urethra, observing for tumours, stones, strictures and the condition of the mucosa. Further information on this procedure is given in Chapter 8.

Planning and implementing care

Effective treatment can be implemented only when the type of incontinence has been correctly diagnosed. This may seem obvious, but patients report instances where their incontinence has been dismissed as trivial, something they have to live with rather than a symptom to be thoroughly investigated (Association for Continence Advice 2000).

Treatments for incontinence include advice on diet, fluid and caffeine intake, pelvic floor muscle exercises, bladder retraining, the administration of antimuscarinic medication, clean intermittent self-catheterisation, relieving underlying medical conditions and surgical intervention. These forms of treatment, together with their application in different forms of incontinence, are described below.

Advice on diet, fluid and caffeine intake

Diet should be reviewed in relation to establishing and maintaining a regular bowel habit. The avoidance of constipation will benefit urinary continence as an overfull bowel can distort the anatomical position of both the bladder and the pelvic floor. Many patients are unclear about what constitutes appropriate fluid intake. Some will restrict fluids in the hope of minimising incontinent episodes, others continually top up their cup or glass, generating such large volumes of urine that the bladder is unable to cope. Six to eight cups or glasses of fluid (approximately 250 mL each) in 24 h is appropriate for most people. There is evidence that caffeine increases the number of episodes of incontinence in those with a diagnosis of urge incontinence (Arya et al 2000, Bryant et al 2002).

Pelvic floor muscle exercises

These exercises are primarily intended to increase the strength of the levator ani muscles and to evoke their contraction to support the bladder during an increase in intra-abdominal pressure. In women, assessment of the ability to 'squeeze' the muscles around the vagina and, where appropriate, teaching them how to exercise to improve their muscle tone can counteract any descent of the pelvic floor and help restore the normal anatomical relationships and sphincter function. Figure 24.5 illustrates the anatomy of the muscles of the pelvic floor in women (Sapsford et al 1997).

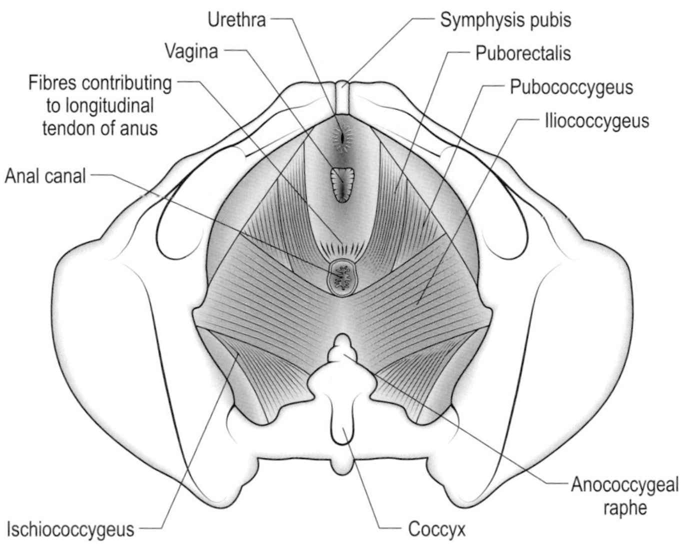

Fig. 24.5 Levator ani, perineal aspect.

Genuine stress incontinence in men or women (see p. 863) is the main problem for which pelvic floor muscle exercises may be used. This type of incontinence occurs when the pelvic floor is unable to counteract a sudden rise in abdominal pressure and allows the urethral sphincter to open, i.e. the intravesical pressure overcomes the intraurethral pressure.

Pelvic floor muscle exercises can also be useful for patients with frequency and urge incontinence. Sitting down when strong 'signals' occur and carrying out pelvic floor muscle contraction can help the patient to overcome the feeling of urgency and encourage the bladder to fill a little more before being emptied in a controlled way.

Pelvic floor muscle exercises are also useful following prostatectomy to stop postmicturition dribble and should be taught preoperatively.

Identifying the pelvic floor muscles Before patients can perform pelvic floor muscle exercises they must be able to identify two specific contractions:

- *the levator ani*, formed of the iliococcygeus, the ischiococcygeus and the pubococcygeus, can be located by imagining the onset of an episode of diarrhoea and the need to tighten the back passage muscle in order to get to the toilet without an accident
- *the pubococcygeus*, the anterior portion of the levator ani (see Fig. 24.5), can be located when passing urine. While in full stream, patients should try to stop, or at least slow, the flow and then try to remember which muscle was used in order to do this. This is only used once to locate the muscle and should not be performed as part of the exercise regimen. Female patients can check their ability to tighten the pelvic floor muscles by placing two fingers in the vagina and squeezing the muscles.

It is essential that patients identify contraction of the correct muscles; bearing down with the pelvic floor will not be of benefit, and may produce adverse results by causing further descent of the pelvic floor.

Motivation and practice In order to encourage compliance, the nurse must ensure that the patient has understood the instructions on performing the exercises and is motivated to practise them. An individual exercise regimen, identifying length of contractions and frequency of repetition, should be developed related to the individual's current muscle strength and opportunities to practise. An unrealistic regimen will be demotivating. Pelvic floor muscle exercises should be performed daily to increase muscle strength and should be performed three to four times weekly in the long term to maintain muscle strength (Laycock et al 2001).

Supplementary techniques Physiotherapists employ a range of equipment and techniques to help patients to overcome stress incontinence. These are detailed in the Chartered Society of Physiotherapy clinical guidelines (Laycock et al 2001).

There are a variety of methods by which the patient can be provided with biofeedback, e.g. digital palpation, manometry or electromyography, which will demonstrate evidence of muscle strength and illustrate any improvement, providing positive reinforcement of the benefit of the exercise regimen.

The use of cones of various weights, which are carried in the vagina, can support the patient in performing pelvic floor muscle exercises. There is no evidence that the use of vaginal cones is more beneficial than pelvic floor muscle exercises alone (SIGN 2004).

Neuromuscular electrical stimulation can be used to initiate muscle contractions, in the absence of a nerve impulse, by stimulating the muscle with a mild electric current. This is beneficial where a patient is unable to perform a voluntary muscle contraction.

Evaluation The success of these conservative approaches to achieving continence may be measured objectively by recording the weight of pads to calculate urine loss, if this is acceptable to the patient, and subjectively by the patient's reports on the perceived improvement in continence or the number of pad changes required per day. The long-term effectiveness of simple interventions such as pelvic floor muscle exercises or bladder retraining was demonstrated by O'Brien and Long (1995) and that of devices by Nygaard (1995).

STOP THINK **24.7** While discussing the rehabilitation of her mother following a mild stroke, Mrs M confides to you that she is occasionally wet after lifting her mother. What is your role here and what advice may be given as to treatment?

Bladder retraining

For the patient with urge incontinence, bladder retraining, in conjunction with antimuscarinic medication, is the main treatment. The aim of this form of treatment is for the bladder to 'learn' to increase its capacity and for the urethral sphincter to maintain its ability to remain closed as the bladder fills, thereby lengthening the intervals between voiding.

Method The treatment begins with a baseline measurement of working bladder capacity, i.e. the amount of urine passed, and frequency of voiding at the time of assessment.

In stages, the patient then learns to hold on for a few minutes more between the bladder signal and going to the toilet. As each lengthened interval is achieved and maintained, new objectives are set for the next few days.

Antimuscarinic medication is a useful adjunct to bladder retraining, as it reduces the initial urge to void and thereby helps to increase bladder capacity. When the patient achieves an acceptable social interval between toilet visits, and an adequate bladder capacity, the medication is then reduced and eventually discontinued. Attempts by the patient to maintain the same regimen as when taking the medication are instigated. If the same interval between passing urine is maintained, the treatment is seen as successful.

Antimuscarinic medication is contraindicated in patients with glaucoma (see Ch. 13). The normal side-effect of a dry mouth should be explained to patients using this medication.

Evaluation Whatever the degree of success of the treatment, toileting regimens will remain individual to each patient. In order to evaluate progress, a further continence chart should be completed after a few weeks' treatment and again towards the end of treatment. Comparison of the charts, showing both voiding intervals and quantities, will allow an objective evaluation to be made as to the success of the treatment.

STOP THINK **24.8** Mrs C needs to pass urine frequently. She tells you that she has had a 'poor' bladder for about 10 years which often wakes her at night, as well as 'keeping her on the run' during the day. After referral for urodynamics and further investigations, it is confirmed that she has urge incontinence. You are requested to instigate her treatment of a course of antimuscarinic medication and bladder training. What plan of action would you implement?

Clean intermittent self-catheterisation

This technique is employed by patients with voiding difficulties caused by conditions such as an atonic bladder or detrusor–sphincter dyssynergia, in which bladder contraction does not synchronise with opening of the urethral sphincter. It has also been used in conjunction with the passing of 'sounds' for treatment of urethral adhesion or prostate enlargement. Adhesions are often due to healing following infections and an enlarged prostate may restrict the diameter of the urethra. Clean intermittent self-catheterisation has also been of particular benefit to individuals with multiple sclerosis, spina bifida (Bardsley 2000), paraplegia and urinary retention due to prostate enlargement.

Intermittent self-catheterisation is a relatively simple treatment for incontinence, or incomplete bladder emptying, which is known to have been used in ancient times. The ancient Egyptians used reeds as catheters and the ancient Chinese, onion stems. The Roman encyclopaedist, Celsus, mentions the use of catheters in his writings (c. 30 BC) and throughout history catheters of a variety of materials are known to have been in use (Stewart 2001).

Assessment of the suitability of intermittent self-catheterisation for a particular patient must include identification of the specific type of incontinence and an evaluation of the manual dexterity, mental ability and motivation of the individual. Children as well as adults have been successful in learning the technique. In some cases it may be appropriate for partners or family members to be taught to carry out the catheterisation.

The procedure of self-catheterisation simulates normal voiding: the bladder is allowed to fill, the clean catheter is introduced and the bladder is then completely emptied. This prevents the build-up of residual urine in the bladder, which otherwise may cause:

- proliferation of bacteria in the bladder
- damage to the nerve endings
- overflow incontinence
- reflux of urine into the ureters and kidneys which may contribute to ascending infection or increase pressure within the upper urinary tract causing renal damage.

Unlike long-term catheterisation, in which aseptic technique is of paramount importance, intermittent catheterisation may seem unhygienic. However, the clean technique is not associated with bladder infection, as the bladder is completely emptied each time a catheter is passed (NHSQIS 2004).

The clean intermittent self-catheterisation technique requires the patient to be able to identify the urethra. A small catheter without a balloon, a nelaton catheter, is introduced into the bladder several times a day, dependent on individual requirements for assisted bladder emptying. There are two types of nelaton catheter available: prelubricated and non-lubricated.

- The prelubricated catheter often requires the patient to soak it in water for 30 s to activate the lubrication. Prelubricated catheters are for single use only.
- The non-lubricated catheter can be used with or without separate lubrication depending on patient preference. Non-lubricated catheters can be rinsed and reused, for a single patient, for up to a week.

Evaluation Most patients find that inserting the catheter becomes easier with each attempt. The success of the treatment can be measured in terms of the improved quality of life it offers to patients who previously were continually wet or who had to visit hospital emergency departments to seek relief from pain caused by failure to empty their bladder.

STOP THINK **24.9** Mrs F, who is 42 years old, has multiple sclerosis. Although she has had symptoms of urge incontinence and frequent bouts of infection, she has now passed into a dyssynergia phase in which large residual volumes of urine occur and clean self-catheterisation is required. She has fairly good manual dexterity. Outline a plan for teaching her self-catheterisation.

Managing symptoms related to underlying medical disorders

Some types of incontinence can be reduced by treating the underlying medical disorder such as constipation, anal fissure and vaginitis.

Relieving constipation Constipation as a causative factor in urinary retention and subsequent incontinence is described on page 879. An investigation of the cause of the constipation must be undertaken, including a review of medication and concurrent conditions. Diet and exercise/mobility should also be assessed.

Preventing constipation Patients who are prone to constipation should be encouraged to be as active as possible. Requests by older patients to go to the toilet should always be responded to as quickly as possible, in order to ensure that the gastrocolic reflex is never ignored. Once on the toilet the patient should be encouraged to sit for as long as is required. In the patient's home, it may be necessary to undertake structural adaptations to make the toilet more accessible or to install a chemical toilet or commode convenient to the patient's bedroom or sitting room.

A lack of privacy, time or comfort in an institutional care setting can easily interfere with the maintenance of good bowel habits. Where patients share facilities, nurses and carers must apply standards that allow patients to retain dignity and privacy.

Constipation can be prevented by the introduction of adequate fibre or roughage into the diet, in conjunction with an intake of approximately 8 cups of fluid a day. A dental check-up may be necessary to ensure that patients will be able to manage the raw or chewy food typical of a high-fibre diet. Individuals who are forced by dental problems to eat only soft foods will be susceptible to constipation, and therefore particular attention should be paid to their fibre intake, with fibre being added to their diet as required (see Ch. 21).

Confusional states For patients with senile dementia or other confusional states, adherence to a regular routine will help to reinforce the need to go to the toilet at particular times during the day. If a high-roughage diet is encouraged and usual patterns of defaecation maintained, usually 30 min after breakfast, a hot drink or other meals, it should be possible to prevent constipation. Spurious diarrhoea can occur in constipated individuals when the mass of faeces breaks down and mucus and faeces flow away, causing faecal incontinence associated with a characteristic, penetrating smell. It is preferable for patients with dementia to be assisted to the toilet at normal intervals rather than to be asked to adapt to new regimens such as using a commode.

STOP THINK **24.10** Mr G has been drawn to your attention because of increasing agitation, exacerbated by what appears as diarrhoea and incontinence of faeces. What aspects of his regimen would be considered in his assessment and what therapies would you implement with his carer to promote continence?

Problems related to bowel evacuation Anal fissures and haemorrhoids need to be soothed and healed in order that constipation caused through pain and avoidance can be prevented. Codeine-based analgesic medication taken over a long period should always be accompanied by a regular laxative to prevent constipation from developing.

Vaginal dryness or vaginitis may be treated with oestrogen creams or oral supplements. Patients should be referred to a doctor if vaginal prolapse or procidentia is evident. For women who are not sexually active and prefer not to have surgery, a ring pessary may be used to correct the uterine displacement. This appliance will need to be changed at intervals of 3–6 months.

Referring patients

It is the responsibility of the nurse to investigate the causes of a patient's incontinence by careful history taking. Nurses in all areas of practice should take responsibility for their patients' continence assessments, as part of a holistic care plan (NMPDU 2002). The findings of the history can then be supplemented with a baseline chart (see p. 867) which records the times that the patient passes urine and/or faeces. Having fully assessed the patient's continence problem, the nurse should be in a position to initiate a plan of care aimed at restoration of continence.

For the nurse who is inexperienced in dealing with the problems of incontinence, a continence advisor or nurse with a specialist interest in continence is a useful resource, and can help the nurse gain confidence to interpret the data obtained from the patient history and the baseline bladder chart.

Should the patient present with a complex history or be unresponsive to the treatment plan, the nurse should arrange referral for specialist assessment from the appropriate professional. This may be a continence advisor, specialist nurse, gynaecologist, urologist, consultant in medicine for older people, physiotherapist, neurologist or psychiatrist.

In a busy surgery or hospital situation, the significance of a patient's incontinence may not be fully appreciated. The nurse, as patient's advocate, should make a case for further investigation, as the individual often feels embarrassed by the problem and is unable to convince the doctor of its impact on their quality of life.

Surgical intervention

Surgery for stress incontinence Although in most cases conservative measures of treatment are used initially, some cases of stress incontinence in women can only be treated by means of surgical intervention. Historically, operations for genuine stress incontinence were carried out under general anaesthetic by the vaginal or suprapubic route, the operation of choice being colposuspension. Work on the insertion of tension-free vaginal tape (TVT) under local anaesthetic has shown that this procedure has a success rate similar to that of the more traditional colposuspension (Ward & Hilton 2002).

Intervention for prostatic enlargement Where the prostate gland partially or completely obstructs the urethra, the bladder will not empty completely and the patient may also experience overflow incontinence. It is essential to assess the patient accurately prior to instigating treatment (Naderi et al 2004). Transurethral resection of the prostate (TURP) is the most common surgical intervention performed for an enlarged prostate. This operation is described in Chapter 9.

Whilst patients with an enlarged prostate gland may have experienced overflow incontinence preoperatively, if damage occurs to the sphincter during the operation, dribbling incontinence may develop postoperatively and in some cases may be permanent. Gentle pressure behind the scrotum on the perineum or bulbospongiosum to drain the urethra following voiding can help to prevent post-micturition dribbling. There is also evidence to support the use of pelvic floor muscle exercises in men (Paterson et al 1997, Theofrastous et al 2002). Absorbent products such as dribble pouches and Y-front pants with a waterproof-backed gusset should be available in hospitals and in the community.

Incontinence within the institutional setting

In all care settings, the nurse should consider the potential impact which their approach to patient care may have on a patient's continence, particularly in settings where older people are cared for (NMPDU 2002). Such care settings tend to have a reputation for poor continence management, although there is evidence that, for example in the acute care sector, incontinent episodes may be seen simply as an inconvenience which interrupts the patient's care (Vinsnes et al 2001, Nazarko 2003a). When this attitude prevails, the patient or care home resident is more likely to be issued with pads or have a catheter inserted, rather than have a detailed assessment of their incontinence carried out, from which an individualised care plan can be developed and rehabilitation planned (Willis 2000).

Heavner (1998), in a review of urinary incontinence in extended care facilities, found that prompted voiding programmes for individual patients could maintain an individual's social continence even where there was a loss of cognitive function. Waters and Easton (1999) identified that whilst nursing staff felt they gave individualised care because they knew what was needed, observations of nurses at work showed a dependency on routine and little choice offered to patients. It was also observed that patients were often left without access to the nurse call system. Under these circumstances it is difficult for patients to continue with their own toilet regimen.

Examples of nursing where continence can be compromised are many and varied: for example, attention to the pelvic floor during labour and delivery, initial care of orthopaedic patients and providing accessible toilets for all patients in outpatient clinics.

Evaluation

The last stage of the problem-solving approach to nursing is to evaluate the care given and assess whether the goals set have been achieved. At this point new problems may come to light, in which case the nursing process will begin again with an assessment for this new problem.

STOP THINK **24.11** Fully assess the next patient suffering from incontinence who is admitted to your ward or who you meet in the community. Outline your strategy for care resulting from this assessment.

Continence advisory services

NHS services

Nurses may find that, within their own health area, there is a well-established continence advisory service which offers support in the promotion of continence in the community and in the hospital setting. Each region in Scotland benefits from at least one continence advisor.

A review of continence services by the Department of Health resulted in a report which recommended models of good continence services and targets for health care teams (DH 2000). These included:

- The development of integrated continence services to provide continence assessment, care planning and evaluation for all individuals with continence problems.
- Specialist continence advice for individuals with complex continence problems.
- The development of protocols and care pathways for the integrated continence service.
- A system to evaluate the care given, including service user involvement.

The targets specified that continence care should be provided to all patients, including children and those with learning difficulties, and cover all care settings, community, care home and acute sector.

Continence advisors

The post of continence advisor has been of key importance in the struggle to improve care for individuals suffering from incontinence. In addition to carrying a small caseload of their own, continence advisors usually work at a strategic level developing continence services across a health board area (Nazarko 2003b). In the larger health board areas in Scotland there are teams of continence nurses with different geographical areas of responsibility or professional areas of expertise. In addition to individual patient care, the teams work to develop the overall standard of continence care by providing education to staff at all levels, in both the NHS and the care home sector. The continence teams also work on public awareness in national campaigns and local initiatives.

Networks have been set up to facilitate communication among, and to give support to, professionals working in the area of continence care. The Association for Continence Advisors (ACA) was formed in 1980. The association, which changed its name in 1990 to The Association for Continence Advice, is multidisciplinary and has over 750 members, including international members and representatives from appropriate manufacturers.

In order to expand the knowledge base of continence advisors and to provide peer support, the ACA organises branch meetings, holds annual conferences and issues four newsletters a year.

The setting up of local networks in some regions has helped continence advisors to disseminate information to nurses at all levels, and across authorities. The aim is to encourage sharing of best practice and to motivate and support nurses who are trying to improve their own knowledge and practice in the field of continence care (Ballantyne 2003).

MANAGING INTRACTABLE INCONTINENCE

For some patients, incontinence will unfortunately be intractable. The key to successful management of these patients' requirements for toileting programmes, aids and equipment is, as always, to determine individual needs and priorities with a view to improving quality of life. The problem-solving approach should again be applied, taking into account:

- personal preference
- lifestyle
- home conditions
- the degree and frequency of micturition or defaecation
- financial considerations.

Aids and equipment

Aids and equipment are formally submitted to evaluation by product trials (Medical Devices Agency 1996a,b, 1997, 1998a,b, Fader et al 2001).

The type of aid that should be recommended for an individual will depend upon the specific type of incontinence experienced. The assessment of a patient's requirements for aids or equipment must be informed by an understanding of the cause of the incontinence.

Aids to enhance mobility and stability, raised toilet seats, portable bidets or commodes and clothes that have been chosen or adapted for ease of access may be helpful to many individuals. Aids to personal cleansing can also be made available to help the patient maintain independence and dignity.

Urinals for women

For women who are, for example, confined to a wheelchair, have arthritis or are taking diuretics, incontinence may result from an inability to get to the toilet in time, and the woman may benefit from using a female urinal. These are listed in the continence products directory (Continence Foundation 2000). Cottenden et al (1999) provide a review of the products in use.

Pads and pants

For men and women who cannot achieve urinary control, a wide range of appliances, pads and pants is available. For up-to-date details on these, the reader is again directed to the Continence Products Directory (Continence Foundation 2000), to PromoCon (see 'Useful websites and addresses', p. 882) or to the nearest NHS continence service, which will be able to provide information on the availability of containment products in their locality. A range of absorbent products are provided through local health services. The availability of aids and the process of collection or delivery vary for each area (Anthony 1997, Morrow 2003).

The type of absorbent product that is appropriate for an individual will be influenced by the laundry facilities available and the role and time available of any carer involved with the patient. During assessment for such aids, the nurse should balance the patient's wishes and the availability of laundry facilities, such as a washing machine, home help or laundry service, with the problems of disposing of soiled waste, for example no outside bin or limited weekly volume of waste allowed for uplift.

The pads available fall into the following categories:

Light incontinence To absorb minimal volumes of urine, small adhesive pads worn with the patient's own underwear or with stretch net pants, or cotton pants with a protective waterproof gusset, can be used.

Medium and heavy incontinence For medium and heavy incontinence, larger waterproof-backed pads can be used with stretch net pants. Where hygiene is a concern or where large amounts of reflex emptying occur, all-in-one adult diapers or nappy-style pads may be appropriate. Waterproof mattress covers are also available to prevent soiling. Reusable bed pads may be appropriate for those who have the necessary laundry facilities to cope with laundering and drying.

Procedure pads are used as an extra protection for furniture during a clinical procedure, e.g. administration of an enema or insertion of a catheter, and should not be used as a containment product for urinary incontinence.

Products for men

Additional equipment designed to enable men to contain urinary incontinence is available on prescription. Sheaths (urodomes) with varying types of adhesive fixings and drainage systems are continually being modified and the range available increased, to allow a more individual approach (Fader et al 2001).

Urethral occlusive devices are available but should be used with caution.

Y-front pants with a padded, waterproof-backed gusset are particularly useful for men with a retracted penis and dribbling problems.

Obtaining further information

Many other aids are available in addition to those mentioned above which may prove helpful to particular patients. During assessment for aids and equipment, it may be advisable to consult an occupational therapist, physiotherapist or continence advisor on the range of supplies available in a particular health area. The patient may wish to investigate aids to daily living on view in regional centres or in specialist outlets.

Financial support and advisory service

Individuals who are incontinent or who care for an incontinent person may be eligible for a number of benefits such as Disability Living Allowance, Attendance Allowance, Invalid Care Allowance or other financial support. Further information can be obtained from local social security offices and post offices and from the website (see 'Useful websites and addresses', p. 882).

A number of voluntary agencies may also be able to offer practical support. For children, the Family Fund can give help with washing machines, tumble driers and bedding. Services such as 'Crossroads' may be available to provide respite care so that carers can have a break from their responsibilities, and in some areas day centres are available for patients to attend.

STOP THINK **24.12** When you are in your local post office or library, take note of any free literature or available benefits. Jot down the reference numbers of leaflets that may be relevant to your patients or build up a collection to refer to as particular questions on benefits arise.

Long-term catheter care

Long-term indwelling catheterisation is used in the management of incontinence only after all other treatment possibilities have been eliminated. It should not be undertaken without due consideration of the patient's lifestyle, preferences and likely level of compliance. The potential effect of long-term catheterisation on sexual relationships should also be considered (Getliffe 2003). Insertion of a suprapubic catheter may be preferable for some patients. The patient should be made aware of what catheter management will entail before the procedure is carried out (NHSQIS 2004).

Catheter care is an important part of the nurse's role in both the hospital and community; an understanding of the principles of catheter selection and drainage system management, together with skill in patient education, are prerequisites for this. The anatomy and physiology of the lower urinary tract system and the selection and management of catheters are outlined in Chapter 8. The following exercise will help readers to review their knowledge.

STOP THINK **24.13** Mr A, who is 69 years old, has been sent home from hospital with a Foley catheter in place. He will need advice and information. Ascertain whether your knowledge base will be adequate to give good management care of his catheter and drainage system by considering the following questions.

(a) State four situations in which catheterisation would be justified.
(b) Define what is meant by a Foley catheter.
(c) When is a large balloon catheter (30 mL) used?
(d) When is a small balloon catheter (10 mL) used?
(e) State four other features which should be considered in the selection of a catheter.
(f) What materials can be used to make catheters?
(g) Can air, saline or other substances be used to fill the balloon of a Foley catheter? Justify your answer.
(h) List five features of drainage bags that are important to patients in selecting the appropriate system.
(i) Describe the options available to a female patient who wishes to have the choice of wearing short skirts or tight trousers over her catheter drainage system.
(j) What conditions are correct for the storage of catheters? What conditions should be avoided?

Preventing urinary tract infection

Urinary tract infection is the most common of all infections acquired in hospital, accounting for 30–40% of the total (Emmerson et al 1996). However, infection in the catheterised patient is not inevitable and can be prevented when the potential entry points of infection are properly managed.

STOP THINK **24.14** In Figure 24.6, can you identify the potential entry points for infection? What techniques can be used to prevent infection at each of these entry points?

Considerable and ongoing research is being carried out on catheter management and, in keeping with the Nursing and Midwifery Council *Code of Professional Conduct* (NMC 2004), all nurses involved in catheter care should keep abreast of new research findings in this area.

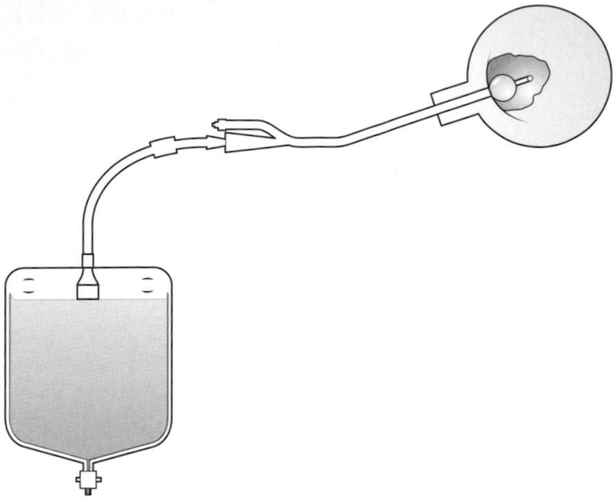

Fig. 24.6 Schematic of urethral catheter (see Stop-Think' 24.14).

Bladder lavage or catheter maintenance solution

Nurses should be clear that there is a difference between bladder irrigation and catheter maintenance or washout. Strictly speaking, irrigation refers to the continuous washing out of the bladder (see Ch. 8). Catheter maintenance solutions are available on prescription as a means of reducing catheter encrustation and debris and are often cited as a way of prolonging the 'life' of a catheter. There is disagreement as to whether these procedures should be carried out at all, as they disrupt the 'closed system' approach to management and cause shedding of cells from the bladder mucosa (Getliffe et al 2000). Research has shown that there may be a role for acidic catheter maintenance solutions in dissolving struvite crystals which encrust catheters (Getliffe et al 2000). However, these must be administered according to an individual treatment plan reflecting the patient's specific urinary pH fluctuations.

Nursing Care Plan 24.1 demonstrates the use of a problem-solving approach in identifying a patient's problems in caring for his catheter. It proceeds from identification of problems to setting goals with the patient and his relatives and then breaking down nursing interventions into their smallest components so that they can be carefully monitored and evaluated.

Supplying catheter equipment

Following the introduction of nurse prescribing (Royal College of Nursing 2000), certain qualified nurses working within the community can now order the supplies required by patients who have a catheter in situ. Patients should be given a list of all of their equipment, including sizes, types and capacity, as well as the name of a reliable pharmacist, retailer or mail order supplier. Appropriate details may be obtained by referring to the *Continence Products Directory* (Continence Foundation 2000) and the *Nurse Prescribers' Formulary* (Royal College of Nursing 2000), which is updated biannually. As noted on page 875, assessment of products is now being undertaken by the Medical Devices Agency (MDA 1996a,b, 1997, 1998a,b, Fader et al 2001).

Emergency help and contact numbers All catheterised patients in the community should be given a 24-h contact

Nursing Care Plan 24.1 Management of an indwelling catheter

Problem	Goal	Nursing action	Evaluation
Day 1 Unable to manage catheter and urine bag due to lack of knowledge and lack of manual dexterity	Day 1 To successfully and confidently manage care of the catheter and urine bags in as safe a manner as possible, by the time of discharge: Day 10	Day 1 Assess patient's ability to cope with buttons and zips	Day 1 While dressing today, patient was able to manage zip, but was slow with buttons
		Day 2 Change leg bag today and explain equipment and procedure	Day 2 Took a great deal of interest in management and asked how the catheter stayed in
		Day 3 Discuss with patient and daughter the general management of the catheter	Day 3 Married daughter visited; says she can visit him every day at home and phone him She thinks he could cope if instruction was given
		Day 3 Arrange a plan of teaching with patient and carer	Day 3 Married daughter coming on Day 4 at 10.00 h for a teaching session
		Day 4 Display of equipment and information session Provide written information	Day 4 Patient and daughter took interest and a number of queries were raised
		Day 4 Extra leg bag change Patient to change leg bag and put on night 'add-on' bag with supervision	Day 4 Managed leg bag Night-time bag put on correctly but forgot to open valve
		Day 5 Night nurse to supervise night-time add-on bag application	Day 5 With prompting, remembered to open valve
		Day 6 Night nurse to supervise removal of night-time bag	Day 6 Remembered to close valve Successful in removal, drainage and disposal
		Day 6 Liaison with district nurse for supervision at home	Day 6 Contacted Sr G. Discussed patient's progress. Will visit Day 7 p.m.
		Day 8 Supply patient with all equipment, written instructions and phone numbers for emergencies	Day 8 Patient read all the information and was able to identify each piece of equipment and how used Given DN's number and info on visit

Continued ▶

Nursing Care Plan 24.1 Management of an indwelling catheter *(Continued)*

Problem	Goal	Nursing action	Evaluation
		Day 9 Discussion with patient and daughter on diet, emergencies, care and storage of equipment	Day 9 Daughter and patient happy about discharge on Day 10 Able to change add-on bag successfully this morning
		Day 10 Discharge 10.00 h	Day 10 Patient discharged, confident about catheter management Has 2 weeks' supply Daughter thanked staff for teaching session

number through which to gain help in an emergency. Practical advice on what constitutes a real problem and on what to do in certain emergencies should be given in writing to patients and carers (Getliffe 2003).

Sexuality

The impact of incontinence on self-esteem and the fear of wetting or soiling during intercourse can understandably have a negative effect on an individual's sex life (White & Getliffe 2003). MacKay and Hemmet (2001), in researching patient perceptions of incontinence, found that 16% of the respondents who considered their incontinence to be a significant problem had told no-one about their symptoms. This reluctance to discuss continence problems coupled with an avoidance of intimacy for fear of urinary leakage will inevitably lead to relationship difficulties.

Although many professionals may not see this aspect of their patient's well-being as a priority, patients who have been sexually active and are suddenly faced with incontinence caused by injury, childbirth or disease, or those who are facing progressive incontinence as a result of chronic disease, will have to make a difficult adjustment to changes in their sexual life. Problems of sexuality and incontinence affect both genders regardless of age (Cassels at al 2003).

The nurse's attitude

Following a review of the nursing literature on human sexuality, as early as 1979 Brower and Tanner concluded that most nursing authors were not concerned with the sexuality of their patients and its implications for nursing care. Booth (1990) confirmed that this is especially the case with respect to older people.

These findings serve to remind us that nurses involved in counselling must examine their own attitudes and feelings relating to the subject of sexuality. Counselling with regard to the implications of incontinence for the individual's sexuality should be initiated only when the patient signals that they are ready to address the issue. However, the nurse may need to introduce the subject and thereby give the patient 'permission' to voice any concerns. Reluctance to discuss questions of sexuality with patients may be due to the nurse's own inexperience or lack of self-awareness (Katz 2003, Wallace 2003). Gregory (2000) warns that there is no justification in encouraging a patient to divulge such personal and sensitive information if the nurse is not able to offer help or direct the patient to the appropriate specialist.

The reader is referred to Katz (2003) or Wallace (2003) for discussion of the issues relating to sexuality. Patient information leaflets discussing incontinence and sexual intercourse are available from Outsiders (see 'Useful websites and addresses', p. 882).

Practical problems and solutions

Certain issues concerning sexuality and incontinence may be dealt with in a practical manner, as outlined in the following.

Nocturnal enuresis is likely to inhibit both social and sexual intercourse and should be treated. The numbers of adults afflicted with nocturnal enuresis is uncertain, due to the hidden nature of the problem, although Hjalmas et al (2004) quote the prevalence of enuresis as 0.5% in otherwise healthy adults aged 18–64.

It is important to chart the patient's pattern of enuresis before treatment is commenced. Again, identifying the underlying cause can direct appropriate treatment. There are three conditions which underlie the diagnosis of enuresis, with patients often having a combination of these:

- a reduced bladder capacity
- an inability to concentrate urine at night
- difficulty in waking when the bladder is full.

Often a form of bladder training is tried initially, whereby the patient learns to hold onto urine longer during the day, thus leading to an increased bladder capacity and increased ability to hold urine at night.

The prescription of desmopressin, a form of the antidiuretic hormone vasopressin, is helpful in reducing urine production at night, but does not cure the problem. This medication is available as a spray. A single intranasal dose taken at night lasts for 10–12 h; this affords control of enuresis without affecting daytime urine production. Prolonged use is not recommended as adverse effects on the nose have been reported as well as water intoxication (NHS Centre for Reviews and Dissemination 1997).

The main treatment for nocturnal enuresis in the teenager and adult is to introduce the use of a personal alarm system to assist with learning to wake in time to void. A small electrode attached to a battery alarm system about the size of a matchbox is pinned to the patient's nightwear. When the first drop of urine touches the electrode, a signal is activated and wakes the patient.

Some patients may benefit from a combination of an alarm and medication to begin the treatment programme and then gradually withdraw both as control is established.

An excellent resource centre dealing with all aspects of enuresis is the Education and Resources for Improving Childhood Continence (ERIC; see 'Useful websites and addresses', p. 882). Many helpful pamphlets are available from the centre for adults as well as for children.

Cystitis involves either an infection or an inflammation of the bladder. The causal bacteria is usually *Escherichia coli*. It occurs most commonly in women, because of the anatomical proximity of the urethra, vagina and anus, and in some women may be linked to sexual intercourse. Incontinence rarely develops, but frequency and pain are present. When this occurs, many couples curtail their sexual activity, which may lead to tension in the relationship.

Careful hygiene, wiping the vulval area from front to back following defaecation and avoiding contact by the penis or fingers with the anus during intercourse may prevent problems. Passing urine before and after intercourse has been found to be helpful. Drinking copious amounts of water to flush the bladder can help when an attack of cystitis occurs. Management of cystitis can also involve antibiotic therapy or self-help techniques (Fihn 2003).

Preparation for intercourse

For many women who are incontinent, orgasm produces further episodes of urine loss. Passing urine before sexual intercourse may help. Protecting the bed and discussing the problem with one's partner can help to make the wetting less of an issue.

Catheterised patients need not avoid intercourse. For men, the catheter may be strapped to the underside of the penis and, in some individuals with a degree of impotence, may also help with rigidity. In women, the catheter may be strapped to the inner thigh or up onto the abdomen (Winson 2001). If clinically appropriate, sexually active patients may opt for a urinary catheter which is inserted suprapubically.

Counselling Open and reflective counselling will help to reveal the extent of any sexual problems experienced by the incontinent patient. If the patient's difficulties are not easily resolved, referral should be made to experts in sexual counselling who are available either in the hospital or in the community, or to other appropriate agencies such as Relate and Outsiders (see 'Useful websites and addresses', p. 882). The nurse should be prepared to furnish information on these organisations and details of how to contact them.

FAECAL INCONTINENCE

While urinary incontinence is more prevalent in the population than faecal incontinence, the latter is the more distressing problem. Faecal incontinence is socially even less acceptable than urinary incontinence and raises strong emotions among carers who have to deal with it. It is a source of discomfort and acute embarrassment for the sufferer, and contributes to feelings of helplessness and a loss of self-esteem.

Perry et al, in their 2002 study, found that approximately 6% of adults living at home aged over 40 had experienced faecal incontinence in the preceding year, although only 0.7% of those classed the faecal incontinence as disabling. It is especially prevalent among older people (Johanson & Lafferty 1996) and those requiring long-term care (Brocklehurst et al 1999). However, cohort research studies are discovering a number of women with damaged levator ani function following vaginal delivery (MacArthur et al 1997).

Faecal incontinence, like urinary incontinence, is a symptom of an underlying pathology and with appropriate assessment and treatment many individuals can be cured (Kenefick 2004).

Normal defaecation

Defaecation is the expulsion of faecal matter from the rectum with the aid of peristaltic movements of the muscular walls of the intestine (see Ch. 4). The rectum is stimulated to empty from impulses received from mass peristalsis, often starting from the gastrocolic reflex. The need for defaecation is felt as a response to distension of the sigmoid colon and the stimulation of the receptors. Further information on normal bowel function can be found in Chapter 4.

Anxiety can produce an urge to defaecate more often and in situations of extreme crisis faecal control can be temporarily lost.

The causes of faecal incontinence must be determined before treatment is instigated. Other than simple constipation, impaction and overflow diarrhoea, the main cause of faecal incontinence is usually damage to the pelvic floor and anal sphincters, resulting in an inability to recognise that the rectum is full or to distinguish between flatus and faeces.

Constipation

The constipated patient may complain of headache, general malaise and lack of appetite. Abdominal discomfort, rectal fullness and cramps may also be reported. During physical examination, the abdomen can be measured for signs of increasing distension (Harari 2004).

In people with a normal bowel, constipation may be caused by any of the following:

- a low-fibre diet
- low fluid intake
- inactivity
- ignoring the signals to defaecate
- pain in the anorectal region from haemorrhoids or fissures, an inability to position oneself comfortably in the necessary position, leading to avoidance of defaecation

- mouth pain or dental problems, leading to intake of soft foods only
- the use of pads for urinary incontinence, leading to neglect of toilet requirements by patient or staff where assistance is required
- intake of opioid analgesics, sedatives or hypnotic medication
- unacceptable toilet conditions
- unfamiliar surroundings or circumstances, leading to loss of habit
- inability to recognise social expectations, as in some cases of learning difficulties, dementia or excessive consumption of alcohol.

Where no obvious cause is found for the constipation, the problem may be due to damage to the pelvic floor and anal sphincter or to some other pathology, such as loss of rectal sensation as a result of surgery, injury or tumour. Other contributing conditions include dehydration resulting from endocrine or metabolic disorders and neurological damage.

Some individuals are prone to diarrhoea. Common causes are infection, inflammation in the bowel or rectum, excessive use of laxatives and the ingestion of certain foods or medicines. Parasitic infection can also cause diarrhoea.

Abnormalities resulting in faecal incontinence

The most common cause of faecal incontinence is damage to the puborectalis muscle and nerves, resulting in a failure of the valve at the anorectal flap or angle and associated lack of control and sensation. This may have been caused by trauma in childbirth (MacArthur et al 1997, Sultan & Kamm 1997), congenital abnormalities or damage sustained during surgery (Norton & Chelvanayagam 2004). Atonic muscles may also preclude adequate pushing to expel the faeces.

In the assessment of faecal incontinence, a history of the complaint and an explanation of what previously constituted a normal habit should be obtained in order to establish the specific type of incontinence. Bleeding, loss of sensation and the presence of mucus are all symptoms that should be investigated. A full description of the incontinence and its frequency are also important to the diagnosis. Liquid leakage is quite different from true diarrhoea.

Following a rectal examination, referral for a plain X-ray, proctoscopy, barium enema and stool culture may be necessary (see Ch. 4).

Interventions may be conservative, involving such measures as changing the diet and making toilets more accessible. Nurse-led clinics providing treatment for faecal incontinence using electrical stimulation have been very successful (Norton & Chelvanayagam 2004). In some cases, however, surgery will be indicated.

Gastrointestinal management of diarrhoea is fully described in Chapters 4, 20 and 21.

For a full account of the treatment available for rectal conditions, see Norton & Chelvanayagam (2004).

REFERENCES

Anthony B 1997 The provision of continence supplies by NHS Trusts. Middlesex University, London

Armstrong L 2003 It's amazing to see life open up for clients. Nursing Times 99(2): 38–39

Arya L A, Myers D L, Jackson N D 2000 Dietary caffeine intake and the risk of detrusor instability. Obstetrics and Gynaecology 96: 85–89

Association for Continence Advice (ACA) 2000 Survey of patients. National Care Audit 1998/9. ACA, London

Audit Commission 1999 First assessment: a review of district nursing services in England and Wales. Audit Commission, London

Ballantyne M 2003 Moving forward and around: cluster group formation. ACA Continence 23(4): 11

Bardsley A 2000 The neurogenic bladder. Nursing Standard 14(22): 39–41

Bayliss V K A, Cherry M, Salter E A 1998 Proposal for the development of care pathways. ACA Continence 18(2): 17–18

Booth B 1990 Does it really matter at that age? Nursing Times 86(3): 50–52

Brocklehurst J C 1993 Urinary incontinence in the community: analysis of a MORI poll. British Medical Journal 306: 832–834

Brocklehurst J C, Dickinson E, Windsor J 1999 Laxatives and faecal incontinence in long term care. Nursing Standard 13: 32–36

Brower H T, Tanner L A 1979 A study of older adults attending a programme on human sexuality: a pilot study. Nursing Research 28(1): 36–39

Bryant C M, Dowell C J, Fairbrother G 2002 Caffeine reduction education to improve urinary symptoms. British Journal of Nursing 11: 560–565

Butler R 1994 Nocturnal enuresis – the child's experience. Butterworth-Heinemann, Oxford

Cassels C, Geront M, Watt E 2003 The impact of incontinence on older spousal caregivers. Journal of Advanced Nursing 42(6): 606–616

Cherry M 2000 Care pathways for urinary continence problems. Nursing Times Plus 96(19): 7–10

Continence Foundation 2000 Continence products directory. Continence Foundation, London

Continence Foundation, InconTact, Association for Continence Advice (ACA), the RCN Continence Care Forum, the Enuresis Resource and Information Centre (ERIC), the Spinal Injuries Association, the Multiple Sclerosis Society 1995 Charter for continence. Continence Foundation, London

Cottenden A, Fader M, Petterson L, Dean G, Brooks R 1999 Selection of female urinals. British Journal of Nursing 8(14): 918–925

Department of Health 2000 Good practice in continence services. DH, London

Edginton A, Shepherd A, Bainton D 1986 'D' is for dignity. Health and Social Services Journal 96: 50–51

Egan M, Playmet K, Thomas T, Meade T 1983 Incontinence in patients in two district general hospitals. Nursing Times 79(5): 22–24

Emmerson A, Enstone J, Griffin M 1996 The second national prevalence survey of infection in hospitals. Journal of Hospital Infection 32(3): 175–190

Fader M, Pettersson L, Dean G, Brooks R, Cottenden A M, Malone-Lee J 2001 Sheaths for urinary incontinence: a randomized crossover trial. British Journal of Urology International 88: 226–236

Fihn S 2003 Acute uncomplicated urinary tract infection in women. New England Journal of Medicine 349(3): 259–266

Freidson E 1970 Profession of medicine. Dodd Mead, New York

Getliffe K A 2003 Catheters and catheterization. In: Getliffe K A, Dolman M (eds) Promoting continence. Baillière Tindall, London

Getliffe K A, Hughes S C, Le Claire M 2000 The dissolution of urinary catheter encrustation. British Journal of Urology International 85: 60–64

Glew J 1985 Incontinence: what every woman should know. Woman Magazine, 9 March: 30–32

Gregory P 2000 Patient assessment and care planning: sexuality. Nursing Standard 15(9): 38–41

Groutz A, Blaivas J, Chaikin D et al 2000 Non-invasive outcome measures of urinary incontinence and lower urinary tract symptoms: a multicentre study of micturition diary and pad tests. Journal of Urology 164(3): 698–701
Haggar V 1995 Strong developments. Nursing Times 91(33): (Continence supplement)
Hald T, Horn T 1998 The human urinary bladder in ageing. BJU International 82(S1): 59–69
Harari D 2004 Bowel care in old age. In: Norton C, Chelvanayagam S (eds) Bowel continence nursing. Beaconsfield Publishers, Beaconsfield
Heath H, Schofield I (eds) 1999 Healthy ageing: nursing older people. Mosby, London
Heavner K 1998 Urinary incontinence in extended care facilities: a literature review and proposal for continuous quality improvement. Ostomy and Wound Management 44(12): 46–53
Hjalmas K, Arnold T, Bower W et al 2004 Nocturnal enuresis: an international evidence-based management strategy. Journal of Urology 171(6): 2545–2561
Horsfield M 1986 Incontinence: a young woman's problem. She magazine, October: 86–87
International Continence Society (ICS) 2002 2nd international consultation on incontinence. ICS, London
Johanson J F, Lafferty J 1996 Epidemiology of faecal incontinence. The silent affliction. American Journal of Gastroenterology 91(1): 33–36
Katz A 2003 Sexuality after hysterectomy: a review of the literature and discussion of the nurse's role. Journal of Advanced Nursing 42(3): 297–303
Kenefick N 2004 The epidemiology of faecal incontinence. In: Norton C, Chelvanayagam S (eds) Bowel continence nursing. Beaconsfield Publishers, Beaconsfield
Laycock J, Standley A, Crothers E et al 2001 Clinical guidelines for the physiotherapy management of females aged 16–65 with stress urinary incontinence. Chartered Society of Physiotherapy, London
MacArthur C, Bick D E, Keighley M R B 1997 Faecal incontinence after childbirth. British Journal of Obstetrics and Gynaecology 104: 46–50
MacKay K, Hemmet L 2001 Needs assessment of women with urinary incontinence in a district health authority. British Journal of General Practice 51(471): 801–804
Mason L, Glenn S, Walton I, Hughes C 2001 Women's reluctance to seek help for stress incontinence during pregnancy and following childbirth. Midwifery 17: 212–221
Medical Devices Agency (MDA) 1996a Disability equipment assessment – catheters for intermittent self-catheterisation. No. A18. MDA, Surbiton
Medical Devices Agency (MDA) 1996b Disability equipment assessment – sterile leg bags. No. A20. MDA, Surbiton
Medical Devices Agency (MDA) 1997 Disability equipment assessment – catheter valves. No. A22. MDA, Surbiton
Medical Devices Agency (MDA) 1998a Disability equipment assessment – enuresis alarms – an evaluation. No. A24. MDA, Surbiton
Medical Devices Agency (MDA) 1998b Disposable, shaped bodyworn pads with pants for heavy incontinence. An evaluation. No. IN.1. MDA, Surbiton
Morrison M, Tappin D, Staines H 2000 "You feel helpless, that's exactly it": parents' and young people's beliefs about bedwetting and the implications for practice. Journal of Advanced Nursing 31(5): 1216–1227
Morrow L 2002 Best Practice Statement: Adults with urinary dysfunction. Nursing Times 98(29): 38–40
Morrow L 2003 The provision of absorbent garments. Nursing Times 99(1): 63
Naderi N, Mochtar C A, de la Rosette J 2004 Real life practice in the management of benign prostatic hyperplasia. Current Opinion in Urology 14(1): 41–44
Nazarko L 2003a The care home perspective. ACA Continence 23(4): 24–26
Nazarko L 2003b Auditing continence services. Nursing Times 99(19): 15
NHS Centre for Reviews and Dissemination 1997 A systematic review of the effectiveness of interventions for managing childhood nocturnal enuresis. CRD report 11. University of York, York
NHSQIS 2004 Urinary catheterization and catheter care. NHS Quality Improvement Scotland, Edinburgh
Norton C, Chelvanayagam S 2004 Conservative management of faecal incontinence in adults. In: Norton C, Chelvanayagam S (eds) Bowel continence nursing. Beaconsfield Publishers, Beaconsfield
Nursing and Midwifery Council (NMC) 2004 The NMC code of professional conduct: standards for conduct, performance and ethics. NMC, London
Nursing and Midwifery Practice Development Unit (NMPDU) 2002 Continence: adults with urinary dysfunction. NMPDU, Edinburgh
Nygaard I 1995 Prevention of exercise incontinence with mechanical devices. Journal of Reproductive Medicine 40(2): 89–94
O'Brien J, Long H 1995 Urinary incontinence: long term effectiveness of nursing interventions in primary care. British Medical Journal 311: 1208
Paterson J, Pinnock C B, Marshall V R 1997 Pelvic floor exercises as a treatment for post-micturition dribble. British Journal of Urology 79: 892–897
Peet S M, Castleden C M, McGrother C W 1995 Prevalence of urinary and faecal incontinence in hospitals and residential and nursing homes for older people. British Medical Journal 311: 1063–1064
Perry S, Shaw C, McGrother C et al 2002 Prevalence of faecal incontinence in adults aged forty years or more living in the community. Gut 50(4): 480–484
Roe B, Doll H, Wilson K 1999 Help-seeking behaviour and social services utilization by people suffering from urinary incontinence. International Journal of Nursing Studies 36(3): 245–253
Rogers J 1998 Promoting continence: the child with special needs. Nursing Standard 12(34): 47–55
Royal College of Nursing 2000 The nurse prescribers' formulary (1999–2000). Nursing Standard 14(16): 16
Royal College of Physicians (RCP) 1995 Incontinence: causes, management and provision. RCP, London
Royal College of Physicians (RCP) 1998 Promoting continence – clinical audit scheme for urinary and faecal incontinence. RCP, London
Sapsford R, Bullock-Saxton J, Markwell S 1997 Women's health: a textbook for physiotherapists, 3rd edn. Saunders, Melbourne
Scottish Intercollegiate Guidelines Network (SIGN) 2004 Management of urinary incontinence in primary care: a national clinical guideline. SIGN, Edinburgh
Shaw C 2001 A review of the psychosocial predictors of help seeking behaviour and impact on quality of life in people with urinary incontinence. Journal of Clinical Nursing 10(1): 15–24
Stewart E 2001 Urinary catheters: selection, maintenance and nursing care. In: Cruickshank J, Woodward S (eds) Management of continence and urinary catheter care. Mark Allan, Bath
Sultan A H, Kamm M A 1997 Faecal incontinence after childbirth. Commentary. British Journal of Obstetrics and Gynaecology 104: 979–982
Theofrastous J P, Wyman J F, Bump R C et al 2002 Effects of pelvic floor muscle training on strength and predictors of response in the treatment of urinary incontinence. Neurology and Urodynamics 21: 486–490
Thomas T M, Plymet K R, Blannin J et al 1980 Prevalence of urinary incontinence. British Medical Journal 281: 1243–1245
Townsend P 1964 The last refuge: a survey of residential institutions and homes for the aged in England and Wales. Routledge and Kegan Paul, London
Van Kessel, Reed S, Newton K, Meier A, Lentz G 2001 The second stage of labour and stress urinary incontinence. American Journal of Obstetrics and Gynecology 184: 1571–1575
Vinsnes A, Harkless G, Haltbakk J, Bohm J, Hunskaar S 2001 Healthcare personnel's attitudes towards patients with urinary incontinence. Journal of Clinical Nursing 10(4): 455–461
Walker I 1987 The one problem we still can't talk about. Living magazine, May: 102–104
Wallace M 2003 Sexuality. Dermatology Nursing 15(6): 570–572
Ward K, Hilton P 2002 Prospective multicenter randomized trial of tension-free vaginal tape and colposuspension as primary treatment for stress incontinence. British Medical Journal 325: 67
Waters K, Easton N 1999 Individualised care: is it possible to plan and carry out? Journal of Advanced Nursing 29(1): 79–87
White H, Getliffe K 2003 Incontinence in perspective. In: Getliffe K A, Dolman M (eds) Promoting continence. Baillière Tindall, London
Willis J 2000 Continence care in acute settings. Nursing Times 96(19): 3–4
Winson L 2001 Catheterisation: a need for improved patient management. In: Cruikshank P, Woodward S (eds) Management of continence and catheter care. Mark Allan, Bath

FURTHER READING

Getliffe K A, Dolman M (eds) 2003 Promoting continence. Baillière Tindall, London
Greenstein B, Gould D 2004 Trounce's clinical pharmacology for nurses, 17th edn. Churchill Livingstone, Edinburgh
Katz A 2003 Sexuality after hysterectomy: a review of the literature and discussion of the nurse's role. Journal of Advanced Nursing 42(3): 297–303
Norton C 1996 Nursing for continence, 2nd edn. Beaconsfield Publishers, Beaconsfield
Norton C, Chelvanayagam S (eds) 2004 Bowel continence nursing. Beaconsfield Publishers, Beaconsfield
Wallace M 2003 Sexuality. Dermatology Nursing 15(6): 570–572
Winder A 2001 Devising an effective general nursing continence assessment tool. British Journal of Nursing 10(14): 935–947

USEFUL WEBSITES AND ADDRESSES

Association for Continence Advice (ACA)
www.aca.uk.com

Continence Foundation
www.continence-foundation.org.uk

Disability benefits
www.disabilitybenefits.co.uk
(*For information on a range of disability benefits*)

Education and Resources for Improving Childhood Continence (ERIC)
www.eric.org.uk

International Continence Society
www.continet.org

NHS Scotland e-library
www.elib.scot.nhs.uk

NHS Quality Improvement Scotland
www.nhshealthquality.org

Outsiders
www.outsiders.org.uk
(*An organisation that supports social inclusion*)

PromoCon Disabled Living
4 Chad's Street
Cheetham
Manchester M8 8QA

Relate
www.relate.org.uk

SLEEP

Andrée le May

25

INTRODUCTION

Sleep is a fundamental element of life. We know that everybody needs sleep and yet people find it difficult to describe exactly what sleep is. We are all intrigued, for instance, by what happens when we fall asleep, why we dream and why our sleep patterns alter. However, despite centuries of observing sleep, extensive and systematic research, and the creation of both physiological and behavioural theories to explain sleep, the mechanisms and functions of sleep still elude us. The aim of this chapter is to enable nurses to understand more about sleep by considering what is meant by sleep, to identify factors that impact on the ability to sleep and to think about the ways in which they can assess a patient's sleeping patterns. Reading this chapter should help nurses feel more confident in providing nursing care that helps patients to overcome some of the problems associated with sleeplessness.

Before reading on, imagine the two scenarios detailed in Box 25.1. In the first, you are lying awake at home at 3 a.m. and in the second, you are awake in hospital. These two scenarios emphasise the importance that we attach to sleep. They also show how, in different situations, sleep means different things to different individuals and is affected by different environmental circumstances, the way we feel and our ability to control how we help ourselves to sleep.

WHAT IS SLEEP?

We spend so much of our lives asleep that one would expect it should be easy to define sleep but, paradoxically, once we are asleep, we remember little about it. One on-line dictionary definition (www.answers.com/topic/sleep) suggests that sleep can be defined as

> *A natural periodic state of rest for the mind and body, in which the eyes usually close and consciousness is completely or partially lost, so that there is a decrease in bodily movement and responsiveness to external stimuli. During sleep the brain in humans and other mammals undergoes a characteristic cycle of brain-wave activity that includes intervals of dreaming.*

This definition seems to reflect what many of us remember from our own experiences of going to or waking from sleep and also our observations of others as they sleep. For the most part, modern scientific researchers have tended to use objective criteria to describe sleep, usually in terms of physiological events occurring during specific stages of sleep. These include changes in the electrical activity of the brain and fluctuations in the secretion of various hormones. However, it is important to bear in mind that it is the individual's subjective experience of sleep that is of greatest importance in an assessment of the quality of sleep. Even when an electroencephalograph (EEG) indicates that sleep

Box 25.1

Thinking about sleep

Scenario one

Imagine you are at home. You went to bed as usual at 11 p.m. but it is now 3 a.m. and you are still awake. There is nothing stopping you sleeping except the gentle workings of your mind: you are warm and comfortable, there is no noise to disturb you and you don't have anything to worry about ... yet you still can't sleep. You know you need to, because you have to get up in the morning and go to work, be level headed and awake ... you toss and turn with frustration then decide to get up and make a drink. You return to bed to sip it and slowly, very slowly, feel the drowsy sleepiness that you've been hoping for wash over you.

Scenario two

Imagine that you are awake during the night in hospital. You are too warm and your bed is unfamiliar. You can hear the constant breathing of the three other people in your bay, the light footsteps of the nurses as they walk past the entrance to the bay and the intermittent ring of the telephone at the nurses' station, all of which keep interrupting the attempts to sleep. You are anxious about the results of the tests that have been taken and are due tomorrow. It seems as if everything is stacked against your sleeping: there is nothing that will help you to sleep without disturbing someone else or ringing for a sleeping pill and it is almost too late in the night to do that. You stare into the darkness willing sleep to overtake you, but it does not.

STOP THINK **25.1**

(a) If you have had sleepless nights, or had difficulty getting off to sleep, in what ways have you tried to deal with your sleeplessness? Try listing these, and then think how successful or otherwise your strategies were.

(b) Consider how patients you have nursed might deal with sleeplessness, and the various factors that might influence their ability to sleep — even the simple options you listed for yourself might be difficult for them to achieve.

For one nursing team's innovative approach to sleep promotion in hospital, see Cmiel et al (2004).

has been long and continuous, if the individual complains of sleeping badly, this cannot be contradicted. Conversely, if an individual habitually sleeps for only 2 h during the night, but feels that this amount is adequate, leaving them rested and refreshed, then there is nothing wrong with their sleep. The most important element of any nursing assessment of sleep is therefore to find out and to respect the patient's experiences and interpretations of their own sleep/waking patterns.

In order to help us to understand patients' sleep difficulties and the implications of these in planning care, some basic knowledge about the structure and function of sleep is useful. A summary of the two distinct types of sleep — non-rapid eye movement (NREM) sleep and rapid eye movement (REM) sleep — and their function is given below (see also Fig. 25.1).

Non-rapid eye movement (NREM) sleep

NREM sleep comprises four stages, first described by Rechtschaffen and Kales (1968) in their seminal work on sleep staging. Each stage is associated with differing electrical activity of the brain.

- *Stage 0 or wakefulness* — the subject is awake with their eyes closed and an EEG would be characterised by generally low-voltage activity.
- *Stage 1 or drowsing* — this is the lightest stage of sleep during which the pupils constrict and dilate at intervals of approximately 1–3 s and the EEG shows mostly low-voltage, mixed-frequency activity. If asked, the subject may report feeling drowsy, but be awake. Even though the subject may feel fully alert, it is likely that observers will note reduced attentiveness. Some simple perceptual distortions, i.e. daydreams, may occur.
- *Stage 2 or light sleep* — this phase of altered consciousness is such that, if awakened, most people recognise that they have been asleep. Body movements begin to diminish and dreams involving a storyline first appear. Dream recall on waking, however, is far less vivid than for the second type of sleep, REM sleep.
- *Stage 3 or slow wave sleep* — when the amplitude of the EEG increases and body movements continue to diminish.
- *Stage 4 or slow wave sleep* — this phase is associated with a high degree of immobility and intense external stimuli are required to rouse a person in this stage of sleep. Large increases in the secretion of growth hormone occur during stage 4.

Note: Stages 3 and 4 are often considered together and termed slow wave sleep (SWS).

Rapid eye movement (REM) sleep

REM sleep, or paradoxical sleep, is characterised by dreaming, muscular relaxation and high levels of physiological arousal. During REM sleep, muscle tone is lower than in any other sleep stage. Blood pressure fluctuates, pulse and respiration rates increase and may become irregular, oxygen consumption increases, premature ventricular contractions may occur and there is penile tumescence in men and increased vaginal secretion in women.

The eye movement which occurs in REM sleep usually consists of rapid darting movements of the eyes under closed lids, occurring in bursts of 3–10 s at intervals of 30–40 s. These do not always occur, and if they are absent this is most likely to be during the first REM period of the night. If subjects are woken up, they often report that they have been dreaming; consequently, REM sleep is frequently referred to as dreaming sleep. In order to identify this phase of sleep, electrodes can be applied to the face to detect electrical activity due to eye movement, and below the chin to detect muscle tone. If all these electrical signals are recorded overnight, the result is a complex series of parallel traces known as a polysomnogram. From this, the

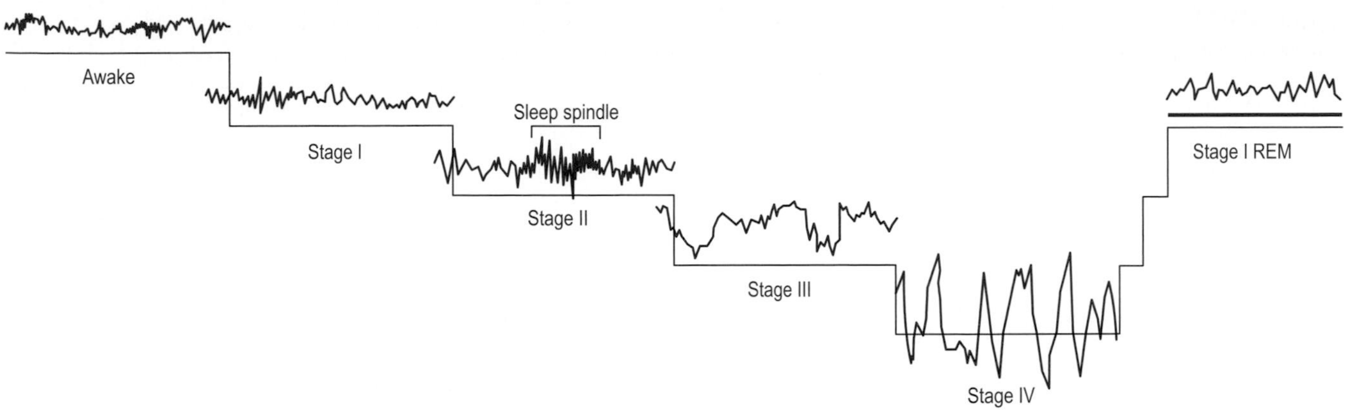

Fig. 25.1 Progressive changes in the EEG following the onset of sleep. (From SLEEP, by J. Allan Hobson. Copyright, 1995 by J. Allan Hobson. Reprinted by permission of W.H. Freeman and Company.)

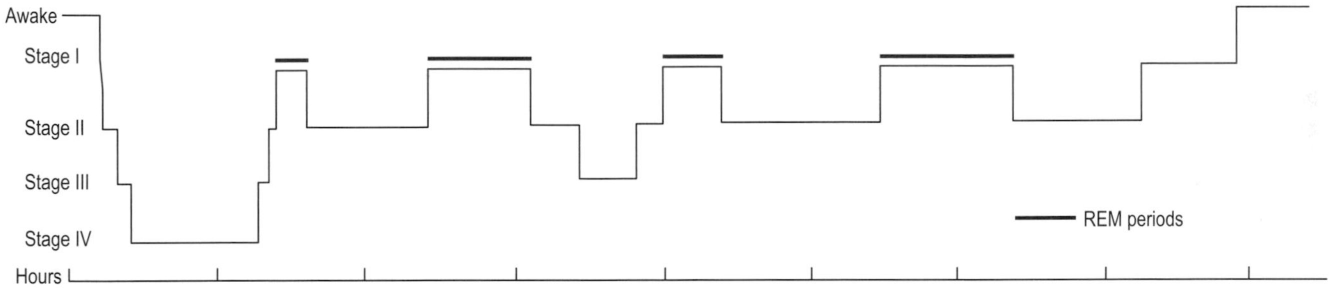

Fig. 25.2 Sleep architecture showing one night's progression of sleep cycles. (From SLEEP, by J. Allan Hobson. Copyright, 1995 by J. Allan Hobson. Reprinted by permission of W.H. Freeman and Company.)

most reliable indicator of REM, i.e. the disappearance of skeletal muscle tone, can be seen.

During a night's sleep both REM sleep and all four NREM stages may occur many times, usually in a cyclical fashion (see Figs 25.1 and 25.2). Sleep usually begins with stage 1 (drowsing) and progresses through stage 2 to slow wave sleep (SWS). This 'deep' sleep is frequently followed by a brief return to stage 2 before an episode of REM. The pattern then repeats, usually starting from stage 2. The duration of this cycle may vary considerably according to age and other factors, but in young healthy adults it lasts approximately 100 min. The first part of the night tends to contain more SWS, while the latter part of the night contains a higher proportion of REM. Interestingly, even during the day, people have been seen to undergo 100-min cycles of alertness and drowsiness, although they are usually unaware of these. During sleep, shifts from stage to stage tend to accompany body movements, with shifts to light sleep tending to occur suddenly, whereas shifts to deep sleep tend to be more gradual.

PHYSIOLOGICAL CONTROL OF SLEEP

Precisely how and why people sleep remains the subject of much research. At present it appears that the brain has several interlinked sleep centres: some relate to the onset and timing of sleep, some to REM sleep, others to NREM sleep and others to wakefulness. In addition, there are several putative, naturally occurring sleep substances, e.g. interleukin-1 and sleep promoting substance (SPS), that seem to be diffused throughout the brain.

Neurological control

The neurological control of sleep is complex and is not yet completely understood. Espana and Scammell (2003), in a useful clinical summary on sleep neurobiology, note that many neurochemically distinct systems interact to regulate wakefulness and sleep. The medulla, pons and midbrain comprise the brain stem (see Ch. 9) and accommodate many of the anatomical structures that govern sleep and wakefulness. It is also suggested that wakefulness is promoted by brain stem and hypothalamic neurones producing neurotransmitters such as acetylcholine, noradrenaline and 5-hydroxytryptamine (5-HT, also called serotonin) as well as dopamine, histamine and orexin/hypocretin. Each of these is capable of increasing wakefulness. In addition, neurones in the pons and preoptic area control both REM and NREM sleep.

Neurotransmitters

The main neurotransmitters implicated in the regulation of sleep and wakefulness are noradrenaline, acetylcholine and 5-HT. Noradrenergic neurones are responsible for the arousal of the cortex observed during wakefulness and REM sleep. Cholinergic cells, i.e. those producing acetylcholine, facilitate REM sleep, while cells producing 5-HT appear to be responsible for the maintenance of NREM sleep and play an important role in the regulation of REM sleep.

Sleep substances

Theories claiming the existence of sleep substances have gained in popularity from the beginning of the 20th century. These are claimed to be naturally occurring substances that accumulate in the central nervous system (CNS) and cause sleep. Several sleep substances have been isolated, but it is not known whether they are central to the regulation of sleep or part of a larger and more complex system.

FUNCTIONS OF SLEEP

Despite enormous research efforts, the only universally agreed reason for sleeping is to avoid being sleepy! Interpretations of research findings vary, but it is generally considered that sleep appears to have a major role in the maintenance and/or restoration of physical and cerebral functioning (Moorcroft 1995). This may include:

- the resetting of physiological systems
- growth
- energy conservation
- modulation of immune functions
- homeostatic restoration of brain function
- maintenance of inherited behaviours and creativity.

It has also been suggested, however, that sleep may be simply an instinctual behaviour, a genetic remnant of earlier days when immobility at night increased our chances of survival.

For comment on the considerable number of hypothetical functions of sleep, see Benington (2001).

SWS and restorative processes

The direct study of sleep and tissue restitution in human subjects presents practical and ethical difficulties. Although it is possible to study people's sleep patterns in sleep laboratories, clearly it would be unacceptable to induce sleep deprivation in people who have sustained injury in order to study the effects of sleep on healing. In these circumstances, it is possible through a rather less direct route to investigate body restoration through the study of circadian variations in the levels of anabolic and catabolic hormones. These regular fluctuations suggest that anabolic processes occur during the sleep period.

In humans, protein synthesis is inhibited by hormones such as cortisol, glucagon and catecholamines, which result in wakefulness and reach their highest levels during the day. During sleep, energy expenditure in the tissues falls and the energy stored within the cells as adenosine triphosphate (ATP) rises to levels which become sufficiently high for protein synthesis to occur. The first episode of night-time SWS has been noted to coincide with peak levels of secretion of human growth hormone (HGH), which stimulates protein and RNA synthesis and amino acid uptake. Consequently, as one seminal overview of research into the functions of sleep suggested, peak tissue-building processes are associated with SWS (Shapiro & Flanigan 1993).

The onset of SWS is also associated with increased immunological activity. Further, SWS is the sleep state which has the highest positive correlation with the length of prior wakefulness and therefore appears to be associated with restorative properties. The evidence from Shapiro and Flannigan (1993) supports the assertion that sleep, and in particular SWS, is essential for tissue restoration.

For further information on sleep and circadian rhythm disorders, together with views on the need to include these subjects within nurse education curricula, see Lee et al (2004).

Functions of REM sleep

The functions of REM sleep are more difficult to explain. Babies have large amounts of REM sleep, whereas older people with chronic brain degeneration have a reduced duration of REM sleep. This implies that REM sleep has a possible role in brain metabolism. Human studies of REM sleep deprivation have not yet produced a clear picture of its effects. There have been tentative suggestions that REM sleep is involved in the integration of emotional experiences and new material into our existing worldviews. It also seems possible that REM sleep is involved in learning and memory, but research has so far failed to provide convincing evidence to support these ideas.

NORMAL SLEEP

No matter what objective recordings of sleep might indicate about its duration, continuity or 'architecture', if the sleeper is satisfied with their sleep, then it may be considered to be normal. A good, restful night's sleep and a good day's refreshed and efficient wakefulness are, of course, interrelated. Even though their relationship is not one of simple cause and effect, each depends on the quality of the other.

Individual requirements for sleep vary enormously. Russo (2005) highlights the differences in sleep required through the life course. For example, adults tend to need an average of 8 h sleep each night, whereas older people generally seem to need less than this, with children and young infants needing more. Some people habitually take a nap during the day. Some are early risers, while others are more active in the evening and tend to go to bed late. Horne and Ostberg (1976), who seminally described such people as 'larks' and 'owls', reported the tendency of individuals to 'morningness' or 'eveningness'. Hospital routines, for instance early or late medication rounds and/or the taking of regular observations, tend to override these individual variations in behaviour, with a possible outcome of disturbed sleep patterns for some (Jarman et al 2002, Cmiel et al 2004).

Factors affecting normal sleep

There are many factors that may naturally affect and may disturb normal sleep, several of which are described below. These include, for example, age and gender, diet, noise, ambient temperature and pain. Each of these influences should be taken into account in nursing assessments of each patient's sleep, since the normal habits and needs of one person may vary from those of another.

Age

Changes in sleep patterns associated with age have been well documented, with neonates usually spending around 18 h asleep in every 24, young adults sleeping for an average of 8 h each night, and older people sleeping for 6 h. Older people tend to sleep less, spend more time in bed, have comparatively less stage 4 and REM sleep, and have more shifts between sleep stages than younger people (Rush & Schofield 1999).

For further information on age-related changes in sleep patterns, see Rush & Schofield (1999).

Problems such as getting to sleep or staying asleep also tend to be more common in older people (Rush & Schofield 1999); however, research reported by Klerman et al (2003) showed that although older people wake up more frequently than younger people, they do fall back to sleep at the same rate as their younger counterparts. These changes have been attributed to age-related loss of neurones and progressive fragmentation of circadian rhythmicity (Hood et al 2004). Older people also have increased amounts of wakefulness after sleep onset. Ancoli-Israel et al (1989) found that 41% of a sample of patients in a nursing home woke frequently due to apnoeic disturbances and leg jerks. Webb and Swinburne (1971) and Ersser et al (1999) attributed a high proportion of night-time awakenings among older people to pain and physical discomforts such as bladder distension and urinary urgency. Awareness of such problems should prompt nurses to alleviate discomfort as far as possible, to encourage regular bowel and bladder habits and ensure that optimum fluid intake is achieved by approximately 6 p.m. For those who enjoy tea or coffee, decaffeinated options should be encouraged for later in the day and evening.

For further information on the effectiveness of strategies to manage sleep in residents of aged care facilities, see Centre for Reviews and Dissemination (2005a).

Older people sustain an absolute and a relative reduction in time spent in stage 4 sleep, which may even disappear in a quarter of those in their sixties. Concurrently, they have an increased total duration of stage 1 sleep and an increase in the number of shifts into stage 1. The total sleep time (TST) is either reduced or unchanged in older people as compared with younger groups, although the time in bed tends to increase. This appears to be because older people spend more time lying in bed at night without attempting to sleep or while unsuccessfully trying to sleep, and lying in bed resting or napping during the day. Obviously, these sleep patterns could be considered abnormal in a younger age group, but should cause less concern amongst older people who are sick in hospital: wards with a large percentage of older patients should consequently adjust their routines to enable older people to continue such sleep habits (Humm 2001).

Maher (2001) discusses ways of assessing and improving disrupted sleep in older people.

For older people and their carers, the knowledge that changes in sleep patterns are commonly experienced and are therefore not necessarily pathological will be reassuring. Although some caution should be exercised, lest treatable problems relating to sleep are overlooked, nurses have an important role to play in educating patients and their carers about the predictable changes that occur in sleep habits with advancing age.

For further information, see Foley et al (1995) and Maher (2004).

STOP THINK **25.2** Discuss with your mentor any changes in sleep patterns that have been experienced by older patients in your care. Consider which may be due to inevitable age-related physiological changes and whether any adverse consequences are likely.

Gender

Research has shown that there are some interesting differences between men and women in terms of their satisfaction with sleep. Men have more disturbances in sleep than women from early adulthood onward (Webb 1982), frequently due to nocturnal penile tumescence occurring during REM sleep. Wever (1984) found that women sleep significantly longer than men, although it is well recognised that women complain of problems with sleeping more than men and that they consume more sleep-inducing drugs. While this difference is evident from early adulthood, it becomes more clearly marked in middle age.

Heredity

Sleep quality and length appear to be influenced by genetic factors. This was demonstrated by Partinen et al's seminal work (1983) in which the sleep of 2238 monozygotic and 4545 dizygotic twin pairs were studied. De Castro (2002), in a study of self-reported sleep patterns in identical and fraternal twins, demonstrated significant genetic influences on the time individuals went to sleep and woke up, how often they woke up during the night, the duration of their sleep and wakefulness and their feelings of alertness both upon waking up and during the day. Familial clustering of narcolepsy (see p. 892) and idiopathic insomnia has also been observed. It is therefore worth noting in a nursing assessment whether there is a family history of sleep difficulties. It may not, however, always be possible to remedy inherited sleep problems by means of nursing interventions.

Body weight

Weight gain is associated with an increased duration of sleep, while weight loss is often associated with shorter sleep. This has been confirmed by several studies of people with anorexia, including one suggesting that anorexia and bulimia were both linked to sleep disorders (Della Marca et al 2004). As body weight falls, so does total sleep, which also becomes more broken and is interrupted by earlier waking. A study of 36 people (Adam 1987) confirmed that both total and percentage REM sleep correlated with body weight, although the reasons for this were not clear.

Exercise

The effect of exercise on normal sleep is not straightforward and research studies have produced conflicting evidence:

some have shown that exercise increases the duration of SWS, whereas some have found no effect and others a negative effect on sleep. Youngstedt et al's (1997) meta-analysis of 38 studies showed that exercise had different effects on different stages of sleep. The changes were somewhat modest, the greatest being an increase of 10 min on SWS. However, most of this research has focused on good sleepers. A randomised controlled trial of depressed older people showed that exercise had a more profound effect on poor than on good sleepers (Singh et al 1997).

Li et al (2004), also in a randomised controlled trial, studied the effectiveness of tai chi in improving sleep quality in older people who had disturbed sleep. Results demonstrated that older people who took part in the 6 month low to moderate intensity tai chi programme reported significantly improved sleep quality on a number of measures, including shorter time to sleep onset and longer sleep duration.

A Cochrane Review of interventions for sleep problems in older age cites one study (Montgomery & Dennis 2005) which found that sleep quality improved after a short (16 week) exercise programme consisting of 30–40 min of walking or low impact aerobics four times a week when compared with no treatment.

It appears that, overall, exercise has a small sleep-promoting effect for many people, provided that it is not taken late in the evening.

Anxiety and depression

Anxiety and depression frequently interfere with sleep. Most people experience these at some time in their lives, associated with, for example, occupational stress, family tension, bereavement, illness or other traumatic event (Lavie 2001). Admission to hospital may be a major cause of anxiety, with all the accompanying worries with regard to illness, investigations or surgery.

For further information on sleep disturbances in people diagnosed with cancer, see Vena et al (2004) and Clark et al (2004); for sleep problems experienced by caregivers of patients with advanced cancer, see Carter (2003).

The increased activity of the sympathetic nervous system due to anxiety results in an increase in plasma noradrenaline levels. This in turn results in sleep changes similar to those seen in older people, who have less stage 4 and REM sleep, and more stage shifts and awakenings, along with elevations of daytime and night-time plasma noradrenaline.

Insomnia due to depression has been associated with raised levels of monoamine oxidase, which catabolises the neurotransmitters noradrenaline and 5-HT, each of which is involved in sleep onset and maintenance. Depressed patients therefore tend to experience difficulty falling asleep, an increased number of awakenings during the night and early morning waking. Nursing staff should encourage depressed and anxious patients to discuss their feelings and, if possible, assist them to deal with underlying difficulties. Alerting medical staff to the apparent existence of anxiety and depression should ensure that the patient receives appropriate medical or psychological treatment.

STOP THINK **25.3** Mr B is a 47-year-old man who had an appendicectomy 3 days ago. His physical recovery has been straightforward, but he is feeling very tired and depressed because he has been finding it difficult to sleep at night. Consequently, he has been reluctant to get up and walk and has been taking short naps throughout the day. Construct a plan of care, giving possible reasons for Mr B's inadequate sleep, suggesting practical nursing interventions and stating the expected outcome of these.

Physical illness

Cardiac and pulmonary diseases often worsen during the night (Redeker & Hedges 2002, Sutherland et al 2003, Redeker et al 2004). For example, the incidence of asthma attacks increases during the latter half of the night, while angina, cardiac dysrhythmias and nocturnal dyspnoea are all likely to worsen during sleep (see Chs 2 and 3). Metabolic disorders such as Cushing's disease, Addison's disease, hyper/hypothyroidism and diabetes mellitus may disrupt normal sleep patterns (see Ch. 5). Diseases that mobilise the immune system, whether viral, bacterial or fungal, may be associated with increased sleepiness (see Ch. 16).

Since many areas of the brain are implicated in sleep regulation, any pathology impinging on these sites can cause problems (see Chs 9 and 28). A rise in intracranial pressure, regardless of cause, increases sleepiness, which in some cases leads to coma and death. Interference with the brain stem or hypothalamus may affect the onset and maintenance of sleep.

Pain

People who live with chronic pain commonly experience sleep problems (see Ch. 19). Pain due to arthritis, cancer and low back injury is often described as intractable. Some types of chronic pain, such as that from peptic ulcers or reflux dyspepsia, have a circadian rhythm of increasing intensity at night. GPs tend to manage such pain by using medication, sometimes by aiming to relieve the cause, but more often providing symptomatic relief by means of analgesics or antacids. Sometimes the use of antidepressants, as adjuvant analgesics, is successful in promoting sleep, since some chronic pain syndromes can be associated with depression.

Nurses are closely involved in giving pain-relieving agents in hospital because of their 24-h, 7 days a week contact with patients. As long ago as 1979, Jones et al studied intensive care patients and found that pain was ranked second in contributing to sleep loss. Pain has been shown to be a major cause of sleep loss in the postoperative period (see Research Abstract 25.1) (Closs 1992, Southwell & Wistow 1995, Closs & Briggs 1997). Postoperative patients have strong views about sleep and pain (Closs 1991; see Box 25.2). If nurses are to be able to help patients cope with pain, they must perform an accurate nursing assessment of quality of sleep and be able to provide suitable interventions (see 'Methods of assessing sleep', p. 892, and Ch. 19).

For further information on the sleep experience of medical and surgical patients, see Tranmer et al (2003).

STOP THINK **25.4** Discuss with your lecturer and your mentor how you can give effective pain relief whilst still ensuring that your patient is not unduly disturbed and gets enough rest. Think about how your care may differ during the day and the night.

RESEARCH ABSTRACT 25.1

A study of patients' and nurses' assessments of sleep in hospital

In this study by Southwell and Wistow (1995), 454 hospital patients completed questionnaires about their sleep. This included patients on medical, surgical, care of older people and acute psychiatric wards. Questionnaires were also distributed to 129 nurses working on those wards. Patients and nurses then answered questions concerning the same nights in hospital.

Half of the patients reported that they could not sleep through the night and were consequently sleep deprived. The main factors which patients reported as disturbing their sleep were discomfort (including beds and pillows and particularly the use of plastic covers on these), pain, noise, being too warm and worries. Half were dissatisfied with both settling and waking times.

There were differences in emphasis between patients' and nurses' views of environmental factors disruptive to sleep. More patients than nurses reported noise outwith the ward, emergencies, patients making a noise, nurses' shoes and nurses talking to one another. More nurses than patients reported treatments, commodes/bedpans, toilets flushing and nurses talking with patients. Nurses were more aware of noise generated by their own work and were largely unaware of the noise they caused by chatting to each other and from their shoes.

In view of the mismatch between nurses' and patients' perceptions, the authors emphasised the need to elicit patients' perspectives on care. However, the two groups were in agreement that patients did not get as much sleep as they needed. It was recommended that nurses, managers and others should take action to ensure that patients' sleep should be disrupted as little as possible. Nurses need to be aware when patients are awake, and take steps to ease pain, discomfort and worries. It is also important to minimise the wide range of possible disturbances during the night.

Southwell M T, Wistow G 1995 Sleep in hospitals at night: are patients' needs being met? Journal of Advanced Nursing 21(6): 1101–1109

Box 25.2

What patients say about postoperative sleep and pain

Effects of tiredness on postoperative pain
- 'The pain is more nagging and it's harder to put up with if you're tired.'
- 'If you're tired, the pain's more draining, more severe, a down-puller. It can actually make you feel depressed.'
- 'If you're tired and in pain, you want to give up quicker. You could have shot me yesterday for all I cared.'

Effects of sleep on pain intensity
- 'If you've slept well, the pain isn't as bad a blow when you waken. If you don't sleep, you wonder when it'll ever end. It's a vicious circle.'
- 'If you're tired you're narky, if you're narky it hurts worse.'
- 'Sleep makes you relax and takes away some of the pain.'

Effects of sleep on coping with pain
- 'It's essential — you can't cope with anything unless you've slept, especially pain.'
- You're not so well able to cope if you're tired, you have a good attitude if you're rested.'
- 'It's impossible to cope properly if you haven't slept well.'

Effects of sleep on recovery
- 'Sleep is the best healer in the world. You know it's going to take longer to get better if you can't get your sleep.'
- 'You've got to get a good sleep before you get anything else. You feel fresh and don't get crabby, you can deal with the pain and everything else and it speeds up your recovery.'
- 'Sleep is a great healer — that's why I don't understand why they wake you up early in the morning. I think, why, what is it for? Certainly not for the patient. It makes you agitated. It's all done to their rules.'

From Closs (1991).

Diet

There has been a long history of research into the effects of diet on sleep. Brezinova and Oswald (1972) investigated the reasons why Horlicks malted beverage seems to enhance sleep. A link was noted between habitual bedtime practices and sleep rather than the content of the Horlicks: those who normally ate little or nothing before bedtime had no improvement in sleep after having Horlicks, while those who usually did have a bedtime drink slept better after Horlicks. Hot milky drinks are provided in some hospitals in the late evening, but these may not suit everyone.

It should be remembered that many people prefer to take an alcoholic 'nightcap' at home, and if they are normally heavy drinkers they will suffer from withdrawal symptoms in hospital if they are not permitted to drink alcohol. Withdrawal from alcohol will result in disturbed sleep, as will withdrawal of hypnotic medication. It should be noted that alcohol is not a good hypnotic, since, although it accelerates sleep onset, it disturbs sleep patterns later on in the night (Williams et al 1983) and can cause early waking due to a full bladder. Drinks such as tea, coffee and coca cola contain caffeine and therefore act as stimulants, disturbing normal sleep patterns. As early as 1976, Karacan et al showed that coffee disturbed sleep, even in those who felt unaffected by it.

Whilst the biochemical effects of diet on sleep are unclear, avoiding stimulants and adhering to dietary routines appear to enhance sleep. Although research in this area has so far been inconclusive, community nurses might be able to help poor sleepers simply by giving them dietary advice, while hospital nurses should allow patients to eat or drink as they would at home prior to bedtime, as far as that is feasible.

STOP THINK **25.5** A middle-aged woman complains to a community nurse that she is having great difficulty in getting to sleep at night. She is extremely anxious about her health and says that this is preventing her from sleeping. She has started taking naps during the day. In addition, she has found no help from taking drinking chocolate or a small drink of alcohol immediately before going to bed. What advice could the nurse give?

Medications

There are many medications that affect sleep, hypnotics being perhaps the best known (see p. 893). In addition, there are many others that have side-effects on sleep, including antidepressants, antihistamines and anticonvulsants. L-dopa and beta-blockers may produce vivid dreams and nightmares, whilst diuretics increase urine production, leading to bladder distension and nocturia. Other medications, e.g. amfetamines, stimulate the CNS, delaying sleep onset and reducing total sleep time.

Sleep position and snoring

Sleep positions have been associated with objective and subjective sleep quality. Poor sleepers appear to spend a greater proportion of their time on their backs with their heads straight and to change position more frequently than better sleepers (Koninck et al 1983). Snoring has been associated with subjects who sleep flat on their backs. Since these symptoms are undesirable for the sleeper, and snoring may disturb others sleeping within earshot, nurses could perhaps encourage and assist poor sleepers to adopt alternative positions for sleeping. Many snorers may have problems such as sleep apnoea (see p. 891) which are amenable to some types of treatment.

Breathing

Hypoventilation and breathing irregularities are common during normal sleep but may sometimes be clinically important. Normal changes include hypoxaemia and hypercapnia due to the slight reduction in metabolic rate that occurs during NREM sleep; in REM sleep irregular breathing is the norm.

Patients at home who have respiratory difficulties might benefit from advice regarding sleep position and the use of pillows to prop themselves up in order to maximise lung expansion and their carers should be advised of this. In hospital, nurses should ensure that anyone with respiratory difficulties, such as postoperative patients or those with chronic obstructive pulmonary disease (COPD) or respiratory tract infections, receives adequate support and assistance, particularly regarding oxygen administration, posture, deep breathing and coughing.

For further information, see Carlsson & Mascarella (2003) and Gay (2004).

Temperature

Sleep patterns are affected by changes in temperature, either in ambient (room) temperature or in body temperature. Kendel and Schmidt-Kessen (1973) pointed out that unclothed and uncovered subjects awoke from cold at an ambient temperature of 26°C and below. Total sleep deprivation has also been shown to alter body temperature, resulting in a decrease in mean daily body temperature and an increase in subjective feelings of cold (Horne 1985).

Fever is associated with a greater number of awakenings, increased total waking time and reduced amounts of SWS and REM sleep. Elevated ambient temperature produces similar results. The duration of the REM phase is shortened in artificially induced fever as well as at high ambient temperature. Zulley (1980) found that the higher the body temperature at sleep onset, the longer the duration of sleep, while REM sleep was negatively correlated with body temperature. These findings suggest that active management of pyrexial patients, perhaps by giving antipyretic medication, such as paracetamol for children, might improve their sleep.

Room temperature should be carefully monitored on general wards so that it may be maintained at a comfortable level, and patients should be encouraged to request more or fewer bedclothes as required. Older people are particularly vulnerable to fluctuations in room temperature, especially at home, since their ability to perceive temperature changes may be diminished. Community nurses are well placed to identify at least some of those individuals susceptible to hypothermia, and have a useful role in advising them about adequate clothing, bedding and heating in the home (see Ch. 22).

Noise

Noise can disturb sleep under all sorts of circumstances. In the home, mothers may wake at the slightest noise from their children, whilst in other circumstances they may sleep deeply through traffic or aeroplane noise. Conversely, those who live near a busy main road may have great difficulty sleeping in a quiet environment. Similarly, town dwellers might have problems sleeping for the first few nights of a quiet country holiday, or a patient who has had a long stay in a noisy hospital ward might have some difficulty readjusting to the quietness of their home environment. Individuals become habituated to the normal circumstances surrounding their sleep.

Zepelin et al (1984) studied subjects aged 18–71 years and found a correlation between a decline in the intensity of noise required to arouse individuals from sleep and increasing age. This reduction was present in all sleep stages but was greatest in stage 4. Ersser et al (1999) also found that noise was one of the most frequently given reasons for older people to have disturbed sleep in hospitals and nursing homes.

In hospital, noise poses a considerable problem, particularly in acute areas (Soutar & Wilson 1986, Aaron et al 1996). Patients' sleep may be disturbed by a wide variety of sounds, including noise made by other patients, nurses talking, footsteps, telephones, traffic, equipment alarms, squeaky doors, trolleys, rattling windows and many others (Closs 1988a, Southwell & Wistow 1995, Simpson et al 1996). While some noise is unavoidable at night, careful maintenance of equipment and precautions such as wearing soft-soled shoes can considerably improve the night-time hospital environment (see Research Abstract 25.2). Where possible, nurses should acquaint the more long-term patients with the unfamiliar sounds on the ward, so that they become accustomed to these noises and develop the ability to sleep through them.

Having observed the detrimental effects of sleep deprivation in their patients, and become more aware of the amount of noise generated by ward activities at night, nurses in a surgical thoracic unit decided to set up a sleep promotion team within their unit, in order to investigate these two related issues (Cmiel et al 2004). The team initiated a quality improvement project, the aims of which were, firstly, to make an objective pre-intervention measurement of noise levels on the ward, using a noise dosimeter. This instrument gave continuous recordings of decibel levels between

RESEARCH ABSTRACT 25.2

Nursing care at night

There is very little research about nursing at night and the impact that good care during this part of the 24 h can have on people. This Swedish study, designed to evaluate nursing care provided at night in one hospital, focused on the perspectives of both patients (n = 356) and nurses (n = 178).

The study used a newly developed questionnaire known as the Night Nursing Care Instrument to gain the views of staff and patients, in order to make comparison between the nurses' assessments and the patients' perceptions of the nursing care provided at night. The researchers found that there were no significant differences between the two groups for areas of medical intervention and evaluation, but the two did differ around areas linked to nursing intervention, including the assessment of the patients' needs for nursing care at night.

The authors concluded by suggesting that night nurses need to improve their ability to assess patients' needs for nursing care at night, particularly in relation to their knowledge of which nursing actions promote patients' rest at night.

Oleni, M, Johansson P, Fridlund B 2004 Nursing care at night: an evaluation using the Night Nursing Care Instrument. Journal of Advanced Nursing 47(2): 25–32

10 p.m. and 7 a.m. Secondly, subjective assessments of noise levels were obtained. In an innovative approach, two registered nurses each spent one night in an acute hospital setting, their bed areas containing the standard equipment and monitoring devices, to which they were connected, in a simulation of a normal patient's situation. Their report contained graphic descriptions of the noise levels and interruptions which disrupted their sleep. Patients were also surveyed about their sleep while in hospital. The sleep promotion team then carefully analysed the data obtained, following which various changes were implemented to improve the night-time environment for patients.

For further information on this quality improvement project, see Cmiel et al (2004).

COMMON SLEEP DISORDERS

Although the existence of sleep disorders has long been recognised, it is only in the past few decades that the seriousness of these has been acknowledged and a greater understanding developed. Epidemiological studies in Europe and the USA have indicated that up to about 40% of these populations reported difficulties in sleeping (Liljenberg et al 1989), with about 17% considering the problem to be serious. Insomnia is the most common complaint and has been defined by the US National Institutes of Health (2004) as 'experience of poor quality sleep, with difficulty in initiating or maintaining sleep, waking too early in the morning, or failing to feel refreshed'. Chronic insomnia is defined as insomnia occurring for at least three nights a week for 1 month or more. General practitioners have reported that around one-third of the subjective complaints made by their patients are of difficulties in sleeping.

Researchers have investigated sleep difficulties for patients at home and in hospital. A large multinational study of approximately 8000 patients in the community who had attended sleep clinics showed that 25% suffered from various types of insomnia, while 39% suffered from excessive daytime sleepiness (Coleman 1983). Smirne et al (1983) investigated sleep disorders of patients in general hospital wards, asking them about their sleep prior to admission. Of 2518 people, 25% reported some kind of sleep disturbance. These figures indicate that sleep presents difficulties for about a quarter of the population, posing a challenge for nurses in all fields of care.

For further information and detail on the grouping of sleep disorders, see The International Classification of Sleep Disorders, Revised: Diagnostic and Coding Manual (2001).

Sleep apnoea syndrome

This problem was first recognised over 25 years ago. The literal meaning of sleep apnoea is cessation of breathing during sleep. Often these episodes are repetitive and each may last up to a minute or even longer. Such apnoeas frequently cause the sleeper to wake, in some cases many times during the night. The main symptom resulting from this disorder is usually daytime sleepiness, although some sufferers complain of insomnia.

There are two main types of sleep apnoea: central sleep apnoea is caused by impaired neurological control of breathing, so that the intercostal muscles fail to contract; obstructive apnoea is the result of an obstruction of the airway, e.g. by large tonsils, a large or oedematous soft palate, fat deposits around the airway, retrognathia (backward displacement of the lower jaw) or micrognathia (a small lower jaw). The cause may be treated if the problem becomes severe. Obesity is common among these patients, in which case weight loss is usually the first approach to relieving the problem. For the more severe cases, continuous positive airway pressure (CPAP; see Ch. 29) during the night may help, while corrective surgery may be required for others.

For further information, see Barthlen (2002) and Centre for Reviews and Dissemination (2005b).

Sleep-induced nocturnal myoclonus

This condition is characterised by repetitive twitching of the legs occurring at regular intervals of 20–60 s. These episodes may last from a few minutes to several hours, and one or both legs may twitch (Barthlen 2002). This does not always disturb the individual, unless they are a light sleeper or the twitching is severe enough to arouse them from 'deep' sleep. Associated with this condition is restless legs syndrome, where an unpleasant, crawling sensation is experienced in the calves or thighs. Nocturnal myoclonus has been associated with the use of tricyclic antidepressant medication and chronic uraemia. Several remedies have been recommended, ranging from reduced caffeine, vitamin E supplementation to medication with ropinirole (Allen et al 2003).

Narcolepsy

This disorder occurs in approximately 4 in 10 000 people and can be described as an imbalance between wakefulness, REM sleep and NREM sleep. Sleep frequently intrudes into wakefulness and this change in conscious state is often triggered by strong emotions such as anger or laughter. It is REM sleep that intrudes, either partially or totally, producing the possibility of four different symptoms, as follows:

- excessive daytime sleepiness
- cataplexy, when only the muscular paralysis of REM occurs: the sufferer may be awake but is paralysed
- sleep paralysis, a type of cataplexy which occurs at sleep onset; paralysis which occurs on waking from REM is benign
- REM dreaming during wakefulness: hypnagogic hallucinations.

Parasomnias/partial arousals

Sleepwalking

This behaviour, when it occurs, commences during SWS, although the sleepwalker appears to be in a part-sleeping, part-waking state. Sleepwalking can be very dangerous: sufferers have been known to walk out of windows and to attack family members. During an episode of sleepwalking, the individual is usually uncommunicative and returns to bed spontaneously, rarely remembering the event the next morning. Sleepwalking is difficult to treat, so it is advisable, if a person does sleepwalk, to take precautions such as locking windows at night.

Night terrors and nightmares

Night terrors also arise during SWS and occur mostly in children. The sufferer often screams and shows signs of panic, such as a dramatic rise in heart rate, respiratory distress and sweating. They may be very difficult to arouse, but usually calm down within a few minutes, usually without waking up. Most people remember nothing about the incident. Nightmares occur during REM sleep and are often remembered very vividly on waking.

THE EFFECTS OF SLEEP DEPRIVATION

Total sleep deprivation, for as little as 48 h, has been shown to result in changes in central nervous system function, such as behavioural irritability, suspiciousness, speech slurring and minor visual misperceptions. Increased suggestibility and/or a reduction in motivation and willingness to perform tasks may also accompany these. In hospital, this could impede a patient's willingness to be up and about and undertake aspects of self-care as well as to communicate. Detrimental psychological effects of sleep deprivation sometimes observed in hospital patients include lethargy, irritability, confusion and, in more extreme cases, delusions and paranoia. Sleep deprivation for individuals in the community could reduce efficiency at work and affect social and family relationships.

A meta-analysis of 19 research studies that addressed the effects of sleep loss (Pilcher & Huffcutt 1996) suggested that the effects of such deprivation might well be underestimated. From a total sample of 1932 people, it was concluded that mood is more affected by sleep deprivation than either cognitive or motor functioning. It was also found that partial or intermittent sleep deprivation produced a greater impairment of cognitive and motor functioning than either short- or long-term sleep deprivation. Both acute and prolonged sleep disturbances, including delirium, have been observed in acute care settings (Cronin-Stubbs 1996). As long ago as 1973, Hartmann assessed sleep requirements by interview and questionnaire and found that stress and illness were virtually always accompanied by an increased subjective sleep need. Taken together, these observations support the hypothesis that sleep aids healing, suggesting that conditions favourable to the promotion of sleep should be created in all areas where patients are suffering from infection or trauma or are recovering following surgery.

METHODS OF ASSESSING SLEEP

Although many researchers have attempted to assess sleep in clinical settings, the methods used have not always been suitable for routine use by nurses (Closs 1988b, Maher 2004). In general, these methods of assessing sleep can be classified into two groups: those which rely on patients' subjective reports of their sleep and those which obtain objective measurements of either physiological events which coincide with sleep or psychological attributes reflecting the effects of sleep. Many of the objective methods of sleep assessment involve the use of expensive and sometimes unwieldy equipment. In most cases, nurses would neither have access to such equipment nor the expertise to use it. In addition, although these methods may be suitable for relatively healthy, stress-free individuals, most hospital patients would probably find such monitoring to be anxiety provoking, restrictive or uncomfortable, which may impact on their ability to sleep. One method which may be used by nurses for assessing sleep is actigraphy. The actigraph, a wristwatch-sized electronic device, is usually worn on the non-dominant wrist and measures sleep through arm movements, as arm movements are known to be linked to wakefulness and not to sleep (Benson et al 2003, Landis et al 2003).

Nursing assessment of sleep

The assessment of sleep is an important and integral part of the general nursing assessment of each patient and is, on an ongoing basis, particularly important to high quality care during the night (see Research Abstract 25.2). While it is appropriate for researchers and clinicians in other disciplines to use sophisticated monitoring equipment, coupled with detailed observations, nurses rely mainly on a combination of their observations of sleep and their communication skills, both questioning patients carefully and listening to what they tell them, in order to make their assessments. Assessment should take into account the patient's age, gender, diet, medical diagnosis and medical/surgical treatments, as well as paying specific attention to issues related to sleep (Fordham 1996) (see also Box 25.3).

Finding out about sleep

Although people are unable to give accurate reports of the actual time it takes for them to fall asleep, or how long they

Box 25.3

Possible questions in the nursing assessment of sleep

- How long have you had a sleep problem?
- What is your usual going to bed and waking routine?
- What treatments, if any, have you used for your insomnia? How successful or otherwise did you find these?
- Do you take a little alcohol to help you sleep, and if so, how helpful or otherwise do you think this is?
- What things do you do to help you get to sleep?
- Do you have difficulty falling asleep and/or do you keep waking in the night? If you keep waking, what do you do to help you get back to sleep?
- What regular exercise do you manage to get?
- How much caffeine do you drink, and at what times during each 24 hours?

Adapted from Maher (2004).

lie awake during the night, they can give reliable accounts of changes in their sleep patterns. Information can be gained from direct questioning, from non-verbal clues, the descriptions provided by relatives and carers, and from the nursing and/or medical records. Where patients are unable to answer direct questions due to age or incapacity, it may be possible to use a relatively new technique which employs a pictorial sleepiness scale on cartoon faces (Maldonado et al 2003).

Encouraging patients, where possible, to talk about themselves, their feelings and their needs is vital to the assessment of sleep. The use of open-ended questions and prompts can facilitate disclosure (Ersser et al 1999, Maher 2001, 2004) (see Box 25.3). Nurses should ask both general questions about sleep, as well as more specific questions that could include details about time of settling down to sleep, time of morning waking, duration of sleep, night-time routines, diet, medication, pain and anxieties. The patient's disclosures should be recorded in the notes so that each nurse participating in their care is aware of their needs.

STOP THINK **25.6** On your clinical placement, observe how and by whom the quality of patients' sleep is assessed.

Body language is also important: patients are less likely to be forthcoming if the nurse speaks from an uncomfortable distance, looking as if they are about to leave for some more important task. Planned nurse–patient interactions can provide ample opportunities for discussion and nursing assessment.

HELPING PATIENTS TO SLEEP

Once an assessment of the patient's sleep has been made, nursing care relevant to these sleeping habits/patterns can be planned. Fordham (1996) highlights several nursing interventions for sleep problems, including:

- *psychological causes* — teaching, counselling and relaxation techniques (see p. 895)
- *physical causes* — control or elimination of symptoms, e.g. nocturia, breathlessness or pain
- *medication-related causes* — assessment of the medication effects and of review with doctors or other prescribers
- *environmental causes* — controlling noise, temperature or light; maintaining dietary rituals as far as possible, e.g. where the person normally eats or what they do during meals, such as watch TV; considering exercise, activity or regularity in terms of sleep/waking patterns
- *scheduling difficulties* — postponement of sleep and discussion of regularity of sleep/wake patterns.

Nurses can also help by providing general information about sleep that enables patients and their carers/partners to have realistic expectations. The importance of including partners in the assessment and planning of care related to sleep disorders cannot be overemphasised since, as Strawbridge et al (2003) point out, a patient's sleep disturbances may impact on their partner's health and well-being.

Cultivating healthy sleep patterns

In addition, nurses can give advice for improving sleep through attention to behaviours and attitudes conducive to healthy sleep patterns. These might include:

- attitudes towards sleep
- the sleep environment
- attention to diet
- sleep scheduling
- pre-sleep activities and routines
- daytime sleep behaviours, e.g. napping.

More specifically, the points given in Box 25.4 should be borne in mind by nurses, on an everyday basis, as they assist patients to cultivate healthy sleep patterns.

Some people will have such serious sleep problems that they will require specialist treatments. If this is the case, the nurse should alert the appropriate professionals. In the community, this may be the GP or clinical psychologist; in hospital, specialist support may be available.

PHARMACOLOGICAL TREATMENTS FOR INSOMNIA

The major treatments available for insomnia are pharmacological, although alternative approaches, e.g. developing good sleep habits, sometimes referred to as 'sleep hygiene', alternative therapies and cognitive–behavioural therapies may be the preferred first line of treatment for many people.

Hypnotic medications

Most hypnotics which are currently prescribed belong to the benzodiazepine group, and include nitrazepam, temazepam and diazepam. Their use is dependent on the type of insomnia and associated symptoms, e.g. anxiety. These hypnotics provide temporary symptomatic relief but are not a cure. The sleep produced by these medicines does not resemble natural sleep: the duration of stage 2 sleep is increased at the expense of REM sleep and SWS. However, even though these medicines change the structure of sleep, most physiological processes associated with SWS

Box 25.4

Information and advice to assist patients to cultivate healthy sleep patterns

- Patients' expectations of sleep should be realistic. Many people think that there is something wrong with their sleep if they do not sleep for 8 h every night. Such incorrect assumptions may in themselves cause anxiety and sleep disturbance. The individual differences in sleep requirements and the normal effects of ageing should be explained clearly in order to encourage realistic attitudes towards sleep.
- Most people experience short episodes of poor sleep for which no particular treatment is needed. There is no evidence that transient insomnia has a detrimental effect on health. Chronic insomnia, i.e. lasting for at least 3 weeks, may require detailed assessment and treatment. If it is clear that the insomnia is transient, nurses may be able to reassure their patients on this point and, in so doing, help them to overcome it by reducing their anxiety about sleep loss.
- People suffering from insomnia tend to stay in bed even when they are unable to sleep. This interferes with their sleep by reducing the psychological association between bed and sleep. They should, if possible, avoid going to bed until they are sleepy, and if they cannot sleep, they should then get up and do something else. For example, they might read, watch television or engage in any other activity that they enjoy, preferably something relaxing.
- Establishing a regular time of waking up in the morning is helpful, even if the previous night's sleep was unsatisfactory. This strengthens the circadian rhythm and should be adhered to at weekends as well as weekdays. A reliable alarm clock or perhaps the assistance of a relative or friend can help to ensure a regular waking time.
- Patients who have difficulty sleeping at night may reduce their night-time sleep drive if they take day-time naps. Avoiding day-time naps also helps to reinforce circadian rhythmicity. Naps may be avoided by planning activities that can coincide with the times that naps are desired, so that there is always an alternative to napping available. If a post-lunch nap is to be missed, for example, the individual could plan to walk the dog or fetch a newspaper at that particular time.
- Poor sleepers should try to reserve the evening hours for relaxation and leisure activities. They should avoid strenuous mental or physical exertion immediately preceding bedtime, with the exception of sexual activity, which may increase relaxation and encourage sleep. The development of calming pre-sleep rituals such as reading can help patients drift off to sleep.
- Hunger and thirst can disturb sleep. If this is a problem, a light snack should be taken at bedtime. This may be anything, provided that it does not contain stimulants. A milky drink and a biscuit or a piece of fruit may be appropriate. There is no evidence to suggest that eating cheese before going to sleep has any adverse effects. Some may wish to keep a drink beside the bed in case they wake up during the night feeling thirsty.
- Many poor sleepers are sensitive to the stimulants found in some foods. It takes at least 8 h to metabolise caffeine, so caffeine-containing beverages and foods should be omitted from the diet after midday. This includes tea, coffee, coca cola and chocolate.
- Sleep is disturbed by the use of nicotine as well as by withdrawal from nicotine. Thus the prevention of disturbed sleep is yet another good reason for not smoking. The role of the nurse as health educator is important here since many people are unaware of any connection between smoking and poor sleep.
- Although small amounts of alcohol hasten sleep onset, larger amounts disturb sleep later on in the night. The detrimental effects of alcohol on sleep can outweigh any benefits. Again, the nurse may have an opportunity to provide health education in this regard, as it is a common misconception that alcohol enhances sleep.
- The sleep-disturbing side-effects of medications such as antihypertensives and anti-asthmatics should be understood. It might be that the patient has not linked their sleep difficulty with their medication. An explanation of such a connection could provide valuable reassurance. If disturbed sleep is accounted for in a rational manner in this way, the patient may perceive it as less of a problem.
- Sudden noises are more disturbing than constant ones. If occasional loud noise is inevitable, using earplugs or masking the disturbing noise with a monotonous background sound such as that made by an electric fan can help.
- Nurses should endeavour to create conditions favourable for sleep. Most people sleep best in a quiet, darkened room on a firm mattress, which is large enough to allow movement and stretching. Individual preferences, however, should be respected as far as is feasible.
- Being too hot or too cold can disturb sleep. Ambient temperature should be comfortable, and the amount and type of bedding adjusted to suit the individual.

continue as usual. It is difficult, therefore, to comment on the difference between the overall quality of sleep induced by hypnotics and that of normal sleep.

The effects of benzodiazepines vary, particularly with regard to their duration of action:

- Nitrazepam has quite long-lasting effects and is used less commonly than other forms, particularly for older people, in whom the medication's 'hangover effect' may cause loss of balance and result in falls.
- Temazepam acts for a shorter duration and has little or no 'hangover' effect.
- Diazepam is used for insomnia which is linked to daytime anxiety and is a long-acting drug which, in a single dose, may treat both insomnia and anxiety.

For further information, see Centre for Reviews and Dissemination (2005c)

Other non-benzodiazepine hypnotics, such as zaleplon, zolpidem and zopiclone, act in a similar fashion to the benzodiazepines. Zaleplon is very short acting, with zolpidem and zopiclone having a longer duration of action. These three medications should not be used for long-term treatment since dependence has been reported in a small number of patients (see *British National Formulary*, www.bnf.org).

Generally, short-acting hypnotics are favoured, since they are less likely to produce hangover effects during the day. While hypnotics are initially effective in inducing sleep, their regular use produces some degree of 'tolerance'. As time goes on, the body requires increasing doses of the medication to achieve the same effect. The effectiveness of most hypnotics is diminished after 3–14 days of use.

Although hypnotics can provide short-term improvement in sleep, long-term use can result in more problems with sleep. After an initial improvement, hypnotics may actually cause tiredness because of the reduction in SWS and REM sleep. When hypnotics are withdrawn, the patient may suffer from rebound insomnia. This involves extreme feelings of edginess, greater difficulty in falling asleep and more intense dreams and nightmares. These symptoms gradually diminish over time. In spite of these drawbacks, the short-term use of hypnotics can be highly beneficial. For example, an anxious patient due to have surgery may benefit greatly from the limited use of hypnotics over, perhaps, 3 or 4 perioperative nights.

For further information and detailed descriptions of medication actions and side-effects, see the latest edition of the *British National Formulary* (www.bnf.org).

Herbal remedies

Although several herbs are claimed to have sleep-inducing properties, either when used as aromatherapy or dropped in bath water, e.g. lavender, geranium or rose oils, or taken as infusions or oral preparations, e.g. chamomile tea or St John's wort, valerian is the only one which has been scientifically evaluated (Centre for Reviews and Dissemination 2005d). Valerian taken orally has been shown to reduce significantly the time taken to fall asleep (Lindahl & Lindwall 1989), to prolong sleep time, increase deep sleep stages and reduce night-time awakening. It is believed that small doses of valerian act in several ways to affect sleep positively through reducing anxiety, exerting a calming influence, relieving stress and relaxing muscles. One of the stated benefits of using valerian is the lack of morning hangover that is commonly associated with other pharmacological preparations. However, noted side-effects include stomach upsets with small doses, and headaches and nausea with larger doses.

For further information on valerian use, see Taibi et al (2004).

Despite the emphasis in the literature on valerian, other unproven herbal remedies may also be effective, not least by virtue of a placebo effect.

PSYCHOLOGICAL AND BEHAVIOURAL TREATMENTS FOR INSOMNIA

While pharmacological treatments of insomnia are palliative, psychological treatments aim to deal with the cause of the sleeplessness. In some cases, insomnia may be attributed to physiological or psychological overactivity. Stress is a common cause of sleep disturbance and can be dealt with by a variety of techniques (see Ch. 17). However, some individuals who suffer from insomnia are constitutionally poor sleepers who are unlikely to respond to any treatment. These people usually have difficulties sleeping throughout their lives, and the process of ageing is likely to reduce further the quality of their sleep. For those whose sleeplessness is associated with physiological or psychological hyperactivity, many non-pharmacological methods of treating insomnia have been attempted, with varying degrees of success. Four of the most widely known — relaxation therapy, paradoxical intention, associative learning technique and cognitive therapy — are discussed below. These therapies are mainly provided by clinical psychologists, whose choice of strategy depends on the cause of the sleeplessness, and on the individual's temperament and personal preference.

For meta-analyses on non-pharmacological interventions for insomnia in older adults, and the identification of effective psychological treatments for insomnia, see Centre for Reviews and Dissemination (2005e and 2005g, respectively).

Relaxation therapy

Emotional problems such as anxiety can be modified using various types of relaxation therapy, which aim to reduce physical and mental tension. Autogenic training (Centre for Reviews and Dissemination 2005f) teaches people to concentrate on sensations of warmth and heaviness in their limbs by repeated suggestion. Progressive muscular relaxation achieves a similar effect by the alternate tensing and relaxing of a series of muscles. These methods have been successful in helping people to fall asleep and in increasing their satisfaction with sleep (Lacks 1987, Richards 1998, Richards et al 2003).

Alternative forms of relaxation

A variety of alternative forms of relaxation have been studied, for example the use of music. In a study of the use of music to promote onset of sleep and sleep maintenance in 52 women over age 70, Johnson (2003) found that its use decreased the time to sleep onset and also the number of night awakenings, thus increasing the women's satisfaction with the quality of their sleep. Lai and Good (2005), in a study of Taiwanese older people who listened to their choice of music prior to going to sleep, found very similar positive results.

Paradoxical intention

Paradoxical intention has been used with success in the treatment of patients who are particularly anxious about their difficulty in falling asleep. This anxiety produces the opposite of the desired effect, making patients too tense to fall asleep. When such individuals are instructed to stay awake all night, their anxiety about falling asleep is reduced, paradoxically allowing them to relax and fall asleep (Ascher 1980).

Associative learning technique

This is a useful technique where the bed and the bedroom have become associated in the patient's mind with sleeplessness. For such people, going to bed is an aversive stimulus that produces an aroused state. Bootzin (1972) devised a method of avoiding all behaviours in the bedroom not associated with sleep, such as reading, eating, watching television or just lying awake. Individuals are instructed to go to bed only when they are sleepy and to get up if they lie awake for more than 10 min. Eventually this re-establishes the psychological association between bed and sleep.

Cognitive therapy

An individual who is plagued by intrusive and repetitive thoughts that keep them awake can be taught to use cognitive refocusing. Usually these are problems and worries which the individual can learn to control, first by recognising that they cannot solve their problems by turning them over and over in their mind at night, and second, by learning to suppress the troubling thoughts, often by concentrating on alternative, benign thoughts. Other techniques employed by cognitive therapists include meditation and guided imagery.

For further information, see Jacobs et al (2004) and Morin (2004).

Increasingly, nurses are learning to provide some of the above therapies, for example relaxation therapy, thus enhancing their already significant contribution to helping patients to sleep. Health visitors are already becoming involved in successful schemes designed to help adults with insomnia (Eaton 1996) and others may also develop such skills. Since sleep is such a fundamental activity of life and is essential to good health, this extension of the nurse's role would seem perfectly legitimate.

CONCLUSION

Despite sleep being a complex and universal behaviour that is prone to disruption by many internal and external influences, it remains an important individual experience. Since everyone needs sleep, every nurse needs to know how patients may be helped routinely to achieve the best sleep possible and how, in specific circumstances, to deal with individual sleep-related problems. Nurses have an important role to play in regulating individual and communal environments, in the hospital, nursing home or the patient's own home, so that they are as conducive as possible to the promotion of good sleep (Fordham 1996). The assessment of individual sleeping needs and of the environment within which patients are nursed should be a routine component of skilled nursing practice. Many difficulties can be overcome by simple changes in lifestyle and by adjustments to the individual's expectations of sleep. Where more serious problems occur, help from other health care professionals should be sought.

REFERENCES

Aaron J N, Carlisle C C, Carskadon M A et al 1996 Environmental noise as a cause of sleep disruption in an intermediate respiratory care unit. Sleep 19(9): 707–710

Adam K 1987 Total and percentage REM sleep correlate with body weight in 36 middle-aged people. Sleep 10(1): 69–77

Allen R, Picchietti D, Hening W et al 2003 Restless legs syndrome; diagnostic criteria, special considerations, and epidemiology. A report from the restless legs syndrome diagnosis and epidemiology workshop at the National Institutes of Health. Sleep Medicine 4: 101–119

Ancoli-Israel S, Parker L, Sinaee R et al 1989 Sleep fragmentation in patients from a nursing home. Journal of Gerontology 44(1): 18–21

Ascher L M 1980 Paradoxical intention. In: Goldstein A, Foa E B (eds) Handbook of behavioural interventions: a clinical guide. Wiley, New York, p 266–321

Barthlen G M 2002 The brain: sleep disorders. Obstructive sleep apnea syndrome, restless legs syndrome, and insomnia in geriatric patients. Geriatrics 57(11): 34–39

Benson K, Friedman L, Noda A et al 2003 The measurement of sleep by actigraphy: direct comparison of two commercially available actigraphs in a non-clinical population. Sleep 27(5): 986–989

Bootzin R R 1972 Stimulus control treatment for insomnia [summary]. Proceedings of the 80th Annual Convention of the American Psychological Association 7: 395–396

Brezinova V, Oswald I 1972 Sleep after a night-time beverage. British Medical Journal 2(5811): 431–433

British National Formulary. Online. Available: www.bnf.org

Centre for Reviews and Dissemination 2005d Valerian for insomnia: a systematic review of randomized clinical trials. NHS Centre for Reviews and Dissemination, University of York, York

Centre for Reviews and Dissemination 2005f Autogenic training: a meta-analysis of clinical outcome studies. NHS Centre for Reviews and Dissemination, University of York, York

Closs S J 1988a A nursing study of sleep on surgical wards. Nursing Research Unit report. Department of Nursing Studies, University of Edinburgh, Edinburgh

Closs S J 1988b Assessment of sleep in hospital patients: a review of methods. Journal of Advanced Nursing 13(4): 501–510

Closs S J 1991 A nursing study of patients' night-time sleep, pain and analgesic provision following abdominal surgery. Nursing Research Unit report. Department of Nursing Studies, University of Edinburgh, Edinburgh

Closs S J 1992 Patients' night-time pain, analgesic provision and sleep after surgery. International Journal of Nursing Studies 29(4): 381–392

Closs S J, Briggs M 1997 Evaluation of an intervention to improve post-operative sleep and pain control in orthopaedic patients at night. Report for the NHS Executive Northern & Yorkshire, University of Hull, Hull

Cmiel C A, Karr D M, Gasser D M et al 2004 Noise control: a nursing team's approach to sleep promotion. American Journal of Nursing 104(2): 40–47

Coleman R M 1983 Diagnosis, treatment and follow-up of about 8000 sleep/wake disorder patients. In: Guilleminault C, Lugaresi E (eds) Sleep/wake disorders: natural history, epidemiology and long term evolution. Raven Press, New York, p 87–97

Cronin-Stubbs D 1996 Delirium intervention research in acute care settings. In: Annual Review of Nursing Research, Vol. 14. Springer, New York, Ch. 3

de Castro J M 2002 The influence of heredity on self-reported sleep patterns in free-living humans. Physiology and Behavior 76(4–5): 479–486

Della Marca G, Farina B, Mennuni G F et al 2004 Microstructure of sleep in eating disorders: preliminary results. Eating and Weight Disorders 9(1): 77–80

Eaton L 1996 Health visitors tackle adult insomnia. Health Visitor 69(8): 312

Ersser S, Wiles A, Taylor H et al 1999 The sleep of older people in hospital and nursing homes. Journal of Clinical Nursing 8(4): 360–368

Espana R, Scammell T 2003 Sleep neurobiology for the clinician. Sleep 27(4): 811–820

Fordham M 1996 Patient problems: a research base for nursing. Churchill Livingstone, Edinburgh

Hartmann E L 1973 The functions of sleep. Yale University Press, New Haven, CT
Hobson J A 1995 Sleep. Scientific American Library, New York.
Hood B, Bruck D, Kennedy G 2004 Determinants of sleep quality in the healthy aged: the role of physical, psychological, circadian and naturalistic light variables. Age and Ageing 33(2): 159–165
Horne J A 1985 Sleep function with particular reference to sleep deprivation. Annals of Clinical Research 17(5): 199–208
Horne J A, Ostberg O 1976 A self-assessment questionnaire to determine morningness–eveningness in human circadian rhythm. International Journal of Chronobiology 4: 97–110
Humm C 2001 Sleep patterns in older people. Nursing Times 97(36): 40–41
Jarman H, Jacobs E, Walter R et al 2002 Allowing the patients to sleep: flexible medication times in an acute hospital. International Journal of Nursing Practice 8(2): 75–80
Johnson J E 2003 The use of music to promote sleep in older women. Journal of Community Health Nursing 20(1): 27–35
Jones J, Hoggart B, Withey J et al 1979 What the patients say: a study of reactions to an intensive care unit. Intensive Care Medicine 5: 89–92
Karacan I, Thornby J I, Anch M et al 1976 Dose-related sleep disturbances induced by coffee and caffeine. Clinical Pharmacology and Therapeutics 20: 682–689
Kendel J, Schmidt-Kessen W 1973 The influence of room temperature on night-time sleep in man (polygraphic night-sleep recordings in the climate chamber). In: Koella W P, Levin P (eds) Sleep. Karger, Basel, p 423–425
Klerman E, Davis J, Duffy J et al 2003 Older people awaken more frequently but fall back asleep at the same rate as younger people. Sleep 27(4): 793–798
Koninck J, De Gagnon P, Lallier S 1983 Sleep positions in the young adult and their relationship with the subjective quality of sleep. Sleep 6(1): 52–59
Lacks P 1987 Behavioural treatment for persistent insomnia. Pergamon Press, New York
Lai H-L, Good M 2005 Music improves sleep quality in older adults. Journal of Advanced Nursing 49(3): 234–244
Landis C, Frey C, Lentz M et al 2003 Self reported sleep quality and fatigue correlates with actigraphy in midlife women with fibromyalgia. Nursing Research 52(3): 140–147
Lavie P 2001 Sleep disturbances in the wake of traumatic events. New England Journal of Medicine 345(25): 1825–1832
Li F, Fisher K J, Harmer P et al 2004 Tai chi and self-rated quality of sleep and daytime sleepiness in older adults: a randomized controlled trial. Journal of the American Geriatrics Society 52(6): 892–900
Liljenberg B, Almqvist M, Hetta J et al 1989 Age and the prevalence of insomnia in adulthood. European Journal of Psychiatry 3: 5–12
Lindahl O, Lindwall L 1989 Double blind study of a valerian preparation. Pharmacology, Biochemistry and Behavior 32(4): 1065–1066
Maher S 2001 Assessing age-related sleep disorders. Nursing Older People 13(3): 27–28
Maher S 2004 Sleep in the older adult. Nursing Older People 16(9): 30–35
Maldonado C, Bentley A, Mitchell D 2003 A pictorial sleepiness scale based on cartoon faces. Sleep 27(3): 541–548
Montgomery P, Dennis J 2005 Physical exercise for sleep problems in adults aged 60+ (Cochrane Review). In: The Cochrane Library, Issue 2. Wiley, Chichester
Moorcroft W H 1995 The function of sleep. Comments on the symposium and an attempt at synthesis. Behavioural Brain Research 69(1–2): 207–210
Oleni M, Johansson P, Fridlund B 2004 Nursing care at night: an evaluation using the Night Nursing Care Instrument. Journal of Advanced Nursing 47(2): 25–32
Partinen M, Kaprio J, Koskenvuo M, Langinvainio H 1983 Genetic and environmental determination of human sleep. Sleep 6(3): 179–185
Pilcher J J, Huffcutt A I 1996 Effects of sleep deprivation on performance: a meta-analysis. Sleep 19(4): 318–326
Rechtschaffen A, Kales A 1968 A manual of standardised terminology, techniques and scoring system for sleep stages of human subjects. US Dept. of Health, Education and Welfare, Bethesda, MD
Redeker N S, Hedges C 2002 Sleep during hospitalization and recovery after cardiac surgery. Journal of Cardiovascular Nursing 17(1): 56–68, 82–83
Redeker N S, Rugiero J S, Hedges C 2004 Sleep is related to physical function and emotional well-being after cardiac surgery. Nursing Research 53(3): 154–162
Richards K C 1998 Effect of a back massage and relaxation intervention on sleep in critically ill patients. American Journal of Critical Care 7: 288–299
Richards K, Nagel C, Markie M et al 2003 Use of complementary and alternative therapies to promote sleep in critically ill patients. Critical Care Nursing Clinics of North America 15(3): 329–340
Rush S, Schofield I 1999 Biological support needs. In: Heath H, Schofield I (eds) Healthy ageing: nursing older people. Mosby, London, p 119–158
Russo M 2005 Normal sleep, sleep physiology and sleep deprivation: general principles. Online. Available: www.emedicine.com/neuro/topic444.htm
Shapiro C M, Flanigan M J 1993 ABC of sleep disorders. Function of sleep. British Medical Journal 306: 383–385
Simpson T, Lee E R, Cameron C 1996 Relationships among sleep dimensions and factors that impair sleep after cardiac surgery. Research in Nursing and Health 19(3): 213–223
Singh N A, Clements K M, Fiatarone M A 1997 A randomized controlled trial of the effect of exercise on sleep. Sleep 20(2): 95–101
Smirne S, Franceschi M, Zamproni P et al 1983 Prevalence of sleep disorders in an unselected in-patient population. In: Guilleminault C, Lugaresi E (eds) Sleep/wake disorders: natural history, epidemiology, and long term evolution. Raven Press, New York, p 61–71
Soutar R L, Wilson J A 1986 Does hospital noise disturb patients? British Medical Journal 292: 305
Southwell M T, Wistow G 1995 Sleep in hospitals at night: are patients' needs being met? Journal of Advanced Nursing 21(6): 1101–1109
Strawbridge W, Shema S J, Roberts R E 2003 Impact of spouses' sleep problems on partners. Sleep 273: 541–548
Sutherland E R, Kraft M, Rex M D et al 2003 Hypothalamic–pituitary–adrenal axis dysfunction during sleep in nocturnal asthma. Chest 123(3)(Suppl): 405S
US National Institutes of Health, cited by Clinical Evidence 2004 Bazian Ltd. BMJ Publishing Group, London
Webb W B 1982 Sleep in older persons: sleep structures of 50 to 60 year old men and women. Journal of Gerontology 37: 581–586
Webb W B, Swinburne H 1971 An observational study of sleep of the aged. Perception and Motor Skills 32: 895–898
Wever R A 1984 Properties of human sleep–wake cycles: parameters of internally synchronised free-running rhythms. Sleep 7: 27–51
Williams D L, McLean A W, Cairns J 1983 Dose–response effects of ethanol on the sleep of young women. Journal of Studies on Alcohol 44: 515–523
Youngstedt S D, O'Connor P J, Dishman R K 1997 The effects of acute exercise on sleep: a quantitative synthesis. Sleep 20(3): 203–214
Zepelin H, McDonald C S, Zammit G K 1984 Effects of age on auditory awakening thresholds. Journal of Gerontology 39(3): 294–300
Zulley J 1980 Timing of sleep within the circadian temperature cycle. Sleep Research 9: 282

FURTHER READING

Barthlen G M 2002 The brain: sleep disorders. Obstructive sleep apnea syndrome, restless legs syndrome, and insomnia in geriatric patients. Geriatrics 57(11): 34–39
Benington J H 2001 Sleep homeostasis and the function of sleep. Sleep 24(7): 750–751
British National Formulary. Online. Available: www.bnf.org
Carlsson B B, Mascarella J J 2003 Changes in sleep patterns in COPD – a new vital sign in the management of people with chronic obstructive pulmonary disease. American Journal of Nursing 103(12): 71–72, 74
Carter P A 2003 Family caregivers' sleep loss and depression over time. Cancer Nursing 26(4): 253–259
Centre for Reviews and Dissemination 2005a Effectiveness of strategies to manage sleep

in residents of aged care facilities. NHS Centre for Reviews and Dissemination, University of York, York

Centre for Reviews and Dissemination 2005b Systematic review on obstructive sleep apnoea; its effect on health and benefit of treatment. NHS Centre for Reviews and Dissemination, University of York, York

Centre for Reviews and Dissemination 2005c Benzodiazepines and zolpidem for chronic insomnia: a meta-analysis of treatment efficacy. NHS Centre for Reviews and Dissemination, University of York, York

Centre for Reviews and Dissemination 2005e Nonpharmacological interventions for insomnia in older adults: a meta-analysis of treatment efficacy. NHS Centre for Reviews and Dissemination, University of York, York

Centre for Reviews and Dissemination 2005g Identifying effective psychological treatments for insomnia: a meta-analysis. NHS Centre for Reviews and Dissemination, University of York, York

Clark J, Cunningham M, McMillan S et al 2004 Sleep–wake disturbances in people with cancer. Part II: evaluating the evidence for clinical decision making. Oncology Nursing Forum 31(4): 747–771

Clinical Evidence 2004 BMJ Publishing Group, London

Cmiel C A, Karr D M, Gasser D M et al 2004 Noise control: a nursing team's approach to sleep promotion. American Journal of Nursing 104(2): 40–47

Edell-Gustaffson U M 2002 Insufficient sleep, cognitive anxiety and health transition in men with coronary artery disease: a self-report and polysomnographic study. Journal of Advanced Nursing 37(5): 414–422

Foley D J, Monjan A A, Brown S L et al 1995 Sleep complaints among elderly persons: an epidemiological study of three communities. Sleep 18: 425–432

Gay P C 2004 Chronic obstructive pulmonary disease. Respiratory Care 49(1): 39–52

Gillin J C, Byerley W F 1990 The diagnosis and management of insomnia. New England Journal of Medicine 322(4): 239–248

Heath H, Schofield I (eds) 1999 Healthy ageing: nursing older people. Mosby, London

Hobson J A 1995 Sleep. Scientific American Library, New York

Jacobs G D, Pace-Schott E F, Stickgold R, Otto M W 2004 Cognitive behavior therapy and pharmacotherapy for insomnia: a randomized controlled trial and direct comparison. Archives of Internal Medicine 164(17): 1888–1896

Jarman H, Jacobs E, Walter R et al 2002 Allowing the patients to sleep: flexible medication times in an acute hospital. International Journal of Nursing Practice 8(2): 75–80

Lee K, Landis C A 2003 Priorities for sleep research during the next decade. Research in Nursing and Health 26(3): 175–176

Lee K A, Landis C, Chasens E R et al 2004 Sleep and chronobiology: recommendations for nursing education. Nursing Outlook 52(3): 126–133

Maher S 2001 Assessing age-related sleep disorders. Nursing Older People 13(3): 27–28

Maher S 2004 Sleep in the older adult. Nursing Older People 16(9): 30–35

Meredith R E 2000 Improving the quality of care provided at night. Professional Nurse 15: 502–505

Morin C M 2004 Cognitive–behavioral approaches to the treatment of insomnia. Journal of Clinical Psychiatry 65(Suppl 16): 33–40

Rush S, Schofield I 1999 Biological support needs. In: Heath H, Schofield I (eds) Healthy ageing: nursing older people. Mosby, London, p 119–158

Taibi D M, Bourguignon C, Taylor A G 2004 Valerian use for sleep disturbances related to rheumatoid arthritis. Holistic Nursing Practice 18(3): 120–126

The International Classification of Sleep Disorders, Revised: Diagnostic and Coding Manual 2001. American Academy of Sleep Medicine, Westchester, IL

Tranmer J E, Minard J, Fox L A, Rebelo L 2003 The sleep experience of medical and surgical patients. Clinical Nursing Research 12(2): 159–173

Vena C, Parker K, Cunningham M et al 2004 Sleep–wake disturbances in people with cancer. Part I: an overview of sleep, sleep regulation, and effects of disease and treatment. Oncology Nursing Forum 31(4): 735–746

USEFUL WEBSITES

National Sleep Foundation
www.sleepfoundation.org

***Sleep* [journal]**
www.journalsleep.org

Sleep Medicine (The Computerized Textbook of Sleep Medicine)
www.users.cloud9.net/~thorpy
(*Lists resources regarding all aspects of sleep including the physiology of sleep, clinical sleep medicine, sleep research and patient information*)

SECTION THREE

NURSING PATIENTS WITH SPECIAL CHALLENGES

THE PATIENT FACING SURGERY

26

Caroline E. Gibson

INTRODUCTION

This chapter aims to give an overview of the nursing care required by patients facing surgery. Discussion will include not only those interventions relevant to the period of hospitalisation, but also the support needed by patients during the diagnostic process and during their eventual rehabilitation at home. Patients undergo many types of surgery for a wide range of reasons, but the principles of care can, to a large degree, be generalised with reference to particular types of procedure. It should be stressed, however, that individuals often react quite differently to a given disease or treatment. What one person may regard as a 'minor' procedure may cause extreme anxiety in another. Nursing staff must be sensitive to each patient's individuality and try to appreciate the significance of the experience of surgery from the patient's own perspective.

STOP THINK **26.1** Think of an intervention or form of treatment you have experienced, such as removal of wisdom teeth, a cervical smear or suturing of a cut. What sort of fears did you have, however irrational they might seem now?

Changing patterns of surgical care

Advances in surgical technology and anaesthesiology have had a dramatic effect in more recent years on the experience of patients undergoing surgery. Previously lengthy operations can be completed more quickly and recovery times are shorter. The recently developed anaesthetic agent, remifentanil, is short acting and can be used in day surgery because it reduces the time from extubation to full recovery (Mason 2002). Many standard invasive surgical procedures are being replaced by laparoscopy, angiographic catheterisation, endoscopy and laser techniques. Minimally invasive surgical interventions include laser treatment to shatter (ablate) renal stones (lithotripsy), arthroscopy is now the method of choice in managing tears of the menisci in the knee and many gynaecological procedures can be carried out laparoscopically, e.g. excision of ovarian cysts and tubal ligation.

Even recovery from major surgical procedures has been accelerated. In the last few years orthopaedic surgeons have developed a 'keyhole' approach to total hip replacement operations (Lucas 2004). The introduction of laparoscopically assisted colonic surgery has reduced most patients' hospital stay from 6–12 days (Retchen et al 1997, Chen et al 1998) to approximately 4–6 days (Lewis et al 2001). There are ongoing trials which aim to revolutionise further the recovery from colonic surgery by revising perioperative care programmes, improving optimal analgesia, introducing early mobilisation and early enteral nutrition (Kehlett & Morgensen 1999, Lewis et al 2001). Results suggest that the postoperative hospital stay may be reduced to 2–3 days. Such advances in perioperative practice and the introduction of minimally invasive surgical approaches have enabled sicker patients to be eligible for surgery.

Day surgery has become possible for many general surgical patients. Since 1986, the amount of day surgery being undertaken has risen by 30% (Mitchell 1997) and UK government targets propose that 75% of all elective surgery should be undertaken as day cases (DH 2000a, Audit Commission 2001). A brief hospital stay increases patient turnover but in turn increases the responsibilities of informal carers and community nurses (Mitchell 2003).

There are increasing numbers of older people in our society and it is estimated that before the end of the current decade over 20% of the population will be aged 65 years or older (Sear 2003). This change in demographics results in greater numbers of older people presenting for surgery (Leung & Dzankic 2001, Sear 2003). Ageing affects all of the body systems. Most affected are the cardiovascular, renal and respiratory systems. Increasing age is mostly associated with a higher risk of developing postoperative complications (Vemuri et al 2004), particularly if the patient has coexisting disease. For example, patients with cardiovascular disease are more at risk of developing myocardial infarction (MI) or arrhythmias following surgery (Sear 2003). Leung and Dzankic (2001) found that approximately 21% of patients over the age of 65 develop one or more in-hospital postoperative complications involving the cardiovascular, neurological or respiratory system.

Nursing staff will also observe a pattern of certain problems requiring surgical intervention in this older population. For example, the severity of appendicitis is increased in the older patient and presentation is often atypical, leading to delayed diagnosis (Pissara 2001). Likewise, the development of diverticular abscesses, associated with a diet high in refined foods and low in fibre, is the leading cause of bowel perforation in older people. Perioperative care of older surgical patients is thus becoming an increasingly important part of nursing practice.

Public expectations of health care have also changed in recent years. Patients increasingly wish to be involved in their own care and to be able to exercise choice in care decisions. The patient facing surgery should be seen as a partner in the care process (DH 2000a, Edwards 2002, Scottish Executive 2003a).

The nature of surgical services is changing rapidly to keep pace with technology and with advances in knowledge and skills. Within surgical wards and departments, nurses are faced with the challenge of providing continuous, individualised care within a more restricted time frame. This is facilitated by the named nurse concept, implemented in its various forms: primary nursing, team nursing or patient allocation (Dooley 1999, Steven 1999). Structured care approaches such as protocols, clinical pathways and algorithms are being used increasingly to organise clinical knowledge and to guide patient care (O'Neill & Dluhy 2000). Mathieson (2000) highlights that nurses in surgical units are constantly facing new techniques and practices which require them to be up to date and receptive to change. Developments in nurse-led initiatives such as orthopaedic assessment units (Sutcliffe & Potter 2002) and nurses carrying out endoscopy (Smith & Watson 2005) will further expand the role of nurses in perioperative care.

PRE-SURGICAL CARE

Classification of surgery

Some patients experience long periods of ill-health or disability before undergoing an operation; others experience sudden illness or injury that necessitates immediate surgery. The degree of urgency of a surgical intervention is a useful criterion for its classification and prioritisation. An older patient with osteoarthritis of the hip who requires a total hip replacement operation would normally not be classified as 'urgent', but would be put on a waiting list and admitted 'electively'. However, if the same patient had fallen and fractured the neck of the femur, repair or, more commonly, total replacement of the hip to prevent further deterioration and ensure a speedy recovery would be regarded as 'essential'.

A given operation may be performed for different classifications of surgery. Surgery for a strangulated hernia will be handled as an emergency, whereas surgery for an irreducible hernia will be considered as essential, and for a reducible one as elective. Patients requiring essential surgery will be admitted to hospital within a week or two of presentation at their outpatient appointment, but elective patients may have to wait for some considerable time. In December 2000 approximately 2% of the UK population were waiting for an operation, some 1 197 000 individuals (DH 2001a).

There has been debate on the usefulness of this focus on waiting times. To say that all patients receive surgery within a given period may meet a standard, but for an individual who requires surgery within several weeks, the standard cannot apply. For those who have to wait longer, the effects can be painful, stressful and expensive (DH 2001a). For those waiting for a hip replacement, a year's wait may be intolerable.

Presenting for surgery

STOP THINK **26.2** Ask a patient who has recently experienced surgery what signs and symptoms first brought the illness to their attention. What was it that made them seek out treatment? How do they define ill-health?

Personal definitions of health and ill-health and the decision to seek treatment are influenced by factors such as previous experience, social context, perceived severity of illness and judgements as to whether treatment would be beneficial. In Case History 26.1(A), Mr W was reluctant to take time off work to seek treatment but came to a point where pain and discomfort made it impossible for him to carry on. In Case History 26.2(A) Mrs B was reluctant to seek help, partly due to her fear of having cancer and partly due to what she felt was an embarrassing symptom. She had also convinced herself that she merely had haemorrhoids and could treat the condition herself.

In Case History 26.3, Mr A had made a voluntary decision to seek treatment based on information obtained through the internet, and from talking with his partner. The accessibility of the internet has meant that more and more of the public use it as a source of information. Patients may present with an increasingly sophisticated level of knowledge about procedures. However, there are no standards guaranteeing the quality of information from the internet. Some of the information Mr A found may not be from a medical source or be research based.

Pathways and progress

Patients may be referred for surgery by different paths. Figure 26.1 represents the progress of Mr W and Mr A

CASE HISTORY 26.1(A)

Mr W

Mr W works for a large construction company. He is married and has three young children. They enjoy a comfortable lifestyle and had bought their own home that year. Mr W has been able to get some overtime work and this helps considerably with the mortgage repayments.

Mr W had been having some pain and swelling in his groin for some time, but it usually resolved on its own over time. However, over the past few weeks the swelling had got worse and was limiting the range of work he could do. He made an appointment with his GP who quickly assessed the extent of his inguinal hernia and made a referral to the local hospital for a surgical opinion. Before leaving the GP's surgery, the practice nurse fitted him with a scrotal support and gave him some simple analgesics.

Three weeks before the scheduled date for surgery, Mr W was invited to the hospital pre-admission clinic where he was seen by a nurse and a doctor. The doctor asked him about his current state of health and examined him, listening to his chest and recording the findings in the medical admission form. The nurse recorded his blood pressure, pulse, took some blood to test for electrolyte abnormalities, levels of urea and full blood count, and asked for a sample of urine to test. The nurse advised Mr W that all of his up-to-date results would be available on the day of surgery, explaining what would happen on that day, and asked him if he had any questions about his proposed operation.

Mr W told the nurse that he was worried about taking time off work and being able to carry on with his job. The nurse reassured him that he would eventually be able to return to a full range of duties once he had completely recovered. The nurse also suggested that if he were able to give up smoking he would have less of the cough that was partly exacerbating his hernia, and that he would have a better chance of a quick recovery after the anaesthetic. Mr W had always found he put on weight when he stopped smoking and was already moderately overweight. They discussed a plan of how he might give up smoking, including the use of nicotine replacement chewing gum and patches. Mr W knew his wife would be very supportive but was less sure of his mates, whom he met in the pub on Friday nights. The nurse gave him a booklet on healthy eating to take home and look at with his wife. He quickly identified that his fried breakfasts and love of chips and beer were major sources of imbalance in his diet. They also talked about how long he should expect to stay in hospital and what sort of work he would be able to do after the operation.

Mr W mentioned his concerns about the effect of the operation on his ability to have sex and whether it would make him sterile. The nurse reassured him on these points and explained that the operation would tighten a track through to his scrotum and would not affect his genitals, although he might be a little tender in the groin for the first week.

through the health care system, and Figure 26.2 that of Mrs B. Patients might enter these pathways at various points; Mrs B, for example, was taken straight to the Emergency Department (ED) by ambulance without seeing her GP. Patients may also be transferred from other wards. For example, a patient on a medical ward may undergo investigations which lead to a diagnosis necessitating surgical treatment and therefore transfer to a surgical ward. A few patients admitted as emergencies may go straight to theatre from the ED and from there to the surgical ward following the operation. Some patients may need to go back to theatre or the intensive therapy unit (ITU) if their condition

CASE HISTORY 26.2(A)

Mrs B

Mrs B is a 78-year-old woman who lost her husband several years ago. Her eldest daughter lives nearby and is very supportive. Mrs B now lives in sheltered housing, which was a relief to her daughter, as she had previously lived in an isolated country cottage. Her sight has been gradually deteriorating in recent years and the arthritis in her fingers and knees limits what she can do. At the time Mrs B became ill, she was pleased that she still had her own home, and enjoyed going to the local day centre twice a week.

One of the care assistants at the day centre was a little concerned that Mrs B did not seem to be enjoying the singing quite so much as before and spent much of the afternoon dozing. Mrs B, being an independent and spirited lady, thanked the young girl for her concern and joked that she wasn't getting any younger and that there was no need to worry about her.

Mrs B thought long and hard that evening. She had been constipated for some time but had put it down to old age. Now she was also passing blood, and although she was frightened that it might be 'something nasty', she had decided that it must be piles. She had bought some ointment and laxatives from the chemist, but was reluctant to go to her GP, who had visited her when she just moved into the area. He was a nice young man, but she did not want him to examine her.

Several weeks later, the driver of the day centre minibus got no reply at Mrs B's door when he called to collect her. Worried that she might have fallen, he called the warden, who had a key to the flat. Mrs B was found still in her bed, in obvious pain and sweating profusely. The warden called an ambulance immediately and then phoned Mrs B's daughter. Mrs B was then taken to the Emergency Department of the local hospital.

deteriorates or requires further intervention. Some hospitals have specialist surgical high dependency unit (HDU) facilities where patients can be closely monitored for the first 24–48 h following their operation. These units usually have a higher ratio of nurses to patients than general ward areas. HDUs are thus often used for patients following major surgery or where pre-existing medical conditions predispose them to complications (DH 2000b, Sheppard & Wright 2000). Occasionally, convalescence or rehabilitation may be required in another ward or hospital, e.g. following amputation or neurosurgery. However, increasingly these services can be provided by community health care teams.

Patients such as M (see Case History 26.4(A)), whose illness is of a chronic nature, may be readmitted to the surgical ward on one or more occasions. Patients with Crohn's disease can present at an early age and may require repeated interventions and admissions to hospital throughout their lives (Pullen 1998). In a busy surgical ward these patients require a sensitive approach. One must not assume that because a patient has been through a procedure before, they will need less support or information than they did the first time. The vast majority of patients are admitted to hospital from home and return to their own homes. Traditionally, the GP has been seen as the gatekeeper to services: the one who will refer the patient for further care from the hospital consultant unless the illness is a sudden emergency or an accident. In Case History 26.2(A) Mrs B was reluctant to visit her GP due to the embarrassment of a possible rectal examination. She could have received advice and support

CASE HISTORY 26.3

Mr A

Mr A is a 41-year-old teacher who lives with his partner and four children. The youngest child is 18 months old. Mr A and his partner did not plan to have any more children. The last pregnancy had been a rather unplanned but welcome event! Mr A looked up some information on sterilisation on the internet on his home computer and was surprised at the amount of information that was available about vasectomy. He had not realised that it could be done as a short outpatient procedure and that it did not necessarily require a general anaesthetic. He discussed it with his partner and they decided that this was the most appropriate course of action.

His GP told them that, in their area, vasectomy could be undertaken at the local Family Planning Clinic and that there was an opportunity to discuss the procedure and decision making in an appointment beforehand. Within a few weeks of the GP's referral to the clinic, a pack of information was sent out to Mr A's home along with a date for a vasectomy counselling appointment. At the clinic he and his partner met a family planning nurse who talked through the details of the procedure with them, including possible complications such as bleeding, infection and recannulation of the vas deferens, the tube connecting the sperm-producing epididymis to the urethra. The nurse ensured that he had no problems with blood clotting and that he was not allergic to lidocaine, a local anaesthetic agent used by the surgeon. Mr A did not know if he had ever been administered lidocaine before, but when the nurse told him that it was often used by dentists to numb the mouth before treatment, he was able to confirm that he had had no problems in the past. The nurse also explained to Mr A about the importance of continuing to use contraception after the procedure until two consecutive samples of ejaculate were found not to contain any sperm cells. It would take approximately 20 ejaculations to clear the sperm duct of stored sperm.

The nurse highlighted that vasectomy was essentially a permanent decision because although reversal operations were possible, the sperm produced following vasectomy were only viable in a small percentage of cases. The nurse therefore asked them to consider their decision in light of possible unforeseen circumstances such as the death of a child or break up of their relationship. They acknowledged that these issues could affect reproductive decision making but that neither of them wanted further children.

The nurse explained that the clinic could carry out vasectomy operations, in patients who were fit and well, and who had not previously had any surgery to the scrotum or surrounding area. Mr A said that he had only had an appendicectomy when he was 16. She reassured him that this would not affect the surgeon's ability to operate in the scrotal area. Based on this consultation, the family planning nurse was able to recommend Mr A for the procedure and gave him an appointment for vasectomy in 11 weeks' time.

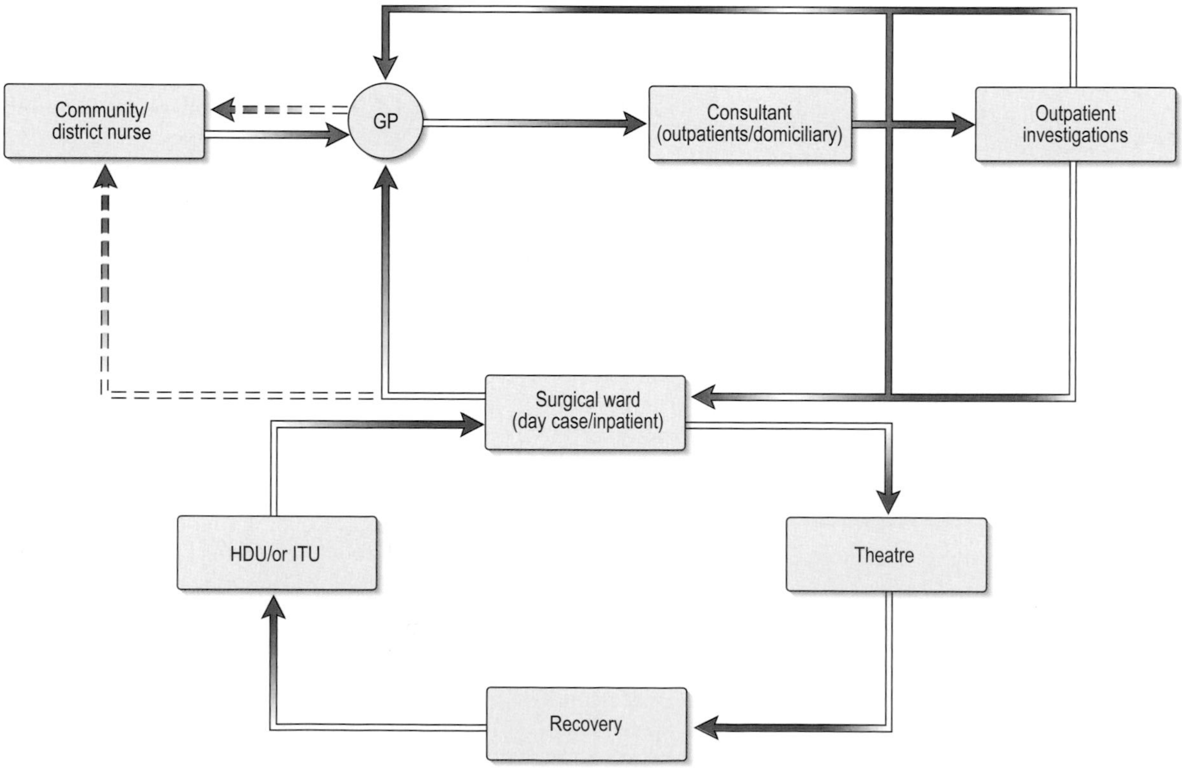

Fig. 26.1 Pathways to essential and elective surgery.

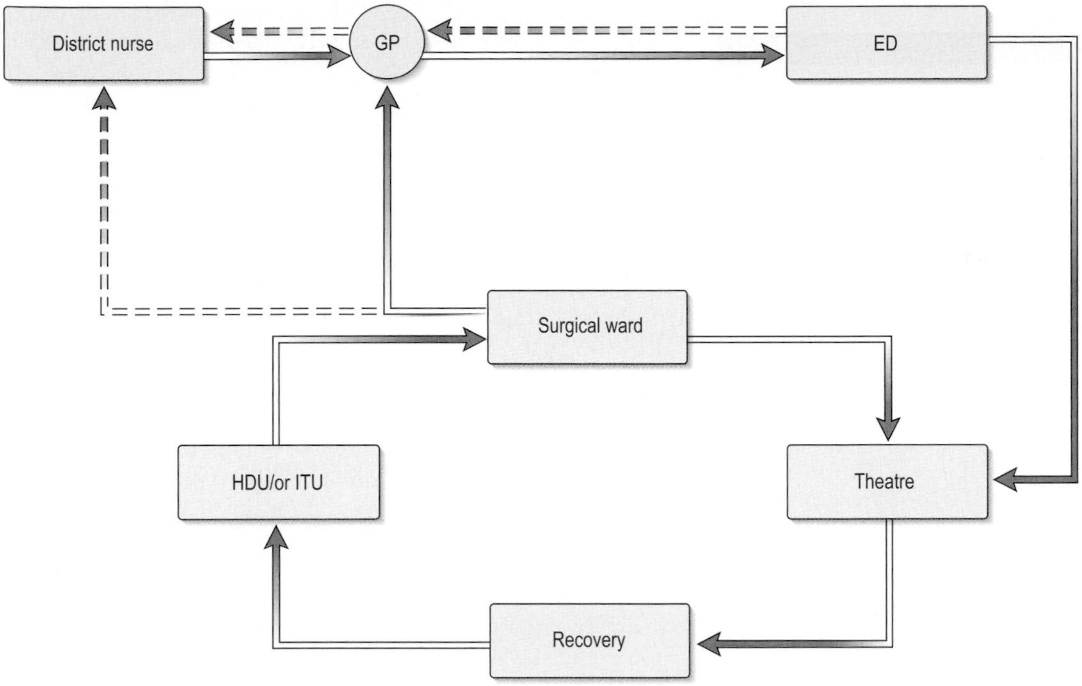

Fig. 26.2 Pathways to emergency surgery.

from the telephone helplines NHS Direct (England and Wales) and NHS 24 (Scotland) (see 'Useful websites', p. 943). These offer 24-h assistance and callers have reportedly found the advice helpful and reassuring (O'Cathain et al 2004).

A substantial morbidity exists among patients on waiting lists for surgery. Mordue (1994) found that around 38% of patients awaiting a cataract operation will experience further deterioration in vision before admission. Patients with gallstone disease requiring elective laparoscopic cholecystectomy make up a significant percentage of those awaiting surgery in the UK (Somasekar et al 2002). Whilst on the waiting list, some patients may suffer recurrent bouts of severe abdominal pain and require emergency hospitalisation (Somasekar et al 2002, Lawrentschuk et al 2003). Waiting for treatment not only causes patients pain, distress and anxiety but can also have expensive consequences, e.g. absence from work and emergency hospital admissions (DH 2001a). Mr W is fortunately supported by his practice nurse, who institutes measures to reduce discomfort and prevent further injury while he waits for treatment.

STOP THINK **26.3** What actions might a community nurse take to improve the health of patients awaiting surgery?

INFORMED DECISION MAKING

The aim of this section is to introduce the issue of informed consent for surgery by discussing nursing responsibilities and highlighting areas for ethical debate.

For a wider discussion on the ethical aspects of consent, see Booth (2002).

The decision to operate

Once the outcome of investigations is known and these have been considered in the light of the patient's presenting signs and symptoms, the surgeon can make a definite or provisional diagnosis and recommend a course of action. This may involve diagnostic, curative or palliative surgery, a combination of these, or no surgical intervention at all. If the patient can be treated as successfully without surgical intervention, then the relevant alternatives will be pursued. Consider the following examples:

- A middle-aged woman is found to have Stage IIA cervical cancer (see Ch. 31) with infiltrating lymph nodes when she undergoes examination under anaesthesia (EUA). It is decided that surgery is not appropriate. She is referred to an oncologist, who prescribes a course of radical radiotherapy.
- Another patient has been referred to hospital for an oesophagoscopy and gastroscopy after complaining of heartburn. He is found to have a hiatus hernia and is prescribed an antacid and gelling agent (Gaviscon). The nurse in the outpatient department gives him advice on sleeping propped up at night, avoiding certain foods, weight reduction and how to take the prescribed medication.
- M (see Case History 26.4(A)) has been making frequent visits over the last few months to see her medical consultant about her vaginal fistula. Despite enteral diets, anti-inflammatory agents and antibiotics, the fistula does not resolve. She is referred to the surgeon and subsequently admitted to the surgical ward.

It may appear from these brief descriptions that it is the medical staff who take the decision on the course of

CASE HISTORY 26.4(A)

M

M is a 23-year-old hotel receptionist who had suffered from Crohn's disease for as long as she could remember. She had been in and out of hospital because of her condition on many occasions. This time she was sent straight up to the ward after her appointment in the outpatient department. The staff nurse who had looked after her on two earlier occasions felt a real friendship with her. When the nurse greeted her on the ward, M burst into tears, explaining how she had developed a horrible faecal discharge from her vagina and that she had been admitted for more investigations. She was pyrexial, looked pale and, with her small frame, appeared extremely fragile. The staff nurse offered her a single room as she was obviously distressed by her uncontrolled diarrhoea.

Once M had telephoned her boyfriend, with whom she had been living for the past year, and had taken time to collect her thoughts, she was visited by the consultant who suggested that a fistula was the cause of the current problem and that the best plan of action would be to close it surgically. M was informed that there was a chance that she would need a defunctioning stoma and spent some time talking to the staff nurse and the night staff about it.

The next day M started her bowel preparation. This consisted of 4 L of Klean-Prep to be taken over the next 24 h. She was not allowed to eat that day but could take extra drinks of clear fluids if she wished. She discussed with her named nurse the use of large pads to absorb leakage from her vagina. She was also given some soft wipes and a tube of barrier cream to avoid excoriation of the perianal area by the diarrhoea.

treatment to be given. However, whereas the doctor decides what treatment appears to be the most appropriate, it is the informed patient who must make the final decision as to what treatment is accepted (Nursing and Midwifery Council 2004). Thus the woman with cervical cancer is offered either radiotherapy or surgery, but is advised by her doctor that radiotherapy would be more suitable in her particular case. The doctor explains that the extent of surgery that would be necessary and the risks and morbidity associated with surgery outweigh the benefits. After being informed of and discussing the survival rates and adverse effects of both forms of treatment, the patient opts for radiotherapy.

Informed consent

'Consent is a patient's agreement for a health professional to provide care' (DH 2001b). When patients undergo any intervention or procedure, they must give consent. Touching someone without their consent and without lawful justification could be construed as trespass, civil assault or battery (Bradshaw 2001, Baxter et al 2002). In practice, it is preferable to obtain verbal rather than written consent from the patient for low-risk procedures, such as a chest X-ray or being given suppositories. However, when a patient is to undergo surgery or any invasive procedure, and when a general or local anaesthetic is required, it is advisable and standard practice to obtain written consent. As the medical team are in charge of these procedures, they are ultimately responsible for obtaining the written consent from the patient. Consent forms are traditionally used within hospitals and clinics to document that the patient and the medical staff have discussed and agreed the proposed treatment (Elliot Penels 1998). However, a signed consent form does not give any indication of what the patient was told, what was consented to or whether there was a meaningful understanding as to what they were agreeing to (DH 2001b). The doctor signing the consent form with the patient has therefore to ensure that:

- the patient understands the information, and not just that it has been given and received
- the extent of the information is sufficient for that patient to make the decision.

The role of the nurse

The nurse has an important role to play in obtaining consent prior to surgery. For a patient to give valid consent, they must comprehend fully what they are consenting to: i.e. their consent must be informed. The nurse can provide the team with knowledge of the individual's need for information and comprehension of the information given (Alderson 1995). The nurse will also provide the patient with information about the procedure and the recovery period, and may be able to clarify points previously discussed between patient and doctor. A strong case is made that doctors, rather than nursing staff, obtain consent for surgery, as nurses will not undertake the actual procedure (Elliot Penels 1998). Where nurses do take consent, they have to meet a medical standard of care and should receive thorough training (DH 2001b). In Mr A's case, specialist family planning nurses provided preoperative information and obtained his consent for his vasectomy. There may also be occasions when the nurse is in charge of a particular procedure and must therefore obtain written consent from the patient. In this instance, providing the information for consent is the nurse's responsibility.

The need for informed consent raises legal and ethical issues for both nurses and patients. The current social climate emphasises consumerism and patients' rights. Patients have an increased desire to be 'partners in care', i.e. to be well informed and to take responsibility for their own health (Coulter at al 1999, Scottish Executive 2003a). Patients have the right to be given an adequate explanation of proposed treatment, including any risks and alternative treatments. Nurses have a vital role to play in ensuring a patient's need for information is met and that full discussion takes place (Anderson & Helms 1995).

However, there may be occasions when the patient is less than fully informed. The depth and complexity of information held by medical staff may be overwhelming for a lay person to absorb and understand. This consideration must be balanced against individual needs and consumer demands. There is now heightened awareness of the need to explain the potential effects of treatments — adverse as well as beneficial (McIlwain 1999). The risks of some procedures are now clearly stated on the consent form itself. Both the chance of occurrence and the severity of potential adverse effects of the procedure must be addressed in considering whether to inform the patient of them. For example, a myelogram carries only a small risk of seizures and loss of power in the limbs, but as the effects would be severe, it is important to inform patients of these risks.

For further information on patients' perceptions of the consent process, see Kay & Siriwardena (2001).

There may be occasions when medical staff deliberately withhold certain information, believing that it would be detrimental to the patient to have this information. This is legal if the doctor is deemed to be acting in the patient's best interests. Our moral principles tell us that one should always tell the truth. However, if knowledge of the truth would have a negative effect upon the patient, then a difficult decision has to be made. If the patient has expressed a desire for full information about the diagnosis, the decision becomes clearer. It would not be legal or ethical to withhold information on the grounds that the patient might refuse treatment if given the full facts.

STOP THINK **26.4** A young woman is told she has ovarian 'cysts' and, although distressed at requiring an oophorectomy and possibly a hysterectomy and so losing the ability to have children, she consents to the operation. Her husband and the surgeon have agreed that she would not cope well with knowing her true diagnosis of ovarian cancer at this time, and so withhold this information from her. She then questions the ward nurses, at first indirectly and then directly with questions such as 'It's cancer, isn't it?' and 'This is going to be the end of me, isn't it?'.

What might you do or say if faced with such a situation in the ward? How might the patient react if you told her you were not able to answer her questions? Discuss the example with your nursing and medical colleagues.

A nurse could face disciplinary action, or even dismissal, for going against the surgeon's expressed wish to withhold information, but this would be unlikely if the nurse was clearly acting in the patient's best interests. Nurses who think that patients are insufficiently informed should discuss their concerns with the surgeon, but not in the presence of the patient (Alderson 1995). Booth (2002) suggests that nurses are in a good position to mediate between doctors and patients, to facilitate two-way communication, and to prevent patients becoming 'passive recipients of [the doctor's] expertise'. However, it is more usual for nursing and medical staff to be sensitive to the individual needs of the patient and to work collaboratively with the patient and family to resolve such moral dilemmas.

In some cases, the patient may be too ill to comprehend what is proposed and thus to give informed consent. Also, within society there are groups of individuals who are 'unable to make decisions for themselves or who cannot communicate these decisions' (Lord Chancellor's Department 1997). This inability is known as 'mental incapacity' (Lord Chancellor's Department 1997). In Scotland, any issue relating to the welfare of an 'incapable adult' is governed by The Adult with Incapacity Act (Scotland) 2000 (Baxter et al 2002). Similar legislation has been introduced recently in England and Wales in the form of the Mental Capacity Bill (O'Dowd 2004). When an adult patient is unconscious or mentally incapacitated, it is necessary to find out whether a family member or friend has been given Power of Attorney, i.e. allowed to make decisions on the patient's behalf, or if the patient has previously indicated their wishes in an advance statement. An 'advance statement' is an expression of the patient's preference for treatment or care, given when they are legally competent. This may include the refusal of certain treatments such as surgical intervention or cardiopulmonary resuscitation (Brooks 1997). Any refusal of treatment must be respected, provided the decision is appropriate in the circumstances. The patient's relatives have no legal right to give or, more importantly, to refuse consent. Lifesaving procedures can be performed without consent using the doctor's clinical privilege (Lord Chancellor's Department 1997). A doctor has the power to take such action as is necessary, but only the minimal amount of treatment should be undertaken to alleviate the particular emergency, and should follow established practice (Elliot Pennels 1998). Good practice would suggest that the relatives are consulted and a decision is made in the patient's best interests (Lord Chancellor's Department 1997).

STOP THINK **26.5** How can nursing staff clarify where decision-making responsibility lies in the following cases?

- A 25-year-old man with Down's syndrome is admitted to the ENT ward for elective tonsillectomy.
- An 81-year-old woman is admitted from a nursing home to the vascular ward with an ischaemic left foot. She has a 5-year history of dementia and is very confused. An embolectomy under local anaesthetic and sedation is proposed.
- A young motorcyclist is admitted to the Emergency Department following a motorcycle accident. He is unconscious and the CT scan reveals a subdural haematoma which requires emergency surgical evacuation.

Similarly, relatives have no legal rights in determining whether information should be given to or withheld from the patient. In fact, the doctor or nurse would be in breach of confidentiality if they were to tell the relatives first, or to tell them at all, without the patient's expressed consent. Where information is withheld from the patient, the patient cannot consent to its being divulged (Nursing and Midwifery Council 2004). There is an NHS code of practice on protecting patient confidentiality (Scottish Executive 2003b).

Resolving dilemmas

When a patient is too ill to be told, or cannot give informed consent, medical and nursing staff must carry out their professional duty to act in the patient's best interests, whilst considering the wishes of the relatives. The *Code of Professional Conduct* (Nursing and Midwifery Council 2004) provides guidelines on professional practice. Nurses are required to follow the Code in terms of acting to safeguard the patient's interests and to work in a collaborative and cooperative manner with other health care professionals.

It is essential that nurses are familiar with the Code and apply it in practice. Guidelines on informed consent have also been produced for doctors and nurses (DH 2001b, General Medical Council 2001).

PREOPERATIVE PREPARATION

Preoperative preparation might begin some time before the patient is admitted to a hospital ward or clinic. Mr W's practice nurse and Mr A's family planning nurse were both involved in preparing their patients for surgery. As this aspect of care has already been considered, this section refers to the immediate preoperative period following admission to hospital.

Patients arrive for admission having experienced very different types of preparation. Mrs B had no preparation at all, being taken to the ED as an emergency. Mr A had already attended the family planning clinic where the vasectomy would be carried out and had discussed the procedure and after-care at length with one of the nurses. Mr W's local hospital has a pre-admission clinic where his admission details were obtained and a full assessment carried out a week before surgery. He was also given the opportunity to ask questions about his proposed operation. He arrived on the ward on the morning of admission having had nothing to eat since going to bed the night before, and only a cup of tea since 6 a.m. The named nurse showed him to a chair where he could wait for a bed to become available. All patients — whether emergency, essential or elective admissions — require appropriate preoperative assessment, information about their care, and safe preparation for anaesthetic and surgery.

Assessment

Assessment of the patient is required to identify any special needs, to highlight potential problems and to provide a baseline against which to measure postoperative progress.

Ideally, the named nurse would admit the patient in order to establish a relationship and to enable direct observation and questioning of the patient. The nurse may also use other sources of information, such as medical or nursing records, the patient's relatives and other health care professionals, to form a complete picture. The way a nurse assesses a patient will vary according to the model used. This might be one developed by the ward nurses or an established nursing model such as Roper et al's (2000) activities of daily living model. But while each nurse's approach to, and description of, the delivery of care may be different, the needs of the patient remain essentially the same. Care pathways have been developed to outline these needs for some types of surgery. They detail the care that a particular group of patients will receive at what point in their stay. Deviations from this pathway are recorded for quality assurance purposes and to enable individual variation in care. This approach to care has led to a reduction in length of hospital stay for some patients and has facilitated a continuance of care in the community for others (Calligaro et al 1996, Schaldach 1997).

Examples of surgical care pathways can be found in Johnson (1997) for patients facing transurethral resection of the prostate gland (TURP), and in Rogers et al (2000) for patients undergoing maxillofacial surgery.

Giving information

Reducing preoperative anxiety and stress is not only desirable on humanitarian grounds, but also promotes recovery. Giving the patient information and emotional support preoperatively is known to reduce pre- and postoperative anxiety substantially (Gammon & Mulholland 1996, Martin 1996). It also has a direct effect on reducing postoperative complications, partly by increasing collaboration between patient and staff. Patients who have received structured preoperative information or teaching have been found to mobilise earlier postoperatively, to have a shorter postoperative hospital stay (Gammon & Mulholland 1996) and to have a reduced need for analgesics postoperatively (Hayward 1975, Shade 1992, Teasdale 1993, Martin 1996) as compared with patients who receive standard ward or unstructured preparation. However, some studies indicate that patients want more information than is given to them (Coulter at al 1999, Thompson et al 2003).

Lack of information has also been found to be a major source of dissatisfaction among day-case patients. Costa (2001) investigated the lived experience of ambulatory surgery patients and suggested that many did not have a clear picture about what to expect preoperatively, postoperatively and throughout their convalescence at home. A small audit of 136 minor day surgery patients by Chowdhury et al (2000) found that 32% of patients did not know their diagnosis, including some receiving surgery for basal cell carcinoma. Nurses and researchers now need to devise approaches to delivering effective preoperative teaching in a reduced time frame and to provide the kind of information most useful to those patients and family members responsible for postoperative care activities at home (Bernier et al 2003). It is important that patients receive information at an appropriate level and on matters that concern them — not simply on what the nurse assumes they will be anxious about.

Cooper (1999) describes the problem of providing adequate preoperative teaching for ophthalmic day surgery patients in a short period of time. She suggests that nurses involve the patient in planning the programme because many adults wish to participate actively in learning, and learn more effectively as a result. This approach may be especially appropriate in the day surgery setting where patients are generally healthy participants who are able to process information and make informed decisions (Lisko 1995). For less able patients, a carer or family member can be involved. However, this approach may not be appropriate in other circumstances, such as emergency surgery, or when anxiety and pain interfere with the patient's ability to participate.

Mitchell (1997) argues that giving patients volumes of information will not lead to a reduction in anxiety for all. Information given should be dependent on the individual patient's preference and need, and be of high quality. Watts and Brooks (1997) studied patients admitted to an intensive care unit following surgery. They found that information about the management of pain, nausea and mouth care was important. This information was thought to reassure patients that they would be closely monitored by a nurse postoperatively and also in terms of bodily comfort. Potential anxiety about using a bedpan or a urine bottle could also be reduced by giving information about the use of urinary catheters.

STOP THINK **26.6** How will this knowledge change the way you would approach giving information to your preoperative patient?

Skilled, systematic and sensitive assessment is essential in determining what is important for the individual.

Sensitive, open questioning can determine what the patient already understands and what they would like to know more about. Simply giving a factual account of what will occur is insufficient. Patients want to know what to expect and how it will feel. They also need the opportunity to discuss their fears and worries. Factual and sensory information, coping strategies and counselling are the essential components of preoperative education. During the admission procedure Mr W told his named nurse that he was afraid of feeling pain during the operation, as he knew he could be awake throughout the procedure. The nurse then described to him what kind of sensations he might expect:

> *Once all the checks and preparations have been completed in the ward, you will be given a tablet that will make you feel a little drowsy and more relaxed. The checks will take place again when you get to theatre and a nurse will stay with you at all times. When you go into theatre, the doctors will put up a screen using green cloth so you won't have to watch what is happening. They will also give you an injection around the top of your leg to begin to numb the area. It feels like a scratch under the skin as they make sure the skin is numb before giving you a deeper dose of anaesthetic. You will probably feel quite sleepy during the procedure, but you may feel the doctor pressing around the area, although there should be no pain or discomfort. You will never lose consciousness and would always be able to tell the doctor if you felt anything. If you would like to listen to some music on the headphones when you are in theatre, let me know before you go up and I can show you what tapes we have. Many people find it takes their mind off things and helps them relax. Remember there is always a nurse with you who you can talk to or ask about things whilst you are in theatre. How do you feel about things now?*

STOP THINK **26.7** Can you identify the information given here in terms of knowledge, sensory information and coping strategies?

When and how information is given will influence its effectiveness. Many patients have difficulty in remembering verbal information. While a personal, verbal explanation is invaluable in that it allows for feedback from the patient, it is difficult to recall over time. Moran and Kent (1995) found that short-stay patients were most often dissatisfied with the extent of information given after the outpatient appointment prior to surgery. They advocate the wider use of pre-admission clinics where nurses can address this problem, and the development of information leaflets and patient-held shared care records to enable full information exchange between hospital, community staff and the patient. Sutcliffe and Potter (2002) highlight preoperative information giving as an important function of the pre-admission clinic because it gives patients time to assimilate information before their surgery. However, Mitchell (1997) argues that because of time limitations the emphasis of these clinics will be on physical assessment and little may be done to reduce the patient's anxiety.

Nelson (1996) found that patients preferred information to be given in a pre-admission programme prior to cardiac surgery. Pre-admission information allows for emotional adjustment over a longer period and enables patients to share information with, and seek support from, their families. Recall of information is also improved when information is given in a more relaxed setting. Beddows (1997) found that patients who were given information in their own homes prior to admission and again on admission were less anxious than those given information on admission only.

Pre-admission booklets for surgical patients can be beneficial in reducing patient anxiety and improving outcomes. Law (1997) found that preoperative information needed to be written as a back-up to verbal advice. Information can also be presented using other media such as video. However, there may always be patients that do not wish to watch information videos about their proposed procedure immediately prior to surgery (Hyde et al 1998). Information leaflets or videos are not, therefore, a substitute for personalised explanation but do provide a constant reference source and can prepare patients to use their contact time with nurses more effectively. This allows the nurse to focus on areas of concern and to devote more time to counselling than to information giving, as in reality it is often difficult to complete both tasks well in the busy preoperative period. Thus, in the example given above (Mr W), the named nurse was able to spend time providing more detailed information and suggesting coping strategies as Mr W had already read about his operation, discussed it at the pre-admission clinic and visited the ward to familiarise himself with the environment.

Preoperative information booklets should be easy to read without being patronising. Print size, reading ease and vocabulary should all be considered and the use of jargon avoided. Markham and Smith (2003) draw attention to the importance of tone in such booklets. A booklet must be comprehensive, as this improves recall and compliance with instructions (Bradshaw et al 1975). Many departments produce their own booklets giving general information about wards and surgery. Some also have leaflets about specific operations which can be given to the patient prior to admission. Preoperative education aims to produce a well-informed consumer, to promote healthy choices and to reduce anxiety. The informed patient is better equipped to make good decisions about their care and to discuss treatment fully and openly with staff. Information also serves to produce a more autonomous patient. One must then respect the view that the well-informed patient has the right to reject advice or treatment against professional judgement for personal reasons (Baxter et al 2002). What the professional advocates may conflict with what the patient wants. Simply informing someone of an objective fact that appears rational (e.g. smoking causes lung cancer) will be insufficient in some cases to promote healthy behaviour or coping mechanisms (Donovan & Ward 2001). It is also important to address the information needs of family members because they may have a role in providing support and care at home (Paavilainen et al 2001).

For additional information on the effects of giving patients preoperative information, see Hughes (2002).

Safe preparation for anaesthesia and surgery

In the admission assessment, the patient's specific needs and potential problems may be identified. The general risks associated with anaesthesia and surgical intervention will also be taken into account in any related medical or nursing procedure. Patients undergoing surgery require medical assessment, the nature of which will depend on the extent of surgery, the age of the patient and on any pre-existing medical conditions. In some centres, an initial assessment is carried out by nursing staff so that patients most in need of anaesthetic review, such as those with poor exercise tolerance, asthma or previous problems during anaesthesia, are seen promptly (Hilditch et al 2003). Mr W was given a chest X-ray to screen for abnormalities of the lungs, a blood test for urea and electrolytes and a full blood count. An ECG was performed to rule out cardiac dysfunction, as it is important to ensure that a patient has no gross abnormalities of the cardiovascular and respiratory systems prior to the administration of an anaesthetic. The anaesthetist noted that Mr W had managed to stop smoking, and that he no longer had a productive cough. Smoking considerably increases the risk of chest infection and atelectasis postoperatively.

Risk of chest infection

All patients receiving a general anaesthetic are at risk of developing a chest infection (Richards & Edwards 2003). Drugs and gases used in anaesthesia dry the respiratory tract and inhibit the action of the cilia. Secretions of mucus become thick and tenacious, causing partial obstruction of the lower airways. Cigarette smoking also damages and paralyses the cilia and leads to excess mucus production. The secretions eventually pool in the base of the lungs and plug the bronchioles. The retained secretions obstruct the lower airways, inhibiting gaseous exchange and providing a source of bacterial infection.

Anaesthesia depresses respiration and, in the deep stage, breathing will actually cease. Artificial ventilation during the operation is at tidal volume and does not fully inflate the lungs (see Ch. 3). Normally, a person will sigh intermittently or increase demands for oxygen by activity, fully inflating the lungs and preventing stagnation and atelectasis. Changes of position, movement and coughing all serve to dislodge excess mucus or fluid, which is then expelled from the lungs as sputum. When under a general anaesthetic the patient will be lying still and unable to cough or sigh throughout the operation. There will also be a period of inactivity postoperatively and perhaps a reluctance to breathe deeply or cough if there is abdominal or thoracic pain. Opiates given for pain relief can also depress respiration (Sheppard & Wright 2000).

Patients should be advised to stop smoking, at least for 2 weeks prior to surgery, if not for good. Haddock and Burrows (1997) found that nurses could have a significant impact on helping smokers to quit before surgery by giving constructive advice and information in the pre-admission stage. All patients, regardless of whether they are smokers or not, must be taught deep breathing exercises and coughing. It can be difficult to teach a patient to contract the diaphragm in order to breathe deeply preoperatively, let alone postoperatively. The tendency is to use intercostal and accessory muscles to lift the rib cage and draw the abdomen in. Although instruction may be the responsibility of the physiotherapist in some wards, it will still require reinforcement from the nursing staff. In this context, the need for early mobilisation can be described to the patient.

For a detailed coughing and deep breathing regimen, see Sheppard & Wright (2000).

Patients should also be informed that they may have oxygen therapy via a mask or nasal cannula postoperatively to help maintain the level of oxygen in their bloodstream while recovering from the anaesthetic (Walker 2003). Oxygen therapy may have a drying effect on the mouth and the mucous membranes of the nose. Patients can be assured that ice chips or a mouthwash will be available to help relieve this.

STOP THINK **26.8** Try some deep breathing exercises yourself. Did you draw in your abdomen and lift the rib cage? Try to breathe using the diaphragm. Place one hand on your abdomen. Breathe in through your nose while you try to feel your abdomen pushing your hand out (as the diaphragm moves downwards and displaces the stomach).

Risk of deep vein thrombosis (DVT) and pulmonary embolism (PE)

An intravascular clot or thrombus is most likely to occur when the following conditions, known as Virchow's triad, exist:

- trauma — damaged endothelium
- stasis — slow blood flow
- hypercoagulable blood.

Thrombus formation is initiated by the activation of factor XII in reaction to exposure to collagen filaments in the damaged endothelium. This results in platelet aggregation, formation of thrombin from circulating prothrombin, and stimulation of the production of insoluble fibrin from fibrinogen (see Ch. 11, p. 482). It has been found that, during surgery, the veins of the lower leg distend by up to 48% (Coleridge Smith et al 1991). This distension leads to subluminal endothelial damage, which can provide a site for clot formation. In the soleal and gastrocnemius veins, the blood flow is highly dependent on exercise, and so these are often the sites of initial thrombus formation following prolonged periods of inactivity and lack of calf muscle pressure to assist venous return. The general adaptation reaction to the stress of surgery (see Ch. 17, p. 695) results in reduced levels of the coagulation inhibitors protein C, protein S and antithrombin III. Fibrin clots may be broken down gradually by the enzyme plasmin in a process called fibrinolysis. However, the thrombus may persist, causing some degree of venous obstruction.

In a small proportion of cases, a fragment of the clot breaks away, forming an embolus. The embolus may travel through the venous system, through the right side of the heart and into the pulmonary arteries. Here it becomes lodged at a point where the arteries become too small to allow the embolus to pass through. The extent of the resultant pulmonary infarct depends on the size of the vessel occluded. Some patients may have no signs or symptoms of either DVT or PE if thrombi are small and infrequent (Dawes 1997) (see Ch. 2). A large PE is a very serious complication. Without treatment there is mortality of approximately 11% of such patients within 1 h of the embolic event and of 30% in those who survive longer than 1 h (Moccia 2000). Early detection and treatment significantly reduce this rate (Campling et al 1995, Gilles et al 1996, British Thoracic Society 1997, Moccia 2000).

After gynaecological surgery, up to 20% of perioperative deaths are attributable to PE (Nicklin & Franzcog 2002). All surgical patients are exposed to a number of risk factors for DVT. Without prophylaxis the overall risk of developing a DVT for surgical patients may be as high as 25–30% and up to 70% for orthopaedic surgery (Dawes 1997, Agu et al 1999). The incidence of DVT in patients undergoing various types of vascular surgery was found to be between 9 and 14% despite standard prophylaxis with anticoagulants (Fletcher & Batiste 1997). In abdominal surgery and neurosurgery the risk has been reported at approximately 5%, again with anticoagulant prophylaxis (Flinn et al 1996, Kakkar et al 1997). During the preoperative assessment, the nurse should assess the patient for the presence of known risk factors (see Box 26.1).

In the UK, the reports of the Thromboembolic Risk Factors Consensus Group (THRIFT 1992) and the Scottish Intercollegiate Guidelines Network Group (2002) make recommendations on the regimens to be used, based on the relative risk of DVT and potential bleeding complications in individual patients. It is now generally accepted that all patients should use graduated elastic compression stockings (GECS) (Jeffery & Nicolaides 1990, Amaragiri & Lees 2001). Although it is not fully understood how GECS work (Arnold 2002, Parnaby 2004), these stockings create a decreasing pressure gradient in the leg from approximately 18 mmHg at the ankle to 8 mmHg at the thigh (full length) or to 14 mmHg at the calf (below-knee length). The gradient increases blood flow in the femoral vein, inhibits stasis of the venous circulation, stops build-up of any nidus of thrombosis formation and prevents the venous distension that causes endothelial damage (Thomas 1999, Parnaby 2004). GECS are inexpensive and reduce the incidence of postoperative DVT by approximately 60% (THRIFT 1992, Williams et al 1996).

The nurse should ensure that a well-designed and well-fitting stocking is applied. Patients can be taught the correct fitting technique and nurses should ensure that patients understand the reason why and the importance of wearing GECS (Parnaby 2004). Stockings are fitted according to calf size and leg length and are available in a wide variety of sizes. If stockings roll down, a constricting band is created which may cause higher pressures, leading to an inverse gradient and delayed venous emptying. Thigh length stockings are suggested to be more effective (Byrne 2001, Scottish Intercollegiate Guidelines Network 2002). However, below-knee stockings have been found to be more comfortable and more accurately applied for patients with few risk factors and who are ambulant (Hui et al 1996, Williams et al 1996). They are also less costly than full-length stockings (Ingram 2003). Small studies comparing below-knee and full-length stockings have suggested that above knee and below knee are equally effective in prophylaxis against DVT (Porteus et al 1989, Hui et al 1996, Williams et al 1996, Parnaby 2004) but Ingram (2003) suggests that the use of below-knee GECS is variable. Every hospital should have DVT prophylaxis guidelines based on best available evidence (THRIFT II 1998) and larger studies are required to clarify this point (Ingram 2003).

Box 26.1

Risk factors for deep vein thrombosis (DVT)

- Age: increased risk in older patients
- Obesity
- Presence of varicose veins
- Previous DVT
- Clotting disorders
- Oral contraceptive pill/hormone therapy
- Immobility
- Pregnancy
- Spinal or epidural anaesthesia
- Surgery, especially major abdominal or orthopaedic surgery

Based on data from Scottish Intercollegiate Guidelines Network (2002) and Parnaby (2004).

Approximately 15–20% of patients are unable to wear GECS because of limb characteristics (Greerts et al 2001), marked leg oedema, severe peripheral arterial disease, dermatitis, severe peripheral neuropathy or other major leg deformity (Scottish Intercollegiate Guidelines Network 2002). The use of GECS is also contraindicated in patients with severe peripheral vascular disease or profound limb ulceration (Parnaby 2004). Patients should wear the stockings prior to surgery and up until discharge (Nicklin & Franzcog 2002).

Other measures that should be encouraged where possible are early activity and hourly leg exercises. The patient should be taught to dorsiflex the foot preoperatively. This will assist venous return by the action of the calf muscle compressing blood in the deep veins. Deep breathing exercises will also aid the respiratory pump, as deep inspiration reduces intrathoracic pressure and hence increases venous return. In addition, ensuring adequate hydration will reduce hypercoagulability.

Intermittent pneumatic compression stockings (IPCS) are mechanical devices that fill with air, periodically compressing the calf and/or thigh muscles of the leg and stimulating fibrinolysis. For patients at high risk of developing DVT, such as those undergoing orthopaedic and cardiac surgery, intermittent pneumatic compression of the legs has been shown to be particularly effective (Capper 1999, Scottish Intercollegiate Guidelines Network 2002), although Arnold (2002) suggests that patients are often reluctant to participate in this treatment. Patients may remove stocking sleeves or disconnect the pump because they find the stockings hot or uncomfortable (Murakami et al 2003). The pumps require connection to an external power source and are frequently disconnected when patients are out of bed or during transfer (Murakami et al 2003). A study by Cornwell et al (2002), investigating the compliance rate with IPCS prophylaxis, found that, out of a total of 1343 observations carried out in patients who were at risk of DVT following trauma, fewer than 20% of patients had their compression devices on, and functioning correctly, during six observations in a 24-h period. It is important that nursing staff exercise vigilance towards any patient receiving IPCS prophylaxis and ensure that the system is fully operational in order to optimise therapeutic effect.

Teaching leg exercises and applying GECS and/or IPCS devices prevent DVT by their action on two aspects of

Virchow's triad, namely stasis and endothelial damage. Hypercoagulability can be avoided to some extent by adequate hydration but will be stimulated by the general adaptation to stress response and by the effects of surgery initiating clotting mechanisms. Medical staff will seek to minimise hypercoagulability with the administration of anticoagulants in the form of prophylactic low dose unfractionated heparin (Breen 2000, Nicklin & Franzcog 2002). Usually 5000 IU are administered subcutaneously every 8 or 12 h and, to be effective, it should be commenced 30 min to 2 h preoperatively (Nicklin & Franzcog 2002). Low dose heparin does not cause full anticoagulation so the risk of bleeding complications is minimal, unless the patient has a clotting disorder. In such a case, administration of anticoagulants must be monitored closely and their value judged carefully against the risk of DVT. A combination of mechanical methods, such as GECS, and pharmacological agents, such as low dose heparin, can reduce the risk of DVT by more than 80% in general surgical patients and by 65% in orthopaedic patients (Parnaby 2004). Small wound haematomas may be more likely to occur in the patient receiving low dose heparin but, when cared for correctly, do not usually pose a threat.

Preoperative fasting

Patients who are to receive a general anaesthetic, heavy sedation or a local anaesthetic with the possibility of proceeding to a general anaesthetic, are all at risk of aspiration pneumonia. When a patient is anaesthetised or unconscious, the swallowing reflex is absent. From the point of induction of the anaesthetic, there is a risk that stomach contents may reflux and be inhaled through the open larynx into the lungs. This inevitably causes respiratory embarrassment and leads to the development of pneumonitis or a diffuse chest infection. In young and healthy individuals pulmonary aspiration is a rare complication of modern anaesthesia (Warner et al 1993, Crenshaw & Winslow 2002). However, because the ability of the respiratory system to protect against aspiration diminishes with age, older patients are more vulnerable to this complication (Cook & Rooke 2003, Rosenthal & Kavic 2004). Risks can be minimised, partly through the administration of certain drugs, but also by fasting the patient of both diet and fluids.

Different foodstuffs pass through the stomach at different rates. Clear liquids are eliminated immediately from the stomach, whereas solids must be broken down (Crenshaw & Winslow 2002). Patients who receive opioids and those with diabetes may also have reduced gastric motility. Gastric emptying is usually complete for most meals in 4–5 h but even fasting patients may have up to 200 mL in the stomach (Dougherty & Lister 2004). Taking this into account, the recommended minimum preoperative fasting period is between 2 and 4 h for fluids, 6 h for a light meal, e.g. tea and toast, and 8 h for a heavier meal. However, a study by Phillips et al (1993) found there was little difference in residual volume when patients were allowed to drink clear fluids up until the time of the premedication (approximately 2 h preoperatively). The patients had no problems with aspiration or regurgitation and they were less thirsty and more comfortable. Murphy et al (2000) found no difference in the rates of aspiration between patients given traditional nil by mouth (NBM) from midnight orders and those who had unlimited clear fluids before surgery. Those fasted for longer had, in fact, clearer gastric contents in the posterior pharynx. A group of Swedish surgeons (Ljungqvist et al 2000) administered a specially developed carbohydrate drink to cholecystectomy and hip replacement patients 2–3 h before surgery. This was thought to result in a less stressful physiological response to the surgical trauma. No adverse effects were reported and patients receiving the supplement had a reduced stay in hospital following surgery.

A classic study by Hamilton Smith (1972) found that patients were often fasted preoperatively for much longer than necessary. Chapman (1996) found that patients continue to be fasted for prolonged periods, with those on a morning list fasted for an average of 12 h and those on the afternoon list for 8 h. This continues to be the case (Jester & Williams 1999, Crenshaw & Winslow 2002). Prolonged fasting is associated with adverse effects (Crenshaw & Winslow 2002). The undesirable results of prolonged fasting are mainly dehydration and electrolyte imbalance. The liver's glycogen stores are sufficient to maintain blood sugar levels for approximately 18 h but even a fast of 6–8 h can reduce the body's ability to cope with stressors such as blood loss or infection (Dean & Fawcett 2002). Patients can experience both physiological and psychological effects including dehydration, headaches, hypoglycaemia, electrolyte imbalance, nausea and vomiting, confusion, irritability and social isolation when missing mealtimes (Jester & Williams 1999). Older patients are particularly vulnerable to fasting. Depending on their pre-existing health status, older people are at risk of dehydration and confusion, potentially rendering them unfit for anaesthesia and surgery (Jester & Williams 1999).

All patients, to some extent, suffer from the effects of fasting, e.g. hunger and a dry mouth. Some might not understand the reasons for fasting and eat or drink against advice, or think that fasting simply means 'no meals' and have snacks instead. Patients must be given adequate information in order to understand why and what they cannot eat or drink, for how long, and be offered choices on how to care for a dry mouth in the meantime, e.g. tooth brushing, chewing gum, sucking ice chips or boiled sweets (Crenshaw & Winslow 2002, Markham & Smith 2003). Markham and Smith (2003) examined written information given to patients preoperatively. They found that much of the information was out of date and did not sufficiently explain why fasting was necessary.

Research is widely available on the appropriate length of preoperative fasting times but normally, in practice, a wide margin of safety is set and patients are fasted for at least 6 h. Apart from that of the first person on the operating list, theatre times are always approximate, as one cannot be entirely sure how long each operation will take. Surgeons may alter the order of patients on the list, but this should not form part of everyday practice. Nurses work to the earliest likely time for theatre, but actual times often prove to be much later. A lack of individualised care leads to the imposition of one fasting time for all patients on the theatre list. A patient on the morning list may be fasted from midnight, but, if last on the list, may not go to theatre until 1400 h. Thus they may have fasted for at least 14 h. Individual fasting times and close liaison with the anaesthetist can resolve such problems. Nursing staff must also feel confident to implement comfort measures in units where NBM has traditionally meant that nothing passes the patient's lips until theatre. If the patient has oral medication prescribed during the fasting time, it should not be routinely withheld; rather, medical staff should be consulted as to whether the drug should be given or not. Tablets can be taken with 30–60 mL of water. Crenshaw and Winslow (2002) highlighted that many patients did not know what arrangements had been made for administration of their medications.

To return to the case histories, Mrs B was to go to theatre as an emergency, so it was not possible to ensure she had fasted for at least 4 h. In this case, her stomach was emptied by aspirating the contents through a nasogastric tube. Mr W came into hospital on the morning of theatre but had received instructions about fasting in his booklet from the pre-admission clinic the week before. He was not sure whether he could have an early morning cup of tea and had asked his named nurse about this during his visit. As theatre would not start until 0930 h he was advised that he might have a drink at 0600 h but nothing after that. In fact, Mr W was third on the list and did not go up to theatre until 1130 h.

STOP THINK **26.9** Observe how long patients are fasted preoperatively in your ward experience. How would you explain to a patient the necessity for fasting prior to theatre?

Skin preparation

The most significant cause of postoperative wound infection is the exposure to nosocomial pathogens (see Ch. 23, p. 840). The risk can be reduced by shortening the length of preoperative stay and the judicious use of standard infection control precautions by the nursing and medical team. The seminal work of Boore (1978) highlighted that by reducing preoperative anxiety, psychological and physiological stress can be reduced and the incidence of postoperative infection lowered.

Hair removal Shaving the skin before theatre has been thought for many years to be an integral part of preoperative preparation. However, shaving leaves small cuts and abrasions that can give rise to infection and delay discharge (Editorial 1983). It is no longer considered to be an appropriate routine preoperative procedure. Hair removal may be justified on humanitarian grounds where sticking plaster is to be used, if the hair occludes the surgeon seeing the anatomy of the operation site, or if adhesive leads, requiring a good skin contact, are to be applied.

If hair removal is necessary, then hair clippers or depilatory cream have been associated with fewer breaches of the skin than shaving (McIntyre & McCloy 1994, Small 1996). Clippers should be sterilised (Small 1996), and a patch test for sensitivity to creams must be carried out before use. Application of depilatories must also be avoided around sensitive mucous membranes in the genital area. When the above procedures cannot be applied, a well-lubricated shave with a sharp razor may be carried out immediately prior to theatre, since there is a link between timing of the shave and subsequent infection. In a classic study, involving analysis of 406 cases, Seropian and Reynolds (1971) found the wound infection rate to be 3.1% when the shave was done just prior to surgery, 7.1% when the shave was done during the 24 h before surgery, and 20% when the shave was done more than 24 h before surgery.

Where hair removal is considered essential, the nurse should ensure that the patient is not especially vulnerable to postoperative surgical infection because of other factors such as a pre-existing skin condition, or an immunocompromised status (Mangram et al 1999). If it is considered appropriate for patients to carry out their own skin preparation, the nurse is responsible for ensuring that they can do this safely and effectively (Small 1996).

Showering In the past, patients have been advised to shower prior to theatre using a skin antiseptic in an attempt to reduce the bacterial count on the skin (Brandberg & Anderson 1980). Although a single preoperative shower is unlikely to reduce the risk of infection, repeated washing with a chlorhexidine-based detergent does reduce the level of resident skin flora (Ayliffe et al 2000). This may benefit patients undergoing cardiovascular or prosthetic surgery (Ayliffe et al 2000). Unfortunately, some patients may have allergies or severe skin reactions to antiseptic solutions and so a patch test before use is essential. Bathing should be avoided where possible, as bacteria may multiply in the warm water and there is a risk of cross-infection from organisms already present in hospital baths. The patient should shower and/or shampoo before transfer to the operating theatre. If the patient is unable to do so, the nurse can wash the surgical site before the patient goes to theatre, or theatre staff can wash the surgical site immediately before application of the antimicrobial skin preparation solution. Removal of superficial soil, debris and transient microbes in this way reduces the risk of wound contamination by decreasing the organic debris from the skin (Anon 1996). It is unnecessary to change bed linen that is clean.

Specific measures

Premedication — 'premed' — is the term used for drugs given to the patient before leaving the ward for theatre. These drugs constitute part of the anaesthetic and are used to prepare the patient to receive a general or local anaesthetic (see Table 26.1). They are often also used to relax the patient and relieve anxiety. However, research by Hyde et al (1998) found that, although patients were often anxious about their surgery, many did not wish to be sedated in the immediate preoperative period. Instead they would rather listen to music, read and be able to move about freely. The premed is prescribed by the anaesthetist after assessing the patient for the administration of the anaesthetic. The prescription may be made for a set time or 'on call', i.e. the anaesthetist will telephone the ward to ask the nurse to administer the prescribed drug once it is clear how long it will take for the patient to be called to theatre. The nurse must ensure that the consent form has been signed, the patient has emptied their bladder and that all other preoperative checks are complete before giving the premed. The patient should then be advised to rest and asked not to get out of bed unsupervised if the premed contains a strong sedative or opioid agent.

Table 26.1 Common premedications

Drug	Usual adult dose	Route	Effects
Diazepam (Valium)	2–10 mg	Oral	Sedative: reduces tension and anxiety. Decreases muscle tone and potentiates non-depolarising muscle relaxants. Induces mental detachment and amnesia
Temazepam	10–20 mg	Oral	Sedative: reduces tension and anxiety. Induces drowsiness
Morphine sulphate	5–15 mg	i.m./s.c.	Opioid analgesic: induces drowsiness, reduces anxiety, induces mental detachment, respiratory depression*, nausea*

*Unwanted/undesirable effect.

Bowel preparation Some patients will require very specific types of preoperative preparation as ordered by medical staff. That most commonly seen is bowel preparation prior to surgery on the gastrointestinal tract or pelvic organs. If a paralytic ileus is anticipated, or the bowel is to be opened (resulting in a risk of infection), then oral laxatives and purgatives, or suppositories and enemas may be used to clear the bowel.

Music Again returning to the case histories, Mr W's anaesthetist prescribed a benzodiazepine sedative (diazepam 5 mg) as a premedication, being aware that Mr W was particularly anxious. Mr W had also borrowed one of the personal stereos from the ward and was enjoying listening to music. While research into the effects of music on anxiety and postoperative pain remain inconclusive, predominantly due to a lack of studies in the area, many patients do find listening to music a helpful distraction at this stage (Good 1996).

Theatre safety

The nurse must carry out preoperative checks before the administration of the premed, as the results of the checks may necessitate a delay in going to theatre. Moreover, the patient should not have received sedative or opioid agents before signing the consent form. Many hospitals have created their own checklists. Examples of criteria for checklists are given in Table 26.2.

Table 26.2 Preoperative checks

Criteria	Action	Rationale
Identification	Prepare two name bands with patient's full name, hospital unit number, date of birth, home address (as a minimum), plus ward and consultant Clearly note allergies on the anaesthetic sheet and on wrist bands as well as the drug Kardex Ensure site is correctly marked with indelible ink	Correct identification of patient Avoidance of all allergens Correct identification of site
Documentation	Ensure that medical notes, nursing notes, signed consent form, X-rays and anaesthetic sheet accompany patient to theatre	Ready availability of all necessary information
Fasting	Check when patient last had anything to eat or drink	Prevention of aspiration pneumonia
Empty bladder	Ask patient to pass urine prior to administering premedication	To prevent damage to full bladder during surgery To enable complete bed rest after premed To prevent postoperative discomfort due to a full bladder
Risk of diathermy burns	Ask patient to remove all jewellery, hair pins and other items containing metal (wedding rings may be covered with tape)	To remove all metal that may concentrate the diathermy current
Prostheses	Ask patient to remove all prostheses, e.g. dentures, hearing aids, contact lenses, false eyes, glasses, etc.	To prevent harm caused by prostheses To prevent loss
Care of valuables	Offer to receive valuables into safekeeping for the patient	Patient will be away from the ward and unfit to be responsible for these valuables
Circulatory assessment	Ask patient to remove all makeup, lipstick and nail varnish	To facilitate observation of colour of skin, lips and nail beds

In order for patients to understand and cooperate with preoperative procedures, adequate explanation and reassurance must be given. However, the nurse should also be aware that some information might cause unnecessary distress. For example, Mrs B did not want to remove her wedding ring. The nurse offered to tape this for her, but Mrs B said that she had never taken it off and that it would be secure. The nurse explained that it was to protect her from the use of electric current to seal blood vessels during the operation.

There are some patients who rely on their hearing aids and/or glasses. In such cases, these can be labelled with adhesive tape and worn by the patient until anaesthetised. Equally they may wish to retain their false teeth until anaesthetised. A note should be made to this effect on the checklist or anaesthetic form.

During the immediate preoperative period, the patient may feel extremely vulnerable and anxious (Costa 2001) — they will be wearing only a flimsy gown; their dentures may have been removed; they may be unable to see well without glasses, and they will feel drowsy from the premed. Anxiety about the impending operation can be high, especially among patients placed in the later part of the operating list (Panda et al 1996). Reassurance by the nurse at this time and, for some patients, distraction can be helpful. Suggestions for managing this period are made by Mitchell (1997) and Hyde et al (1998) and include having a family member stay with the patient. The patient should be encouraged to rest.

Nursing Care Plan 26.1 summarises the preoperative care given to Mr W.

PERIOPERATIVE SAFETY

Caring for the patient in theatre

The patient arrives in the operating theatre accompanied by a nurse from the ward and a porter or operating department assistant (ODA). Patients may be brought to the theatre on a trolley or on their bed from the ward. Once the patient transfers to the theatre table, the bed is taken to a holding area. The patient is then transferred straight back onto the bed at the end of the operation. This reduces the discomfort of transferring from trolley to bed in the ward, and reduces the amount of patient lifting by nurses, porters and ODAs.

The anaesthetic or theatre nurse receiving the patient goes through the preoperative check again (as in Table 26.2). The ward nurse will then usually return to the ward. If the patient is especially nervous or confused, it can be comforting if a nurse who knows them well can stay until the induction of anaesthesia. All patients must be supervised by a nurse in this pre-induction time, as the patient may have received premedication and is in an extremely stressful and unfamiliar environment. It is now common practice for theatre nurses to visit their patients preoperatively to carry out a nursing assessment, to introduce themselves and to give any information required about patient care in theatre (Crawford 1999, Scott et al 1999).

In emergency cases, the theatre nurse may continue the preoperative preparation. For example, Mrs B's daughter arrived at the hospital as these preparations were being carried out. She was escorted to theatre by the ED nurse and saw her mother for a few minutes in the anaesthetic room before she was anaesthetised. The theatre nurse briefly explained what was happening, and once Mrs B was asleep, made a cup of tea for her daughter and let her make a telephone call from the Charge Nurse's office. The theatre nurse then telephoned the named nurse, who sent a clinical support worker to take Mrs B's daughter to the ward.

For further reading on family involvement in perioperative nursing of patients undergoing emergency surgery, see Paavilainen et al (2001).

The roles of theatre staff are summarised in Box 26.2. The anaesthetist will visit the patient preoperatively in the

Box 26.2

The roles of the theatre staff

The anaesthetic nurse
- Receives the patient in the reception area of the anaesthetic room
- Checks patient in, deals with any irregularities
- Helps to relieve patient anxiety
- Assists in the induction (and maintenance) of anaesthesia
- Performs emergency preparation of patients for theatre
- Uses and checks anaesthetic equipment
- Maintains patient safety and comfort

The anaesthetist
- Visits the patient preoperatively:
  — to assess fitness for anaesthesia
  — to provide information and reassurance
  — to prescribe a premedication
- Induces and maintains anaesthesia
- Monitors patient's condition during surgery
- Provides supportive treatment, e.g. fluid replacement, PO_2 level maintenance, correction of arrhythmias
- Initiates postoperative analgesia

The circulating nurse
- Assists with the provision of equipment
- Maintains nursing records
- Positions the patient
- Ensures safety with regard to instruments and swabs
- Cleans and sterilises equipment
- Observes, measures and records vital signs

The scrub nurse
- Positions the patient
- Provides appropriate sterile equipment
- Assists the surgeon
- Protects the patient's dignity
- Prevents diathermy and pressure injuries
- Ensures safety with regard to instruments and swabs
- Manages the high-risk patient

The recovery room nurse
- Maintains patency of the airway
- Observes patient for level of consciousness and safety
- Observes vital signs: colour, respiration, temperature (core and peripheral), pulse, blood pressure, fluid intake and output, wounds and drainage, specific checks as required
- Assesses pain and nausea and administers analgesics and antiemetics
- Reassures the patient and provides a quiet environment
- Provides total patient care
- Provides documentation and facilitates communication

Nursing Care Plan 26.1 Preoperative care for Mr W (see Case Histories 26.1(A) and 26.1(B))

Nursing considerations	Action	Rationale	Evaluation
Anxiety due to: • **hospital environment** • **diagnosis/prognosis** • **anaesthesia and surgery**	• Ensure Mr W is informed of and understands diagnosis, procedure, likely postoperative progress	To reduce anxiety and promote recovery	Anxiety is reduced to an acceptable level
	• Provide opportunity to discuss fears and anxieties		
	• Enhance or supplement coping mechanisms (e.g. use of personal stereo)		
Haemorrhage and shock*	• Record vital signs as baseline	To make data available for postoperative comparison	Staff are prepared to deal with bleeding and shock is prevented
	• Encourage intake of fluids until 4 h before theatre	To maintain good fluid balance	
	• Ensure blood tests and blood grouping completed	To ensure availability of blood products in case transfusion is necessary To ensure good haemoglobin status	
Wound infection*	• Have Mr W shower preoperatively • Provide clean theatre gown	To reduce superficial soiling, skin debris and transient microbes	No infection occurs
Chest infection*	• Teach deep breathing and coughing exercises	To inflate lungs fully and clear stagnating secretions	No infection occurs
	• Continue to support Mr W in not smoking	Patient is under stress and may return to inappropriate coping mechanisms	
Deep vein thrombosis*; pulmonary embolism*	• Teach leg exercises and stress importance of early mobilisation • Fit and apply graduated compression stockings • Teach deep breathing exercises (see above)	Contraction of calf muscle and graduated external compression; increase blood flow in the femoral vein and promote venous return	Thrombosis and embolism are prevented
Aspiration pneumonia*	• Have Mr W fast 4 h (fluids) and 6 (food) preoperatively from 06.00 h	Stomach must be empty prior to anaesthesia; Mr W may need general anaesthetic	Vomiting is prevented
Theatre safety	• Complete checklist prior to administration of premedication (see Table 26.2)	See Table 26.2	Patient is safely prepared for anaesthetic and surgery

*Potential problem.

ward to assess the patient's ability to tolerate the anaesthetic and give information and reassurance. A premedication will be prescribed if required.

If the patient is to have minimally invasive surgery or investigations, e.g. colonoscopy, endoscopic retrograde cholangiopancreatography (ERCP) or cardiac catheterisation, a general anaesthetic may not be used. Instead, the patient may be sedated by medication such as diazepam or midazolam which have amnesic properties, helping the patient to be less aware of what is happening and to remember very little about the procedure. In this situation, an anaesthetist may not necessarily be present but would be available should the need arise to proceed to a general anaesthetic or should other supportive treatment be required. The nurse may act as the surgeon's assistant and take part of the responsibility for monitoring the patient's condition. Some specialist nurses may conduct endoscopies independently. In main theatres, at least two nurses as well as the anaesthetist and surgeon will be present. One nurse acts as the circulating nurse, the other as the scrub nurse. The scrub nurse wears sterile gloves and will provide instruments for the surgeons, assist where necessary and ensure safety with equipment during the operation (see Box 26.2).

The emphasis of the nursing role in theatre is on patient safety and teamwork. Each professional has an important part to play in the patient's passage through theatre. As the team members develop trust and understanding amongst themselves, it may be difficult initially for the student to appreciate the communication links in place, especially when staff have half their faces covered with a mask.

Environmental safety

The environment in the operating theatre is designed to minimise the risk of exogenous infection to the patient. Some of the measures used to ensure safety are as follows:

- Clean filtered air is pumped into clean areas. Air pressure is higher inside the theatre than outside, in order to maintain an air flow from the theatre to the outside. This prevents potentially contaminated air from the rest of the hospital moving into the theatres.
- Humidity is controlled through the ventilation system to prevent static electricity build-up and the risk of sparks, as flammable gases may be in use. Staff are required to wear antistatic shoes (usually clogs or boots). All equipment must have antistatic rubber wheels or covers.
- Clean and dirty areas are delineated by doors or a line on the floor. All personnel moving into clean areas must be clean and appropriately dressed (see below). All items brought into clean areas must be clean. All dirty items leaving theatre should do so via dirty areas. It is essential that staff are aware which are the dirty and the clean areas and corridors. The use of sticky mats at the main entrance to theatre was thought to reduce contamination from the feet of staff entering. This has now been shown to be ineffective and the practice has been discontinued. Similarly, no evidence exists that overshoes reduce bacterial counts on the theatre floor. However, shoe covers may protect members of the surgical team from exposure to blood and body fluids (Mangram et al 1999).
- The numbers and movements of staff inside theatres are kept to an absolute minimum to reduce the number of skin scales shed and mixing of air (Mangram et al 1999).
- All staff entering clean areas are appropriately dressed. Clean theatre dresses or trouser suits are worn. Hair is completely covered by a bonnet-style cap and all jewellery, especially on the hands, is removed. Masks are worn inside the theatre to reduce airborne organisms. Masks, once applied, should be handled only by the tapes as the main fabric of the mask becomes contaminated with moisture and microorganisms which can then be transmitted to and by the hands.
- Practice varies as to whether staff leave the theatre area wearing theatre clothing. Some hospitals restrict staff to the theatre area when dressed in theatre clothing, while others allow for the wearing of gowns over scrub suits when personnel leave the theatre suite (Mangram et al 1999, Editorial 2003, Kaplan et al 2003).
- A sterile field is created around the patient. The patient and trolleys in this area are all covered with sterile drapes. The surgeon and scrub nurse wear sterile gloves and gowns to work within the sterile field.

Safety of the patient

The patient's safety in theatre is further ensured by the following precautions:

- Transfer to operating table and positioning are carried out with extreme care. The preoperative visit by the theatre nurse enables the assessment of any potential problems, especially in relation to joint mobility and the risk of developing pressure ulcers. Surgical patients are particularly at risk of developing pressure ulcers during the perioperative phases of their care because of the combination of immobility while surgery is carried out and circulatory and metabolic changes resulting from anaesthesia and surgical trauma (Scott et al 1999). Patients who have epidural anaesthesia may have reduced sensation in the lower extremities and impaired leg movement because of the effects of the anaesthetic mixture on the motor nerve pathways in the spinal cord. These patients are especially at risk of heel pressure ulcers because they may fail to change the position of their legs in bed, or feel the sensation of discomfort. Special types of pressure-relieving mattresses and overlays are used with high-risk patients. An overlay is placed directly on the mattress. Air, foam, gel or water are commonly used in overlays (Armstrong & Bortz 2001). Once patients are anaesthetised, they may lose muscle tone. Care should be taken with all limbs; for example, if the arm is left to hang over the edge of the table, irreparable damage to the brachial plexus may result. The nurse must also be aware when positioning patients on the operating table of limitations in movement that may result from previous joint replacement surgery; for example, hip flexion may be restricted in patients with a total hip replacement prosthesis (McEwen 1996).
- The diathermy pad is carefully positioned. A self-adhesive pad may be used and the pad is usually placed under the buttocks or strapped to the thigh to ensure good contact over the entire surface. A poor contact by

only part of the surface may concentrate the current, causing it to leave a burn.

- Swabs, needles and instruments used during theatre are counted and checked throughout and at the end of the operation by the scrub and circulating nurses. This ensures that all items used are accounted for and none left inside the patient.
- Allergies to drugs, skin antiseptics and dressings are assessed preoperatively by the theatre nurse and anaesthetist, so the use of any allergens can be avoided. For example, although not fully understood, allergy to latex is present in increasing numbers of patients (Yuill et al 2003).
- The patient's skin is cleaned at the start of the procedure. Alcoholic solutions containing chlorhexidine, povidone–iodine or triclosan are quick acting and produce a rapid reduction in skin flora and the risk of endogenous infection (Ayliffe et al 2000). Once applied, alcoholic solutions must be allowed to dry completely lest they ignite on contact with diathermy. Some surgeons also use a sterile plastic adhesive drape over the skin (Incisa-drape) through which to make the incision. This prevents the surgeons' and nurses' sterile gloves being contaminated with the patient's skin flora.
- Prophylactic antibiotics may be given (usually intravenously) during the operation, or the site of the surgery may be irrigated with an antibiotic solution. These measures are usually taken only if there is a specific risk of contamination, or if contamination from an abscess or the gastrointestinal tract is already present.
- During surgery the patient is at risk of primary haemorrhage. When an incision is made, the patient will bleed until a clot is formed or until the pressures within the vessel and the cavity into which it is bleeding have equalised. Bleeding during surgery is minimised by the use of clamps and ligatures, local pressure or diathermy to seal small vessels. Topical haemostatic agents such as cellulose and collagen may also be used. To facilitate the surgeon's vision, the site of operation is kept free of blood by swabbing or suctioning. The circulating nurse may weigh the swabs or note the volume of blood in the suction bottle to estimate 'total blood loss'.
- Special procedures must be followed for the care of patients identified as carriers of certain infectious diseases — commonly blood-borne diseases with a high morbidity and mortality (see Ch. 11). To prevent cross-infection and to reduce risks involved with cleaning and spillages, disposable equipment may be used where possible (see Ch. 16). In many hospitals, such procedures are now followed for all patients as it is often not known whether a patient is a carrier of an infectious disease. The surgeon and scrub nurse may wear two pairs of gloves, and the patient may not be taken into the recovery room after the operation, in case of further blood loss, but recovered in theatre instead. The patient should be at the end of a theatre list to enable recovery in theatre and to allow thorough cleaning and disinfection of the theatre before it is used again.

In summary, the safety of the patient in theatre is the prime responsibility of all members of the theatre team.

For further information on patient safety in theatre, see the National Association of Theatre Nurses' 1998 publication, *Principles of Safe Practice in the Perioperative Environment.*

Anaesthesia

An anaesthetic is used to block any sensations of pain during surgery. It may be applied locally or regionally to the area of surgery or generally throughout the body. A brief introduction to the use of anaesthetics is given here.

For further information on medications used in anaesthesia, see Waller et al (2001) and Chapters 17–20 and 27.

Local anaesthesia

Local anaesthesia blocks transmission of pain from the region operated upon. In some cases, only the sensory receptors may be blocked; this is more correctly termed local analgesia. A local anaesthetic, e.g. lidocaine, is often combined with adrenaline to constrict blood vessels and delay absorption of the anaesthetic into the bloodstream. This reduces the amount of local anaesthetic required and prolongs its action. Types and common uses of local anaesthetics are summarised in Table 26.3. Epidural or spinal anaesthetics may be used when a general anaesthetic could be harmful or is undesirable, e.g. in older patients with arteriosclerosis or diabetes, in patients with respiratory disorders and in patients with hypertension. An infusion of epidural anaesthetic agents can also be continued after surgery to provide effective postoperative analgesia (see p. 929). The procedure causes hypotension and so should be avoided in patients with this condition.

Care must be taken to prepare the patient psychologically in order to reduce anxiety and ensure cooperation. Psychological support should continue throughout the operation and the nurse should ensure that the patient's vision of the procedure is adequately screened.

Both Mr W and Mr A were conscious during their operations as they were carried out under local anaesthetic. Mr W's anaesthetist had prescribed a sedative for him which was administered an hour before going to theatre. Both patients were reassured and informed of progress throughout the operation by the surgeon and the nurse.

General anaesthesia

General anaesthesia is characterised by loss of consciousness, analgesia and muscle relaxation. These effects occur according to the stage of anaesthesia, as follows:

Stage 1 The pain is reduced or relieved, but the patient is still conscious. Heavy sedation can produce 'dissociative anaesthesia' and some muscle relaxation, while local analgesics supplement pain control as necessary. The patient may remain drowsy but conscious throughout the procedure.

Entonox (50% oxygen with 50% nitrous oxide) can be self-administered during childbirth or painful procedures to achieve stage 1 anaesthesia for pain control. This application is discussed with other methods of pain relief in Chapter 19.

Stage 2 Consciousness is lost, but the patient may exhibit wild movements and irrational behaviour. With i.v.

Table 26.3 Local anaesthetics

Method of administration	Effect	Example of drugs and their uses
Topical: solution or cream applied to skin or mucous membranes	Blocks local sensory nerve receptors	Lidocaine, benzocaine Minor ENT procedures Insertion of cannulae
Infiltration: injection into surgical site	Blocks local sensory nerve receptors	Lidocaine, procaine Removal of skin moles Insertion of Hickman line Drainage of abscess
Nerve block: injection close to relevant nerve trunk	Blocks conduction of sensory impulses to central nervous system	Lidocaine with adrenaline Brachial plexus procedures on the arm (Bier's block) Intercostal blocks for pain relief
Epidural: injection into space outside the dura	Blocks nerves as they enter the spinal cord	Lidocaine, bupivacaine Rectal or pelvic surgery Caesarean section
Spinal: injection into the subarachnoid space below the second lumbar vertebra	Blocks preganglionic fibres (motor and sensory) Position of patient determines distribution of drug and spinal nerves affected	Lidocaine, bupivacaine Amputation Abdominal surgery

induction of anaesthesia, this stage is passed through very quickly and may be more in evidence when the patient is recovering from anaesthesia.

Stage 3 Breathing becomes regular and there is relaxation of the muscles along with loss of reflexes. This is the level of surgical anaesthesia. The degree of muscle relaxation required to facilitate surgery can be achieved by deepening this stage but this has undesirable side-effects such as fall in cardiac output, respiratory depression and liver damage. To overcome this problem, muscle relaxants can be administered to enable a relatively light anaesthetic to be used and so reduce the risks of anaesthesia in older people and those with cardiovascular and respiratory complications. This has also aided the development of day-case surgery.

Premedication can be used to relieve anxiety, induce a state of analgesia, reduce bronchial and salivary secretions, prevent vasovagal stimulation (mainly bradycardia) and make the patient less aware and somewhat drowsy. Usually, a sedative or anxiolytic is given orally (see Table 26.1).

The induction of anaesthesia is usually achieved with a short-acting i.v. agent administered with a short-acting muscle relaxant (see Tables 26.4 and 26.5). This rapidly produces surgical anaesthesia, in which the patient is unable to maintain their own airway (due to lack of reflexes) and the muscles of breathing are paralysed. An endotracheal tube is passed through the relaxed larynx and artificial ventilation is maintained throughout the operation. For emergency patients who have not fasted, the anaesthetist may decide to use rapid sequence induction with cricoid pressure (Hurford 2000). Pressure is applied to the cricoid cartilage in the throat as the patient becomes unconscious (Frakes 2003). Pressure on the cricoid cartilage will mechanically occlude the oesophagus and reduce the likelihood of aspiration of any regurgitated gastric contents.

For further information on rapid sequence intubation, see Stewart (1999).

Anaesthesia can be maintained during surgery, usually by means of inhaled anaesthetics and a longer-acting muscle relaxant. At the end of the operation, the anaesthetic gas is discontinued and the effects of the muscle relaxant are reversed with the appropriate drug. The patient gradually regains consciousness, passing through stages 2 and 1 of anaesthesia and regaining muscle tone, which enables

Table 26.4 General anaesthetics

Method of administration	Effect	Example of drugs and their uses
Intravenous: for induction	Sedation, surgical anaesthesia Respiratory depression Some cause hypotension	Thiopental, etomidate, ketamine, propofol, remifentanil Induction of anaesthesia Short surgical procedures, EUA, dental extraction
Inhalation: for maintenance of anaesthesia	Surgical anaesthesia Some cause hypotension, nausea and vomiting	Halothane, nitrous oxide, isoflurane Maintenance of anaesthesia Wide range of surgical procedures

Table 26.5 Muscle relaxants

Name of drug	Effect	Use
Suxamethonium (depolarising): binds and blocks acetylcholine receptors	Skeletal flaccid paralysis Increased K^+ release Rarely: prolonged apnoea and malignant hyperpyrexia	Short acting (15 min) Induction, manipulations, ECT No drug available to reverse effects
Atracurium, pancuronium and rocuronium (non-depolarising) Prevents acetylcholine gaining access to receptor site	Skeletal flaccid paralysis Can cause hypotension	Longer acting (30–45 min) Maintenance of relaxation during anaesthesia or controlled ventilation Reversed by neostigmine (anticholinesterase — raises levels of acetylcholine)

independent breathing. During this time, the patient is transferred to the recovery room.

Recovery from anaesthesia

Once surgery is completed, the patient will normally be kept in the recovery room until the immediate effects of the anaesthetic have worn off. The patient should be able to maintain their own airway and be considered stable before transfer back to the ward. In some cases the patient will be transferred directly to the intensive therapy unit (ITU) while continuing to be intubated and their respiration is maintained by artificial ventilation. Alternatively, the patient may be ventilated in the recovery room overnight, hereby avoiding unnecessary admission to ITU.

Whilst the patient is still unconscious, the nurse must ensure that the airway is kept open. This can be achieved by placing the patient in a lateral or semi-prone position, tilting the head backwards and pulling the mandible forwards, or inserting a Guedel airway. If a Guedel airway is used, it can be left in position until, as reflexes return, the patient expels it spontaneously. There is a risk of aspiration pneumonia should the patient vomit while regaining consciousness; therefore, suction equipment must be available. Anaesthetics, muscle relaxants, narcotics and severe pain itself can cause nausea and vomiting. Pain must be adequately controlled and antiemetics may be required.

The nurse should observe the patient's level of consciousness and be aware that a stage of excitement (stage 2) may occur. Close observation and the use of side rails may be required. Many patients will be prescribed oxygen until fully awake, in order to maintain PO_2 while there is still some respiratory depression due to anaesthesia. The patient should be encouraged to commence deep breathing and leg exercises as soon as consciousness is regained.

As the patient regains consciousness, the nurse should bear in mind that hearing is usually one of the first senses to return. Verbal reassurance that the operation is over should be given. It may be appropriate to return hearing aids and spectacles at this point. The patient should be allowed to rest as quietly as possible during this period and will usually fall asleep after regaining consciousness. Close and frequent observation of vital signs is required for the early detection of changes in the patient's condition. During the recovery period patients are especially at risk of reactionary haemorrhage as their blood pressure rises. Hypotension is often induced during surgery due to anaesthetic agents. A ligature or clot may become dislodged, leading to signs of haemorrhage and hypovolaemic shock (see p. 718). Observation of wound dressings and wound drainage will also aid assessment of the patient in the recovery period.

In surgery, the patient may have had a large surface area exposed, leading to loss of body heat. A high risk of hypothermia, a core temperature of less than 36°C, exists in older patients, in surgery where the peritoneal cavity is opened or when large amounts of unwarmed irrigation fluids are used (Scott et al 1999). Shivering will have been suppressed, due to the use of skeletal muscle relaxants. The environmental temperature in theatres is therefore kept fairly high, but patients may still have a low body temperature. As well as feeling uncomfortable, the patient may also suffer adverse effects on postoperative recovery. A drop of 2°C during colorectal surgery has been shown to triple wound infection rates and to lead to an increased length of stay (Kurz et al 1996). Shivering in the recovery period increases oxygen demand and is distressing and painful for the patient (Scott et al 1999). Extra blankets, forced air system (e.g. Bare Hugger) and warming of i.v. fluids can be used, but the nurse must be wary of warming the patient too quickly, as this can lead to peripheral vasodilatation and a consequent fall in blood pressure.

Pain control begins before, or as, the patient regains consciousness. A patient such as Mr W may have the operation site infiltrated with more local anaesthetic at the end of surgery. Adrenaline may also be given to cause vasoconstriction and so localise the effects. This type of analgesic for herniorrhaphy has been found to provide good pain control and reduce recovery time to around 3 h for day-case surgery patients (Morris 1995). The anaesthetist may also prescribe some opioid analgesics and a simple oral analgesic for the patient's return to the ward.

Mrs B was commenced on an i.v. infusion of morphine which she was able to administer herself using a patient-controlled analgesia system (PCA, see p. 930). Many patients will receive their first dose of analgesic in the recovery room via the rectal, i.m., s.c. or i.v. route. The patient's pain should be controlled before leaving the recovery room. In a partially conscious patient, a sudden rise in blood pressure and restlessness may indicate the presence of pain. The nurse must also be aware that opioid analgesics may cause a fall in blood pressure and respiratory depression, and that severe pain in itself can lead to shock and shallow breathing.

The patient may spend several hours in the recovery room and will, in many respects, require the same care as an unconscious patient (see Ch. 28). Most patients will require attention at least to the mouth, as mucous membranes will be dry due to oxygen therapy, fasting and perhaps dehydration, as well as to pressure areas. The recovery room nurse will document the care given and provide a summary to the ward nurse who collects the patient. In this way, continuity of care can be achieved. The role of the recovery room nurse is summarised in Box 26.2.

For further reading on patient assessment in recovery, see Starritt (1999).

POSTOPERATIVE CARE

All patients require close observation during the immediate postoperative period in order to detect any complications. This close observation may be continued for hours or days for the patient requiring intensive nursing care, or perhaps for an hour or two if a local infiltration of anaesthetic or a very light general anaesthetic has been used. The next stage of postoperative care focuses on recovery and repair and on the active prevention of complications. Rehabilitation will be achieved at a different pace and to differing levels by each patient. The patient with a hip replacement may find that their joint pain is almost immediately reduced postoperatively and that their functional ability is far better than before the operation. Some patients may not be able to achieve the desired level of recovery and others may be seeking palliation rather than cure.

For purposes of clarity, this section will focus on the postoperative recovery, repair and rehabilitation most commonly experienced during the hospital stay, while the section on 'Rehabilitation' focuses on continued care after discharge from hospital. It is recognised, however, that many patients will still be recovering from the effects of the anaesthetic after discharge following day surgery. This can take up to 24 h to be eliminated from the body. Examples of postoperative care are given in Nursing Care Plans 26.2 and 26.3.

Shock and haemostasis

Shock is discussed here with specific application to the care of surgical patients. For a wider discussion of the types and mechanisms of shock and their signs and symptoms, see Chapter 18.

When the patient returns from theatre to the ward, they require frequent observations for signs of impending shock or haemorrhage. As blood pressure continues to rise, there is a continued risk of reactionary haemorrhage for the first 24 h. Hypovolaemic shock may also occur due to a slow, continuous loss of fluid; this might be a slowly bleeding vessel or the pooling of fluid in the gastrointestinal tract during the paralytic ileus that occurs as a consequence of surgery. The loss of fluid may be detected as soakage on the dressing or blood in the wound drains, but if the patient is bleeding into a body cavity or losing fluid into the gut it may be less obvious. Distinction should also be made between hypovolaemic and other forms of shock, i.e. cardiogenic, septic, anaphylactic and neurogenic.

- Cardiogenic shock is caused by failure of the heart to pump and maintain adequate cardiac output. Possible causes following surgery may be pulmonary embolus, causing massive resistance to the output from the right side of the heart, fluid overload and concomitant heart failure, anaesthetic depression of cardiac output or myocardial infarction. Patient signs and symptoms and measurement of central venous or pulmonary wedge pressures along with other vital signs can help the nurse to distinguish between hypovolaemic and cardiogenic shock.
- Secondary haemorrhage can occur 1–7 days postoperatively due to vessel erosion by infection or from a long, slow bleed. The patient may collapse suddenly and will usually need to return to theatre. Fortunately, this is not a common problem.
- The patient may also be at risk of:
  - — neurogenic shock, usually due to severe pain
  - — anaphylactic shock, usually due to drug reactions
  - — septic shock, from infections following surgery.

The aim of nursing observations in the first 24 h following surgery is to detect changes that might indicate the initial stages of compensation to hypovolaemic shock. As the circulating volume falls, the nurse may see increased loss of blood on dressings or in wound drainage bags or bottles. There will be a slight rise in heart rate to maintain cardiac output but systolic blood pressure may remain unchanged, or even rise slightly. Peripheral vasoconstriction to conserve blood supply to vital organs, i.e. brain, heart and lungs, and the eccrine response may lead to a pale, clammy appearance. The vasoconstriction of the veins maintains diastolic (end) volume and therefore increases stroke volume. This, along with increased cardiac contractility, maintains blood pressure to at least pre-shock levels. As the brain is extremely sensitive to hypoxia, the respiratory rate may be increased and the patient may also appear restless.

If the blood or fluid loss continues, then these mechanisms may eventually fail to compensate effectively, leading to further vasoconstriction of the arterioles to increase peripheral resistance. There is also reduced parasympathetic activity to increase heart rate and stroke volume, resulting in increased cardiac output. At this point the heart rate increases further and blood pressure begins to fall. Urine output decreases rapidly, due to decreased renal perfusion over and above the effects of increased antidiuretic hormone (ADH) and aldosterone (see p. 359), as blood flow is conserved to maintain the brain, heart and lungs as a priority.

The patient appears breathless, centrally cyanosed and may be quite confused due to hypoxia. The signs and symptoms of the initial compensation and failing compensation are summarised in Box 26.3.

Shock must be detected at the first level of compensation and not when the classic picture of falling blood pressure and rising pulse occurs and a crisis ensues. If a patient is allowed to continue at the first level of compensation, all but the vital organs will be deprived of oxygen and newly anastomosed tissue will have an increased tendency to breakdown and infection due to prolonged vasoconstriction and hypoxia.

Nursing Care Plan 26.2 Care for Mrs B on her third postoperative day (see Case History 26.2(A) and 26.2(B))

Nursing considerations	Action	Rationale	Evaluation
Abdominal pain	• Discontinue i.v. opioid PCA • Undertake hourly pain assessment • Administer regular oral analgesics as prescribed • Offer s.c. opioid analgesic, up to 1-hourly as prescribed for 'breakthrough' pain and 10–20 min prior to activity • Reassess pain after 20 min to ascertain effect of analgesic • Involve Acute Pain Specialist Nurse if pain is unrelieved by prescribed analgesics • Record respiratory rate hourly • Ensure that Mrs B is positioned comfortably • Encourage her to support wound on moving • Apply heat pad for 'wind pains'	To prevent pain and foster recovery by enabling Mrs B to cough, exercise, rest and sleep comfortably	Mrs B is sufficiently pain free to cooperate with therapy
Fluid and electrolyte imbalance	• Encourage intake of oral fluids and supplemented drinks • Monitor oral intake, supplement with i.v. infusion if intake below 1000 mL/24 h • Observe pulse and BP 6-hourly • Observe for dyspnoea • Record all fluid intake and output • Observe for nausea, vomiting and diarrhoea	To detect any sign of dehydration and electrolyte imbalance early	Fluid and electrolytes maintained at satisfactory levels
Postoperative ileus	• Observe for passage of flatus/faeces in stoma bag	To detect return of normal peristalsis	Mrs B is comfortable until normal peristalsis returns
	• Administer antiemetics as prescribed	To prevent nausea and dehydration	
	• Give oral fluids and supplemented drinks as tolerated	To facilitate recommencement of oral nutrition at early opportunity	
	• Observe for abdominal distension, nausea and vomiting	To observe for signs of unresolved ileus	
Retention of urine	• Record urine volumes on fluid balance chart 6-hourly	To ensure adequate urinary output	Diuresis is adequate
	• Report volumes of <180 mL in 6 h		
	• Observe urine for signs of infection, i.e. cloudy appearance, malodour	To detect early catheter-related urinary tract infection	

Continued

Nursing Care Plan 26.2 Care for Mrs B on her third postoperative day (see Case History 26.2(A) and 26.2(B)) *(Continued)*

Nursing considerations	Action	Rationale	Evaluation
Wound infection	• Check wound daily for colour, exudate and surrounding inflammation (redness) • Record axillary temperature 6-hourly • Observe exudate from wound drain. Remove drain according to medical staff's instructions • Recommence oral nutrition at early opportunity, e.g. supplemented milky drinks	To detect early signs of infection and promote healing	Wound is kept free of infection
Pressure ulcers*	• Use a pressure-relieving mattress overlay • Assist Mrs B to change position in bed 2-hourly, do not have her lie on left shoulder • When Mrs B is sitting up, have er stand hourly to relieve pressure • Consider parenteral nutrition if unable to recommence oral intake (see Ch. 21)	To prevent loss of skin integrity	Mrs B does not develop pressure ulcers
Chest infection*	• Keep Mrs B as upright as possible in bed • Encourage her to sit out of bed and help her to mobilise for short distances • Humidify oxygen therapy • Assist her hourly with deep breathing exercises, with spirometer • Assist with chest physiotherapy twice daily • Encourage coughing and expectoration • Observe any expectorate produced for signs of infection (greenish/yellow sputum) and send sample for culture and sensitivity • Observe temperature and respiration	To prevent build-up of secretions To detect early any chest infection and treat appropriately	No shortness of breath Sputum is clear
Deep vein thrombosis and pulmonary embolism*	• Assess daily for calf tenderness and inflammation • Use graduated elastic compression stockings (GECS), full length • Encourage hourly leg exercises while in bed or sitting in chair • Encourage early activity, e.g. walking in ward twice daily with nurse • Encourage Mrs B to sit out of bed for 1–2 h periods as able • Encourage a good fluid intake	To detect early signs of thrombus and encourage good circulation	No detection of DVT

Continued

Nursing Care Plan 26.2 Care for Mrs B on her third postoperative day (see Case History 26.2(A) and 26.2(B)) *(Continued)*

Nursing considerations	Action	Rationale	Evaluation
Pain in knees and left shoulder	• Ensure Mrs B's position is comfortable • Administer analgesics as prescribed • Apply heat pad • Assist with passive exercise and gentle massage	To alleviate pain and prevent stiffness	Mrs B's comfort is maintained at acceptable level
Inability to maintain own hygiene	• Encourage Mrs B in self-care tasks • Assist with washing only for areas she cannot reach, i.e. back and lower half • Assist with oral hygiene • Change and wash GECS daily • Give psychological support when Mrs B changes nightclothes in view of stoma's effect on body image (see Nursing Care Plan 26.3)	To promote return to independence To help Mrs B maintain dignity	Mrs B is able to resume self-care and cope with changed body image

Nursing Care Plan 26.3 Stoma care plan for Mrs B (see Case History 26.2(A) and 26.2(B))

Nursing considerations	Action	Rationale	Evaluation
Patient's lack of knowledge about her colostomy	• Explain the reasons for the colostomy, liaising with medical staff • Assess Mrs B's level of understanding and her wish for knowledge • Include Mrs B's daughter in teaching • Provide a colostomy booklet for Mrs B to read and to use as a guide for teaching • Give basic information about appliances • Discuss the effects of colostomy on lifestyle • Check Mrs B's retention of information from previous sessions	To provide a sound basis for good stoma care	Mrs B acquires an understanding of the rationale of stoma care
Anxiety about stoma formation and change in body image	• Encourage Mrs B to voice fears; provide reassurance in the form of accurate information • Support Mrs B in her grief, provide privacy, passive listening, counselling, touch • Provide support for daughter	To provide an outlet for anxiety	Mrs B is better able to adjust to her new situation

Continued ▶

Nursing Care Plan 26.3 Stoma care plan for Mrs B (see Case History 26.2(A) and 26.2(B)) *(Continued)*

Nursing considerations	Action	Rationale	Evaluation
Lack of skill and confidence to care for the colostomy	• Implement the following stages: – encourage Mrs B to look at stoma; give reassurance – show her how to check and clean stoma, then supervise as she does this – discuss the range of appliances available, and guide her in making a suitable choice – show Mrs B how to fit appliance and teach skin care – encourage her to fit appliance under supervision and to check and clean stoma independently – encourage her to care for stoma independently	To build confidence by helping Mrs B to succeed at each stage	Mrs B achieves independence in colostomy care
Inability to cope with the stoma at home*	• Liaise with community stoma nurses about support at home prior to discharge • Give advice and information on the following as appropriate: diet; fluid and electrolyte balance; alcohol consumption; clothing; prescriptions; flatus control; disposal of appliances; travel; pursuing hobbies and interests; intimate relationships; local colostomy association; attitudes of loved ones • Provide on discharge: supply of equipment; prescription care; prescription exemption form	To prepare Mrs B for her discharge home	The transition from hospital to home care is smooth; Mrs B feels that she is able to cope

* Potential problem.

The nurse should report any significant changes to the nurse in charge of the patient's care, who may then decide to call in the medical staff. Actions to correct shock must be taken swiftly and must be appropriate to the cause and presentation. For example, raising the foot of the bed to aid venous return could have disastrous effects in patients undergoing gastrointestinal surgery. If there is bleeding or large volumes of fluid due to paralytic ileus or obstruction in the abdomen, these contents would fall against the diaphragm, impeding respiratory and cardiac function. Equally, aggressive fluid replacement in older patients can lead to heart failure, arrhythmias and cardiogenic shock.

Once assessed, oxygen therapy will be started or increased to reduce hypoxia. In hypovolaemic shock the lost fluid must be replaced or returned to the circulation. Some patients may have large amounts of fluid available in the body, as in paralytic ileus or peripheral oedema, but in the wrong body compartment. This fluid can be drawn back into the circulation by treating the cause and by raising the osmotic pressure of the circulation.

Crystalline fluids can be given intravenously but are soon lost from the circulation. Colloids such as plasma protein substitutes (PPS) or Gelofusine are given as plasma expanders. These raise the osmotic pressure and draw extracellular fluid into the circulation (Kavanagh et al 1995). Interstitial fluid also moves into the capillaries as hydrostatic pressure falls in response to lowered blood pressure and arteriolar constriction. In haemodynamic shock, rapid transfusion of blood may be required and should be given through a blood warmer (see p. 726). Central venous pressure measurements are of great value in assessing the volume of blood returning to the heart and the heart's

Box 26.3

Signs and symptoms of shock, by stages

Initial compensation

- Appears clammy, pale
- Peripheral cyanosis
- Appears restless; may complain of feeling generally unwell
- Falling urine output but may remain above 30 mL/h
- Increase in pulse rate
- Slight rise in systolic blood pressure
- Increased soakage of blood on wound dressings and in wound drains

Failing compensation

- Appears cold, clammy
- Central cyanosis
- Appears confused, often agitated, and then increasingly drowsy
- Urine output falls below 30 mL/h
- Tachycardia
- Fall in blood pressure
- Large volumes of blood may be lost

ability to pump (see Ch. 18). A central venous catheter may be inserted as an emergency in a patient whose shock proves difficult to manage. Nursing Care Plan 26.4 illustrates the type of nursing care required to detect the early signs of shock.

Fluid and electrolyte balance

Most patients experience some loss of fluid during surgery which may be compounded by electrolyte disturbances resulting from the illness itself or trauma during surgery. Preoperative dehydration due to excessive fasting should be avoided (see p. 912). Patients having a general anaesthetic will be fasted postoperatively until they are fully conscious and cough and swallowing reflexes have returned. Some may be required to fast for longer than this if there is a paralytic ileus or after facial or laryngeal surgery. These patients require fluid and electrolyte replacement via the i.v. route to meet normal demands and some require over and above this volume to replace fluid lost at theatre.

Fluid and electrolyte balance can be significantly affected by the physiological response of the body to the stress of surgery. Glucocorticoid secretion increases reabsorption of sodium and water in the renal nephrons with a reciprocal loss of potassium and hydrogen ions. Elevated levels of ADH also increase water reabsorption and high aldosterone levels increase sodium reabsorption further. The net effect is to increase the extracellular fluid volume and reduce urine output. Consequently, it would not be unusual for a well-hydrated patient to retain fluid and have a high positive fluid balance for the immediate postoperative period (Bove 1994).

As a result of trauma to the tissues during surgery, the intracellular electrolyte potassium is released. This is excreted in part-exchange for retained sodium. Potassium levels will be closely monitored by medical staff in patients who have undergone major surgery and appropriate replacement with i.v. fluids given.

Many surgical patients complain of thirst and a dry mouth postoperatively. This is due partly to dehydration, to the drying effects of oxygen therapy and to the anti-cholinergic effects of drugs given during anaesthesia. As a result, thirst is an unreliable measure of hydration.

Metabolic and stress responses

Surgery and general anaesthesia are major stressors which result in the 'general adaptation syndrome' (Selye 1976). The psychological effects of stress are often seen as anxiety and withdrawal in surgical patients and are addressed in detail in Chapter 17. The importance of adequate pre-operative education and counselling in minimising stress is discussed on page 908.

The physiological effects of stress can be reduced by minimising anxiety both pre- and postoperatively. In the immediate postoperative period, and up to 4 days after a major operation, the patient utilises protein (normally spared) as a source of energy along with fats and carbohydrates. The amino acids act as a source of glucose for the brain. Blood glucose levels can be elevated, resulting in glycosuria. This will be a cause for concern and careful monitoring is required in diabetic patients and in those receiving parenteral nutrition. It is important that patients are in a nutritional state sufficient to withstand this period of catabolism and negative nitrogen balance. If the patient has a poor nutritional status, and/or is undergoing major surgery with or without prolonged fasting, parenteral nutrition is generally indicated.

Well-nourished patients can tolerate catabolism and some starvation for approximately 7–10 days after major surgery (Everitt & McMahon 1994). Many become anabolic after 24–48 h and begin to rebuild proteins, while hormones released in stress decrease. A large diuresis and negative fluid balance may be seen at this point. Chapter 21 describes nursing interventions to improve the nutritional status of the patient and provides a complete discussion of parenteral nutrition.

Surgical trauma to the gastrointestinal tract causes temporary paralysis of the smooth muscle known as post-operative or temporary paralytic ileus (Field 2002, Holte & Kehlet 2002). This is manifest by the absence of bowel sounds and cessation of peristalsis. Bowel sounds are high-pitched gurgling noises caused by liquid and air moving through the gastrointestinal tract (Field 2002). Traditionally a period of fasting was commonplace following gastro-intestinal surgery involving an intestinal anastomosis (Holte & Kehlet 2002). Oral intake was restricted during this time to reduce the demands on the anastomosis, allowing it to heal, and to prevent postoperative nausea and vomiting (Lewis et al 2001). Neither eating nor drinking was allowed until bowel sounds had returned or other signs of gastric motility were apparent, such as passing of flatus or stool. In fact, conclusions in *Consensus in Clinical Nutrition* (Everitt & McMahon 1994) suggested that, following major surgery, nutritional support would not be considered in well-nourished patients unless it was expected that it would be more than 7–10 days before they could eat (Beier-Holgersen & Boesby 1996).

Nursing Care Plan 26.4 Immediate postoperative care plan for M (see Case History 26.4(A) and 26.4(B))

Nursing considerations	Action	Rationale	Expected outcome
Shock due to haemorrhage and pain*	• Observe TPR and BP ½-hourly • Observe for pallor, sweating and confusion • Record urine output hourly • Give O_2 therapy at 4 L/min as prescribed • Implement pain control (see below) • Check wound and drains ½-hourly • Maintain circulatory volume as prescribed	To ensure pulse is maintained at 65–90, BP at 100/65 to 140/95, urine output at ≥ 30 mL/h	Shock does not develop
Abdominal pain	• Provide patient-controlled analgesia as prescribed • Record respiratory rate hourly • Assess effectiveness of analgesia using appropriate assessment tool • Ensure comfortable positioning • Encourage M to support wound while moving	To control pain and enable deep breathing exercises to be performed	Pain is kept at an acceptable level
Fluid and electrolyte imbalance*	• Provide i.v. infusion as per chart; change giving set after 24 h • Observe for dyspnoea, irregularities in CVS • Record all fluid intake and output • Observe for nausea, vomiting and diarrhoea	To maintain circulatory volume	Fluid and electrolytes maintained at satisfactory levels
Nausea and vomiting	• Allow only sips of water or ice chips for first 4 h postoperatively • Regular assessment of nausea • Administer antiemetics promptly and regularly as prescribed	To detect and treat any nausea or vomiting in the postoperative period	Any nausea experienced in postoperative period is recognised and treated effectively
Loss of bladder tone	• Observe and record urine output; urinary catheter with 10 mL balloon inserted in theatre • Perform catheter care morning and evening • Maintain asepsis of closed drainage system	To prevent urinary retention and infection	Diuresis satisfactory Infection of urinary tract does not develop
Wound infection*	• Check wound and drains ½-hourly • Do not disturb dressing until 48 h postoperatively • Observe vaginal loss twice daily	To promote healing and prevent infection	Wound begins to heal normally

Continued

Nursing Care Plan 26.4 Immediate postoperative care plan for M (see Case History 26.4(A) and 26.4(B)) *(Continued)*

Nursing considerations	Action	Rationale	Expected outcome
Pressure ulcers*	• Carry out assessment of M's skin for risk of pressure ulcers • Change M's position according to comfort needs and prior to hyperaemia of skin • Observe for reddening of pressure areas • Ensure skin is clean and dry • Use pressure-relieving mattress	To safeguard skin integrity	M does not develop pressure ulcers
Deep vein thrombosis and pulmonary embolism*	• Administer subcutaneous heparin as prescribed • Use TED stockings below knee • Assist with leg exercises hourly • Have patient sit out of bed on first postoperative day	To encourage good circulation, especially venous return	No thrombosis or embolism
Chest infection*	• Nurse M as upright as possible • Assist with deep breathing exercises hourly • Encourage coughing and expectoration • Assist with chest physiotherapy	To prevent build-up of secretions and resulting infection	Chest remains clear
Inability to maintain personal hygiene	• Assist M to wash and change into own nightclothes when appropriate • Provide bed bath with complete assistance on first postoperative day • Provide oral hygiene as required • Change and wash TED stockings daily	To assist M in maintaining dignity and regaining independence	M's comfort and hygiene maintained
Anxiety about outcome of surgery	• Reassure M about the outcome of the operation • Repeat information as required if she is drowsy post anaesthetic	To reduce anxiety	M is encouraged about prospects for the future

* Potential problem.

There is growing evidence of the importance of early nutrition after surgery (Lewis et al 2001). Research suggests that early enteral feeding can improve the quality of healing at the anastomosis site and reduce septic complications while being tolerated well (Lewis et al 2001). Moreover, some studies suggest that early oral feeding can reduce the duration of temporary ileus to 1–2 days (Holte & Kehlet 2002, Di Fronzo et al 2003).

Most patients who have abdominal surgery may commence oral fluids on the first postoperative day (Field 2002, Feo et al 2004) and progress to normal diet over the first 2–3 days. Field (2002) recommends a proactive approach, starting by giving patients milky drinks rather than water, which has no nutritional value. Nurses should be vigilant for any symptoms which suggest that the postoperative ileus has not resolved, such as abdominal distension, nausea and vomiting. Such patients may need a nasogastric tube to be inserted in order to decompress the stomach contents and decrease tension on the anastomosis. Further oral intake should be withheld and referral to the nutrition team may be indicated if it becomes apparent that feeding will be delayed for more than 7 days (Field 2002).

Pain

Postoperative pain deserves close attention in nursing practice, research and education. Issues relating to pain specifically in the postoperative period are discussed here. The reader is also referred to Chapter 19, where broader but equally pertinent issues are addressed. Being in pain has been and remains the major preoperative concern of many patients (Biley 1989, Macintyre & Ready 2001). While thoracic and abdominal operations tend to cause most pain, Mitchell (2003) suggests that pain management is a considerable issue for day surgery patients in the first 24 h postoperatively.

Despite advances in pain management, recent studies suggest that between 75 and 80% of patients still report moderate to severe pain postoperatively (Macintyre & Ready 2001, Manias 2003). The Royal College of Surgeons and College of Anaesthetists Working Party in 1990, and the Audit Commission in 1997 reported that health professionals working in acute care environments are not effectively managing and relieving pain. More alarmingly, they also suggested that nurses lacked the knowledge and commitment to achieve satisfying postoperative pain control (Sheppard & Wright 2000).

Pain control after surgery is a prime concern on humanitarian grounds alone. Sherwood et al (2003) highlight that patients often expect to experience pain, and may express satisfaction with pain management even if they are in pain, postoperatively. However, pain is not a 'natural, inevitable, acceptable or harmless consequence of surgery' (Macintyre & Ready 2001). It has significant effects on other aspects of the patient's recovery. Good pain control allows for early activity, so minimising problems of immobility such as chest infection, urinary tract infection, deep vein thrombosis, pressure ulcers and muscle wasting. Pain after surgery has been cited as one of the main reasons for poor sleep (Closs 1992, Dawson et al 1999). Older patients are at an increased risk of the postoperative complications described above, and their subsequent recovery will be influenced by pain management.

Ineffective pain relief in the postoperative period can have serious psychological consequences for patients facing subsequent surgery and is also associated with the development of chronic pain (Perkins & Kehlet 2000, Macintyre & Ready 2001). Macrae (2001) suggests that the development of chronic postsurgical pain is common, resulting in distress and disability for many patients. A variety of surgical procedures are associated with the development of chronic pain including thoracic, breast and gall bladder surgery and amputations (Perkins & Kehlet 2000). Chronic pain is reported in 5–13% of patients undergoing dental surgery and in 5–33% of men following vasectomy (Macrae 2001). The causes of chronic postsurgical pain are not clear. Some pain specialists believe that patients who suffer from certain conditions such as irritable bowel syndrome, Raynaud's disease and migraine headaches are more at risk of chronic pain after surgery. These conditions may be related to changes in the nervous system, and such changes may result in amplification of painful sensations (Macrae 2001). Nurses should be aware that uncontrolled postoperative pain can develop into a chronic condition and must ensure that pain is managed optimally.

According to Lovett et al (1994), nurses have two specific roles in the management of postoperative pain: pain assessment and provision of the means to alleviate the pain. Assessment is the cornerstone of care and accurate and systematic assessment of pain is essential. Sjostrom et al (2000) found that nurses consistently underrated patients' postoperative pain and made little use of pain assessment tools. Visual analogue scales, verbal numerical rating scales and other assessment techniques are valuable (Macintyre & Ready 2001) but have limitations (see Ch. 19, p. 747). Findings by Manias (2003) suggest that linear scales can be problematic where patients' first language is not English.

Postoperative pain can vary according to the site of the incision, being greater with midline, subcostal and intercostal incisions (see Fig. 26.3). The small incisions required for laparoscopic technique usually cause the least discomfort. However, patients can suffer extreme 'wind pain' following laparoscopic surgery which is disproportionate to the size of the incision, and 35–63% of patients complain of shoulder tip pain (Hong & Lee 2003). Pain following laparoscopic surgery occurs as a result of stretching of the peritoneum and irritation of the diaphragm by the CO_2 used to establish inflation of the abdomen to allow visualisation of the internal organs (Wills & Hunt 2000). This pneumoperitoneum can persist for a number of days postoperatively and patients undergoing laparoscopy will require information and advice on how to control any pain following discharge.

Thoracic and abdominal drain sites can also cause pain, at both change of dressing and during removal of the drains (Critical Care Extra: Critical Questions 1999) and may require short-term pain relief (Sheppard & Wright 2000). Inhalation of Entonox works rapidly and allows patients to have a degree of control over their pain relief during short procedures (Sheppard & Wright 2000). One source of

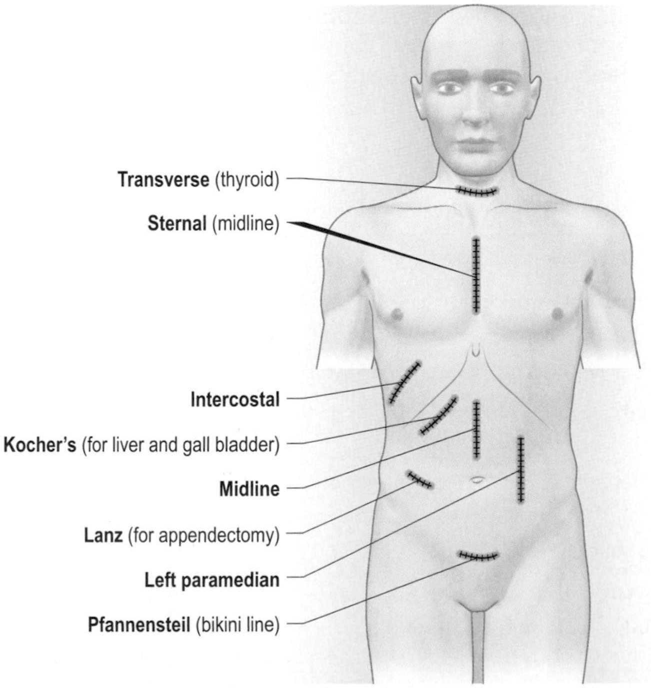

Fig. 26.3 Some incision lines used in surgery.

controversy in pain management concerns the assessment of pain as part of the diagnostic process. The location and nature of the pain, especially abdominal pain, is an important diagnostic aid, which can result in medical staff withholding analgesics until a full assessment has been carried out and a provisional diagnosis has been made. Town (1997) asserts that early pain management will not obscure diagnosis of patients who have acute abdominal pain. Instead, it is likely to decrease diffuse pain and splinting, the muscle contraction and rigidity to avoid pain, and will help the surgeon to localise the pain during the physical examination, facilitating diagnosis.

Controlling pain in the immediate postoperative period is the responsibility of the anaesthetist and, increasingly, of the acute pain team.

For a review of the role of the acute pain team, see McDonnell (2003).

The anaesthetist visits the patient preoperatively to discuss the prevention and relief of pain and to make a full assessment of the individual's needs.

Opioid analgesics are the mainstay of postoperative pain control. Some commonly used analgesics are given in Table 26.6. Traditionally, i.m. injection has been the most commonly used method of administration, but is not always the most effective (Macintyre & Ready 2001). In addition, patients may fear the discomfort of the injection itself. Injection of the analgesic via a small cannula or 'butterfly' via the s.c. route avoids the need for repeated skin punctures and the rate of absorption of morphine into the circulation is similar to that following an i.m. injection (Macintyre & Ready 2001). Recent 'Best Practice Guidelines' recommend that this method of administration replace i.m. injection (NHS Quality Improvement Scotland 2004a). Subcutaneous morphine can be administered hourly if required. The nurse should explain to the patient that the opioid is not absorbed to therapeutic levels immediately, so they should ask for an analgesic at the first indication of discomfort; the patient should be advised not to wait until the pain is unbearable (suffering the ill-effects of this pain) as they may continue to suffer for a further 15–20 min until the injection takes effect.

Other methods of pain control aim to prevent large fluctuations in plasma levels. Continuous infusions of opioid analgesics can be given through the i.v., s.c. or epidural route. Intravenous infusion can be advantageous as it enables the rate of infusion to be altered immediately, according to the patient's respiratory rate, as opioid drugs may depress respirations if too large a dose is given.

Patient-controlled analgesia (PCA)

PCA allows the patient to control the administration of small boluses of i.v. analgesic (see Ch. 19). A special infusion pump is set to give a specific volume of solution (and therefore a set dosage according to the dilution of the drug) when the patient presses a hand-held button. The machine is programmed to provide a bolus only after a certain length of time has elapsed (lockout) and a maximum total number of boluses over a specified time period.

PCA can be very effective. Mackintosh and Bowles (1997) found that patients using PCA postoperatively gained significantly greater relief of pain than those receiving i.m. injections. However, patients given a PCA without sufficient explanation beforehand, or inadequately educated staff to support them while using the device, still may not achieve optimal pain relief (Macintyre & Ready 2001). Some patients are unable to understand the function of the system and press the button inappropriately. Therapeutic levels of opioid can fall while the patient is sleeping, leading to awakening in pain. Some patients develop association nausea when they press the button and antiemetic medication should be prescribed and administered appropriately (Dawson et al 1999).

Intravenous opioids should be given carefully to older patients. It should not be assumed that they have higher pain thresholds, but they may receive slightly lower doses of analgesics as their clearance and metabolism of analgesics are slower (Gagliese et al 1999). Intravenous doses of analgesic medications should also be given more slowly as peak blood concentrations after a single i.v. medication will be

Table 26.6 Analgesics commonly used in postoperative pain control*

Method of administration	Example of dug used	Example of types of surgery
Epidural infusion	Bupivacaine and lidocaine, fentanyl and bupivacaine mixture, diamorphine	Major pelvic or lower abdominal, e.g. colectomy
Intravenous or subcutaneous infusion	Diamorphine, morphine sulphate, fentanyl	Major pelvic or abdominal, e.g. gastrectomy
Intramuscular injection	Morphine sulphate, tramadol, codeine	Many types, e.g. total hip replacement Specifically used in neurosurgery
Nerve blocks and local anaesthetic	Lidocaine with adrenaline	Thoracic surgery, wound areas can be infiltrated after surgery
Sublingual	Buprenorphine	Many types of major and minor surgery
Oral	Diclofenac sodium (Voltarol), tramadol, co-codamol, paracetamol	Many products are available Used in continued recovery and rehabilitation or alone after minor surgery

*For further reading, see Macintyre & Ready (2001).

higher due to reduction in cardiac output in the older patient.

Epidural analgesia (EA)

EA is becoming increasingly common following major surgery, e.g. following radical prostatectomy or colonic surgery (Kehlett & Morgensen 1999). Major surgery places patients at significant risk of postoperative complications because of the effects on the lungs of prolonged anaesthesia and the creation of large incision sites. Patients may be unable to cough or deep breathe postoperatively because of severe wound pain. EA is an effective form of postoperative pain relief for this group of patients because a solution of local anaesthetic and/or opiate is infused into the epidural space in the spine. This blocks the dermatomal nerves supplying the area of the wound (Greenland 1995). Such patients may have little or no sensation of pain at all in the immediate postoperative period (Richardson 2001) and are able to carry out breathing exercises and get out of bed shortly after surgery, thus minimising the risk of complications. EA is also associated with decreased levels of postoperative anxiety (Caumo et al 2001). There are, however, a number of complications associated with EA and for this reason patients should be cared for in areas where staff have special skills and knowledge in this form of pain relief, such as a high dependency unit.

For further reading on the use of epidural analgesics, see Greenland (1995) and Cox (2002).

All opioid agents have similar side-effects, e.g. central nervous system and cardiovascular depression, and the risk of addiction and the possibility of nausea and vomiting.

Fear of respiratory depression can lead to doctors underprescribing and nurses underadministering (Hunt 1995). Opioid agents (except buprenorphine) can be reversed with naloxone should respiratory depression occur. It should also be remembered that respiration will, in fact, be hindered by inadequate pain control (see p. 929). The fear of addiction from the administration of opioids is largely unfounded. When opioids are administered only in the postoperative period less than 1% of patients will develop problems of addiction (Sheppard & Wright 2000).

The amount of opioid a patient requires can be reduced by the use of other medications and local anaesthetic agents. This is known as the multimodal approach. The use of non-steroidal anti-inflammatory drugs (NSAIDs) such as diclofenac sodium and ibuprofen, used in conjunction with opioids in the perioperative stage, can result in a 20% reduction in opioid analgesic requirements (Sheppard & Wright 2000), but are associated with undesirable side-effects including bleeding, renal failure and gastric ulceration. The role of one of the most common analgesics, paracetamol, should not be overlooked. Paracetamol can be used alone to treat mild pain, or in combination with opioids, because of its morphine-sparing properties. It can be given orally or via the rectal route and an i.v. preparation has recently become available (Hahn et al 2003). Medications used in association with an opiate are most effective if given regularly, rather than 'as required' or 'PRN' doses (Sheppard & Wright, 2000). Other drugs may also be utilised; for example, hyoscine butylbromide (Buscopan), which has an anticholinergic effect causing smooth muscle relaxation, can be useful in the treatment of intestinal colic (Sheppard & Wright 2000). In day surgery, where side-effects such as respiratory depression, sedation and nausea can delay discharge, opioid-sparing strategies are particularly important (Rawal 1998).

The variety of causes of postoperative pain and discomfort and the wide range of nursing interventions available clearly demonstrate that the nurse has a key role to play in alleviating postoperative pain (see Table 26.7 and Case Histories 26.1(B), 26.2(B) and 26.4(B)). A sensitive individualised approach to patient care will also improve the management of postoperative pain, as one experienced nurse can get to know the patient well. Detailed knowledge of the patient and their reaction to pain assists in planning and evaluating care, while the close relationship between nurse and patient instils trust and confidence. This not only reassures the patient, but also has a placebo effect that supplements the analgesic administered. The therapeutic contribution of the nurse in relation to pain control is addressed in detail in Chapter 19. The nurse's knowledge of pain assessment, measurement and relief, and knowledge of the psychological impact of surgery and pain, together with assertiveness and communication skills, are all vital

CASE HISTORY 26.1(B)

Mr W *(cont'd from Case History 26.1(A), p. 903)*

Mr W had had his incision site for inguinal hernia repair infiltrated with lidocaine at the end of the operation. He did not experience any pain on return to the ward and was up and about that evening. He had some difficulty with lower back stiffness and pain, but found some relief from a gentle back massage by one staff nurse who had taken a course in this technique. The staff nurse also used some aromatherapy oils to help him relax and get to sleep that evening. Mr W did not require any analgesics until the following morning, when he took some co-codamol before getting up. After being seen by medical staff he got ready to go home. He had already bought some paracetamol to take at home as instructed in his pre-admission booklet.

CASE HISTORY 26.2(B)

Mrs B *(cont'd from Case History 26.2(A), p. 903)*

Mrs B was surprised to be given a handset with a button to control her pain (patient-controlled analgesia, PCA). She found this difficult to press because of the stiffness in her hands. The Acute Pain Nurse Specialist exchanged the handset for one she was able to squeeze which made things easier. Mrs B had not been told much about this kind of pain relief preoperatively because she had gone to theatre overnight as an emergency, but her named nurse explained that she could give herself pain-relieving medication every time she wanted, and before she planned to move or cough. Mrs B was a bit nervous that she could accidentally give herself too much of morphine, but the nurse reassured her that this was unlikely to happen because of the lock-out facility on the pump. At first Mrs B pointed the handset towards her abdomen every time she used it, but her named nurse explained that the handset was connected to a pump which delivered the medication directly into her vein.

Table 26.7 Some specific causes of postoperative pain and discomfort

Cause	Suggested nursing action
Joint, neck and back pain and stiffness	Prevent overextension of the neck at intubation point. Exert care in assessment and positioning of patients with rheumatoid arthritis and osteoarthritis. Assist with frequent change of position and passive exercises. Administer analgesics (NSAIDs can be given as suppositories as well as orally). Provide massage, heat pads.
Anastomotic leak (in GI surgery)	Identify patients at risk preoperatively, i.e. immunocompromised (e.g. steroid use), malnourished and those with low cardiac output, and observe such patients closely. Observe for signs and symptoms of peritonitis, gradual or sudden onset of abdominal pain and shock, pyrexia, shallow breathing, abdominal distension, obvious change in drain output. Alert nurse in charge of the patient and/or medical staff immediately. Anastomotic leak typically presents 5–7 days after initial surgery.
Nasogastric (NG) tube	Keep nasal passages clean, lubricate with petroleum jelly. Ensure tape is secure, clean and does not obscure view. Support the weight of the tube and/or bag by taping or pinning it to nightclothes (this also helps to prevent the tube being pulled out by sudden movement). Pass NG tubes while the patient is under anaesthetic where possible.
Wound drains	Wound drains with softer tubes cause less pain. Sudden or severe pain at a drain site should be reported. (In cases of anastomotic leak or haemorrhage, relieve weight of drainage bags by regular emptying, if appropriate.) Secure drains well with tape to prevent pulling on the securing suture. Label tubes if there is more than one. (The exit may become obscured from view by securing tape.) Provide analgesic cover prior to drain removal. Encourage patient to use relaxation techniques to reduce muscle tension.
Sutures, clips, staples	Sutures should not normally be a cause of pain. Deep tension sutures, wounds under tension (e.g. perianal) or clips catching on nightclothes can cause discomfort. Check wounds daily for signs of infection. Teach patient to support wound when coughing and moving. Cover clips with a light dressing to prevent catching. Provide reassurance and encourage use of relaxation techniques on suture removal.
Dressing changes	These should not be painful for the vast majority of patients, provided good practice is followed. Irrigate wounds with warm saline to clean and use non-adherent wound care products. Wounds tend to become painful when granulating, as nerve endings are exposed. Any adherent dressings should be soaked to aid removal. Excess hair around site may be removed in theatre to prevent adherence (see p. 913). Analgesics ranging from paracetamol to a general anaesthetic may be required for some dressings. Entonox can be extremely useful in providing short-acting pain relief during dressing changes.
Urinary retention	Observe urine output in uncatheterised patients having pelvic or abdominal surgery, or reduced mobility postoperatively. (Urinary catheters should be inserted in theatre if their need can be predicted.) Observe for a palpable bladder and rising blood pressure. (These signs may also be present in a catheterised patient if the catheter blocks up; measurement of specific gravity of the urine indicates if urine output is truly falling as urine becomes more concentrated.) Ensure privacy and comfortable positioning of patient when bedpans or bottles are being used. Discuss continued retention with medical staff and perform residual catheterisation if necessary, leaving the catheter in situ. Blocked catheters should be irrigated or changed. (See Ch. 24 for care of patients with urinary catheters.)
Colic and wind	When the patient's paralytic ileus is resolving, strong pains and spasmodic muscle contractions may be experienced. Pockets of gas may also have collected in the GI tract and may cause distension. Early and frequent activity can reduce these pains. With approval of medical staff, peppermint water can be given, or, if appropriate, peppermint oil can be used in aromatherapy. Drinks of warm water may also give some comfort. Antispasmodic drugs such as hyoscine butylbromide (Buscopan) can be prescribed, but can cause a return of the ileus and constipation and precipitate tachycardia. Heat pads and gentle massage (by experienced hands) can be helpful.

elements of the ability to provide effective postoperative pain control.

Nausea and vomiting

In the past, the use of ether as an anaesthetic agent led to a 75% incidence of postoperative nausea and vomiting (PONV) (Thompson 1999). Modern-day anaesthetics have fewer side-effects yet PONV continues to be a common postoperative complication experienced by 20–30% of patients (Jolley 2001). Some studies report PONV as the most unpleasant symptoms for patients, even more so than pain (Chimbria & Sweeney 2000). The causes of PONV are multifactorial and complex, but include patient-related factors (Janknegt et al 1999), the nature of surgery undergone (Jolley 2000) and the anaesthetic agent used (Jolley 2001) (see Box 26.4).

CASE HISTORY 26.4(B)

M *(cont'd from Case History 26.4(A), p. 906)*

M had undergone two operations over the last few years for her Crohn's disease. She did not like having injections to control the pain and had become more frightened and anxious about pain with each operation. The anaesthetist decided she would be a good candidate for patient-controlled analgesia (PCA) and spent some time teaching her about this preoperatively. M kept her infusion until she was able to manage her pain control with a simple compound analgesic. She made a quick postoperative recovery and said she had experienced far less pain than with her previous operations. She had also felt reassured that pain relief would be there as soon as she needed it.

Box 26.4

Risk factors for postoperative nausea and vomiting (PONV)

- Obesity
- Age: older age is associated with a decreased risk of PONV
- Female gender
- Prior history of travel sickness
- High preoperative anxiety
- Type of surgery
- Anaesthetic agent used

Based on data from Jolley (2001).

Women are three times more likely to experience PONV than men (Jolley 2001). Gynaecological and abdominal procedures have an increased risk because of mechanical disturbance to the gut during surgery (Jolley 2000). In orthopaedic surgery, the use of opioids in extradural infusions has been linked to the high incidence of PONV (Alexander & Fennelly 1997). Patients undergoing gynaecological and orthopaedic procedures have an incidence of above 40% (Jolley 2000). Patients receiving thiopental as an induction agent are more likely to experience PONV than those who receive propofol (Jolley 2001) and spinal and regional blocks are less likely to cause PONV than general anaesthetics. There is some evidence to suggest that smokers are at less risk of PONV (Chimbria & Sweeney 2000).

PONV is exacerbated when patients have pain and inadequate pain relief (Thompson 1999). Quinlan (2002) reports that relief of postoperative pain is usually associated with relief of nausea. Unfortunately, PONV is also a common side-effect of opioid analgesics.

A period of prolonged starvation can cause PONV but so also can inadequate preoperative fasting and the collection of secretions in the stomach. Paralytic ileus can lead to the accumulation of a large quantity of gastrointestinal secretions. Following some surgery, e.g. partial gastrectomy, patients may have some bleeding into the stomach postoperatively which can induce nausea.

Postoperative hypotension is another common cause of PONV which can be avoided by helping patients to move in bed or sit up slowly. Jolley (2000) advocates the use of a risk assessment tool by nurses and anaesthetists. Thomas et al (2002) compared two PONV risk assessment tools and found nurses greatly underestimated the actual incidence of PONV.

Although it remains unclear which risk factors, in combination or alone, are most likely to lead to PONV (Thompson 1999), the effect of unresolved PONV is not insignificant. Patients are at risk of complications such as aspiration, dehydration, electrolyte imbalance and pain. Patients may also suffer psychological effects such as distress, shame and embarrassment (Jolley 2001). This has been shown to heighten anxiety prior to subsequent surgery. Assessment and management should be performed using a tool or treatment algorithm. The cause of PONV should be identified and an appropriate antiemetic used prophylactically and regularly. Studies show that of 75% patients prescribed antiemetics, only 56% were administered any medication (Ernst 1994). Caution must be taken with the administration of metoclopramide as this promotes gut motility and should be avoided in a patient who has obstructed. Ming et al (2002) found that PONV can be reduced by the use of acupressure bands on the wrist. Small studies have evaluated the use of complementary therapies such as inhalations (Tate 1997, Merritt et al 2002) and ginger root preparations (Visalyaputra et al 1998) but so far have been inconclusive. It is important, however, that patients be made aware preoperatively that PONV is not an inevitable outcome of anaesthesia, and that medication can and will be provided.

Sleep

Closs (1992) argued that surgical patients have very disrupted sleep patterns. In addition to factors affecting the sleep of all hospital patients, surgical patients are exposed to pain, general discomfort and restricted positioning. Postoperative patients may experience hypoxia and hypercapnia due to anaesthetic sedation or shock, severely compromising CNS control of sleep patterns (see Ch. 25). Opioids can alter normal sleep patterns (Dawson et al 1999). Typically, patients report dropping off to sleep and feeling they have slept for hours, only to find that just a few minutes have passed. Some patients will be distressed by this and nursing staff can support and reassure them, explaining that this is a common but temporary side-effect of the analgesic. It is important to ascertain whether the patient has stopped using their PCA or asking for analgesics in an effort to relieve this symptom, because this will cause an exacerbation of pain. For many patients, the presence of a nurse during this wakeful period may be all that is required. In the postoperative period, frequent observations and recordings are necessary, often into the first postoperative night. These disturbances, along with the general noise generated by procedures, new admissions and emergency action that may occur, all add to the disruption of patients' sleep.

Sleep is especially important for the postoperative patient as the all-important protein synthesis for optimal recovery takes place predominantly during sleep and rest. Growth hormone is secreted during periods of rapid eye movement (REM) sleep. Sleep and rest are therefore essential, not only for a feeling of well-being, but also for anabolism and tissue repair. Older patients are especially vulnerable as they have fewer physiological reserves and may have concurrent and chronic illness. Equilibrium is disturbed by lack of sleep and this may be related to development of delirium in some postoperative older patients (Bowman 1997).

Pain control and general comfort measures are paramount in promoting a good night's sleep. Bowman (1997) noted the impact made when nurses modified the environment to promote sleep, and suggests that warmth and effective pain control facilitate natural sleep in older patients.

The measurement of O_2 saturation via pulse oximetry can be useful to indicate night hypoxia in vulnerable patients, e.g. those who have had thoracic or abdominal surgery; however, oximeters require careful use to prevent undue disturbance. Nursing observations should be minimised to safe levels and noise reduced where possible.

Elimination

Postoperative constipation is a common problem which arises as a consequence of immobility, the use of opioid analgesics and dehydration. Conversely, diarrhoea can occur as postoperative temporary ileus resolves, but normal bowel function should resume spontaneously in a few days. Patients may experience colicky pain due to flatus and muscle spasm; this can be reduced by increasing mobility and offering peppermint water (see Table 26.7). Ensuring adequate hydration and early activity help prevent constipation before it becomes necessary to resort to oral laxatives.

Urinary retention may occur due to immobility, the relaxation of bladder muscle tone caused by anaesthesia, or as the result of temporary ileus following abdominal or pelvic surgery. When urinary retention is anticipated, the patient should be catheterised in theatre to minimise discomfort. Otherwise, patients should be given the opportunity for privacy and assistance to assume a normal position to pass urine where possible. If retention leads to distension of the bladder and discomfort, or is a cause for concern, urinary catheterisation may be carried out.

Once the temporary ileus resolves, as detected by return of bowel sounds or passage of flatus or faeces, the urinary catheter is usually removed. If the catheter is used for monitoring in haemodynamic shock, or in retention due to immobility, it can be removed when monitoring is no longer required or the patient is sufficiently active to pass urine successfully.

Use of urinary catheters should be avoided where possible due to the associated risk of infection (Winn 1996, NHS Quality Improvement Scotland 2004b). The postoperative patient may also be at risk of urinary infection without catheterisation, as a result of immobility when a small volume of concentrated urine may remain in the bladder for prolonged periods, providing a medium for the growth of bacteria.

Following some surgical procedures on the bladder, for example transurethral resection of the prostate (TURP), continued blood loss and clot formation may obstruct the urethra. To prevent this, patients are catheterised with a three-way/triple lumen catheter and continuous bladder irrigation given to wash out potentially obstructing clots or debris (see Ch. 8).

Wound care

Wound care is given with the aim of promoting healing and minimising the risk of infection (see Nursing Care Plan 26.4). Buggy (2000) argues that 9–27% of patients undergoing colorectal surgery acquire a wound infection. Methods of promoting healing depend on the individual patient's circumstances. Factors that should be considered, especially with the surgical patient, are prolonged hypoxia due to shock, dehydration or local pressure, protein calorie malnutrition, and the local wound dressing. Factors to be considered in all patients with regard to wound healing are discussed in Chapter 23.

Prevention of infection begins in the preoperative period with reduction of anxiety, and skin and, if necessary, bowel preparation (see p. 914). Asepsis in theatre reduces the threat of exogenous infection (see p. 915). Tissue perfusion of the incision site during surgery is thought to be an important factor in influencing wound healing (Buggy 2000). Good tissue perfusion ensures that oxygen, neutrophils, nutrients for cellular regrowth and systemically administered antibiotics are carried to the incision site. However, tissue perfusion during surgery may be diminished because blood loss and manipulation of body structures aggravate the stress response, causing vasoconstriction of the skin, gut and renal vessels. The anaesthetist aims to reduce the impact of the stress response by maintaining the patient's tissue perfusion during the operation. This is done by increasing oxygen delivery during and after surgery, administering optimal fluid replacement therapy and avoiding hypothermia (Buggy 2000).

The use of wound drains and aseptic technique, along with precautions against haematoma formation, will help to reduce wound infections postoperatively. However, some patients will be more at risk of infection than others, depending on the type of surgery and on exposure to endogenous bacteria (see Table 26.8). In the immediate postoperative period, the wound and any drains in the operation site must be checked frequently for signs of bleeding. To assess the degree of soakage on a wound dressing, a ballpoint or felt-tipped pen can be used to mark the margin of the soakage. Any advancing margin can then be easily detected. Volume markings on drainage bottles and bags give a clear indication of the amount of blood or fluid lost. Large volumes of bloodstained fluid may be due to the fluid used to wash out a cavity but this should still be reported. Wound dressings should not be changed if they become soaked with blood; instead, fresh pads should be added on top to promote clot formation beneath both dressings. To disturb dressings on the first or second postoperative day also increases the risk of infection. The patient's nutritional status and wound healing are necessarily closely linked. Patients who are malnourished preoperatively are at risk of delayed healing and have increased susceptibility to wound or systemic infection. Early postoperative nutritional support clearly improves healing (Collins 1996) (see p. 928).

Wound drains

The aim of wound drains is to drain blood and inflammatory exudate, to prevent haematoma formation and infection, and to give an indication of blood loss. Some drains may have suction applied to collapse the space left in the

Table 26.8 Risk of infection in different types of surgery*

Type of surgery	Percentage of patients with infected wounds (% risk)	Example of types of operation
Clean: hollow organs not opened, no preoperative inflammation or infection	2–5	Inguinal hernia repair, mastectomy, total hip replacement
Clean contaminated: hollow organs (not bacteriologically clean, e.g. respiratory and urinary tract) opened	5–10	Transurethral resection of prostate, pneumonectomy, elective cholecystectomy
Contaminated: in areas known to be heavily contaminated, e.g. lower GI tract or in the presence of infection	10–50	Large bowel surgery, traumatic wounds, abscesses

*For further reading, see Mangram et al (1999) and Ayliffe et al (2000).

tissues after an operation. Drains can also indicate when an anastomosis has broken down by discharging blood, digestive or faeculent fluid and, when an abscess has resolved, the cessation of discharge of pus. Some examples of the more common types of wound drain are given in Figure 26.4.

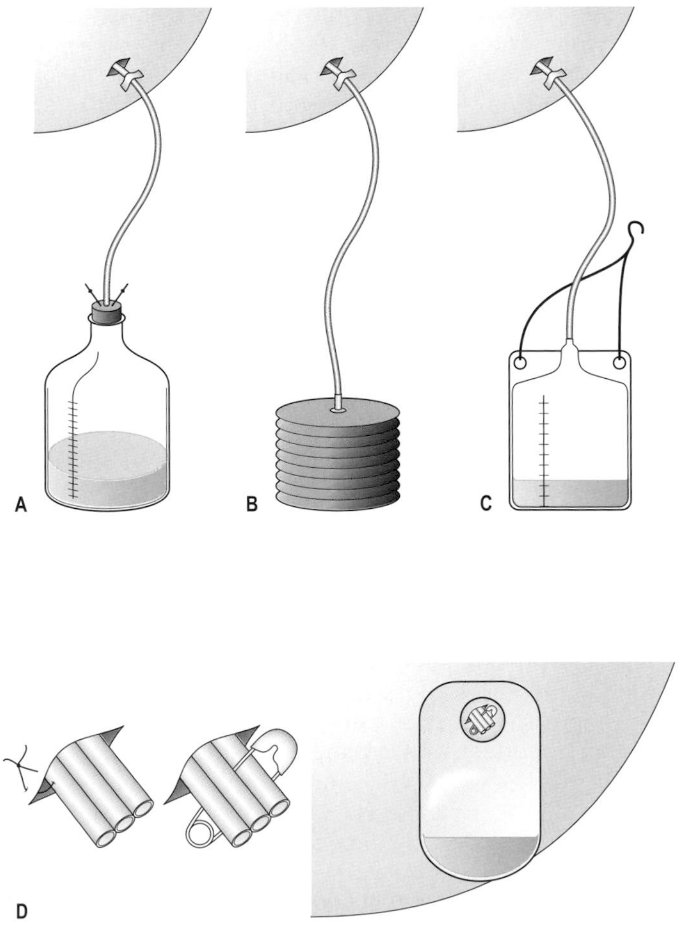

Fig. 26.4 Some types of wound drain A: Redivac drain (prongs come together as vacuum is lost). B: Concertina-type drain. C: Simple tube/Penrose drain. D: Corrugated drain: secured by a suture and then a safety pin as the drain is shortened to prevent it from falling back into the patient. Fluid drains down the channels and into a bag.

To prevent infection, the entry site should be dressed aseptically and a closed drainage system maintained. If bags or bottles need to be changed, e.g. when the vacuum is lost or the receptacle is full or heavy, then asepsis must be maintained and sterile equipment used.

The decision to remove the drain is made by the doctor when there is minimal or no further drainage. Non-vacuum drains may be shortened before removal to encourage the space left behind to collapse and granulate, otherwise a cavity might be left that could fill with fluid and give rise to an abscess. Before a drain is removed, the procedure should be explained to the patient and careful assessment performed as analgesics may be required (Critical Care Extra: Critical Questions 1999). Relaxation exercises can help to reduce the patient's anxiety and muscle tension. Vacuum drains should have their suction released and the securing sutures removed. Shortened drains should be secured to prevent them slipping below the skin surface; alternatively, a large, sterile safety pin can be passed through the tube to prevent this from occurring. Drains that do not move smoothly may be eased by rotating the tube slightly. Traction should not be applied to drains if they are fixed or tethered. Such cases must be referred to the medical staff.

After the first 24 h, the wound and drains should be checked to ensure optimal healing is occurring. As stated previously, wound dressings should not be disturbed for the first 48 h to reduce the risk of infection. However, most infections typically do not appear until at least 3 days postoperatively. Regular temperature monitoring may also detect signs of infection. Patients discharged within the first 2 days after an operation should be taught how to recognise a wound infection and know how to report it. Mr A was advised to inspect his scrotal suture area for redness, oozing or swelling postoperatively. He was advised to inform his GP if symptoms occurred. Community and practice nurses may continue checks on patients with wounds who have been discharged home early.

After 48 h, wounds healing by 'primary intention' have laid down a layer of epithelium across the wound. The wound is effectively sealed from exogenous infection and may be left exposed, which allows for easy observation. Dressings are not necessary unless the wound has been closed with clips or staples that may catch on clothing or there is continued discharge from the wound. Some wounds may be left to heal by 'secondary intention' due to lack of

Box 26.5

Examples of factors that may predispose patients to delayed wound healing

Mrs B (see Case History 26.2)
- High risk of wound infection due to:
  - perforated bowel
  - unprepared bowel
- Anaemia (preoperative)
- Malnutrition and dehydration (preoperative) and fasting (postoperative)
- Prolonged shock (postoperative)
- Immunosuppression (due to cancer and prolonged stress)
- Age

M (see Case History 26.4(A) and 26.4(B))
- Steroid therapy (pre- and postoperative)
- Contamination of wound (bowel opened and infection present)
- Low body fat/protein reserves
- Pre-existing inflammatory condition

tissue to close the wound or to the presence of infection in the tissues, where closure may well lead to abscess formation. Care of such of wounds is discussed in Chapter 23.

Wounds heal at different rates according to growth rate and blood supply of the local tissues and the patient's general physical condition (see Box 26.5). Clips would be removed from a thyroidectomy incision line at 2–3 days postoperatively, whereas Mrs B's abdominal sutures were not removed until 10 days postoperatively. There is an increasing trend towards the use of absorbable continuous sutures where good healing is expected. This is especially useful when the patient is to be discharged home in the first few days. Most patients are also relieved to hear that their sutures do not have to be removed. Patients discharged home with non-absorbable sutures in situ may be referred to the community or practice nurse for their removal and some cosmetic procedures or facial wounds may be closed using adhesive preparations (Davies 1994).

For a description of some common types of suture and their removal, see Jamieson et al (2003).

Potential complications

Virtually all surgical patients will be at some risk of developing deep vein thrombosis (DVT), pulmonary embolism (PE), chest infection and atelectasis. Prevention is the mainstay of care and is described on pages 910–912. Preventive measures such as leg and breathing exercises, thromboembolic deterrent (TED) stockings and s.c. heparin are all continued throughout the postoperative recovery. Early mobilisation contributes significantly to the prevention of these complications. Mrs B's care exemplifies the type of proactive preventive measures required (see Nursing Care Plan 26.3). As with pain, pressure ulcers may deter patients from optimal return to normal activity.

Obese, immunocompromised and older patients are at risk of wound dehiscence, the separation and opening of the wound. Nursing management for a patient whose abdominal wound dehisces is to apply sterile pads which have been saturated with normal saline to prevent the abdominal organs from drying and becoming damaged. Assistance from the surgical team is required rapidly. Reassurance and support of the patient is vital as this can be both distressing and frightening and further surgical intervention is likely. Lewis et al (2001) and Candido (2002) suggest that surgical dehiscence is a major complication of abdominal surgery, carrying with it considerable mortality and morbidity.

For case studies explaining the management of wound dehiscence, see Candido (2002).

Communication

When a patient recovers from a general anaesthetic, the first sense to return is that of hearing. Care of the patient in the recovery room can be enhanced by having aids to communication, such as their hearing aid and glasses, available. A number of patients, especially older people or the very ill, may become and remain confused postoperatively (Bowman 1997). This may be due to the effects of the anaesthetic or to systemic illness. Efforts must be made to detect and treat the cause, and nursing measures to reorientate and minimise confusion should be taken. The use of anticholinergic drugs that cross the blood–brain barrier, such as atropine and hyoscine, should be avoided in older patients as they may cause confusion. Opioid analgesics are undoubtedly the cause of delirium in some patients and non-opioid analgesics, such as diclofenac sodium, might be employed.

Patients with provisional diagnoses are often anxious to speak to the doctor about findings in theatre and their prognosis. When information is not immediately given, a moral dilemma may exist for nursing staff (see p. 907). Patients are often reluctant to raise all their concerns with the consultant or registrar, possibly surrounded by an entourage of junior doctors and medical students on ward rounds. The nurse has an important role to play in clarifying the patient's understanding and answering questions where possible or referring the patient's queries to others. The nurse will require to support both patient and family at this anxious time, particularly if samples have been sent to pathology for diagnosis.

Good communication among professionals in the postoperative period is essential. Medical and nursing staff must rely on one another for information and advice in order to provide a coordinated plan of care. Other health professionals, such as physiotherapists and dietitians, also have an important role to play in a patient's postoperative recovery.

Body image

Body image is the mental picture we hold of our body and its functions. This is influenced not only by physical appearance but also by our attitude towards ourselves (Bredin 1999). Gibson (2001) suggests that body image consists of three essential components:

- body reality — an individual's actual physical appearance

- body ideal — how an individual wishes their body to be
- body presentation — an individual's efforts to find a compromise between body reality and ideal.

Body image forms part of our total self-concept and, as such, can have enormous impact on psychological, sociocultural and physical concepts of self. Body image can be altered by a change in physical appearance, such as when a patient undergoes amputation of a limb (Gibson 2001), or when something causes an individual to change their attitude towards their body, for example following a diagnosis of cancer (Bredin 1999), or a combination of both these factors. If this alteration leads to a negative self-concept, educational and psychological support will be necessary to help the patient regain a positive self-concept. Mr W's body image became very positive after his operation as his appearance was restored in line with cultural values such as youth, health, beauty, intactness and vigour. His ability to provide for his family was restored and he felt he would be seen by his workmates as able to cope with all aspects of his job again. Fortunately, the practice nurse had already provided education to correct his misconception about the operation's effect on his sex life and fertility.

M needed much psychological support from her named nurse. She understood how a vaginal fistula had formed and how it could be treated, but felt that her sexual relationships and ability to have children might be affected. She could not come to terms with the continuous loss of fluid through her vagina and having to wear large incontinence pads. She associated wearing the pads with babies and the debilitated older patients she had seen in the wards previously. She felt everyone could see the pads and could detect an unpleasant odour. The named nurse provided a 'listening ear' for M so that she could talk about her fears and her relationship with her new boyfriend. The nurse also comforted and reassured her.

Mrs B recovered from the anaesthetic to find herself attached to lines and tubes, loosely draped in a hospital gown and, worst of all, wearing a colostomy bag. As Mrs B went to theatre as an emergency, there was no time to prepare her for this. At first, she was acutely distressed by the stoma and refused to look at it. She was only able to begin to accept it and learn about it once she learned that, in her particular case, it could be reversed in several months' time. Her attitude towards her body was also influenced by knowing that she had had cancer. Mrs B saw cancer as stigmatising and she felt that everyone would know she had a bag and why. Her self-esteem was severely threatened. Mrs B's stoma care plan (see Nursing Care Plan 26.3, p. 924) outlines the care planned by the named nurse to help her cope with this threat.

For information on the physical and psychological management of patients undergoing stoma surgery, see Black (1997) and Borwell (1997).

Mrs B had a considerable need for education but required support, often given non-verbally through touch or simply by having someone with her before she was able to assimilate the information. The stoma nurse visited Mrs B in hospital to offer expert advice, to begin to establish a relationship and to plan her home care following discharge. The therapeutic role of the nurse in offering psychological support should not be underestimated (Jenkinson 1996).

It is not only patients with obvious outward structural changes in appearance who experience a change in body image. Perceived or actual alterations in function can change individuals' body image and self-concept, such as patients who experience changes in libido and sexual functioning following hysterectomy (Walsgrove 2001).

DISCHARGE PLANNING

Discharge plans aim to provide a smooth transition from hospital to home for continued patient care, often called seamless care, and should be considered from the time of admission. However, decreasing lengths of hospital stay have reduced the time available for nurses to meet patients' post-discharge needs. Inadequate discharge planning can lead to patients being readmitted because they are unprepared for self-care (Maramba et al 2004). Communication is fundamental to the process of collaborative discharge planning. However, Anderson and Helms (1995) found that information passed to the community carers on discharge was of poor quality and often late. Maramba et al (2004) suggest that a designated discharge coordinator who implements a discharge protocol can facilitate this process by providing consistent advice and initiating referrals.

In a busy surgical ward there is often an urgent need for beds, which can lead to hasty and poorly planned discharge. All patients are referred to their GP on discharge from hospital by the surgeon (see Figs 26.1 and 26.2). The nurse will decide whether the patient also needs to be referred to the community nurse. Referrals can be made for nursing interventions ranging from wound care to providing psychological support for the patient and family where there is a poor prognosis. If patients are able to attend the health centre or clinic for wound dressing procedures, then arrangements for an appointment can be made before discharge. It should be remembered, when starting a patient on a course of treatment, that not all wound dressing materials are available in the community.

However, as indicated, information for community nurses is not merely procedural or task centred; the patient's emotional state, mobility, social circumstances and informational needs are also included. Raiwet et al (1997) argue that care maps covering the whole patient care episode, including community care, can facilitate continuity of care. A personal telephone call, a copy of the care plan on discharge, or a visit by the community nurse to the ward can all be useful. Mrs B's stoma nurse had visited her in hospital on several occasions prior to discharge and had liaised closely with her named nurse to ensure she was well prepared to go home.

Forward planning and continuous responsibility as an element of primary nursing may help nurses to achieve the goal of effective discharge preparation. This has been given greater significance by the growth of day surgery where the necessity for discharge planning is heightened, and responsibilities are often taken by lay carers (Mitchell 2003).

Discharge education

Patient teaching for discharge begins on or before the day of admission to hospital. Mr W had received a booklet at his preoperative visit which helped him plan for convalescence at home. He also had learned, from his practice nurse, about healthy diet, interventions to help him stop smoking and about expected function and return to work.

For further reading on patient education, see Naidoo & Wills (2000) or Ewles & Simnett (2003).

Patients require specific information to continue their recovery from surgery, but the opportunity for more general health education should also be taken. The opportunity to teach patients about their care on discharge may be limited, as with day-case patients, or more prolonged, as during an inpatient stay after major surgery. Information may also be given to relatives, with consent from the patient, to enable them to continue support at home (Mitchell 2003). Heseltine and Edlington (1998) implemented a telephone follow-up service which allowed nurses to respond to patients' questions about pain relief and to clarify any points in their postoperative recovery. This also allowed an audit of patient satisfaction with the care they received, and of the follow-up service. Mr A received only a local anaesthetic to his groin area. He was advised to use cold packs for 5–10 min on the local area for the first 1–2 days postoperatively. He was advised that some local swelling and bruising was common but that any sign of bleeding or extensive swelling should be referred to his GP. The family planning nurse suggested that if he required to contact his GP he should highlight that he had undergone vasectomy surgery that day.

Some patients may be quite unsure, or have misconceptions, about how they should progress during their recovery at home. In day case surgery it is essential that patients understand that the anaesthetic may take a full 24 h to be eliminated from the body. Therefore they must not drive home from hospital, should be accompanied for the first 24 h after surgery and should not drive to work the following morning. Some individuals expect to feel fully fit and to be able to care for themselves immediately on discharge. According to Correa at al (2001), following day surgery, patients may be 'home ready' but not 'street ready'. Advice may be given such as:

- Do not drink alcohol.
- Do not drive a motor vehicle.
- Have a responsible adult stay overnight with you.
- Do not make important decisions for 24 h following a general anaesthetic, regional anaesthetic and/or i.v. sedation.

Nurses should be aware that there is a high rate of failure to follow such recommendations, but cooperation is always enhanced if patients can understand the importance of this advice. Many will feel a little insecure without the presence of the nurse and feel anxious about their health (Mitchell 2002). Cooper (1999) suggests that taking home tape recordings made of their consultation for ready reference may be helpful for some.

Mrs B was to return home for several months before the surgeon would consider reversing her colostomy. She had to be independent in caring for her stoma and so required staged teaching and much support (see Nursing Care Plan 26.3). She had a booklet to reinforce the teaching given by the nurses, which also acted as a focus for discussions of the stoma with her daughter. The stoma nurse had given Mrs B a telephone number and promised to visit her in her own home in the next week.

All patients should be clear about seeking advice or treatment from the most appropriate source on discharge. Referral to community nurses and GPs, when possible, establishes continued support and may be preferable to telling patients just to ring the ward.

REHABILITATION

Rehabilitation of the patient does not take place exclusively in either hospital or home, but is nonetheless an increasing focus of care in the community setting. The needs of patients in terms of recovery from surgery do not differ dramatically from the time they leave hospital to their arrival at home. Discharge from hospital is therefore a stage in patient care, involving transfer of care from one setting to another. The plan of care for the discharged patient may thus address similar factors to that of the patient who continues recovery in hospital. Many interventions described in the sections on postoperative care will be equally relevant to the patient in hospital or at home.

Rehabilitation can be a lengthy process, requiring continued support by community nurses, or a short event with minimal professional intervention. There are increasingly sophisticated services such as community high dependency nursing teams who can provide care for ventilated patients in the long term. Mrs B was visited by the health visitor to assess whether she needed any additional support at home. She was also visited regularly by the stoma care nurse whom she had first met in hospital. Mr A recovered well at home and was able to undertake all of his normal daily activities. As his surgery was on Friday, he 'took it easy' over the weekend, avoiding any lifting or exertion such as carrying shopping bags, or golf clubs, and vacuum cleaning. His incision site and surrounding area were tender but this responded well to paracetamol 1 g, taken every 6 h. He avoided aspirin or ibuprofen in case of bleeding problems. His stitches were absorbable, eliminating the need to attend his GP surgery, and he sent semen samples to the hospital at 11 and 15 weeks as arranged. After the second sample Mr A was informed by the laboratory that his results were 'all clear' and that he could discontinue contraception. At work Mr W talked to an occupational health nurse about resuming a full range of duties.

The demands made by postoperative patients upon the community nursing services have increased greatly in recent years. This is partly due to an ageing population making greater demands on the service. Older people are known to be vulnerable on discharge and are more likely to have contact with community nurses (Dash et al 1996). The trend towards day case surgery and early discharge (see p. 901) places more responsibility for postoperative care in the hands of community health care workers. A phenomenological study by Edwards (2002) provides an insightful glimpse into the difficulties experienced by a group of older patients following elective orthopaedic surgery. One patient felt the nurses had 'washed their hands' of after-care. Edwards (2002) advocates flexible support such as telephone helplines run by specialist nurses and 'drop in' clinics, e.g. NHS Direct or NHS 24 (see 'Useful websites', p. 943).

Jester and Turner (1998) describe a 'hospital at home' scheme which facilitated early discharge into the care of a multiprofessional care team.

Trends towards increased day surgery have been driven partly by public demand. In 1991, the Audit Commission reported that 80% of day case patients preferred this option. A number of studies (Otte 1996, Heseltine & Edlington 1998, Hunt et al 1999) support this. An increasing number of patients are therefore recovering from surgery at home.

Patients undergoing surgery require a range of care from nurses in both the hospital and community settings, in both the pre- and postoperative periods. Whilst care can often appear to be focused on performing tasks in a standardised manner, it has been proposed in this chapter that patients enter the surgical experience for a wide variety of reasons with differing health care needs. The nurse is ideally placed not only to coordinate and humanise the surgical experience, but also to facilitate a safe and speedy recovery in an individualised manner.

REFERENCES

Agu O, Hamilton G, Baker D 1999 Graduated compression stockings in the prevention of venous thromboembolism. British Journal of Surgery 86: 922–1004

Alderson P 1995 Consent to surgery: the role of the nurse. Nursing Standard 9(35): 38–40

Alexander R, Fenelly M 1997 Comparison of ondansetron, metoclopramide and placebo as premedicants to reduce nausea and vomiting after major surgery. Anaesthesia 52(7): 695–698

Amaragiri S V, Lees T A 2001 Elastic compression stockings for prevention of deep vein thrombosis (Cochrane Review). In: The Cochrane Library, Issue 3. Wiley, Chichester

Anderson M, Helms L 1995 Communication between continuing care organisations. Research in Nursing and Health 18: 49–57

Anon 1996 Recommended practice for skin preparation of patients. Association of Peri-operative Registered Nurses' Journal 64(5): 813–816

Armstrong D, Bortz P 2001 An integrative review of pressure relief in surgical patients. Association of Peri-operative Registered Nurses 73(3): 645, 647–648

Arnold A 2002 DVT prophylaxis in the perioperative setting. British Journal of Perioperative Nursing 12(9): 326–332

Audit Commission 1997 Anaesthesia under examination. Audit Commission, London

Audit Commission 2001 Day surgery: review of national findings, No 4. TSO, London

Audit Commission and the National Health Service in England and Wales 1991 Measuring quality: the patient's view of day surgery. HMSO, London

Ayliffe G A, Fraise A P, Geddes A M et al (eds) 2000 Control of hospital infection: a practical handbook, 4th edn. Oxford University Press, New York

Baxter C M, Brennan M G, Coldicott Y G M 2002 The practical guide to medical ethics and law. MPG Books, Bodmin

Beddows J 1997 Alleviating preoperative anxiety in patients: a study. Nursing Standard 11(37): 35–38

Beier-Holgersen R, Boesby S 1996 Influence of post operative enteral nutrition on post surgical infections. Gut 39(6): 833–835

Bernier M J, Sanares P C, Owen S V et al 2003 Pre-operative teaching received and valued in a day surgery setting. Association of Peri-operative Registered Nurses, Journal 77(3): 563–582

Biley F C 1989 Perceptions of stress in pre-operative patients. Journal of Advanced Nursing 14(7): 575–581

Boore J R P 1978 Prescription for recovery. Royal College of Nursing, London

Booth S 2002 A philosophical analysis of informed consent. Nursing Standard 16(39): 43–46

Bove L A 1994 How fluids and electrolytes shift after surgery. Nursing 94: 34–39

Bowman A M 1997 Sleep satisfaction, perceived pain and acute confusion in elderly clients undergoing orthopaedic procedures. Journal of Advanced Nursing 26(3): 550–564

Bradshaw M 2001 Guidelines to consent for examination or treatment to support the Countess of Chester Hospital Consent to Treatment Policy. Countess of Chester Hospital NHS Trust, Chester

Bradshaw P W, Ley P, Kinnay J 1975 Recall of medical advice, comprehensibility and specificity. British Journal of Sociology and Clinical Psychology 14: 55–62

Brandberg A, Anderson I 1980 Whole body disinfection. Royal Society of Medicine International Congress and Symposium, Series 23. Academic Press, London

Bredin M 1999 Mastectomy, body image and therapeutic massage: a qualitative study of women's experience. Journal of Advanced Nursing 29(5): 1113–1120

Breen P 2000 DVT: what every nurse should know. Registered Nurse 63(4): 58–63

British Thoracic Society 1997 Pulmonary embolism: treatment guidelines. Thorax 52(Suppl 4)

Brooks G 1997 Advance directives, current legal and ethical issues. Nursing in Critical Care 2(1): 25–28

Buggy D 2000 Can anaesthetic management influence surgical wound healing? Lancet 356(9227): 355–357

Byrne B 2001 Deep vein prophylaxis: the effectiveness and implications of using below knee or thigh length graduated compression stockings. Heart and Lung 30(4): 277–283

Calligaro K D, Miller P, Dougherty M J et al 1996 Role of nursing personnel in implementing clinical pathways and decreasing hospital costs for major vascular surgery. Journal of Vascular Nursing 14(3): 57–61

Campling E A, Devlin H B, Hoile R W, Lunn J N 1995 The report of the national confidential enquiry into perioperative deaths. NCEPOD, London

Candido L C 2002 Treatment of surgical wound dehiscence. Dermatology Nursing 14(3): 177–178, 181

Capper C 1999 External pneumatic compression therapy for deep vein thrombosis prophylaxis. British Journal of Theatre Nursing 9(3): 109–111

Caumo W, Schmidt A P, Schneider C N, Bergmann J 2001 Risk factors for postoperative anxiety in adults. Anaesthesia 56(8): 720–728

Chapman A 1996 Current theory and practice: a study of preoperative fasting. Nursing Standard 10(18): 33–36

Chen H H, Wexner S D, Weiss E G, Iroatulam A J 1998 Laparoscopic colectomy for benign colorectal disease is associated with a significant reduction in disability as compared with laparotomy. Surgical Endoscopy 12: 1397–1400

Chimbria W, Sweeney B P 2000 The effect of smoking on postoperative nausea and vomiting. Anaesthesia 55(6): 540–544

Chowdhury M, Varma S, Roberts D L et al 2000 Audit of patient satisfaction with surgical services. British Journal of Dermatology 143(57)(Suppl): 107–108

Closs S J 1992 Patients' night-time pain, analgesic provision and sleep after surgery. International Journal of Nursing Studies 29(4): 381–392

Coleridge Smith P D, Hasty J H, Schurr J H 1991 Deep vein thrombosis: effects of graduated compression stockings on distension of the deep veins of the calf. British Journal of Surgery 78: 724–726

Collins C M 1996 Nutrition and wound healing. Care of the Critically Ill 17(3): 87–90

Cook D J, Rooke G A 2003 Priorities in perioperative geriatrics. Anesthesia and Analgesia 96(6): 1823–1836

Cooper J 1999 Teaching patients in post operative eye care: the demands of day surgery. Nursing Standard 13(32): 42–46

Cornwell E E, Chang D, Velmahos G et al 2002 Compliance with sequential compression device prophylaxis in at-risk trauma patients: a prospective analysis. American Surgeon 68(5): 470–473

Correa R, Menezes R B, Wong J et al 2001 Compliance with post operative instructions. A telephone survey of 750 day surgery patients. Anaesthesia 56(5): 481–484

Costa M J 2001 The lived peri-operative experience of ambulatory surgery patients. Association of Peri-operative Registered Nurses' Journal 74(6): 874–881

Coulter A, Entwhistle V, Gilbert D 1999 Sharing decisions with patients: is the information good enough? British Medical Journal 318(7179): 318–322
Crawford B 1999 Highlighting the role of the perioperative nurse: is perioperative assessment necessary? British Journal of Theatre Nursing 3(4): 12–15
Crenshaw J, Winslow E 2002 Preoperative fasting. Old habits die hard: research and published guidelines no longer support the routine use of 'NPO' after midnight but the practice persists. American Journal of Nursing 102(5): 36–44
Critical Care Extra: Critical Questions 1999 Patients' experience of tube removal. American Journal of Nursing 99(8): 24
Dash K, Zarle N C, O'Donnell L, Vince Whiman C 1996 Discharge planning for the elderly: a guide for nurses. Springer, New York
Davies J E 1994 Tissue adhesive: use and application. Emergency Nurse 2(2): 16–18
Dawes P J D 1997 Thromboembolic prophylaxis and ENT surgery. Clinical Otolaryngology 22(1): 1–2
Dawson L, Brockbank K, Carr E et al 1999 Improving patients' postoperative sleep: a randomised control study comparing subcutaneous with intravenous patient controlled analgesia. Journal of Advanced Nursing 30(4): 875–881
Dean A, Fawcett T 2002 Nurses' use of evidence in preoperative fasting. Nursing Standard 17(2): 33–37
Department of Health 2000a The NHS plan: creating a 21st century NHS. TSO, London
Department of Health 2000b Comprehensive critical care planning and managing critical care capacities. Detailed models can provide information for making good decisions. TSO, London
Department of Health 2001a Inpatient and outpatient waiting in the NHS. Report by the Comptroller and Auditor General. HE 221 Session 2001–2002. National Audit Office, London
Department of Health 2001b Good practice in consent implementation guide: consent to examination or treatment. TSO, London
Di Fronzo A L, Nader Y, Kaushal P et al 2003 Benefits of early hospital discharge in elderly patients undergoing open colon resection. Journal of the American College of Surgeons 197(5): 747–752
Donovan H S, Ward S 2001 A representational approach to patient education. Journal of Nursing Scholarship 33(3): 211–216
Dooley F 1999 The named nurse in practice. Nursing Standard 13(34): 33–38
Dougherty L, Lister S 2004 The Royal Marsden Hospital manual of clinical nursing procedures, 6th edn. Blackwell, Oxford
Editorial 1983 Preoperative depilation. Lancet 1: 311
Editorial 2003 The role of covering gowns in reducing rates of bacterial contamination of scrub suits. Obstetrical and Gynaecological Survey 58(9): 582–583
Edwards C 2002 A proposal that patients be considered honorary members of the health care team. Journal of Clinical Nursing 11(3): 340–348
Elliot Pennels C 1998 Consent and adults. Professional Nurse 13(4): 252–253
Ernst E M C 1994 The economics of quality care: postoperative nausea and vomiting. Direct Publishing Solutions, Cookham
Everitt N, McMahon M 1994 Nutrition in the surgical patient. In: Heatley R V, Green J H, Losowsky M S (eds) Consensus in clinical nutrition. Cambridge University Press, Cambridge
Feo C, Romanini B, Sortini D et al 2004 Early oral feeding after colorectal resection: a randomised controlled study. Australian and New Zealand Journal of Surgery 74(5): 298–301
Field J 2002 Feeding patients after abdominal surgery. Nursing Standard 16(48): 41–44
Fletcher J P, Batiste P 1997 Incidence of deep vein thrombosis following vascular surgery. International Angiology 16(1): 65–68
Flinn W R, Sandager G P, Silva M B et al 1996 Prospective surveillance for perioperative venous thrombosis. Archives of Surgery 131(5): 472–480
Frakes M A 2003 Rapid sequence induction medications: an update. Journal of Emergency Nursing 29: 533–540
Gagliese L, Katz J, Melzack R 1999 Pain in the elderly. In: Wall P D, Melzack R (eds) The textbook of pain, 4th edn. Churchill Livingstone, Edinburgh
Gammon J, Mulholland C W 1996 Effect of preparatory information prior to elective total hip replacement on post-operative physical coping outcomes. International Journal of Nursing Studies 33(6): 589–604
General Medical Council 2001 Standards of practice, 3rd edn. GMC, London
Gibson J 2001 Lower limb amputation. Nursing Standard 15(28): 47–55
Gillies T E, Ruckley C V, Nixon S J 1996 Still missing the boat with fatal pulmonary embolism. British Journal of Surgery 83: 1394–1395
Good M 1996 Effects of relaxation and music on postoperative pain: a review. Journal of Advanced Nursing 24: 905–914
Greenland S 1995 A review of the uses of epidural analgesia. Nursing Standard 9(32): 32–35
Greerts W H, Heit J A, Claget C P et al 2001 Prevention of venous thromboembolism. Chest (Suppl) 119(1): 132–175
Haddock J, Burrows C 1997 The role of the nurse in health promotion: an evaluation of a smoking cessation programme in surgical pre-admission clinics. Journal of Advanced Nursing 26(6): 1098–1110
Hahn T W, Morgensen T, Land C et al 2003 Analgesic effect of IV paracetamol: possible ceiling effect of paracetamol in postoperative pain. The ACTA Anaesthesiological Foundation 47(2): 138–145
Hamilton Smith S 1972 Nil by mouth. Royal College of Nursing, London
Hayward J 1975 Information: a prescription against pain. Royal College of Nursing, London
Heseltine K, Edlington F 1998 A day surgery post-operative telephone call line. Nursing Standard 13(9): 39–43
Hilditch W G, Asbury A J, Crawford J M 2003 Preoperative screening: criteria for referring to anaesthetists. Anaesthesia 58(2): 117–124
Holte K, Kehlet H 2002 Postoperative ileus: progress towards effective management. Drugs 62(18): 2603–2615
Hong J Y, Lee I H 2003 Suprascapular nerve block or a piroxicam patch for shoulder tip pain after day case laparoscopic surgery. European Journal of Anaesthesiology 20(3): 234–238
Hui A C, Heras-Palon C, Dunn I et al 1996 Graded compression stockings for prevention of deep vein thrombosis after hip and knee replacement. Journal of Bone and Joint Surgery 78: 550–554
Hunt K 1995 Perceptions of patients' pain: a study assessing nurses' attitudes. Nursing Standard 10(4): 32–35
Hunt L, Luck A J, Rudlin G et al 1999 Day case haemorrhoidectomy. British Journal of Surgery 86(2): 255–258
Hurford W E 2000 Techniques for endotracheal intubation. International Anesthesiology Clinics 38(3): 1–28
Hyde R, Bryden F, Asbury A J 1998 How would patients prefer to spend the waiting time before their operations? Anaesthesia 53(2): 192–195
Ingram J E 2003 A review of thigh length versus knee length anti-embolism stockings. British Journal of Nursing 12(14): 845–851
Janknegt R, Pinckaeris J W, Rohof M H et al 1999 Double blind comparative studies of droperidol, granisetron and granisetron plus dexamethasone as prophylactic antiemetic therapy in patients undergoing abdominal, gynaecological, breast or otolaryngological surgery. Anaesthesia 54(11): 1059–1068
Jeffery P C, Nicolaides A N 1990 Graduated compression stockings in the prevention of deep vein thrombosis. British Journal of Surgery 77(4): 380–383
Jenkinson T P 1996 The nurse as significant other for surgical patients. Professional Nurse 11(10): 651–652
Jester R, Turner D 1998 Hospital at home: the Bromsgrove experience. Nursing Standard 12(20): 40–42
Jester R, Williams S 1999 Pre-operative fasting: putting research into practice. Nursing Standard 13(39): 33–35
Jolley S 2000 Post-operative nausea and vomiting: a survey of nurses' knowledge. Nursing Standard 14(23): 32–34
Jolley S 2001 Managing post operative nausea and vomiting. Nursing Standard 15(40): 47–53
Kakkar V V, Boeckl O, Boneu B et al 1997 Efficacy and safety of a low-molecular-weight heparin and standard unfractionated heparin for prophylaxis of postoperative venous thromboembolism: European Multicenter Trial. World Journal of Surgery 21(1): 2–9
Kaplan C, Mendiola R, Ndjatou V et al 2003 The role of covering gowns in reducing rates of bacterial contamination of scrub suits. Obstetrical and Gynaecological Survey 58(9): 582–583
Kavanagh R T, Radhakrishnan D, Park G R 1995 Crystalloids and colloids in the critically ill patient. Care of the Critically Ill 11(3): 114–119
Kehlett H, Morgensen T 1999 Hospital stay of 2 days after open sigmoidectomy with multimodal rehabilitation programme. British Journal of Surgery 86(7): 968–969
Kurz A, Sessler D, Lenhardt R 1996 Perioperative normothermia to reduce the incidence of surgical-wound infection and

shorten hospitalization. New England Journal of Medicine 334(19): 1209–1215
Law M 1997 A telephone survey of day surgery eye patients. Journal of Advanced Nursing 25: 355–363
Lawrentschuk N, Hewitt P M, Fracs P M 2003 Elective laparoscopic cholecystectomy: implications of prolonged waiting times for surgery. Australian and New Zealand Journal of Surgery 73(11): 890–893
Leung J M, Dzankic S 2001 Relative importance of pre-operative health status versus intraoperative factors in predicting post-operative adverse outcomes in geriatric surgical patients. Journal of the American Geriatrics Society 49(8): 1080–1085
Lewis S J, Egger M, Sylvester P A, Thomas S 2001 Early enteral feeding versus 'nil by mouth' after gastrointestinal surgery: systematic review and meta analysis of controlled trials. British Medical Journal 323(7316): 773–776
Lisko S A 1995 Development and use of videotaped instructions for pre-operative education of the ambulatory gynaecological patient. Journal of Post Anaesthesia Nursing 10(6): 32–48
Ljungqvist O, Nygren J, Thorel A, Hansel J 2000 Pre-operative nutrition therapy: novel developments. Scandinavian Journal of Nutrition 44: 3–7
Lord Chancellor's Department 1997 Who decides? Making decisions on behalf of mentally incapacitated adults: a consultation paper. Lord Chancellor's Department, London
Lovett P E, Stanlon S L, Hennessy D et al 1994 Pain relief after major gynaecological surgery. British Journal of Nursing 3(4): 159–162
Lucas B 2004 Nursing management issues in hip and knee replacement surgery. British Journal of Nursing 13(13): 782–787
Macintyre P E, Ready L B 2001 Acute pain management. A practical guide. Saunders, London
Mackintosh C, Bowles S 1997 Evaluation of a nurse led acute pain service. Can clinical nurse specialists make a difference? Journal of Advanced Nursing 25: 355–363
Macrae W A 2001 Chronic pain after surgery. British Journal of Anaesthesia 87(1): 88–98
Mangram A J, Horan T C, Pearson M L et al 1999 Guideline for prevention of surgical site infection. American Journal of Infection Control 27(2): 97–134
Manias E 2003 Pain and anxiety management in the postoperative gastro-surgical setting. Journal of Advanced Nursing 41(6): 585–594
Maramba P J, Richards S, Larrabee J H 2004 Discharge planning process: applying a model for evidence-based practice. Journal of Nursing Care Quality 19(2): 123–129
Markham R, Smith A 2003 Limits to patient choice: examples from anaesthesia. British Medical Journal 326(7394): 863–864
Martin D 1996 Pre-operative visits to reduce patient anxiety: a study. Nursing Standard 10(23): 33–38
Mason P 2002 Remifentanil. Intensive and Critical Care Nursing 18(6): 355–357
Mathieson A 2000 Factors affecting the use of research in practice. Professional Nurse 15(6): 406–407
McEwen D 1996 Intraoperative positioning of surgical patients. Association of Peri-operative Registered Nurses Journal 63(6): 1059–1079
McIlwain J C 1999 Clinical risk management: principles of consent and patient information. Clinical Otolaryngology 24(4): 255–261
McIntyre F J, McCloy R 1994 Shaving patients before operation: a dangerous myth? Annals of the Royal College of Surgeons of England 76: 3–4
Merritt B A, Okyere C P, Jasinski D M 2002 Isopropyl alcohol inhalation: alternative treatment of post-operative nausea and vomiting. Nursing Research 51(2): 125–128
Ming J C, Kno B I T, Lin J G 2002 The efficacy of acupressure to prevent nausea and vomiting in post-operative patients. Journal of Advanced Nursing 39(4): 343–351
Mitchell M 1997 Patients' perception of preoperative preparation for day surgery. Journal of Advanced Nursing 26(2): 356–363
Mitchell M 2002 Guidance for the psychological care of day case surgery patients. Nursing Standard 16(40): 41–43
Mitchell M 2003 Impact of discharge from day surgery on patients and carers. British Journal of Nursing 12(7): 402–407
Moccia M 2000 Using the ECG to identify pulmonary embolism. Dimensions of Critical Care Nursing 19(3): 27–31
Moran S, Kent G 1995 Quality indicators for patients' information in short stay units. Nursing Times 91(4): 37–40
Mordue A 1994 Thresholds for treatment in cataract surgery. Journal of Public Health Medicine 16(4): 393–398
Morris J 1995 Monitoring post-operative effects in day surgery patients. Nursing Times 91(10): 32–34
Murakami M, Tandace L, Cindrick-Pounds L et al 2003 Deep venous thrombosis prophylaxis in trauma, improved compliance with a novel miniaturised pneumatic compression device. Journal of Vascular Surgery 38(5): 923–927
Murphy G S, Ault M L, Wong A Y, Szokol J W 2000 The effect of a new NPO policy on operating room utilization. Journal of Clinical Anesthesia 12(1): 48–51
Nelson S 1996 Pre-admission education for patients undergoing cardiac surgery. British Journal of Nursing 5(6): 335–340
NHS Quality Improvement Scotland 2004a Best Practice Statement: Postoperative pain management. Online. Available: www.nhshealthquality.org
NHS Quality Improvement Scotland 2004b Best Practice Statement: Urinary catheterisation and catheter care. Online. Available: www.nhshealthquality.org
Nicklin J L, Franzcog C 2002 Thromboembolic complications in gynaecologic surgery. Clinical Obstetrics and Gynaecology 45(2): 545–552
Nursing and Midwifery Council (NMC) 2004 Code of professional conduct: standards for conduct, performance and ethics. NMC, London
O'Cathain A, Sampson F, Munro J et al 2004 Nurses' views of using computerized decision support software in NHS Direct. Journal of Advanced Nursing 45(3): 280–286
O'Dowd A 2004 Analysis. Nursing Times 100(27): 12–13
O'Neill E S, Dluhy N M 2000 Utility of structured care approaches in education and clinical practice. Nursing Outlook 48(3): 132–135
Otte D I 1996 Patients' perspectives and experiences of day case surgery. Journal of Advanced Nursing 23(6): 1228–1237
Paavilainen E, Seppanen S, Asted-Kurki P 2001 Family involvement in perioperative nursing of adult patients undergoing emergency surgery. Journal of Clinical Nursing 10(2): 230–237
Panda N, Bajaj A, Pershad D et al 1996 Pre-operative anxiety, effect of early or late position on the operating list. Anaesthesia 51(4): 344–346
Parnaby C 2004 A new anti-embolism stocking: use of below-knee products and compliance. British Journal of Perioperative Nursing 14(7): 302–307
Perkins F, Kehlet H 2000 Chronic pain as an outcome of surgery: a review of predictive factors. Anesthesiology 93(4): 1123–1133
Phillips S, Hutchinson S, Davidson T 1993 Preoperative drinking does not affect gastric contents. British Journal of Anaesthesia 70(1): 6–9
Pissara P H 2001 Recognising the various presentations of appendicitis. Dimensions of Critical Care Nursing 20(3): 24–27
Porteus M J, Nicholson E A, Morris L T et al 1989 Thigh length versus knee length stockings in the prevention of deep vein thrombosis. British Journal of Surgery 76: 296–297
Pullen M 1998 Supporting patients with Crohn's disease. Nursing Times 94(39): 63
Quinlan S 2002 Sick and tired. Nursing Standard 17(13): 24
Raiwet C, Halliwell G, Andruski L, Wilson D 1997 Care maps across the continuum. Canadian Nurse 93(1): 26–30
Rawal N 1998 Postoperative pain management in day surgery. Anaesthesia 53(2) (Suppl): 50–52
Retchen S M, Penberthy L, Desch C et al 1997 Perioperative management of colonic cancer under Medicare risk programs. Archives of Internal Medicine 157: 1878–1884
Richards A, Edwards J 2003 A nurse's survival guide to the ward. Churchill Livingstone, Oxford
Richardson J 2001 Postoperative epidural analgesia: introducing evidence based guidelines through an education and assessment process. Journal of Clinical Nursing 10(2): 238–245
Roper N, Logan W, Tierney A 2000 The Roper–Logan–Tierney model of nursing: the activities of living model. Churchill Livingstone, Edinburgh
Rosenthal R A, Kavic S M 2004 Assessment and management of the geriatric patient. Critical Care Medicine 32(4) (Suppl): S92–S105
Royal College of Surgeons and College of Anaesthetists 1990 Report of the working party on pain after surgery. Royal College of Surgeons, London
Schaldach D E 1997 Measuring quality and cost of care: evaluation of an amputation clinical pathway. Journal of Vascular Nursing 15(1): 13–20

Scott E, Earl C, Leaper D et al 1999 Understanding perioperative nursing. Nursing Standard 13(49): 49–54
Scottish Executive 2003a Partnership for care: Scotland's health. White Paper. TSO, Edinburgh. Online. Available: www.scotland.gov.uk/library5/health/pfcs-00.asp
Scottish Executive 2003b NHS code of practice on protecting patient confidentiality. TSO, Edinburgh
Scottish Intercollegiate Guidelines Network (SIGN) 2002 Prophylaxis of venous thromboembolism. SIGN, Edinburgh
Sear J 2003 Implication of aging on anaesthetic drugs. Current Opinion in Anaesthesiology 16(4): 373–378
Selye H 1976 The stress of life, 2nd edn. McGraw-Hill, New York
Seropian R, Reynolds B M 1971 Wound infections after preoperative depilatory versus razor preparation. American Journal of Surgery 121: 251–254
Shade P 1992 PCA: can client education improve outcomes? Journal of Advanced Nursing 17: 408–413
Sheppard M, Wright M 2000 Principles and practice of high dependency nursing. RCN/Baillière Tindall, Edinburgh
Sherwood G D, McNeil J A, Stark P I et al 2003 Changing acute pain management outcomes in surgical patients. Association of Peri-operative Registered Nurses' Journal 77(2): 374–395
Sjostrom B, Dahlgren L O, Haljamae H 2000 Strategies used in post operative pain assessment and their clinical accuracy. Journal of Clinical Nursing 9: 111–118
Small S 1996 Preoperative hair removal: a case report with implications for nursing. Journal of Clinical Nursing 5(2): 79–84
Smith G D, Watson R 2005 Gastrointestinal nursing. Blackwell Publishing, Oxford
Somasekar K, Shankar P J, Foster M E, Lewis M H 2002 Costs of waiting for gall bladder surgery. Postgraduate Medical Journal 78(155): 668–671
Steven A 1999 Named nursing: in whose best interest? Journal of Advanced Nursing 29(2): 341–347
Sutcliffe A, Potter A 2002 Multidisciplinary preadmission clinics for orthopaedic patients. Nursing Standard 16(21): 39–42
Tate S 1997 Peppermint oil: a treatment for post-operative nausea. Journal of Advanced Nursing 26(3): 543–549
Teasdale K 1993 Information and anxiety: a critical reappraisal. Journal of Advanced Nursing 18: 1125–1132
Thomas R, Jones N S, Strike P 2002 The validity of risk scores for predicting post-operative nausea and vomiting when used to compare patient groups in a randomised control trial. Anaesthesia 57(11): 1119–1128
Thomas S 1999 Graduated compression and the prevention of deep vein thrombosis (part 1). Journal of Wound Care 8(1): 41–43
Thompson H J 1999 The management of postoperative nausea and vomiting. Journal of Advanced Nursing 29(5): 1130–1136
Thompson K, Melby V, Parahoo K et al 2003 Information provided to patients undergoing gastroscopy procedures. Journal of Clinical Nursing 12(6): 899–911
THRIFT 1992 Thromboembolic Risk Factors Consensus Group. Risk of and for prophylaxis for venous thromboembolism in hospital patients. British Medical Journal 305: 567–574
THRIFT II 1998 Second Thromboembolic Risk Factors Consensus Group. Risk of and prophylaxis for venous thromboembolism in hospital patients. Phlebology 13: 87–97
Town J 1997 Bringing acute abdomen into focus. Nursing 97(5): 52–57
Vemuri C, Wainess R M, Dimick J B et al 2004 Effect of increasing patient age on complication rates following intact abdominal aneurysm repair in the United States. Journal of Surgical Research 118(1): 26–31
Visalyaputra S, Petchpaisit N, Somcharoen K et al 1998 The efficacy of ginger root in the prevention of postoperative nausea and vomiting after outpatient gynaecological laparoscopy. Anaesthesia 53(3): 506–510
Walker J A 2003 Care of the post-operative patient, Part 1. Professional Nurse 18(11): 615–616
Walsgrove H 2001 Hysterectomy. Nursing Standard 15(29): 47–55
Warner M A, Warner M E, Weber J G 1993 Clinical significance of pulmonary aspiration during the perioperative period. Anesthesiology 78(1): 56–62
Watts S, Brooks A 1997 Patients' perceptions of the pre-operative information they need about events they may experience in the intensive care unit. Journal of Advanced Nursing 26(1): 85–92
Williams A M, Davies P R, Sweetnam D I S et al 1996 Knee length versus thigh length graduated compression stockings in the prevention of deep vein thrombosis. British Journal of Surgery 83: 1553
Wills V L, Hunt D R 2002 Pain after laparoscopic cholecystectomy. British Journal of Surgery 87(3): 273–284
Winn C 1996 Basing catheter care on research principles. Nursing Standard 10(18): 38–40
Yuill G M, Sanya D, Yuill S L 2003 A national survey of the provision for patients with latex allergy. Anaesthesia 58(8): 775–777

FURTHER READING

Ayliffe G A, Fraise A P, Geddes A M, Mitchell K (eds) 2000 Control of hospital infection: a practical handbook, 4th edn. Oxford University Press, New York
Black P 1997 Practical stoma care. Nursing Standard 11(47): 49–53
Booth S 2002 A philosophical analysis of informed consent. Nursing Standard 16(39): 43–46
Borwell B 1997 Psychological considerations of stoma care nursing. Nursing Standard 11(48): 49–53
Candido C L 2002 Treatment of surgical wound dehiscence. Dermatology Nursing 13(3): 177–181
Cox F 2002 Making sense of epidural analgesia (NT Plus: Pain supplement. Postoperative pain management). Nursing Times 98(32): 56–58
Ewles L, Simnett I 2003 Promoting health: a practical guide, 5th edn. Baillière Tindall, Edinburgh
Garden O J, Bradbury A W, Forsythe J 2002 Principles and practice of surgery, 4th edn. Churchill Livingstone, Edinburgh
Gibson J E 1997 Focus of nursing in critical and acute settings: prevention or cure. Intensive and Critical Care Nursing 13: 163–166
Greenland S 1995 A review of the uses of epidural analgesia. Nursing Standard 9(32): 32–35
Griffiths R V 1999 Anaesthesia: breathing management. British Journal of Theatre Nursing 9(11): 537–539
Hughes S 2002 The effects of giving patients pre-operative information. Nursing Standard 16(28): 33–37
Jamieson E M, McCall J M, White L A 2003 Clinical nursing practices: guidelines for evidence-based practice, 4th edn. Churchill Livingstone, Edinburgh
Johnson S 1997 Pathways of care. Blackwell Science, Oxford,
Kay R, Siriwardena A K 2001 The process of informed consent for urgent abdominal surgery. Journal of Medical Ethics 27: 157–161
Macintyre P E, Ready L B 2001 Acute pain management. A practical guide. Saunders, London
Mangram A J, Horan T C, Pearson M L et al 1999 Guideline for prevention of surgical site infection. American Journal of Infection Control 27(2): 97–134
Markanday L (ed) 1997 Day surgery for nurses. Whurr, London
McDonnell A, Nicholl J, Read S M 2003 Acute pain teams in England: current provision and their role in post-operative pain management. Journal of Clinical Nursing 12(3): 387–393
Mottram A 2001 Pre-registration student nurses' perceptions of the day surgery unit. Ambulatory Surgery 9(2): 103–107
Myers C 1997 Stoma care nursing: a patient centred approach. Arnold, London
Naidoo J, Wills J 2000 Health promotion: foundations for practice. Baillière Tindall, Edinburgh
National Association of Theatre Nurses 1998 Principles of safe practice in the perioperative period. NATN Publications, Harrogate
Paavilainen E, Seppanen S, Asted-Kurki P 2001 Family involvement in perioperative nursing of adult patients undergoing emergency surgery. Journal of Clinical Nursing 10(2): 230–237
Rogers S N, Naylor R, Potter L 2000 Three years' experience of collaborative care pathways on a maxillofacial ward. British Journal of Oral and Maxillofacial Surgery 38: 132–137
Salter M (ed) 1997 Altered body image: the nurse's role. Wiley, Chichester
Sheppard M, Wright M 2000 Principles and

practice of high dependency nursing. RCN/Baillière Tindall, Edinburgh
Smith S 1996 Discharge planning: the need for effective communication. Nursing Standard 10(38): 39–41
Starritt T 1999 Back to basics: patient assessment in recovery. British Journal of Theatre Nursing 9(12): 593–595
Stewart C E 1999 Airway management with rapid sequence intubation: Part 1. Online. Available: www.emsmagazine.com/articles/airwayart.html
Sutherland E 1996 Day surgery – a handbook for nurses. Baillière Tindall, London
Waller D G, Renwick A G, Hillier K 2001 Medical pharmacology and therapeutics. Saunders, Edinburgh

USEFUL WEBSITES

NHS 24 (Scotland)
tel: 08454 242424
www.nhs24.co.uk

NHS Direct (England and Wales)
tel: 0845 4647
www.nhsdirect.nhs.uk

NHS Quality Improvement Scotland
www.nhshealthquality.org

THE PATIENT WHO EXPERIENCES TRAUMA

27

Lorrie Lawton

INTRODUCTION

Every year, 15 million patients attend Emergency Departments (ED) in England and Wales (Audit Commission 2001). They present with a wide variety of injuries or conditions, some that may be considered as life threatening and others that are relatively minor. This means that nurses working within an ED environment are required to have a broad knowledge base and a wide range of skills to enable them to meet the needs of all patients. This chapter considers this diverse nature of emergency nursing. As many of the medical and surgical conditions have been discussed in other chapters of this book, this chapter will focus on the concept of trauma. It will outline the process of triage, which includes the concept of 'see and treat'. This concept is based around the principle that the first clinician is able to treat and discharge the patient (Heyworth & Holt 2002).

Two case studies will be used to highlight the principles of emergency nursing care and will examine what is meant by trauma, by exploring the range of injuries that may be encountered by an ED nurse, whilst highlighting key principles of care. The case studies will focus on:

- the care of a patient who has multiple injuries and who therefore requires immediate resuscitation
- the care of a patient who attends with a minor injury and who is assessed, diagnosed, treated and discharged independently by a nurse.

Whilst trauma accounts for a large proportion of ED work, it is important to consider other distinct areas of practice that require specific skills to enable the nurse to meet both the patient's and the family's physical and psychosocial needs. Bereavement is an extremely sensitive and emotional area of emergency nursing, as relatives and friends have had no opportunity to anticipate or prepare themselves for their sudden loss. Principles of caring for families during their crises will be explored with specific reference to the loss of a baby as a result of sudden infant death syndrome (SIDS). It is also important to acknowledge the ED staff's personal needs during these difficult periods, and the concept of critical incident stress debriefing (CISD) will be outlined.

The Emergency Department provides an interface between the community and the hospital setting. Operating an 'open door' philosophy confronts the ED nurse with many practical and ethical challenges, which are often linked to wider sociological and political issues. Strategies that may be adopted to prevent incidents of violence and aggression will be discussed and the Emergency nurse's responsibility to the law highlighted. The dynamic nature of the ED environment means that the workload is often unpredictable and Emergency nurses have to be prepared for the unexpected. For this reason, a section of this chapter is devoted to the key aspects of an Emergency Department's response to disasters, which involve large numbers of casualties. Also considered is the subsequent psychological impact this may have on the survivors, their families, the witnesses and the rescuers and health care workers involved, both at the scene of the disaster and within the hospital environment. Throughout the chapter, the importance of patient and family involvement in the planning and delivery of nursing care will be emphasised.

Trauma

Trauma may be defined as any physical wound or injury. It can be caused by a variety of accidents, but may also be self-inflicted or result from acts of violence. The impact of traumatic events on victims, witnesses and staff may also cause psychological problems long past the event itself (Van Der Kolk 1998) (see 'Post-traumatic stress disorder', p. 962).

The severity of the wound or injury may be as minor as a simple graze, which can be self-treated within the home environment, or one which requires more specialised treatment in a hospital Emergency Department. Conversely, the trauma victim may present with life-threatening multiple injuries, such that they are vulnerable to imminent death within the initial hours following the traumatic event. In England alone, 873 000 people are admitted to hospital each year via Emergency units, following an injury (Department of Health 2003a). Trauma is the main cause of death in young people. Annually in the UK, 14 500–18 000 deaths occur as a result of trauma, with 60 000 patients being admitted to hospital each year as a result of a road traffic collision (RTC) (Bonnett et al 2003). Whilst there has been legislation to reduce the number of accidents, e.g. the wearing of seat belts for car users, helmets for motorcyclists, drink driving laws (Hill 1990) and the Health and Safety at Work Act (Health and Safety Commission 1974, still extant), society can still view risk-taking behaviour as a positive characteristic so that these measures are not always adhered to (Brannon & Feist 2004). Despite this, statistically there has been a reduction in the incidence of trauma, but still the cost to the health and social services of caring for injured people is £1.2 billion/year (Department of Health 2002a). It is for this reason that Emergency nurses must be able to meet the immediate needs of patients who attend with both life-threatening and less serious conditions.

Reception in the Emergency Department

The ED is designed to accommodate patients who arrive by a variety of means and who present with a diversity of problems. Within the NHS it is generally accepted that the general practitioner (GP) is the primary source of medical care through which patients are referred to hospital facilities and specialist practitioners. Those who require acute specialist care will more often than not be admitted through the ED and will be seen and assessed by the relevant medical or surgical team. However, patients present to the ED via other channels. With the knowledge that they can gain immediate access to hospital facilities without GP referral, many individuals self-present to the ED. Other patients are referred via occupational health services and schools. Generally, more seriously ill or injured patients will arrive via the local ambulance service by road transport; however, there is an increase in the use of helicopters within the United Kingdom to transfer seriously injured or ill people to hospital (Black et al 2004). Usually these patients arrive singly, but on occasion, as in the case of RTCs that involve several vehicles, there will be many patients arriving at one time, often with injuries of differing severity.

For this reason the ED environment must be flexible. The physical division of any department facilitates this. There are usually two points of access to the ED, one for ambulance patients, which provides direct access into the clinical area, and one for other patients which leads into a reception and waiting area. In most units there are separate areas allocated to treat patients with minor injuries and areas that contain individual examination cubicles for those who require a more thorough examination. All departments have a designated resuscitation area for those patients who present with life-threatening conditions. Larger departments may have separate plaster areas, theatres for minor operations and specially equipped cubicles for eye and dental problems. In departments where children are seen, it is recommended that there are separate waiting areas and cubicles which are suitably decorated and equipped to meet the needs of children (Royal College of Nursing 2003).

Although the concept of triage, which involves the nursing assessment of the patient's illness or injury to determine a priority of care, is still utilised in some emergency departments, the process of 'see and treat' is now being used more widely throughout the country (Cooke et al 2002). The key principles of 'see and treat' are that upon arrival in the Emergency Department patients are seen, treated and referred or discharged by one clinician. This clinician may be a member of the nursing team. Therefore, the nurse must be able to make autonomous clinical decisions about treatment, investigations and discharge. More seriously ill patients, or those who require more in-depth assessment or treatment, should be taken to, and treated in, a separate area (Department of Health 2002b).

In order for members of the nursing team to be able to practise 'see and treat' competently, they need to have excellent interpersonal as well as clinical and diagnostic skills, thus allowing the pertinent information to be collated. For medicolegal reasons this information needs to be documented in a clear and logical manner (Nursing and Midwifery Council 2004). One way to organise this information is by using a model, which means that all nurses working within its framework use the same guidelines (Sbaih 1992). One framework that can be used is based upon the medical model (Talley & O'Connor 2000) (see Box 27.1).

In order to make a correct diagnosis, the most important skill that a nurse needs to develop is one of obtaining a clear and concise history from the patient. The nurse initially must establish why the person has attended the Emergency Department. This will establish the presenting complaint (PC). It is then important to determine the history of the presenting complaint (HPC), i.e. how the injury occurred, known as the mechanism of injury. The mechanism of injury will assist the nurse in making a provisional diagnosis and enable a decision to be made on which investigations are required, e.g. X-rays and the administration of analgesics. Working within protocols allows nurses, on reaching the limit of their expertise, to refer on to another clinician, either an Emergency Nurse Practitioner (ENP) or doctor.

Box 27.1

Medical model used in assessing minor trauma

PC	—	presenting complaint
HPC	—	history of presenting complaint
PMH	—	past medical history
DH	—	drug history including allergies
SH	—	social history, including living arrangements and activities of daily living
O/E	—	on examination — includes all the major systems
CVS	—	cardiovascular system
CNS	—	central nervous system
RS	—	respiratory system
MS	—	musculoskeletal system
GIT	—	gastrointestinal tract
GUS	—	genitourinary system
IMP	—	impression of information gained
DD	—	differential diagnosis based upon the information gained
Plan	—	what investigations, e.g. X-rays etc., are needed to confirm or refute the differential diagnosis. Also includes the treatment that is needed

Adapted from Talley & O'Connor (2000).

Box 27.2

Trimodal distribution of death following trauma

First peak
Mortality during this peak occurs very shortly after the time of injury and usually at the scene of the incident. The person's injuries are so grave that no resuscitative intervention would be successful. The primary way of avoiding such deaths is through accident prevention programmes such as drink driving campaigns and seat belt legislation.

Second peak
Mortality occurs hours after the incidence of trauma and patients may die from airway, breathing and circulatory problems. Many of these deaths are preventable during this period, which is commonly known as the 'golden hour' — the period during which the patient is in the resuscitation room of an Emergency Department.

Third peak
Mortality occurs days or weeks following the initial incident and patients may die from multi-organ failure, acute respiratory distress syndrome (ARDS) or sepsis.

Adapted from Bonnett et al (2003).

Many benefits of the 'see and treat' process have been identified:

- There is a significant reduction in the time that each patient has to wait (Cooke et al 2002). This therefore improves the patient's experience within the ED, by improving the flow through the department and reducing the number of steps that the patient goes through.
- There is also an indication that this has improved job satisfaction for nursing staff (Department of Health 2002b). However, in order for the 'see and treat' process to be in place, considerable educational resources must be available to enable the nursing staff to learn about the process of assessment, the requesting of X-rays and the administration of analgesics. Specific protocols must also be written, to allow the 'see and treat' nurse to have clear parameters within which to work.
- The process of 'see and treat' can be used in conjunction with a simplified triage system. For example, if there is an influx of patients, they will go through the 'see and treat' process, following which a priority allocation can be given to each patient to be seen by either the ENP or a doctor. The Manchester Triage (Manchester Triage Group 1997) is seen nationally as an effective system of prioritisation.

IMMEDIATE TREATMENT OF EMERGENCIES

In 1988, The Royal College of Surgeons of England identified that approximately one-third of emergency-related deaths were preventable and were often due to hypoxia, continuing haemorrhage and missed diagnosis. Bonnett et al (2003) describe a 'trimodal distribution' of death which identifies three peaks following trauma when casualties die as a result either of their injuries or of subsequent events (see Box 27.2). For these reasons it is important that any ED is fully prepared to receive any patient, no matter how severely injured, at any time of the day or night.

It is also vital that there is a predetermined system, such as the advanced trauma life support (ATLS) protocols (American College of Surgeons 2004), to guide personnel through the initial assessment of the patient, enabling them to identify any life-threatening conditions quickly and to treat them appropriately. Patients admitted with such life-threatening injuries will be cared for in a resuscitation area which is designed to have the necessary equipment readily available and the space to enable a trauma team, consisting of nurses, doctors and a radiographer, to care for the patient efficiently and effectively (see Fig. 27.1).

The trauma team

Effective staffing is as important as the organisation of equipment. Having too many people in the resuscitation room may be as problematic as having too few, as overcrowding can lead to confusion and delays. A trauma team consists of an integrated group of nurses and doctors who are needed to ensure that there is an efficient and organised resuscitation approach. There should be a system of identifying, from the total nursing staff in the department, a group of at least three nurses who will contribute to the team in the resuscitation room. Both a nurse and a doctor lead the team.

The aim of resuscitation is to stabilise the patient, identify injuries and initiate a definitive management plan. It has been shown that the most efficient resuscitation will occur if a 'horizontal organisation' approach is adopted (Bonnett et al 2003). This is when each member of the team carries out individual tasks simultaneously rather than sequentially. This reduces the time taken to resuscitate a patient and

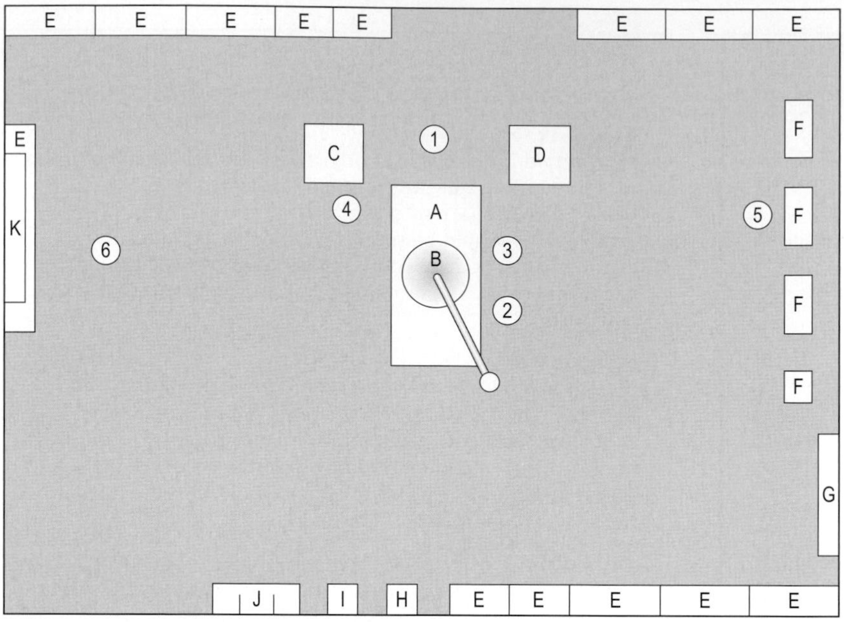

Fig. 27.1 Organisation of the resuscitation room.

initiate life-saving procedures, which will improve the patient's chances of survival. For this to be successful, each member of the team must be aware of his or her precise role, which will have been designated by the team leaders. The size of the team will depend on the size of the individual department. As well as the designated nurses, there will be either an ED consultant or a senior doctor from the ED and an anaesthetist and surgeon on call. An example of the responsibilities of each nursing team member can be seen in Box 27.3.

On the patient's arrival at the ED, an initial history will have been received from the ambulance crew, but further information may become available with the arrival of relatives or friends. Collecting this information should, where possible, be the responsibility of a fourth nurse who can act as liaison between the trauma team and the patient's family or friends. The paramedics routinely leave a copy of their clinical documentation for the patient with the ED.

The advanced trauma life support (ATLS) system

To care effectively for seriously injured patients, they must be rapidly assessed, their injuries identified and any life-threatening conditions immediately treated. Within the ED environment, this includes completing a primary and, where possible, a secondary survey to ensure a full assessment is made. Within the primary survey, an ABCDE process is followed to ensure that logical and sequential treatment priorities are identified:

A — Airway maintenance, with protection of the cervical spine
B — Breathing and ventilation
C — Circulation, with haemorrhage control
D — Disability, which involves a neurological assessment
E — Exposure of the patient, ensuring that the environment is optimal to prevent further hypothermia.

If any life-threatening condition is identified during the process, it is treated before moving on to the next stage, e.g. if the patient is found to have a compromised airway, this is stabilised before the patient's breathing and ventilation are assessed.

Box 27.3

Responsibilities of nursing members of a trauma team

Nurse One
This nurse will coordinate the team, as well as assisting the other nurses by preparing appropriate equipment as necessary for procedures, and recording any clinical observations and laboratory findings.

Nurse Two
This nurse is often referred to as the airway nurse and has two key responsibilities: first, to assist the anaesthetist in securing and maintaining the patient's airway, whilst protecting the patient's cervical spine; second, to establish a rapport with the patient, giving psychological support whilst in the resuscitation room. Ideally, all information to the patient should be relayed through this nurse.

Nurse Three
This nurse may be referred to as the circulating nurse. Her responsibilities include removing the patient's clothes, attaching the patient to monitors and measuring the patient's clinical vital signs. Subsequently, this nurse will ensure that i.v. access has been established and will be responsible for the patient's fluid requirements. This nurse will also assist with any procedures, e.g. catheterisation, insertion of a chest drain.

The secondary survey is only started when the primary survey is complete and the patient's condition is stabilised. If the patient is critically injured, this secondary survey may not take place in the ED, as the patient is likely to require surgical intervention to stabilise their condition. However, if the patient's condition does permit, then the secondary survey involves a full head-to-toe examination and gives the nurse the opportunity to complete a thorough set of clinical observations, including neurological observations.

The resuscitation room

It is important that the resuscitation area is designed to complement both the assessment principles (e.g. the ATLS protocols) which are to be applied when examining the patient and the team who have to work within its environment. Usually staff are given some warning via their local ambulance service that a patient with severe or life-threatening injuries will be admitted shortly. This may mean that there is little time for preparation before the patient is rushed into the department. It is vital that the resuscitation area is always prepared for such emergencies and it is the nurses' responsibility at all times to ensure that all areas are fully stocked and, at the beginning of each shift, that the equipment is in working order. It is also vital that health and safety issues are considered to prevent any further harm occurring to the patient and to prevent staff becoming inadvertently injured during the haste of a resuscitation. This includes the availability of plastic aprons, disposable gloves and protective goggles for all staff.

Most resuscitation rooms have spacious trolley areas for the team to work in. A policy of keeping 'a place for everything and everything in its place' should be followed, so that staff can learn the location of every item and find anything that is needed immediately. Certain items may be prepared in advance. For example, the cardiac monitor may have its chest electrodes attached, and receivers with the most commonly used blood sample bottles, corresponding forms and large syringes may be kept ready. Clipboards with the usual documentation may also be prepared in advance. As well as the technical life-saving equipment, it is important to ensure that sharps boxes and clinical waste bins are strategically placed so that nurses or doctors do not have to walk far to dispose of their needles and clinical waste. Furthermore, patients vary in size and weight. It is therefore necessary to have a range of appropriate sizes of all equipment stored within the resuscitation area. The arrangement of the resuscitation room and its cupboards should not be changed unless all staff are informed.

Staff must continually update their knowledge of the procedures that may be performed. It is easy to forget skills that are used infrequently, but patients' lives may depend on the rapidity with which certain measures are undertaken. When equipping the resuscitation area it is useful to consider the above-mentioned ABCDE assessment process.

Airway maintenance with protection of cervical spine

Equipment that will help to clear and maintain a patient's airway should be readily available at the head end of the patient trolley. On arrival, the patient's airway should be examined for any type of obstruction and appropriate steps taken to clear it if necessary. Piped suction with a rigid catheter attached will facilitate this process. If the patient is unable to fully maintain their airway, the airway nurse can try several manoeuvres. Manual procedures such as a jaw thrust or chin lift can be done in the immediate instance, but doing this will mean that the nurse is unable to assist the rest of the team. Using adjuncts such as oropharyngeal or nasopharyngeal airways will free the nurse and may be all that is required in the patient who has an altered level of consciousness. The best place to store this equipment is attached to the wall at the head of the patient.

For patients who have more serious injuries, it may be necessary to protect their airway definitively. This is done by an anaesthetist who will intubate the patient using a laryngoscope and endotracheal (ET) tube. Again, if this has to be done as a life-saving measure, the equipment must be to hand. Occasionally it will be necessary to sedate and paralyse the patient to facilitate this process. The anaesthetist will require a range of drugs and the airway nurse should be familiar with the current drugs used and have them ready for immediate use. Once the ET tube is in place, a mechanism for ventilation will be required which must be attached to a high percentage of oxygen via a piped oxygen supply. Ideally, all this equipment should be pre-prepared for rapid use. In patients who have sustained massive facial injuries, a surgical airway may be the only way to oxygenate them adequately. This requires specialist equipment, which, again, should be pre-prepared and ready for immediate use.

Patients who present with multiple injuries have often been involved in high-velocity accidents, e.g. RTCs or falls from a height. It is vital that the patient's cervical spine is protected in in-line immobilisation until the trauma team is sure that the neck is uninjured. This requires the nurse either to support the patient's neck manually or to place a semi-rigid collar around it. Further support is then achieved by placing a sandbag at each side of the patient's face and applying tape across the forehead to the sides of the trolley. The airway nurse must be vigilant in observing the patient for any signs of nausea or vomiting. With the spine immobilised, the patient is unable to move. If vomiting is likely, the team would have to log roll the patient (see p. 951) to protect the spine and assist the patient with suction apparatus.

Breathing and ventilation

The patient's respiration rate must be measured and recorded; this should include the rate, depth and use of any ancillary muscles. However, it is also important to note how effectively the patient is ventilating, i.e. that there is effective gas exchange taking place at the alveolar capillary membrane. All patients who have sustained significant injuries should receive a high flow of oxygen. This can be delivered via a mask with a reservoir bag (non-rebreather oxygen mask) with a flow rate of 12–15 L/min (American College of Surgeons 2004). By the addition of a reservoir bag the patient will receive up to 90% oxygen concentration compared to only 50% oxygen concentration with an ordinary oxygen mask (Resuscitation Council (UK) 2000). Using pulse oximetry enables the nurse to monitor continually the patient's oxygenation saturation of arterial blood so a pulse oximeter should be situated by the trolley side. Usually this is part of an extensive system that monitors the patient's heart rate, blood pressure, respiration rate and oxygen saturation continuously and simultaneously.

There are six immediately life-threatening chest conditions: airway obstruction, cardiac tamponade, tension pneumothorax, massive haemothorax, open chest wound and flail chest (Bonnett et al 2003). If a patient has sustained any of these injuries, immediate treatment will be required and the necessary equipment for chest drain insertion (see Ch. 3, p. 98) or pericardiocentesis (aspiration of fluid from the pericardial sac) must be easily accessible. This type of equipment is usually pre-packed in sterile trays ready for use at a moment's notice. It is the nurse's responsibility to become familiar with the contents of these trays in order to assist the medical staff with any necessary procedures.

Box 27.4

Differing types of intravenous access

Access via peripheral veins
- Veins in the forearm
- External jugular vein
- Femoral vein

Access via the central veins
- Internal jugular vein
- Subclavian vein

Other types of access
- Intraosseous access via proximal tibia
- Cutdown using long saphenous vein of the leg

Adapted from Resuscitation Council (UK) (2000).

Circulation, with haemorrhage control

In severely traumatised patients, the most common circulatory problem is hypovolaemia (see Ch. 18). Any overt bleeding should be controlled by direct pressure using absorbent dressings and bandages. Emergency treatment consists of restoring the circulatory volume as rapidly as possible by the administration of i.v. fluids. One method of estimating the amount of fluid a patient has lost, or is continuing to lose, is to monitor clinical vital signs. This includes regular measurement and recording of the patient's heart rate, blood pressure and respiration rate, which can be done using the technical equipment described above.

Simply observing the patient's skin colour can provide some indication of the degree of shock present, whilst talking to the patient will indicate their current mental status. The greater the blood loss, the paler the patient will look, and as oxygen availability decreases in the blood supply, the patient will become increasingly confused and perhaps agitated (Bonnett et al 2003). Once 50% of total blood volume is lost, the patient will become unconscious. A further guide is the patient's urine output. A catheterisation tray should be readily available and, if the patient has been catheterised, the urine output should be measured at regular intervals using a urometer. The normal urine output for an adult is 30–50 mL/h.

To prevent any deterioration as a result of hypovolaemia, the circulating nurse should ensure that two wide-bore peripheral cannulae are inserted simultaneously into large veins such as the antecubital fossa found at the elbow joint. In some EDs, it is the nurse who has developed the clinical skills to carry out this procedure, ensuring that enough blood is withdrawn for the necessary laboratory investigations to assess the patient's condition. To facilitate this process, sample bottles, forms and large syringes should be prepared and a policy should be in place for the quick transport of samples to the laboratory. Once the peripheral lines have been established, replacement fluids, either crystalloids or colloids, warmed via a warming cabinet to approximately 39°C (American College of Surgeons 2004), must be administered. If the patient appears severely compromised, it may be necessary to use a mechanical pump, e.g. the Level One Blood Warmer, to infuse the fluid more quickly. However, by the time the patient reaches hospital, their peripheral circulation may be 'shut down' (see Ch. 18). This occurs in hypovolaemia as a result of the body's attempt to preserve the vital organs by constricting the peripheral blood vessels and redirecting the available blood to the major organs. Therefore it may be impossible to insert an i.v. cannula in a surface vessel and it may be necessary to perform an i.v. cutdown procedure. This involves making an incision in the skin and subcutaneous tissues and locating a deeper vein in which to insert a cannula. Again, the necessary equipment should be ready (see Box 27.4 for differing types of intravenous access).

In order to monitor the patient's progress, it is important that all findings are recorded at regular intervals. In the initial stages of the resuscitation this may be as frequently as every 5 min. The appropriate charts should be available for the recording of vital signs and fluid balance.

Disability: neurological assessment

It is important that a rapid assessment is made of the patient's neurological status using the AVPU scale. On arrival, it is easy for the airway nurse to determine if the patient is **Alert**, i.e. eyes open and responding, or if they respond only to **Voice**. If the patient does neither of these, then the nurse needs to assess if the patient responds to **Painful** stimuli. If not, the patient is considered to be **Unresponsive**. Concurrently, the nurse should use a torch to assess the patient's pupils to see if they are equal in size and react to light. Again this should be documented as a baseline for future comparison. For a more in-depth neurological assessment, the nurse should proceed to use the Glasgow Coma Scale (see Ch. 28).

Exposure, ensuring environmental control

Whilst the patient's dignity should be preserved as much as is possible, it is essential that all clothing is removed so that the entire body can be examined from head to toe, front and back, to ensure that no injuries are missed. It is important to remember that exposure can cause rapid body heat loss, so it is vital that the resuscitation room temperature is warm enough to preserve the patient's body temperature. The use of warmed blankets, which must be

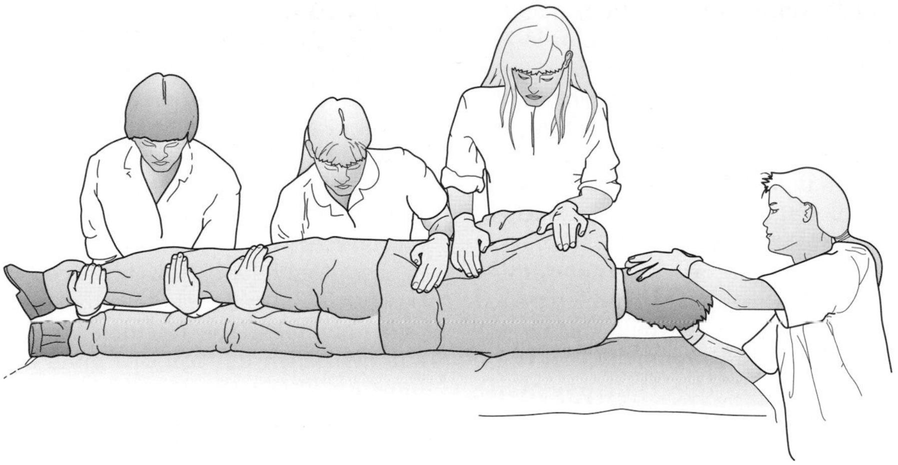

Fig. 27.2 The log roll technique. (Reproduced with kind permission from Lisa Hadfield-Law, Oxfordshire.)

replaced between any procedure or examination, will also prevent further temperature drop. The log roll technique (see Fig. 27.2) should be used to enable full examination of the patient's spine. To ensure total spinal immobilisation, a coordinated approach, using a team of at least four people, is required. The leader of the team will manually immobilise the patient's cervical spine, whilst the three assistants will control the patient's thorax, pelvis and legs.

STOP THINK **27.1** Find out from your mentor or lecturer how to carry out a log roll safely and effectively. Practise this with your fellow students in your clinical laboratory.

A PATIENT WITH MULTIPLE TRAUMA

Assessment and immediate treatment

In Case History 27.1, the ambulance team have informed the Emergency Department by radio patch of J's condition and given an estimated time of arrival of 10 min. The trauma team and radiographer have been summoned and the resuscitation room prepared. Due to the nature of the accident, the paramedics, having safely removed his helmet, immobilised J on a spinal board with full cervical spine immobilisation.

On arrival, J is transferred onto a trolley, which allows X-rays to be taken without moving him. At the same time the paramedics provide an immediate verbal handover outlining the nature of the accident, i.e. speed, involvement of any other vehicles or any other injured patients, and an overview of J's clinical condition during his transportation to hospital. The paramedics later provide a written handover of the incident.

Once transferred, the airway nurse assesses J's airway. She notes that J is now more alert and trying to remove the oropharyngeal airway that is causing him to gag. His airway is clear and there is no overt evidence of facial injuries. J is responding to her voice. Whilst reassuring him, she applies an oxygen mask with reservoir bag attached to 15 L/min of oxygen. She continues to explain to J what is happening to him. Meanwhile the circulating nurse removes J's clothes by carefully cutting them. This allows her to attach the monitor, which will record J's pulse, blood pressure and oxygen saturation, whilst one of the doctors looks, listens to and feels J's chest. The nurse counts J's respiration rate, noting the depth of each breath. All clinical observations are passed to the team leader who records them on a trauma chart. J's breathing appears rapid (24 breaths/min) and laboured and, on inspection, it is found that the left side of his chest is not inflating. His oxygen saturation is 91% despite the high-flow oxygen administration. Palpation of the chest wall reveals swelling and crepitus on the left side, indicating possible fractured ribs and a possible pneumo/haemothorax. To ensure adequate gaseous exchange and tissue perfusion, a chest drain must be inserted (see Ch. 3). This will also prevent mediastinal shift. Whilst the equipment is being prepared by the team leader and the radiographer is taking chest X-rays, the circulating nurse (see Box 27.3) ensures that two wide-bore cannulae are inserted in J's arms and 2 L of Hartmann's solution, warmed to 39°C, are administered rapidly. The blood taken from one of these lines is sent directly to the laboratories for a full blood count, urea and electrolytes, and group and cross-match for at least 6 units of blood. The equipment is prepared and the chest X-ray confirms a haemothorax and three fractures of the lower ribs on the left side. The chest drain is inserted using local anaesthetic and strict asepsis. Its placement is confirmed by X-ray and by visible oscillations in the drainage tube. The amount of blood drained from the chest is carefully measured and recorded. Continued observation of respiratory rate,

CASE HISTORY 27.1

J

J is an 18-year-old man who has been knocked off his motorcycle while travelling at high speed. He was wearing a crash helmet but is unconscious when brought into the department by ambulance. He has an oropharyngeal airway in situ and has been given oxygen by the paramedics. His left leg is splinted from the groin to the toes and a closed fracture of the femur is suspected. The police who were called to the scene of the accident have succeeded in finding identification and are now trying to contact J's family.

rhythm and depth reveals that J's respiration rate has improved (18 breaths/min), with fairly good expansion on both sides. His oxygen saturation is increasing (now measuring 95%). His colour is pale but not cyanosed.

(Note — motorcyclists often wear expensive leather protective clothing. Conscious patients will frequently forbid this clothing to be cut, preferring to suffer pain rather than have their leathers damaged. In a situation such as the one described here, the clothing must be cut to prevent further injury. Care should be taken, however, to cut clothing along the seams if at all possible, so that it can be repaired later. However, the patient's condition will dictate the urgency with which clothing should be removed.)

As J's breathing has stabilised, the circulating nurse is able to palpate J's radial pulse. She notes its rate, which is rapid (120 beats/min); rhythm, which is regular; and strength, which is thready. At the same time she notes that J's skin is cool, clammy and pale. The monitor displays that J is also hypotensive, with a blood pressure of 70/30 mmHg. These recordings show evidence of hypovolaemia (see Ch. 18). There is no overt sign of haemorrhage, although there appears to be an obvious closed fracture to J's left femur and right wrist. J's clinical findings indicate that he may be bleeding internally. Simultaneously, the radiographer has completed pelvic X-rays, and these show no fracture. However, there is bruising over the left upper quadrant of J's abdomen and he is tender on palpation. A ruptured spleen is suspected, as this is often associated with left lower rib fractures. As the spleen is a highly vascular organ, the likelihood is that J has lost a considerable amount of blood into the abdominal cavity. A nurse contacts the general surgeon on call. Further assessment is carried out while the team waits for the surgeon.

Whilst the circulating nurse has been attending to J's circulatory status, the airway nurse has determined that J continues to respond to her voice. He knows who he is, where he is and what month it is. He is complaining of severe pain in his left leg and right wrist. His pupils are checked and found to be equal, within normal limits (2–5 mm) and both react to light. The nurse informs the medical team leader of J's distress, who then decides to apply a Thomas splint to J's left leg and administer an i.v. opioid, e.g. morphine, to relieve J's pain, plus an antiemetic to prevent any nausea or vomiting. The splint will provide some pain relief as it realigns the fractured bone. Pre- and post-application of the splint, J's dorsalis pedis pulse is checked and is easily palpable.

Using members of the medical and nursing team, J is now 'log rolled' so that his back and spinal column can be examined (see Fig. 27.2). Since his known major injuries are on the left side, he is rolled to the right. Spinal injury has not yet been ruled out, so great care is taken to keep his spine in anatomical alignment. The spinal column is palpated for loss of normal continuity and abnormal curves or 'dips'. J is asked to indicate any areas of pain. No abnormality is detected and J reports no back pain. After preparing J, and prior to passing a urethral catheter (American College of Surgeons 2004), a rectal examination is performed to check for a high riding or absent prostate gland, which may indicate urethral damage. Other signs of urethral damage include blood around the external urinary meatus and scrotal haematoma in the male patient.

The cross-matched blood has now arrived and the rapid transfusion of two units of whole blood is commenced. The appropriate care and observations for a patient having a blood transfusion are maintained (see Ch. 11). The urinary catheterisation set is ready, and after explaining why it is important to monitor J's urine output, the catheter is inserted and a urometer attached. A plaster of Paris (POP) backslab is applied to support J's wrist. The surgeon arrives and agrees that J needs immediate transfer to theatre for a laparotomy. Once this has been done and J's condition has further stabilised, the orthopaedic surgeon will reduce and immobilise the fractures more definitively while J is still anaesthetised. The operating staff are informed and a theatre will be prepared. A ward is identified for J's subsequent transfer, but in the meantime J's clinical condition continues to be monitored at 15-min intervals.

Care of relatives

J's mother, Mrs S, has now arrived in the department. She has been met by the senior nurse of the ED and brought to the relatives' room. Ideally, each department should have a quiet room where the family and friends of seriously ill or injured patients may wait. This room should have comfortable chairs as waiting may often be long, facilities for making tea or coffee, and a telephone, so that other family members or friends can be contacted (British Association for Accident and Emergency Medicine and Royal College of Nursing 1995). A nurse should, if at all possible, stay with the relatives. People who are in a strange and, in this case, threatening environment are often unsure of how to behave and what is expected of them. They may have questions to ask, such as where the toilets are located, but may be reluctant to leave the room they have been shown into in case they miss some vital information about their loved one. They may also feel that if they come out and ask questions they are depriving their relative of a key member of staff who is essential to the team. Clearly, much anxiety and distress can be avoided if a member of staff remains with the family. Where pressures of work or staff shortages make this impossible, the family should be reassured that their relative is being constantly monitored and is never left alone. They should also be introduced to a nurse, usually Nurse One of the trauma team, who will act as their contact. The family should also be told where this nurse can be found, and encouraged to voice any queries or problems. This nurse should be responsible for seeing the relatives every 15 min or so in order to bring them up to date with developments.

Mrs S has not had the opportunity to contact her husband, as she has come straight to the hospital with the police. She is offered the use of a telephone to get in touch with him but requests that a member of staff does this for her instead. She is given details about her son's condition. These details are truthful, conveying the seriousness of J's condition. It is neither helpful nor compassionate to reassure people falsely in such circumstances. They need time to adjust their feelings in order to cope with what may be very bad news. If relatives are falsely reassured that everything will be all right, they will understandably feel cheated, and trust will be lost, if the outcome is not a happy one. At the same time, all hope should not be destroyed. In encounters such as this, it is essential that the nurse is an experienced communicator, since there is a fine line to be drawn between giving false hope and causing unnecessary anguish. Relatives also have needs at such a stressful time, which the nurse must assess before embarking on lengthy explanations. Mrs S, for example, may have preferred to wait until her husband arrived before being given any information. Breaking bad news thus requires distinct skills, which nurses must learn and practise.

The police have already told J's mother of the circumstances of the accident. Traffic police investigate all RTCs to determine if there are any legal implications of the accident. The police are frequently used as a liaison for the relatives and are a valuable resource for the ED staff. Mrs S wishes to 'know the worst' about J's condition and is now informed of his injuries and the treatment he has received so far. The fact that he has a chest drain and is receiving i.v. fluid is explained, so that she is not alarmed by the presence of this equipment. Mrs S is told that a surgeon has been called and that J is at present being prepared for theatre, but that she may see him if she wishes. The trauma team need not interrupt their treatment of J to allow his mother to see him. The team's first priority is, obviously, the patient's physical condition, and they may become so caught up in this that other considerations are forgotten. Often, all that is necessary to reassure relatives and patients is that they can see each other briefly. Family members may be more content if they can see that the patient is actually alive, and it can comfort the patient to know that the family is present. As Mrs S is keen to see her son, she is taken to the resuscitation room accompanied by the same nurse. She is encouraged to stand by the airway nurse and speak to her son. Everything that is happening is explained to both J and Mrs S. The surgeon has now arrived and J's mother returns to the relatives' room with the nurse to wait for her husband. She asks if J's brother, sister and girlfriend should be contacted, and is told that it may, in fact, do everyone good if they are all together at this time of family crisis.

J's vital signs continue to be recorded at regular intervals. It is found that his pulse and blood pressure have stabilised, remaining at 100 beats/min and 90/50 mmHg, respectively. The doctor now has time to spend with J's family, who have now arrived, and explain in more detail the implications of J's injuries. Meanwhile, in the resuscitation room, all documentation is assembled. J's clothing and valuables have already been placed in property bags and are now given to his mother. Departments differ as to policy for dealing with property; some record details in a property book, while others leave this task to the admitting ward.

In certain circumstances, notably in cases of violent assault such as shootings, stabbings or rape, the victim's clothes should be carefully bagged, recorded and given to the police for forensic examination. This may also apply in the case of hit-and-run accidents. It is preferred that items are bagged separately, so that one item does not contaminate another. If property is given to the police, it is important that a police officer signs the property book as receiver of the property and that the nurse who hands it over also signs so that future queries from any source can be readily answered.

J is now ready to be taken to theatre (see Ch. 26). His family and girlfriend are called to accompany him. They will be able to talk to him along the way and to say their goodbyes when he reaches theatre. The theatre staff are informed that J's family are going to wait, so that they can be kept informed of his progress and be notified when he is returned to the recovery ward. The family is taken to a relatives' room beside the wards, and theatre staff are told where they can be contacted.

It is likely that J will make a full recovery; however, what would have happened if he had died in the Emergency Department? The following section deals with the nurse's role in supporting relatives who are bereaved by the sudden death of a loved one.

DEATH IN THE EMERGENCY DEPARTMENT

A very difficult dilemma for the ED staff may arise when they begin to realise that resuscitative measures are not going to succeed. If staff know that the resuscitation attempts are likely to be futile and the family has arrived, it is important that the relatives are gently made aware of the situation by the nurse caring for them, who can outline the gravity of the situation. This provides the family with time, even just a few minutes, to internalise the seriousness of the situation. The decision to stop resuscitation efforts is a difficult one, and one that should be made after considering individual team members' views. If the relatives have arrived in the ED, it may be possible to offer them the option of seeing their loved one to say goodbye before the resuscitation efforts are stopped.

All bereavement is traumatic, but sudden death is recognised as one of the most traumatic of experiences (Wright 1996). The deceased was usually last seen alive and well and the fact that they are now dead is very difficult for loved ones to comprehend, as they have had no opportunity to prepare for grief. Feelings of guilt may also prevail if the bereaved person begins to reflect upon things not said or done when the loved one was still alive. Caring for distressed relatives in these circumstances is one of the most draining of nursing interactions (Cudmore 1998) and it is important that the nurse is prepared for a wide range of emotional reactions. It is also important that the nurse is aware of the individual's religious and cultural beliefs, particularly concerning the disposal of the body following a sudden death. Each Emergency Department should have direct access to religious ministers from different faiths who can either offer advice or, if the family members request it, be present to support them during this difficult period.

If relatives wish to see their loved one, nurses can do much to help. If possible, those parts of the body that are exposed should be washed. One or (if possible) both of the deceased's hands should be left outside the sheets. The head of the trolley should be slightly raised, otherwise the face may seem distorted when the family first sees the body. False teeth should be replaced for the same reason and the hair combed or smoothed. Where there are severe head injuries, bandages should be left in place and perhaps covered with a clean outer layer. A nurse should initially accompany the relatives, and, if they seem hesitant, can indicate that it is all right for them to touch the body, perhaps by doing so personally or by asking the family members if they wish to hold the loved one's hand. The nurse should then offer to withdraw. Not everyone will want to be left alone, but some may have private words of parting to say and should be given the opportunity to do so. Where a whole family is present, this chance should be given to each person individually. One family member may not feel able to ask for this for themselves, but when it is suggested by the nurse, they may gratefully accept. Relatives should also feel free to hug or kiss the body; in the case of a dead child, the parents should be able to take the child in their arms. This seems to help people to cope with the denial stage of grieving, especially in cases of sudden death (Kubler-Ross 1984).

Following this period, some relatives may find it difficult to leave the department and may need some assistance. Part of the concluding process may be to give the relatives information relating to the immediate future. Relatives should be made aware that where death has occurred as the result of trauma, under legal requirements a postmortem is always required and there will probably be an inquest at a later date. Providing a card with the departmental telephone number allows the relatives to ask further questions. It is particularly helpful to provide the name of the liaison nurse who cared for them as this provides some continuity. At the same time, it is important to determine how the relatives are going to get home and arrange transport if necessary. On their departure it is wise to inform the family GP, who may offer assistance. Families may also be directed to a variety of support groups such as CRUSE or Compassionate Friends (see 'Useful websites and addresses', p. 964). Most groups have local branches and it is helpful if the department can supply their addresses and telephone numbers. Many organisations produce leaflets or other information that may be beneficial to the bereaved.

Organ donation

In situations where it has become clear that resuscitation will not be successful, it may be possible to approach the family regarding the question of organ donation. Organs and tissues which may be used for transplantation may come either from the 'beating heart' donor — when the patient will usually be admitted to an intensive care unit until brain stem death tests are completed (see Ch. 28) — or from patients who have died, i.e. when cessation of circulatory and respiratory function has occurred within the ED. In both instances, the subject may be broached in the ED, so that the family have time to consider their decision. However, it is important that nurses have a sound knowledge base about the different aspects of donation and transplantation, together with an awareness of their own fears surrounding death, to give them greater confidence in communicating with potential donors. This may seem a cruel intrusion at a time of great grief, but in the long term the donation of the organs of the deceased may help the family to come to terms with their tragedy. By helping someone else to live, their loved one's death may come to seem less futile (Dolan 2000).

Sudden infant death syndrome

The parents of babies who have died from sudden infant death syndrome (SIDS) are particularly vulnerable. This is when an apparently healthy baby has died unexpectedly for no apparent reason (Foundation for the Study of Infant Deaths 2004). The parents will be asked to identify their baby in the presence of a police officer, before the postmortem examination. This may produce great anxiety and distress, as the parents may feel that they are being accused of causing their child's death. The police are very sensitive to this situation and extremely supportive of parents, but if staff forewarn the parents of this formality they can be saved much anguish. A further supportive measure that may be offered to these parents is to take a photograph of their baby and/or a lock of the baby's hair or a hand/footprint. Sometimes this is not wanted at the time, but the parents should be reassured that they can collect it at any time in the future. Most importantly, parents need to be given the opportunity to be with and hold their baby. They are going to need help and support at this difficult time and should be given information on how to contact the Foundation for the Study of Infant Deaths (see 'Useful websites and addresses', p. 964).

Staff grief

It is very difficult for staff to have worked hard to save a life but without success. Feelings of inadequacy and failure may arise, especially when the patient is young or when the circumstances of the accident seem senseless. Repeatedly caring for patients and relatives in these circumstances may take its toll, both emotionally and physically, which means that the caregivers themselves may become casualties. It is important, therefore, to consider the grief that will be felt by staff who have been involved with the patient and/or the relatives. There should be a forum for expressing feelings and anxieties within the department. One method is a 'defusing' session which can be described as a short type of crisis intervention for staff involved in such an incident (Wright 1996). It allows staff to talk with one another about the experience in a relaxed atmosphere and provides an opportunity to give all staff the key information relating to the whole episode of the incident. This ventilation of feelings and re-run of events can be of benefit in two ways: it can allow staff to express their emotions, and it can highlight defects in the system or ways of improving practice in the future.

For particularly distressing incidents, a more formal type of debriefing may be required. Critical incident stress debriefing (CISD) (Cudmore 1998) is a session which may be facilitated by someone who has knowledge of counselling skills. It usually takes place 24–48 h after the event and follows a structured format that focuses on the emotional consequences for staff involved in these types of resuscitation. Most importantly, staff should be prepared to help them cope with these types of stresses. Knowledge about stress and coping mechanisms will help staff to recognise their own limitations and to know when they themselves need help.

A PATIENT WITH MINOR TRAUMA

Development of the emergency nurse practitioner role

Emergency Departments and minor injury units (MIUs) have seen the development of an enhanced nursing role.

Within the emergency environment these nurses are often referred to as emergency nurse practitioners (ENPs). To date, over 60% of EDs offer a service which includes the role of an ENP (Marr et al 2003). One of the fundamental rationales for these rapid developments is the need to reduce waiting times for patients who have suffered minor trauma (Sakr et al 1999). Nurses who practise in this role will have received formal post-basic education in:

- holistic assessment
- physical diagnosis
- prescription of treatment
- promotion of health.

They will also be working within pre-arranged guidelines as recommended by the Royal College of Nursing (2002). A generally accepted definition of a nurse working within this role describes the practitioner who is able, without reference to a doctor, to see a patient and elicit data which enable the nurse to reach a diagnostic conclusion and make decisions about the patient's treatment (Hunt & Wainwright 1994, Cable 1995). Despite this definition, there are no nationally accepted boundaries of practice for ENPs to work within. The *Code of Professional Conduct* (Nursing and Midwifery Council 2004), which provides guidelines for any nursing role expansion, requires that the nurse accept full responsibility and accountability for any nursing actions. It further requires that any developments within nursing practice must maintain the continuity of patient care whilst meeting the needs and serving the interests of the patient. These guidelines are broad and unspecific, but have enabled Emergency Departments and MIUs to develop the ENP role to meet the needs of patients presenting with minor injuries. Generally, ENPs are able to see, assess, diagnose and treat or refer patients who present with injuries that are considered to fall under the umbrella title of minor trauma. This ensures that the ENP is working within the *Code of Professional Conduct* by using expanded skills to ensure the continuity of care and, in many cases, to treat the patient's entire injury episode (Nursing and Midwifery Council 2004). Examples of some common areas of practice can be seen in Box 27.5.

Box 27.5

Common areas of practice within the emergency nurse practitioner role

- Assessment, examination and treatment of uncomplicated
  - lacerations and wounds
  - hand/wrist/arm/shoulder injuries
  - lower limb injuries
  - minor scalds and burns
  - specified dental, ophthalmic and ENT problems
- Assessment, examination and referral of the above, when there is evidence of any neurovascular or tendon injury or other complications that require specialist intervention
- The requesting of X-rays
- The removal of foreign bodies
- The issue of specified drugs, e.g. tetanus toxoid, antibiotics, analgesics, within identified protocols

Adapted from Royal College of Nursing (2002).

Assessment and treatment

In Case History 27.2, Mrs N is seen by the 'see and treat' nurse who assesses her injury using the medical model shown in Box 27.1. Mrs N is able to provide the history of the presenting complaint and describes how her finger was cut whilst she was washing up some dishes. The water was fairly clean, as she had just put some glasses in to soak. She felt the wound had bled a fair amount since the accident happened approximately 30 min ago and became concerned because the wound looked deep and began to bleed again every time she bent her finger.

On examining the wound, the 'see and treat' nurse obtains objective information, i.e. there appears to be no evidence of neurovascular compromise as Mrs N's finger is pink and warm to touch and she can feel light touch at the end of her finger. The bleeding can now be described as a controllable minor haemorrhage. The 'see and treat' nurse then obtains further drug and past medical history. Mrs N states that she is usually fit and well and has no other illness or conditions that may complicate this injury. Using this information, the 'see and treat' nurse considers the severity of her condition and decides that, within her limit of expertise and training, she can initiate the request of an X-ray to determine if there is any glass in the wound and administer an analgesic such as paracetamol for pain, if needed. The 'see and treat' nurse documents her assessment on the medical notes (see Fig. 27.3) and, using the Manchester Triage system, allocates a prioritisation category to Mrs N.

In the interim period it is important that the 'see and treat' nurse ensures that no further harm is caused, and because of the possibility of swelling and the potential of impairing the circulation to Mrs N's finger, the nurse removes Mrs N's wedding ring into safe keeping. A pressure dressing is applied to the finger and Mrs N's arm is held elevated by the patient or may be placed in a high arm sling to stop the bleeding and prevent any further swelling. Mrs N is then sent to the X-ray department for an X-ray of her finger. Her husband returns home to care for the children.

Once Mrs N has had her X-ray she is called through to the treatment area by the ENP, who continues to gather a thorough history and complete a more extensive assessment of the injury, an outline of which can be seen in Box 27.6. Using a more in-depth examination technique, the ENP confirms that there is no neurovascular damage and that the finger can be moved within its full range of movement, which indicates that there is no injury to the underlying tendons.

CASE HISTORY 27.2

Mrs N

Mrs N is a 44-year-old mother of four. She lives with her family and her husband has brought her to the Emergency Department. Whilst washing up, she 'cut' her left ring finger on a broken glass. This has produced a wound that is still bleeding.

MRS. N. Patient's label here		Date 29/03/06 Time triaged 12.07	Triage nurse stamp A. B., STAFF NURSE			
Presenting complaint LACERATION LEFT RING FINGER	Discriminator BLEEDING		Page 136	Area MINORS	Category GREEN	Estimated wait 1 HOUR

Dr / ENP Nurse stamp LORRIE LAWTON Emergency Nurse Practitioner		Allergies NONE KNOWN	Urinalysis N/A	Referred to N/A	Childhood immunisations N/A	Time Ametop N/A	Time U.Bag N/A
Time seen by Dr / ENP 12.25	Tetanus last injection 3 YEARS AGO		HCG N/A	Contact time N/A		Weight N/A	CPR N/A

HISTORY & ASSESSMENT

Pain score 0 min _____ 5 _____ 10 max

P.C. LACERATION TO LEFT RING FINGER.

HPC – Washing up in clean water (APPROX. 30 mins ago)
Cut left finger on broken glass. Since then difficult to stop bleeding, especially when bending finger.

O/E: laceration over joint of finger. Circulation and sensation intact.
No active bleeding

PLAN:
① Remove wedding ring
② Offer Paracetamol 1gm orally for pain – Refused.
③ Apply temporary dressing – dry. High arm sling
④ X-ray left ring finger to exclude foreign body
⑤ Refer to ENP for further treatment

Staff Nurse A.B.
'See & Treat' Nurse

OBSERVATIONS	
T	
P	
R	
BP	
Sats air	
Sats O_2	
O_2 % given	
Cap refill	
BM	
Pupils	
VA (left)	
VA (right)	
GCS	
PFR (pre)	
PFR (post)	

ENP Assessment:
44 yr old female shop assistant. Right-handed
History as above:
O/E:

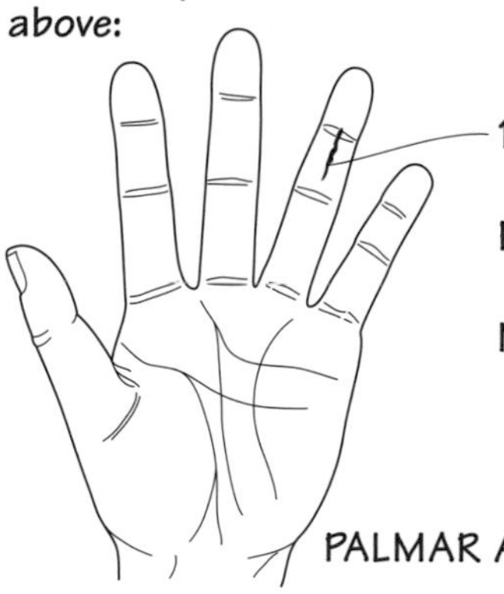

1.5 cm long laceration, approx. 0.25 cm deep over MIPJ
Edges of wound jagged not easily opposed
No deep structures seen

PALMAR ASPECT

Written advice given:

Relatives aware of admission? Yes ☑ No ☐

Property
Given to relatives initials: N/A
Given to ward initials: N/A

DRUGS / TREATMENTS

Date	Drug / treatment	Dr's initials	Nurse's initials	Time

Fig. 27.3A Triage Sheet for Mrs N. Completed documentation (for Mrs N). DH, drug history; ENP, emergency nurse practitioner; FB, foreign body; FDP, flexor digitorum profundus; FDS, flexor digitorum superficialis; FROM, full range of movement; Imp, impression; MIPJ, middle interphalangeal joint; O/E, on examination; PMH, past medical history; SH, social history.

HMR 4 A (Code 90-535)

.... HOSPITAL

HISTORY SHEET

Unit No.

SURNAME (Block Letters) MRS. N.

FIRST NAMES

DATE	CLINICAL NOTES (Each entry must be signed)
29/03/06 12.25	O/E Cont'd: No bony tenderness F.R.O.M. – against resistance F.D.P. & F.D.S intact Sensation – normal 2 point discrimination 4 mm. Finger warm and pink. Capillary Refill < 2 sec. Not actively bleeding PMH – None. Normally fit & well DH – None. No allergies. ATT 3yrs ago SH – Mother of 4 children Works as shop assistant part-time Imp: Laceration L ring finger on glass Plan: ① Review X-ray – No foreign body seen ② Clean, explore and suture wound Treatment: Lignocaine 1% – 2.5 mls infiltration Wound explored. No F.B. seen, tendons intact Wound cleaned with Normal Saline Wound closed – 3 x 4'0 ethilon™ sutures Dry dressing and high arm sling applied Removal of sutures – 10 days as over joint Advice: Re signs of infection Re removal high arm sling within 24 hours Husband contacted G.P. letter sent LH Lawton ENP. 29/03/06

Fig. 27.3B Triage Sheet for Mrs N. *Cont'd*

Box 27.6

Key factors to consider in the assessment of wounds: history, examination, investigations

History
- How did the injury occur?
- When did the injury occur?
- In what environment did it occur?

Examination
- What size is the wound?
- What type of wound is it?
- How deep is the wound?
- What is the associated neurovascular status?

Investigations
- X-ray for any foreign bodies
- Consider the possibility of infection — bacteriology

If there were evidence of damage to the vessels, nerves or tendons, the ENP would refer Mrs N to the relevant medical specialist team, e.g. the plastic surgery team or orthopaedic team who specialise in hand injuries. The ENP reviews the X-ray requested by the 'see and treat' nurse and determines that there is no glass visible. Despite this, it is still important that the wound is explored thoroughly under local anaesthetic. Mrs N is transferred to the minor theatre where she is asked to lie on a trolley. The wound that she has sustained can be described as a laceration. The edges are jagged and the wound crosses over a joint, so it gapes open every time Mrs N bends her finger. Because of this Mrs N requires some form of primary wound closure, the purpose of which is to approximate the wound edges accurately, thus creating the right conditions to enable an epithelial covering to form over the defect and result in a thinner scar line (Wardrope et al 1999). The most common methods of wound closure used within EDs are plastic adhesive strips (Steri-Strips), staples, tissue glue and sutures. Whilst the first three of these methods are less invasive for Mrs N, they are normally used for wounds where the edges come together easily and preferably not over a joint. In Mrs N's case the wound edges are jagged and do not oppose easily, and therefore the most appropriate method to ensure adequate wound closure is to insert sutures which will keep the edges firmly opposed during the healing process.

The ENP first infiltrates the wound with 2.5 mL 1% lidocaine using a needle and syringe; this is the most common local anaesthetic used in the ED (Wardrope et al 1999). Adrenaline can be added to the local anaesthetic. However, as adrenaline has a vasoconstrictive action and is useful on wounds which are bleeding, e.g. scalp lacerations, it should never be used on digits, or on the nose or penis, because of the risk that it could cause ischaemia and necrosis. It is important that approximately 5 min is allowed to ensure that the full effect of the local anaesthetic is achieved, so the ENP prepares the equipment that is needed to insert the sutures into the wound. Having checked local anaesthesia has been achieved, and following aseptic procedures throughout, the wound is cleaned using a warmed sodium chloride solution and the ENP explores the wound carefully. Not only is it necessary to explore the wound for any contamination or foreign bodies, but it is also important to examine the underlying structures to ensure that they are fully intact. There is no evidence of any foreign bodies and the wound is not contaminated. The ENP then inserts four interrupted sutures, using an aseptic technique, while explaining all these actions to Mrs N. Once this is completed and the ENP is sure that there is no further bleeding, a dry, non-adhesive dressing is applied to ensure that the wound is kept clean and dry. Again, Mrs N is asked to keep her arm elevated or it may be placed in a high arm sling for 24 h to minimise any swelling and prevent any further bleeding. The ENP explains the need to remove the sling after 24 h in order to prevent stiffness of the shoulder. The ENP has ascertained that Mrs N has recently had a tetanus vaccination and so does not require this cover. Since 2003, the tetanus vaccination has also contained a low dose of diphtheria vaccine (Td). This is based upon WHO recommendations (Department of Health 2003b) because there is evidence of an increase in the occurrence of diphtheria internationally, particularly in the older population.

Due to the implementation of the 'see and treat' system, Mrs N has received a rapid and seamless assessment of her wound, the required investigations have been rapidly initiated and treatment carried out. This has enabled Mrs N to be seen in a more timely fashion, enabling her to return home quickly.

Health education and discharge advice

For ED staff, the main involvement in health education activity is in primary health education, concerning accident prevention, and secondary health education, involving first aid and discharge advice (McConnell 1997). The aim of health education in the ED is to empower patients to take responsibility for their recovery and future health status. Patients require practical, achievable solutions to help them cope with their injury. Discharge advice can, if understood and followed, hasten the patient's recovery and prevent complications, but may require the patient to change some aspects of their usual daily activities.

As well as completing a full physical assessment, it is important that the ENP complete a psychosocial assessment. In the case of Mrs N, she has good family support and her children are old enough to contribute to the running of the family home. It is important that Mrs N keeps this finger clean and dry for at least 48 h after primary suture to allow epithelial cover over the wound (Wardrope et al 1999). She will need to keep the sling on for approximately 24 h. This may have been difficult if she had young children to care for, and no one to help her with, for example, the cooking and washing up. Mrs N should also be warned against driving until her injured finger is completely healed. Were she to do so, she might not have complete control of the steering wheel. In addition, if she were to be involved in an accident even through no fault of her own, normal car insurance would be unlikely to provide cover for her if it became known that she had an injured finger. It is important that she can get transport home. If necessary, she should be given the opportunity to telephone her husband to ask him to collect her. Mrs N should be told that if, during the healing period, the wound becomes increasingly painful or swollen, she should contact her GP or practice nurse for a review of her wound, as she may be developing an infection. In most parts of the UK information leaflets have been superseded by the use of computerised discharge plans for ED patients; these are not only quick and easy to use but also allow patients to be given printed, individualised instructions (McKenna 1994). Mrs N is given instructions that remind her to have the sutures removed in 10 days' time (Wardrope et al 1999) and the signs and symptoms of potential infection are reiterated. The sutures are left in for 10 days as the wound is over a joint. This allows extra healing time and reduces the risk of the wound opening again once the sutures are removed. Mrs N is advised to have the sutures removed by the practice nurse at her GP's surgery and either to visit the surgery or return to the Emergency Department if she has any problems. The ENP completes the relevant documentation (see Fig. 27.3) which includes a discharge letter to Mrs N's GP so that there is a complete record of Mrs N's medical history.

AGGRESSION AND VIOLENCE IN THE EMERGENCY DEPARTMENT

Our changing society

Emergency nursing is a challenging and rewarding area in which to work. The dynamic nature of the job means that one never knows what will happen next. One minute the nurse may be required to comfort an elderly gentleman who has unexpectedly lost his partner of 50 years, and the next to support a mother who has unexpectedly gone into labour and is about to deliver her baby. Likewise, caring for patients with minor injuries ranges from caring for a child who has sustained a fall, to irrigating a patient's eyes as a result of a chemical splash incident whilst at work. As a result, nurses are able to practise a wider range of skills than is perhaps used in other clinical settings.

However, there are drawbacks to operating an 'open door' policy. It means that nurses will be required to care for patients with a range of conditions and problems. The nature of these events may put the individual concerned into a sudden state of crisis that may produce various types of stress reaction. These include intense emotions, e.g. fear, anxiety, confusion and loss of control, all experienced as a result of the uncertainty of the situation. On occasion, this may display itself in the form of aggression and, in extreme cases, physical violence. The Zero Tolerance Zone campaign (Department of Health 1999) defines violence as 'any incident where staff are abused, threatened or assaulted in circumstances related to their work, involving an explicit or implicit challenge to their safety, well-being or health'. In 2000/01 there were over 84 000 reported incidents of violence or abusive behaviour to staff within the NHS (Department of Health 2002c).

Harkness (1997) (see Research Abstract 27.1) identified two frequently influential factors with regard to the occurrence of violence: the presence of alcohol or other drugs, and levels of perceived frustration of the aggressor. Within the ED environment, patients are often treated for injuries that are alcohol related or that have been self-inflicted, e.g. drug overdoses. Added to this is the frustration experienced by many patients over long waiting times. As a result of government initiatives such as *The Patient's Charter* (Department of Health 1991), patients are more aware of their rights, and sometimes their expectations to be seen and treated quickly exceed what the ED can provide. However, the zero tolerance policy within the NHS has highlighted the rights of staff to work in a safe environment. The NHS now takes a more proactive stance in preventing violence and aggression within the workplace and will actively seek prosecution, with the assistance of the police, of patients who attack staff. Therefore, it is important that nurses working in this environment are able to anticipate possible situations and prevent them from escalating to a point where potential harm may be caused.

RESEARCH ABSTRACT 27.1

A study of violence at work

Violence in the workplace is a growing concern for both employers and employees. A study which considered two service sector groups, including hospital staff, investigated the incidence of violence, observed the nature of violent incidents and observed the antecedents of any reported violent incidents, the actual behaviour and how the incident ended. Key findings identified that 24% of hospital staff had experienced aggressive physical contact and 69.8% had experienced verbal abuse in the preceding 12 months. Antecedents included patients' questioning medical/nursing procedures, and individuals thought to be under the influence of alcohol. The most common methods of bringing an incident to a close included reassurance, discussion and walking away, although in 18% of cases hospital security was called and in 3% the police were called to intervene. The report concluded that training can help to equip an employee to be more competent in a range of situations.

Harkness L 1997 Part of the job? A study of violence at work. Occupational Health Review 65: 25–27

Defusing a potentially aggressive situation

Nurses should remember that aggression is seldom directed towards them personally. It is important that they are able to recognise the factors that influence aggression in the ED situation. These include a lack of information either about the condition of a relative or about the excessive waiting times. Waiting rooms that have poor facilities can contribute to an individual's level of frustration, e.g. a telephone box that does not work, uncomfortable seating and an unwelcoming decor. The attitude of staff to patients, particularly if it appears judgemental and unsympathetic, may contribute to the development of a confrontation between patient or relative and nurse.

However, it must be acknowledged that not all aspects of aggression are avoidable within the ED environment. Sometimes the aggression is a result of metabolic disorders which cause acute confusional states, e.g. hypoxia or diabetes mellitus, or a result of head injury. In these situations the patient has no control over their actions. However, there are usually warning signs, such as those given in

Box 27.7

Warning signs of aggression

Emotional
- Individual appears agitated and tense
- Individual's voice increases in volume and pitch, apparent in the abrupt response to questions
- Individual may use sarcasm and obscenities when talking to staff

Behavioural
- Body posture may reveal muscular tension in face and limbs
- Individual may be making fists with hands, banging fists or hitting out at objects

Physiological
- Pupils may be dilated, although this may be difficult to observe

Adapted from Morcombe (1999).

Box 27.7, and it is essential that nurses are able to recognise these if they are to prevent the situation escalating. Other strategies that help to defuse difficult situations include the use of good verbal and non-verbal communication and the adoption of a calm, non-threatening approach.

Adopting appropriate body posture

Trying to resolve situations within large groups often increases the aggression so it is preferable to invite the aggressive individual to a separate area. Ideally this should be in a private place, but this should not compromise the safety of the member of staff. Adopting an oblique posture is less confrontational and, if standing, the nurse should take a position with feet slightly apart and body weight on the slightly flexed back leg. The nurse should be aware of the individual's personal space and remain at least an arm's length away. These actions serve two purposes: they are less threatening and they allow a quick escape should the need arise (Morcombe 1999). The nurse must demonstrate genuine interest in what the individual has to say. Direct eye contact may be interpreted as being provocative, but completely avoiding eye contact may be perceived as dismissive and suggestive of disinterest, so it is better to focus away from the face, just below the larynx area.

Listening to aggressive patients

The nurse should listen carefully to the complaint and offer an explanation. It is difficult not to shout back when being shouted at, but it is more effective if the pitch, tone and volume of the nurse's voice remain within a normal conversational range (Morcombe 1999). The nurse should be sensitive to the individual's circumstances and a sympathetic approach may avoid the escalation of the aggressive confrontation. If the individual is confused for any reason, the nurse may have to repeat what is being said several times before being understood. If possible, a plan of action should be agreed with the individual to resolve the situation. It is unwise to give false information or agree on solutions that are unachievable, as this will result in trust being lost and may cause further aggression at a later stage.

Avoiding physical danger and attack

Unfortunately there are times when, despite all the strategies, violence does occur and it is vital that the nurse considers this possibility in all encounters with aggressive patients. For this reason, nurses should never place themselves in a situation where they are trapped in an enclosed area. If interviewing an aggressive individual alone in a private room, the nurse should ensure that the area is free of objects that may be used as weapons and that the door is not lockable. Potential weapons include equipment such as scissors and stethoscopes carried by the nurse which, if grabbed, could be used to threaten. The safety of the staff and the other patients is of paramount importance. If it appears that violence is going to erupt, the nurse should slowly back away from the situation and not attempt to restrain the individual. Help should be summoned using agreed departmental procedures. All EDs have panic buttons that, when activated, summon help either from other ED staff or security officers, or are connected directly to the local police station. Until help is available, the nurse should make every attempt to avoid physical contact. This may involve the use of hospital equipment to create space between the nurse and the aggressive individual. It is preferable that hospital equipment is damaged rather than people hurt.

It is important that, following any incident of aggression or violence, whether verbal or physical, an incident form is completed and that this is reviewed by the hospital's health and safety officer or risk management team. This monitors the escalating problem and may reveal patterns of aggression in the workplace, thereby allowing preventive strategies to be formulated. These may include extra education opportunities for the staff or an increase in staffing levels. If it is apparent that there is an increase in violent and aggressive situations, statistical evidence is useful when making a bid to management staff for more security staff or better protection.

STOP THINK **27.2** Find out about the procedure to follow in your hospital/health centre should a member of staff be injured. What documentation is required? Who should complete it and where should any forms be sent?

Emergency nursing and the law

Due to the nature of ED work, nurses are, on occasion, required to work in close collaboration with the local police force. Victims of crime and those who have committed an offence may require hospital treatment and the medical findings are used as evidence in a court of law. If a death has occurred under suspicious circumstances, the police may require that forensic evidence be collected to assist them with their enquiries. This sometimes creates a conflict in the nurse's professional practice. All patients are entitled to confidentiality in respect of information pertaining to them and it is the nurse's responsibility to ensure that this right is respected (Nursing and Midwifery Council 2004). However, there are exceptions to this which particularly arise within the ED environment, e.g. if a person has been involved in a RTC then the law requires that any relevant information should be given to the police. Other examples are outlined in Box 27.8. As part of this process, the nurse may be required to make a statement which will form part

Box 27.8

Exceptions to the duty of confidentiality

- Consent of a patient
- Best interests of the patient
- Court orders
  - — subpoena
  - — The Civil Procedure (Modification of Supreme Court Act 1981) Order 2004
- Statutory duty to disclose
  - — Misuse of Drugs Act (1971) (Modification) Order 2001
  - — Prevention of Terrorism Act (2002)
  - — Public Health Act (1984)
  - — Road Traffic Act (1999)
- Public interest

of the police investigation, especially if witnessing an event such as a violent incident within the department. It should be noted, however, that it may be several years before a case, whether criminal or civil, comes before the courts and the nurse is asked to write the statement. For this reason it is important that careful attention is paid to accurate documentation within the patient's nursing and medical records.

MAJOR INCIDENTS

There is no one standard definition of a major incident. For the purpose of guidance, the National Health Services Executive (1998) states that:

> *A major incident can have a huge impact on one part of the health service, while leaving others relatively unaffected. In a similar way, an NHS major incident is not necessarily a major incident for other emergency services, such as police, or local authority services and vice versa.*

This definition is deliberately non-specific, because what constitutes a major incident for a small rural hospital may have minimal impact in a large inner city hospital. Similarly a large-scale disaster may affect only one hospital or may require the services of several hospitals within a region. The purpose of emergency planning for such situations within the NHS is to ensure that all the emergency services are able to work collaboratively and provide an effective response to any type of incident.

Major incident planning

In this era of global terrorism the approach to dealing with and preparing for major incidents has not only had to be re-thought (Hayward 2003) (see also www.ukresilience.info) but, with each new incident, e.g. the July 2005 London bombings, re-appraised. It is essential that every hospital has a major incident plan, including a chemical decontamination plan. The ED plays a major role in this, as it is required to provide the initial and rapid response. A National Audit Office survey (2002) found that while many hospitals were not prepared for 'mass casualties', they were better prepared for major incidents (Crouch 2003).

To enable the ED to manage effectively in such a situation, it is vital that the department has the support of all other services within the hospital. Extra equipment will be needed, patients will have to be moved quickly and it should be anticipated that more staff will be needed than usually work on a shift. For this reason it is important that all hospital departments, including portering, catering staff, cleaning staff, as well as other clinical support areas, are involved in the development of the major incident policy. The essence of any plan is that it is flexible enough to cater for any situation, which may include chemical contamination incidents or a large number of patients with multiple or thermal injuries.

In the event of an incident, the ED will be notified by the police or the local ambulance service, which will inform the ED of the type of incident that they are dealing with. The ED will have to prepare quickly to receive the predicted number of patients. This is achieved by clearing the department as quickly as possible and restocking principal areas with extra equipment, such as decontamination equipment if dealing with a chemical incident, whilst calling in extra staff. The ED may be asked to provide an on-site mobile medical team (MMT). The MMT is formed from ED personnel, supported by an anaesthetist, usually from intensive care. Each MMT is made up of four members: an experienced doctor to act as the team leader, an anaesthetist, a senior ED nurse and a second experienced nurse (Eaton 1999). It is vital that these staff are adequately equipped with correct personal protective equipment (PPE) (Hayward 2003) as they will be required to support the ambulance service in difficult and potentially dangerous environments (see Box 27.9). Casualties are predominantly brought into the department by ambulance, although the 'walking wounded' will often be brought in by local people not involved in the incident. However, if there is a chemical incident no casualties should leave the scene of the incident until they have been thoroughly decontaminated by the Fire Service. Inevitably, some casualties may 'slip through the net' and will require immediate decontamination on arrival in the department.

Due to the volume of patients, it is important that careful attention is paid to adequate identification of all individuals. The police documentation team, which is based in the hospital, will operate a 'casualty bureau', where all

Box 27.9

Personal protective equipment for a mobile medical team

- Good quality helmet, with chinstrap, light and Perspex visor; it should be green with 'nurse' in white
- Pair of fire-retardant overalls with kneepads
- High visibility tabard and jacket, marked front and back with wearer's designation, such as 'nurse' or 'doctor'; it must have reflective strips and be green in colour
- Leather boots with steel cap toes that are fire, oil and acid resistant
- Heavy duty and latex gloves

Adapted from Keane & King (2001).

information regarding the patients is collated. Members of the public can contact the bureau for further information regarding casualties. The ED staff will have to keep this unit updated with details of patients. Many relatives will arrive at the hospital seeking information and, as in all public interest events, the media will require regular press statements. It is important that this does not interrupt the staff's care of the patients. The hospital will need to ensure that adequate facilities and support staff are in place to care for friends and relatives waiting to see the injured, whilst establishing separate communication networks for the media. Once all the casualties have been cared for and transferred to other areas for their definitive care, the ED must resume its customary work as soon as possible.

Because of the relative infrequency of major incidents and the pattern of staff changes, it is recommended that hospitals carry out regular major incident exercises, together with the ambulance and other emergency services, so as to ensure a rapid and effective response (National Health Service Executive 1998).

STOP THINK **27.3** Where is the major incident and chemical decontamination plan held in your hospital? Ask your mentor or lecturer if you may see it and have an opportunity to discuss its content, perhaps during a seminar.

Post-traumatic stress disorder

It has become apparent in recent years that the survivors of major incidents may suffer from a range of long-term psychological and physical symptoms, often unrelated to injuries sustained at the time. These may include feelings of desperation, helplessness, guilt at having survived where others have died and shame at the loss of control. The survivors may also experience anger, feelings of loss and profound sadness, and may be unable to put the incident out of their minds. Physical symptoms may include insomnia, nausea, diarrhoea, dizziness and palpitations, to name only a few (Sowney 1996; see also Ch. 17). It is important for survivors to realise that these manifestations are normal reactions to a terrible tragedy and that they are not 'losing their minds'. However, if these symptoms persist and start interfering with the individual's normal life then it may be that they are suffering from what has been described as 'post-traumatic stress disorder'. In these instances, some of the victims will require prolonged counselling in order to come to terms with their feelings and anxieties, and members of their families may also need to be included in counselling sessions.

Witnesses of disasters may also be deeply affected. Following the Lockerbie air disaster in 1988, when, as a result of a terrorist bomb, a Pan American aircraft disintegrated over this small town in Scotland, killing 259 passengers and 11 town residents, more than 100 residents were referred to community psychiatric nurses. O'Byrne (1989) reported: 'The brush with death had forced many of the town's inhabitants to re-evaluate what they were doing with their lives'. Close media coverage of such events may give those who were not involved, but who were bereaved as a result of the incident, the feeling that they were present when it happened. These people may also experience the feelings of guilt suffered by the actual survivors. This will naturally involve the families of the victims but may also include a much wider range of people. One example of this was when more than 200 people drowned in the Zeebrugge car ferry disaster in 1987 — 160 off-duty crew members of the *Herald of Free Enterprise*, some of whom had changed duties with their shipmates, were among the circle of people requiring counselling and support (Johnston 1989).

Rescue workers, ED staff and other personnel involved in the event are also vulnerable to serious emotional disturbances following such incidents (Collins 2001). Even with good deployment of staff, disasters provoke an 'all hands on deck' situation. Staff may need to be called in from off duty, and others will volunteer after hearing about the incident on the news. Staff will be required to work long hours under difficult conditions, especially if they are part of an on-site team. Some victims will not be saved and this may produce feelings of inadequacy or guilt. Because of the need for the department to return to normality as soon as possible so that it can deal with other patients, there may be insufficient time for staff to rest and recover before returning to more routine jobs. A rush of adrenaline will keep everyone going at the time, but afterwards they may display sheer exhaustion and emotions ranging from anger to guilt or deep sorrow.

It is apparent that following major incidents a range of facilities must be made available to staff (Robson et al 1995, Nutt et al 2000). The nature of these facilities may differ from place to place, but they should include educational programmes and a support network for all staff, and should ideally be in place before any such incidents occur. Where these networks are available and accepted, staff may be less inclined to feel stigmatised if they make use of them when the occasion arises. Now that it is recognised that staff of all disciplines who are involved in disaster situations may suffer from post-traumatic stress disorder, it is essential that provision should be made in disaster planning for the support of these carers following a traumatic event.

CONCLUSION

This chapter has explored the diverse nature of emergency nursing and various aspects of the experiences of patients who attend the ED with trauma. The concept of trauma covers a wide range of injuries, from patients who present as acute emergencies, suffering from life-threatening conditions and multiple trauma, incorporating multisystem injury, to others who present with relatively minor injuries. The roles of nurses working within the ED multidisciplinary team — whether as part of the department's trauma team, as the 'see and treat' nurse or as Emergency Nurse Practitioners — are also explored. The chapter highlights the areas of practice that require specific skills to enable the nurse to meet both the physical and psychosocial needs of individual patients and of their families.

REFERENCES

American College of Surgeons 2004 Advanced trauma life support program for physicians, 7th edn. American College of Surgeons, Chicago

Audit Commission 2001 Accident and emergency acute hospital portfolio. Review of national findings. Online. Available: www.audit-commission.gov.uk

Black J, Ward M, Lockey D 2004 Appropriate use of helicopters to transport trauma patients from incident scene to hospital in the United Kingdom: an algorithm. Emergency Medical Journal 21: 355–361

Bonnett R, Gwinnutt C, Driscoll P 2003 Trauma resuscitation. The team approach, 2nd edn. Taylor and Francis, London

Brannon L, Feist J 2004 Health psychology: an introduction to behavior and health, 5th edn. Wadsworth, London

British Association for Accident and Emergency Medicine (BAAEM) and Royal College of Nursing (RCN) 1995 Bereavement care in A&E departments: report of the working group. RCN, London

Cable S 1995 Minor injuries clinics: dealing with trauma. British Journal of Nursing 4(20): 1177–1182

Collins S 2001 What about us? The psychological implications of dealing with trauma following the Omagh bombing. Emergency Nurse 8(10): 9–13

Cooke M, Wilson S, Pearson S 2002 The effect of a separate stream for minor injuries on accident and emergency department waiting times. Emergency Medical Journal 19: 28–30

Crouch D 2003 Thinking the unthinkable. Nursing Times 99(13): 22–27

Cudmore J 1998 Critical incident stress management strategies. Emergency Nurse 6(3): 22–27

Department of Health 1991 The Patient's Charter: a summary. HMSO, London

Department of Health 1999 Zero tolerance policy. DH, London. Online. Available: www.nhs.uk/zerotolerance

Department of Health 2002a Personal Social Service expenditure and unit costs, England 2000–01. TSO, London

Department of Health 2002b See and treat. DH, London. Online. Available: www.modern.nhs.uk/emergency

Department of Health 2002c 2000/2001 Survey of reported violent or abusive incidents, accidents involving staff and sickness absence in NHS trusts and health authorities, in England. DH, London. Online. Available: www.nhs.uk/zerotolerance/survey/index.htm

Department of Health 2003a Hospital episode statistics England, financial year 2002–03. TSO, London

Department of Health 2003b Replacement of single adsorbed diphtheria vaccine for adults with combined tetanus/low dose diphtheria vaccine (Td tetanus with low dose diphtheria). DH, London. Online. Available: www.dh.gov.uk

Dolan B 2000 Care of the bereaved. In: Dolan B, Holt L (eds) Accident and emergency theory into practice. Baillière Tindall, London

Eaton C 1999 Essentials of immediate medical care. Churchill Livingstone, Edinburgh

Foundation for the Study of Infant Deaths (FSID) 2004 What is cot death? Online. Available: www.sids.org.uk

Harkness L 1997 Part of the job? A study of violence at work. Occupational Health Review 65: 25–27

Hayward M 2003 Pre-hospital response to major incidents. Nursing Standard 17(30): 37

Health and Safety Commission 1974 Health and Safety at Work Act 1974. HMSO, London

Heyworth J, Holt L 2002 See and treat. Emergency Service Collaborative. DH, London

Hill M 1990 Trauma prevention: puzzlement or possibility? American Association of Occupational Health Nurses (AAOHN) Journal 38(10): 465

Hunt G, Wainwright P 1994 Expanding the role of the nurse: the scope of professional practice. Blackwell Science, Oxford

Johnston J 1989 Haunted by memories. Nursing Times 85(11): 56–58

Keane C, King G 2001 The varying standards of Mobile Medical Team equipment held by London hospitals. Emergency Nurse 9(4): 12–15

Kubler-Ross E 1984 On death and dying. Tavistock, London

Manchester Triage Group 1997 Emergency triage. BMJ, London

Marr S, Steele K, Swallow V et al 2003 Mapping the range and scope of emergency nurse practitioner services in the Northern and Yorkshire Region: a telephone survey 2003. Emergency Medical Journal 20: 414–417

McConnell D 1997 Health promotion for A&E practice. Emergency Nurse 5(7): 19–22

McKenna G 1994 The scope for health education in the accident and emergency department. Accident and Emergency Nursing 2(2): 94–99

Morcombe J 1999 Interpersonal approach to managing violence and aggression. Emergency Nurse 7(1): 12–15

National Audit Office 2002 Facing the challenge: NHS emergency planning in England. Report by the Comptroller and Auditor General, HC 36 session 2002–2003: 15 November 2002. NAO, London

National Health Services Executive (NHSE) 1998 Planning for major incidents: the NHS guidance. NHSE, London

Nursing and Midwifery Council (NMC) 2004 NMC code of professional conduct: standards for conduct, performance and ethics. NMC, London

Nutt D, Davidson J, Zohar J 2000 Post-traumatic stress disorder: diagnosis, management and treatment. Taylor and Francis, London

O'Byrne J 1989 Talking through the pain. Nursing Standard 3(25): 12

Resuscitation Council (UK) 2000 Advanced life support course. Provider manual, 4th edn. Resuscitation Council (UK), London

Robson R, Mitchell J, Murdoch P 1995 The debate on psychological debriefings. Australian Journal of Emergency Care 2(4): 6–7

Royal College of Nursing (RCN) 2002 Nurse practitioners – an RCN guide to the nurse practitioner role, competence and programme accreditation. RCN, London

Royal College of Nursing (RCN) 2003 Children and young people nursing: a philosophy of care. Guidance for nursing staff. RCN, London

Royal College of Surgeons of England 1988 The management of patients with major injuries: report of a working party. Royal College of Surgeons of England, London

Sakr M, Angus J, Perrin J et al 1999 Care of minor injuries by emergency nurse practitioners or junior doctors: a randomized controlled trial. Lancet 354: 1321–1326

Sbaih L 1992 Accident and emergency nursing: a nursing model. Chapman and Hall, London

Sowney R 1996 Stress debriefing: reality or myth? Accident and Emergency Nursing 4: 38–39

Talley N, O'Connor S 2000 Clinical examination, 3rd edn. Blackwell Science, Oxford

Van Der Kolk B 1998 The psychology and psychobiology of developmental trauma. In: Stoudermire A (ed) Human behavior: an introduction for medical students, 3rd edn. Lippincott-Raven, New York

Wardrope J, Smith J, Edhouse J 1999 The management of wounds and burns, 2nd edn. Oxford University Press, Oxford

Wright B 1996 Sudden death: a research base for practice, 2nd edn. Churchill Livingstone, Edinburgh

USEFUL WEBSITES AND ADDRESSES

The Compassionate Friends
www.tcf.org.uk

Crisis Counselling, Training, Education, Support (CRITEC)
Accident and Emergency Department
Leeds General Infirmary
Great George St
Leeds LS1 3EX
Tel: 01132 926498
Fax: 01132 922810

CRUSE
www.crusebereavementcare.org.uk

London Prepared (Anti-terrorism information)
www.londonprepared.gov.uk

The Foundation for the Study of Infant Deaths
www.sids.org.uk

UK Resilience (contains links to official reports and useful information for health professionals for major/chemical incidents)
www.ukresilience.info

Zero Tolerance Policy
www.nhs.uk/zerotolerance

THE UNCONSCIOUS PATIENT

Lesley Pemberton
Catheryne Waterhouse

28

INTRODUCTION

The unconscious patient presents a special challenge to the nurse. Medical management will vary according to the original cause of the patient's condition, but nursing care will be constant. The unconscious patient has no control over themselves or their environment and is therefore dependent upon the nurse to accept responsibility for the management of their activities of living and for monitoring their vital functions.

A high quality of nursing care is of crucial importance if the patient is to relearn to perceive self and others, to communicate, to control their body and their environment and to self-care. The responsibility placed on the nurse is considerable and can be a source of anxiety, even for experienced nurses. It is essential that the nurse has a firm understanding of the mechanisms causing altered states of consciousness, as well as a sound knowledge of the potential and actual physiological, psychological and social problems that these patients face. Skills training, exploring attitudes and using support systems can all help the nurse to overcome anxiety and take up the challenge.

To nurse an unconscious patient back to recovery must be one of the most rewarding aspects of nursing; however, even with all the medical advances made recently, not all patients can hope for complete recovery. Some may not survive and others may be left with a residual mental and/or physical handicap. These patients and their families will need considerable emotional support and reassurance. The nurse, who is with the patient more than any other member of the multidisciplinary team, is in the best position to give this support.

Defining consciousness

Normal conscious behaviour is dependent on intact brain function, specifically on intact cerebral hemispheres and an intact reticular activating system (see below). Impaired, reduced or absent consciousness implies the presence of brain dysfunction and demands urgent medical attention if potential recovery is to be expected. In order to appreciate the importance of altered states of consciousness, a basic understanding of the physiology of consciousness is required.

Hickey (2002) defines consciousness simply as 'a state of general awareness of oneself and the environment' and includes the ability to orientate toward new stimuli. The individual is wakeful, alert and aware of their personal identity and of the events occurring in their surroundings. Deep coma can be defined as the opposite — unrousable and unresponsive to external stimuli — and there may be varied states of altered consciousness in between the two extremes. The difference between sleep and coma is that, in sleep, the individual can be aroused by external stimuli, whereas in a coma this cannot be done. Consciousness therefore depends on whether the person can be aroused to wakefulness. Different stages of consciousness will be discussed later in this chapter.

ANATOMICAL AND PHYSIOLOGICAL BASIS FOR CONSCIOUSNESS

The reticular formation (RF) and the reticular activating system (RAS) are responsible for collating and transmitting motor and sensory activities and controlling sleep/waking cycles and consciousness (see Fig. 28.1 and Ch. 25).

The reticular formation (RF)

The RF is a network of neurones in the central core of the brain stem (Waugh & Grant 2001). These neurones connect with the spinal cord, cerebellum, thalamus and hypothalamus. The RF is involved in the coordination of skeletal muscle activity, including voluntary movement, posture and the maintenance of balance. It is also concerned with automatic and reflex activities and has links with the limbic system. All sensory pathways, including those of the special senses, link into the RF (Fitzgerald 1996). Neurones that produce aminergic neurotransmitters are embedded within the RF. Some of these have a stimulating effect and some an inhibitory effect on other neurones, although their exact functions are not yet fully understood.

The reticular activating system (RAS)

The RAS is a physiological component of the RF and the neurones which project (or radiate) to ocular motor nuclei and to the cerebral cortex via the thalamus and hypothalamus. It is concerned with the arousal of the brain in sleep and wakefulness (Marieb 2004).

Two main parts of the RAS have been identified (Guyton & Hall 2000):

- the mesencephalon
- the thalamus.

The mesencephalic area is composed of grey matter in the upper pons and midbrain of the brain stem. Stimulation of this area causes a diffuse flow of nerve impulses which pass upwards through the thalamus and hypothalamus. The impulses then radiate out to wide regions of the cerebral cortex (see Fig. 28.1). This causes a generalised increase in cerebral activity and general wakefulness.

Stimulation of the thalamus activates localised areas of the cerebral cortex. Signals from specific parts of the thalamus initiate activity in specific parts of the cortex, rather than activating the whole cortex. This selective stimulation prevents the cortex from receiving too much information at once and may play a part in directing one's attention to specific mental activities.

The reticular nucleus, which receives impulses from the RF, surrounds the front and sides of the thalamus. It is this nucleus that sends inhibiting messages back to thalamic nuclei via the neurotransmitter gamma-aminobutyric acid (GABA). In animal experiments, it has been demonstrated that thalamocortical neurones are inhibited by the reticular nucleus during sleep (Fitzgerald 1996).

In order to function, the RAS must be stimulated by input signals from a wide range of sources. These are transmitted via the spinal reticular tracts and various collateral tracts from all the modalities of sensation, e.g. the specialised auditory and visual tracts (see Ch. 9). The RAS is also affected by signals from the cerebral cortex, i.e. the RAS may first stimulate the cerebral cortex, and the cortical areas responding to reason and emotion may 'modify' the RAS, either positively or negatively, according to the 'decision' of the cerebral cortex. The RAS filters information to prevent sensory overload (Marieb 2004).

When an individual is in a deep sleep, the RAS is in a dormant state. However, almost any type of sensory signal can immediately activate the RAS and waken the individual,

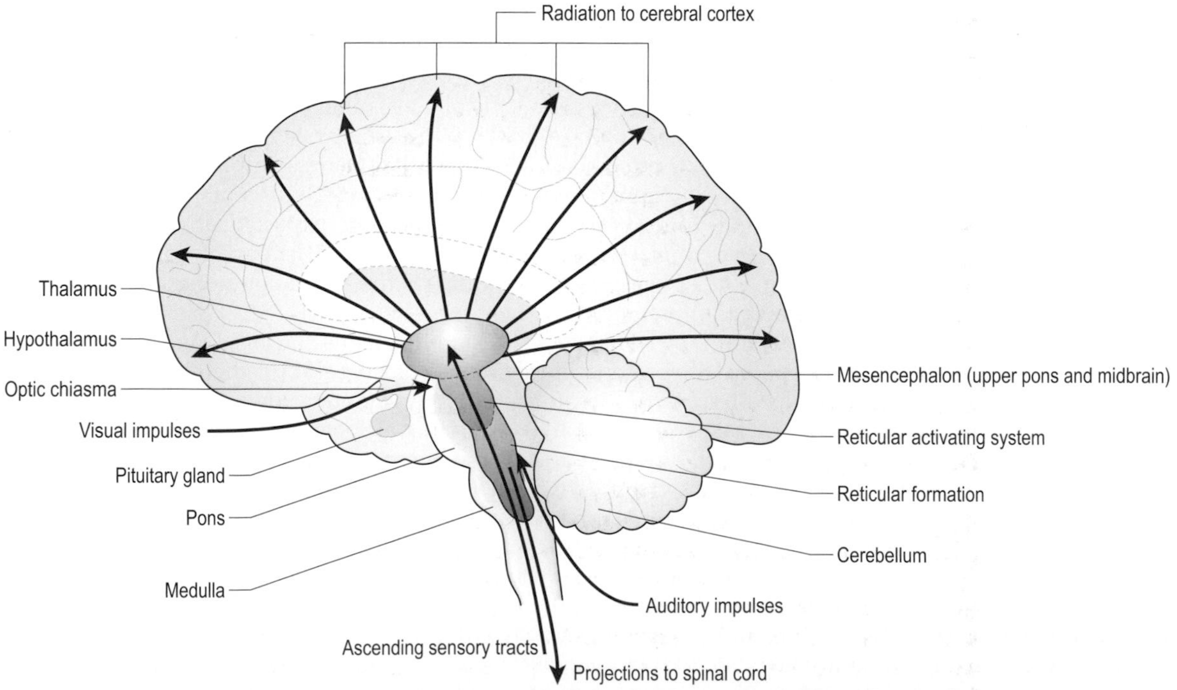

Fig. 28.1 The mid-sagittal section of the brain, showing the reticular activating system and related structures.

e.g. pain stimulus or unaccustomed noise. This is called the 'arousal reaction' and is the mechanism by which sensory stimuli wake us from deep sleep (Guyton & Hall 2000) (see Ch. 25).

Sleep is induced by a hormone called melatonin. This is synthesised from serotonin in the pineal gland. The normal arousal from sleep occurs as it gets light. Daylight is detected by the retina of the eye, which sends impulses to the suprachiasmatic nucleus of the hypothalamus. This activates sympathetic nerve fibres that inhibit the secretion of melatonin in the pineal gland. There is also evidence from animal experiments that histamine, produced in the posterior hypothalamic area, activates the cerebral cortex. Lesions in this area can cause excessive sleepiness or even coma (Fitzgerald 1996).

There are numerous pathways to both mesencephalic and thalamic portions from the sensory and motor cortex and from cortical areas that deal with the emotions. Whenever any of these areas becomes excited, impulses are transmitted into the RAS, thus increasing the activity. This is termed a 'positive feedback response'.

The feedback theory

Guyton and Hall (2000) claim that the cerebrum regulates incoming information by a positive feedback mechanism (Fig. 28.2). A second feedback cycle that stimulates proprioceptors in skeletal muscles is also shown in Figure 28.2.

After a prolonged period of wakefulness, the synapses in the feedback loops become increasingly fatigued, reducing the level of stimulation and activity directed to the reticular activating system, thereby inducing a state of lethargy, drowsiness and eventually sleep (Guyton & Hall 2000).

Figure 28.2 illustrates a number of activating pathways passing from the mesencephalon upward. Conversely, if all pathways are activated simultaneously, a high level of consciousness ensues.

The return to consciousness demonstrates that the RAS is still functioning and capable of screening and discrimination.

The content of consciousness

The content of consciousness refers to the sum of cognitive and affective mental functions. It is dependent upon relatively intact functional areas within the cerebral hemispheres that interact with each other as well as with the RAS.

Injury to, or disease of, the cerebral hemispheres, resulting in diffuse damage, can inhibit or block the signals from the RAS and consciousness cannot be completely maintained. The damaged cortex is unable to interpret the incoming sensory impulses and therefore cannot transmit them to other areas for action.

Localised damage to the cerebral hemispheres can also diminish the content of consciousness to a lesser degree. For example, a patient who has suffered a stroke, causing aphasia, may appear awake and alert. Their inability to understand or to use language, however, decreases their full awareness of self and their environment. Such localised defects are not generally regarded as a true altered state of consciousness, but this example highlights the difficulties in defining true conscious behaviour.

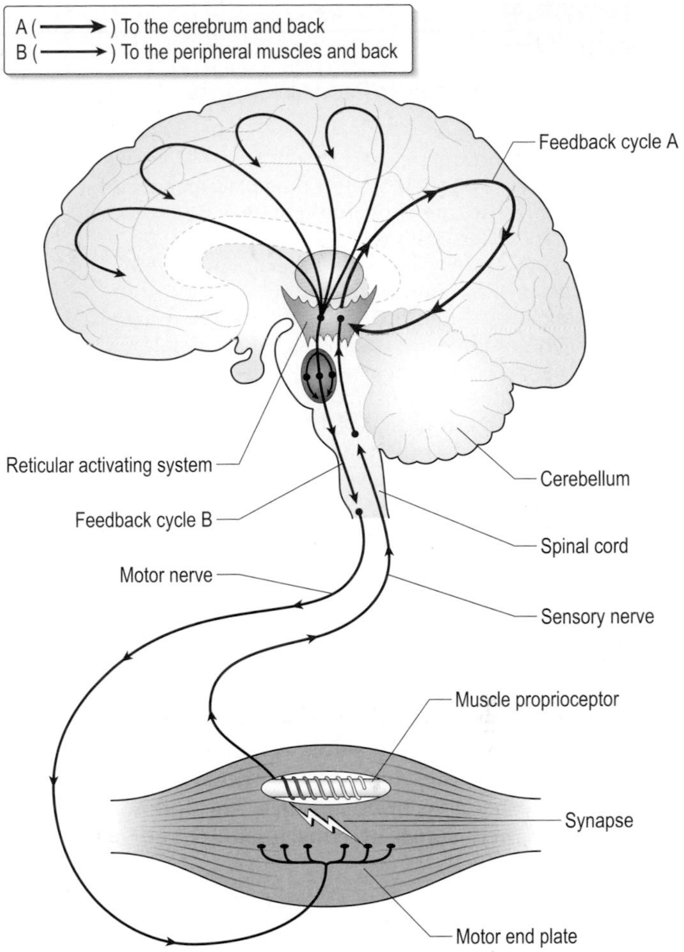

Fig. 28.2 The feedback mechanism, showing two feedback cycles passing through the RAS. In cycle A, the RAS excites the cerebral cortex and the cortex in turn re-excites the RAS. This initiates a cycle that causes continued intense excitation of both regions. In cycle B, impulses are sent down the spinal cord to activate skeletal muscles. Activation of the muscle stimulates proprioceptors to transmit sensory impulses upward to re-excite the RAS. Consciousness results when the RAS, in turn, stimulates the cerebral cortex.

STATES OF IMPAIRED CONSCIOUSNESS

There is no international definition of levels of consciousness but, for assessment purposes, differing states of consciousness can be considered on a continuum between full consciousness and deep coma (Hickey 2002) (see Box 28.1). Consciousness cannot be measured directly but can be estimated by observing behaviour in response to stimuli. The Glasgow Coma Scale (GCS) (Teasdale 1975) is widely used as an assessment tool and helps to reduce subjectivity during assessment. The GCS is explained on pages 970–974.

Signs of deterioration in a patient's level of consciousness are usually the first indications of further impending brain damage. The nurse must be able to assess and observe the patient accurately so that appropriate intervention can be instituted if the level of consciousness changes. Sleep is considered a normal phenomenon and is discussed in Chapter 25.

Box 28.1

Continuum of levels of consciousness

- *Full consciousness* — awake, alert, orientated, cognitive (mental) functioning intact
- *Confusion* — disorientated to time/place/person, short attention span, memory problems, may be agitated/restless/irritable
- *Lethargy* — orientated, slow speech, slow mental processes, slow motor activities
- *Obtundation* — rousable with stimulation, responds verbally with one or two words, follows simple commands, very drowsy
- *Stupor* — quiet, minimal movement, generally unresponsive except to vigorous stimuli, responds in normal way to painful stimuli
- *Coma* — unrousable, no verbal sounds, inappropriate or no response to stimuli

It is difficult to classify levels of consciousness exactly, but this is a useful guide to help to describe various levels.

Adapted from Hickey (2002).

Impaired states of consciousness can be categorised as acute or chronic. Acute states are potentially reversible, whereas chronic states tend to be irreversible as they are caused by destructive brain lesions. The following definitions of impaired states of consciousness can be used as broad guidelines to describe the patient's condition. Individual patients are unlikely to exhibit all the stages noted on the continuum (see Box 28.1), even if they pass from full consciousness to coma or vice versa. Deterioration or improvement will depend on a number of factors such as type, extent and site of injury, age, previous state of health, length of coma and whether or not the altered level of consciousness is a result of acute or chronic insult. Common causes of unconsciousness are illustrated in Figure 28.3.

Acute states of impaired consciousness

Intracranial diseases and metabolic disease, such as hypoglycaemic coma, renal and hepatic disorders or drug overdose, cause acute states of impaired consciousness, including:

- reduced awareness
- delirium
- illusions
- hallucinations
- delusions
- stupor
- coma.

Reduced awareness

Reduction in awareness reflects generalised brain dysfunction, as seen in systemic and metabolic disorders (see Fig. 28.3). These disorders interfere with the integrity of the RAS, thus affecting the arousal response.

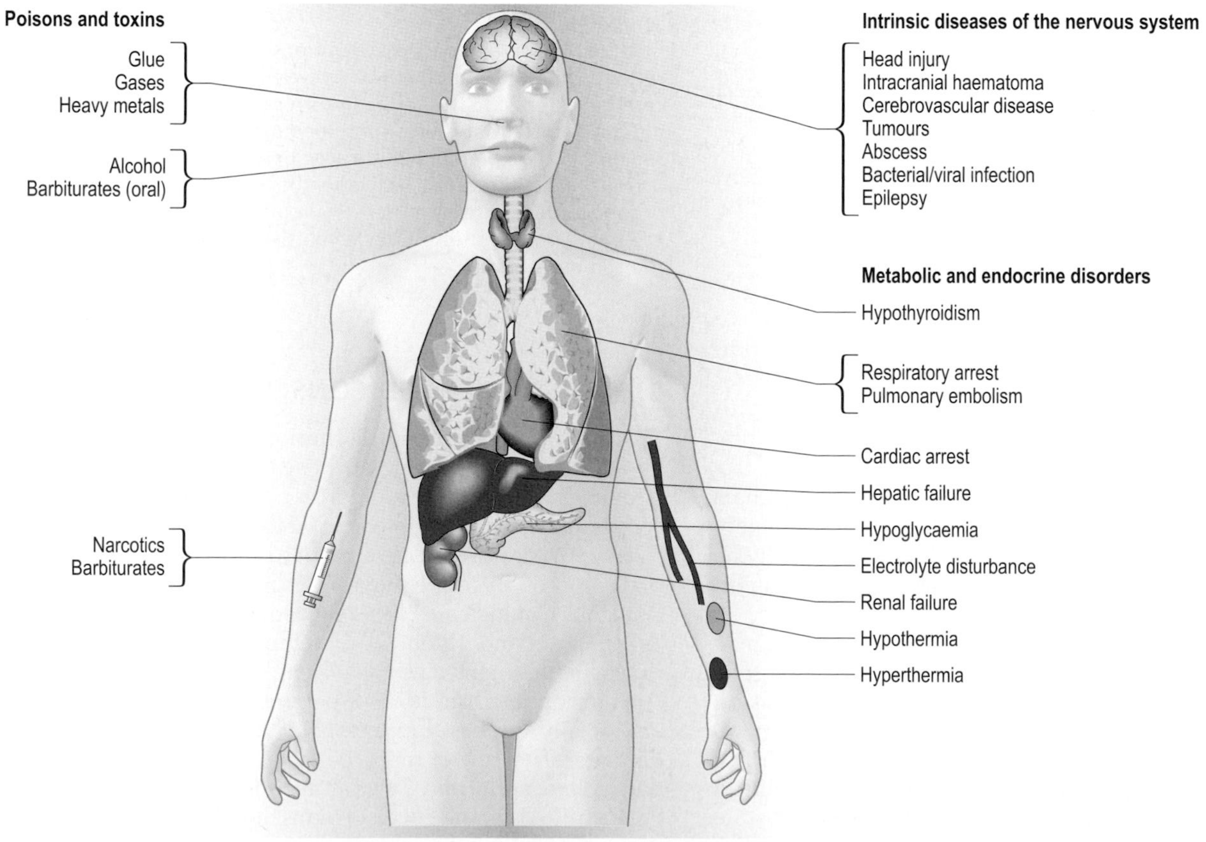

Fig. 28.3 Common causes of unconsciousness.

In the early stage, the patient may exhibit signs of hyperexcitability and irritability, alternating with drowsiness. This may progress to a confused state and increased levels of disorientation. The patient is bewildered and often has difficulty in following commands.

Initially, subtle changes may occur in the patient's behaviour. Minor disturbance of consciousness can easily go undetected if attention is not paid to what the patient says and does. If a normally placid and cooperative patient becomes irritable and aggressive, this denotes a behaviour change that requires further investigation. Similarly, comments from a relative such as 'she does not seem to recognise me today' should alert the nurse to the fact that something is not quite right with the patient. Martin (1994) suggests that nurses who are expert in the care of head-injured individuals can identify cues which indicate behavioural, cognitive, motor and sensory changes even in mild head injury.

Any change in the patient's behaviour must be reported to the appropriate nursing or medical staff, particularly if the patient has not previously exhibited any of these signs. The patient's nursing care plan will also need to be evaluated and new goals for care set.

Cognitive disabilities, e.g. poor concentration and memory changes, may only become apparent when a patient returns home. These can cause emotional distress for both the patient and family if they go unheeded and help is not provided. Hemingway and McAndrew (1998) suggest that the community mental health nurse could have a role in supporting people with acquired brain injury, and their families, in the early stages following injury and through to long-term community care.

Delirium

Delirium is a fluctuating mental state characterised by confusion, disorientation, fear and irritability. The patient is usually loud, talkative, offensive, suspicious and agitated. This behaviour reflects generalised brain dysfunction due to interference with the RAS, affecting arousal. The causes and manifestations of delirium are listed in Box 28.2.

Box 28.2

Causes and manifestations of delirium

- Toxic disorders of the nervous system, e.g. acute poisoning by:
  - metals
  - gases
  - drugs
  - alcohol
- Metabolic disorders, e.g.:
  - renal failure
  - hepatic failure
  - encephalitis
- Severe head injury
- Psychological manifestations
  - illusions
  - hallucinations
  - delusions

Illusions are defined as misinterpretations of sensory material in the patient's environment. A shadow on the wall is seen as an animal or a person, for example, or noises are misinterpreted as voices of strangers who have come to do harm.

Hallucinations are defined as seeing or hearing something in the absence of the relevant sensory stimuli; for example, the patient will hear voices when no-one is present or see objects that do not exist in their environment. Other senses, such as touch, taste or smell, can be affected; with acute disorders of the brain, however, hallucinations are usually visual.

Delusions are defined as persistent misperceptions that are firmly held by a person, even though they are illogical or contrary to reality.

Illusions and hallucinatory experiences are common in temporal lobe epilepsy (see Ch. 9). Perceptual disturbances and delusions can also occur in patients exposed to sensory deprivation or overload, e.g. in intensive care units or in sleep deprivation (Phipps et al 1999, Jones et al 2001, Hewitt 2002). Therefore, when undertaking an assessment, it is important to consider the environment as well as the patient's physiological state.

Stupor

The term stupor describes a state whereby the patient is quiet and tends not to move, except in response to vigorous and repeated noxious stimuli (Hickey 2002).

Coma

Coma is an impaired state where the patient is totally unaware of themselves and their environment. It may vary in degree and, in its deepest stages, no reaction of any kind is obtainable.

For further reading, see Hickey (2002), Chapter 8.

Chronic states of impaired consciousness

The chronic states of impaired consciousness are:

- dementia
- vegetative
- locked-in syndrome.

Dementia

This condition is caused by a generalised and progressive loss of cortical tissue from the brain. Mental functions decline progressively. There is global deterioration of memory, thinking, motor performance, emotional responsiveness and social behaviour; however, arousal remains intact.

As the condition develops, speech may become hesitant with eventual aphasia. Behaviour becomes increasingly unreasonable and often disruptive, until control of basic and vital processes is disorganised. There are numerous causes of progressive dementia. The most prevalent type is Alzheimer's disease.

Dementia is usually an irreversible condition. However, there are some occasions when the decline in cognitive functions can be halted and even partially reversed, e.g. in normal pressure hydrocephalus, which can be treated by insertion of a ventricular shunt (Dalvi 2004, Wilson & Islam 2004; see also Life NPH in 'Useful websites', p. 988).

Vegetative

Vegetative state (VS) is a term used to describe a condition that can occur following brain injury, where there is severe damage to the cerebral cortex. In a vegetative state, the patient has sleep/waking cycles and will open their eyes when awake. The thinking, feeling part of the brain is destroyed, although many reflex responses may remain. Physiologically, the brain stem is functioning but the cerebral cortex is not. Patients can survive for many years in this condition and require full-time care. 'Continuing vegetative state' describes the patient's condition prior to confirmation of 'permanent vegetative state' (PVS). The British Medical Association recommended 'that the diagnosis of irreversible PVS should not be considered or confirmed (and therefore treatment not be withdrawn) until the patient has been insentient for 12 months' (British Medical Association 1996). The Royal College of Physicians (2003) issued new guidance on the diagnosis and management of patients in a vegetative state, as assessment, management and legal requirements had changed.

There is ongoing debate, both in the UK and abroad, about the moral, ethical and legal issues surrounding the care and treatment of these individuals (Multi-society Task Force Report on PVS 1994, Day et al 1995, British Medical Association 1996, Grubb et al 1996, Smith 1997, Royal College of Physicians 2003). Cases such as those of Bland in England (Airedale NHS Trust v. Bland E 1993), Cruzan in the USA (Cruzan 1990) and Johnstone in Scotland (Law Hospital NHS Trust v. The Lord Advocate and Others 1996) brought the dilemma of 'the right to die' and withdrawal of treatment to media, and thus public, attention. Research into the views of doctors and nurses in Europe on PVS was conducted by a project committee headed by Professor Andrew Grubb (Grubb et al 1996).

Locked-in syndrome

This condition results in paralysis of voluntary muscles without interfering with consciousness and cognitive functions. The patient is unable to speak and is sometimes unable to breathe spontaneously, the latter requiring artificial ventilation. The patient is, however, able to control vertical eye movements and blinking and may be able to use these movements to develop a simple communication system. It is important to remember that the patient is aware of their surroundings, even if appearing to be mentally and physically inert.

The pathological basis for this condition is damage to the pons in the brain stem, which may result from cerebral vascular disease or trauma.

For further information on PVS and locked-in syndrome, see Randall (1997), Smith (1997) and the Report of a working party of the Royal College of Physicians (2003). The ongoing and wider debate about an individual's 'right to die' can also be followed on various media and the internet — see also www.justice4diane.org.uk.

STOP THINK **28.1** What implications may there be for the patient and family if PVS is misdiagnosed?

ASSESSMENT OF THE NERVOUS SYSTEM

Nurses must be competent to monitor the conscious level for signs of deterioration, improvement or stability and they must understand what the observations mean. The need to assess conscious level may arise at any time in any ward in any hospital. In seminal work, Teasdale (1975) noted that ambiguities and misunderstandings can result when passing on information about the patient's level of consciousness to other staff. There was clearly a need for a standardised system of assessing the conscious level, so that different nurses and doctors would make similar observations on the patient at any one time. In 1974, Teasdale and Jennett developed the Glasgow Coma Scale (GCS), a process used throughout the UK and worldwide as part of the neurological assessment and ongoing observation of the patient (see Fig. 28.4). Its use provides the detail from which to determine any change in the patient's level of consciousness, i.e. is it static, improving or deteriorating, so that appropriate action can be taken expeditiously (Waterhouse 2005). The National Centre for Clinical Excellence (NICE) (2003) has published guidelines for the management of patients with head injury, which stipulate the use of the GCS for all head-injured patients (see also Ch. 9).

The Neurological Observation Chart

The Glasgow Coma Scale

In monitoring the patient's conscious level, the functional state of the brain is assessed as a whole. The nurse observes and describes three aspects of the patient's behaviour:

- eye opening
- verbal response
- motor response.

Each of these is independently assessed and recorded on a chart (see Fig. 28.4). Each aspect shows a variety of possible responses. The patient's response is recorded by placing a dot in the appropriate square. The dots are joined to form a graph, making the chart easier to read. The decision about the time intervals between recording the assessments will be based on the patient's condition. The best response for each of the three aspects is recorded as a numerical score. In the case of eye opening, the best response would score a 4, the best verbal response would score a 5 and the best motor responses would score a 6. The lowest response for each of the three parameters is a score of 1.

The scores can be added together to give a total which could range from 3 to 15. The higher the score, the better the patient's condition; a score of 8 or less is generally considered to indicate that the patient is in a coma. However, it is important to consider each of the three aspects (eye opening, verbal response and motor response) separately as well as together. A patient may be blind, deaf, mute or have paralysis unrelated to their current condition and these other conditions would affect the scores. In some wards/hospitals, the numerical scores are not recorded. It is also worth noting that, although the GCS is widely used, there may be some slight variations in the layout of the assessment chart in different hospitals.

The Neuroscience Nurses' Benchmarking Group (NNBG) (see 'Note', p. 988) has set the standard for the assessment

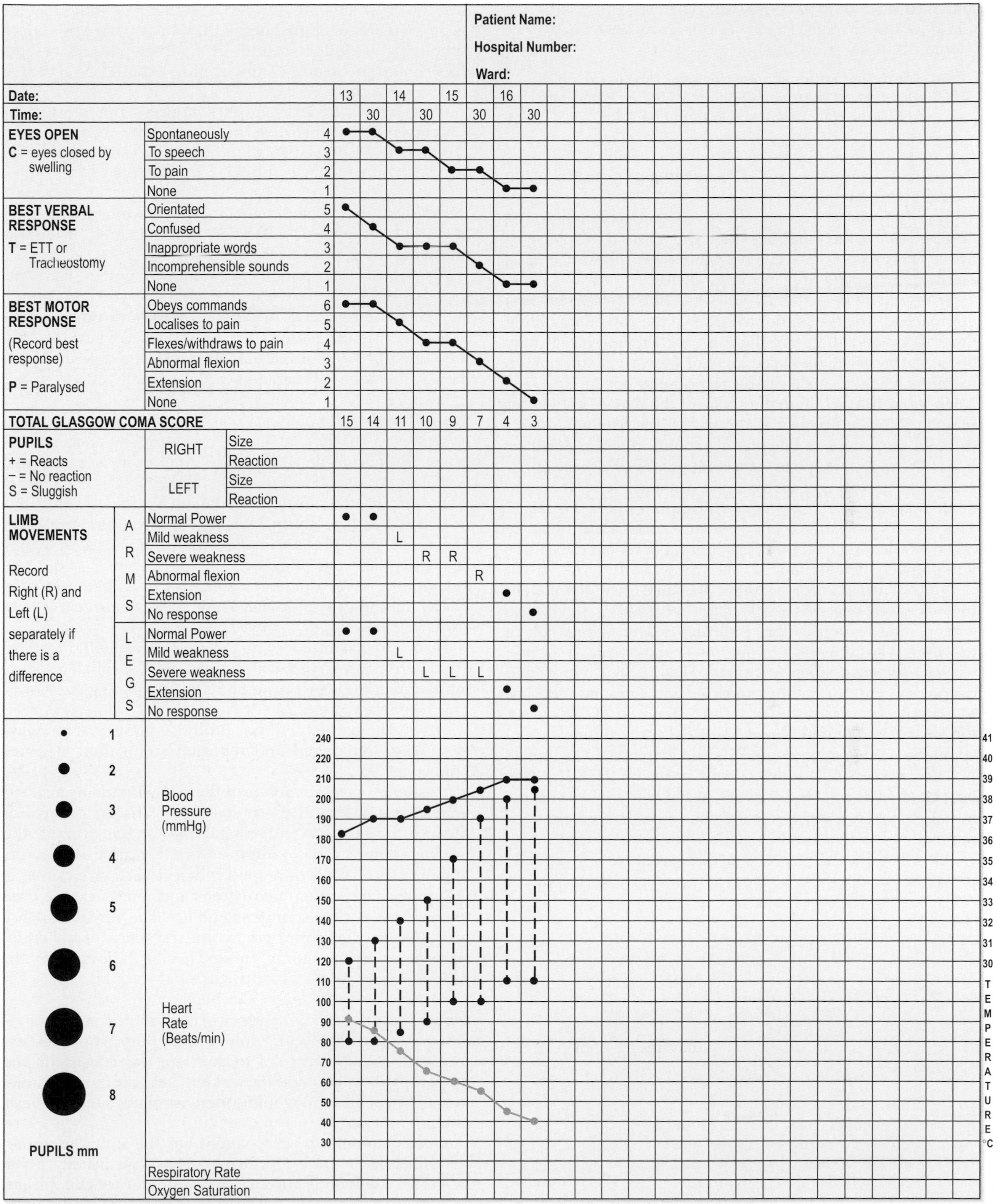
Patient Name:
Hospital Number:
Ward:
Date:
Time:
13 14 15 16
30 30 30 30
EYES OPEN
C = eyes closed by swelling
Spontaneously 4
To speech 3
To pain 2
None 1
BEST VERBAL RESPONSE
T = ETT or Tracheostomy
Orientated 5
Confused 4
Inappropriate words 3
Incomprehensible sounds 2
None 1
BEST MOTOR RESPONSE
(Record best response)
P = Paralysed
Obeys commands 6
Localises to pain 5
Flexes/withdraws to pain 4
Abnormal flexion 3
Extension 2
None 1
TOTAL GLASGOW COMA SCORE
15 14 11 10 9 7 4 3
PUPILS
+ = Reacts
− = No reaction
S = Sluggish
RIGHT
LEFT
Size
Reaction
LIMB MOVEMENTS
Record Right (R) and Left (L) separately if there is a difference
ARMS
Normal Power
Mild weakness
Severe weakness
Abnormal flexion
Extension
No response
L
R R
R
LEGS
Normal Power
Mild weakness
Severe weakness
Extension
No response
L
L L L
1 2 3 4 5 6 7 8
PUPILS mm
Blood Pressure (mmHg)
Heart Rate (Beats/min)
240 220 210 200 190 180 170 160 150 140 130 120 110 100 90 80 70 60 50 40 30
41 40 39 38 37 36 35 34 33 32 31 30
TEMPERATURE °C
Respiratory Rate
Oxygen Saturation

Fig. 28.4 The Neurological Observation Chart.

and recording of a patient's neurological status using the Glasgow Coma Scale (Fairley & Cosgrove 1999, Shah 1999, Mooney & Comerford 2003).

For further information on the use of the Neurological Observation Chart and GCS in practice, see Woodward (1997a–d), NICE (2003) and Waterhouse (2005).

Eye opening The degree of stimulation required to make the patient open their eyes is observed and recorded using the following categories.

Spontaneously The patient opens their eyes when first approached, which implies that the arousal response is active. This response is given a score of 4. Allowance must be made if the patient is in a natural sleep.

To speech The patient's eyes are not open when first approached. The nurse should speak to the patient by calling their name and then ask them to open their eyes. It may be necessary to increase the level of the verbal stimulation to gain a reaction. A successful response scores 3.

To pain Initially, a gentle shake of the patient's shoulder may be sufficient to elicit a response. If the patient still fails to open their eyes, a peripheral painful stimulus must be used. Pressure is applied to the lateral inner aspect of the second or third finger using a pen or pencil, held at a right angle against the finger, for a maximum of 30 s (Fig. 28.5). This response scores 2 on the coma scale. Care must be taken not to exert pressure on the patient's cuticle as this will damage the nail bed.

None If the painful stimulus does not cause the patient to open even one eye, then this is recorded as having no eye-opening response. This indicates a deep depression of the arousal system and is scored as 1 on the scale.

Possible assessment problems The patient who is in a deep coma with flaccid eye muscles will show no response to stimulation. If the eyelids are drawn back, however, the eyes may remain open. This is very different from spontaneous eye opening and should be recorded as 'none'.

The nurse needs to be aware if the patient has any hearing deficits as, if the eyes are closed, this could affect the initial response. Congenital deficits of the eye or previous removal of the eye should also be taken into account.

After trauma or surgery, eyelid swelling occasionally prevents eye opening, as does tarsorrhaphy where upper and lower eyelids are sutured together. A condition such as ptosis (palsy of cranial nerve III) will also have this effect, although this seldom results in complete closure of both eyes. Enforced closure of the eyelid(s) should be recorded as 'C' on the chart.

Opening of the eyes implies arousal, but it must be remembered that this does not necessarily mean that the patient is aware of their surroundings. This can be misleading and be a source of false optimism in relatives.

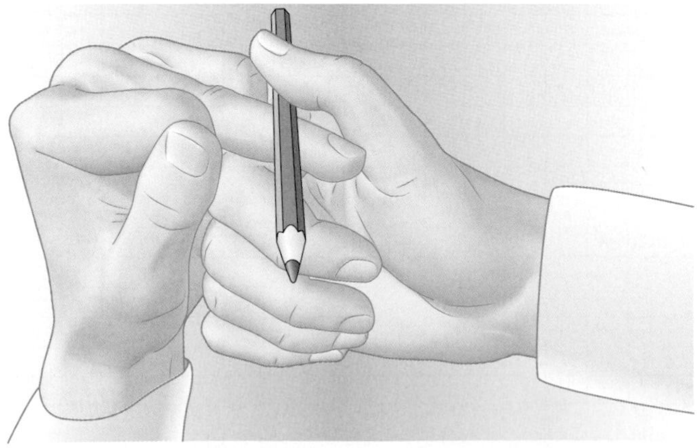

Fig. 28.5 Applying a peripheral painful stimulus: fingertip stimulation. (Adapted from Teasdale 1975.)

Verbal response The patient's best achievement in respect of verbal response is observed and recorded using the following categories.

Orientated The patient is orientated if they can state their name, where they are and what the year and month are. This is orientation in person, place and time, respectively, and is given a score of 5. Questions can be varied but they must be kept simple; for example, the date and even the day are not easily remembered, especially after a period in hospital.

Confused If the patient is capable of producing phrases or sentences but the conversation is rambling and inappropriate to the questions about orientation, it is a confused verbal response and scores 4.

Inappropriate words The patient will speak only one or two words, usually in response to physical stimulation. The words and phrases make little or no sense and may be obscenities. On occasion, the patient may shout out obscenities or call a person's name for no apparent reason. These all indicate a lower level of responsiveness and score 3.

Incomprehensible sounds The patient will moan or grunt in response to physical stimulation. The verbal response may contain indistinct mumbling but no intelligible words. This response scores 2.

None The patient will not produce any verbal response even when prolonged and repeated stimulation is given. This scores 1.

Possible assessment problems The patient may be unable to understand the nurse's questions or commands because they do not understand the language or have a hearing defect. The patient's verbal response may be impaired as a result of a speech defect such as dysphasia. If appropriate, written instructions and replies can be used to assess the patient's language ability. The verbal response may also be compromised by the presence of an endotracheal or tracheostomy tube. This is indicated on the patient's chart as 'T'.

Motor response The patient's best motor response is observed (see Fig. 28.6). Only upper limb responses are recorded, as leg responses to pain are less consistent and inappropriate spinal withdrawal reflexes occur more readily in many patients who would otherwise show a total absence of brain function.

Obeys commands The patient has the ability to appreciate instructions (see Fig. 28.6A). These are usually given by verbal commands such as: 'Put out your tongue, please' or 'Lift up your arms, please'. If the patient obeys these instructions, a score of 6 is given.

Localises to pain This is the response to a central painful stimulus. If the patient does not obey commands, the NNBG guidelines advocate the application of pressure over the supraorbital ridge. The nurse's hand rests gently on the patient's forehead and the flat of the nurse's thumb is placed on the patient's supraorbital ridge under the eyebrow. Pressure is gradually increased for a maximum of 30 s. The response is recorded as 'localising to pain' if the patient moves their arm across the midline, to the level of the chin, in an attempt to locate the source of the pain (see Fig. 28.6B). In the presence of facial fractures or gross orbital oedema, the trapezium pinch is an effective alternative. The patient's shoulder is exposed and the trapezius muscle is squeezed between the nurse's fingers and thumb (Frawley 1990). Localisation to pain will score 5.

During the course of the day, the patient may display a localising response to other sources of irritation, e.g. attempts to remove their oxygen mask, nasogastric tube or urinary catheter.

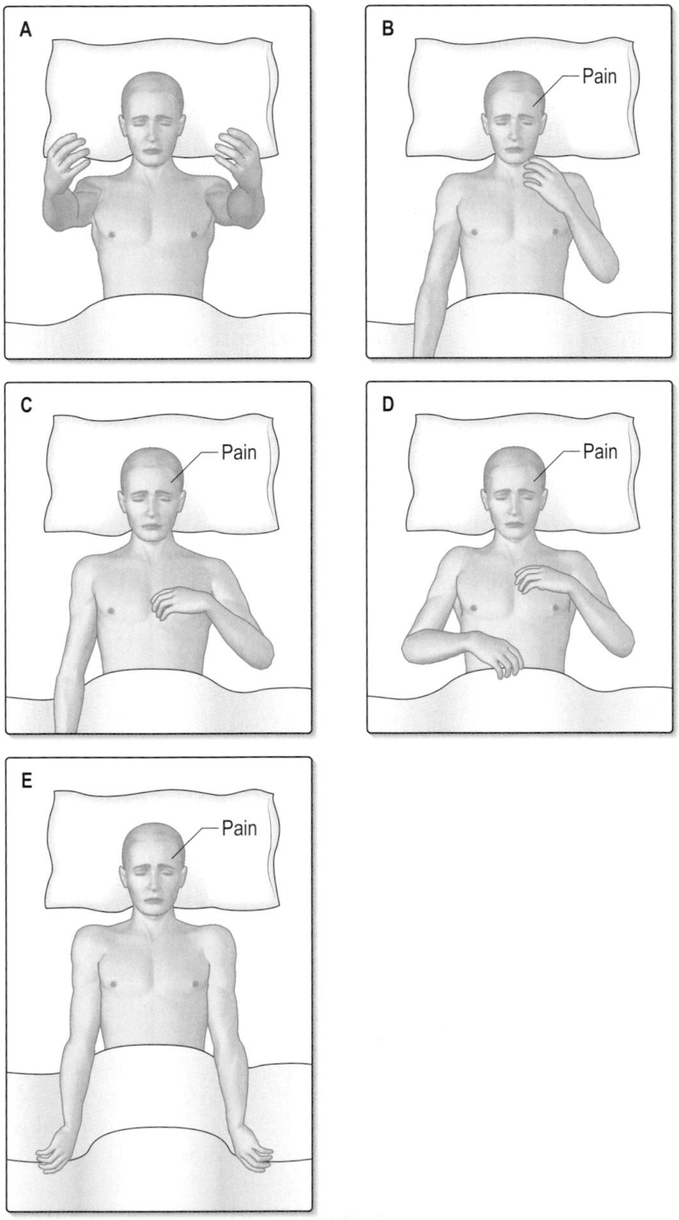

Fig. 28.6 Motor responses. A: Obeys commands ('lift up your arms'). B: Localising to pain. C: Flexing to pain. D: Abnormal flexion. E: Extending to pain.

Flexion to pain Following the application of a central painful stimulus, the patient responds by bending their elbow and withdrawing their hand, but no attempt to localise is made (see Fig. 28.6C). This is 'flexion to pain' and scores 4.

Abnormal flexion This involves the patient bending their elbow with adduction of the upper arms and spastic flexion of the wrist and fingers, otherwise known as decorticate posturing (see Fig. 28.6D). Abnormal flexion is scored as 3.

Extension to pain After painful stimulation, the patient responds by rigid extension, i.e. straightening the elbows and hyperpronation of the forearms, otherwise known as decerebrate posturing. The response usually includes spastic hand and wrist movements, with an inward rotation of the shoulders and forearms (see Fig. 28.6E). The legs are generally straight, with the feet pointing outwards. This response scores 2.

None This response is only recorded when sufficient painful stimulus has been applied to the patient to provoke a response and no detectable movement has been observed. This will score 1 on the scale.

Decortication and decerebration Painful stimuli can initiate abnormal postures if motor nerves are interrupted at specific cerebral levels. A patient with severe brain damage may exhibit one or a combination of these postures without any stimulation.

Possible assessment problems Variations in the motor response may occur during the assessment. Therefore, it is the best response that should be scored; for example, if the patient localises to pain on the left side but flexes to pain on the right, the localising response is recorded. Asymmetrical responses are significant, indicating that a focal neurological deficit is present, but overall brain function is more accurately reflected by the level of best response on the better side (see 'Limb movement' below).

When applying a painful stimulus, it is important to explain to the patient and relatives what you are about to do and why you are doing it, otherwise they may feel that unnecessary trauma is being inflicted.

Recording other measurements

The Neurological Observation Chart is used to record additional measurements (see Fig. 28.4) as follows:

- vital signs
  - — blood pressure
  - — heart rate (pulse)
  - — respirations
  - — temperature
- pupil size and reaction
- limb movements.

Vital signs

Blood pressure and pulse The famous Canadian neurosurgeon Harvey Williams Cushing (1869–1939) noted that a rise in intracranial pressure (ICP) led to a rise in blood pressure (elevated systolic pressure and widening pulse pressure) and a slowing pulse (see Ch. 9), termed 'Cushing's response'. However, this is a very late sign of raised ICP, and the Glasgow Coma Scale will show evidence of deterioration much earlier.

Changes in the blood pressure and pulse can indicate injury or disease elsewhere in the body; for example, falling blood pressure and a rapid and weak pulse are indicative of haemorrhage and shock (see Ch. 18).

Respiration Conditions that impair consciousness may also cause respiratory changes. The pattern and rate of respiration may be directly affected by brain damage. The rate of respiration is recorded on the chart, but it is also important for the nurse to observe the depth, rhythm and characteristics of respiration. Deep lesions in the cerebrum tend to produce a periodic pattern such as Cheyne–Stokes respiration. Lesions affecting the pons and medulla cause more irregular patterns. If the patient is being ventilated, abnormal respiratory patterns will not be evident.

Temperature Impaired brain function seldom causes significant changes in body temperature, unless there has been direct damage to the temperature-regulating centre in the hypothalamus (see Ch. 22), when the temperature can rise rapidly. Each rise in degree of temperature increases the brain's metabolic rate, and must be treated urgently to prevent further neurological deterioration. A gradual elevation in temperature is likely to be an early sign of infection in the lungs or urinary tract, or in a wound.

Pupil size and reaction

The size of both pupils is measured by comparing them with a series of circular millimetre measures on the chart (see Fig. 28.4) or by descriptive terms (Hickey 2002). Reaction to light is recorded by a plus (+); no reaction is recorded by a minus (–). Pupil reactions should be assessed in dim surroundings, using a small bright flashlight. To elicit the direct-light reflex, the nurse holds both of the patient's eyelids open in turn, brings the light in from the outer side of the eye and shines it directly into the eye. This should cause a brisk constriction of the pupil, and withdrawal of the light should produce brisk dilatation of the pupil. The size and reaction are observed and recorded on the chart. The shape of the pupils should also be assessed.

Abnormal pupillary size and reaction can indicate brain dysfunction and/or raised ICP. It is important to note any changes, particularly if they occur in conjunction with other changes in the neurological observations.

For further information on the Glasgow Coma Scale and other neurological observations, see Hickey (2002), Chapter 8, NICE (2003), Department of Health (2005) and Waterhouse (2005).

Limb movement

Disturbances of limb movement indicate localised (focal) brain damage and vary according to the site and extent of the damage; for example, the right arm and leg will be affected by a lesion in the left cerebral hemisphere. Diffuse brain damage will result in a greater disturbance of movement.

When no localised brain damage is suspected, such as in metabolic or drug coma, the best motor response on the coma scale is usually sufficient for monitoring responses. When localised brain damage is suspected, an additional detailed assessment of each limb is necessary (see Fig. 28.4).

The nurse examines the arms and legs for movement and strength, and compares the right and left sides. When the two sides are the same, recordings are made in the standard manner (see p. 971). When differences exist, right and left are recorded independently, noting 'R' for right and 'L' for left. Responses can be elicited by verbal commands, such as asking the patient to grip the nurse's hand as tightly as possible, to lift up their arms or to bend their knees. To test strength, the nurse may need to provide some form of resistance, such as pressing down on the patient's knee when the patient is trying to bend it.

Painful stimuli may be applied to the appropriate limb if verbal comments fail to elicit a response.

CAUSES OF UNCONSCIOUSNESS

The major causes of unconsciousness are shown in Figure 28.3.

Unconsciousness occurs when the RAS is damaged or its function is depressed so that there is an interruption of the normal arousal mechanisms. This may be caused by a primary or secondary insult to the nervous system: primary insults are commonly caused by intrinsic diseases of the brain; secondary involvement is most often caused by metabolic, endocrine or toxic conditions, where the critical insult is manifested elsewhere in the body.

Information on some of the conditions that can result in loss of consciousness can be found in Chapters 5 and 9.

EMERGENCY CARE OF THE UNCONSCIOUS PATIENT

Whatever the cause of unconsciousness and wherever the event occurs, the patient's life depends on the knowledge and skills of those who find and care for them. The first aid and care that the patient receives until consciousness is regained, if this is achievable, will help to determine the outcome (see Box 28.3).

A hospital emergency

In hospital, an individual can be rendered unconscious by any of the causes shown in Figure 28.3. The person does not necessarily need to be a patient; visitors and members of staff are also at risk from events such as cardiac arrest, cerebrovascular accident or falls resulting in head injury. The measures a nurse should take on finding someone collapsed are as follows:

1. Shout for assistance and press the emergency call button.
2. Move the person into a wider space if this is possible.
3. Following the ABC principles (see p. 34), initiate cardiopulmonary resuscitation (CPR) if the individual is not breathing and the carotid pulse is absent. The cardiac arrest team should be called at this point.
4. If the person is breathing and a pulse is present, place them in a semi-prone (recovery) position. However, if spinal injury is suspected, do not move the person or place them in the semi-prone position without keeping

Box 28.3

First aid for someone who is unconscious

N.B. If alone, the first action normally is to seek help.

1. Check the victim's breathing and pulse. If they are not breathing and a pulse is not felt in the carotid artery, turn them onto their back and initiate cardiopulmonary resuscitation (see Ch. 2). If possible, get help to do this.
2. Clear the victim's airway if necessary. Remove dentures or dental plates, if possible, and keep them in a safe place.
3. Call for help. If outside the hospital setting, send someone to telephone for an ambulance. Make sure that the person knows the location and has some details of the victim. Ask the person to return to confirm that the telephone call has been made.
4. If the victim is breathing and has a pulse, loosen their clothing at the neck, chest and waist. Keep bystanders away from the victim. If necessary, and if possible, move them to a safer place.
5. Check for any other injuries or bruises and stem any bleeding.
6. Place the victim in the semi-prone or recovery position, as follows:
   (a) Kneel beside them and place their arms alongside their body.
   (b) Cross the victim's ankle furthest away from you over the one nearest to you.
   (c) Cushion their head with your hand.
   (d) Place your other hand on the victim's hip furthest from you and roll them gently towards you.
   (e) Maintain a clear airway by grasping under their jaw and moving their chin upwards and backwards. This extends the neck and prevents the victim's tongue from blocking their throat.
   (f) Pull up the arm nearest to you so that the point of the elbow is in line with the victim's shoulder.

   This position prevents the victim's tongue from falling into the back of their throat and blocking the airway. It also allows fluid, such as blood or vomit, to drain from their mouth.

   Note: The position is contraindicated in victims with suspected spinal injury, when movement risks further damage to the spinal cord (see Chs 10 and 27).
7. Stay with the victim until the ambulance arrives. Give a detailed account of events to the paramedics. This should include how the victim was found and what resuscitative measures were taken.

the head, neck and spine in alignment. In the hospital setting it may be possible to obtain a cervical collar or spinal board if necessary. Stay with the person until assistance arrives and they can be moved to an appropriate place for further treatment and investigation.

Planned admission

When an unconscious patient is to be admitted to hospital, the following measures must be taken:

- Remove the top bedclothes and the head of the bed to facilitate easy access to the patient.
- Check that the oxygen supply and suction apparatus are functioning and that there is an adequate supply of relevant equipment.
- The necessary equipment should be available for immediate use:
  (a) a resuscitation trolley containing the following:
  — Guedel airways (usually size 3 or 4 for an adult)
  — Ambu bag with universal catheter mount. If the patient is unable to breathe spontaneously, they must be ventilated manually via an endotracheal tube, using an Ambu bag, until they can be transferred to an intensive care unit
  — laryngoscope and selection of endotracheal tubes, sizes 6.5–10.00 mm
  — lubricating jelly; strapping or tape; 5 mL syringe to inflate the endotracheal tube cuff
  — emergency drug box or pack
  (b) an intravenous infusion stand
  (c) equipment for passing a nasogastric tube to aspirate the stomach contents
  (d) a neurological examination tray
  (e) the appropriate charts and admission forms.

Priorities of nursing management

The following checklist itemises the priorities of nursing management in an emergency situation, in order to sustain the patient's vital functions:

1. Maintenance of a clear airway
   (a) the patient's position
   (b) artificial airways
   (c) suction
   (d) oxygen
   (e) nasogastric tube.
2. Assessment of the central nervous system
   (a) Glasgow Coma Scale
   (b) vital signs
   (c) pupillary reactions
   (d) limb movements.
3. Maintenance of fluid balance
   (a) intravenous infusion
   (b) catheterisation of the urinary bladder, if necessary.

Care of relatives Measures to sustain the vital functions of the patient must take priority. Anyone accompanying the patient must also be considered, and a nurse who is not involved in the immediate care of the patient should be allocated to care for them. The nurse should provide them with written information regarding hospital procedures and explain the investigations related to the patient's condition. At the same time, the nurse may be able to gather the patient's biographical data and other information to help in planning the patient's care.

Medical management

An unconscious patient is a medical emergency, unless the unconscious state represents the terminal state of a progressive and not specifically treatable disease. Although life support measures have priority, the cause of the unconscious state must be determined before the appropriate treatment can be given. These life support measures include establishment of an adequate airway, control of haemorrhage, and fluid or blood replacement. When the patient has ingested an overdose of drugs, gastric lavage may be indicated, but is only performed under advice from the National Poisons Information Service (see 'Useful websites').

The patient must be intubated before gastric lavage is carried out, to minimise the risk of aspiration of fluid into the lungs.

STOP THINK **28.2** What are the guidelines and protocols in the Emergency Department of your hospital for management of unconscious patients suspected of ingesting drugs or toxic substances?

The medical history

The doctor or an experienced nurse will need to gain further information about the patient. If an appropriate person has accompanied the patient to hospital, it is important that this person does not leave until the doctor or nurse has had an opportunity to ask them about the patient's medical history and the circumstances preceding and surrounding the onset of the unconscious state.

The physical examination

The general physical examination of the unconscious patient will include special attention to the patient's:

- vital signs
- pattern of respiration
- signs of trauma
- skin colour and texture
- breath odour.

The signs and symptoms listed in Table 28.1 can provide clues to the cause of the unconscious state.

The neurological examination of the patient will include assessment of the cranial nerves, motor and sensory function, and the patient's reflexes. A nurse should be present at the initial neurological assessment so that any future changes in the patient's condition can be monitored in relation to their initial state.

Laboratory tests

Laboratory tests for unconscious patients usually include a complete blood count, blood glucose levels and blood urea, and electrolyte estimation. Blood gas analysis is obtained when the patient's respiratory and/or cardiovascular state are compromised. Screening tests of blood and urine are carried out if drug intoxication or ingestion of poison or alcohol is suspected. The patient's urine may be checked for glucose, acetone, blood and infection.

Radiological studies and imaging

Radiological investigations are carried out once the patient has been resuscitated and their condition stabilised. Skull and cervical spine X-rays are obtained when head trauma is obvious or is suggested from neurological signs; possible injury to the cervical spine should always be suspected in cases of head trauma.

If other injuries are apparent or suspected, X-rays will be taken as appropriate. Angiography, computed tomography (CT) or magnetic resonance imaging (MRI) scans may be undertaken if further investigation is considered to be necessary, and in some hospitals facilities to undertake positron emission tomography (PET scan) are available and may be used.

Table 28.1 Clues to the cause of unconsciousness on general physical examination

Sign or symptom	Possible cause
Elevated temperature	Infection Heat stroke
Subnormal temperature	Dehydration Excessive intake of alcohol Barbiturate intoxication Hypothyroidism Exposure to the cold
Bleeding from the mouth	Epileptic seizure Trauma
Pulse irregularities	Hypoxia from inadequate cardiac output
Slow, regular respirations	Hypothyroidism Morphine or barbiturate intoxication
Cheyne–Stokes respiration	Bilateral cerebral dysfunction Late stages of increased intracranial pressure Severe cardiopulmonary disease
Ataxic, irregular (cluster) respirations	Lesions of the brain stem — signifies impending apnoea
Breath odour	Excessive intake of alcohol Hepatic dysfunction Renal dysfunction Ingested poisons Diabetes mellitus
Skin	
Jaundice	Hepatic dysfunction
Cyanosis	Cardiopulmonary problems
Rash	Infection; reaction to medication
Needle puncture marks	Drug abuse
Hypertension	Raised intracranial pressure Intracranial haemorrhage
Hypotension	Blood loss Septicaemia Myocardial infarction Pulmonary embolism

Further investigations

Further investigations may be undertaken to aid diagnosis, e.g.:

- electroencephalogram (EEG)
- lumbar puncture (LP)
- electrocardiogram (ECG)
- Doppler (ultrasonic) studies.

NURSING MANAGEMENT OF THE UNCONSCIOUS PATIENT

The Roper et al activities of living model as applied by Holland et al (2003) is used to illustrate the nursing management of the unconscious patient (see also Ch. 9).

Breathing

Oxygen is essential for the survival of all body cells. Irreversible damage to the brain cells will occur if they are deprived of oxygen, even for a few minutes. Consequently, all activities of living and life itself are entirely dependent on breathing, and the establishment and maintenance of a patent airway are essential for the unconscious patient.

Any obvious potential obstructions to the airway, such as dentures or dental plates, should be removed. The nurse also needs to be aware of the presence of loose teeth, caps or crowns, as these could become detached and obstruct the airway. Bleeding into the oropharynx from head or facial injuries may also cause obstruction. Vomiting presents another hazard. The insertion of a nasogastric tube in the initial stages of coma will facilitate the emptying of the stomach, thus helping to avoid the potential aspiration of gastric contents into the respiratory tract.

Position of the patient

Unconscious patients, unless their condition contraindicates, should be nursed in a semi-prone or lateral recumbent position with the head of the bed tilted slightly upwards (10–30°). This prevents the tongue from obstructing the airway, encourages the drainage of respiratory secretions and saliva and therefore reduces the danger of aspiration into the lungs. Patients who have sustained a head injury will also benefit from head elevation to aid cerebral venous drainage and help to reduce intracranial pressure (Hickey 2002) (see Ch. 9). Pillows positioned at the patient's back and between the knees will help to maintain the position. If the patient has any spinal injuries, there may be some variation in positioning and extra care must be taken when carrying out any procedures (see Ch. 10).

Artificial airways

The unconscious patient's cough reflex is depressed or absent, so they are unable to cough and clear their own airway. The use of artificial airways and suctioning may be required.

Oropharyngeal airway The Guedel airway is the oropharyngeal airway most commonly used in UK hospitals. This has the advantage of relatively easy insertion and is available in varying sizes to facilitate the needs of individual patients. The airway is designed to lie over the tongue and permit the passage of air into the pharynx (see Fig. 28.7). It keeps the patient's tongue from obstructing the throat and it has a hollow centre that allows the patient to breathe through the device. It also allows easier access to facilitate suction of the oropharynx and trachea. An oropharyngeal airway can stimulate the gag and cough reflex, causing the patient to retch or cough, in which case a nasal pharyngeal airway may be tolerated better as this is passed through the nose and does not exert a stimulus on the rear part of the tongue.

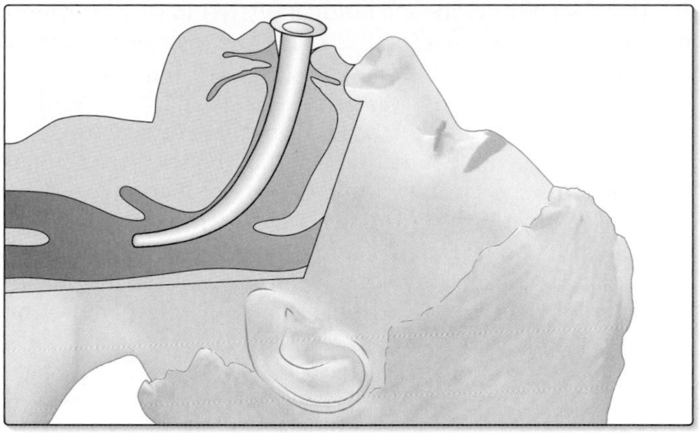

Fig. 28.7 A Guedel airway in situ.

Endotracheal tube An endotracheal tube is indicated if either the Guedel or nasal pharyngeal airway proves inadequate or when mechanical ventilation is required. The tube is made of plastic and has an inflatable cuff (see Fig. 28.8). The tube is normally inserted through the mouth by a doctor or a nurse who is competent to carry out the procedure. It is then passed into the trachea to the point just above the bifurcation of the bronchi. This permits deep suctioning. Breath sounds are determined immediately after insertion to make certain that the tube is properly positioned and is not obstructing one of the primary bronchi. The cuff of the tube is then inflated with air. The inflated cuff provides an airtight seal around the outside of the tube, particularly when mechanical ventilation is required. It also prevents the aspiration of material from the digestive tract. The tube is secured in position externally using hypoallergenic tape or tied with ribbon gauze. It is the nurse's responsibility to check the patency and position of the tube at regular intervals.

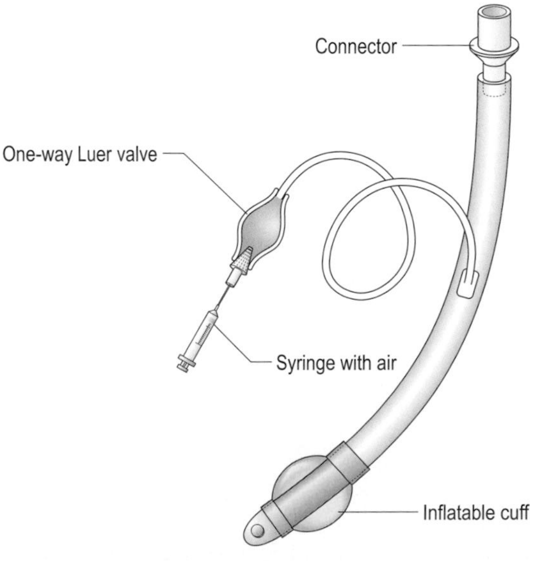

Fig. 28.8 Endotracheal tube.

An endotracheal tube is not usually left in place for more than 5–7 days because of the increased risk of erosion to the tracheal wall.

Tracheostomy tube A tracheostomy, a surgical opening in the anterior wall of the trachea, may be used to facilitate breathing and is usually indicated if intubation needs to be prolonged, or if there are difficulties in inserting an endotracheal tube. The tracheostomy tube bypasses the nose, pharynx and larynx, enabling air to flow directly into the lungs, thus reducing dead space and therefore the effort required by the patient to breathe, and facilitates suctioning of bronchial secretions (see Ch. 14).

A variety of different types and sizes of tracheostomy tube are available, made of silver, plastic or nylon, and the tubes may be cuffed or uncuffed. In the acute area, cuffed tubes are used more frequently because they are made with high volume, low pressure, soft cuffs to reduce the risk of pressure trauma to the trachea.

Most tubes consist of three parts: an obturator inside the tube to keep it rigid during insertion, an outer cannula and an inner cannula. The advantage of a tube with an inner cannula is that this can be removed every 2–4 h for cleaning, and then replaced. This prevents the potential danger of obstruction with secretions. The procedure can also be carried out without disturbing the outer tube. This reduces the frequency of outer tube changes, thus minimising the risk of trauma to the stoma and trachea.

Infection is a potential problem and the tracheal stoma should always be treated as an open wound (see Ch. 23). The incidence and severity of infection may be minimised by keeping the wound area free of secretions that collect around the tube. The stoma is cleansed using an aseptic technique, and a sterile absorbent, non-adherent dressing may be applied.

The NNBG (see 'Note', p. 988) recommends the following for best nursing practice:

- use proprietary stoma dressings which should be changed at least once a day
- change tracheostomy tubes in line with manufacturer's guidelines
- inflate the cuff slowly with air, in 0.2–0.5 mL increments, using a 10 mL syringe
- measure the amount of air in the cuff using a pressure gauge. Pressures should be maintained between 15 and 25 cm H_2O unless otherwise directed by medical staff (Dikeman & Kazandijan 1995)
- if a pressure manometer is unavailable, listen for air leaks with a stethoscope over the thyroid cartilage until no airflow is detected from around the cuff (Ganner 2001).

Suctioning

Suctioning is carried out to remove potentially dangerous secretions from the oropharynx, trachea and bronchi. The nurse's assessment of the patient's colour, respiratory rate and pattern will indicate how often this is required. Suction must be applied if one or more of the following occurs:

- signs of cyanosis
- increased and irregular respirations
- noisy, gurgling respirations.

The following equipment is required:

- a piped source of vacuum pressure, indicating calibrated pressures, or a portable suction device
- a collection jar and disposable connecting tubing
- disposable plastic sterile suction catheters of the correct size for the patient, usually 12–14 French gauge for an adult; the catheter should be no more than one-half the diameter of the tracheostomy/endotracheal tube
- non-sterile examination gloves
- sterile disposable plastic gloves
- sterile normal saline
- a sterile bowl
- masks.

The use of a closed suction catheter system and disposable suction equipment is recognised as good practice.

Procedure Each hospital will have its own policy regarding suctioning, but the procedure described below is based on good practice and provides a general example (Buglass 1999, Laws-Chapman et al 2000).

1. Explain the procedure to the patient.
2. Assemble the equipment needed — masks are advocated in some areas for the nurse's protection.
3. Turn on the suction device to 80–120 mmHg.
4. Wash hands and pour the sterile normal saline into a sterile bowl.
5. Patients who are dependent on oxygen should continue with their therapy until immediately prior to inserting the suction catheter.
6. Put on a pair of non-sterile examination gloves for your own protection.
7. Open the pack containing the sterile catheter and put a plastic sterile glove on the dominant hand.
8. Attach the catheter to the connecting tube, taking care not to contaminate the catheter.
9. Remove oxygen mask/nasal cannula from the patient.
10. Insert the catheter into the airway without applying suction.
11. Advance the catheter as far as it will easily pass, until resistance is met.
12. Withdraw the catheter 1 cm. Continuous suction is applied as the catheter is slowly withdrawn (Glass & Grap 1995, Laws-Chapman et al 2000).
13. Remove secretions within a time limit of 15 s.
14. Use the catheter once only and then wrap it around the gloved hand. Remove the glove with the catheter inside and discard both.
15. Rinse the suction tubing through with sterile water.
16. Give the patient at least 60 s to recover before suctioning again. Give oxygen again, if required.
17. If all the secretions have not been removed, repeat the procedure using a new sterile glove and sterile catheter.
18. Use a new catheter to suction the patient's mouth and nose at the end of the procedure if necessary. Nasal suction is contraindicated if the patient has sustained a frontal skull fracture or has nasal leakage of cerebrospinal fluid (CSF rhinorrhoea). The passage of a suction catheter through the nose could lead to damage to brain tissue and infection.

19. If a piped disposable system is not available, empty the collection jars and disinfect them at least once every 24 h during regular use; cleaning should be according to local policy.

Some policies advocate the instillation of 5–10 mL of sterile normal saline into the airway, immediately before suctioning, in order to loosen the secretions; however, the value of this technique is questioned (Raymond 1995, Ackerman 1996). Ackerman argues that this practice can irritate the mucosa and has little or no value in thinning, mobilising or removing dried secretions. The preferred option is the use of a saline nebuliser which will deliver tiny droplets of moisture to the alveoli to optimise humidification and mucociliary transport.

Humidification

Normally the air drawn into the lungs is warmed, moistened and filtered through the nose and upper respiratory tract. If the patient has an endotracheal or tracheostomy tube in situ, the air entering the lungs is dry and so a humidifier must be used, otherwise irritated mucous membranes and dried tenacious secretions will soon result.

Oxygen

The amount of oxygen prescribed depends on the respiratory status of the patient and the laboratory evaluation of their arterial blood gases. A specimen of arterial blood is taken to ascertain the pH and partial pressures of oxygen (P_aO_2) and carbon dioxide (P_aCO_2). Ideal values should be: pH, 7.36–7.44; P_aO_2, 11–15 kPa; P_aCO_2, 4.6–5.9 kPa. Deviations from normal may be corrected by an increase or decrease in the amount of oxygen delivered. Mechanical ventilation may be indicated to ensure adequate oxygenation.

RESEARCH ABSTRACT 28.1

The unconscious experience

A small pilot study was carried out in the USA (Podurgiel 1990) involving patients who had been unconscious and returned to consciousness and nurses who had talked to such patients. The study describes how people consistently reported on four particular states:

- near-death — at peace, leaving the body, seeing a light, returning to life
- unconsciousness — no perception of external environment
- semi-consciousness — aware of external and own internal environment but unable to communicate
- dreams and nightmares.

There appeared to be movement back and forth between these states, rather than progressive stages, and patients were able to respond emotionally to what was happening to them. Warm, caring, personal contacts were noted as positive. Some procedures and negative statements the patients overheard had a more detrimental effect.

Podurgiel M 1990 The unconscious experience: a pilot study. Journal of Neuroscience Nursing 22(1): 52–53

The ventilated patient is cared for in an intensive therapy unit or a high-dependency unit.

There are various methods of administering oxygen and the doctor's prescription will include instructions about the rate of flow, duration of therapy and type of equipment to be used. The nurse must monitor the administration of oxygen and observe the patient for complications. (Ch. 3 gives a more detailed account of the administration of oxygen and mechanical ventilation.)

Nursing and physiotherapy

The prevention of respiratory complications is a priority in the nursing management of the unconscious patient, but infection may occur despite every precaution being taken. Antibiotics can be effective against organisms but the patient could drown in their own purulent secretions unless these are removed. Effective respiratory management is dependent on the skill and cooperation of the nurse and physiotherapist.

Communicating

The patient

Research undertaken by Podurgiel (1990), albeit with small numbers, explored patients' experiences and recollections of impaired consciousness (see Research Abstract 28.1). There is much anecdotal evidence of patients recalling, with startling accuracy, conversations they have overheard whilst unconscious. It can be concluded therefore that conversations not intended for the patient should not be held in their presence, as unguarded or misinterpreted expressions can cause distress.

It is imperative that the nurse explains clearly and simply to the patient every aspect of their care, whether it is related to procedures being carried out, the associated equipment or to the patient's progress. The explanations and reassurances should be repeated whenever a procedure is carried out. With the advent of ICP monitoring, several studies were undertaken to determine the effects of verbal and physical interactions on ICP (Treloar et al 1991, Chudley 1994). Some interactions were shown to cause a rise in ICP, some a decrease and some no change. However, authors of such studies advocated a need for further research.

Once the patient has come through the acute phase of the illness, recovery may be helped through the use of sensory stimulation. For example, common smells, distinctive flavours, soft or harsh fabrics, visual stimuli and certain sounds, such as favourite music, may be used.

The family and others significant to the patient

Relatives and other visitors may be bewildered and frightened when they see the unconscious patient, together with the associated equipment, particularly for the first time. Time should be spent with them before they see the patient in order to explain what is happening and what the patient looks like. A brief explanation of the immediate environment and the function of any equipment should be provided. Relatives and others significant to the patient should be encouraged to speak to and touch the patient. The family should be given an opportunity to ask any questions and to speak with the doctor and nurse in charge about the patient's progress. Many misconceptions about coma have developed, particularly through the media. The nurse should therefore explore the relatives' or significant others' understanding of the patient's condition and try to correct any misconceptions.

STOP THINK **28.3** Can you think of any of these misconceptions? How might you correct them?

For further information, see Johnson & Roberts (1996) and Hemingway & McAndrew (1998).

Rest and sleep

Providing adequate rest and sleep for a patient is one of the most difficult challenges confronting the nurse, and it is doubtful whether it is ever overcome, given the associated hospital background noise. (More information on sleep can be found in Ch. 25.)

It must be borne in mind that, in the unconscious patient, the RAS, the system that is normally responsible for the sleep/waking cycle, is impaired. Therefore it could be assumed that a normal sleep/waking pattern is not possible in the unconscious patient. However, patients whose level of consciousness fluctuates may experience periods of sleep and periods of wakefulness even though they may not be responsive to external stimuli. Podurgiel (1990) reported that some patients recalled dreams and nightmares (see Research Abstract 28.1). As noted earlier in this chapter, patients in vegetative states also exhibit sleep/waking cycles.

Treloar et al (1991), Chudley (1994) and Hickey (2002) mention the need to provide rest periods for patients between nursing and other activities. However, there does not appear to be any conclusive evidence in the literature about the need for sleep and rest in the patient with an altered level of consciousness. Nurses should consider this potential need when planning care. It could be detrimental to patients to be stimulated constantly by nurses undertaking frequent observations and procedures, along with other members of staff who are attending to the patient.

Eating and drinking

The unconscious patient will be unable to eat or drink in the normal way and will need to receive nourishment and fluids by an alternative method. An adequate fluid intake helps to prevent dehydration, which can cause drying and thickening of secretions, making suctioning difficult and creating a breeding ground for bacteria.

In any very stressful situation, whether physical or emotional, calorie intake may need to be increased to meet an increased metabolic rate. For example, a severely head-injured patient may require 30–35% additional calories/day in the acute stages (Segaran & Glynn 2002).

Fluids

The most common method of administering fluids to an unconscious patient is intravenously, either peripherally or via a central line. Intravenous (i.v.) fluids are also given to:

- administer medications, such as antibiotics
- administer additional electrolytes, such as potassium, to correct imbalances.

Intravenous fluids are normally prescribed by medical staff, following estimation of the patient's serum electrolyte levels, which are measured on a daily basis. Fluids are usually prescribed for the following 24 h; however, in seriously ill patients, prescriptions may be adjusted more frequently. It is essential that the correct fluids are administered at the prescribed rate to maintain fluid balance and metabolic needs. Fluids may be restricted if cerebral oedema is suspected (see Ch. 9).

The patient may also have an arterial line, which looks very similar to an i.v. cannula and could easily be mistaken for one. An arterial line must be clearly identified and multiple lines and ports can be labelled with different colours to distinguish them.

An infusion pump will be used to ensure accurate flow rates in the seriously ill patient (see Chs 20 and 21 for more information).

Nutrition

Provision of adequate nutrition is important in the unconscious patient. Malnourishment will result in weakening of the body's immune system and loss of muscle mass and energy, both of which are essential for recovery. The patient's nutritional status must be reappraised at regular intervals.

Daily nutritional requirements are usually calculated on the basis of body weight, gender, height and age. However, weight may need to be an estimation as it may not be possible to weigh the unconscious patient, unless a bed with an integral weighing scale is available.

Nasogastric feeding The easiest and most economical way to provide an alternative means of feeding is via a nasogastric tube. Nasogastric tube feeding is the most frequently used method of providing nutritional support in the unconscious patient, provided that the patient's alimentary tract is functional. With the help and advice of the dietitian, the patient's nutritional requirements should be assessed and the appropriate dietary solutions prescribed.

Occasionally, it may be necessary to use an orogastric instead of a nasogastric tube, e.g. if the patient has a nasal injury, CSF rhinorrhoea or blockage of the nose.

Care must be taken when inserting an intragastric tube via the nose or mouth of an unconscious patient as insertion is more difficult if the patient is unable to sit up or cooperate. There is also a higher risk of aspiration of stomach contents into the trachea and lungs if the patient is in the lateral recumbent position. The patient must be observed carefully for any sign of aspiration which will compromise respiration. Suction equipment must be at hand and ready for use at all times.

Parenteral nutrition

Parenteral feeding is delivered either through a central venous line or a peripherally inserted central line (PIC line) (see Ch. 21). Unconscious patients who may benefit from parenteral nutrition include:

- multiple trauma patients, particularly if there are gastrointestinal and/or facial injuries
- malnourished patients

- patients with sepsis or multisystem failure
- patients with inflammatory bowel disease which is extensive and life threatening
- patients in prolonged coma who are unable to tolerate intragastric feeding.

Percutaneous endoscopic gastrostomy feeding

Whenever possible, it is preferable to deliver food directly into the gut to prevent the risk of translocation of bacteria from the unused gut. Long-term feeding is better achieved by using a percutaneous endoscopic gastrostomy (PEG) tube. This is easier to manage than intragastric or parenteral feeding and relatives/carers can be taught how to administer feeds through the tube. PEG tubes are particularly useful if the patient is later cared for at home.

When the patient recovers consciousness, it is essential to ensure that gag, cough and swallowing reflexes are present before giving oral fluids or food. The speech and language therapist (SALT) may assess the patient for any swallowing difficulties. (For further information on enteral feeding and parenteral nutrition, see Ch. 21.)

Elimination

The normal means of elimination of urine and faeces are altered by confinement to bed, and the ability of the patient to control elimination is impaired due to their altered level of consciousness.

The unconscious patient will not be able to indicate when they need to pass urine or defaecate, although they may become restless. Despite the acknowledged dangers of urinary tract infection and urinary calculi, if the patient is unconscious, early catheterisation will be required. This helps to retain the patient's dignity, avoid the embarrassment of incontinence and prevent skin breakdown. Catheterisation will be undertaken on admission if an accurate measurement of urinary output is required (Cioffi 2000, McArthur-Rouse 2001). A closed urine collection system helps to reduce the risk of infection. Local protocols should be followed with regard to catheter care (see Ch. 8).

Once the initial acute period is over and the patient is stabilised, many male patients will be able to manage with external penile collection devices such as uri-sheaths. There is no ready solution for the management of defaecation. The patient's bowel movements should be monitored, particularly if being tube fed. Hospital protocols should be followed for the prevention and management of constipation and diarrhoea (DH 2001). If necessary, prophylactic stool softeners may be administered in order to produce a regular stool. It is important for the patient to avoid straining to defaecate as this will raise intracranial pressure.

Personal cleansing and dressing

The unconscious patient is dependent upon the nurse to attend to all aspects of personal cleansing and dressing, but still has the right to have these procedures performed in privacy. This is especially important when performing intimate procedures such as the provision of personal hygiene in the menstruating female or in giving urinary catheter care.

Bathing in bed is necessary for any totally dependent patient, but when turning the unconscious patient there is a danger that the airway may become compromised and the patient's chest movement may be impeded. To avoid this, turning should be planned and requires a minimum of two nurses to execute it safely. If a mechanical hoist is available, the patient can be bathed using this. Bathing, hair and nail care should all be performed as often as necessary. Hair washing may be difficult and, if the use of a wet shampoo is impossible, a dry shampoo may be used. Nails should be kept short and clean. Male patients may require a daily facial shave and an electric razor is recommended. If the patient has a moustache/beard, this should be trimmed as necessary.

As unconscious patients do not blink, the corneas become dry; in some unconscious patients, the eyelids may remain open. Eye care is therefore carried out on a regular basis to prevent damage to the cornea.

The eye and surrounding area are cleaned with sterile normal saline, followed by the instillation of artificial tear drops. If the patient's eyelids do not close naturally, tape may be applied. If tape is used, the delicate skin of the eyelid must be observed closely for excoriation. This can be minimised by using hypoallergenic tape and regularly altering the position of the tape. Alternatively, the eyes could be protected by gauze pads, eye shields or eye patches. If the area around the eyes is swollen or bruised, ice packs or compresses may be used. Local protocol should be followed.

Oral hygiene should be maintained following initial and ongoing assessment of the individual patient (Turner 1996, DH 2001) (see also Ch. 15). A number of authors note that mouth care tends to be based on traditional and ritualistic practices rather than being scientifically or research based (Moore 1995, Holmes 1996, Pearson 1996). These authors and others note that evidence suggests that a toothbrush is the most effective tool, whereas foam sticks tend to be popular amongst nurses for cleaning a patient's mouth (Buglass 1995).

The unconscious patient who has an artificial airway or endotracheal tube in place may present with particular problems such as a dry mouth and difficult access to the oral cavity.

When possible, the use of a small, soft toothbrush to clean the teeth, tongue and gums with a small amount of fluoride toothpaste and plain water will be of benefit. Many oral care products are available; for example, chlorhexidine gluconate 0.2% 5 mL in 100 mL has an antimicrobial effect and can help to remove debris, tenacious mucus and reduce plaque formation (Buglass 1995). Petroleum jelly may be used to prevent dry lips, although there appears to be no research evidence as to its effectiveness (Holmes 1996, Turner 1996). Dentures can be stored dry, after being cleaned, and should be cleaned again and rinsed in cold water before reinsertion. Some nurses may prefer to store a patient's dentures in water or a proprietary denture solution, particularly if relatives request this. Dentures should be stored in a covered container that is labelled with the patient's name and hospital number. Local protocols should be followed.

The *Essence of Care* initiatives (DH 2001), developed from the commitment made in the *Making a Difference* document

(DH 1999), highlighted the need for further research to improve standards and practice for a patient's personal and oral hygiene requirements. The guidance is to address this through local initiatives.

Maintaining a safe environment

The unconscious patient is physically vulnerable to many threats, such as pressure ulcers and infection, and nursing staff must always be alert to the need to maintain a safe environment.

Prevention of pressure ulcers

The prevention of pressure ulcers is important for the comfort of the patient and is good practice. Regular alteration of the patient's position and relief of pressure are paramount, particularly in the unconscious patient, who may be immobile (see Ch. 23).

STOP THINK **28.4** Apart from direct pressure on the skin, what other factors can contribute to the development of pressure ulcers? Can you think of any additional hazards that may lead to tissue damage in the unconscious patient?

Infection

The unconscious patient is particularly at risk of infection occurring in the chest and bladder. Wounds and drains, e.g. external ventricular drains, are also potential sites for infection. Gram-negative bacillary pneumonia causes 40–60% of respiratory infections that are acquired in institutionalised settings (see www.mold-help.org/pulmonary infections). Most people are resistant to this organism, which is constantly present in the environment, but certain factors contribute to the breaking down of physiological and immunological defences. The unconscious patient is exposed to many of these, including endotracheal intubation and the presence of invasive lines such as i.v. cannulae and urinary catheters. Antibiotic-resistant infections have become a problem in many hospitals. For example, methicillin-resistant *Staphylococcus aureus* (MRSA) is a potentially life-threatening organism, particularly in vulnerable patients. In areas where patients are at high risk of acquiring MRSA, routine screening of staff will be determined by local policy (Mackenzie 1997, Royal College of Nursing 2004a) (see also Ch. 16, p. 663).

The mechanism of infection Infection will occur if a sufficient number of microbes reach the lower respiratory tract or urinary bladder. The likelihood of infection occurring depends on the virulence of the organism, the susceptibility of the patient, the cleanliness of the environment and the hygiene of other people in contact with the patient. Ironically, the original source of the Gram-negative bacilli is often the patient themselves. Infection can spread from the digestive tract, its usual and commensal location, into the lungs or bladder. Endotracheal or tracheostomy tubes, which bypass the normal protective mechanism of the nose, encourage the spread of infection, and a depressed cough reflex enables pooling of secretions within the lungs, resulting in stasis. Urinary catheterisation provides a ready entry route for bacteria to the bladder. Preventive measures, in which the nurse plays a major role, include:

- unit design, e.g. facilities for hand washing, facilities for cleaning and disposal of equipment, provision of single/isolation rooms
- a control-of-infection policy which is meticulously followed
- aseptic techniques.

The nurse needs to be aware of and conscientious about implementing standard infection control precautions and local policies with regard to prevention and treatment of infection (see Ch. 16). Hand washing is acknowledged to be the single most effective intervention to promote infection control in the clinical setting (Voss & Widmer 1997, Royal College of Nursing 2004b).

Medication

The hazards of administering medication to patients are well documented, but the risks are increased in the unconscious patient for two reasons:

- The routes that are used carry a greater risk for the patient. The simpler and safer oral route is contraindicated. Other methods of administration have to be utilised, including i.m. injections, i.v. infusions, via an intragastric tube and per rectum.
- The patient cannot confirm their identity, so the nurse must ensure that the correct medication is being given to the correct patient via the correct route and in the correct dose.

The types of medication most commonly used in the unconscious patient include analgesics, anticonvulsants, antibiotics and laxatives, depending upon their condition and individual requirements.

Motor and sensory loss or impairment

The motor and sensory loss experienced by unconscious patients may be drug induced or part of the underlying disease process. Whatever the cause, the nursing intervention remains the same.

Motor loss See 'Mobility' below.

Sensory loss The sensory system is part of the body's defence system and the unconscious patient is unable to process sensory information. It is imperative that the patient is not exposed to extremes of temperature, particularly in a localised area of the skin, e.g. if heating or cooling devices are used.

Care must be taken when moving and positioning the patient as they will not be aware of friction or pressure. The patient may have a reduced or absent sensation of pain or, if experiencing pain, may be unable to communicate that feeling.

Seizure

The main role of the nurse (or onlooker) when the unconscious patient, or indeed anyone, has a seizure is to ensure that the patient does not harm themselves. First aid, as recommended by Epilepsy Action (British Epilepsy

Box 28.4

First aid for seizures

What to do when someone has a seizure

With some seizure types very little first aid may be needed. For example, in a partial seizure, guiding someone away from danger may be all that is necessary.

DO ...

- Protect the person from injury — move any sharp or hard objects. Guide the person away from danger if they are having a partial seizure.
- Cushion the person's head if they fall down.
- When the convulsive part of the seizure is at an end, place the person in the recovery position. This will help their breathing.
- Be quietly reassuring.
- Stay with the person until they have regained full consciousness.
- Go over any missed events.

DO NOT ...

- Try to restrain the person having the seizure.
- Put anything into the person's mouth or force anything between the teeth.
- Try to move the person unless they are in danger.
- Give the person anything to drink until they have fully regained consciousness.

It is not usually necessary to call for an ambulance when someone has an epileptic seizure. However, it may be necessary in the following circumstances unless a doctor can attend straight away.

Call for an ambulance if ...

- It is the person's first seizure, the cause of which is uncertain and needs investigation.
- Injuries have occurred during the seizure, e.g. a cut that needs stitching.
- A generalised seizure shows no signs of stopping after 5 min or 2 min longer than is usual for that person.
- A second seizure occurs without the person regaining consciousness.

Status epilepticus

A prolonged seizure or series of seizures without regaining consciousness is called 'status epilepticus' and is a medical emergency.

Lack of normal respiratory movements combined with extreme muscular contractions during a seizure throws stress on the cardiovascular system. The continuing lack of oxygen may lead eventually to brain damage.

Status epilepticus is usually convulsive, but sometimes it can be non-convulsive, i.e. absence or complex partial status. This will need intervention, although the urgency is not as great. Status epilepticus is a rare occurrence, except in a very few patients with difficult to control epilepsy.

When status epilepticus occurs, a doctor will usually give an intravenous injection of diazepam at the scene of the seizure or in hospital. Other intravenous compounds may be used as an alternative.

Diazepam can now also be given in the form of a rectal application. It can be administered by a trained, competent and willing individual, who has received permission from the person or the parents of the person with epilepsy.
It is reassuring for some parents to feel they can use this treatment at home. Ultimately it is safer and quicker in an emergency situation and allows the person with epilepsy to lead a broader lifestyle and participate in a wider range of activities.

(The above is based on the availability and use of diazepam in the UK — practice in other countries may vary.)

Reproduced with kind permission from Epilepsy Action, from which further information on seizures can be obtained (see 'Useful websites').

Association) (see 'Useful websites'), for someone having a seizure is outlined in Box 28.4. Further information about epilepsy can be found in Chapter 9.

Mobility

The nursing management of mobility and activity remains the same, whatever the cause of the unconsciousness. Lack of attention to mobility could lead to the development of:

- contractures
- muscle atrophy
- pressure ulcers
- postural hypotension
- deep vein thrombosis
- hypostatic pneumonia.

Any one of these hazards will delay the patient's rehabilitation and result in additional pain and discomfort.

Whilst the patient remains dependent, the nurse is responsible, together with the physiotherapist, for ensuring that the patient maintains a full range of movement.

Correct positioning is important and the following should be considered:

- body alignment, especially if spinal injury is suspected
- use of aids such as pillows, foam pads or splints, if required, to help to support the patient
- avoidance of pressure, e.g. an arm trapped under the body, the pinna of the ear bent forward, bedclothes too tight
- avoidance of friction when moving the patient
- changing the patient's position; this should be done frequently — at least every 2 h is recommended
- careful handling of joints and paralysed or weak limbs
- safety — e.g. if the patient is restless, padded bed rails may be required.

Safety/restraint

Some patients experience confusion and can become aggressive as they recover consciousness and many patients in critical care environments may undergo changes to their normal behaviour. This may be due to their underlying illness and pathology, medication, sensory deprivation or the unfamiliar environment. Health care teams face difficult decisions about identifying strategies to prevent the patient inadvertently dislodging tracheostomy tubes, invasive lines or dressings. Providing diversional therapy, involving the patient's family and friends or providing one-to-one nursing supervision may distract the patient. Balancing the best interests of the patient to ensure safety and promoting the patient's well-being may be difficult, but it is the responsibility of all nurses who must adhere to their *Code of Professional Conduct* (Nursing and Midwifery Council 2004). When all other alternative therapies have failed, and only as a last resort, short-term restraint may be necessary, following communication and discussion with the patient and their relatives (Department of Health and Welsh Office 1999, DH 2001, Royal College of Nursing 2004c). The Mental Health Act, article 5, relating to restraint, was amended in 2004.

Recovery from coma

A multidisciplinary approach is essential to facilitate early mobilisation of the patient. Patients who have been nursed in bed for just a few days often experience dizziness and light-headedness due to postural hypotension when they sit up for the first time.

STOP THINK **28.5** What are the causes of postural (orthostatic) hypotension?

The patient recovering from coma may also have some motor weakness and sensory loss, which makes them feel insecure. Many units now have adjustable or electronically operated beds that will enable the patient to adopt a more natural sitting position in bed. This will help the patient to get used to the position and will give them a psychological boost.

On first raising the patient to a sitting position, the nurse should check the patient's vital signs and colour, and ask whether they are experiencing any untoward symptoms. If they are, the mobility programme should be implemented at a slower rate.

Initially, the patient may be unsure and apprehensive about the prospect of getting out of bed. Repeated explanations of what is expected of them will provide the necessary reassurance. The patient may need to practise sitting on the side of the bed whilst the nurse and physiotherapist assess balance and head and trunk control. If there are no ill-effects, the patient can progress to sitting out of bed for a short period. The nurse should continue to observe the patient's colour and vital signs. If the patient's status is not compromised, the length of time and frequency of sitting out of bed can be increased gradually. Highly dependent patients with motor loss or impairment may require a specialist chair that will provide additional support and security. The physiotherapist will normally carry out an assessment of the patient prior to provision of this equipment.

Once in the chair, anything which the patient is able to use, such as a call bell, drinks, radio or newspapers, should be readily available to them. The amount of time that the patient is up in the chair should be noted; it is more beneficial for the patient to sit up for several short intervals rather than for one long period (see Ch. 34).

An individualised mobility rehabilitation programme should be devised in conjunction with the physiotherapist.

Controlling body temperature

Body temperature must be maintained within a relatively constant range to sustain life, i.e. 36–37.5°C. It is controlled by the heat-regulating centre in the hypothalamus, which acts like a thermostat (see Ch. 22). Pyrexia, an abnormally high temperature, is more commonly seen in the unconscious patient than is hypothermia, an abnormally low temperature, although hypothermia may be the primary cause of unconsciousness (see Ch. 22).

Pyrexia may be due to damage to the heat-regulating centre in the hypothalamus or to an infective process or metabolic disorder. The danger is that, for each degree of temperature over the normal range, the cerebral metabolism significantly increases, adversely increasing the brain's oxygen demands, which may have serious implications for recovery.

The nursing interventions remain similar, irrespective of the cause of pyrexia. In the acute stages it is important to monitor the patient's temperature continually with an electronic probe, sited over the patient's skin, rectally or into the patient's bladder. The use of mercury-in-glass thermometers is now contraindicated for health and safety reasons.

Dying

Skilled care of the unconscious patient often saves life, but some patients will die despite all measures taken. Active treatment may have been continued right up until the last moment or it may have been decided that no further active intervention would benefit the patient. The emphasis would then move from curative to palliative care. If the patient is on a mechanical ventilator it may be that they fulfil the criteria required for assessing brain stem death.

Brain stem death

Some patients in apnoeic coma can suffer severe and irreversible brain damage but continue to have their blood pressure, heart beat and respirations artificially maintained for a period of time by ventilation, drug therapy and other life support interventions. Some, however, will never recover and the brain stem death criteria have been developed to identify such patients, in order that therapy can cease.

Brain stem death may be clinically diagnosed by following a set of guidelines issued by the Working Group of the Conference of Medical Royal Colleges and their Faculties (1976, with revisions in 1979) and according to the concept of death endorsed by the Working Group of the Royal College of Physicians in 1995. These guidelines consist of a number of tests that can be applied only after a series of preconditions have been fulfilled (see Fig. 28.9).

Preconditions include positively diagnosed structural brain damage that is irremediable and that the patient is unresponsive and on a ventilator. The examiners, both doctors, must satisfy themselves that any reversible causes of coma have been eliminated, including:

- drug intoxication, e.g. as the result of an overdose or the administration of a neuromuscular blocking agent to facilitate passage of an endotracheal tube
- primary hypothermia

Diagnosis to be made by two doctors, one a Consultant and the other a Consultant or Specialist Registrar.

Diagnosis should not be considered until at least 6 hours after the onset of Coma;
12-24 hours will be more usual.

NAME: .... UNIT NO. ....

PRE-CONDITIONS

Nature of irremediable brain damage	Time of event leading to coma
Dr A	....
Dr B	....

Do you consider that Apnoeic Coma is due to:

	Dr A	**Dr B**
Depressant Drugs		
Neuromuscular Blocking (relaxant) drugs		
Hypothermia		
Metabolic or Endocrine Disturbances		

TESTS FOR ABSENCE OF BRAIN STEM FUNCTION

Is there evidence of:

	Dr A	**Dr B**
Pupil reaction to light		
Corneal reflex		
Eye Movements with Cold Caloric Test		
Cranial Nerve Motor Responses		
Gag reflex		
Respiratory movements on disconnection from Ventilator to allow adequate rise in $PaCo_2$		

Date and time of First Testing..

Date and time of Second Testing..

Dr A	**Dr B**
Signature	Signature ....
Status	Status ....

Fig. 28.9 Criteria for the diagnosis of brain stem death (Allan 1987). (Reproduced with kind permission from *Professional Nurse*, where this figure first appeared in 1987.)

- metabolic or endocrine imbalances such as uncontrolled diabetes.

Testing brain stem function Once satisfied that the preconditions have been fulfilled, testing of brain stem function can be performed. Two doctors should carry out the tests. Usually one is the consultant responsible for the patient and the other is of at least senior registrar status. If organ donation from the patient is being considered, neither doctor must be a member of the transplant team. The doctors may carry out the tests separately or together. There are six parts to the test:

1. The pupillary response to light is tested, using a bright torch. Absence of response indicates loss of function, although the examiner should be satisfied that a non-responsive pupil is not due to the instillation of paralytic eye drops or damage to cranial nerve III.
2. The integrity of the corneal reflex is tested by drawing a wisp of cotton wool across the exposed cornea. Absence of a blink response indicates loss of function, although the examiner should be satisfied that the presence of corneal oedema is not preventing the normal blink response.
3. Cranial nerve motor responses are tested at several sites, including the head and face, in case the patient has a cervical cord injury. Again, no response indicates loss of function, although spinal reflexes can remain intact even in a brain-dead patient (Pallis & Harley 1996).

4. The cough and gag reflexes are tested by moving the endotracheal tube back and forth or by applying suction and observing the patient's throat muscles for movement. No response would indicate loss of the pharyngeal and laryngeal reflexes.
5. Absence of the oculovestibular reflex rules out the existence of normally functioning anatomical pathways within the brain stem and is a very sensitive test of brain stem function. It is tested by syringing 20 mL of ice-cold water into the patient's ears in turn and noting any eye movement in response. This is called 'cold caloric testing'. Before testing, the examiner should use an auriscope to look directly at the tympanic membrane to ensure that it is intact and that there is no obstruction preventing the water from making contact with the membrane.
6. The final test is that for apnoea. Arterial blood gases are checked and P_aCO_2 should be 5.33–6.00 kPa (40–45 mmHg). The patient is disconnected from the ventilator after providing a continuous flow of 100% intratracheal oxygen for 10 min. The patient's chest wall is observed closely for any respiratory movement and the P_aCO_2 is allowed to rise above threshold level to stimulate breathing, usually to at least 6.65 kPa (50 mmHg). The time taken to achieve this will vary, but is no more than 10 min for most patients.

The ventilator is then reconnected and the entire process is repeated after a minimum time lapse of 30 min (in practice, usually 24 h) before the patient is declared brain dead. Although the second set of tests is not required by law, for medicolegal purposes the completion of the second testing determines the time of death. After consultation with the relatives, the patient is normally disconnected from the ventilator by medical staff.

In some countries, further neurophysiological tests are recommended, such as electroencephalography, evoked cerebral potentials and cerebral perfusion, to confirm the clinical diagnosis (Haupt & Rudolf 1999).

Previously, it may have been indicated that the patient wished to donate organs and/or tissues for transplantation. If the next of kin is in agreement, following the usual preliminary procedures and consultation with the hospital administrator and local coroner, the patient would remain ventilated until the organs were removed (Great Britain Parliament 1961, amended 1989, United Kingdom Parliament 2004). The doctor or transplant coordinator must obtain permission from the patient's next of kin before taking organs and tissues. The transplant coordinator will offer counselling to the patient's relatives and/or those who have a significant relationship with the patient.

For further information on brain stem death, see Pallis & Harley (1996); on issues in organ donation and transplants, see www.uktransplant.org.uk; on organ shortage, see Meeting the Organ Shortage (1999); and on organ transplantation, see NHB Organ Transplantation (www.nap.edu).

STOP THINK **28.6** Discuss with your lecturer and mentor the ethical and legal implications in procuring organs/tissues for transplant or medical research.

Physical and psychological care

The patient The principles of care for the dying unconscious patient are the same as those for all patients requiring palliative care (see Ch. 33). The unconscious patient must be treated with dignity and sensitivity even though they are unable to respond.

The family A sensitive and coherent strategy for caring for the relatives is needed. The nurse should know what information has been given to the relatives by other members of staff, including doctors. This will enable the nurse to reaffirm what has been said and avoid confusing the family members at a time when their ability to process information is drastically reduced. They need to see and feel that the patient, even if unconscious and unresponsive, is still being treated as a person, through the humane, caring attitude of the nurse (Sque et al 2003).

Some relatives may be helped by being encouraged to perform simple acts of care for the patient such as bathing them or, providing their head is not shaved or bandaged, combing their hair. This reduces their feelings of passivity and helplessness in the strange, alien world of the hospital and in a situation in which they are unlikely to be able to draw on previous experience.

Psychologically, this is a traumatic and emotionally distressing period for the patient's family, friends and/or those who have a significant relationship with the patient. They have perhaps spent the last few days (and in some cases, much longer than that) with the patient, in the unfamiliar technical surroundings. They may be relieved that an ending has been achieved or may find it difficult to accept the death, particularly if the patient has been artificially ventilated.

The support of a religious advisor may be appreciated. The nurse can contact the hospital chaplain/religious advisors if the relatives need assistance with this, or if the patient has previously spoken of it. Bereavement counselling and support should be offered as well as practical information (preferably written) about registering the death and other formalities.

CONCLUSION

Inevitably, this chapter has focused on the care of unconscious people in hospital because, at the present time, only a small minority is cared for at home. This may change in the future, at least to some extent, as new technology is developed. Where the outcome is death, some families may cope more easily with the stress and sadness in the familiar surroundings of the home. Wherever the location of care, it is important for nurses to be sensitive to the fundamental changes the unconscious patient has wrought in the lives of those who know them as a responsive human being. Not only is the patient totally reliant upon the nurse, but the family and/or carers also require a great deal of support.

As noted at the outset of this chapter, caring for the unconscious person is a major challenge for nurses. Whatever the outcome, be it death, permanent disability or complete recovery, meticulous attention to nursing observations and care is vital.

REFERENCES

Ackerman M H 1996 A review of normal saline instillation: implications for practice. Dimensions of Critical Care Nursing 15(1): 31–38

Airedale NHS Trust v. Bland E 1993 AC 789. House of Lords, London

Allan D 1987 Criteria for brain stem death. Professional Nurse 2(11): 357–359

British Medical Association 1996 Treatment decisions for patients in persistent vegetative state. British Medical Association, London. Online. Available: www.bma.org.uk

Buglass E A 1995 Oral hygiene. British Journal of Nursing 4(9): 516–519

Buglass E A 1999 Tracheostomy care: tracheal suctioning and humidification. British Journal of Nursing 8(8): 500–504

Chudley S 1994 The effect of nursing activities on intracranial pressure. British Journal of Nursing 3(9): 454–458

Cioffi J 2000 Nurses' experience of making decisions to call emergency assistance to their patients. Journal of Advanced Nursing 32: 108–114

Cruzan N B 1990 Cruzan v. Director, Missouri Department of Health. 110 S Ct 2841. US Supreme Court, Washington DC

Dalvi A 2004 Normal pressure hydrocephalus. Online. Available: www.emedicine.com

Day L, Drought T, Davis A J 1995 Principle-based ethics and nurses' attitudes towards artificial feeding. Journal of Advanced Nursing 21: 295–298

Department of Health 1999 Making a difference: strengthening the nursing, midwifery and health visiting contribution to health and health care. DH, London

Department of Health 2001 The essence of care. DH, London

Department of Health and Welsh Office 1999 Mental Health Act 1983 Code of Practice. DH, London

Dikeman K J, Kazandijan M S 1995 Communication and swallowing management of tracheostomised and ventilator-dependent adults. Singular Publishing, San Diego

Epilepsy Action (British Epilepsy Association) 2004 First aid for seizures. Online. Available: www.epilepsy.org.uk

Fairley D, Cosgrove J 1999 Glasgow coma scale: improving nursing practice through clinical effectiveness. Nursing in Critical Care 4(6): 276–279

Fitzgerald M J T 1996 Neuroanatomy – basic and clinical, 3rd edn. W B Saunders, London

Frawley P 1990 Neurological observations. Nursing Times 86(35): 29–34

Ganner C 2001 The accurate measurement of endotracheal tube cuff pressures. British Journal of Nursing 10(17): 1127–1134

Glass C A, Grap M J 1995 Ten tips for safer suctioning. American Journal of Nursing 95: 51–53

Great Britain Parliament 1961 The Human Tissue Act, Chapter 54. HMSO, London

Great Britain Parliament 1989 The Human Tissue Act. HMSO, London

Grubb A, Walsh P, Lambe N et al 1996 Survey of British clinicians' views on management of patients in persistent vegetative state. Lancet 348: 35–40

Guyton A C, Hall J E 2000 Textbook of medical physiology, 10th edn. W B Saunders, London

Haupt W F, Rudolf J 1999 European brain death codes: a comparison of national guidelines. Journal of Neurology 246(6): 432–437

Hemingway S, McAndrew S 1998 Acquired brain injury: identifying emotional and cognitive needs. Royal College of Nursing Continuing Education Article 923. Emergency Nurse 5(10): 29–38

Hewitt J 2002 Psycho-affective disorder in intensive care units: a review. Journal of Clinical Nursing 11: 575–584

Hickey J V 2002 The clinical practice of neurological and neurosurgical nursing, 5th edn. Lippincott, Williams and Wilkins, New York

Holland K, Jenkins J, Solomon J, Whittam S 2003 Applying the Roper–Logan–Tierney model in practice: elements of nursing. Elsevier, Edinburgh

Holmes S 1996 Nursing management of oral care in older patients. Nursing Times 92(9): 37–39

Jones C, Griffiths R D, Humphries G 2001 Memory, delusions and the development of acute post-traumatic stress disorder – related symptoms after intensive care. Critical Care Medicine 29(3): 573–580

Law Hospital NHS Trust v. The Lord Advocate and Others 1996 Scottish Council of Law Reporting, Edinburgh

Laws-Chapman C, Rushmer F, Miller R et al 2000 Suction guidelines pack. St. George's Healthcare NHS Trust. Portex Ltd, Hythe, Kent

Mackenzie D 1997 MRSA: the psychological effects. Nursing Standard 12(11): 49–53

Marieb E N 2004 Human anatomy and physiology, 6th edn. Addison Wesley Longman, San Francisco

Martin K M 1994 When the nurse says 'He's just not right': patient cues used by expert nurses to identify mild head injury. Journal of Neuroscience Nursing 26(4): 210–218

McArthur-Rouse F 2001 Critical care outreach services and early warning systems: a review of the literature. Journal of Advanced Nursing 36: 696–704

Mold-Help. Online. Available: www.mold-help.org/pulmonary infections

Mooney G P, Comerford D M 2003 Neurological observations. Nursing Times 99(17): 24–25

Moore J 1995 Assessment of nurse-administered oral hygiene. Nursing Times 91(9): 40–41

Multi-society Task Force Report on PVS 1994 Medical aspects of the persistent vegetative state. New England Journal of Medicine 330: 1499–1508, 1572–1579

National Centre for Clinical Excellence (NICE) 2003 Head injury: triage, assessment, investigation and early management of head injury in infants, children and adults. Clinical Guideline 4. NICE, London

Neuroscience Nurses' Benchmarking Group (NNBG). Online. Available: www.bann.org.uk

Nursing and Midwifery Council (NMC) 2004 The NMC code of professional conduct: standards for conduct, performance and ethics. NMC, London. Online. Available: www.nmc-uk.org

Pallis C, Harley D H 1996 ABC of brainstem death, 2nd edn. BMJ Publishing Group, London

Pearson L S 1996 A comparison of the ability of foam swabs and toothbrushes to remove dental plaque: implications for nursing practice. Journal of Advanced Nursing 23: 62–69

Phipps W J, Sand J K, Marek J F (eds) 1999 Medical–surgical nursing: concepts and clinical practice, 6th edn. Mosby, St Louis

Podurgiel M 1990 The unconscious experience: a pilot study. Journal of Neuroscience Nursing 22(1): 52–53

Raymond S J 1995 Normal saline instillation before suctioning. Helpful or harmful? A review of the literature. American Journal of Critical Care 4(4): 267–269

Royal College of Nursing 2004a Methicillin resistant Staphylococcus aureus (MRSA). Guidance for nursing staff. Working Well Initiative. Royal College of Nursing, London. Online. Available: www.rcn.org.uk/publications

Royal College of Nursing 2004b Good practice in infection control. Guidance for nursing staff. Working Well Initiative. Royal College of Nursing, London. Online. Available: www.rcn.org.uk/publications

Royal College of Nursing 2004c Restraint revisited – rights, risk and responsibility. Guidance for nursing staff. Royal College of Nursing, London

Royal College of Physicians 2003 The vegetative state – guidance on diagnosis and management. Royal College of Physicians, London

Segaran E, Glynn K 2002 Nutrition and severe head injury. Complete Nutrition 2(4)

Shah S 1999 Neurological assessment. Nursing Times 13(22): 49–56

Smith S 1997 The outer edge of consciousness. Nursing Times 93(39): 28–32

Sque M, Long T, Payne S 2003 Research notes on organ donation. Nursing Standard 17(34): 21

Teasdale G 1975 Acute impairment of brain function: assessing conscious level. Nursing Times 71(24): 914–917

Teasdale G, Jennett B 1974 Assessment of coma and impaired consciousness. Lancet 2: 81

Treloar D M, Nalli B J, Guin P, Gary R 1991 The effect of familiar and unfamiliar voice treatments on intracranial pressure in head-injured patients. Journal of Neuroscience Nursing 23(5): 295–299

Turner G 1996 Oral care. Royal College of Nursing Continuing Education Article 330. Nursing Standard 10(28): 51–54

United Kingdom Parliament, House of Commons session 2003–2004 Human Tissue Bill. Online. Available: www.the-stationery-office.co.uk

Voss A, Widmer A F 1997 No time for hand washing? Hand washing versus alcohol rub: can we afford 100% compliance.

Infection Control and Hospital Epidemiologist 18(3): 205–208
Waterhouse C 2005 The Glasgow Coma Scale and other neurological observations. Nursing Standard 19(33): 56–74
Waugh A, Grant A 2001 Ross and Wilson's anatomy and physiology in health and illness, 9th edn. Elsevier, Edinburgh
Wilson J, Islam O 2004 Normal pressure hydrocephalus. Online. Available: www.emedicine.com
Working Group of the Conference of Medical Royal Colleges and their Faculties in the UK 1976 Diagnosis of death. British Medical Journal ii: 1187–1188
Working Group of the Conference of Medical Royal Colleges and their Faculties in the UK 1979 Diagnosis of death. British Medical Journal i: 3320
Working Group of the Royal College of Physicians 1995 Criteria for the diagnosis of brainstem death. Code of practice. Journal of the Royal College of Physicians (London) 29: 381–382

FURTHER READING

British Medical Association 1996 Treatment decisions for patients in persistent vegetative state. British Medical Association, London. Online. Available: www.bma.org.uk
Department of Health 2005 The National Health Service framework for long-term conditions. DH, London
Dougherty L, Lister S 2004 The Royal Marsden Hospital manual of clinical nursing procedures, 6th edn. Blackwell Science, Oxford
Haupt W F, Rudolf J 1999 European brain death codes: a comparison of national guidelines. Journal of Neurology 246(6): 432–437
Hemingway S, McAndrew S 1998 Acquired brain injury: identifying emotional and cognitive needs. Royal College of Nursing Continuing Education Article 923. Emergency Nurse 5(10): 29–38
Hickey J V 2002 The clinical practice of neurological and neurosurgical nursing, 5th edn. Lippincott, Williams and Wilkins, New York
Johnson L H, Roberts S L 1996 Hope facilitating strategies for the family of the head injury patient. Journal of Neuroscience Nursing 28(4): 259–266
Meeting the organ shortage 1999 Health and quality of Life. Online. Available: www.social.coe.int
National Centre for Clinical Excellence (NICE) 2003 Head injury: triage, assessment, investigation and early management of head injury in infants, children and adults. Clinical Guideline 4. NICE, London
NHB organ transplantation: medical and ethical issues in procurement. Institute of Medicine, National Academies Press, Washington DC. Online. Available: www.nap.edu
Pallis C, Harley D H 1996 ABC of brainstem death, 2nd edn. BMJ Publishing Group, London
Randall P 1997 A stranger in the family. Nursing Times 93(39): 32–33
Report of a working party of the Royal College of Physicians 2003 The vegetative state – guidance on diagnosis and management. Royal College of Physicians, London
Smith S 1997 The outer edge of consciousness. Nursing Times 93(39): 28–32
Waterhouse C 2005 The Glasgow Coma Scale and other neurological observations. Nursing Standard 19(33): 56–74
Woodward S 1997a Practical procedures for nurses No. 5.1. Neurological observations – 1: Glasgow Coma Scale. Nursing Times 93(45) Suppl 1–2
Woodward S 1997b Practical procedures for nurses No. 5.2. Neurological observations – 2: Pupil response. Nursing Times 93(46) Suppl 1–2
Woodward S 1997c Practical procedures for nurses No. 5.3. Neurological observations – 3: Limb responses. Nursing Times 93(47) Suppl 1–2
Woodward S 1997d Practical procedures for nurses No. 5.4. Neurological observations – 4: Case studies. Nursing Times 93(48) Suppl 1–2
www.justice4diane.org.uk
www.uktransplant.org.uk

NOTE

The Neuroscience Nurses' Benchmarking Group (NNBG)
The NNBG was established in 1995. It consists of nurses from a number of neuroscience units in the UK and Eire, and membership is open to any neuroscience nurse who is interested. The group meets every few months to share ideas and information. A benchmarking system is used 'to identify and achieve continual improvement in best nursing practice'. Literature reviews, research and evidence-based practice are discussed to reach a consensus between the members on best practice relating to a specific aspect of nursing. The specific nursing activity is then 'tested' against the benchmark in the nurses' own areas of practice and comparisons made at the next meeting. The benchmarks are not static and are reviewed in the light of changing practice and updated as necessary. Further information about the NNBG and its benchmarks can be found on the British Association of Neuroscience Nurses website (see 'Useful websites', below).

USEFUL WEBSITES

British Association of Neuroscience Nurses
www.bann.org.uk

British Brain and Spine Foundation
Freephone helpline: 0808 808 1000
www.bbsf.org.uk

Epilepsy Action
Freephone helpline: 0808 800 5050
www.epilepsy.org.uk

Head and brain injuries: Equip (Electronic Quality Information for Patients)
www.equip.nhs.uk/topics/neuro/injury.html

Headway – the brain injury association
Freephone helpline: 0808 800 2244
www.headway.org.uk

Life NPH (Normal Pressure Hydrocephalus)
www.allaboutnph.com

National Poisons Information Service
www.npis.org

Organ/tissue donation and transplants
www.uktransplant.org.uk

UK Clinical Ethics Network
www.ethics-network.org.uk

THE CRITICALLY ILL PATIENT

29

Catriona E. Smith

INTRODUCTION

The term 'critically ill' is used to describe people who have acute, life-threatening conditions but who might recover if they are given prompt, appropriate, effective and often highly technical nursing and medical care. Critically ill patients, the conditions from which they suffer and the care and treatment they need are so varied that elements from every chapter in this book are relevant to their care.

Patients who present in a critically ill state can be considered in three main categories:

- those who have never before had a significant illness and who have suffered a sudden, acute life-threatening event, e.g. extensive trauma, severe burns, near drowning, major childbirth complications or deliberate self-harm
- those who suffer from chronic illness, perhaps involving frequent previous hospital admissions, e.g. chronic obstructive airways disease (COAD) or chronic pancreatitis, and who present as critically ill as a combination of their chronic illness with a life-threatening event
- those who have become critically ill as a result of surgery — in some cases, the life-threatening situation is not expected, while in others, postoperative intensive care is a recognised necessity.

Increasingly, the major health issues and inequalities in our society will be underlying factors, with varying degrees of significance in the presentation of the critically ill patient, e.g. drug, alcohol and other substance abuse or dependence, smoking, poor dietary habits, lack of exercise and mental health concerns. Because most of these patients will be nursed in specialised units, such as an intensive care unit (ICU), their treatment and nursing care will be viewed primarily within that context. Criteria for admission to an ICU vary from hospital to hospital, but in most general ICU settings the main admission criteria are the patient's respiratory status and its maintenance. Intensive care has been defined as 'a service for patients with potentially recoverable diseases who can benefit from more detailed observation and treatment than is generally available in the standard wards' (Spiby 1989). In some hospitals there now exist critical care outreach teams. This new and steadily growing service can address the need for early intervention at ward level and may avert the need for admission to ICU, and can also follow up patients discharged from ICU (Odell et al 2002). However, where admission to ICU is necessary, duration of stay will vary greatly, from the overnight ventilatory support that may be required postoperatively, to months of intensive therapy vital to such as multiple trauma victims. In recent years there has been considerable progress in the management of many acute life-threatening conditions and consequently there has been a substantial growth in both the number and size of such units.

The nursing care of the critically ill patient is an extensive area of care and one that will not be covered fully in this chapter. It is therefore expected that those interested in this field will refer both to relevant chapters within this textbook and to more specialised texts and journals.

The Mead model for nursing

The primary responsibility of the nurse in the ICU setting is to provide care to patients with life-threatening illnesses who require continuous monitoring and life support, embracing a holistic approach. Any model used to guide intensive care nursing must therefore be flexible and allow for creativity. This chapter introduces the model for nursing developed by staff at St Thomas' Hospital, London (Mead ward), which was devised specifically to guide the nursing care of critically ill patients. Although developed two decades ago, the Mead model for nursing is still in use in a large number of ICUs. Adapted from Roper et al's (1996) activities of living (AL) model, the Mead model places the patient at the centre of all activities. Those factors which influence the ALs are given a higher profile and are used as a framework for care. Unlike Roper et al's model, the Mead model places explicit emphasis on the physical aspects of critical care nursing, such as the status of the respiratory, cardiovascular, neurological and other body systems. Generally, it is these physical needs that must take priority, often reflecting the patient's reason for admission. However, the Mead model also addresses the important contextual factors that can affect the patient, their care and the eventual outcome of that care (see Nursing Care Plan 29.1).

Nursing Care Plan 29.1 The Mead model

Name: Mr H **DOB**: 10/12/30 **Date**: 24/05/06

DIAGNOSIS: Repair of abdominal aortic aneurysm (AAA), ischaemic heart disease, peripheral vascular disease, respiratory failure, acute renal impairment

24 HOUR SUMMARY

Second day postop following AAA repair: respiratory function improving, continues on dopamine for renal impairment

Assessment	Day/night	Goals and planned care
RESPIRATORY SIMV: 10 × 700, ASB: 20, PEEP: 5, F_iO_2: 0.6 S_aO_2: 95–97%, RR: 15–20 Air entry R=L, quiet bases Minimal obtained on tracheal suction ABGs: PO_2 9.6, PCO_2 6.2		*Goal*: To optimise gaseous exchange and tissue perfusion *Plan*: Continue with ventilatory support; assist with physiotherapy and the clearance of secretions; position for optimal lung expansion; repeat ABGs
CARDIOVASCULAR HR: 95–110, irregular with ventricular ectopics BP: 180/95–210/100 Temperature: 37.5–38°C K+: 4.3, Hb: 8.9 Peripherally cool, feet mottled with pedal pulses present		*Goal*: To promote and maintain cardiovascular stability *Plan*: Monitor vital signs hourly, reporting any abnormalities; control hypertension with GTN infusion; transfuse with 2 units of RCC; continue with antibiotic therapy; monitor K+, 12-lead ECG
RENAL Hourly urine output: 25–55 mL/h CVP: +12–14 cm Maintenance fluid running at 30 mL/h + previous hour's urine output, slight peripheral oedema Urea: 12.5, Creatinine: 210 Dopamine infusion: 4 mg/mL, at 3 mL/h		*Goal*: To optimise renal function and maintain adequate hydration *Plan*: Record hourly urine output; continue with dopamine infusion at 3 mL/h; monitor urea and electrolytes; involve renal physicians if necessary; continue with maintenance fluids as prescribed
NEUROLOGICAL GCS: 9, PEARL, size 3 Sedated on midazolam 2 mL/h (1 mg/mL) Morphine at 3 mL/h (1 mg/mL) Pain score: 0–1 Sedation score: 3		*Goal*: To maintain neurological integrity and maintain pain-free *Plan*: Assess neurological status at regular intervals; monitor sedation and pain scores hourly; continue with sedation and analgesia as is

Continued

Nursing Care Plan 29.1 The Mead model *(Continued)*

NUTRITION/GI 4-hourly NG aspirates minimal, on free drainage 50–85 mL/h bile-coloured fluid, no bowel sounds present, blood sugars: 6–12 mmol/L, i.v. antacid prescribed BD, no bowel movements	*Goal*: To optimise nutritional support and maintain GI integrity *Plan*: Aspirate NG tube 4-hourly; discuss on ward round about commencing enteral feeding as per protocol; monitor blood sugars 4–6-hourly, assessing the need for insulin therapy
HYGIENE/MOBILITY/WOUND CARE Pressure areas intact, feet mottled, especially left big toe, mouth dry due to open mouth breathing, eyes slightly sticky, tolerates side lying, abdominal wound left intact, minimal leakage	*Goal*: To promote and maintain personal hygiene and maintain skin integrity *Plan*: Give all care as required; assess pressure area score daily; assess wound and re-dress as per wound care protocol
PSYCHOSOCIAL Mr H appears to be a very anxious man. His wife and their two sons and their families keep in close touch and visit on a regular basis	*Goal*: To minimise the stress/anxiety of the ICU environment *Plan*: Offer adequate reassurance and encouragement and explain all procedures prior to them being carried out; keep Mr H's family well informed as to his condition

ABG, arterial blood gases; ASB, assisted spontaneous breathing; CVP, central venous pressure; ECG, electrocardiograph; F_iO_2, inspired oxygen fraction; GCS, Glasgow Coma Scale; GTN, glyceryl trinitrate; HR, heart rate; K+, potassium; NG, nasogastric; PEARL, pupils equal and reacting to light; PEEP, positive end-expiratory pressure; RCC, red cell concentrate; RR, respiratory rate; SIMV, synchronised intermittent mandatory ventilation.

PROGRESS/EVALUATION REPORT

Day: Tuesday **Time**: 19.30	**Night** **Time**
Ventilatory settings unchanged; gaseous exchange slightly improved, maintaining S_aO_2 95–97%; spontaneous respiratory effort minimal 2–5 breaths; tracheal secretions now mucopurulent; specimen sent to bacteriology Tolerated manual hyperinflation with physiotherapy HR remains irregular, rate 100–135; BP 180 systolic/90 diastolic; continues on a GTN infusion; remains pyrexial; antibiotics discontinued; WBC up to 12.6 Transfused 2 units of RCC; 12-lead ECG shows AF, started on i.v. digoxin; K+ checked at 16.00: 3.9 Peripheral circulation remains the same; seen by the surgeons who seem content with his progress Urine output: 65–100 mL/h, on dopamine 3 mL/h CVP: + 10 to + 14 cm; remains slightly oedematous peripherally; maintenance fluids as before; urea and creatinine remain elevated; renal physicians to be consulted GCS 9, PEARL size 3; morphine at 3 mL/h and midazolam at 2 mL/h; responds to speech, and will obey commands NG aspirates nil; commenced on enteral feed at 25 mL/h, to continue as per enteral feeding protocol; blood sugars stable; i.v. antacid discontinued; no bowel movements All care given as required; pressure areas intact; abdominal wound left exposed, as no leakage Mr H requires a lot of reassurance Mr H's wife and sons visited this afternoon for a short while; they seemed pleased with his progress	

The aim of using this care plan format is to provide a structured framework for application of the nursing process (assessment, planning, intervention and evaluation) and to document this in such a way as to help others to find out about a patient's individual care easily, without working through less relevant information, much of which is documented elsewhere, e.g. 24-h chart, drug prescription chart. The development of the Mead model for nursing demonstrates that the nurse should be free to select from a model those elements that are appropriate to a specific type of patient care.

For further reading on nursing models in ICU, see Robb (1997).

MEETING THE PHYSICAL NEEDS OF THE CRITICALLY ILL PATIENT

RESPIRATORY NEEDS AND CARE

Intensive care units became established when life could be supported and maintained by means of artificial ventilation and therefore the care of ventilated patients is paramount to intensive care nursing (Woodrow 2001). While many disease processes may lead to the need for mechanical ventilation (see Box 29.1), it is most clearly indicated in the treatment of patients with severe respiratory failure who do not respond to conventional forms of medical treatment. Mechanical ventilation is the artificial support of or assistance with breathing when adequate gaseous exchange and tissue perfusion can no longer be maintained (see Ch. 3). Modern ventilatory equipment and techniques enable therapy to be directed specifically at a wide range of respiratory disorders and can do far more than just maintain vital functions.

Box 29.1

Causes of respiratory failure

Acute respiratory failure without respiratory distress
- Central airway obstruction
- Decreased level of consciousness
  - — head injury
  - — sepsis
  - — drug overdose
- Neuromuscular pathway impairment
  - — Guillain–Barré syndrome
  - — myasthenia gravis
  - — postoperative diaphragmatic paralysis
  - — trauma
- Cardiovascular impairment
  - — acute myocardial infarction
  - — cardiogenic shock

Lung parenchymal disease
- Asthma
- Pneumonia
- Adult respiratory distress syndrome (ARDS)

Acute or chronic respiratory failure
- Exacerbation of chronic obstructive airways disease (COAD)
- Chronic neuromuscular disease

Adapted from Weilitz (1993).

Nursing priorities and management

Goal: to ensure optimal gaseous exchange and tissue perfusion.

Plan:

- monitor and maintain safe ventilatory support
- assist with physiotherapy and the removal of tracheal secretions
- wean from ventilatory support when appropriate.

Monitoring respiratory function and maintaining safe ventilation

It is the nurse's responsibility to understand both normal and abnormal respiratory function, therapeutic modes of ventilation, how to maintain safe ventilatory support and how to respond appropriately to any problems that might occur. Ashworth, in 1990, suggested that advanced technology is only as good as those who use it and Woodrow (2001) states that nursing care should focus on the person rather than the machines.

STOP THINK **29.1** Describe the general principles of respiratory physiology.

Ventilators

Consideration of the patient's specific needs and diagnosis will determine the most appropriate mode of ventilation. Positive pressure ventilators are those most commonly used, and the positive pressure, volume-controlled ventilator is that most widely seen in general ICUs. This type of ventilator exerts positive pressure on the airway, delivering a predetermined volume of gas and allowing limits to be set for pressure and time. Specific considerations in the choice of ventilator include:

- the delivery of accurate predetermined oxygen concentrations of 21–100%
- a variety of modes (see Table 29.1)
- the delivery of preset volumes, despite lung characteristic changes
- the facility to monitor respiratory variables
- the appropriate alarm limits with electrical and gas safety features and a back-up system
- minimal circuit resistance allowing effective spontaneous breathing modes
- cost and user-friendliness
- reliable sterilisation and maintenance of the ventilator parts (Berston & Soni 2003)
- the use of heated bacterial filters
- the effective and safe provision of humidification and nebulised drugs.

Modes of ventilation are as follows (see Table 29.1):

- intermittent positive pressure ventilation (IPPV)
- synchronised intermittent mandatory ventilation (SIMV)
- biphasic positive airway pressure (BiPAP)
- assisted spontaneous breathing/pressure support (ASB/PS)

Table 29.1 Modes of mechanical ventilation

Mode	Advantages	Disadvantages	Uses
IPPV — also referred to as volume control, it delivers a preset volume of air at a certain rate regardless of the patient's own attempts to breathe (Berston & Soni 2003)	Complete control over ventilation; improves CO_2 elimination and improves oxygenation	Provides only full ventilation; sedation and/or paralysing agents required for the patient to tolerate it; barotraumas; decreases cardiac output; water retention; atelectasis; reduced lung compliance	Failure of ventilation (e.g. neuromuscular disease) To facilitate CO_2 excretion To reduce cerebral blood flow in patients with cerebral oedema secondary to head injury To reduce the work of breathing in patients with cardiorespiratory failure (Hillman & Bishop 1996)
SIMV — the patient's positive pressure breaths are synchronised with the inspiratory effort. If no inspiration time is sensed, a mandatory breath is delivered at a predetermined interval (Hinds & Watson 1996)	Provides both partial and full ventilation support; minimises mean airway pressure; allows spontaneous unassisted breathing; synchronises positive pressure breaths with the patient's effort (Hillman & Bishop 1996)	General hazards of artificial ventilation	As above, SIMV provides the most therapeutic mode of ventilation
BiPAP is a pressure controlled system similar to CPAP with periods of deflation, can range from full ventilation to pure spontaneous breathing (Hormann et al 1994)	It allows the patient to breathe more comfortably through invasive ventilation conditions, improving lung conditions and reducing damage associated with barotraumas	Initially used only for weaning. Is now recognised as suitable irrespective of the degree of pulmonary failure or underlying disease	Significantly reduces the need for sedatives and can be delivered non-invasively like CPAP
ASB/PS — not found on older models of ventilators, this mode senses each breath and assists breathing with a preset amount of positive pressure	Aids the transition from ventilation support to spontaneous breathing; can be used on its own or in conjunction with ventilator breaths (SIMV mode)	Does not control ventilation	Facilitates weaning Used to encourage spontaneous breathing
PEEP occurs when, instead of allowing airway pressures to reach atmospheric pressure between breaths, an end expiratory pressure is applied, enabling diffusion of more O_2 from the alveoli into the pulmonary capillaries and thus optimising gaseous exchange. Not used on its own (Hillman & Bishop 1996)	Improves oxygenation; recruits alveoli for ventilation	Decreases venous return; decreases cardiac output; can cause pulmonary barotraumas; decreases extrathoracic organ blood; increases the work of breathing; pulmonary overdistension	Patients with ARDS, LVF, pulmonary oedema, atelectasis or profound hypoxaemia may benefit greatly from the addition of some PEEP
CPAP is an option which delivers gas to the airways at a constant pressure, allowing for inspiratory pressure as well as providing PEEP. Can be used on its own	Recruits alveoli; low intrathoracic pressures compared with full ventilation; improves oxygenation; increases lung compliance; decreases the work of breathing; decreases cardiac preload and can be delivered via the ventilator or through a face mask, avoiding the need for intubation	Potentially has the same disadvantages as PEEP and artificial ventilation; however, pressures are lower and so, therefore, are the risks	Used to support spontaneous breathing

ARDS, acute respiratory distress syndrome; ASB/PS, assisted spontaneous breathing/pressure support; BiPAP, biphasic positive airway pressure; CPAP, continuous positive airway pressure; IPPV, intermittent positive pressure ventilation; LVF, left ventricular failure; PEEP, positive end-expiratory pressure; SIMV, synchronised intermittent mandatory ventilation.

- positive end-expiratory pressure (PEEP) — used as an adjunct to IPPV, SIMV and ASB/PS
- continuous positive airway pressure (CPAP).

Weaning modes (in order of decreasing ventilatory support), as indicated above, are:

- SIMV/ASB
- BiPAP
- ASB
- CPAP.

During the weaning phase, patients may alternate between these modes until they are able to cope continually on a reduced mode, ultimately achieving spontaneous breathing.

Assessment of respiratory function

This focuses heavily on physical examination and together with the patient's underlying medical condition, age and weight, will determine the prescribed mode of ventilation. Monitoring and maintaining safe ventilation is crucial and, once the patient is intubated (see Ch. 28) and receiving ventilation support, constant and thorough observations are required as there are many associated complications (see Box 29.2) (Hillman & Bishop 1996, Juniper & Garrard 1997).

Nursing priorities for maintaining safe ventilation

Chest auscultation This should be performed at the start of a shift, as a baseline, and thereafter at the discretion of the nurse. It can offer a wealth of information about the patient's air entry — from an expiratory wheeze requiring treatment with a bronchodilator, to areas of reduced air entry due to secretion retention, consolidation or pulmonary oedema. Using a systematic approach, this can spotlight trouble early and assure appropriate intervention (Cox & McGrath 1999).

Maintaining a patent airway This involves endotracheal suctioning and while it is essential to keep the airway clear of secretions, it is also just as important not to oversuction and thereby cause unnecessary trauma, irritation and hypoxia (Wood 1998, Day et al 2002).

Humidification The oxygen used to ventilate the patient must be warmed, humidified and filtered artificially as the endotracheal tube bypasses the natural processes of the nasal passages. Exposing the lungs and airways to cold gas has a number of potentially harmful effects: it can increase mucus viscosity, depress ciliary activity and obstruct the airways due to the build-up of the tenacious secretions. Temperature-controlled water humidifiers may be used; however, disposable heat moisture exchange filters (HMEF) are now more widely seen, primarily because they are cheaper, disposable and reduce the risk of infection (Beaumont 1998).

Ventilator and endotracheal (ET) tubes The ventilator tubes must not be allowed to become kinked which would reduce the desired respiratory effect. Patient comfort must be balanced with the safe and secure position of the ET tube in the patient's mouth. This is achieved by tying a crepe bandage or non-allergic adhesive tape, to decrease the risk of raised intracranial pressure in the case of a patient with a head injury, around the patient's mouth, in order to prevent movement of the ET tube. Care should be given to the pressure prevention and the position of the ET tube can be changed daily to facilitate this. Ventilator tubes must not be allowed to drag, pulling on the ET tube and thereby applying pressure to the lips. Ventilators usually have an 'arm' which will support the weight of the tubes. It is important that the tubes slope downward from the patient towards water traps, so preventing water from condensation entering the ET tube and the lungs. When turning the patient, care should always be taken to ensure that ET and ventilator tubes are guarded and supported.

Endotracheal cuff pressures These need to be checked regularly using an endotracheal cuff manometer. While cuff pressures of 30 mmHg are recommended, pressures of 17–23 mmHg have been shown to be adequate. Complications arising from prolonged excessive ET cuff pressures include tracheal oedema, loss of mucosal cilia, ulceration, ruptured tracheo-oesophageal fistula, stenosis, necrosis, sore throat and hoarseness (Wood 1998). Prevention of these complications is part of the rationale behind re-siting the airway and the fashioning of a tracheostomy after 12–14 days of oral intubation.

Level of sedation If patients are too alert, when the mode of ventilation used prevents/reduces their opportunity to trigger a break, e.g. IPPV, they may fight against the work of the ventilator, so preventing the desired therapeutic treatment being carried out; in these cases, sedation becomes necessary. Other patients may clamp down on the tube, preventing ventilation and clearance of secretions. It is also not uncommon for patients to bite through the ET tube completely. On the other hand, oversedation will inhibit patient progress, if weaning from the ventilator and spontaneous breathing are the goals. Maintaining the appropriate balance in sedation is important.

Box 29.2

Potential complications of mechanical ventilation

- Damage to the airways/lung parenchyma
- Barotrauma, tension pneumothorax, disconnection/occlusion of the endotracheal tube
- Mechanical failure
- Subcutaneous emphysema
- Hypo/hyperventilation
- Pulmonary oedema/pleural effusions
- Nosocomial hospital acquired infection (HAI), consolidation
- Low cardiac output
- Cardiovascular depression
- Arrhythmias
- Water retention
- GI haemorrhage, aspiration of stomach contents, paralytic ileus
- Impairment of CNS, kidneys and liver function
- O_2 toxicity
- Altered body image
- Sleep deprivation
- Tracheal injury

Ventilator observations Continual observations should include the patient's colour to check if well perfused or cyanosed; oxygen saturations (S_aO_2); level of consciousness, i.e. if on sedation, whether drowsy due to CO_2 retention; and chest movements, i.e. are both lungs being ventilated? It is essential that the fraction of inspired oxygen (F_iO_2), the prescribed ventilatory setting, the expired minute volume, the patient's tidal volume, airway pressures and respirations (spontaneous and ventilator breaths) are all recorded hourly allowing for continual respiratory assessment and the early detection and treatment of any problems.

Vital signs Changes in a patient's vital signs can immediately indicate problems with ventilation. Blood pressure, heart rate and rhythm, temperature, and respiratory rate and pattern should all be closely monitored.

Arterial blood gases (ABGs) Regular analysis of ABGs (see Ch. 3) will most accurately reveal a patient's respiratory progress or deterioration and the adequacy of ventilatory support.

Inhaled nitric oxide (NO) administration Nitric oxide has a powerful and often beneficial vasodilatory effect on the body (Woodrow 1997). It is used in ICU primarily to treat pulmonary hypertension, a known feature of acute respiratory distress syndrome (ARDS). For intensivists, its therapeutic properties of dilating pulmonary vasculature, reducing pulmonary vascular resistance and optimising gaseous exchange are of major significance. However, it is often seen as a last resort, as its potential toxicity necessitates that nurses responsible for its safe delivery are fully aware of the doses and dangers associated with its use, both to patient and staff; nitric oxide can form nitrogen dioxide, a highly toxic environmental pollutant. Closed suction systems should therefore always be used (Ismail-Zade & Oduro-Dominah 1997, Powroznyk & Latimer 1997, Woodrow 1997). There is no evidence that NO improves final outcome.

Assisting with physiotherapy and the removal of tracheal secretions

Physiotherapists are invaluable members of the multidisciplinary team. Their main role, in relation to the respiratory needs of the critically ill patient, is to aid the clearance of tracheal secretions, so preventing alveolar collapse, atelectasis or consolidation of the lungs, and generally optimising ventilatory efficiency through good positioning, manual hyperinflation and ET suctioning. Modern physiotherapy methods are both prophylactic and therapeutic (Juniper 1999).

Positioning

Depending on where the pulmonary abnormality is, the patient should be positioned to maximise the matching of ventilation and perfusion. In a case of a left lower lobe collapse, it may be helpful to nurse the patient on the right side, thereby optimising the treatment to the affected area. Regularly turning patients will not only assist in the prevention of pressure ulcers but also facilitate pulmonary postural drainage, and adopting a semi-recumbent position may reduce the risk of aspiration and consequently acquired ventilator-associated pneumonia (Woodrow 2000).

When a patient's oxygenation remains poor, despite high oxygen delivery and high PEEP levels, it may be decided to turn the patient to the prone position. Studies have shown that significant and dramatic improvements in arterial blood oxygenation can be achieved through the use of the prone position (Thomas 1997, Gosheron et al 1998, Ball et al 1999), especially in the treatment of patients with ARDS. For patients with ARDS, fluid tends to fill the alveoli, predominantly in the posterior lung bases, due to the effects of gravity and the usual supine positioning. These patients exhibit improved oxygenation when positioned prone because this position allows increased perfusion of the better ventilated antero-apical regions. Physiotherapy will be severely limited in this situation.

Once positioned and ready for physiotherapy with the most affected lung uppermost, manual hyperinflation (hand ventilation) is likely to be the method adopted, unless the patient's condition proves too unstable to tolerate it.

Hand ventilation (manual hyperinflation)

This is a manual form of positive pressure ventilation which is not without severe adverse effects (see Box 29.3). It is used primarily to stimulate a cough in patients with either a poor or absent cough reflex, or when there is atelectasis or excessive bronchial secretions. It may also be necessary when there is a ventilator fault, or more obviously during cardiopulmonary resuscitation, or as part of the treatment of those with raised intracranial pressure. It may also be the method used during short transfers from theatre to ICU (Robson 1998).

Endotracheal suction

Together with hand ventilation, ET suctioning is a procedure used to facilitate the clearance of secretions when a patient's normal cough mechanism is either inadequate or disrupted, e.g. where there is underlying respiratory or neurological disease or when the cough reflex is suppressed by sedation, muscle relaxants or anaesthetic agents during IPPV. Its purpose is the removal of pulmonary secretions, thereby avoiding any of the problems associated with their retention, such as increased airway pressures, pneumothorax,

Box 29.3

Some adverse effects of hand ventilation

Respiratory effects
- Pneumothorax
- Loss of the effect of PEEP
- Bronchospasm
- Decreased respiratory drive
- Rebreathing CO_2

Cardiovascular effects
- Decreased blood pressure due to decreased venous return caused by the IPPV of hand ventilation
- Increased blood pressure due to inadequate sedation or inadequate hand ventilation
- Vagal stimulation (causing bradycardia)

Box 29.4

Potential hazards of endotracheal suctioning

- Tracheal mucosal damage
- Hypoxaemia
- Atelectasis
- Arrhythmias
- Infections
- Excessive coughing
- Stress response
- Pain
- Aspiration of stomach contents

cardiovascular instability, lobar consolidation, ventilation–perfusion mismatch, pneumonia, hypoxaemia and atelectasis (Day et al 2002).

Endotracheal suction can produce complications and carries with it hidden risks (see Box 29.4). In order to minimise these risks, certain principles should be adhered to; these are discussed in Chapter 28. Infection control measures may necessitate that closed suction systems be used to minimise risk to both staff and patients.

For further reading on performing endotracheal suction, see White (2001).

Weaning from ventilatory support

Weaning is the term employed for the gradual transition from mechanical to spontaneous ventilation (self-ventilation). It should be individually tailored and begun as soon as it is established that the patient is physically capable of maintaining respiration. Often nurse-led, weaning is most successful when the underlying clinical condition predisposing the patient to require ventilation support has first been corrected. Such factors as a disturbed acid–base balance, electrolyte abnormalities, arrhythmias or altered state of consciousness may severely hinder the chances of successful weaning.

Before attempts are made to wean a patient, certain criteria must be met (Crocker 2002, Martensson & Fridlund 2002). These are:

- a stable physiological status
- a stable psychological status
- an adequate nutritional status.

The main underlying principle in weaning is that of 'minimising the work of breathing'. Box 29.5 sets out how this may be done.

Close monitoring is essential during the weaning process. Should signs of poor tolerance to weaning be evident (see Box 29.6), ventilation support may need to be resumed.

STOP THINK **29.2** Discuss the measures used to wean a patient from ventilatory support.

Extubation

When spontaneous respiration is successfully maintained, the next step is the removal of the ET tube, a procedure known as extubation (see Box 29.7). Prior to this procedure, ABGs, oxygen saturations, tidal volumes, respiratory rate and pattern, vital signs, any evidence of tiring, and the presence of a gag reflex together with a strong cough reflex must all be reviewed. Extubation should not be considered unless the patient can cough, swallow and protect the airway, and is sufficiently alert to cooperate. If possible, a planned extubation early in the day is ideal, with more staff on duty. Emergency equipment should be available in case rapid reintubation is necessary.

Box 29.5

Minimising the work of breathing in relation to weaning from ventilatory support

The nursing aims should be to:

- Prepare the patient psychologically
- Treat the underlying disease
- Reduce airway secretions
- Position for optimal lung expansion
- Reverse bronchospasm
- Maintain haemoglobin levels within normal limits
- Maintain cardiovascular stability
- Correct fluid and electrolyte imbalances
- Limit CO_2 production
- Maintain arterial blood gases within normal limits (all other aspects considered)
- Ensure optimal nutritional support
- Facilitate sleep
- Ensure neurological integrity
- Optimise pain control.

Box 29.6

Indicators of poor tolerance to weaning

- Respiratory rate increases, exceeding 45/min, or 10 above the baseline, climbing over three consecutive half-hours
- Heart rate increases, exceeding 130 beats/min
- Hypoxia develops
- Hypercarbia develops
- Conscious level deteriorates
- Systolic blood pressure increases or decreases 20 mmHg
- Diastolic blood pressure increases or decreases 10 mmHg
- Poor tidal volumes (250–300 mL)
- Significant arrhythmias
- Significant changes to arterial blood gas analysis
- Shallow breathing/use of accessory muscles
- Desaturation (S_aO_2 decreases to an unacceptable level)
  - — 100–95%: acceptable
  - — 95–90%: acceptable*
  - — 90–80%: requires to be treated*
  - — 75%: life-threatening
- Cyanosis
- Profuse sweating
- Altered breath sounds

*Depending on past medical history, e.g. COAD.

Box 29.7

Extubation procedure

1. Position the patient well, preferably as upright as possible, for optimal lung expansion.
2. Explain the procedure to the patient, as this will minimise anxiety and maximise cooperation.
3. Any sedation in use should be discontinued prior to extubation as it may hinder successful unassisted spontaneous breathing.
4. Clear the airway, both oral and tracheal, via endotracheal (ET) suction.
5. Deflate the cuff on the ET tube, cut the tape securing the ET tube, repeat ET suction and removal of the suction catheter, and then remove the ET tube.
6. Immediately substitute ET tube with an appropriate percentage of O_2 via a face mask.
7. Be aware of the patient's vital signs.
8. Record oxygen saturations with the face mask in situ.
9. Clear any oral secretions.
10. Ask the patient to cough and encourage regular deep breathing post-extubation.
11. Listen, by auscultation, to air entry.
12. Pain control may need to be reassessed following extubation, especially in the case of postoperative patients.

Adapted from Rippe et al (1995) and Hinds & Watson (1996).

CARDIOVASCULAR NEEDS AND CARE

The cardiovascular system is a closed system with haemodynamic pressures existing within the heart and arterial system. Pressure changes occur because of altered circulating volume, vessel resistance or blood viscosity and because of changes in the efficiency of the cardiac pump. In intensive care settings, monitoring systems are essential in order to evaluate any potentially fatal physiological derangements and to allow timely treatment to correct any abnormalities. The cardiovascular system can be monitored by the measurement of volume, flow, pressure and resistance in different areas. Chapter 18 covers haemodynamic monitoring and should be referred to in relation to this section.

Nursing priorities and management

Goal: to maintain haemodynamic stability and optimal perfusion.

Plan:

- monitor heart rate and rhythm
- monitor arterial blood pressure
- monitor central venous pressure
- monitor pulmonary artery pressure
- monitor temperature.

Monitoring heart rate and rhythm

The amount of information which can be gleaned from a three-lead ECG and, more importantly, a 12-lead ECG must never be underestimated and a sound understanding of the heart's electrical activity facilitates this. Cardiac arrhythmias are commonplace in patients in ICU. In general, hypoxia, shock, electrolyte abnormalities, sepsis, vagal stimulation from ET suctioning, irritation from central venous or pulmonary artery catheters, and medication are responsible for the majority of cardiac arrhythmias; however, some will be the result of myocardial ischaemia in patients with underlying heart disease. Accordingly, where possible, the nurse needs to be aware of any cardiac impairment the patient may have. Monitoring should be continuous, to enable early detection and prompt treatment of underlying problems. For details on the conduction pathways of the heart, arrhythmias and their management, see Chapter 2.

Monitoring arterial blood pressure

Patients admitted to the ICU generally have an arterial line inserted for the accurate measurement of arterial blood pressure and the provision of easy access to arterial blood for blood gas analysis. Common sites for the insertion of arterial lines are (in order of preference):

- radial artery
- brachial artery
- femoral artery
- dorsalis pedis artery.

(See Ch. 18 for information on the insertion of arterial lines.)

Arterial blood pressure monitoring is necessary:

- in those patients who are haemodynamically unstable, requiring inotropic support
- for those who have cardiopulmonary failure
- when a non-invasive blood pressure is unobtainable.

Together with the systolic and diastolic arterial pressure, the mean arterial pressure (MAP) is also recorded. This gives the measurement of perfusion pressure over the majority of the cardiac cycle. A MAP of 65–85 mmHg is generally the acceptable range. Below 50 mmHg is not desirable as it is inadequate to perfuse vital organs and tissues. Complications associated with arterial lines can and do arise (see Box 29.8).

Monitoring central venous pressure (CVP)

Central venous access is generally preferred over peripheral access, with the obvious benefit of being able to assess the patient's circulating blood volume as well as allowing the administration of intravenous medication that can only

Box 29.8

Complications associated with arterial lines

- Infection/potential sepsis
- Haemorrhage due to disconnection of the line
- Air embolism
- Vascular occlusion/thrombosis (distal circulation should be assessed regularly)
- Ischaemia
- Poor reading
- Spasm of the artery

be infused centrally, i.e. all inotropes, specific antibiotics/antifungals and certain electrolyte supplements. Monitoring the CVP also allows for the assessment of the tone of the vascular system and the ability of the right side of the heart to accept and expel blood, itself influenced by left ventricle function (see Ch. 18 for the insertion, reading and care of CVP). The trend of readings, along with other clinical information, is more important than any one reading on its own.

Monitoring pulmonary artery pressure

A pulmonary artery catheter is an important tool in the care of the critically ill patient, enabling the rapid treatment of potentially life-threatening cardiac dysfunctions. It enables the assessment of the functioning of the left ventricle and very often becomes part of the monitoring profile in situations causing either circulatory failure or acute respiratory failure. Its use is considered when information is required about fluid status, cardiovascular function or oxygen delivery (Bridges 2000). It provides information which guides the therapy of those patients on mechanical ventilation, circulatory assist devices or inotropic medication (see Ch. 18 for information on insertion of and care of pulmonary artery catheters).

The pulmonary artery wedge pressure (PAWP), or 'wedge', gives a more accurate indication of the fluid status of the patient. Elevated PAWPs may arise as a result of volume overload, left ventricular failure (LVF), mitral stenosis or regurgitation and cardiac tamponade, whereas abnormally low readings may relate to hypovolaemia.

The frequency of haemodynamic measurements depends on the patient's condition and, as with all invasive monitoring, actions should be supported by clinical findings (see Box 29.9).

Doppler monitoring

Oesophageal Doppler monitoring is now increasingly favoured in ICU, primarily because it offers a reduced risk of morbidity and mortality in comparison to the pulmonary artery catheter, as it is less invasive. An ultrasound probe is placed in the oesophagus running parallel with the descending aorta. The Doppler then measures the velocity of the blood flow in the descending aorta (Edwards 1998).

Box 29.9

Haemodynamic cardiac profile — normal readings

- Pulmonary artery pressure (PAP)
  — systolic: 15–25 mmHg
  — diastolic: 8–15 mmHg
- Pulmonary artery wedge pressure (PAWP): 6–12 mmHg
- Cardiac output (CO): 4–8 L/min
- Cardiac index (CI): 2.5–4.2 L/min per m^2
- Systemic vascular resistance (SVR): 900–1600 dyn/s per cm^5 (this measurement relates to the resistance to flow in the whole systemic circulation)
- Mixed venous oxygen saturations (S_vO_2): 65–75%

Adapted from Coombs (1993).

This form of monitoring is not suitable for all types of patient. It is most useful as a guide in deciding when, what and how much fluid replacement to give in cases of hypovolaemia. The pulmonary artery catheter may still be required for absolute measurements of CO, PAWP, S_vO_2 and SVR (see Box 29.9), especially in cases of severe sepsis.

STOP THINK **29.3** How could an atypical pneumonia cause multisystem failure in a 65-year-old woman admitted to ICU following a respiratory arrest in a medical high-dependency unit? Discuss her nursing care and what haemodynamic monitoring may be necessary.

Inotropic medication

A pulmonary artery catheter is often inserted in order to determine inotropic therapy, as it clarifies whether there is a pressure problem, i.e. reduced blood pressure, a problem with the flow, i.e. decreased cardiac output, or a problem with oxygen delivery and consumption. Cardiac contractility can become impaired, either as a direct result of cardiogenic shock, or secondary to hypovolaemic and septic shock. In such cases, inotropic medication such as adrenaline, dopamine and dobutamine, which improve cardiac contractility, are frequently used to support the patient until such time as definitive treatment is administered or the patient recovers (Hillman & Bishop 1996). Administration is always via a central vein and the effects of inotropic therapy are monitored closely. Different combinations of inotropic medication may be advocated in order to achieve the desired effect. It is common practice to titrate inotropic therapy against MAP, generally aiming for a MAP of between 65 and 85 mmHg; inotropic medication is always titrated down 1 mL at a time before discontinuation.

Monitoring temperature

Despite a wide variety of heat-producing metabolic processes and the range of ambient temperatures to which the human body may be exposed, core body temperature is maintained with remarkable stability. However, critical illness can disturb temperature control, producing body temperatures at either end of the spectrum, i.e. hypothermia (<35°C) or hyperthermia/hyperpyrexia (<38.5°C) (Ch. 22 explores temperature maintenance in depth).

For further reading on the management of hypothermia, see McGowan (1999).

RENAL/FLUID BALANCE NEEDS AND CARE

The kidneys are very sensitive organs and it is not uncommon for an abrupt decline in renal function to occur in the presence of other systemic illnesses. This is particularly so if the cardiovascular or respiratory systems become compromised. Renal function is especially susceptible to the effects of underperfusion and hypoxaemia. In the critically ill patient, acute renal failure (ARF) is a relatively common complication resulting from severe hypotension or drug toxicity, or more frequently as a consequence of overwhelming sepsis and multisystem organ failure (MSOF). However, it is usually multifactorial. According to Hinds and Watson (1996), 'ARF can be defined as a sudden (and usually reversible) failure of the kidneys to excrete the waste products of metabolism, and may be broadly categorised as prerenal, renal or postrenal'. The treatment of ARF is predominantly one of support until recovery occurs.

STOP THINK **29.4** Discuss the key regulatory functions of the renal system.

Nursing priorities and management

Goal: to maintain indices of renal function within the patient's own normal limits.

Plan:

- monitor and maintain optimal fluid and electrolyte balance
- provide necessary and appropriate renal replacement therapy.

Monitoring and maintaining optimal fluid and electrolyte balance

In the susceptible patient, the primary goal must always be the prevention of renal impairment. This involves knowledge of the causes of ARF and meticulous monitoring and assessment of the patient. The causes of ARF fall into the three categories mentioned above: prerenal, renal and postrenal (see Ch. 8, p. 388); the first two are largely responsible for the development of ARF, but elements of all three may coexist in the critically ill patient. ARF can be divided into phases, or stages (see Ch. 8, p. 388), as follows:

- the onset phase — the time between the precipitating episode and oliguria or anuria developing
- the oliguric phase (diminished urine output) — can last from 7 to 21 days
- the diuretic phase — characterised by an increase in urine output over several days
- the recovery phase — follows the gradual improvement of kidney function and usually occurs over 3–12 months.

Systemic manifestations may accompany the development of renal insufficiency, as outlined in Box 29.10 (Henke & Eigsti 2003).

Box 29.10

Systemic manifestations of acute renal failure

Respiratory
- Pulmonary oedema
- Suppressed cough reflex
- Kussmaul respiration (see Ch. 5, part 2)

Cardiac
- Congestive cardiac failure/overload
- Arrhythmias
- Uraemic pericarditis

Vascular
- Hypertension
- Fluid overload, increased CVP, decreased urine output
- Electrolyte imbalance
- Metabolic acidosis

Haematopoietic
- Anaemia (as a result of reduced erythropoietin production)
- Coagulopathy (platelets have a reduced life span due to the uraemic toxins)
- More prone to infections (as a result of uraemic toxins)

Neuromuscular
- Electrolyte imbalance
- Uraemic encephalopathy

Gastrointestinal
- GI bleeding
- Nausea
- Uraemic halitosis
- Bowel changes

Skin integrity
- Purpura rash (due to coagulopathy)
- Yellowness (uraemia)
- Dry skin (due to decreased sweat production as a result of uraemic toxins)

Nursing priorities in monitoring and maintaining optimal fluid and electrolyte balance

Urine output In addition to the monitoring of all fluid intake, hourly urine output volumes must be recorded, together with an accurate 24-h fluid balance, of all fluid gains and losses. While a urine output of 400 mL or less (oliguria) over a 24-h period is indicative of ensuing renal failure, it is also acknowledged that ARF can occur in the absence of oliguria (non-oliguric ARF).

Urea and electrolytes Daily assays of urea and electrolytes will indicate the degree of renal insufficiency present. Urea, creatinine and some electrolyte levels rise with developing ARF, leading to varying degrees of metabolic acidosis. It should be noted, however, that elevated urea on its own may indicate, merely, that the patient is dehydrated.

The nurse must know the normal plasma values for urea, creatinine and the more common electrolytes and the significance of any deviations, as some electrolyte abnormalities can produce life-threatening arrhythmias.

Fluid therapy Intravenous fluid therapy should be considered carefully in the management of the critically ill patient. This is particularly so in conditions of sepsis, ARDS or systemic inflammatory response syndrome (SIRS). In such situations, the permeability of capillary endothelial cells increases and the vessels become 'leaky', allowing large protein particles to pass into the interstitial space and thus reducing the capillary osmotic pressure. This facilitates the movement of water together with further protein molecules into the interstitial space, depleting intravascular volume and impairing gaseous exchange. This results in peripheral oedema and, within the lungs, results in pulmonary oedema, causing hypoxaemia and consequently diminished oxygen delivery and consumption by peripheral tissues. Vascular volume must be restored. The three main groups of volume-expanding fluids are crystalloids, colloids and blood:

- Crystalloids are made up of non-ionic solutes such as sodium chloride added to water; they do not contain oncotic particles and will therefore eventually move out of the vascular compartment (see Ch. 20). These fluids, unlike colloids, are cheap to produce and are not associated with immunologically mediated reactions.

- Colloids, which contain oncotic particles, generating oncotic pressure, are mainly confined to the intravascular space, at least when first administered.
- Blood and blood products also exert an oncotic pressure due to the large protein particles they contain and so are less likely to contribute to interstitial oedema.

Clinical assessment A careful clinical assessment is necessary, observing for signs of worsening pitting oedema, notably at the ankles and sacrum. Chest auscultation may reveal widespread coarse crackles and suggest fluid overload and pulmonary oedema.

Cardiovascular status directly affects renal perfusion. It is recommended that the MAP is above 60 mmHg for renal perfusion to be ensured (Kishen 2002). Regular monitoring of the CVP, cardiac output and PAWP will indicate whether fluid input or inotropic support is required. The presence of peaked T waves is suggestive of a rising plasma potassium level.

Nephrotoxic medication The use of nephrotoxics, e.g. gentamicin and non-steroidal anti-inflammatory drugs (NSAIDs), should be avoided in those with impending renal failure or in those whose renal function is precarious (Hillman & Bishop 1996).

Immediate management of diminishing renal function

- Optimise fluid balance either by giving a fluid challenge if vital signs indicate hypovolaemia or by using diuretic therapy if there are clinical signs of fluid overload. Furosemide, a potent loop diuretic, is the drug of choice.
- Correct electrolyte imbalances as necessary.
- Maintain haemoglobin within the normal range.
- Assess nutritional input, with particular attention to appropriate protein and carbohydrate content. Generally, nutritional support is provided via the enteral route unless otherwise contraindicated. The dietitian will make an important contribution to the team approach to care.
- Remove any known causative factors, e.g. nephrotoxic drugs.
- Exclude obstruction, e.g. make sure that the urinary catheter has not become blocked with sediment.

If this is not enough to resolve renal impairment, then continuous renal replacement therapy (CRRT) will be required.

Renal replacement therapy

In unresolving ARF, the management focuses on supportive renal replacement therapy and the control of metabolic derangements arising from renal failure. Rapid commencement of CRRT is essential in situations where the patient is severely hyperkalaemic, grossly overloaded or suffering from uraemic complications or pericarditis, or where ARF has been drug induced. Forni and Hilton (1997) assert CRRT to be an effective and efficient way of controlling the problems caused by ARF and, while not providing a 'cure', it enables the critically ill patient to be supported pending recovery from the underlying disease process or injury.

Caring for patients with CRRT is deemed part of the professional practice of experienced nurses working in the ICU. They require a thorough knowledge of the reasons for its use, the equipment involved, the problems that can arise and how to respond to them.

Haemofiltration

Traditionally, the recognised form of treatment for critically ill patients with ARF was peritoneal dialysis or haemodialysis. However, dialysis has not always produced a beneficial outcome as haemodialysis often induces severe hypotension and peritoneal dialysis impairs ventilation. For some decades now, there has been increasing use of a less aggressive form of renal replacement therapy — haemofiltration. This is a relatively straightforward form of CRRT by which excess fluid and solutes are removed by passing the patient's blood through a haemofilter. By creating a positive pressure gradient within this haemofilter, fluid removal from the blood by ultrafiltration is facilitated. For the clearance of solutes, a large amount of fluid must be filtered. To prevent dehydration, replacement fluids must be carefully monitored (Urwin & Fletcher 2000, Urwin et al 2001).

Continuous venovenous haemofiltration (CVVH) This is generally the mode of choice in haemofiltration, as it allows the slow, steady removal of fluid volume. It also gives the venous system time to compensate for fluid lost from the interstitial spaces. Most importantly, it avoids the rapid shift of solutes and electrolytes, thereby preventing the risk of cardiovascular instability. It is the only safe line of treatment in the management of ARF in those with haemodynamic instability and/or MSOF, where the removal of fluid and waste products is vital. A further advantage of CVVH is that it does not require arterial access. Access for CVVH is via a double-lumen catheter, often referred to as a Quinton line. This line is inserted into a main vein — the femoral, subclavian or internal jugular. When not in use, the lumens of this line are injected with heparinised saline to maintain line patency and prevent clot formation and the release of emboli.

Molecular adsorbent recycling system (MARS) is a membrane-based blood purification system, also referred to as bioartificial liver support. It works directly with the CVVH in supporting liver function in severe liver failure, providing time for detoxification, hepatic regeneration or donor availability, and is used in patients with fulminant hepatic failure (FHF), e.g. after paracetamol and other drug overdoses (Karnik & Freeman 1998, Stange et al 2002).

Nursing responsibilities in haemofiltration

Fluid balance Accurate measurement of input and output of fluid is essential, and renal replacement therapy is reviewed daily by the renal physicians. The nurse responsible for the patient should adjust filtration rates in accordance with the medical prescription.

Vital signs The recording of vital signs is imperative. At the start of CVVH, the patient's blood pressure may fall, as blood is removed from the circulating volume. However, this can be pre-empted and is readily corrected by giving volume expanders.

The patient's temperature is also altered. It is generally believed that body temperature drops by 1°C with CVVH in process. It is therefore not uncommon for a patient to become moderately hypothermic. To prevent this, replacement fluid should be warmed to a suitable temperature. It should be noted that CVVH may mask developing sepsis, as a recorded temperature of 37°C may equate to a patient temperature of nearer 38°C.

Urea, electrolytes and ABGs Regular assessment of urea, electrolytes and ABGs is necessary in order to assess acid–base balance. Electrolyte supplements are often required and potassium is usually given in replacement fluid being administered via the filter. Initially, no potassium may be required as hyperkalaemia may be the very reason for commencing haemofiltration. Other electrolyte supplements such as calcium and phosphate can be administered intravenously or nasogastrically. Lactate-free filtrate solute is also available when lactate acidosis is a problem.

Monitoring the activated clotting time (ACT) The ACT is the time it takes for a small sample of blood to clot. It is of particular importance if the patient is receiving heparin as anticoagulation therapy while on the haemofilter. Heparin, the anticoagulant of choice, is administered to prevent clotting of the extracorporeal circuit (Urwin et al 2001). Patient coagulation, and therefore the demand for heparin, will vary greatly depending on the underlying disease process. However, a concentration of 250 IU/mL at a rate of 1–6 mL/h is normally administered. Some patients will not be able to tolerate the effects of heparin, as it is known to disrupt the intrinsic coagulation cascade and promote platelet aggregation. This is seen particularly in liver failure. In such cases, prostacyclin can be used as it preserves platelet function and number. It does, however, have strong side-effects, noticeably vasodilatation, causing facial flushing and significant hypotension. ACT is not required with prostacyclin as the normal clotting process is not so severely altered.

Preventing infection Preventing infection and maintaining asepsis are vital. Patients on haemofiltration are often immunocompromised and therefore are more susceptible to infection. Residual catheterisation is performed every 2–3 days, preventing stasis of urine in the bladder, a potential source for infection. If urine volume is 250 mL or more, the catheter is normally left in situ, as this can be indicative of the return of renal function.

Patient safety Maintenance of patient safety is the nurse's responsibility. If access is via the femoral vein, the limb should be carefully observed to ensure optimal perfusion is maintained (Woodrow 1993). Furthermore, the prevention of air emboli, infection or haemorrhage, as a consequence of heparin use, should be borne in mind.

Psychological care Providing psychological support and reassurance to the patient receiving CVVH is all-important, true indeed for any procedure carried out on the critically ill patient. Extended body image is an issue not widely written about, but some, e.g. Smith (1989), have studied its implications in relation to the critically ill patient with particular reference to the ventilation tubing and dialysis lines. The nurse responsible for the patient undergoing CVVH must be aware of and sensitive to this issue.

High-volume haemofiltration (HVHF) and haemodialysis

When a patient's stability is restored, HVHF or haemodialysis may then become an option. It facilitates the rapid clearance of waste products over a period of 3–4 h. Daily, or alternate-day, treatment may be necessary until the kidneys recover completely. Full renal recovery is entirely possible in patients with no prior history of renal impairment.

NEUROLOGICAL NEEDS AND CARE

A number of conditions predispose critically ill patients to altered states of consciousness. These include (Goldhill & Withington 1997):

- intracranial pathology, such as intracranial haemorrhage, cerebral hypoxia, tumours and abscesses
- systemic disease affecting the cerebral blood supply or oxygenation, such as sepsis, metabolic encephalopathy, hypoglycaemia, hepatic failure (hepatic encephalopathy), renal failure, pancreatitis, respiratory failure or hypo/hyperthermia
- exogenous agents, such as drugs and toxins, and drug withdrawal.

Neurological functioning is an important part of the overall clinical assessment and continuous care of those being nursed in the ICU. The use of a standardised neurological assessment tool such as the Glasgow Coma Scale (GCS) is essential, enabling early detection of any deterioration and facilitating prompt treatment (see Ch. 28). In addition, invasive neurological monitoring of intracranial pressure (ICP), which facilitates the monitoring of the cerebral perfusion pressure (CPP), is often indicated in patients who demonstrate a GCS of 8 or less and/or a grade 3 or 4 encephalopathy (see Box 29.11). As with the majority of clinical observations, it is the trend that is of greatest significance when monitoring ICP and CPP.

Nursing priorities and management

Goal: to maintain neurological status.
Plan: monitor neurological function.

Box 29.11

Grades of encephalopathy

1	Mild confusion, poor concentration, but fully coherent when awake
2	Increasingly confused, disoriented, yet remains rousable
3	Very drowsy, may be agitated or aggressive when roused to command
4	Responsive to painful stimuli, not rousable to command. May display signs of pupil and limb changes, abnormal breathing and extensor plantars

Monitoring neurological function

The Glasgow Coma Scale is the standard tool used in assessing neurological function. It is an objective way of measuring levels of consciousness (LOCs) and is set out in detail in Chapters 9 and 28. However, Price et al (2000) looked at the appropriateness of the GCS in ICU and concluded that it has limited use as an assessment tool as many therapeutic interventions, such as ventilation, may obscure the real LOC.

Cerebral function analyser monitor (CFAM) This comprises a visual display unit and printer which allows the continual monitoring and display of cerebral activity. This activity is picked up by five electrodes: two are situated over each hemisphere and one ground electrode allows both hemispheres to be compared. This system is better than the conventional EEG. It is used continuously by the bedside to assess whether the patient is appropriately sedated and commonly used with patients receiving paralysing agents in order to detect whether or not they are having seizures.

Computed tomography (CT) scan In relation to neurological functioning, CT scanning is usually performed in order to detect cerebral haematomas, oedema, infarctions, atrophy, hydrocephalus and tumours.

ICP monitoring Intracranial pressure is the pressure exerted by the intracranial contents against the skull. Normally, brain tissue constitutes 80%, cerebrospinal fluid (CSF) 10% and blood volume 10% of the intracranial contents. It becomes necessary to monitor the ICP in the critically ill when a patient displays signs of raised ICP manifested as severe encephalopathy (see Box 29.11). For patients who do not progress any further than a grade 1 or 2 encephalopathy, the prognosis is good. Severe head injuries remain the most common cause of raised ICP, but it may also occur in patients presenting with problems such as hepatic encephalitis due to fulminant hepatic failure (Hawker 1996), increasingly seen nowadays as the consequence of paracetamol overdose.

For a case study on paracetamol poisoning, see Leighton (1995).

ICP monitoring can be used to help minimise neurological damage in those patients predisposed to neurological problems, as such monitoring will demonstrate neurological changes before they present clinically and thus greatly assist clinical observation. For further discussion of raised ICP, see Chapter 9 (p. 406).

Cerebral perfusion pressure (CPP) The value of monitoring the ICP is that it allows the CPP to be calculated. This is done by subtracting the ICP measurement from the mean pressure of circulating blood within the cranial cavity (i.e. CPP = MAP – ICP). Generally the aim is to maintain CPP above 70 mmHg, thus preventing underperfusion of the cerebral tissue.

Jugular bulb oximetry (S_jO_2) This is an uncommon invasive monitoring system, but may be used to provide information about global cerebral oxygen consumption (Chatfield & Rees-Pedlar 2001).

The immediate management of elevated ICP

The level at which treatment of raised ICP will be necessary depends on the patient's condition, but is often set at around >15 mmHg. Medication of choice includes mannitol 20% initially and then subsequent administration of furosemide, which both enhances its effect and produces a faster diuresis. It is important to be aware of the patient's renal status prior to administration of these medications, i.e. is there a significant degree of renal impairment? In order to counteract any sudden electrolyte changes due to induced diuresis, plasma protein substance (PPS) is also part of the treatment protocol. This line of treatment can be considered at 4- to 6-hourly intervals. If ineffective, barbiturate therapy may be necessary. Barbiturates exert their effect on ICP by reducing cerebral oxygen consumption and thereby producing vasoconstriction and reduction in ICP. Another useful agent is thiopental which lowers ICP by reducing metabolism to a minimum as well as lowering blood pressure by reducing venous and arterial tone, thus reducing cerebral perfusion (Stanley & Hancox 2001).

Nursing activities and ICP

- ET suction should be carried out only as required, i.e. in response to secretions. Retention of secretions will increase ICP, just as frequent suctioning can be detrimental. The maintenance of adequate ventilatory support is essential as hypercapnia and hypoxia will increase cerebral vasodilatation, causing raised ICP. It may be necessary to continually monitor the end-tidal CO_2 (Frakes 2001).
- Secure the ET tube with adhesive tape, thus not restricting cerebral drainage.
- Ensure good head alignment, elevating the head of the bed to promote cerebral drainage.
- Keep all nursing procedures to a minimum.
- Check pupils hourly and following all nursing and medical procedures.
- Maintain an accurate fluid balance chart. Monitor and be aware of electrolyte levels, e.g. both hypo- and hypernatraemia can contribute to raised ICP.
- Prevent cerebral ischaemia and maintain CPP above 60 mmHg.
- Provide adequate nutritional support. Patients with ICP problems are often in a hypercatabolic state.
- Assess the need and extent to which pressure area care is appropriate.

STOP THINK **29.5** Describe the nursing care of a patient following an overdose of tricyclic antidepressants.

SEDATION AND PAIN CONTROL

Nursing priorities and management

Goal: to maintain the optimal level of sedation and pain control.

Plan: assess the need for sedation and analgesics.

Assessing the need for sedation and analgesics

Pain has been identified as a major problem for patients in the ICU. Pain is a subjective experience and the control of pain will require regular assessment and clear documentation. The challenge is to provide the most appropriate form of pain relief. Pain control is covered extensively in Chapter 19 and therefore this section will focus primarily on the assessment of sedation required.

Most patients admitted to the ICU will, at some point during their stay, require sedation and/or analgesics (Arbour 2000). Views and practice have changed considerably over the years from the belief that patients should be heavily sedated and unaware of their surroundings to the current preferred state of lighter sedation while maintaining an optimal state of comfort (Shelley 1998). Many units now operate some form of sedation protocol. Patient comfort may be achieved by creating a supportive environment, through constant reassurance and explanation prior to all procedures, together with the maintenance of some sort of diurnal rhythm. However, medication may be required to produce the respiratory depression necessary to facilitate adequate ventilation, to aid tolerance of the presence of the ET tube or to decrease anxiety in general. Shelley (1998) suggested that patient comfort is a better term than sedation, as sedation is only one of the desired effects.

Sedation and analgesics can be administered continually or as a bolus, the prescribed regimen being tailored to the needs of each patient. The nurse must constantly assess the sedation level (a number of sedation scaling systems exist — see Box 29.12) and therefore should display a sound knowledge of the issues surrounding sedation in the ICU, i.e. sensory overload, sensory deprivation, ICU psychosis and psychological support. The goal of sedation is to decrease anxiety, fear and restlessness and to increase cooperation and compliance. Optimal sedation should enable the patient to be rousable on stimulation but able to sleep/rest when undisturbed — keeping the patient comfortable is a balance between under- and oversedation (Shelley 1998).

Patient comfort

Four main groups of drugs can be enlisted to enhance patient comfort:

Sedatives Benzodiazepines are probably the most commonly used medications in ICUs, with midazolam used widely. Its has sedative, anxiolytic and amnesic properties and has a short half-life. However, it is largely hepatically metabolised and renally excreted and therefore could accumulate should these organs be impaired (Bion & Oh 2003).

Box 29.12

Sedation scale

0	Asleep, no response to tracheal suction
1	Rousable, coughs with tracheal suction
2	Awake, spontaneously coughs or triggers the ventilator
3	Actively breathes against the ventilator
4	Unmanageable

From Cohen & Kelly (1987).

Propofol, administered either as a bolus or continuous infusion, has anaesthetic properties and is commonly used to sedate patients who require short periods of mechanical ventilation. It is widely used as it provides a controllable level of sedation which is easily maintained and recovery is rapid, allowing weaning from the ventilator to progress.

Analgesics Morphine provides safe analgesia but should be used with caution in those with liver and renal impairment. NSAIDs and local analgesics in the form of nerve blocks may also be considered.

Alfentanil is a valuable analgesic used in the ICU, especially when short-term supplementation is required. It is short-acting with a short half-life.

Neuromuscular blocking agents The use of these agents has been reduced, partly as a result of the more effective use of sedatives, but also because of improved ventilator design. A muscle relaxant will be administered initially to most patients admitted to ICU, in order to facilitate intubation and line insertion, e.g. suxamethonium has a rapid onset and offset action, but is not suitable for prolonged administration (Goldhill & Withington 1997). Longer administration may be required to aid ventilation control, reduce O_2 consumption in patients who have developed ARDS, and lower ICP in head injury — in such cases, a neuromuscular blocking agent such as atracurium is often used.

Antidepressants (e.g. amitriptyline) Antidepressants are often prescribed in those showing depressive behaviour, often patients who have been critically ill for weeks, where weaning from the ventilator is slow, or those with previous depressive illness. As well as improving mood, antidepressants can help to normalise the sleep pattern.

For further reading on sedation and the critically ill patient, see Kress et al (2002).

NUTRITIONAL/GASTROINTESTINAL NEEDS AND CARE

The nutritional status of patients in hospitals has been the topic of much research over the years. It is well recognised that critical illness in general is associated with a massive increase in catabolic hormone production leading to a rise in basal metabolic rate. If not addressed appropriately, malnutrition in such patients can contribute to immunosuppression, increased postoperative complications, delayed wound healing and consequently longer stays in hospital, all of which may adversely affect their outcome (Leary et al 2000a,b). Chapter 21 covers nutritional support thoroughly and should be studied in relation to nutrition and the critically ill.

It is now believed that the gut has an extremely important and active role to play in the treatment of the critically ill patient (Singer & Carr 1996). Well recognised for its role in absorbing and digesting nutrients, the gut also has a vital function as a barrier to microorganisms and endotoxins. This defence mechanism is preserved by the normal epithelial cells and is supported by a series of immunological mechanisms. In the critically ill, this barrier is often severely compromised and as a result the bowel, which acts as a reservoir for organisms, facilitates the process of gut translocation of bacteria. This practice allows the transfer of endotoxins and pathogens into the portal and systemic circulation and may add to the risk of sepsis (Leary et al 2000a,b). Consequently, it is imperative that, where possible, optimal gastrointestinal function should be maintained. In the past, nutritional support was often not considered an immediate priority in the management of critically ill patients, but it is now widely acknowledged that early assessment and optimal nutritional support are vital components in the overall treatment of such patients and where possible such nutritional support should be via the enteral route (Maitnel & Blackburn 2003).

Nursing priorities and management

Goal: to minimise weight loss and maintain normal gastrointestinal (GI) function.

Plan:

- establish nutritional support
- maintain GI integrity.

Establishing nutritional support

Nurses are responsible for assessing nutritional needs, administering nutritional therapy, monitoring its effects and complications, and evaluating its effectiveness. There are basically two clinical routes for maintaining nutritional support: parenteral and enteral (see Ch. 21).

Parenteral nutrition

In the past, parenteral nutrition (PN) was the accepted form of nutritional support for the critically ill. However, evidence now suggests that using the parenteral route may not only increase the risk of sepsis from complications associated with its administration (see Ch. 21), but also, because gut function is not maintained, result in mucosal atrophy and the facilitation of bacterial translocation (Buckley & McFie 1997, Maitnel & Blackburn 2003). Microorganisms and endotoxins cross into the blood, resulting in sepsis. Systemic inflammatory response syndrome (SIRS) follows and can lead to multisystem organ failure, as illustrated in Figure 29.1.

PN, which requires administration via a large central vein, is an unnatural method of feeding, however justified, in certain situations, where the use of the gut is either impossible or inadequate. Because of the well-recognised complications arising from PN administration, as well as its cost, enteral feeding is preferred in the treatment and support of the critically ill patient.

Serum electrolytes Monitoring electrolyte levels to prevent imbalances is essential. This in fact pertains to both routes of nutritional support, but is especially the case in PN. It is necessary to check regularly the patient's blood glucose level, monitoring for hypo/hyperglycaemia and consequently assessing the need for insulin therapy. Patients requiring inotropic therapy in the form of adrenaline also need their blood sugar levels monitored closely, as adrenaline, especially at higher doses, affects the utilisation of glucose from the cells. Insulin resistance is frequently a

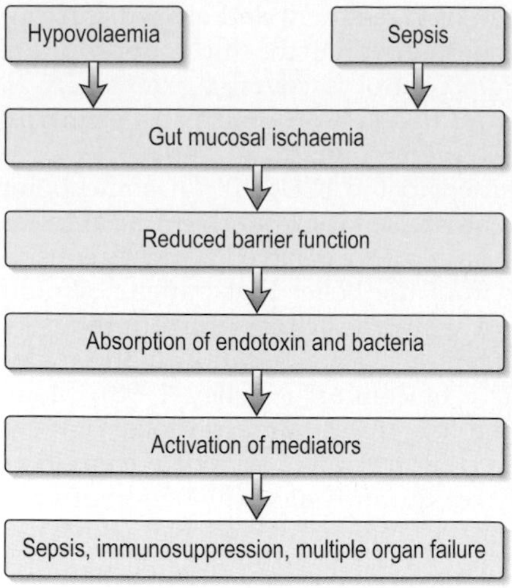

Fig. 29.1 The role of the gut in multiple organ failure.

feature of critical illness and studies have concluded that the use of insulin to maintain blood sugar levels no higher than 110 mg/dL reduces morbidity and mortality in critically ill patients in the ICU, irrespective of whether or not they had a history of diabetes mellitus (Van den Berghe et al 2001, Bradley 2002).

Enteral nutrition

Besides being relatively inexpensive and safe to use (Leary et al 2000a,b; see also Ch. 21), enteral nutrition (EN) offers a protective effect on the GI tract and should be utilised early and often, reducing the risk of bacterial translocation and maintaining mucosal integrity. EN is also believed to maintain the autoregulation of blood flow to the gut. Most patients in the ICU can be fed enterally, the only absolute contraindication being true gut failure. Relative contraindications include bowel anastomosis distal to the feeding tube, pancreatitis or small bowel disease. Gut function may be decreased and an ileus may develop as a result of IPPV or the use of opiates; however, the small bowel retains motility and absorptive functions in most critically ill patients. Feeding is usually via the nasogastric or nasoenteral route — nasoduodenum or nasojejunum — however, a jejunostomy tube may be fashioned.

For further reading on nasogastric intubation, see Dougherty & Lister (2004).

Feeding via the enteral route On introducing enteral feeding, a protocol should be followed and this, together with competent nursing practice and perseverance, will enable most critically ill patients to be fed by this method. Lack of bowel sounds is not a contraindication to enteral feeding (Leary et al 2000a,b). As patients who are ventilated often swallow less air than normal, therefore reducing their main source of gas, bowel sounds do not always correlate with gastric absorption. The feed should be administered using an infusion pump at a constant rate, helping to reduce the incidence of diarrhoea, and nasogastric aspiration carried out every 4 h to monitor feed absorption. A number of standard formula feeds exist and, while usually satisfactory for most patients, special feeds may be required to meet the excessive metabolic demands of the critically ill. Some examples of special properties are:

- high-protein, low-osmolarity feeds
- fibre/bulking agents
- low-carbohydrate, high-fat content — for those producing too much CO_2, inhibiting weaning from the ventilator
- low-protein, high-calorie content with reduced potassium — for those with renal or liver impairment
- constituents targeted specifically at critically ill patients — e.g. multiple trauma, sepsis, general states of catabolic stress — include omega-3 fatty acids and glutamine. Glutamine, in particular, is thought to increase the gut's ability to accept nutrients during critical illness (Verity 1996), enhancing gut mucosal integrity. This enables proliferation of both lymphocytes and macrophages, correlating with a boost in the immune system.

STOP THINK **29.6** Identify physiological changes caused by inadequate nutritional support.

Maintaining GI integrity

As well as providing nutritional support, the assessment and alleviation of GI problems must be given due consideration. These can range from delayed gastric emptying, abdominal distension, diarrhoea or constipation to the presence of stress ulcers (see Ch. 4).

Delayed gastric emptying

This may be alleviated through the use of a wide variety of pharmacological agents, e.g. metoclopramide which will stimulate gastric emptying and erythromycin which has been demonstrated to increase gastric motility (Bradley 2001a, Oudemans-van Straaten 2003). In extreme cases, when pharmacological agents are not enough, feeding via a distal tube, e.g. into the jejunum, may be considered. In this way the need for gastric emptying integrity is bypassed.

Abdominal distension

This is associated with the malabsorption of enteral feed and, in this case, feeding should be reduced or stopped for a few hours and the enteral feeding regimen reviewed.

Diarrhoea or constipation

This is not uncommon in the critically ill patient. However, it cannot be assumed automatically to be the result of enteral feed intolerance. Many factors can induce diarrhoea, not least antibiotic therapy or infection, *Clostridium difficile* being a common causative agent.

Rarely is feeding stopped because of feed-induced diarrhoea. On occasions, contamination of the feed may be the root cause, highlighting the need for an aseptic technique during the handling of feeding equipment. At the other end of the spectrum, it is also necessary to review the need for aperients.

Stress ulceration

This may develop due to damage to the mucosal layer, often during a period of ischaemic anoxia as part of a shocked state (see Ch. 28). In addition, impaired production of gastric mucus, reduced epithelial renewal, disturbed acid–base balance, reflux of bile acids and the presence of uraemia all predispose the patient to gastric ulceration (Bradley 2001b, Tucker & Dexter 2003).

Enteral feeding acts as prophylaxis; however, in patients being supported by PN, prophylactic medication should be prescribed. Antacids and H_2-receptor blockades are thought to be equally effective as prophylactic agents for stress ulcers.

HYGIENE AND MOBILITY NEEDS AND WOUND CARE

Caring for the critically ill patient requiring mechanical ventilation is both a medical and nursing challenge. Many patients in the ICU setting are fully dependent on the provision of all care. Meticulous nursing care is required in order to maintain optimal body tissue integrity and organ function. Individualised care tailored to the needs of the patient is a prerequisite with regular assessment and evaluation of the effectiveness of care chosen.

Nursing priorities and management

Goal: to provide optimal personal hygiene and to maintain skin integrity.

Plan:

- maintain personal hygiene, preventing infection
- maintain skin integrity and promote wound healing
- promote and maintain normal tone, power and movement of the musculoskeletal system.

Maintaining personal hygiene and preventing infection

Personal hygiene

Assisting with the maintenance of personal hygiene not only promotes comfort and dignity, but also represents an opportunity for thorough assessment of the patient, including skin integrity, any potential sites of infection, e.g. inflamed cannula insertion sites, and the peripheral circulation. The nurse should maintain the dignity of the critically ill patient at all times.

Oral hygiene

Most seriously ill patients will encounter oral problems, some specific to the disease and others associated with the medication. There is, for example, an increased risk of mouth ulcers, dry, cracked oral mucosa or yeast growth in those with diabetes mellitus, acute or chronic breathing difficulties and thyroid dysfunction.

Furthermore, with the use of certain antibiotics, diuretics or morphine and procedures such as intermittent suction, the potential for oral hygiene problems is heightened. Knowledge of the factors which contribute to poor oral health is important in order to maintain hygiene (Thurgood 1994) (see Ch. 15 for further detail on oral hygiene).

Eye care

Eye care is a very necessary procedure for those patients who are unconscious, paralysed or sedated, who lack a blink reflex, have an inability to close their eyes or who experience dry eyes. Eye care facilitates maintenance of healthy eyes, comfort and the prevention of infection (Lloyd 1990).

Effective eye care is vital to prevent particular ocular complications such as:

- exposure keratopathy — incomplete closure of the eyelid
- dry eyes
- infection, e.g. conjunctivitis
- 'ventilator eye' (oedematous eyes); for explanation, see below
- corneal ulcerations.

(Ch. 13 discusses the disorders of the eye in depth.)

The critically ill patient is more susceptible than most patients to developing ocular problems, for the following reasons:

- Mechanical ventilation leads to the retention of body fluid, which in turn leads to increased venous pressure, producing oedematous eyes, often referred to as 'ventilator eye' (Lloyd 1990).
- Medication used during intubation can lead to raised intraocular pressure, predisposing the patient to ocular damage.
- Paralysing and sedating agents prevent patients from carrying out important physiological eye protection mechanisms. The blink mechanism is diminished, whereby tears are no longer effectively dispersed over the eye, if indeed they are produced at all. Tear production and dispersion are important in the prevention of infection and the maintenance of the structural integrity of the eye. In addition, those patients being ventilated artificially are at risk of eye infections arising from poor ET suctioning procedures, whereby cross-contamination from droplets sprayed out of the ET tube during suction can occur.
- The side-effects of some drug therapies are known to contribute to dry eyes, including atropine, antihistamines and tricyclic antidepressants.
- The patient who is critically ill will often be immunocompromised and thus more susceptible to infection. As with all procedures pertaining to patient care, strict and thorough handwashing must be maintained.

Maintaining skin integrity and promoting wound healing

A sound knowledge of the factors involved in successful wound healing and those that adversely affect its progress are necessary (see Ch. 23). The main types of wound encountered in the ICU are surgical wounds (see Chs 23 and 26), traumatic wounds and pressure ulcers (Chs 23 and 30).

For further reading on the effect of septic shock upon wound healing, see James (2001).

Pressure ulcers

Prevention is always better than cure and this is certainly the case when it comes to pressure ulcers. However, with the critically ill patient, the main priority is ultimately to maintain haemodynamic stability and optimise ventilation, and in some cases this may be jeopardised by turning or rolling the patient. Therapeutic beds are regularly required for the maintenance of skin integrity. Recent years have witnessed many developments in the design of specialised beds, from temperature regulatory devices to beds specifically for cardiac or respiratory patients providing rotation and percussion, as well as devices to assist with the movement of patients and the nursing of patients in the prone position.

There is also a risk of tissue damage due to pressure from equipment, such as an ET tube pressing on the lip, a tightly taped three-way tap or tube pressing on the skin, or even an overinflated tube cuff, which has been shown to cause necrosis through the tracheal wall to the oesophagus.

Pressure ulcers may delay recovery, pose increased infection risks and entail much discomfort for the patient. Assessment of the patient's risk of developing a pressure ulcer should be undertaken daily using a standardised tool such as the Waterlow pressure sore prevention/treatment policy (see p. 851).

Promoting and maintaining normal tone, power and movement of the musculoskeletal system

As well as regularly positioning the patient to optimise air entry, ventilation and maintain skin integrity, passive and active exercises should be carried out. In patients who have limited movement or who are unable to move at all, a regimen of passive movements can be implemented which will progress to active/assisted movements as the patient's condition improves. This can counteract effects of bed rest, e.g. deep venous thrombosis (DVT), contractures and foot drop.

MEETING THE PSYCHOSOCIAL, CULTURAL AND SPIRITUAL NEEDS OF THE CRITICALLY ILL PATIENT

PSYCHOSOCIAL NEEDS

Anyone who becomes critically ill is first and foremost a person; 'patient' is only one of their current subsidiary roles in life. It is sometimes difficult to remember this when immersed in life-saving procedures on the body of someone unknown.

Critical illness may be caused by trauma, infection or other pathophysiological state, possibly complicated, at least initially, by major surgery, and may affect any, or all, of the body systems and vital organs. Malfunction of one organ or system is likely to affect others and progress to multiple organ failure. Patients may be fully conscious and able to talk and move, or totally unconscious and/or paralysed. Each person has a unique combination of age, gender, personality, ethnic origin, social and cultural background, general health and other experiences, which may result in different physical and psychological responses (Clark 1987).

Nursing priorities and management

Goal: to support the patient psychologically, interacting in order to minimise the stress of the ICU environment.

Plan:

- provide adequate information, reassurance and encouragement
- prevent sensory overload or sensory deprivation
- maintain natural biorhythms/sleep patterns.

Providing adequate information, reassurance and encouragement

Nichols (1993) identified informational care, emotional care and counselling as the essential components of good psychological care in illness. All are dependent on optimal communication. Similarly, 'reassurance' and 'encouragement' are often identified as important to nursing, particularly in intensive care, but they are often not defined in practical terms. The difficulties of communicating with intubated patients and the theoretical reasons why communication is essential have long been known, e.g. Ashworth (1980). Good communication may enable patients to see monitoring equipment as helpful rather than frightening, even if they do not always remember being told about it. Support for each patient is most likely to be optimised when nurses, visitors and the patient collaborate to achieve effective and sensitive communication.

For further reading on maintaining confidentiality and information giving, see Lissemann (2000).

Preventing sensory overload/sensory deprivation

The sensory environment of an ICU is abnormal, compared with the environment in which people usually live, and can be disturbing even to those who are healthy. The sounds of ventilators, tracheal aspiration, equipment warning signals, the movement of trolleys and the like all combine to provide an auditory environment which may both bewilder and provoke anxiety. Patients may also experience other unusual stimuli, such as bright lights and strange equipment, and sensations of heat or cold, of being handled by other people, and of being attached to tubes and wires. There may also be a fear of falling out of bed during a change of position while paralysed, discomfort from tapes holding the ET tube in situ, and pain. Sometimes there is a lack of body privacy and a sense of humiliation. Boredom, powerlessness and fear that essential machinery might fail are commonly reported (Offord 1998, Bemun et al 2003).

Critically ill patients may suffer sensory overload or sensory deprivation, or a combination of both. Many years ago, Goldberger (1966) identified five areas of investigation related to sensory alteration which bear mention here:

- reduction of stimulus input variables — an absolute reduction in the variety and intensity of stimuli
- reduction of stimulus variability — the quantity of stimuli is the same but there is reduced patterning, imposed structuring and homogeneous stimulation. When light is diffuse, sound is muffled and body sensations are non-distinct and difficult to interpret; this is referred to as perceptual deprivation
- social deprivation — isolation from people and familiar environment
- confinement — immobilisation or restriction of movement
- increased sensory input — input via a number of senses at greater intensity than normal.

All of these can be found in individual or collected accounts of the experience of critically ill patients, as can accounts of nightmare auditory and visual hallucinations, delusions and paranoid feelings about staff and the environment (Heath 1989).

Patients may also experience depersonalisation, disturbed body image and extension of body boundaries, so that they regard machinery such as the ventilator as part of themselves (Smith 1989). One factor which is important in determining a patient's responses to a critical care environment is the nature of the human environment. Psychological as well as physical stimuli can be stressful and cause physiological reactions that may be harmful to critically ill patients. Such stimuli may result from deficiencies in the human environment. Nurses are an important part of the sensory and human environment of patients, and vice versa. Nurses affect the internal environment and responses of patients, and are in turn affected by them (Ashworth 1980). Many ex-patients say that a caring staff member, usually a nurse, who they trusted, was essential to their confidence and sense of security.

For further reading on nurses' experiences of assessing and dealing with patients' psychological needs, see Price (2004).

Psychological and behavioural problems

Mental health problems in the ICU can be divided into three categories:

- organic brain disorder, e.g. dementia, delirium
- psychological reaction to illness, i.e. depressive illness
- previous mental illness.

Delirium is common among critically ill patients within the general ICU setting; postanaesthetic states, hypoxia, systemic infections, drug intoxication, alcohol withdrawal and metabolic derangement also contribute to states of delirium. Symptoms vary considerably and, prior to medical intervention, the patient should be assessed clinically, establishing haemodynamic stability and, where possible, the probable cause of delirium (Roberts 2001).

Haloperidol is usually the medication of choice but should not be given before first assessing the patient's vital signs, clinical condition and the underlying cause of their behaviour.

Maintaining natural biorhythms/sleep

Human beings have biological or circadian rhythms that are normally related to the sleep/wake cycle, including fluctuations in body temperature, blood pressure, heart rate and plasma levels of various hormones (see Ch. 25).

In ICUs, there is always a concern that activity and lighting may be more or less constant because of the need for constant observation and frequent treatment, leading to lack of sleep for patients and disturbance of their biological rhythms, and also contributing to the sensory–perceptual alterations and delirium known to affect a considerable proportion of critically ill people. Diminishing the amount of light, noise and disturbance as far as possible at night can help to minimise such potential problems. It is clear that nursing requires the application of sound knowledge, judgement and skill. Practice must be sensitive, relevant and responsive to the needs of the individual and nowhere more so than when preventing sleep deprivation.

CULTURAL NEEDS AND SPIRITUAL CARE

Nursing priorities and management

Goal: to meet the spiritual and cultural needs of the patient and family.

Plan: ensure that the spiritual beliefs of the patient and family are upheld.

Spiritual health relates to having a sense of meaning, hope and purpose in life, not simply to having a religious faith. Cultural and personal values are relevant to purpose in life and should be considered in assessment and care.

Some critically ill patients lose hope and 'give up', ceasing to fight for life, particularly when ill for days or weeks, and this can contribute not only to their current physical and emotional experience but also to the outcome of the illness. Anything a nurse can do, either directly or with the help of the patient's family or friends, to help the patient draw on their usual resources and sources of support must be helpful (Hupcey 2001). Helping people to continue the practices important to them in life can enable them to do so, and there are a variety of ways of doing this. Many former patients have indicated that faith can be an important part of a person's life and a comfort in a crisis (Ashworth 1987).

The role of family and friends

Family and friends play an important role in relieving social isolation, depersonalisation and disorientation for patients. Yet family and friends are unable to be of maximum help to patients unless they themselves are assured of any necessary help from the nurses in the form of access, information and emotional support. Nurses have a great influence on the extent to which family and friends can support the sick patient during intensive care, after transfer to a ward and then home. Some of the major expressed needs that have been identified from a number of studies are the need to reduce anxiety, the need for information, the need to be near the patient and the need to be helpful.

For further reading on the needs of family members of ICU patients, see Wilkinson (1995).

SUMMARY

Care of the critically ill patient is a diverse and ever-expanding field, as medicine and technology collaborate to support patients through life-threatening situations. It is often viewed only as a highly technical arena. However, the same general principles of care apply, be it in an ICU, a general hospital ward or the community setting. To be effective, nurses must have a sound knowledge and understanding of physiology and other sciences, of how the body works in health as well as in illness; of technical equipment and its functions and of how people behave in, and respond to, health and illness. The expertise, however, is to be able to use this knowledge to generate competent skills and the judgement necessary to achieve the best possible outcomes for patients and their families.

This chapter has only touched on some of the fundamental concerns surrounding the nursing care of the critically ill patient. It has to be said that, as medicine strides forward to maintain life in increasingly fragile states, it does indeed create its own ethical dilemmas, and while it is not possible to cover these issues in this chapter, it is important to consider the ethical implications that critical care nursing may encounter.

REFERENCES

Arbour R 2000 Sedation and pain management in critically ill adults. Critical Care Nurse 20(5): 39–56

Ashworth P 1980 Care to communicate. Scutari, Harrow

Ashworth P 1987 The needs of the critically ill patient. Intensive Care Nursing 3(4): 182–190

Ashworth P 1990 High technology and humanity in intensive care. Intensive Care Nursing 6(3): 150–160

Ball C, Adam J, Boyce S, Robinson P 1999 Clinical guidelines for the use of the prone position in ARDS. Intensive and Critical Care Nursing 17: 94–104

Beaumont T 1998 How to guides: Humidification and filtration. Intensive and Critical Care Nursing 14(3):

Bemun I, Wright M, Ingram D, Ley A 2003 An investigation of patients' memories in intensive care. Care of the Critically Ill 19(2): 49

Berston A D, Soni N (eds) 2003 Oh's intensive care manual, 5th edn. Butterworth-Heinemann, Edinburgh

Bion J F, Oh T E 2003 Sedation in intensive care. In: Berston A D, Soni N (eds) Oh's intensive care manual, 5th edn. Butterworth-Heinemann, Edinburgh

Bradley C 2001a Drug therapy review: erythromycin as a gastrointestinal prokinetic agent. Intensive and Critical Care Nursing 17(2): 117–119

Bradley C 2001b Drug therapy review: stress ulcer prevention – the controversy continues. Intensive and Critical Care Nursing 17: 58–59

Bradley C 2002 Drug therapy review: insulin therapy in critically ill patients. Intensive and Critical Care Nursing 18(2): 128–129

Bridges E J 2000 Monitoring pulmonary artery pressures: just the facts. Critical Care Nurse 20(6): 59–78

Buckley P M, McFie J 1997 Enteral nutrition in critically ill patients: a review. Care of the Critically Ill 13(1): 7–10

Chatfield D, Rees-Pedlar S 2001 Jugular venous oxygen saturation: is it relevant to the nurse? Nursing in Critical Care 6(4): 187–191

Clark S 1987 Nursing diagnosis: ineffective coping. I. A theoretical framework: II. Planning care. Heart and Lung 16(6): 670–685

Cohen A, Kelly D R 1987 Assessment of alfentanil by intravenous infusion as long-term sedation in intensive care. Anaesthesia 42: 545–548

Coombs M 1993 Haemodynamic profiles and the critical care nurse. Intensive and Critical Care Nursing 9: 11–16

Cox C L, McGrath A 1999 Respiratory assessment in critical care units. Intensive and Critical Care Nursing 15: 226–234

Crocker C 2002 Nurse led weaning from ventilatory and respiratory support. Intensive and Critical Care Nursing 18(5): 272–279

Day T, Farnell S, Wilson-Barnett J 2002 Suctioning: a review of current research recommendations. Intensive and Critical Care Nursing 18(2): 79–89

Edwards S 1998 Determining hypervolaemia using trans-oesophageal Doppler monitoring. Nursing in Critical Care 3(4): 176–181

Forni L G, Hilton P J 1997 Continuous hemofiltration in the treatment of acute renal failure. New England Journal of Medicine 336(18): 1303–1309
Frakes M A 2001 Measuring $ETCO_2$: clinical applications and usefulness. Critical Care Nurse 21(5): 23–35
Goldberger L 1966 Experimental isolation: an overview. American Journal of Psychiatry 122: 774–782
Goldhill D R, Withington P S 1997 Textbook of intensive care. Chapman and Hall, London
Gosheron M, Leaver G, Forster A, Harnsworth A 1998 Prone lying – a nursing perspective. Intensive and Critical Care Nursing 14(3): 89–92
Hawker F H 1996 Intensive care management of fulminant hepatic failure. In: Dellinger R P, Burchardi H, Dobbs G J, Bion J (eds) Current topics in intensive care, No. 3. WB Saunders, London, Ch. 9
Heath J V 1989 What the patients say. Intensive Care Nursing 5(3): 101–108
Henke K, Eigsti J 2003 Renal physiology: review and practical application in the critically ill patient. Dimensions of Critical Care Nursing 22(3): 125–133
Hillman K, Bishop G 1996 Clinical intensive care. Cambridge University Press, Melbourne
Hinds C J, Watson D 1996 Intensive care: a concise textbook. WB Saunders, London
Hormann C, Baum M, Putensen C, Mutz N J, Benzer H 1994 Biphasic positive airway pressure (BIPAP) – a new mode of ventilatory support. European Journal of Anaesthesiology 11: 37–42
Hupcey J 2001 The meaning of social support for the critically ill patient. Intensive and Critical Care Nursing 17(4): 206–212
Ismail-Zade I, Oduro-Dominah A 1997 Nitric oxide: update on basic science and clinical implications. Intensive and Critical Care Nursing 13(4): 130–134
Juniper M 1999 Ventilation associated pneumonia: risk factors, diagnosis and management. Care of the Critically Ill 15(6): 198–201
Juniper M C, Garrard C S 1997 The chest X-ray in intensive care. Care of the Critically Ill 13(5): 198–200
Karnik A, Freeman J 1998 Acute liver failure. Care of the Critically Ill 14(5): 148–154
Kishen R 2002 Managing acute renal failure in the critically ill: where are we today? Care of the Critically Ill 18(6): 170–171
Leary T, Fletcher S, Fellows I 2000a Enteral nutrition – Part 1: Its use early and often. Care of the Critically Ill 16(1): 22–26
Leary T, Fletcher S, Fellows I 2000b Enteral nutrition – Part 2: Its use early and often. Care of the Critically Ill 16(2): 50–52
Lloyd F 1990 Eye care for ventilated or unconscious patients. Nursing Times 86: 36–37
Maitnel S K, Blackburn G L 2003 Feeding the critically ill patient. Journal of Parenteral and Enteral Nutrition 27(5): 383–384
Martensson I E, Fridlund B 2002 Factors influencing the patient during weaning from mechanical ventilation: a national survey. Intensive and Critical Care Nursing 18(4): 219–229
Nichols K 1993 Psychological care in the physical illness, 2nd edn. Chapman and Hall, London
Odell M, Forster A, Rudman K, Bass F 2002 The critical care outreach service and the early warning system on surgical wards. Nursing in Critical Care 7(3): 132–135
Offord R J 1998 Patients' experiences of being critically ill or severely injured and cared for in an intensive care unit in relation to the ICU syndrome. Intensive and Critical Care Nursing 14(6): 294–307
Oudemans-van Straaten H M 2003 Measures to promote motility of the gut with special attention to the colon. Care of the Critically Ill 19(1): 2–3
Powroznyk A V V, Latimer R D 1997 Progress in monitoring and delivery of inspired nitric oxide therapy. British Journal of Intensive Care 7(4): 149–154
Price T, Miller L, deScossa M 2000 The Glasgow coma scale in intensive care: a study. Nursing in Critical Care 5(4): 170–173
Rippe J M, Irwin R S, Fink M P, Cerra F B, Curley F J, Heard S O (eds) 1995 Procedures and techniques in intensive care medicine. Little Brown, New York
Roberts B L 2001 Managing delirium in adult intensive care patients. Critical Care Nurse 21(1): 48–55
Robson W P 1998 To bag or not to bag. Manual hyperinflation in intensive care. Intensive and Critical Care Nursing 14(1): 239–243
Roper N, Logan W, Tierney A J 1996 The elements of nursing: a model of nursing, based on a model of living, 4th edn. Churchill Livingstone, Edinburgh
Shelley M P 1998 Sedation in the ITU. Intensive and Critical Care Nursing 14(3): 85–88
Singer M, Carr C 1996 Early enteral feeding: benefits and mechanisms. In: Dellinger R P, Burchardi H, Dobbs G D, Bion J (eds) Current topics in intensive care, No. 3. WB Saunders, London, Ch. 6
Smith S 1989 Extended body image in the ventilated patient. Intensive Care Nursing 5(1): 31–38
Spiby J 1989 Intensive care in the UK: report from the King's Fund panel. Anaesthesia 44: 428–431
Stange J, Hassanein T I, Mehta R, Mitzner S R, Bartlett R H 2002 Molecular adsorbents recycling system as a liver support system based on albumin dialysis: a summary of preclinical investigations, prospective, randomized, controlled clinical trials and clinical experience from 19 centers. Artificial Organs 26(2): 103–110
Stanley I R, Hancox D 2001 Initial management of severe head injuries: is cerebral perfusion pressure maintained? Care of the Critically Ill 17(5): 166–167
Thomas C 1997 Use of the prone position: the ventilation/perfusion relationship in ARDS. Intensive and Critical Care Nursing 13(3): 95–100
Thurgood G 1994 Nurse maintenance of oral hygiene. British Journal of Nursing 3(7): 332–353
Tucker S, Dexter T 2003 Stress ulcer prophylaxis in the ITU. Care of the Critically Ill 19(2): 46–48
Urwin S, Fletcher S 2000 Haemofiltration I. Care of the Critically Ill 16(6): 205–208
Urwin S, Leary T S, Fletcher S 2001 Haemofiltration II. Care of the Critically Ill 17(3): 99–104
Van den Berghe G, Wouters P, Weekers F et al 2001 Intensive insulin therapy in critically ill patients. New England Journal of Medicine 345(19): 1359–1367
Verity S 1996 Nutrition and its importance to intensive care patients. Intensive and Critical Care Nursing 12(2): 71–78
Weilitz P B 1993 Weaning a patient from mechanical ventilation. Critical Care Nurse 13(4): 33–40
Wood C 1998 Endotracheal suctioning: a literature review. Intensive and Critical Care Nursing 14(1): 124–136
Woodrow P 1993 Resource package: haemofiltration. Intensive and Critical Care Nursing 9: 95–107
Woodrow P 1997 Nitric oxide: some nursing implications. Intensive and Critical Care Nursing 13: 87–92
Woodrow P 2000 Will nursing ICU patients in the semi-recumbent position reduce rates of nosocomial infection? Nursing in Critical Care 5(4): 174–178
Woodrow P 2001 Intensive care nursing. Routledge, London

FURTHER READING

Dougherty L, Lister S 2004 The Royal Marsden Hospital manual of clinical nursing procedures, 6th edn. Blackwell Publishing, Oxford (www.blackwellroyalmarsden.com)
Hinds C J, Watson D 1996 Intensive care: a concise handbook, 2nd edn. WB Saunders, London
Hunter J D 2002 Rhabdomyolysis. Care of the Critically Ill 18(2): 52–54
James C 2001 A case study on the influence of septic shock upon wound healing. Nursing in Critical Care 6(5): 93–100
Jones J 1995 Ethical dilemmas in intensive care: a case history. Intensive and Critical Care Nursing 11(1): 32–35
Kress J P, Pohlman A S, O'Connor M F, Hall J B 2000 Daily interruption of sedative infusions in critically ill patients. New England Journal of Medicine 343(11): 814–815
Kress J P, Pohlman A S, Hall J B 2002 Sedation and analgesia in the intensive care unit. American Journal of Respiratory and Critical Care Medicine 166(8): 1024–1028
Leighton H 1995 Paracetamol poisoning: a case study. Intensive and Critical Care Nursing 11(6): 280–282
Lissemann I 2000 Maintaining confidentiality and information giving in intensive care. Nursing in Critical Care 5(4): 187–193
Manji M, Bion J 1997 Transporting the critically ill patient. In: Goldhill D R, Withington P S (eds) Textbook of intensive care. Chapman and Hall Medical, London, Ch. 6
McGowan J 1999 Management of

hypothermia in adults. Nursing in Critical Care 4(2): 59–62
McMahon K 1995 Multiple organ failure: the final complication of critical illness. Critical Care Nursing 15(6): 20–28
McMahon-Parkes F, Cornock M 1997 Guillain–Barré syndrome: biological basis, treatment and care. Critical Care Nursing 13(1): 42–48
Mulnier C, Evans T 1995 Acute respiratory distress in adults (ARDS). Care of the Critically Ill 11(5): 182–186
Pace N, McLean S A 1996 Ethics and the law in intensive care. Oxford University Press, Oxford
Price A M 2004 Intensive care nurses' experiences of assessing and dealing with patients' psychological needs. Nursing in Critical Care 9(3): 134–142
Ridley S 2002 Functional outcome after critical illness. Care of the Critically Ill 18(2): 44–47
Robb Y A 1997 Have nursing models a place in intensive care units? Intensive and Critical Care Nursing 13: 93–98
Somerville G, Wilkinson D 1997 How to guides: temperature maintenance. Care of the Critically Ill 13(2):
Sutcliffe A 2001 Hypothermia (or not) for the management of head injury. Care of the Critically Ill 17(5): 162–165
van der Hulst R R W J, Van der Kreel B K, von Meyenfeldt M F et al 1993 Glutamine and the preservation of gut integrity. Lancet 341: 1363–1365
Waterlow J A 1995 Pressure sores and their management. Care of the Critically Ill 11(3): 121–125
White P 2001 'Just going to give you a little cough': reflection on performing endotracheal suction in one intensive care patient. Nursing in Critical Care 6(2): 83–87
Wilkinson P 1995 A qualitative study to establish the self perceived needs of the family members of patients in a general intensive care unit. Intensive and Critical Care Nursing 11(1): 77–86

THE PATIENT WITH BURNS

Breeda McCahill

30

INTRODUCTION

Imagine for a moment having lost everything: your loved ones; your home and possessions, including mementoes from the past; your health and ability to function normally; your appearance — in other words, yourself. This not infrequently occurs when people are victims of a house fire.

Most people are burned more than once in their lifetime but few have any conception of the horror associated with severe burns injury. Extensive burns injury is catastrophic, both physically and psychologically, for the patient and their family. It is also one of the most challenging and arduous types of injury to treat. In order to help the patient and their family to achieve optimum function, the responsibility of care must be distributed throughout the multidisciplinary team. However, the nurse, being the only professional in 24-h attendance, will play an especially important role. Nurses also attend to many patients whose burns are not extensive, providing care in the community, in emergency departments (ED) and in general surgical wards. This chapter aims to provide information which will help the nurse care for patients with burn injuries in any of these settings.

PREVENTION OF BURN INJURIES

Burns are frequently described in the literature as being among the most serious of injuries because of the long-term problems which are often associated with them. Advances in treatment and improved facilities have led to a reduction in mortality rates, but the morbidity resulting from burns is such that prevention must be viewed as the responsibility of all health care personnel.

One of the main aims identified in the constitution of the International Society for Burn Injuries (ISBI 1979) is 'to disseminate knowledge and to stimulate prevention in the field of burns'. Many studies have since emphasised that, in order to be effective, burn prevention programmes should involve assessment of the incidence of burn injuries, followed by planning, implementation and evaluation of appropriate interventions (Liao & Rossignol 2000).

Assessment

This includes identifying the extent of the problem, its causative agents and any predisposing factors.

The extent of the problem

Department of Trade and Industry data (1999) revealed that, in the UK, 112 000 people attend emergency departments annually suffering from the effects of burn injuries, with a further 250 000 presenting at GP services; approximately 7765 people require hospital admission and 211 people die each year as a result of burn injury. However, due to advances in treatment, burn mortality rates have fallen over the last two decades (Pereira et al 2004). Although statistical data on burn mortality are generally available, the incidence of burn morbidity is difficult to estimate. Van Loey et al (2001) identify the problem as being substantial in terms of the ensuing psychological and physical difficulties experienced by the patient.

Causative agents

Studies report that either scalds or flame burns are the most common type of burn injury. Contact burns (from touching hot objects) also have a high incidence. Chemical and electrical burns occur less frequently.

The Office of the Deputy Prime Minister (2003), which is responsible for collating fire statistics, identifies the most common cause of death in domestic fires as careless handling of fire and hot substances, mainly smokers' materials. Non-fatal burn casualties result from the misuse of equipment or appliances, most commonly cooking appliances (see Case History 30.1). In the case of scalds, the electric kettle is recognised as a major cause of injury, usually in children of pre-school age (Sheller & Thuesen 1998). Hot water in plumbing systems is also a considerable cause for concern in countries where there is no legislation governing the upper limit of plumbed water temperature. Although many authorities advocate a temperature of 50°C (which would take 2–3 min to cause a burn), because of altered sensation and reduced mobility in older people, this figure has been reduced to 43°C in residential accommodation for older people (Stone et al 2000) (see Box 30.1 for advice on reducing the risk of scalds).

Predisposing factors

Epidemiological studies identify toddlers as being at greatest risk of burn injuries, with scalds accounting for most of these. Adult high-risk groups include those with epilepsy (Josty et al 2000) and those who smoke tobacco, drink alcohol in excess and take prescribed psychotropic medications (Duggan & Quine 1995) (see Case History 30.2). Haum et al (1995) found that patients with positive blood alcohol levels had a significantly higher fatality rate than those with negative blood alcohol levels. Older people have also been identified as being more susceptible to burn injury and as having a higher mortality rate following injury (Sarhadi et al 1995). Studies agree that males of all ages are at higher risk than females.

The common denominator of predisposition to burn injury appears to be a combination of reduced awareness of danger and decreased mobility.

CASE HISTORY 30.1

Ms C

Ms C, aged 24, returned home after a night out with her friends and, feeling hungry, decided to have some chips. She put the chip pan on the stove, leaving the fat to heat whilst she got ready for bed. Smelling smoke, she rushed back to the kitchen to find the saucepan in flames. In her panic she tried to douse the flames by smothering them with a dry towel, which promptly caught fire. She then remembered to put the lid on the saucepan and turn off the stove. Her screams alerted the neighbours, who phoned for an ambulance. Ms C was rushed to the nearest casualty department, where, on examination, she was found to have a total of 8%, mainly superficial, burns to her hands, forearms, chest and face.

Box 30.1

Reducing the risk of scalds

- Water does not have to be close to boiling point to cause severe injury.
- A cup of freshly made tea or instant coffee takes 20 min to reach a temperature which will not damage the skin and 15 min if milk is added (Mercer 1988). The same study found that the contents of a newly boiled kettle containing 1.5 L of water will take 1 h to reach a safe temperature.
- Water at a temperature of 66°C will cause a full-thickness scald after 2 s contact and, at 60°C, after 6 s (Moritz & Henriques 1947). Walker (1990) and Adams et al (1991) advocate the reduction of plumbed hot water temperatures to 50–55°C, and to 43°C in residential accommodation for older people (Stone et al 2000).
- Setting the hot water thermostat to a lower temperature will help to reduce fuel bills.

CASE HISTORY 30.2

Mr M

Mr M, aged 47, regularly abused alcohol and was a heavy smoker. One evening, after a bout of heavy drinking, he fell asleep, dropping his cigarette onto the horsehair sofa on which he was resting. The material smouldered, but did not immediately burst into flames or produce toxic fumes. Mr M was lying on his left side with his right hand resting on the sofa. He was eventually found by his brother, who dragged him off the sofa, extinguished the flames and called for an ambulance. On admission to the burns unit, Mr M was found to have sustained full-thickness burns to the left side of the face and chest. There was no circulation through his left hand and arm (which required above-elbow amputation) and the fingers of his right hand were burned down to the bone. The total body surface involved was estimated at 20%.

Planning and implementation

Planning for a burns prevention programme must be realistic. While it is impossible to modify certain risk factors, e.g. gender and age, having identified the groups most at risk, it should be possible to alter some of the related predisposing factors.

In the past, burn prevention programmes were based on education of the public, but recent studies indicate that, on its own, this is not an effective method.

McLoughlin (1995) recommended the use of the 'public health model' which considers three factors: the host or person at risk, the agent and the environment. With regard to the host, Adams et al (1991) found that recognition of potential danger did not alter the behaviour of adult high-risk groups. There are already numerous health education campaigns aimed at persuading the public not to smoke and to drink alcohol in moderation. It seems unlikely that those who do not comply would be influenced by the knowledge that smoking and drinking increase their risk of burn injuries. Tones and Tilford (2001) point out that, unlike the promotion of commercial products, which is based on enhancing pleasure, promising immediate gratification, health promotion usually urges people to stop doing something which they find pleasurable in the hope of long-term benefit. They also state that the public have a right not to be unreasonably frightened. Blatant shock tactics are therefore considered unacceptable and are likely to make people 'switch off'. More subtle, but potentially potent, messages may be conveyed, e.g. by incidental reference in popular television series.

Identification of the burn agent or energy source results from epidemiology studies. The agent may be a result of poor design of equipment, such as the hot water jug which has a higher centre of gravity than a kettle, or a stove or radiator which produces a high surface temperature. Once the problem has been recognised, modification of design may be sufficient to eradicate the danger.

Product modification may be carried out voluntarily by manufacturers; however, legislation is often required. Since 1990, it has been against the law to sell new or re-upholstered soft furnishings which are padded with foam that is not combustion-modified or which are covered with fabric that does not resist ignition tests for both smouldering cigarettes and match-like flames. Currently, cigarettes contain an additive which allows them to smoulder for 28 min, and in many developed countries there is interest in introducing a regulation to reduce the ignition propensity of cigarettes (Harper & Dickson 1995, McLoughlin 1995).

Previous legislation and regulations include the prohibition of the sale of highly flammable children's nightwear and the requirement that all new gas or electric fires and radiant oil-burning stoves are fitted with a fireguard which passes British Standards specifications.

With regard to the environment, probably the greatest single factor in reducing death and injury by fires in the home has been the introduction of smoke detectors/alarms. In North America, their installation into both new and established domestic properties is legally required. In the UK, legislation is more arbitrary and installation into established properties is voluntary. Because of their sensitivity, smoke detector alarms may be set off by cooking fumes, e.g. burning toast, and there have been numerous reports of people consequently removing the batteries from smoke detectors from properties where they have been installed. Some detectors have a temporary 'silence' button which may solve the problem of false alarms; however, as the ceiling is the recommended site for mounting, the detector may be out of easy reach.

It must be recognised that the groups at highest risk of injury from burns, i.e. older or disabled people, may be less able than others to buy the new, safer soft furnishings and heating appliances. Smoke detectors may be bought for as little as £5, but their fitting, although simple for the able-bodied, may be impossible for older or disabled individuals.

Health care workers, therefore, not only have a responsibility to disseminate information on the prevention of burn injuries, but also must work closely with other interested groups such as the Fire Brigade, The Royal Society for the Prevention of Accidents (see 'Useful websites', p. 1027) and both local and national government offices in order to lobby for more effective legislation and regulations. Nurses working in the community have the opportunity to observe the environment and to give specific advice relating to burns prevention.

For further information on prevention and health promotion, see Ewles & Simnett (2003) and Sidell et al (2003).

FIRST AID TREATMENT OF BURNS

Burn injuries result from the transfer of energy from a source of heat to vulnerable tissues. The higher the temperature of the heat source and the longer it is in contact with the tissues, the greater will be the destruction.

The first priority of first aid treatment is to remove the individual from the source of heat. If the causative agent is electricity, it is important to switch off the supply, if possible, or to use non-conducting material to rescue the person.

Frequently, there is a continuing source of heat in the form of the individual's clothing, which may be on fire or saturated by a hot liquid. The most effective way to remove this continuing heat source is to throw cool liquid, which is neither flammable nor corrosive, over the affected material, thus dousing the flames or reducing the temperature of the scalding liquid. If no such cool liquid is immediately to hand, rapid removal of hot saturated clothing will arrest the heat transfer. Where clothing is on fire, it is important to stop the person running around as this will fan the flames. The person assisting should lie the victim on the ground and use heavy material such as a coat or blanket to smother the flames. If chemicals are the causative agent, prompt sluicing with copious amounts of water will dilute the strength of the agent and limit the penetration of the chemical into the skin, where it will continue to cause damage for many hours. Hojer et al (2002) demonstrate the advantage of taking this universal first aid measure rather than taking time searching for specific neutralising agents. In the clinical situation, a useful means of identifying whether a chemical is acid or alkaline is to apply a Multistix, normally used for urine testing, as this will give a pH reading.

Having taken steps to remove the heat source from the skin, the next measure is to cool the superheated tissues. The easiest means of doing this is to place the affected part in cold water. For the face, however, cold soaks should be applied. The application of ice or chilled water below 5°C is contraindicated, as Sawada et al (1997) found that this was associated with increased likelihood of tissue damage, possibly due to vasoconstriction. There is no doubt that continued cooling helps to reduce pain from the burn wound, but if a large area of the body surface is involved there is a risk of hypothermia.

Ellis and Rylah (1990) advised against using cold soaks or ice packs during the transfer of patients to hospital, especially if the journey was to take some time. For example, a 10-year-old girl sustained 12% burns on her back when her shirt-tail came into contact with a gas flame. Her brother, with whom she was playing, threw the contents of a jug of lemonade over the flames; then she was placed in a bath by her mother, who repeatedly scooped cold water over the burned area. She then wrapped her daughter in a clean sheet and took her to the local hospital. From there, the child was transferred to a specialist unit, a journey of more than 1 h. During the period of transfer she was lying prone on a stretcher lined with incontinence pads, absorbent surface up. The escorting nurse carried out the instructions, which were to continually irrigate the saline soaks which had been placed on the girl's back with cold saline from a cool-pack. When the patient arrived at the specialist unit, the rectal temperature was recorded at 34.8°C. Tsuei and Kearney (2004) have noted a high mortality rate related to trauma patients who have a core temperature of less than 35°C at the time of their admission to hospital. Fortunately, in the case described, the child survived. Patients with extensive burns clearly have problems in retaining body heat. The use of space blankets or other heat-retaining coverings is advised during the period of transfer.

Many burns units in the UK are now advising that the temporary wound dressing of choice is polyvinyl chloride film, e.g. clingfilm (Lawrence 1996a). The reasons for this are as follows:

- the film is sterile on the inner rolled surface
- it does not adhere to the wound surface and cause pain on removal
- it conforms closely to the body contours and excludes air, thus reducing pain
- a succession of personnel can view the wound without removal of the transparent film.

This kind of material is often available in the home but, if not, a clean cloth should be used as a temporary cover. The use of ointments, lotions and powders should be avoided as they may change the appearance of the wound and thus impair the assessment of the burn.

Practice and treatment room nurses often see people with severe sunburn that, unsuccessfully self-managed, has become infected. This can also happen with other types of burns, as in Case History 30.3.

To summarise, first aid treatment of burn injuries consists of:

- separating the individual from the source of injury
- immersion of the affected part in cold water for 10 min or application of cold soaks to the face
- application of polyvinyl chloride (cling) film or a clean cloth to the wound; cold soaks may be used for wounds which are not extensive.

ASSESSING THE SEVERITY OF BURN INJURIES

The majority of patients with burn injuries do not require hospital inpatient care. The UK National Burn Injury Referral Guidelines (2001) recommend that when deciding whether to refer patients to a burn unit, consideration should be given to the complexity of the burn injury rather than simply to the size of the burn wound. The categories of patients for whom admission or referral to a regional burns unit is advisable include:

- those under 5 years or over 60 years
- those whose burns exceed 5% of the body surface area
- those with burns on functionally important areas such as face, hands, feet, perineum, joints or flexor surfaces
- those with electrical or chemical burns
- those with infected wounds or evidence of infection
- those with small, full-thickness burns which would benefit from early excision and grafting
- those whose injury limits their capacity to care for themselves at home
- those with associated injuries, e.g. smoke inhalation, crush injuries, fractures
- those with other medical conditions, e.g. epilepsy, diabetes mellitus, cardiac limitation
- where there is doubt, either suspected non-accidental injury or uncertainty about the depth of the burn.

For patients who do not fall into any of these categories, relief of pain and local treatment of the burn wound are generally all that is required. Both interventions will be described later in the chapter (see p. 1022).

The UK guidelines also suggest that in the post-acute phase of burn injury, practice nurses and district nurses should refer patients whose burn has not healed within 14 days, as any resulting scarring may have significant impact on the subsequent physical and psychological rehabilitation of the patient.

Assessment of the severity of the burn injury involves estimation of:

- the extent of body surface area involved
- the depth of tissue damage
- the probability of associated respiratory tract injury.

Knowledge of the circumstances of the accident, e.g. whether electricity was involved, and information about the individual's general health and domestic situation will help in deciding whether the patient may, or may not, be managed by the primary health care team.

Extent of burn

Whenever body tissues are traumatised, the inflammatory response is stimulated, resulting in increased circulation to the area (hyperaemia) and increased movement of fluids from intravascular to interstitial compartments. If this occurs in a small area, i.e. over less than 5% of the body surface, the effects are localised. However, when a larger percentage of the body surface is injured, there is a massive shift of fluids into the tissues with a corresponding reduction in circulating volume. It is generally accepted that children with burns involving more than 10%, and adults with burns of more than 15%, of body surface area will suffer from hypovolaemic shock unless there is prompt intravenous replacement of fluid (see Ch. 18).

In order to estimate the percentage of body surface affected, the simplest and most easily remembered method is the long established 'rule of nines' introduced by Wallace

CASE HISTORY 30.3

Miss K

Miss K, aged 53, suffers from diabetes and lives alone. One morning she awoke to find that she had blistering on her left lower leg. She assumed this had been caused by contact with her hot water bottle. As there was no pain, she did not contact her doctor but dressed the burn herself, using an antiseptic cream and a bandage. A week later she attended the local health centre as the wound was now very inflamed and producing pus.

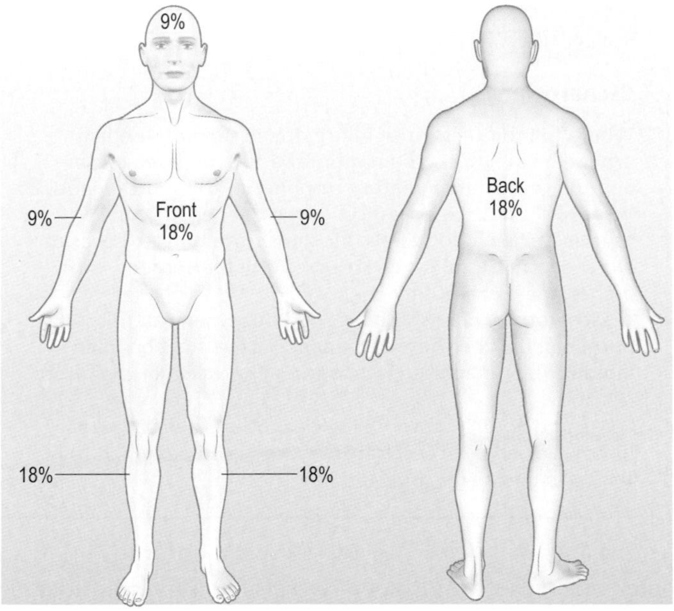

Fig. 30.1 Wallace's rule of nines.

in 1951 (see Fig. 30.1). In this method, the head and upper limbs each equal 9%, while the anterior trunk, the posterior trunk and the lower limbs each equal 18%. The remaining 1% is usually applied to the perineum. Another rapid approximation of the percentage can be made by using the palmar aspect of the patient's hand (with fingers together) as 1% of the body surface area.

The rule of nines should never be used for estimating burn percentage in young children as it does not allow for the different proportions of head and lower limbs in infants and toddlers. Under the age of 1 year the child's head equals 19% of the body surface area and the lower limbs are correspondingly smaller. A more accurate chart which allows for the changing proportions of different age groups and which shows percentages applicable to smaller, more specific areas of the body surface is the Lund and Browder (1944) burn chart (see Fig. 30.2). This is generally in use in specialist units and is available in EDs throughout the country.

Burn depth

The depth of a burn influences the rate at which the wound will heal spontaneously. The longer the wound takes to heal, the greater the probability of infection and the worse the scarring and loss of function (see Ch. 23). There are a number of methods of classifying burn depth. In the UK, the most popular is to differentiate between partial-thickness and full-thickness skin destruction. Partial-thickness burns involve the epidermis and part of the dermis. Full-thickness burns destroy the epidermis and all of the dermis. Full-thickness burns may also involve deeper structures such as fat, muscle and bone. Partial-thickness burns are classified as 'superficial' or 'deep', depending on the amount of dermis involved. As a general rule, deep partial-thickness and full-thickness burns require surgical enhancement of healing in the form of skin grafting.

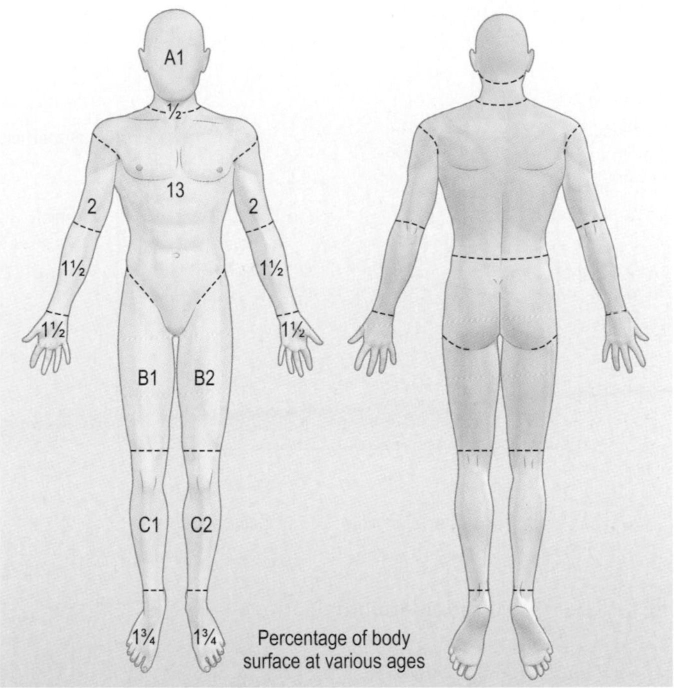

Percent of areas affected by growth

	0	1	5	10	15	Adult age
A = ½ head	9½	8½	6½	5½	4½	3½
B = ½ one thigh	2¾	3¼	4	4¼	4½	4¾
C = ½ one leg	2½	2½	2¾	3	3¼	3½

To estimate the total of the body surface area burned, the percentages assigned to the burned sections are added. The total is then an estimate of the burn size.

Fig. 30.2 The Lund and Browder burn chart.

As may be seen from Figure 30.3, the more superficial the injury, the greater the number of surviving epithelial sources from which cells will undergo mitosis and migrate across the wound surface; thus a more superficial burn heals more rapidly and causes less wound contraction. The effects of superficial partial-thickness burns and full-thickness burns are described below and in Table 30.1.

Superficial partial-thickness burns

These burns are very painful as the sensory nerve endings are stimulated by the injury or exposed to air. They are characterised by oedema, blister formation and serous exudate where the blisters burst. The blistering results from the increased permeability of the capillary walls, with fluid leaking into the interstitial spaces and from the wound surface. This fluid collects into blisters beneath the non-germinating layers of the epidermis. Heat radiates from the wound surface due to arteriolar dilatation and increased blood flow and as part of the inflammatory response. This also causes the typical bright pink appearance of the wound, which will blanch on pressure. On removal of the pressure the hyperaemia is restored.

Full-thickness burns

These burns are painless, as the sensory nerve endings have been destroyed. There is no blister formation and the

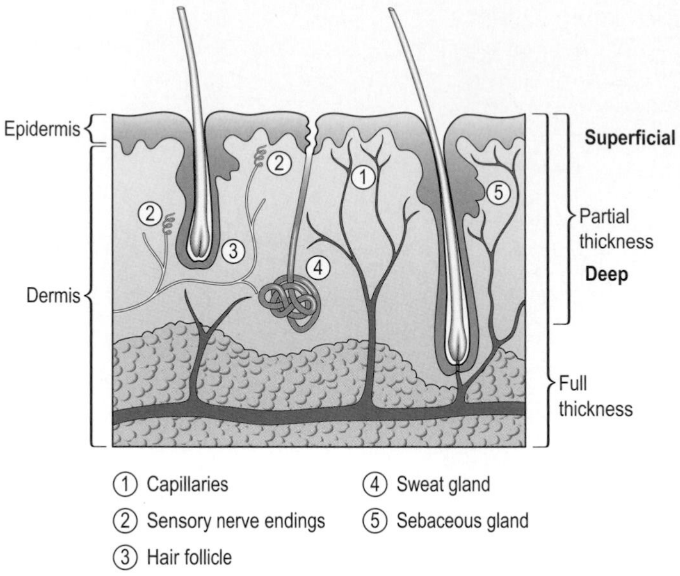

Fig. 30.3 Classification of burn depth.

wound surface is dry. There is no overt oedema, the wound surface is cool to the touch and the colour may be white, brown or bright red with no blanching on pressure. These characteristics are all due to the fact that there is no surviving circulation within the dermis. The brown or red colour is due to the release of haem pigments from destroyed red blood cells. The area may appear translucent with thrombosed vessels being apparent. It is important to recognise that there is an inflammatory response in the deeper tissues affected, but this is masked by overlying necrotic tissue. High temperatures (>60°C) cause coagulation of the tissue proteins and water is lost from the cells, interstitial spaces and blood vessels, resulting in a degree of contraction of the affected tissues. Destruction of the dermis renders the skin inelastic and the texture becomes firm and leathery. This destroyed tissue is known as eschar (see Box 30.2).

Box 30.2

Escharotomy

Where full-thickness burn injury occurs circumferentially around a limb, the combination of a firm inelastic eschar and the covert inflammatory response in the subcutaneous tissues will cause compression of the deeper structures, especially the blood vessels. Incisions through the eschar to allow decompression are carried out by the surgeon and are termed escharotomy.

Escharotomy may also be carried out when full-thickness burn injury of the chest and upper part of the abdomen inhibits rib or diaphragmatic movement, causing respiratory difficulty.

Nursing note. Monitoring of circulation to distal parts of limbs involved or of respiratory ease is required when full-thickness burns are suspected in either site.

Deep partial-thickness burns

As the depth of destruction in this type of burn is between those of superficial partial-thickness and full-thickness burns, the presenting signs and symptoms are between the extremes in sensation, blistering, temperature and colour.

Problems in assessment

The assessment of burn depth is not an exact science, although much work has been carried out to make it more so in recent years. The use of a hypodermic needle to test for

Table 30.1 Indications of burn depth

Depth	Signs and symptoms	Related anatomy/physiology
Superficial partial-thickness burns	Very painful	Sensory nerve endings in the dermis are stimulated by the injury and/or exposed to air
	Oedema, blister formation, serous exudate where blisters have burst	As a result of the inflammatory response, the capillary walls are more permeable and fluid leaks into the interstitial spaces of the dermis, collecting below the non-germinating layers of the epidermis or exuding from the wound surface
	Wound surface warmer than unburned skin	Also due to the inflammatory response; arteriolar dilatation causes increased blood flow
	Wound appears bright pink and blanches with pressure	Due to increased blood flow. Pressure greater than capillary blood pressure occludes the flow of blood
Full-thickness burns	Painless, no sensation	Sensory nerve endings in the dermis are destroyed
	Wound surface dry. No blistering	Cessation of blood flow through dermal capillaries
	No overt oedema	Necrosis of dermis renders it inelastic
	Wound surface cooler than unburned skin	Cessation of blood flow through dermal capillaries
	Wound colour may be white, brown, translucent showing thrombosed vessels, or bright red (does not blanch on pressure)	Cessation of blood flow through dermal capillaries. Brown or red appearance is caused by release of haem pigments from destroyed red blood cells

pinprick sensation was first described by Bull and Lennard-Jones (1949), and Settle (1996) admits that, although not an absolute test for viability, it is still useful. Pape et al (2001) found that laser Doppler imaging may be used successfully in aiding assessment of burn depth; however, this option is not readily available outwith specialist burn units. Frequently, assessment of burn depth is dependent on the visual characteristics of the wound, the information given regarding the circumstances of the accident, the agent involved and the first aid measures carried out.

Burn-associated respiratory tract injury

Inhibition of respiratory function may result from thermal injury to the skin of the trunk and neck. Covert oedema formation below the leathery, inelastic eschar of circumferential full-thickness burns causes pressure on the deeper structures. In deep burns of the neck, this may cause compression of the trachea and, if there is involvement of the chest and upper abdomen, will inhibit expansion of the thoracic cavity. Decompression by escharotomy will be required (see Box 30.2).

Inhalation of smoke and hot toxic gases is frequently associated with burn trauma. The potent synergistic effects of burns and smoke inhalation are noted by Beeley and Clark (1996), who state that for victims of smoke inhalation who are unburned and alive on arrival at hospital the mortality rate is low, whereas for those who are also burned the mortality rate associated with the extent of burn is substantially increased.

The main causes of inhalation injury are:

- intoxication and hypoxaemia
- thermal damage to the airways
- respiratory tract injury due to irritants.

Intoxication and hypoxaemia

Intoxication and hypoxaemia most commonly result from inhalation of carbon monoxide and/or hydrogen cyanide produced by burning plastics.

Carbon monoxide (CO), produced by the combustion of carbon and organic materials in a limited oxygen supply, has an affinity for haemoglobin many times that of oxygen. Therefore, following inhalation of CO there is displacement of oxygen on the haemoglobin molecules and the production of carboxyhaemoglobin (COHb) with resulting generalised hypoxia. The symptoms of CO poisoning are related to the concentration of the inspired gas and to COHb levels and are recognised as mild headache, dizziness, confusion, irritability, nausea, vomiting and fainting. At higher levels there will be convulsion, coma, respiratory failure and death. Diagnosis is suggested by the typical cherry pink appearance of the patient and confirmed by checking COHb levels. The formation of carboxyhaemoglobin can be reversed by the administration of high concentrations of oxygen.

Hydrogen cyanide is rapidly absorbed through the lungs and binds readily to the cytochrome system, inhibiting cell function and resulting in metabolic acidosis. It causes loss of consciousness, neurotoxicity and convulsions. However, over a period of time it is gradually metabolised by the liver enzyme rhodenase (Australia & New Zealand Burn Association Ltd (UK) 1996).

Thermal damage

The upper airway may be damaged by the inhalation of hot gases, hot vapours or combustible gas mixtures. Mucosal oedema will narrow the lumen of the airway. The diagnosis is suspected where there is a history of explosion, burns of the face, singed nasal hairs, erythema and ulceration of the oropharynx. Hoarseness and inspiratory stridor may present later. As signs of upper airway obstruction may take several hours to become apparent, constant supervision is required.

Hot, dry air seldom causes burns of the airway below the level of the epiglottis as the respiratory tract has an excellent heat exchange capability. Injury to the lower airway is most commonly caused by inhalation of toxic chemicals.

Inhalation of irritant chemicals

The combustion of various materials produces a wide spectrum of irritant chemicals, including chlorine, ammonia, formaldehyde and phosgene. The extent of the resultant damage to the respiratory system will be determined by the density of the smoke and the duration of exposure. Patients who are asleep or under the influence of drugs or alcohol at the time of the fire will tend to have a longer exposure time, as will those who have restricted mobility, e.g. older or disabled people.

When irritant chemicals bound to carbon particles settle on the respiratory endothelium, the following reactions occur:

- the inflammatory response — this causes increased secretions and narrowing of the lumen of the trachea, bronchi and bronchioles
- inflammation of the alveolar capillary membrane — this interferes with gaseous exchange, and capillary exudate will leak into the alveoli
- bronchospasm — this causes further narrowing of the lumen of the airway
- chemical denaturation of all protein, which leads to:
  - necrosis and ulceration of the epithelial tissue, with an increase in cellular debris
  - cessation of ciliary activity, inhibiting removal of secretions and cellular debris
- loss of surfactant production by type II alveolar cells.

Surfactant normally lowers the surface tension of the walls of the alveoli, thus preventing collapse, and also prevents the transudation of fluid from capillaries into the alveoli. Loss of surfactant production will therefore lead to atelectasis (see Ch. 3).

In summary, the pathophysiological results of the inhalation of irritant chemicals may include tracheobronchitis, pulmonary oedema, atelectasis and airway obstruction. These are frequently compounded by infection.

In cases where the patient survives long enough for admission to hospital, the respiratory damage related to inhalation of smoke may take several hours or even days to become manifest. Suspicion should be aroused where:

- the fire occurred within an enclosed space, especially at night
- there is a history of exposure to smoke, especially if the patient required bodily rescue
- the patient's breath and clothing smell of smoke

- there is inflammation of the conjunctivae
- carbon particles are present in clothing, wounds, nose, mouth and sputum.

Other injuries

The appearance of a patient with extensive burns may be so visually dramatic as to distract the assessor from checking for other, less obvious, injuries. Fractures, internal injuries and spinal cord damage may have been sustained, especially if the burn was a result of a road traffic accident, an explosion or high tension electricity, or if the patient jumped from a burning building.

THE PATIENT WITH EXTENSIVE BURNS

Early problems and nursing care

The patient with extensive burns has multiple problems, the relative urgency of which will vary during the perhaps very prolonged period following injury. There is increasing awareness that extensive burn injury causes a systemic inflammatory response syndrome (SIRS) in which there is widespread disorganisation of the immune system, eventually resulting in multiple organ dysfunction syndrome (MODS) (Sparkes 1997). Sparkes attributes this to a lipid protein complex associated with burned skin.

During the first 36–48 h, however, the most life-threatening problem, except where inhalation injury is present, will be burn shock. The subject of shock is covered in Chapter 18, but a summary of events which have particular relevance to burns injury is given here (see Table 30.2).

The initial physiological response to a burn injury results in plasma loss from the circulation (see p. 1022). This is accompanied by:

- *Gross oedema* of the affected tissues.
- *Hypovolaemia* — as in all types of shock, this results in decreased circulation to the skin, muscle and internal organs. Cerebral and coronary perfusion, being of greatest priority, are temporarily maintained.
- *Haemoconcentration* — unlike the hypovolaemia which results from haemorrhage, the loss of plasma alone from the intravascular compartment causes an increase in the ratio of blood cells to plasma in the circulation, a raised haematocrit. This increases the viscosity of the blood, further reducing the flow through the capillaries.

In addition to suffering from burn shock, the patient may be emotionally shocked, in great pain and have extensive destruction of the skin and, possibly, deeper structures. There may be associated injuries, especially inhalation of smoke, and a pre-burn illness may be present.

Haemoglobinuria may develop in patients who have been badly burned. This is described in Box 30.3.

Table 30.2 **Pathology and related clinical features of burn shock**

Pathological condition	Clinical signs and symptoms
Hypovolaemia	Thirst Rapid, weak pulse Hypotension Peripheral and splanchnic vasoconstriction
Peripheral vasoconstriction	Pale skin and mucosa Extremities feel cold Patient complains of feeling cold
Reduced perfusion of kidneys	Oliguria, anuria Impairment of renal function Metabolic acidosis Renal failure may occur
Red cell haemolysis	Haemoglobinuria Renal failure may occur
Reduced perfusion of lungs	Rapid, shallow breathing Air hunger — gasping
Reduced perfusion of gastrointestinal tract	Reduced absorption and intestinal stasis Vomiting, loss of electrolytes Paralytic ileus, lack of bowel sounds Bacterial translocation through mucosa
Hypoxaemia/electrolyte imbalance	Restlessness, disorientation, confusion May lead to coma and death

Box 30.3

Haemoglobinuria

This is a potential complication of extensive burn injury which may result in acute renal failure.

As haemoglobin has the molecular weight of 68 000 mmol, it may be filtered through the glomerulus and pass into the renal tubules. Under normal circumstances, haemoglobin is not free in plasma, because when erythrocytes degenerate they are processed by the mononuclear phagocytic system. If pathogenic haemolysis does occur intravascularly, the haemoglobin is usually combined with the plasma protein haptoglobin, a mechanism for iron conservation, which forms a molecular complex too large to pass through the glomerulus.

However, if intravascular haemolysis is extensive, there will be exhaustion of the haptoglobin and therefore free haemoglobin will be present in plasma. The reason why haemolysis occurs in extensive thermal injury appears to be more complicated than the direct effect of heat on the erythrocytes (Yuan et al 1988). Studies indicated that one of the mechanisms involved is the release of toxic oxygen metabolites, e.g. superoxide and hydrogen peroxide from activated neutrophils (Hatherill et al 1986). The red blood cell changes include increased osmotic fragility and decreased membrane deformability (Endoh et al 1992). Brady et al (1996) noted that there is uncertainty as to the means by which free haemoglobin, and myoglobin from damaged muscle, causes damage to the renal tubules and suggest that it may be due to metabolites of the compounds, other toxins from red blood cells/muscle or the coexistence of other renal insults such as hypovolaemia.

The emergency department

To those unfamiliar with burns, the patient with extensive burns may not appear to be critically ill. The loss of plasma from the circulation is less rapid than haemorrhage from ruptured vessels and the patient may appear quite well. Inexperienced staff should consult with the regional burns unit to ensure that treatment is appropriate to the severity of the injury.

The Australia and New Zealand Burn Association Ltd (UK) (1996) identifies the following principles of primary assessment and management by medical personnel:

A Airway maintenance and cervical spine control
B Breathing and ventilation
C Circulation; cardiac status, with control of haemorrhage if present
D Disability, neurological status
E Exposure with environmental control; evaluation of extent and depth of injury, including removal of jewellery and keeping the patient warm
F Fluid resuscitation; i.v. fluid replacement, including introduction of a urinary catheter for monitoring output, and insertion of a nasogastric tube.

These are followed by X-ray of the cervical spine, chest and pelvis to exclude associated injury.

After life-threatening conditions have been excluded or treated, the secondary survey should be commenced. This includes a patient history, description of incident and complete examination.

Except in instances where nurses are specially educated, the role of nursing staff is to assist with the above procedures, to support the patient and their relatives and to keep meticulous records of fluid balance and of medications given.

Transfer of the patient with extensive burns

The patient should be prepared for transfer with the application of a temporary wound dressing, preferably clingfilm, and covered with a space blanket or layers of ordinary blankets. As described earlier, there is a high risk of hypothermia, especially during transfer, and wet dressings should not be used. If there are airway problems the patient must be accompanied by an experienced nurse, as well as by a member of the medical staff. Monitoring of vital signs and maintenance of the intravenous fluids are usually carried out by the nurse. The speed of travel is frequently rapid, which will make the task of monitoring and recording fluid balance and vital signs very difficult; nonetheless these records are important and, along with the ED file, should be given to the staff of the burns unit on arrival.

Admission to a regional burns unit

The burns unit staff are usually informed in advance of the imminent admission of a patient with extensive burns. The time between their notification and the actual arrival of the patient, depending on the distance from the referral centre, is used to prepare the environment and the necessary equipment.

Reception of the patient

When the patient arrives at the unit, they should be greeted sensitively and orientated as to place, as many regional burns units receive patients from a wide catchment area. One nurse should be designated to receive the patient from the escorting nurse. Where possible, the patient should be reassured and given a simple explanation of what is being done at every stage of the admission procedure and thereafter, throughout their stay in the unit. The appearance and smell of the burn wounds may be very upsetting, not only for the patient but also for inexperienced staff. It is important for staff to appear calm and confident, thus helping to reassure the patient.

The receiving staff must wear protective clothing, e.g. waterproof gowns, plastic aprons or tabards and gloves. This is to protect staff against contact with wound exudate and blood and the patient against wound contamination (Weber et al 2004).

The patient should be received into a single room warmed to a temperature of 28°C, as heat loss from the inflamed wounds, in addition to evaporative heat loss from the wound exudate, can be extensive.

Maintaining the airway

If the patient has inhalation injury, endotracheal intubation and assisted ventilation may have been instituted in the ED or may be required at the time of admission to the unit. In any case, all nursing care and observations relative to this treatment must be carried out (see Ch. 3).

Constant observation of respiratory rate and ease, and of the colour of unburned skin and mucosa, must be carried out and recorded. Humidified air or oxygen administered by face mask or nasal catheter may be required.

Weighing the patient

If possible, an accurate body weight in kilograms should be obtained as this is one of the baseline measurements on which the volume of fluid replacement is calculated. Estimation of weight is sometimes carried out but, unless the person doing so is experienced in this, gross over- or undertransfusion may result. In many units the patient is weighed on a special bed or sling, still covered in the blankets and temporary dressings used for the transfer; these are then gently removed and the patient laid on and covered with sterile sheeting, e.g. linen, foam or clingfilm. The original coverings are then weighed and their weight subtracted from the total in order to get a naked weight. It is important to record the weight immediately as the exact figure may easily be forgotten, especially if there is a great deal of activity in the room.

Wound assessment

The medical staff will estimate the depth of the burn wounds and chart their position and extent. Colour photographs may also be taken for recording purposes. In addition to being useful baseline records of wound appearance and distribution, the photographs may, with the patient's permission, be used in evidence in criminal or civil proceedings. Whilst the wounds are exposed, the nurse can take swabs for bacteriological examination from each wound site, e.g. right hand, left hand, chest, neck. This reduces the possibility of wound contamination and the discomfort and possible loss of dignity suffered by the patient during repeated removal of the coverings. The initial wound swabs usually show no bacteriological contamination but provide a useful baseline for further monitoring. The wounds are then covered with a temporary dressing. Specific care will be carried out once the patient's condition has been stabilised.

Bacteriology swabs from nose and throat are also obtained in order to identify commensals which may act as wound pathogens.

Analgesics

It is unusual for patients to complain of pain at this stage, even if their wounds are of partial thickness. If pain is felt, however, intravenous analgesics, usually in the form of morphine, are administered by infusion pump, giving an initial dose and then at an hourly rate of 20–30 mcg/kg. The intramuscular route is never used if the patient is in shock, as the medication will not be absorbed owing to the peripheral vasoconstriction.

Intravenous fluid replacement

Once an accurate body weight has been obtained and the percentage area of the burn estimated, the medical staff will calculate the volume of intravenous therapy required. There are a number of different formulae in current use but most depend on these two parameters for calculation of the volume to be infused. Regulation of the rate of flow and recording of the volume transfused, as well as care of the intravenous site, is the responsibility of the nurse. A volumetric intravenous pump provides accuracy for the infusion of volumes required in each period which may be very large.

Monitoring urine

If this has not been carried out in the ED, an indwelling urinary catheter is passed, the bladder emptied and the urine volume measured. A specimen is tested for specific gravity and analysed using a Multistix. The appearance is noted. A urimeter which allows hourly measuring and sampling whilst maintaining a closed system is attached to the catheter. Settle (1996) emphasised the importance of monitoring renal function through regular, frequent measurement of volume and composition of the urine. A volume of 0.5–1.0 mL/kg body weight hourly is generally accepted as indicating that intravenous fluid replacement is satisfactory, although urine concentration, measured by specific gravity or osmolality, must also be estimated in order to assess renal function.

The appearance of the urine is monitored for indications of haemoglobinuria (see Box 30.3) and, if this is present, for indications that it is diminishing. It is important that the nurse inform the medical staff at the first indication of haemoglobinuria, as it is usual for a solution of sodium bicarbonate and an osmotic diuretic, e.g. mannitol, to be prescribed in order to clear the pigments.

Monitoring vital signs

Pulse If the patient is shocked, the pulse will be rapid and weak. This, combined with generalised oedema, can make manual counting very difficult and mechanical aids such as the pulse oximeter are normally used. It should be remembered, however, that the pulse oximeter will only give pulse rate.

Blood pressure Where all four limbs have been burned, it is not usual practice to record blood pressure. Indeed, even if one limb is unaffected it has been considered more important to ensure effective intravenous replacement than to repeatedly constrict the vessels with a blood pressure cuff. Bainbridge et al (1990), however, found that it is possible to monitor mean arterial pressure by using oscillometric automatic blood pressure monitors with the cuff applied over bulky dressings and this method is useful for monitoring blood pressure in limbs with burns.

The routine measurement of central venous pressure or arterial pressure is not recommended in most UK burns units because of the risk of systemic infection associated with such invasive techniques, especially if the site of entry of the catheter is close to the burn wound. Settle (1996) advised that invasive monitoring should be employed if there has been a delay in starting fluid replacement or if severe respiratory, renal or cardiac impairment exists. However, Schiller and Bray (1996) found that the routine use of the pulmonary artery catheter in patients with extensive burns facilitated optimum levels of fluid replacement and was associated with a significant decrease in overall mortality.

Temperature A good indicator of the state of peripheral perfusion is the difference between core and shell temperatures (see Ch. 22, p. 813). In the normal person, under warm conditions, the temperature of a toe is 1–4°C lower than rectal temperature, but in the patient suffering hypovolaemic shock the vasoconstriction is such that the difference may be as much as 15°C. Temperature monitoring is usually facilitated by the use of thermistor probes in preference to the repeated insertion of a rectal thermometer. In some units, a specially designed probe is inserted into the external auditory meatus in preference to using the rectum (see Ch. 22, p. 820). If thermistor probes are not available, it is possible to gauge the shell temperature by feeling the temperature of the peripheries, especially the toes or the tip of the nose.

In addition to monitoring the difference between a normal core temperature and changes in the shell temperature, measuring the core temperature will, of course, also indicate a trend towards hyperpyrexia or hypothermia (see Ch. 22).

Oral intake

Because of the reduction in gastrointestinal tract perfusion which results from hypovolaemia, it is necessary to restrict the volume of oral fluids initially, even if the patient is very thirsty, until it has been established that there is no nausea or vomiting. If there is persistent vomiting, a nasogastric tube is passed and is either allowed to drain freely or aspirated hourly before small amounts of water are given. In some units, a nasogastric tube is passed routinely in all patients with burns greater than 35% of the body surface. However, studies have shown that early (within 6 h) introduction of intragastric feeding is beneficial in reducing both gastrointestinal ulceration (Raff et al 1997a) and mortality (Raff et al 1997b).

Box 30.4

Complications of burn injuries

In some patients with extensive burns, recovery from the initial injury may be complicated by severe episodes of conditions such as severe sepsis, adult respiratory distress syndrome (ARDS) and/or disseminated intravascular coagulation (DIC), causing them to fluctuate between a satisfactory and a critical condition, perhaps for many weeks. This is especially distressing for the relatives who are trying to cope with the altered appearance of their loved one and who can be given no assurance of eventual recovery; their hopes are raised and dashed repeatedly by their own observations of the patient's condition. Less life-threatening complications include gastrointestinal ulceration and haemorrhage, systemic infection of the respiratory system or urinary tract, wound infection, and wound contraction and scar formation.

Patient behaviour

In addition to recording clinical measurements as described above, it is useful for the nurse to keep a record of the patient's behaviour, noting for example, restlessness, confusion, distress or apathy, as these, along with the measured recordings, will give a more complete picture of the patient's condition. If there is cause for concern, monitoring of neurological status is facilitated by use of the Glasgow Coma Scale (see Ch. 28).

The post-shock phase

After the first 36–48 h following injury, the fluid in the interstitial spaces is reabsorbed into the circulation and, although there is continuous fluid loss through exudate and evaporation from the wound surface, there is normally no longer a need for intravenous replacement of fluids. Unless complications arise (see Box 30.4), the intermediate stage of management will have been reached.

Nursing management during the intermediate stage of burn injury recovery follows the basic principles of burn care whatever the extent of body surface involved. Thus nursing priorities include:

- pain relief (see p. 1022)
- hydration and nutrition
- prevention of infection and local wound care
- psychosocial support for patients and relatives (see p. 1025).

Hydration and nutrition

Until wound closure is complete, there will be continuous loss of the water, protein and electrolytes which comprise the wound exudate (see Ch. 20). In addition, nutritional requirements will be increased because of the elevation in the metabolic rate resulting from trauma, as well as the cellular requirements of wound healing. In patients whose burn area is less than 20% of the body surface, oral intake of a normal diet, perhaps supplemented with high-protein, high-calorie drinks, should be all that is required. However, dietary intake should be monitored to allow assessment by the dietitian and the patient should be weighed weekly. The patient should be encouraged to take fluids and the fluid balance should be monitored and charted.

In more extensive burns, metabolic requirements will be greatly increased, making enteral nutrition via a nasogastric tube necessary. As a fine-bore tube is used to facilitate patient comfort and reduce trauma, there may be difficulty aspirating gastric contents to ensure correct placement; X-ray confirmation of the position of the tube will therefore be required. There are a number of proprietary preparations of enteral feeds available and the dietitian will prescribe the type, volume and rate of administration for each individual. Many manufacturers of enteral feeds produce their own giving sets and volumetric pumps; their instructions should be followed in the use of this equipment. Diarrhoea, nausea and vomiting may complicate enteral feeding. Raff et al (1997a) advise that, rather than commencing with diluted feeds, patient tolerance is best developed by introducing the feed at a slow rate and gradually increasing this until the required rate is reached. If there is a problem with using the nasogastric route, percutaneous endoscopic gastrostomy (PEG) may be performed; Kreis et al (2002) found that the placement of PEG tubes through wound areas did not precipitate wound complications. Parenteral nutrition is reserved for patients who are unable to achieve adequate nutrition by the preferred enteral route (see Ch. 21) because of the danger of infection associated with the introduction of central lines; peripheral lines are usually impractical because of the limited availability of peripheral veins.

Prevention of infection

Both non-specific and specific mechanisms of the immune system are impaired in patients with extensive burns (see Ch. 16).

Because of the large areas of skin destruction and the presence of exudate and necrotic tissue, burn wounds rapidly become colonised with bacteria. It has been found that most of the bacteria are acquired from other contaminated patients or equipment in the ward or unit and therefore meticulous attention must be paid to the prevention of cross-infection (Tredget et al 2004) (see Ch. 16). When possible, the patient should be nursed in a single room and standard infection control precautions implemented. Once the patient's wound becomes colonised with an organism, it will soon be found on their bedclothes, personal clothing and on the surface of dressings. Protective clothing must be worn whenever the patient is attended to; this normally consists of plastic tabards or water-resistant gowns. Disposable water-resistant gowns are expensive but are necessary in the care of patients with major burns, as bodily contact between nurse and patient extends well beyond the confines of an apron when handling and moving procedures are carried out or when dressings are being changed. The wearing of masks and caps is usually not necessary, except when the wound is exposed. Gloves should be worn during any direct contact with the patient and the immediate surroundings; clean rather than sterile gloves may be used for most procedures, apart from those requiring an aseptic technique. Adherence to good handwashing practice requires frequent emphasis (Weber et al 2004).

The bacteriological status of the wounds should be monitored regularly by obtaining wound swabs during dressing changes.

THE BURN WOUND

As for any wound, the aim of management is to provide the optimum environment for the natural healing processes to take place (see Ch. 23). However, most burn wounds involve larger areas of the body surface than is common in other types of wound and this presents many problems in wound management.

Most burn wounds exude copious amounts of fluid. This is evident in superficial partial-thickness wounds from the outset. In deeper wounds, the surface is initially dry and, depending on the depth of tissue destruction, it may take days before the eschar becomes saturated with fluid leaking from the damaged capillaries in the deeper tissues. The volume of exudate has been calculated to be as much as 5200 g/m^2 per day in some burn wounds (Lamke et al 1977) and the evaporative water loss may be as much as 20 times the rate of that from normal skin (Quinn et al 1985).

Unless the superficial partial-thickness burn wound becomes infected, or is subjected to further trauma, it should re-epithelialise in 7–10 days. As migration of the epithelial cells occurs, the exudate will gradually diminish. Bayley (1990) described the major aim in burn wound care to be obtaining wound closure as soon as possible. In order to meet this goal, management must entail:

- meticulous cleansing and debridement of devitalised tissue in order to prevent infection
- facilitating re-epithelialisation or granulation in preparation for any necessary wound grafting
- reducing scarring and contractures
- promoting patient comfort.

Pain relief

It is generally agreed that patients with burns experience the greatest pain during therapeutic procedures (Patterson et al 2004). Pain-relieving strategies used in wound care include:

- the administration of morphine and other similar opioids timed to ensure optimum cover during the procedure
- patient-controlled analgesia by inhalation methods, e.g. Entonox
- relief of anxiety through explanation, and if necessary hypnosis and other psychological coping strategies.

The degree of discomfort the patient experiences will be strongly related to the skill of the dresser and to their ability to recognise and appreciate the individual's pain threshold and tolerance (see Ch. 19). Examples of useful pain assessment tools are given in Chapter 19.

Wound cleansing and debridement

The following procedures must be carried out using strict aseptic technique. If carried out correctly, they can be very time consuming and, where wounds are extensive, will require a number of staff. In some units, patients with extensive burns will have dressings changed under general anaesthesia with the involvement of a full surgical team.

A number of different methods are currently in use for burn wound cleansing. As long as the wound surface comprises non-viable tissue, the method of choice may be to use saturated gauze or foam pads, although physical cleansing is contraindicated in wounds which are granulating or epithelialising. Depending on the size and site of the wound, less traumatic methods include irrigation via a syringe, showering or immersion in a special tub. There is still debate over the type of solution to be used. Although the use of warmed sterile normal saline is generally advocated for wound cleansing, a survey of UK burns units established that antiseptics such as chlorhexidine acetate and povidone–iodine are also used for the initial cleansing of burns; however, as no rationale is given for the use of the antiseptics, it is best to adhere to local policy (Edward-Jones et al 2000). What is important for both patient comfort and to limit heat loss, especially when the wounds are extensive or on the trunk, is to ensure that the solution used is warmed to body temperature.

Following cleansing, loose devitalised tissue is trimmed using sharp scissors. Specialists vary in their approach to the management of blisters: Flanagan and Graham (2001) advise that they be left intact, whereas DuKamp (2001) advocates this approach only if the blister does not restrict joint movement, recommending aspiration of the blister with a needle and syringe in this instance. In contrast, components of blister fluid have been found to inhibit the healing process (Rockwell & Erlich 1990) and to promote wound contraction (Wilson et al 1997). It would therefore appear that evacuating the fluid from intact blisters, allowing the 'roof' of the blister to come into contact with the wound surface and act as a biological dressing, is the most logical approach. However, all authors agree that this subject warrants further research and investigation.

As hair harbours bacteria, it should be clipped short in the area of the wound and a surrounding margin of approximately 5 cm. Shaving is not advised as it can be painful and cause further wound trauma. Long hair which may encroach on the wound should be restrained with elastic bands or adhesive tape.

Promotion of re-epithelialisation or granulation and the prevention of wound contamination may be facilitated either by exposing the wound or by applying dressings.

Exposing the burn wound

This method is currently most commonly used for burns of the face and occasionally for burns of the perineum. The aim of the exposure method is to provide a dry, intact scab under which re-epithelialisation will take place. Relevant nursing management is described in the section dealing with burns of the face (see p. 1023).

Dressing the burn wound

One of the main problems presented by the burn wound is the copious amount of exudate it produces. This strongly influences the choice of dressing material used. Many modern materials are designed to create the optimum environment for healing, i.e. warmth and moisture, whilst removing excess exudate. This may be accomplished by highly absorbent materials, such as alginates, hydrocolloids or hydrophilic foams, or by materials which allow rapid transmission of water vapour. These types of dressing can be used successfully in burns which are of a relatively small area, but a substantial margin must be in contact with unburned skin to prevent leakage of exudate. Thus their use is often not feasible for large wounds.

For extensive burns, no material has yet been found to exceed the benefits of conventional dressings (Lawrence 1996b). These comprise an inner layer of mesh, usually impregnated with paraffin or water-miscible cream, which may or may not provide a base for antibacterial agents; layers of cotton gauze (Fowler 1994); cotton wool or Gamgee. The materials may be retained with cotton conforming bandages, or on the trunk by stitching or stapling. The aim of conventional dressings is to allow exudate to filter through the layers and for water to evaporate from the surface of the dressing, thus preventing maceration of the wound. It is important, therefore, that the surface of the dressing is not occluded with a non-porous material, such as many of the adhesive tapes used to retain bandages. Other non-porous materials which may come into contact with the surface of the dressing include plastic mattress and pillow covers; such contact should be avoided by the use of foam wedges, slings and special mattresses or beds. If the outer surface of the dressing does become moist, the outer layers only are changed under aseptic conditions. To change the whole dressing unnecessarily exposes the burn to contamination from the atmosphere and may disrupt healing if the innermost layer has become adherent.

The frequency of scheduled dressing changes depends on the depth and state of the wound and on the properties of any medication incorporated in the innermost layer. Superficial partial-thickness burns may have their dressings left undisturbed for 7–10 days, the estimated time of healing, unless there are indications for investigating the wound, such as signs of infection. More frequent changes, daily, every second day or twice weekly are required in deeper burns as the presence of necrotic tissue increases the likelihood of bacterial growth. In such cases, antibacterial agents are normally used. For many years, silver sulfadiazine cream, in the UK Flamazine, was a popular antibacterial application for burn wounds throughout the developed world. However, because of its tendency to change the appearance of the wound and to macerate non-viable tissue, making surgical excision difficult, silver sulfadiazine with cerium nitrate (Flammacerium) is used as an alternative. In addition to its antibacterial effects, Sparkes (1997) found that cerium nitrate inhibits the release of toxins from the burn eschar. Interest is also being expressed in other silver-containing wound products including Aquacel Ag (Caruso et al 2004) and Acticoat (Dunn & Edward-Jones 2004).

The ideal wound cover is the patient's own skin in the form of an autograft which 'takes' to provide wound closure. Other types of skin graft, i.e. from other humans, an allograft, or from animals, a xenograft, provide only temporary cover except in the case of identical twins. Sheets of epidermal cells (keratinocytes) may be cultured from the patient's own skin but it may take some weeks before sufficient material is available and research indicates that, for optimum survival and growth when applied to the wound, they require a collagen-based carrier (Shakespeare 1993). Loss et al (2000) have now successfully demonstrated effective results using Integra, a bilaminate skin substitute, with cultured epidermal autografts.

Care of burn wounds prior to skin grafting

The necrotic tissue has to separate from the wound bed before granulation tissue, suitable for skin grafting, is produced. This process of separation may take many weeks and is aided by judicial trimming of loose slough at each dressing change. In relatively small wounds, the process may be accelerated through the use of hydrogels or hydrocolloids.

Surgical removal of necrotic tissue may be carried out, usually within the first 4 days following injury. The tissue is either excised with a scalpel or shaved down to a viable (bleeding) surface with a skin grafting knife. This procedure can result in extensive blood loss, and multiple transfusions may be required. The freshly prepared wound bed is usually skin grafted immediately, but if the bleeding is difficult to control, the skin grafts will be harvested and stored in order that they can be applied without a second operation, usually within the following 48 h.

A skin graft 'takes' by the ingrowth of capillaries from the wound into the graft, a process which takes only a few days. This will be disrupted if there is any blood, serum or pus preventing contact between graft and wound. Other factors which can cause disruption of the graft include any shearing of the graft/wound interface and the presence of β-haemolytic *Streptococcus*, group A (*Strep. pyogenes*) which produces streptokinase, an activator of plasmin which is fibrinolytic. Sometimes the surgeon will choose not to apply a dressing to a newly grafted area. Nursing staff will be responsible for ensuring that there is no collection of fluid under the graft. This is done by gently rolling a rolled-up swab from the centre to the margins of the graft, thus expressing any blood or serum. An aseptic technique is employed and great care is required to prevent the graft shearing on its bed.

The skin graft donor area is a very superficial wound and, as a result, can be very painful. For the first 48 h or so it produces large amounts of bloodstained exudate and is usually dressed with calcium alginate followed by a conventional dressing, which is managed in the same way as that covering a superficial partial-thickness burn. The speed of re-epithelialisation depends on the depth of dermis removed along with the epidermis but is normally between 10 days and 2 weeks.

Ideally, the dressing is left intact until it falls off. Injudicious early investigation will cause further trauma, delay healing and lead to risk of infection.

The alginate dressing dries out as epithelialisation occurs but readily regains its gel consistency when soaked with normal saline.

Care of special areas

The face The most common method of managing facial burns is that of exposure. Bulky absorptive dressings which extend well beyond the wound margin are liable to encroach on the facial features, which should not be covered.

The face becomes very oedematous and the head should be elevated as soon as the patient's condition allows. Drying out of the exudate is encouraged in order to produce a thin scab. The longer the wound exudes, the greater is the build-up of serum; this will produce a thick crust which may never completely dry out and is more likely to crack.

Rapid drying may be facilitated by regular aseptic application of well wrung-out saline swabs which quickly absorb the exudate and are then removed; barely damp material absorbs liquid more effectively than dry material. Careful use of a hair dryer on a cool setting will also speed the drying process but care should be taken that the patient is able to achieve complete closure of the eyelids before such air flow is directed at the face.

Once the scab has formed, it will be similar to a cosmetic face mask and greatly restrict facial movement. Because of this it is usual practice in some units to apply a thin layer of liquid paraffin to facial burns (Hudspith & Rayatt 2004), in particular to the areas around the eyes and mouth, as mobility of these areas is most important The resultant stickiness may allow adherence of debris and it is important to cleanse these areas gently with saline on a regular basis.

Oedema of the periorbital region can cause closure of the eyelids. This is very frightening for the patient, who may think the blindness is permanent. The nurse should warn the patient that eyelid closure may occur but reassure that the swelling will lessen in a few days. Eye drops or ointment will be prescribed in order to reduce the possibility of conjunctivitis. The use of artificial tears will make the patient more comfortable.

Oedema of the lips may cause eversion of the oral mucosa, which should not be allowed to dry out. The skin of the lips should be kept lubricated with yellow soft paraffin and care must be taken when oral hygiene is performed. The use of a soft toothbrush, by patient or nurse, will help to maintain normal mouth care and, if the patient is unable to eat, regular mouthwashes should be given. If oral intake is allowed, the patient may experience difficulty in drinking from a normal cup; a feeding cup with a spout is preferable to using a straw as the patient may find it difficult to exert just the right pressure to allow suction without collapsing the straw.

Oedema of the ears may cause them to jut out at right angles to the head, making them more susceptible to further trauma. If the pinna produces exudate, this is liable to trickle into the external auditory meatus, where it will collect and dry out at the level of the ear drum, reducing the patient's ability to hear. This may not be detected until some time later, in which case it may prove very difficult to evacuate the plug. It is easy to avert this problem by inserting a small piece of gauze just at the opening of the meatus to absorb the exudate, changing it as necessary. The ears may be dressed lightly with a conventional dressing or have gauze spread with an antibacterial ointment, e.g. Flamazine, gently applied. The ears will be very painful when touched and it is useful to elevate the head slightly off the pillow, using either a well-padded foam ring or a foam wedge, as this will reduce the possibility of the ears coming in contact with the pillow.

The lower nostrils should be kept free of exudate build-up by regular cleansing with a dampened cotton bud. If exudate dries on the nasal hairs, the crust will occlude the nostrils and its removal will be very painful indeed. This problem may be prevented by the application of a light smear of soft yellow paraffin just inside the nostrils.

The beard in male patients also becomes incorporated in the crust as it grows. This does not usually present problems until the scab is separating from the newly epithelialised facial skin; in the case of deep burns, the hair follicles will be destroyed and no hair growth will occur. Once the scab starts to lift it may be rehydrated using a moisturising lotion or hydrogel; this causes swelling of the scab, which will then no longer fit the contours of the face, and softens it to allow painless removal. Many men prefer to keep their beard for a time, but if they wish to be clean-shaven, the use of an electric razor is preferable as it causes less trauma to the skin.

Scab removal As the scab lifts on the rest of the face, loose areas should be trimmed with care. There may be a strong temptation on the part of both nurse and patient to remove as much as possible, as the satisfaction of revealing nice pink skin can prove irresistible. However, it must be borne in mind that removing adherent crust causes trauma and may increase the possibility of scar formation. Newly epithelialised skin needs to be moisturised regularly with a bland cream to keep it from drying out (see Box 30.5).

Box 30.5

Care of newly healed skin

Care of newly healed skin consists of washing with mild soap, rinsing well, patting dry and applying a moisturising cream. Newly healed skin does not produce sufficient sebum to prevent it from drying out nor cracking on the surface; neither does it produce enough melanin to prevent burning if exposed to sunlight. It must therefore be protected by covering with clothing or by high protection factor sun creams for at least a year.

The hands Burns involving the majority of the hand are most commonly treated by the application of polythene bags or gloves, with or without the addition of an antibacterial cream, in order to facilitate movement and thus prevent joint stiffness and allow the patient a degree of independence. Because the polythene does not allow evaporation of water, the wound environment is very moist and the non-burned skin will become macerated. As large volumes of exudate will collect, it is usual, before applying the bag, to apply several layers of gauze around the wrist to absorb some of the exudate. The bags should be changed on a daily or more frequent basis, and the hand gently cleansed at each change. Minor burns to the hand are treated with lighter dressings, which should not restrict mobility.

Limbs In order to reduce oedema formation, burned limbs are elevated and exercised on a regular basis, unless freshly laid skin grafts preclude movement.

Joints Wound contraction is an integral part of the healing process, but excessive contraction leads to dysfunction and deformity. As flexor surfaces are more liable to contract, joints must be correctly positioned, with compensatory hyperextension especially of the wrists and neck. Physiotherapy should be carried out regularly, with adequate analgesic cover, to maintain a full range of movement of all joints. However, splinting may be necessary to arrest or correct contracture formation.

Scar formation

Scar formation is part of the maturation phase of the healing process. In wounds healing by secondary intention, the scar often appears red and is raised above the level of the surrounding skin (hypertrophic). Hypertrophic scarring is a well-known complication following burn injury and the resulting disfigurement causes great distress. The most common means of prevention is the application of external pressure, usually effected by the use of specially designed elasticated garments which can be made to fit any anatomical part. The garments should be worn, apart from bathing and skin care, for 24 h/day; treatment should continue for at least 9 months and a pressure of at least 24 mmHg is necessary for the treatment to be effective. Patients are provided with at least two sets of garments, which are alternately washed and worn.

Elastic garments are not very effective for applying pressure to concavities on the body surface, especially on the face around the nose and mouth. For treatment of these areas, a rigid, or semi-rigid, transparent face mask can be made. One technique which does not rely on pressure to reduce the hypertrophy and redness of scars is the use of silicone gel sheets (Mustoe et al 2002). These need to be retained in place with light bandages or adhesive tape and must be removed regularly for washing as they are reusable for a few applications. The sheets are relatively expensive and tend to be used only when problems arise in pressure therapy. A cheaper and more practical method described by Davey (1997) is the use of adhesive tapes such as Mefix applied directly onto florid scars, with the application of Silastic elastomer on areas when early thickening is detected.

PSYCHOLOGICAL EFFECTS OF BURN INJURIES

The disfigurement and impaired function which result from wound contracture and scar formation are generally accepted as the major sequelae of burn injuries, causing great distress and psychological problems for the patient and their loved ones. This, however, describes the long-term view and does not take into account that, for the patient and their family, the psychological effects start at the time of injury.

Partridge (1990) gives a graphic account of his experiences when he sustained burns in a road traffic accident and notes that 'being on fire is unforgettable, you will recall those seconds with crystal clarity for the rest of your life'. Many patients voice their relief at being alive in the immediate period following the accident, but as the implications of their injury sink in, their emotions and behaviour may begin to go through a series of changes.

Bereni-Marzouk et al (1981) described four psychological phases experienced by patients hospitalised following burn injuries:

- critical
- stabilisation
- recovery
- pre-discharge.

This categorisation will be adopted in the following discussion of the problems commonly encountered by individuals with burn injuries.

The critical phase

During the early stages of treatment, the patient will be preoccupied by bodily feelings and by the care provided by nursing and medical staff. If the wounds are extensive and complications arise, the patient will require constant attendance, perhaps for lengthy periods of time, which may result in intensive care psychosis (see Ch. 29, p. 1007). Topf et al (1996) emphasised the need for nursing staff to be aware of the harmful effects of the experience of intensive care, and the importance of providing communication and controlling environmental factors in order to promote sleep and sensory balance. Nightmares associated with the accident are common at this stage, as are fears of dying. A constant presence, reassurance and reorientation may be necessary.

Stabilisation

When the patient reaches this stage, anxiety related to survival is replaced with fears for the future, both short and long term. In the short term, stress is related to anticipation of pain and many patients become depressed or are hostile towards the nursing staff. They may regress in their ability to cope with activities of living and demand care and attention. This is perhaps the most difficult phase for the unit staff to cope with. Pain control helps to reduce patient anxiety related to wound care, and physiotherapy and monitoring of pain should continue throughout the period of hospitalisation.

Although there is a tendency to expect that there will be more pain the greater the injury and that pain will reduce in time, in their study Choiniere et al (1989) found no correlation between pain scores and the time elapsed following injury, or between pain scores and size of burn.

Longer-term anxieties include the fear of disfigurement and of losing function and former roles. Nursing staff can help the patient come to terms with their changed situation by being honest and supportive and allowing them to grieve. The first look in the mirror should not be accidental but a planned occasion with the patient making the choice whether to be alone or to be accompanied by nursing staff or loved ones. Although the patient may have some idea of their changed appearance from watching the reactions of visitors, the true extent of disfigurement may only be seen on first looking in a mirror. Some patients have glimpsed their reflection in the spectacles of attendant personnel, in darkened windows or in plate glass doors and later reported that they were able to deny their appearance, attributing it to a flaw in the glass.

If the hands are not injured, the patient may gauge contour and textural changes through touch, but the reality of their changed appearance will still be a great shock.

Manifestations of hostility may range from refusal to cooperate with treatment, through cursing and swearing, to actual bodily assault. Sometimes the hostility is directed only towards certain nurses and the patient may manipulate the situation to create discord among the staff. Care should be planned to ensure a consistent approach by all staff and it may be necessary to reallocate staff. If the patient's behaviour is uncooperative to the extent that it will interfere with recovery, behaviour modification techniques may be in order. A contract may be drawn up specifying the type of behaviour expected of the patient and describing the rewards which will be given or withheld accordingly.

Regression in physical ability may also be managed by behavioural modification, with the patient being set easily achievable tasks, such as pouring a drink from their own water jug and being encouraged to feel a sense of achievement on doing so. Many patients regress when there is a sudden, unexplained reduction in the amount of nursing care they receive. Explanation about their improving condition, and patient involvement in identifying needs and planning the reduction of care can help to alleviate this problem.

Recovery

This phase is marked by the patient beginning to rediscover former interests and pleasures. The patient may, for example, take more notice of the activity in the unit and of the other patients. When possible, mixing with the other patients should be encouraged; the patient's involvement in small tasks, such as distributing newspapers, will also aid independence and self-esteem. When disfigurement is highly visible, such as on the face and hands, the patient may not wish to mix with others and will require a great deal of support from staff as well as from family and friends. Griffiths (1989) offered the following list of coping strategies which the nursing staff can explore with the patient:

- Do not give in to fear.
- Learn to control fear and anxiety.
- Practise positive self-talk.
- Concentrate on relevant pieces of information.
- Do not interpret discomfort as rejection.
- Find your own way of acknowledging the disfigurement.
- Congratulate success.

The pre-discharge phase

Patients frequently experience ambivalence about leaving the safe confines of the unit where they are known and accepted. The actual discharge may be graduated by the introduction of progressively longer visits home and by giving the patient the opportunity to discuss the pleasures and problems encountered. Williams and Griffiths (1991) emphasise the patient's need for practical advice in the form of staff-led discussions during the period prior to or immediately following discharge from hospital in order to reduce the psychological sequelae of burn injuries. Liaison with the primary health care team will ensure continuity of care, and involvement of the social work department and occupational therapists in the community will provide financial and practical help in the resumption of home life.

After discharge

It is possible that the patient will need to return to hospital for clinic appointments and, later on, for plastic surgery to improve appearance and function, a process which may involve many operations over a number of years. Many patients suffer long-term psychological problems including depression, anxiety and other post-traumatic stress symptoms. In 2001, Van Loey et al, in a survey of European hospitals, found that the provision of continuing support was inadequate and there is no evidence that this has improved with regard to the NHS; it would therefore appear that there is a growing need for voluntary groups such as Changing Faces (see 'Useful websites').

No matter how high the standard of care provided, the patient who suffers extensive burns may never return fully to their former physical or emotional functioning — a fact which can only serve to emphasise the need for greater effort in the field of burn prevention.

REFERENCES

Adams L E, Purdue G F, Hunt J L 1991 Tap-water scald burns: awareness is not the problem. Journal of Burn Care and Rehabilitation 12(1): 91–95

Australia and New Zealand Burn Association Ltd (UK) 1996 Emergency management of severe burns course manual. UK version for The British Burn Association

Bainbridge L C, Simmons H M, Elliot D 1990 The use of automatic blood pressure monitors in the burned patient. British Journal of Plastic Surgery 43: 322–324

Bayley E W 1990 Wound healing in the patient with burns. Nursing Clinics of North America 25(1): 205–221

Beeley J M, Clark R J 1996 Respiratory problems in fire victims. In: Settle J A D (ed) Principles and practice of burns management. Churchill Livingstone, Edinburgh

Bereni-Marzouk T, Giacalone L, Thieulard L et al 1981 Behavioural changes in burned adult patients during their stay in hospital. Burns 8(5): 365–368

Brady H R, Brenner B M, Lieberthal W 1996 Acute renal failure. In: Brenner B M (ed) The kidney, Vol II, 5th edn. W B Saunders, Philadelphia

Bull J P, Lennard-Jones J E 1949 The impairment of sensation in burns and its clinical application as a test of the depth of loss. Clinical Science 8: 155

Caruso D M, Foster K N, Hermans M H E, Rick C 2004 Aquacel Ag in the management of partial thickness burns: results of a clinical trial. Journal of Burn Care and Rehabilitation 25(1): 89–97

Choiniere M, Melzack R, Rondeau J et al 1989 The pain of burns: characteristics and correlates. Journal of Trauma 29(11): 1531–1539

Davey R B 1997 The use of contact media for burn scar hypertrophy. Journal of Wound Care 6(2): 80–82

Department of Trade and Industry 1999 Burns and scald accidents in the home. Government Consumer Safety Research. Online. Available: www.dti.gov.uk

Duggan D, Quine S 1995 Burn injuries and characteristics of burn patients in New South Wales, Australia. Burns 21(2): 83–89

DuKamp A 2001 Deroofing minor burn blisters – what is the evidence? Accident and Emergency Nursing 9(4): 217–221

Dunn K, Edward-Jones V 2004 The role of Acticoat with nanocrystalline silver in the management of partial thickness burns. Burns 30(Suppl 1): S1–9

Edward-Jones V, Dawson M M, Childs C 2000 A survey of toxic shock syndrome (TSS) in UK burns units. Burns 26(4): 323–333

Ellis A, Rylah L T A 1990 Transfer of the thermally injured patient. British Journal of Hospital Medicine 44: 206–208

Endoh Y, Kawakami M, Orringer E P et al 1992 Causes and time course of acute haemolysis after burn injury in the rat. Journal of Burn Care and Rehabilitation 13: 203–209

Ewles L, Simnett I 2003 Promoting health. A practical guide, 5th edn. Baillière Tindall, Edinburgh

Flanagan M, Graham J 2001 Should burn blisters be left intact or debrided? Journal of Wound Care: 10(2) 41–45

Fowler A 1994 Burns care and management. Journal of Tissue Viability 4(1): 3–9

Griffiths E 1989 More than skin deep. Nursing Times 85(40): 34–36
Harper R D, Dickson W A 1995 Reducing the burn risk to elderly persons living in residential care. Burns 21(3): 205–208
Hatherill J R, Till G O, Bruner L H, Ward P A 1986 Thermal injury, intravascular haemolysis, and toxic oxygen products. Journal of Clinical Investigation 78(3): 629–636
Haum A, Perbix W, Hack H J et al 1995 Alcohol and drug abuse in burn injuries. Burns 21(3): 194–199
Hojer J, Personne M, Hulten P, Ludwigs U 2002 Topical treatments for hydrochloric acid burns: a blind controlled experimental study. Journal of Toxicology 40(7): 861–866
Hudspith J, Rayatt S 2004 First aid and treatment of minor burns. British Medical Journal 328(7454): 1487–1489
International Society for Burn Injuries (ISBI) 1979 Constitution. Online. Available: www.worldburn.org
Josty I C, Narayanan V, Dickson W A 2000 Burns in patients with epilepsy: changes in epidemiology. Epilepsia 41(4): 453–456
Kreis B E, Middelkoop E, Vloemans A F, Kreis R W 2002 The use of a PEG tube in a burn center. Burns 28(2): 191–197
Lamke L O, Nilsson G E, Reithner H L 1977 The evaporative water loss from burns and the water vapour permeability of grafts and artificial membranes used in the treatment of burns. Burns 3: 159–165
Lawrence J C 1996a First aid measures for the treatment of burns and scalds. Journal of Wound Care 5(7): 319–322
Lawrence J C 1996b Dressings for burns. In: Settle J A D (ed) Principles and practice of burns management. Churchill Livingstone, Edinburgh
Liao C C, Rossignol A M 2000 Landmarks in burn prevention. Burns 26(5): 422–434
Linares A Z, Linares H 1990 Burn prevention: the need for a comprehensive approach. Burns 16(4): 281–285
Loss M, Wedler V, Kunzi W et al 2000 Artificial skin, split thickness autograft and cultured autologous keratinocytes combined to treat a severe burn injury of 93% T.B.S.A. Burns 26(7): 644–652
Lund C C, Browder N C 1944 The estimation of areas of burns. Surgery, Gynaecology and Obstetrics 79: 352–354
McLoughlin E 1995 A simple guide to burn prevention. Burns 21(3): 226–229
Mercer N S G 1988 With or without? A cooling study. Burns 14(5): 397–398
Moritz A R, Henriques F C 1947 Studies of thermal injury: the relative importance of time and surface temperature in the causation of cutaneous burns. American Journal of Pathology 23: 695–699
Mustoe T A, Cooter R D, Gold M H et al 2002 International clinical recommendations on scar management. Plastic and Reconstructive Surgery 110(2): 560–571
National Burn Injury Referral Guidelines 2001 National Burn Care Review Committee, Standards and Strategy for Burn Care, p 68–69
Office of the Deputy Prime Minister 2003 Fire statistics, United Kingdom – 2001. ODPM, London
Pape S A, Skouras C A, Byrne P O 2001 An audit of the use of laser Doppler imaging (LDI) in the assessment of burns of intermediate depth. Burns 27(3): 233–239
Partridge J 1990 Changing faces: the challenge of facial disfigurement. Penguin, London
Patterson D R, Hoflund H, Espey K et al 2004 Pain management. Burns 30(8): 10–15
Pereira C, Murphy K, Herndon D 2004 Outcome measures in burn care. Is mortality dead? Burns 30(8): 761–771
Quinn K J, Courtney J M, Evans J H et al 1985 Principles of burn dressings. Biomaterials 6(6): 369–377
Raff T, Germann G, Hartmann B 1997a The value of early enteral nutrition in the prophylaxis of stress ulceration in the severely burned patient. Burns 23(4): 313–318
Raff T, Hartmann B, Germann G 1997b Early intragastric feeding of seriously burned and long-term ventilated patients; a review of 55 patients. Burns 23(1): 19–25
Rockwell W B, Erlich H P 1990 Should burn blister fluid be evacuated? Journal of Burn Care and Rehabilitation 11(1): 93–95
Sarhadi N S, Kincaid R, McGregor J C, Watson J D 1995 Burns in the elderly in the South East of Scotland: review of 176 patients treated in the Bangour burns unit (1982–91) and burns inpatients in the region (1975–91). Burns 21(2): 91–95
Sawada Y, Urushidate S, Yotsuyanagi T, Ishita K 1997 Is prolonged and excessive cooling of a scalded wound effective? Burns 23(1): 55–58
Schiller W R, Bray R C 1996 Haemodynamic and oxygen transport monitoring in management of burns. New Horizons 4(4): 475–482
Settle J A D 1996 General management. In: Settle J A D (ed) Principles and practice of burns management. Churchill Livingstone, Edinburgh
Shakespeare P 1993 Burn wound healing. Journal of Tissue Viability 3(1): 16–21
Sheller J L, Thuesen B 1998 Scalds in children caused by water from electric kettles: effect of prevention through information. Burns 24(5): 420–424
Sparkes B G 1997 Immunological responses to thermal injury. Burns 23(2): 106–113
Stone M, Ahmed J, Evans J 2000 The continuing risk of domestic hot water scalds to the elderly. Burns 26(4): 347–350
Tones K, Tilford S 2001 Health promotion: effectiveness, efficiency and equity. Nelson Thornes, Cheltenham
Topf M, Bookman M, Arrand D 1996 Effects of critical care unit noise on the subjective quality of sleep. Journal of Advanced Nursing 24(3): 545–551
Tredget H, Shankowsky R, Rennie R et al 2004 Pseudomonas infections in the thermally injured patient. Burns 30(1): 3–26
Tsuei B J, Kearney P A 2004 Hypothermia in the trauma patient. Injury 35(1): 7–15
Van Loey N E E, Faber A W, Taal L A 2001 A European hospital survey to determine the extent of psychological services offered to patients with severe burns. Burns 27(1): 23–31
Walker A R 1990 Fatal tapwater scald burns in the USA, 1979–86. Burns 16(1): 49–52
Wallace A B 1951 The exposure treatment of burns. Lancet i: 501–504
Weber J, McManus A and the Nursing Committee of the International Society for Burn Injuries 2004 Infection control in burn patients. Burns 30(8): 16–24
Williams E E, Griffiths T A 1991 Psychological consequences of burn injury. Burns 17(6): 478–480
Wilson A M, McGrouther D A, Eastwood M, Brown R A 1997 The effect of burn blister fluid on fibroblast contraction. Burns 23(4): 306–312
Yuan Y, Fang Z Y, Zhang Z H 1988 Changes in the rate of haemolysis during the early stage after burns in the rabbit. Burns 14(5): 365–368

FURTHER READING

Ewles L, Simnett I 2003 Promoting health. A practical guide, 5th edn. Baillière Tindall, Edinburgh
Sidell M, Jones L, Katz J et al (eds) 2003 Debates and dilemmas in promoting health, 2nd edn. Palgrave Macmillan, Basingstoke

USEFUL WEBSITES

British Association of Skin Camouflage
www.skin-camouflage.net

Changing Faces
www.changingfaces.org.uk

The Royal Society for the Prevention of Accidents (RoSPA)
www.rospa.org.uk

THE PATIENT WITH CANCER

Bernadette M. Byrne

31

INTRODUCTION

Cancer touches all of us at some stage in our lives — personally, through friends, acquaintances or the media. It is a disease with a profound effect on every aspect of life, whether physical, psychological, social or spiritual. There are two principal reasons for this. First, cancer is still associated with suffering and death. Second, despite improvements in cure rates, many uncertainties persist concerning the nature and causes of cancer and the methods of prevention and cure. This uncertainty serves to perpetuate various myths and fears surrounding the disease, some of which are described in Box 31.1.

STOP THINK **31.1** (a) What words come to mind when you think of the word 'cancer'?
(b) Ask the same question of a few friends, or a member of your family. How do their responses compare with yours?
(c) Is their overall attitude one of optimism or of pessimism?

Cancer is a serious social problem, costing much in human and financial terms. One in three people in the UK risk developing cancer in their lifetime, with one in four deaths being attributable to cancer, which has now overtaken heart disease as the UK's number one killer (SHS 2005, Cancer Research UK 2005a,b). Globally, by 2020, there are likely to be 20 million new cancer patients each year, double that identified by Oliver in 1999. While statistics appear to present a bleak picture, people in the UK are surviving cancer, with death rates falling since the 1970s (Kmietowicz 2004). This provides clear evidence for a more positive approach by nurses and other health professionals, which will foster realistic hope in their patients. With existing knowledge and advancing technology, the WHO cancer programme hopes to prevent up to 50% of cancers in the next 20 years (Sikora 1999).

Before reading further, consider your own knowledge and attitudes towards cancer by carrying out the following exercise.

STOP THINK **31.2** Consider the following statements. Decide whether they are true, partly true, or false:

(a) Everyone with cancer dies from the disease.
(b) Cancer is the cause of the highest number of deaths per year in the UK.
(c) Cancer is the result of a person's lifestyle.
(d) Cancer is hereditary.
(e) Certain personality types are more prone to cancer than others.
(f) Some forms of cancer are contagious.
(g) Most persons with cancer are disfigured in some way by the disease.
(h) Cancer patients can enjoy many years of normal, productive life.
(i) A cancerous growth is a collection of cells that are foreign to the body.
(j) The side-effects of all cancer treatments are particularly severe.
(k) Everyone with cancer suffers pain at some point during the disease.

Oncology as a specialty

Since the mid-1990s, cancer has been a high priority on the UK political and health care agenda in response to variable patterns of care and the then relatively low survival rates in comparison with mainland Europe. Several fundamental changes have been made to the organisation and provision of cancer services initiated by the publication of the Calman–Hine/Calman report (DH 1995). The vision of the Calman report was to focus care around the patient and their family, care being delivered in specific designated cancer centres and cancer units by coordinated services in

Box 31.1

Sociohistorical perspectives

In medieval times, cancer was believed to be contagious, caused by lack of cleanliness and even by a form of demon possession (Nery 1986).

Society
The cultural legacy of historical beliefs is the aura of fear and shame that surrounds the disease even today. Skott (2002), using patient narratives, from a sociocultural perspective, examines the highly metaphorical language in which the cancer disease process and treatment are described — such as the cancer 'eating' away tissues or of an 'invasion' by an 'alien army' of 'colonising' cells.

This tendency to view cancer symbolically is also evident in the causes to which many patients attribute their disease, ranging from divine retribution to a stressful life event, a fall or physical blow, dirt or, very commonly, personal failing (Walker 1990).

Cancer stigma
Stigma is a process of negative social judgements (Flanagan & Holmes 2000) which, according to seminal work by Goffman, 'reduce the person in our mind from a whole and usual person to a tainted and discounted one' (Goffman 1963). This is illustrated in a recent study where patients with lung cancer perceived that others held the belief that they were 'dirty', 'disgusting', 'blameworthy' and automatically assumed to be smokers. One individual imagined others viewing him as a 'leper' (Chapple et al 2004).

For individuals with cancer, insurance cancellations or refusal, job discrimination and problems with reintegration into school or the workplace are manifestations of the persistent social stigma of cancer.

In favourable circumstances, most people are not conscious of these underlying social attitudes. However, a person with cancer may soon become painfully aware of the degradation and isolation which accompanies the disease. Family and friends may struggle to maintain a supportive relationship, as excessive fear and dread may give rise to avoidance or overprotective behaviour.

Analysis of media coverage reveals a tendency to emphasise the tragic nature of cancer (Macmillan Cancer Relief Fund 1999). However, the media are in a powerful position to provide accurate, balanced and comprehensive sources of information to replace such negative attitudes with a more realistic public awareness. Cancer still remains a relatively taboo subject, as anyone who tries to discuss it in social gatherings will discover.

Patients and their families bring these attitudes and beliefs into their cancer experience. Assessment of their perception of the situation is an essential first step in the provision of supportive care.

partnership with each other. The report recommended a seamless service, integrating primary, secondary and tertiary care, with real commitment to psychosocial as well as medical needs. It also provided the opportunity to think about cancer control, early screening and detection programmes.

Building on this framework, subsequent policy documents have influenced the progression of cancer services (DH 2000a,b, SEHD 2003). Comprehensive long-term strategies have been developed to shape cancer services, looking at all aspects of the patient's cancer journey, promoting high standards of equitable care and investing in equipment and the cancer workforce. Cancer networks have been identified as the organisational model for implementing these strategies, through the development of shared protocols and pathways of care, and the promotion of working partnerships between health professionals, the voluntary sector, local authorities and users of the service across a geographical area (Kunkler 2000). Mapping the patient's journey allows everyone involved to see the process from the patient's perspective, thus providing continuity and avoiding fragmentation of care.

There is acknowledgement of the need for investment in education, research and professional development for all health care professionals and for the promotion of core skills in communication, teamwork and palliative care. Students and newly qualified health care professionals need to understand the multidisciplinary nature of cancer management within and outside the hospital, appreciating the roles of all those providing patient care (DH 1995, RCN 1996a,b).

These initiatives clearly demonstrate the value of the nurse in cancer care and recognise the need for specialist cancer care education (DH 2000c, RCN 2003). With the development of the roles of the advanced nurse practitioner and nurse specialist, it is imperative that the expertise required of all nurses at ward level and in primary care is not forgotten.

The cancer process

The process of cancer or carcinogenesis has many stages and occurs over time. Cancer develops when cells grow and divide uncontrollably outside the normal cell regulatory mechanisms. These cells have no specific tissue function, but are able to spread from the site of origin to distant tissues. In the last three decades, molecular biology has made great progress in unravelling the steps involved in this process of cell transformation and is improving our ability to classify, diagnose and treat cancer. There still, however, remain many unanswered questions.

A critical component in understanding the cancer process and rationale for treatment is a knowledge of the structure and function of cells, the role of DNA and the reproductive cell cycle; for further reading, see Martini (2004) or Tortora & Grabowski (2005).

When a cell divides, a chain of chemical signals controls the process. The links are proteins such as growth factors, receptors, cytoplasmic message-carrying proteins and cell nucleus regulatory proteins. Specific genes in the cell DNA express these proteins during protein synthesis. The basic cause of cancer is damage to one or more of these genes. Such damage may occur from either errors in DNA replication during mitosis or exposure to environmental agents. In the transformation to a cancerous growth, there is a progressive series of mutations of genes regulating cell division and differentiation.

Exciting research into these cell regulatory genes has recognised that 'proto-oncogenes' promote cell division ('on switch') and 'tumour suppressor genes' inhibit cell division ('off switch'). One such tumour suppressor gene, p53, is now recognised to have mutated in at least 50% of human cancers (Brown 1999). Normally, the protein from a p53 gene halts the cell cycle in the G_1 phase at a control checkpoint before DNA replication occurs. This allows the cell to repair any DNA damage identified. If, however, genomic damage is excessive, the cell undergoes a programmed cell death (apoptosis). For this reason, p53 is often referred to as the 'guardian of the genome'. When p53 mutates, cells do not repair defective DNA and continue to replicate. Changes in p53 are not a direct cause of cancer, but cells lacking p53 are at high risk of malignant transformation (Yarbro 2000, Lee & Yielding 2003). Cancer cells therefore grow in an erratic and uncoordinated way because of an alteration in cell regulatory mechanisms. As tumours grow by repeated cell divisions, their rate of growth is often defined in terms of 'doubling time'. Tumours vary greatly in their doubling time but, contrary to popular belief, their growth is not as rapid as that of certain normal tissues. For a tumour growth to exceed 1 or 2 mm, it requires a blood supply for survival; therefore a capillary network from the surrounding host tissue is initiated by proteins or angiogenic factors, e.g. fibroblast growth factor (FGF) and tumour necrosis factor (TNF) (Fidler 1997, Franks & Teich 1997).

At any one time, a tumour consists of a mixture of cells, some dividing or growing, some dying or dead. Tumour cells appear to have the capacity to develop various strains within one tumour, each with different properties and, unfortunately, different levels of resistance to anticancer treatments.

Tumour pathology

Malignant and benign tumours The word 'cancer' is a general term used to describe all malignant neoplasms, i.e. a new growth of tissue, or tumour. A tumour may be benign or malignant, although this distinction is not always clear. Brain tumours, for example, may be benign in nature, e.g. meningioma, but because of their location within a limited space may prove to be fatal.

Benign tumour cells are usually well differentiated, i.e. they resemble the host tissue, are slow growing and do not invade surrounding tissue or form metastases in distant tissue. Once removed, they rarely recur. Malignant tumours have the opposite properties, albeit to varying degrees. A malignant tumour poses a threat to life mainly because of its ability to proliferate destructively into surrounding tissue and to metastasise to other parts of the body.

The molecular biology of cancer is profoundly changing the approach to identifying cancer by tissue analysis (histology). A definitive cancer diagnosis is made by the examination of tissue and cell (cytology), samples under a microscope combined with molecular technology such as DNA analysis and immunohistochemistry (IHC). This technology aims to identify tumours by recognising unique molecular alterations occurring in specific tumour types and provides a more sophisticated method of classifying tumours (Harris 2005). IHC, for example, has been invaluable in determining a primary tumour (Costa & Cordon-Cardo 2001).

Identification of the steps involved in carcinogenesis has led directly to the discovery of molecular tumour markers (see Table 31.1). Among the cancers for which molecular diagnostics has had the greatest impact is chronic myeloid leukaemia (CML). The marker of this disease is the Philadelphia chromosome, which is detectable in 95% of cases (Pasternak et al 1998). In addition to diagnosis, prognosis has in many cases been enhanced by the identification of such markers. For example, in 20–30% of breast and ovarian tumours, the oncogene HER-2/neu is overexpressed and is a reliable indicator of poor prognosis (Loud et al 2002). The protein expressed by this gene has now become a therapeutic target to improve treatment outcomes.

Histology reports therefore communicate both diagnostic and prognostic information by referring to the degree of differentiation of tumour cells, their capacity to invade, the degree of vascularity (blood supply) and now the molecular analysis. Well-differentiated tumour cells bear considerable resemblance to the original tissue in structure and function.

Table 31.1 **Examples of molecular genetic markers used in cancer diagnosis and prognosis**

Cancer	Genetic marker	Principle application
Chronic myeloid leukaemia	Philadelphia chromosome t(9;22)(q34;q11) [BCR/ABL]	Primary diagnosis, detection of residual disease after treatment
Non-Hodgkin's lymphoma:		
Follicular	t(14;18)(q32;q21) [BCL2/IGH]	Primary diagnosis, detection of residual disease after treatment
Burkitt's	t(8;14)(q24;q32)	As above
Neuroblastoma	MYCN amplification	Prognosis
Breast cancer	HER2-neu/ERB2 amplification	Prognosis
Familial cancers		
Breast	BRCA1, BRCA2	Diagnosis of hereditary predisposition
Colon	APC, MSH2, MLH1	As above
Wilms' tumour	TP53 mutation	As above
Retinoblastoma	RB mutation	As above

These tumours are usually slower growing and are less likely to spread (metastasise), usually responding well to treatment. Undifferentiated cells, however, are very different from the original tissue, almost unrecognisable. These tumours grow and disseminate more rapidly, and may be more resistant to treatment.

Tumours may be classified, not only by their biological behaviour, but also traditionally by their tissue of origin. Most tumours retain sufficient characteristics of the normal differentiated cell to allow recognition of the type of tissue from which they were derived which is the basis for the classification of tumours by tissue type (see Table 31.2). Tumours of one organ may be of various tissue types with differing behaviours and prognoses. For example, an adenocarcinoma of the lung behaves in a much less malignant way than small cell carcinoma of the lung, the latter carrying a much poorer prognosis.

Cancer is therefore not one disease but many, each type behaving in a very different way. This must be taken into account in all discussions about cancer and in all relationships with cancer patients.

The spread of cancer (see Fig. 31.1)

The term 'carcinoma in situ' refers to a cancer before it has become invasive. The exact manner in which invasion occurs is unknown but is thought to be due partly to physiological changes occurring in tumour cell membranes which reduce their adhesion to other cells. Tumours also produce proteolytic enzymes (protein-dissolving), which may assist the invasion of normal tissue. Malignant cells also seem to lose 'contact inhibition', failing to recognise their boundaries and to cease growth on meeting a different tissue type. For example, tumours of glandular lung tissue may continue invasion through the pleura to the chest wall. Once local invasion has occurred to any degree, metastases may develop in distant tissue. Metastatic spread (dissemination) may occur in one of four ways:

- via the lymphatic system
- via the bloodstream
- via serous cavities
- via the cerebrospinal fluid (CSF).

Lymphatic spread Tumour cells may invade the lymphatic vessels and grow in clumps and cords, establishing themselves en route in local lymph nodes. This is termed 'regional spread'. It eventually causes lymph node swelling, which may be painful, and may prevent local tissue fluid drainage, causing lymphoedema, for example, in the affected arms of some patients with breast cancer. Ultimately, distant lymph nodes may also be involved.

Table 31.2 Classification by tissue type of malignant tumours

Tissue of origin	Malignant tumour
Epithelial	**'Carcinoma'**
Squamous: surface epithelium, cell lining covering body cavities, organs and tracts	Squamous cell carcinoma, e.g. lung, skin, stomach
Glandular: glands or ducts in the epithelium	Adenocarcinoma, e.g. breast, lung, colon
Transitional cells: bladder lining	Transitional cell carcinoma, e.g. bladder
Basal cells: skin layer	Basal cell carcinoma ('rodent ulcer')
Liver	Hepatocellular carcinoma
Biliary tree	Cholangiocarcinoma
Placenta	Choriocarcinoma
Testicular epithelium	Seminoma, teratoma, embryonal carcinoma
Endothelial cells	Angiosarcoma
Mesothelial: covering the surface of serous membranes	Mesothelioma, e.g. pleura, peritoneum
Connective tissue	**'Sarcoma'**
Bone	Osteosarcoma
Cartilage	Chondrosarcoma
Fatty tissue	Liposarcoma
Fibrous tissue	Fibrosarcoma
Lymphoid tissue	Lymphomas
Bone marrow	Leukaemias, e.g. ALL, CML
Muscle	**'Myosarcoma'**
Smooth muscle	Leiomyosarcoma
Striated muscle	Rhabdomyosarcoma
Cardiac muscle	Cardiac sarcomas
Neural	
Meninges	Meningeal sarcoma
Glia	Glioblastoma multiforme
Neurones	Neuroblastoma, medulloblastoma
Germ cells	
Testes or ovary	Teratoma, germ cell

ALL, acute lymphoblastic leukaemia; CML, chronic myeloid leukaemia.

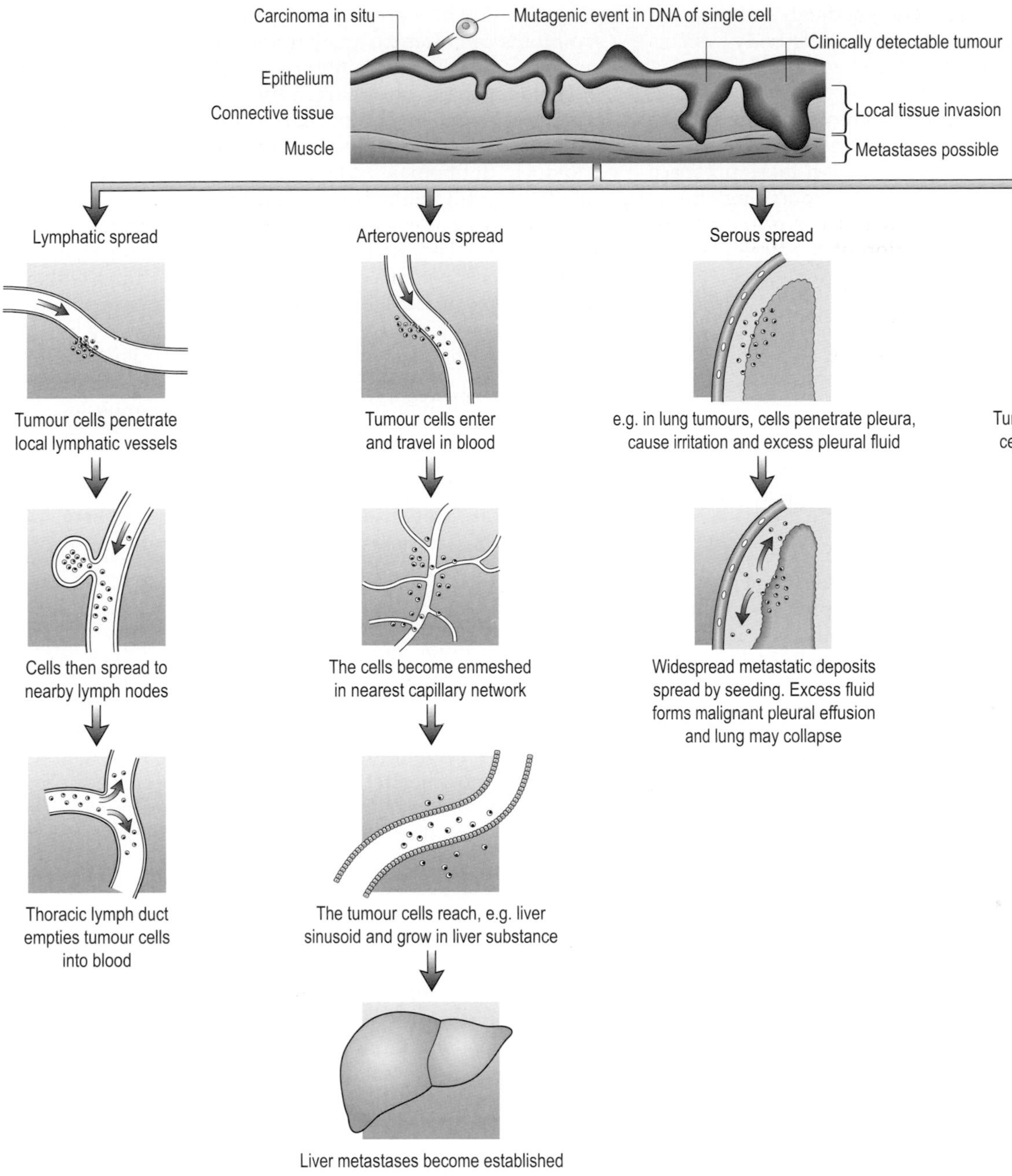

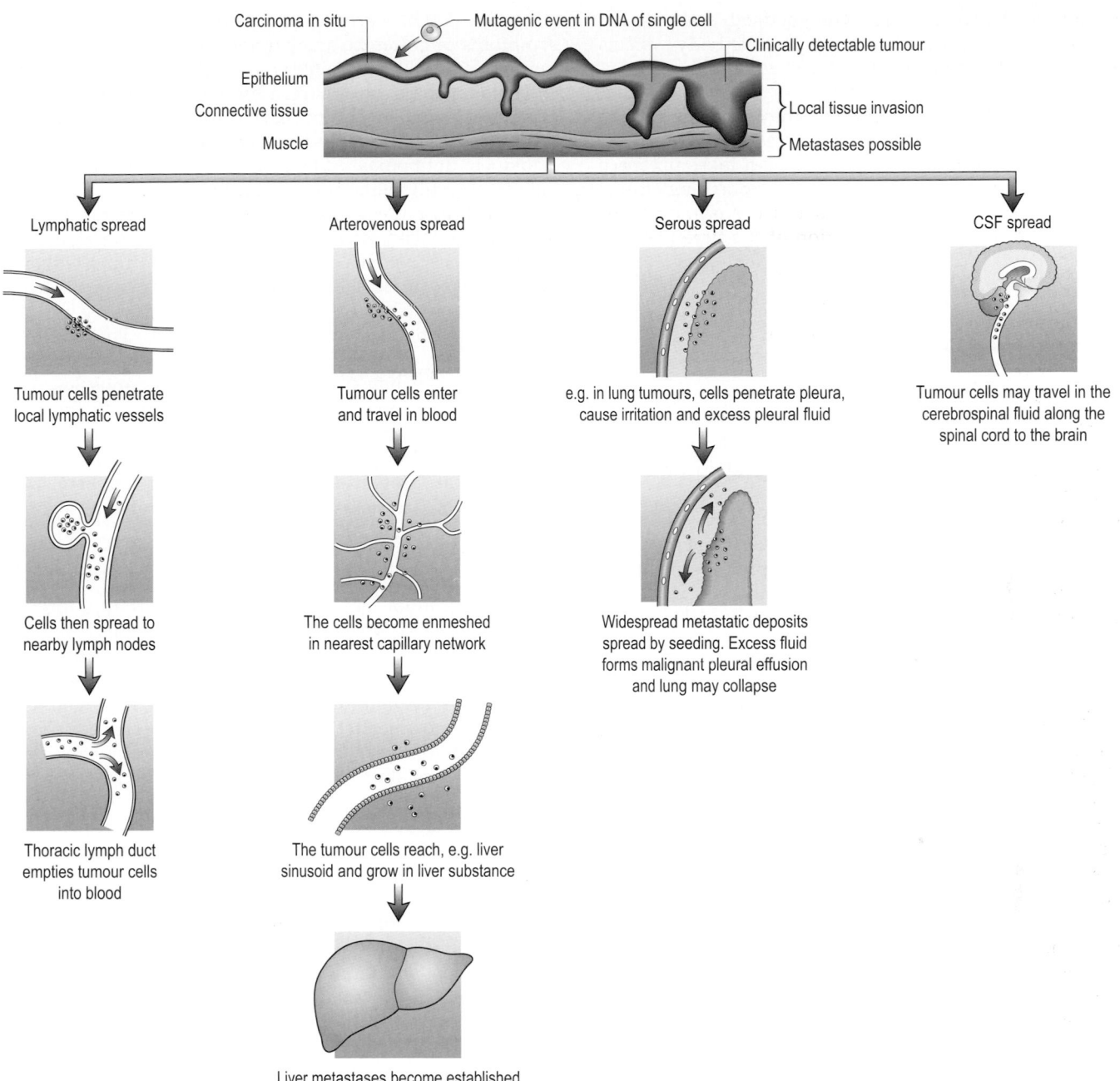

Fig. 31.1 The cancer process.

Arteriovenous spread Tumour cells enter blood vessels near the primary tumour or are shed into the blood via the thoracic lymph duct. They then become enmeshed in the next capillary network they encounter. Hence cancer of certain organs has a certain pattern of spread; gastrointestinal tumours, for example, typically spread via the portal venous system, initially to the liver.

Serous cavity spread Serous membranes, e.g. the pleura or the peritoneum, may be invaded by tumours, either locally from the primary tumour or from nearby metastases. Resulting irritation causes excess serous fluid to be produced, which can distribute cancer cells widely in the serous cavity. This process is called 'seeding'. The excess fluid forms malignant pleural effusions or ascites.

CSF spread Similarly, tumour cells may spread directly in the CSF. Some brain tumours metastasise along the spinal cord in this fashion.

The most common sites of metastatic deposit are the lungs, bones, brain and liver. Two-thirds of patients develop metastases; in half of these, dissemination occurs before diagnosis, and often even before symptoms arise.

The effects of cancer

The manifestations of cancer depend directly or indirectly on the location, size and type of tumour involved and on the extent of any metastases. The medical and nursing problems associated with cancers of particular body systems are covered in preceding chapters.

Direct tumour effects Symptoms may be due to the following direct tumour or metastatic effects.

Occupation of limited space Because it takes up space within the body, the tumour can cause the following effects:

- obstruction of ducts and tracts, e.g. the oesophagus, causing dysphagia
- compression of major blood vessels, e.g. tumours at the apex of the lung or metastatic mediastinal lymph nodes may compress the superior vena cava, causing ischaemia, oedema of the head, neck and right arm, and dyspnoea
- compression of neighbouring tissues and organs, e.g. brain metastases may cause pressure and local oedema, which can compromise brain function and level of consciousness, depending on the area of brain tissue involved
- pressure on regional nerves, causing pain and/or paralysis, e.g. metastases in the spinal vertebrae may compress the spinal cord and result in pain or loss of sensation and paralysis from the level of the lesion downward (spinal cord compression, one of the significant oncological emergencies)
- invasion and replacement of normal tissue, e.g. gastric tumours often spread diffusely across the gastric mucosa, compromising digestive function.

Haemorrhage Tumours may invade small local blood vessels, causing chronic bleeding and anaemia. Occasionally haemorrhage may be sudden and fatal, as when a major blood vessel such as the carotid artery is eroded.

Ulceration Tumour tissue growth may outstrip local blood supply, causing necrosis, or ulceration, of part of the tumour and adjacent normal tissue. This ulceration may be internal or external. Advanced breast tumours may result in surface ulceration. Due to their appearance, these lesions are often termed 'fungating'.

Infection This is very common, being seen as the cause of death in 50% of patients with metastatic cancer. Increased susceptibility to infection is caused by malnutrition, cancer treatments and, sometimes, by metastatic invasion of the bone marrow, compromising haemopoiesis. Eroded or ulcerating tumours are prone to local infection, which may then become systemic.

Metabolic imbalances These are numerous and tumour-specific and, in advanced disease, may become widespread. Tumours of the pancreas may cause disturbance in glucose metabolism. Liver metastases may alter ability to metabolise essential medication and renal tumours cause progressive renal failure, leading to fluid and electrolyte imbalance.

Hypercalcaemia is a common and serious manifestation of advanced cancer of the breast, bone, lung and kidney and is caused by bone destruction due to metastases or by the tumour's production of substances causing bone dissolution.

Indirect tumour effects These are sometimes termed 'paraneoplastic' effects (or syndromes) and may be the presenting features before diagnosis in 10–15% of patients (Haapoja 2000). Early detection is important as these symptoms can often be ameliorated even when the primary tumour cannot be controlled.

The syndromes result from the secretion of substances, usually proteins, by the primary tumour or its metastases. These substances include hormones, growth factors, cytokines, antibodies and other immune products, which indirectly result in a multitude of disorders (see Fig. 31.2).

Almost all patients with cancer will experience at least one paraneoplastic effect. For example, approximately two-thirds of cancer patients suffer some degree of cancer cachexia. This complex syndrome has been termed 'a physical fading of wholeness' (Costa 1977). It involves progressive and extreme weight loss and muscle wasting. The resulting weakness can be very severe and death may eventually ensue due to exhaustion of the respiratory muscles. This is most common in patients with gastrointestinal and lung tumours. The causes are multifactorial; however, research has demonstrated increased basal metabolic rate and disturbed fat, protein and carbohydrate metabolism, with accompanying anorexia, altered digestion and absorption of nutrients (Tisdale 2000, Inui 2002).

Prognosis and the cause of death The risk of disease recurrence cannot be discounted with certainty until a period of several years has elapsed. This length of time depends on the type of cancer and varies from 3 to 20 years, so for practical purposes a limit of 5 years is often used to estimate survival rates. The term 'cure' is, however, used cautiously; most health care professionals prefer the phrase 'complete remission'. However, these concepts are often open to interpretation, creating ambiguity and lack of understanding (Chapman et al 2003). It is therefore important for health care professionals to clarify their meaning for patients.

This uncertain outlook can probably be explained by the fact that malignant cells, which are often undetectable by current diagnostic techniques, frequently persist despite treatment and in time cause local recurrence of the tumour and/or metastases. Many factors intervene, however, such that no patient's prognosis can be calculated with certainty.

It may seem obvious that any of the effects of cancer (described on p. 1033) may result in or contribute to death. While this is the case, the immediate cause of death is often uncertain, and in these situations it is generally presumed to be the subtle interplay of the failure of different body systems. The issue of whether or not cognitive and emotional states can influence long-term survival remains controversial, with evidence so far being inconsistent (Petticrew et al 2002). However, Brown et al (2003) suggest that the cancer diagnosis and physical effects of the disease may predispose to distress which, if maintained over time, enhances disease progression.

It is now widely accepted that quality of life in cancer patients may be improved by psychological interventions (Meyer & Mark 1995, Goodwin et al 2001). Prolongation of life, however, is more controversial, but this has opened up an area known as psycho-immunology. There has been increasing speculation in the psychosocial literature on whether intervention groups can lead not only to good outcomes with respect to mood but also to improved chances of survival (Fox 1995, Greer 1995). Preliminary evidence from research by Spiegel et al (1989) and Fawzy

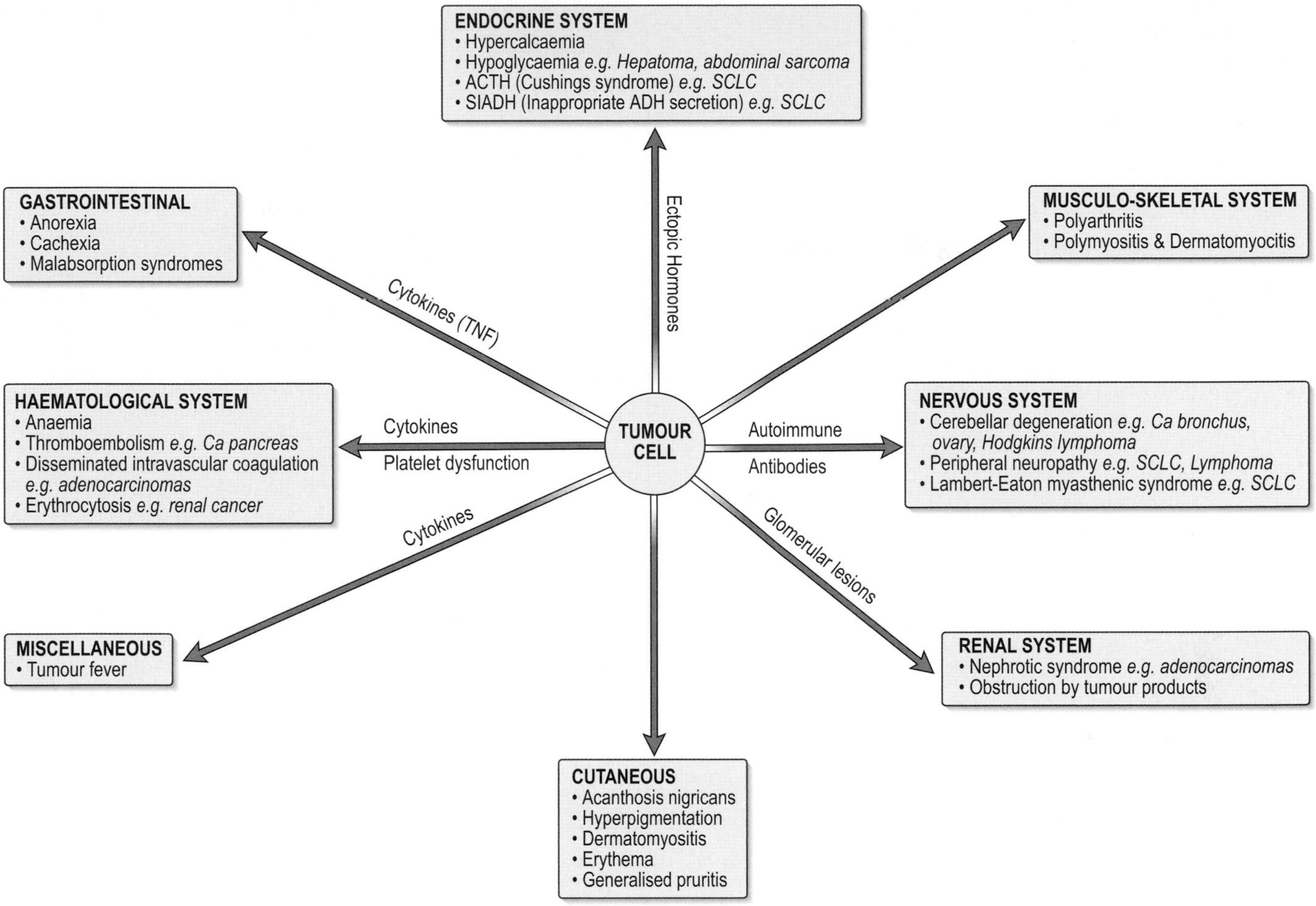

Fig. 31.2 Paraneoplastic syndromes. (Adapted from Haapoja 2000.)

et al (1993) indicated that cancer support groups may foster positive changes in immune function, which may influence tumour growth rate, thus promoting survival. However, at the 10-year follow-up, the survival benefits of the intervention had weakened, though not entirely disappeared. It is difficult to prove this type of relationship, and attributing physical deterioration to the patient's emotional state is not justified (Petticrew et al 2002). Research has also indicated that social deprivation and life crises may have a negative impact on prognosis (Barraclough 1998). A good social support system and elements of spirituality and religious belief appear to be consistent predictors of improved quality of life (Creagan 1997). As the expected time of death is often uncertain, a specific prediction of prognosis is therefore unwise and may even lead to loss of hope.

STOP THINK

31.3 Consider patients you have cared for who have died from cancer. Do you know what was the immediate cause of death? Ask a doctor involved if you are unsure. Is the doctor certain of this cause? Were psychological and social factors important?

31.4 It is common for relatives to want to know the details and exact cause of death of the patient. Discuss with other students why you think this need is so common. Relate any experiences of being with the recently bereaved. What do you think is the nurse's role in the face of this uncertainty? What are the ethical issues involved?

Epidemiology of cancer

Epidemiological studies have given rise to theories about the possible causes of different forms of cancer and hence to strategies for cancer prevention and for the screening of high-risk population groups for early-stage, treatable disease. Figure 31.3 shows the incidence of the 10 most common causes of cancer mortality in the UK.

In the developed world, populations are ageing and age is one of the major risk factors for developing cancer. More than 65% of all people diagnosed with cancer are over 65 years old (Cancer Research UK 2005a). Although cancer is very rare in children, it is now the most common cause of death (after accidents) in those under 15 years, despite the fact that childhood tumours respond to treatment far more readily than those in adults (Cancer Research UK 2004a).

For a discussion of the specialist treatment of paediatric and adolescent cancer care, see Baggott et al (2002).

The incidence of cancer in the UK is one of the highest in the Western world (see Ch. 35). Predominantly, cancer is a disease of the rich, although the pattern is shifting and many developing countries will triple their cancer incidence over the next decade (IARC/WHO 1998, Parkin et al 2002).

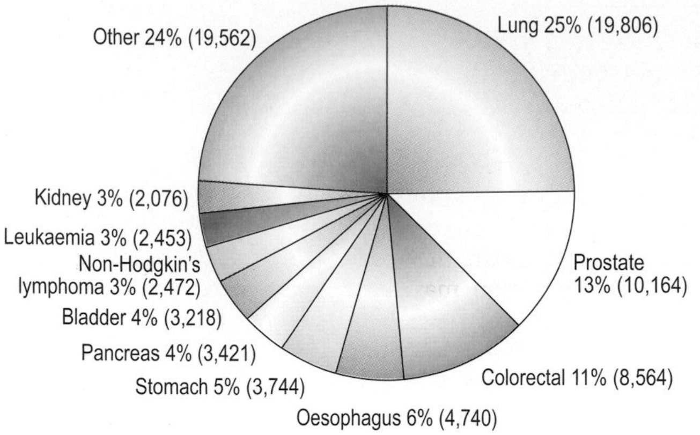

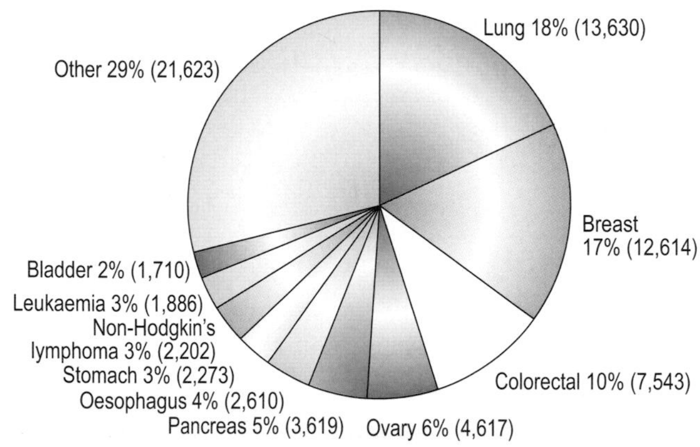

Fig. 31.3 The 10 most common causes of cancer deaths in the UK in 2003. A: Men; total number of cancer deaths = 80 220. B: Women; total number of cancer deaths = 74 327. Variations in the cancer mortality between the sexes reflect, as well as anatomical differences, different behavioural and environmental factors. Although lung cancer represents 22% of all cancers, there is a downward trend which reflects the fall in tobacco consumption since the first two World Wars. However, as smoking increases, particularly among teenage girls, and without effective tobacco control measures, this decreased mortality may be reversed in the future. (Reproduced with permission from Cancer Research UK 2005.)

The greater incidence in Western society may be partly attributed to the more sophisticated screening, diagnostic and reporting procedures. Also with the eradication of smallpox, polio and other diseases, life expectancy is greater. Western diet, industrial pollution and behaviours such as smoking and excessive alcohol consumption are chief environmental causes of cancer.

Geographical variations in the incidence of cancer provide fascinating clues to the causes of the disease. In Mozambique a high incidence of liver cancer is thought to be associated with aflatoxin from mould found on stored peanuts. Since the introduction of more appropriate storage practices, the incidence of liver cancer has been falling (Souhami & Tobias 2005). The Japanese have a low incidence of breast cancer but a high incidence of stomach cancer. However, within one or two generations, Japanese immigrants to Hawaii showed the American pattern of a high incidence of breast cancer and a moderate incidence of stomach cancer (Haenszel & Kurihera 1968). This seminal study and other similar studies indicate that geographical variations in cancer incidence are attributable to environmental rather than genetic factors; however, there may be an interaction with genetic disposition.

Epidemiological investigation of genetic predisposition to cancer is growing rapidly as developments in molecular biology make it possible to study genetic markers in large populations. The completion of the Human Genome Project (see Box 31.2) is accelerating the discovery of such markers (Peters et al 2001, Loud et al 2002).

Box 31.2

Human Genome Project

In the mid-1980s, it was first suggested that the fundamental problem of cancer could be addressed by studying the sequence of the entire human genome. Initiated in 1988, the specific aim of the International Human Genome Project (HGP) was to map the estimated 50 000–1 000 000 genes determining the sequence of nucleotides that make up the human genome. With the initial sequencing and analysis now complete, demonstrating 30 000 genes, the availability of this information is helping to unlock biological processes, allowing the translation of this knowledge into cancer care. Major opportunities are developing for identifying those at risk of developing cancer and the ability to detect cancer early (screening), and for more effective cancer treatments (pharmacogenetics).

From its inception, it was recognised that acquiring and using genetic knowledge would have profound implications for both the individual and society. Therefore, the analysis of the ethical, legal and social implications associated with the availability of this information is a major component of the HGP.

A series of articles highlighting the explosion of information and technology in this genetic revolution and its implications for oncology nursing are detailed in 'Further reading' (p. 1070) and include Calzone & Masny (2004), Greco & Mahon (2004), Jenkins (2004), Kwitkowski & Daub (2004), Loud & Hutson (2004), Lowrey (2004), Rieger (2004) and Vadaparampil et al (2004).

The causes of cancer

Most cancers develop through the interaction of genetic and environmental factors and it is difficult to separate the two completely. Although all cancers have a genetic origin at the cellular level, this does not mean all cancer is inherited. Genetic is a general term used when discussing genes or chromosomes. Genetic changes or mutations may be either *somatic* (acquired) or *germline* (inherited).

- *Germline mutations* are those present in the egg or sperm of a parent that can be passed to the offspring through

fertilisation. The mutation is present in every cell of the body.
- *Somatic mutation* is when an individual body cell, postconception, acquires a gene alteration. If not repaired, the mutation is passed on to all future cells through mitosis. These clonal changes are unique to the cells in that particular tissue and are not inherited.

Many questions remain to be answered regarding the exact mechanisms involved in the cellular mutations that lead to cancer. However, epidemiological studies have identified certain causative factors, termed 'carcinogens'. Knowledge of identified carcinogens is essential for:

- the development of prevention and screening strategies
- the provision of accurate information for patients, allaying the myths surrounding cancer causation.

Carcinogenesis is multifactorial and factors may enhance or inhibit the process. Stages include:

- *initiation* — a mutagenic event occurs in the DNA of a single cell; this may, for example, be radiation-induced
- *promotion* — repeated exposure to carcinogenic agents may or may not cause this initiated cell to proliferate to form a tumour.

A long latency period may exist between carcinogen exposure and cancer development. Carcinogenic factors and substances can be divided into those that are intrinsic and those that are extrinsic to the individual.

Intrinsic factors

Heredity Inherited cancers contribute 5–10% of all cancers. Several genes have now been identified that are responsible for predisposing individuals to develop certain cancers. For example, childhood tumours such as retinoblastoma are due to inherited chromosomal abnormalities. Cancers that occur with increased frequency in families are components of various hereditary cancer syndromes, e.g. hereditary non-polyposis colon cancer (HNPCC).

Cancer susceptibility genes such as BRCA1 and BRCA2 have been identified in breast and ovarian cancer. Women who inherit a mutation in these genes may face a 50–85% lifetime risk of developing breast cancer including an increased risk for ovarian cancer (Calzone & Biesecker 2002). Testing for these particular genes and others is now available commercially. (See Ch. 6 for more details regarding genetics and the implications for individuals with cancer).

Hormones Excessive amounts of certain hormones are thought to promote some tumours. Early menarche, late menopause and nulliparity are all associated with a high incidence of breast cancer, implying that prolonged exposure to oestrogen is a causative factor (Toniolo et al 1995). Results of the Million Women Study (2003) in the UK have confirmed that use of combined oestrogen plus progesterone hormone replacement therapy (HRT) increases the risk of breast cancer. This risk increase is duration dependent, declining when HRT is discontinued and, by 5 years, the risk level is the same as that of a non-user (Million Women Study Collaborators 2003). Endometrial cancer risk increases with exposure to 'unopposed' oestrogen, i.e. oestrogen only HRT, obesity, the sequential use of oral contraceptives and a late menopause. High levels of gonadotrophins are associated with an increased risk of ovarian cancer (Henderson & Bernstein 1997) and high testosterone levels have been related to prostate cancer (Ross et al 2003).

Immunity Individuals with impaired immunity are more prone to cancer than others; for example, people with AIDS have a high incidence of Kaposi's sarcoma (see Ch. 37). This does not mean that cancer is an infectious disease. Immunosuppression may predispose to certain infections, which may then contribute to the cancer process.

Pre-existing disease Any tissue subjected to constant irritation or to some disease process has an increased susceptibility to malignant change. Hence, ulcerative colitis may precede colonic carcinoma.

Age The rising incidence of cancer with age is thought to be attributable to:

- prolonged exposure to carcinogens
- decreased resistance to carcinogens
- hormonal changes that occur with age.

Extrinsic factors

The fact that 70% of cancers occur in epithelial cells that are constantly exposed to external, ingested or inhaled substances implies that extrinsic factors related to lifestyle and the environment are important in carcinogenesis. These factors may be considered under the following headings:

- physical agents
- chemical agents
- viruses
- diet.

Physical agents

Radiation is known to cause cellular mutations and cancer. Survivors of the atomic bomb explosions in Hiroshima and Nagasaki experienced a high incidence of leukaemia and skin cancer. Early research has shown an apparent increase in the incidence of leukaemia among the children of fathers working in the nuclear industry, possibly due to germ cell mutations (Gardner et al 1990). Repeated exposure to therapeutic doses of radiation is not thought to be harmful, although stringent precautionary regulations should be followed for the protection of all exposed workers. Therefore, it is not routine discharge of radioactivity by the nuclear industry that should be feared, but rather the catastrophic event, such as occurred at Three Mile Island in 1979 and at Chernobyl in 1986. In the former accident, radioactive noble gases were released into the atmosphere. By the worst estimate, there will be one radiation-induced cancer death in the 2 million people living around the reactor. Chernobyl, however, released much of its radioactive core into the atmosphere and will account for an increase of 2–3% in related cancer deaths (Hall 1997).

UV light There is overwhelming evidence that repeated exposure to solar UV light is the primary cause of basal and squamous cell carcinoma. Data establishing a direct causal relationship with sunlight are more complex, but suggest a promotional role of sunlight in the cause of melanoma. Fair-skinned or freckled individuals who are unable to manufacture sufficient protective melanin are particularly at risk (see Ch. 12).

Chemical agents Ninety per cent of all lung cancer cases can be attributed to tobacco smoking. The temporal relationship between smoking and lung cancer was defined in the 1950s by studies undertaken by Doll and Hill (1954). Cigarette smoking has now clearly been identified as a major cause of cancers of the mouth, pharynx, larynx, bladder and pancreas, whilst contributing to many others. Risk is more dependent on duration of smoking than on consumption. Smoking 20 cigarettes a day for 40 years is eight times more hazardous than smoking 40 cigarettes a day for 20 years. People who stop smoking even well into middle age avoid most of their subsequent risk of lung cancer and stopping before middle age avoids more than 90% of the risk attributable to tobacco (Peto et al 2000). It is also evident that non-smokers are at risk from exposure to other people's smoke: one-quarter of lung cancer cases in non-smokers are estimated to be due to passive smoking (Trichopoulus et al 1981, DH 1998a,b, IARC 2004).

Excessive alcohol, ingested over long periods of time, contributes to cancers of the mouth, pharynx, oesophagus and liver. Those who drink spirits as opposed to wine and beer and those who smoke as well as drink are particularly at risk (see Ch. 36).

Many other chemicals, whether inhaled, ingested or absorbed through the skin, have been shown to cause cancer. Lung cancer in non-smokers is most prevalent in large cities where traffic fumes and chimney smoke raise atmospheric levels of polycyclic hydrocarbons, the same chemicals present in cigarette smoke.

Other carcinogenic chemicals present occupational hazards. Some of these, but by no means all, are now subject to government control or ban. These controlled substances, and associated cancer sites, include:

- asbestos (lung, mesothelium and larynx)
- vinyl chloride (liver)
- certain chemical dyes (bladder)
- arsenic (lung and skin)
- some hardwood dusts (nasopharynx).

Viruses Although cancer is not contagious, viral infections account for one in seven human cancers worldwide (Poeschla & Wong-Staal 1997). The Epstein–Barr virus causes a systemic infection that may precede Burkitt's lymphoma, a malignant disease common in parts of Africa. Patients with chronic hepatitis B are more susceptible than others to liver cancer. The human papilloma virus, which may be sexually transmitted, is associated with cervical cancer and *Helicobacter pylori* is estimated to cause 60% of cases of stomach cancer in the USA (Cole & Rodu 2001).

Diet Epidemiological studies that isolate diet as a causal factor in the development of cancer are extremely problematic to undertake. Nevertheless, dietary factors have been implicated as a major cause of the high incidence of cancer in the West. Countries where the average diet is high in fat and protein appear to have a high incidence of breast cancer, and low-fibre diets are thought to contribute to bowel cancer. Some food additives have been found to be carcinogenic and have been removed from the market, although many others have not yet been fully investigated.

Cancer prevention and screening

Prevention of human cancers is a major focus of research and education. The principal hope lies in the rigorous application of prevention and screening programmes. The goal of primary prevention is to reduce the risk of the healthy population developing cancer. Secondary prevention aims to detect early-stage, curable, cancer. Primary prevention is therefore the most effective and economic method of controlling cancer.

Nurses now have a much wider role, incorporating health promotion, health education and disease prevention as well as the care of those who are ill. This wider role is reflected in their initial and post-basic education. Many health visitors, district nurses and practice nurses working in community health centres offer innovative health promotion programmes, as well as screening for ill-health. Antenatal care, well-woman or well-man clinics, family planning centres and other health screening clinics all provide opportunities for the promotion of cancer prevention. In clinical practice, nurse specialists are now incorporating cancer awareness and prevention in their roles, with many involved in local and national initiatives such as cancer site-specific awareness weeks and health promotion in schools.

Primary prevention

Primary cancer prevention is true health promotion and includes such activities as:

- identifying risk factors in individuals or groups
- counselling high-risk individuals to promote behaviour modification
- genetic screening
- implementation of new cancer prevention programmes, e.g. smoking cessation, healthy eating.

Walker (1990) argued that cancer prevention programmes that use fear of the disease to motivate compliance may be counterproductive. Media reporting of cancer risk development requires cautious interpretation and should be put into perspective by reference to the original studies on which they are based. It is important to remember, for example, that substances that are carcinogenic in animals are by no means always so in humans. Moreover, everyday exposure to some of the substances implicated is so minimal as to make risk insignificant. Some of these media scares do little to promote health; fear of cancer, after all, is one of the most common reasons why people avoid screening or fail to present with symptoms.

Health promotion programmes Box 31.3 lists actions that people can take to reduce their risk of cancer. Arguably, observing these guidelines will result in a healthier lifestyle with a low risk of many health problems including cancer. Health promotion programmes should explore practical and realistic ways of assisting people to integrate such generally healthy behaviours into their daily lives.

Box 31.3

Lifestyle and cancer — how to reduce your risk

Two-thirds of all cancers are linked to lifestyle and could be prevented.

- Breathe clean air. Stub out cigarettes — the longer you give up cigarettes, the more you reduce your cancer risk.
- Drink sensibly — all alcohol in moderation following recommended guidelines.
- Eat healthily — a diet low in fat and rich in fruit, vegetables and fibre.
- Be active — exercise moderately for at least 30 min five times a week. Avoid being overweight.
- Protect yourself in the sun — don't burn and follow recommended advice for protection.
- Take care with chemicals or radiation exposure — follow Health and Safety instructions.
- Be body aware — know your body and what is normal for you.
- Know the early signs of cancer — see your doctor about unusual lumps, moles, bleeding or other persistent symptoms.
- Go for screening — early changes can be picked up and the chance of successful treatment maximised.
- Practise safe sex — using a condom decreases the chance of passing on a virus.

Adapted from Cancer Research UK (2002).

Health education programmes have some measure of success (Ewles & Simnett 2003). The Community Intervention Trial for Smoking Cessation (COMMIT) funded by the National Cancer Institute (NCI) was designed to test the effectiveness of a 4-year community-based intervention programme to help smokers achieve and maintain cessation. The programme had a positive effect on light to moderate smokers, but no significant impact on the heavy smokers' group (COMMIT Research Group 1995). These results are both positive and disappointing. However, it has provided important information regarding future cessation programmes. Dissemination of knowledge, it appears, is not in itself sufficient to motivate changes in behaviour.

Several government publications have taken on 'The Cancer Challenge', with measures to promote a 'pro-health' culture (Scottish Office 1999, DH 2000a, SEHD 2003). Projects have been developed to assist smokers to quit, particularly in areas with high levels of deprivation, prisons, the army, and working men's clubs. Political action has included a comprehensive ban on tobacco advertising, reduction of smoking in public places and the workplace, the setting up of new 'stop smoking clinics' and a smokers helpline, nicotine replacement patches and bupropion (Zyban) available on prescription, as well as a major health education campaign in schools aimed at preventing youngsters from starting to smoke (DH 2000a, SEHD 2003).

Through working partnerships with the community and the food industry, strategies to promote healthy eating include a national 'Five a Day' programme, improving accessibility to affordable fresh fruit and vegetables, and advocating five portions of these daily. The national School Fruit Scheme ensures that fruit is available each day at school for children 4–6 years of age. However, if an impact is to be made, continuing legislation is required regarding the control of tobacco sales, occupational exposure to carcinogens and regulation of food additives.

Attitudes Many factors other than knowledge deficit are known to affect a person's health attitudes. Psychologists have developed a Health Belief Model (Strecher & Rosenstock 1997) to predict an individual's preventive health behaviour and account for some of the factors which determine attitudes to health and illness.

The Health Belief Model states that an individual feels vulnerable to a disease if they believe they are susceptible to developing it and believe the disease to be serious. Preventive action will be taken only after the individual has balanced the benefits of that action against its physical, psychological and financial costs (Fernsler & Miller 2000).

Despite being taught about the risks of smoking, teenage smokers may consider themselves to be young and healthy and therefore not 'at risk'. Young people in general are motivated by short-term rather than long-term rewards. Smoking in some subcultures and families is associated with attributes such as maturity or rebelliousness, which the young person and their peer group may value. Later, the physical addiction to nicotine becomes a coping mechanism for life's stresses and social deprivation. For such people, possible avoidance of lung cancer is not worth the cost of surrendering the immediate gratification and social status offered by smoking.

Clearly, consideration of the wider causes of individual behaviour would lead those involved in health promotion to an awareness of the social and political action necessary. Most cancers are more common in lower socioeconomic groups than in more affluent groups, yet uptake of preventive and screening services is lower in the former. The causes of social deprivation need to be considered alongside individual behaviour. Preventive services must be readily accessible and based on the expressed needs of the community, e.g. on the principle of client-centred care (DH 1998c).

The concepts of health and ill-health are open to wide interpretation. An essential aspect of communication is that everyone understands and attaches the same meaning to language used. If adherence to health care programmes is to be achieved, nurses need to understand an individual's personal health beliefs and how information is interpreted (Wilkinson 1999).

STOP THINK

31.5 Using the Health Belief Model, consider the factors that would be taken into account by a community or practice-based nurse working in liaison with an area health promotion officer in devising a cancer prevention programme in the following community health centres:

(a) An inner city practice in which 50% of the population are first- and second-generation immigrants from the Indian subcontinent. The remaining 50% consist of students in rented housing, young professional people in their first jobs and homes, and workers in a local petrochemical industry.

(b) A new town practice covering a large area of farmland. The new town housing estates accommodate a large percentage of single, unemployed parents. The nearest large hospital is 20 miles away.

Discuss this as a group. Also consider how community nurses in each centre might incorporate cancer prevention into their practice.

Secondary prevention: screening

The prognosis of patients with most types of cancer is very much improved if the tumour is detected at an early stage. Often, complete cure can be assured if pre-cancerous tissue can be identified and treated, as in the case of cervical intraepithelial neoplasia (CIN).

Cancer screening issues The development of accurate and cost-effective methods of screening at-risk sections of the population is problematic for several reasons. The test must have both a high degree of sensitivity, reducing the risk of false-negative results, and specificity, reducing the psychological trauma and expense of treating false-positive results. It must be possible to identify an at-risk group, otherwise the cost of screening becomes prohibitive. Finally, and most problematically, it must be determined whether detecting the cancer type at an early stage will actually prolong life (Segnan et al 2004). In the case of small cell lung cancer, for example, early detection with existing tests would simply mean that patients would have an earlier knowledge of their diagnosis, but still live for the same number of years (see Ch. 3).

Two standard screening methods concern cancers affecting women:

- breast cancer screening
- cervical screening.

Breast cancer screening Despite recent debates about the quality of over 40 years of trials, it is generally agreed that there is a clear benefit and reduction in mortality from breast cancer from screening women over the age of 50 years by mammography every 2 years (IARC 2002). Accepted screening techniques include mammography and clinical breast examination, although Baxter (2001) has concluded that breast self-examination is of no benefit in routine screening. Controversy still surrounds the value of screening women of 40 years or younger, consequently professional clinical judgement and a woman's choice should guide decision-making. The denser breast tissue of premenopausal women makes mammograms difficult to interpret in this age group. In future, genetic screening and new technologies such as digital mammography may be of benefit.

Cervical cancer screening Cervical cancer is among the most common of female cancers in developing countries. Since the introduction of the Pap (Papanicolaou) smear test over 20 years ago, there has been a steady decline in mortality rates in the UK (Cancer Research UK 2005b). New guidelines in the USA suggest that smears should be taken from 3 years after the onset of vaginal intercourse, which for some women in the UK is below the age at which screening is offered, i.e. 25 years (Smith et al 2003). However, some GPs may offer early screening as part of their consultation with women regarding sexual health.

Initially, uptake of the service by groups at highest risk, i.e. women over the age of 40, of lower socioeconomic status and in minority ethnic groups, was poor. Barriers to cervical screening include lack of sensitivity and trust in health professionals; possible feelings of guilt and embarrassment may be exaggerated by judgemental attitudes, a lack of privacy and supportive care in clinics (Fitch et al 1998). It is important for staff working in screening services to have well-developed interpersonal and communication skills to alleviate any fears or anxieties. In addition, clinic schedules should allow time for giving support.

Intervention strategies based on individual respect, health care provider relationships and inclusion of significant others may increase adherence to cancer screening guidelines (Steven et al 2004). For example, the recent provision of culturally sensitive information to women in minority ethnic groups has been successful, as evidenced by improved service uptake (DH 2000a).

There has been controversy regarding the reliability of screening tests and accurate detection of abnormal smears. However, the introduction of liquid-based cytology, and the potential to detect human papilloma virus in the same sample, are thought to reduce the number of inadequate smears (Uyar et al 2003).

Screening for other cancers Screening programmes for other cancers are now under scrutiny, including:

- colon cancer
- prostate cancer
- ovarian cancer
- lung cancer.

Colon cancer The natural history of colon cancer with the relatively long time from biological onset to the development of cancer makes it a good candidate for screening. A UK pilot for colorectal cancer screening tested the value of the faecal occult blood (FOB) test for early detection and mortality reduction (Scholefield et al 2002) and, as a result, a national bowel screening programme is to begin in 2006 (Birmingham 2004). Further trials are also being conducted looking at the role of flexible sigmoidoscopy in diagnosis (Boyle et al 2003). The proposed screening interval is 2 years for those aged 50–69 years. Campaigns by Colon Cancer Concern have been initiated to promote a greater awareness of the early warning signs of colon cancer. Emerging future technologies to improve sensitivity include virtual colonoscopy and DNA testing of stools.

Prostate cancer There is at present no consensus regarding the most appropriate screening method. There are three main screening modalities: digital rectal examination (DRE), serum prostate-specific antigen (PSA) and transrectal ultrasonography (TRUS). There are wide ranges in the estimates of sensitivity and specificity. Interest in PSA (a blood test) emerged in the late 1980s when it was shown that, post-prostatectomy, previously abnormal PSA levels reduced by half (Catalona et al 1991). However, PSA may be elevated in men with non-cancerous conditions. There is currently no evidence that prostatic screening improves clinical outcomes; in fact, there are issues of uncertainty surrounding the appropriateness and type of treatment for men with early-stage prostatic cancer, since it has a long asymptomatic latency period. It is therefore important to consider that there might be an adverse psychological impact as a result of prostate screening although, for those men at risk, it may provide some reassurance (Cantor et al 2002).

To address some of these concerns, a prostate risk management programme has recently been introduced which sets out initiatives to improve men's understanding of the benefits and limitations of PSA testing (NHS Cancer Screening Programme 2004). Working in conjunction with CancerBACUP (see 'Useful websites'), a booklet explaining the PSA test has been produced.

Ovarian cancer Transvaginal ultrasound and detection of a raised cancer antigen (CA125) in the blood provide two possible techniques for the screening of ovarian cancer. However, as with PSA, CA125 may be elevated in non-malignant conditions. A UK collaborative trial of ovarian cancer screening (UKCTOCS) aims to answer the question of whether or not early detection will save lives. The effectiveness of different screening technologies will be examined and a report is expected in 2010.

Women known to have a high familial risk of developing ovarian cancer are offered annual screening as part of a national familial ovarian cancer screening study.

Lung cancer It has been shown that low dose spiral CT scanning can identify lung cancer in high risk but asymptomatic individuals (Gohagan et al 2005). Whilst this may be a useful screening test, evidence is required to substantiate a link with decrease in mortality.

Screening in the future With the discovery of susceptibility genes, cancer prevention will become a more prominent area of cancer care. The provision of psychological support during screening and for decision making regarding treatment in cases with a positive diagnosis requires considerable knowledge, skill and sensitivity on the part of nurses and team colleagues.

STOP THINK **31.6** Consider the role of (a) school nurses and (b) occupational health nurses in the primary and secondary prevention of cancer. Try to arrange to spend a day with one of these practitioners, and identify the elements of their role which could be further expanded to fulfil this function.

CASE HISTORY 31.1(A)

D

D, a 22-year-old student, discovered a testicular swelling but chose to ignore it, initially because he misinterpreted it as a sports injury, and later because he felt embarrassed. Nine months later he presented to the student health centre because he was becoming breathless far more readily than usual and suffered a constant backache. These symptoms were due to lung metastases and referred pain caused by metastases in the para-aortic lymph nodes.

CASE HISTORY 31.1(B)

D *(cont'd from Case History 31.1(A))*

D was admitted to a surgical ward, where a biopsy under anaesthesia was performed. A frozen section taken for histology showed a testicular teratoma. A left orchidectomy was then performed.

Following postoperative recovery, D was taken to an oncology ward for staging. D lived too far away to travel to the department each day, otherwise the necessary tests could have been performed while he was an outpatient. The tests were carried out and their results were as follows:

- chest X-ray: showed multiple lung metastases
- thoracic CT scan: confirmed lung metastases
- abdominal CT scan: showed a large para-aortic lymph node and no liver metastases
- blood samples for full blood count, urea, creatinine and electrolytes, liver function and tumour markers (AFP and HCG).

These tests showed that D had stage IV testicular teratoma; however, even extensive disease is curable with cisplatin-based chemotherapy (Souhami & Tobias 2005). Accordingly, this was the treatment course chosen.

Creatinine clearance is calculated from the serum creatinine to establish baseline measurements for subsequent assessment of any nephrotoxicity induced by platinum compounds.

CASE HISTORY 31.2

Mrs F

Mrs F is 45, married and has three grown-up children. She is very health conscious and presents herself every 3 years for a cervical smear at the occupational health centre of her workplace. On this occasion, she is informed that her smear is positive. Subsequent colposcopy reveals carcinoma in situ, i.e. a pre-invasive cancer of the cervical cells that is curable by cone biopsy or laser therapy.

MEDICAL INTERVENTION AND THE NURSE'S ROLE

Diagnosis and staging

Patients present with cancer in a wide variety of ways. Consider the different physical and psychosocial care needs of the three patients in Case Histories 31.1–31.3.

Patients may present at any point in the disease process, ranging from the premalignant to the metastatic phase. Staging is the process whereby the extent of the disease is established; this involves a varied number of tests for each patient (see the appropriate chapter for a given tumour site). Diagnosis and staging are carried out in a variety of settings, depending on the patient's presenting signs and symptoms. This process can be long, complex and tedious for the patient, raising many issues of uncertainty. However, accurate staging of the extent of the disease is vital for the following reasons:

- Certain modes of treatment are known to be effective at specific disease stages. For example, thoracic surgery for Mr H (see Case History 31.3) would be inappropriate given the dissemination of his disease. Staging spares the human and financial cost of inappropriate treatment.
- Prognosis can be estimated according to the disease stage and cell differentiation (see p. 328).

CASE HISTORY 31.3

Mr H

Mr H is a 76-year-old widower. A heavy smoker, he has suffered from chronic bronchitis for 30 years. His respiratory symptoms have seemed more troublesome lately, but it is pain in the ribs and back (due to bone metastases) which finally cause him to consult his GP. These pains are initially considered to be arthritic in nature, causing further delay in the eventual diagnosis of disseminated small cell bronchogenic carcinoma.

Box 31.4

Summary of the TNM staging system for lung cancer

T (primary tumour)

TX	Positive cytology only
Tis	Carcinoma in situ
T1	Tumour ≤3 cm in diameter. No proximal invasion
T2	Tumour >3 cm in diameter, within 2 cm from carina or invading the visceral pleura or partial atelectasis
T3	Tumour of any size extending into the chest wall, diaphragm, pericardium, mediastinal pleura or within 2 cm of carina, total atelectasis
T4	Tumour of any size with invasion of mediastinal organs or vertebral body, malignant pleural effusion

N (lymph nodes)

N0	Nodes negative
N1	Positive nodes in ipsilateral hilar nodes
N2	Positive ipsilateral, mediastinal and subcarinal nodes
N3	Positive contralateral mediastinal or hilar nodes, scalene or supraclavicular nodes

M (distant metastases)

M0	No metastases
M1	Metastases present

The disease is then staged using the above information, as follows:

Stage IA	T1	N0	M0
Stage IB	T2	N0	M0
Stage IIA	T1	N1	M0
Stage IIB	T2	N1	M0
	T3	N0	M0
Stage IIIA	T1–3	N2	M0
Stage IIIB	T4	Any N	M0
Stage IV	Any T	Any N	M1

Adapted from Sobin & Wittekind (2002).

Box 31.5

UK staging system of testicular tumours

Stage I	Tumour confined to testes
Stage II	Pelvic and abdominal lymph node involvement
Stage III	Mediastinal and/or supraclavicular lymph node involvement
Stage IV	Distant metastases, e.g. lung

- Staging information is valuable for cancer research, for statistical analysis and in considerations of the patient's eligibility to enter a trial of a new treatment.

The TNM system

The most common internationally used method of defining disease stages is the TNM system (Sobin & Wittekind 2002), in which:

- T denotes the size or extent of local invasion of the primary tumour
- N refers to the spread to local lymph nodes
- M refers to the presence of metastases.

Box 31.4 illustrates the use of the TNM system in carcinoma of the lung. Some types of cancer — usually those that are disseminated at presentation — cannot be effectively staged with the TNM system and have necessitated the development of other systems. Box 31.5 shows the staging system generally used in the UK for testicular tumours. During the course of their illness, patients may be restaged in order for their response to treatment, or the extent of disease recurrence, to be assessed. Case History 31.1(B) illustrates the experience of staging for a patient with testicular cancer.

Psychological impact of diagnosis and staging

Confirmation of diagnosis It is very common for patients to be aware that they have cancer before they are told formally of their diagnosis. This awareness derives from their experience of symptoms, tests and, in some cases, surgery and from the non-verbal communication of staff or relatives. How to inform patients in *full* of their diagnosis, and when this should be done are ongoing issues of ethical debate (see Box 31.6).

Even if they suspect their diagnosis, patients often cling to hope or use denial as a coping mechanism (Stephenson 2004). These are the early emotional reactions experienced by people facing any actual or potential life crisis or loss, as described by Kübler-Ross in her seminal text (1973).

For further reading, see Niven (1999).

For most patients, confirmation of their fears comes as a devastating shock; this is often followed for varying periods by a normal stress reaction, which may include anxiety, depression, insomnia and poor concentration. This stressful time is one of great emotional confusion, during which the individual attempts to adjust to a shattered world. Relatives and friends also experience a conflict between their desire to be supportive and their fear of impending change and loss. The following words summarise the feelings of one patient immediately after she was told of her diagnosis (Evans 1989):

> *Then he mentioned cancer. I suddenly went numb, rooted to the spot. The only thing that I could think of was that I was going to die. With that one word he had shattered my well-ordered world. I felt my life was closing in on me. I wanted to cry but the tears would not come. I wanted to laugh but it was not funny. Shock and fear invaded my*

Box 31.6

Informing patients of their diagnosis: ethical considerations

Two ethical principles are central to the discussion of whether it is always right to tell a patient the whole truth about their diagnosis: these are the principles of autonomy and of beneficence (for a fuller discussion, see Thomson et al 2000).

Autonomy
Patients have a right to autonomy, or self-determination. They cannot make decisions about their treatment or the future if they are not fully aware of their diagnosis. However, research has suggested that denial as a coping mechanism is sometimes necessary for the preservation of well-being during a crisis, allowing an individual time to mobilise the resources to cope with the seriousness of their disease (Moyer & Levine 1998). Unlike 30 years ago, patients are now normally told their diagnosis, with a discussion of prognosis — often a medical uncertainty — and the level of information is tailored to the individual's needs. There is no evidence to suggest that acceptance correlates positively to survival in cancer (Creagan 1997, Spiegel 2001).

Beneficence
The principle of beneficence obligates health care professionals to prevent harm and 'do good' for their patients. It may seem obvious that to tell lies or withhold the truth is wrong. Patients may suffer severe psychological problems if they continue to feel unwell despite the optimistic messages they receive from others, and may even blame themselves for their symptoms. They may also lose trust if and when they discover the 'conspiracy'.

Discussion
The matter is seldom as simple as the choice between lying and truth-telling, and each case must be considered individually. Relatives may ask that their family member be protected from the *whole* truth. However, respect for the patient's autonomy should, whenever possible, override such a request, but the relatives and patient need to be supported when such information is given, and their issues and concerns addressed.

Tension can arise within the health care team when medical staff fail in their responsibility to disclose appropriate information to those patients who clearly wish to know more. Other staff — nurses in particular — who spend more time with patients become frustrated in their attempts to meet the psychological needs of individuals who lack awareness of the reality of their situation. There must be an open staff forum for the discussion of such problems.

In most cancer centres, the issue is not whether, but how and when, to inform patients of diagnosis and prognosis. A study by Schofield et al (2003) shows that practices linked to lessening anxiety include preparing the patient for a possible cancer diagnosis, having significant others present at diagnosis, being given as much information as desired in understandable language, having questions answered, talking about feelings and being given reassurance. It would seem appropriate that a nurse is present at such discussions because they can follow up the conversation and help the patient to strike a balance between realistic hope and the acceptance of reality.

mind. Did I really hear correctly what he had said? I wondered what on earth I was going to do. I turned to my husband and looked into his eyes, hoping to find the much needed help and support. All I could see was my own disbelief, horror and fear mirrored back at me. I knew I was on my own.

At the same time, this patient expressed relief at having a label for her symptoms and knowing that treatment could now proceed.

Disease recurrence The discovery that the disease has recurred after a symptom-free period may provoke even greater psychological disturbance, for the patient's hopes of cure have been disappointed. In any event, most newly diagnosed or re-diagnosed patients will be anxious to proceed with treatment as soon as possible, and many will become frustrated with the staging process. The period of waiting for test results, whether at initial diagnosis or at recurrence, is one of great anxiety; the patient is often afraid of the verdict but nonetheless desperate to know it.

Psychological support Aside from providing the necessary nursing care prior to and following each test, the nurse must act as communicator. It is important to know why each test is being performed and what it will entail for the patient so that explanations and reassurance can be provided. Findings suggest that a substantial proportion of the lay public do not understand phrases often used in cancer consultations. For example, in one study, only 52% understood that the phrase 'the tumour is progressing' was not good news and less than a third understood what was meant by 'seedlings' (Chapman et al 2003). The nurse, acting as facilitator, should ensure that the doctor explains test results and their significance to the patient as soon as possible. Many fears for the future, both rational and irrational, arise at this time. These need to be discussed openly, and it is the nurse who is most suitably placed to do this.

STOP THINK **31.7** (a) Consider D's needs for information and emotional support during the staging process (see Case History 31.1(B)). Devise a care plan showing how you would meet these needs.
(b) Mr H (see Case History 31.3) has been discharged home following palliative radiotherapy to his ribs and spine. One day he asks his district nurse how long it will be before his strength returns. Consider the other questions he may be implying by asking this. What information would the nurse need and what might be the reply?

Aims of treatment

Cancer treatments can be described in terms of the following categories:

- curative — often termed 'radical' treatment
- palliative — given with the intention of controlling the disease and distressing symptoms.

The transition from radical to palliative therapy need not be presented to the patient as a major or sudden change of direction, as this may lead to feelings of abandonment and hopelessness. Often, several forms of treatment are given in combination; this is termed 'multimodal therapy'. Usually one therapy is the primary therapy while the others are termed 'adjuvant' therapies, as in the case of adjuvant radiotherapy following breast surgery.

Response to treatment

Changes in the size of a tumour following treatment are termed 'response rates'. These may be *complete* — the tumour has disappeared; *partial* — the tumour has decreased by at least 50%; *minimal or stable* — there is very little change in tumour volume; *progressive* — 25% increase in tumour volume. A good tumour response does not necessarily prolong the patient's survival, but it may, in any event, significantly improve quality of life. Unfortunately, cancer treatments can have considerable side-effects, which may seriously reduce quality of life. Thus, the decision to treat a patient must be based upon a careful balancing of the costs and benefits of treatment and should, ideally, be taken jointly by the health care team and the patient.

Treatment modalities

The principal forms of cancer treatment are:

- surgery
- radiotherapy
- chemotherapy – both cytotoxic chemotherapy and biological response modifiers (BRM).

Surgery

Surgery is the oldest form of treatment for cancer and remains the most successful method of achieving long-term survival for patients with various types of localised tumour. Surgical removal of tumours of the skin (non-melanoma), thyroid gland, uterus, colon and rectum (early stage) are associated with an excellent chance of cure. Certain other tumours, particularly those disseminated at presentation such as small cell carcinoma of the lung, are inoperable.

Surgical procedures are not always performed with curative intent. Surgery may be used adjuvantly with other treatments, e.g. in the resection of diseased bone after radical chemotherapy for osteosarcoma. Palliative surgery can improve the quality of the patient's remaining life; for example, a stent insertion or bypass of the common bile duct can be performed to relieve jaundice in cancer of the head of the pancreas or in cholangiocarcinoma.

Psychological support Surgical techniques, pre- and post-operative nursing care, and the psychological problems associated with undergoing surgery are discussed in Chapter 26. The patient with cancer has all of the usual problems of the surgical patient to contend with, together with the stigma of cancer and the fear and uncertainty of an unknown outcome. Frequently, it is during the perioperative period on a general surgical ward that the patient is told of the diagnosis. There is a need for the nurses on these wards to be aware of the particular problems and needs of the cancer patient.

Radiotherapy

Radiotherapy is the use of ionising radiation to destroy cancer cell populations. Approximately half of all patients with cancer receive radiotherapy during the management of their disease.

Radiation physics and biology are complex topics, which are subject to intense research and development. More comprehensive accounts can be found in Dow et al (1997) and Faithful & Wells (2003).

There are two kinds of radiation:

- particle radiation, e.g. alpha particles, beta particles, electrons, protons, neutrons which have a mass, limiting their depth of penetration
- ionising electromagnetic radiation, i.e. gamma (γ) rays and X-rays — these are similar to light, radio or microwaves, but have a very much higher energy level and are deeply penetrating.

Alpha particles are of low energy; they can be absorbed by a sheet of paper and are too weak to kill cancer cells. Electrons are of higher energy and can penetrate anything up to the density of wood. In radiotherapy, electrons are used to treat superficial areas located a few centimetres underneath the skin, for example as a 'booster' treatment to the scar line postoperatively in breast cancer to prevent local recurrence. Gamma rays are short, very powerful waves that require lead or concrete to absorb them. They are emitted from the nuclei of radioactive elements, e.g. caesium and cobalt, and are able to penetrate deeply into the body tissues (Hilderley 2000).

The most common form of radiotherapy now is the X-ray. These rays are artificially generated when a stream of electrons bombard against tungsten metal targets, releasing energy in the form of X-rays.

Radioactivity Understanding ionising radiation requires a basic understanding of atomic and molecular structure. All matter is made up of atoms, which consist of a central nucleus containing positively charged protons and uncharged neutrons, orbited by negatively charged electrons, equivalent in number to the protons. The negatively charged electrons (–) orbit the nucleus, being held in place by the attractive force of the positively charged protons (+); hence a stable state is maintained (see Fig. 31.4).

However, as the number of protons increases, an excess number of neutrons are required in order to hold the nucleus together. This imbalance causes the spontaneous disintegration of the nucleus with an associated emission of charged particles and radiation energy.

Some elements exist in a variety of states, depending on the number of neutrons in the nucleus. These are termed the isotopes of an element. Two isotopes of iodine, for example, are ^{127}I and ^{131}I. The latter is a radioisotope, i.e. it is unstable, because the nuclei of its atoms have a disproportionate number of neutrons. Radioisotopes may be naturally occurring, such as radium-226 (^{226}Ra), which is now seldom used in radiotherapy, or artificially manufactured by bombarding elements with neutrons in a nuclear reactor, e.g. cobalt-60 (^{60}Co).

The effects of radiation Cellular response to radiation is not yet fully understood. Radiation causes ionisation of atoms and molecules. The main target of radiation is DNA, which is altered *directly* by ionisation of its own molecules or *indirectly* by changes in the chemical environment of the cell, caused by ionisation of other molecules, particularly

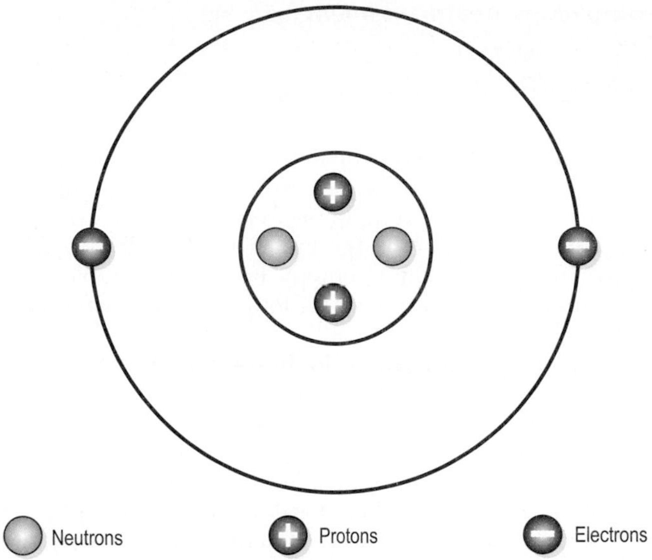

Fig. 31.4 The stable atom. The nucleus of this atom is stable because the number of neutrons and protons are in balance. The neutrons counteract the electrostatic forces pushing the protons apart.

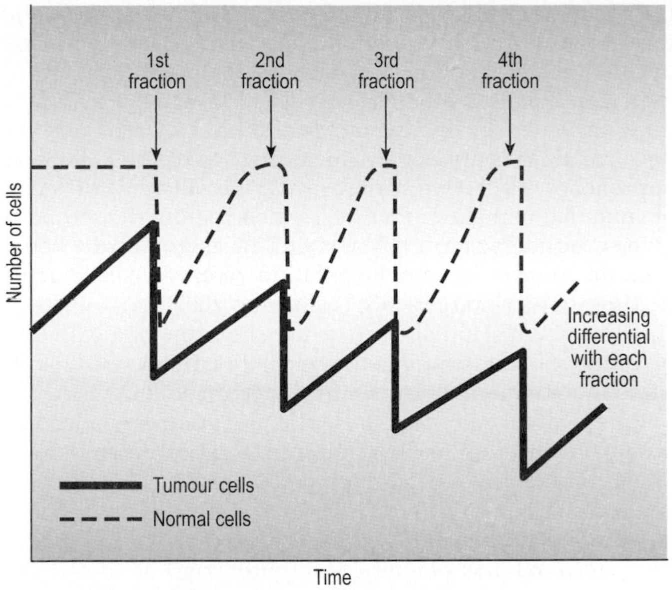

Fig. 31.5 The difference between normal and tumour cell kill and recovery in radiotherapy. Normal cells have the capacity to recover to their previous population level more rapidly than malignant cells. Therefore, successive treatments given after normal cell population recovery but before malignant cell population recovery will result in minimal damage to normal tissue but successive reductions in tumour size.

water. The latter results in a free radical in the cell, a very reactive atom with an unpaired electron, which triggers chemical changes. This ultimately stimulates a chain of events that leads to biological damage, irreparably damaging DNA, which retards cell metabolism and causes cell death. Cells are therefore more sensitive to radiation-induced damage at certain phases of the cell cycle, e.g. G_2 and M phase.

To revise your knowledge of the cell cycle, see Martini (2004) or Tortora & Grabowski (2005); for further information regarding the radiobiological basis of radiotherapy, see Adamson (2003).

Radiosensitivity of a given tumour is closely related to cell proliferation activity. As malignant cells are constantly dividing, they are all radiosensitive, although to varying degrees. Unfortunately, rapidly dividing healthy cells, such as those of the skin, the epithelium of the gastrointestinal and urinary tracts, the gonads and the bone marrow, are also vulnerable to radiation damage; this accounts for the unwanted side-effects of radiotherapy. Figure 31.5 explains the difference between the radiation responses of tumour cells and normal cells. In theory, all tumour cells could be eradicated by radiotherapy. However, the often narrow difference between the dose required to produce lethal damage to the tumour and that which causes irreversible damage to normal tissue (therapeutic ratio), makes it difficult to achieve optimal dosing without causing unacceptable side-effects.

Radiotherapy is prescribed as an 'absorbed dose'. The unit used is the gray (Gy), where 1 Gy = 1 joule as absorbed by 1 kg of body tissue. The dose prescribed will vary, depending on several factors such as the volume and site of the area to be treated, sensitivity of the surrounding normal tissue, radiosensitivity of the particular tumour and also treatment intent, i.e. curative or palliative.

Sources of radiation Radiotherapy is given in a variety of ways, according to tumour type and stage and, occasionally, the patient's condition. Teletherapy (from the Greek téle — 'far'), sometimes called 'external beam therapy', is the most common method of treatment. Brachytherapy (from the Greek brachys — 'short') is administered via radioactive sources placed within a body cavity or tumour bed.

Teletherapy External beam radiotherapy is administered by machines, which are categorised according to the level of energy of radiation produced and depth of penetration (kilovoltage, orthovoltage, megavoltage, cobalt machine). The 'linear accelerator' or 'linac' is the predominant teletherapy equipment in use throughout the world. Machines delivering lower voltages are still used to treat superficial lesions, such as skin carcinomas. The total prescribed radiation dose, if administered in one session, may be far too toxic to normal tissue and possibly even fatal to the patient. Hence treatment is often administered in daily 'fractions' of the total dose, so as to take advantage of the four Rs of radiobiology — repair, reproduction, redistribution and reoxygenation. Repair of sublethal cell injury generally occurs within 24 h, but possibly in as little as 30–90 min. Normal cells can therefore repair between daily doses of radiation. Tumour cells may do so initially but become less capable as treatment is protracted.

The standard fractionation schedule is a daily single dose five times a week. Alternative fractionation schemes continue to receive attention as the search continues to achieve greater cell kill and tumour control. Two strategies have been developed involving multiple fractions per day: hyperfractionation and continuous hyperfractionation accelerated radiotherapy (CHART). Hyperfractionation is the use of several smaller than standard doses given two to three times daily. The accumulative daily and total doses are usually greater than for conventional treatment. Accelerated hyperfractionation refers to an overall shortened treatment time, achieved by increasing the number of fractions per day, treating continuously including weekends. In both approaches, 6 h between doses must be allowed for repair of sublethal damage from the first dose before the second is given (Saunders et al 1997). CHART has significantly better tumour control but implementation requires considerable changes in working practice (Adamson 2003).

The patient's initial visit to the department involves a planning session (simulation) which, if complex, may necessitate more than one visit. Extreme accuracy in devising the unique plan for each patient is vital, the aim being adequate dosage to the tumour and minimum exposure of healthy tissues and organs. Localisation of the tumour is made using an X-ray simulator which mimics the treatment machine, and information from CT or MRI scans. This information is then used by the planning computer staff to determine a beam configuration that conforms precisely to the target organ or site. Patient immobilisation is important, particularly for patients with head and neck tumours. A close fitting individualised Perspex shell is made in the mould room, which is worn throughout treatment. Some individuals may find this claustrophobic.

Intensity modulated radiation therapy (IMRT) harnesses the latest advances in digital, diagnostic imaging, information processing and beam-shaping technologies to enable clinicians to determine and deliver an optimal treatment plan whereby beams can be shaped to avoid surrounding tissue (Staehelin 2003).

In most centres, the treatment field, or reference points, are marked out on the patient's skin using small permanent tattoos. Traditionally these had been defined using ink marks, which were not to be washed off.

Brachytherapy This form of treatment is less common than teletherapy. It is the temporary or permanent placement of a radioactive source (isotope), either in close proximity to or within a tumour. It offers the advantage of delivering a continuous dose of radiation to a specific tumour volume. The most common methods used include interstitial implants, intracavitary treatment and systemic therapy. In an interstitial implant, the radioactive source is contained in the form of a needle, seed, wire or catheter that is implanted directly into the tumour (e.g. iridium — breast, prostate, head and neck cancer). In intracavitary treatment, the radioactive source is placed directly into the body cavity by remote control and held in place by a prepositioned applicator (e.g. caesium — cervical, endometrial, vaginal and lung cancer). In systemic therapy an unsealed radioactive source is given orally or intravenously (e.g. iodine — hyperthyroidism).

Stereotactic radiotherapy has been developed to deliver a precise dose of radiotherapy to a small area (millimetres). It is a complex and highly specialised treatment, initially used for the treatment of benign brain tumours of poor surgical risk.

For more details of stereotactic radiotherapy, see Kreth et al (1995); if caring for patients receiving brachytherapy, refer to a specialist text, e.g. Dow et al (1997) or Faithful & Wells (2003).

Radiotherapy treatment intent may be:

- curative (radical)
- adjuvant/long-term control
- palliative.

The goal of radiotherapy in early stage cancer is curative as in the treatment of radiosensitive tumours such as skin cancer, Hodgkin's lymphoma, cervical cancer, cancer of the larynx and seminoma (germ cell tumour, testicular in origin). Treatment is often lengthy with considerable side-effects but the good prognosis for long-term survival makes it worthwhile.

Adjuvant radiotherapy Radiotherapy is commonly used as adjuvant treatment to ensure local control, usually either pre- or postoperatively, or, increasingly, with chemotherapy e.g. breast, prostate, colon and rectal cancer.

For those cancers in the later stages where cure or eradication is not possible, local control ranging from months to years may be the treatment goal. Usually more than one treatment modality is advocated. In order to improve the therapeutic ratio, concurrent radiotherapy and chemotherapy regimens are being used. Chemotherapeutic agents such as cisplatin, 5-fluorouracil (5-FU), doxorubicin or mitomycin C are given alongside radiotherapy in cancers of the cervix, anus, head, neck and lung to achieve a greater cell kill.

Palliative radiotherapy constitutes 50% of all radiotherapy treatments given (Blyth et al 2001) and involves a shorter course of treatment at much lower doses than either radical or adjuvant therapy. Its aim is to achieve symptom relief with minimum side-effects, ensuring that quality of life is maximised. Again, radiotherapy is effective primarily in the control of local problems, such as local recurrence of breast cancer, pain, compression of adjacent structures by metastases and bleeding, e.g. haemoptysis in carcinoma of the lung or rectal bleeding in carcinoma of the rectum. Spinal cord compression and superior vena cava obstruction, for example, often present as emergencies, and the treatment is usually immediate radiotherapy.

Large field radiotherapy Occasionally, radiotherapy is given to much larger areas of the body. Total body irradiation is used for some patients with leukaemia to eradicate all tumour cells from chemotherapy-resistant tissues. This treatment must be followed by bone marrow transplant to restore bone marrow function (see Ch. 11). Hemi-body (half body) radiation provides effective palliation for patients with extensive bone metastases, as are common, for example, in prostatic cancer.

The decision making and planning surrounding any course of radiotherapy involve a team approach. Informed consent is essential as is patient and carer education. Incorporation of the principles of physics, radiobiology, dosimetry, treatment technique, anatomy, physiology, psychosocial and patient/family care requires a multidisciplinary approach.

Radiation protection There is much fear and misconception amongst both professionals and lay people about the dangers of radiation exposure. Indeed, radiation is potentially extremely hazardous, and exposure to high doses can cause all of the side-effects itemised in Table 31.3, together with cell mutations that may lead to carcinogenesis, or to congenital abnormalities if pregnant women are exposed.

Every institution dealing with radiation is legally obliged to appoint a radiation protection officer, to follow stringent guidelines for radiation monitoring to provide education for staff and patient protection. If these are adhered to, radiation damage risk is negligible. Staff most at risk are those working constantly with unsealed sources. Staff working in areas of potential radiation exposure should wear badges in which radiographic film records exposure if it occurs.

STOP THINK **31.8** Arrange to visit a radiotherapy department. Where is it located in the hospital, how is it designed, and why? Ask what types of machine are in use and what kind of treatment each is used for. Ask who the radiation protection officer is, and ask to see a copy of the local policy. Try to imagine how a patient might feel arriving at the department for their first treatment. Compare your impressions with that of another student.

Side-effects of radiotherapy Side-effects occur when normal tissue is irradiated. Manifestation of side-effects varies greatly from patient to patient, depending on the location and amount of tissue being irradiated, the dose and its fractionation, and the patient's physical and psychological state. Treatment techniques are constantly being developed to improve accuracy of delivery and minimise side-effects. Patients may suffer from systemic side-effects such as fatigue, lethargy, nausea, anorexia and headaches. Such a cluster of symptoms, termed 'radiation sickness', may be due to the circulation of tumour breakdown products. In general, however, radiotherapy affects only those tissues in the area being irradiated. For example, a patient receiving treatment for bladder carcinoma, as opposed to radiotherapy to the brain, will not lose the hair on their head.

Side-effects may be 'early' (acute), occurring 10–14 days after commencement of treatment, continuing for a period of weeks following treatment completion. Long-term or 'late' side-effects usually present 18 months to 2 years after treatment. Acute problems manifest in areas of rapid cell growth and division and are usually reversible. The nursing management of the most common of side-effects forms a major part of the nursing role in the radiotherapy department and is discussed in Table 31.3.

Late side-effects occur as, due to DNA damage, slowly dividing cells fail to replicate. Problems are most often a consequence of damaged vasculature and are usually permanent. Examples include the distressing symptoms of fibrosis of the lung, chronic bowel inflammation, and lymphoedema resulting from lymph node damage. Monitoring of late side-effects is important for patients attending follow-up outpatient clinics.

Psychological and supportive care Radiotherapy patients are often perceived as the self-caring 'walking wounded'. Their needs are often less obvious as treatment is mostly on an outpatient basis with the added stress of daily travel to and from the department (Wells 1998a). It is important to remember that radiotherapy treatment is not always an isolated event but usually precedes or follows other forms of cancer treatment. Although it brings its own problems and side-effects, its impact needs to be considered in the context of the patient's overall experience. That experience may be affected by existing psychosocial, physical and functional needs related to other existing disease or to financial or social constraints. A particularly vulnerable time for a patient is at the end of treatment, when side-effects are often at their peak and professional support is not always accessible. Patients may experience considerable uncertainty and vulnerability (Wells 1998b).

Myths and fears As Rotman et al (1977) pointed out several decades ago, few therapeutic modalities in medicine induce more misunderstanding, confusion and misapprehension than radiotherapy. Several studies over the years have shown that patients have many fears and anxieties, with some experiencing psychological distress, and more often than not feeling they are given insufficient information pre- and post-treatment (Eardley 1985, Poroch 1995, Mills & Sullivan 1999). A seminal study carried out in the 1970s found that more than 60% of patients receiving radiotherapy experienced mild to moderate anxiety or depression prior to starting treatment. Many expressed fears related to the machines, the radioactivity and being burned or scarred (Peck & Boland 1977).

For many patients, the news that they are to receive radiotherapy comes soon after knowledge of their diagnosis when they are already coping with multiple stressors and feelings of loss. Myths and fears compound these stresses. Hammick et al (1998) examined patients' knowledge and perceptions of radiotherapy and radiation. Outside of medical usage, radiation was commonly perceived in terms of the atom bomb. Media coverage often highlighted problems in terms of overdosages, burns and permanent damage. From observations in clinical practice it is apparent that media reports do influence patients' anxiety levels regarding treatment. This became evident at the time of publicity surrounding patients belonging to RAGE (Radiation Action Group Exposure), where women had developed long-term toxicity as a result of radiotherapy to the brachial plexus following treatment for breast cancer. Health care professionals need to be aware that patients may have many anxieties following public information releases and that it is important to place these reports into perspective. As Mackenzie (1996) points out, it is not surprising that patients find it confusing that radiation, which is known to cause cancer (e.g. following Chernobyl in 1986), can be both curative and survivable.

The nurse's role Nurses can do much to alleviate the patient's fears and anxieties, helping to make the experience of radiotherapy more tolerable. Supportive care relies on the understanding of the impact of cancer and its treatment viewed from the perspective of the patient. A thorough needs assessment is fundamental to enable effective interventions to support the patient and their family throughout treatment. Dennison and Shute (2000) piloted a simple checklist for use in the outpatient setting to identify quickly issues of concern for patients regarding their illness, treatment, symptoms, finances, social support and relationships. Outpatient nurses reviewed the completed checklists prior to the consultation so that appropriate support and specialist referrals could be initiated. As a result, patients found that communication and relationships with staff improved, allowing them greater involvement in their care.

Table 31.3 Nursing management of the side-effects of radiotherapy

Irradiated body part/organ	Radiation effect	Nurse intervention	Rationale
General	Fatigue	Forewarn patients of the likely occurrence during and after radiotherapy. Provide appropriate information about the experience and pattern of symptoms	To foster independence, encouraging energy-saving activities
		Assess and promote self-care strategies. Refer to appropriate allied health care professional as necessary	To prevent feelings of social isolation, low mood and to decrease anxiety levels
		Assess baseline fatigue levels prior to treatment starting	To monitor changes over time and need for further intervention
		Check for physical, biochemical and psychological causes of fatigue	Electrolyte imbalances/anaemia may be corrected. Appropriate psychological support can be given
		Encourage patients to maintain a daily record of fatigue levels and the relationship to activities	Enhances the ability to control activities or plan ahead, goal setting and prioritising
Skin Particularly areas where the skin is thin, moist, e.g. skin folds, axilla, groin, breast and perineum. Fair skin is especially sensitive	Three-stage reaction: 1. Erythema: redness, heat, itchiness	No metal-containing skin preparations	Metal may intensify radiation reactions
		Gentle washing with warm water and gentle drying, no rubbing	Friction causes irritation. Ink marks must not be washed off
		Application of simple moisturiser, e.g. aqueous cream	Soothing and minimises friction, keeps skin supple
		If itchy, an antihistamine cream may be prescribed. Apply 1% hydrocortisone	To alleviate discomfort and itch
		Avoid exposure to the sun and extremes of heat and cold	UV light may intensify any reaction
		Encourage non-constrictive clothing in lightweight, natural fabrics: no tight or elastic clothing	Reduces sweating and friction
	2. Dry desquamation: dryness, scaliness, tight feeling, pain on movement	1% hydrocortisone or lanolin cream (centres vary in their recommendations)	Soothing emollient and/or anti-inflammatory
		Expose skin to fresh air or cool fan	Cooling has a short-term analgesic effect
		For moderate to severe reaction, or if skin folds involved, consider application of hyperfix, ensuring it is removed with baby oil	Preventive measure and promotes wound healing as is permeable. Removing with oil ensures the skin is not damaged
	3. Moist desquamation: blisters, loss of surface epithelium, pain, susceptibility to infection. Occasionally progresses to necrosis	A break in treatment may be required	To prevent further skin breakdown and discomfort
		Analgesics	
		Observation for signs of infection	Infection exacerbates skin damage and may become systemic
		Use of hydrogel/hydrocolloid/ alginate dressings	To promote wound healing
		Dressing plan: assessment, dressings, evaluation using wound care principles	To record any changes, evaluating the effectiveness of the intervention applied
Scalp	Alopecia (in treatment field only). Loss of any body hair occurs from weeks 2–3	Reassure the patient that hair will usually grow back in 2–3 months, although it may be of a different texture and colour	Hair loss poses a very stressful threat to body image, especially for women
		Organise provision of a wig	
		Wearing of scarf/turban at night	Prevents distress of hair on pillow
Brain	Cerebral oedema (within week 1 of treatment): altered mental state, restlessness, irritability, headaches, nausea, ↑ BP, ↓ P, ↓ respirations, ? raised intracranial pressure (see Ch. 9)	Administer prescribed steroids	Anti-inflammatory
		Observe and report alterations in mental status	Enables prompt medical intervention
		Ensure patient safety	

Table 31.3 Nursing management of the side-effects of radiotherapy *(Continued)*

Irradiated body part/organ	Radiation effect	Nurse intervention	Rationale
Mouth	1. Mucositis due to damaged, sloughed oral mucosa. Opportunistic infection may ensue, e.g. *Candida albicans*	Comprehensive dental review prior to treatment	To identify potential infection risks and carry out any necessary dental work, giving time for wound healing
		Regular use of an oral assessment tool	To monitor any changes, evaluating interventions
		Teaching and encouraging frequent routine systematic oral hygiene, initiated prior to treatment if possible	To reduce the amount and severity of mucositis and encourage compliance. Also to minimise the risk of infection
		Use of a soft toothbrush, fluoride toothpaste and regular normal saline mouthwashes	To minimise damage to the oral mucosa and prevent build-up of plaque
		Use of antibacterial/antifungal preparations, e.g. chlorhexidine, nystatin	To prevent or treat infection
		Regular analgesics: topical, e.g. benzydamine, and systemic including opiates	Oral pain is excruciating and always to the forefront of consciousness
		Use of cellulose film-forming agents to line the mucosa, e.g. Gelclair	Forms a thin protective film which relieves pain and discomfort
		Observe for signs of dehydration and inadequate nutrition, liaising with the dietitian (NCI 2003)	Prompt parenteral hydration and dietary supplements or enteral feeding may be commenced
	2. Xerostomia (dry mouth) due to altered salivary gland function. May be permanent. Causes difficulty in chewing, swallowing and talking	Frequent mouth rinses with normal saline and sodium bicarbonate	Comforting, aids swallowing, buffering of oral environment
		Frequent sips of water	Lubrication of mucosa
		Use of artificial saliva	
		Moist soft diet	Easier to tolerate
		Avoidance of spices, alcohol, smoking, extremes of temperature	These are mucosal irritants
	3. Taste changes due to xerostomia and damaged tastebuds	Assist patients to experiment with other foods	To maintain nutritional intake
	4. Dental decay due to xerostomia and radiation gingivitis	Pre-treatment dental referral	Any caries will be exacerbated by radiation and form foci for infection
		Avoidance of high sugar content foods and fluids	Sugar alters natural slightly alkaline pH of mucosal environment and demineralises teeth
Neck area	1. Pharyngitis, laryngitis, causing pain, hoarseness, loss of voice, dry cough and occasionally respiratory stridor	Discourage smoking	Mucosal irritant
		Encourage patient to rest voice	
		Observe respiratory status and colour	Medical intervention in the form of steroids or even a tracheostomy may be necessary
		Linctus as a cough suppressant	Prevents mucosal irritation caused by coughing
		Topical analgesics prior to food, e.g. aspirin gargles, anaesthetic throat spray; systemic analgesics	Promotes comfort and aids swallowing
	2. Oesophagitis (upper one-third) causing dysphagia	Maintain nutrition. Soft diet, referring to the dietitian for supplements. Avoid irritant foods, strong alcohol and smoking	These patients are often already malnourished
Thorax	1. Oesophagitis (lower two-thirds) causing 'heartburn'	As above; also administer antacids prior to food. Some antacids also contain topical anaesthetics	Lines oesophagus and prevents pain and trauma of swallowing and from gastric acid reflux

Continued

Table 31.3 Nursing management of the side-effects of radiotherapy *(Continued)*

Irradiated body part/organ	Radiation effect	Nurse intervention	Rationale
Thorax *(cont'd)*	2. Pneumonitis due to inflammation of bronchioles and alveolar lining. May cause dyspnoea, productive cough and haemoptysis	Discourage smoking	Irritant
		Observe for signs of infection: pyrexia, purulent sputum	Enables prompt commencement of antibiotics
		Oxygen as prescribed (see Ch. 3)	
		Assessment and management of breathlessness (Corner et al 1995)	Patient comfort and integrated approach to managing this distressing symptom
	3. Dyspepsia, nausea and vomiting (less severe than with abdominal radiation)	(see below)	
Abdomen and pelvis	1. Nausea and vomiting due to inflammation of gastrointestinal epithelium; also a generalised radiation reaction	Encourage a small meal 3 h before treatment and light snacks after	Some patients are unable to eat after treatment due to nausea
		Regular antiemetics: systematically try various kinds and routes	Regular administration required to prevent and relieve nausea
		Distraction/relaxation techniques	There may be a contributing psychological factor in nausea (Holmes 1996)
		Monitor fluid and food intake	To avoid dehydration
	2. Diarrhoea, possibly accompanied by rectal bleeding	Maximise privacy	
		Administer antimotility medication as prescribed	
		Low-residue, bland diet, low fat	Better tolerated by damaged mucosa
		Observe for dehydration	Avoid dehydration
		Maintain high fluid intake	
		Observe perianal skin: gently apply barrier cream after washing if necessary	To prevent skin excoriation
	3. Cystitis due to inflammation of urinary tract. Predisposition to urinary tract infection	Encourage high fluid intake (3 L daily)	Prevents stasis of urine and sloughed epithelium
		Encourage and/or assist with personal hygiene	Helps prevent ascending urinary tract infection
		Regular collection of urine specimens for microbiology	Enables prompt antibiotic treatment of urinary tract infection
	4. Altered sexual function (degree depends on exact treatment site and dosage)	Psychological support and counselling	Loss of any degree of sexual function is very threatening to most people's self-image; opportunity to talk this through is vital
		Include partner in discussion if patient wishes	To gain understanding and support and minimise body image problems
		Assess the need for psychosexual counselling	To maintain a healthy relationship and sexuality
	Men:		
	Erectile dysfunction (usually temporary)	Psychological support	To explore possible options to help with erectile difficulties
		May need referral to erectile dysfunction clinic for discussion re: access to vacuum constriction devices, penile prosthesis, pharmacological intervention	
	Sterility (usually permanent)	Offer sperm banking if appropriate	To enable sperm to be used for artificial insemination
	Decreased sexual desire/libido	Monitor hormone levels	To improve libido and promote healthy sexuality
		Testosterone replacement therapy	
		Patient/couple education and psychological support	

Table 31.3 Nursing management of the side-effects of radiotherapy *(Continued)*

Irradiated body part/organ	Radiation effect	Nurse intervention	Rationale
	Women:		
	Sterility (if ovaries are irradiated). May be temporary or permanent	Advise continued contraception during and for several months after treatment	Fertility is not always immediately affected and any pregnancy may not be viable
	Dyspareunia due to vaginal fibrosis and dryness	Advise use of water-based vaginal lubricant	To promote comfort and ease of penetration
		Use of barrier contraceptives, e.g. condom during intercourse	There may be a burning sensation associated with semen and this will help to decrease irritation
		Education and use of vaginal dilators during (if tolerated) and for up to 2 years after treatment	To prevent vaginal stenosis and post-coital bleeding, facilitating future sexual intercourse and internal examination
	Loss of libido	Patient/couple education and psychological support, sensitively explaining that this is usually temporary	To maintain healthy sexual relationships
	Premature menopause (if ovaries irradiated)	Inform of possibility and potential menopausal symptoms Discuss possible strategies in managing the hot flushes, osteoporosis, etc. Hormone replacement therapy should be discussed with the individual in light of media highlighted risks and benefits	To help women manage menopausal symptoms

Supportive care may also involve simple behavioural strategies such as simply being there, actively listening, talking, preserving the patient's individuality and providing information (see Research Abstract 31.1). Forming a relationship with the patient and answering questions have also been shown to have a positive effect on patients' coping strategies (Poroch 1995, Hinds & Moyer 1997).

Information is seen as crucial, relieving anxiety and promoting a sense of control (Poroch 1995, Mills & Sullivan 1999, Van der Molen 1999). Nurses are responsible, therefore, for becoming accurately informed themselves — about radiotherapy in general, and about each patient's individual treatment plan and likely side-effects in particular.

Studies indicate that patients tend to prefer verbal information backed up with written material (Slevin et al 1996, Hammick et al 1998). Good practice advocates that written information should be accompanied by verbal explanation wherever possible. The last few years have therefore seen the development of a comprehensive patient information strategy by support agencies such as CancerBACUP, Macmillan and Tenovus (see 'Useful websites'), alongside telephone information helplines and publication of in-house material. Managed clinical networks are also involved in the development of information, ensuring patients receive accurate information at the appropriate time across all care settings. The use of other methods of providing effective information such as audio and visual tapes is also being explored (Hagopian 1996, Harrison et al 2001). The media have been shown to be important contributors to knowledge and to help with decision making, although some sources are trusted more than others (Balmer 2005). The internet has many sites providing high quality information and in this latter study was seen as a valuable tool.

Studies have also shown that the vast majority of patients want as much information as possible to enable them to prepare for treatment, decrease their fears and anxieties, and increase their understanding of treatment. Information requested includes:

- how treatment works
- the effectiveness of treatment
- likely side-effects
- preventive and self-care strategies
- impact of treatment on their lives and their families (Fieler et al 1996, Barnett et al 2004, Skalla et al 2004).

With so much emphasis on information and ever-increasing resources, it is not surprising that some patients report informational overload, problems with retention and confusion (Skalla et al 2004). A patient-centred approach is therefore vital, with information being tailored to the individual's needs.

Nurses in Europe, in comparison with their American colleagues, have been slower to realise their contribution to radiotherapy care. However, this is changing. Both nurses and therapy radiographers are developing advanced practitioner roles through which innovative approaches to care are increasingly evident. The central components of these roles include assessment, education, knowledge, prevention of side-effects, psychosocial support, liaison with other health care professionals and rehabilitation. Employment of both nurse specialists and therapy radiographers to provide information and counselling

RESEARCH ABSTRACT 31.1

Support is regarded as an essential aspect of nursing care, enabling patients to cope with stressful situations. A Canadian qualitative study explored how patients and their caregivers describe their experiences and perceptions of support during radiotherapy treatment. Twelve patients and five family caregivers were interviewed whilst the patient was receiving radiotherapy or 4–6 weeks post-treatment.

Both patients and caregivers repeatedly described support as ordinary, everyday words and deeds. Three main types of support were encountered: 'being there', 'giving help' and 'giving information'. Forms of support included being encouraged where possible to take part in everyday life, for example:

- going out for a coffee or walk, help with shopping, gardening, etc. (physical)
- being encouraged to verbalise fears, concerns and feelings, providing diversions and laughter (emotional)
- support through the prayers of family, friends and congregations (spiritual).

Interestingly it was family and friends who were perceived to be the main source of support for all types, also shown more recently by Wengstrom and Haggmark (2001), whereas nurses provided a professional source of support in providing information and advice.

Support also appeared to be related to the way in which it was given rather than meeting a specific need. Nurses who were seen to be making an effort were noticed and appreciated. Participants also commented that support was most likely to be of value if it occurred in the context of a relationship.

These findings illustrate that support is a multifaceted concept as perceived and interpreted by patients. Although this study was small, it highlights that nurses are able to provide support beyond that which is informational and affirming. As the authors point out, provision of support promotes feelings of self-worth, maintains identity and ensures that the person is treated as an individual rather than just a patient receiving radiotherapy.

Hinds C, Moyer A 1997 Support as experienced by patients with cancer during radiotherapy treatments. Journal of Advanced Nursing 26: 371–379

services, practitioner-led review and follow-up clinics, telephone follow-up and nursing interventions for side-effects can make a positive contribution to patient care (Colyer & Hlahla 1999, Campbell et al 2000, Collins 2001). The future holds many challenges for nurses, radiotherapists and oncologists working together in this field towards a collaborative, coordinated and supportive approach to care.

For further reading on supportive care in radiotherapy, see Faithful & Wells (2003).

STOP THINK **31.9** Use the above information together with supplemental reading to devise an explanation of external beam radiotherapy and its effects that would be suitable to give to a patient prior to treatment. Draw upon available patient literature, such as that published by CancerBACUP (see 'Useful websites'), and your own impressions during your visit to the radiotherapy department. Avoid technical terms and emotive words such as 'burn' or 'blast', and bear in mind that patients need to know what they will actually experience.

Systemic treatment: chemotherapy

The word 'chemotherapy' literally means 'treatment with chemicals' and therefore can refer to any form of medication therapy.

Cytotoxic (literally 'poisonous to cells') chemotherapy involves the use of medication to disrupt the cell cycle and thus ultimately kill malignant cells.

How cytotoxic chemotherapy works Cytotoxins are termed 'antiproliferative'; like radiation, they are toxic to dividing cells, both healthy and malignant. There are many different types of cytotoxic agents, which have various modes of action and therefore work at different phases in the cell cycle.

For a description of the cell cycle, see Tortora & Grabowski (2005).

Cytotoxic drugs are usually classified according to their chemical structure, cell cycle activity and primary mode of action. The classic categories include:

- alkylating agents
- antimetabolites
- antitumour antibiotics
- plant alkaloids.

The action of each of these is described in Box 31.7.

Modes of cytotoxic chemotherapy treatment Cytotoxic chemotherapy differs from radiotherapy in that it is a systemic rather than a localised treatment modality. It is therefore particularly useful for the treatment of haematological malignancies, which are usually disseminated or metastatic in nature. These drugs were first identified in the 1940s, and their use has since become widespread. Despite their great potential, results have been disappointing to date because it has been mainly the rarer tumours that have responded well. Childhood leukaemia is particularly responsive, with approximately 70% of children being cured. Complete responses are also being achieved in adults with Hodgkin's lymphoma. Very few solid tumours are as responsive, the exception being some childhood tumours and testicular teratoma, in which cure rates of 80–90% have been achieved. However, these potentially curable malignancies represent a mere 5% of patients with cancer (Souhami & Tobias 2005).

Adjuvant and palliative chemotherapy For the most part, chemotherapy is used:

- as the sole, or most important, treatment
- as a means of reducing the size of the tumour to aid the success of subsequent surgery or radiotherapy, i.e. 'debulking' of tumours, such as those of the head, neck and bladder
- following radiotherapy or surgery to eliminate remaining tumour cells or micrometastases; adjuvant

Box 31.7

Classification of cytotoxic agents

Alkylating agents
Alkylating agents are highly reactive and are cell cycle non-specific. Their primary mode of action is to join together or cross-link the two strands of DNA, preventing them from separating and therefore replicating. Cyclophosphamide is an example of a cytotoxic which acts in this way. Another group of alkylating agents are platinum-based compounds, e.g. cisplatin and carboplatin, which cause interstrand and intrastrand linkages.

Antimetabolites
These are cell cycle specific, exerting their effect in the S phase. They are structural analogues of normal intracellular metabolites essential for cell function and replication and so are used to disrupt cellular metabolism. Methotrexate, for example, inhibits the enzyme necessary for the conversion of folic acid to folinic acid. Folinic acid is necessary for the formation of purines and pyrimidines, components of DNA. Folinic acid rescue, in the form of folinic acid replacement, is necessary 12–24 h after the administration of methotrexate to prevent the death of too many healthy cells. Other antimetabolites include 5-fluorouracil (5-FU) and cytosine arabinoside.

Plant alkaloids
Many plants and plant extracts continue to be screened to identify new cytotoxic agents. To date these include the vinca alkaloids, taxanes and topoisomerase inhibitors.

Topoisomerase inhibitors (etoposide, teniposide, irinotecan and topotecan) interfere with DNA replication by binding to DNA and the topoisomerase enzymes. Mitotic inhibitors include vincristine, vindesine and vinblastine, which are cell cycle specific acting in the mitosis phase. They bind to microtubule proteins, blocking spindle formation and preventing cell separation. The taxanes (docetaxel and paclitaxel), on the other hand, promote assembly of the microtubule which results in a very stable microtubule that is non-functional.

Antitumour antibiotics
Some classes of antibiotic have been found to be cytotoxic. In general, they are cell cycle non-specific and interfere with DNA function, although several other mechanisms of action may occur, such as alteration of the cell membrane or inhibition of certain enzymes. The most widely used is doxorubicin because it has a broad spectrum of activity; others include mitoxantrone and bleomycin.

Cytotoxic agents are constantly being researched and developed. There are several which do not fit into the above categories and whose action may not be fully understood.

postoperative chemotherapy is commonly used for cancer of the breast or ovary to improve disease-free survival
- to treat a relapse after initial treatment
- for palliation of symptoms — some tumours are partially chemoresponsive, so that treatment may relieve symptoms and improve the quality of, and possibly lengthen, life
- for investigation of the usefulness of a new medicine.

Combination chemotherapy, which uses a variety of agents, has been found to be far more effective than single-agent chemotherapy. At any given time, the cells of one tumour will be at different phases of the cell cycle: a combination of agents acting on those various phases will therefore kill more cells than a single agent. A lower dose of each agent is given, thus reducing the side-effects of each. Tumour cells unfortunately have the capacity to acquire resistance to single agents, and therefore giving intermittent high doses of drugs, alternating drugs and minimising the intervals between treatments are the major factors used to prevent acquired drug resistance.

Administration of chemotherapy Chemotherapy is usually given in 'intermittent' doses, sometimes called 'pulses' or 'cycles', the principle being similar to that of fractionation in radiotherapy. Chemotherapy is toxic to rapidly dividing healthy cells, although these have the capacity to recover more quickly than tumour cells. A graph similar to Figure 31.5 could be drawn to illustrate this principle. Hence, most chemotherapy is organised into 'regimens', sometimes called 'protocols', particularly if the treatment is part of a research trial.

Chemotherapy may be administered systemically or regionally and by several routes.

Systemic chemotherapy The goal is to provide a concentration of the drugs that is sufficient to achieve a therapeutic cytotoxic effect without causing too much toxicity to normal cells. Routes of administration include oral, subcutaneous, intramuscular and intravenous. Intravenous administration may be delivered either as a 'bolus' or infusion. Continuous infusions may be delivered using a medication delivery pump via a vascular access device (VAD) such as a skin-tunnelled catheter (STC), a totally implanted port (TIP) or a peripherally inserted central catheter (PICC).

These devices have permitted safe and reliable access to the venous system and patients are now able to spend longer periods at home while receiving continuous infusions of chemotherapy. The development of such devices has enhanced the lives of cancer patients but their use poses challenges for patients and health care professionals. Concerns include psychosocial issues, care of the device to prevent potential complications, and management of any complications which may occur. Some of these complications may be life threatening and require immediate and effective intervention.

For more information about VADs, see Weinstein (2001). This text covers appropriate usage, insertion techniques and the management of associated complications, both common and rare.

Regional chemotherapy The goal of regional chemotherapy is localisation of effects by delivering chemotherapy drugs directly into blood vessels supplying the cavity containing the tumour or into the tumour itself. Such routes include intrahepatic, intra-arterial, intrapleural, intraperitoneal and intrathecal.

Many patients receive chemotherapy as outpatients, on a day unit, and so need a considerable amount of support and teaching in order to be able to cope with the side-effects they experience at home. There is agreement that this

Box 31.8

Safe administration of chemotherapy

Cytotoxic agents can be dangerous if they are not handled appropriately. A joint proposal to develop national guidelines for the administration of chemotherapy was initially funded by the NHS Executive (1995). From this, the Royal College of Nursing (1998) and the Scottish Cancer Care Pharmacy Group (2000) have issued guidelines for the safe use of cytotoxic chemotherapy in the clinical environment. These guidelines are to assist practitioners in defining and demonstrating high standards of practice, reducing unacceptable variations.

Extravasation

Some cytotoxic agents, e.g. doxorubicin and vincristine, are termed 'vesicants' and can cause severe burns and tissue damage if they leak from the vein into the subcutaneous tissue. Figure 31.6 shows the possible result of extravasation. If extravasation is suspected, the infusion should be stopped and an experienced clinician informed immediately. There are various antidotes available, but more scientific research is required (for more details, see How & Brown 1998, Jones & Coe 2004, NEIS 2004).

Staff protection

There has been concern for many years regarding the potential exposure and subsequent effects in health care workers. Sufficient scientific evidence exists, however, to support the need for staff handling these medications to do so with extreme caution. It is known that at therapeutic doses these substances can cause carcinogenesis, cell mutations and fetal damage. Staff handling cytotoxic medicines should be educated about exposure risks, safe handling procedures and appropriate clothing, i.e. wearing aprons and latex gloves, as risk management strategies have been shown to minimise exposure (Ziegler et al 2002). More research is required to evaluate occupational surveillance. A register for those at risk should be kept and safe practice needs to be regularly audited. Chemotherapeutic agents should be prepared in a specially designed pharmacy unit (laminar air flow/isolator). Staff should always wear gloves when handling oral preparations and should mop up spillages immediately, using large amounts of water and wearing protective clothing. Spillage kits should be available in all the areas where chemotherapy is administered. On seeing the precautions necessary, patients may be alarmed that such dangerous substances are required to control their disease. They should be reassured that these measures are necessary to protect those who are constantly dealing with cytotoxic agents.

Handling body fluids

Many cytotoxic agents are excreted unchanged in urine and faeces and both should be treated as hazardous for at least 48 h. However, Cass and Musgrove (1992) highlighted that some excreta may be contaminated for as long as 7 days. It is therefore important to wear gloves when handling the body fluids of patients receiving chemotherapy, and also to teach patients and their families to take appropriate precautions.

requires specially prepared chemotherapy nurses to fulfil this role (RCN 1998) (see Box 31.8).

Side-effects of chemotherapy As seen with the examples given in Table 31.4, each cytotoxic agent causes different side-effects, varying in intensity with dosage and method of administration. Nursing management of the potential side-effects requires an in-depth knowledge of the common and uncommon toxicity profiles of each agent given in the regimen (Fischer 2003).

Physical and emotional responses to chemotherapy vary greatly between patients. Studies by Sitzia and Wood (1998) and Tanghe et al (1998) have shown that nurses' interpersonal skills and manner influence patients' coping mechanisms. In both studies, nurses underestimated the distress caused by chemotherapy and overestimated the patients' ability to cope. Nurses reported common side-effects, such as alopecia and nausea and vomiting, as being the most distressing toxicities for patients. However, interestingly, a large number of patients reported more subjective symptoms such as fatigue, mood disturbances, altered appetite and restlessness as a source of distress. These findings have implications for nurses assessing patient side-effects and delivering appropriate therapeutic interventions. The following is a brief summary of some of the potential physical side-effects of chemotherapy.

Myelosuppression is not only the most common dose-limiting toxicity of chemotherapy but also potentially the most lethal. To understand the potential damage that chemotherapy may cause to the bone marrow, it is helpful to review normal blood cell development (see Ch. 11). The suppression of the production of blood constituents by the bone marrow occurs to varying degrees after almost all types of cytotoxic chemotherapy. Cell cycle specific agents (e.g. antimetabolites, natural products) tend to cause a rapid decline to a low point (nadir) in the marrow cells, usually 7–10 days after drug administration, although with some drugs the nadir may be reached earlier. Cell cycle non-specific drugs (doxorubicin, cisplatin) have nadirs around 10–14 days, while the nitrosureas' nadir is 26–30+ days. Such factors need to be considered in the planning of treatment regimens. The resultant three problems of leucopenia/neutropenia, anaemia and thrombocytopenia are far more severe in the case of chemotherapy for haematological malignancies (see Ch. 11). Since the prime function of neutrophils is phagocytosis, neutropenia eliminates one of the body's prime defences against bacterial infection. The longer the nadir period, the greater the frequency and severity of infections which are invasive or due to overgrowth of pathogenic microbes. Thrombocytopenia is usually delayed and, if active bleeding occurs, transfusions of platelets may be given. For all patients, myelosuppression may compound other side-effects such as stomatitis.

In view of the significant problems associated with bone marrow suppression, attention has been focused on the therapeutic use of haemopoietic growth factors such as granulocytic colony-stimulating factor (GCSF) (Cappozzo 2004). Studies have shown that these factors can significantly reduce or prevent myelosuppression induced by chemotherapy (Trillet-Lenoir et al 1993, Gatzemeier et al 2000).

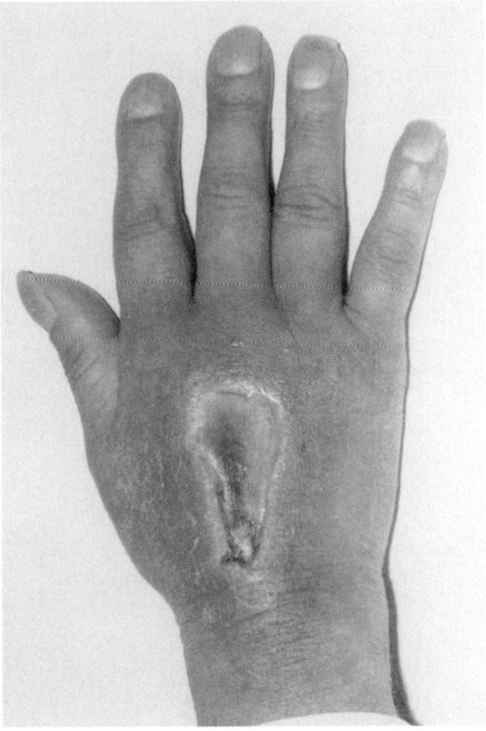

Fig. 31.6 Skin damage caused by extravasation of vesicant cytotoxins. This photograph shows a moderate degree of damage; in some cases there may be nerve and blood vessel damage, progressing to necrosis and requiring skin grafting or even amputation. The key factor in avoiding this situation is vigilant, regular observation of cannulation sites during injection or infusion. The patient should also be asked to report any altered sensation in the area, e.g. coldness, heat, tingling, pain, numbness or swelling. Should extravasation occur, the infusion should be stopped immediately, area marked with a pen, cannula aspirated, a doctor informed and an experienced professional consulted for advice. There is a lack of research to guide treatment for extravasation; however, all centres administering chemotherapy should have a local management policy. For national monitoring, a green card should be completed and sent to the National Extravasation Information Service (Allwood et al 2002, NEIS 2004). It is most important to avoid concentrating only on the affected limb whilst ignoring the stress generated for the patient in this situation.

With the support of GCSF, higher doses of chemotherapy may be given, whilst minimising the effects on the bone marrow.

Therapeutic interventions for myelosuppression are aimed at the prevention and active treatment of infection and bleeding.

Stomatitis/mucositis induced by chemotherapy is significantly associated with myelosuppression and regarded as the main dose-limiting factor in radical treatment regimens (Trotti 2000). It is the result of a two-stage process: First, some cytotoxic agents have a direct effect on the oral mucosa, causing thinning and ulceration within 4–7 days of administration. Patients may experience mild erythema and oedema along the mucocutaneous junction of the lip, mouth dryness and a burning sensation in the lips (Dose 1995). Nausea, vomiting and a reduced food and fluid intake compound this effect, making the mucosa an ineffective barrier to opportunistic infection. Within 10–16 days, myelosuppression causes the already compromised mucosa to be even more susceptible to infection and haemorrhage. Nursing care is similar to that for the patient with radiation stomatitis, described in Table 31.3, see page 1049. Regular thorough assessment and care of the oral mucosa is a vital part of a supportive care strategy (Miller & Kearney 2001). A meaningful and validated assessment tool should be used at least daily and more often if mucositis is severe. It will contain questions about eating, swallowing, pain, erythema and will include an ulceration score (Sonis et al 1999, Eilers & Epstein 2004).

5-Fluorouracil (5-FU) commonly causes mucositis. Oral cryotherapy or sucking on crushed ice during the administration of 5-FU has been shown to reduce the frequency and severity of resulting mucositis. However, further clinical evaluation of this approach is needed (Casanu et al 1994).

The literature suggests many pharmacological regimens for oral care but often the evidence base is weak. Oral care interventions should aim to provide adequate pain relief, prevent or treat infection and promote healing. Advances in molecular biology are again creating new opportunities for novel therapies (Peterson et al 2004).

For further reading, see the series of articles in Seminars in Oncology Nursing 2004, Volume 20(1), by Brown & Wingard; Daniel et al; Eilers & Epstein; Epstein & Schubert; Peterson et al; and Sonis.

Nausea and vomiting induced by chemotherapy can be particularly troublesome, especially with agents such as adriamycin and cisplatin. These drugs activate the chemoreceptor trigger zone (CTZ) in the brain, which in turn stimulates the centre in the brain stem that controls nausea and vomiting. It is important to remember that persistent nausea is often more unbearable than vomiting, which may relieve nausea. The problem may be severe enough to trigger 'anticipatory vomiting' at the sight of the hospital or any stimulus associated with chemotherapy. During the past decade, with the advent of new antiemetics such as the 5-HT_3 antagonists, for example ondansetron and granisetron, the management of chemotherapy-related nausea and vomiting has vastly improved. However, studies continue to show that nurses are markedly underestimating this side-effect and patients report the negative impact such symptoms have on their quality of life (Fawcett & Dean 2004, Grunberg et al 2004, Miller & Kearney 2004). These medications have their own side-effect profile, including constipation and headaches. Steroids such as dexamethasone potentiate the effect of these antiemetics and are most effective in delayed emesis. Again they have their own toxicity profile, such as indigestion, hyperactivity and mood disturbance, and may mask signs of infection in myelosuppressed patients. Relaxation, meditation and sedatives such as lorazepam have also been found to be helpful for some patients.

Alopecia is caused by some agents, e.g. adriamycin, taxanes, topoisomerase inhibitors, and may range from slight thinning to complete hair loss. Several factors contribute to the severity of hair loss including the specific drug, dose and schedule. It usually occurs approximately 2 weeks after therapy has started and is temporary, with hair regrowth occurring about 6 weeks after the completion of treatment.

Table 31.4 Cytotoxic agents and common side-effects

Cytotoxic agent	Action	Common use	Potential side-effects
Capcitabene	Prodrug, antimetabolite	Breast cancer Colorectal cancer	Myelosuppression Mucositis Palmar–plantar syndrome Diarrhoea Mild nausea
Cisplatin	Action uncertain Similar to alkylating agent	Wide spectrum Cancer of the testes, ovary, cervix, endometrium, bladder, head and neck, lymphomas, small cell lung	Severe nausea and vomiting Metallic taste Diarrhoea (HD) Myelosuppression Hearing changes/loss (due to damage to VIIIth cranial nerve) Peripheral neuropathy Renal impairment
Cyclophosphamide	Alkylating agent	Wide spectrum Cancer of the breast, ovary, bladder, small cell lung Acute leukaemias	Nausea and vomiting (HD) Myelosuppression Haemorrhagic cystitis Alopecia (HD) Infertility (especially in men)
Cytosine arabinoside (Ara-C)	Antimetabolite	Acute myeloid leukaemia Acute lymphoblastic leukaemia (low dose may be given subcutaneously)	Severe nausea and vomiting (HD) Myelosuppression Flu-like symptoms Mucositis Corneal ulceration
Doxorubicin (Adriamycin)	Antitumour antibiotic (interferes with nucleic acid synthesis in the S-phase)	Wide spectrum Lymphomas Cancer of the breast, ovary, stomach, sarcomas, small cell lung	Severe mucositis Severe nausea and vomiting Cardiotoxicity (dose limiting) Myelosuppression Alopecia Vesicant if extravasated
Etoposide (Vepesid, VP16)	Mitotic inhibitor arresting cell cycle at G_2-phase	Testicular cancer, small cell lung, lymphoma Acute lymphocytic leukaemia	Myelosuppression Mucositis (HD) Alopecia Hypotension if infused rapidly
Fludarabine (Fludara)	Purine metabolite	Chronic lymphocytic leukaemia Low-grade non-Hodgkin's lymphoma	Myelosuppression Nausea and vomiting Flu-like symptoms Central nervous system toxicities (HD)
5-Fluorouracil (5-FU)	Antimetabolite	Breast, colorectal and GI, head and neck cancers	Myelosuppression Diarrhoea Mucositis Mild nausea Vein discoloration
Irinotecan (Campto, CPT-11)	DNA topoisomerase inhibitor, spindle poison	Colorectal cancer	Myelosuppression Nausea and vomiting Alopecia Delayed diarrhoea Acute cholinergic syndrome
Methotrexate	Antimetabolite (folic acid antagonist)	Wide spectrum Breast cancer Osteosarcoma Choriocarcinoma Acute lymphocytic leukaemia Non-Hodgkin's lymphoma	Myelosuppression Diarrhoea Mucositis Mild nausea Renal failure (HD)

Table 31.4 Cytotoxic agents and common side-effects *(Continued)*

Cytotoxic agent	Action	Common use	Potential side-effects
Paclitaxel (Taxol)	Plant alkaloid Tubulin spindle poison	Ovarian and breast cancer	Myelosuppression Alopecia Hypersensitivity — urticaria, abdominal cramping, rash, anaphylaxis Peripheral neuropathy; numbness, tingling and loss of function Myalgia/arthralgia — joint and muscle pains
Vincristine (Oncovin)	Vinca alkaloid Spindle poison, blocks mitosis in M-phase	Wide spectrum Sarcoma, lung, breast cancer Acute lymphocytic leukaemia Lymphoma	Myelosuppression Alopecia Peripheral neuropathy; numbness, tingling and loss of function Vesicant if extravasated

HD, high dose.

Hair may grow back a different texture and colour, to which patients should be alerted. Patients should be offered the choice of a wig before they experience hair loss in order to enable close matching to their own hair. Promoting a positive self-image by offering advice to minimise hair loss and about the use of fashion accessories is important, as the psychological impact of alopecia should not be underestimated (Munstedt et al 1997, Batchelor 2001).

Scalp cooling techniques have been developed with varying degrees of success (Macduff et al 2003, Massey 2003). Earlier scalp cooling techniques involved wetting the scalp and applying ice packs, but more sophisticated refrigeration systems are now available which offer a more uniform cooling at a constant rate (Protiere et al 2002, Massey 2003). Observations from clinical practice suggest that scalp cooling can slow down the rate of hair loss when used with single-agent drugs with a short half-life at low dosages, e.g. adriamycin, cyclophosphamide, docetaxel. It may also be effective with such regimens as FAM (5-fluorouracil, adriamycin, mitomycin C) and CMF (cyclophosphamide, methotrexate, 5-fluorouracil).

Sexual dysfunction may occur due to vascular changes and hormonal imbalance. Amenorrhoea and menopausal symptoms may be induced due to ovarian failure and follicle destruction. Women under 35 years of age have a greater chance of resumption of the menses on completion of treatment; however, this may not occur for 6–12 months.

Infertility may occur, depending on the agent, its dosage, the patient's age and gender, and other as yet unknown factors. Infertility may be temporary or permanent. Alkylating agents such as cyclophosphamide, chlorambucil and the nitrosurea compounds are certain to induce infertility. This variability must be stressed when patients are informed about potential side-effects. Barrier methods of contraception are encouraged, as the exposure of an unborn fetus to cytotoxic agents may result in deformities or an unviable fetus (Chasle & How 2003).

In certain circumstances, some patients may receive counselling for sperm banking or oocyte harvesting. These options raise emotional and ethical dilemmas which may compound patients' existing stress concerning their diagnosis and treatment. This is an area of nursing that provides new challenges in terms of psychological support for patients and their partners.

Other side-effects It is not possible to address all the potential side-effects of chemotherapy in this chapter. However, apart from the more common ones mentioned above and those in Table 31.3, it is important to remember the more generalised effects, e.g. fatigue, anorexia, general malaise, mood disturbances and lack of concentration. Ream and Richardson's (1999) nursing research focused attention on fatigue and the need to develop positive interventions such as energy conservation.

For further information, see Holmes (1997) and Dodds (2001).

Biological response modifiers

Biological therapy, often referred to as the fourth treatment modality, involves the therapeutic use of substances known to occur naturally in the body. Most of these are involved in some way in the immune response, controlling cell-mediated and humoral responses; hence some of these new developments are termed 'immunotherapies'. The theory behind these new treatments is that it may be possible to manipulate the immune system such that it recognises tumour cells as antigens and causes the body to reject them.

Biological therapies were prematurely hailed as 'miracle cures' for all cancer types. In fact, the response of the immune system to tumours has been found to be far more subtle and complex than the response to microbes, and results have been far from dramatic. Nevertheless, several substances, mostly created by recombinant DNA technology, have been developed. Although research is still at a very early stage, tumour response, however transient, has been achieved for some cancer types.

Cytokines are substances released from an activated immune system. Interferon α_{2a}, for example, is an activator of natural killer cells and protects host cells against viruses. It has been found to maintain remission in hairy cell leukaemia and is being used with some success in certain patients with renal cell carcinoma and AIDS-related Kaposi's sarcoma. Side-effects include flu-like symptoms and mood disturbances, which may be very unpleasant. Other similar substances include tumour necrosis factor (TNF) and interleukin 2.

Haemopoietic growth factors include GCSF which stimulate the proliferation of leucocytes. Used appropriately, these factors may reduce the number or degree of myelosuppressive episodes, prevent treatment delays and allow high doses of treatment to be given (stem cell transplantation). Erythropoietin is another stimulating factor used in the treatment of anaemia. The number of blood transfusions may be reduced and symptoms of fatigue minimised, thus enhancing quality of life.

Monoclonal antibodies A limiting factor in effective cancer therapy is its current lack of specificity. During the 1980s, significant strides were made in the field of antibody therapy, which promotes specific targeting of cells through an antigen–antibody response. Tumours have been found to possess antigens on their surface, and monoclonal antibodies to these antigens can now be manufactured in laboratories. Examples of monoclonal antibodies used in the clinical setting are rituximab (MabThera) and trastuzumab (Herceptin). Rituximab is directed against the CD20 antigen expressed in over 90% of B cell lymphomas and chronic lymphocytic leukaemia (CLL). Trastuzumab is directed against the human epidermal growth factor HER2-neu (c-erb2) proto-oncogene. In clinical studies, HER2 protein overexpression and gene amplification have been associated with a higher frequency of tumour recurrence and a reduction in overall survival time. Trastuzumab is presently used as a single agent for the treatment of women with metastatic breast cancer whose tumours overexpress the HER2-neu protein. Trials are ongoing to determine its value in the adjuvant setting (Miles 2001).

Cancer vaccines Based on the antibody–antigen response mechanism, several vaccines have been developed for use in melanoma and trialled with encouraging responses. A cancer vaccine for the human papilloma virus (HPV16 and 18), a risk factor for cervical cancer, has recently been developed with positive trial outcomes (Harper et al 2004). More research is required in this area to determine the therapeutic value of such vaccines (Mitchell 1998).

Side-effects These therapies have quite different toxicity spectra from those of chemotherapy, such as flu-like syndromes with patients frequently experiencing fever, chills, headache, malaise, arthralgia and fatigue, severe enough to be dose-limiting factors. These symptoms can disrupt and impact on a patient's lifestyle quite significantly. It is important for nurses to be aware of this in order to support their patients, initiating appropriate interventions such as premedication and energy saving techniques.

For further reading, see the following comprehensive articles on new biological cancer treatments in Seminars in Oncology Nursing 2003, Volume 19(3), by Gale; Liu; Mautner & Huang; Muehlbauer & Schwartzentruber; and Schmidt & Wood.

STOP THINK **31.10** Choose a patient who is about to receive combination chemotherapy. Find out whether the doses or medications in the regimen are low or high. List the side-effects you may expect to see and those that actually occur. For information, consult the manufacturers' instructions, your hospital pharmacy cytotoxic manual and texts on chemotherapy, e.g. Holmes (1997), Allwood et al (2002) and Fischer (2003).

Psychological support during systemic therapy (see Box 31.9). There is increasing recognition, supported by research, that chemotherapy, particularly the highly toxic regimens, can cause short- and long-term side-effects that can lead to psychological distress and thus affect an individual's quality of life (Amir & Ramati 2002, Del Mastro et al 2002). In a recent study in Scotland, nurses reported that patients were often anxious, distressed or frightened and emphasised that patients required individualised, clear information about their disease and treatment. Psychological, social and financial support for themselves and their families was also seen to be important. Nurses perceived that patients required more psychological support at the beginning and at the end of treatment, which may be difficult times for patients. The importance of talking and providing information was seen as an essential intervention for meeting patients' psychological needs (Arantzamendi & Kearney 2004). As with radiotherapy, the key to effective support for these patients is an understanding of the impact of chemotherapy on the patient and their family, a thorough needs assessment and an individualised plan of care.

Nurses in most oncology centres and some cancer units have their own patient caseload where care priorities include assessment of treatment toxicities, cannulation, administration of bolus and intravenous chemotherapy, and

Box 31.9

Chemotherapy: the patient's perspective

The need for information and emotional support during chemotherapy varies according to the patient's perception of the treatment. The following responses by patients to the discovery that they required chemotherapy (cited in Tierney et al 1989) reflect this variability.

Negative feelings

I can't tell you how terrified I am ... it's like being put into a dark room ... you've no idea what to expect and you're really frightened.

The word 'chemotherapy' sends shivers up my spine — you hear so much about how awful it is.

Mixed feelings

I do want it, but I don't. I feel really nervous ... Butterflies in my tummy all the time ... and then I tell myself not to be silly ... You'll manage, I say.

Positive feelings

I'm making myself feel positive because I intend to do everything possible to survive. That never occurred to me before ... the idea of survival ... but your priorities change when you are faced with a disease like this.

coordinating the chemotherapy/BRM regimens in collaboration with the clinician. The continuity of care engendered by this approach allows a trusting supportive relationship to be built between nurse and patient.

A more recent development in the UK is home chemotherapy. Specialised nurses, who may be hospital- or community-based, deliver chemotherapy to patients in the comfort of their own homes (Watters 1997). Some projects are nurse-led pilot schemes, others are being set up in collaboration with intravenous access companies in the private sector (Pattison & Macrae 2002).

STOP THINK **31.11** The patient receiving palliative chemotherapy may find travelling exhausting and feel that staying at home is far preferable to spending precious time in hospital. With new services developing to include chemotherapy administered in the patient's home, what potential problems can you foresee for the patient, the family and the nurse? On balance, do you think this is a worthwhile and cost-effective scheme?

Non-cytotoxic chemotherapy

Agents other than cytotoxic drugs are used to control, but as yet not to cure, cancer. Tumours that arise in tissues under the control of hormones have been found to respond to hormone manipulation. This may mean surgical removal of the ovaries (oophorectomy) or testes (orchidectomy) to reduce the growth stimulus to tumours of the breast or prostate provided by oestrogen and testosterone, respectively. In the last 30 years, similar control has been achieved by the use of medication such as tamoxifen. Tamoxifen blocks the action of oestrogen by binding to oestrogen receptor sites on the tumour cells. However, more recently, tamoxifen has been superseded by the use of aromatase inhibitors such as anastrozole in post-menopausal women. They work on the cancer cells differently from tamoxifen, not by blocking the effect of oestrogen, but by preventing its production.

Steroid hormones, such as prednisolone and dexamethasone, are also widely used, the former in conjunction with cytotoxic medication as primary treatment, usually for lymphomas, and the latter for its anti-inflammatory action in symptom control and the control of emesis.

Symptom control forms a major part of both the nursing and medical roles in oncology (see Ch. 33).

Clinical trials

Despite an enormous amount of worldwide investment in research, cancer remains on the whole an incurable disease.

Most cancer centres are involved in multiple research trials, and nurses should be familiar with the format of these trials in order to understand the implications for patients and for their nursing care and to consider the ethical dilemmas which arise around all experimental therapy.

Following laboratory testing, new treatment methods are tested on consenting patients by means of a series of trials termed phase 1, 2 and 3 trials. During phase 1, the maximum tolerable dose is established and information is obtained about the drug's toxicity profile; phase 2 trials discover which type of cancer is most responsive; and finally, phase 3 trials discover the extent to which the treatment improves survival. In phase 3 trials, patients from the target group are randomly selected to receive either the new treatment or the best established one. Survival rates are then compared.

New approaches to established radiotherapy and chemotherapy treatments are constantly being tested in this way. In addition, some centres are involved in trials of totally new modes of treatment.

Complementary therapy

As treatment outcomes of conventional medicine are uncertain, and as cancer may become a chronic illness affecting every area of life, there is increasing interest in complementary therapies. Based on the connection between body and mind, these therapies focus on a more 'holistic' approach to health in which the individual is encouraged to take control of their own life, both mentally and physically. Such therapies include homeopathy, acupuncture, therapeutic touch, massage, aromatherapy, relaxation techniques, yoga, hypnotherapy, nutrition, self-help groups and stress management.

Little research exists to justify the use of any of these therapies as alternatives to orthodox treatments (Fitch et al 1999) and evidence for the value of complementary therapy is conflicting. However, evidence is accumulating that some interventions may contribute positively to both psychological and physical health outcomes. Data from eight randomised controlled trials in a Cochrane Review of the use of massage and aromatherapy for symptom relief in patients with cancer found short-term benefits. The authors conclude that longer follow-up studies are required to determine whether these benefits persist (Fellowes et al 2004).

Recent discoveries of neurotransmitters connecting the brain, body and immune system suggest a physiological basis for improved outcomes. It is also possible, however, that the extra time, attention and caring mediated by therapists in the course of complementary treatments are factors in the patient's feeling of well-being. It is well established that, when patients feel in control, they have better coping skills, emotional well-being, physical health, immune function and, most importantly, experience subjectively a better quality of life (Gerits & De Brabander 1999, Henderson & Donatelle 2003, Link et al 2004).

It is important that health professionals respect an individual's beliefs and choices, recognising the potential benefits of a combined approach to cancer treatment. In order to avoid potential harm, only certified practitioners with knowledge of interactions or contraindications should deliver complementary therapies. Recent surveys confirm that a substantial proportion of patients are using herbal medicines, which have the potential to cause adverse reactions (Werneke et al 2004, Molassiotis et al 2005). For efficacy and safety, it is helpful for patients and clinicians to discuss any planned complementary therapy.

NURSING PRACTICE IN CANCER CARE

The cancer nurse

Cancer and its treatment have a unique impact on an individual's life. Although the physical problems experienced by cancer patients may be similar to those of patients with many non-malignant conditions, the combination of these problems with the chronic nature of cancer, the highly toxic effects of treatment and the profound psychological impact of the disease mean that cancer nurses require specialised knowledge and skills. Cancer nursing as a specialty has been in existence for many years in the UK and is continually developing. The last decade has recognised the increasing diversity of the role of the cancer nurse and the particular contribution in providing seamless care throughout the cancer journey. Key skills in cancer nursing are those that help the cancer patient and their carers to adapt to the reality of living with cancer while maximising quality of life.

Hospital–community liaison

Cancer is a chronic illness characterised by remissions, exacerbations and progressive physical changes. More patients with cancer are living longer. Health professionals caring for cancer patients should view care as a continuous process whether it takes place in the hospital or in the community setting. Supporting the patient through the cancer journey requires the skills of all members of the multiprofessional team in conjunction with the patient and family. If care is to be a truly continuous process then the importance of sharing the care between hospital and community must be acknowledged (Owen & Black 1996). Shared care protocols, a relatively new concept in cancer care, came about in response to the recognition of unfulfilled needs of patients receiving active treatments at home, e.g. immunotherapy or continuous chemotherapy infusions. Such protocols promote the philosophy of continuity of care between hospital and community. Effective communication and discharge planning are essential to optimal care. Without proper coordination and integration of services, the cancer patient's 'journey' through the health care system can be a bewildering and demoralising experience. The example of Mr A in Case History 31.4 illustrates the need for good discharge planning and liaison between hospital and community nurses.

Cancer patients spend most of their lives at home, interrupted by short hospital admissions. As a result, much of the psychological and physical adjustment to cancer takes place at home. Community initiatives and services are set up to support patients, their families and other carers from diagnosis to terminal illness, helping patients in decision making and achieving optimal independence and quality of life.

Cancer care in any setting can be very satisfying; it can also be stressful and nurses working in this specialty need to develop healthy and effective coping strategies (see Box 31.10).

Cancer care in the community

Community nursing staff are involved in cancer care during five phases:

- prevention programmes
- diagnosis
- treatment-related support
- rehabilitation following initial cancer treatment
- palliative care.

GPs, practice nurses, community nurses, liaison nurses and health visitors are generally involved in prevention schemes. Some health visitors may visit patients recently discharged from hospital in order to assess how they and their families are coping and their needs for care and emotional support. District nurses coordinate and carry out a needs assessment for patients throughout their time in the community. In some areas, new initiatives are being developed to support patients in the community at diagnosis and during treatment with the introduction of community cancer care nurses with specialist oncology knowledge and skills (Gorman et al 2000). Towards the later stages of the disease, symptoms may become more problematic and place more strain on carers; at this stage, Macmillan, Marie Curie or community palliative care nurses who have close links with the hospice and hospital-based palliative care teams, may become involved. These nurses have specialist skills in managing complex symptoms, providing psychosocial support and planning care in conjunction with the

CASE HISTORY 31.4

Mr A

Mr A, a 58-year-old head teacher, is married with two children: a daughter in Australia and a married son with two small children who lived nearby.

He presented to his GP with urinary hesitancy and frequency. Examination and subsequent referral to a urologist revealed a T3 adenocarcinoma of the prostate (a locally invasive tumour with no metastases). A biopsy of the tumour and a bone scan were performed with Mr A as an outpatient. Mr A opted for 4 weeks of radical radiotherapy rather than a prostatectomy. Because he lived in a small town 50 miles away from the nearest radiotherapy department, he became an inpatient, going home at weekends. During his recovery at home, a health visitor visited twice.

Two years later, 1 week after his retirement, rib pain necessitated a further bone scan. This showed metastatic deposits in the ribs and spine. At Mr A's local hospital, a bilateral orchidectomy was performed to reduce hormonal stimulation of tumour growth. Mr A was then readmitted to the radiotherapy department. One week of palliative radiotherapy and the commencement of opiate analgesics enabled discharge and 6 months of reasonably independent life.

However, a fall whilst Mr A was gardening resulted in the collapse of the third thoracic vertebra, with resultant severe pain and paraplegia due to spinal cord compression. High dose steroids initially, emergency radiotherapy and intensive physiotherapy restored some function, but Mr A was now confined to a wheelchair and had no bladder or bowel control.

Mrs A was fit and very determined to cope at home with the help of her son and his wife. Prior to Mr A's discharge, the community occupational therapy department oversaw the installation of a wheelchair ramp, bath aids and a hoist in the A's bungalow. District nurses visited regularly and referred Mr A to social services to provide support with washing and dressing. The Macmillan nurse provided psychological support and complex symptom management, linking Mr A in with the local hospice.

Within 6 weeks a further admission, this time to the local hospital, was necessary due to hypercalcaemia, which was treated with intravenous bisphosphonates for several months. Gradually Mr A's condition deteriorated and he was generally too weak to get out of bed. District nurses now visited him twice a day, and the Macmillan nurse visited regularly for pain and symptom control. It was arranged for Marie Curie nurses to care for Mr A at night, in order to give the family a rest. Mr A died peacefully at home with his family.

Box 31.10

Stress in cancer nursing

In 1988, Speck stated that the most important ethical choice made by cancer nurses is whether or not to engage in 'an intense, personalised involvement' with their patients in response to human need. A degree of emotional involvement is inevitable, and even necessary, to achieve excellence in cancer care. But such involvement, particularly as it may be terminated by the patient's death, results in considerable occupational stress. This emotional involvement is simultaneously a great asset and a point of vulnerability for nurses (Cunningham 2000).

The picture that emerges from the research and literature related to stress, burnout and the emotional labour of cancer nursing is mixed (Magnusson & Robinson 2000). A focus group found that patient care or contact was the greatest source of job satisfaction for cancer care workers. Oncology was felt to be a special environment because of the type of relationship established with patients and their families. However, over a third of participants demonstrated high levels of emotional exhaustion and low levels of personal accomplishment (Grunfeld et al 2005).

The constructive expression of emotions is as important as stress control. Establishing an environment of trust and mutual respect where it is safe to admit to colleagues feelings of inadequacy, grief and guilt, and even personal fears about cancer and death, is beneficial in relieving stress. Such support should also be provided on an organised basis in the form of support groups and counselling services, as formal support groups are often catalysts for social support, problem solving and task sharing (Tschudin 1996). Reflective practice, clinical supervision and mentorship are also important concepts that enable and empower individuals within their nursing practice.

Nurses continue to describe emotionally charged areas of care as being the most difficult and stressful; however, Wilkinson et al (2002) have shown that an integrated approach to communication skills improves nurses' expertise in this area.

An active life and supportive relationships outside of work are also vital in maintaining a realistic perspective on life. Without external interests, it may be easy for the nurse to imagine that cancer is far more prevalent than it is. Fields et al (1997) introduced stress reduction therapies such as a 10-minute massage, listening to music, visual imagery and social support group sessions and found that nurses experienced increased vigour and decreased anxiety and fatigue.

A commitment to continuing education by nursing management is essential in stress control. However, as Tschudin (1996) concludes: 'nurses themselves need to take on more direct responsibility for their own psychological care', and in campaigning for support and education.

district nurse and other members of the primary care team. The fostering of links with the Macmillan service as early as possible, when a patient is still able to discuss their hopes, fears and goals, assists in the establishment of a supportive relationship (see also Ch. 33).

The role of the district nurse The role of community staff is one of partnership with the patient and their family, who constitute the main 'unit of care'. Providing information, support and advice is often as important as assistance with physical care.

Another major role of the district nurse involves co-ordination of the primary care team and integration of statutory and non-statutory services. Because of the nature of cancer, the need for these services is considerable. The statutory services available include all of those necessary for the care of the chronically ill in the community (see Ch. 32).

Non-statutory services in the community Non-statutory services for cancer patients are particularly comprehensive in their provision and include the following.

Support and self-help groups Such groups can reduce the isolation of the cancer experience. The sharing of feelings and experiences provides emotional support, fosters hope and encourages a sense of self-worth and purpose. Many local groups exist for patients and/or their carers.

Support and information centres Empowerment of individuals, thereby allowing them to help themselves, is the basis of psychoeducational intervention programmes advocated by Fawzy et al (2000). Information, emotional support, relaxation and stress management are provided in thoughtfully designed environments for those affected by cancer, including carers, partners, relatives and friends. Programmes have been developed to provide opportunities for people to live and cope with a cancer diagnosis. Maggie's Cancer Caring Centres and Macmillan Information Centres are just two examples. Many other UK cancer support centres provide similar assistance and access to complementary therapists.

Counselling services Counselling may be necessary to assist the patient and their family to adapt emotionally to cancer and can help to relieve anxiety and depression. The Cancer Counselling Trust provides this service by telephone and in person and CancerBACUP advises about other local counselling services.

Financial aid The Cancer Relief Macmillan Fund (CRMF) can provide financial aid to meet the cost of aids, appliances, heating, bedding, holidays and other special needs.

Nursing services The Marie Curie organisation provides nursing staff, including a night nursing service, to allow carers some respite or sleep.

See 'Useful websites'.

Nursing frameworks for cancer care

No one framework or model of nursing can be suitable for every cancer patient or care setting. Integrated care pathways are an example of a framework which aims to integrate evidence-based practice through a documented plan of anticipated care for a group of patients with a particular diagnosis or set of symptoms. Each professional involved in the patient's care has a clearly defined role and the plan of care leads each patient towards a desired goal (Middleton & Roberts 2002). In palliative care for example, the Liverpool Care of the Dying Pathway transfers a hospice model of care into other health care environments (Ellershaw & Wilkinson 2003).

It is important to adapt and combine models and approaches to provide a workable framework of care for each patient.

Family coping

A cancer diagnosis can have a drastic effect on the patient's family and loved ones in the following ways:

- Cancer can disrupt patterns of familial and other interpersonal interaction. Those who are close to the patient are usually perplexed as to how to relate to the person in the most helpful way. Reactions vary from overprotection and excessive vigilance to distancing behaviour and even the complete breakdown of relationships. Many patients, especially in the early stages of the disease, may feel that they have to be the strong one emotionally, supporting and holding the family together. Under such strain it is no wonder that cancer can, and does, precipitate partnership and marital breakdown. Most at risk are those whose relationship is already unstable. In a study by Barraclough (1998), however, a majority of married people stated that they actually felt closer to their partners in the few months following a cancer diagnosis.
- Cancer disrupts planning for the future. An experience with cancer may last for many years. The uncertainty involved disrupts family plans and dreams for holidays, retirement, parenthood and so forth. Roles within the family change, particularly if the patient is a breadwinner or parent. Such change is stressful and can undermine the patient's sense of self-worth and purpose. Loss of income and increased expenditure due to the illness can create financial strain.
- Cancer alters the interaction of the family with external groups. Patients and their families may become isolated as a result of the social stigma of cancer, financial hardship and any residual disability. For some, however, involvement in self-help groups and cancer charities expands social interaction.

Nursing interventions After assessment of family dynamics and needs, the following nursing interventions may help to alleviate some of the above problems:

- Providing regular information about the patient's status and plans for care, preferably facilitating open communication between the patient and their family, which is associated with lower anxiety levels (Edwards & Clarke 2004). Shared information helps to promote a positive attitude and improves adaptation and communication within the hospital setting and at home.
- Encouraging relatives to express their feelings of fear, loss, guilt and exhaustion.
- Encouraging realistic, mutual goal-setting, e.g. the timing and planning of holidays.
- Encouraging family members to adapt the patient's role within the family to maintain a sense of belonging and worth, e.g. by exchanging physical tasks for clerical ones.
- Referring families promptly to the social work department for financial assistance and, if necessary, rehousing.
- Recognising signs of exhaustion in carers, giving them 'permission' to take time off and arranging respite care or hospital/hospice admission for the patient if necessary.
- Encouraging continued social involvement, suggesting appropriate activities if necessary.
- Suggesting referral to a psychologist or marriage guidance counsellor if family relationships appear to be breaking down.

Nutrition

In most societies, food and drink have sociological, psychological and cultural significance. They are an important source of enjoyment and social interaction with adequate nourishment symbolising health and well-being. Up to 85% of cancer patients, due to a variety of complex factors, are malnourished (Shaw 2002).

Cancer cachexia (see p. 1034) is a multifaceted syndrome not yet fully understood (Inui 2002). The associated weight loss can have a very negative effect on a patient's body image and sexuality; it represents a major source of concern for both patient and family, often acting as a barometer of the patient's condition.

Malnutrition in cancer patients is associated with a poor prognosis, reduced response to anticancer treatments and prolongation of treatment side-effects (Holmes 1996). Causes of malnutrition and weight loss in cancer patients include the following:

- Reduced food intake due to:
  - — anorexia: due to multiple causes, e.g. release of cytokines such as TNF and interleukin-1 are thought to delay gastric emptying, thus delaying digestion, suppressing the appetite and causing satiety (Shaw 2002)
  - — taste changes: may occur in any cancer patient (Foltz 2000); they are most common following radiotherapy to the head or neck due to destruction of salivary tissue. These changes involve a lowered threshold for bitter tastes, and therefore aversion to meat; raised threshold for sweet tastes, and hence many foods taste bland and 'cardboard-like'; alteration of the taste of tea and coffee
  - — early satiety: metabolic abnormalities directly related to tumour burden may result in early satiety, a premature feeling of fullness, usually progressing over the day
  - — other symptoms: such as pain, nausea, vomiting and drowsiness
  - — physical difficulties: due to oral prostheses or badly fitting dentures; also to the tumour and treatment, e.g. oesophageal obstruction, chemotherapy-induced mucositis
  - — anxiety and depression.
- Malabsorption due to:
  - — resection of tumours of the gastrointestinal tract, leading to decreased enzyme production and increased transit time
  - — impairment of nutrient absorption resulting from chemotherapy and abdominal radiotherapy.
- Excess expenditure of nutrients, due to:
  - — in many patients, raised basal metabolic rate, partly due to the demands of the tumour

— excessive loss of body protein due to vomiting, diarrhoea, haemorrhage, oedema, and exudates from stomas, fistulae and ulcerations.

Nursing interventions Actions that the nurse can take to help the patient overcome or manage difficulties with eating and drinking include the following:

- Use at regular intervals of a screening tool such as MUST (malnutrition universal screening tool) to assess the patient's current nutritional status and potential for further deterioration (Malnutrition Advisory Group 2003). Weekly weighing is adequate; more frequent weighing may cause the patient to become anxious and demoralised by continued weight loss.
- Identifying the major factors that contribute to the nutritional deficit.
- Referring 'at-risk' patients to a dietitian.
- Referring to a speech and language therapist those patients with an identified swallowing or aspiration problem.
- Referring to an occupational therapist to assist with functional or practical difficulties.
- Referring to a social worker for a care package to assist with shopping and meal preparation.
- Enlisting the help of relatives and friends to offer the patient's favourite foods whilst respecting autonomy. However, it is important to explain that there are very real reasons for the patient's reluctance to eat. Provision of dietary information, recipes and self-care measures may be helpful.
- Offering frequent, small, high calorie attractive meals and snacks throughout the day; negotiating with the catering department for flexibility in portion size and for a supply of nutrient-rich foods to be kept at ward level.
- Encouraging patients to take fluids in the form of high-energy drinks; discouraging drinking at mealtimes, to avoid early satiety.
- Decreasing satiety by the avoidance of high fat foods which delay gastric emptying; the use of prokinetics, e.g. metoclopramide, may promote gastric emptying.
- Reassuring the patient that taste changes are to be expected and may disappear in time; offering taste-enhancing herbs, spices, marinades (unless mucositis a problem) and alternatives to tea and coffee.
- Supporting the patient if there is further weight loss despite sufficient calorie intake, due to disruption of normal metabolism.
- Using gentle exercise, relaxation or modest amounts of alcohol to stimulate the appetite.
- Controlling other symptoms. Antiemetics and analgesics, topical and systemic, should be administered 30 min before meals.
- Encouraging regular mouthwashes before and after meals.
- Providing dietary supplements which may be nutritionally complete supplements, or calorie supplements. These may be fruit juice, milk or yoghurt based. Research into the use of fish oils as a nutritional supplement may prove useful for the future (Barber 2001).
- Eliminating nauseating environmental stimuli at mealtimes, such as bedpans, odours and disturbing procedures.
- If intake is consistently inadequate and/or weight loss continues, commencing other forms of feeding: nasogastric if absorption is adequate; parenteral if not.
- Once the patient is well, encouraging a healthy, well-balanced diet, similar to that recommended for preventing cancer (see Box 31.3). It is also important to assist patients to make an informed choice by providing appropriate information regarding the nutritional value, ease, practicality, availability and cost of alternative diets.

Expressing sexuality

Following treatment for cancer, up to 50% of patients who were sexually active before the illness report some reduction in sexual interest or activity (Barraclough 1998). Health care professionals in general fail to take the initiative in addressing their patients' sexual problems within the context of treatment for chronic and life-threatening illness. The reticence of some nurses may be due to embarrassment, but a lack of relevant knowledge and counselling skills has also been reported (Guthrie 1999, White 2002).

Sexuality involves more than sexual intercourse. It includes self-image in relation to gender, role behaviour within a partnership, and many forms of love and affection between partners. Partners are also affected by the experience of cancer and in some cases report higher levels of psychological distress and psychosexual concerns than patients (Carlson et al 2000). A cancer patient's sexuality may be altered for many reasons, including:

- the physical effects of the tumour, e.g. lesions of the spinal cord may interfere with the nerve pathways necessary for sexual sensation or motor function
- symptoms caused by the tumour, e.g. pain, immobility, nocturia, dysuria, rectal bleeding and fatigue can all contribute to a decrease in desire for sexual intimacy
- the physical effects of treatment, e.g. hormone manipulation may alter sexual function; surgery may alter the anatomy, for example a prostatectomy may cause pelvic nerve damage resulting in impotence; pelvic irradiation may reduce vaginal lubrication causing dyspareunia, i.e. painful intercourse
- body image problems, e.g. postmastectomy or following stoma formation; less obvious changes may also contribute, e.g. varying degrees of weight loss or hair loss
- anxiety and depression related to the cancer diagnosis resulting in low self-esteem.

Nursing interventions The nurse can provide support for the cancer patient experiencing problems with the expression of sexuality in the following ways:

- Initiating discussion in order to give the patient 'permission' to voice their concerns. Once the discussion is initiated, the patient will indicate whether or not they wish to pursue the topic.
- Anticipating problems before treatment: explaining how long they will last and that they are to be expected; describing measures that can be used to relieve them

(see Table 31.3 for examples of interventions for radiotherapy patients).

- Opening discussion with non-threatening subjects such as contraceptive advice or the alterations in partnership roles due to illness. This will aid progression to potentially more personal issues.
- Discovering and using the patient's own language in relation to their sexuality.
- Ensuring that anxiety and depression are treated and body image problems addressed. Severe body image problems may require de-sensitisation therapy by a psychologist.
- Involving partners in discussion and physical care as appropriate.
- Facilitating the privacy of couples in hospitals.
- When appropriate, discussing ways in which a couple may share sexual pleasure that does not involve intercourse. CancerBACUP and Cancer*Index* provide information that describes such methods (see 'Useful websites').
- Referring patients and partners with severe problems for psychosexual counselling as appropriate.

Communicating

From the cancer patient's perspective, patient-focused communication can be the most important aspect of treatment, in part because of its capacity to exacerbate or allay the fear that often accompanies cancer (Fallowfield & Jenkins 1999). Communication encompasses three areas of activity, which may be described as:

- cognitive — the giving and receiving of information
- emotional — the feeling and expression of psychological responses
- spiritual — the expression and feeling of thoughts relating to existential issues beyond the self.

Although this division can help in identifying specific nursing activities, the three areas are interrelated. Providing information in a sensitive, caring manner affords emotional support, and many people do not consciously make the distinction between the emotional and spiritual dimensions.

Cognitive activity The patient's need for information in relation to diagnosis and treatment has been examined in earlier sections of this chapter. To this discussion the following observations may be added:

- Knowledge is power: power that enables independence, choice, autonomous decision making and realistic goal-setting for patients and their families. Information promotes the patient's sense of control over their life.
- Studies of patients' perceived needs rank information as a key component for coping with cancer (Peck & Boland 1977, Eardley 1986, Van der Molen 1999).
- Lack of information can deepen a depressive reaction to a cancer diagnosis.
- Specific information about diagnosis and prognosis can encourage active participation by patients in their own care, and in fact generates rather than negates hope (Cassileth et al 1980, Skalla et al 2004).
- Patients have traditionally expected their needs for information to be met by doctors, and their needs for support to be met by nurses. However, in practice, particularly with the evolution of specialist nurses, this is changing. Patients will choose the person they wish to obtain information from depending on their needs.
- Studies show that patients seldom take the initiative in seeking information, mainly because staff appear busy and unavailable (Wells 1998b).
- Nurses, by their behaviour and non-verbal communication, may indicate they are too busy to answer questions at that particular time. They may also feel they lack the information the patient is seeking, or fear that information-giving may lead to an emotional unburdening by the patient, for which they may lack the personal resources necessary to cope.
- Patients and their families need information on the cause of the cancer, the possible course of the disease, treatment options, the role of the health care team, available services and sources of further information.
- Patients vary greatly in their desire for, and receptivity to, information. For example, patients who actively deny their cancer are unlikely to listen to information about community nursing support on discharge, and patients with a fatalistic attitude may not be interested in information about self-help groups or complementary therapy.

Nursing interventions The following advice may assist the nurse to meet the patient's communication needs:

- Be equipped with the information that the patient needs. Be assertive in obtaining this information from other members of the health care team so that a consistent 'story' is given to the patient.
- Be present at as many interactions between the patient and the doctor as possible. Afterwards reinforce messages and ensure that the patient has understood.
- Find out what the patient already knows and has been told, and what they want to know. In general, follow the patient's agenda.
- Discover the patient's principal fears and give information to correct any misconceptions.
- Bear in mind that when receiving information most people remember only three specific points; the first three points made are those most likely to be remembered.
- Avoid jargon: 'your white cell count will fall', for example, may mean nothing to most patients. Information about how they will feel and what they will experience is most important to patients.
- Document information given, together with an estimation of the patient's retention and reaction.
- Be prepared for the patient to forget or deny receiving the information given.
- Reinforce verbal information with written information. CancerBACUP and many oncology centres produce patient literature on a wide range of subjects.
- Be prepared for information-giving to lead to emotional issues. Allow time for this or promise to return at an arranged time — and do so.
- Give the patient and their relatives the same information. Give each the opportunity to receive this information both together and separately, so that

personal anxieties can be expressed privately and within the family group.

Emotional activity Enabling patients and their families to cope with the emotional impact of cancer demands effective listening skills and is an essential component of counselling (see Box 31.11). The following considerations should be borne in mind by the nurse in addressing the cancer patient's emotional needs:

- During any stage of the disease, the cancer patient is suffering the effects of various actual or potential losses. These may include loss of a body part or function, loss of self-image, loss of work or leisure activities, loss of family or social role, loss of control over life, loss of goals and dreams for the future and, ultimately, loss of life itself. Loss is the predominant factor in all sadness and depression.
- There are many uncertainties involved in cancer; uncertainty leads to anxiety.
- While the majority of cancer patients adjust emotionally and cope reasonably well with loss and uncertainty, several studies document the prevalence of psychological distress and even psychiatric illness among this client group (Maguire 1985). A study by Zabora et al (2001), examining the prevalence of psychological distress in 14 cancer sites (n = 4496), found the overall prevalence rate of distress to be 35.1%.
- A great deal of this emotional turmoil, anxiety and depression passes undetected and unrelieved (Fallowfield et al 2001). Rates of depression have been reported to be as high as 75% in several psychiatric studies (Mathieson & Stam 1995). Maguire (1985) calculated that only one-fifth of patients with severe emotional problems were helped effectively. Subsequent research has focused on prediction and early detection of affective disorders, through screening and improving communication skills of health professionals as well as therapeutic interventions (Maguire 1995).
- Emotional support is not a luxury in nursing care. Emotional distress may result in somatic symptoms such as confusion, immobility, insomnia and pain. As previously suggested, long-term distress may exacerbate disease progression (Brown et al 2003).
- The growth of complementary therapies in cancer care represents a recognition that healing is a much wider concept than that of cure; indeed, healing can take place even in the absence of a medical cure. Healing involves psychological adaptation to living with cancer, a process of coming to terms with one's situation.
- Patients' reactions to cancer vary greatly, depending on personality, past experience and learned coping strategies.

Box 31.11

Communication skills: an example

This is an example of how one nurse offered her support to a young woman with acute leukaemia and her family. Notice the importance of following the patient's agenda and responding to the situation as it developed, rather than imposing a preconceived structure for communication (cited by Benner & Wrubel 1989):

While waiting for confirmation of the diagnosis, I did a lot of listening. I listened to the expression of shock, fear and guilt. I did not negate their concerns or try to offer false assurances.

It was clear that one of the most useful things I could do for this distraught family, who were in a strange and overwhelming place, was to assist them, little by little, in gaining control over their experiences. This involved helping them to anticipate and be prepared for what was to come, for how it might feel or look physically or emotionally. It also involved helping them to continue in their usual roles as much as possible, and engaging them in the decisions affecting Lara's care.

Although she knew that she had less than a 50% chance of survival, Lara concentrated on the here and now: the pain associated with frequent i.v.s, bone marrows and lumbar punctures; the embarrassment of hair loss; the isolation from her friends; and the nausea and vomiting associated with her chemotherapy. I followed her lead by responding to her immediate concerns.

I used a variety of approaches in working with her, depending on what kind of day she was having. Sometimes we would just joke around; other times we would talk about more serious issues — not just her illness but her personal life, as well as my own.

I was always open with her, accepted her feelings, and never made light of them. I did not assure her that 'it would get better soon' or that 'I knew how she must be feeling' because I truly did not know whether she would get better or how she actually felt.

Lara was just plain miserable. All I could do with her was listen, acknowledge how awful it must be, and honestly say that she must feel like crying. Permission to cry was all she needed to let the tears flow. One day, she looked me directly in the eyes and said, 'I'm so sick, am I going to die?'. Although it was a matter of seconds before I answered, it seemed like hours as my mind groped for the right words. I did not avert my gaze and answered from my heart: 'I'm afraid Lara, you are so sick that you could die'.

Nursing interventions The following strategies can be employed to give patients support as they adjust emotionally to their illness and treatment:

- Many patients cover up a great deal of their distress and assume that nurses do not have time to listen to them. Be alert to clues to this distress, such as constant information-seeking, manipulative behaviour and unrealistic goal-setting.
- Give the patient 'openings' to state what is on their mind, e.g. by concluding an information-giving session by asking them how they feel about the information, or by remarking upon a worried or sad expression.
- Do not be afraid of saying the wrong thing. A desire to understand and an attitude of concern are the important factors (Hinds & Moyer 1997).
- Learn and apply interviewing techniques used in counselling, e.g. reflecting back a patient's question or statement. This gives the patient the chance to realise what has been said and to expand on it, and the nurse time to reflect on what is meant. Constant reflection of questions, however, will irritate patients. Once the

patient's main concerns have been established, it may be time to give direct answers.

- Resist giving 'pat' answers and false reassurances. Many of the dilemmas faced by cancer patients have no ready solution. Do not be afraid to admit that answers cannot be given to all the patient's questions about the future. Try, however, to leave the patient with some hope: help the patient to identify something positive in their situation on which to focus.
- Assist the patient to identify realistic goals in order to foster hope. These goals should originate from the patient but often need an objective person to identify them. Examples may be the goal of fighting the disease, of living until a daughter's wedding or returning to work part-time.
- A certain degree of worry and sadness is to be expected. Be alert to signs of disabling anxiety (somatic stress symptoms, lack of concentration, feelings of panic) or depression (a 'flat' mood, an exaggerated feeling of guilt and self-blame, suicidal ideation). If these are noted, refer the patient to a psychologist or psychiatrist. Anxiolytic and antidepressant medication and various forms of psychological therapy may be required before other forms of counselling therapy can be effective (Strong et al 2004).
- Patients may react to their disease with denial, anger, bargaining, depression and acceptance (Kübler-Ross 1973). Counselling cannot force the patient to move from one stage to another, but it does allow them to express feelings and perhaps make progress. The nurse should give patients permission to express their feelings in any safe way they choose and should not feel a sense of failure when a patient becomes emotionally distraught. The expression of emotions is therapeutic and is an important part of psychological adaptation.
- Supporting patients and their families through the cancer experience is very demanding emotionally. It is important for nurses to recognise the resultant stress in themselves and their colleagues and to seek and offer active support (see Box 31.10).

Spiritual activity A full consideration of the cancer patient's quality of life must recognise the spiritual dimension of the experience, which might be described, in the most basic terms, as the search for meaning and purpose. Cancer has been described as 'a modern metaphor for human confrontation with existential uncertainty' (Goldberg & Tull 1983). Because spirituality involves the contemplation of things that affect us but lie beyond our control, cancer has the capacity to precipitate a spiritual crisis.

For many in modern society, the spiritual needs for love, hope, creativity and purpose are met in relationships with others and in their engagement with the material world. The person faced with a cancer diagnosis may feel such needs with particular acuity and may be assisted by interventions similar to those described in the section on emotional activity (p. 1065).

For some, whether or not death is imminent, a cancer diagnosis creates a greater urgency to come to terms with concepts of God, the meaning of life, the problem of human suffering and the possibility of an afterlife. For others, religious conviction will provide a framework for such questioning and a vehicle for spiritual expression.

Nursing interventions In acknowledging and addressing the cancer patient's spiritual needs, the nurse should bear in mind the following considerations:

- Spiritual issues are often not expressed as such by the patient. They may be expressed as anger and disbelief, doubts about self-worth, feelings of guilt and a fear of death. These feelings should be recognised as possibly stemming from spiritual questioning. The nurse should listen non-judgementally to the patient's views and acknowledge that some questions can never be answered.
- Patients of all faiths should be assisted to worship according to their custom. Nurses who share the patient's faith may find that a few minutes of shared prayer may be of more benefit than an hour of counselling.
- Even the most religious patients may express feelings of doubt, despair and anger against their God. This does not necessarily mean that they are losing their faith, but could indicate that they are grappling with it. The nurse should acknowledge the patient's distress and, if the patient wishes, enlist the help of a spiritual counsellor or minister.
- Not everyone with cancer is dying. However, almost all cancer patients consider the possibility of death at some point. If patients verbalise this possibility, and the timing is appropriate, they should not be denied the chance to begin the very necessary process of anticipatory grief. At the same time, all reasonable hope for the short-term future should be fostered and the patient's quality of life in the present should be enhanced by all means possible.

New directions for cancer care

Seminal work by Slevin et al (1990) pointed out that those who do not have cancer, whether they are lay people or professionals, have very little concept of the experience of cancer or of how the cancer patient perceives quality of life, their future and the decisions that must be made. Cancer is a chronic illness and more patients are living with their disease than previously. These patients, as survivors, have needs and expectations — physical, psychosocial and spiritual. Cancer patients may survive but they may not necessarily thrive. In this situation, cancer rehabilitation is paramount to support patients in effectively managing their illness on a day-to-day basis.

This millennium will see an increase in self-care, with individuals, families and communities playing a larger role in determining and meeting their own health needs. The internet has empowered patients by providing access to information about their disease and treatment, and opening up communication links with fellow patients. Advances in molecular biology may lead to the identification of high-risk groups and better targeted prevention as well as treatment. New challenges lie ahead for nurses in all fields for role development, research and education to support patients and their families through the cancer experience.

REFERENCES

Adamson D 2003 The radiobiological basis of radiation side effects. In: Faithful S, Wells M (eds) Supportive care in radiotherapy. Elsevier, Edinburgh

Allwood M, Stanley A, Wright P 2002 The cytotoxic handbook, 4th edn. Radcliffe Medical Press, Oxford

Amir M, Ramati A 2002 Post-traumatic symptoms, emotional distress and quality of life in long-term survivors of breast cancer: a preliminary research. Anxiety Disorders 16: 191–206

Arantzamendi M, Kearney N 2004 The psychological needs of patients receiving chemotherapy: an exploration of nurse perceptions. European Journal of Cancer Care 13(1): 23–31

Balmer C 2005 The information requirements of people with cancer. Cancer Nursing 28(1): 36–44

Barber M D 2001 Cancer cachexia and its treatment with fish oil enriched nutritional supplementation. Nutrition 17(9): 751–755

Barnett G C, Charman S C, Sizer P et al 2004 Information given to patients about adverse effects of radiotherapy: a survey of patients' views. Clinical Oncology 16: 479–484

Barraclough J 1998 Cancer and emotion. A practical guide to psycho-oncology, 3rd edn. Wiley, Chichester

Batchelor D 2001 Hair and cancer chemotherapy: consequences and nursing care – a literature study. European Journal of Cancer Care 10(3): 147–163

Baxter N 2001 Preventive healthcare, 2001 update: should women be routinely taught breast self examination to screen for breast cancer? Canadian Medical Association Journal 164(13): 1837–1846

Benner P, Wrubel J 1989 The primacy of caring: stress and coping in health and illness. Addison-Wesley, Menlo Park, CA

Birmingham K 2004 A national bowel screening programme. Cancer Nursing Practice 3(10): 4

Blyth C M, Anderson J, Hughson W et al 2001 An innovative approach to palliative care within a radiotherapy department. Journal of Radiotherapy in Practice 2: 85–90

Boyle P, Autier P, Bartelink H et al 2003 European code against cancer and scientific justification: third version. Annals of Oncology 14(7): 973–1005

Brown K, Levy A R, Rosberger Z, Edgar L 2003 Psychological distress and cancer survival: a follow up study 10 years after diagnosis. Psychosomatic Medicine 65(4): 636–643

Brown M A 1999 Tumour suppressor genes and human cancer. Advanced Genetics 36: 45–135

Calzone K A, Biesecker B B 2002 Genetic testing for cancer predisposition. Cancer Nursing 25(1): 15–25

Campbell J, German L, Dodwell D 2000 Radiotherapy out-patient review: a nurse led clinic. Clinical Oncology 12(2): 104–107

Cancer Research UK 2002 Patient information leaflet: Lifestyle and cancer – how to reduce your risk. CRUK, London

Cancer Research UK 2004 Childhood cancer. Information Resource Centre. CRUK, London

Cancer Research UK 2005a Cancer stats: incidence – UK. CRUK, London. Online. Available: www.cancerresearchuk.org/cancerstats

Cancer Research UK 2005b Cancer stats: mortality – UK. CRUK, London. Online. Available: www.cancerresearchuk.org/cancerstats

Cantor S B, Volk R J, Cass A K et al 2002 Psychological benefits of prostate screening: the role of reassurance. Health Expectations 5(2): 104–113

Cappozzo C 2004 Optimal use of granulocyte-colony-stimulating factor in patients with cancer who are at risk for chemotherapy induced neutropenia. Oncology Nursing Forum 31(3): 569–576

Carlson L E, Bultz B D, Speca M, St Pierre M 2000 Partners of cancer patients. Part I: Impact, adjustment and coping across the illness trajectory. Journal of Social Oncology 18(2): 39–63

Casanu S, Fedeli S L, Catalano G 1994 Oral cooling (cryotherapy): an effective treatment for the prevention of 5 fluorouracil induced stomatitis. Oral oncology. European Journal of Cancer 30B(4): 234–236

Cass Y, Musgrove C F 1992 Guidelines for safe handling of excreta contaminated by cytotoxic agents. American Journal of Hospital Pharmacy 49: 1957–1958

Cassileth B R, Zupkis R V, Sutton-Smith K et al 1980 Information and participation preferences among cancer patients. Annals of Internal Medicine 92(6): 832–836

Catalona W J, Smith D S, Ratliff T L et al 1991 Measurement of prostate-specific antigen in serum as a screening test for prostate cancer. New England Journal of Medicine 324: 1156

Chapman K, Abraham C, Jenkins V et al 2003 Lay understanding of terms used in cancer consultations. Psycho-Oncology 12(6): 557–566

Chapple A, Ziebland S, McPherson A 2004 Stigma, shame and blame experienced by patients with lung cancer: a qualitative study. British Medical Journal 328(7454): 1470–1473

Chasle S, How C 2003 The effect of cytotoxic chemotherapy on female fertility. European Journal of Oncology Nursing 7(2): 91–98

Cole P, Rodu B 2001 Analytic epidemiology: cancer causes. In: DeVita V T Jr, Hellman S, Rosenberg S A (eds) Cancer. Principles and practice of oncology, 6th edn. Lippincott, Williams and Wilkins, Philadelphia

Collins D 2001 Telephone follow-up clinics. Macmillan Voice 17: 11–12

Colyer H, Hlahla T 1999 Information and support radiographers: a critical review of the role and its significance for the provision of cancer services. Journal of Radiotherapy in Practice 1: 117–124

COMMIT Research Group 1995 Community Intervention Trial for Smoking Cessation (COMMIT) II : changes in adult cigarette smoking prevalence. American Journal of Public Health 85(2): 193–200

Corner J, Plant H, Warner L 1995 Developing a nursing approach to managing dyspnoea in lung cancer. International Journal of Palliative Nursing 1(1): 5–11

Costa G 1977 Cachexia: the metabolic component of neoplastic disease. Cancer Research 37: 2327–2335

Costa J, Cordon-Cardo C 2001 Cancer diagnosis: molecular pathology. In: DeVita V T, Hellman S, Rosenberg S A (eds) Cancer: principles and practice of oncology, 6th edn. Lippincott, Williams and Wilkins, Philadelphia

Creagan E T 1997 Attitude and disposition: do they make a difference in cancer survival? Mayo Clinic Proceedings 72(2): 160–164

Cunningham M L 2000 Thriving as an oncology nurse. In: Yarbro C H, Frogge M H, Goodman M, Groenwald S L (eds) Cancer nursing: principles and practice, 5th edn. Jones and Bartlett, Boston

Del Mastro L, Costantini M, Morasso G et al 2002 Impact of two different dose-intensity chemotherapy regimens on psychological distress in early breast cancer patients. European Journal of Cancer 38: 359–366

Dennison S, Shute T 2000 Identifying patient concerns: improving the quality of patient visits to the oncology out-patient department – a pilot study. European Journal of Oncology Nursing 4(2): 91–98

Department of Health 1995 A policy framework for commissioning cancer services: a report by the Expert Advisory Group on Cancer to the Chief Medical Officers of England and Wales. HMSO, London

Department of Health 1998a Report of the Scientific Committee on tobacco and health. TSO, London

Department of Health 1998b Smoking kills. TSO, London

Department of Health 1998c A first class service: quality in the new NHS. TSO, London

Department of Health 2000a The NHS cancer plan: a plan for investment, a plan for reform. DH, London

Department of Health 2000b The NHS plan. DH, London

Department of Health 2000c The nursing contribution to cancer care: a strategic programme of action in support of the national cancer programme. DH, London

Doll R, Hill A B 1954 The mortality of doctors in relation to their smoking habits. A preliminary report. British Medical Journal 1: 1451–1455

Dose A M 1995 The symptom experience of mucositis, stomatitis and xerostomia. Seminars in Oncology Nursing 11(4): 248–255

Dow K H, Bucholtz J D, Iwamoto R R et al 1997 Nursing care in radiation oncology. W B Saunders, Philadelphia

Eardley A 1985 Patients and radiotherapy. 1. Expectations of treatment. 2. Patients' experience of treatment. Radiography 51: 324–326

Eardley A 1986 What do patients need to know? Nursing Times 82(16): 24–26

Edwards B, Clarke V 2004 Psychological impact of a cancer diagnosis on families:

the influence of family functioning and patients' illness characteristics on depression and anxiety. Psycho-Oncology 13(8): 562–576
Eilers J, Epstein J B 2004 Assessment and measurement of oral mucositis. Seminars in Oncology Nursing 20(1): 22–29
Ellershaw J, Wilkinson S (eds) 2003 Care of the dying: a pathway to excellence. Oxford University Press, Oxford
Evans J 1989 The cancer experience: a patient's view. In: Pritchard A P (ed) Cancer nursing: a revolution in care. Macmillan, London
Ewles L, Simnett I 2003 Promoting health: a practical guide, 5th edn. Baillière Tindall, Edinburgh
Faithful S, Wells M 2003 Supportive care in radiotherapy. Elsevier, Edinburgh
Fallowfield L, Jenkins V 1999 Effective communication skills are the key to good cancer care. British Journal of Cancer 35: 1592–1597
Fallowfield L, Ratcliffe D, Jenkins V et al 2001 Psychiatric morbidity and its recognition by doctors in patients with cancer. British Journal of Cancer 84(8): 1011–1015
Fawcett T N, Dean A 2004 The causes of cancer-related fatigue and approaches to its treatment. Professional Nurse 19(9): 503–507
Fawzy F, Fawzy N, Hyun C et al 1993 Malignant melanoma: effects of an early structured psychiatric intervention, coping, and affective states on recurrence and survival six years later. Archives of General Psychiatry 50: 681–689
Fawzy F, Fawzy N, Canada A 2000 Psychoeducational intervention programs for patients with cancer. Psychologische Beitrage 42(1): 95–118
Fawzy F, Canada A, Fawzy N 2003 Malignant melanoma: effects of a brief structured psychiatric intervention on survival and recurrence at 10 year follow up. Archives of General Psychiatry 60(1): 100–104
Fellowes D, Barnes K, Wilkinson S 2004 Aromatherapy and massage for symptom relief in patients with cancer. The Cochrane Database of Systematic Reviews, Issue 3: CD002287
Fernsler J I, Miller M 2000 Factors affecting health behaviour. In: Yarbro C H, Frogge M H, Goodman M, Groenwald S L (eds) Cancer nursing: principles and practice, 5th edn. Jones and Bartlett, Boston
Fidler I J 1997 Molecular biology of cancer: invasion and metastases. In: DeVita V T et al (eds) Cancer: principles and practice of oncology. Lippincott-Raven, Philadelphia
Fields T, Quintino O, Henteleff T et al 1997 Job stress reduction therapies. Alternative Therapies 3: 54–56
Fieler V K, Wlasowicz G S, Mitchell M L et al 1996 Information preferences of patients undergoing radiation therapy. Oncology Nursing Forum 23(10): 1603–1608
Fischer D S 2003 The cancer chemotherapy handbook, 6th edn. Mosby Yearbook, St Louis
Fitch M I, Greenberg M, Cava M et al 1998 Exploring the barriers to cervical screening in an urban Canadian setting. Cancer Nursing 21: 441–449
Fitch M I, Gray R E, Greenberg M et al 1999 Nurses' perspectives on unconventional therapies. Cancer Nursing 22(3): 238–245
Flanagan J, Holmes S 2000 Social perceptions of cancer and their impacts: implications for nursing practice arising from the literature. Journal of Advanced Nursing 32(3): 740–749
Foltz A T 2000 Nutritional disturbances. In: Yarbro C H, Frogge M H, Goodman M, Groenwald S L (eds) Cancer nursing: principles and practice, 5th edn. Jones and Bartlett, Boston
Fox B H 1995 Some problems and some solutions in research on psychotherapeutic interventions with cancer patients. Supportive Cancer Care 3: 257–263
Franks L M, Teich N M (eds) 1997 Introduction to the cellular and molecular biology of cancer. Oxford University Press, Oxford
Gardner M J, Snee M P, Hall A J et al 1990 Results of case control study of leukaemia and lymphoma in young people near Sellafield nuclear plant in West Cumbria. British Medical Journal 300: 423–429
Gatzemeier U, Kleisbauer J F, Drings P et al 2000 Lenograstim as support for ACE chemotherapy for small cell lung cancer: a phase III, multicentre, randomized study. American Journal of Clinical Oncology 23(4): 393–400
Gerits P, De Brabander B 1999 Psychosocial predictors of psychological, neurochemical and immunological symptoms of acute distress among breast cancer patients. Psychiatry Research 85(1): 519–528
Goffman E 1963 Stigma: notes on the management of a spoiled identity. Prentice Hall, Englewood Cliffs, NJ
Gohagan J K, Marcus P M, Fagerstrom R M et al 2005 Final results of the lung screening study, a randomized feasibility study of spiral CT versus chest X-ray screening for lung cancer. Lung Cancer 47(1): 9–15
Goldberg R J, Tull R M 1983 The psychosocial dimensions of cancer: a practical guide for health care providers. Free Press, New York
Goodwin P J, Leszcz M, Ennis M et al 2001 The effect of group psychosocial support on survival in metastatic breast cancer. New England Journal of Medicine 345(24): 1719–1726
Gorman D R, Mackinnon H, Storrie M et al 2000 The general practice perspective on cancer services in Lothian. Family Practice 17(4): 323
Greer S 1995 Improving quality of life: adjuvant psychological therapy for patients with cancer. Supportive Cancer Care 3: 248–251
Grunberg S M, Deuson R R, Mavros P 2004 Incidence of chemotherapy-induced nausea and emesis after modern antiemetics. Perception versus reality. Cancer 100: 2261–2268
Grunfeld E, Zitzelsberger L, Ciristine M et al 2005 Job stress and job satisfaction of cancer care workers. Psycho-Oncology 14(1): 61–69
Guthrie C 1999 Nurses' perceptions of sexuality relating to patient care. Journal of Clinical Nursing 8: 313–321
Haapoja I S 2000 Paraneoplastic syndromes. In: Yarbro C H, Frogge M H, Goodman M, Groenwald S L (eds) Cancer nursing: principles and practice, 5th edn. Jones and Bartlett, Boston
Haenszel W, Kurihera M 1968 Studies of Japanese migrants: 1. Mortality from cancer and other diseases among Japanese in the United States. Journal of the National Cancer Institute 60: 545–571
Hagopian G 1996 The effects of informational audiotapes on knowledge and self-care behaviours of patients undergoing radiation therapy. Oncology Nursing Forum 23(4): 697–700
Hall E J 1997 Etiology of cancer: physical factors. In: DeVita V T et al (eds) Cancer: principles and practice of oncology. Lippincott-Raven, Philadelphia
Hammick M, Tutt A, Tait D M 1998 Knowledge and perception regarding radiation in patients receiving radiotherapy: a qualitative study. European Journal of Cancer Care 7(2): 103–112
Harper D M, Franco E L, Wheeler C et al 2004 Efficacy of a bivalent L1 virus-like particle vaccine in prevention of infection with human papillomavirus types 16 and 18 in young women: a randomised controlled trial. Lancet 364: 1757–1765
Harris A L 2005 Editorial. British Journal of Cancer 92(1): 1–2
Harrison R, Dey P, Slevin N J et al 2001 Randomised controlled trial to assess the effectiveness of a videotape about radiotherapy. British Journal of Cancer 84(1): 8–10
Henderson B E, Bernstein L 1997 Etiology of cancer: hormonal factors. In: DeVita V T et al (eds) Cancer: principles and practice of oncology. Lippincott-Raven, Philadelphia
Henderson J W, Donatelle R J 2003 The relationship between cancer locus of control and complementary and alternative medicine use by women diagnosed with breast cancer. Psycho-Oncology 12(1): 59–67
Hilderley L J 2000 Principles of radiation therapy. In: Yarbro C H, Frogge M H, Goodman M, Groenwald S L (eds) Cancer nursing; principles and practice, 5th edn. Jones and Bartlett, Boston
Hinds C, Moyer A 1997 Support as experienced by patients with cancer during radiotherapy treatments. Journal of Advanced Nursing 26: 371–379
Holmes S 1996 Radiotherapy: a guide for practice. Asset Books, Surrey
Holmes S 1997 Cancer chemotherapy: a guide for practice. Asset Books, Surrey
How C, Brown J 1998 Extravasation of cytotoxic chemotherapy from peripheral veins. European Journal of Oncology Nursing 2(1): 51–58
International Agency for Research on Cancer (IARC) 1998 Cancer in five continents. Electronic database for cancer, IARC/WHO, Lyon
International Agency for Research on Cancer (IARC) 2002 IARC handbooks of cancer prevention: Breast Cancer Screening 7: 100–101. IARC Press, Lyon
International Agency for Research on Cancer (IARC) 2004 Tobacco smoking and involuntary smoking. IARC monographs on the evaluation of carcinogenic risks to humans; 83. IARC, Lyon
Inui A 2002 Cancer anorexia–cachexia syndrome: current issues in research and management. Canadian Cancer Journal Clinics 52(2): 72–91
Jones L, Coe P 2004 Extravasation. European Journal of Oncology Nursing 8(4): 355–358

Kmietowicz Z 2004 British cancer death rates fell by 12% between 1972 and 2002. British Medical Journal 328(7435): 303
Kreth F, Faist M, Wernke P C et al 1995 Interstitial radiosurgery of low grade gliomas. Journal of Neurosurgery 82(2): 418–429
Kübler-Ross E 1973 Death, the final stage of growth. Prentice Hall, New York
Kunkler I 2000 Managed clinical networks: a new paradigm for clinical medicine. Journal of the Royal College of Physicians of London 34: 230–233
Lee W M F, Yielding N M 2003 Molecular basis of cancer. In: Warrell D A, Cox T M, Firth J D, Benz E J (eds) Oxford textbook of medicine, 4th edn. Oxford University Press, Oxford
Link L B, Robbins L, Mancuso M E 2004 How do cancer patients who try to take control of their disease differ from those who do not? European Journal of Cancer Care 13: 219–226
Loud J, Peters J, Fraser M et al 2002 Applications of advances in molecular biology and genomics to clinical cancer care. Cancer Nursing 25(2): 110–122
Macduff C, Mackenzie T, Hutcheon A et al 2003 The effectiveness of scalp cooling in preventing alopecia for patients receiving epirubicin and docetaxel. European Journal of Cancer Care 12: 154–161
Mackenzie C 1996 Patients' perceptions of radiotherapy treatment. In: Patterson A, Price R (eds) Current topics in radiography. W B Saunders, London
Macmillan Cancer Relief Fund 1999 Public attitudes and knowledge of cancer in the UK: an analysis of six months of the British press. Cancer Relief Macmillan Fund, London
Magnusson K, Robinson L 2000 The practice base of cancer nursing. In: Kearney N, Richardson A, Di Guilio P (eds) Cancer nursing practice: a textbook for the specialist nurse. Churchill Livingstone, Edinburgh
Maguire P 1985 The psychological impact of cancer. British Journal of Hospital Medicine 34(2): 100–103
Maguire P 1995 Psychosocial interventions to reduce affective disorders in cancer patients: Research priorities. Psycho-Oncology 4: 113–119
Malnutrition Advisory Group 2003 The 'MUST' report. Nutritional screening of adults: a multidisciplinary responsibility. Executive summary. British Association for Parenteral and Enteral Nutrition, London
Massey C S 2003 A multicentre study to determine the efficacy and patient acceptability of the Paxman scalp cooler to prevent hair loss in patients receiving chemotherapy. European Journal of Oncology Nursing 8(2): 121–130
Mathieson C M, Stam H J 1995 Renegotiating identity: cancer narratives. Sociology of Health and Illness 17(3): 283–306
Meyer T J, Mark M M 1995 Effects of social intervention with adult cancer patients: a meta-analysis of randomised experiments. Health Psychology 14: 101–108
Middleton S, Roberts A 2002 Integrated care pathways: a practical approach to implementation. Butterworth-Heinemann, Oxford
Miles D 2001 HER2 as a target for the therapy of breast cancer. In: Mansel R, Smith I E, Kunkler I, Miles A (eds) The effective management of breast cancer. UK key advances. Aesculapius Medical Press, London
Miller M, Kearney N 2001 Oral care and patients with cancer: a literature review. Cancer Nursing 24(4): 241–254
Miller M, Kearney N 2004 Chemotherapy-related nausea and vomiting – past reflections, present practice and future management. European Journal of Cancer Care 13: 71–81
Million Women Study Collaborators 2003 Breast cancer and hormone replacement therapy in the million women study. Lancet 362(9): 419–427
Mills M E, Sullivan K 1999 The importance of giving information for patients newly diagnosed with cancer: a review of the literature. Journal of Clinical Nursing 8(6): 631–642
Mitchell M 1998 Perspectives on allogeneic melanoma lysates in active specific immunotherapy. Seminars in Oncology 25(6): 623–635
Molassiotis A, Fernandez-Ortega P, Pud D et al 2005 Use of complementary and alternative medicine in cancer patients: a European survey. Annals of Oncology 16: 655–663
Moyer A, Levine E G 1998 Clarification of the conceptualization and measurement of denial in psychosocial oncology research. Annals of Behavioural Medicine 20: 149–160
Munstedt K, Manthe Y N, Sachsse S et al 1997 Changes in self concept and body image during alopecia induced cancer chemotherapy. Supportive Cancer Care 5: 139–143
National Cancer Institute (NCI) 2003 Oral complications of chemotherapy and head/neck radiation PDQ. Cancernet. Online. Available: http://cancernet.nci.nih.gov
National Extravasation Information Service (NEIS) 2004 Online. Available: http://www.extravasation.org.uk/home.html
Nery R 1986 Cancer: an enigma in biology and society. Croom Helm, London
NHS Cancer Screening Programme 2004 Online. Available: www.cancerscreening.nhs.uk/prostate
NHS Executive 1995 A policy framework for commissioning cancer services. DH, London
Oliver G 1999 WHO programme on cancer control: developing a global strategy for cancer, a review. European Journal of Cancer Care 8(1): 10–11
Owen J, Black C 1996 Supportive and shared care. In: Hancock B (ed) Cancer care in the community. Radcliffe Medical Press, Oxford
Parkin D M, Whelan S L, Ferlay L et al 2002 Cancer in five continents. VIII. International Agency for Research on Cancer, Scientific publication no. 155. Lyon
Pasternak G, Hochhaus A, Schultheis B, Hehlmann B 1998 CML: molecular and cellular aspects. Journal of Cancer Research in Clinical Oncology 124: 643–646
Pattison J, Macrae K 2002 Home chemotherapy: NHS and independent sector collaboration. Nursing Times 98(35): 34–35
Peck A, Boland J 1977 Emotional reactions to radiation treatment. Cancer 40: 180–184
Peters K, Menaker T, Wilson P et al 2001 The Human Genome Project: an update. Cancer Nursing 24(4): 287–292
Peterson D E, Beck S L, Keefe D M K 2004 Novel therapies. Seminars in Oncology Nursing 20(1): 53–58
Peto R, Darby S, Deo H et al 2000 Smoking, smoking cessation and lung cancer in the UK since 1950: combination of national statistics with two case-control studies. British Medical Journal 321: 323–329
Petticrew M, Bell R, Hunter D 2002 Influence of psychological coping on survival and recurrence in people with cancer: systematic review. British Medical Journal 325(7372): 1066–1069
Poeschla E M, Wong-Staal F 1997 RNA viruses. In: DeVita V T et al (eds) Cancer: principles and practice of oncology. Lippincott-Raven, Philadelphia
Poroch D 1995 The effect of preparatory patient education on the anxiety and satisfaction of cancer patients receiving radiation therapy. Cancer Nursing 18(3): 206–213
Protiere C, Evans K, Camerlo J et al 2002 Efficacy and tolerance of a scalp cooling system for prevention of hair loss and the experience of breast cancer patients treated by adjuvant chemotherapy. Supportive Care in Cancer 10(7): 529–537
Ream E, Richardson A 1999 Continuing education. From theory to practice: designing interventions to decrease fatigue in patients with cancer. Oncology Nursing Forum 26(8): 1295–1305
Ross R K, Makridakis N M, Reichard J K et al 2003 Prostate cancer: epidemiology and molecular endocrinology. In: Henderson B E, Pender B, Ross R K (eds) Hormones, genes and cancer. Oxford University Press, Oxford
Rotman M, Rogow L, Delean G et al 1977 Supportive therapy in radiation oncology. Cancer 39: 744–750
Royal College of Nursing (RCN) 1996a A structure for cancer nursing services. RCN, London
Royal College of Nursing (RCN) 1996b Guidelines for good practice in cancer nursing education. RCN, London
Royal College of Nursing (RCN) 1998 The administration of cytotoxic chemotherapy – clinical practice guidelines. Recommendations. RCN, London
Royal College of Nursing (RCN) 2003 A framework for adult cancer nursing. RCN, London
Saunders M, Dische S, Barrett A et al 1997 Continuous hyperfractionation accelerated radiotherapy (CHART) versus conventional radiotherapy in non small cell lung cancer; a randomised multicentre trial. Lancet 350: 161–165
Schofield P, Butow P N, Thompson J F et al 2003 Psychological responses of patients receiving a diagnosis of cancer. Annals of Oncology 14: 48–56
Scholefield J H, Moss S, Sufi F et al 2002 Effect of FOB screening on mortality from colorectal cancer: results from a randomized controlled trial. Gut 50: 840–844
Scottish Cancer Care Pharmacy Group 2000 Guidelines for the safe use of cytotoxic chemotherapy in the clinical environment.

The Association of Scottish Trust Chief Pharmacists, Edinburgh
Scottish Health Statistics (SHS) 2005 Overviews of cancer in Scotland. Online. Available: www.isdscotland.org
Scottish Executive Health Department (SEHD) 2003 Cancer in Scotland: action for change – where we are now. SEHD, Edinburgh. Online. Available: www.scotland.gov.uk/library3/health/csac-04.asp
Scottish Office 1999 Towards a healthier Scotland – A White Paper on health. TSO, Edinburgh. Online. Available: www.scotland.gov.uk/library/documents-w7/tahs-00.htm
Segnan N, Armardi P, Sancho-Garnier H 2004 Screening. Evidence-based cancer prevention: strategies for NGOs – a UICC handbook for Europe. Online. Available: www.uicc.org
Shaw C 2002 Therapeutic aspects of nutrition in cancer patients. In: Souhami R, Tannock I, Hohenberger P et al (eds) Oxford textbook of oncology, Vol 1. Oxford University Press, Oxford
Sikora K 1999 Cancer – a global problem. Cancer Topics 10(12): 17–19
Sitzia J, Wood N 1998 Study of patient satisfaction with chemotherapy nursing care. European Journal of Cancer Care 2(3): 142–153
Skalla K A, Bakitas M, Furstenberg C T et al 2004 Patients' need for information about cancer therapy. Oncology Nursing Forum 31(2): 313–319
Skott C 2002 Expressive metaphors in cancer narratives. Cancer Nursing 25(3): 230–235
Slevin M L, Stubbs L, Plant H et al 1990 Choices in cancer treatment: comparing the views of patients with cancer with those of doctors, nurses and the general public. British Medical Journal 300: 1458–1460
Slevin M L, Nichols S E, Downer S M et al 1996 Emotional support for cancer patients: what do patients really want? British Journal of Cancer 74: 1275–1279
Smith R A, Cokkinides V, Eyre H J 2003 American Cancer Society guidelines for the early detection of cancer 2003. CA Cancer Journal Clinics 53(1): 27–43
Sobin L H, Wittekind C (eds) 2002 TNM classification of malignant tumours, 6th edn. Wiley-Liss, New York
Sonis S, Eilers J P, Epstein J B et al 1999 Validation of a new scoring system for the assessment of clinical trial research of oral mucositis induced by radiotherapy or chemotherapy. American Cancer Society 85(10): 2103–2113
Souhami R, Tobias J 2005 Cancer and its management, 5th edn. Blackwell Science, Oxford
Speck P W 1988 Ethical issues in cancer care. In: Webb P (ed) Oncology for nurses and health care professionals, 2nd edn. Harper and Row, London
Speigel D 2001 Mind matters – group therapy and survival in breast cancer. New England Journal of Medicine 345: 1747–1768
Spiegel D, Kraemer H C, Bloom J R et al 1989 Effect of psychosocial treatment on survival of patients with metastatic breast cancer. Lancet 2(8668): 888–891
Staehelin R 2003 Intensity modulated radiation therapy – a breakthrough in oncology. Business Briefing: European Pharmacotherapy. Online. Available: www.varian.com
Stephenson P S 2004 Understanding denial. Oncology Nursing Forum 31(5): 985–988
Steven D, Fitch M, Dhaliwal H et al 2004 Knowledge, attitudes, beliefs and practices regarding breast and cervical cancer screening in selected ethnocultural groups in Northwestern Ontario. Oncology Nurses Forum 31(2): 305–311
Strecher V J, Rosenstock I 1997 The health belief model. In: Glanz K, Lewis F, Rimer B (eds) Health behaviour and health education, 2nd edn. Jossey-Bass, San Francisco, p 41–59
Strong V, Sharpe M, Cull A et al 2004 Can oncology nurses treat depression? A pilot project. Journal of Advanced Nursing 46(5): 542–548
Tanghe A, Evers G, Pandoens K 1998 Nurses' assessments of symptom occurrence and symptom distress in chemotherapy patients. European Journal of Oncology Nursing 2(1): 14–26
Thomson I E, Melia K M, Boyd K M 2000 Nursing ethics, 4th edn. Churchill Livingstone, Edinburgh
Tierney A J, Taylor J, Closs S J 1989 A study to inform nursing support of patients coping with chemotherapy for breast cancer. Nursing Research Unit, University of Edinburgh, Edinburgh
Tisdale M J 2000 Metabolic abnormalities in cachexia and anorexia. Nutrition 16(10): 1013–1014
Toniolo P G, Mortimer L, Zelenuich-Jacquotte A et al 1995 A prospective study of endogenous oestrogens and breast cancer in postmenopausal women. Journal of the National Cancer Institute 87(3): 190–197
Trichopoulus D, Kalandidi A, Sparros L et al 1981 Lung cancer and passive smoking. International Journal of Cancer 27(1): 1–4
Trillet-Lenoir V, Green J, Manegold C et al 1993 Recombinant granulocyte colony stimulating factor reduces the infectious complications of cytotoxic chemotherapy. European Journal of Cancer 29A: 319–324
Trotti A 2000 Toxicity in head and neck cancer: a review of trends and issues. International Journal of Radiation Oncology, Biology, Physics 47(1): 1–12
Tschudin V (ed) 1996 Nursing the patient with cancer, 2nd edn. Prentice Hall, Hemel Hempstead, Herts
Uyar D S, Eltabbakh G H, Mount S L 2003 Positive predictive value of liquid based and conventional cervical Papanicolaou smears reported as malignant. Gynaecologic Oncology 89: 227–232
Van der Molen B 1999 Relating informational needs to the cancer experience: information as a key coping strategy. European Journal of Cancer Care 8: 238–244
Walker A 1990 The problems of patients with cervical cancer. In: Faulkner A (ed) Excellence in nursing: the research route: oncology. Scutari, London
Watters C 1997 The benefits of providing chemotherapy at home. Professional Nurse 12(5): 19–21
Wells M 1998a What's so special about radiotherapy nursing? European Journal of Oncology Nursing 2(3): 162–168
Wells M 1998b The hidden experience of radiotherapy to the head and neck: a qualitative study of patients after completion of treatment. Journal of Advanced Nursing 28(4): 840–848
Wengstrom Y, Haggmark C 2001 Coping with radiation therapy. Strategies used by women with breast cancer. Cancer Nursing 24: 264–271
Werneke U, Earl J, Seydel L et al 2004 Potential health risks of complementary alternative medicines in cancer patients. British Journal of Cancer 90: 408–413
White I 2002 Facilitating sexual expression: challenges for contemporary practice. In: Heath H, White I (eds) The challenge of sexuality in healthcare. Blackwell Science, Oxford
Wilkinson J A 1999 Understanding patient health beliefs. Professional Nurse 14(5): 320–322
Wilkinson S, Gambles M, Roberts A 2002 The essence of cancer care: the impact of training on nurses' ability to communicate effectively. Journal of Advanced Nursing 40(6): 731–738
Yarbro J 2000 Milestones in our understanding of cancer. In: Yarbro C H, Frogge M H, Goodman M, Groenwald S L (eds) Cancer nursing; principles and practice, 5th edn. Jones and Bartlett, Boston
Zabora J, Brintzenhofeszoc K, Curbow B et al 2001 The prevalence of psychological distress by cancer site. Psycho-Oncology 10: 19–28
Ziegler E, Mason H J, Baxter P 2002 Occupational exposure to cytotoxic drugs in two UK oncology wards. Occupational and Environmental Medicine 59: 608–612

FURTHER READING

Adamson D 2003 The radiobiological basis of radiation side effects. In: Faithful S, Wells M (eds) Supportive care in radiotherapy. Elsevier, Edinburgh
Baggott C R, Patterson-Kelly P, Fochtman D et al (eds) 2002 Nursing care of children and adolescents with cancer, 3rd edn. Association of Paediatric Oncology Nurses/Saunders, London
Bomford C K, Kunkler I H 2003 Walter and Miller's textbook of radiotherapy. Radiation physics, therapy and oncology, 6th edn. Elsevier, Edinburgh
Brown C G, Wingard J 2004 Clinical consequences of oral mucositis. Seminars in Oncology Nursing 20(1): 16–21
Calzone K A, Bowles B 2002 Genetic testing for cancer predisposition. Cancer Nursing 25(1): 15–25
Calzone K A, Masny A 2004 Genetics and

oncology nursing. Seminars in Oncology Nursing 20(3): 178–185
Daniel B T, Damato K L, Johnson J 2004 Educational issues in oral care. Seminars in Oncology Nursing 20(1): 48–52
Dodds M J 2001 Managing side effects of chemotherapy and radiation therapy. UCSF Nursing Press, San Francisco
Dow K H, Bucholtz J D, Iwamoto R R et al 1997 Nursing care in radiation oncology. W B Saunders, Philadelphia
Eilers J, Epstein J B 2004 Assessment and measurement of oral mucositis. Seminars in Oncology Nursing 20(1): 22–29
Ellershaw J, Wilkinson S (eds) 2003 Care of the dying: a pathway to excellence. Oxford University Press, Oxford
Epstein J B, Schubert M M 2004 Managing pain in mucositis. Seminars in Oncology Nursing 20(1): 30–37
Faithful S, Wells M 2003 Supportive care in radiotherapy. Elsevier, Edinburgh
Fischer D S 2003 The cancer chemotherapy handbook, 6th edn. Mosby Yearbook, St Louis
Gale D M 2003 Molecular targets in cancer therapy. Seminars in Oncology Nursing 19(3): 193–205
Greco K E, Mahon S 2004 Common hereditary cancer syndromes. Seminars in Oncology Nursing 20(3): 164–177
Groenwald S L, Frogge M H, Goodman M et al 1995 A clinical guide to cancer nursing: a companion to cancer nursing, 3rd edn. Jones and Bartlett, Boston
Holmes S 1996 Radiotherapy: a guide for practice. Asset Books, Surrey
Holmes S 1997 Cancer chemotherapy: a guide for practice. Asset Books, Surrey
How C, Brown J 1998 Extravasation of cytotoxic chemotherapy from peripheral veins. European Journal Oncology Nursing 2(1): 51–58
Jenkins J 2004 Genomics: offering hope for oncology care. Seminars in Oncology Nursing 20(3): 209–212
Kreth F, Faist M, Wernke P C et al 1995 Interstitial radiosurgery of low grade gliomas. Journal of Neurosurgery 82(2): 418–429
Kwitkowski V E, Daub J R 2004 Clinical applications of genetics in sporadic cancers. Seminars in Oncology Nursing 20(3): 155–163
Liu K 2003 Breakthroughs in cancer gene therapy. Seminars in Oncology Nursing 19(3): 217–226
Loud J T, Hutson P S 2004 The art and science of cancer nursing in the genomic era. Seminars in Oncology Nursing 20(3): 143–144
Lowrey K 2004 Legal and ethical issues in cancer genetics nursing. Seminars in Oncology Nursing 20(3): 203–208
Martini F H (ed) 2004 Fundamentals of anatomy and physiology, 6th edn. Pearson Education, San Francisco
Mautner B, Huang D 2003 Molecular biology and immunology. Seminars in Oncology Nursing 19(3): 154–161
Middleton L, Dimond E, Calzone K et al 2002 The role of the nurse in cancer genetics. Cancer Nursing 25(3): 196–206
Middleton L, Peters K 2001 Genes and inheritance. Cancer Nursing 24(5): 357–369
Muehlbauer P M, Schwartzentruber D J 2003 Cancer vaccines. Seminars in Oncology Nursing 19(3): 206–216
Niven N 1999 Health psychology for health care professionals. Churchill Livingstone, Edinburgh
Otto S E (ed) 2001 Oncology nursing, 4th edn. Mosby, St Louis
Peters J, Loud J, Dimond E et al 2001 Cancer genetics fundamentals. Cancer Nursing 24(6): 446–461
Peterson D E, Beck S L, Keefe D M K 2004 Novel therapies. Seminars in Oncology Nursing 20(1): 53–58
Rieger P T 2004 The biology of cancer genetics. Seminars in Oncology Nursing 20(3): 145–154
Schmidt K V, Wood B A 2003 Trends in cancer therapy: role of monoclonal antibodies. Seminars in Oncology Nursing 19(3): 169–179
Sonis S 2004 Pathobiology of mucositis. Seminars in Oncology Nursing 20(1): 11–15
Tannock I F, Hill R P (eds) 1998 The basic science of oncology, 3rd edn. McGraw-Hill, New York
Tortora G J, Grabowski S R 2005 Principles of anatomy and physiology, 11th edn. Harper Collins, New York
Vadaparampil S T, Permuth-Wey J, Yeomans-Kinney A 2004 Psychosocial aspects of genetic counselling and testing. Seminars in Oncology Nursing 20(3): 186–195
Varmus H, Weinberg R A 1993 Genes and the biology of cancer. Scientific American Library, New York
Vooght S 1996 A study to explore the role of a community oncology nurse specialist. European Journal of Cancer Care 5(4): 217–224
Weiger W, Smith M, Boon H et al 2002 Advising patients who seek complementary and alternative therapies for cancer. Annals of Internal Medicine 137(11): 889–903
Weinstein S M 2001 Plumer's principles and practice of intravenous therapy, 7th edn. Lippincott, Philadelphia
Yarbro C H, Frogge M H, Goodman M, Groenwald S L (eds) Cancer nursing: principles and practice, 5th edn. Jones and Bartlett, Boston

USEFUL WEBSITES

CancerBACUP
www.cancerbacup.org.uk
A comprehensive site offering clear, up-to-date cancer information for patients, their families and also health care professionals.

CancerHELP UK
www.cancerhelp.org.uk
Clearly sets out information on different cancers, lifestyle issues, treatments and prevention.

Cancer*Index*
www.cancerindex.org
Guide to internet resources for cancer; provides over 100 pages and more than 1000 links to cancer-related information that is regularly updated.

Macmillan Cancer Relief
www.macmillan.org.uk
Provides expert information and advice. Also provides a list of helpful organisations and publications.

Maggie's Centres
www.maggiescentres.org
Charitable organisation supporting all those affected by cancer through provision of information psychological support relaxation and stress management in uplifting environments.

National Cancer Institute
www.cancer.gov
American site with cancer information, treatment options, genetics and clinical trials. Information for patients and/or health professionals.

National Electronic Library for Health
www.nelh.nhs.uk
Provides access to best current knowledge offering reliable up-to-date information with links to NHS Direct.

Oncology Nursing Society
www.cancersymptoms.org
Up-to-date information on cancer symptoms such as anorexia, pain, depression, neutropenia including interventions in their management.

Tenovus
www.tenovus.com
Charitable organisation that funds research, prevention/education, counselling and care for cancer patients and their families.

THE CHRONICALLY ILL PERSON

32

Erica S. Alabaster

INTRODUCTION

Medicine's traditional cure orientation has long influenced health service development, resulting in chronic illness assuming low priority. In these terms, working with those for whom there is no prospect of full recovery carried little prestige and represented the antithesis of skilled practice. However, the opportunity to focus on care, a concept central to nursing, attests to the importance of nurses' commitment in this area. Changes in demography and morbidity, shifting emphasis to community care and evolving roles mean that nurses encounter in all settings chronically ill people who are living with an array of conditions, occupying differing stages of disease processes and experiencing a variety of life circumstances.

The range of knowledge and skill needed to meet the challenges of promoting and restoring optimum health, in its broad bio-psycho-social and spiritual senses, among this disparate client group cannot be underestimated. Nursing involvement is influenced by the application of a diagnostic label, but directed by what is meaningful to the individual and interdisciplinary input. The role is, therefore, collaborative in nature and must be formulated within context, which includes the nature of chronic illness, its prevalence, its impact on personal experience and functioning, and the relationship between individuals, their carers and care agencies. Perhaps the best place to begin is to consider how chronic illness has been defined.

THE NATURE OF CHRONIC ILLNESS

Terminology

An analysis of the terminology used is an essential starting point for any discussion of chronic illness. Its multifaceted nature means that defining chronicity is extremely difficult. Nevertheless, a number of attempts have been made to describe illnesses that are 'long term and have a profound influence on the lives of sufferers' (Locker 2003). The way in which key terms are applied may reveal assumptions held about the causation and prognosis of enduring conditions and about the individuals who experience them. For example, the North American definition offered by the Commission on Chronic Illness in 1954 (cited by Daly 1993) focuses on disease and refers to chronic illness as being a deviation from the norm, both raising questions as to what constitutes a 'normal' state as well as suggesting that people with such conditions are 'less than normal'. More recently, Curtin and Lubkin (1998) contend that from a nursing perspective:

> *Chronic illness is the irreversible presence, accumulation, or latency of disease states or impairments that involve the total human environment for supportive care and self-care, maintenance of function, and prevention of further disability.*

This reflects growing concern with attending to the whole person within their own context.

'Illness' and 'disease'

It is important to note that some definitions of chronic illness are orientated towards disease rather than illness. A distinction is made between these two terms by some writers such that 'disease' is a medical conception of pathological abnormality as indicated by its presenting features, whereas 'illness' is the subjective response by the individual to feeling unwell (Crumbie & Lawrence 2002, Armstrong 2003). Although it is possible to feel ill without having a disease, and vice versa, 'illness' and 'disease' do not constitute discrete phenomena but, rather, operate at different levels of human experience (Greaves 1996). Their relationship is dependent on the nature and severity of the disease process and on coexisting psychosocial variables. Chronic illness is generally associated with the presence of a protracted disease process which is not amenable to treatment, is responsible for impairment or disability and, so, has a sustained influence on the functioning and lifestyle of the individual. From this perspective, the relationship between disease and illness is characterised by its complexity.

'Impairment', 'disability' and 'handicap'

Biomedical classifications of disease do not necessarily account for the psychological and social consequences which accompany the conditions identified. For example, Dickens et al (2003) consider that depression experienced by women with rheumatoid arthritis is related to social stress, rather than the severity of their physical problems. The terms 'impairment', 'disability' and 'handicap' are commonly employed with reference to chronic illness and are applied in a variety of ways, whether their definitions are stated explicitly or merely implied.

- 'Impairment' is generally used to describe any disturbance of the body's structure and function (Field & Kelly 2003). Impairment may also be influenced by extrinsic factors such as the manner in which the presenting condition is managed. Pressure ulcers, constipation, urinary tract infections and other complications of restricted mobility are examples of these.
- The word 'disability' can be used to identify any long-term or permanent loss or reduction in functional capacity. This may also be defined in relation to behaviour, such as that arising from the individual's inability to perform activities which are expected of them (Nettleton 1995). The level of disability experienced by an individual reflects the severity and duration of impairment, taking into account concurrent disease, illness and the effects of the ageing process. People interested in the study of chronic illness should consider the notion of disability since this presents an opportunity to discuss a range of behavioural responses without concentrating on the diseases concerned. This recognises the reality of disability as something that is lived and experienced physically and psychologically (Marks 1999).
- The term 'handicap' may be applied when limitation of activity persists as a residual effect of impairment, even following rehabilitative efforts to restore function. Handicap stems from extrinsic factors and is not, therefore, merely the presence of disability and impairment, but the social, economic and environmental consequences of these. It is helpful to think of handicap in terms of social disadvantage and deprivation in so far as individuals are prevented from participating in prescribed roles and relationships. Handicap can have different implications for individual experience depending on the way in which social, cultural and economic values are applied to restricted role behaviour (Locker 2003). In this way, 'handicap' can be interpreted as both more and less than 'disability'.

SOCIETAL ATTITUDES TOWARDS ILLNESS AND DISABILITY

Attention is clearly directed towards associations between aspects of lifestyle and some chronic illnesses; for example, smoking is linked with lung cancer and a high dietary intake of saturated fats with coronary heart disease. General awareness of these relationships may result in the individual being judged to be the cause of their own disease and related suffering (Rosenberg 1997). There is also an implication that the individual has failed to respond to preventive health education campaigns. Attribution of personal blame is shown to have a strong moral influence where a link can be alleged between disease and sexual behaviour, such as that between HIV/AIDS and promiscuity (Pitts 1996, Brandt & Rozin 1997). Current beliefs concerning the origin of chronic illness and disability appear, therefore, to reflect a combination of moral ideology and scientific principles.

STOP THINK **32.1** Given the association between cigarette advertising and tobacco consumption (Charlton et al 1997, MacFadyen et al 2001) and that tobacco companies appear to be accepting the addictive nature of their products, can individuals be blamed for their behaviour? What other forces influence personal health choices?

Disability and unemployment

The individual's economic survival in a pre-industrial society largely depended on their capacity to engage in physical labour. Those who were restricted by the effects of protracted illness or impairment would thus have had a limited function within their social group. This, together with their likely dependency on others, could result in the perception that disabled people were of less value than their able-bodied counterparts.

In an industrialised society, however, technological developments and diversification of working practices should create opportunities for those with a wide range of disabilities to gain employment. Nonetheless, disabled people seeking to enter the labour market encounter discrimination. It has been argued that the Disability Discrimination Act (1995) has not addressed this because it defines disability using a medical rather than a social model (Reid 1997), is riddled with ambiguity (Jacklin 1997) and does not assure full civil rights (Mahony 1997).

Governmental response to poverty is influenced by the way impoverished people are viewed by other members of society. The assumption that those living with chronic illness experience economic difficulties because their inability to obtain employment results directly from their incapacity is not held universally. Some believe instead that such individuals are malingerers who choose not to work (Scambler 2003a, Spinney 2003). When this interpretation predominates, programmes for the alleviation of poverty concentrate on motivating individuals by reforming attitudes and implementing workfare-style schemes, so such programmes may appear to be punitive rather than benevolent.

Stigma

As Goffman (1963) points out in his seminal text, the word 'stigma' was originally used with reference to visible signs inflicted with the intent of branding individuals (including slaves or criminals) unfit for participation in normal social interaction. These signs had moral and judgemental implications, such that the disgrace and shame of the stigma assumed more importance than its physical presence (Saylor & Yoder 1998).

The stigma attached to a chronic illness relates to deviation from the perceived norm and depends on the part of the body affected, the degree to which effects of the condition are visible and application of a diagnostic label. To be labelled chronically ill is to be made exceptional and, in many cases, marginalised. People with a chronic illness are engaged in constant effort to make themselves acceptable and their stigmatising condition often assumes primacy in establishing their social identity and relations with others. Case History 32.1 gives some insight into the stigmatisation that may be suffered by an individual with an obvious skin condition. People with less visible conditions such as epilepsy experience 'felt stigma'. Their burden of constantly concealing a discreditable part of themselves in order to pass as normal and avoid being found out is added to by difficulties in gauging which details to share with whom, so that relationships can be maintained (Radley 1994, Pierret 2003). Family members also experience stigma by association and this impacts on their response to the affected individual and their contact with others.

STOP THINK **32.2** Have you ever been aware of being embarrassed or uncomfortable when you were with someone with an obvious skin disorder? What were your reactions?

CASE HISTORY 32.1
Mrs I

Mrs I is 44 years old and is employed as a part-time receptionist. She lives in a terraced house with her husband and their three teenage children. Mrs I has had psoriasis for some years, involving much of her body surface.

Although prescribed treatment has controlled features of this condition to some extent, Mrs I has periods of exacerbation. Reddened raised patches sometimes appear on her face, and her scalp is often affected. Medical opinion varies as to whether this is actually due to psoriasis or to seborrhoeic dermatitis. Mrs I feels this distinction to be largely academic because neither condition is curable and the outcome for her remains the same. At present her scalp is covered in a thick, hardened layer of scales. When these areas are detached, her scalp surface weeps and becomes painful. Scales are also deposited continually on her clothing and in her immediate vicinity.

Mrs I finds that living with a skin condition is made more difficult by the reaction of others. She is often conscious that people stare at her and look at her affected skin rather than making eye contact during conversations. Mrs I remembers that when her children were small, one of them tried to prevent her from attending a school play. After a long discussion he admitted that it was because he was embarrassed by her appearance. Mrs I thinks that some people regard her condition to be contagious or to be caused by poor personal hygiene. She considers that this explains why passengers on the bus she takes to and from work rarely occupy the space next to her until the vehicle becomes crowded. Such behaviour still makes her uncomfortable but she has learned to accept it as something she must live with.

Mrs I feels that she has developed effective methods of coping with the problems resulting from her disorder. Since her job involves meeting the public, she has learned to project an outgoing and friendly image which she feels is stronger than the visual impression which her condition creates. She avoids wearing dark clothes likely to make her fallen scales more obvious and purchases her clothing by mail order or from shops which do not have communal changing rooms. She has learned by trial and error which chemicals or cosmetics irritate her skin and excludes them from the household. She takes her own prescribed shampoo to the hairdressers and never uses biological washing powder. Her friends and relations are aware that only selected toiletries are welcome as birthday and Christmas presents. Mrs I has also adapted her treatment regimen to account for exacerbations of her condition. She applies some creams only when she feels that she needs to, rather than at prescribed intervals. As some preparations require careful application due to possible staining of clothes and localised burning (see Ch. 12), Mrs I tries to restrict their use to days when she is not rostered to work. To prevent unnecessary soiling, she reserves specific bed linen for occasions when she needs to leave scalp ointment on overnight.

Public awareness campaigns

Groups have been established to raise public awareness of problems encountered by individuals with chronic conditions. In the USA, veterans of the First World War were successful in exerting large-scale efforts to obtain privileges and opportunities for disabled servicemen returning to civilian life (Dimond & Jones 1987). The amount of popular support such programmes receive depends upon whether the situations to which they are related are viewed positively. This can be illustrated with reference to American veterans of the Vietnam War, who endured stigmatisation by association with a controversial and unpopular conflict (Figley & Leventman 1990).

Other groups draw attention to named conditions and their effects on individual experience. Independent from formal health agencies, these organisations function as a resource for chronically ill people, their families and professionals, lobby to influence health and social policy, and raise funds for facilities and research. Groups operating without the active participation of individuals with chronic conditions risk calling attention to assumed, as opposed to actual need. In addition, activists within the disabled people's movement assert that national fundraising events merely reinforce the notion that an automatic relationship exists between disability and charity. Members of these groups believe that disabled people should avoid passivity and the socialised dependency which results. Their practice of self-advocacy, use of direct action and insistence upon parity rather than charity contrasts sharply with the conventional image of 'the disabled' as recipients of care (see

'Useful websites', p.1093, for the British Council of Disabled People's website).

THE PREVALENCE OF CHRONIC ILLNESS

The prevalence of chronic illness or disease is difficult to establish, given the many definitions and interpretations offered by various agencies. Some indication may, however, be derived from a review of studies which account for such variables as demography and disability. The data are not definitive because reporting and collection methods are inconsistent.

Improvements in public health in the UK during the last century resulted in the near-eradication of some infectious diseases, while others have been largely controlled by vaccination programmes (Galbraith & McCormick 1997). In addition, once contracted, infectious diseases are generally amenable to treatment. Chronic rather than infectious disease therefore remains the major cause of premature death and disability (Griffiths & Brock 2003).

It must not be assumed that infection has been eliminated from Western societies, nor that chronic disease cannot be infectious (Radley 1994). AIDS is the result of infectious disease, yet to contract it means living with a chronic illness.

Patterns of infection are also subject to continual change worldwide. The speed at which this occurs reflects the acceleration of human, social, technical, environmental and population change. This has resulted in the appearance of new diseases, such as severe acute respiratory syndrome (SARS) (Donnelly et al 2003, WHO 2003), and the re-emergence of others. For example, notifications of tuberculosis have risen by nearly a fifth in the UK since 1993 with an increase in drug-resistant isolates and it has become more common than measles or whooping cough (Office for National Statistics 2003a). This is in part due to improvements in the system of notification, but the increase of pulmonary tuberculosis is genuine and associated with socioeconomic deprivation. Almost half of overall notifications are from immigrant communities and are most prevalent among young South Asians (Galbraith & McCormick 1997). Observations such as this have led to members of marginal groups, including political asylum seekers, being viewed pejoratively as the cause of disease and thus a threat to wider society (Pitts 1996). Further, this gives rise to 'port health' thinking, leading to unreasonable fears of infection from abroad and a restrictive view of minority ethnic health issues (Smaje 1995).

The continuing decline in mortality from infectious disease is reflected in an increased expectation of life for all age groups, a trend which is predicted to continue (Charlton 1997). This has implications for the number of people afflicted by chronic disorders because the proportion of the population considered to be impaired or handicapped rises with advancing age. Confirmation of this relationship can be found in data from the annual General Household Survey (GHS) involving a sample of 21 180 people aged 16 years and over (Office for National Statistics 2003b). Respondents were asked whether they had any long-standing illness, disability or infirmity and, if they had, to state whether it served to limit their activities in any way. A long-standing illness was reported by 32% and a limiting long-standing illness by 19%. A comparative measure of acute illness was obtained by enquiring whether participants had limited their usual activities as a result of illness or injury within the 2-week period prior to the interview. Only 14% of the sample fell into this category. The report concludes that in the period 1972–2001, rates of long-standing illness have increased steadily. Although the reporting of such disorders rose from 22% in those aged 16–44 years to 63% in those aged 75 years or more, demographic distribution means that fewer older men were found in this category.

Respondents declaring long-standing illness most frequently identified musculoskeletal, circulatory and respiratory disorders as its source. Among these disorders, musculoskeletal conditions were the most common. Circulatory problems were the second most common form of chronic illness identified; these were reported by 1.9% of adults aged 16–44 years and approximately 33% of those aged 75 years or older. Mortality from these disorders declined during the latter half of the last century (Office for National Statistics 2003a) but still accounted for around 30% of all deaths in England and Wales at the millennium (Griffiths & Brock 2003).

The GHS reveals social inequality in that those connected with routinised and manual occupations were most likely to report long-standing and limiting illnesses. The prevalence of these was also highest among economically inactive respondents. There is striking similarity between the proportions of men and women experiencing various forms of chronic illness, with the following two exceptions among those aged 75 years and above. First, 26% of men stated that they had a long-standing musculoskeletal disorder, compared with 35% of their female counterparts. This could be partly due to the higher proportion of much older women who fall into this age category. Second, 10% of males considered themselves to be suffering from respiratory disease, whereas only 7% of women characterised themselves in the same way. Differences in lifetime smoking behaviour are reflected here, although occupational factors may also be significant (Dunnell 1997).

The number of conditions identified per person increased with advancing age, being 1.3 for those aged 16–44 years and 1.8 for those aged 75 years and above. The findings of these surveys support the notion that, while chronic illness is widespread and involves a variety of conditions, only a proportion of those affected are appreciably disabled. A survey carried out in 1995 on behalf of the Department of Health revealed that, amongst adults aged 16 years and over, serious disabilities were most likely to be caused by arthritis and rheumatism, diseases of the nervous system, particularly Parkinson's disease and multiple sclerosis, and circulatory disease/stroke (DH 1997a).

STOP THINK **32.3** Given that chronic illness is so widespread, think again about the meaning of health for different people. Can people with chronic disease be 'healthy'?

Cancer was reported as the cause of their disability by 2% of respondents (DH 1997a). Cancer mortality has fallen during the last 40 years in men under 70 years and women under 50 years of age as a consequence of improved treatment and reduced risk (Swerdlow et al 2001). Data from the GHS show that neoplasms and benign growths are the cause of long-standing illness in 1% of adults.

CASE HISTORY 32.2

Mrs F

Mrs F is 64 years old. She has been widowed for 9 years and has lived with cancer for the last 8. Mrs F can recall clearly the moment when she feels her life changed. She had dropped her soap whilst bathing and, when bending to retrieve it, she noticed a lump in her left breast. For a time it seemed to her that the world stood still, her immediate fear being of the likely diagnosis. Mrs F knew what her course of action should be but she postponed visiting her GP for a week. She felt as though hearing someone else voice her suspicions would make things worse and that somehow the lump would be more real.

Within a short time, Mrs F underwent a series of investigations and a lumpectomy. It seemed that she was on a merry-go-round and could not get off. Each appointment with a hospital department led to another and she joked that her social diary had never been so full. Once surgery was over Mrs F was unsure of herself. Her life was under immediate threat. She did not know how she was supposed to feel or what was normal behaviour in this abnormal situation. The sense of threat lessened as the period between follow-up appointments increased. Despite the surgeon's optimism, Mrs F feared the disease returning. Her medication regimen acted as a constant reminder but as time passed she wondered if she dared to believe that she was safe. Feeling it important to do something to occupy her time, Mrs F enrolled in adult education classes and began work for a local children's charity.

Two years later, further surgery was advised to remove diseased axillary lymph nodes. A course of radiotherapy followed. Mrs F coped by fitting appointments around her charity work but found that her condition was less easy to ignore than before. She was tired, her skin was sore and she found it difficult to use her left arm. Again, the medical team appeared optimistic. Mrs F wondered if they were telling her the truth and found herself looking for clues in their words and mannerisms. She recognised that the disease now posed more problems than ever. Until now she had described herself as healthy.

Mrs F gained some reassurance as the time between follow-up appointments increased as before and scans did not reveal further metastatic spread. The doctors always seemed to define survival in terms of a 5-year period. This assumed great importance for Mrs F. She felt as though it represented an almost magical goal, beyond which her existence was assured. In the meantime she managed her medication regimen and the side-effects of additional treatment. Every previously innocent ache, pain or cough she experienced took on a new meaning. Was it her arthritis, a chest infection or had the disease spread?

Increasing back pain led to Mrs F relinquishing her charity work and to the recent diagnosis of bony metastases. She was offered a place at a hospice day centre but refused. Mrs F felt that accepting it confirmed that the cancer was now bigger than she. She also did not relish making new acquaintances there and then wondering who would be missing when she next attended. Mrs F thought the outcome of her illness was certain but was still unsure of what would happen on the way.

STOP THINK **32.4** Read Case History 32.2 and also refer to Chapter 31. Do all cancers result in chronic illness?

FEATURES OF CHRONIC ILLNESS

While analysing the prevalence of long-standing disease is useful in predicting the demand for support services, it gives no indication of the impact of such conditions on daily life. Incongruously, overemphasis on diagnosis and disease entities conceals both the psychological and social problems common to chronically ill people and the uniqueness of each person's experience. In their seminal work, Strauss et al (1984) developed a framework to enable the experience of chronic illness to be understood more clearly and empathically. To provide a basis for this, the seven features of chronic illness outlined below were identified. Only when they are aware of these features can nurses begin to appreciate the profound effect chronic illness has on individuals, their families and health workers.

Chronic illnesses are long-term by nature

The time span for the treatment of acute illness contrasts markedly with that for chronic disease. Once treatment is initiated, the resolution of acute illness is generally achieved within a short period of time and life is resumed as before. The protracted nature of chronic illness results in repeated interactions between individuals and service providers, perhaps over a period of months or years. This leads to individuals gaining familiarity with the organisations providing support and the personnel with whom they come into contact, and has implications for the development of complex social relationships between patients and carers. For example, Curtin and Lubkin (1998) liken chronic illness to an unexpected guest who announces an indefinite stay and becomes part of the household.

Although diagnostic labels often come as a relief, because they explain symptoms and validate individuals' feelings that 'something isn't right' (Locker 2003), labelling also represents a defining moment in the trajectory from person to patient. For example, after being told she had Addison's disease, one woman told of a heightened sense that 'things would never be the same again'.

Adulthood is a dynamic period usually associated with autonomy and control. It is a time of life in which the individual expects to nurture others, rather than to be nurtured. The limitations imposed by illness and a need for protracted care conflict with these expectations and can be damaging to the individual's self-esteem. People with chronic illness may be encouraged to relinquish whatever control they still possess in favour of control by the health professionals (Daly 1993), though this stance has been vigorously questioned, for example in patient-focused rehabilitative care (Wilson 2002). Ironically, failure to accept this may be regarded as active opposition to adopting the role of patient and can result in the individual acquiring a reputation for being 'difficult'. Frequent service usage or long-term admission to hospital do not necessarily enhance relationships between patients and health professionals, despite the opportunity it presents for interpersonal development in the course of continued interactions (Stockwell 1972, Johnson 1997, Jiwa 2000).

Chronic illness is uncertain

Living with chronic illness means living with uncertainty. Obtaining a diagnosis may be a lengthy and complicated process due to the ambiguity of symptoms experienced and insidiousness of onset. Difficulty in establishing a prognosis with any degree of certainty is also a source of stress for all concerned, since only the progress of the disease itself gives sufficient information to suggest a likely timescale of events for a particular individual (Strauss et al 1984).

Adulthood is also associated with the achievement of socially and culturally specified tasks such as leaving the parental home, finding a partner and rearing a family (Schaie & Willis 2001). The restriction, discomfort and possible dependence which accompany chronic illness may force the individual to forgo these and adopt an alternative lifestyle. Biographical disruption leads to grieving for previously taken-for-granted opportunities, ambitions and loss of self. The difficulty that individuals with a degenerative illness may have in visualising the future is illustrated in Case History 32.3.

Fear of dependence, which in itself causes uncertainty, is a fundamental human concern in cultures valuing self-reliance and economic and physical independence. For instance, following a diagnosis of Parkinson's disease, this problem is shared to an extent by medical staff who must decide how much information to give regarding the likely course of the disorder and difficulties of treatment. Although it is seen as important to provide patients with sufficient data to enable them to exert maximum control over their new situation, doctors question their own professional commitment in situations where purely medical solutions have only a limited effect (Pinder 1992).

Fluctuations in symptoms, and energy to manage them, make it impossible to forecast the occurrence of 'good days' and 'bad days' and this is compounded because a 'good day' can turn abruptly into a 'bad day' and vice versa. Uncertainty is also present because of the inherently episodic nature of many chronic illnesses, in which recurrent unpredictable crises occur, followed by periods of remission or control. Since the onset and duration of these crises cannot be anticipated, individuals and their carers must be vigilant for indications of impending difficulty and ready to respond at any time. Pre-empting the sudden imposition of change results in the restriction and reorganisation of lifestyle. Social uncertainty thus exists for people with chronic illness and their families, who find it difficult to plan their activities in either the long or short term and may be excluded from full participation in community life as a result (Strauss et al 1984). Fluctuation in chronic conditions influences the way in which individuals perceive themselves and are perceived by others. The invisibility of symptoms in some conditions can cause people to question the reality of their experience and those around them to doubt that it exists (Aylett & Fawcett 2003, Foley & Sarnoff 2003). For example, where health workers and family members 'all say "but you look so good for someone who has MS" … if they can't see it, there really isn't anything wrong with me' (Doss 2002). This also means that the pervasive consequences of living with a protracted disorder are disregarded. Individuals are believed to be directly affected by the disease only when it becomes noticeable, and variation in ability during periods of crisis and remission is misunderstood. Paradoxically, uncertainty can be a positive experience in chronic illness. For example, in Mishel's (1993) study of people receiving renal dialysis, higher levels of uncertainty correlated with adherence to the regimen, while lower levels were related to non-adherence.

CASE HISTORY 32.3
S

S is 28 years old and works as a cook in an independent school for girls. She has been in this employment since leaving college and lives on the premises. Her social life revolves largely around sporting activities, an interest shared with her boyfriend, A.

S was diagnosed as having multiple sclerosis (MS) 2 years ago when she was admitted to hospital following a fall while playing tennis. She had been experiencing difficulty in focusing her eyes for some time but had thought that this was due to overwork. She had also begun to find it difficult to coordinate her movements and became known for dropping and spilling things. These events were explained when the diagnosis was made and S found it strange that she had lived with the condition for so long without realising that something was seriously wrong.

After the diagnosis was confirmed, S felt compelled to search the internet to find out more about the condition and what it would mean to her. She resolved that her approach would be to get on with living despite the disease. Within a short period, however, her balance deteriorated and walking became difficult. She also found that she tired easily. S responded by opting out of strenuous activities. Having valued her physical fitness, she began to experience frustration at her loss of ability and function. She felt as though her body had betrayed her and she did not like to be seen walking with a stick. When S developed frequency and urgency of micturition, she began to avoid visits to public places where toilets would be difficult to reach or where queues were likely.

In private, S found herself increasingly reduced to tears of frustration and despair, believing that no one else could understand her experience. She chose not to share these feelings. She had always been able to manage her life independently and wanted to appear to be continuing to do so. S's boyfriend, A, tried to support her as much as possible, but maintaining a positive stance at all times was hard. His friends advised him not to remain in the relationship, purely because of his concern for S, and his feelings for her were sometimes confused. He wondered if her reluctance to visit public venues was actually her way of avoiding him because she wanted their relationship to end.

S was preoccupied by questions about her future. How long would she be able to continue in her present post? Would it be possible to seek alternative employment? Giving up her job would mean giving up her home. Her parents wanted her to live with them but S was anxious to retain her autonomy and knew that her mother would try to protect her too much. However, it was her future with A that was her greatest concern. S loved him and had hoped that their relationship would lead to marriage. She wanted children of her own and already felt that time was running out. S felt it impossible to confront A about such a commitment, fearing that he would perceive this as pressure to make an immediate decision and that as a result she may lose him altogether. Her sad conclusion was that with MS she could no longer be sure of anything.

STOP THINK

32.5 In Case History 32.3, S obviously believes that her life course is being undermined and she has many anxieties about her long-term goals. Anxiety is a distressing experience in itself, but could interfere with her ability to function. If you were caring for S, how would you help her to deal with her situation? What role could an MS specialist nurse have played from the time of diagnosis?

For more information, see Multiple Sclerosis Trust/Royal College of Nursing (2003) and UK Multiple Sclerosis Specialist Nurse Association et al (2003).

Chronic illnesses require proportionately greater efforts at palliation

In view of the remote prospect of effecting a cure in chronic illness, the control of elements which influence quality of life assumes primary importance. More emphasis is placed on palliative measures, e.g. alleviating pain and discomfort, providing symptomatic relief and addressing problems created by the restriction of activity. Palliation is of greater significance than in acute illness because people with long-term disease must learn to live with both the features of their condition and the side-effects of treatment (Strauss et al 1984). The cooperation of patients, their families and close associates is necessary to achieve this. Since symptoms such as constant pain and nausea can compromise the individual's ability to engage in a variety of activities, their treatment is seen as desirable even though it will have little effect upon the disease process.

Decisions as to which palliative measures are selected for individual treatment are influenced by availability, acceptance by the medical profession, their perceived benefit to the patient and financial constraints. Improvements in quality of life following palliation are difficult to measure objectively, and this has implications for the allocation of resources.

Individuals have considerable resources of their own and many use these to try to resolve health problems before seeking professional help or as an adjunct to it, particularly if statutory agencies cannot provide palliation or the side-effects of treatment are unacceptable. The use of complementary therapies is common amongst people who feel that conventional medicine has nothing further to offer (Watkins 1996, Cant & Sharma 1999). This not only represents an assumption of responsibility for their own well-being but a desire to achieve control over unpredictable illness (Montbriand & Laing 1991). Furthermore, in contrast with conventional care, there is a possibility of accessing person-centred treatments which are inherently pleasurable.

Coping strategies can be learned through experience and membership of self-help groups (Field & Kelly 2003). Although self-help groups provide a means of empowering individuals and can complement formal services, they also reflect a subversive readiness to assert the value of experiential knowledge and to question that of medicine (Scambler 2003b). The UK government's 'Expert Patients' initiative stems from a recognition that traditional cure-oriented services have not dealt comprehensively with problems faced by chronically sick people and that partnership enhances self-management, giving patients greater mastery over their lives (DH 2001a). It is intended to introduce user-led training programmes in England and feed these into the forthcoming National Service Framework (NSF) for long-term health conditions and other disease-specific frameworks. Examples of these for diabetes may be found across the UK (DH 2001b, Scottish Executive Health Department 2002, Welsh Assembly Government 2002, CREST 2003).

STOP THINK

32.6 In a study exploring attitudes towards patient expertise in chronic illness Thorne et al (2000) found that: 'Whether or not they had any actual expert advice to offer, patients reported that many professionals cling to the role of expert within the health care encounter. In the case of type 1 diabetes mellitus (see Ch. 5, part 2), this occurred despite clear evidence of established patient sophistication in self-care decision-making'. Why may members of the health care team retain the expert role when working with people with chronic illness?

Chronic diseases are multiple diseases

The systematic and degenerative effects of many chronic diseases are such that the failure of one organ or physiological system leads eventually to the involvement of others. In addition, long-term disability related to an existing chronic condition is likely to generate further disease. This can be illustrated with reference to complications associated with diabetes mellitus. These include vascular damage, which may result in renal and visual dysfunction, and an increased risk of myocardial infarction. Impaired circulation to the lower limbs also predisposes to the development of gangrene, the onset of which is, in turn, influenced by degeneration of the nervous system and greater susceptibility to infection (Crumbie 2002a). Amputation of an affected limb results in further alteration of physical, psychological and social functioning. Clearly, the disabling effects of chronic conditions are not merely confined to features of the disease process, but are compounded by the consequences of treatment used.

Efforts to adjust to the reduction in activity, imposed by chronic disease, are complicated by the multiplication of symptoms and the increasing disability that results (Strauss et al 1984). For example, chronic pain not only inhibits movement but also correlates with atrophy in the brain's prefrontal cortex and impairs decision making (Melton 2004). To be confronted with the inevitability of deterioration is a substantial psychological challenge to individuals and their carers, acting as an additional source of stress. Individuals fearing the prospect of total disability might regard any development of their disease with anxiety and anger, directing these emotions towards close associates and health workers. Carers are confronted with difficulties in dealing with this, at the same time as they face increased demands placed on them to compensate for the individual's failing abilities. These demands may include seeking information about services, learning new skills and accommodating more physical activity when managing care. This has a considerable impact because care giving is carried out in the context of other competing demands, such as employment, marriage and child rearing (Bull & Jervis 1997).

Health care professionals can be perceived by individuals as being incapable of resolving certain problems or, in the case of problems resulting from treatment, actually being responsible for them. This has obvious implications for the quality of nurse–patient relationships, which in order to be genuinely therapeutic must be characterised by mutual trust and cooperation.

Chronic diseases are disproportionately intrusive

A significant aspect of living with a chronic illness is the 'daily grind' of monitoring and managing its features (Locker 2003). Such work is unrewarding, unrelenting and inescapable. As one person with chronic fatigue syndrome (CFS) explained: 'For one wonderful moment when you wake up you forget. But there it is, again. It's the hardest work I've ever done and there's no time off'. This prompts a fundamental shift from the self and life that 'used to be' towards recognition and acceptance of a 'new normal' (Harpam 1997, Fennell 2003). Adaptation is central to wellness but is far from straightforward, particularly because 'good adaptation' is judged by others (Radley 1994). The emotional burden involved can be added to by shame and guilt at failing to recover or adjust as quickly as expected. Individuals can feel responsible for not doing better, in the light of images of chronically ill people as 'brave', with an innate capacity to tolerate adversity, or assumptions that they must simply adjust to the obvious (LeMaistre 1996). Pressure can be added where media portrayals of triumph over tragedy create models of behaviour which individuals feel they must live up to. For example, a man with lymphatic cancer recalled: 'Everything tells you to think positively. So, when the tumour came back I thought it was my fault. I hadn't thought positively enough'.

In episodes of acute illness it is both feasible and acceptable to gain temporary exemption from normal social obligations. This is not always possible, however, for those with chronic illness who must restructure daily life such that persistent features of their condition and periods of crisis can be accommodated. It may be difficult for these people and their families to enjoy a sense of continuity, as their capacity to pursue various activities will vary unpredictably over time. It is unsurprising that individuals become sick and tired of feeling sick and tired (Donaghue & Siegel 2000). Parson's (1951) conceptualisation of the sick role makes sense of illness as a social state, but its applicability is questionable in long-term illness, since an obligation to recover is implied. The sick role does, however, facilitate access to helpful resources and chronically sick people are expected to adhere to medical advice in the same way as those who are acutely ill (Field & Kelly 2003).

Chronic illness often imposes changes to normal domestic routines to allow for physical limitations and requirements of treatment regimens. Structural alteration of accommodation may also be required to install equipment and reassign room space to allow access to household facilities. These adaptations, together with alterations in appearance and behaviour associated with the long-term disease, will impact on other members of the household and affect familial relationships.

Chronic illness will also have economic implications. Even if not totally disabled, continued employment might be impossible because of the demands which the condition and its treatment make upon time, strength and stamina. Difficulty in adhering to work schedules and periods of absence during relapses can give the impression that chronically ill people are unreliable. Individuals may be assigned to less demanding positions and be overlooked for promotion because they are perceived to have a poor prognosis and are thus not deserving of the investment of training for more advanced work (Taylor 1995). Gaining employment may be problematic in itself; the prospect of incapacity and variable function may be seen by the employer to represent risk and hidden costs, including lost production and redeployment of other workers. Despite there being advantages in disclosing health status to an employer, it is understandable that people with chronic illness are often reluctant to do so because it affects their workplace identity. For example, a woman with multiple sclerosis maintained her silence for 8 years to avoid being 'stuck with the MS label, to become Sukie with MS as opposed to just Sukie' (Freeman 2002). Disclosure can also lead to an individual's competence being doubted. This diminishes self-esteem, giving rise to guilt and fear of letting others down and can result in chronically ill people sensing that they have to work harder than others to prove their worth.

Chronic illness affects the individual's ability to participate in social activities. The degree to which these are impeded will depend to some extent on whether the individual has learned to deal with the features of the disease process. For example, fear of frequent episodes of loose stools and odour are major social concerns for people with ulcerative colitis (Robinson 2004). The management of these features is particularly difficult in settings where toilet facilities are not readily available. Individuals may respond either by withdrawing from interaction or by planning outings carefully, using known routes and venues with accessible lavatories. Anxiety regarding the accidental emission of diarrhoea during sexual encounters can be met by avoiding intimate relationships, instituting strategies such as keeping an unobtrusive towel at the bedside or having spontaneous sexual encounters to avoid anticipatory preoccupation with the disorder.

The nature of chronic disease is such that it impinges on domestic, work-related and recreational activities. This is liable to result in involuntary social isolation affecting individuals and their close associates (Biordi 1998). People who are chronically ill require sustained support to manage their conditions and treatment regimens. Their families' daily activities are often centred around meeting these needs, and it may no longer be possible for them to pursue interests which they once enjoyed together. Providing long-term care changes relationships and compels those who have acquired reluctantly an unexpected caring role to make fundamental changes to their entire way of life.

Chronic diseases require a wide variety of ancillary services

There is an abundance of statutory and voluntary agencies in the UK concerned with the care and support of people with long-term illness. Statutory support is provided in the main by the National Health Service, the Department of Work and Pensions and the local authority social services. Care within institutional and domestic settings requires the close collaboration of a wide range of representatives of these agencies, such as nurses, therapists, doctors, social workers, civil service employees and home care workers. This collaboration can be difficult to achieve, given the number and variety of staff necessary to meet an individual's needs, and problems are sometimes compounded by poor interagency coordination and frequent transfers between care settings (Howkins 1995).

The definitions adopted by formal agencies to categorise individuals and allocate resources are not generally compatible with the experience of chronically ill people. For example, assessment to determine eligibility for benefits and support services may fail to acknowledge variation in function during episodes of crisis; if the assessment is performed during a period of relative wellness, the type and level of support required at other times may not be apparent to the assessor.

Some people do not obtain support because they perceive the organisation of services to be complex or somewhat arbitrary. Ineffective communication presents an obstacle when individuals who are entitled to benefits lack information or have difficulty interpreting the information they are given. In addition, some families may be reluctant to seek or accept help because to do so would be at variance with their cultural values regarding responsibility and self-sufficiency.

Systems for the organisation and provision of care are complex, with variation between UK constituent countries. Cross-party commitment to the concept of community care since the 1960s has been formalised in legislation, such as the National Health Service and Community Care Act 1990 (DH 1990) and Community Care (Direct Payments) Act 1996 (HMSO 1997), and is a feature of the government's modernisation agenda. The latter also aims to improve interagency working so that integrated health and social care is user focused (DH 1997b, 1998a,b, 2001c). This reflects trends towards casting the service user as consumer (Alabaster et al 2000). Key reforms implemented from the 1990s include splitting the commissioning and provision of care and dominance of the market by the private and voluntary sectors. Related initiatives, including the introduction of unified health and social assessments, have enabled the development of creative and flexible care packages. The responses of many agencies remain ineffective, however, due to differences in priorities and practices, as exemplified in the differential provision of 'free' nursing and personal care in care home and domestic settings in the UK constituent countries. Funding of health and social care are devolved functions but varying degrees of devolution have resulted in diverse governmental responses (Scottish Executive 2001a, Northern Ireland Assembly 2002, Age Concern England 2003, Long-term Care Commission 2003, Welsh Assembly Government 2003).

Differing priorities and practices have significant implications for quality of life. For example, giving priority to people who have complex needs and are at risk of admission to residential care means withdrawing low-level support from others who, in turn, become more dependent on their informal carers. An emphasis on personal or physical care also results in classifying social needs as lesser wants (Means et al 2003). Carers are entitled to a separate assessment of their needs but this may not occur, as many partners and family members take caring as the natural order of things and it is expected that they have assumed the role willingly (DH 1997a). People with long-term illness and their families may not, therefore, receive the kind of help which they believe would be of greatest benefit to them (Pitkeathley 1991, Finkelstein & Stuart 1996).

Chronic illness is expensive

The direct and indirect costs of chronic illness are high. While expensive technological intervention is not always required, support is ongoing and increases in intensity as the individual's condition progresses. Chronically ill people make repeated contact with health agencies to monitor the effectiveness of treatment and rehabilitation programmes. This involves regular encounters with members of primary and secondary health care teams. Individuals are likely to experience multiple pathology as a result of systemic and degenerative disease and, since contemporary medical services are organised by area of specialisation, they need to attend a variety of clinics. Someone with diabetes mellitus, for example, may require referral to a physician in renal medicine, an ophthalmologist and a vascular surgeon.

The long-term prescription of medication to control or palliate features of chronic conditions has significant financial and ethical implications. Rationing of health care has become more explicit in the face of growing demand and the increased availability of treatment options, coupled with pressure to reduce expenditure (British Medical Association 2002, Ham & Robert 2003). Limited resources mean that decisions regarding treatment options are concerned with identifying the potential benefit to the individual and justifying whether such expenditure on a single patient is warranted. For example, lipid-lowering drugs used to reduce the risk of dying from coronary artery disease in men with hypercholesterolaemia at the beginning of the 21st century cost £162 500 per life saved (Ferner & Mann 2001).

Treatment intended to inhibit the development of underlying disease, but which does not necessarily cure or save lives, can also be costly. For example, individuals with ambulatory relapse-remitting multiple sclerosis, i.e. a pattern of disease characterised by at least two attacks of neurological dysfunction over the preceding 2-year period, followed by complete or incomplete recovery, can be prescribed interferon beta-1a or b, to be administered by injection (Kita & Goodkin 2000, Sweetman 2002). This may decrease the frequency of relapses and prevent the accumulation of neurological damage, although evidence that it improves clinical disability is equivocal (Weiner et al 1997, Rice et al 2003). Treatment in the UK is prescribed to between 2 and 5% of suitable patients (Coles 2001) at a net annual cost at the time of writing of £7260–£12 068 per person (Joint Formulary Committee 2003). Clinical governance should aid people with chronic illness by eradicating inequalities in care and raising standards, though frameworks and working practices differ among UK countries (Ward 2002). The Healthcare Commission carries out clinical governance reviews in England and Wales which consider the implementation of NSFs and guidance from the National Institute for Clinical Excellence (NICE). Such guidance is provided in Scotland by NHS Quality Improvement Scotland and the Scottish Intercollegiate Guidelines Network, while the Northern Irish approach is under development. NICE recommendations are intended to inform professionals' decisions without overriding patients' individual circumstances and the Institute states that people should not be denied access to treatments while these are undergoing appraisal (NICE 2003). The extended time taken to appraise beta-interferon use in multiple sclerosis and provisional opinion that prescription should not be offered to new patients has, however, been criticised. Delays in implementing a UK-wide risk-sharing scheme, whereby a cohort of patients is monitored and manufacturers paid less should the drugs fail to meet expectations, resulted in prolonging the 'postcode lottery' and in frustrating individuals who feared that progression of their symptoms in the meantime would disqualify them from receiving treatment (MS Society 2003). Balancing the interests of stakeholders, including doctors, the pharmaceutical industry and self-help groups lobbying for access to treatment is a complex process.

Additional medications may need to be introduced to the regimen as illnesses evolve and to compensate for side-effects of treatment or medication already prescribed. Changes in the treatment programme may be initiated by episodes of crisis. This, and the increased use of support services during such times, is a source of considerable expense.

Repeated periods of admission for acute hospital care may be necessary to achieve management of crises. Interdisciplinary involvement is essential in view of the effect that chronic illness has on all aspects of the individual's life. Cost containment in health care has led to a reduction in the length of stay in acute care hospitals; however, the presence of acute illness superimposed on a chronic condition inevitably results in a longer stay (Daly 1993).

The cost of chronic illness in comparison with that of acute illness is very high in respect of lost employment, reliance on state benefits and social exclusion.

STOP THINK **32.7** Where resources are limited, it could be argued that efforts should be directed towards patients for whom improvement can be assured rather than those who are chronically ill or disabled (Hinsliff 2004). Why should patients with a chronic illness be given equal consideration?

For further exploration of related ethical issues, see Thompson et al (2000).

A FRAMEWORK FOR UNDERSTANDING THE EXPERIENCE OF CHRONIC ILLNESS

The features of chronic illness detailed above are reflected in the framework presented by Strauss et al (1984) for understanding the experience of ongoing ill health. This framework is built around the five components outlined in the following.

Key problems

Any disease has the potential to create multiple problems for individuals and these are liable not only to disrupt routine activities but also to lead to social isolation and attendant psychological and familial difficulties. For example, people with multiple sclerosis and their associates may have difficulty adjusting to the effects of variation in ability and fatigue experienced. It can be difficult for them to make firm arrangements to attend social gatherings, and friends may eventually hesitate to extend invitations when the affected individual withdraws repeatedly from events due to fatigue. Family members may begin to experience regret and resentment as outings and social activities are curtailed.

Basic strategies

Patients and their associates need to develop a repertoire of methods or techniques for overcoming key problems. For instance, individuals with diabetes mellitus can learn to adjust their behaviour and treatment regimen when attending social occasions where food and drink are offered. Their selection of type and quantity of food may be guided by their treatment regimen, rather than purely by desire. If they do not wish to bring their condition to the attention of others at this time, they might avoid alcoholic drinks on the pretext of wanting to 'keep a clear head'. Conversely, they may choose to amend the timing and dosage of insulin injections to allow for indulgence in the food and drink which they actually prefer. Creative non-adherence (Taylor 1995) to treatment schedules or 'intelligent cheating' (Pressly 1995) is common in chronic illness and can result in errors; however, such mindful adaptation reflects individuals' assertion of control and successful renegotiation of life situations in their own context.

Agents

Employing basic strategies can require the assistance of family members, friends, acquaintances or strangers. These 'agents' may function in various ways, for example by assisting in the maintenance of a treatment regimen or protecting the individual from harmful effects of the disorder. Someone who has epilepsy may need help from colleagues such that, should an unexpected seizure occur in the workplace, the individual is eased to the ground and away from dangerous machinery (see Ch. 9).

Organisational or family arrangements

The strategies adopted to address key problems require the coordinated effort of the individual and the agents involved. The establishment and maintenance of arrangements rely on trust, skilled interaction, sufficient resources and realistic negotiation of the roles, responsibilities and expectations of all concerned. Someone who is housebound due to longstanding arthritis may be able to enlist family members and neighbours to do shopping, pick up drug prescriptions and collect benefit monies. The continued success of such arrangements will depend on each person involved having a clear appreciation of what actually is required, as well as an understanding of their own contribution to the wellbeing of the individual, in the context of the help given by others.

Consequences

The strategies and arrangements adopted by chronically ill people and their associates may be successful in resolving key problems but can have implications for the agents taking part, thus creating further problems. For example, the paced schedule of activities that enables individuals with chronic obstructive pulmonary disease (COPD) to accommodate oxygen deprivation and recovery times between tasks may present little opportunity for flexibility. Events such as a visit to the hairdresser's can disrupt well-established routines, with implications for both the individual and carer alike. Both parties are also faced with developing a lifestyle structured by the demands of the presenting condition, within which spontaneity has no place (see Research Abstract 32.1). Adopting the roles of carer and cared for also have an inevitable impact on relationships, changing established patterns of engagement. Marriott's (2003) insight into the all-consuming consequences of caring

RESEARCH ABSTRACT 32.1

Carers of the chronically ill

The Office for National Statistics (2002) used data obtained from the General Household Survey (GHS) to explore trends in caring and revealed the following:

- 21% of households contained a carer
- Women were more likely to be carers than men — 18% compared with 14%
- 8% of 16–29 year olds have caring responsibilities, compared with 24% of 45–64 year olds and 16% of those aged 65 years and above
- Almost a third of married or co-habiting women aged 45–64 were carers
- A third of carers were the only support for the main person cared for
- 21% had been caring for someone for at least 10 years
- 28% of carers spent at least 20 hours a week on their caring responsibilities and 1% 50 hours or more
- Half of those spending 20 hours or more a week on caring were looking after someone needing constant attention and who could not be left for a few hours
- 35% of those devoting at least 20 hours per week to caring reported a limiting long-standing illness, rising to 47% among older carers
- 39% reported that their physical or mental health had been affected as a result of caring
- 41% of people being cared for received visits from health, social and voluntary services; those living with their carers were less likely to receive services than those living in different households.

for a spouse with Huntington's disease and the 'emotional whirlpool' entered into, is helpful in coming to understand the stresses imposed; for example, the conflict experienced when carers sense that their lives are no longer their own but feel that it is selfish to resent this.

The elements in Research Abstract 32.1 provide a means of thinking about the experience of chronic illness from the perspective of the people concerned. Living with chronic illness is influenced by a range of interacting physical, psychosocial and spiritual elements. It is only through exploring these that the meaning for each individual can be truly appreciated.

For more information about the social psychology of chronic illness, see Livneh & Antonrak (1997).

STOP THINK **32.8** 'Chronic illness is a lonely experience. It makes for a sense of uniqueness that often leads to a feeling of separateness and alienation. It tends to foster a perception that you are in a world of your own and cannot join the ranks of mainstream culture' (Klein & Landau 1992). Refer to this, or any self-help guide or website for people with a chronic illness. Has this helped you to understand the experience of living with a chronic condition? If so, in what way? Why is the use of self-help groups of particular value to people with chronic illness?

NURSING INTERVENTION

Developments in the location and organisation of care

Nurses encounter adults with chronic illness in a range of community and institutional settings including the person's own home, care homes and hospitals providing acute, intermediate or continuing care. Statutory and other agencies have responded to the shift in provision to community care by attempting to meet rising demand and provide user-focused services, while accounting for the shortcomings of long-term institutionalisation (Benjamin 1997). Ironically, the payment of care home fees through social security benefits favoured institutional care (Leathard 2000). Domiciliary care is viewed as resource effective, while also being preferable for and preferred by individuals.

People with chronic illness have diverse needs which sometimes cross, or fall between, traditional service boundaries, resulting in inappropriate and fragmented provision. Moving into long-term care is generally seen as the last resort for people with chronic illness but can come as a relief where, for example, an inflexible care package has been in place. Nurses have an important role in supporting individuals and their carers in considering care options, adjusting to new environments, grieving for their past life and constructing a future (Jarrett 2003). The quality of daily life while in long-term care will depend upon the extent to which staff recognise residents' adult status, enable them to exercise choice in their activities, avoid socialised dependency and help them to preserve links with the wider social world. All of this should be aided by the introduction of standards for care homes (DH 2001d, Scottish Executive 2001b, Welsh Assembly Government 2004) which are, arguably, more stringent than those applied to statutory agencies. Regional anomalies regarding the nature of nursing care and 'postcode funding' have led to delayed admissions, care home fees rising to compensate for shortfalls and the closure of some establishments.

Trends in service provision mean that nurses are more likely to encounter chronically ill people who are living in their own homes. Community nursing is an essential component of home care and visits can continue over a period of years in this context. Carers' needs have not always been a focus of nursing intervention; however, developments favouring partnership may change this and result in nurses acting as co-experts with the carers. In addition, NHS reforms are diverting resources towards primary care and nurses' involvement in primary care groups/trusts (PCGs/ PCTs), or community health partnerships (CHPs) in Scotland, provides a platform for their promotion of the worth of working with family units in this setting (McClure 2001).

Acute hospital care occurs in relation to the establishment of diagnoses, periods of crisis during which features of the illness are exacerbated and when the disease process necessitates stabilisation or palliation. Such contact is therefore intermittent and recurrent. It should also be borne in mind that hospitalisation may result from the development of unrelated health problems. Disease management in the form of integrated care pathways has particular relevance in chronic illness because it presents a structured means of planning and delivering coordinated, patient-oriented care as part of a sequential journey, instead of as a series of separate episodes. There is, however, a danger that rigid adherence to protocols may actually prevent individuals having a say in their treatment (Hunter 2000).

The foundation for the nursing role

While the contribution of health professionals is crucial during diagnosis, in relapses and in the establishment of treatment regimens, individuals and their associates are primarily responsible for handling the condition on a daily basis.

A significant minority of chronically ill people are unable to function independently and responsibility for their support frequently rests with family members. The nursing role is therefore far from restricted to the delivery of direct care. For example, the cognitive and physical capacities of individuals and their carers to develop required practices must first be assessed. It is also vital to ensure that the information that they need to implement care regimens at home has been successfully communicated (see Case History 32.4). In pursuing the goal of optimum self-management, the nurse must also be prepared to adopt a flexible approach to care. During some phases of long-term illness it may be necessary to act for patients and carers, while on other occasions support will be focused on monitoring the performance of self-care activities, imparting knowledge, teaching practical skills or giving emotional support to facilitate coping behaviour. This means that nurses need to be committed to forming and maintaining collaborative, empowering relationships (McWilliam et al 1997, Crumbie 2002b).

The notion of empowerment has particular value for people living with chronic illness; however, they are likely to have lost power, control and confidence in their own abilities, through the psychological effects of the illness or institutionalisation. Empowerment is an enabling process that enhances personal control and facilitates the process of recreating self. This strategy will, however, present difficulties for those nurses who feel that sharing information and skill constitutes a threat to their control of the caring situation or somehow undermines their professional role.

32.9 After reading Case History 32.4, how do you think communication could have been enhanced to prevent the problems which occurred when Mr P was learning about his diabetes? The community nurse recognised the need to respond to Mr P's difficulties with language by involving a link worker. A number of different people could have been asked to perform this role in the hospital setting:

(a) a young female family member
(b) any member of the local South Asian community
(c) a member of the hospital catering staff who speaks the same language as Mr P
(d) a community link worker employed for this purpose on a sessional basis.

What are the advantages and disadvantages of using each of the above as an interpreter? You may like to think about issues relating to culture, age, gender, varieties of Asian language, availability and confidentiality.

CASE HISTORY 32.4

Mr P

Mr P is 62 years old and lives with his wife and their son V in a suburban area of a large city. The family own and manage a successful video rental business and are active within the local South Asian community.

Mr P usually enjoys good health but had been feeling unwell during recent months, experiencing frequency of micturition and an increased thirst. He was eventually persuaded to visit his general practitioner and was admitted to hospital on the GP's advice. A diagnosis of diabetes mellitus was made and medical staff decided that control could be achieved through a combination of prescribed oral hypoglycaemic agents and dietary management (see Ch. 5, part 2). In the days which followed, stabilisation of blood glucose levels was achieved. Nursing staff and the ward dietitian spent time with Mr P explaining the nature of his condition and his future role in its management. He seemed to listen carefully to what was said but did not ask questions of the staff. It was believed that this was an expression of his quiet and reserved nature which had been in evidence since admission. The dietitian was anxious to speak to Mrs P about her husband's dietary requirements, but the latter was not able to visit the hospital during office hours. Mr P said that he had discussed his condition with his wife and was confident that he would be able to cope after discharge. He was very much looking forward to returning home.

The responsibility for Mr P's nursing care was transferred to staff outside the hospital by way of the community liaison nurse. When the community nurse, N, visited to assess the level of support which would be needed, she was greeted by V. He told her that both he and his mother were concerned about Mr P, who now appeared to be little better than he had been before admission to hospital. N checked Mr P's blood glucose level and found it to be higher than expected. In an attempt to discover the likely cause of this problem she asked Mr and Mrs P what they knew of the condition and to describe the treatment regimen.

It soon became clear that Mr P had misunderstood the information given to him in the hospital. He felt that the staff had been kind and concerned for his welfare, but he had observed them to be busy and did not wish to detain them unnecessarily by asking what he feared were trivial questions. He also confided that he was a little deaf and could not always hear what was said to him. The nurses had spoken quietly and quickly but Mr P had been too embarrassed to ask them to repeat all the information given. Although his working knowledge of English is good, Mr P uses this as his second language in daily life. Unfamiliar vocabulary presented during his admission had not enhanced communication with hospital staff. N discovered that Mr P believed he should reduce only the amount of sugar in his diet. Apart from this his food intake was unaltered, being predominantly foods high in fat and with a high glycaemic index. N recognised that the specific support she could give was limited and decided to offer the family contact with a community link worker and Diabetes Specialist Nurse.

The complexity of long-term illness and its impact on individual lifestyle and functioning have already been emphasised. It is all too easy for nurses to make assumptions about the problems experienced by individuals on the basis of medical diagnosis alone. There are additional implications arising from classifying people as 'chronically ill'. The overuse of this label can give the impression of a homogeneous group for whom care can be planned unilaterally.

Using frameworks and models to guide practice

The case has already been made that, although a variety of characteristics are shared by people with chronic illness, there is considerable diversity in the way ongoing ill-health affects individuals. It is therefore advantageous to adopt an approach to nursing which explicitly recognises the uniqueness of each individual and enables the totality of their situation to be understood. The use of a formalised framework to guide practice is also valuable in that it presents a systematic prescription for action and encompasses a sound theoretical base.

A variety of models has been constructed to articulate beliefs about the essential components of nursing practice and the underpinning concepts and theories. These conceptual models are intended to provide a descriptive representation of the reality of practice and consideration of the concepts of person, environment, health and nursing is generally regarded as central to them (Fawcett 2000). The selection of a particular model largely depends on the extent to which it reflects the nursing team's own personal values and what they perceive their work goals to be. Several possible advantages can be gained when a team agrees as to their model of choice; not least among these are consistency and continuity of nursing action.

While a number of models have relevance for nursing adults with chronic illness, the three models discussed below may be of particular interest to nurses entering this field of care.

Orem's self-care model

It is likely that the self-care deficit nursing theory (SCDNT) put forward by Orem (2001) would be favoured by nurses who consider its emphasis on client autonomy and motivation to be consistent with the aim of helping individuals to accept responsibility for themselves. This might seem appropriate, given the role chronically ill people play in managing their condition. Its concern with independent action is, however, more complex than face value suggests. The concept of self-care must be seen in the context of the model's other components, in order for the underlying theory to be understood and the whole operationalised.

Self-care is the contribution people make to their own continued existence and involves practising activities to maintain health and well-being (Gast 1996). Nurses assist patients and their associates to achieve self-care, taking individual ability and need into account. Following negotiation with all parties concerned, care is organised in terms of one of three nursing systems. These are wholly compensatory, i.e. the nurse may perform activities for the individual; partly compensatory, i.e. the nurse may assist the individual in carrying out shared activities; or supportive–educative, i.e. the nurse may help the individual to develop the ability to act on their own behalf. The decision to use a nursing system or a combination of systems is not static but changes in response to patient need over time.

Orem's model therefore presents some advantages for the care of chronically ill people in a variety of settings. The importance of partnership with both patient and carers is acknowledged and their involvement in planning nursing interventions considered essential. Attention is given to the notion that they are active in learning to live with the effects of the condition and it is assumed that they are motivated to do so. The variation in nursing activity necessary to address the range of problems likely to be experienced during the course of long-term illness is also accounted for.

Roy's adaptation model

Another model, which may be applied when nursing chronically ill individuals, is that devised by Roy (Roy & Andrews 1999). This takes the view that human behaviour is influenced by an interrelated set of biological, psychological and social systems. Each of these systems is directed towards achieving a state of relative balance which will, as far as possible, promote regularity of function and the ability of each person to adapt positively to environmental stimuli. Roy identifies three types of stimuli to which individuals are exposed: focal, contextual and residual. A focal stimulus is something which has an immediate effect on the person; a contextual stimulus is a contributory circumstance; and a residual stimulus arises from beliefs or attitudes relating to past experiences. Maladaption occurs where the effect of any stimulus exceeds someone's capacity to make a positive response. This results in a threat to continued health and well-being. Roy's model accepts that individuals possess a unique capacity to deal with stimuli, such that people react differently when faced with the same events. The ability to adapt thus varies from person to person.

Nursing intervention is needed when an individual's usual methods of coping with stressors prove ineffective. The nursing role centres on promoting adaptation, both in maintaining health and during periods of illness, and is concerned with the manipulation of stimuli so that patients are able to respond in a positive way. This model also has value for care in long-term illness in a variety of settings. Its focus is congruent with the belief that it is desirable for people to develop the ability to live with the effects of their condition and that they should collaborate in their care. Nurses are encouraged to consider factors which influence the individual's total situation, not merely the immediate problems confronting the person. In this way it is possible for nurses to appreciate the effects of the disorder on the patient's personal functioning over time and how the person feels about this. The model assists nurses in identifying successful coping mechanisms which have been used in the past and elements likely to impede future adaptation, so that intervention may be planned with realisable goals. Care can therefore be tailored in relation to individual resources.

The Roper–Logan–Tierney (RLT) model

A more detailed examination will be made here of the model for nursing put forward by Roper et al (2000). This model has been widely adopted in the UK and is thus one with which many nurses are familiar. In addition, it is based on ideas drawn directly from practice and articulated in terms which are readily understood. This representation of the reality of practice is such that the model can be identified as being 'for real nurses, nursing real people' (Newton 1991). Examples of how it may be applied have already been given in earlier chapters.

The authors based their model for nursing on a model for living, demonstrating that health status and lifestyle are closely related. An awareness of this relationship helps nurses to perceive that their role is broadly concerned with health maintenance as well as being disease orientated. Roper et al's portrayal of an uncomplicated view of nursing is a deliberate attempt to provide a flexible framework which can be applied across settings. The stated purpose of this model is to equip practitioners with a means to plan and deliver individualised care. This refers mainly to nurse-initiated activity, but acknowledges the contribution of other members of the health care team. The model also offers a method of thinking about the beliefs, aims and practice of nursing in general terms.

The RLT model for nursing comprises the following five components:

- the activities of living (ALs)
- life span
- the dependence/independence continuum
- factors influencing the ALs
- individualising nursing.

These will now be considered in turn with reference to the care of adults with chronic illness.

Activities of living Roper et al (2000) identified 12 activities of living as follows:

- maintaining a safe environment
- communicating
- breathing
- eating and drinking
- eliminating
- personal cleansing and dressing
- controlling body temperature
- mobilising
- working and playing
- expressing sexuality
- sleeping
- dying.

Living can be described as a fusion of the ALs, and which individuals experience and carry out differently (Holland et al 2003). Although the ALs present a framework for assessment when applying the model to practice, there is a danger that some nurses may use it simply as a 12-point checklist to guide this and subsequent aspects of care. The model's other dimensions may be overlooked as a result (Price 1991) and this would both restrict its usefulness and yield a limited understanding of the needs of patients and their families.

The focus of nursing intervention in this model is on assisting individuals in the prevention, resolution and management of problems identified in relation to the ALs. Problems are defined as actual or potential, as nurses are concerned not only with problems which actually exist but also with preventing the development of others.

The performance of any of the ALs requires the co-ordination of a complex pattern of behaviour. The ability to communicate, for example, relies on a number of skills, including the reception and interpretation of information and the formulation and transmission of appropriate verbal and non-verbal responses. This is influenced by many variables, such as the efficiency of physiological and psychological functions. There is thus considerable scope for errors to occur and it is likely that people with chronic illness will experience a wide range of associated problems. For instance, some individuals may not understand or express ideas verbally following a stroke, while others find no difficulty in this area but are unable to articulate words clearly (see Ch. 9). In either case, individuals will be limited in their ability to make their thoughts and feelings known and this will cause frustration for all concerned.

Speech deterioration also takes place in, for example, Parkinson's disease (see Ch. 9). In this condition, communication may be further inhibited by memory impairment and loss of facial expression. The latter provides the listener with poor feedback and results in the absence of important non-verbal cues. Alteration in physical appearance can also present a barrier to communication. People may be embarrassed when they encounter disfigurement and avoid casual social contact with someone whose appearance disturbs them. In addition, they may make unfair assumptions about the individual's mental state. Wheelchair users often comment that people tend to speak over their heads to anyone who happens to be accompanying them, even when it would be more appropriate for them to be addressed directly.

It is common for people with chronic illness to find that disruption in the performance of one AL leads to difficulty in the performance of others. For instance, someone who has COPD and experiences shortness of breath may discover that their capacity to walk, eat and drink, communicate and attend to personal hygiene is also compromised. The restriction in mobility associated with arthritis can also interfere with the performance of workplace, domestic and recreational activities. For example, the purchase of food can prove problematic due to an inability to carry shopping, and the preparation of meals may be made difficult by reduced physical dexterity.

Life span This component of the model represents the passage through life from conception to death. The progression along the life span is marked by continual change as the individual moves through a series of developmental stages, each of which is associated with the expression of different levels of physical, cognitive and social function. As mentioned previously, adulthood is a period generally characterised by self-reliance which centres around occupational and family interests. There is, of course, great diversity in the lifestyle and behaviour exhibited by individuals during this life stage. Chronological age does not give the nurse sufficient information to appreciate the likely impact of chronic illness. Rather, the nurse will need to gain an understanding of the developmental tasks which the individual has already achieved, those aspired to and the value placed on them by the individual and by those close to them.

Obtaining this kind of information would reveal the existence of actual or potential problems requiring nursing intervention. For example, a woman who has multiple sclerosis (MS) and wishes to become pregnant, may have to confront issues such as sexual dysfunction, the impact of discontinuing disease-modifying or other medication due to her pregnancy, and whether her functional impairment would present difficulties in meeting the needs of an infant. Once the nurse recognises this as a source of emotional distress it can be accounted for in the care planning process; for example, the woman's need for accurate, evidence-based information may be met by referral to an MS specialist nurse (Watkiss & Ward 2002).

The dependence/independence continuum This component acts as a reminder that individuals are not always able to perform each of the ALs independently (Holland et al 2003). Some people have yet to acquire the necessary skills or do not have the means to develop them, whilst others lose abilities which they once had, possibly as a result of illness or trauma.

No single measure reflects the capacity for independent function in all ALs, since it can be argued that few, if any, people are truly self-sufficient. In addition, the concepts of dependence and independence have meaning only when considered in relation to each other. For these reasons, any form of assessment will have a subjective bias which is determined by the nurse's interpretation of each individual's abilities in comparison with clinical, developmental and social norms (Newton 1991). For example, assumptions about the inevitability of universal deterioration with age and chronic illness need to be questioned. Health professionals must not fall into the trap of labelling or stereotyping older people. Take, for example, the case of a practice nurse performing an 'over 75 years' assessment of a frail woman who has chronic arthritis. Prior to the patient's arrival, the nurse assumed the encounter would focus on support and services for health needs. To her astonishment she found herself discussing the Open University's services for disabled students; her client was planning to gain a degree!

The interactive nature of the ALs was mentioned earlier with reference to the way difficulty in carrying out one activity can affect adversely the performance of others. This has implications for the maintenance of independent action in chronic illness. In recognition of this, it is essential that attention is paid to each of the ALs when assessing a patient's dependence/independence status.

Factors influencing the activities of living Individual differences can be identified in the way in which the ALs are performed, regardless of the point reached in the life span or the level of dependence held. Knowledge of five influential factors assists nurses in taking an holistic view of a patient's situation:

- biological
- psychological — incorporating intellectual and emotional factors
- sociocultural — incorporating spiritual, religious and ethical factors
- environmental
- politico-economic — incorporating legal factors.

These factors, acting singly or in combination, influence each of the ALs to some degree. It is not always easy to distinguish the influence of one group of factors from that of another since they are interrelated and share several areas of concern.

Consideration of these factors during assessment provides the basis for a deeper understanding of the cause of difficulties experienced by individuals as well as indicating likely outcomes. This has particular relevance for people with chronic illnesses given the timescales involved, the multiple effects of these disorders and the cycle of deterioration associated with them. For example, knowledge of normal anatomical structure and physiological function enables the nurse to appreciate the effects of disease processes. This is useful both in guiding immediate action to alleviate existing problems and in devising care to prevent the onset of anticipated complications. An exploration of psychological status will reveal what the individual comprehends about the condition. The capacity and motivation to acquire further information and develop the skills necessary for self-management can also be identified.

The behaviour exhibited in everyday life in relation to the promotion of health and the management of chronic illness has strong social and cultural determinants. The nurse should attempt to understand how the condition has affected the individual's accustomed roles and in what respect this has influenced relationships with others. A male manual worker who has disabling back pain, for instance, may perceive that his role as head of the family group is threatened when he is no longer able to continue employment and requires help from his partner to perform basic living activities.

Environmental factors such as noise, climate and atmospheric pollution can affect the performance of each of the ALs in protracted illness. People with COPD experience worsening of their symptoms during periods of poor air quality and find it difficult to obtain adequate sleep if their home is located in a noisy neighbourhood. The structure and layout of buildings in which activities are performed are also of relevance here. Someone who suffers from arthritis and lives in a top-floor flat without a lift may not be able to negotiate the stairs easily in order to leave the building. This would further reduce their mobility, limiting opportunities for social interaction and activities such as shopping for clothes and food. Access to health centres can be made difficult if they are sited at some distance from available public transport or situated on a steep incline. This may deter individuals from attending appointments and result in inadequate monitoring of treatment regimens and a lack of attention to some features of their illness. Admission to hospital is a source of anxiety to people for whom the environment is unfamiliar. The distance between facilities and the need to share bathing and sleeping accommodation may interfere with the individual's routine performance of a number of ALs.

The organisation of all public services is subject to political and economic influences. These factors therefore have a significant effect on the manner in which people conduct their daily lives. Despite the high direct and indirect costs of chronic illness (see p. 1081), it is not always given priority in resource allocation. This has implications for staffing levels and the provision of equipment, and hence for the level of support patients are offered as they strive to attain optimum functioning and independence. Poor resourcing has additional implications for individual lifestyles. If a chair of a suitable height cannot be obtained for someone who has arthritis, resulting in an inability to rise to a standing position, it will not be possible for the individual to exercise or get to the toilet independently.

Individualising nursing As noted previously, the way each person carries out the ALs is unique. Such individuality arises from the complex interaction between the components described above and is apparent in the frequency, location and timing of activities, rationale for the use of particular practices, and the knowledge, beliefs and attitudes of the person concerned. An appreciation of this provides the foundation for individualised nursing. The process of nursing is used as a vehicle to translate Roper et al's theory into practice and to systematise the delivery of care (Holland et al 2003).

APPLYING THE ROPER–LOGAN–TIERNEY MODEL USING THE NURSING PROCESS

Assessment

This stage of the nursing process is a dynamic and ongoing activity, rather than a single event associated with the first encounter between nurse and patient. In protracted illness, an initial assessment is important because it presents a structured method of data collection which will create a total picture of the individual and thus provide a baseline against which change can be measured (see Case History 32.5). It must be acknowledged, however, that in ongoing illness circumstances are seldom static and therefore continued assessment is essential.

Collection of data pertaining to biography, health and the ALs is needed to ensure nursing needs are assessed effectively. It is likely that these elements will be closely related in chronic illness; for example, the perception of the individual's health status which the individual and the carers have can shape the performance of some ALs. Efforts should therefore be made to obtain a comprehensive assessment at any stage of the nurse–patient relationship.

A number of issues warrant attention during the assessment of chronically ill people, regardless of the setting concerned. Some are related directly to the disease process and include the type and duration of the presenting condition, methods already used for managing symptoms and the extent to which strategies have been developed to cope with the uncertainty generated. Details of the treatment regimen should also be collected to help the nurse ascertain how the individual deals with incorporating this into daily life.

Review of biographical data provides an opportunity for nurses to explore the individual's previous lifestyle and to appreciate the changes imposed by long-term illness in this context. The impact of these changes should be reviewed with reference to the ALs while the other components of the model are borne in mind. It is suggested that all the activities should be considered so that for each individual their specific relevance can be established and relationships between them identified. For example, some people may be concerned that their condition hastens the prospect of dying, while others may instead express profound grief at the loss of social function which has resulted from the gradual relinquishment of personal and occupational roles.

The Roper, Logan and Tierney model (2000) prompts nurses to pay attention to the individual's abilities as well as disabilities in carrying out the ALs through reference to the dependence/independence continuum. Any equipment used to assist independence can be identified and the involvement of support services and carers can be explored. This part of the assessment may well help to determine whether the individual has a realistic idea of personal abilities.

Although much of the data required for assessment may be obtained from the patient, other sources of information must not be ignored. The views of both formal and informal carers should be elicited to build up a more detailed impression of behaviour and events. For example, when a man with motor neurone disease (MND) is admitted to hospital for respite care, a community nurse might communicate an observation that during recent months there has been a marked deterioration in the relationship between

CASE HISTORY 32.5

H

H is a 19-year-old nursing student who was diagnosed in early adolescence as having epilepsy. Since leaving home to take up his studies, H has become more acutely aware that he is in some way 'different' from other people. Although realising the importance of informing teaching and placement staff of his condition, should any seizures occur whilst he is working with equipment or patients, H feels as if he is introducing himself as an epileptic first and an individual second. He believes that people are more likely to remember him by his diagnosis rather than his personal qualities.

H's epilepsy had been well controlled by prescribed medication but recently he has become tired, vague and forgetful. He has experienced seizures in the student residences and in the hospital canteen and feels angry that he seems to be losing control of himself.

Although H's medication was changed following a visit to the outpatient department, the seizures have continued. Their onset is unpredictable and H finds that he is increasingly anxious about the uncertainty of his situation. He spends much of his time wondering when the next seizure will occur. He has not taken sick leave because he fears that this would detract from his image, which he considers to be already tarnished by his condition.

H has stopped riding his bicycle and limits his excursions to journeys within a small radius of the hospital campus. His friends do not seem to understand this change in behaviour. H had always been the first to suggest visits to the pubs and clubs in the city centre. They respond by going out without him and suggest that he is taking himself too seriously. H feels isolated and is annoyed by having to think before doing anything.

When he next visits the outpatient department H's unstable condition results in admission to hospital for monitoring of his seizures. U, H's allocated nurse, finds him to be aggressive during her initial assessment. As they talk, H tells her that he has always made every effort to take his medication at prescribed intervals and yet his difficulties persist. He thought that he had recognised the problems his current situation presents for his safety and had adjusted his activities accordingly. He now feels as though he were somehow being punished for this. H considers that he has done everything in his power to help himself and he expresses resentment towards hospital staff because he believes that they have failed him. H is also concerned that he will not be able to continue to cope with the demands of his studies. His sole ambition is to become a nurse. From what he says, U becomes aware that H has lost confidence and lacks self-esteem. Her assessment reveals that H's condition has more implications for his care than had at first been obvious.

the patient and his partner, although the couple strenuously deny that this has taken place. This could then be interpreted with reference to the features of MND and the key problems associated with this, and accounted for in the plan for care.

Planning

Care is planned to address the actual and potential problems identified in the course of assessment. The priority accorded to each problem depends upon the situation in which the individual is placed, though life-threatening problems assume precedence over those with a less immediate impact. Aside from this, priority setting in chronic illness should always be negotiated by the nurse, patient and main carer. An open discussion is useful in clarifying the meaning of each problem to the individual, determining how problems are related to each other and creating a shared awareness of difficulties. This helps to foster collaborative relationships and enhances the motivation of all concerned.

STOP THINK **32.10** Sometimes a care plan has been well established prior to any nursing involvement at home or in hospital. In Case History 32.5, H had established his, with the previous help of his family. What might the implications of this be for H and his carers when the nurse as a professional carer becomes involved?

The aim of the care plan is to assist the patient in preventing, solving, alleviating or managing problems as far as is possible by using best practice. Goals are set for each actual and potential problem and appropriate activities devised to attain them. In chronic illness it is particularly important that goal-setting is realistic in terms of the individual's capacity to achieve such goals and is consistent with personal values and priorities. Both short- and long-term goals can be specified. However, given the instability of chronic illness, the selection of broad objectives for eventual achievement, such as acceptance of the condition and total self-management, might be inappropriate. It is preferable to simplify these by dividing them into a series of short-term goals so that progress can be achieved. This provides patients with a stimulus and sense of purpose (Holland et al 2003). Goals must also be expressed in measurable terms so that their attainment is obvious to patient and carer.

Care plans should describe prescribed nursing interventions and patient participation in detail. This offers a means of ensuring continuity of care and is of particular value in chronic illness; for example, it can help to prevent confusion when an individual is learning to develop a routine for renal dialysis in a domestic setting. It also articulates nursing's contribution to interdisciplinary planning, for instance with reference to integrated care pathways.

Implementation

The actions proposed in the care plan are realised in this phase of the nursing process. It is tempting to believe that the majority of nurses will experience little difficulty in this area because they are familiar with the idea of carrying out practical activities. While there may be some truth in this assumption, there is a tendency for ease of performance to conceal the depth of knowledge and the complex array of skills needed to meet the needs of chronically ill people effectively.

The delivery of care in relation to the ALs should be consistent with the way in which individuals usually behave, whether or not they normally require assistance. As in Orem's (2001) model, this may require the nurse to act for the patient, to supplement and develop the person's self-care capability or to help in the development of an understanding of the promotion of health. In order to determine the emphasis to be placed on each of these activities in a given situation, nurses must be sensitive to the individual's experience of chronic illness in the light of the factors considered in the first part of this chapter, while being aware of the possibilities of their nursing role.

The development of a therapeutic relationship with patients and their carers is a sound basis from which to work. It is important for nurses to gain their patients' trust and to recognise that, under normal circumstances, they have the responsibility for managing their daily lives and features of the disease process. In both hospital and domestic settings, nurses must be mindful of their role in enabling these individuals to retain control of their situation rather than expecting them to conform to alien norms and expectations.

In chronic illness, nursing intervention is far from restricted to the delivery of physical care, although the value of this should not be underestimated. Assisting another person in carrying out any activity, such as washing and dressing, requires more than the ability to reproduce simple practical actions. Nurses need to be prepared to help patients to express their needs and, if necessary, to adopt the role of advocate in liaising with formal and informal carers. The promotion of health and self-care capability requires an understanding of an individual's developmental level as well as of effective teaching techniques. This involves the use of refined communication skills, as does the role of counsellor and supporter to both the patient and the family.

When helping an individual to adapt to the presence of a protracted degenerative disease and the difficulties which this can cause, the nurse should present explanations honestly, yet positively, to foster realistic hope for the future. Non-verbal communication, principally that of touch, can be a helpful way to strengthen a caring relationship, providing this is culturally appropriate. Extending traditional nursing skills in relation to touch has significant benefits for people with chronic illness. The provision of massage, for example, can be of value in assisting them in dealing with stress, enhancing self-worth, achieving palliation and facilitating sympathetic reconnection with a body that has 'let them down' (Vickers 1996).

Evaluation

The effectiveness of nursing interventions can be judged by evaluating whether or not goals have been achieved. This phase of the nursing process lends meaning to those which precede it. The extent to which goals have been achieved should be measured objectively where possible. For example, successful self-management of insulin-dependent diabetes can be demonstrated by HbA1c measurement and a pattern of stability in blood glucose readings (Coates & Boore 1995). It is also possible to identify movement on the dependence/independence continuum in response to teaching programmes or how patients cope with symptoms.

The evaluation of some aspects of care is, however, largely dependent on subjective data. For instance, it is difficult to measure to what extent a patient has adapted to the idea of having a chronic disease. Evaluation in this area could be guided instead by discussion with the individual and interpreting responses in terms of known elements, such as interest in the management of the condition or avoidance of discussion of the illness and its related problems.

The achievement of any goal for care relies on a variety of situational variables. It is therefore sometimes difficult to identify whether or not nursing strategies have been successful. The contribution of staff and material resources, efforts made by carers and the emotional status of the patient can all influence outcome. Nurses should be prepared to recognise that not all interventions they initiate will be effective for each individual, even if they have been used with success on previous occasions. This acts as a stimulus for reassessment, from which revised problem statements and new goals for care can be generated.

The importance of the nurse's own self-evaluation must not be forgotten. Caring for chronically ill people engenders considerable emotional labour for a number of reasons. Nurses sometimes find it difficult to work within the boundaries of their occupational role where over time relationships develop with individuals and their families. They can find it difficult to accept the inevitability of the patient's decline and to have a meaningful role where medicine deems that nothing more can be done (Alabaster 2003). It is also possible that they will identify with the patient, particularly if they occupy the same stage of the life span. Some nurses will be unable to form close protracted relationships with particular patients due to differences in personality, culture and attitude. Individual nurses must recognise that they cannot be all things to all people. Exposure to another's traumatic experience is a source of vicarious stress and the cumulative impact of working with chronic illness adds dimensions to this. Nurses should be supported in developing strategies to manage their own experience of sharing difficult journeys in often restrictive service environments and be offered genuine opportunities for clinical supervision and reflection (Rolfe et al 2001).

CONCLUSION

Nurses encounter people with chronic illnesses in a variety of settings. Effective care requires not only a full understanding of the patient's particular condition, but also a grounding in human and physical sciences so that the experiences of the individual and the family can be interpreted accurately. The nursing role is collaborative in nature and involves the expression of technological, clinical and interpersonal skills. In the long term, emphasis is placed on caring, a concept fundamental to nursing but which has often been overshadowed by other considerations. Working with individuals with chronic illnesses presents nurses with the opportunity to reaffirm their unique contribution to health care.

Finally, it is suggested that a good foundation for the development of an effective nursing role is for the nurse, and indeed the interdisciplinary health care team, to avoid thinking about the individual in need of intervention as a chronically ill person but, rather, as a person who happens to have a chronic illness.

REFERENCES

Age Concern England 2003 Continuing NHS health care, 'free' nursing care and intermediate care, Factsheet 20. Age Concern England, London

Alabaster E S 2003 Same old, same old: an interpretive analysis of nursing students' experiences of working with older people. PhD thesis, University of Wales, Cardiff

Alabaster E S, Allen D, Fothergill A et al 2000 User involvement in user-focused research? Nursing, Health and Social Care Research Centre, University of Wales College of Medicine

Armstrong D 2003 Outline of sociology as applied to medicine, 5th edn. Butterworth-Heinemann, Oxford

Aylett E, Fawcett T N 2003 Chronic fatigue syndrome: the nurse's role. Nursing Standard 17(35): 33–37

Benjamin A E 1997 Home-care politics in the 1990s. In: Fox D M, Raphael C (eds) Home-based care for a new century. Blackwell/Milbank Memorial Fund, Malden, Ch. 3

Biordi D 1998 Social isolation. In: Lubkin I M (ed) Chronic illness: impact and interventions, 4th edn. Jones and Bartlett, Sudbury, Ch. 8

Brandt H M, Rozin P (eds) 1997 Introduction. In: Morality and health. Routledge, London

British Medical Association 2002 BMA response to the interim report of the health trends review. Available online: www.bma.org.uk

Bull M J, Jervis L L 1997 Strategies used by chronically ill older women and their caregiving daughters in managing posthospital care. Journal of Advanced Nursing 25(3): 541–547

Cant S, Sharma U 1999 A new medical pluralism? Alternative medicine, doctors, patients and the state. UCL Press, London

Charlton J 1997 Trends in all-cause mortality: 1841–1994. In: Charlton J, Murphy M (eds) The health of adult Britain 1841–1994 (1). Office for National Statistics. TSO, London, Ch. 3

Coates V E, Boore J R P 1995 Self-management of chronic illness: implications for nursing. International Journal of Nursing Studies 32(6): 628–640

Coles A 2001 Multiple sclerosis. In: Scalding N (ed) Contemporary treatments in neurology. Butterworth-Heinemann, Oxford, Ch. 6

CREST 2003 Executive summary of the report of the Northern Ireland task force on diabetes: a blueprint for diabetes care in Northern Ireland in the 21st century. CREST, Belfast

Crumbie A 2002a Diabetes. In: Crumbie A, Lawrence J (eds) Living with a chronic condition. Butterworth-Heinemann, Oxford, Ch. 6

Crumbie A 2002b Patient–professional relationships. In: Crumbie A, Lawrence J (eds) Living with a chronic condition. Butterworth-Heinemann, Oxford, Ch. 1

Crumbie A, Lawrence J (eds) 2002 Introduction. In: Living with a chronic condition. Butterworth-Heinemann, Oxford

Curtin M, Lubkin I 1998 What is chronicity? In: Lubkin I M (ed) Chronic illness: impact and interventions, 4th edn. Jones and Bartlett, Sudbury, Ch. 1

Daly B J 1993 Managing the hospitalized chronically ill. In: Funk S G, Tornquist E M, Champagne M T, Wiese R A (eds) Key aspects of caring for the chronically ill: hospital and home. Springer, New York, Ch. 3

Department of Health 1990 National Health Service and Community Care Act 1990 (c19). HMSO, London

Department of Health 1997a On the state of the public health 1996. TSO, London
Department of Health 1997b The new NHS: modern, dependable. TSO, London
Department of Health 1998a Modernising social services: national priorities guidance 1999/00–2001/02. TSO, London
Department of Health 1998b Modernising social services: promoting independence, improving protection, raising standards. TSO, London
Department of Health 2001a The expert patient: a new approach to chronic disease management for the 21st century. DH, London
Department of Health 2001b The National Service Framework for diabetes. DH, London
Department of Health 2001c Health and Social Care Act 2001. DH, London
Department of Health 2001d The care home regulations 2001. DH, London
Dickens C, Jackson J, Tomenson B, Hay E, Creed F 2003 Association of depression and rheumatoid arthritis. Psychosomatics 44(3): 209–215
Dimond M, Jones S L 1987 Chronic illness across the life span. Appleton-Century-Crofts, Norwalk, CT
Disability Discrimination Act 1995 HMSO, London
Donaghue P J, Siegel M E 2000 Sick and tired of feeling sick and tired: living with invisible chronic illness, 2nd edn. Norton, New York
Donnelly C A, Ghani A C, Leung G M et al 2003 Epidemiological determinants of spread of causal agent of severe acute respiratory syndrome in Hong Kong. Lancet 361(9371): 1761
Doss C 2002 Quotation. In: 'But you look so good'. National Multiple Sclerosis Society of America. Online. Available: www.nationalmssociety.org/brochures-but%20you%20look.asp
Dunnell K 1997 Are we healthier? In: Charlton J, Murphy M (eds) The health of adult Britain 1841–1994 (2). Office for National Statistics. TSO, London, Ch. 25
Fawcett J 2000 Analysis and evaluation of contemporary nursing knowledge: nursing models and theories. Davis, Philadelphia
Fennell P A 2003 Managing chronic illness using a four-phase treatment approach: a mental health professional's guide to helping chronically ill people. Wiley, New York
Ferner R, Mann R D 2001 Drug safety and pharmacovigilance. In: Page C, Curtis M, Sutter M, Walker M, Hoffman B (eds) Integrated pharmacology, 2nd edn. Mosby, Edinburgh, Ch. 6
Field D, Kelly M P 2003 Chronic illness and physical disability. In: Taylor S, Field D (eds) Sociology of health and health care, 3rd edn. Blackwell, Oxford, Ch. 7
Figley C R, Leventman S (eds) 1990 Strangers at home: Vietnam veterans since the war. Brunner/Mazel, New York
Finkelstein V, Stuart O 1996 Developing new services. In: Hales G (ed) Beyond disability: towards an enabling society. Open University/Sage, London, Ch. 17
Foley F, Sarnoff J 2003 Taming stress in multiple sclerosis. National Multiple Sclerosis Society of America. Online. Available: www.nationalmssociety.org/Brochures-TamingStress1.asp
Freeman H 2002 Should you reveal your health status? The Guardian, April 20th
Galbraith S, McCormick A 1997 Infection in England and Wales 1838–1993. In: Charlton J, Murphy M (eds) The health of adult Britain 1841–1994 (2). Office for National Statistics. TSO, London, Ch. 15
Gast H L 1996 Orem's self-care model. In: Fitzpatrick J J, Whall A L (eds) Conceptual models of nursing: analysis and application, 3rd edn. Appleton and Lange, Stamford, Ch. 7
Goffman E 1963 Stigma. Penguin, Harmondsworth
Greaves D 1996 Concepts of health and disease. In: Greaves D, Upton H (eds) Philosophical problems in health care. Avebury, Aldershot, Ch. 5
Griffiths C, Brock A 2003 Twentieth century mortality rates in England and Wales. Health Statistics Quarterly 18. Office for National Statistics, London
Ham C, Robert G 2003 Reasonable rationing: international experience of priority setting in health care. Open University Press, Buckingham
Harpam W S 1997 When a parent has cancer. Harper Collins, New York
Her Majesty's Stationery Office 1997 Community Care (Direct Payments) Act 1996 (c30). Stationery Office, London. Online. www.opsi.gov.uk/acts/acts1996/1996030.htm
Holland K, Jenkins J, Solomon J, Whittam S 2003 Applying the Roper–Logan–Tierney model in practice. Churchill Livingstone, Edinburgh
Howkins E 1995 Collaborative care: an agreed goal, but a difficult journey. In: Cain P, Hyde V, Howkins E (eds) Community nursing – dimensions and dilemmas. Arnold, London, Ch. 4
Hunter D J 2000 Disease management: has it a future? British Medical Journal 320: 530
Jacklin J 1997 Disability Discrimination Act 1995: an enabling act or a discriminating law? Online. Available: http://freespace.virgin.net/steven.jacklin/ddacont.html
Jarrett L 2003 Attitudes to long-term care in multiple sclerosis. Nursing Standard 17(17): 39–43
Jiwa M 2000 Frequent attenders in general practice: an attempt to reduce attendance. Family Practice 17(3): 248–251
Johnson M 1997 Nursing power and social judgement. Ashgate, Aldershot
Joint Formulary Committee 2003 British national formulary (46). British Medical Association/Royal Pharmaceutical Society of Great Britain, London
Kita M, Goodkin D E 2000 Multiple sclerosis. In: Rakel R E (ed) Conn's current therapy. WB Saunders, Philadelphia
Klein R A, Landau M G 1992 Healing the body betrayed: a self-paced, self-help guide to regaining psychological control of your illness. Chronimed, Minneapolis
Leathard A 2000 Health care provision: past, present and into the twenty-first century, 2nd edn. Stanley Thornes, Cheltenham
LeMaistre J 1996 After the diagnosis. Ulysses Press, Berkeley
Locker D 2003 Living with chronic illness. In: Scambler G (ed) Sociology as applied to medicine, 5th edn. Baillière Tindall, London, Ch. 6
Long-term Care Commission 2003 Long-term care: statement by Royal Commissioners. Online. Available: www.ltc-commissioners.org.uk/4554.html
Mahony C 1997 An act of contrition. Nursing Times 93(30): 18
Marks D 1999 Disability: controversial debates and psychosocial perspectives. Routledge, London
Marriott D 2003 The selfish pig's guide to caring. Polperro Heritage Press, Polperro
McClure L 2001 Family caregivers and community nurses: co-experts in care? In: Hyde V (ed) Community nursing and health care: insights and innovations. Arnold, London, Ch. 5
McWilliam C L, Stewart M, Brown J B et al 1997 Creating empowering meaning: an interactive process of promoting health with chronically ill older Canadians. Health Promotion International 12(2): 111–123
Means R, Richards, S, Smith R 2003 Community care: policy and practice, 3rd edn. Palgrave Macmillan, Basingstoke
Melton L 2004 Aching atrophy. Scientific American 290(1): 15–16
Mishel M H 1993 Living with chronic illness. In: Funk S G, Tornquist E M, Champagne M T, Wiese R A (eds) Key aspects of caring for the chronically ill: hospital and home. Springer, New York, Ch. 6
Montbriand M J, Laing G P 1991 Alternative health care as a control strategy. Journal of Advanced Nursing 16(3): 325–332
MS Society 2003 Risk sharing scheme: how will it work? What's the latest? MS Matters, January–February
National Institute for Clinical Excellence (NICE) 2003 General information on the work of NICE. Online. Available: www.nice.org.uk/cat.asp?c=57703
Nettleton S 1995 The sociology of health and illness. Polity Press, Cambridge
Newton C 1991 The Roper–Logan–Tierney model in action. Macmillan, Basingstoke
Northern Ireland Assembly 2002 Report on the Health and Personal Social Services Bill (NIA Bill 06/01), Session 2001/2002 third report. Committee for Health, Social Services and Public Safety. Online. www.niassembly.gov.uk/health/reports
Office for National Statistics (ONS) 2002 Carers 2000. TSO, London
Office for National Statistics (ONS) 2003a Social trends 33. TSO, London
Office for National Statistics (ONS) 2003b General household survey. TSO, London
Orem D E 2001 Nursing: concepts of practice, 6th edn. Mosby, St Louis
Parsons T 1951 The social system. Routledge and Kegan Paul, London
Pierret J 2003 The illness experience: state of knowledge and perspectives for research. Sociology of Health and Illness 25(3): 4–22
Pinder R 1992 Coherence and incoherence: doctors' and patients' perspectives on the diagnosis of Parkinson's disease. Sociology of Health and Illness 14(1): 1–22
Pitkeathley J 1991 Seen but not heard? Nursing Times 87(42): 22
Pitts M 1996 The psychology of preventive health. Routledge, London

Pressly K B 1995 Psychosocial characteristics of CAPD patients and the occurrence of infectious complications. ANNA Journal 22(6): 563–572
Price B 1991 Preface. In: Newton C (ed) The Roper–Logan–Tierney model in action. Macmillan, Basingstoke
Radley A 1994 Making sense of illness: the social psychology of health and disease. Sage, London
Reid T 1997 Caught in the act. Nursing Times 93(28): 12–13
Rice G P A, Incorvaia B, Munari L, Ebers G, Polman C, D'Amico R, Filippini G 2003 Interferon in relapsing–remitting multiple sclerosis (Cochrane Review). In: The Cochrane Library, Issue 4. Wiley, Chichester
Robinson L 2004 Living with constant surprises. Online. Available: www.nac.org.uk
Rolfe G, Freshwater D, Jasper M 2001 Critical reflection for nursing and the helping professions: a user's guide. Palgrave Macmillan, Basingstoke
Roper N, Logan W, Tierney A J 2000 The Roper, Logan and Tierney model of nursing. Churchill Livingstone, Edinburgh
Rosenberg C 1997 Banishing risk: continuity and change in the moral management of disease. In: Brandt H M, Rozin P (eds) Morality and health. Routledge, London, Ch. 3
Roy C, Andrews H A 1999 The Roy adaptation model, 2nd edn. Appleton and Lange, Stamford
Saylor C, Yoder M 1998 Stigma. In: Lubkin I M (ed) Chronic illness: impact and interventions, 4th edn. Jones and Bartlett, Sudbury, Ch. 5
Scambler G (ed) 2003a Deviance, sick role and stigma. In: Sociology as applied to medicine, 5th edn. Baillière Tindall, London, Ch. 13
Scambler G (ed) 2003b Health and illness behaviour. In: Sociology as applied to medicine, 5th edn. Baillière Tindall, London, Ch. 3
Schaie K W, Willis S L 2001 Adult development and aging, 5th edn. Prentice Hall, Englewood Cliffs, NJ
Scottish Executive 2001a Report of the Chief Nursing Officer for Scotland's group on free nursing care. Scottish Executive, Edinburgh
Scottish Executive 2001b Draft national care standards: services for adults. Online. Available: www.scotland.gov.uk/library3/social/dncsa-00.asp
Scottish Executive Health Department 2002 Scottish diabetes framework. Scottish Executive Health Department, Edinburgh
Smaje C 1995 Health, 'race' and ethnicity: making sense of the evidence. King's Fund Institute, London
Spinney L 2003 Lying with intent. The Guardian, May 29th. Online. Available: www.guardian.co.uk/life/feature/story/0,13026,965634,00.html
Stockwell F 1972 The unpopular patient. Royal College of Nursing, London
Strauss A L, Corbin J, Fagerhaugh S, Glaser B G, Maines D, Suczek B, Weiner C L 1984 Chronic illness and the quality of life. Mosby, St Louis
Sweetman S C (ed) 2002 Martindale: the complete drug reference, 33rd edn. Pharmaceutical Press, London
Swerdlow A, dos Santos Silva I, Doll R 2001 Cancer incidence and mortality in England and Wales: trends and risk factors. Oxford University Press, Oxford
Taylor S E 1995 Health psychology, 3rd edn. McGraw-Hill, New York
Vickers A 1996 Massage and aromatherapy: a guide for health professionals. Chapman and Hall, London
Ward L 2002 Clinical governance. In: Crumbie A, Lawrence J (eds) Living with a chronic condition: a practitioner's guide to providing care. Butterworth-Heinemann, Oxford, Ch. 3
Watkins A D 1996 Contemporary context of complementary and alternative medicine: integrated mind–body medicine. In: Micozzi M S (ed) Fundamentals of complementary and alternative medicine. Churchill Livingstone, Edinburgh, Ch. 4
Watkiss K, Ward N 2002 Multiple sclerosis: pregnancy and parenthood. Nursing Standard 17(3): 45–53
Weiner H L, Olek M J, Hohol M J, Khoury S J, Dawson D M, Hafler D A 1997 Rational therapy in multiple sclerosis. In: Russell W C (ed) Molecular biology of multiple sclerosis. Wiley, Chichester, Ch. 17
Welsh Assembly Government 2002 Diabetes NSF standards (Wales). Welsh Assembly Government, Cardiff
Welsh Assembly Government 2003 A guide to NHS funded nursing care in care homes: updated draft guidance November 2003. Welsh Assembly Government, Cardiff
Welsh Assembly Government 2004 National minimum standards for care homes for older people (revised March 2004). Welsh Assembly Government, Cardiff
Wilson A 2002 A rehabilitation framework for patient-focused care. Nursing Standard 16(50): 38–44
World Health Organization 2003 Communicable disease surveillance and response (CSR): update – severe acute respiratory syndrome (SARS). Online. Available: www.who.int/csr/sars/archive/2003_03_16/en/

FURTHER READING

Brykczynska G (ed) 1997 Caring: the compassion and wisdom of nursing. Arnold, London
Carers UK 2002 Without us…? Calculating the value of carers' support. Carers UK, London
Charlton A, While D, Kelly S 1997 Boys' smoking and cigarette-brand-sponsored motor racing. Lancet 350(9089): 1474
Ewles L, Simnett I 2003 Promoting health: a practical guide, 5th edn. Baillière Tindall, London
Hinsliff G 2004 Doctors told Nadia to let her child die. The Observer, January 4th
Jasper M 2003 Beginning reflective practice: foundations in nursing and health care. Nelson Thornes, Cheltenham
Livneh H, Antonrak R F 1997 Psychosocial adaptation to chronic illness and disability. Aspen, Gaithersburg
MacFadyen L, Hastings G, MacKintosh A M 2001 Cross sectional study of young people's awareness of and involvement with tobacco marketing. British Medical Journal 322: 513–517
Multiple Sclerosis Trust/Royal College of Nursing 2003 Competencies for MS specialist nurses. Multiple Sclerosis Trust, Letchworth; RCN, London
Snyder M, Lindquist R 2002 Complementary/alternative therapies in nursing, 4th edn. Springer, New York
Thompson I E, Melia K M, Boyd K M 2000 Nursing ethics, 4th edn. Churchill Livingstone, Edinburgh
Thorne S E, Nyhlin K T, Paterson B L 2000 Attitudes towards patient expertise in chronic illness. International Journal of Nursing Studies 37(4): 303–311
UK Multiple Sclerosis Specialist Nurse Association, Royal College of Nursing, MS Research Trust 2003 Specialist nursing in MS – the way forward: the key elements to developing an MS specialist nurse service. Multiple Sclerosis (Research) Charitable Trust, Letchworth; Royal College of Nursing, London

USEFUL WEBSITES

British Council of Disabled People
www.bcodp.org.uk

Carers UK with the Worshipful Company of Information Technologists (WCIT) and the Invest to Save partnership
www/carersonline.org.uk

Department of Health National Service Framework
www.dh.gov.uk/Policy And Guidance/Health And Social Care Topics

Invisible Disabilities Advocate
www.myida.org/ida.htm

US National Center for Chronic Disease Prevention and Health Promotion
www.cdc.gov/nccdphp/index.htm

Website offering a variety of personal experiences of health and illness
www/dipex.org

World Health Organization
www.who.int/health_topics/chronic_disease/en/

THE PATIENT RECEIVING PALLIATIVE CARE

33

Helen A. S. Dougan
Margaret M. Colquhoun

INTRODUCTION

Palliative care is the term given to the approach adopted when cure is unlikely and it is expected that the patient will die in the foreseeable future. People of all ages die, in a range of settings — at home, in hospitals, in nursing homes and in hospices. They die of many different diseases. Some die suddenly and some die slowly. Palliative care has been developed to help those who are dying slowly or, as is often said, living with dying. Led by the hospice pioneers, this approach to care has a recent and inspiring history (Gamlin 2001, Davies & Seymour 2002, Doyle et al 2004).

Many reasons have been given as to why this specialty developed quickly and comprehensively in the UK in the late 20th century. Among the most notable are:

- the improvements in medical care, which have lengthened the time from diagnosis to death
- the promotion of honesty and openness between doctor, patient and family regarding a life-threatening diagnosis and prognosis
- the intolerance of the physical and mental suffering witnessed by those caring for patients with cancer.

The World Health Organization (WHO) provides a useful definition of palliative care (Sepulveda et al 2002):

> *Palliative care is an approach that improves the quality of life of patients and their families facing the problems associated with life-threatening illness, through the prevention of suffering by means of early identification and impeccable assessment and treatment of pain and other problems, physical, psychological and spiritual.*

The need to apply evidence-based knowledge to the care of people dying from diseases other than cancer has long been recognised. This important area of development in palliative care is detailed in a number of publications (Addington-Hall & Higginson 2001, Hockley & Clark 2002, Doyle et al 2004).

At its best, palliative care is teamwork where the patient and family are part of the interdisciplinary team. The care is individual, sensitive, non-judgemental, detailed and time-consuming. Patients and their families are met where they are, i.e. the health professional should have no preconceived ideas about them; there is no such being as a typical dying patient. It is a style of care in which the successful outcome has been redefined to mean a good death — a death that meets the expectations of the patient first and foremost, but also those of the family, close friends and the health professionals.

Delivering good palliative nursing care requires knowledge and a wide range of skills and it draws on life experience, self-awareness and motivation. It requires the nurse to understand and respect the roles of all the interdisciplinary team members and to work together with them to achieve a comprehensive and consistent approach to care. It is a daily challenge, which can be harrowing and stressful; however, the ultimate reward of facilitating a good death is very satisfying and worth striving for.

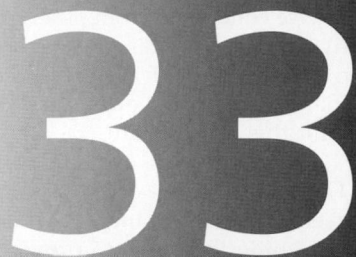

In the UK and many other countries, specialist palliative care nurses, sometimes known as Macmillan nurses, and specialist palliative care teams are well established in the community, in some hospitals and in the hospices. These specialists provide expertise for patients and families with problems that are difficult to manage. They frequently advise colleagues from other areas of health care. The palliative approach to care, however, is the right of all patients, no matter what their diagnosis, lifestyle or age. It is essential, therefore, that all nurses develop knowledge and skills to offer this style of care.

In this chapter, a model for palliative care is presented. The model is flexible in that it can be adapted to suit each individual and their circumstances, and therefore can guide the nurse to provide person-centred and family-centred care. The style of record keeping used within a health care setting is often very personal to the interdisciplinary team; it may have been designed or adapted to their satisfaction. Therefore, the suggested model does not have a set written format; it may be used along with the established documentation.

The text has been structured by applying the model to the case studies of three patients. The first patient's care is used to outline the application of the model without exploring the necessary detailed knowledge required to implement the care. In contrast, the care of the second and third patients is given in more detail. Issues of communication, psychological theory, pathophysiology and symptom control are discussed, illustrating the application of theory to practice. A nurse's formal reflection, using the reflective cycle described by Gibbs (1988), is presented in relation to Case Study 2 (see Box 33.3, p. 1109).

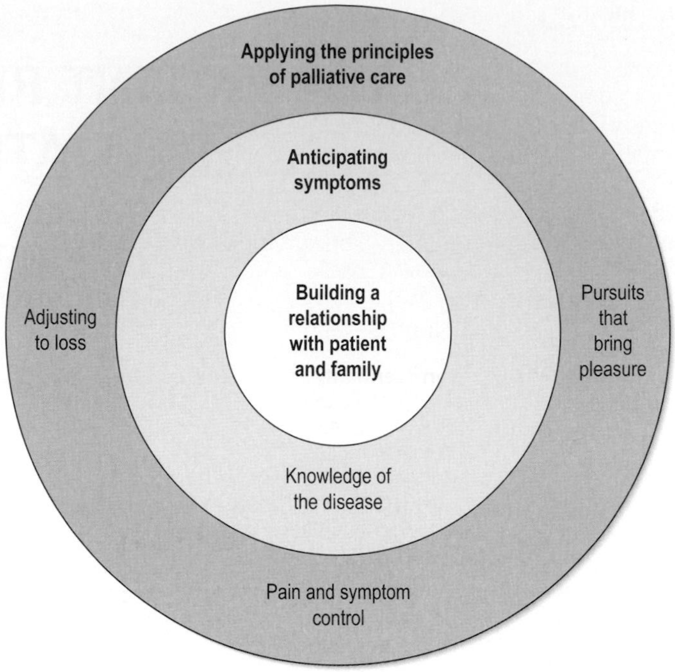

Fig. 33.1 A model for palliative care.

A MODEL FOR PALLIATIVE CARE

In the busy world of health care, the sheer volume of information available to the nurse in relation to palliative care could be overwhelming. This is not a narrow specialty where the range of in-depth knowledge and specific skills is limited to a particular organ and its pathology. The knowledge base for palliative nursing care is necessarily broad and derived from many disciplines. The very diversity of the population who may benefit from palliative care demands a structured model which, although fixed in its parts, is totally flexible in its content.

The model in Figure 33.1 is presented as a guide for the clinical nurse in the early 21st century. This nurse, in the climate of continuous lifelong learning, is envisaged as a critical thinker, i.e. one who challenges assumptions and looks for creative and workable solutions to problems, who critically reads literature and appraises research and, in partnership with the interdisciplinary team, implements reflective, evidence-based practice.

The three salient features of the model are presented. The order of their application should be interchangeable depending on individual circumstances. They are:

- *Building a relationship* with the patient and family to explore their experience with the life-threatening illness and to become informed as to their functioning, i.e. their roles, bonds and coping strategies, as well as to ascertain their needs, priorities and wishes
- *Anticipating the symptoms* that may occur by using knowledge of pathophysiology and disease management
- *Applying the principles* of palliative care:
  — employing good control of symptoms
  — facilitating adjustment to losses and changes in lifestyle, for both patient and family
  — providing support to carry out pursuits that give pleasure for as long as possible.

Central to the model is the quality of life of the patient and family. When a patient requires palliative care, immediate problems are often overwhelming physical suffering, such as pain or nausea and vomiting. It is essential that these problems are tackled and the symptoms reduced before exploring the patient's psychosocial concerns.

Before embarking on the case studies, each aspect of the model will be considered in more detail.

Building a relationship and developing a profile

Communication is an essential feature of palliative care. This includes verbal, non-verbal and written communication with the patient and family and within the interdisciplinary team. Particular emphasis is therefore placed on this aspect of the model at the outset.

When it is recognised that the intention of a patient's care has become palliative, this often means subjecting the person to information-seeking interviews. However, one of the most commonly reported problems in the last few months of life is fatigue (Sweeney et al 2004), and patients often complain that too many people ask them the same questions (Faulkner 1998). Therefore, effective communication within the team must be developed to protect these tired, frail patients, without compromising opportunities for them to share their fears, problems and concerns (Kinghorn 2001).

Combined interdisciplinary written documentation in the form of patients' notes is being adopted by many teams.

In addition, interdisciplinary team meetings are being held regularly at which the many different facets of patient and family problems may be discussed and shared goals set.

Patients and families need to feel secure that confidentiality will be maintained concerning matters revealed to the health care team. It is often believed that patients realise that they are being cared for by a team of staff and that they therefore implicitly agree that information given to one may be shared within the team. This should not be assumed. It is useful at times to remind patients and families that information is shared within the team and to emphasise that they do not have to talk about areas they prefer to keep private.

The ethics of confidentiality are beyond the scope of this text; readers wishing to explore this important area in more detail may refer to Randall & Downie (1999).

To implement the model, a great deal of information needs to be gathered in relation to the patient and the family. This section gives an example of a named nurse building a relationship and developing a profile.

Before embarking on an interview with the patient, the named nurse should ascertain what information is required, recognising that the patient profile will very likely be added to throughout the illness. The patient's notes should be read, as they may contain a great deal of the required information regarding diagnosis, treatment and other problems. However, it is wise to remember that the problems as perceived by the referring doctor or nurse, or the team currently caring for the patient, may be different from those causing the greatest concern to the patient (Heaven 1995, Davy & Ellis 2000). Communication with other members of the team may reveal that another interview is planned on the same day, and the team members may agree to sit down with the patient together. If not, one of the interviews should be postponed until the following day to prevent overtiring the patient.

An ideal situation for an assessment interview will be one in which privacy is provided without interruption. The nurse will give good eye contact, display warmth and respect, and the patient's physical comfort will be attended to. Skilful questioning will be utilised and blocking behaviour curbed. Many authors discuss sound communication and counselling skills (Faulkner 1998, Davy & Ellis 2000, Stein-Parbury 2000, Kinghorn 2001).

The patient should be engaged in a conversational interview (Brown 1995) by being encouraged to talk about their main current problems. It is then useful to enquire about how each problem affects the patient's life and about their expectations of getting help with these problems, i.e. what are the patient's goals? Should the patient concentrate on physical concerns, it is useful to indicate that feelings are also important. From this conversation, the named nurse should be able to appraise the patient's understanding of their illness (Heaven 1995, Kinghorn 2001). The patient may become tired or distressed during the interview, in which case the nurse must enquire if the patient wishes to stop. The distressed patient should not be abandoned. A cup of tea might be appreciated and the mood lightened by moving the conversation away from the difficult topic.

The framework in Box 33.1 is suggested as a means of helping the patient to communicate fully about specific physical or emotional problems (Heaven 1995).

Box 33.1

Assessing a specific problem

To assess a problem fully, be it physical or emotional, it is useful to structure your questions using the following framework:

- Nature — what is it like?
- Location (for a physical problem) — Show me where you get it
- Severity — what is it like at its worst?
- Frequency — how often do you get this?
- Duration — how long does it last?
- Triggers — what starts it up? what makes it worse?
- Alleviating factors — what helps?
- Impact on life — how does this affect your day-to-day life?
- Impact on feelings — how does this affect how you are feeling in yourself?

Adapted from Heaven (1995).

Having given the patient the opportunity to discuss their concerns, it is useful to move on to include the family. A family tree or genogram is a good method for gathering information in a form that is easily shared within the team (see Fig. 33.2). Compiling the genogram may encourage the

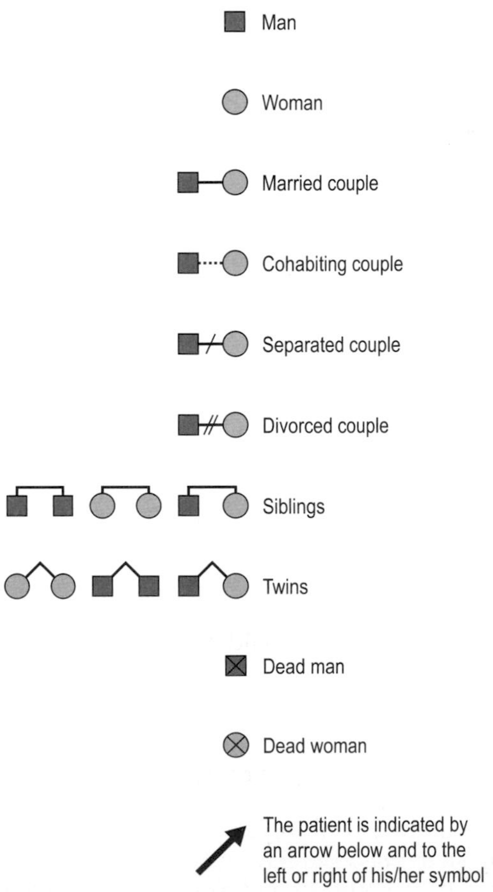

Fig. 33.2 A genogram is a code for recording a family, using the symbols shown. (Adapted from McGoldrick & Gerson 1985.)

patient to talk about roles, relationships and personalities and to identify issues of concern. In addition, it demonstrates an interest in the patient's family, thus reinforcing the principle that family support is an integral part of palliative care (Murray Parkes et al 1996, Davy & Ellis 2000).

Following the interview, the named nurse will clearly and succinctly document the information and communicate any immediate issues to the appropriate team member.

Anticipating symptoms

Consideration now needs to be given to the nature of the life-threatening illness and any other existing medical problems from which the patient may suffer. For example, if caring for a person with cancer, the named nurse needs to know how that disease may spread (see Ch. 31). If the person has AIDS, it will be important to have an understanding of opportunistic infections or HIV-related malignancies that may occur (see Ch. 37). Complications of advanced disease can often be anticipated and, in some cases, effective management instigated. This can result in an improved quality of life for the patient and is therefore an important aspect of good palliative care. The named nurse may wish to update knowledge of the specific disease process; the chapters in the first section of this book are a rich source of relevant information.

The named nurse is now in a position to prepare a summary of the patient's main problems, expectations and priorities and of the patient's understanding of the illness and the problems that may occur.

Applying the principles of palliative care

Once the named nurse has developed a profile and identified the actual and potential problems that the patient may have, a plan of care can be devised. This will be done with the patient, the family and the interdisciplinary team. In the plan, the principles of palliative care will be applied.

Pain and symptom control

The key components of good symptom control in palliative care are well described (Twycross & Wilcock 2001, Faull & Woof 2002, Regnard & Hockley 2004). In summary, the interdisciplinary team must work with the patient to:

- make a thorough assessment of each symptom
- discuss causes and treatment options
- plan symptom management in the light of the patient's expectations and priorities.

Attention to detail is also important, as is continuous review of the situation, because of the progressive nature of disease. All of this must be underpinned by an understanding of the pathophysiology of the symptom.

Facilitating adjustment

Making the adjustment from thinking of oneself as a relatively healthy person who will die someday in the future, to thinking of oneself as an ill person who is dying right now, is a very big step. Theorists have described the potential emotions and behaviours of people in this situation (Barraclough 1999, Houldin 2000). Many variables influence the responses of the dying patient and the family, the most notable being personal characteristics, level of social support, past experience of illness and death, age, culture, religious belief and the characteristics specific to the illness.

Loss is an abiding feature in the life of a person who is dying — loss of future, loss of role, loss of independence. This period in the palliative care patient's life has been compared to bereavement. Many of these patients perceive that those who are dying are shunned by health professionals because they cannot be cured. The nurse caring for the dying person needs to be acutely aware of this and must demonstrate the importance of the individual by displaying interest and respect, e.g. by consulting the patient about needs, wants and priorities and thereby helping to maintain self-esteem.

It has been suggested that a useful starting point for understanding an individual's response to a life-threatening illness is to consider the question: 'What does this illness mean to this person?' (Barraclough 1999).

Supporting pursuits that give pleasure

Supporting the patient in carrying out pursuits that bring pleasure plays a vital part in maintaining hope and improving quality of life (Houldin 2000, Chaplin & McIntyre 2001). This might be anything, from moving a patient's bed out into the hospice garden to enjoy the summer sunshine, to enabling a very frail patient to attend the performance of a much loved play. The named nurse in palliative care needs actively to seek these opportunities.

Case Study 1 will briefly illustrate the model.

CASE STUDY 1 — MRS A

Building a relationship, developing a profile and anticipating symptoms

Mrs A was admitted to the community hospital the previous day. She was admitted by her general practitioner (GP) because of pain and rectal bleeding. The named nurse spends time building a relationship and developing a profile of the patient and her family:

- *Main problems* — the patient identifies these as a foul rectal discharge with some bleeding, pain at times in her perineal area and a sensation of wanting to empty her bowels continuously (tenesmus). In addition, her husband, who has suffered a stroke, is already in the same hospital.
- *Expectations* — Mrs A is pleased to be in the hospital — 'my husband is so well looked after, and I am so tired and weary'. She does not expect that the smell will go away but she is sure the staff will not let her suffer.
- *Priorities* — the things that are most important to her are seeing her family, her faith, playing the piano, and having her clothes on during the day.
- *Understanding of illness* — Mrs A speaks openly about her cancer. She admits that she put off going to the doctor because of caring for her husband. When she was told her diagnosis, it was a relief to have it out in the open. It was a shock for the family and she is still trying to help them to come to terms with it, especially her eldest daughter.
- *Anticipated symptoms* — because of her diagnosis of advanced rectal cancer, her main anticipated problems

are pain, difficulty with defaecation, possible development of fistulae between the bowel, bladder and the vagina and a small risk of catastrophic rectal haemorrhage.

Having obtained this information, the named nurse will liaise with the other members of the interdisciplinary team, in particular the family doctor, who will have completed a medical examination. A care plan will then be written. Towards the end of life, a patient's condition may change rapidly, and therefore the care plan should be reviewed daily and updated promptly.

Applying the principles of palliative care

The care plan for Mrs A, structured by the three principles of palliative care, will include the following.

Pain and symptom management

- Stop the prescribed co-codamol 30/500 and commence 4-hourly oral morphine (normal release formulation) to enable titration of the optimum daily dose of morphine required to control perineal pain, plus commence paracetamol 6-hourly. Also, begin amitriptyline as an adjuvant analgesic for the tenesmus. For a detailed discussion of pain management, see pages 1103–1105.
- Continue the prescribed combined softening and stimulant oral laxative, co-danthramer.
- Ensure that emergency drugs have been prescribed, to be given in case of a catastrophic haemorrhage.
- Offer a daily bath to soothe the perineal area.
- Install air freshening unit in her room.

Adjustment to loss and change

- Ensure that openings are given to Mrs A to talk about her feelings should she so wish. Mrs A has requested some time with her priest and this has been organised for today. A family meeting has been arranged for Friday at 15.00 h.
- Make it possible for the family to spend time together in privacy.

Pursuits that give pleasure

- Put arrangements in place for Mrs A to play the piano in the sitting room in the late afternoon; she may wish her visitors to accompany her.
- Ensure that the timing of help with personal hygiene does not prevent Mrs A going to the Sunday service in the chapel.

To demonstrate its flexibility, the model will now be applied more fully to two further case studies. The detailed content will include evidence-based theory and practice, providing a transferable body of knowledge as a basis for palliative nursing care practice in hospital, hospice, home or nursing home.

CASE STUDY 2 — MS M

Day 1 Ms M is a 39-year-old mother and company director who is separated from her husband. She has advanced breast cancer with metastases to bone, liver and brain. Ms M has been admitted to the hospice at her own request, having had a short admission 6 months previously for pain management. The referral from the GP requested admission for escalating pain, nausea and vomiting, and general deterioration in her condition.

On admission, Ms M is very pale and quiet. She is accompanied by her mother who looks distressed. Neither of them appears to recognise S, the named nurse who cared for them on the previous admission. Quietly and without speaking much, S, displaying warmth and concern in her non-verbal communication, settles the new patient into her bright comfortable single room. Together, she and one of the medical staff talk with Ms M about her immediate physical problems. The doctor carries out a brief examination. Having administered a s.c. injection of the analgesic diamorphine and an i.m. injection of the antiemetic cyclizine (local practice may be to give cyclizine s.c.), S leaves Ms M to rest. The doctor will return later to take a medical history and carry out a full physical examination. Some time is spent with the patient's mother listening to her concerns and reassuring her before arranging for a friend to take her home.

Using the model, S has started to build a relationship with the patient and her family. It is not appropriate at this stage to tire the patient with a psychosocial interview. Pain and symptom control must take priority. The provision of good palliative nursing care requires knowledge of the patient's disease, including the anticipated problems, as well as knowledge of pain management.

The anticipated symptoms of advanced breast cancer

In common with many patients suffering from advanced disease, patients with breast cancer may complain of insomnia, fatigue, anorexia, constipation or sore mouth. They may be at risk from pressure ulcers and infections. The causes of these problems are many and varied; observant and vigilant nursing care may alleviate or prevent these conditions. There are, however, symptoms associated specifically with advanced breast cancer and its spread. Fortunately, many of these can be anticipated and some can be managed to prevent unnecessary suffering.

Bone is generally considered the most common site for disseminated breast disease (Hoskin & Makin 2003, McIllmurray 2004), followed by metastases to lung, liver and brain. It is important to remember that this is metastatic spread of the original disease. For example, when a patient with adenocarcinoma of the breast is diagnosed as having metastases in the femur, she has breast cancer in the bone, not a primary bone cancer.

Bone metastases

The bones most commonly affected by metastases are the ribs, vertebrae and pelvis, followed by the long bones, in particular the humerus and the femur. Patients often have metastases in more than one site.

The problems that may arise as a result are localised or neuropathic pain (see Ch. 19), pathological fracture, spinal cord or nerve root compression and bone marrow infiltration. In the past, hypercalcaemia would have been included in this list. Although this serious paraneoplastic disorder is associated with bone metastases, it is not now thought to be due directly to bone destruction. It will therefore be discussed separately.

The clinical diagnosis of bone metastases may be confirmed radiologically. It is not unknown, however, for the X-ray to appear relatively normal, contradicting the clinical examination, and therefore a bone scan may be required to confirm the diagnosis. Radiotherapy, orthopaedic surgery, chemotherapy and hormone therapy are all used to manage this complication of cancer. Until these therapies can be organised, analgesics may give some relief.

A single dose of radiation is usually effective in relieving localised bone pain, although around 15–20% of patients will fail to respond to radiotherapy (Hoskin & Makin 2003). Patients should be warned that it can take 2–4 weeks for a response to be noticed. Side-effects from the treatment are usually minor. Hemibody radiotherapy is a useful treatment for scattered bone pain, but because of the associated potential toxicity, it has to be considered on a holistic basis for a patient with far-advanced disease.

Radiotherapy is generally an effective method of relieving bone pain and facilitating healing of a pathological fracture. It may be used as the sole treatment or in conjunction with surgery. Orthopaedic surgery in the form of surgical internal fixation of a long bone is an effective method of either preventing a pathological fracture or quickly relieving the severe pain when a fracture has occurred.

Chemotherapy may be a useful treatment for bone metastases, when the primary tumour is chemosensitive, and may be given in conjunction with local radiotherapy. Hormone therapy is often beneficial to relieve the pain of bone metastases in patients with hormone-sensitive cancer of the breast.

Spinal cord compression is a very serious complication of bone metastases in the vertebrae. Bone metastases will be the cause in approximately 85% of patients with this condition (Twycross & Wilcock 2001). The tumour may encroach on the spinal cord, causing paralysis. This serious condition most commonly affects the thoracic vertebrae. However, for a significant minority, the site will be the lumbar region, and a smaller group will be at risk from quadriplegia because of tumour in the cervical vertebrae. Disease in more than one site is common. Spinal cord compression can be prevented, and therefore anticipation of this condition is of major importance.

Patients who are at risk of this complication, including patients with a diagnosis of breast cancer, must be warned to seek help immediately if they become aware of any of the following symptoms:

- a history of increasing back pain, which may radiate and be worse on movement and lying down
- sciatic-type pain in the lower back
- muscle weakness, which may make climbing stairs difficult and tripping-up common
- the sensation of weakness, or a loss of feeling, in the lower limbs or buttocks
- urinary hesitancy or retention, sphincter disturbance with incontinence of urine or faeces, or constipation (Twycross & Wilcock 2001).

In addition, neck pain, pain radiating to the shoulders and arms, or general weakness in the upper body should not be overlooked as this may be indicative of a cervical cord lesion.

Diagnosis is made on clinical examination and confirmed by an urgent magnetic resonance imaging (MRI) scan. Management must be considered immediately, as the progression to paralysis can be very rapid with significant implications for deterioration in the quality of life. Oral or i.v. corticosteroids would be commenced to reduce any peritumour inflammation (Twycross & Wilcock 2001). Analgesics such as oral morphine may also be required to provide some comfort for the patient.

Local radiotherapy is very effective and is usually the treatment of choice. However, some patients may benefit from surgery to stabilise the spine.

Lung metastases

The most common radiological abnormalities of lung metastases are multiple opacities in the lower lobes of the lungs. Lymphangitis carcinomatosis, the infiltration of the pulmonary lymphatics by tumour, may also be a problem. The severity of symptoms will depend on the number, site and size of the metastases. Dyspnoea may be caused by invasion of lung tissue, lymphangitis, pleural effusion or infection. Pain may also be caused by the pleural involvement. Haemoptysis and cough may be due to lobular collapse (Hoskin & Makin 2003).

Patients with breast cancer who have dyspnoea due to bronchial obstruction may respond to chemotherapy, radiotherapy or hormone therapy if these treatment options have not already been exhausted.

Respiratory symptoms are common in patients with advanced illness, with and without cancer (see Ch. 3). The management of acute breathlessness in chronic obstructive pulmonary disease is discussed in Case Study 3.

Liver metastases

Liver metastases indicate widespread dissemination of the disease and are therefore a poor prognostic sign. They may present as stretched capsule pain due to liver enlargement or be noticed on clinical examination of the abdomen. The diagnosis can be confirmed by ultrasound examination. As in the previous sites of secondary tumour discussed above, chemotherapy may be an option for the patient with breast cancer.

The enlarged liver may be the cause of a 'squashed stomach syndrome' with resultant nausea, vomiting, reduced gastric emptying and oesophageal reflux. The patient might also complain of dyspnoea, peripheral oedema and ascites. Liver function may be adequate until far on in the illness when jaundice and pruritus may occur (see Ch. 4).

Corticosteroids are very useful in relieving the pain of a liver enlarged with advanced cancer. Cancerous cells are frequently surrounded by inflamed oedematous tissue; a corticosteroid such as dexamethasone will reduce this swelling and therefore the overall dimensions of the tumour. The result is some relief of the pain (Regnard & Hockley 2004).

Brain metastases

On occasion, secondary cancer in the brain is the presenting sign of a patient's cancer. It is, however, more commonly a sign of widespread disseminated disease with a poor prognosis. The main symptom of a severe headache is the result of local pressure produced by the tumour, associated haemorrhage or oedema of the surrounding brain tissues. The headache is often described as being like a tight band around the head, which is sometimes worse in the morning. It may be associated with visual disturbances, nausea and vomiting, confusion and altered consciousness.

Other signs and symptoms will depend on which area of the brain is affected, with many patients having tumours in multiple sites. Suspicion should be raised when the patient appears to have cognitive impairment, i.e. confusion, memory loss or personality change, or if suffering from seizures, motor or sensory loss, or difficulty with balance.

The diagnosis may be confirmed by a brain scan. However, if the patient is very frail, a corticosteroid such as dexamethasone for a few days may help to confirm the diagnosis by relieving the symptoms. Radiotherapy to the whole brain is the usual method of treating cerebral metastases for patients who are strong enough and have a prognosis of longer than a few weeks. Corticosteroids will be given to the patient to relieve the symptoms until the radiotherapy has an effect and to treat the potential increase in cerebral oedema, which may be a temporary result of the therapy. The patient must be gently warned of the likely hair loss.

Paraneoplastic disorders

These are generally thought to be due to substances produced by the tumour or by other cells in the body in response to the tumour. Some paraneoplastic disorders are life threatening and many have a detrimental effect on the patient's quality of life. Therefore, when implementing this model of palliative care for a patient with a specific cancer, reference must be made to an oncology text (Hoskin & Makin 2003). The paraneoplastic disorder most commonly associated with breast cancer is the metabolic disorder of hypercalcaemia.

Hypercalcaemia is an easily managed disorder and therefore knowledge of its symptoms is important in anticipating this life-threatening condition (Twycross & Wilcock 2001, Hoskin & Makin 2003). Untreated hypercalcaemia can have a miserable effect on the patient's quality of life.

There was a time when it was believed that the high calcium in the blood was due to the mere presence of bone metastases. This theory has been superseded; it is now recognised that many patients with bone metastases do not develop hypercalcaemia and that some patients without bone metastases do. A simple outline of the present understanding will be given, as will the symptoms and management of the condition.

It would seem that various substances released from tumour cells cause tumour-induced hypercalcaemia. The most common of these is the parathyroid-related protein (PTHrP — not to be confused with the parathyroid hormone). PTHrP causes the reabsorption of calcium from bone and renal tubular reabsorption of calcium.

A high serum calcium will cause an osmotic diuresis, leading to polyuria, dehydration and thirst. The action on smooth muscle and the central nervous system may cause constipation, confusion and nausea. As this is a biochemical imbalance, it can stimulate the chemoreceptor trigger zone (CTZ) in the brain to cause vomiting.

The symptoms associated with rising calcium levels may therefore include the following: fatigue, lethargy, weakness, anorexia, thirst, nausea, vomiting, constipation, polyuria, delirium, drowsiness or coma. Death may be preceded by renal failure and/or cardiac arrhythmia in severe untreated hypercalcaemia.

Immediately a clinical diagnosis is made, treatment will begin by rehydration with i.v. normal saline. The drug treatment of choice is a bisphosphonate such as i.v. pamidronate, which should normalise the serum calcium concentration within a week. This drug inhibits osteoclast activity and therefore inhibits bone reabsorption. It does not block PTHrP-mediated renal tubular reabsorption of calcium (Twycross & Wilcock 2001).

The effect on the patient is often dramatic. However, the condition will recur and the treatment will need to be repeated regularly for the remainder of the patient's life. This management alone may relieve the many symptoms associated with the condition, but until this reversal comes about, vigorous pain and symptom management will be necessary.

Building a relationship and developing a profile

Day 2 Ms M has had a settled night requiring further s.c. diamorphine at 04.00 h with good effect. Today her pains will be assessed and titration of analgesics will be commenced. Simultaneously, other physical problems will be addressed, but attention is first given to total pain and suffering (see p. 1102). It is known that pain and other symptoms are often difficult to manage because of psychological and emotional concerns. Therefore S, the named nurse, has determined to carry out an initial interview with Ms M today, and later will arrange to spend time with Ms M's mother.

S refreshes her memory by reading the patient's notes. Ms M's genogram constructed on the previous admission is useful (see Fig. 33.3). She is also aware of the detailed clinical examination carried out by the consultant physician earlier this morning. To enable her to implement the model, S will need to collect information from the patient, so that an up-to-the-minute patient-centred care plan can be written. Ensuring the patient's comfort and that they will

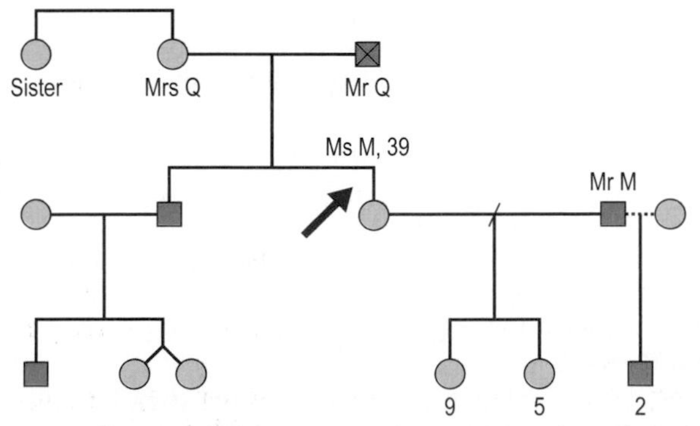

Fig. 33.3 Genogram for Ms M.

not be interrupted, S gently encourages Ms M to talk about her situation and her feelings.

Gradually responding to S's warm approach, Ms M confides that she has underestimated the emotional pain of leaving her children and that she is very worried about her mother. Ms M goes on to explain that her daughters, aged 5 and 9, have moved in on a permanent basis with their father, his new partner and their 2-year-old son. This seemed to be the most practical solution as he is a good dad and really loves them. It was, however, a terrible wrench: 'I cried and cried and really upset Mum. My mother is used to me being strong; all this is difficult for her'.

Ms M continues by repeating that she knew that this was the best for her children, and that their father's new partner is a real 'earth mother' type. She jokes about this having its good and bad points; that she as a career woman would have brought them up to be strong, independent women like herself. 'However, they know I am dying, we have talked and cried about it and read the right books. I have tried my best to prepare them.'

Note that S asks Ms M what her main problems, expectations and priorities are. She does not ask her directly about her understanding of the disease or the anticipated problems, as that would have been insensitive. S is able to document the information from the conversation; other members of the team will be consulted to add to this section of the assessment:

- *Main problems* — the patient initially identifies these as uncontrolled pain, nausea and vomiting, and sheer exhaustion. Following the above conversation, she admits to emotional pain, but wishes it to be recorded that she would only talk to S about it.
- *Expectations* — having had her pain alleviated on a previous admission, she hopes that the doctor will be able to help her again. She trusts him and is comforted by his determination; she knows he will not give up on her. She also expects to go home again.
- *Priorities* — Ms M identifies that she needs to rest. She requests not to be disturbed in the mornings until at least 10 o'clock. Getting her assets put in trust for her daughters has been a lengthy procedure. Fortunately, her lawyer and business partner will come to the hospice for final signatures sometime in the week, and then she will be able to relax. It is very important for Ms M to see her daughters; she has, however, instructed her husband that the girls are only to visit at the weekend, as she does not want to prejudice their schooling. Her mother and her aunt will be in every day. They are her main carers and have a need to visit. Other people have been asked by Ms M not to come.
- *Understanding of illness* — having read widely in relation to her disease, including searching the internet, Ms M has been involved in the decisions at every stage of her illness. She assures S that it has been a conscious decision to come to the hospice, as she liked what she had read about palliative care units. She is also aware of the complications that might come about because of her disease.
- *Anticipated symptoms* — because of her diagnosis of advanced metastatic breast cancer, Ms M's main anticipated problems are pain at multiple sites, hypercalcaemia, anaemia and spinal cord compression. Because she is receiving morphine, constipation must be prevented.

Having obtained this information, S ensures that Ms M is not upset and is comfortable before writing up the assessment and the care plan. Ms M thanks S for listening to her, saying with a wry smile: 'It has helped to talk, but I will not be making a habit of it'.

Later in the day, S spends some time talking with Mrs Q, the patient's mother. From this conversation, she is made aware that the patient and her mother had a strained relationship before the daughter's illness. Mrs Q had at times found her daughter's forceful personality difficult, although she is very proud of her. She was very upset when the marriage broke down and continues to admire her son-in-law for his gentle, loving nature and his good parenting skills.

She cries when she tells S of how the last few weeks have been so much better. It has been like 'having her little girl again', as she has helped her to shower and dress, and she talked about the past. Now she feels so useless and is dreading the next few weeks.

S gently asks who Mrs Q has to talk to, having noticed on the genogram that she has a sister. She is very relieved when Mrs Q speaks warmly of the support her sister is providing and the importance of her friends in the church.

S reminds Mrs Q that the hospice staff are available to help families as well as patients. She also decides to ask Ms M how she would feel about her mother coming in some days to help with her physical care.

Before moving on to care planning, the reader will realise that knowledge of suffering, pain assessment and management, as well as managing nausea and vomiting, are necessary to implement this patient's care.

Suffering

Pain and suffering are terms that are sometimes used as if they had the same meaning; this demonstrates a deep misunderstanding of human suffering. Physical pain can usually be controlled or reduced, whereas suffering is a much more complex phenomenon, encompassing emotions and psychosocial concerns that may elude control (Roy 1998, Houldin 2000).

Patients and families may suffer because of unresolved issues from the past. There may be guilt, remorse, loss of hope and fear of the future. People who are dying have lost control over their future, have suffered multiple losses in relation to their previous lifestyle and are often witnessing their decline into total dependence on others. In addition, they may be suffering through observing the effect their imminent demise is having on their family, and may be worried about how their survivors will cope. The family members are suffering by watching their loved one's decline, feeling useless and unable to help. Previous bad experiences of poor symptom control in the dying may be the cause of considerable anxiety.

Coping styles have attracted much interest in the literature. There is no doubt that some people cope much more effectively than others in stressful situations. Some individuals are flexible in being able to change their lifestyle to their new circumstances, to seek information, to be involved in the decision making, to maintain hope and to preserve their self-worth. Others become helpless and hopeless and go into a steep decline (Barraclough 1999, Chochinov & Breitbart 2000, Folkman & Greer 2000).

Many factors are involved. These are as diverse as personality, the manner in which the bad news was broken, and the social support available. A previous coping style is not always useful in relation to facing a life-threatening illness. This can be very distressing for patients and families as they struggle to cope with the fearful situation. Changing coping styles is not generally an option. What is recommended is to provide extra coping strategies to enable the individuals to achieve some relief from the suffering.

Realising the enormity of suffering, by both patient and family, can be daunting in palliative care. However, some help can be offered. By building up a relationship with the patient and the family, the nurse may gain some insight into what would be useful.

Daily communication with the family is a good method of giving support. The family members should never feel they have to search for someone to talk to, or that the nurse or doctor is too busy. A conscious effort must be made to give the family members respect by memorising their names and displaying warm body language towards them. Listening to their concerns is often useful, as is exploring who they have outwith the family to give support. Practical solutions may help, such as providing privacy for the patient and family to talk and for Ms M's mother to be involved in her daughter's physical care.

Mind and body are inextricably linked. The stresses caused by suffering may evoke physiological effects on the body. Complementary therapies may therefore be of great benefit to patients. Relaxation, massage, music therapy and other distractions may help to relieve the stresses of dying and should be available alongside mainstream medicine (Cassileth & Schulman 2004).

Whenever the patient seems to be very anxious or down, or when the usual pain management does not appear to be having the desired effect, the nurse caring for the dying must consider whether all avenues have been explored to assist the patient with the suffering. This may mean referring the patient to a social worker, counsellor, chaplain or a clinical psychologist.

The health care team may also suffer. Realising that clinical skills and knowledge are insufficient to relieve the patient's suffering may cause considerable distress (Bernard & Creux 2003). A culture of support must be developed by those caring for the dying, to enable them to realise, through maturity and experience, that there are limits to what can be achieved in relieving the suffering of some individuals.

Roy (1998) supports this, urging the health care team to 'realise your limits, there are some kinds of suffering that are so bound up in another person's uniqueness that they cannot be spoken away by other human beings, no matter how compassionate their words might be'.

Anxiolytic medications such as the benzodiazepines, e.g. temazepam, lorazepam and midazolam, are frequently prescribed in palliative care. They can help the patient sleep at night and get some relief from inner torment (Twycross & Wilcock 2001).

In getting to know Ms M, S recognises that the patient has trust in her hospice doctor because of her previous good experience of being helped with her pain. She also recognises that this is a woman who has what the psychologists call a 'high internal locus of control' (Murray Parkes et al 1996), i.e. she has a need to continue to have some control over her circumstances. S will therefore ensure that Ms M is consulted and informed as to any decisions being made about her care. S is also realistic in knowing that she cannot take away the profound sadness that her patient feels at the loss of her future as a mother. She can empathise with her and provide her with openings to talk about it and pleasurable distractions, but she cannot remove that suffering.

One area of suffering that can generally be helped is the management of physical pain. When physical pain is relieved or reduced to a level acceptable to the patient, other areas of suffering can be explored. Before moving on to this section of the chapter, the reader is advised to read Chapter 19.

Pain assessment

Despite the complexity of pain, a vast amount of knowledge is available to manage pain effectively. However, pain that is not identified will not be treated, and pain will not be treated vigorously enough if its severity is underestimated (Vallerand 1997, Farrer 2001).

It has now been well accepted that the patient's self-report is the most reliable indicator of pain (McCaffery & Pasero 1999). Self-report of pain, however, is rarely an option in the confused or non-verbal older patient. Behaviour becomes the main method of assessing pain in these individuals (Lefebvre-Chapiro 2001). In addition, of course, there are many personality, attitudinal and cultural reasons why people do not reveal their pains. These range from being loath to admit to an increase in pain, as this may signify progression of their disease, to being unwilling to admit that the doctor's best efforts have been to no avail.

Patients who are dying have more than one pain, and therefore the nurse committed to helping the patient must systematically and regularly assess and document information about these pains.

The following information should be documented in relation to each pain:

- location
- severity
- radiation
- type (dull/acute)
- when started
- aggravating factors
- alleviating factors.

The nurse, having assessed the patient's pain, should then discuss this with the medical staff. It is essential this be done in an informed manner by giving a detailed description of the pain as outlined above. It is poor practice when requesting medical attendance to give the blank statement that the patient is in pain.

Pain management

An accurate diagnosis of new pains derived from observation, discussion and physical examination must be undertaken by a physician. This is essential, as the new pains may

Box 33.2

Analgesic medications commonly used for cancer pain

Step 1 — Non-opioids for mild pain
Paracetamol or non-steroidal anti-inflammatories (NSAIDs)

Step 2 — Opioids for mild to moderate pain
Codeine often combined with paracetamol, e.g. co-codamol 30/500

Step 3 — Opioids for moderate to severe pain
Normal release — Oramorph or Sevredol
Controlled release — MST Continus or MXL
Diamorphine by subcutaneous injection

require laboratory or radiological investigations and other treatments as well as analgesics.

Analgesic medications, given regularly to prevent the recurrence of pain, are central to effective pain management. It is essential that an adequate, regular dose is calculated and administered, enabling the patient to be as comfortable as possible without being drowsy. A list of those commonly used for cancer pain is given in Box 33.2.

Adjuvant medications are frequently given along with analgesics in the effective management of pain (see Ch. 19). Some pains do not respond well to the analgesics codeine, morphine and the other medications that are known collectively as opioids. Bone pain and neuropathic pain commonly require adjuvant therapy. A list of adjuvant analgesics is in Table 33.1.

Principles have been established by the World Health Organization (WHO 1986, 1996) to guide medical staff in the management of chronic pain. In addition, the Scottish Intercollegiate Guidelines Network (2000) publication on *Control of Pain in Patients with Cancer* is readily available online. Registered nurses must have a sound knowledge of these principles and guidelines to promote good interdisciplinary understanding and patient confidence.

Table 33.1 Adjuvant analgesics commonly used for cancer pain

Medication	Example	Indications
Non-steroidal anti-inflammatory	Diclofenac	Bone pain, soft tissue infiltration
Corticosteroids	Dexamethasone	Raised intracranial pressure Nerve compression Soft tissue infiltration Hepatomegaly
Tricyclic antidepressants Anticonvulsants	Amitriptyline Gabapentin	Nerve compression or infiltration, paraneoplastic neuropathies
Bisphosphonates	Pamidronate	Bone pain

An adjuvant may be given in conjunction with an analgesic from any step on the ladder.

The WHO analgesic ladder

The key principles of the WHO approach are that analgesics be given by the mouth, by the clock and by the ladder.

By the mouth This convenient and easy route of administration should be the method of choice for as long as possible. When the patient can no longer tolerate oral medicines, the s.c. route is frequently used by setting up a syringe driver.

By the clock Morphine solution is effective for 4 h. Therefore, it *must* be administered regularly every 4 h. The exceptions to this are the controlled-release preparations, such as MST Continus.

Persistent pain must be prevented; it is inhumane to allow pain to return before administering the next dose. In an inpatient setting, care must be taken, therefore, that the patient does not have to wait on a routine drug round for this analgesic. A more accurate timing of drug administration may be achieved if it is given directly by the patient's named nurse or deputy, or by self-medication.

By the ladder Having taken a careful history and carried out a physical examination, the doctor will now be in a position to prescribe medication for the patient's pains. This may be a combination of analgesics and adjuvant therapies.

If the patient's management starts on step 1 of the ladder (mild pain), paracetamol may be given until the ceiling of 4 g in 24 h has been reached, i.e. the upper dose limit of this drug. If it does not control the pain then a drug on step 2 (mild to moderate pain) will be prescribed. Co-codamol 30/500, a combination of the step 2 opioid codeine and paracetamol, is commonly used. It is referred to as co-codamol 30/500 as each tablet contains codeine 30 mg and paracetamol 500 mg. It will be given up to the ceiling of two tablets 6-hourly. When that ceases to control the patient's pain, the step 2 opioid is stopped and a drug on step 3 (moderate to severe pain) will be prescribed. It is essential to note that paracetamol may be continued simultaneously with a step 3 opioid. The decision to use a step 3 opioid should be based on patient need, not the prognosis. The outdated practice of saving morphine for the last few weeks of life is misinformed.

A normal-release oral preparation of morphine, such as Oramorph or Sevredol tablets, will be prescribed, with the intention of establishing a regime that will relieve the pain without causing oversedation. This is known as titration. A common starting dose of normal-release morphine is 5–10 mg, except in the older person or the cachectic patient when 2.5 mg might be the starting dose. It will be prescribed to be taken 4-hourly round the clock, i.e. at 06.00, 10.00, 14.00, 18.00, 22.00 and, if awake, at 02.00 h.

Should the patient be in pain between doses, a breakthrough dose equivalent to the standard 4-hourly dose will be given. If a breakthrough dose is given, the timing of the next regular dose must not be altered. For example, if a patient has Oramorph at 06.00 h and requires a breakthrough dose at 09.00 h, the dose due at 10.00 h will still be given on time. An adjuvant medication may be given in conjunction with an analgesic from any step on the ladder.

Some common side-effects might be expected when a patient commences on step 3 opioids. Transitory effects may be sleepiness and nausea; these usually pass in a few days. More troublesome are constipation and a dry mouth. Constipation must be treated prophylactically; a laxative such as co-danthramer must be prescribed at the same time as the opioid.

Occasionally intolerable side-effects such as opioid toxicity, intractable constipation or a poor response to morphine might cause the physician to prescribe an alternative opioid, such as oxycodone or fentanyl. This is referred to as opioid switching or rotation (Farrer 2001, Twycross & Wilcock 2001).

When the dose of morphine has been stable for 24–48 h, the patient may be prescribed the daily dose of morphine in a controlled-release preparation. For example, on her first admission, Ms M was stabilised on 10 mg of morphine 4-hourly, i.e. 60 mg daily. She was therefore discharged home on 30 mg of MST Continus 12-hourly. She was also instructed to take a sixth of her daily dose, i.e. 10 mg of normal-release morphine mixture for breakthrough pain if required.

Around 80–90% of pain due to cancer can be relieved with oral analgesics and adjuvant medications following the WHO guidelines. The remaining percentage of pain can be difficult to manage (Portenoy et al 2004).

For detailed information on difficult pain problems, see Scottish Intercollegiate Guidelines Network (2000) and Twycross & Wilcock (2001).

Fear of addiction

One barrier to effective pain control in palliative care is the fear that patients, families and some health care professionals have of addiction to opioids. This fear is unfounded when the patient has physical pain. The confusion frequently arises when the patient on opioids requires increasing doses to relieve the physical pain.

An understanding of the terms 'addiction', 'tolerance' and 'dependence' is useful to reassure the patient and family. Addiction, i.e. psychological dependence, is usually seen in individuals who are taking morphine in the absence of physical pain. In contrast, tolerance is an involuntary physiological response to opioids when, having taken the opioids for some time, the patient requires larger doses to benefit from the same analgesic effect. Physical dependence is another physiological response, which these patients may show when an opioid is suddenly stopped (Twycross & Wilcock 2001).

Tolerance and physical dependence are not the same as addiction. Less than 1% of patients receiving opioids for physical pain over many months will develop addiction. However, 75–100% of patients receiving opioids for some months will develop tolerance and physical dependence (American Pain Society 1992). Other authors consider that the requirement for increasing doses is due to disease progression and not pharmacological tolerance (O'Neill & Fallon 1998).

Assessing and managing Ms M's pain

Until recently, Ms M completed a pain diary on a daily basis.

She found it a useful method of monitoring her pain management and of communicating with her doctors. In the last week, however, she has been too exhausted to continue this activity. She is therefore pleased that both the hospice physician and S are systematically assessing her pains.

The doctor, using a body chart and writing directly into the patient's notes, has thoroughly documented the patient's description of her pains along with the findings of the physical examination.

S has learned from past experience that very ill patients sometimes overlook communicating a feature of their pain when faced with a formal enquiry. She has therefore decided to carry out a pain assessment while bedbathing Ms M. Carefully observing the patient's non-verbal communication, S asks Ms M to talk about her pains as she helps her to wash. She also encourages Ms M to use her hands to identify where she is sore.

Ms M identifies three pains. First, she rubs the upper right quadrant of her abdomen and states that a feeling of extreme pressure builds up from deep inside her body. It has been getting steadily worse over the last few weeks, especially if she tries to lie on her right side. S recognises this as visceral pain because of a liver enlarged with metastases and a stretched liver capsule. Ms M has been prescribed the opioid analgesic diamorphine by s.c. injection and the adjuvant medication dexamethasone (a corticosteroid) for this pain. Before admission, Ms M was trying to take MST Continus 60 mg 12-hourly for this pain; however, nausea and vomiting affected concordance.

For guidance on transferring patients from oral morphine to subcutaneous diamorphine, see Scottish Intercollegiate Guidelines Network (2000) and the Lothian Palliative Care Guidelines (Lothian NHS Board 2004).

Second, Ms M places her hands around her head and describes the tight band of headache that is frequently worse on waking in the morning. The dose of dexamethasone already prescribed for her liver pain has been increased to reduce the cerebral oedema caused by cerebral metastases. In addition, paracetamol 4 g in 24 h will now be prescribed to help relieve this headache. The doctor has discussed with Ms M the role of palliative radiotherapy in treating this problem, if she can bear losing her hair again.

Third, Ms M grimaces as the skin over her right femur is washed. When encouraged, she points with her finger to a specific area of pain in the bone that is causing discomfort. Extensive bone metastases were a considerable problem almost 1 year previously when they were successfully managed with hemibody radiotherapy. Ms M is upset as she recognises that this may be a recurrence of bone metastases. S listens and gently reassures her that the paracetamol being commenced for her headaches may also relieve bone pain. In addition, there is a group of analgesics known as non-steroidal anti-inflammatory drugs (NSAIDs), which can bring considerable relief. Having left her patient refreshed and comfortable, S carefully documents a detailed pain assessment in the patient's notes. She then seeks out the doctor to discuss the pain in Ms M's right femur.

Managing nausea and vomiting

Nausea and vomiting are common, very distressing symptoms in palliative care. The pathophysiology of nausea and vomiting is complex and incompletely understood. There is no WHO antiemetic ladder to guide the interdisciplinary team, but efforts have been made to identify a logical approach to these symptoms (Twycross & Back 1998, Mannix 2004). This involves:

- understanding the pathophysiology
- assessment
- explanation
- individualising the plan of care
- attention to detail.

An understanding of the pathophysiology of nausea and vomiting (Campbell & Hately 2000, Twycross & Wilcock 2001, Mannix 2004) is important to allow the named nurse to actively participate in planning care and to explain care to patients and their families.

In order for vomiting to occur, the body needs to have detectors to identify the need to vomit, a coordinating centre and effectors which make the vomiting take place. The main detectors of the need to vomit are in:

- the gastrointestinal tract
- the chemoreceptor trigger zone (CTZ), a specialised area of the brain on the floor of the fourth ventricle
- the inner/middle ear
- the higher brain centres.

Messages from each of these detectors are transmitted to the vomiting centre in the medulla, which coordinates vomiting. Transmission from the gastrointestinal tract to the vomiting centre is via the vagus nerve. As this nerve innervates other tissues, vomiting may be stimulated by disease or trauma to other organs, e.g. the pharynx, liver or bladder. Direct stimulation of the vomiting centre by pressure, trauma or disease may also cause vomiting.

In advanced cancer, therefore, the vomiting centre can be activated in a number of ways:

- Vagal stimulation caused, for example, by gastric or bowel distension, liver capsule stretch, mediastinal disease or genitourinary problems
- Stimulation from the CTZ caused by chemical abnormalities in the blood, e.g. uraemia, hypercalcaemia, drugs or bacterial toxins
- Stimulation from the inner/middle ear due to infection, movement or local tumour
- Stimulation from higher central nervous system centres by anxiety, fear or revulsion
- Direct stimulation from raised intracranial pressure (Regnard & Comiskey 1995, Mannix 2004).

Many neurotransmitter receptors have been identified as playing a part in these vomiting pathways (Mannix 2004) and understanding of this is developing. What is important in terms of patient care is to appreciate that particular antiemetics are thought to block messages about the need to vomit at specific points along the vomiting pathways. It is this action which produces improvement or control of nausea and vomiting. Some of the commonly used antiemetics in palliative care act centrally at the vomiting centre, vestibular centre and/or the CTZ. Some act peripherally in the gastrointestinal tract and some act at both levels (Twycross 1999). Specific antiemetics may therefore be selected for specific causes of nausea and vomiting.

- *Cyclizine* acts centrally at the vomiting centre and in the inner or middle ear, and is therefore useful in managing the vomiting associated with raised intracranial pressure or motion.
- *Haloperidol* acts centrally at the CTZ and is an effective antiemetic for chemical causes of nausea and vomiting, such as hypercalcaemia or opioid-induced vomiting.
- *Metoclopramide* has its principal site of action peripherally in the gastrointestinal tract, where it acts by improving gastrointestinal motility. It may therefore be used to treat motility problems such as gastric stasis or 'squashed stomach syndrome'.
- *Levomepromazine* is a broad-spectrum antiemetic that has activity at the vomiting centre, vestibular centre and CTZ. It is useful in vomiting of uncertain or mixed origin and when other antiemetics have failed. In situations where an antiemetic is required and a degree of sedation is appropriate, levomepromazine may be prescribed.
- *Ondansetron* and *granisetron*, although very effective in the vomiting associated with cancer chemotherapy, have yet to find a place in the management of nausea and vomiting from other causes in palliative care (Mannix 2004).

Careful assessment of nausea and vomiting is crucial. Working with the patient, the team puts together a detailed picture of these symptoms. Recent guidelines emphasise the importance of the clinical picture in assessing and managing nausea and vomiting (Bentley & Boyd 2001, Lothian NHS Board 2004). Information about the onset, nature, pattern and severity of the nausea and vomiting is required. The doctor's comprehensive physical examination of the patient is another important source of information. Blood tests may be organised to check serum urea, calcium and electrolyte levels. In the process of care, the named nurse may acquire an understanding of the meaning of this symptom to the patient.

Management of nausea and vomiting involves identifying the cause(s) of the symptoms and discussion with the patient. Only in this way can care be truly individualised. The named nurse is central to this process. Reversible causes, such as pain, oral infection or raised intracranial pressure, should be treated.

The interdisciplinary team may consider non-pharmacological measures as part of the plan. The potential benefits of non-pharmacological approaches such as transcutaneous electrical nerve stimulation (TENS), acupuncture and guided mental imagery are acknowledged in the literature (Mannix 2004), but more research is required. An appropriate antiemetic should be selected, either while reversible causes are treated or in the longer term. Because of the progressive nature of advanced disease, regular review of symptom control must be planned.

The challenge for the interdisciplinary team in caring for Ms M is to use these principles to tailor symptom management to Ms M's problems, expectations, priorities and wishes. A detailed history and physical examination are undertaken by the palliative care consultant. Blood tests are organised to measure urea, electrolytes and serum calcium levels. S, the named nurse, learns from Ms M that during the week prior to admission, Ms M felt pressured by her mother to eat at mealtimes: 'It seemed so important to her that I should eat. Like a mother coaxing a child to clear her plate. She means it for the best ...'.

Identifying the cause(s) is vital to managing nausea and vomiting. In advanced disease, there may be more than one cause. For Ms M some likely causes might be:

- raised intracranial pressure due to cerebral metastases
- 'squashed stomach syndrome' because of an enlarged liver
- hypercalcaemia
- anxiety about pleasing her mother by eating at mealtimes.

The blood tests are satisfactory and the serum calcium is normal. The interdisciplinary team decide that Ms M's vomiting is most likely to be associated with her cerebral metastases. Cyclizine, an antiemetic directed principally at the vomiting centre, is selected. Cyclizine 50 mg i.m. (local practice may be to administer this drug s.c.) is given to Ms M shortly after admission, as the oral route is best avoided until vomiting settles. The corticosteroid dexamethasone is increased to treat the raised intracranial pressure. It is acknowledged by Ms M and the team that not feeling pressured to eat may in itself improve the symptoms. The importance of Ms M deciding when and what she wants to eat is documented in the care plan.

On review next day, Ms M has not felt sick or been sick since admission. When this symptom is discussed with Ms M, she makes it clear to S and the doctor that she does not want to start taking an antiemetic regularly if it is not required. It is agreed with Ms M that cyclizine be prescribed on an 8-hourly as-required basis in the meantime. S or her deputy is to discuss this with Ms M on each shift and it is to be reviewed with the doctor each day.

Attention to detail is the key in assessing Ms M's nausea and vomiting, in planning its management with her and in reviewing its effectiveness.

The assessment and management of nausea and vomiting in palliative care are addressed in more detail in Mannix (2004) and Regnard & Hockley (2004). In particular, discussion of the complex issues of managing nausea and vomiting in intestinal obstruction, not addressed here, can be found in Regnard & Hockley (2004) and Ripamonti & Mercadente (2004).

Applying the principles of palliative care (a care plan for Ms M)

It is useful to be aware that every day in this hospice ward, the named nurse or her deputy ensures that the patient's activities of living are met and reviewed and that care is tailored to the individual patient's capability on that day. A pressure area assessment, mouth assessment, manual handling assessment and a record of the care given are documented daily for the purposes of good team communication and to facilitate audit. In addition, however, the care plan for Ms M is structured by the three principles of palliative care. This part of her care plan, for the third day of her present admission, is given below.

Pain and symptom management

- Set up a syringe driver at 11.00 h loaded with diamorphine 40 mg and dexamethasone sodium phosphate 10 mg, scheduled to be delivered in 24 h; see prescription sheet. (It is good practice to check local drug information sources for compatibility of drugs used as a subcutaneous infusion.)
- Check accuracy of delivery every 4 h by measuring the length of the solution remaining and checking that the indicator light is flashing.
- Check site of the 25G 'butterfly' cannula inserted subcutaneously in the left upper arm 4-hourly.

These medications are being given to relieve deep pain in the right upper quadrant of the abdomen (from the liver) and a tight band of headache. Constant attention should therefore be given to assessing these pains to ensure medication efficacy. When able to tolerate oral medications, the NSAID diclofenac may be prescribed for bone pain. If that is the decision, a gastroprotective medication such as omeprazole will also be prescribed.

- Administer one bisacodyl and one glycerine suppository as prescribed, as she is unable to tolerate co-danthramer at present and is complaining of rectal discomfort.
- Do not disturb until 10.00 h, as she is very tired.
- Encourage Ms M to decide when and what to eat. A supply of her favourite foods is kept in the patients' fridge in the kitchen. Topping up of this supply will be organised by Ms M. The antiemetic cyclizine 50 mg is prescribed, orally, i.m. or s.c. on an 8-hourly as-required basis. This is to be reviewed each shift.
- Support the patient to perform her own mouth care with toothbrush and toothpaste.

Adjustment to loss and change

- Ms M is a highly organised person who has coped with her illness and impending death in a practical fashion, by being informed and involved. She has made careful arrangements for those who will survive her. She is very private regarding her feelings. However, she has spoken to S about her profound sadness. It is important to her that she is seen to be coping bravely. S will provide her with opportunities to talk should she wish to. Ms M's estranged husband and her daughters are being helped by counselling arranged by their family doctor.
- Ms M is expecting her lawyer at 14.00 h today. This is an important meeting for which she requires to conserve energy. She would very much like to be helped to sit out in a chair and to be wearing a smart outfit.

Facilitating pursuits that give pleasure

- Ms M likes to have her radio tuned to Classic FM and does not watch television. She enjoys picking up and sending her own e-mail. She can do this in the day hospice if taken by wheelchair.
- It is very important for Ms M to get her *Financial Times* every day. As she is very tired, encourage one of the volunteers to ask her if she would like it read to her.
- Ms M's daughters are in a school concert this week. She is determined to go to the school and give the girls a surprise on Thursday afternoon. Having been seen at sports day last month in a wheelchair, she is sure she will not embarrass her daughters. A nursing auxiliary has agreed to go with Ms M. They will be taken in the

hospice people carrier, which will wait for them, enabling them to return at any time.

This care plan is constantly being updated as the patient's circumstances change. Good written documentation is essential for good communication within the team and with the patient and family. It is an important element in high-quality care.

S's reflection

Good staff support systems must be in place to enable nurses like S to cope with caring for dying patients and their families. In the hospice ward in which she works there is a good culture of support. The senior staff make it explicit that they value their staff by involving them in important decisions, providing a pleasant working environment and granting generous study leave. The nurses and other members of the interdisciplinary team are quick to recognise when difficult situations are being encountered by their colleagues. They help each other by being flexible and by being available to listen to worrying concerns.

In addition to this, a system of formal clinical supervision is in place. S uses a reflective diary to prepare herself for her monthly supervision. She also uses a formal model to help her learn from experience when an incident from work is very troubling. One such incident happened during this week in relation to caring for Ms M. S broke down and cried when handing over to the patient's named nurse on night duty. Naturally, her colleague was very sympathetic; recognising that S was very tired she listened to her and then encouraged her to go home to her family.

S was concerned at her behaviour and decided to try to make some sense of it by analysing the incident using Gibbs' (1988) reflective cycle (see Fig. 33.4). This reflection (see Box 33.3) is written in the first person.

S wrote this reflection on her day off. She found it a very cathartic experience. However, she felt relieved following the exercise and decided that she must care for herself more vigilantly. She therefore immediately arranged to go swimming and out for lunch with a friend.

S will take this reflection to clinical supervision next week, as the wise counsel of the very experienced home care sister who is her supervisor is a major part of her professional support system.

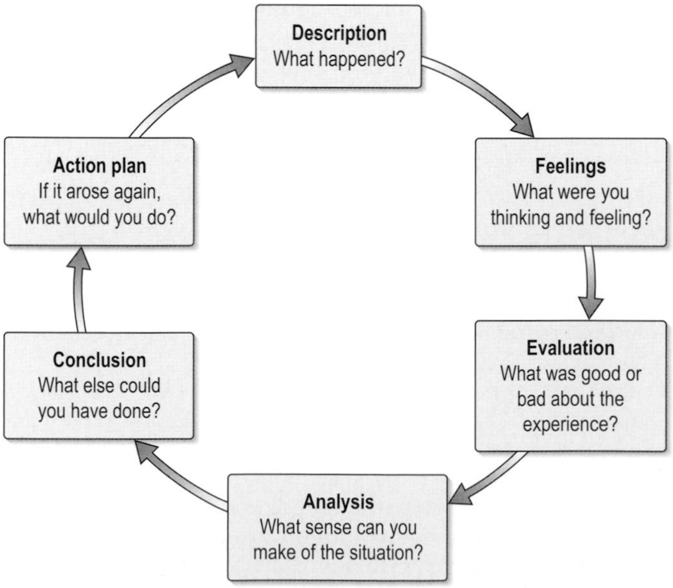

Fig. 33.4 The reflective cycle. (Adapted from Gibbs 1988.)

CASE STUDY 3 — MR Z

Mr Z is being cared for at home by his wife, daughter-in-law and the primary care team. At the age of 75, this retired gardener wants to die in his own home surrounded by his family. He is very fortunate that his GP and the district nurses in the practice have extensive experience in palliative care. They occasionally seek help from the local hospice but that has been less necessary in recent years.

Mr Z knows and is known to his doctor well, as his chronic obstructive pulmonary disease (COPD) has caused a gradual deterioration in his health for 6 years. Recently M, the district nurse, has been visiting the house regularly to dress Mrs Z's varicose leg ulcer. She has discussed Mr Z's steady deterioration with Dr J and, along with the patient and family, has made plans for the patient's end-of-life care at home. M is concerned, however, that this will not be possible as Mrs Z, who is a few years older than her husband, is also in poor health.

Working closely with the social services, equipment has been installed to ensure patient comfort and carer safety. This comprises a hospital bed, hoist, a wheelchair and sliding sheets. Oxygen equipment, including a regular supply of cylinders, has been in place for a year. Fortunately, the house is all on the ground level, a walk-in shower was installed to replace the bath some years ago, and Mr Z has an upright adjustable armchair.

Although M knows this patient and family well, she recognises the importance of going back to the model of palliative care (see Fig. 33.1) to ascertain that all aspects of care are being addressed.

Building a relationship and developing a profile

In reconsidering the relationship the primary care team have built up with the family, M studies the genogram that Dr J has drawn of Mr Z in the patient's notes (see Fig. 33.5).

Mr and Mrs Z have two sons and a daughter, having lost a third son in childhood. Their sons are both married and their daughter is divorced. All three have had two children of their own, so the Zs have six grandchildren. The oldest grandchild, whose wedding 3 years ago was the last social event Mr Z enjoyed, has recently had her first child.

The sons and their respective wives all live in the same neighbourhood as Mr and Mrs Z. They are all patients of the same health centre and are regarded as a very close supportive family. Their sister lives in Minnesota; she has not been home since the wedding.

This family is pulling together in stressful circumstances. They have open clear communication, flexible boundaries and roles, and yet they all have clearly designated responsibilities. Mr Z is always consulted on family matters. Although frail and the centre of care and attention, he is

Box 33.3

S's reflective account

Description — what happened?
On Thursday evening, when handing over to the night staff, I managed to get to my last patient, Ms M, when I could not continue as I started to cry. This had never happened before. I do occasionally cry at work, but it is normally done discreetly. It had been a very busy day, part of a difficult week. Two of my patients had died, one of whom I had known for many months. His family were extremely distressed at the end, especially his mother — after all he was only 35. I was glad I was on duty at the time as I had come to know them well.

After that family had gone home in the early afternoon, I had been auditing part of our admission standard. This involved accessing patients' notes from 6 months ago. The colleague who was supposed to help me with the audit was off sick. I went ahead without her because the secretary had looked out the notes, a considerable amount of work. Many of the patients whose notes had to be read have died since then; it was therefore a sad task.

Later in the evening one of my patients, Ms M, was talking about her daughters' excitement at performing in the school concert. It reminded me of when my daughters were young and I showed her a picture of my older daughter's graduation last month. Afterwards I wished I had not, as I saw the sadness come over her. I quickly changed the subject and some minutes later left the room.

I was tired when the night staff came on duty; however, that is a common experience. What was uncommon was for me to break down and cry.

Feelings — what were you thinking and feeling?
I was very embarrassed. My immediate thought was that my colleagues would think I was not coping. It was a distressing experience, especially as I cried all the way home and into the night. I felt better the next morning and was very grateful I was again on the late duty, as it gave me time to recover.

I know I am good at my job, and feel valued for my maturity and experience. I felt that I handled the young man's death well and really helped his family cope. Doing the audit was awful; I should have realised how it was affecting me and stopped. I have done a similar exercise before but always with a colleague.

I felt rotten at my lack of self-awareness in relation to Ms M. I know that her greatest source of emotional pain is in not being part of her daughters' future. Their graduation is potentially part of that. I like and admire Ms M and I do think she trusts me to do my best for her. I would be very upset to lose that trust. I also feel very guilty that I may have hurt her.

Evaluation — what was good and bad about the experience?
The good was that M, the night nurse I was handing over to, is a particularly valued colleague. She is wise and always helpful. On this occasion, she said, 'It is surprising we don't all break down more often, especially at the end of a harrowing day when we are exhausted like you are'. I felt supported and relieved to be going home.

The bad was my momentary lack of self-awareness, which meant that I might have reminded a patient of her emotional pain; also, that I left her room without giving her the opportunity to talk about it. Although in retrospect that was probably wise — because of my tiredness, talking at a deep emotional level with a patient would have been ill advised.

Analysis — what sense can you make of the situation?
That I have very high expectations of myself and therefore get very upset if I do not always get things right. That I need to continue to develop my self-awareness, particularly in recognising and taking appropriate action when I am stressed, such as in doing the audit unsupported. Also, that I need to be more vigilant with my communication, especially when tired.

That helping Ms M means a lot to me, I respect and admire her. I would be very upset if I lost her trust. I also feel I have a good understanding of her profound sadness, as I have had the joy of seeing my own two daughters into adulthood. Perhaps that was why I let her see the photograph.

Conclusion — what else could you have done?
I could have been open with Ms M and apologised for being insensitive. However, would that have benefited the patient or me? Ms M has acknowledged her emotional pain and indicated that she does not generally find it useful to talk about it. Perhaps I am being overly sensitive, as on the following day she asked me about my girls and asked me to bring in more pictures. She also indicated that she had asked her mother to bring in the photograph albums of her daughters so we could share them.

In relation to the audit, when I found it distressing I should have stopped and consulted the audit coordinator.

Action plan — if it arose again, what would you do?
I would indicate to the night staff that I had had a very emotional day and would be grateful if they would not be 'nice' to me as I might break down! I would give a brief report without any deep discussion and then I would go home. I would, of course, reassure them that a detailed report on each patient had been documented. In future, if an audit partner is off sick I will cancel the audit.

still the head of the family. The younger son is beginning to take on his father's role, as he is looked on as the family representative when decisions have to be made. The older son, a quiet man, occupies himself by ensuring that heavy physical tasks are attended to. Mrs Z is the coordinator and the communicator, although recently she has been very forgetful. The relationships within the family are warm and affectionate; they are tolerant of each other's idiosyncrasies.

M recognises these traits as being those of a well-functioning family (Bloch et al 1994, Davies et al 1994). She is aware, however, that the stress of nursing a dying relative at home has the potential to destabilise any family. Therefore, the primary care team must provide constant support, education and reassurance to enable this family to complete its task.

A district nurse is required to have a wide knowledge base in many areas of health care. This depth of knowledge cannot always be easily remembered. M acknowledges this and has therefore developed her information-seeking skills, frequently using the local nursing library and accessing the internet. In relation to this family, she recognises the need to revise her knowledge of the disease process of COPD to enable her to anticipate the symptoms Mr Z may suffer from at the end of life.

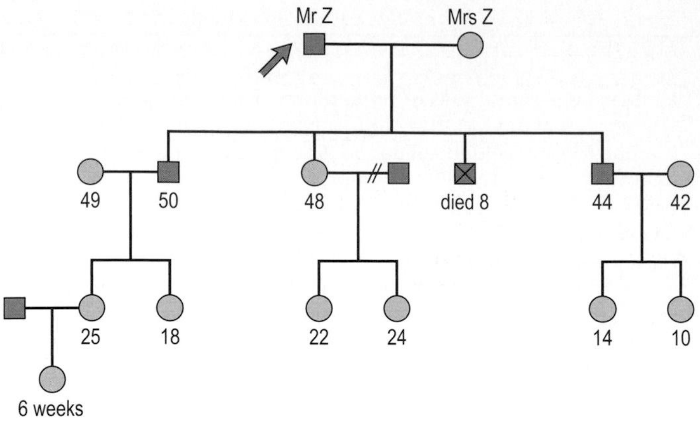

Fig. 33.5 Mr Z's genogram.

The anticipated symptoms of advanced COPD

Although there are many types of advanced pulmonary disease, of which Mr Z's diagnosis of COPD is one, the final problems are very similar (see Ch. 3). These are respiratory failure, cardiac failure and infection (Herbst 1996, Shee 2001). COPD is a broad classification for a number of conditions in which there is a chronic obstruction to airflow entering and leaving the lungs. Usually these conditions are bronchitis, an excessive secretion of mucus within the airways, and emphysema, an increase in the size of the air sacs distal to the terminal bronchioles with a loss of alveolar walls and elastic recoil of the lungs.

Advanced COPD often progresses to produce hypertrophy and failure of the right ventricle (right-sided heart failure). This is the result of the lungs being deprived of oxygen, which causes hypoxaemia, decreased arterial saturation, and hypercapnia, increased carbon dioxide in the blood, resulting in ventilatory insufficiency. This in turn leads to increased resistance in the pulmonary circulation with subsequent pulmonary hypertension. It is the pulmonary hypertension that leads to the right-sided heart failure (Smeltzer & Bare 2003).

The anticipated symptoms of advanced COPD are extreme breathlessness and a productive cough. An increase in the decline of the patient's forced expiratory volume (FEV) has been shown to be a useful indicator of the terminal phase of the patient's illness (Leach 2004). In addition, a drop in body weight due to increased metabolism from the effort of breathing and difficulty in maintaining an adequate nutritional intake indicates a poor prognosis (Herbst 1996). Other symptoms that should be anticipated include generalised muscle weakness and osteoporosis due to prolonged steroid therapy, pain from the osteoporosis, and chest pain due to ischaemic heart disease. Pulmonary embolism is also a risk due to immobility.

As the right ventricle fails, it should be anticipated that venous congestion and impaired sodium excretion might cause oedema in the peripheral tissues. Venous congestion of the abdominal organs may cause anorexia and nausea, and hepatic congestion may cause abdominal pain from an enlarged liver. In addition, there may be distended neck veins, ascites or a pleural effusion. Headache, confusion and stupor may come about because of carbon dioxide retention.

The medical management of COPD includes the use of long-term oxygen. Studies done in the 1980s in both the UK and the USA (Shee 1995) demonstrated that the use of long-term oxygen and cessation of smoking were the only actions that prolonged life in these chronically ill patients. However, physiotherapy, including a gentle exercise programme and breathing exercises, is thought to improve the patient's quality of life.

Exacerbations of chest infections are usually treated with antibiotics. Inhaled medications, such as the bronchodilators salbutamol and terbutaline, as well as the anticholinergic drug ipratropium bromide, are useful in relieving breathlessness, if they are administered correctly. The nurse must educate the patient and family in how to do this; an explanation of this method of delivering medication is given in Chapter 3.

Inhaled or oral corticosteroids may be prescribed for their anti-inflammatory effect. Oral corticosteroids may be prescribed to promote a feeling of well-being and increase the appetite (Shee 2001).

Severe breathlessness frequently responds to normal-release oral morphine. It should be started at a low dose (Leach 2004). There is a slight risk that some patients may develop carbon dioxide retention, respiratory acidosis. Therefore, a patient with advanced COPD who is commenced on morphine should be observed for headache and disorientation. It is useful to remember that a laxative must be prescribed when opioids are commenced.

A low dose of an anxiolytic such as lorazepam may partially relieve breathlessness by helping the patient to relax. Diuretics and a reduction of oral fluids to 1500 mL a day can help to relieve oedema (Leach 2004).

Monday In preparation for a team meeting on Tuesday at which the Z family will be discussed, M revised the pathophysiology of COPD in her local nursing library. She now feels prepared to seek information from Mr Z on which to plan care, i.e. based on his needs and priorities. She finds Mrs Z preoccupied making a fancy dress costume with her granddaughter, and takes the opportunity to speak to Mr Z on his own. M has structured her information-seeking guided by the headings suggested earlier in this chapter. In a short period, M skilfully gathers wide information to develop a profile and care plan. One potential problem she is aware of is constipation.

Constipation is a very common problem for patients in the palliative phase of illness. It can cause abdominal pain and embarrassment. It may lead on to other serious problems such as faecal impaction, overflow diarrhoea, urinary dysfunction, nausea, vomiting and even confusion (Atkinson & Virdee 2001). Careful assessment, management and documentation of this symptom may make the difference between the patient staying at home and hospital admission. The nurse's role in this is crucial.

In patients with advanced disease, many factors may work together to cause constipation. Sometimes constipation is disease related. For example, in the patient with cancer, the site of the tumour or the presence of hypercalcaemia may be a cause. Eating very small helpings of food with little roughage, drinking considerably less than before and restricted mobility may all contribute to the development of constipation. When opioids are added to this scenario, constipation becomes a certainty. Opioids have a number of effects on the bowel. They reduce peristalsis, inhibit fluid secretion (Regnard & Hockley 2004), increase sphincter tone and diminish sensitivity to rectal distension (Sykes 2004). In this way, the patient can quickly become constipated, struggling to expel small, dry, hard stools.

Anticipation and assessment of this symptom form the basis for effective management. In other words, the district nurse does not wait until the patient complains of constipation, but is constantly alert to this possibility, reviewing the situation at each visit. As part of holistic assessment of the patient, the nurse needs to take a careful and sensitive history. This will include enquiry about:

- previous bowel habit
- the most recent stool (when it was passed, what it was like, any problems experienced)
- intake of diet and fluid
- concordance with laxative regimen
- other medications taken
- accessibility and acceptability of toilet arrangements.

Most important of all, the nurse needs to explore sensitively the patient's perception of the problem, i.e. his priorities and expectations. Where constipation is suspected, abdominal and digital rectal examinations are indicated (Sykes 2004). Depending on local policy and practising within the *Code of Professional Conduct* (Nursing and Midwifery Council 2004), a nurse may perform a digital examination of the rectum. A plain X-ray of the abdomen may be useful in assessing constipation (Sykes 2004).

The management of constipation is about more than prescribing and administering laxatives (Atkinson & Virdee 2001). It involves attention to the relief of pain and other symptoms, to fluids and diet and to adapting toilet facilities. Especially in the community, education of the patient and family may allow the patient to remain in control of this very personal and private aspect of care. Most patients in palliative care will, however, require a laxative. An understanding of laxatives is vital, especially for the district nurse who may also be a nurse prescriber (Campbell et al 2001).

Oral and rectal laxatives may be classified as predominantly peristalsis-stimulating or predominantly stool-softening agents. Danthron and senna are predominantly stimulants. An example of an oral stool softener is docusate. Bulking agents are rarely used in palliative care because they are unpalatable, require to be taken with a large volume of fluid and may complete an incipient intestinal obstruction. There is evidence to suggest that the combination of a stimulant and stool softener (e.g. co-danthrusate or co-danthramer) gives the most favourable results, at an acceptable dose, with a minimum of unwanted side-effects (Sykes 2004). The dose should be titrated against patient response.

As the majority of patients prefer oral to rectal measures (Sykes 1997, cited in Atkinson & Virdee 2001), the nurse should endeavour to keep the use of enemas and suppositories to a minimum. All rectal measures act, to a greater or lesser extent, by stimulating the anocolonic reflex. Enemas and suppositories, however, can also be classified as stimulants or softeners. For example, the stimulant bisacodyl suppository is useful for evacuating soft stool from the rectum. A microenema or phosphate enema may be effective in softening and evacuating more solid stool. Arachis oil enema or glycerine suppository may be used to soften hard stool, where this needs to occur before further treatment to evacuate the bowel will be possible. When rectal treatment is given, the doctor should review the oral laxative prescription and increase the dose if appropriate. Many teams will have devised a multidisciplinary protocol for the use of oral and rectal laxatives.

The management of constipation in palliative care patients is addressed in more detail in Regnard & Hockley (2004) and Sykes (2004).

Mr Z has never in his life had problems with constipation. When Dr J prescribed an opioid for Mr Z's increasing breathlessness, he simultaneously prescribed the laxative co-danthramer suspension 5 mL at night (a combined softener and stimulant). M emphasised to Mr Z and his wife the importance of taking this regularly (as prescribed), rather than waiting to see if constipation developed. Mr Z indicated that he could not bear the taste of the laxative, so M arranged for the doctor to change the prescription to co-danthramer one capsule at night. She also warned Mr Z that his urine may turn pink as result of taking co-danthramer, as this is a recognised side-effect of the laxative (Regnard & Hockley 2004).

While gathering information for the profile, M asks Mr Z about his bowels. He says that although he has been taking the 'medicine', his bowels have not moved for 3 days. Until now, his bowels have moved daily. At first he was glad, because 'it's such an effort with this breathlessness' and he rationalised that as he was 'not really eating' it did not matter. However, people eating very little can still become constipated, because desquamation, gut secretions and bacteria mean that waste is still produced in the bowel (White 1995). M explains this to Mr Z. On further sensitive questioning, M learns that the last stool passed was small, as he 'hadn't the puff to push more out'. Mr Z is now beginning to experience rectal discomfort.

Together they discuss some options. M explains that a rectal examination would allow her to give appropriate treatment. Rectal examination is within the scope of M's professional practice and there is a local multidisciplinary protocol on the use of rectal laxatives in the community. As rectal examination is an invasive procedure, M carefully and thoughtfully discusses and negotiates the need for this with Mr Z. Because he is tired from his conversation with M, they agree that she will come and help with his care first thing tomorrow. If it is still required, she can treat his constipation then.

Tuesday morning Before attending the multidisciplinary meeting, M goes to Mr Z's house. While assisting his daughter-in-law to wash Mr Z in bed, she notices that his abdomen is quite soft. There is no reason to suspect an intestinal obstruction. Gentle rectal examination reveals that his rectum is loaded with fairly hard faeces. A microenema is given as indicated on the protocol. M documents this in his notes, and shortly afterwards she helps Mr Z to the toilet and his bowels move well. It is clearly an enormous effort for Mr Z to get to the toilet. He acknowledges that a commode may be useful, but 'not yet'. M decides to place an order for a commode to be ready if required. She also makes a note to discuss Mr Z's laxative prescription with Dr J at the meeting later. A small increase in oral laxative may be worth considering. Such discussion between the nurse and doctor is crucial in caring for the palliative care patient with constipation in the community (Doyle & Jeffrey 2000).

Before the extended multidisciplinary meeting, M writes the following summary into the patient's notes in preparation for updating the interdisciplinary care plan.

Main problems Extreme breathlessness is Mr Z's main problem. It has been getting steadily worse for years. He now requires help with washing, dressing and going to the toilet. He uses continuous oxygen administered with nasal cannulae, which he describes as 'his lifeline'.

Eating is a problem, as he does not have the energy to lift the food to his mouth and his dentures are loose. He finds it embarrassing but his wife is now feeding him her good home-made soups and his favourite puddings. He is, however, still losing weight and that is upsetting as he already thinks he looks like 'a bag of bones'.

Breathlessness is also making it difficult to empty his bowels. It is very exhausting and therefore he has been pleased that recently bowel movements are infrequent. He has rationalised that this is because he is not eating. He has in fact become constipated and the reasons for this have been explained to him.

Expectations Mr Z expects that soon he will not be able to get out of bed except when the nurses come and use the hoist. This is causing him some concern as the bedroom window looks out onto a brick wall whereas the sitting room has large windows onto the garden.

Doctor J has promised him he will die at home. That is all he is hoping for now. He is sure that everyone will rally round and he will try not to be too much bother to anyone: 'One day soon I will just stop breathing. I wouldn't say this to the family but it will be a relief, I am worn out with all of this being ill'.

Priorities Mr Z has a beautiful garden, which he laid out over 30 years ago. It is maintained by his older son, who lives with his wife and grown-up family in the next street. Mr Z tells M that watching the garden throughout the seasons is still his greatest pleasure. He impresses on her his need for the garden, although now he is just a spectator, not the worker he used to be. He jokes about how he used to rush back to it from the family holidays. Mr Z chuckles as he reminisces about this and then becomes serious again, anxious that M understands why he must die at home.

He insists that his only other pleasure is being with the family when they all gather round in the evening. This is why he wants to be able to continue to sit in his chair in his own sitting room.

Understanding of illness Mr Z demonstrates a full understanding of his illness. He has shared with M how he expects to die. The actual process of dying does not appear to be worrying him; what he is concerned about is where the last days of his life will be spent.

Anticipated symptoms Because of Mr Z's diagnosis of COPD and his long-term incapacity, he has many actual and potential problems. His skin is very friable due to long-term use of steroids, and recently he has lost 2 stones in weight. Nocturnal dyspnoea affects his sleep. His main anticipated physical symptoms are increasing oedema of the lower limbs, pressure ulcers, sore mouth, constipation, pain in the chest and/or the right upper quadrant of the abdomen. Disease progression may lead to chest infection, pulmonary embolism and respiratory and/or cardiac failure.

Mr Z may also become very anxious and frightened and may have a respiratory panic attack. He has previously attended a nurse-led clinic to promote self-management of these problems (Syrett & Taylor 2003).

Applying the principles of palliative care

Pain and symptom management

- *Support the family in helping Mr Z to take his medication regularly.* He is continuing to take the bronchodilators salbutamol and ipratropium by nebuliser, oral prednisolone 10 mg daily and furosemide 80 mg daily for ankle oedema. Mr Z has continuous oxygen by nasal cannulae at 2 L/min via an oxygen concentrator. For 2 weeks he has been taking oral morphine 2.5 mg 4-hourly to ease his severe breathlessness. This has been a useful addition to his pharmacological management, easing the dyspnoea, especially at night.
- *Monitor Mr Z's pain control.* Mr Z insists that he has no pain. However, he did admit that his chest felt more relaxed since commencing on the morphine and he is not breathing so rapidly.
- *Monitor Mr Z's bowel function.* The laxative co-danthramer suspension 5 mL has been changed to co-danthramer one capsule at night, as Mr Z hates the sickly taste of the liquid preparation. Rectal treatment by means of a microenema was given for constipation. The need to increase the oral laxative will be discussed with Dr J at the meeting. A commode has been ordered, so that it is ready when Mr Z wants it.

Adjustment to loss and change

- *Support Mr Z and his family in their ongoing adjustment to loss and change.* Mr Z has suffered many losses throughout his long illness. He appears to have adjusted to his increasing incapacity in a positive fashion, although when he could no longer work in his garden he was angry with the doctors and could not believe there was not a cure for his illness.

  Mr Z states that he is not a religious man but a man of the soil, observant of the life cycle as well as of the seasons. He is sorry he will not see the snowdrops again but he recognises that his life span is ending. He has had a good life and has few regrets although he is worried about how his wife will cope with his death. She has suffered from depression regularly throughout her life and was in hospital on two occasions, once after they lost a son. The other occasion was when her elderly mother died.

Pursuits that give pleasure

- *Encourage and support Mr Z to live at home with his family during this final illness.* Mr Z has impressed on all of the health care team that being in his own home surrounded by his family looking out on his beautiful garden gives him the greatest pleasure. He cannot concentrate on television and is too weary to read.

Obtaining a wheelchair 3 months ago from the social services has been a great success, as Mr Z can again be out in the garden, with the help of his family.

Tuesday (cont'd) Mr Z is the subject of a case conference at which the extended primary care team are present; Mr Z's younger son is also in attendance. Dr J leads the meeting, ensuring that all present have the opportunity to contribute. Two main issues arise which require discussion with the patient.

M tentatively raises the issue of moving Mr Z's hospital bed from the master bedroom into the sitting room. This is accepted as sensible by the son, but he is not sure what his father's reaction will be to the suggestion. Mr Z has slept in the same room as his wife for over 50 years. The son agrees to discuss the move with Mr Z.

The son informs the team that his father has been incontinent of urine regularly in the mid-morning for a few weeks, but he will not tell the nurses. Dr J suggests that he would talk with Mr Z about this 'man to man' and suggest a urinary catheter.

M suggests that it is time for the care assistants to assist the family with the patient's personal care on a daily basis.

When the son leaves the meeting to go back to work, Dr J takes the opportunity to introduce to the team the concept of an 'integrated care pathway for the dying patient', being piloted by the neighbouring health centre. He indicates that Mr Z would be a suitable patient for this multiprofessional document which replaces existing documentation with a template based on evidence-based guidelines relating to the care of the dying (Ellershaw & Wilkinson 2003).

Wednesday Dr J visits Mr Z in the late morning, a time when patients' respiratory problems are often at their least troublesome. He finds Mr Z in his bed in the sitting room; the family made the move with their parents' consent on the Tuesday evening. After a short useful discussion, Mr Z thanks the doctor for his help and readily agrees to have a urinary catheter inserted. Dr J is very concerned that Mrs Z is looking very tired and frail. He records her blood pressure, which is slightly raised, and takes some blood for a full blood count.

M calls in the early evening on her way home to teach the sons catheter care, including emptying the closed system bag.

Friday The older son pays an early morning call to his father, sharing a cup of tea before his mother rises. This is a routine for father and son, especially in summer time. Before leaving to go to work, the son becomes aware that his mother is not around, and on going to waken her he finds that she has died in the night. Shocked and unsure what to do, he is relieved when he sees M's car drawing up at the gate.

M immediately arranges for Dr J to come to the house. When he has certified Mrs Z as dead, the doctor, district nurse and the son sit down together to make plans for sharing the bad news. The son and Dr J will speak to the immediate family. M will tell Mr Z.

M is very aware of the need for this communication to be sensitive and structures her approach following the framework advised by Buckman (1992). She starts by 'firing the warning shot': 'You know how your wife has been looking so tired and frail lately. Well, Dr J had noticed and did some tests on her. I am afraid I have a shock for you'. At this point M hesitates to ensure that Mr Z had heard and understood her communication. The patient nods his head. M continues, gently telling him in 'bite-sized pieces' what happened that morning. Mr Z reaches out towards her, holds her hands but says nothing. They sit for a few minutes. M then asks, 'What can I do for you?'. After a long silence, Mr Z says: 'It is for the best. She has gone before me'. After another long silence and a few tears, he asks to see his son, and M leaves them together.

Monday, week 2 It has been a busy weekend for the Z family as they try to come to terms with Mrs Z's sudden death. There is a sense of unreality about what has happened as they arrange for the funeral, care for Mr Z and support each other. Many emotions and feelings are being experienced in this initial period of grief, as the impact of the event becomes a reality (Murray Parkes et al 1996, Worden 2003).

Wednesday, week 2 The Z's daughter arrived from the USA on Tuesday. She is causing some anxiety in the household, as she is very critical of her father's care, indicating that such an ill man should be in hospital. At the sons' request, Dr J and M have an appointment to see her in the health centre this morning. The health care team will have to employ patience and understanding towards a family member who may be very insulting in her attitude about their care. This reaction has been described by Jenkins and Bruera (1998) as the 'daughter-from-California syndrome'. It refers to the reactions and behaviour of an absentee member of the family who returns during a serious illness.

Four characteristics are described:

- shock at the extent of the patient's deterioration
- unrealistic expectations regarding treatment options, because of lack of involvement in treatment decisions
- guilt about being absent at such an important time
- reassertion of role through conflict.

Friday, week 2 M has timed her visit to Mr Z to coincide with the time of his wife's funeral, knowing that it will be an emotional time, a time in which she can demonstrate her support by being there. Most of the family have gone to the crematorium. M enters by the garden, as she has many times before. Standing in the door, she witnesses an intimate family picture. The eldest granddaughter is sitting by the bed breast feeding her baby, and her husband is at the other side of Mr Z's bed reading from the Psalms.

On approaching the bed, M realises that Mr Z is dying. His peripheral circulation is failing, he is covered in a drenching sweat, his skin feels cold and clammy and his extremities are blue. There is a Cheyne–Stokes pattern of breathing and he appears to be unconscious. M speaks to him but there is no response. She then concentrates on explaining to the young couple that their grandfather is dying. By the time the family return from the funeral, Mr Z has died — as he had wished, in his own home.

Wednesday, week 3 On the day following Mr Z's funeral, M and Dr J have arranged to meet the family to offer their condolences, answer any questions regarding their parents' deaths and offer bereavement support.

Bereavement Talking with the health professionals who have become known and trusted by the family during the final illness may help the family in this early phase of grief to accept the reality of the loss. Discussing the death and answering questions can help to dispel anger and prevent needless guilt arising. It can give the family the opportunity to criticise the care provided. Relatives rarely feel able to do this when the patient is alive. It can also give the family the opportunity to thank the health professionals and therefore finish the experience of living with the terminal illness and move into the adjustment period of the bereavement (Murray Parkes et al 1996).

Case review

Part of the primary care team's support system is to hold a debriefing meeting following difficult situations. M and Dr J are pleased to hold such a meeting following the deaths of Mr and Mrs Z.

The interdisciplinary team members discuss the patients' illnesses and the care and management provided. The postmortem carried out on Mrs Z concluded that she had suffered a stroke.

A lively discussion is held postulating the possible outcome had intervention been offered before the event. The successful conclusion to Mr Z's final illness allows the team to feel satisfied. M and Dr J are supported by their colleagues' praise for the organisation and hard work, which enabled Mr Z to die at home in very difficult circumstances.

Bereavement assessment is discussed. A leaflet containing information about the help available both in the health centre and from Cruse bereavement care has been left with the family. M is going on holiday for 2 weeks and has arranged to meet the family for a bereavement visit on her return.

CONCLUSION

Working in a hospice, one is often asked: 'What is so special about palliative care?'. This chapter has endeavoured to answer that question by demonstrating how this approach to care can be utilised in a hospital ward, in a hospice and in the home. It is never appropriate to say that 'there is nothing more that can be done'; what can be done is to implement a palliative care model, the focus being on the quality of life of the patient and the family in the time that they have left together.

REFERENCES

Addington-Hall J M, Higginson I J 2001 Palliative care for non-cancer patients. Oxford University Press, Oxford

American Pain Society 1992 Principles of analgesic use in the treatment of acute pain and cancer pain, 3rd edn. American Pain Society, Illinois

Atkinson J, Virdee A 2001 Promoting comfort for the patient with symptoms other than pain. In: Kinghorn S, Gamlin R (eds) Palliative nursing – bringing comfort and hope. Baillière Tindall, Edinburgh

Barraclough J 1999 Cancer and emotion. A practical guide to psycho-oncology, 3rd edn. Wiley, Chichester

Bentley A, Boyd K 2001 Use of clinical pictures in the management of nausea and vomiting: a prospective audit. Palliative Medicine 15: 247–253

Bernard M, Creux F 2003 Suffering – a problem that also affects nurses. European Journal of Palliative Care 10(2): 77–81

Bloch S, Hafner J, Harari T et al 1994 The family in clinical psychiatry. Oxford University Press, Oxford

Brown S J 1995 An interviewing style for nursing assessment. Journal of Advanced Nursing 21: 340–343

Buckman R 1992 How to break bad news. Papermac, London

Campbell T, Hately J 2000 The management of nausea and vomiting in advanced cancer. International Journal of Palliative Nursing 6(1): 18–25

Campbell T, Draper S, Reid T et al 2001 The management of constipation in people with advanced cancer. International Journal of Palliative Nursing 7(3): 110–119

Cassileth B R, Shulman G 2004 Complementary therapies in palliative medicine. In: Doyle D, Hanks G, Cherny N et al (eds) Oxford textbook of palliative medicine, 3rd edn. Oxford University Press, Oxford

Chaplin J, McIntyre R 2001 Hope. In: Kinghorn S, Gamlin R (eds) Palliative nursing – bringing comfort and hope. Baillière Tindall, Edinburgh

Chochinov H, Breitbart W 2000 Handbook of psychiatry in palliative medicine. Oxford University Press, Oxford

Davies B, Reimer J C, Martens N 1994 Family functioning and its implications for palliative care. Journal of Palliative Care 10(1): 29–36

Davies S, Seymour J 2002 Historical and policy contexts. In: Hockley J, Clark D (eds) Palliative care for older people in care homes. Open University Press, Buckingham

Davy J, Ellis S 2000 Counselling skills in palliative care. Cromwell Press, Trowbridge

Doyle D, Jeffrey D 2000 Palliative care in the home. Oxford University Press, Oxford

Doyle D, Hanks G, Cherny N et al (eds) 2004 Oxford textbook of palliative medicine, 3rd edn. Oxford University Press, Oxford

Ellershaw J, Wilkinson S 2003 Care of the dying: a pathway to excellence. Oxford University Press, Oxford

Farrer K 2001 Pain control. In: Kinghorn S, Gamlin R (eds) Palliative nursing – bringing comfort and hope. Baillière Tindall, Edinburgh

Faulkner A 1998 Effective interaction with patients, 2nd edn. Churchill Livingstone, Edinburgh

Faull C, Woof R 2002 Palliative care. Oxford University Press, Oxford

Folkman S, Greer S 2000 Psychological wellbeing in the face of serious illness when theory, research and practice inform each other. Psycho-oncology 9: 11–19

Gamlin R 2001 Palliative nursing: past, present and future. In: Kinghorn S, Gamlin R (eds) Palliative nursing – bringing comfort and hope. Baillière Tindall, Edinburgh

Gibbs G 1988 Learning by doing: a guide to teaching and learning methods. Further Education Unit, Oxford

Heaven C 1995 Communication skills in palliative care. The Cancer Research Campaign, Psychological Medicine Group, Christie Hospital, Manchester

Herbst L H 1996 Prognosis in advanced pulmonary disease. Journal of Palliative Care 12(2): 54–56

Hockley J, Clark D (eds) 2002 Palliative care for older people in care homes. Open University Press, Buckingham

Hoskin P, Makin W 2003 Oncology for palliative medicine, 2nd edn. Oxford Medical Publications, Oxford University Press, Oxford

Houldin A D 2000 Patients with cancer: understanding the psychological pain. Lippincott, Williams and Wilkins, Philadelphia

Jenkins C, Bruera E 1998 Conflict between families and staff. In: Bruera E, Portenoy R K (eds) Topics in palliative care. Oxford University Press, New York, Vol 2

Kinghorn S 2001 Communication in advanced illness. In: Kinghorn S, Gamlin R (eds) Palliative nursing – bringing comfort and hope. Baillière Tindall, Edinburgh

Leach R 2004 Palliative medicine and

non-malignant end stage respiratory disease. In: Doyle D, Hanks G, Cherny N et al (eds) Oxford textbook of palliative medicine, 3rd edn. Oxford University Press, Oxford
Lefebvre-Chapiro S 2001 The DOLOPLUS 2 scale – evaluating pain in the elderly. European Journal of Palliative Care 8(5): 191–194
Lothian NHS Board 2004 Lothian palliative care guidelines. NHS Lothian, Edinburgh
Mannix K A 2004 Gastrointestinal symptoms. In: Doyle D, Hanks G W C, Cherny N et al (eds) Oxford textbook of palliative medicine, 3rd edn. Oxford University Press, Oxford
McCaffery M, Pasero C (eds) 1999 Assessment. In: Pain: clinical manual, 2nd edn. Mosby, St Louis
McGoldrick M, Gerson R 1985 Genograms in family assessment. Norton, New York
McIllmurray M 2004 Palliative medicine in the treatment of cancer. In: Doyle D, Hanks G W C, Cherny N et al (eds) Oxford textbook of palliative medicine, 3rd edn. Oxford University Press, Oxford
Murray Parkes C, Relf M, Couldrick A 1996 Counselling in terminal care and bereavement. British Psychological Society, Leicester
Nursing and Midwifery Council (NMC) 2004 Code of professional conduct. NMC, London
O'Neill B, Fallon M 1998 Principles of palliative care pain control. In: Fallon M, O'Neill B (eds) ABC of palliative care. BMJ Books, London
Portenoy R K, Forbes K, Lussier D et al 2004 Difficult pain problems: an integrated approach. In: Doyle D, Hanks G W C, Cherny N et al (eds) Oxford textbook of palliative medicine, 3rd edn. Oxford University Press, Oxford
Regnard C, Comiskey M 1995 Nausea and vomiting. In: Regnard C, Hockley J (eds) Flow diagrams in advanced cancer and other diseases. Edward Arnold, London
Regnard C, Hockley J 2004 A guide to symptom relief in palliative care, 5th edn. Radcliffe Medical Press, Abingdon
Roy D 1998 Editorial. The relief of pain and suffering: ethical principles and imperatives. Journal of Palliative Care 14(2): 3–5
Scottish Intercollegiate Guidelines Network 2000 Control of pain in patients with cancer, a national clinical guideline (SIGN 44). Online. Available: www.sign.ac.uk
Sepulveda C, Marlin A, Yoshida T et al 2002 Palliative care: The World Health Organization's global perspective. Journal of Pain and Symptom Management 24(2): 91–96
Shee C D 1995 Palliation in chronic respiratory disease. Palliative Medicine 9: 3–12
Shee C D 2001 Respiratory disease. In: Addington-Hall J M, Higginson I J (eds) Palliative care for non-cancer patients. Oxford University Press, Oxford
Smeltzer S C, Bare B G 2003 Brunner and Suddarth's textbook of medical surgical nursing, 10th edn. Lippincott, Philadelphia
Stein-Parbury J 2000 Patient and person, 2nd edn. Harcourt, Sydney
Sweeney C, Neuenschwander H, Bruera E 2004 Fatigue and asthenia. In: Doyle D, Hanks G, Cherny N et al (eds) Oxford textbook of palliative medicine, 3rd edn. Oxford University Press, Oxford
Sykes N P 2004 Constipation and diarrhoea. In: Doyle D, Hanks G, Cherny N et al (eds) Oxford textbook of palliative medicine, 3rd edn. Oxford University Press, Oxford
Syrett E, Taylor J 2003 Non-pharmacological management of breathlessness: a collaborative nurse–physiotherapist approach. International Journal of Palliative Nursing 9(4): 150–156
Twycross R 1999 Guidelines for the management of nausea and vomiting. Palliative Care Today VII(IV): 32–34
Twycross R, Back I 1998 Nausea and vomiting in advanced cancer. European Journal of Palliative Care 5(2): 39–45
Twycross R, Wilcock A 2001 Symptom management in advanced cancer, 3rd edn. Radcliffe Medical Press, Abingdon
Vallerand A H 1997 Measurement issues in the comprehensive assessment of cancer pain. Seminars in Oncology Nursing 13(1): 16–24
White T 1995 Dealing with constipation. Nursing Times 91(14): 57–60
Worden J W 2003 Grief counselling and grief therapy, 3rd edn. Brunner-Routledge, Hove
World Health Organization 1986 Cancer pain relief. WHO, Geneva
World Health Organization 1996 Cancer pain relief with a guide to opioid availability, 2nd edn. WHO, Geneva

FURTHER READING

Davy J, Ellis S 2000 Counselling skills in palliative care. Cromwell Press, Trowbridge
Faull C, Woof R 2002 Palliative care. Oxford University Press, Oxford
Kinghorn S, Gamlin R (eds) 2001 Palliative nursing – bringing comfort and hope. Baillière Tindall, Edinburgh
Lothian NHS Board 2004 Lothian palliative care guidelines. NHS Lothian, Edinburgh
Mannix K A 2004 Gastrointestinal symptoms. In: Doyle D, Hanks G W C, Cherny N et al (eds) Oxford textbook of palliative medicine 3rd edn. Oxford University Press, Oxford
Randall F, Downie R S 1999 Palliative care ethics, a good companion, 2nd edn. Oxford Medical Publications, Oxford University Press, Oxford
Regnard C, Hockley J 2004 A guide to symptom relief in palliative care, 5th edn. Radcliffe Medical Press, Abingdon
Ripamonti C, Mercadente S 2004 Pathophysiology and management of malignant bowel obstruction. In: Doyle D, Hanks G W C, Cherny N et al (eds) Oxford textbook of palliative medicine, 3rd edn. Oxford University Press, Oxford
Scottish Intercollegiate Guidelines Network 2000 Control of pain in patients with cancer, a national clinical guideline (SIGN 44). Online. Available: www.sign.ac.uk
Sykes N P 2004 Constipation and diarrhoea. In: Doyle D, Hanks G W C, Cherny N et al (eds) Oxford textbook of palliative medicine, 3rd edn. Oxford University Press, Oxford
Twycross R, Wilcock A 2001 Symptom management in advanced cancer, 3rd edn. Radcliffe Medical Press, Abingdon

USEFUL WEBSITES

Palliative care formulary
www.palliativedrugs.com

South East Scotland Cancer Network (SCAN)
www.scan.scot.nhs.uk

THE PATIENT IN NEED OF REHABILITATION

34

Glynis Pellatt

INTRODUCTION

This chapter will address the rehabilitation requirements of two categories of patient: those in whom some recovery is expected, the aim being to achieve optimal improvement in function by applying specific therapeutic techniques, and those with progressive and chronic conditions where more emphasis is placed on social, psychological and environmental factors than on specific interventions (Nolan et al 1997).

Rehabilitation is an issue of considerable political and health care team interest, both nationally and internationally (DH 2001a, WHO 2001). The National Service Framework for Older People (DH 2001a) requires effective rehabilitation services, with nurses playing a pivotal role within the interprofessional team and it has been argued (Edwards 2002) that the scope for the nursing contribution to rehabilitation has widened considerably. Although Henderson's (1966) assertion that nurses are 'rehabilitators par excellence' has often been quoted to support the view that nurses have a unique role in rehabilitation care, Nolan et al (1997) consider that nursing has not yet fulfilled its potential in the field of rehabilitation. Pre- and post-registration nurse education should enable nurses to develop the competencies that will enable them to reach their potential within the rehabilitation setting (Low 2003). This chapter aims to address competency in rehabilitation nursing by presenting general principles that nurses can apply to a range of practice situations.

Evidence-based practice

Evidence-based knowledge about illness and disability is necessary to enable patients to take an active part in their care and to enable health care professionals to develop appropriate care interventions (DH 1996). It is both ethically and professionally desirable that nursing care is based on current, research-based and accessible information. The Nursing and Midwifery Council's *Code of Professional Conduct* (2004, para. 6.5) states: 'You have a responsibility to deliver care based on current evidence, best practice and, where applicable, validated research when it is available'. Therefore nurses are required to be research-minded to enable them to evaluate current health care research and implement the findings in their practice.

What is rehabilitation?

There are many definitions of rehabilitation, but little agreement on any one definitive definition. Rehabilitation has been defined as being concerned with the restoration of an individual's social, physical and emotional functions and abilities to their prior level (Gibbon 1992). Other definitions view rehabilitation as enabling an individual to reach the optimal level of functioning they are able or motivated to achieve (Davis & O'Connor 1999, Edwards 2002). Chamberlain (1997) has suggested that whereas disability limits choice, rehabilitation can restore choice to a disabled person. However, it has to be recognised that not all patients can achieve full recovery as many have complex health problems which will prevent this from happening. Wade (2002) points out that rehabilitation is a way of thinking rather than a way of doing. Barnes and Ward (2000) suggest that rehabilitation is an individual, active and dynamic process, the basic nature of which is to work with a disabled person and the family in a partnership. O'Kelly (1997), who suffered a stroke at a relatively early age, and while fully involved in his professional career, states:

> *Rehabilitation is an active process in which disabled people work together with professional staff, relatives and members of the wider community, to achieve their optimum physical, psychological, social and vocational well-being.*

CASE HISTORY 34.1
Mrs J

Mrs J is a 35-year-old woman who has been newly diagnosed with multiple sclerosis. She has two children at junior school. Her husband is a lorry driver. She works as a waitress in a café. Her most prominent problem is fatigue and muscle weakness that gets worse as the day progresses, but is relieved by rest. She is keen to return to work as soon as possible.

Rehabilitation should therefore focus on helping patients achieve their own goals (see Case History 34.1). Smith (1999a) suggests that the aims and characteristics of rehabilitation are as follows:

- Reduction of disability and handicap
- Independence
- Empowerment
- Problem solving
- Client centredness
- 'Holistic' approach
- Educational process.

The approach to a patient with an acute illness differs from the approach to the care of a patient with a chronic illness. This is because a chronic illness places new demands on patients, which may limit their self-care abilities (Neal 2001) (see also Ch. 32). However, the individual who survives an acute illness may experience disability and chronic ill health. For example, a person who has a stroke may experience three different care environments — emergency, acute and rehabilitation — each with a different intervention focus (Burton 2000a). In an acute care setting, a major focus of the nurse's role is the physical care of the patient. As rehabilitation progresses, nurses steadily and intentionally reduce the physical care provided. However, they simultaneously increase the team's emotional and psychological support as the patient copes with the process of rehabilitation (Sheppard 1994).

In recent years, there has been a shift towards a more patient-centred approach to rehabilitation. This philosophy advocates patient autonomy and independence with patients empowered to be actively involved in their care (Preston 1994, Wilson 2000). In this patient-centred philosophy the individual becomes the expert in taking control of and managing their own care. Goal planning has been seen as a way of increasing patients' involvement in rehabilitation (Duff et al 1999, Playford et al 2000). It is a part of the care process that involves both the interprofessional team and the patient in identifying the patient's needs. Both parties negotiate and establish goals based on individual need (Kennedy et al 1996).

STOP THINK **34.1** Review Case History 34.1 and reflect on what the nurse's role would be in supporting this patient in her desire to return to work. Discuss this with your mentor on your community placement.

Who needs rehabilitation?

Rehabilitation skills are inherent in evidence-based nursing practice and have been described for specific conditions elsewhere in this book. The purpose of this chapter is to focus on those patients whose health condition causes continuing disability and consequent activity limitations.

World Health Organization international classification of functioning, disability and health (ICF)

In May 2001, the World Health Assembly approved a new international classification of functioning, disability and health (ICF) (WHO 2001). In contrast to the previous WHO international classification of impairments, disabilities and handicaps (WHO 1980), which focused narrowly on the impact and consequences of disease and, according to Gray (2001), suggested a linear causal relationship among these three consequences, the ICF takes a multiperspective approach and provides 'a classification of people's health characteristics, within the context of their individual life situations and environmental impacts' (WHO 2001). The ICF has two parts, each with two components (see Fig. 34.1):

- Part One deals with functioning and disability. The term 'functioning' encompasses all body functions and structures, activities and participation, whereas the term 'disability' encompasses impairments of body functions and structures, activity limitations and participation restrictions. The ICF points out that the term 'impairment' does not necessarily mean a disease is present. It is a broader and more inclusive term, e.g. the loss of a limb is an impairment of body structure but is not a disease.
- Part Two deals with environmental factors, e.g. the physical, social and attitudinal environment for each individual, and with personal factors, e.g. gender, race, culture, age and lifestyle. These factors combine to

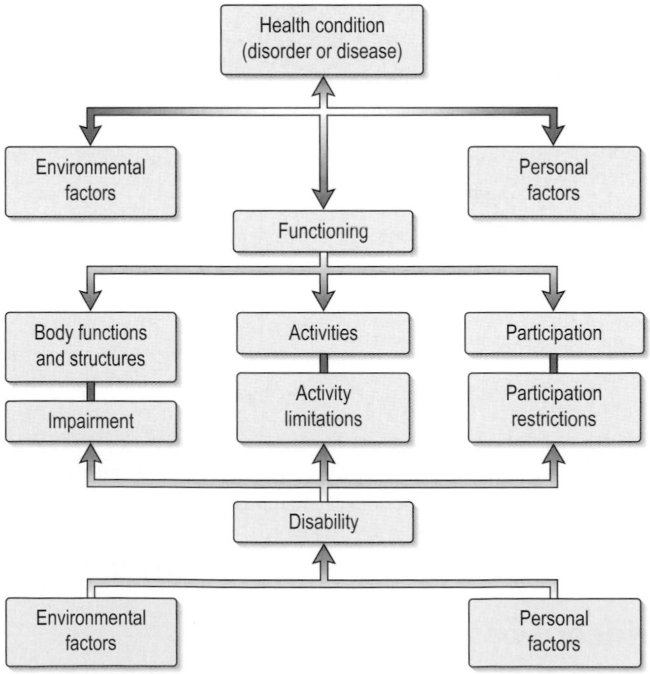

Fig. 34.1 Interactions between the components of the international classification of functioning, disability and health. (Adapted from WHO 2001, with permission.)

constitute the all-important context in which individuals live with their health condition, and which impacts on all aspects of their functioning and disability.

The ICF (WHO 2001) was designed in an attempt to find a common language with which to code and classify functioning, disability and health, and thus permit international comparisons. More than 50 countries took part in its compilation, including people with disabilities and related organisations, leading to a feeling of 'ownership' by all its users. Through its use, the World Health Organization hopes that disability advocacy will be fostered and more interventions will be identified which can improve levels of participation. It is acknowledged (WHO 2001) that more research is needed to evaluate the application of the ICF to practice, and Grimby and Smedby (2001) suggest various ways in which this could be fruitfully explored.

For more detail on the ICF, and examples of the application of ICF concepts to individuals (Annex 4), see WHO (2001).

THE PSYCHOLOGY OF DISABILITY

The effects of illness and disability on the psychological status of a patient may be intense. As nurses are with the patient 24 h per day, they are in a unique position to observe and assess a patient's behaviour and to provide first line psychological support (Thomas 1999, Pellatt 2003) (see Research Abstract 34.1). To enable nurses to carry out this important role, an understanding of the psychology of disability will provide the basis for the sustained therapeutic relationship which is crucial in the rehabilitation process. By being aware of the psychological responses of individuals to trauma and disability, nurses can differentiate between what is an expected or normal response and that which requires referral to a professional with different, more developed skills (Tripp 1999).

RESEARCH ABSTRACT 34.1

Perceptions of the nursing role in spinal cord injury rehabilitation

One section within a large ethnographic study (Pellatt 2003) aimed to identify how nurses and patients perceived the nursing role in spinal cord injury rehabilitation. Semi-structured interviews were carried out with 14 spinal cord injured patients and 14 registered nurses from a large spinal cord injury unit. Patients had a range of levels of injuries and were either in the rehabilitation stages of being a new injury or had been injured for some years. The nurses had been qualified for at least a year, had undertaken a post-registration course in the specialty and had a role in decision-making processes as named nurses and/or key workers.

The findings suggest that patients value the nursing contribution as a means of emotional and physical support, but that they do not necessarily see nursing input as rehabilitation. Nurses see their role as multifaceted, but identify difficulties in crossing over from an acute care philosophy to a rehabilitation philosophy.

The implications for practice are that the roles and responsibilities of nurses should be more clearly defined for patients. Nurses need to develop self-awareness and explore ways of working that empower patients to make decisions about their care.

Pellatt G 2003 Perceptions of the nursing role in spinal cord injury rehabilitation. British Journal of Nursing 12(5): 292–299

Stigma

The concept of stigma is an important factor in the consideration of the social situation of people with disabilities. An appreciation of the dynamics of a stigmatised illness can help nurses understand the social and psychological aspects of their patients' lives. Originally, the term stigma referred to physical blemishes, which were perceived by the ancient Greeks to signify something unusual or bad about the moral status of an individual (Sim 1990). Goffman's seminal work (1968) describes stigma with reference to an individual deemed to be socially unacceptable due to a failing or handicap, which marks them out as a tainted person. There are two types of stigmata — those that are immediately apparent to others, such as the use of a wheelchair or obvious scarring, and those that are not immediately visible or apparent to others, such as epilepsy. The stigmatised person is perceived to deviate from what society regards as normal (Faugier & Sargeant 1997). People without stigma may generalise from a particular disability to an assortment of disabilities or imperfections. This may lead to people speaking to a person in a wheelchair as if that person does not understand, to shout at someone who is blind or to speak to the companion of a person with a disability rather than to the person with the disability (Joachim & Acorn 2000). In many countries and cultures, physical appearance affects how people feel about themselves and also how others perceive them. People with chronic illness or disability may have conditions that alter their appearance, e.g. a person who has suffered a hemiplegic stroke. Others may have a change in appearance that, although not immediately visual to others, is felt by them to be stigmatising, such as a colostomy.

Stigma has also been viewed in terms of dependency. Illness may mean that an individual is in the dependent position of receiving care without being able to contribute in return (Sim 1990).

Some people with a disability have argued that their contact with nurses and other health care professionals tends to be disabling. French (1994) pointed out that research findings on whether the attitudes of health professionals towards stigmatised individuals are more or less positive than those of the general public tend to conflict. However, the weight of evidence suggests that the attitudes of health care professionals are not very different from those of the general public and may become more negative as professional education proceeds. Scullion (1999), in a study of student nurses, found that disability was conceptualised as a form of deviation, a condition of dependency or a concept that was difficult to define.

It is important that nurses realise that patients' self-concept reflects the reactions of others to them. Negative attitudes held by nurses towards stigmatised groups can adversely affect their care. Contact with chronically ill or disabled patients may give rise to a variety of emotions but how these emotions are displayed will impact on the patient's care. Expression of distaste will be hurtful, and pity may be perceived as patronising and reinforce the person's sense of inferiority. Professional detachment may lessen rapport and accentuate the social distance experienced by the stigmatised person (Sim 1990). To avoid this, Lucke (1999) has identified that nurses and other health care professionals need to be committed to forming caring relationships with patients. A caring relationship is one in which professionals share their knowledge and experience with patients, thus communicating respect and value for the patient.

Grief

The impact of sudden disability has been described as similar to that of bereavement. In her seminal text, Kubler-Ross (1969) described a model of grief that encompassed five interdependent emotional stages:

- Denial
- Anger
- Bargaining
- Depression
- Acceptance.

This model has also been adopted for describing the stages that individuals undergo when they experience a severe illness or disability (Wilson & Fletcher 2002). However, it is important to recognise that the five stages may occur simultaneously, may overlap, or may not occur at all. It is also important to be aware that an individual's cultural background and religious beliefs will influence reactions to loss and grief (Holland & Hogg 2001).

Morse (1997) has developed a five stage model, *Responding to Threats to Integrity of Self*, which describes a person's responses to illness or injury. The theory is one of recovery and rehabilitation. The stages are as follows:

- *Vigilance* — where the individual suspects that something is wrong: a feeling of dis-ease or illness or the checking for the extent of injury after an accident
- *Disruption* — where the individual attempts to hold on to life, i.e. enduring to survive
- *Enduring to live* — where the individual develops strategies to help bear the pain, maintain control and gradually consider the implications of the injury or illness, i.e. striving to regain self
- *Suffering* — where the individual begins to struggle with grief, what has been lost and the altered future, i.e. striving to restore self
- *Learning to live with the altered self* — where the individual learns to live with the changes that have occurred, such as paralysis, an amputation or fatigue.

Nurses have an important role to play in helping patients as they go through the stages of grief and adapt to change. It is vital that nurses facilitate both the setting and achievement of goals by the patient. Rehabilitation should focus on what the patients can achieve, not on what they cannot do, but at the same time should recognise each patient's own limits. Nurses can empower patients by enabling them to recognise new possibilities (Wade G 1998). For example, patients in Lucke's (1999) study identified that caring nurses and therapists created an atmosphere in which they were able to identify that they were still able to have meaningful relationships with their partners and children despite having a disability. A Swedish study of people with muscular dystrophy identified that participants trusted rehabilitation staff whom they perceived to be supportive, committed and knowledgeable. This enabled them to develop problem-solving skills and to capitalise on the things that they were able to do (Natterlund & Ahlstrom 1999).

Stress and coping

Stress is discussed in depth in Chapter 17.

People use different strategies to cope with stress. According to Engel (1964) stress caused by illness and injury may be due to:

- loss or threat of loss of anything that is of great importance to an individual
- real or threatened injury to the body
- frustration of drives.

How an individual copes with the demands of illness or injury depends on the method used to cope with stress (Groomes & Leahey 2002). The most common ways of coping are:

- *problem focused*, where people with disabilities collect information about treatments or take action such as modifying the house to enable wheelchair access
- *emotion focused*, where people with disabilities aim to reduce the impact of the stress response by controlling their emotions or conversely venting frustration, anger or despair; the individual may exhibit resigned acceptance or coming to terms with the disability
- *avoidance*, where people with disabilities focus on small, manageable components of a situation or focus on the perception that there are others worse off than them.

Research has suggested that an individual's ability to set flexible but durable goals will influence their psychological adjustment to physical disability (Brillhart & Johnson 1997, Elliott et al 2000). However, the loss of control experienced by people with chronic illness and disability may cause anxiety and depression (Kennedy et al 2003). This may in turn lead to helplessness and dependency (Mahat 1997) (see Case History 34.2), which may be factors in the motivation of patients to participate in their rehabilitation (Maclean & Pound 2000).

CASE HISTORY 34.2

Mr S

Mr S is 75 years old and has suffered a stroke that has left him with a left-sided weakness. He has been admitted to a rehabilitation unit from an acute ward and has expressed surprise that he is expected to participate in his own care as the nurses in the other ward did everything for him.

34.2 Review Case History 34.2. Consider the role of the nurse in enabling Mr S to understand the rehabilitation process and to participate as a partner with the nursing staff.

The rehabilitation team has an important role to play in supporting patients as they work through the psychological processes associated with disability and chronic illness. They need to be positive, encouraging and willing to empower patients to become actively involved in their rehabilitation. Nurses need to be aware that they may inadvertently encourage patients to adopt a passive role by doing things for them in order to complete their care more quickly (Maclean et al 2000). For the person with disability, social support supplied by family and friends acts as a buffer against the stressors caused by the disability (Davidhizar 1997). The supportive role of the patient's family and friends, and the support that they need to undertake that role, should be recognised and facilitated by the rehabilitation staff.

RESEARCH ABSTRACT 34.2

The nursing role in stroke rehabilitation

A study undertaken by Burton (2002b) describes the nursing role in stroke rehabilitation and three factors which shape that role. The method used was reflective enquiry to collect data that were grounded in the realities of clinical practice. The study took place in a 24-bedded rehabilitation unit, and 13 qualified nursing staff participated by completing reflective accounts of clinical incidents that had been important to them. A total of 35 incidents were collected for analysis.

Three role categories were identified: the nurse as care giver; the nurse as facilitator of personal recovery, which involved helping, comforting, teaching and working with the patient and family; and the nurse as manager of multidisciplinary provision.

The findings suggest that nurses have a key role in stroke rehabilitation but need to build on and develop new partnerships with patients and carers.

Burton C 2000b A description of the nursing role in stroke rehabilitation. Journal of Advanced Nursing 32(1): 174–181

THE PROCESS OF REHABILITATION

The interprofessional team

It has been recognised that an interprofessional team approach to rehabilitation is more effective than when individuals work in isolation or as a unidisciplinary group (Seaman 1999). Evans et al (1995) argue that patients who receive an interprofessional rehabilitation service are more likely to survive, have greater functional ability and have a better chance of returning home than those who do not. An interprofessional team brings together separate but interlinked professional skills. Team members share a common goal and common objectives and work together to achieve that goal (Engel 1994). The membership of the interprofessional team may vary considerably; however, a successful team is thought to have five important attributes (Miller et al 1999):

- A central purpose that transcends disciplinary boundaries
- All members understand each other's roles and recognise where roles overlap
- Members appreciate other disciplines' knowledge — how it is gained and used
- Members value different perspectives, can accept changes in authority and status and are willing to accept challenges
- Members are able to resolve conflict by understanding the difference between accountability and responsibility of different team members and knowing what is expected of them.

The skills required by a rehabilitation team will vary depending on the needs of the person with a disability. However, the core skills required by all teams will include assessment and management of impaired physical mobility, dexterity, communication, eating and swallowing, cognition, continence, tissue viability and emotional well-being, as well as counselling skills. Medical knowledge of diagnosis, prognosis, drug treatment and its complications must be readily accessible. In addition, team members need team-related skills such as communication, good information recording, public relations, teaching, evaluation and monitoring of outcomes, and research and development (Harvey 1997) (see Research Abstract 34.2).

It has been suggested that rehabilitation programmes aim to change an individual's behaviour in ways that support improved physical, social and psychological functioning (Kennedy & Hamilton 1999). It could be argued that the identification and setting of appropriate goals is one of the skills that characterises rehabilitation professionals (Wade D 1998). Goal planning involves all members of the interprofessional team. In the first stage of the process the patient and the named nurse together complete a needs assessment checklist. This checklist is composed of benchmarks for quality of care and expectations of independence. Categories of assessed need include activities of daily living, bladder, bowel and skin management as well as social and psychological issues (Duff et al 1999). By using a needs assessment and goal planning approach to rehabilitation, patients are able to think about their personal needs and therefore increase their involvement in and control over the rehabilitation process. It also enables staff to recognise what the key issues are for a particular patient. It is important, when assessing the category of independence, that no distinction is made between verbal and physical independence, so as to enable all patients to have the potential to achieve 100% independence. Even if unable to achieve a task physically, if patients are able to instruct others how to do it for them, they are considered verbally independent.

When using a needs assessment and goal planning programme, the patient is allocated a key worker who can come from any professional discipline in the team. The key worker coordinates the goal planning meetings and works with the patient and the interprofessional team to establish and identify needs, clarify goals and set targets. Goal planning meetings normally take place every 2–3 weeks, with the goals being reviewed and additional goals set. As confidence in the process is gained, the patient is able to take over from the key worker and coordinate the process for themselves (Foley 1998).

In the community, the concept of 'need' was central to the implementation of the NHS and Community Care Act (DH 1990). Professional groups were required to develop systems for needs assessment that promoted the views of the client. This has meant, for example, that community nursing services are responsible for the development of appropriate methods of identifying clients at risk or in need of intervention (Carney et al 1996). However, whichever tools are used to assess need, it is vital that assessment is not seen as a single event (Cowley et al 1996) and that the views of clients and their carers are taken into account (Tranter & Sullivan 1996).

Outcome of the rehabilitation process

There has been considerable emphasis by professionals on the attainment of the physical goals of rehabilitation. Where they are appropriate, physical goals are important and there are several quantitative tests available to measure functional outcomes. It has been suggested that the financial climate of health care requires both efficient and effective rehabilitation that has measurable outcomes. Functional gain is an easily observable indicator of successful rehabilitation (Nolan & Nolan 1998). However, these functional measurements have been criticised as being generically applied to all patients, without taking account of the context in which the patient's rehabilitation is taking place. The implication of this is that they can be used across many settings with no consideration being given to the meaning in context of the functional outcomes for the individual patient (Williams 1996). For example, although a patient may be able to get dressed in the morning in the hospital setting, it may take them so long to dress unaided once they are at home that they are unable to get to their place of work on time. This will prevent the individual from earning a living and force them to rely on benefits.

In addition, reliance on functional outcomes which do not address the value of qualitative aspects of people's lives, such as satisfying and meaningful relationships, suggests that people with severe disability have less potential than those with less disability.

Rehabilitation is therefore concerned with both qualitative and quantitative aspects of life. It involves not only preventing complications, but also providing therapy and, for example, the fitting of adaptive equipment, and psychological assessment and counselling (Glass 1999, Thomas 1999).

ROLES

The role of the patient

Patients should be regarded as co-workers in the rehabilitation process and their contribution should be regarded as equally important as that of health care professionals (McLeod 1995, DH 2001b). One of the patient-focused outcomes in the government's document *Essence of Care* (DH 2001c) is that patients have control over their own health care. This document provides benchmarks for best practice, one of which states that 'patients/clients and practitioners are working in partnership to establish their responsibilities in meeting self-care needs'.

The notion of patients having expertise in the management of their conditions has been encouraged by the government in its document *The Expert Patient: A New Approach for Chronic Disease Management for the 21st Century* (DH 2001b). The aim is to enable individuals with chronic illness to self-manage their illness, based on empowerment and assertiveness. However, there is conflicting evidence about patients' expectations of their role in the rehabilitation process. In some studies, patients did not expect to be involved actively in the planning and implementation of rehabilitation (Sheppard 1994, Abbott 1999). Other studies suggest that patients do recognise the importance of their own role in rehabilitation (David 1995, Brillhart & Johnson 1997). Proot et al (2002) suggest that patients use the strategies of 'taking responsibility' and 'initiative' to facilitate their autonomy in the rehabilitation process, encompassing:

- cooperation
- anticipating
- problem solving
- taking stock of the situation
- investing own effort
- refusing, i.e. deciding to decline.

Lucke (1999) cites patients with spinal cord injury who see being able to take charge of rehabilitation as an outcome of good relationships between themselves and rehabilitation team members.

It is important that health care professionals recognise the fact that rehabilitation may be hard work for patients. Patients have described rehabilitation as a mental and physical struggle (Sheppard 1994, Maclean et al 2000). In a Canadian study of spinal cord injured patients, the rehabilitation phase was described by patients as doing 'hard labour in jail' (Carpenter 1994) (see Box 34.1). However, there are strategies that health care professionals can use to enhance the rehabilitation experience for patients by enabling them to take control of the process, such as:

- providing information
- supporting patients in activities of living (ALs), e.g. dressing
- promoting mobility
- communicating with patients
- guarding against a paternalistic approach
- enhancing patient choice
- working in partnership with patients and their families.

By adopting these strategies the rehabilitation team can challenge patients to solve their own problems and act in a more consultative role (Proot et al 2002) (see Case History 34.3).

The role of the nurse

The role of the nurse in rehabilitation has suffered from a lack of clarity. However, the role is multifaceted and Long et al (2001) (see Research Abstract 34.3) have identified six core elements:

- Assessment
- Coordination and communication

Box 34.1

An experience of rehabilitation

It was a lovely hot sunny day. The sea looked so inviting. I was 16 and on holiday with my Mum, Dad and younger brother. There was a causeway jutting out into the sea and my brother and I had been jumping into the water from it all day. However, this time I must have jumped differently, as I went into the sea head-first. I felt my head hit the sand and felt a crack in my neck. I couldn't move, I couldn't feel anything, I thought I was going to drown. Luckily my brother realised something was wrong and screamed to my Mum and Dad who were nearby. They and some other people dragged me out of the water and called an ambulance. I was taken to the local hospital where they diagnosed a fracture/dislocation of my sixth and seventh cervical vertebrae. This left me with limited use in my arms and no sensation or movement in my trunk and legs. They applied skull traction to my head to keep the spine still. At that time I don't think I really realised what had happened to me; I remember Mum being in tears and that I had tubes and things in me but that's about all.

Soon afterwards I was transferred to a spinal cord injury centre. It was here that the impact of what had happened hit me. The staff were very honest with us about the fact that I was unlikely to recover any more movement or sensation. They were very supportive and explained everything that they did to me in those early stages. I was shattered. I couldn't see any future for me. All around me were people in wheelchairs so it soon dawned on me that this was how things would be. However, I found it very comforting to have people in a similar situation beside me — they were experiencing similar feelings and could tell me what it was like to go through the different stages of rehabilitation.

I was kept on bed rest for 10 weeks, during which time I had physiotherapy and the occupational therapist made splints for my hands to prevent them contracting up. Then a collar was made for me and I was ready to get up in a wheelchair for the first time. I was so excited as I had seen other patients whizzing about in their wheelchairs. The nurses got me up in the wheelchair and stayed with me, but I was so disappointed. I felt terrible, so weak and dizzy. I was put back into bed after 20 min. However, gradually I got up for longer periods of time. I went to physiotherapy and occupational therapy. I had hydrotherapy, which was really scary at first as I kept remembering being in the water, unable to move or breathe. It was incredibly hard work and sometimes I felt so tired, but I was determined to work as hard as possible so that I could get home. I practised what I had learnt in the departments and with the nurses on the ward. I gradually got stronger and stronger until I was able to wash and dress. I had a suprapubic catheter to prevent urinary incontinence and I learned to manage my bowels. All the staff pushed and encouraged me, and made sure I and my family learned as much about my condition as possible so that we could teach others when I went home.

In the meantime some alterations had been carried out on our house, which luckily was a bungalow, so that when I was discharged home I was able to get into my bedroom and the bathroom. When I went home I was able to manage most things for myself, but I had a district nurse who looked after my catheter and was there if we needed anything, from equipment to advice. I knew I could always contact the spinal unit and attended outpatients for check-ups. I went back to school and got my 'A' levels and I then went to university and got my degree. I also learned to drive, so I drive an adapted car with hand controls.

I now work as a journalist on a local newspaper. I have moved into my own adapted flat. In my spare time I play wheelchair rugby, although I don't think I'll make the Olympic team! I have a great circle of friends that I go out with to pubs and clubs. I have been very lucky in having a supportive family who have let me do things at my own pace and did not try and cushion me from the realities of living in the world with a disability. They have always been there for me.

CASE HISTORY 34.3

S

S is 18 years old and has sustained a fracture of her 7th cervical vertebra resulting in limited arm function and no sensation or movement in her legs. She has been learning how to transfer from her wheelchair on to the toilet using a lateral transfer board (sliding board) with a physiotherapist. It is the weekend and she wishes to practise the technique before her next physiotherapy session on Monday.

STOP THINK **34.3** Review Case History 34.3 and consider the role of the nurse in helping S to practise what she has been taught in her therapy sessions.

- Technical and physical care
- Therapy integration and therapy 'carry-on', i.e. enabling patients to practise what they have learnt to do with therapists and giving them support and encouragement to undertake these tasks at weekends and evenings
- Emotional support
- Involving the family.

It should be noted that some nurses will undertake aspects of all these roles at any one time, whereas others may be involved in only one or two areas.

Assessment

Nurses will carry out an initial assessment from which the nursing care plan is developed. A range of models and frameworks is available to enable nurses to structure a holistic assessment of the patient's rehabilitation needs and goals, and to plan appropriate interventions to meet those needs and goals (Johnston 1996). However, the choice of model will be defined by the setting within which the rehabilitation nursing takes place. The most important aspect of whichever model is used is that of patient-centred care, partnership between patients and nurses being central to the delivery of effective rehabilitation. For example, Orem's (2001) model is widely used in rehabilitation settings to determine self-care activities and to assess activities that require nursing input that is wholly compensatory, partially compensatory or supportive of educational needs.

RESEARCH ABSTRACT 34.3

The role of the nurse in the rehabilitation team

This research aimed to explore how nurses identified the physical, social and emotional needs of patients and carers, and the nurse's desired and actual role in contributing to meeting those needs, from the perspective of the nurse, other professionals, patients and carers (Long et al 2001). The research also investigated pre- and post-registration education and development in preparing nurses for this role and keeping up to date in rehabilitation. Data were collected using a two-phase design:

1. an ethnographic study of three contrasting case study areas: fractured neck of femur, rheumatoid arthritis and stroke, to which 49 participants were recruited
2. national expert workshops with four groups: users, carers and carer organisations; nurses; interprofessional team members; and educationalists.

A comparative analysis of the nurse's role across the three case study areas suggested that the nurse's role in rehabilitation is dependent on the needs with which patients present. The nurse is often seen as someone who 'does for' a patient; however, nurses aimed to get patients to do things for themselves. Nurses sometimes felt that patients equated rehabilitation with therapy. Six core nursing roles were identified:

- *Assessment* — nurses performed an initial assessment from which the nursing care plan was devised and referrals to other team members made
- *Coordination and communication* — included gathering, synthesising and disseminating information, liaison, negotiation and discharge planning
- *Technical and physical care* — perceived as 'routine' roles by nurses and other team members
- *Therapy integration and therapy 'carry-on'* — involved creating an environment that was therapeutic and facilitated rehabilitation through addressing emotional, social and physical barriers to rehabilitation; it also involved the nurse building on the work of therapists
- *Emotional support* — where nurses assist patients to come to terms with, and understand the ramifications of, their condition
- *Involving the family* — nurses were often seen as the first port of call when seeking advice or information.

The authors found that nurses in rehabilitation settings felt undervalued and under-recognised as a specialty by their own profession. Their colleagues from other professions perceived nurses as being task orientated and disempowering in their approach to patient care. Nurses were often not able to attend team meetings and this affected team communication.

Pre-registration education was not considered as providing adequate preparation for a rehabilitation role and nurses felt that there was a need for better access to specific post-registration education to enable them to participate in the rehabilitation process.

The authors identified that nurses need to have a full understanding of the philosophy, models and principles that underpin rehabilitation. Rehabilitation therefore should be integrated into nursing education so that, on completion of their pre-registration education, nurses can work effectively in rehabilitation settings. They can subsequently develop specialist rehabilitation skills at post-registration level. Generic themes such as communication, coordinating care and problem solving could be taught interprofessionally. Work-based learning would enable the development of skills and knowledge pertinent to the local setting.

The authors conclude that to enable nurses to play their full role in rehabilitation, client expectations need to be modified by education, explanation and information from 'doing for' to 'helping you do it yourself'. They suggest that higher education institutions and service providers need to work in partnership to produce nurses who can provide a quality service and that there should be an interprofessional approach to rehabilitation education.

Long A, Kneafsey R, Ryan J et al 2001 Teamworking in rehabilitation: exploring the role of the nurse. The English National Board for Nursing, Midwifery and Health Visiting, London

If Orem's model of nursing is adopted, the assessment will include the patient's self-care requisites and 'basic conditioning factors'. Basic conditioning factors are both external and internal to the individual, such as age, developmental state, pattern of living and the availability and adequacy of resources. Because injury or chronic illness places many new and different demands on the patient, there may be a wide range of self-care limitations. The assessment should cover a wide range of areas and be undertaken in partnership with the patient (Burks 1999, Orem 2001).

Coordination and communication

Nurses are present with patients 24 hours a day, 7 days a week, and therefore there is considerable scope for nurses to coordinate the functions of the multidisciplinary team (Aylett & Fawcett 2003). The involvement of multiple personnel and departments means that that there is a need to prevent fragmentation so that the care the patient receives is as integrated as possible (Johnson 1995). Nurses are able to provide information relating to a patient's progress, coping and emotional health (Burton 2000b) (see Research Abstract 34.3). Nurses can clarify goals and promote decision making as part of their coordinating role. However, this role requires a detailed knowledge of interprofessional working. It also requires a high level of communication skills, diplomacy and assertiveness. Rehabilitation nurses also need to have knowledge of service delivery systems to enable them to carry out this role (Nolan & Nolan 1998).

The need to cover a 24-h service means that nurses have to work shifts and this can impede communication, as team meetings to discuss a patient's progress are often arranged for the Monday–Friday, 9am–5pm work pattern (Pellatt

2003). Low (2003) points out that if the team agrees that nurses are coordinators of patients' care, then nurses must be empowered to fulfil that role effectively (see Research Abstract 34.3).

Technical and physical care

Within this role, nurses are described by Kirkevold (1997) as conserving function. This entails maintaining normal functions, preventing complications and trauma, and meeting the patient's basic needs such as personal hygiene and elimination.

Nolan and Nolan (1998) have identified the knowledge that nurses need in order to deliver skilled physical care as:

- detailed knowledge of physiology, related anatomy and pathology of relevant conditions, e.g. stroke and multiple sclerosis
- knowledge of normal anatomy and physiology
- knowledge of a range of therapeutic interventions
- knowledge of a range of measurement indices and their operational bases.

Technical skills required by nurses in rehabilitation settings, in both hospital and the community, cover a wide range, including all the activities of daily living. For example, a patient may require urinary catheterisation, administration of medication, wound dressing and management of nasogastric and percutaneous endoscopic gastrostomy (PEG) tubes to meet nutritional needs (Kneafsey et al 2003).

Key areas of concern in maintaining the physical and mental well-being of patients include those discussed below (Baillie 2001, Long et al 2001). Some require primarily the demonstration of practical skills by the nurse, whereas others require psychosocial skills or, more frequently, a blend of both.

Care of the skin A variety of pressure ulcer risk assessment scales is available (see Ch. 23). A benchmark of best practice, as outlined in the *Essence of Care* (DH 2001c), is that all patients identified as being at risk should undergo a screening process that progresses to further assessment. The patient in need of rehabilitation may have mobility problems and any neurological impairment will increase the risk of skin damage and pressure ulcer formation, particularly if sensation is poor or absent. There may also be psychological factors that will increase the risk of pressure ulcer development, e.g. the patient's coping strategy and the stage reached in adapting to the disability or illness (Graham 1997). The rehabilitation programme therefore needs to be tailored to the individual rather than the individual having to adjust to the rehabilitation programme. Pressure ulcers can have serious consequences and greatly impede the rehabilitation process, so effective preventive measures are essential. These measures include provision of a suitable support surface that does not impede mobility, use of correct moving and handling techniques, adequate nutrition, education, pain management and skin care (Pellatt 2001). The National Institute for Clinical Excellence (NICE) has published guidance on preventing pressure ulcers and the use of pressure-relieving devices (NICE 2003).

Continence There is a high incidence of continence problems in patients undergoing rehabilitation (Pellatt 2001). Assessment of mobility problems and the level of manual dexterity are important. Nurses should have knowledge about specialist services, such as those provided by a continence advisor and by support organisations, so that they can advise and refer patients as appropriate. Continence management requires careful assessment of each individual and knowledge of appropriate strategies and products. Continence care for the rehabilitation patient should be based on the best evidence available (Baillie & Arrowsmith 2001). A detailed discussion of continence can be found in Chapter 24.

Nutritional care A detailed discussion of nutrition can be found in Chapter 21. Rehabilitation patients may have a number of problems with eating, drinking and feeding themselves, due for example to paralysis, poor coordination or tremor. Patients may have an altered level of consciousness or may be suffering from severe fatigue. Conditions such as stroke may affect a patient's ability to swallow — dysphagia (Child & Higham 2001). Some patients may be unable to speak — aphasia — and therefore be unable to articulate their food preferences and/or cultural dietary requirements (Bowie 1999).

Hygiene Helping patients to wash and dress has been recognised as a fundamental function of the rehabilitation nurse (Pellatt 2003). Problems of paralysis, altered sensation and cognitive changes may affect the patient's ability to carry out this very personal aspect of care. The patient should be assisted to maintain their personal hygiene including oral hygiene and shaving. If the patient usually uses deodorants, aftershave or make-up, then helping to continue this routine will add to the patient's feeling of well-being and self-esteem (Major 2001).

Sexual health Sexuality encompasses a whole range of aspects of a person's life. It includes not just the sexual act but how a person dresses, behaves and interacts with others. An injury or chronic illness may impact on a person's sexual health, due to both physical and psychosocial limitations and barriers, but this does not mean, as is sometimes thought, that they are asexual beings (Smith 1999b). In the rehabilitation patient, alterations in sexual function may be due to any of the following:

- Impaired physical mobility — which may limit transfers on to a bed, cause difficulties in dressing or undressing, or in attending to personal hygiene
- Increased or decreased sensation — when sensation is altered, the pleasure derived from stimulation may not be perceived in some of the body's erogenous zones (Smith 1999b)
- Pain — which may limit positioning of the body and may cause depression
- Bowel and bladder incontinence — which causes embarrassment and worry
- Fatigue — one of the side-effects of brain injury, stroke, rheumatic disease and multiple sclerosis which may lead to lack of energy and enthusiasm for sex
- Changes in libido — some stroke patients, for example, experience decreased sexual interest

- Genital sexual dysfunction — patients with diabetes mellitus, spinal cord injury and multiple sclerosis may have erectile dysfunction or impotence (Astbury-Ward 2000)
- Decrease in fertility — men may suffer from decreased fertility due to a reduced sperm count after spinal cord injury and some brain injuries. Semen quality and motility are reduced secondary to recurrent urinary tract infections, elevated deep scrotal temperature (caused by the position of the legs when seated in a wheelchair), medication, prostatic fluid stasis, spermatozoan contact with urine due to retrograde ejaculation, testicular denervation and changes in seminal fluid due to endocrine abnormalities (Sipski & Alexander 1992, McDonald & Sadowsky 2002, Naderi & Safarinejad 2003)
- Medication — analgesics, used for treating pain, that depress the central nervous system, antispasmodics, antihypertensives and some tranquillisers can cause a range of sexual problems (Greco 1996)
- For some patients, notions of self-worth and sense of identity focus on the dysfunctional or disfigured part of the body (Price 1996) to the detriment of their sexual health.

The rehabilitation nurse must be prepared to address sexuality and sexual health with patients on an individual basis. To do so effectively, knowledge and skills in counselling and intervention techniques are essential. Nurses require sensitivity to support patients as they work through their grief and anxieties and help them to find ways of focusing on other qualities, skills and personal appearance (Nolan & Nolan 1998).

Although it could be said that nurses, because of their 24-h care of the patient, are ideally placed to discuss sexual health with patients, Smith (1999b) argues that they are not fully addressing the rehabilitation patient's sexual health needs. However, nurses should be able to recognise where there is a need for a patient to receive specialist sexual health advice and discuss this with the patient and the rehabilitation team, prior to referral.

Therapy integration and therapy 'carry-on'

Nurses play an important role in reinforcing the input of therapists in rehabilitation by assisting the patient to incorporate the skills learned in episodic therapy sessions into the rest of their day. In so doing, nurses are able to assess progress on a 24-h basis and feed back information to the rehabilitation team. For example, a physiotherapist may teach a patient how to transfer from a wheelchair on to the toilet, using a lateral transfer board (sometimes called a sliding board). The rehabilitation nurse will then support and encourage the patient to practise this manoeuvre on a daily basis early in the morning, late at night and at weekends so that the patient is confident and competent by the time of discharge home. Nurses have been described as 'closing the circle', ensuring that rehabilitation is a continuous process (Johnson 1995), but this role can cause tensions, if some nurses perceive themselves as 'jacks of all trades' (Hill & Johnson 1999), expected to take on roles when other professionals are not available. However, the continuation and integration of therapy has an important therapeutic value for patients, as it enables them to translate the development of physical skills into activities of daily living (Burton 2000a).

Emotional support

The 24-h contact that nurses have with patients can be an important source of emotional support (Pellatt 2003). An empathetic approach allows nurses to understand patients' underlying needs and emotions in order effectively to support them when undergoing rehabilitation. Empathy is the ability to see the world from another person's point of view and involves being non-judgemental and non-evaluative. To achieve this, nurses need to imagine how it feels to be that person. Shaw (1996) has likened the nurse–patient relationship to the rapport that two people develop when they share a journey and go their separate ways at the end.

During the rehabilitation process emotional support is necessary to help patients develop strategies to work through the grieving process. Unless they have gone through this process it may be difficult for them to accept any rehabilitation intervention. However, grieving takes time and patients' physical recovery cannot wait for this to be experienced. For successful physical recovery, rehabilitation must start immediately and sensitive support is important if, at this point, a patient is not emotionally ready for it (Hill & Johnson 1999).

Patients have identified that nurses provide emotional support when they convey a sense of commitment and are ready to take the time to listen to what they have to say. Nurses who are sensitive to patients' wishes and enable them to speak about their situation in peace and quiet are a source of support (Natterlund & Ahlstrom 1999). A basic responsibility for the nurse is to establish a trusting relationship with the patient. This will enable the nurse to facilitate a normal grieving process, to promote hope and to prevent depression as patients come to terms with the extent of their disability or the implications of their illness (Kirkevold 1997). A caring relationship between nurse and patient will contribute to patients' feelings of well-being and this contributes to mood, motivation and self-esteem, which in turn can empower patients to move forward in their rehabilitation (Lucke 1999).

Providing a caring, supportive relationship requires emotional work on the part of the nurse (James 1992). Emotional work is the mental work required to manage one's feelings: the aim is to reflect positive feelings both in one's behaviour and in encouraging a patient's feelings of self-worth and security. The nurse in a rehabilitation setting must develop social skills such as listening, acknowledging the other's perspective, identifying and acting on behavioural cues, and speaking clearly. These are activities that can be enhanced by self-awareness and educational programmes (McQueen 2000).

Involving the family

Stressor change affecting one family member also affects the other family members and lack of family involvement in the patient's rehabilitation process can lead to failure to achieve rehabilitation goals (Dean-Baar 1996). Involvement of family members is therefore vital, both for the patient and the family, who need to be included and informed about

> CASE HISTORY 34.4
> **Mrs D**
>
> Mrs D is 64 years old. She is married and has two daughters, both of whom live nearby but have their own families. She has rheumatoid arthritis, which causes her pain and considerable limitation of mobility. She is concerned that she is becoming more dependent on her family and the condition is affecting her social activities and her family relationships.

what is happening. Support from the family enables the patient to make choices and to carry out a range of activities. However, Holland and Hogg (2001) point out that roles and responsibilities in families will vary in different circumstances and cultures. The patient may, for example, be part of a close and extended family, while others may be from a single parent family. The way in which members give, or are able to give support, can impact on the patient's autonomy, positively or negatively. While families can be an important source of information about a patient, with regard to their previous life and customs, some families are overprotective and therefore constrain the patient's autonomy and progress to maximal independence. Nurses therefore need to work in partnership with families as well as the patient and educate them together in identifying goals and objectives, assisting the patient appropriately and being involved in the discharge planning process (Proot et al 2002) (see Case History 34.4).

STOP THINK **34.4** Review Case History 34.4 and identify what support may be available for Mrs D and her family.

THE WAY AHEAD

As the 21st century progresses, there will be a considerable increase in the number of people, particularly older people, with chronic illness and disability (DH 2001a). There has been a move away from long-term care, with a drive towards earlier hospital discharge (Kneafsey et al 2003), and this is likely to continue. A report by the Audit Commission (1997) concluded that there was too little investment in preventive and rehabilitative services, which led to unplanned admissions of older people which, in turn, caused premature admission to long-term residential care. The report recommended investment in prevention and rehabilitation, the aim being to enable more people with chronic illness and disability to live at home. The National Service Framework for Older People Standard 3: Intermediate care (DH 2001a) states:

> *Older people will have access to a new range of intermediate care services at home or in designated care settings, to promote their independence by providing enhanced services from the NHS and councils to prevent unnecessary hospital admission and effective rehabilitation services to enable early discharge from hospital and to prevent premature or unnecessary admission to long-term residential care.*

The community nurse therefore has an important role in the provision of community rehabilitation and in particular may be the main contact for older people and their carers in the community (Kneafsey et al 2003).

Inadequacies in service provision in the community have been highlighted by both nurses and patients (Long et al 2001), and it is felt that there may be a lack of specialist interprofessional care. When they are discharged home, patients may need services such as physiotherapy, occupational therapy, podiatry, social work and specialist nursing. They may require aids such as wheelchairs and house adaptations, and their carers may require physical help and support.

There is considerable scope for community nurses to act as care coordinators (Aylett & Fawcett 2003) or as care managers to provide support that will help maintain the patient's dignity and prolong independence, thus preventing hospital admission and readmission.

The community nurse's role is to:

- monitor the patient's well-being
- support both patient and family
- initiate intervention as required
- liaise with colleagues in social services and in the other health care professions.

To fulfil these roles effectively, the nurse must have detailed information about the patient's continuing rehabilitation programme (Casley 1997).

Long-term health maintenance

The issue of where rehabilitation ends, if it does end, and where long-term health maintenance begins is viewed differently by professionals and users of rehabilitation services. Davidhizar and Shearer (1997) prefer the term 'high level wellness' that includes psychosocial functioning. However, as individuals with a disability or chronic illness grow older it is important that long-term health maintenance is considered. Studies carried out in the UK and USA over the last 50 years with people with a spinal cord injury suggest that as they age, they are likely to develop complications such as respiratory problems and urinary tract infections (Frankel et al 1998, Lammertse 2001). Equally, wheelchair users are at risk of developing musculoskeletal problems and degenerative changes in their shoulders as they age (Crewe 1991, Waters & Sie 2001) (see Case History 34.5).

> CASE HISTORY 34.5
> **N**
>
> N is 20 years old and has a paraplegia injury, which means he has no sensation or movement from the waist down since a car accident a few months ago. He is keen to learn everything he possibly can about his condition so that he can prevent any complications occurring when he goes home.

The concept of a 'disability career' was identified by Safilios-Rothschild (1970). The career spans the first instant that symptoms or an accident are experienced, to the final stage when no further effort is made to change the extent of the residual disability. Disabled people follow different pathways as they pass through a series of definable stages during this disability 'career'. The Disability Movement has, however, questioned whether disabled people need the services of professionals at each of these stages (Craddock

1996, Oliver 1996). Problems arise when disabled people are defined as 'ill'. This can mean that disabled people's lifestyles are broken down into segments when their care needs are being assessed. The reality is that, for some disabled people, their problems are associated with illness, but many disabled people are fit and healthy (Finkelstein & French 1993). If an independent living approach is adopted, the focus of support will move away from an emphasis on impairment and treatment to the importance of removing external barriers and encouraging self-direction.

Kneafsey et al (2003) suggest that three concepts should inform the community nurse's practice:

- The restoration and achievement of an optimal level of functioning in roles which the patient and carer value
- The goal of independent living
- User and carer autonomy.

STOP THINK **34.5** Review Case History 34.5. What sort of information and health promotion advice will N need from the rehabilitation nurse to enable him to prevent possible complications at home?

CONCLUSION

This chapter has shown that the nurse's role in rehabilitation is diverse. Nurses are in a position to have a considerable impact on the rehabilitation process. However, rehabilitation is in itself a multidimensional concept that is difficult to define. What is clear is that rehabilitation must be a partnership between the patient and health care staff and include the family where appropriate. Nurses have a key role to play in facilitating autonomy and participation of patients in the setting of rehabilitation goals that are meaningful and of importance to the patient.

STOP THINK **34.6** (a) Investigate rehabilitation provision in your locality. Visit a disabled living centre or an employment retraining centre.

(b) Study the role of a specialist rehabilitation nurse, e.g.:
- stoma nurse
- stroke coordinator
- multiple sclerosis specialist nurse
- breast care nurse
- spinal injury liaison nurse
- neurorehabilitation nurse.

(c) Study disability experientially, e.g.:
- wear special lenses that simulate a visual impairment
- go shopping in a wheelchair
- eat, using only one hand — your left, if you are right-handed; your right, if you are left-handed
- try washing and dressing using only one hand.

(d) Assess the ease of access to public buildings, transport and shops in your locality by accompanying a wheelchair user.

(e) Attend a multidisciplinary team meeting.

(f) Attend a case conference.

REFERENCES

Abbott S 1999 Planning and implementation of care: the patient's role. British Journal of Therapy and Rehabilitation 6(8): 398–401

Astbury-Ward E 2000 The erectile dysfunction revolution. Nursing Standard 15(11): 34–40

Audit Commission 1997 The coming of age: improving care services for older people. Belmont Press, Northampton

Aylett E, Fawcett T 2003 Chronic fatigue syndrome: the nurse's role. Nursing Standard 17(35): 33–37

Baillie L 2001 Learning practical nursing skills: an introduction. In: Baillie L (ed) Developing practical nursing skills. Arnold, London, p 1–30

Baillie L, Arrowsmith V 2001 Meeting elimination needs. In: Baillie L (ed) Developing practical nursing skills. Arnold, London, p 175–243

Barnes M, Ward A 2000 Textbook of rehabilitation medicine. Oxford University Press, Oxford

Bowie I 1999 Assessment in rehabilitation. In: Davis S, O'Connor S (eds) Rehabilitation nursing. Foundations for practice. Baillière Tindall, Edinburgh, p 83–116

Brillhart B, Johnson K 1997 Motivation and the coping process of adults with disabilities: a qualitative study. Rehabilitation Nursing 22(5): 249–256

Burks K 1999 A nursing practice model for chronic illness. Rehabilitation Nursing 24(5): 197–200

Burton C 2000a Re-thinking stroke rehabilitation: the Corbin and Strauss chronic illness trajectory framework. Journal of Advanced Nursing 32(3): 595–602

Burton C 2000b A description of the nursing role in stroke rehabilitation. Journal of Advanced Nursing 32(1): 174–181

Carney O, McIntosh J, Worth A et al 1996 Assessment of need for health visiting. Research Report, Glasgow Caledonian University, Glasgow

Carpenter C 1994 The experience of spinal cord injury: the individual's perspective – implications for rehabilitation practice. Physical Therapy 74(7): 614–629

Casley S 1997 Rehabilitation nursing. In: Goodwill C, Chamberlain M, Evans C (eds) Rehabilitation of the physically disabled adult, 2nd edn. Stanley Thornes, Cheltenham

Chamberlain M 1997 Introduction. In: Goodwill J, Chamberlain M, Evans C (eds) Rehabilitation of the physically disabled adult, 2nd edn. Stanley Thornes, Cheltenham

Child K, Higham S 2001 Assessing and meeting nutritional needs. In: Baillie L (ed) Developing practical nursing skills. Arnold, London, p 103–142

Cowley S, Bergen A, Young K et al 1996 Establishing a framework for research: the example of needs assessment. Journal of Clinical Nursing 5(10): 53–61

Craddock J 1996 Response of the occupational therapy profession to the perspective of the disability movement, Part 1. British Journal of Occupational Therapy 59(1): 17–22

Crewe N 1991 Ageing and severe physical disability: patterns of change and implications for services. International Disability Studies 13(4): 158–161

David J 1995 Patients' views on rehabilitation. Journal of Cancer Care 4: 57–60

Davidhizar R 1997 Disability does not have to be the grief that never ends: helping patients adjust. Rehabilitation Nursing 22(1): 32–35

Davidhizar R, Shearer R 1997 Helping the client with chronic illness achieve high-level wellness. Rehabilitation Nursing 22(3): 131–134

Davis S, O'Connor S 1999 Models and theories. In: Davis S, O'Connor S (eds) Rehabilitation nursing. Foundations for practice. Baillière Tindall, Edinburgh

Dean-Baar S 1996 Outcome directed teaching and learning. In: Hoeman S (ed) Rehabilitation nursing: process and application, 2nd edn. Mosby, St Louis, p 130–143

Department of Health 1990 NHS and Community Care Act. HMSO, London

Department of Health 1996 The National Health Service: a service with ambitions. HMSO, London

Department of Health 2001a National Service Framework for Older People. DH, London

Department of Health 2001b The expert patient: a new approach to chronic disease management for the 21st century. DH, London

Department of Health 2001c Essence of care. DH, London

Duff J, Kennedy P, Swalwell E 1999 Clinical

audit of physical rehabilitation: patients' views of goal planning. Clinical Psychology Forum 129(1): 34–38
Edwards A 2002 A rehabilitation framework for patient-focussed care. Nursing Standard 16(50): 38–44
Elliott T, Uswatte G, Lewis L et al 2000 Goal instability and adjustment to physical disability. Journal of Counselling Psychology 47(2): 251–252
Engel C 1994 A functional anatomy of teamwork. In: Leathard A (ed) Going interprofessional. Routledge, London, p 64–67
Engel G 1964 Grief and grieving. In: Schwartz L, Schwartz S (eds) The psychodynamics of patient care. Prentice-Hall, New York
Evans R, Connis R, Hendricks R et al 1995 Multidisciplinary rehabilitation versus medical care: a meta-analysis. Social Science and Medicine 40(12): 1699–1706
Faugier J, Sargeant M 1997 Stigma: its impact on professional responses to the needs of marginalized groups. NT Research 2(3): 220–229
Finkelstein V, French S 1993 Towards a psychology of disability. In: Swain J, Finkelstein V, French S et al (eds) Disabling barriers – enabling environments. Sage, London, p 26–33
Foley A 1998 A review of goal planning in the rehabilitation of the spinal cord injured person. Journal of Orthopaedic Nursing 2(3): 148–152
Frankel H, Coll J, Charlifue S et al 1998 Long-term survival in spinal cord injury: a fifty year investigation. Spinal Cord 36(4): 266–274
French S 1994 Attitudes of health professionals towards disabled people. Physiotherapy 80(10): 687–693
Gibbon B 1992 The role of the nurse in rehabilitation. Nursing Standard 6(36): 32–35
Glass C 1999 Spinal cord injury: impact and coping. BPS Books, Leicester
Goffman E 1968 Stigma. Penguin, London
Graham A 1997 The development of pressure sores in patients with spinal cord injury. Journal of Wound Care 6(8): 393–395
Gray J 2001 Discussion of the ICIDH-2 in relation to occupational therapy and occupational science. Scandinavian Journal of Occupational Therapy 8(1): 19–30
Greco S 1996 Sexuality, education and counselling. In: Hoeman S (ed) Rehabilitation nursing: process and application, 2nd edn. Mosby, St Louis, p 594–627
Grimby G, Smedby B 2001 Editorial: ICF approved as the successor to ICDH. Journal of Rehabilitation Medicine 33(5): 193–194
Groomes D, Leahey M 2002 The relationships among the stress appraisal process, coping disposition, and level of acceptance of disability. Rehabilitation Counselling Bulletin 46(1): 15–24
Harvey A 1997 Working in teams. In: Goodwill J, Chamberlain A, Evans C (eds) Rehabilitation of the physically disabled adult, 2nd edn. Stanley Thornes, Cheltenham, p 53–65
Henderson V 1966 Basic principles of nursing care. International Council of Nurses, Geneva
Hill M, Johnson J 1999 An exploratory study of nurses' perceptions of their role in neurological rehabilitation. Rehabilitation Nursing 24(4): 152–157
Holland K, Hogg C 2001 Cultural awareness in nursing and health care. Arnold, London
James N 1992 Care = organisation + physical labour + emotional labour. Sociology of Health and Illness 14(4): 488–509
Joachim G, Acorn S 2000 Stigma of visible and invisible chronic conditions. Journal of Advanced Nursing 32(1): 243–248
Johnson J 1995 Achieving effective rehabilitation outcomes: does the nurse have a role? British Journal of Therapy and Rehabilitation 2(3): 113–118
Johnston M 1996 Models of disability. Physiotherapy Theory and Practice 12(3): 131–141
Kennedy P, Hamilton L 1999 The needs assessment checklist: a clinical approach to measuring outcome. Spinal Cord 37(2): 136–139
Kennedy P, Henderson J, Gallagher S 1996 Improving goal attainment with spinal cord injured patients. Journal of the Association for Quality in Health Care 3(4): 145–150
Kennedy P, Duff J, Evans M et al 2003 Coping effectiveness training reduces depression and anxiety following traumatic spinal cord injuries. British Journal of Clinical Psychology 42(1): 41–52
Kirkevold M 1997 The role of nursing in the rehabilitation of acute stroke patients: toward a unified theoretical perspective. Advances in Nursing Science 19(4): 55–64
Kneafsey R, Long A, Ryan J 2003 An exploration of the contribution of the community nurse to rehabilitation. Health and Social Care in the Community 11(4): 321–328
Kubler-Ross E 1969 On death and dying. Macmillan, New York
Lammertse D 2001 Maintaining health long-term with spinal cord injury. Topics in Spinal Cord Injury Rehabilitation 6(3): 1–21
Long A, Kneafsey R, Ryan J et al 2001 Teamworking in rehabilitation: exploring the role of the nurse. English National Board for Nursing, Midwifery and Health Visiting, London
Low G 2003 Developing the nurse's role in rehabilitation. Nursing Standard 17(45): 33–38
Lucke K 1999 Outcomes of nurse caring as perceived by individuals with spinal cord injury during rehabilitation. Rehabilitation Nursing 24(6): 1–13
Maclean N, Pound P 2000 A critical review of the concept of patient motivation in the literature on physical rehabilitation. Social Science and Medicine 50: 495–506
Maclean N, Pound P, Wolfe C et al 2000 Qualitative analysis of stroke patients' motivation for rehabilitation. British Medical Journal 321(7268): 1051–1054
Mahat G 1997 Perceived stressors and coping strategies among individuals with rheumatoid arthritis. Journal of Advanced Nursing 25(6): 1144–1150
Major C 2001 Meeting hygiene needs. In: Baillie L (ed) Developing practical nursing skills. Arnold, London, p 143–173
McDonald J, Sadowsky C 2002 Spinal-cord injury. Lancet 359(9304): 417–426
McLeod E 1995 Patients in interprofessional practice. In: Soothill K, Mackay L, Webb C (eds) Interprofessional relations in health care. Edward Arnold, London, p 331–348
McQueen A 2000 Nurse–patient relationships and partnerships in hospital care. Journal of Clinical Nursing 9(5): 723–731
Miller C, Ross N, Freeman M 1999 Shared learning and clinical teamwork: new directions in education for multiprofessional practice. English National Board for Nursing, Midwifery and Health Visiting, London
Morse J 1997 Responding to threats to integrity of self. Advances in Nursing Science 19(4): 21–36
Naderi A, Safarinejad M 2003 Endocrine profiles and semen quality in spinal cord injured men. Clinical Endocrinology 58(2): 177–184
National Institute for Clinical Excellence (NICE) 2003 Pressure ulcers: prevention and pressure-relieving devices. Online. Available: www.nice.org.uk
Natterlund B, Ahlstrom G 1999 Experience of social support in rehabilitation: a phenomenological study. Journal of Advanced Nursing 30(6): 1332–1340
Neal L 2001 Using rehabilitation theory to teach medical–surgical nursing to undergraduate students. Rehabilitation Nursing 26(2): 72–75
Nolan M, Nolan J 1998 Rehabilitation: scope for improvement in current practice. British Journal of Nursing 7(9): 522–526
Nolan M, Booth A, Nolan J 1997 New directions in rehabilitation: exploring the nursing contribution. English National Board for Nursing, Midwifery and Health Visiting, London
Nursing and Midwifery Council (NMC) 2004 Code of professional conduct: standards for conduct, performance and ethics. NMC, London
O'Kelly D 1997 Rehabilitation – the different strokes way. Different Strokes Annual Review, London
Oliver M 1996 Understanding disability: from theory to practice. Macmillan, Basingstoke
Orem D 2001 Nursing: concepts of practice, 6th edn. McGraw-Hill, New York
Pellatt G 2001 Caring for the person with impaired mobility. In: Baillie L (ed) Developing practical nursing skills. Arnold, London, p 334–360
Pellatt G 2003 Perceptions of the nursing role in spinal cord injury rehabilitation. British Journal of Nursing 12(5): 292–299
Playford E, Dawson L, Limbert V et al 2000 Goal-setting in rehabilitation: a report of a workshop to explore professionals' perceptions of goal setting. Clinical Rehabilitation 14(5): 491–497
Preston K 1994 Rehabilitation nursing: a client-centred philosophy. American Journal of Nursing 94(2): 66–70
Price B 1996 Illness careers: the chronic illness experience. Journal of Advanced Nursing 24(2): 275–279
Proot I, Abu-Saad H, Van Oorsouw G et al 2002 Autonomy in stroke rehabilitation: the perceptions of care providers in nursing homes. Nursing Ethics 9(1): 36–50
Safilios-Rothschild C 1970 The sociology and social psychology of rehabilitation. Random House, New York

Scullion P 1999 Conceptualising disability in nursing: some evidence from students and their teachers. Journal of Advanced Nursing 29(3): 648–657
Seaman A 1999 Team-working in rehabilitation nursing. In: Smith M (ed) Rehabilitation in adult nursing practice. Churchill Livingstone, Edinburgh, p 175–194
Shaw E 1996 Severe head injury: the primary nurse's key role within the rehabilitation team. British Journal of Therapy and Rehabilitation 3(10): 561–563
Sheppard B 1994 Patients' views of rehabilitation. Nursing Standard 9(10): 27–30
Sim J 1990 Physical disability, stigma and rehabilitation. Physiotherapy Canada 42(5): 232–238
Sipski M, Alexander C 1992 Sexual function and dysfunction after spinal cord injury. Physical Medicine and Rehabilitation Clinics of North America 3(4): 811–828
Smith M 1999a The nature of rehabilitation. In: Smith M (ed) Rehabilitation in adult nursing practice. Churchill Livingstone, Edinburgh, p 1–30
Smith M 1999b The nurse as promoter of sexual health. In: Smith M (ed) Rehabilitation in adult nursing practice. Churchill Livingstone, Edinburgh, p 123–137
Thomas D 1999 Psychological implications and assessment following illness and injury. In: Smith M (ed) Rehabilitation in adult nursing practice. Churchill Livingstone, Edinburgh, p 91–104
Tranter G, Sullivan S 1996 Whose shout? Health Service Journal 106(5501): 31
Tripp S 1999 Providing psychological support. In: Smith M (ed) Rehabilitation in adult nursing practice. Churchill Livingstone, Edinburgh, p 105–122
Wade D 1998 Evidence relating to goal planning in rehabilitation. Clinical Rehabilitation 12(4): 273–275
Wade D 2002 Rehabilitation is a way of thinking, not a way of doing. Clinical Rehabilitation 16(5): 579–581
Wade G 1998 A concept analysis of personal transformation. Journal of Advanced Nursing 28(4): 713–719
Waters R, Sie I 2001 Upper extremity changes with SCI contrasted to common aging in the musculoskeletal system. Topics in Spinal Cord Injury Rehabilitation 6(3): 61–68
Williams G 1996 Representing disability: some questions of phenomenology and politics. In: Barnes C, Mercer G (eds) Exploring the divide: illness and disability. Disability Press, Leeds, p 194–212
Wilson C 2000 Rehabilitation: philosophy into practice. Elderly Care 12(1): 8–10
Wilson C, Fletcher P 2002 Dealing with colon cancer. One woman's emotional journey. Clinical Nurse Specialist 16(6): 298–305
World Health Organization 1980 International classification of impairments, disabilities and handicaps (ICIDH). WHO, Geneva
World Health Organization 2001 International classification of functioning, disability and health (ICF). WHO, Geneva

FURTHER READING

Craddock J 1996 Response of the occupational therapy profession to the perspective of the disability movement, Part 1. British Journal of Occupational Therapy 59(1): 17–22
Devlieger P 1999 From handicap to disability: language use and cultural meaning in the United States. Disability and Rehabilitation 21(7): 346–354
Kneafsey R, Long A, Ryan J 2003 An exploration of the contribution of the community nurse to rehabilitation. Health and Social Care in the Community 11(4): 321–328
National Institute for Clinical Excellence 2003 Pressure ulcers: prevention and pressure-relieving devices. Online. Available: www.nice.org.uk
O'Kelly D 1997 Rehabilitation – the different strokes way. Different Strokes Annual Review, London
World Health Organization 1980 International classification of impairments, disabilities and handicaps (ICIDH). WHO, Geneva
World Health Organization 2001 International classification of functioning, disability and health (ICF). WHO, Geneva

USEFUL WEBSITES

Age Concern
www.ace.org.uk

Community rehabilitation team network
www.crtnetwork.co.uk

Database of individual patients' experience
www.dipex.org

Department for Transport
www.mobility-unit.dft.gov.uk

Dial UK
www.dialuk.org.uk

Disability Information Services
www.diss.org.uk

Disabled Living Foundation
www.dlf.org.uk

Limbless Association
www.limbless-association.org

Multiple Sclerosis Society
www.mssociety.org.uk

Royal Association for Disability and Rehabilitation (RADAR)
www.radar.org.uk

The Society for Research in Rehabilitation
www.srr.org.uk

Spinal Injuries Association
www.spinal.co.uk

The Stroke Association
www.stroke.org.uk

Transport for London – Access and Mobility
www.londontransport.co.uk/tfl/ph_mobility.shtml

THE OLDER PERSON

Roger Watson

35

INTRODUCTION

Old age has always been a possibility but it is now an increasing probability — at least in the developed world (Kirkwood 1999). Medical, social and economic advances of the last century have largely eradicated a range of 'killer' diseases which robbed people of life in their childhood or early adult years. Infectious diseases, for example, and the widespread use of antibiotics — one of the major medical 'spin-offs' of the Second World War — have accounted for a dramatically decreased mortality from infections which would previously have proved fatal (Christiansen & Grzybowski 1993). Concomitantly, nutrition has improved, people generally live in better housing and health and safety has become more important in the workplace. Some of the more dangerous occupations such as coal mining have been made safer or have largely disappeared due to changing economic circumstances.

The outcome of the above changes is that more people are living longer: Figure 35.1 shows a striking difference in the age profile between the 1990s and approximately 100 years ago; Figure 35.2 shows that life expectancy at birth in Europe and North America has increased over the second half of the last century and that this is expected to continue; Figure 35.3 shows how this has had an impact on the number of people aged over 65 years, mainly in the developed world. This has social and economic consequences (Masson 1990) which impinge upon the health services and upon nursing.

Consequences of an ageing population

More people are living longer. As explained above, this has been due in part to the eradication of many diseases and improvements in the treatment of other diseases. However, there has been a resultant increase in the prevalence of diseases that are, largely, associated with old age (Armour & Cairns 2002). These include cancer, heart disease and dementia.

Socially and economically, the changing demographic profile of the population, with an increasing proportion of older people, is challenging for society. The likely impact on health and nursing services — and how this should be addressed — was recognised in the UK when the Royal Commission on Long Term Care (1999) reported to the UK government at the end of the last century. The increasing, but not inevitable, likelihood of developing particular diseases with age demands health service resources at the primary and secondary levels. The economic consequences are obvious, as a sector of the population which is not, generally, economically active and which in fact may be economically demanding due to retirement and pension payments, requires an increasingly larger slice of the economic cake (Masson 1990, Heller 1998). This is compounded by the fact that towards the end of the last century there has been a trend of earlier retirement (Posner 1995) as shown in Figure 35.4. These are facts which must be faced and not avoided by governments, planners and health services. They are not meant to cast a shadow over the fact

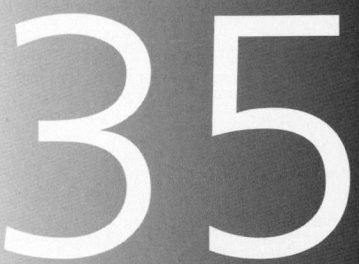

	1880s	1990s
Born alive	1,000,000	1,000,000
Alive at 5 years	736,818	991,350
Alive at 25 years	684,054	984,230
Alive at 35 years	568,993	977,500
Alive at 45 years	502,915	963,960
Alive at 65 years	309,020	830,990
Alive at 75 years	161,164	612,740
Alive at 85 years	38,575	286,950
Alive at 95 years	2,153	45,450
Alive at 100 years	223	8,710

Fig. 35.1 Survival in England and Wales in the 1880s and 1990s. (Adapted from Kirkwood 1999.)

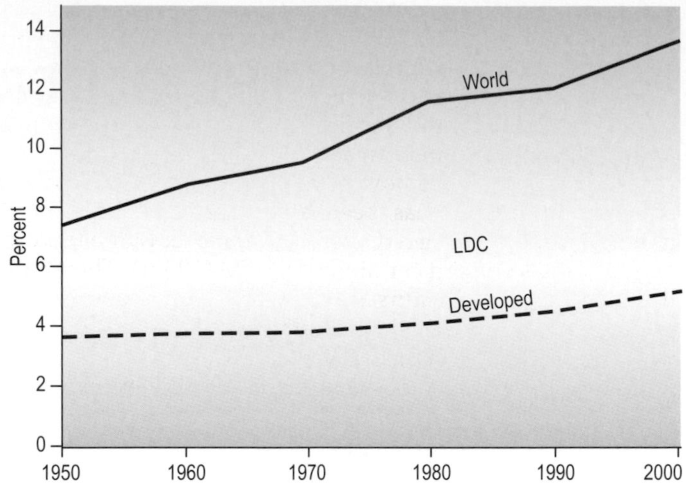

Fig. 35.3 The increasing percentage of the population 65 years or over. (Reproduced from Posner 1995, with permission from The University of Chicago Press.)

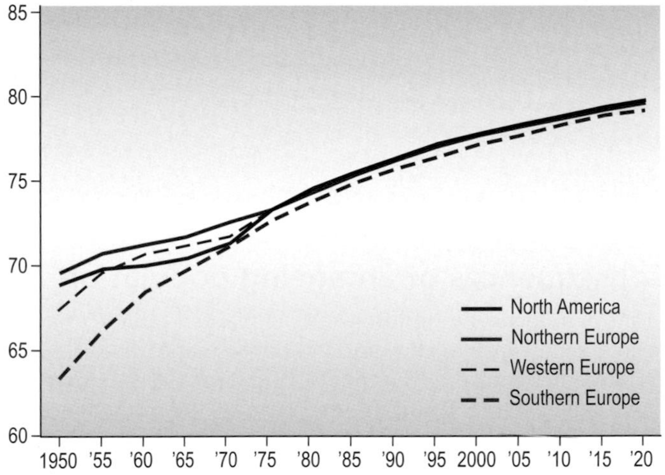

Fig. 35.2 The increasing life expectancy at birth. (Reproduced from Disney 1996, with permission from The MIT Press.)

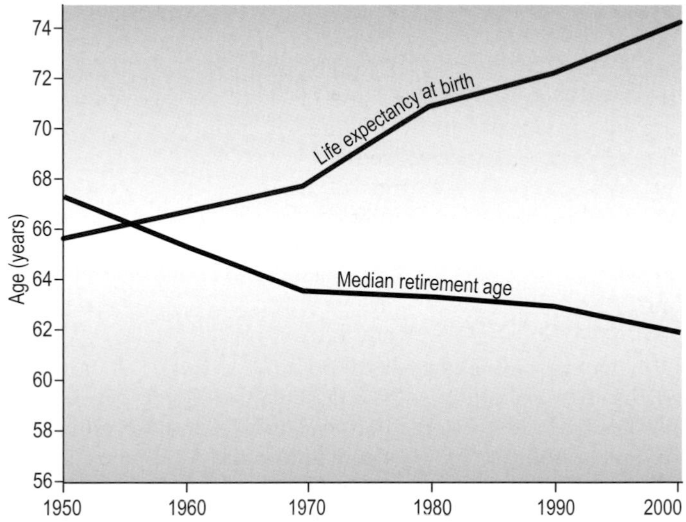

Fig. 35.4 The changing profile of life expectancy and retirement. (Reproduced from Posner 1995, with permission from The University of Chicago Press, Chicago.)

that more people are living longer; the 'burden' of an ageing population is often referred to in the literature (Warnes 1993) but this longevity is an indicator of success in health and social terms, even if governments and planners in the developed world have been taken by surprise (Olshansky et al 1993).

35.1 Older people have been referred to as 'our neglected assets' (Help the Aged 2004). What positive contributions socially and economically do older people make in society? As you meet older people with health care problems and deficits, are you aware of the positive contributions that may be part of their life experience?

It is the job of governments to introduce policies to cope with the changing demographic profile and it is the job, increasingly, of nurses, to work with individual older people who have health needs. Clearly, nurses are not the only people to work with older people and the role of other members of the multidisciplinary team will be referred to throughout the chapter. The other members of the multidisciplinary team include doctors, social workers and therapists but, however large the team of people working with an older person, it should be the older person who is the focus of the team and not any particular discipline.

WORKING WITH OLDER PEOPLE

Nurses increasingly work with older people whether or not they specialise in this area (SNMAC 2001). Some nurses choose to work exclusively with older people in hospitals and the community (Watson 1993a). However, with the increasing proportion of older people in our society, unless the choice is made to specialise in working with children or in maternity care, nurses will increasingly meet older people in general medical and surgical wards, in the community and in many specialist areas. For example, in hospitals, two-thirds of beds are now occupied by people aged over 65 years and there has been an increase in emergency admissions of people aged over 75 years, over half of whom suffer from ill-defined conditions (SNMAC 2001). Therefore, the vast majority of nurses will work with older people and most other nurses should understand the implications of ageing and develop the skills which are necessary to work with older people. The possible causes and the implications of ageing will be considered later in the chapter but, in this section, the skills that nurses need to work with older people are explored.

In one sense, older people are no different from other people nurses come into contact with in the course of their work, despite the negative images that are often used to portray older people in our society (Carrigan & Szmigin 2000). Like any patient, the older person requires sensitivity, tact and professionalism. In relation to the media and advertising, one could be mistaken for assuming that the best things in life are only available for younger people (Loretto et al 2000). Advertising of clothes, cars and cosmetics, albeit that many of these are designed to hide the signs of ageing, are conveyed as purely of interest to younger people. If the subject of an advertisement is not about pensions and retirement issues, the target audience is almost exclusively younger people (Carrigan & Szmigin 2000). Television and films focus on younger people, often presenting them in a positive light, while older people are often portrayed more negatively. Nurses are part of society and it is understandable that they too may have negative images of older people. Such images will not be dispelled by propaganda on behalf of older people but by evidence and an understanding of the ageing process and the facts about ageing. Nurses should avoid, in particular, holding and conveying stereotypes. One popular stereotype, for instance, is that older people are either no longer interested in sex or are incapable of sexual relations. Thankfully, there is plenty of evidence to the contrary (Kaye 1993, Araujo et al 2004), but the stereotype persists.

STOP THINK **35.2** Identify current media descriptions and media images of older people. Are these negative or positive? How do nurses and other professional colleagues refer to older people in day-to-day work conversations? Is ageism an issue in health care?

In 1998, with specific reference to the care of older people in acute wards in general hospitals, the Health Advisory Service 2000 produced a pivotal report entitled *Not Because They Are Old* (HAS 2000 1998). The HAS report can be described as 'pivotal' because it gave rise to two further influential reports which will be discussed in this chapter. One of these, on the nursing contribution to the care of older people (SNMAC 2001) will be described here and the other, the *National Service Framework for Older People* (DH 2001a), which outlines UK government policy with regard to the care of older people, will be discussed later. *Not Because They Are Old* catalogued the lamentable level of care which many older people experience in hospital and some of these areas of concern are shown in Box 35.1.

Box 35.1

Areas of concern identified by HAS 2000 (1998) in relation to the care of older people

- Poor satisfaction with care
- Delays in admission
- Poor physical environments in wards
- Shortages of equipment and supplies
- Staff shortages
- Poor quality food and drink
- Lack of help with feeding and nutrition
- Lack of privacy and dignity
- Negative interactions between staff and patients
- Communication problems with patients and staff

Amongst other things, the HAS 2000 report recommended that older people themselves and their relatives must be more involved in the care of older people in hospital, there must be more clarity about who is responsible for the nutrition of older people in hospital and that better education is needed for staff, including nurses, about the specific needs of older people in hospital.

As a response to the need for better education of nurses highlighted by HAS 2000, in 2001 the Standing Nursing and Midwifery Advisory Committee (SNMAC) commissioned research into the care of older people, as it related to nurse education, and produced a report *Caring for Older People: A Nursing Priority — Integrating Knowledge, Practice and Values* (SNMAC 2001). This report highlighted deficiencies in the care of older people and in the education of nurses about the care of older people. Amongst other things, SNMAC noted the points listed in Box 35.2.

Box 35.2

Issues in the care of older people identified by the Standing Nursing and Midwifery Advisory Committee (2001)

- Older patients and their carers are the least satisfied of all groups with the care that they receive from the NHS when they are acutely ill.
- Older people now comprise two-thirds of all patients in acute settings.
- The nursing care of older people is highly skilled and physically and emotionally taxing.
- The care of older people is mainly deficient in fundamental aspects of nursing, failing far too often to meet their basic needs for food, fluid, rest, activity and elimination.
- Course curricula must be revised to ensure that much more attention is given to caring for older people, for example, to disability, rehabilitation, palliation, and the treatment of chronic illnesses, as well as the fundamental skills of nursing. Media portrayals of the profession, particularly in recruitment campaigns, need to reflect that the majority of patients requiring acute care are older people.

SNMAC identified that one of the core skills lacking in the nursing care of older people was communication. They also identified that the 'fundamental skills' required in the care of older people such as bathing, help with using the toilet and assistance with feeding were tasks often delegated to unqualified staff. To provide good nursing care for older people, nurses need to have skills which include an understanding of the ageing process and of the multiple pathologies and diseases of old age. Nursing assessment, care planning and care pathways for older people should include physical and psychological needs, mental health needs and prioritisation of complex needs. Nutrition and medication management, including self-medication, were also identified as necessary skills. Nurses also need to understand the role of the multidisciplinary team including physiotherapy, occupational therapy and dietetics and the part these other professions play in the care of older people.

In terms of nurse education, the adult branch of nursing, to which this chapter is relevant, should be 'reoriented' (SNMAC 2001) to highlight the needs of older people. Specifically, recruitment campaigns need to reflect the care of older people and 'challenge the stereotype of nursing older people as unskilled and unrewarding'. This can be achieved by emphasising such things as the independence of older people, the success of rehabilitation and that palliative care, when no further curative treatment is available, can improve quality of life for older people. The SNMAC report is the platform for the philosophy and detail of the present chapter. In addition, other bodies such as Help the Aged (1999) have addressed the issue of the dignity and privacy of older people who are in acute hospitals and the United Kingdom Central Council for Nursing, Midwifery and Health Visiting (1994) addressed similar issues in the care of older people living in nursing homes.

In summary, one of the fundamental attributes required by the nurse working with older people is to treat them as individuals and not as a homogeneous group (Watson 2003). Each older person has a unique history and a unique perspective on life; older people are not less intelligent than their younger counterparts and they do not appreciate being treated as such. The older person must be at the centre of the nursing care of older people. The next section will examine the ageing process and the evidence for changes associated with it, and will evaluate the extent to which older people require specialised care.

THE PROCESS OF AGEING

That ageing takes place is beyond dispute (BSRA 2004), despite the efforts of people to deny this or to hide the effects of the ageing process. Most of what is considered ageing is quite superficial. Aspects of the ageing body, such as the loss of elasticity in the skin leading to wrinkling and the loss of hair colour and thinning of the hair — all the aspects which obsess us most and which, as a result of that obsession, ensure large profits for the cosmetics industry — have little or no clinical significance (BSRA 2004). They are external indicators that ageing is taking place but, without the application of cosmetics, people age very differently. Some people retain their hair into old age, others become grey haired prematurely and others seem not to suffer from wrinkling of the skin to the same extent. Of course, environmental factors may play a part in the appearance of ageing. For example, sun-bathing, a popular pursuit of the young to make their bodies more acceptable to others, often the opposite sex, is almost guaranteed to lead to premature ageing of the skin (Rutishauser 1994).

There are other features of ageing which are less superficial, such as increasing kyphosis of the spine leading to a more stooped posture and a decline in height (Christiansen & Grzybowski 1993), partially associated with the loss of skeletal tissue (bone and cartilage) which results from ageing (see p. 1136). There are, however, myths about ageing, for example, that older people are less intelligent or lose their memories. These myths need to be exposed, as they will below.

Why do we age?

Before looking at the ageing process in some detail it is worth pondering, briefly, what the purpose of ageing is, if indeed it has a purpose. Why do we age? Why do we not remain as youthful looking as we were at maturity, say in our early 20s, for the whole life span? This question is hard to answer biologically. Most nursing students, when asked why we age, will answer that it is necessary to age and die to make way for future generations. This is possibly true but it does not answer why we age. Ageing alone does not necessarily cause death, as the extreme longevity of some individuals demonstrates. Certainly, ageing may lead to death but there are many alternative ways to die which would be sufficient to make way for the next generation. It is thought that ageing may confer some biological advantages for our species in the sense that, biologically, we invest more energy in maintaining vitality during the years that we are reproductive and, as we grow older and our reproductive potential declines, less energy is invested in maintaining vitality, which leads to ageing (Kirkwood 2001). This kind of thinking has led to the development of one of the most credible theories of ageing: the 'disposable soma theory' which, essentially, postulates that the somatic cells (body cells) are disposable from the perspective of maintaining the species and exist to ensure that our gametes (sperm and egg cells) can be brought together at fertilisation to produce new members of our species (Kirkwood 2001). However, we can merely speculate about why we age; it is more relevant to consider how we age and what this leads to in terms of the effects of ageing on the human body.

How do we age?

The question of how we age refers to the underlying biological mechanisms that lead to the outward signs of ageing and other physiological changes that take place in the body. The precise mechanisms of ageing are not known and theories abound. However, some of the theories refer to outcomes of ageing rather than mechanisms. As we age, the body does, to some extent, wear out and this is encapsulated in the 'wear and tear' theory of ageing (Kirkwood 1999). There are clear aspects of 'wear and tear' in the body as we age: in the weight-bearing joints of the body, the knees and hips, it is almost inevitable that osteoarthritic changes will take place but these will not necessarily be debilitating, unless the process is very advanced or is exacerbated by the older person being very overweight, for example. This constitutes 'wear' but there are also people who accumulate sports injuries in their younger and more active years, especially of the joints, which may stay with them into old age and this constitutes 'tear'. The ligaments and tendons of the body, which are composed of collagen, become less flexible as we age, and this is also responsible for the wrinkling of the skin of which collagen is a major component. The stiffening of collagen is due to chemical processes which increase the amount of chemical cross-linking between the collagen strands (Christiansen & Grzybowski 1993) and this stiffening of ligaments and tendons compounds the weakening of the muscular system and the thinning of bones.

Almost all of the systems of the body become less efficient with age and the unifying physiological process of homeostasis becomes less able to correct physiological deficits and restore the former balance in the systems of the body; this is described in the 'homeostatic imbalance theory' (Herbert 1992). However, these theories are based on observations and are just as likely to be the result of the process of ageing rather than underlying mechanisms in themselves. Other theories of ageing, such as those based on the reduction in somatic cell doubling with age (Christiansen & Grzybowski 1993) and those related to the harmful and cumulative effects of oxygen, are also likely to be based on outcomes rather than mechanisms.

Another observation about ageing is that the immune system becomes less efficient. It protects us less well and even loses its ability to distinguish self from non-self, leading it to attack somatic cells. This has led to a theory of ageing based on autoimmunity (Christiansen & Grzybowski 1993). However, while there are some age-associated diseases which are autoimmune, for example, type 2 diabetes and rheumatoid arthritis, this, again, may be an outcome of ageing rather than an underlying mechanism.

The 'state of the art' in research into ageing points to mechanisms operating at the genetic level (Kirkwood 2002). As our somatic cells divide and duplicate during mitosis, part of this process is the replication of DNA and this process is always accompanied by some errors in replication called mutations. Enzymes exist in cell nuclei that can detect and repair most mutations; however, this process is not perfect and some mutations will always appear in the DNA of newly divided cells. It is reckoned, despite the highly conservative nature of DNA replication, that no two somatic cells are identical. DNA is the template, through the process of transcription, for RNA which in turn is used in the process of translation to order the sequence of amino acids during protein synthesis and proteins are involved in every aspect of the functioning of the human body: structural, metabolic and regulatory (Watson 2005). In this way, with the accumulation of errors in DNA as we age, it is logical that there will be an accumulation of errors in protein molecules and that this will lead to inefficiency in every aspect of the function of the human body. Ageing, therefore, is viewed as an accumulation of errors in the protein of the body and this, eventually, leads to increasing inefficiency and all of the obvious, and less obvious, signs of ageing (Kirkwood 2002). It is also observed that, as cells age, a region at the end of the DNA molecule called the telomere becomes shorter (Ahmed & Tollefsbol 2001). Telomeres may have some protective role towards DNA in chromosomes and shortened telomeres have been found in people with progeric syndromes which lead to premature ageing (Dyer & Sinclair 1998).

Ageing is considered to be about 25% heritable (Kirkwood 2002). In other words, the rate at which we age and, indeed, our longevity is related to genetic factors transmitted from our parents. On the other hand, it is hard to extricate the inherited from the environmental and there are other factors which may accelerate the ageing process. One of the biochemical mechanisms thought to be related to ageing is that of the toxic effects of oxygen and free radicals, the highly reactive molecules in the body (Goyns 2002). The fact that these molecules are damaging is possibly related to ageing, as there are mechanisms that protect us from the harmful effects of these molecules. However, free radicals in the body are increased, for example, by smoking (Christiansen & Grzybowski 1993) and our ability to deal with free radicals may be dependent upon some dietary factors such as eating sufficient fresh fruit and vegetables. Despite this speculation about the causes of ageing and related factors, it should be noted that there is no 'cure' for the ageing process. The pharmaceutical industry sells many products on the basis that they can reverse or arrest the effects of ageing. However, apart from a few topical applications that can reduce wrinkling of the skin, there is nothing that can arrest or reverse the underlying causes; these are simply not well enough understood and are, possibly, not amenable to 'treatment'. Ageing is not, in itself, a disease (BSRA 2004).

What happens to us as we age?

Some of the superficial aspects of ageing have already been mentioned, but these have little or no clinical significance. In fact, it should be understood that ageing, as well as being an inevitable process, is also quite natural and that ageing in itself is not pathological or an indicator that someone is or will become ill (BSRA 2004). On the other hand, there are some age-associated diseases and it is relevant to see how these are related to the underlying process of ageing.

As we age we generally have less ability, as previously mentioned, to maintain homeostasis. This is not a problem under circumstances where, from the physiological perspective, the body is not unduly stressed. However, in conditions of extreme temperature or dehydration, for example, an older person will usually be less able to adapt than a younger person (Watson & Fawcett 2003) and this will be particularly important when an older person has an infection.

Cardiovascular and respiratory systems

Most systems of the body show signs of ageing. The cardiovascular system ages in terms of cardiac output (Horan 1992) and elsewhere in the cardiovascular system there is increased deposition of atheromatous plaques in the blood vessels (Christiansen & Grzybowski 1993), leading to less adaptability and a tendency to increased blood pressure (see Ch. 2). The heart and blood vessels become less responsive to adrenaline and noradrenaline ('down-regulation') which means that the homeostatic mechanisms for maintaining blood pressure become less efficient (Collins 1998).

One tangible outcome of this is a tendency towards postural hypotension (Watson & Fawcett 2003) whereby a sudden change in position from sitting to standing is less well tolerated and blood pressure remains low, leading to dizziness or even fainting due to cerebral insufficiency.

In tandem with these changes in the cardiovascular system there are changes in the respiratory system such that it becomes less efficient at extracting oxygen from the blood (Horan 1992). This is not usually a problem but it does lead to exercise intolerance. The older person may well be able to go about their normal level of activity as these systems have considerable reserve capacity but will, for instance, be less able to run to catch a bus than they were when they were younger. Clearly, these changes will be compounded by changes in the musculoskeletal system (see Ch. 10).

Another consequence of changes in the cardiovascular system, through a combination of arterial disease and raised blood pressure, is a greater tendency in older people to suffer from cerebrovascular accidents, more commonly known as stroke (DH 2001a). Stroke essentially leads to the deprivation of a blood supply and, thereby, of oxygen to a region of the brain. The effect of a stroke can range from being fatal, through severe and permanent disability to full recovery. Deterioration in the blood supply to the brain can also lead to more chronic cerebrovascular disease which may lead to ischaemic dementia (McKeith & Fairbairn 2001), transient ischaemic attacks (Slack 1999) or to a fully evolved stroke.

Musculoskeletal system

With age our muscles atrophy, tendons and ligaments become less flexible and the skeleton becomes weaker due to the fact that less bone material is laid down in the skeleton (Christiansen & Grzybowski 1993). This is particularly marked in postmenopausal women but also in some men who may suffer from osteoporosis (NIH Consensus Development Panel 2001). The combined effects of osteoporosis and thinning of the cartilaginous discs between the vertebrae lead to a more stooped posture and this, in conjunction with the atrophy of skeletal muscle, of which the diaphragm is one, contributes to the reduced efficiency of the respiratory system (Christiansen & Grzybowski 1993).

Digestive system

The digestive system, because it is largely composed of smooth muscle which atrophies with age, shows some decline in motility with age and also some decline in its absorptive capacity (Christiansen & Grzybowski 1993) (see Ch. 4). However, these changes are minimal and they should not lead to any significant changes with ageing. Many older people complain of constipation and older people use greater amounts of laxatives than younger people (Harari et al 1993). However, this may not necessarily be associated with the ageing process. It is quite common for older people to be edentulous (Clay 1999) but this situation is likely to decline as dental care and diets improve. Dentists are now more likely to adopt a conservative and restorative approach than to remove teeth at the first signs of decay.

Renal system

The renal system is one which shows significant changes with ageing (Christiansen & Grzybowski 1993). However, the kidneys, in common with all the other systems of the body, have considerable reserve capacity and a decline in filtration rate is unimportant except in illness and in the administration of medication. This will be considered in more detail later in the chapter.

Endocrine system

With age, there are changes in the endocrine system which, along with the nervous system, is one of the main homeostatic regulators of the body (Watson & Fawcett 2003) (see Ch. 5). While the absolute levels of hormones in the body are relatively unaffected, the changes lead to decreased responsiveness of the endocrine system, both through the 'axes' between effector organs and their endocrine glands and in the responsiveness of tissues, due to the 'down-regulation' of hormone receptors in the tissues. This can be seen in the phenomenon of postural hypotension, referred to earlier, and also in the fact that older people take longer to acclimatise when they move between climates of extreme temperature (Schofield 2000). This latter phenomenon is due to the fact that acclimatisation is achieved by changes in the levels of circulating thyroxine: levels of thyroxine increase in cold climates and decrease in warmer climates. With age, the pituitary–thyroid axis is less sensitive to these changes, leading to slower acclimatisation in older people (Schofield 2000).

Immune system

The changes in the immune system that occur with age are complex. The overall levels of immunoglobulins remain relatively stable with ageing but the composition of these immunoglobulins changes and more immature T cells are produced (Christiansen & Grzybowski 1993). This may lead to decreased defences against infections and also to the phenomenon in some older people whereby they do not necessarily exhibit pyrexia when they have a bacterial or viral infection (Horan 1992). Instead, the presence of an infection may only be noticed when it is quite advanced, when confusion and drowsiness may occur.

As mentioned above, in old age, the immune system may become less able to distinguish 'self' from 'non-self', leading to autoimmunity whereby the immune system begins to attack its own tissues. Type 2 diabetes is, for example, a disease with autoimmune components and is definitely associated with ageing. The immune system also plays a key role in keeping cancer cells under check via immune surveillance which becomes less effective with age (Redmond & Aapro 1997) (see also Chs 16 and 31).

Nervous system

Despite misconceptions, the nervous system remains relatively unchanged with ageing (Christiansen & Grzybowski 1993). There are very few changes of any note in the central nervous system and some changes in the peripheral nervous system. The psychological aspects of ageing will be considered separately.

With age, the speed of nervous conduction slows and reaction times, measured in milliseconds, decline (Deary 2001). However, these are merely observations and have little, if any, impact on the life of an older person and have no clinical relevance. Except in degenerative neurological conditions, such as Alzheimer's disease, there is no widespread loss of nervous tissue with age.

In the peripheral nervous system there are changes but not all of these are associated with nervous tissue. For example, there is an inevitable decline in vision as we age and this is due to changes in the eye, rather than in the neural conduction system from the eye to the brain. With age it is common for the lens to become more opaque (Wolf 2004) and some older people suffer from cataracts which, if untreated, severely limit their vision. In the ear, the bones which transmit sound waves from the outer to the inner ear — the malleus, incus and stapes — tend to become fused together, thereby reducing their ability to transmit sound, leading to reduced hearing (Christiansen & Grzybowski 1993). This does not mean that all older people are blind and deaf but this reduction in hearing and vision has to be taken into account when considering their care and support.

Other aspects of the peripheral nervous system which change with age are taste and pain perception (Christiansen & Grzybowski 1993). It is not uncommon to hear older people complain that they do not enjoy their food as much as they used to and to see them enhance their food with copious amounts of salt, for example. This can have consequences for nutrition as will be discussed below. That older people suffer from pain must be made clear, but Seers (1999) argues that they have a reduced acuity to pain sensation. This means that, while they feel pain, they sometimes have difficulty in locating it and describing it and, as a result, many older people suffer from vague aches and pains. It appears, therefore, that the senses decline somewhat with age and this can lead to a decline in the ability to sense extremes of heat and cold. This can be potentially dangerous, leaving older people more vulnerable, for example, to hypothermia (Watson 1993b) (see Ch. 22).

Psychological aspects of ageing

Contrary to popular myth, there are very few psychological changes with ageing. Older people are no less intelligent, are no less able to remember and recall and are no more stubborn than their younger counterparts. The facts are plain; other than in neurodegenerative conditions such as dementia, memory and intelligence remain relatively intact with age and the personality we are born with is usually the one we take into old age. There is some loss of short-term memory with ageing (Ponto 1999) but this does not usually interfere with leading a normal life. Some older people do suffer from age-associated memory impairment (Deary 1995); however, it is unclear as whether or not this is a precursor to dementia. Intelligence, measured using standard IQ tests, does not decline with age. There is some change in intelligence, with a decline in fluid intelligence (e.g. problem solving) and an increase in crystallised intelligence (the application of learning to new problems), but these changes do not have a significant impact on daily living (Ponto 1999).

There is an abundance of theories related to psychological ageing and this abundance demonstrates that, in fact, very little is known about the psychological changes, if any, that accompany ageing. One of the most popular theories, based on the seven stages of ageing, was proposed by Erikson (Ponto 1999). According to this theory and others that are closely related to it (Ponto 1999), there are identifiable stages in the psychology of ageing during which the ageing person either manages or fails to come to terms with their life before moving on to the next stage, with the ultimate stage of ageing leading to the older person either being at peace with life and reconciled to what they have, or have not, done and experienced. The problem with such theories, while they make interesting frameworks for literature about ageing, is that they lack any empirical evidence. Clearly, people age and gain experience and, sometimes, wisdom regarding the life course and their own part in it, but it is not uncommon to hear older people, and people at almost any stage in their life, say that they feel no different as they age. Apart from the obvious physical signs of ageing, they think, react and often act in old age as they did when they were younger (Thomson 1993). Such testimony does not support theories which depend on stages of ageing.

Two juxtaposed, but popular, theories have dominated the psychosocial theories of ageing in recent years and these are, respectively, the activity theory of ageing (Ponto 1999) and the disengagement theory of ageing (Ponto 1999). Both theories acknowledge changes with ageing; the former that as people age they give up certain activities and take up others and the latter, that as people age they give up activities and gradually withdraw from life and from society. While there is evidence to support both theories, it is unlikely that these are really psychosocial ageing theories but rather explanations for observations of ageing as experienced by different people. Withdrawing from life and society is almost inevitable as people age; they leave work, family and friends move away and die and they become physically less able to participate in certain activities. However, such a view of ageing is derived from economically developed societies where retirement is the norm. In some parts of the world older people do not or cannot retire. They remain economically active into advanced years and never have the opportunity to withdraw or to take up other activities in old age, hobbies and travel being prime examples in developed countries (International Labour Organisation 1990).

DISEASES AND OLD AGE

Old age and disease are not synonymous but, as alluded to above, some diseases are more common in old age. The British Society for Research on Ageing has addressed the issue of biological ageing directly (BSRA 2004), defining ageing as 'a normal biological process that increases the frailty of otherwise healthy organisms'. The effect of ageing is to 'compromise(s) a creature's ability to cope with physiological stress producing an increased likelihood of long-term sickness and death'. The BSRA document dispels the myth that there is no identifiable 'ageing process', a view adhered to until recently by many in the medical community. Ageing, therefore, is not in itself an illness nor 'the sum of symptoms of the diseases from which the older person suffered'. Rather, there is an underlying biological process, which is entirely normal, and the study of this process is worthy in itself and not just in relation to those degenerative diseases that are associated with old age. Ageing, however, 'is thus an independent but potent risk factor for the development of many diseases and imposes serious quality of life issues in its own right.

Table 35.1 Breast cancer incidence by age

Age	Incidence
Up to 25	One in 15 000
Up to 30	One in 1900
Up to 40	One in 200
Up to 50	One in 50
Up to 60	One in 23
Up to 70	One in 15
Up to 80	One in 11
Up to 85+	One in 10
Lifetime risk	One in 9

Source: Cancer Research UK (2005).

The relationship of the ageing process to disease is akin to that between a worn part and a broken part'.

One of the diseases, while not exclusively associated with ageing, but which increases markedly in prevalence with age is cancer (Redmond & Aapro 1997) as shown in Table 35.1. Cancer is, essentially, a genetic disease in the sense that it originates in mutations in DNA which lead to uncontrolled growth of affected tissues, with disastrous consequences for the organs that are affected. With age, the likelihood of genetic mutations increases and the mechanisms, including surveillance by the immune system, that keep mutated cells in check become less effective with age. Some cancers of old age are sex-specific, namely prostate cancer in males and breast cancer, albeit not absolutely specific to women, in females (Redmond & Aapro 1997).

Cardiovascular disease increases with age and this is due for the most part to the deposition of fatty plaques in the arteries. This leads to an increase in heart disease with age, expressed as angina and heart failure, and also to cerebrovascular disease and arterial disease elsewhere in the body. The phenomenon of autoimmunity has already been referred to and this is implicated in the age-associated disease, type 2 diabetes.

Dementia, caused mainly by Alzheimer's disease and cerebrovascular changes, is definitely associated with age (Harvey 2001). While dementia, leading to profound memory loss and decline in cognitive function, is not inevitable with age, by the age of 90, one in two people will suffer from some degree of dementia (www.alzheimers.org.uk).

The impact of dementia goes beyond the individual older person with dementia; it takes a considerable toll on those who live with the person, usually family members. The government has pursued policies of care in the community since the late 1980s and this, combined with the changing age profile of society, has led to more older people with dementia being cared for at home, in the community (Nolan et al 2002). This has meant that carers 'have moved from the margins of social policy' (Nolan et al 2002), and they now occupy a more central role. There is now a much greater emphasis on the involvement of carers of people with dementia and, indeed, of people with dementia themselves in participation in service delivery and development (Killeen 2001).

Frailty and multipathology

The discussion of ageing so far has presented what is known about the biological and psychological aspects of growing old. Some diseases which are more common with age have also been described. However, this is quite a superficial explanation of why older people need nursing care; in fact, the reasons for this are quite complex and are often unrelated to a single medical diagnosis and more related to the poorly defined concept of frailty (Markle-Reid & Browne 2003) which results from the common occurrence of multipathology in older people. It is very uncommon for older people not to have some manifestation of pathology and it is common that older people suffer from a range of disorders (Ruzicka 1997). None of these disorders is, in itself, life threatening but the total effect of several of these disorders may cause a significant strain on a person who is already compromised by the process of ageing, such that they lose their independence. This, rather than a single diagnosis, is what prompts the need for nursing care. For example, an older person may suffer from mild heart failure, rheumatoid arthritis or osteoarthritis, type 2 diabetes and some degree of memory loss. Each of these is not serious enough to require help with activities of daily living and even the combination can be coped with, but a serious incident, such as a fall or a chest infection, may tip the balance towards loss of independence and, thereby, dependence on nursing care.

The reasons why older people require help with their activities of daily living was conceptualised by Isaacs (1981) in the four giants of geriatric medicine, also known as the four I's shown in Box 35.3. These four factors concisely describe the manifestations of multipathology and, furthermore, they describe a vicious circle of circumstances that compound each other. The four I's also have in common the fact that none is easily treatable and all require human helpers to enable the older person to cope. This serves to emphasise the role of the nurse in working with older people.

The four I's are interrelated: if an older person falls, they may become immobile either as a result of injury related to the fall, e.g. fractured neck of femur, or due to fear of a subsequent fall; immobility may lead to incontinence and also to sensory deprivation and confusion. Certainly, immobility will lead to muscle atrophy and this may prevent the older person from becoming fully mobile again. Incontinence will be considered again below.

Box 35.3

The four 'giants' of geriatric medicine identified by Isaacs (1981)

- Immobility
- Instability
- Incontinence
- Mental impairment

STOP THINK **35.3** In relation to older people who have difficulty with mobility, explore with them the effect of this on their lives.

It can be seen, therefore, that an older person who presents to the doctor with one of the four I's represents a very complex case. To treat the presenting cause is difficult, if not impossible. Treating the many underlying causes may require the prescription of a range of medications and this leads to another common phenomenon in older people — polypharmacy.

Polypharmacy

Polypharmacy is the prescription of more than four medications at the same time (DH 2001b). For the older person, the prescription of any medication has to be considered carefully. Due to the decline in glomerular filtration, older people require lower doses of most medications to achieve the desired effect (McGavock 2003). The therapeutic range of most medications is reduced such that lower doses are required to have the desired effect but also to avoid unwanted side-effects. The situation is compounded when more than one medication is prescribed, as older people are also more prone to adverse medication interactions whereby the administration of one medication either reduces the effect of another or enhances its effect and side-effects. While the prescription of medications remains largely a medical responsibility, monitoring the effects and side-effects of medications is a major nursing responsibility.

STOP THINK **35.4** Identify a number of older people living at home who have been prescribed several medications. Analyse the particular risks to these older people from polypharmacy.

Medications and older people

The problems which older people may have with medications arise as a result of the normal ageing process, the multipathology from which many older people suffer and difficulties in adhering to medication prescriptions. Of course, the problem often arises with prescribers who may not understand these difficulties sufficiently and who do not take enough care in their prescribing practices.

The main problem associated with ageing, already referred to, is the decreased filtration capacity of the kidneys. The effect of this is to alter the distribution of medications in the body — the pharmacokinetics (McGavock 2003) — such that for any given dose there is usually a higher level in the blood of an older person than in a younger person.

The down-regulation of cell receptors for hormones referred to earlier also affects medication receptors and this means that some tissues become less sensitive to certain medications, referred to as pharmacodynamics (McGavock 2003). For example, the tissues of the cardiovascular system, the blood vessels and the heart muscle, become less sensitive to adrenaline and noradrenaline (Collins 1998). However, older people are more sensitive to some other medications; for example, the cardiovascular system becomes less sensitive to adrenergic medications and the central nervous system becomes more sensitive to phenothiazines.

There is no general rule, but it can be seen that medication prescribing for older people requires considerable skill. For example, there will always be a tendency to lower medication dosages — that is a general rule — but where these medications are less effective there may be a tendency to increase the dose. The combined effect of pharmacokinetics and pharmacodynamic changes in older people will generally narrow the therapeutic index of the medication: there will be a narrow range within which the medication will work without leading to side-effects. The *British National Formulary* gives specific guidance in relation to prescribing medication to older people and this is summarised in Box 35.4.

Some of the other normal effects of ageing may become more significant for older people who are prescribed medications. The older person, who is likely to be taking more than one medication, may suffer from reduced hearing and poorer memory which may lead to difficulty in understanding a complicated medication regimen (Watson 2002). Poor vision may compound this due to difficulty in reading

Box 35.4

Guidelines for the administration of medications to older people

- First always question whether a drug is indicated at all.
- LIMIT RANGE. It is a sensible policy to prescribe from a limited range of drugs and to be thoroughly familiar with their effects in the elderly.
- REDUCE DOSE. Dosage should generally be substantially lower than for younger patients and it is common to start with about 50% of the adult dose. Some drugs (e.g. long-acting antidiabetic drugs such as glibenclamide and chlorpropamide) should be avoided altogether.
- REVIEW REGULARLY. Review repeat prescriptions regularly. In many patients it may be possible to stop some drugs, provided that clinical progress is monitored. It may be necessary to reduce the dose of some drugs as renal function declines.
- SIMPLE REGIMENS. Elderly patients benefit from simple treatment regimens. Only drugs with a clear indication should be prescribed and whenever possible given once or twice daily. In particular, regimens which call for a confusing array of dosage intervals should be avoided.
- EXPLAIN CLEARLY. Write full instructions on every prescription (*including* repeat prescriptions) so that containers can be properly labelled with full directions. Avoid imprecisions like 'as directed'. Child-resistant containers may be unsuitable.
- REPEATS AND DISPOSAL. Instruct patients what to do when drugs run out, and also how to dispose of any that are no longer necessary. Try to prescibe matching quantities.

If these guidelines are followed most elderly people will cope adequately with their own medicines. If not, then it is essential to enrol the help of a third party, usually a relative or a friend.

Reproduced with permission from the Joint Formulary Committee 2005.

NB: For the latest guidelines, refer to the current edition of the *British National Formulary*; the BNF is updated twice yearly.

labels and instructions and this, combined with reduced manual dexterity, either due to muscle atrophy or arthritis, may lead to problems opening medication packages (Watson 2002). Clearly, a great deal can be done to alleviate medication-related problems for older people and, in the UK, a National Service Framework, published as part of the *National Service Framework for Older People*, deals specifically with medicines and older people (DH 2001b).

- At the point of prescribing, clear, concise instructions should be given regarding medication prescription and this should be enhanced with written instructions — in clear large type — which the older person can take home.
- Pharmacists can provide packages with labels which have large writing and medicines in packages which are easily opened.
- Childproof containers are particularly problematic for some older people but, of course, additional precautions are required by older people who may be living with young children; packages that are not childproof must be kept out of their reach.

A range of professions is involved in ensuring that older people derive the most benefit from their prescribed medications and nurses have a key role to play with older people at home and in hospital. A detailed consideration of medications and older people and the strategies to help them is beyond the scope of this chapter but one major initiative is helping older people to learn about their medications while in hospital and to learn to self-administer these. This involves being able to allow older people to keep their medications while in hospital (Heath & Webster 1999). Secure storage is essential and accurate recording is required but this should ensure that older people can return home and be more independent with their medications.

Medication interactions and side-effects

Medication interactions are, of course, not unique to older people; when more than one medication is administered to anyone then there is the possibility of a medication interaction. As older people tend to take more medications, their chance of having a medication interaction is increased.

Some of the problems older people suffer from, including the 4 I's, may be caused by adverse medication reactions. Such reactions are more likely in older people due to the narrowed therapeutic index of medications and some classic adverse reactions include confusion, depression, falls, postural hypotension, constipation, urinary incontinence and Parkinsonism. The medications responsible are shown in Table 35.2 (Offerhaus 1997).

Table 35.2 **Medications causing adverse reactions in some common disorders of older people**

Confusional states	Depression	Falls	Postural hypotension	Constipation	Urinary incontinence	Parkinsonism
Hypnotics	Methyldopa	Hypnotics	All antihypertensives	Codeine	Loop diuretics	Antipsychotics
Tranquillisers		Tranquillisers	Diuretics	Dextro-propoxyphene	Hypnotics	Medication for vertigo
Antidepressants	Beta-blockers	Antidepressants	Antianginal medication	Narcotic analgesics	Tranquillisers	Methyldopa
Antipsychotics	Tranquillisers	Antipsychotics	Beta-blockers	Diuretics	Antipsychotics	
Anticholinergics (centrally acting)	Levodopa	Antihistamines	Hypnotics	Anticholinergics	Prazosin	Metoclopramide
Non-steroidal anti-inflammatory drugs	Corticosteroids	Carbamazepine	Tranquillisers	Disopyramide	Labetalol	
Levodopa		Phenytonin	Antidepressants	Verapamil		
Bromocriptine		Glyceryl trinitrate	Antipsychotics	Nifedipine	Beta-blockers	
Antidiabetics (hypoglycaemia)		All medication liable to produce postural hypotension	Antihistamines	Antipsychotics	Lithium*	
Corticosteroids			Levodopa	Antidepressants	All medication liable to produce faecal impaction	
Digitalis glycosides		—			—	
Anticonvulsants						
Cimetidine						

*Because of polyuria.

Reproduced from Offerhaus 1997, with permission from the World Health Organization.

Box 35.5

Medicines and older people: issues identified by the Department of Health (2001b)

- Many adverse reactions can be prevented
- Some medicines which could benefit older people are under-used
- Medicines are not taken because older people and their carers have not been involved in making decisions about their treatment
- Medicines are wasted due to some repeat prescription practices
- GPs change medication after older patients are discharged from hospital
- Primary and secondary care communication is poor
- Labels on some medications are inadequate
- Getting to the surgery or the pharmacy can be a problem for some older people
- The contribution that carers could make in helping older people with their medication is often not addressed
- Medication review could reduce costs
- Some long-term medications could be withdrawn without adverse effects

Box 35.6

Questions the older person could be asked during a medication review

- How long have you been taking/using this medicine?
- Is the medicine in its original container?
- What is the purpose of this medicine?
- Do you know how to take the medicine, when and how often?
- Do you have a daily routine for taking this medicine?
- Do you have any side-effects from this medicine?
- Do you have any medicine allergies?
- Do you buy (or has anyone else bought for you) any non-prescription medicines from the chemist or any other shop such as a supermarket?
- Has anyone (such as a friend or neighbour) given or 'lent' you any medicines, vitamins, herbal or homeopathic products to use?
- Do you use/take any other form of medication or home remedies or products prescribed by any other source of advice?
- Any other similar questions that may be important in individual cases

Reproduced with permission from the Department of Health (2001a).

The *National Service Framework: Medicines and Older People* (DH 2001b) was produced for some of the reasons summarised in Box 35.5. One of the main recommendations from the NSF was for medications review for older people and a framework for this, including the questions that should be asked of older people, was outlined. Questions, which are very relevant to nursing practice, are shown in Box 35.6.

Box 35.7

National Service Framework standards

- Standard one: rooting out age discrimination
- Standard two: person-centred care
- Standard three: intermediate care
- Standard four: general hospital care
- Standard five: stroke
- Standard six: falls
- Standard seven: mental health in older people
- Standard eight: the promotion of health and active life in older age

Reproduced with permission from the Department of Health (2001a).

THE NATIONAL SERVICE FRAMEWORK FOR OLDER PEOPLE

The care of older people is currently guided by the *National Service Framework for Older People* produced by the UK Department of Health in 2001 (DH 2001a). The NSF provides an overarching framework which deals with attitudes to the care of older people, primary and secondary care and, as described earlier, with specific aspects of the care of older people such as medicines. The NSF is presented as eight standards shown in Box 35.7.

Standard one

The first standard: rooting out age discrimination, sets the tone for the NSF and also hopes to set the tone for the care of older people in the UK. Essentially, with regard to NHS services, these should be provided 'regardless of age' with clinical decisions being made on the basis of the health of an older person and not on the basis of their age. The concept, once familiar in the care of older people, that any older person has had 'a good innings' and does not deserve further treatment is no longer acceptable (Watson & Buswell 2001) — if indeed, it ever was.

Standard two

Person-centred care, which is the focus of the second NSF standard, is a key concept in the care of older people and has long been championed by nurses working and researching in this area. The NSF promotes this by saying that older people must be treated as individuals and that they should be able to make choices about their care. Standard two also promotes the idea of a single assessment procedure which crosses the primary–secondary care interface and also spans health and social care. The objective here is to provide less fragmented pathways of care to older people by providing and sharing information across different settings.

Standard three

One of the objectives in caring for older people is to promote their independence and to provide care as close to home as possible. This has been seen over the last 20 years with the advent of care in the community initiatives (Henwood 1992); there is often a gap in care between hospital and home which is evident when an older person is able to leave hospital but not quite ready to manage on their own at home and this should be addressed through intermediate care, the focus of standard three of the NSF.

Intermediate care is a controversial subject and the concept itself almost defies definition (Andrews et al 2004). Across the UK there are as many different models of intermediate care as there are services delivering it and it has become the focus of research in recent years. Intermediate care may be anything from district nursing care, meals delivery or having a carpenter visit to make alterations such as adding handrails, which will help the older person to be independent (Andrews at al 2004). The point behind intermediate care is that it should be person-centred and based on the needs of the older person; it should also be time limited, perhaps to a number of days or weeks after which, if the older person continues to require such care, it is no longer intermediate and other care services, social and health, are required.

Standard four

It is recognised that the care of older people in general hospitals can be poor and this was reported in some detail in the landmark report entitled *Not Because They Are Old* (HAS 2000 1998). Older people are often, frankly, neglected in general hospitals in emergency departments, outpatient departments and in wards. This has been alluded to earlier in the chapter but the report by HAS 2000 highlighted prolonged waits in inappropriate surroundings leading to disorientation and development of pressure ulcers, and inadequate care on general wards with poor attention to nutrition, all of which may result in older people leaving hospital with more problems than those with which they entered. Standard four of the NSF addresses this issue directly and specifies that there should be specialist teams to provide advice on the care of older people in hospital and that a consultant in geriatric medicine should be available. Also, nurses should have appropriate education for the care of older people and attention should be given to the maintenance and improvement of the older person's health while in hospital, making use of a wide range of services.

Standard five

Stroke is a particular problem in older people due to changes in the vascular system of the brain and the NSF provides a separate standard (standard five) for this. Standard five includes, for example, stroke prevention and delivery of services by specialist stroke teams, including rehabilitation and long-term support.

Standard six

Another problem that is more common in older people is falls and this is related to one of the four 'giants of geriatric medicine' (Isaacs 1981), namely, instability. Falls lead to injury and are usually indicative of some underlying problem. Falls which result in injury may lead to immobility and the NSF standard six recommends the development of programmes to prevent falls in older people, improvements in the care of older people who have fallen and the prevention and treatment of osteoporosis. The National Institute for Clinical Excellence (2004) has published a clinical guideline related to falls in older people.

Standard seven

The mental health of older people includes the full range of mental health problems suffered by younger people, but depression and dementia are particularly common. Services across the UK vary widely for older people with mental health problems and the NSF specifies key interventions in standard seven for the promotion of good mental health, early recognition and management of mental health problems and the availability of specialist services for older people. In relation to this standard, it is recognised that those caring for older people with mental health problems at home require information, advice and support.

Standard eight

The NSF concludes with standard eight which relates to the much neglected area of health promotion and active living for older people. Pointing out that dependency and disability are not inevitable aspects of growing old, the NSF cites evidence that risk factors in later life can be modified and that there is no reason to withhold health promotion from older people. Specific interventions relate to heart disease, mental health and cancer and the NSF recognises that such programmes must be tailored for older people, taking into account cultural and ethnic diversity (RCN 1998). Interventions should be aimed at diet and nutrition, physical activity and immunisation, for example, annual winter protection from 'flu.

STOP THINK **35.5** Community nurses such as health visitors, district nurses and general practice nurses meet older people at home, in health centres and other community settings. Compare the contribution of these nurses to health promotion and care of older people.

SPECIFIC ISSUES IN THE CARE OF OLDER PEOPLE

It has been emphasised throughout this chapter that old age is not, in itself, a pathology and that old age is not inevitably associated with physical and mental problems. Nevertheless, it has also been demonstrated that there is some association between old age and some physical and mental problems and the nurse working with older people needs to understand these. The range of potential problems that could be covered is large but this section will focus on two specific areas: nutrition and incontinence.

Nutrition and older people

Older people generally suffer from more problems with nutrition than younger people (Copeman 1999) and it is especially the case that older people in hospital suffer greatly from nutritional problems (Tierney 1996). Mainly, although not exclusively, older people suffer from undernutrition which leads to weight loss and vulnerability to secondary problems of infection, skin breakdown, poor recovery from illness and from surgical procedures (Watson 2003). The reasons why older people suffer from poor nutrition are varied and encompass not only some of the biological problems which may be associated with age, such as lack of teeth and a reduced sense of smell and taste, but also such things as being immobile or less mobile due to a fall (Copeman 1999). This may prevent the older person from being able to prepare food or from being able to shop for appropriate food. However, there are also social and economic reasons why older people may become poorly nourished. Generally speaking, older people in retirement have reduced incomes compared to their working years and this may lead them to reduce their food intake or to eat foods that are less nutritious than they require (Copeman 1999). Older people with cognitive impairment related, for example, to dementia are particularly at risk of undernutrition (Watson 1997), especially in the terminal stages, but weight changes can become apparent very early, for example, in Alzheimer's disease (Barrett-Connor et al 1996).

The most important requirement for nurses caring for older people, with regard to nutrition, is to understand that problems can arise (see Ch. 21). Nurses have a considerable responsibility in hospital and at home to detect if an older person is suffering from undernutrition and towards this end they should be able to assist in the assessment of the nutritional status of older people. Usually, it is sufficient for the nurse to be able to screen for nutritional problems and then to pass this information to the doctor or the dietitian. However, the nurse, especially in hospital, has a major responsibility for helping older patients to eat and drink; whatever dietary supplements are prescribed by the doctor or dietitian, they will be completely ineffective if the older person with malnutrition cannot eat, drink or swallow. It is beyond the scope of this chapter to provide comprehensive guidance on the nutritional care of older people but excellent guidance, along with recommended dietary intakes and strategies to help older people to eat, has been published by Age Concern (see Box 35.8) (Copeman 1999). Other authors have outlined assessment strategies for dietary intake (Green & McDougall 2001) and fluid requirements (Woodrow 2002) in older people.

Box 35.8

Recommendations for food consumption by older people

- Dietary energy intakes of older people should tend to the generous, except for those who are obese
- Older people should derive their dietary intakes from a diet containing a variety of nutrient-dense food
- An active lifestyle, with prompt resumption after episodes of intercurrent illness, is recommended as contributing in several ways to good health
- Steps should be taken to increase the awareness by health professionals of the importance of both overweight and underweight in older people
- Intakes of fibre comparable to those of the general population are advised for most older people
- The statutory fortification of yellow fats other than butter with vitamins A and D should continue
- Older people should be encouraged to increase their dietary intakes of vitamin C
- Older people, in common with those of all ages, should be advised to eat more fresh vegetables, fruit and wholegrain cereals
- Older people should be encouraged to adopt diets which moderate their plasma cholesterol levels
- Older people should be encouraged to consume oily fish and to maintain physical activity to reduce the risk of thrombosis
- A daily intake of 6 g of salt is advised
- The calcium intakes of older people in the UK should be monitored
- Doorstep deliveries of milk for older people should be maintained
- All older people should be encouraged to expose some skin to sunlight regularly during summer; if not possible, vitamin D supplements should be given
- Health professionals should be aware of the often inadequate food intake of older people in institutions
- Assessment of nutritional status should be a routine aspect of history taking and clinical examination when an older person is admitted to hospital

Reproduced with permission from Copeman (1999).

Continence and older people

First of all, the myth must be dispelled that older people commonly suffer from incontinence. People can suffer from incontinence at any age but, as with many physical problems, there is an association between incontinence and ageing (Norton 1999). When referring to incontinence, it is usually urinary incontinence that is being implied; faecal incontinence is relatively rare. Urinary incontinence is more prevalent in women than in men but the frequency of incontinence rises in both men and women with age (Heath & Watson 2003). Urinary incontinence can lead to multiple problems that span the psychological, the social and the physical. People find urinary incontinence profoundly embarrassing and can become socially isolated as a result, with the condition completely dominating their lives (White & Getliffe 2003).

Urinary incontinence (see Ch. 24) can arise for several reasons but can usually be classified (Williams et al 1995) as follows:

- detrusor dysfunction arises from an inability to suppress spontaneous contractions of the bladder leading to voiding of urine
- stress incontinence arises through incompetence of the pelvic floor muscles and, while this is common in women following childbirth, it can arise in men following pelvic surgery
- outflow obstruction arises when there is something blocking outflow of urine from the bladder, for example, it may arise in constipation, prostate hyperplasia or as a result of a tumour, and this leads to urine overflowing periodically under the pressure in the bladder
- neurogenic bladder arises when the peripheral nervous supply to the bladder has been damaged; a common cause of this is dementia.

Urinary incontinence in older people is difficult to resolve unless the cause is obvious and easily obviated, such as an obstruction to outflow which can be removed or a urinary tract infection which can be treated. Nurses should understand the possible associations between ageing and urinary incontinence. In the absence of effective treatments, nurses should approach older people suffering from urinary incontinence with sensitivity, tact and the hope — in the absence of a cure — that life with urinary incontinence can be made more bearable (see Ch. 8).

Once again, it is beyond the scope of this chapter to provide detailed guidance regarding the management of urinary incontinence but it should be noted that a variety of appliances, some specific to men and some to women, are available and that technology in this area has vastly improved in recent years with the introduction of highly absorbent gels which help to keep the person with incontinence dry and free from odour.

PROMOTING THE DIGNITY AND INDEPENDENCE OF THE OLDER PERSON

It is hoped that the need to respect the dignity and independence of older people has been promoted thus far in this chapter. However, it is important finally to specify some areas of care where this can be promoted. There is no point in pretending that old age is a positive experience for everyone. Nevertheless, is behoves the nurse to have as positive an attitude towards ageing as possible and this will not, necessarily, be engendered only by working with older people. Reading around the subject of old age is very important and Hepworth (2000) in *Stories of Ageing*, for example, has studied how old age is portrayed in literature: often it is sad, sometimes amusing but always interesting to see how others view this, almost inevitable, stage of life. It is also important to realise that health promotion applies in old age as much as it applies in younger years (Bernard 2000) and, through empowerment and action, many older people have been able to take control of their lives in adverse circumstances and make a valuable contribution to health and social policy.

Consent

Often, however, nurses work with older people who are vulnerable; they may be in poor physical health and confused. This does not mean that their rights can be overridden, even in the apparent pursuit of the best interests of the older person; action taken must not lead to an affront to dignity. Wherever possible, the consent of an older person to treatment or even a seemingly innocuous nursing intervention is required (DH 2001c); specifically, treatment, including life-saving treatment, cannot be forced on an older person without consent. In particular, restraint should not be applied unnecessarily to an older person who is confused and who may be wandering or aggressive due to confusion. Clearly, patient and staff safety are paramount considerations but restraint has such harmful consequences (Strumpf et al 1998) that it should only be applied under very controlled conditions for which the Royal College of Nursing (1999) has produced relevant guidelines.

Related to restraint is the issue of elder abuse. This has been known about for many years but is becoming more widely acknowledged (CDNA 2003, British Geriatrics Society 2005). Nurses should be able to recognise signs of abuse and know what action to take.

CONCLUSION

This chapter has explored some aspects of the care of older people. More comprehensive texts should be consulted, many of which are referred to in this chapter (Matteson et al 1997, Heath & Schofield 1999, Redfern & Ross 1999). Likewise, there are specific areas of the care of older people which can be studied in greater depth such as nutrition (Copeman 1999), incontinence (Getliffe & Dolman 2003), intermediate care (Wade 2004) and dementia (Cantley 2001). As a nurse working with adults you will inevitably encounter older people in the course of your practice. You will have much to offer each older person you meet and, in turn, they will have much to offer you.

REFERENCES

Ahmed A, Tollefsbol T 2001 Telomeres and telomerase: basic science implications for aging. Journal of the American Geriatrics Society 49: 1105–1109

Andrews J A, Manthorpe J, Watson R 2004 Involving older people in intermediate care. Journal of Advanced Nursing 46: 303–310

Araujo A B, Mohr B A, McKinlay J B 2004 Changes in sexual function in middle-aged and older men: longitudinal data from the Massachusetts Male Aging Study. Journal of the American Geriatrics Society 52: 1502–1509

Armour D, Cairns C 2002 Medicines in the elderly. Pharmaceutical Press, London

Barrett-Connor E, Edelstien S L, Corey-Bloom J, Wiederholt W C 1996 Weight loss precedes dementia in community-dwelling older adults. Journal of the American Geriatrics Society 44: 1147–1152

Beers M H, Berkow R 2002 The Merck manual of geriatrics, 3rd edn. Merck, New Jersey

Bernard M 2000 Promoting health in old age. Open University Press, Buckingham

British Geriatrics Society 2005 Abuse of older people. BGS, London

British Society for Research on Ageing (BSRA) 2004 Scientific aspects of ageing: response to the House of Lords Science and Technology Committee enquiry. BSRA, London

Cancer Research UK 2005 Breast cancer incidence by age. Cancer Research UK, London

Cantley C 2001 A handbook of dementia care. Open University Press, Buckingham

Carrigan M, Szmigin I 2000 Advertising in an ageing society. Ageing and Society 20: 217–234

Christiansen J L, Grzybowski J M 1993 Biology of aging. Mosby, St Louis

Clay M 1999 Neglected areas: dental health, foot care and skin care. In: Heath H, Schofield I (eds) Healthy ageing. Mosby, London

Collins K J 1998 The autonomic nervous system. In: Pathy M S J (ed) Principles and practice of geriatric medicine, 3rd edn. Wiley, London

Community and District Nursing Association (CDNA) 2003 Responding to elder abuse. CDNA, London

Copeman J 1999 Nutritional care of older people. Age Concern Books, London

Deary I J 1995 Age associated memory impairment: a suitable case for treatment? Ageing and Society 15: 393–406

Deary I J 2001 Intelligence: a very short guide. Oxford University Press, Oxford

Department of Health 2001a National Service Framework for Older People. DH, London

Department of Health 2001b Medicines and older people: implementing medicine-related aspects of the NSF for older people. DH, London

Department of Health 2001c Seeking consent: working with older people. DH, London

Disney R 1996 Can we afford to grow older? MIT Press, Boston

Dyer C A E, Sinclair A J 1998 The premature ageing syndromes: insights into the ageing process. Age and Ageing 27: 73–80

Getliffe K, Dolman M 2003 Promoting continence: a clinical research resource, 2nd edn. Baillière Tindall, London

Goyns M H 2002 Genes, telomeres and mammalian ageing. Mechanisms of Ageing and Development 123: 791–799

Green S, McDougall T 2001 Assessing dietary intake in older people. Nursing Older People 13(6): 27–28

Harari D, Gurwitz J H, Minaker K L 1993 Constipation in the elderly. Journal of the American Geriatrics Society 41: 1130–1140

Harvey R J 2001 Epidemiology of presenile dementia. In: Hidges J R (ed) Early-onset dementia: a multidisciplinary perspective. Oxford University Press, Oxford

Health Advisory Service 2000 1998 Not because they are old. HAS 2000, London

Heath H, Schofield I (eds) 1999 Healthy ageing. Mosby, London

Heath H, Webster C 1999 Pharmacology and medications. In: Heath H, Schofield I (eds) Healthy ageing. Mosby, London

Heath T, Watson R 2003 Mostly male. In: Getliffe K, Dolman M (eds) Promoting continence: a clinical research resource, 2nd edn. Baillière Tindall, London

Heller PS 1998 Aging in the Asian tiger economies. Finance and Development 35(2): 26–29

Help the Aged and The Orders of St John Trust 1999 Dignity on the ward: promoting excellence in care. Good practice in acute hospital care for older people. Help the Aged, London

Henwood M 1992 Through a glass darkly. King's Fund Institute, London

Hepworth M 2000 Stories of ageing. Open University Press, Buckingham

Herbert R 1992 The normal aging process reviewed. International Nursing Review 39: 93–96

Horan M A 1992 Introduction – presentation of diseases in old age. In: Brocklehurst J C, Tallis R C, Fillit H M (eds) Textbook of geriatric medicine and gerontology. Churchill Livingstone, Edinburgh

International Labour Organisation 1990 No retirement for the ageing poor. ILO Information 26(4): 4

Isaacs B 1981 Ageing and the doctor. In: Hobman B (ed) The impact of ageing. Croom Helm, London

Joint Formulary Committee 2005 British National Formulary, 49th edn. British Medical Association and Royal Pharmaceutical Society of Great Britain, London. Online: Available: www.bnf.org

Kaye R 1993 Sexuality in later years. Ageing and Society 13: 415–426

Killeen J 2001 Involving people with dementia and their carers in developing services. In: Cantley C (ed) A handbook of dementia care. Open University Press, Buckingham

Kirkwood T 1999 Time of our lives. Phoenix, London

Kirkwood T 2001 The end of age. Profile Books, London

Kirkwood T 2002 Evolution of ageing. Mechanisms of Ageing and Development 123: 737–746

Loretto W, Duncan C, White P J 2000 Ageism and employment: controversies, ambiguities and younger people's perceptions. Ageing and Society 20: 279–302

Markle-Reid M, Browne G 2003 Conceptualizations of frailty in relation to older adults. Journal of Advanced Nursing 44: 58–68

Masson P R 1990 Long-term macroeconomic effects of aging populations. Finance and Development 27(2): 6–9

Matteson M A, McConnell E S, Linton A D 1997 Gerontological nursing: concepts and practice. Saunders, Philadelphia

McGavock H 2003 How drugs work. Radcliffe Medical Press, Oxford

McKeith I, Fairbairn A 2001 Biomedical and clinical perspectives. In: Cantley C (ed) A handbook of dementia care. Open University Press, Buckingham

National Institute for Clinical Excellence (NICE) 2004 The assessment and prevention of falls in older people. Clinical Guideline 21. NICE, London

NIH Consensus Development Panel on Osteoporosis Prevention, Diagnosis and Therapy 2001 Osteoporosis prevention, diagnosis and therapy. Journal of the American Medical Association 285: 758–795

Nolan M, Ingram P, Watson R 2002 Working with family carers of people with dementia. Dementia 1: 57–93

Norton C 1999 Eliminating. In: Redfern S J, Ross F M (eds) Nursing older people, 3rd edn. Churchill Livingstone, Edinburgh

Offerhaus L 1997 Drugs for the elderly, 2nd edn. World Health Organization, Geneva

Olshansky S J, Carnes B A, Cassel C K 1993 The aging of the human species. Scientific American 268(4): 18–24

Ponto M T 1999 The psychology of human ageing. In: Redfern S J, Ross F M (eds) Nursing older people, 3rd edn. Churchill Livingstone, Edinburgh

Posner R A 1995 Aging and old age. University of Chicago Press, Chicago

Redfern S J, Ross F M 1999 Nursing older people, 3rd edn. Churchill Livingstone, Edinburgh

Redmond K, Aapro M S 1997 Cancer in the elderly: a nursing and medical perspective. Elsevier, Amsterdam

Royal College of Nursing (RCN) 1998 The nursing care of older people from black and minority ethnic communities. RCN, London

Royal College of Nursing (RCN) 1999 Restraint revisited: rights, risk and responsibility. RCN, London

Royal Commission on Long Term Care 1999 With respect to old age. TSO, London

Rutishauser S 1994 Physiology and anatomy: a basis for nursing and health care. Churchill Livingstone, Edinburgh

Ruzicka S A 1997 Nursing diagnoses influenced by setting of care. In: Matteson M A, McConnell E S, Linton A D (eds) Gerontological nursing: concepts and practice. Saunders, Philadelphia

Schofield I 2000 Promoting travel health for older people. Elderly Care 12(2): 15–19

Seers K 1999 Pain and older people. In: Redfern S J, Ross F M (eds) Nursing older people, 3rd edn. Churchill Livingstone, Edinburgh

Slack J 1999 Mobility. In: Heath H, Schofield I (eds) Healthy ageing. Mosby, London

Standing Nursing and Midwifery Advisory Committee (SNMAC) 2001 Caring for older people: a nursing priority — integrating knowledge, practice and values. DH, London

Strumpf N E, Robinson J P, Wagner J S, Evans L K 1998 Restraint-free care: individualized approaches for frail elders. Springer, New York

Thomson P 1993 'I don't feel old': the significance of the search for meaning in later life. International Journal of Geriatric Psychiatry 8: 685–692

Tierney A J 1996 Undernutrition and elderly hospital patients: a review. Journal of Advanced Nursing 23: 228–236

United Kingdom Central Council for Nursing, Midwifery and Health Visiting 1994 Professional conduct – occasional report on standard of nursing in nursing homes. UKCC, London

Wade S 2004 Intermediate care of older people Wiley, London

Warnes R A 1993 Being old, old people and the burdens of burden. Ageing and Society 13: 297–338

Watson R 1993a Caring for elderly people. Baillière Tindall, London

Watson R 1993b Hypothermia in the elderly. Elderly Care 5(6): 41–46

Watson R 1997 Undernutrition, weight loss and feeding difficulty in elderly patients with dementia: a nursing perspective. Reviews in Clinical Gerontology 7: 317–326

Watson R 2002 Medications and older people. Nursing Older People 12(6): 21–26

Watson R 2003 Nursing older adults. In: Brooker C, Nicol M (eds) Nursing adults: the practice of caring. Mosby, Edinburgh

Watson R 2005 Anatomy and physiology for nurses. Elsevier, Edinburgh

Watson R, Buswell C 2001 End of 'a good innings' and the start of something better? Nursing Older People 13(4): 34–35

Watson R, Fawcett T N 2003 Pathophysiology, homeostasis and nursing. Routledge, London

White H, Getliffe K 2003 Mostly male. In: Getliffe K, Dolman M (eds) Promoting continence: a clinical research resource, 2nd edn. Baillière Tindall, London

Williams K, Roe B, Sindhu F 1995 An evaluation of nursing developments in continence care. National Institute for Nursing, Oxford

Wolf N 2004 How does one define aging in relation to pathology? Lifespan: The Journal of the British Society for Research on Ageing 12(2): 1–9

Woodrow P 2002 Assessing fluid balance in older people: fluid needs. Nursing Older People 14(9): 31–32

FURTHER READING

Banning M 2004 Enhancing older people's concordance with taking their medication. British Journal of Nursing 13(11): 669–674

Clarke A, Hanson E J, Ross H 2003 Seeing the person behind the patient: enhancing the care of older people using a biographical approach. Journal of Clinical Nursing 12(5): 697–706

Dewar B, Tocher R, Watson W 2003 Enhancing partnerships with relatives in care settings for older people. Nursing Standard 17(40): 33–39

Getliffe K, Dolman M (eds) 2003 Promoting continence: a clinical research resource, 2nd edn. Baillière Tindall, London

Help the Aged 2004 Older people: our neglected assets. Help the Aged, London

Hubbard G, Tester S, Downs M 2003 Meaningful social interactions between older people in institutional settings. Ageing and Society 23(1): 99–114

Jamieson A, Harper S, Victor C (eds) 1997 Critical approaches to ageing and later life. Open University Press, Buckingham

Meyer J, Sturdy D 2004 Exploring the future of gerontological nursing outcomes. Journal of Clinical Nursing 13(Suppl 2): 128–134

Reed J, Stanley D, Clarke C 2004 Health, well-being and older people. The Policy Press, Bristol

Squire A 2002 Health and well-being for older people. Baillière Tindall, Edinburgh

Walker A, Hennessy C H (eds) 2004 Growing older. Open University Press, Maidenhead

Webster J 2004 Person-centred assessment of older people. Nursing Older People 16(3): 22–27

USEFUL WEBSITES

Age Concern
www.ageconcern.org.uk

Alzheimer's Society
www.alzheimers.org.uk

Better Government for Older People
www.bgop.org.uk

British Society for Research on Ageing
www.bsra.org.uk

Cancer Research UK
www.cancerresearchuk.org

Help the Aged
www.helptheaged.org.uk

National Service Frameworks
www.dh.gov.uk/PublicationsAndStatistics/fs/en

Royal Bank of Scotland Centre for the Older Person's Agenda: Scottish Hub for Access to Research and Evidence
www.qmuc.ac.uk/opa/share

SUBSTANCE USE

Philip D. Cooper

36

INTRODUCTION

STOP THINK

36.1 In preparation for reading this chapter, carry out the following exercise:

(a) List as many legal and illegal substances you can think of. Beside each, briefly write your feelings, positive or negative, relating to these substances. For example, are they acceptable/attractive/frightening?

(b) Write a brief description of your feelings in relation to:
- illegal substance use and substance users
- alcohol use and problem drinkers
- tobacco use and smokers
- legal substances (e.g. prescribed medication, tea, coffee) and their users.

This chapter provides an introduction to substance use and outlines the important contribution that nurses can make to the care of people with substance use problems. The term 'substance use' refers to legal substances, i.e. alcohol, tea, coffee, tobacco and prescribed medications, and currently illegal substances, i.e. cannabis, cocaine, opiates and opioids. Whatever the nature of substance use, it must be considered in the context of the individual's personal history and circumstances; stereotypes of the substance user must be abandoned in favour of a more individualised and holistic understanding of the person. Not all substance use is problematic. As in all areas of nursing, interventions on behalf of the individual with substance use problems must be based on thorough assessment and should involve the individual and the family, as partners in care.

Because substance use may have physical, mental, emotional, social and economic implications for the individual, multiagency collaboration and approach to treatment is essential to ensure all dimensions of the person's situation are considered, as adjustments necessary to resolve a substance use problem are made (DH 2002a). Prochaska and DiClemente's (1986) seminal integrative model of change and Miller and Rollnick's (2002) motivational interviewing are outlined as approaches that will be relevant to nurses.

The importance of early identification cannot be overemphasised. To assist nurses in all fields in recognising the signs, and understanding the long-term effects of excessive or inappropriate substance use, the second half of the chapter outlines the physical, social, spiritual and psychological effects of using a range of legal and illegal substances. Alcohol use is discussed at some length, given the high prevalence of alcohol-related problems in the UK; emphasis on alcohol use and associated problems is reflected in the Scottish Alcohol Plan (Scottish Advisory Committee on Alcohol Misuse 2002) and the Alcohol Harm Reduction Strategy for England (Prime Minister's Strategy Unit 2004). However, Saunders and Marsh (1999) suggest that it is misleading to consider alcohol and drug use as separate entities, given the many similarities between their social, psychological and medical implications.

In view of the wide range of psychoactive substances that can be obtained by legal or illegal means, and the wide range of therapies that are available to individuals who seek help, this chapter cannot hope to be comprehensive. Readers are directed to the 'Further reading' list (p. 1167) when pursuing any topics of special relevance to their area of practice.

'Understanding drug use' is an interactive CD-ROM that provides an excellent overview of substance use problems and helps to put problematic substance use in perspective. Contact: The Drug and Alcohol Coordinator, Southern Public Health Unit, Bunbury, Western Australia (tel: +61 (08) 9792 2500; e-mail: raquel.willis@health.wa.gov.au).

For an overview of alcohol use, see Cooper (2000).

Definitions

Dependency

Drug dependency is described by the World Health Organization (WHO 2004a) as 'a cluster of cognitive, behavioural and physiological symptoms indicating that the individual continues the use of the substance despite significant substance-related problems'.

Dependency may be psychological or physical, or both, and is clinically defined by at least three of the following:

- A strong desire or sense of compulsion to take the substance
- Difficulties in controlling substance-taking behaviour in terms of its onset, termination or levels of use
- A physiological state of withdrawal
- Evidence of tolerance
- Progressive neglect of alternative pleasures or interests
- Persistent use despite clear evidence of overtly harmful consequences (WHO 2004a).

Thus, dependency may develop when an individual becomes physically, socially or psychologically reliant on a substance, such that life without it becomes intolerable. Dependency is not automatic. Saunders and Marsh (1999) argue that any substance can be used without the user becoming dependent on it.

During the 1960s, many experts attempted to clarify the distinction between addiction and habituation. These two terms were subsequently abandoned in favour of dependence. It is therefore safe to assume that 'dependence' and 'addiction' refer to the same thing. However, an increasing number of professionals working within the substance use field believe that such labels as dependence and addiction are, at best, unhelpful in the treatment setting.

Other terms

Drug The WHO Expert Committee on Drug Dependence describes the word 'drug' as 'a term of varied usage'. As a medicinal product, 'drug' can refer to 'any substance in a pharmaceutical product that is used to modify or explore physiological systems or pathological states for the benefit of the recipient' (WHO 1985). In addition, the term is used to refer to non-prescribed and illicit substances that include alcohol, tobacco and caffeine.

Tolerance and cross-tolerance are generally understood in pharmacology, the former as 'a decrease in response to a drug dose that occurs with continued use', and the latter as 'the development of tolerance to another substance, to which the individual has not previously been exposed, occurring as a result of acute or chronic intake of a substance'.

Substance misuse This is 'the result of a psychoactive substance, drug or alcohol, being consumed for a purpose other than that for which it was intended, and that causes physical, social and psychological harm' (Rassool 1998). However, it could be argued that many people consume substances, e.g. alcohol, intentionally for social reasons and that such intentional use can result in physical, social or psychological harm. Many illicit substances, e.g. ecstasy, are manufactured specifically to help individuals enjoy a social occasion. Therefore the user is consuming the substance for the purpose for which it was intended. The smoker with a diagnosis of lung cancer will have experienced physical harm as a result of using tobacco for the purpose intended. These individuals have not 'misused' but 'used' substances in a manner that could be harmful or hazardous. The term ***substance use*** may therefore be a more appropriate term to apply to individuals who use drugs or alcohol and it is the term that will be used throughout this chapter. Substance use could be described as a continuum ranging from low risk use, through harmful and hazardous use to dependence. Not all individuals will remain static on the continuum nor will all progress to dependence. Individuals may move back and forth along the continuum during their substance-using career in response to personal and/or social circumstances.

Detoxification is a process of removing from the body the substance on which the individual is physiologically dependent. During this process, medication may be prescribed and the individual is assisted in making lifestyle adjustments such that the substance is no longer needed. Detoxification is increasingly undertaken in the home environment. Only severe cases, in which complications have been identified, require hospitalisation (Cooper 1994).

Withdrawal symptoms These are best described as psychological and/or physiological reactions to the reduction or complete withdrawal of the substance of use. How long withdrawal lasts depends on the previous use of the substance and on the nature and extent of both physiological and psychological dependence (Cooper 1994).

A MODEL FOR CHANGING ADDICTIVE BEHAVIOURS

In 1984, a seminal conference held in Scotland aimed to 'develop a more comprehensive model of change for the treatment of addictive behaviours' (Prochaska & DiClemente 1986). It was agreed that any model developed should be applicable to the many different ways in which people change, ranging from those requiring maximum intervention (hospitalisation) to those needing minimal intervention, e.g. self-help manuals (Prochaska & DiClemente 1986). This model had to be applicable to the variety of dependency behaviours that individuals wish to change and, at the same time, to advance the understanding of how people change their behaviours, from the stage at which a problem is recognised to the point at which it is resolved.

Prochaska and DiClemente (1986) proposed a model of change, which is now widely accepted. This model provides a framework that assists professionals in organising their knowledge and in making case management decisions. Prochaska and DiClemente felt that this model should take account of the person who self-changes as well as the individual progressing through therapy and that it should be applicable to the wide range of dependency problems that exist. In addition, it should help the therapist to synthesise the various treatment methods presently available.

The Prochaska and DiClemente (1986) model is 'three-dimensional', integrating changes, together with processes and levels of change. The model comprises four stages — pre-contemplation, contemplation, action and maintenance — which may be conceived of as cyclical, thus allowing the individual to join or leave the process of change at any given stage (see Fig. 36.1). This model is also referred to as 'the integrative model of change' or 'the motivation to change model'. Its stages are described as follows:

- *Pre-contemplation stage* — at this stage the individual is not aware of dependency. This could be because of ambivalence, denial or selective exposure to information. As the individual becomes aware of the problem, progression to the next phase is made possible.
- *Contemplation stage* — at this point the individual admits that something is wrong and begins to think seriously about behaviour change. This stage may last for a few weeks to many years, and some individuals never progress beyond this point.
- *Action stage* — here, the individual makes a commitment to alter the problematic behaviour. This is a brief stage; when the decision has been made the individual progresses to the next stage.
- *Maintenance stage* — at this point, new behaviour is strengthened and develops into self-efficacy; the individual's feeling of being in control is maximised. This stage affords the exit point to termination.

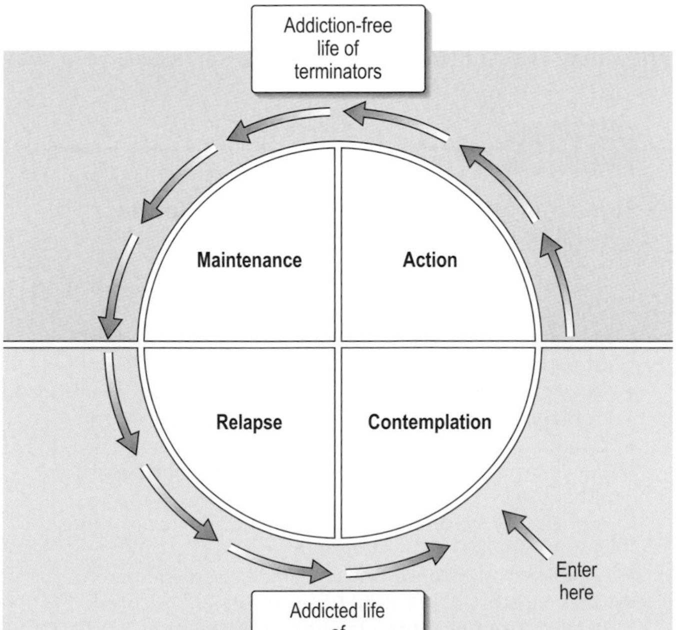

Fig. 36.1 The integrative model of change. (Reproduced with permission from Prochaska & DiClemente 1986.)

At the maintenance stage, the individual may temporarily lapse as a result of the extreme effort required to maintain the change in behaviour. Occasionally this extends to relapse, in which case the individual often goes back to the pre-contemplation stage before rejoining the cycle. Prochaska and DiClemente (1986) suggest that 84% of 'relapsers' progress back into the contemplation stage. In addition, it has been indicated that the typical self-changer makes three revolutions of the change cycle before exiting into a relatively dependency-free life (Schacter 1982, Prochaska & DiClemente 1983). However, some individuals do become arrested at one particular stage.

It is essential that the individual and the professional are in agreement as to which stage of change is relevant at a given time. Any resistance to therapeutic interventions often comes as a direct result of the therapist and client working at different stages of the change process. Prochaska and DiClemente (1986) explain the importance of this as follows:

> *The more directive, action-orientated therapist would find a client who is at the contemplation stage to be highly resistant to therapy. From the client's perspective, however, the therapist may be seen as wanting to move too quickly ... A therapist who specialises in contemplating and understanding the causes of problems will tend to see the client who is ready for action as resistive to the insight aspect of therapy. The client would be warned against acting impulsively. From the client's perspective ... the therapist might be warned against moving too slowly.*

In applying the Prochaska–DiClemente integrative model of change in their interventions with substance-using individuals, nurses should never hesitate to seek help and advice from more experienced or knowledgeable practitioners. Nurses should strive to be well informed about all aspects of substance use. Nurses of all levels and specialties have contact with individuals with substance use problems and therefore need to be aware of the physical, social, psychological and legal consequences of dependency and the implications of these for the individual, the family and the nurse (Prime Minister's Strategy Unit 2004).

THE ROLE OF THE NURSE

Although our understanding of substance use has improved in recent years, there remains a tendency for nurses and other professionals to fail to identify substance-using individuals. The Scottish Advisory Committee on Alcohol Misuse (2002) and the Prime Minister's Strategy Unit (2004) suggest a multidisciplinary approach is essential and expound the need for shared care as an effective intervention for those with substance use problems.

Inadequate preparation in pre/post-registration nursing education is a barrier to providing effective management and interventions for these individuals. However, the Alcohol Harm Reduction Strategy for England (Prime Minister's Strategy Unit 2004) makes specific recommendations regarding the need for pre/post-registration education and training for all health professionals in the early identification of alcohol problems. Nurses may feel unable or reluctant to engage with substance-using individuals for a number of reasons:

- *Role legitimacy* – nurses are uncertain as to whether, or how far, harmful substance use falls within their remit

- *Role adequacy* – nurses perceive a lack of knowledge and skill in identifying and responding to substance-using clients
- *Role support* – nurses feel that they would have insufficient access to or support from specialist services should they identify a harmful substance user (Cooper 1994).

For some professionals, increased knowledge and understanding of substance use may challenge their own values, attitudes and beliefs. Their own use of alcohol or drugs may be questioned, giving rise to negative attitudes towards substance use. Such attitudes may impact on the quality of care provided. The individual who uses substances is often viewed as not motivated to change, manipulative and self-destructive (Banerjee et al 2002). Professionals may find it difficult to work with someone who is perceived as a demanding individual. Nurses must be aware of their own attitudes towards substance use and of how this impacts on standards of care.

In their interactions with individuals with a substance use problem, it is important for nurses to recognise that the substance used is but one part of the problem. Each person presents with unique concerns that may cause, contribute to or interact with the development of the presenting state. Individuals experiencing substance use problems often change their behaviour as a direct result of crisis, such as a change in an important relationship, an accident or illness, redundancy, a birth or a death. Such events can curtail, neutralise or enhance the nurse's endeavours with an individual (Davidson 1991) and must be taken into account in the formulation of treatment and intervention. During interactions with the person, the nurse should be prepared to:

- identify the individual with a substance use problem
- recognise the types of problems experienced by the individual
- assist the individual in the process of acknowledging, exploring and understanding substance use
- appreciate the individual's own perception of substance use
- consider with the individual the treatment and intervention options
- facilitate achievement of the person's chosen goal(s)
- acquaint the individual with available services and facilities
- act in a non-judgemental way
- provide nursing interventions in withdrawal
- provide understanding and support should relapse occur.

STOP THINK **36.2** The following exercise may help the reader to imagine themselves in the problem substance user's place. For 1 week, stop using your favourite substance, e.g. tea, coffee, alcohol, chocolate, tobacco. At the end of the week, make a few notes on the following:

(a) How easy did you find it to live without the substance?
(b) Was your mood affected? If so, in what way? Did you experience cravings?
(c) What strategies did you use to avoid temptation?

Identifying substance use

The early identification of substance use is important in providing appropriate intervention or accessing relevant support. Box 36.1 lists various signs and symptoms that can indicate the existence of a substance use. However, there is a danger that some of these may be dismissed as being attributed to the primary illness. For instance, an individual in an acute mental health unit may exhibit increasing symptoms of psychosis, restlessness and anxiety in the hours following admission. This may be misdiagnosed and treated according to a primary diagnosis of acute psychotic disorder. Alternatively, an individual who arrives in a surgical ward in the morning, in preparation for an operation, may become overanxious and agitated by the evening, which may be interpreted as preoperative apprehension. It is possible that both individuals may have alcohol-related problems. Therefore, during assessment, nurses should be aware that not every feature listed necessarily applies to a given individual, nor does the existence of any one feature demonstrate or exclude conclusively a substance use problem.

Whilst the use of alcohol and drugs has increased over the past few decades, not all individuals who use substances will develop related problems. Many individuals limit their use to weekends. During the week, nurses, for example, hold positions of responsibility and trust and their weekend substance use does not appear to impact on their ability to complete daily tasks. The majority of individuals use substances responsibly and are aware of the effects and consequences of such use.

Substance use is often time limited. When responsibilities change at home (relationships/children) and at work (promotion), most individuals adjust their substance use. Although there are health risks associated with this type of use, the damage is less severe and disabling than through prolonged, repeated use. For a small minority, however, their substance use will continue and dependence may occur. They may use substances as a means of release or a way

Box 36.1

Signs that may alert the professional to the existence of a substance-using client

- Physical health problem, e.g. vitamin deficiency, gastritis, infections, ulcers
- Mental health problem, e.g. anxiety, depression, suicide attempts
- Symptoms of substance use, e.g. tremor, shakes, sweating
- Problem at work, e.g. lateness, absenteeism, accidents
- Criminal offences
- Family problems, e.g. neglect, child disturbance, marital disharmony
- Requests for help, e.g. from the client, family or other professional
- Evidence of substance use, e.g. smell, used equipment
- Known history of substance use
- Family history of substance use
- Other, e.g. complaints of fatigue, lethargy, insomnia, restlessness

of coping with memories of traumatic childhood events, difficult family or marital relationships or work-related stress. For these individuals the accurate early identification of problems and the provision of timely interventions are essential.

Approaching a substance use problem

If assessment identifies a substance use problem, further exploration of the substance use should be raised in a non threatening manner. While the individual may initially be evasive or defensive, at least there has been a demonstration of concern and a first approach. The subject should not be laboured but the nurse should be tactful and sensitively try to make progress at each contact. The nurse is not a judge, but a facilitator, educator and carer.

Bedside conversations in large wards do not facilitate confidentiality. Curtains round a bed do not block out sound. Nurses should consider where and how they would want to be approached if they were in the same situation and apply the standards of confidentiality that would be expected for themselves in their interactions with others.

If nurses are unsure about how to proceed, they should seek advice and support. Local agencies may be helpful, as may colleagues who have similar individuals on their caseloads. Mutual support is essential in all areas of nursing.

Assessment

Intervention should only be undertaken following a full and systematic assessment of the individual's and the family's needs. If treatment is to be effective and therapeutic, a complete picture of the person's substance use must be obtained. Moreover, a clear understanding of the person's chosen treatment goals is essential. Is the aim to reduce use, to change to a less harmful substance, to control use, withdrawal or total abstinence?

Many individuals with substance use problems 'sound out' a service before committing to care. Therefore, any information given on treatment options should be clear and to the point, and communicated both verbally and in written form. Assessment should include details of past and present substance use. In preparation, the individual could be asked to complete a diary similar to that shown in Figure 36.2. The following factors should always be considered in any assessment:

- psychological state
- work, social and cultural factors
- problematic effects of use
- motivation for treatment
- family psychodynamics
- relevant personal factors
- physical state and complications.

Brief intervention

Brief intervention is an approach less intensive than that of traditional methods. It can range from 5–10 min of information-giving, to three to five individuals, or group, sessions involving motivational interviewing techniques. Brief intervention is usually opportunistic, i.e. the primary reason for contact with the nurse is not related to substance use. Brief intervention is aimed at non-dependent substance users whose consumption is harmful but who are not experiencing consequential major health problems. However, it can be offered to those expressing concern or seeking advice about use. Brief intervention is motivational and should encourage the individual to conclude that a reduction in use, or less harmful use, is beneficial. It should aid individuals in identifying their own goals in order to reduce or modify substance use. Information, written and verbal, should be provided regarding the health risks associated with the particular substance use and any advice given should be tailored to individual needs.

Bien et al (1993) identified six elements shown to be effective in brief intervention, described as the FRAMES model:

- **F**eedback — assessment and evaluation of the problem
- **R**esponsibility — emphasising personal choice
- **A**dvice — explicit advice on changing behaviour
- **M**enu — aiding the development of alternative goals and strategies
- **E**mpathic interviewing — a non-confrontational reflective approach
- **S**elf-efficacy — instilling optimism that chosen goals can be achieved.

All nurses, whether working in hospital or community, should be capable of offering this intervention. The World Health Organization (2001) offers an excellent manual on brief intervention in primary care that includes guidance for clinicians, an education brochure and self-help book (see Box 36.2 for information offered in brief intervention).

Prevention

Whether or not an individual develops a substance use problem depends on the social resources available. It is vital that the problems and experiences that can set the stage for substance use problems are recognised by health and social care professionals and that relevant agencies persevere in improving and developing preventive strategies at both local and national levels.

In recent years, campaigns such as 'No Smoking Day' and 'Drinkwise Day' have had some effect. Most health authorities now have a drug and alcohol advisory service, as well as a health promotion officer dealing with HIV/AIDS-related issues (see Ch. 37). Initiatives such as outreach programmes and needle exchange schemes have proved valuable in the early identification of substance users (see p. 1175).

Nurses and substance use

It is important that nurses are aware of the high levels of stress that they may experience in their professional lives, which can make them vulnerable to substance use problems (Coombs 1996). It is very hard for a nurse to broach this subject with a colleague suspected of substance use. It is equally as difficult for the nurse with a substance use problem, as it is for any other person, to admit to this and ask for help because of the negative attitudes and stigma still

Day	Time drinking commenced and ended	Type and amount consumed	Mood prior	Mood after	Number of units consumed
Monday					
Tuesday					
Wednesday					
Thursday					
Friday					
Saturday					
Sunday					
Totals					

Fig. 36.2 Sample form for an alcohol use diary.

Box 36.2

Brief intervention

Information offered in brief intervention to a problem drinker in a primary care or acute ward setting:
The nurse has identified an individual at possible risk of harmful alcohol use. This may be through conversation during routine procedures or as a direct/indirect result of the person's attendance/admission to the clinical area.

Accurate assessment
The Fast Alcohol Screening Test (FAST) enables the nurse to assess the need and level of intervention required if alcohol use is hazardous. FAST consists of four questions and is completed in 1 min. A score of 3 or more indicates a risk of alcohol-related harm. To obtain a clearer picture of the extent of a person's alcohol use, a drinking diary could be completed (see Fig. 36.2). A drinking diary highlights the frequency, levels, patterns and triggers to an individual's alcohol consumption on a 'typical' week that can subsequently be explored. From the drinking diary the individual can be taught how to calculate the weekly alcohol consumption in units (also referred to as 'standard drinks'). The risk levels and appropriate interventions required are as follows:

- *Low risk*: men <21 and women <14 units/week — general preventive strategies; it is important to note that the recommendations suggest low risk and ***not*** no risk
- *Moderate risk*: men 21–50 and women 14–35 units/week — brief intervention strategies
- *High risk*: men >50 and women >35 units per week — specialist agency referral
- *Binge drinking*: men >8 units and women >6 units/drinking session — information specific to binge drinking and intervention as above depending on level of consumption.

Providing information
During brief intervention, the nurse offers practical advice and information, tailored to meet the needs of the individual. Information on weekly and daily drinking is provided, in addition to how to calculate units. Offering information on the consequences of harmful alcohol use should be considered, paying attention to the harm associated with intoxication, binge drinking and excessive use (see Box 36.4). The individual is aided to consider the positive and negative consequences of alcohol consumption in relation to social, physical, psychological and spiritual needs. Practical advice can be given on how to reduce alcohol consumption. Examples include changing strength of drinks from a higher to a lower alcohol content, drinking more slowly, alternating alcoholic and non-alcoholic drinks, eating food (e.g. crisps), engaging in other activities whilst drinking to slow consumption (e.g. playing pool, darts or cards), or setting limits on consumption. It is useful to consider alternative activities to drinking that the individual may find enjoyable.

Written material to complement and build on, if necessary, the information provided during an intervention should be offered. Appropriate contact details of local alcohol services should be provided where necessary. If referral to a specialist agency is required and the individual agrees, the nurse may make contact to arrange a full assessment or provide written details.

associated with substance use in today's society. The nurse with a substance use problem may ask the following questions (Cooper & Faugier 1993):

- Will my colleagues find out details of my problem and treatment?
- If I cannot look after myself, how can others be entrusted to my care?
- Will treatment for a substance use problem be noted on my record and limit my professional development?
- How will I relate to the nurses who are caring for me?
- Will I be suspended, disciplined or asked to leave?
- Will I be considered responsible enough to continue in my profession if I accept help?
- How will I convince others that I can be trusted to hold drug cupboard keys?
- How can I impress on senior managers and nursing colleagues that any future time off from work is not due to the substance use?
- How will I arrange regular time off to keep my counselling appointments?

How nurses can get help

The nurse who has acknowledged a substance use problem should check to see whether the employer has an alcohol and drug workplace policy. If a nurse feels that substance use problems, of any kind, are affecting working life, then seeking help before formal measures by the employer become necessary is imperative. It is possible to approach the Occupational Health Service or an outside agency in confidence. If the problem has been brought into the open by a warning from an employer, then the workplace policy will be invoked and the nurse referred to Occupational Health for further support and treatment. The nurse should make sure that the policy is duly followed. Although probably under a contract, by which improvement in work performance is required, the policy is usually in the nurse's favour, protecting job security whilst undertaking agreed therapy, and providing adequate time off to attend counselling and treatment sessions.

DUAL DIAGNOSIS

The term dual diagnosis is applied to individuals who experience a coexisting mental health and substance use problem (drugs or alcohol). This term is not a diagnostic label but rather it signifies an individual with a coexisting mental health and substance use disorder who has complex needs rather than two distinct problems (Banerjee et al 2002). Dual diagnosis encompasses a diverse group of individuals with differing types of mental disorder, with varying degrees of severity, who may be using one or more psychoactive substances in varying frequencies and in varying amounts (Ryrie & McGowan 1998).

The Department of Health (2002b) identify four possible mechanisms that may lead to a dual diagnosis:

- A primary psychiatric illness precipitating or leading to substance misuse
- Substance misuse worsening or altering the course of a psychiatric illness
- Intoxication and/or substance dependence leading to psychological symptoms
- Substance misuse and/or withdrawal leading to psychiatric symptoms or illness.

It is estimated that approximately one-third of the UK mental health population has a substance use problem and that 50% of individuals seen by drug and alcohol services have some form of mental health problem (Banerjee et al 2002). Individuals with a severe mental illness are more than twice as likely as the general population to have an alcohol disorder and those who have an alcohol problem at some point during their lifetime more than double their likelihood of experiencing mental health problems (Regier et al 1990).

Clenaghan (2000) considers there are a number of theories as to why people with a mental health problem use substances. Such theories include:

- for the same reasons as others in the community use alcohol or drugs
- as an attempt to alleviate the symptoms of mental illness
- to reduce the side-effects of medication.

Concern for this group of individuals has increased in recent years and current service provision appears unable to address their needs adequately. Individuals with a dual diagnosis, when compared to those with a mental health problem alone, are more likely to have:

- increased risk of suicide
- more severe mental health problems
- homelessness and unstable housing
- increased risk of being violent
- increased risk of victimisation
- more contact with the criminal justice system
- family problems
- history of childhood abuse (sexual/physical).

They are also:

- more likely to slip through the net
- less likely to be compliant (Banerjee et al 2002).

The Department of Health (2002a) offers a treatment model within which different approaches may be required at differing stages. The model aims to aid clinicians in acknowledging the long-term nature of interventions with dual diagnosis individuals and in identifying and offering appropriate and timely interventions. The model consists of four stages:

- *Engagement* — the development and maintenance of a therapeutic clinician–client relationship that is empathic, non-judgemental and non-confrontational
- *Persuasion* — draws on the principles of motivational interviewing, exploring ambivalence and motivation to change
- *Active treatment* — can only take place if goals are realistic and set by the client
- *Relapse prevention* — educating clients about their early warning signs; anxiety management and coping skills training.

Readers with a special interest in the area of prevention are referred to Keene (1997) and Watson (2000).

SUBSTANCE USE: SOME FACTS

LEGAL SUBSTANCES

Caffeine

> *The sufferer is tremulous and loses his self-command; is subject to fits of agitation and depression. He loses colour and has a haggard appearance. As with other agents, a renewed dose of the poison gives temporary relief, but at the cost of future misery.*
>
> *(Cited in Pickles 1991)*

Coffee, tea, colas, 'energy' drinks and some analgesics contain caffeine, a substance that has a stimulating effect upon the central nervous system. The existence of a caffeine withdrawal syndrome is now accepted. Silverman et al (1992) stated that 'caffeine withdrawal can produce severe symptoms, and health care professionals should be aware of the problem'. Participants in their double-blind study underwent physical and psychological tests during a period of normal diet followed by a period of caffeine-free diet. Half the group, who received a caffeine supplement during the second period, reported no significant change. The other half, given placebo drugs, recorded more headaches, increased use of analgesics and greater fatigue. Depression and anxiety scores were also abnormally high in this group. Drinking more than eight cups of coffee per day is likely to induce symptoms of withdrawal. Caffeine intake above 300 mg/day has been associated with low birth weight and miscarriage. This increased risk is possibly due to the extended half-life of caffeine in pregnant women from 4–6 h to 18 h and the cumulative effect of this (COT 2001). The equivalent of 300 mg of caffeine is three average mugs of coffee, six average cups of tea, eight regular colas and eight standard 50 g chocolate bars.

Tobacco

Nicotine is the drug in tobacco that causes addiction (USDHHS 1989). The World Health Organization (2003) refers to tobacco consumption as the 'global tobacco epidemic'. There were about 5 million tobacco-related deaths worldwide in 2003, an increase of over one million from 1990. Smoking tobacco is globally and regionally recognised as one of the top 10 risks in terms of the burden of disease it causes (WHO 2002) and is the world's leading preventable cause of death (WHO 2003).

It takes between 10 and 19 s for the chemicals contained in tobacco smoke to produce an effect within the brain (Royal College of Physicians 2000). The primary effect of nicotine is that it appears to stimulate the release of dopamine in the brain (Taylor Hays 2000), a chemical similar to adrenaline, which is responsible for emotional response and pleasure. Nicotine's positive effects include reduced stress and anxiety, relaxation, the enhancement of cognitive function, weight control (USDHHS 1989) and mood modulation (Nissell et al 1995). The rapid decline of these effects, however, encourages further use, and dependence develops quickly. If tobacco use is stopped abruptly, restlessness, irritability, anxiety, nervousness, impaired cognitive function and concentration, and craving may be experienced.

Tobacco use is on the rise and every second a smoker will die of tobacco-caused disease (WHO 2003). Around 120 000 people die each year from smoking-related causes in England alone (Royal College of Physicians 2002). In 1998, Raw et al estimated the health cost of tobacco-related illnesses as up to £1.7 billion a year. In 2002, 10% of 11–15 year olds were regular smokers (DH 2003).

Consequences for health

The high cost of tobacco use to the nation's health is clearly demonstrated in Table 36.1. Tobacco use is also thought to be a contributing factor in the development of pancreatic cancer, peripheral vascular disease, respiratory infections, cancer of the lungs, mouth and throat, coronary heart disease, and increased severity of asthma (WHO 2004b).

Women and smoking A total of 30% of women smoke during pregnancy, a figure that has remained consistent for at least a decade (Owens & Penn 1999). Women from lower socioeconomic backgrounds are at increased risk from tobacco use with 43% of women in social groups C2DE smoking during pregnancy, compared to 15% from groups ABC1 (Owens & Penn 1999). It has been suggested that pregnant women who smoke run the risk of spontaneous abortion, low birth weight and infant death (Bloch 2000). Reports have suggested a close link between smoking and sudden infant death syndrome (SIDS) (Mitchell et al 1992, 1993).

The incidence of cancer of the cervix is high among women who smoke heavily (Health Education Authority 1996) and, as in the general population, women who smoke increase their risk of coronary heart disease, stroke, blood clots, pulmonary embolism, circulatory disease, and raised blood pressure and cholesterol levels (Health Education Authority 1996).

Smoking has also been associated with reduced fertility in both men and women (British Medical Association 2004).

Passive smoking

Children and adolescents exposed to passive smoking have been quoted as being at risk of the adverse effects of smoking. Impaired respiration, chest infections and asthma in children are more often associated with parental smoking

Table 36.1 Estimated incidence of tobacco-related death in the UK in 1997

Disease	Number
Lung cancer	29 200
Ischaemic heart disease	24 300
Chronic obstructive pulmonary disease (COPD)	23 700
Other cancers: buccal cavity, oesophagus, larynx, bladder, kidneys and cervix	15 900
Aortic aneurysm and atherosclerotic peripheral disease	5800
Peptic ulcers	2000

Adapted from Royal College of Physicians (2000).

than with any other causative factor (Pagliaro & Pagliaro 1996).

People who are subjected to the smoke of others in the home have a 24% increased risk of developing lung cancer (Hackshaw et al 1997) and a 23% increased risk of developing heart disease (Law et al 1997). The effects of tobacco smoke on non-smokers can include nose, throat and chest irritations, breathing difficulties, coughing, red and runny eyes, headaches, dizziness, nausea, lack of concentration and decrease in lung function. Those with long-term health problems such as asthma, chronic bronchitis, allergies and heart problems are especially at risk.

Cessation aids

It has been suggested that 68% of male and 65% of female smokers would like to stop (Office for National Statistics 2002). However, pharmacological and psychological dependence often prevents them from doing so. The NHS Cancer Plan (DH 2000) identified that a third of all cancers were related to smoking and set a target to reduce smoking among manual groups from the 1998 figure of 32% to 26% by 2010 and outlined a plan of how this would be achieved (see Box 36.3).

A combination of pharmacological therapy and behavioural intervention is the most effective treatment for nicotine dependence (Taylor Hays 2000). Pharmacological interventions include nicotine replacement therapies such as transdermal patches, gum, lozenge, nasal spray, inhaler and sublingual tablet in addition to bupropion (Zyban), a non-nicotine medication. Behavioural interventions include specialist interventions in the form of smoking cessation clinics, counselling and group work, and opportunistic brief interventions by non-specialist practitioners. Information provided in a successful brief intervention should include the setting of a definite stop date, problem-solving skills training and relapse prevention training (Taylor Hays 2000).

Changing to a low tar brand of cigarette has not been shown to reduce the risk of developing tobacco-related harm. This is due to the smoker consuming the tobacco more vigorously than the machine used in the laboratory for testing tar levels and adapting their smoking behaviour, consciously or otherwise, so as to increase nicotine intake. Nicotine intake per cigarette has been shown to be up to eight times greater than the machine-smoked yields (Jarvis et al 2001).

Box 36.3

Tobacco control strategy

- Commitment to ban tobacco advertising
- New specialist NHS smoking cessation services
- Nicotine replacement therapy is available on prescription from GPs (DH 2001)
- Nicotine replacement therapy to be made available on general sale rather than only through pharmacies or on prescription — available since May 2001 (DH 2001)
- Bupropion (Zyban) available on prescription from primary care
- Updated guidance on smoking for health care professionals and commissioners from the Health Development Agency
- A best practice code to enforce the law against cigarette sales to children under 16
- A new media campaign and an NHS smokers' help line

From Department of Health 2000, 2001.

The Health Education Authority produces booklets that the nurse may find useful.

Action on Smoking and Health (ASH) produce a set of information sheets (see 'Useful websites and addresses', p. 1167).

Alcohol

STOP THINK **36.3** For a 1-week period, keep a daily diary of your alcohol consumption, using the format given in Figure 36.2. When you have read the following section, refer to your diary as you discuss with your colleagues your reactions to and reflections on your own alcohol use.

Alcohol is the most popular psychoactive substance in society, consumed by approximately 90% of the UK adult population. One of the first recorded uses of alcohol was in 3500 BC by the Egyptians and alcohol's effects on man are recorded in the Bible. Plato is reported to have written:

> *When a man drinks wine he begins to be better pleased with himself and the more he drinks the more he is filled full of brave hopes, and conceit of his powers, and at least the string of his tongue is loosened, and fancying himself wise, he is brimming over with lawlessness and has no more fear or respect and is ready to do or say anything.*

When used in moderation, alcohol is a social 'lubricant', lowering inhibitions and facilitating social interaction. However, binge drinking, excessive, heavy and prolonged use, has serious consequences for health.

Over the past 70 years, alcohol consumption has more than doubled in the UK (Royal College of Physicians 2001) and continues to increase. It is estimated that one in three men and one in five women drink above the weekly recommended limits (Prime Minister's Strategy Unit 2003). The economic cost in industry is estimated to be up to £6.4 billion/year from absenteeism and loss of productivity (Prime Minister's Strategy Unit 2003). The cost to the NHS per year from alcohol-related injury and illness is estimated to be approximately £3 billion, up to 12% of its total spending (Royal College of Physicians 2001). The total cost of alcohol-related harm in England is up to £20 billion per year and includes harm to health, crime and antisocial behaviour, loss of productivity and social harm such as family breakdown (Prime Minister's Strategy Unit 2004). The highest risk groups are those aged between 16 and 35 and young women aged 16–24, whose average weekly consumption has increased by 93% since 1992 (Office for National Statistics 2004). Drinking culture in the UK promotes occasional but heavy drinking sessions. 'Binge drinking' is the term applied to describe this pattern of consumption and is of increasing concern. Binge drinking accounts for 40% of male and 22% of female drinking occasions (Prime Minister's Strategy Unit 2003).

Alcoholic drinks mainly comprise water and ethanol (alcohol) and are produced by the fermentation of fruits, vegetables or grain. Congeners are added to give the drink its distinctive flavour, taste and smell.

Units of alcohol

One unit (or 'standard drink') of alcohol contains approximately 8 g of absolute alcohol. This is based on a standard measure of an average-strength drink, i.e. half a pint of beer, lager or cider, a single measure of spirits, e.g. whisky, gin, vodka, a standard glass of wine, a small glass of sherry or a measure of vermouth (or aperitif). Therefore, if a total of 2 pints of average-strength lager and a small sherry were consumed, the total number of units consumed would be 5. However, since many varieties of alcoholic drinks of varying strengths are available, it is difficult to estimate how much alcohol an individual has consumed. Table 36.2 gives an approximate guide to the calculation of unit consumption for drinks of various strengths.

What is less harmful?

It has been suggested that the following units represent maximum levels for 'less harmful' weekly consumption. Consumption above these levels can be expected to lead to increased health problems:

- For men: up to 21 units; not exceeding 4 units/day
- For women: up to 14 units; not exceeding 3 units/day.

Alcohol absorption and elimination

Alcohol is one of the quickest-acting orally administered substances. It is also a toxic substance. The only organ capable of eliminating alcohol from the body is the liver. Alcohol passes chemically unchanged from the stomach into the blood supply within 5 min. Adding carbonated drinks, alternating alcohol with carbonated drinks, drinking on an empty stomach and drinking quickly may speed up absorption.

It takes approximately 30 min for alcohol levels to peak in the blood and 1 h for the liver to eliminate 1 unit. Any other alcohol taken during this time will accumulate in the blood, awaiting processing. Therefore, if 8 units are consumed (e.g. 4 pints of lager or 4 double spirits) the liver will take approximately 8–9 h to eliminate all the alcohol.

Table 36.2 Calculation of unit consumption for alcoholic drinks of various strengths

Type of drink	Measure	Number of units
Export beer	1 pint 1 can*	2.5 2
Strong beer or lager	1 pint 1 can*	4 3
Extra strong beer or lager	1 pint 1 can*	5 4
Strong cider	1 pint	4
Spirits	1 bottle	30
Table wine	1 bottle 1 L bottle	7 10
Sherry	1 bottle	13
Low-alcohol beers and lager	1 pint	0.66
Low-alcohol cider	1 pint	0.5

*1 can = 3/4 pint.

Health consequences of excessive alcohol use

Binge drinking, excessive, chronic or inappropriate alcohol use can lead to a wide range of health problems affecting virtually all parts of the body (see Fig. 36.3). In addition to the possible consequences of intoxication, binge drinking, excessive regular use and dependence (see Box 36.4), alcohol consumption, even at moderate levels, can interfere with the effects of many prescribed drugs such as oral contraceptives, antibiotics, anti-inflammatory agents, tranquillisers, antidepressants and diuretics. The habitual overuse of alcohol is associated with a number of psychosocial problems.

Long-term use and withdrawal

Tolerance develops quickly with regular use. Physical as well as psychological dependence can occur. Sudden withdrawal can be accompanied by unpleasant symptoms such as sweating, increased anxiety, tremor, headache, thirst, nausea and occasional vomiting. Delirium tremens and convulsions may also be experienced, but are rare.

Those who have suffered severe withdrawal symptoms in the past or who, following assessment, appear to be at risk, will need a supervised withdrawal (Cooper 1994). Contrary to popular belief, it is possible for someone with an alcohol problem to return to 'normal' social drinking or controlled drinking.

Box 36.4

Alcohol use: associated harm

Consequences of intoxication

- Accidents
- Acute poisoning
- Acute gastritis
- Drug overdose
- Epileptic-type seizures
- Head injury
- Suicidal behaviour

Consequences of excessive regular use

- Anxiety
- Cancer of the mouth/throat
- Depression
- Fatty liver
- Liver cancer
- Liver cirrhosis
- Pancreatitis
- Peripheral neuritis
- Phobic illness
- Sexual impotence
- Stomach haemorrhage

Consequences of dependence

- Alcoholic psychosis
- Anxiety
- Delirium tremens
- Depression
- Hallucination
- Paranoid states
- Polydrug abuse
- Withdrawal: epileptic seizures

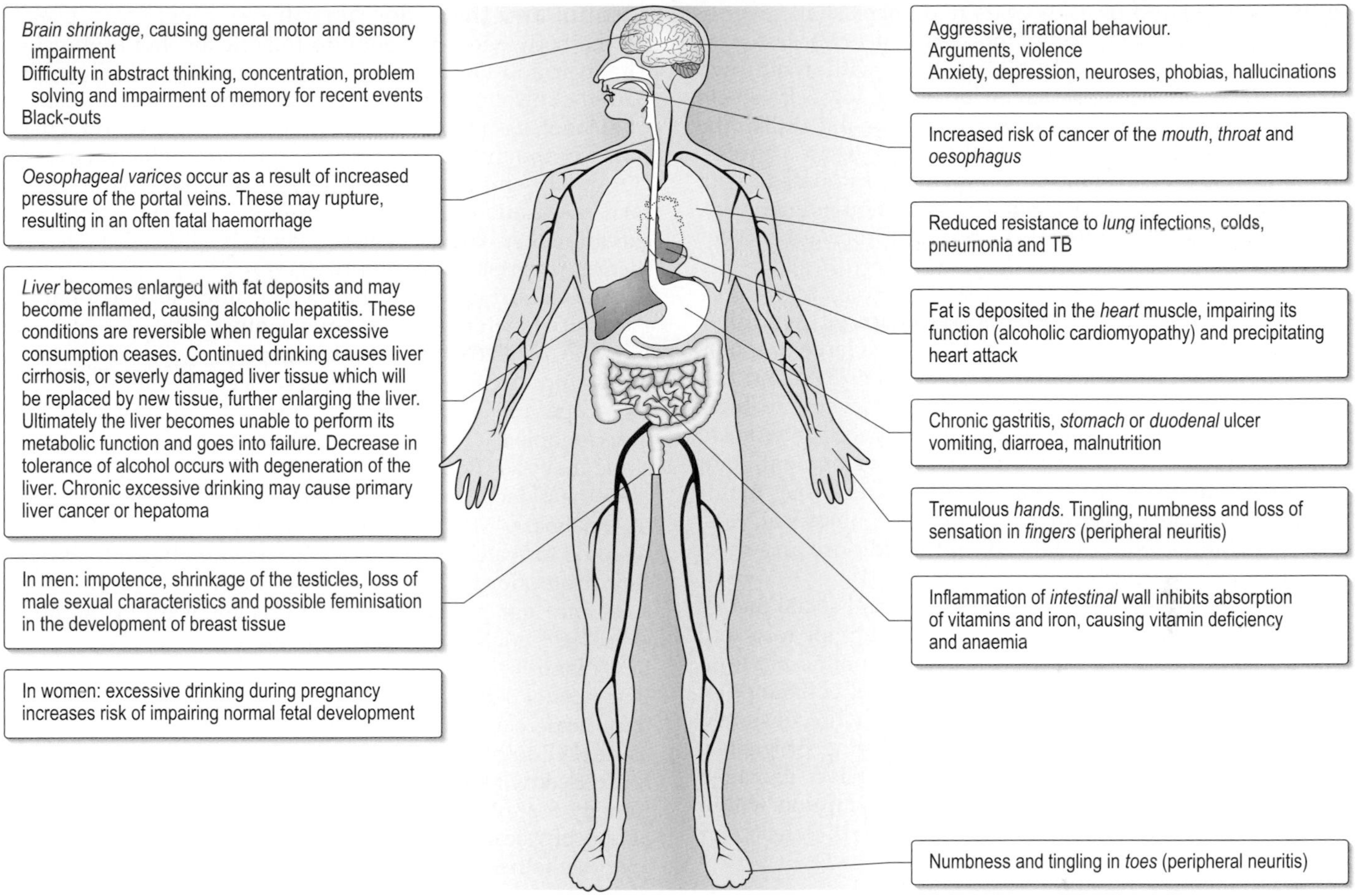
Brain shrinkage, causing general motor and sensory impairment
Difficulty in abstract thinking, concentration, problem solving and impairment of memory for recent events
Black-outs
Oesophageal varices occur as a result of increased pressure of the portal veins. These may rupture, resulting in an often fatal haemorrhage
Liver becomes enlarged with fat deposits and may become inflamed, causing alcoholic hepatitis. These conditions are reversible when regular excessive consumption ceases. Continued drinking causes liver cirrhosis, or severly damaged liver tissue which will be replaced by new tissue, further enlarging the liver. Ultimately the liver becomes unable to perform its metabolic function and goes into failure. Decrease in tolerance of alcohol occurs with degeneration of the liver. Chronic excessive drinking may cause primary liver cancer or hepatoma
In men: impotence, shrinkage of the testicles, loss of male sexual characteristics and possible feminisation in the development of breast tissue
In women: excessive drinking during pregnancy increases risk of impairing normal fetal development
Aggressive, irrational behaviour.
Arguments, violence
Anxiety, depression, neuroses, phobias, hallucinations
Increased risk of cancer of the *mouth*, *throat* and *oesophagus*
Reduced resistance to *lung* infections, colds, pneumonia and TB
Fat is deposited in the *heart* muscle, impairing its function (alcoholic cardiomyopathy) and precipitating heart attack
Chronic gastritis, *stomach* or *duodenal* ulcer vomiting, diarroea, malnutrition
Tremulous *hands*. Tingling, numbness and loss of sensation in *fingers* (peripheral neuritis)
Inflammation of *intestinal* wall inhibits absorption of vitamins and iron, causing vitamin deficiency and anaemia
Numbness and tingling in *toes* (peripheral neuritis)

Fig. 36.3 Consequences of excessive consumption of alcohol.

Teenage drinking

The issue of teenage drinking in the UK has given rise to a certain degree of public alarm. Newspaper articles condemn the behaviour of the young drinker and demand that underage drinking be stopped. However, there is little available evidence to suggest that the majority of teenagers do anything other than drink sensibly, or, indeed, that heavy consumption at an early age leads to excessive or chronic alcohol use in later life (Alcohol Concern 2004).

Children in our society encounter alcohol at an early age. However, Coggans and McKellar (1995) suggest that 'despite the apparent high levels of alcohol-related disorders involving young people in recent years there is nothing new about the phenomenon'. The authors continue by suggesting that alcohol-related hooliganism has been with us for centuries!

Young people tend to be introduced to alcohol by their parents. Most, from an early age, accept alcohol as part of everyday life. While excessive alcohol use is a real problem for some teenagers, what is needed is not a demand for total abstinence among young people, which would be unenforceable in practice, but increased education on the risks of binge drinking, inappropriate or excessive alcohol use — including the links with HIV/AIDS, promiscuous behaviour and teenage pregnancy — and other substance use (Cooper 2000). Teenagers should be allowed to develop their own concepts about the appropriate use of alcohol in a straightforward and, most importantly, informed manner. A failure to be open in our approach to the subject of alcohol use may only serve to entice young adults to explore this 'forbidden' territory in a spirit of rebellion.

STOP THINK **36.4** Do you think that there is a widespread teenage drinking problem in the UK? If so, how could you as a nurse help to prevent drinking problems among young people?

Women and alcohol use

It is generally acknowledged that alcohol-related problems amongst women are increasing (Plant 1997). Compared with men, women's health is more likely to be affected at lower levels of alcohol intake. This occurs mainly because women have less body water than men, and therefore alcohol is less diluted within the body (Morgan 1992). There are key physical differences in the way a woman's body copes with alcohol. Factors concerning the female reproductive system can influence metabolism and play an integral part in alcohol-related harm (Plant 1997).

Women present to caring agencies with the same alcohol-related problems as men, e.g. gastritis, duodenal ulcers, peripheral neuritis, cancer of the mouth, throat or oesophagus, amnesic episodes and suicidal behaviour. However, women who drink excessively have a greater risk of acute inflammation of the liver than men. Moreover, any damage to the liver in child-bearing years may increase in severity even after cessation of alcohol intake (Plant 1997).

Women present to helping agencies with their own specific set of problems, which include guilt, low self-esteem and depression. This requires sensitive nursing skills. The individual needs to feel sufficiently at ease with a professional to disclose substance use problems. In order to gain the woman's confidence, the nurse must be non-judgemental, supportive and well informed about appropriate sources of help.

Alcohol in pregnancy There is a recognised syndrome in babies of women who regularly consume large amounts of alcohol in pregnancy. Jones and Smith (1973) called this 'fetal alcohol syndrome'. They recorded several features commonly found in babies of alcohol-dependent women, including growth deficiencies, delayed development, joint and heart abnormalities, microcephaly and fine motor dysfunction. Facial features included asymmetrical ears, receding chin, receding forehead, upturned nose and short palpebral fissure length.

Plant (1997) suggests that there are several social factors that may influence birth defects, including tobacco and alcohol consumption and general socioeconomic environment. Investigating specific levels of alcohol consumption during pregnancy, Plant found that 'women who consumed 10 units of alcohol on a single occasion during pregnancy were more likely than other women to have damaged offspring'. However, levels of alcohol consumption within the accepted limits are not associated with birth defects.

STOP THINK

36.5 Test your factual knowledge by answering the following questions.

(a) On average, how much (i) wine, (ii) spirits, (iii) beer, (iv) lager would you need to drink to be over the legal limit for driving?
(b) Which parts of the body are affected by alcohol, and what are the effects?
(c) What organ in the body breaks down alcohol?
(d) After drinking 1 pint of ordinary beer, how long will it take before the alcohol in it is completely burned up by the body?
(e) Which of these is an effective way of sobering up?
- Drinking a cup of strong black coffee
- Taking fresh air
- Taking physical exercise
- Taking a cold shower
- Making yourself sick.

(f) What level of daily consumption is considered to lead to the possibility of alcohol dependence?
(i) 4 pints of beer
(ii) 8 glasses of wine
(iii) 2 single measures of whisky
(iv) 2 double measures of rum
(v) 6 glasses of fortified wine
(vi) 3 pints of lager.
(g) Is the recommended safe limit of drinking for women lower or higher than that for men?
(h) Equal amounts of alcohol have a greater effect on a young person than on the average adult male.
Why is this?
(i) What can speed up the effect of alcohol?

Alcohol and the older person

As the body ages, its ability to tolerate alcohol diminishes. The liver and kidneys become less efficient, and the elimination of alcohol from the body becomes slower. The effect of alcohol on reflexes, balance, self-control and judgement may compound existing health problems, increasing the risk of falls and other accidents. Equally, many older people take medication such as hypnotics, analgesics and anti-inflammatory drugs which, when mixed with alcohol, increase the risk of health problems.

Age can bring with it many difficulties such as financial hardship, loneliness, isolation, insomnia, pain and susceptibility to cold. (Note that a 'hot toddy' will not warm a person up. Alcohol dilates the blood vessels, allowing heat to escape and increasing the risk of hypothermia.) Many older people eat unbalanced diets and have a poor appetite; some may sacrifice food for alcohol.

Some older people may use alcohol to block out feelings of loneliness. Many of these individuals will find it hard to come forward for help, and it can sometimes be difficult for professionals to recognise alcohol and/or other substance use problems among this client group (Graham et al 1998, McKee 2000). The relatives of an older person may dismiss such drinking as a minor foible or take the view that alcohol helps them to cope. Nurses working in this field may hear relatives and carers expressing sentiments such as 'It will do her no harm' or 'What else has she got to live for?'. Even GPs have been known to suggest alcohol as a remedy for insomnia in older people. This can be unwise, as the physical, social and psychological effects of alcohol are often felt among this client group at a relatively low level of consumption.

Treatment Older people who have come forward for help, or who have been identified as having an alcohol-related problem, often feel guilt and shame. In many cases, information on the sensible use of alcohol is all that is required to relieve anxiety and enable the person to adopt healthier drinking habits. It is important to remember, however, that age does not make someone less able to make decisions about their own life. If the individual does not wish to reduce or modify consumption, that is a personal choice. Professionals have a responsibility, nonetheless, to ensure that the individual has adequate information on which to base informed decisions.

The Alcohol Harm Reduction Strategy

(Prime Minister's Strategy Unit 2004)

This highlights the increasing concerns of drinking behaviour among young people aged 16–35 and especially of women aged 16–24 years. The strategy aims to reduce consumption among these groups by implementing national guidelines on improving education and training for all professionals in the identification and management of individuals with alcohol-related problems. The report emphasises the need for increased service provision, improved access to services, the implementation of clear integrated care pathways and multiagency collaboration. It further highlights the importance of improving education programmes to increase young people's knowledge of alcohol, its use and effects, the associated harms and to promote sensible drinking.

CASE HISTORY 36.1

A personal account

My drinking took off in my early twenties. I saw myself as a failure in love, a failure in my career and I blamed my father for everything. With so much hate in my head, I had to have something to ease the pain and so I used alcohol … as the anger inside increased.

After a while … I couldn't feel comfortable without the aid of a drink. It began to take over my life and the terrible craving began. As the anger inside got worse, so did my need for alcohol. Current resentments were coloured and magnified by the anger from the past and all I could do was escape from my misery ... I was cruel to my family and a 'mouse' to the outside world … I hated myself for being such a fraud.

I was breathalysed and banned twice for drink driving. I lived in a state of perpetual fear, unable to function without a drink, vowing to stop drinking and then drinking again. Totally out of control. I was a mess with no peace of mind and no self-esteem at all.

Sometimes I think of [my] addiction as a train that will not stop. The train seemed so comfortable when you first got on. Soft velvet seats, plenty of room to spread your legs and the fare was reasonable too. It started slowly, increasing in speed as the weeks and months rolled by. For some strange reason the train wouldn't stop, it just kept on going, faster and faster … The plush seats were threadbare after a while. The ticket collector wore a frown and the weather was dark clouds and rain the whole time. For some strange reason I wanted to stop, yet I wanted to keep on going. The train was my life and I was not to blame. I longed to see my family again without the noise of the train. I had to shout at them all of the time because of the noise … I tried to explain that I *need* the train more than anything else in the world, then said I'd get off as soon as I could …

Any obsession is hard to break … People have to be desperate before they go on their hands and knees for help. For many years I denied my drinking was out of control … I would swear off the stuff every morning yet pick up a drink the same afternoon and carry on drinking for the rest of the day. It was a terrible treadmill. I couldn't escape, yet I kept kidding myself that somehow, someday, my problem would just go away … I used to sit in a room on a Sunday afternoon, away from my wife and sons, feeling alone and apart, just waiting for the pubs to open. Always there was a desperate need to drink and once I had one I could never drink enough …

I variously blamed my wife, my mother-in-law, my boss and my ill fortune in life for my drinking ... but I was the problem and my drinking had nothing to do with anyone else. For years I was blind to my own shortcoming and forever bemoaning the faults of others. I could see nothing wrong with the way I behaved. I desperately struggled to keep my family in order who seemed to be falling apart. The truth is I was the one who was falling apart and I just couldn't see it …

I was lucky. One day I answered the door to a health visitor who, I assumed, had come to see my hopeless, incompetent wife. Straightaway the woman confronted me and asked if I would go for help with my drinking. I had never seen the woman before in my life but the shock was so great that I agreed there and then to seek help for my problem. Had I known my interfering mother-in-law had arranged it all and that it was her intervention that saved my life there would have been hell to pay. Thankfully the truth was kept from me until I was able to take it with equanimity! The fact is she was a lovely caring woman but I just couldn't see it at all …

(Neville D. Lewis 2002, with permission)

Comment

Neville commenced a sustained period of abstinence and attended local groups for support and treatment. Through counselling he addressed issues surrounding his anger and the feelings toward his father and experienced 'spiritual enlightenment' that he found helpful. Neville is now able to drink alcohol socially, drinking in a way he finds relaxing, with his friends, and not as a means of managing his anger. For the past 13 years Neville has avoided intoxication by remaining within the recommended daily and weekly drinking limits.

For a personal account of alcohol addiction, see Case History 36.1.

Safe drinking recommendations

(DH 1995, WHO 1996)

- As a rule do not consume more than two standard drinks per day.
- Have *at least* two alcohol-free days per week.
- Consistent drinking of 4 standard drinks per day for men and 3 per day for women is *not* advised as a sensible drinking level because of the progressive health risks.
- Sensible limits should not be saved up for one drinking session.
- Avoid drinking to intoxication.
- Some individuals, because of lower body weight, composition, metabolism or during pregnancy and whilst breast feeding, should consume lower levels of alcohol.
- The intake of up to 2 units per day can have a moderate protective effect against heart disease for men over 40 and postmenopausal women. However:
  - — non-drinkers should not be advised to start drinking for their health, and
  - — those individuals who consume up to the 2 standard drinks per day should not be encouraged to increase their consumption to reduce the risk of heart disease.

STOP THINK **36.6** On the basis of the information given in this section, how would you define 'the sensible use of alcohol'? Can alcohol in any way be beneficial?

Anxiolytics and hypnotics

In 2001, approximately 25 million prescriptions for anxiolytics and hypnotics were prescribed in the UK (Prescription Prescribing Agency 2001). Among consumers of these drugs, women form the larger group, although there is a steady increase in prescriptions for men, which appears to be associated with unemployment and poor employment prospects. The most common group of prescribed anxiolytics and hypnotics are the benzodiazepines: diazepam, lorazepam and temazepam. It is estimated that 174 000 adults aged 16–59 years used benzodiazepines in England in 2002/2003 (Condon & Smith 2003).

Seivewright (1998) has noted that tranquilliser (anxiolytics and hypnotics) withdrawal carries with it serious physical and psychological risks. Once dependent, abrupt cessation is dangerous. Therefore, it is essential that any withdrawal is gradual, perhaps over years. Because the symptoms of withdrawal often mirror the symptoms of the original complaint, dependence often goes unidentified until the substance is reduced or stopped or until tolerance develops. Withdrawal symptoms are similar to phobic anxiety states and may include fear, agoraphobia, suicidal feelings and panic attacks.

The Royal College of Psychiatrists' (1997) report on benzodiazepines recommends their primary use in the short-term treatment of severe anxiety and related symptoms, where the individual is experiencing significant distress or problems in social functioning. The report states that to reduce the risk of dependence, benzodiazepines should not be prescribed regularly for more than 1 month; the report advocates their use on an 'as required' basis every few days. For insomnia, the report recommends limiting use to 2–4 weeks at the lowest dose.

Effects

The effects of hypnotics and anxiolytics commence within 1 h of administration and last up to 12 h. They include:

- relief from tension
- a sense of calm and relaxation
- decreased self-control, alertness, power of observation and level of dexterity
- control of anxiety
- short-term memory loss
- lowered inhibitions
- release of aggression
- the onset of sleep.

With intoxication, the individual may experience dysarthria, ataxia, nystagmus and emotional lability.

It is not clear how long it will take an individual to become dependent, although an increase in anxiety has been noted after 4 weeks' use. By 6 months, the risk of dependency is greatly increased. Psychological dependence is common.

Tolerance can develop with both therapeutic and non-therapeutic use and withdrawal symptoms may occur even with therapeutic doses (see Box 36.5). Whilst these are not potentially fatal, they can be very unpleasant and have been described by some as worse than those experienced in heroin withdrawal.

Support during withdrawal

As withdrawal symptoms commence even after a small reduction in dosage, the withdrawal process needs to be undertaken gradually. It may take several months or years for the person to be able to live comfortably without the substance.

Support, whether given individually or in a group, is essential. Nurses should be aware of the unpleasantness associated with withdrawal and the fear and emotional stress this process is likely to cause the individual and the family.

For useful information on the process of tranquilliser withdrawal, see Seivewright (1998).

Box 36.5

Common tranquilliser withdrawal symptoms

- Convulsions
- Dry retching
- Hand tremor
- Headaches
- Increased tension/anxiety
- Irritability
- Loss of feeling/emotion
- Mental confusion
- Muscle pain/stiffness
- Nausea
- Nightmares
- Palpitations
- Panic attacks
- Personality change
- Profuse sweating
- Rebound insomnia
- Weight loss

Volatile substances

Many solvents, glues, gases and volatile substances are readily available in homes, shops, offices and factories. Under normal use, they are reasonably safe. However, they are sometimes inhaled specifically for their depressant effect on the central nervous system. The Scottish Executive (2003) describe three kinds of volatile substance use among young people:

- experimental — by those who want to know what it is like
- recreational — by those who use volatile substances more frequently, usually in a group
- problematic — regular, long-term use.

An average of 73 premature deaths per annum is associated with volatile substance use (Field-Smith et al 2004), with 14% of 11–15 year olds claiming to have tried a volatile substance (Boreham & McManus 2003). Substances of use are adhesives, cleaning fluids, aerosols and fuels, with the primary substance of use being butane lighter fuel which accounted for 59% of solvent-related deaths in 2001 (Field-Smith et al 2004). In addition to being relatively easy to obtain, these solvents offer a cheap alternative to alcohol and other drugs.

Effects of solvent inhalation

Effects commence within 7 s of inhalation and last for approximately 30 min. Continual sniffing maintains the effect, with most users reporting elevation of mood and hallucinations (WHO 2004a). As the level of intoxication is reduced, the user experiences nausea and headache. With the repetition and deep inhalation, overdose may result, causing loss of control, disorientation and unconsciousness. On cessation, recovery usually follows quickly. Concentration of the substance and intensification of effects can be achieved by placing a plastic bag over the head. This method brings with it the danger of asphyxiation.

It is not easy to identify use, as the presenting problems may appear to be similar to behaviour associated with 'normal' adolescent development, e.g. moodiness, aggression, loss of appetite, disinterest and aloofness. With regular use, tolerance may develop. Whilst physical dependence does not appear to occur, evidence suggests there is an increased risk of psychological dependence for some users (WHO 2004a).

Dangers of excessive and frequent use

It is important for the substance user to avoid exertion, as this may affect the function of the heart and increase sensitivity. Any exercise may lead to collapse and death.

Other dangers include damage to the liver, lungs, kidneys, heart and central nervous system, as well as death by suffocation, accidents, direct toxic effect on the heart and inhalation of vomit. Gas squirted directly into the mouth can cause suffocation.

Britton and Noor (2003) identify a range of approaches to prevention and intervention that are adopted in relation to solvent and other drug use:

- maintaining the user's confidentiality
- collecting information
- accurate assessment and identification of needs
- providing information and education appropriate to needs
- offering activity substitution: individual or group
- providing individual counselling or therapy
- encouraging parental/carer education and involvement in treatment
- offering family counselling or therapy
- organising self-help groups
- organising community action
- educating professionals.

STOP THINK **36.7** As a nurse who may at some stage come into contact with solvent users, consider which method or combination of methods listed above would be most effective, and why? What other measures can you think of? How would you introduce them?

ILLEGAL SUBSTANCES

Illicit drug use in the UK has steadily increased since the 1950s (Handford & Colenso 1998). This is reflected in the number of persons found guilty, cautioned, given a fiscal fine or dealt with by compounding (an administrative sanction used by Customs involving a financial penalty) for drug offences, which rose from 13 400 in 1978 (Home Office Statistical Bulletin 1979) to 113 050 in 2002 (Ahmad & Mwende 2004). Thirty-six per cent of adults aged 16–59 admit to having used an illicit drug (Condon & Smith 2003), an increase of 8% since 1994. The high risk groups are those aged 16–29 with 50% reporting illicit drug use, an increase of 7% since 1994. Young males aged 20–29 are 1.4 times more likely than females to use illicit drugs, with 63% and 60% of males aged 20–24 and 25–29 respectively reporting substance use (Ramsey et al 2001). Since 1998, cocaine, crack, ecstasy and Class A drug use has significantly increased (Aust et al 2002). Cannabis, reclassified to Class 'C', is the most commonly used prohibited substance, with 44% of 16–29 year olds having imbibed (Ramsey et al 2001). More than 5 million British people regularly use cannabis, 2.4 million ecstasy, and 2 million amfetamines and cocaine (The Observer 2002). There may be some evidence to suggest that drug use is associated with frequency of drunkenness, with 59% of binge drinkers (18–24 years old) reporting drug use in the past year compared to 33% of non-binge drinkers (Richardson & Budd 2003).

Opiates and opioids

Opiates are derived from the sap of the opium poppy (*Papaver somniferum*). They are narcotic analgesics. Their synthetic equivalents are collectively known as opioids.

Heroin

Heroin ('H', 'smack') is a narcotic made from morphine, injected ('shooting' or 'mainlining') or smoked over tinfoil through a small tube ('chasing the dragon'). The purity of the drug is often unknown, and consequently accidental overdose can easily occur and may be lethal. Heroin users who share needles and syringes ('works') are at risk of septicaemia, hepatitis and HIV/AIDS (see Ch. 37).

The effects of heroin include euphoria, drowsiness and a sense of well-being and raised self-esteem. Tolerance develops quickly, demanding increased intake to achieve the desired effect. Physical and psychological dependence may follow. Contamination of the substance often leads to severe allergic reactions, which may be exacerbated by poor diet and self-neglect. This degenerative process may lead to death if medical care is not available. Withdrawal is unpleasant and is often described as being 'like a severe dose of flu'. Other problems include constipation and vomiting. Complaints of diarrhoea, abdominal cramps and muscle spasm are common. Although it has been suggested that withdrawal from heroin is easier to achieve than withdrawal from nicotine, alcohol or methadone, it should be attempted gradually, using reducing doses of methadone as a heroin substitute.

Stimulants

Amfetamines (Amphetamines)

Amfetamine ('speed', 'billy') is usually found in powder form that can be 'snorted' (sniffed), 'bombed' (swallowed), smoked (through a pipe) or injected. The effects, intensity and duration depend on the route of administration and dosage but usually last around 3–6 h.

Amfetamine is a stimulant that activates or excites the central nervous system and is similar in function to the body's own natural stimulants, adrenaline and noradrenaline. Amfetamine increases energy levels, but as the body replaces the energy used, the user feels tired, depressed and hungry, i.e. the opposite of how the amfetamine makes them feel.

Medically, amfetamines are used in the treatment of depression, obesity and attention deficiency disorders. Amfetamine is more physically toxic than cocaine. The liver can struggle to break down amfetamines in large doses, which can result in liver damage and failure. The combined use of amfetamine and alcohol is therefore not advised, due to the increased risk of liver damage. In low doses, amfetamines increase heart rate, blood pressure, respirations and body temperature. The user will experience alertness, wakefulness, improved confidence and elevation of mood. At higher doses, amfetamine can induce dizziness, nausea/vomiting, cardiac arrhythmia, paranoia, confusion and insomnia/sleep disturbance.

Cocaine

Cocaine ('coke', 'charlie') is an alkaloid derived from the coca plant, a shrub native to South America. This white crystal-like powder is a powerful but short-acting central nervous system stimulant. Cocaine stimulates the release of dopamine in the brain, a chemical that is thought to be involved in emotional responses and pleasure. Dopamine is also thought to be involved in the gross, automatic movements of skeletal muscles. Cocaine can be sniffed ('snorted'), injected or smoked (in the form of 'crack'). When cocaine is treated with baking powder and water, it forms into tiny chalk-like lumps or 'rocks' and is referred to as 'crack'.

The effects of cocaine peak within 15–30 min and then gradually decrease. The user experiences an elevation in mood, increased alertness, concentration and energy. This physiological arousal and euphoria lead to an indifference to pain and fatigue. Normal requirements for food are decreased. Large doses may lead to agitation, anxiety, hallucinations and erratic behaviour.

Dependence is usually psychological. The individual may complain of depression, fatigue and inability to cope. Chronic use may cause restlessness, nausea, sleeplessness, paranoia, hyperexcitability and depression. Repeated sniffing also leads to erosion of the nasal membrane and respiratory problems.

Hallucinogens

Hallucinogens (psychedelics, psychotomimetics or psychotogens) include lysergic acid diethylamide (LSD), hallucinogenic mushrooms and cannabis. The prime effect of these substances is the alteration of perceptual functions of the brain.

Cannabis

It is generally believed that, when used occasionally, cannabis has no long-lasting effects and is safer than alcohol. Cannabis, a preparation of the hemp plant, is available in three forms:

- 'grass', a dried leaf (marijuana)
- resin, a compact block ('hash')
- oil, the most highly concentrated form.

Cannabis is essentially a depressant with hallucinogenic properties. Cannabis contains around 60 chemicals known as cannabinoids, which stimulate naturally occurring cannabinoid receptors found in the brain and parts of the body. These receptors are thought to have a role in pain perception/management, motor coordination, cognition, memory and reward, amongst others. The main psychoactive chemical in cannabis is known as tetrahydrocannabinol (THC).

Cannabis is usually mixed with tobacco and smoked (as a 'joint') and this is the most popular method of administration. The effects commence after 2–3 min and can last up to 4–6 h, depending on strength and dose. Smoking cannabis is the most physically damaging method of use and carries the highest progressive health risks. The main health hazards appear to derive from those associated with tobacco use, although damage may occur to the airway and respiratory system when cannabis is used without tobacco, due to the smoke and high level of heat required to burn cannabis. The advantage of smoking cannabis is the user's control over the dosage, being able to discontinue use when the desired effect is achieved. Cannabis may also be ingested in cakes, meals and hot drinks. The effects when eaten are more powerful and intense than when smoked and the user has little control over the effects once ingested. The immediate effect is one of relaxation, talkativeness and hilarity. Intensification of sound and colour may also be experienced. There is a reduction in short-term memory function and in motor skill. Concentration is poor. High doses of cannabis can lead to confusion, anxiety/panic, paranoia and depersonalisation.

Learning to use cannabis is an acquired skill. The inexperienced user may experience nausea, dizziness, impaired vision and disorientation (a 'whitie' or 'colonel whitie') due to being unable to identify correctly the adequate dosage. However, the user soon learns, through repeated use and discussion with peers, how to regulate the dosage to achieve and maximise the desired effect.

In recent years, the medicinal use of cannabis has increasingly been researched.

For current knowledge and research into the medicinal use of cannabis, see Mathre et al (2001–2003), Cannabis – the whole story, parts 1–7.

The therapeutic use of cannabis is now strongly associated with pain management for individuals with cancer, AIDS, arthritis, spinal cord injury, peripheral neuropathy, migraine, central post-stroke pain and multiple sclerosis, in movement disorders such as Parkinson's and Huntington's disease and in insomnia. At present, such use is illegal according to UK law. However, the debate rightly continues around legalisation for specific medical use. One would eventually hope that common sense will prevail and legalisation will follow. Until the law is changed, significant numbers of these groups are denied effective legal clinical intervention.

Lysergic acid diethylamide (LSD)

LSD ('trips', 'acid') is a derivative of ergot, a fungus commonly found on rye and other grasses. An exceedingly potent substance, only minute doses of LSD are required to achieve a hallucinogenic effect.

The short-term user experiences a 'trip', in which hilarity, elation, heightened self-awareness, hallucinations (visual, auditory, olfactory and tactile), disturbance of perception, increase/decrease of passage of time, disorientation, disassociation from the body, anxiety and paranoia may occur. Physiological effects include increases in heart rate, body temperature and blood pressure. At low doses, LSD increases respirations; however, at higher doses it will depress the respiratory system. These experiences commence within 1 h following ingestion and peak 2–6 h later, gradually fading after 8–12 h depending on dosage.

Excessive and long-term use can cause prolonged psychological reactions and re-experiencing of past 'trips' ('flashbacks'). However, LSD is not known to cause physical dependence.

'Magic' mushrooms

There are approximately 12 varieties of mushroom that contain hallucinogenic chemicals. The most common of these mushrooms is *Psilocybe semilanceata* ('liberty cap').

'Magic' mushrooms contain two active ingredients, psilocybin and psilocin. The mushrooms may be crushed, eaten fresh, brewed in a tea or cooked in soup. The user experiences effects similar to those of LSD. Commencing within 30 min, the effects peak at approximately 3 h and last 4–10 h.

Dependence, withdrawal and overdose are unlikely, the primary danger to health lying in the possibility that the individual may pick and consume a poisonous mushroom by mistake. Symptoms of poisoning include vomiting, diarrhoea, stomach cramps, watery eyes and mouth, twitching or 'fits' and respiratory problems.

Methylenedioxymethamfetamine (MDMA, Ecstasy, E)

MDMA is a stimulant drug with hallucinogenic properties. It stimulates the production of serotonin, a naturally released chemical in the brain that affects mood. This increase in serotonin leads to an increase in an individual's mood (euphoria). Once the MDMA is eliminated from the system, the body has difficulty in replacing lost serotonin quickly. Less serotonin is released with each electrical impulse and fewer serotonin receptors are activated. This produces feelings of depression, restlessness, irritability, sleep disturbance and anxiety. It is thought that prolonged repeated use of Ecstasy may cause permanent reductions in serotonin production leading to lasting alterations in mood (mood swings, dysthymia and depression). Other possible effects of long-term or excessive use can include anxiety, insomnia, lasting memory impairment, suppression of the immune system and liver damage.

MDMA usually comes in tablet form, occasionally powder form that is 'snorted', and the effects usually begin after 20–60 min and last between 3 and 6 h. The effects and duration depend on dosage and purity of the drug. The effects at low doses include increased heart rate, blood pressure and energy, dilated pupils, loss of appetite, blurred vision and tightening of jaws. The user may experience feelings of warmth and empathy, enhanced sense of communication and increases in perception and sensual experience. Higher doses can lead to hyperthermia, hypertension, hyponatraemia (abnormally low blood sodium levels due to dehydration), cardiac arrhythmia, anxiety, confusion/disorientation, hallucinations and paranoia.

STOP THINK

36.8 Take 30 min to write down your feelings, attitudes and experiences relating to cannabis. Once you have completed this task, read the articles by Mathre and colleagues (2001–2003) on Cannabis – the whole story, parts 1–7. These articles attempt to put the use of cannabis into perspective. Once you have completed your reading, spend 30 min repeating the above writing exercise/task and see how and/or if your opinions have changed and why you think this is.

36.9 Consider the evidence for and against the main aspects of substance legislation. Discuss the following quotations. How convincing are the arguments? Should all substances be legalised? Explain your reasoning.

(a) 'Prohibition, which worked in the 50's ... simply cannot work now as it goes against the grain of social change ... Since present policies have failed, and in my view have no chance of succeeding, it is surely time to devise some new approach that would take drug supply out of criminal hands and bring it within a legal framework. Carefully tailored regimes for each drug, taxation used to finance much more research, education and treatment ...' (Morris 2001).

(b) 'Drug problems will not be beaten out of society by yet harsher laws, lectured out of society by yet more hours of "health education", or treated out of society by yet more drug experts. There is a place, however, for legislation and education and treatment.' (Royal College of Psychiatrists 1987).

SUPPORT AGENCIES

Outreach workers

There are three main kinds of outreach worker in the field of substance rehabilitation. Some, mainly nurses, are employed professionals. Others are unpaid or paid scripted users or ex-users. Whatever their background, the aim of these workers is to facilitate access to caring services for individuals who want to deal with a substance use problem. An example of how outreach work might be carried out is given in Box 36.6.

Professional outreach workers

These workers are usually nurses; some have dual qualifications in general and mental health nursing. They work independently of the alcohol and/or drug advisory service and their main function is to provide health education and health delivery at the 'grass roots' level. Advice on general care issues, substance use and safe practice is given with the aim of increasing the number of substance users coming forward to seek professional help.

Existing scripted users: unpaid

These outreach workers already live, work and socialise with other users. Their aim is to deliver a health promotion message, e.g. harm minimisation and HIV/AIDS advice, and to promote the idea that local agencies are 'user friendly'.

Ex-users and existing users: paid

In most cases employed by alcohol and/or drug advisory services, these individuals are detached youth workers

Box 36.6

Outreach work: an example

The outreach worker may go to a pub or dance club. During the evening, the worker may meet up with an existing contact, who during the course of a conversation may introduce the worker to an associate who would like to talk (this form of contacting is often referred to as 'snowballing'). This individual may be experiencing substance use problems or problems with their GP. In the case of a health care problem, the worker may be able to facilitate 'harm minimisation' (see below). For example, the user may be advised to go for a health check or for HIV/AIDS and hepatitis B and C testing, or may be informed about how to obtain clean 'works'. In some cases, the worker undertakes these tasks, dealing with the problem on street level.

As the user's trust develops, the worker may bring a colleague along to a meeting or encourage attendance at a clinic. This process gradually leads to a deeper level of care and involvement with the community drug team.

dealing with all welfare aspects of substance use. Their aim is to increase levels of understanding, to give information on safer substance-using practices and to encourage attendance at substance clinics for appropriate interventions.

Harm minimisation

Harm minimisation is a form of intervention that has given rise to much controversy. It is a process by which substance users are advised on safe methods of substance use, rather than being urged to abstain. The user is offered blood tests and health checks, is given advice on safer using practices and is supplied with clean paraphernalia and condoms. The underlying philosophy is that while it may be impossible to eradicate the illegal use of substances, it is nonetheless beneficial for individuals and society to make existing substance use as safe as possible (see Ch. 37).

Needle exchange schemes Usually operated by drug and/or alcohol advisory services, these schemes aim to distribute clean needles, syringes and containers (paraphernalia) with a view to preventing the sharing of equipment and thus reducing the spread of infection. These schemes allow for access to paraphernalia, health promotion materials and advice, e.g. on cleaning of equipment and on safe sexual practice.

Some pharmacists, GPs and community psychiatric nurses offer this service. Needle exchange schemes also facilitate the safe disposal of used paraphernalia and help to maintain the link between the user and agencies.

Voluntary and professional agencies

Local services

Most health districts have a drug and/or alcohol advisory service, usually staffed by specialist nurses, social workers and administrators. Other professionals such as health promotion officers, occupational therapists, doctors/consultants and probation officers may be attached to the team.

These teams offer help, advice, information, health education, treatment and counselling for the substance user, the family or close associates and health care professionals. Some districts have a similar, voluntary service staffed by trained counsellors. Many voluntary services provide a range of alternative therapies, e.g. acupuncture and/or massage, as part of the treatment package. Contact with these services can be made via the Yellow Pages, citizens' advice bureaux, occupational health, community mental health and primary care teams. Some regional alcohol and/or drug treatment units still operate, offering outpatient and inpatient treatment, usually on a 6-week basis. However, access to these may be difficult to obtain and usually requires a doctor's recommendation.

National bodies

Technical information and advice relating to voluntary services may be obtained by making contact with the following organisations (see 'Useful websites and addresses', p. 1167):

- Alcohol Concern
- Drugscope
- Nursing Council on Alcohol (NCA)
- Re-Solv
- The Addictions Forum.

Support groups

Statutory and voluntary drug and/or alcohol advisory services may offer group therapy in a variety of formats. Membership of these groups may be open or closed, and may be for men only, women only or mixed. Some aim for total abstinence, others for controlled use. Some groups are set up to provide support for family members.

- 'Drinkline' is organised on lines similar to 'Weightwatchers'. Total abstinence is not a requirement.
- Alcoholics Anonymous (AA) and Narcotics Anonymous (NA) are self-help organisations offering individual and group support. Total abstinence is required.
- Al-Anon, Al-Ateen and Families Anonymous are run on similar lines to AA and NA groups and provide self-help for the families and friends of substance users.
- Tranquilliser support groups have also been established to offer support and encouragement to individuals during the often long and difficult process of withdrawal.

Additional programmes undertaken by drug and/or alcohol advisory services may include group psychotherapy, social skills training, relaxation, family therapy, education and prevention, and telephone support. Most teams are able to access intensive residential courses, 'dry' hostels and other care facilities. Each of these offers a particular philosophy of care. The service provider usually agrees admission following assessment.

STOP THINK **36.10** The Department of Health (1999) suggests that all workers should have knowledge of the services and facilities available to them and how to access these. Produce your own 'resource catalogue' using the information and addresses contained within this chapter. In addition, to increase your familiarity with the services available in your own health district, carry out the following project:

(a) Research all local resources that may assist you in the care of your patient, whether this would be with advice, help, information or statistics. Don't forget self-help groups and counselling services such as the Samaritans, as well as mother-and-toddler groups, which may provide much-needed support for a mother under stress.

(b) Prepare a file card or computer database on each group, listing the contact name, address, telephone number and type of help offered.

CONCLUSION

This chapter has attempted to provide an introduction for the nurse to the many issues surrounding the care of individuals who use substances and who may or may not have a problem with that use. While work with these individuals can constitute a specialism within nursing, the need for nurses in every field to be aware of the signs and the consequences of substance use cannot be overemphasised (Prime Minister's Strategy Unit 2004).

Substance use problems occur in every age group and social class. Within the family, substance use problems may have serious implications not only for the individual directly affected, but also for the spouse or partner and children. Indeed, the nurse may first identify the existence of substance use not through contact with the substance user, but through interactions with family members (see Case History 36.1). It is vital that nursing interventions, undertaken in response to substance use, are based on an assessment not only of the individual but also of the family circumstances.

As in many areas of nursing, prevention and education show the way forward (Watson 2000). When averting or changing from substance use, be that use problematic or otherwise, individuals must be given adequate information on which to base free and informed decisions. Nurses working with substance users may find that, in order to be more responsive to the needs of the individual, they must venture beyond traditional clinical settings into outreach work. In any event, interventions will demand a holistic approach in which the unique identity of the individual is paramount, and in which all aspects of physical, mental and social well-being are addressed by the cooperative efforts of a multidisciplinary and multiagency team.

Nurses are in a privileged position by virtue of their close and frequent contact with the individual. They are often seen as the 'human face' of community and hospital health services and are perceived to be 'on the patient's side' — practical, approachable and down-to-earth. As a result, nurses are well placed to listen to, support, advise and inform, and nursing the substance-using individual can offer a particularly challenging and rewarding context for the practice of these invaluable skills.

STOP THINK **36.11** Now that you have read through the chapter, repeat exercise 36.1, taking note of the following:

- Have your feelings changed? If so, in what way? What new information influenced this change?
- Are there any areas that you feel you need to investigate further? If so, what are these and what sources could you use?

REFERENCES

Ahmad M, Mwende L 2004 Home Office statistical bulletin: drug seizure and offender statistics, United Kingdom 2001 & 2002. Home Office Research, Development and Statistics Directorate, London

Alcohol Concern 2004 Factsheet 1: Young people's drinking. Alcohol Concern, London

Aust R, Sharp C, Goulden C 2002 Prevalence of drug use: key findings from the 2001/2002 British crime survey. Home Office Research Study 182. Home Office Research, Development and Statistics Directorate, London

Banerjee J, Clancy C, Crome I 2002 Co-existing problems of mental disorder and substance misuse (dual diagnosis): an information manual 2002. Royal College of Psychiatrists Research Unit, London

Bien T H, Miller W R, Tonigan J S 1993 Brief interventions for alcohol problems: a review. Addiction 88(3): 315–333

Bloch M 2000 Women's health and tobacco: a global view. Journal of Substance Use 5(Suppl): 165–170

Boreham R, McManus S (eds) 2003 Smoking, drinking and drug use among young people in England in 2002. National Centre for Social Research and the National Foundation for Educational Research. TSO, London

British Medical Association (BMA) 2004 Smoking and reproductive life: the impact of smoking on sexual, reproductive and child health. British Medical Association, Board of Science and Education & Tobacco Control Resource Centre, London. Online: Available: www.bma.org.uk

Britton J, Noor S 2003 First steps in identifying young people's substance related needs. Drugs Strategy Directorate, Home Office, London

Clenaghan P 2000 Mental health and mental illness. In: Cooper D B (ed) Alcohol use. Radcliffe Medical Press, Oxford, Ch. 9

Coggans N, McKellar S 1995 The facts about alcohol, aggression and adolescence. Cassell, London

Condon J, Smith N 2003 Prevalence of drug use: key findings from the 2002/2003 British Crime Survey. Home Office Research study 229. Home Office Research, Development and Statistics Directorate, London

Coombs R H 1996 Addicted health professional. Journal of Substance Misuse 1(4): 187–194

Cooper D B (ed) 2000 Alcohol use. Radcliffe Medical Press, Oxford

Cooper D B 1994 Alcohol home detoxification and assessment. Radcliffe Medical Press, Oxford

Cooper D B, Faugier J 1993 Substance misuse. In: Wright H, Giddey M (eds) Mental health nursing – from first principle to professional practice. Chapman and Hall, London

COT (Committee on Toxicity of Chemicals in Food, Consumer Products and the Environment) 2001 Statement on the reproductive effects of caffeine. COT Statement 2001/06. COT, London

Davidson R 1991 Facilitating change in problem drinkers. In: Davidson R, Rollnick S, MacEwan I (eds) Counselling problem drinkers. Tavistock, London, p 3–20

Department of Health 1995 Sensible drinking: the report of an inter-departmental working group. HMSO, London

Department of Health 1999 Drug misuse and dependence – guidelines on clinical management. DH, London

Department of Health 2000 The NHS cancer plan: a plan for investment, a plan for reform. DH, London

Department of Health 2001 The NHS cancer plan: making progress. DH, London

Department of Health 2002a Updated drug strategy 2002. Drug Strategy Department, DH, London

Department of Health 2002b Mental health policy implementation guide: dual diagnosis good practice guide. DH, London

Department of Health 2003 Statistical bulletin: statistics on smoking: England 2003. Online. Available: www.publications.doh.gov.uk/public/sb0321.htm

Field-Smith M E, Butland B K, Ramsey J D et al 2004 Trends in death associated with abuse of volatile substances, report No. 17. Department of Community Health Sciences, St George's Hospital Medical School, London

Graham K, Clarke D, Bois C et al 1998 Depressant medication use by older persons in the broader social context relating to use of psychoactive substances. Journal of Substance Misuse 3(3): 161–169

Hackshaw A K, Law M R, Wald N J 1997 The accumulated evidence on lung cancer and environmental tobacco smoke. British Medical Journal 315: 980–988

Handford C, Colenso L 1998 Altered minds: the report of the Channel Four citizens' commission on drugs. Channel Four Television, London

Health Education Authority (HEA) 1996 Health update: smoking. HEA, London

Home Office Statistical Bulletin (HOSB) 1979 Statistics of the misuse of drugs in the United Kingdom 1978. Home Office Statistical Department, London

Jarvis M J, Boreham R, Primatesta P et al 2001 Nicotine yield from machine-smoked cigarettes and nicotine intakes in smokers: evidence from a representative population survey. Journal of the National Cancer Institute 93(2): 134–138

Jones K L, Smith D W 1973 Recognition of the foetal alcohol syndrome in early infancy. Lancet 2: 999–1001

Law M R, Morris J K, Wald N T 1997 Environmental tobacco smoke exposure and ischaemic heart disease: an evaluation of the evidence. British Medical Journal 315(7114): 973–980

Mathre M L 2001a Cannabis series – the whole story, part 1: overview. The Drug and Alcohol Professional 1(1): 3–7

Mathre M L 2001b Cannabis series – the whole story, part 2: current research findings on

cannabis and cannabinoid therapies. The Drug and Alcohol Professional 1(2): 4–11
Mathre M L 2002 Cannabis series – the whole story, part 5: research and development of cannabis preparations and delivery systems. The Drug and Alcohol Professional 2(4): 4–8
Mathre M L 2003a Cannabis series – the whole story, part 6: Potential risks related to acute chronic use of cannabis. The Drug and Alcohol Professional 3(1): 3–6
Mathre M L 2003b Cannabis series – the whole story, part 7: differentiating between medical use and recreational/social use, abuse and addiction. The Drug and Alcohol Professional 3(3): 5–10
Mathre M L, Byrne A 2002 Cannabis series – the whole story, part 3: the US cannabis prohibition and beyond. The Drug and Alcohol Professional 2(1): 4–9
Mathre M L, Krawitz M 2002 Cannabis series – the whole story, part 4: medicinal use of cannabis pre-prohibition. The Drug and Alcohol Professional 2(2): 3–7
McKee E 2000 Alcohol and the older person. In: Cooper D B (ed) Alcohol use. Radcliffe Medical Press, Oxford
Miller M R, Rollnick S 2002 Motivational interviewing: preparing people for change, 2nd edn. Guilford Press, New York
Mitchell E A, Taylor B J, Ford R P K et al 1992 Four modifiable and other major risk factors for cot death: the New Zealand study. Journal of Paediatric Child Health 28(Suppl 1): 3–8
Mitchell E A, Ford R P, Stewart A W et al 1993 Smoking and the sudden infant death syndrome. Paediatrics 91(5): 893–896
Morgan M 1992 Resume of paper 3: 'The medical background'. In: Royal College of General Practitioners (ed) Women and alcohol. HMSO, London
Morris K 2001 The failure of prohibition: a personal view. The Drug and Alcohol Professional 1(2): 12–17
Nissell M, Nomikoss G G, Svensson T H 1995 Nicotine dependence, midbrain dopamine systems and psychiatric disorders. Pharmacology and Toxicology 76: 157–162
Office for National Statistics (ONS) 2002 Living in Britain 2001: results from the 2001 general household survey. TSO, London
Office for National Statistics (ONS) 2004 Living in Britain: results from the 2002 general household survey No 31. TSO, London
Owens L, Penn G 1999 Smoking and pregnancy: a survey of knowledge, attitudes and behaviour 1992–1999. Health Education Authority, London
Pagliaro A M, Pagliaro L A 1996 Substance use among children and adolescents: its nature, extent and effects from conception to adulthood. Wiley, New York
Pickles Judge J 1991 A futile war. 'Byline' BBC1
Plant M L 1997 Women and alcohol: contemporary and historical perspectives. Free Association Books, London
Prescription Prescribing Authority (PPA) 2001 Practice prescribing and spending on mental health drugs. PPA, Newcastle
Prime Minister's Strategy Unit (PMSU) 2003 Strategy unit alcohol harm reduction project: interim analytical report. Cabinet Office, London
Prime Minister's Strategy Unit (PMSU) 2004 Alcohol harm reduction strategy for England, March 2004. Cabinet Office, London
Prochaska J O, DiClemente C C 1983 Stages and process of self-change of smoking: towards an integrative model of change. Journal of Consulting and Clinical Psychology 51(3): 390–395
Prochaska J O, DiClemente C C 1986 Towards a comprehensive model of change. In: Miller W R, Heather N (eds) Treating addictive behaviours: processes of change. Plenum, London
Ramsey M, Baker P, Goulden C et al 2001 Drug misuse declared in 2000: results from the British crime survey, Home Office research study 224. Home Office Research, Development and Statistical Directorate, London
Rassool G (ed) 1998 Substance use and misuse: nature, context and clinical interventions. Blackwell Science, Oxford
Raw W, McNiell A, West R 1998 Smoking cessation guidelines for health professionals. Thorax 53(Suppl 5): S1–38
Regier D A, Farmer M E, Rae D S et al 1990 Co-morbidity of mental disorders with alcohol and other drug abuse: results from the epidemiological catchment area (ECA) study. Journal of the American Medical Association 264(19): 2511–2518
Richardson A, Budd T 2003 Alcohol, crime and disorder: a study of young adults, Home Office research study 263. Development and Statistics Directorate, London
Royal College of Physicians (RCP) 2000 Nicotine addiction in Britain. A report of the Tobacco Advisory Group of The Royal College of Physicians, London
Royal College of Physicians (RCP) 2001 Alcohol – can the NHS afford it? Recommendations for a coherent alcohol strategy for hospitals. A report of the Working Party of The Royal College of Physicians February 2001. RCP, London
Royal College of Physicians (RCP) 2002 Protecting smokers, saving lives: the case for a tobacco and nicotine regulatory authority. Tobacco Advisory Group of The Royal College of Physicians, London
Royal College of Psychiatrists 1987 Drug scenes: a report on drugs and drug dependency. Gaskell, Oxford
Royal College of Psychiatrists 1997 Benzodiazepines: risks, benefits and dependence: a re-evaluation. Council Report CR59 January 1997. Royal College of Psychiatrists, London
Ryrie I, McGowan J 1998 Staff perceptions of substance use among acute psychiatric inpatients. Journal of Mental Health Nursing 5: 137–142
Saunders B, Marsh A 1999 Harm reduction and the use of currently illegal drugs: some assumptions and dilemmas. Journal of Substance Use 4(1): 3–9
Schacter S 1982 Recidivism and self cure of smoking and obesity. American Psychologist 37: 436–444
Scottish Advisory Committee on Alcohol Misuse (SACAM) 2002 Plan for action on alcohol problems. Scottish Executive Health Department, Edinburgh
Scottish Executive 2003 Volatile substance abuse: know the score. Scottish Executive, Edinburgh
Seivewright N 1998 Current opinion: theory and practice in managing benzodiazepine dependence and misuse. Journal of Substance Misuse 3(3): 170–177
Silverman K, Evans S M, Stragin E C et al 1992 Withdrawal syndrome after the double-blind cessation of caffeine consumption. New England Journal of Medicine 327(16): 1109–1114
Taylor Hays J 2000 Tobacco, nicotine and addiction. Journal of Substance Use 5(Suppl): 159–164
The Observer 2002 ICM research poll: drugs uncovered. The Observer Sunday Supplement 21/04/02
USDHHS (US Department of Health and Human Services) 1989 Reducing the health consequences of smoking: 25 years' progress. A report of the Surgeon General, US Department of Health and Human Services, Public Health Services, Center for Disease Control, Center for Chronic Disease Prevention and Health Promotion, Office of Smoking and Health. DHHS Publication (CDC) 89:8411. USDHHS, Washington, DC
Watson H E 2000 Alcohol: prevention, identification and health promotion. In: Cooper D B (ed) Alcohol use. Radcliffe Medical Press, Oxford
World Health Organization (WHO) 1985 The use of essential drugs. Publication TRS722. WHO, Geneva
World Health Organization (WHO) 1996 Alcohol and primary health care. WHO, Copenhagen
World Health Organization (WHO) 2001 Brief intervention for hazardous and harmful drinking: a manual for use in primary care. Department of Mental Health and Substance Dependence. WHO, Geneva
World Health Organization (WHO) 2002 World health report 2002: reducing risks, promoting healthy life. WHO, Geneva
World Health Organization (WHO) 2003 World health report 2003: shaping the future. WHO, Geneva
World Health Organization (WHO) 2004a Neuroscience of psychoactive substance use and dependence. WHO, Geneva
World Health Organization (WHO) 2004b Building blocks for tobacco control: a handbook. WHO, Geneva

FURTHER READING

Advisory Council on the Misuse of Drugs 1995 Volatile substance abuse. HMSO, London

Banerjee J, Clancy C, Crome I 2002 Co-existing problems of mental disorder and substance misuse (dual diagnosis): an information manual 2002. The Royal College of Psychiatrists Research Unit, College Research Unit, London

Cameron D 1995 Liberating solutions to alcohol problems: treating problem drinkers without saying no. Jason Aronson, Northvale, NJ

Cameron D 2000 Alcohol use in perspective. In: Cooper D B (ed) Alcohol use. Radcliffe Medical Press, Oxford

Cooper D B 1994 Alcohol home detoxification and assessment. Radcliffe Medical Press, Oxford

Cooper D B (ed) 2000 Alcohol use. Radcliffe Medical Press, Oxford

Cooper D B, Cooper P D 2001 Helping people with alcohol problems. Professional Nurse 16(8): 1276–1280

Department of Health 2002 Tackling crack: a national plan. Drugs Strategy Directorate. TSO, London

Department of Health 2003 Alcohol use: how much does it cost? Department of Health Strategy Unit, London

Graham K, Clarke D, Bois C et al 1998 Depressant medication use by older persons in the broader social context relating to use of psychoactive substances. Journal of Substance Misuse 3(3): 161–169

Heather N, Robertson I 1997 Problem drinking, 3rd edn. Oxford University Press, Oxford

Keene J 1997 Drug misuse: prevention, harm minimisation and treatment. Chapman and Hall, London

Mathre M L 2001a Cannabis series – the whole story, part 1: overview. The Drug and Alcohol Professional 1(1): 3–7

Mathre M L 2001b Cannabis series – the whole story, part 2: current research findings on cannabis and cannabinoid therapies. The Drug and Alcohol Professional 1(2): 4–11

Mathre M L 2002 Cannabis series – the whole story, part 5: research and development of cannabis preparations and delivery systems. The Drug and Alcohol Professional 2(4): 4–8

Mathre M L 2003a Cannabis series – the whole story, part 6: Potential risks related to acute chronic use of cannabis. The Drug and Alcohol Professional 3(1): 3–6

Mathre M L 2003b Cannabis series – the whole story, part 7: differentiating between medical use and recreational/social use, abuse and addiction. The Drug and Alcohol Professional 3(3): 5–10

Mathre M L, Byrne A 2002 Cannabis series – the whole story, part 3: the US cannabis prohibition and beyond. The Drug and Alcohol Professional 2(1): 4–9

Mathre M L, Krawitz M 2002 Cannabis series – the whole story, part 4: medicinal use of cannabis pre-prohibition. The Drug and Alcohol Professional 2(2): 3–7

McKee E 2000 Alcohol and the older person. In: Cooper D B (ed) Alcohol use: the handbook. Radcliffe Medical Press, Oxford

Miller M R, Rollnick S 2002 Motivational interviewing: preparing people for change, 2nd edn. Guilford Press, New York

Pagliaro A M, Pagliaro L A 1996 Substance use among children and adolescents: its nature, extent and effects from conception to adulthood. Wiley, New York

Preston A 1996 The methadone briefing. ISDD, London

Prime Minister's Strategy Unit 2004 Alcohol harm reduction strategy for England, March 2004. Cabinet Office, London

Rassool G H, Gafoor M 1997 Addiction nursing: perspectives on professional and clinical practice. Stanley Thornes, London

Royal College of General Practitioners 1992 Women and alcohol. HMSO, London

Royal College of Physicians 2000 Alcohol: can the NHS afford it? RCP, London

Scottish Advisory Committee on Alcohol Misuse (SACAM) 2002 Plan for action on alcohol problems. Scottish Executive Health Department, Edinburgh

Scottish Intercollegiate Guidelines Network (SIGN) 2003 The management of harmful drinking and alcohol dependence in primary care: a national clinical guideline. SIGN, Edinburgh

Seivewright N 1998 Current opinion: theory and practice in managing benzodiazepine dependence and misuse. Journal of Substance Misuse 3(3): 170–177

Slattery J, Chick J, Cochrane M et al 2003 Prevention of relapse in alcohol dependence. Health Technology Assessment Report 3. Health Technology Board for Scotland, Glasgow

Stimmel B 1997 Pain and its relief without addiction. Haworth Medical Press, New York

Stratton K, Howe C, Battaglin F (eds) 1996 Fetal alcohol syndrome: diagnosis, epidemiology, prevention and treatment. Institute of Medicine and National Academy Press, Washington, DC

Watson H E 2000 Alcohol: prevention, identification and health promotion. In: Cooper D B (ed) Alcohol use: the handbook. Radcliffe Medical Press, Oxford

World Health Organization (WHO) 2001 Brief intervention for hazardous and harmful drinking: a manual for use in primary care. Department of Mental Health and Substance Dependence. WHO, Geneva

World Health Organization (WHO) 2001 Ecstasy: MDMA and other ring-substituted amphetamines. Department of Mental Health and Substance Dependence. WHO, Geneva

USEFUL WEBSITES AND ADDRESSES

Action on Smoking and Health (ASH)
www.ash.org.uk

Alcohol Concern
www.alcoholconcern.org.uk

Council for Involuntary Tranquilliser Addiction
www.patient.co.uk/showdoc/26738750/

Drinkline: 0800 567 123

Drugscope
www.drugscope.com

Ethnic community languages AIDS Helpline: 0800 917 2227
Minicom: 0800 521 361
1st Floor Cavern Court
8 St Mathew Street
Liverpool L2 6RE

GamCare (National Association for Gambling Care)
www.gamcare.org.uk

Medical Council on Alcohol
www.medicouncilalcol.demon.co.uk

National AIDS Helpline: 0800 567 123

National Drug Helpline – Talk to Frank: 0800 77 66 00
www.talktofrank.com

Nursing Council on Alcohol (NCA)
www.nursingcouncilonalcohol.org

QUIT
www.quit.org.uk

Re-Solv (The Society for the Prevention of Solvent and Volatile Substance Abuse)
www.re-solv.org

Smokers' Quitline: 0800 00 22 00
Bengali: 0800 00 22 44
Gujarti: 0800 00 22 55
Hindi: 0800 00 22 66
Punjabi: 0800 00 22 77
Urdu: 0800 00 22 88
Turkish & Kurdish: 0800 00 22 99

Terrence Higgins Trust
www.tht.org.uk

The Addictions Forum
Professor Moira Plant
Alcohol and Health Research Centre
University of the West of England
Glenside Campus (Room 1EO1)
Blackberry Hill
Stapleton
Bristol BS16 1DD

Women's Alcohol Centre
www.womeninlondon.org.uk/wac.htm

THE PERSON WITH HIV/AIDS

John Atkinson

37

INTRODUCTION — THE 21ST CENTURY GLOBAL CONTEXT

It may seem strange that 16 years since work on the first edition for this book started, there continues to be a chapter devoted to one infectious disease. Nurses around the world now deal with other diseases, some newly emergent, like severe acute respiratory syndrome (SARS) (Waters 2003), and others with a more enduring presence in our care such as hepatitis C (Gungabissoon 2003) and methicillin-resistant *Staphylococcus aureus* (MRSA) (RCN 2004). However, there is still much to learn from human immunodeficiency virus (HIV) and acquired immune deficiency syndrome (AIDS). At their appearance nearly 25 years ago, fever hospitals and the specialist qualification of fever nurse were being disbanded in affluent and so-called 'developed' countries. Young, fit people did not die of infectious disease in great numbers and perhaps a degree of hubris and of complacency had set in. AIDS changed all that.

Since AIDS was first recognised, great advances have taken place in the treatment of people with HIV and its related illnesses. Undoubtedly, the main advance is in the expansion and sophistication of combination (multiple) therapies. In the early days of the emergence of the disease, people diagnosed with AIDS would live only weeks or months, whereas the improved therapies have led to the survival of some patients for over 10 years and some over 20 years, and to many more patients being cared for outside hospital.

The reader is directed to the British HIV Association website and their HIV treatment guidelines (British HIV Association 2003) and to the United Nations 2004 Report on the global AIDS epidemic (UN 2004).

In terms of new endeavour, emphasis is now on the practical implementation of treatment for the vast numbers of people with HIV and its related illnesses in financially poor and developing countries, particularly in Africa. Progress is slow, but gathering momentum. The World Health Organization's (2003a) '3 by 5' campaign, which aimed to treat 3 million people by 2005, is in stark contrast to previous ideals and policies, whose counsel of despair was that only prevention was a possibility in non-affluent countries. Jong-wook Lee, Director-General of the World Health Organization (WHO), speaking of the '3 by 5' initiative, states:

> *Lack of access to antiretroviral therapy (ART) is a global health emergency … To deliver antiretroviral treatment to the millions who need it, we must change the way we think and change the way we act.*
> *WHO 2003b*

Another advance has been the development of the legal and regulatory framework between countries and within the workplace, in relation to people with HIV and their abilities, rights and duties regarding travel and employment. Dimond (2003) discusses the law, HIV and employees, and the All-Party Parliamentary Group on AIDS (2003) examines migration and HIV (Singh 2003). In the UK, the main policy theme is that people with HIV should be able to travel and work without interference or harassment and, in most circumstances, have their confidentiality maintained.

The story of AIDS emerged in the USA where five men died of *Pneumocystis carinii* pneumonia (PCP), a rare infection (Shilts 2000). The only characteristics they had in common were their young age, their gender and the fact that they were homosexual. Later that year a patient with similar symptoms and characteristics died in a London hospital (Adler 2001). The condition we now call acquired immune deficiency syndrome (AIDS) had arrived. In 1983–84, in France and the USA, the causative agent, a virus from the family of retroviruses (see p. 1171), was isolated. This virus was found to infiltrate and destroy human helper T lymphocytes, which promote both the ability of B-lymphocyte-derived plasma cells to produce antibodies and the activation of killer T lymphocytes, the $CD8^+$ cytotoxic cells, which are able to attack and kill those cells infected with viruses. The viruses which cause AIDS are known as the human immunodeficiency viruses.

This chapter will present the main historical features of the advent of HIV/AIDS, along with a profile of the retrovirus. It will address the social and economic implications of HIV/AIDS and the effect of the disease on patients and their carers. Testing will be highlighted, together with concomitant ethical and practical dilemmas. The final sections of the chapter will consider the clinical manifestations of HIV/AIDS, giving details of the treatments currently available. The contribution of nurses to the care of individuals with HIV/AIDS will be discussed. Whilst reading this chapter, the reader should remember that the person with HIV/AIDS will spend most of their time at home and not in hospital or other formal care settings.

By setting HIV/AIDS, at the outset, in a wide social context, this chapter intends to emphasise that HIV/AIDS is both a clinical and a sociopolitical issue. It is hoped that nurses, armed with the information provided by this chapter, will be able to develop a knowledgeable and empathetic mode of practice with people who have HIV and related problems.

Definitions

In order to use the correct terminology relating to HIV/AIDS, it is helpful to understand how this terminology developed.

The syndrome

The only clinical factor linking the original patients with AIDS was the fact that they were so profoundly immunosuppressed, that microorganisms which generally inhabit the body harmlessly took the opportunity to replicate wildly, disseminate and cause clinical illness, e.g. *Pneumocystis carinii* pneumonia (PCP). Until that time, this infection was seen only occasionally, in patients who were immunosuppressed with diseases such as leukaemia or whose immunity was suppressed as a side-effect of medication. These types of illness and neoplastic events, which only manifest themselves in persons who have a severely compromised immune system, are referred to as 'opportunistic diseases' and they are the hallmark of the syndrome now referred to as AIDS. As this immunosuppressed state was not a primary, e.g. congenital, but a secondary immunodeficiency, it was called acquired immune deficiency (the main linking clinical factor) syndrome, i.e. a group of recognised clinical signs. In time it would be recognised that this particular immunodeficiency was secondary to specific viral infection.

Human immunodeficiency virus (HIV)

The retroviruses, now called human immunodeficiency viruses, were isolated and designated the causative agents of AIDS. A blood test which could detect antibodies to HIV following infection was developed in 1985. An individual who becomes infected with HIV will respond by producing antibodies in a process known as seroconversion. When a person is found to have HIV antibodies, they are said to be HIV antibody-positive or, less correctly, HIV-positive (HIV+) and are considered to be infected with HIV.

Since the discovery of HIV, a major strain variation within the species human immunodeficiency viruses — HIV 2 — has been identified. It is most commonly found in certain countries on the west coast of Africa and in west India. HIV 2 is less able to be transmitted from an infected mother to her child, i.e. vertical transmission, and infection with HIV 2 is generally associated with a longer incubation period to an AIDS-defining illness (Adler 2001).

AIDS diagnosis

A patient is diagnosed as having AIDS only if they are HIV antibody-positive and have one of the designated infections or diseases associated with AIDS. The classification of these diseases devised by the Centers for Disease Control (CDC 1987) in the USA is used globally. Also current is the *World Health Organization Clinical Staging System for HIV Infection and Disease* (WHO 2003c, see Box 37.1). This system attempts to address some of the anomalies which the CDC system presented. A helpful explanation of the staging system is given in Pratt (2003).

It is important to understand the following relationship between HIV antibodies and AIDS. Everybody who has AIDS is HIV antibody-positive, but not everybody who is HIV antibody-positive has AIDS. It should also be pointed out that an individual who has a positive HIV antibody status may sometimes become ill without being diagnosed as having AIDS. This may be because they have not yet contracted one of the infections or diseases on the classified list but are ill for some other reason, or because they are experiencing side-effects of, for instance, antiretroviral treatment.

Nurses will meet many people who have at some time been diagnosed as having AIDS but who are presently well. A patient may have an AIDS-defining illness, be treated for it, recover and no longer be considered to have AIDS. This is increasingly common as people with the syndrome survive longer. When the author began working in the field, death 18 months to 2 years after diagnosis was the 'norm'. Now one may meet individuals who have survived 10–20 years. Thus the term AIDS as an 'illness label' can be unhelpful, and even misleading, because it does not necessarily reflect how the person is at a given moment. For nurses in particular, the term has little relevance. It is more helpful to consider the term 'persons living with HIV infection' rather than AIDS or HIV patients. The term conveys

Box 37.1

WHO staging system for HIV infection and disease in adults and adolescents

Clinical stage I

1. Asymptomatic
2. Persistent generalised lymphadenopathy

Performance scale 1: asymptomatic, normal activity

Clinical stage II

3. Weight loss, <10% of body weight
4. Minor mucocutaneous manifestations, e.g. seborrhoeic dermatitis, prurigo, fungal nail infections, recurrent oral ulcerations, angular cheilitis
5. Herpes zoster within the last 5 years
6. Recurrent upper respiratory tract infections, e.g. bacterial sinusitis

And/or performance scale 2: symptomatic, normal activity

Clinical stage III

7. Weight loss, >10% of body weight
8. Unexplained chronic diarrhoea, >1 month
9. Unexplained prolonged fever (intermittent or constant), >1 month
10. Oral candidiasis (thrush)
11. Oral hairy leukoplakia
12. Pulmonary tuberculosis within the past year
13. Severe bacterial infections, i.e. pneumonia, pyomyositis

And/or performance scale 3: bedridden <50% of the day during the last month

Clinical stage IV

14. HIV wasting syndrome, as defined by the Centers for Disease Control and Prevention[a]
15. *Pneumocystis carinii* pneumonia
16. Toxoplasmosis of the brain
17. Cryptosporidiosis with diarrhoea >1 month
18. Cryptococcosis, extrapulmonary
19. Cytomegalovirus disease of an organ other than liver, spleen or lymph nodes
20. Herpes simplex virus infection, mucocutaneous >1 month, or visceral any duration
21. Progressive multifocal leukoencephalopathy
22. Any disseminated endemic mycosis, i.e. histoplasmosis, coccidioidomycosis
23. Candidiasis of the oesophagus, trachea, bronchi or lungs
24. Atypical mycobacteriosis, disseminated
25. Non-typhoid *Salmonella* septicaemia
26. Extrapulmonary tuberculosis
27. Lymphoma
28. Kaposi's sarcoma
29. HIV encephalopathy, as defined by the Centers for Disease Control and Prevention[b]

And/or performance scale 4: bedridden >50% of the day during the last month

Note: both definitive and presumptive diagnoses are acceptable.
[a]HIV wasting syndrome: weight loss of >10% of body weight, plus either unexplained chronic diarrhoea (>1 month) or chronic weakness and unexplained prolonged fever (>1 month).
[b]HIV encephalopathy: clinical findings of disabling cognitive and/or motor dysfunction interfering with activities of daily living, progressing over weeks to months, in the absence of a concurrent illness or condition other than HIV infection which could explain the findings.

Reproduced with permission from the World Health Organization (2003c).

a continuum from the moment of infection to end-stage disease and death with early, middle and late events and issues affecting individuals.

Issues surrounding terminology

HIV/AIDS has become a deeply politicised disease phenomenon. The nurse, as educator and advocate, must be sensitive to the sociopolitical issues surrounding HIV/AIDS and its description. The patient has the right to expect that nurses will use terminology that is appropriate and technically correct, promotes well-being, is not stigmatising and does not give offence.

Although the term AIDS has limited clinical usefulness, it is still the term commonly used by the media and the public. Also common are the terms 'the AIDS virus' and 'the HIV virus'. Neither is strictly correct and nurses should use 'HIV' instead.

It is now generally accepted that 'person/s living with AIDS' (PLWA) or HIV is a more acceptable term than 'AIDS patient'. The latter term is inappropriate as an individual may live a normal life for long periods without recourse to medical or nursing care. Calling an individual a 'victim' raises questions of guilt or innocence and, along with 'sufferer', implies that they are powerless to help themselves.

VIRUSES AND NORMAL IMMUNOLOGY

The reader is referred to Chapter 16 for an outline of normal immunology.

Viruses

Viruses are not complete organisms. They can survive only as part of 'host' cells. Unlike bacteria, fungi, protozoa and other infective agents, all of which are complete and independently viable, viruses cannot replicate (multiply/reproduce) by themselves. They are also very small and cannot be seen by a light microscope. Viruses are made up of a core of nucleic acid, i.e. DNA or RNA, never both, and are enveloped in a protein shell.

Retroviruses

These viruses, to which HIV belongs, contain RNA. They have the ability to infiltrate the DNA of the host cell and implant their genetic material there, after which the host cell will have the capability to reproduce HIV.

DNA is present in all organisms. It plays a central part in heredity and, because of its structure, the two interwoven strands of nucleotides, connected by hydrogen bonds, can replicate, carrying the genetic blueprint to the next generation of cells. RNA is made up of a single strand of nucleotides and is involved in protein synthesis. It provides the genetic blueprint of some viruses, including HIV. HIV infects a variety of cells that contain the $CD4^+$ host cell receptors, including T lymphocytes of the helper subset. The presence of additional host cell receptors is known to be necessary in order for HIV to attach itself to, and infect a cell.

The importance of this disruption of the T lymphocytes must be understood within the context of the normal immune response (see Ch. 16). The various types of white blood cell have interlinking but quite distinct cell-mediated responses to seek and destroy invading microorganisms

Box 37.2

The normal immune response

Warning
In response to the invading microorganism, helper T cells orchestrate defences by releasing chemicals which stimulate other cells of the immune system.

Preparation
Activated by these chemical signals, other kinds of T cells (cytotoxic cells and lymphokine producers) begin to proliferate, while B lymphocytes multiply and become plasma cells which start to manufacture antibodies.

Attack
Activated T cells and antibodies are released into the circulation, where they specifically target and destroy the invading organism.

Stand down
Once the foreign organism is routed and the infection is under control, the activity of the immune system is reduced, perhaps partly through the action of suppressor T lymphocytes.

and malignant cells. For a stage-by-stage summary of this process, see Box 37.2. Given the essential role played by helper T cells in the immune system, it is clear that their invasion and destruction by HIV will have devastating results.

For further information on retroviruses, see Chapters 2 and 3 in Pratt (2003).

THE TRANSMISSION OF HIV

Modes of transmission

The first stage of HIV infection occurs when the individual is infected with HIV through an exchange of body fluids and/or blood with an infected individual. Sexual contact and blood-to-blood contact are known as 'horizontal' methods of transmission, i.e. they move 'across' from one individual to another.

Transmission through sexual contact

Unprotected vaginal or anal intercourse is the most common means by which HIV can be transmitted from an infected to a non-infected person. It is difficult to determine absolutely whether other intimate sexual activities, e.g. oral sex, can transmit the virus as they do not often occur in isolation. However, some individual cases have been reported (Rothenberg et al 1998). There is much debate in the scientific and secular worlds about which sexual activities are the most 'dangerous'. Until recently, anal sex was considered to be most risky. Also, women were thought to be more at risk from penis/vagina sex than men. More recent findings are leading to a re-examination of these assumptions, and the scientific debate is not conclusive (Stine 2000).

It is important, therefore, to inform patients that they may be at risk from any intimate sexual contact.

Transmission through blood and blood products

Blood transfusions The spread of HIV in Western countries that have sophisticated blood transfusion services has been greatly reduced since the rigorous screening of donors was instituted in most countries in 1985. In the UK it is now reckoned that there is a risk factor of less than one transmission in a million units of blood. This means fewer than three transmissions a year.

The best-known recipients of blood products are those suffering from haemophilia and those with other blood-clotting disorders. Before 1985, many thousands of such individuals became infected through blood products. Since 1985, these products have been heat treated. The treatment is totally successful but reduces the efficacy of the products, such that more of them are required.

Blood transmission through sharing of equipment HIV transmission can occur through the sharing of syringes, needles and other blood-giving equipment. In Western countries this commonly occurs through the illicit, intravenous (i.v.) use of drugs. Here the probability of infection is often increased by the user 'flushing' the syringe with their blood before injection. In poorer countries, it also occurs where there is reuse of medical equipment and insufficient sterilising facilities. The mode of transmission is the same in both cases.

Percutaneous 'needlestick' injuries There have been very few proven cases of infection by this mode. A study of 3000 incidents where individuals were exposed to HIV puts the risk of seroconversion from a contaminated needlestick at 0.3%. Only 92 cases of occupational infection with HIV have been reported worldwide (Sistrom et al 1998, Babcock & Fraser 2003, Nursing and Midwifery Council 2003a).

Transmission through skin piercing procedures Transmission is certainly a theoretical risk from procedures such as tattooing (Greif et al 1999), and cases have been reported of transmission by body piercing (Armstrong 1998) and skin grafting.

Transmission through other bodily fluids Infection with HIV takes place only when there is sufficient concentration of the virus. Infection through saliva, for instance, is therefore considered unlikely. Worldwide retrospective studies have shown that the number of workers contracting the virus through urine, faeces or saliva, for example, has been extremely small (Jeffries 1997).

Mother-to-child transmission

This form of transmission is known as 'vertical' transmission, i.e. 'from' an infected mother to her child in the womb or during delivery, when the mother's blood and the child's blood become mixed. There is a possibility that transmission through amniotic fluid and ('horizontally') through breast milk may also take place (Gibb et al 2003).

From birth until 11–18 months, the baby will carry the mother's antibodies including HIV. Therefore, all babies born to HIV-infected mothers are found to be HIV antibody-positive. At about 11–18 months, the baby will lose the mother's antibodies and go on either to being HIV antibody-negative, i.e. not carrying the virus, or to developing their own antibodies, i.e. being infected in their own right. A few of these babies go on to become HIV antibody-negative but positive to another test which isolates antigen (particles of the actual virus), so that they are carrying the virus but not the antibodies.

For further information, see Newberry & Kelsey (2003).

At the beginning of the HIV epidemic it appeared that approximately 50% of children born to HIV antibody-positive mothers became infected in their own right. In countries where there are good antenatal facilities and the mother remains well throughout pregnancy, the rate of transmission from mother to child is dramatically lower. If the mother's immune system is robust, if she is treated in the last trimester and has an early elective caesarean section, transmission is reduced to less than 1% (De Cock et al 2000, WHO 2000).

Stages of HIV infection

The dormant or asymptomatic stage

In HIV-related illness, two main processes take place in the infected person's body:

- HIV destroys the helper T cells and replicates itself
- The body's immunity is inexorably weakened and is attacked by other infections. The body becomes increasingly unable to combat these attacks.

Since viruses cannot multiply by themselves, they need to use the cell-building material of their host cells in order to reproduce themselves (see Fig. 37.1). When HIV enters the bloodstream, it attaches itself to the outer cell membrane of the helper T lymphocyte. Following this, it breaks into the cell and releases its genetic blueprint, which has the ability to replicate itself.

The disease process may then go no further for several months or even years. The person is infected with HIV and may or may not have produced antibodies. This may take 3 months or more. If they have seroconverted and started to produce antibodies, they may or may not have become ill. If they did become ill with acute seroconversion illness (CDC phase A), the usually mild and very common flu-like symptoms were probably not recognised by the individual or their physician as a sign of HIV infection. The helper T-lymphocyte blood count will still be normal and therefore the immune system will remain unaffected. The patient will continue to be well. This stage, often called the dormant stage, is referred to as 'Clinical stage one: 1 – Asymptomatic' in the World Health Organization staging system (WHO 2003c).

In time, the infected T cells will start to replicate new HIV retroviruses. Although it is unclear what triggers this process, it seems that, if an individual keeps generally well and leads a healthy lifestyle, the stage at which HIV starts to replicate and destroy the T cells may be delayed. A clearer finding is that, in conditions of deprivation and poor health, the illness seems to progress more quickly.

The replication stage

The first process At some point after HIV has been incorporated into the helper T lymphocyte, it begins to replicate itself within the cell walls using the cell's own material. The new viruses aggregate, start to destroy the outer cell membrane and break out of the helper T cell, encased in membrane stolen from the host cell and clinging onto the remnants of the cell. This is known as 'budding' (see Fig. 37.1). At this stage, the host cell dies. The new viruses then disperse throughout the bloodstream, infecting other helper T lymphocytes, and the process begins again.

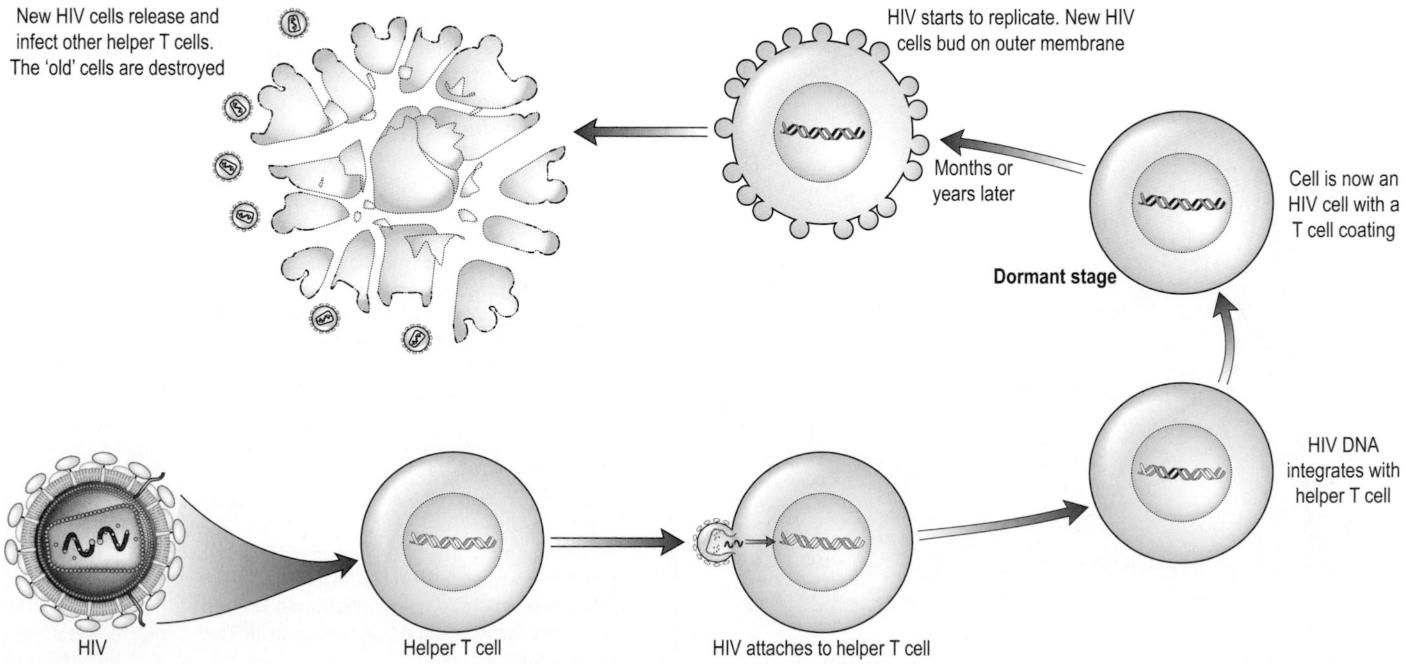

Fig. 37.1 The human immunodeficiency virus in action.

The second process begins when helper T cells have been infected to the degree that the number of normal, healthy helper T cells begins to fall markedly. At this point the body's immune response to other infections will begin to be compromised. From the clinician's viewpoint, this is a significant stage, as the depletion of normal helper T cells can be measured in a blood sample ($CD4^+$ T cell count, see Appendix 1).

Also significant is the ratio between the helper T lymphocytes and the cytotoxic T lymphocytes, which is thought to assist in the 'stand down' phase of the normal immune response (see Box 37.2). Normally, the ratio is 1.5 helpers to 1.0 suppressor cytotoxic cells; however, as the number of healthy helper cells decreases, this ratio changes. This will have a detrimental effect on the immune system. It is also one of the diagnostic signs used to confirm the presence of HIV-related illness. In other forms of immune deficiency illnesses, both helper and suppressor cell levels fall, and so the ratio between them remains roughly the same.

As the helper T cell level falls, the body will become more susceptible to other infections. The individual may at first experience rather vague symptoms, progressing to debilitating but not life-threatening conditions and finally to serious illness and death. Information on the specific diseases which may appear is given later in the chapter.

A typical profile of HIV infection is shown in Figure 37.2. How HIV/AIDS actually manifests itself will vary dramatically from one person to another. Many people with extremely low helper T cell counts may seem healthy; others with what should be a 'good' count will be extremely ill. The nurse must rely on observations of and discussions with the patient in assessing their condition, rather than on abstract clinical indicators alone.

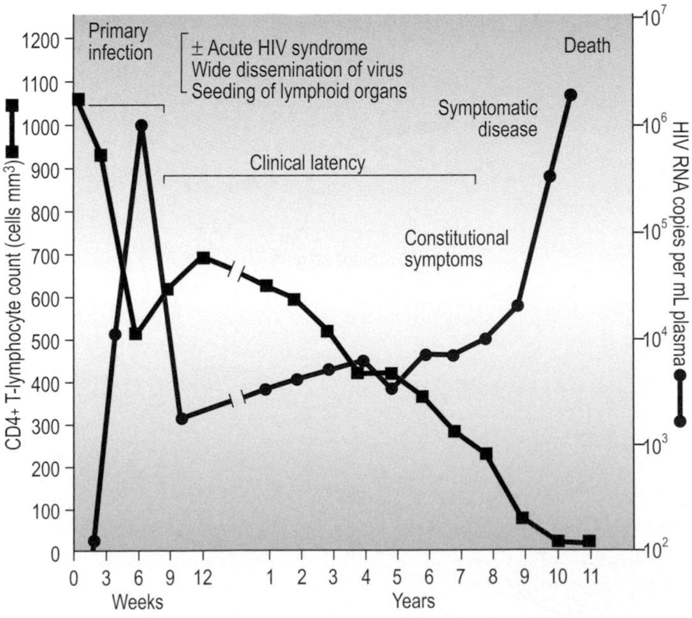

Fig. 37.2 The course of HIV infection. (Adapted from Pratt 2003.)

POLITICAL AND SOCIAL IMPLICATIONS OF HIV/AIDS

AIDS has been referred to as 'the real global terrorist' of the present and compared to the great plagues of the past in that it appears to be spreading unchecked and has, as yet, no cure. Like other infectious diseases which have reached epidemic or pandemic proportions, HIV/AIDS has given rise to a great deal of fear and stigmatisation. In formulating health and social policies in response to AIDS, governments have a duty not only to safeguard the health and well-being of their populations as a whole, but also to protect the rights of those individuals affected by the disease.

The foundation for political and social responses to HIV/AIDS is provided by the work of epidemiologists, who define the disease, describe its typical progression and determine its national and international incidence. Also relevant is its prevalence within particular groups. On the basis of these findings, predictions are made as to the future impact of the disease (Barker & Rose 1998). Armed with this knowledge, nursing, medical and scientific practitioners, along with the individuals and groups affected, endeavour to raise awareness of HIV/AIDS and to lobby governments to take appropriate action.

Although cases of HIV infection were known in 1981, it was not until 2 or 3 years later that HIV appeared officially to be recognised as a threat to the whole community. Various media campaigns were instigated from 1985 onwards and the first full debate in the UK was held in the House of Commons in November 1986 (Hansard 1986).

Some of the questions and issues raised by the epidemiology of HIV/AIDS are listed in Box 37.3.

Box 37.3

Questions and issues raised by HIV/AIDS

- In developing countries, particularly Africa, HIV affects mainly heterosexual people. In the West, with some notable exceptions, the prevalence appears to be overwhelmingly among homosexual men and intravenous drug users. Why is the pattern so different, given that HIV is now present in all sections of the population in the West?
- In many cities in the USA and Africa, the prevalence of HIV among young heterosexuals is rising dramatically. It is now the most common cause of death in this group. Will this happen everywhere?
- Given that there is no cure for AIDS, just how effective are education and prevention policies? Some countries, notably the USA, have strict entry laws. What is the case for stringent political action, e.g. restricting the movements of known HIV-positive individuals?
- Is there a case for testing as many people as possible anonymously to get a more accurate profile of what is going on so that policymakers are better able to provide proper services?
- Is the nurse's primary responsibility to the individual patient and to their confidentiality and wishes? If so, what responsibility does the nurse have to protect the public at large? Can both responsibilities be met at the same time?

Political challenges

The most intractable problem presented by HIV to policy makers is the length of time it takes for the disease to manifest itself after an individual becomes infected. This has the following profound epidemiological implications:

- Most people who are infected are not aware of it until they become ill.
- The government figures published regularly related to people with AIDS do not reflect the prevalence of HIV at that moment. They give, at best, an idea of the prevalence 5–10 years ago.
- It is more difficult to gauge specifically who is at risk, although some 'high-risk' activities can be identified, e.g. i.v. drug use, unprotected sexual intercourse.

It is therefore vital that data on AIDS are as specific as possible. In England and Wales, the Health Protection Agency, and in Scotland, Health Protection Scotland (see 'Useful websites', p. 1189) collect, collate and distribute information on the incidence and prevalence of HIV and AIDS.

Until January 1991, the number of reported AIDS cases in the UK was published monthly. The main figure quoted was the cumulative total, i.e. the overall number known since reporting started. Since the implementation of the AIDS (Control) Act 1987 and other measures, it has been possible to gather more specific, local information from hospitals, clinics and health authorities. There is now an annual breakdown of HIV seropositive incidence, cases of AIDS, gender, high-risk activity, e.g. drug use, and age. Internationally, data collection has been improved by the coordination of research projects and the collation of information and there is an annual global AIDS medical conference.

STOP THINK **37.1** Obtain national and local AIDS/HIV-related statistics from the Health Protection Agency (England and Wales) or Health Protection Scotland. Analyse trends over the last 5 years.

The impact of HIV/AIDS on health and social services

Although qualified nurses tend to work exclusively in either a hospital or a community setting, it is important to consider HIV in relation to the full range of services available to the (typically young) person living with HIV, particularly in the light of innovations in medication in the mid-1990s and the longer life expectation. The settings in which care is given to individuals with HIV/AIDS may be categorised as follows:

- Hospital care
  - — inpatient ward or hospice
  - — day care
  - — outpatients
- Community care
  - — treatment room: health centre/clinic
  - — home: with a district nurse, health visitor or other practitioner
  - — home: self-care or with family/partner/friends
  - — outreach: residential, e.g. hostels, prisons, caravans
  - — outreach: non-residential, e.g. drop-in centres, street work.

Hospital care At first, HIV care was delivered almost exclusively in the hospital inpatient setting. This was an expensive, labour-intensive and often arguably a 'patient-unfriendly' option. Individuals would spend many days or weeks in hospital per year, sometimes feeling relatively well but requiring, for example, i.v. therapy. The hospital setting is still used for seriously ill patients. However, day care units are now used extensively and often have flexible hours to facilitate patients' work commitments. Day care units and outpatient departments are used as places of treatment, monitoring, counselling and group work as well as traditional consultation.

Community care Most procedures, including continuous i.v. therapy, can now be performed in the patient's home. The author looked after a young person who, having been in prison, was frightened at the thought of being in hospital. Even though the patient lived in a very poor area, in a crowded home with young children, a high standard of nursing care was possible, including the successful care of a gangrenous ulcer. This patient very rarely went into hospital.

Outreach care is now a well-developed area of health and nursing delivery, particularly in relation to HIV and drug misuse, providing drop-in centres where counselling, medical cover, family planning and antenatal care with direct access to the hospital services are available.

HIV has an enormous social impact on both the individual and carers. In order to provide the best possible care, it is essential to have an integrated, multidisciplinary service that addresses social as well as clinical concerns, particularly in discharge planning and follow-up (Pratt 2003). Creating an environment which enables an effective but confidential service is difficult, especially as more agencies become involved in care. The best principle to adopt is a 'need to know' policy of information disclosure, involving the patient at every stage. This sometimes causes problems, as many professionals, quite wrongly, think they have a 'blanket' right to know a patient's details.

Manpower implications

The two main effects that HIV has had on health service manpower are:

- change and extension of roles
- increased workloads and accompanying costs.

Role change has been seen both in hospital and in the community. By the 1970s it was felt that infectious disease nursing as a 'specialty' was no longer needed and infectious diseases hospitals were increasingly used for other purposes. Now infectious disease facilities have once again become necessary. Special provision for people with HIV/AIDS has been built, requiring the supply and educational preparation of a large number of new staff. To date there has been no audit of how many nurses in the UK have been deployed in this field. However, each health authority publishes an annual report on activities and services under the 1987 AIDS (Control) Act.

Costs

Since 1995–96 and the first edition of this text, these implications have changed, particularly as individuals receive combination therapies (see p. 1186) from an earlier stage in their illness, with the result that many remain in better health for longer periods. This has a considerable impact on financial resources but has lessened the need for specialist inpatient facilities. Hospital admissions, mainly for the treatment of devastating opportunistic infections, increase costs considerably. Newer treatments, although expensive, are seen to be cost-effective as they delay the onset of the advanced stages of HIV disease (AIDS) for which care is very expensive (Adler 2003). More people are therefore able to stay well for longer although, despite some remarkable survival stories, the long-term influence of combination therapy (see p. 1186) on the infected population is unknown (Stine 2000). As highlighted in the Introduction, the move to establish combination therapy in poor and developing countries magnifies these challenges considerably (Lo & Bayer 2003, Mandela 2003, WHO 2003b)

Increased workloads

In the community, HIV has had the effect of creating new fields of work for health care practitioners. District nurses, whose main workload lies in caring for older people, now have younger people on their caseloads with a variety of clinical needs.

Increased input by social services is needed by most affected people, at one stage or another, as their situation changes. Typically the individual is young, independent and employed, perhaps living alone, paying a mortgage or rent, and may have no regular partner. As the disease progresses, these circumstances may change rapidly. In units where there is no resident social worker, the nurse may need to act as advisor and advocate in helping the patient to obtain benefits, housing, domestic assistance, meal supplements and other services. For these nurses, the key to success is to identify the appropriate services, without divulging the patient's personal details, and then, with the patient, to approach them for help. Without careful management, this extension of the nursing role can result in staff being 'spread too thinly'.

If one compares HIV therapy with another long-term disease and treatment, e.g. diabetes mellitus and insulin, where many individuals being treated from a young age may expect to live a fully functional life with normal longevity, the situation with HIV is still uncertain, especially as other factors, such as virus mutation with new disease patterns, manifest themselves (Shaw & Mahoney 2003). These patterns include drug resistance.

Statistics from the Health Protection Service show the cumulative total of cases reported for HIV and AIDS up to 2004. Although the greatest proportion of people affected has been homosexual men, the most rapid increase is among heterosexuals. In the UK, heterosexual transmission outstripped homosexual transmission in 2004.

STOP THINK **37.2** What are the current statistics on new AIDS cases?

Social implications

The social impact of HIV/AIDS is felt in two ways: on society as a whole, and on the individual as a social being. Here the wider societal implications are first considered.

Consider the following quotation (Connor & Kingman 1989):

> *At least one American senator was heard to say 'somewhere along the way we are going to have quarantine'.*

This typifies the way in which epidemics are often viewed by the makers of social policy. When the management of an epidemic is seen as being analogous to the management of acute illnesses in clinical practice (Barker & Rose 1998), the following equation is made:

The organism + the individual = the disease + the population = the epidemic.

In this view an intervention must be made to prevent the transformation of 'organism' into 'epidemic'. Theoretically, the options are:

- to kill the organism
- to make the organism inoperative
- to ameliorate the effects of the organism on the individual
- to separate the individual from the organism
- to separate the individual from the population
- to separate affected groups from the rest of the population.

Looking at disease in this way, the reader may see the role of antibiotics and disinfectants to kill the organism, immunisation to make the organism inoperative, symptom control to ameliorate the effects, infection control and health education to separate the individual from the organism, quarantine to separate the individual from the population and banishment/leper colonies to separate groups from the population.

It may be seen that HIV does not present many options. There is no antibiotic at present and no vaccine. As HIV takes a long time to manifest itself and has no very clear presenting features, quarantine and isolation of potential and actual 'victims' are difficult. At present, only the amelioration of the effects, health education and infection control, including, in this case, the use of condoms, are available in the 'battle' against this epidemic.

These options may seem as being very limited, and therein lies the key to public reaction to HIV and AIDS. In the eyes of society, those who have been appointed to protect the population from disease have not come up with a satisfactory solution for HIV/AIDS. This has led to a reaction of fear and a willingness to stigmatise and even scapegoat those with HIV.

Fear It is important for the nurse to appreciate the complex nature of fear. For example, the knowledge that one cannot 'catch' HIV by shaking hands may not be enough to dispel someone's fear of such contact, for along with the fear of actual physical contamination may be the fear of the very idea of the disease. HIV is particularly frightening because there are very few factors which separate an individual from the virus. This in itself may lead people to distinguish their own behaviour from that of individuals affected by HIV in the hope of confirming their own 'immunity', as in: 'I can't get HIV because I'm not homosexual'. At the same time, this implies that individuals with HIV/AIDS are themselves to blame and that if everyone in society conformed to certain patterns of behaviour then everything would be all right.

Stigmatisation Scapegoats are those chosen by society to take the blame for evil or misfortune. The selection of a scapegoat is either arbitrary or based in prejudice. This is clear in the case of HIV, which can infect anyone, particularly the sexually active. In the Western world, the virus happens to have affected large numbers of homosexual men first, followed by i.v. drug users. In other areas of the world, its epidemiology has followed other patterns. In any event, the appearance of the virus among one group or another has been a matter of historical accident only and has no inherent moral significance. Nonetheless, people with HIV have been stigmatised officially, e.g. by being refused insurance, employment or entry into certain countries, and unofficially, e.g. by physical and verbal abuse. Individuals affected often become isolated, and because they expect abuse they may start to avoid social interaction, thus compounding their isolation and stigmatisation.

Whether the person involved is a gay man, a drug user, a patient's mother or a child in the playground, fear and stigmatisation can have devastating consequences. A thoughtful nurse often makes all the difference.

Effects on the individual The psychological impact of HIV/AIDS is similar to that of other life-limiting illnesses. For a fuller discussion of the psychological implications of life-limiting illness and of palliative care the reader is referred to Chapter 33.

The sick role Individuals diagnosed as being ill are often implicitly or otherwise 'given permission' to behave in certain ways. Conditions which are seen as 'self-inflicted' tend to elicit less sympathy than others. The author has worked with a patient who, while receiving treatment for a malignant illness, became infected with HIV through a blood transfusion. The patient described to carers the shift in attitude which he then perceived. While the diagnosis was 'cancer', a great deal of sympathy was given. When the diagnosis became 'HIV', the sympathy was considerably less.

A patient who eventually becomes ill may think that they are to blame for not keeping fit enough and may feel guilty when forced to leave work or abandon former social roles. The difficulties are compounded when the person, e.g. a young drug user who prostitutes, has a disordered or chaotic lifestyle. Combined with all of their other problems, a positive HIV diagnosis can be devastating.

It is often difficult for the patient to inform relatives of their diagnosis, thus becoming cut off from a potential source of support and practical help. The nurse can often help the patient and the family to achieve a mutually acceptable resolution, but must bear in mind that whereas a family caring for someone with, say, cancer may get support and practical help from neighbours and others, HIV often sets the scene for isolation, guilt, prejudice and despair. This can happen in any terminal illness, but is often a particular problem in HIV.

Philosophical issues for nurses

The problems the patient experiences, as a stigmatised member of society, demand that nurses who seek to help are very clear about their own attitudes and professional philosophy. Central to any philosophy of nursing practice is the patient's right to 'quality health care in an atmosphere of human dignity without regard to age, ethnic or national origin, sex or sexual orientation, religion or presenting illness' (Pratt 2003). Coupled with this is the duty of nurses to look after all patients.

Models of care

The so-called 'medical model' on which much of nursing practice is based, tends not to provide a satisfactory approach to illnesses for which there is no cure. This model works best when the illness can be reduced to a few constituent parts, which can then be treated, eliminated or made ineffective. HIV and AIDS offer little scope for such an approach, although the search for a 'cure' continues. The reductionist medical model tends to be less effective with multifaceted problems, especially those such as AIDS which are heavily influenced by sociopolitical factors.

Western care systems are based on humanist and utilitarian philosophies whereby the individual is respected and recognised as being capable of independent moral judgement and action. While most people accept this sentiment, there is always difficulty in its application, as it tends to be put into practice only when the individual asserts their rights (Downie & Telfer 1980, Scott et al 2003). Those who have difficulty expressing their rights or who are considered as less worthy than others to do so are often treated as second-class citizens. Many people with HIV fall into these categories. Moreover, professionals and society at large may impose what may be called 'existential assumptions' upon a situation. One patient who is thought to be 'going somewhere' or to have 'been someone' may be considered to be more 'worthwhile' than another patient who is 'going nowhere'. So the death of a 'promising' young pianist, say, is considered sadder than the death of a young prostitute. This attitude pervades care delivery as some professionals prioritise their care using these value judgements as well as formal clinical signs (Bishop & Scudder 1990).

Western models of care tend to hold that one person's rights and liberties must not impinge upon another's and that one may not interfere with a person, even for their own good, unless they are violating the rights of other people (Scott et al 2003). In the case of people who are considered members of a 'minority', these principles often work against their right to high-quality care.

Another possible reaction is for the professional to look at a patient in difficulty and say, 'Who am I to interfere with this person's right to choose to live like this?' as if the young, homeless, ill, drug user has made the same kind of choices and been afforded the same opportunities as, for example, the student nurse. This attitude is seen in specific cases where patients are 'left alone', and in general where whole groups of people are either ignored or given the minimum of care. In a study of homeless men in hostels, Atkinson (2000) describes this minimum care.

Finally, Western care models are structured on materialistic rationalism whereby only what is 'rational' is accepted as being 'real'. The reader is invited to consider how limiting this view is as an approach to someone whose mind, body and spirit are in turmoil. By being too rational, the nurse may become cut off from the patient's real lived experience. The author undertook a study of cancer patients' experience of their 'journeys' through their treatment. A fascinating insight emerged, as often what the patient experienced and needed from the nurse was different from what the nurse thought. One patient expressed this …

> *The nurse was ever so good. She told me how the treatment would attack the cancer in great detail, but she didn't tell me whether I would wet myself on the way home.*
>
> *Atkinson et al (2002)*

TESTING AND SCREENING

AIDS/HIV testing involves analysis for HIV antibodies. Testing for the actual virus, i.e. testing for HIV core antigen, particles of the virus, is used for clinical prognosis and management, not generally for diagnostic purposes. Blood samples are used at present for all forms of testing, although urine and saliva tests are being developed, especially for use in screening.

Screening The term 'screening' is generally used, in the context of HIV, to refer to the process by which blood samples undergo laboratory analysis by enzyme-linked immunosorbent assay (ELISA). This procedure is carried out on several samples at once and is used to find out the prevalence of HIV antibodies in a batch of samples. The process may stop here, as in the case of anonymous prevalence surveys. The screening assay has a 'built-in' false-positive rate which ensures that there are no false-negative readings. The analysts know the percentage false-positive rate of the assay and so, when confronted with a batch of positive results, can make a mathematical adjustment to get an accurate picture of the prevalence of HIV in the group.

Individual testing While ELISA is an efficient method of mass screening, it is far from satisfactory for testing an individual, for whom a false-positive result would be devastating. Therefore in individual testing, the sample first undergoes ELISA, and then immunoblotting or the Western blotting method, accurate to within thousandths of 1%, to confirm the diagnosis. This method is more complex and is available only in sophisticated laboratories. In poorer countries, samples may undergo repeated ELISA procedures instead of Western blotting to achieve maximum accuracy in difficult circumstances.

Timing

Generally, HIV antibodies are produced between 3 weeks and 3 months after the individual becomes infected with HIV. The timing of a diagnostic test is important. Individuals who have a test which proves negative are often advised to come back for a repeat test. Because of this uncertainty and the personal impact of a positive result, HIV antibody testing should take place only with pre- and post-test counselling.

Forms of testing

There are various forms of HIV testing, some of which have become controversial. All types are defined here so that the reader can differentiate between them and enter into the continuing debate over their efficacy, need and ethics.

Named voluntary testing with pre- and post-test counselling This form occurs when an individual seeks a test following a specific high-risk activity or contact, or when the individual, for reasons of their own, wants to know their sero status. It is available at genitourinary clinics and HIV units, and from some GPs and other community practitioners. People found to be positive are, with their consent, referred to medical/nursing services. Professionals and others agree that this form is the most acceptable, both practically and ethically.

Named voluntary testing with minimal or no counselling Many people go for testing without being given the opportunity to discuss the implications of a positive or negative result. On being found positive, individuals may not be referred to health services. Others, on being found negative, think that they are 'safe' and need not worry or make behavioural changes. It may be seen, therefore, that this form of testing has drawbacks for the individual and is not advisable.

Conditional named 'voluntary' testing Increasingly, organisations, countries giving work permits, and insurance companies are asking applicants to have an HIV antibody test before gaining entry or obtaining services. The clinical value of these tests is doubtful as they are taken in isolation, often without counselling.

Patients on transplant and other medical waiting lists and those attending infertility clinics are often tested as a condition of entry onto waiting lists. This is done mainly in a hospital setting.

Also, an HIV antibody test is increasingly used as part of a battery of tests to determine a diagnosis, especially for ill patients admitted with unusual or vague symptoms or for patients who appear to be from 'high-risk' groups. Nurses must be particularly careful in these cases. It is their legal duty, as well as that of the doctor, to ensure that every patient gives their informed consent for the test. This may be difficult if the patient is very ill. However, this does not change the nurse's legal and professional accountability (Nursing and Midwifery Council 2003b).

Local anonymous HIV seroprevalence surveys These surveys are carried out by hospital departments who use part of blood samples, given for other purposes, to screen for HIV seroprevalence in a given locality or patient group. This is perfectly legal as long as the patients are informed that this procedure may be carried out. The sample has to be made anonymous and the result is not given to the patient.

Controversy has arisen surrounding this form of testing, particularly when the results are published in medical journals and the media. This is because relatively small numbers of patients are highlighted. For example, 1000 or so pregnant women may be screened, of whom 15 are shown to be HIV antibody-positive. Some publications may break this down even further and state that, of these 15, eight came from a particular place. This narrows down the numbers so much that many people are of the opinion that it compromises anonymity.

National Anonymous Survey of the Seroprevalence of HIV This is an ongoing survey directed by the Department of Health and organised by the Health Protection Agency. As in local surveys, surplus blood from patient samples is used. Again the patients do not have to give specific consent, but they must be informed that their blood may be used. This is done via a multilingual poster campaign and through the nursing and medical professions. The samples are made anonymous, but certain pieces of information, such as gender, age and geographical area, remain with the sample. The various governmental and professional organisations concerned, including nursing and midwifery, meet in a special forum to monitor and improve the project. The results are published nationally with a breakdown of regions and other groups.

Advantages and disadvantages of anonymous testing

Voluntary, informed testing with counselling allows the HIV seropositive individual to be referred to the appropriate services. Ethically and practically, this form is best for patient and professional carer alike. However, in the public perception, the risk of HIV appears to centre around minority groups. Most people do not feel they are at risk. Of those who do feel some risk, most do not think they need to be tested.

Anonymous testing is the compromise that has emerged to satisfy, on the one hand, the need of professionals to find out how many people are, or are likely to be, affected and, on the other, the personal and civil liberties of individuals. Some professionals argue that not enough political effort has been made to increase the uptake of voluntary named testing. As HIV care improves, it is becoming clearer that the earlier an individual knows the diagnosis and is referred to medical and nursing services, the better.

This presents one of the ethical dilemmas of anonymous testing. As the number of anonymous positive samples increases, it will become apparent that, for instance, X number of pregnant women and their babies are affected, but nothing can be done for them because they are unknown. Another objection made by some is that testing babies is an underhand way of testing mothers and that as the number of known but unnamed HIV-positive babies increases, the government will be forced to establish Draconian measures such as mandatory testing for all mothers. Many professionals would argue, however, that the more we know about national and local prevalence, the more we can target services.

In these matters, the rights of the individual must be balanced against the rights of the community. Nurses are bound to uphold the rights of the individual, but they also have a duty towards the community. These obligations are not mutually exclusive, but require that the issues are considered from every viewpoint. The professional bodies provide guidelines on many of the more contentious issues. It may be fair to say, however, that nurses should generally 'err' on the side of the individual patient, for the nurse is sometimes their only advocate (Nursing and Midwifery Council 2003b)

Targeted screening Until the National Survey, screening took place almost exclusively in specialist areas and among particular groups who were considered 'high risk'. Although the information gleaned from this work was useful, it was incomplete, yielding little knowledge about the population at large. Moreover, HIV would always seem to affect mainly homosexuals or drug users if most of the samples continued to be taken from those groups.

'Opt out' testing In some areas of the UK, this has been introduced as part of antenatal screening and sexually transmitted infection screening. The client has to say they do not wish the test, otherwise it will be carried out.

Counselling

While a comprehensive guide to counselling cannot be presented here, the following offers a few basic principles:

- Counselling is a helpful tool, among other tools, which may be used to assist the patient. It is not an end in itself. One person with AIDS half-jokingly remarked: 'Nurses are so keen to counsel me, it seems they forget I have practical needs. Sometimes I feel I'm being counselled to death!'.
- Counselling is not advice-giving. Patients often ask: 'What would you do, nurse?', but the nurse must seriously consider the relevance of their reply. Advice of the 'If I were you …' type is rarely appropriate.
- Counselling is not about getting the patient to do the 'right' thing; for example, a young, pregnant, HIV-seropositive woman cannot be 'counselled' to have, or not to have, an abortion.
- Counselling is about helping someone come to their own decisions.
- Counselling is an exploration made by two people of issues and problems. The counsellor is an equal partner whose personal opinion is very often not relevant, although it may come up in the course of the conversation.
- It is difficult to counsel and do something else. On many occasions nurses gain the patient's confidence in the process of delivering clinical and personal services. This is a good entry into the counselling relationship, as is the provision of accurate information. To achieve the equality necessary, it is advisable to be in a neutral place on an eye-to-eye level. This is difficult if the patient is lying down with few clothes on with the nurse standing over them!
- Good counselling does not have to take a long time. Some practitioners think counselling is 'rather fancy' and too time-consuming for the busy clinical situation. This is not the case. Effective counselling can be

achieved in half an hour or less, especially if the counsellor gives the individual their undivided attention.
- Know your limitations. During a session it may become apparent to the counsellor that they are getting into areas where one or both parties feel they cannot cope or are out of their depth. There is no shame in this. Seek appropriate help. No one is supposed to have all the answers.

Pre- and post-test counselling

Nurses are often asked to give pre- and post-test counselling. It is essential that the nurse is proficient in attempting this. Courses are now available in many authorities. Counselling in other clinical areas, especially oncology, genetics and palliative care, can provide very good experience. The counsellor must have sound clinical knowledge, as unusual questions which are worrying the patient will often be encountered.

Pre-test counselling will involve the following:

- Establishing why the individual wants to be tested. Many people come armed with misconceptions. Clinical factors must also be established. A patient of the author's came seeking the test and a termination of pregnancy. She thought her partner was HIV-positive and that her baby would die of AIDS. When she was investigated it was found that she was, in fact, not pregnant. Her partner's HIV status was not known, but because she had been worrying, she had imagined the very worst.
- Exploring the 'pros and cons', for that individual, of having the test. Is it appropriate? Should they wait for 3–6 months? Have they been at risk?
- Considering the implications of a positive result. Most people come for a negative result, in order to be reassured.

Most dedicated test centres offer a next day, and some a same day, result service. Ideally the same counsellor should give the person the result, but in the hospital setting the result is often given by the doctor.

If the result is negative, it is important that the individual knows how to avoid risk in the future and whether it is advisable to come back for a repeat test in, for example, 6 months' and 1 year's time. If the result is positive, the counsellor may want to be accompanied by a colleague who can be on hand to assist. There is no good way of divulging such devastating news. Experts in the field often say that every time they have to do so, it is different and that it does not get easier.

STOP THINK **37.3** When helping a person in distress with a condition such as HIV, black-and-white answers seldom fit. Here are some true situations. How can you help?

Remember: What you think is 'right' may not help you or the patient.

(a) A patient is found to be HIV-positive. He understands the 'duty' he has to tell his partner but does not know how to do it and 'cannot go through with it'. How do you help him?
(b) A patient who is demonstrating signs of serious illness has been advised to have the HIV test. She does not want to and asks you as the nurse to help her. What do you do?
(c) A colleague of yours receives a needlestick injury from a suspected drug user. There is pressure to test the drug user to see if he has HIV. What is your view of the matter?
(d) A patient with HIV tells you that he is scared of becoming ill and wants to die now. Is he depressed? Is there any hope? How do you cope when you can't say 'It'll be all right'?
(e) A patient tells you of a 'high-risk' activity he has engaged in. You want to help him. How do you reassure him without lying? On the other hand, how do you tell him the truth without panicking him or making him behave rashly?

In all of these situations, where do your 'loyalties' lie? To whom are you accountable or responsible — the patient, the public, the government, yourself, your profession?

HEALTH EDUCATION AND PROMOTION IN HIV

Caplan's (1961) classic model describes health education and promotion as having three parts:

- *primary* — preventing occurrence of the disease; providing education, raising awareness, giving information
- *secondary* — detecting disease early; screening, performing individual testing
- *tertiary* — preventing deterioration of individuals affected, giving support.

These general aims must be responsive to the physical, mental, emotional, spiritual and societal needs of the individual (Catalan 1999, Ewles & Simnett 2003).

Health promotion in HIV/AIDS entails more than raising general public awareness through mass media campaigns. It can also involve such activities as providing assertiveness training for individuals affected and helping them to learn self-care and nurturing skills. HIV awareness also has implications for the workplace, raising concerns about working practice and hiring policies. Legal and ethical issues must also be grappled with by nurses working with people who are involved in illicit drug use and prostitution and who consequently face particular difficulties.

To become equipped to operate on so many levels, the reader is urged to read not only 'mainstream' publications on health promotion, such as Ewles and Simnett (2003), but also books which demonstrate particular perspectives. Stine (2000) presents not only the clinical reality but also provides extracts from the media about experience, politics and ethical dilemmas. These may help the reader to take a more analytical view of large-scale media campaigns.

Elements of health promotion

Targeting the 'audience'

The way in which HIV educators convey their message sometimes seems to contradict the message itself. For example, the maxim that 'there are no high-risk groups, only high-risk activities' is generally 'targeted' at drug users, prostitutes and gay men, which may amount to ideological double talk.

The labelling of whole groups as being 'at risk' is not precise. A gay man, for example, is not at risk if he refrains from unprotected sexual intercourse. An i.v. drug user who does not share injecting equipment is also not at risk from HIV, although impure street drugs are themselves a risk. These individuals are not at risk merely because they can be labelled 'gay' or 'drug user'; rather, people are at risk if they undertake a high-risk activity.

Advertisers and health educators, however, record that certain groups have certain behaviour patterns in common. It makes sense, therefore, to target these groups with certain services and messages, always remembering that general patterns will not fully reflect the complexity of individuals.

Initiatives vary and take on cultural differences around the world, from the 'light touch' of fun days and health awareness messages on beer mats, to in-depth and detailed information provided for particular groups of individuals displaying high-risk behaviour, e.g. pregnant women who use illicit drugs intravenously. It should be remembered that individuals move through different groups. A good example in this context is the young, adult holidaymaker whose behaviour, during most of the year, would not be considered at risk but who may be considered high risk when on holiday. Several initiatives around the world address this issue.

The right medium and the right message

Leaflets are frequently used in various kinds of information campaigns because they are very simple to distribute. Most people in the UK can read, and by means of leaflets, information can be placed unequivocally in the hands of the target audience. Unfortunately, research over the years has shown that people tend not to read unsolicited leaflets. While they can be an excellent written adjunct to a spoken session, leaflets are of limited use 'cold'.

The first public message from the UK government came in the form of an open letter from the Chief Medical Officer at the Department of Health, warning of the risks of HIV. This message was published in all the national newspapers. Following this, there was a leaflet drop to every household in the UK and a poster and television campaign. The commercials and posters carried the slogan 'Don't die of ignorance' but did not go into clinical detail. They were designed to raise awareness. The National AIDS Helpline was set up where people could, and still can, phone free to speak to a trained telephone counsellor.

Although the early health promotion approaches did prompt some reduction in high-risk behaviour, research subsequently showed that general messages warning of danger and giving non-specific information were of limited efficacy. Over the years, mass media messages have therefore become much more specific, aiming at particular individuals and behaviour groups.

Although HIV education through the mass media has some degree of effectiveness, this kind of communication, no matter how expert, always has a high degree of 'wastage'. Even the most successful television advertising campaigns can only expect to 'reach', i.e. to elicit sales from, 2% of the adult population. However, as long as this form of health promotion is successful in influencing the behaviour of some people for their own benefit and that of the larger community, mass media information campaigns must continue to constitute a vital part of the battle against HIV.

STOP THINK **37.4** Some people feel that health promotion needs to change radically as its HIV-related messages, such as those about 'safer sex', are not getting through to those at risk. What is your evaluation of current HIV-related health messages?

The nurse's role

Given the limitations of mass communications in influencing behaviour, nurses must take every opportunity to make general messages relevant to the patients in their care. Nurses have always been involved in assisting patients to understand their treatment, and in answering their questions in terms that can be understood. In doing so, they require sound clinical knowledge together with an understanding of the patient's needs, lifestyle and expectations, as obtained from the nursing assessment.

One of the nurse's greatest advantages as a health educator lies in the opportunities to be with the patient for long periods of time in a position of trust. Many other health care professionals see the patient only during short visits and often have to work harder to establish a rapport (Bishop & Scudder 1990). Nevertheless, the nurse may still experience difficulty in discussing sexual matters and sexuality with patients. Public campaigns are restricted by legislation and 'public taste', and it may be left to the nurse to provide more explicit information. Personal value judgements, embarrassment and questions of status may present obstacles. Answering questions on, for example, oral sex from a person of a different sexual persuasion to oneself may be difficult. Speaking to an underage person who is sexually active may be embarrassing and raise ethical questions. Many practitioners become expert at putting up verbal and non-verbal barriers so that such discussions are avoided.

Despite this potential for awkwardness or discomfort, it is clear, given the devastating effects of HIV, how important it is for nurses to fulfil their obligations as health educators. It is strongly suggested that the reader find an expert practitioner who can act as a role model and mentor. Attending an education course may also help. It is not suggested the nurse must necessarily change their opinion about certain issues or that they must agree with what each patient has to say. However, caring must be unconditional, answering to the patient's needs regardless of the nurse's personal values.

A mentor can also help the less experienced practitioner to deal with difficult, sometimes ethical, issues. Patients sometimes give the nurse information about past actions which places the nurse in a difficult position. In such cases, nurses at all levels should seek advice, whilst ensuring that patient confidentiality is maintained. Under the Nursing and Midwifery Council guidelines (2004), the nurse is judged both on confidentiality and on the accounts given of personal actions in a difficult situation. To give an example, the author once looked after an HIV antibody-positive 15-year-old individual who was having penetrative sex with an underage female partner who lived with her parents. The situation was discussed and acted upon, keeping the confidentiality of all parties. The 15-year-old was assisted to approach the partner and her parents accompanied by nursing staff. Although, in this case, the medical consultant had the power to make an approach without consent, sensitive work with the patient made this unnecessary and a good working relationship was maintained.

Nurses, particularly those working as health advisors within sexual health services, have an extremely important role in HIV. Partner notification work, for example, requires a sensitive and expert approach.

Health educators are sometimes faced with the dilemma that encouraging safe practice and encouraging someone to break the law seem to amount to the same thing. For example, nurses are now involved in giving drug users clean needles and syringes. This practice has government and professional support. Is it correct, however, for the nurse to tell the patient how to inject safely or to use one form of drug instead of another? (see Ch. 36). In the face of a bleak prognosis, the practitioner may see no option but to fall back on the pragmatic principle of 'harm reduction' rather than to insist upon an ideal. In such a situation the nurse should seek guidance and support from management (Crouch 2003, Johnson 2003, Donovan 2004).

Group work Nurses are increasingly becoming involved in working with groups, particularly in the community. These may be self-help groups or people attending a clinic for a particular service. Whether the nurse personally sets up the group, or 'piggy-backs' a service onto an existing group, the results can be significant. By speaking to a small number, answering questions members of the group want to ask and offering individuals the opportunity to speak in private afterwards, the nurse can make health education messages personally relevant.

For further information on the formal and informal intricacies of setting up groups, agendas and action plans, see Ewles & Simnett (2003).

CLINICAL MANIFESTATIONS AND MANAGEMENT OF HIV/AIDS

People with HIV disease rarely get all of the diseases associated with AIDS (see Box 37.1), and often those that do occur manifest one at a time. The precise course of the illness is virtually impossible to predict. A number of patients of the author seemed so close to death in late 1987 that it seemed cruel to persist with medication; however, between 2000 and 2004, the author has seen or heard news of some of them, although others have died.

The treatment of AIDS is a rapidly developing field. This section will therefore present a matrix of available approaches that can be used by the nurse as a conceptual and practical framework as the medical and nursing management of HIV/AIDS advances.

Approaches to nursing care

Pratt (2003) provides detailed strategies and philosophies for ward and service management. The author has used a process based on Roy's adaptation model (Andrews & Roy 1997) which takes into account the following aspects of the patient's illness experience:

- physiological adaptation — clinical signs, disease process
- self-concept adaptation — anxiety, aggression, grief, social belonging
- role function adaptation, e.g. as a parent, a partner, a worker — sense of failure, sense of conflict
- interdependency adaptation — loneliness, rejection, social interaction.

These four 'adaptive modes' are placed in the context of three 'stimuli':

- focal, e.g. the surrounding facilities, services available; other people
- contextual, e.g. space available, distance to toilet, room temperature
- residual, e.g. personal beliefs, prejudices, personal qualities.

The nurse applying this model, having identified a clinical problem, e.g. the patient's sudden inability to walk, will consider not only the medication and treatment but also the patient's ability to function and adapt. This is then put alongside the practicalities of the stimuli. Are the facilities at home suitable? How far is it to the toilet? Can the patient cope with a commode in the front room? Will they let their partner look after them?

Roy's model is also useful as it helps the nurse consider all the adaptations needed to make an individual service effective. Does the present service or nursing procedure need to change? Does the environment suit the patient? Does the patient need to modify their lifestyle? How can the nurse foster the necessary changes? The adaptation model encourages a flexible approach by nurse and patient in both hospital and community care settings.

People with HIV may present with seemingly minor problems which cannot always be diagnosed or predicted. For example, an individual may suffer weight loss, difficulty in swallowing, anorexia, night sweats, lethargy, mouth ulcers, diarrhoea and/or constipation. In addition to this, they may become depressed and desperate, as such conditions, even if not in themselves life threatening, can be very distressing. A patient of the author's had, over 2 years, contracted two serious bouts of PCP. He had borne these very well. However, he became severely depressed some time later when he was back at work. Having contracted oral thrush, he could not swallow properly and was losing weight. This made him feel powerless and he said it was worse than the 'serious' illnesses. Such examples serve to remind the practitioner that the seriousness of a condition cannot be judged strictly by clinical criteria. Moreover, by taking notice of even the smallest signs and taking action, nurses can help many patients remain alive. Many HIV-related conditions, if diagnosed early, respond well to treatment.

Infection control

For general principles of infection control, the reader is referred to Chapter 16. The essence of infection control with HIV is to use standard infection control precautions (SICPs) to protect the patient who will be at increased risk of health care associated infection (HAI) (Wilson 2001). Care should be taken with all body fluids, and gloves and aprons should be used for intimate procedures. Because of the damaged immune system, the patient may be more at risk from the nurse than the other way round.

For further information on HIV-related infection control, see Chapter 14 in Pratt (2003).

In the home, basic hygiene is to be encouraged and clothes and bedding should be washed in a washing machine. Disposal of medical waste should be carried out in accordance with local nursing policies and procedures. Needles and syringes found in the street are the responsibility of the Environmental Health Department, although health care professionals finding them have a duty to minimise the risk of injury to themselves and others where possible.

CONDITIONS, TREATMENTS AND SPECIFIC NURSING INTERVENTIONS

What follows is a description of the main presenting infections, conditions and treatments associated with HIV and AIDS (see Box 37.1).

For further information, the following are recommended: Pratt (2003) for discussion of nursing strategy; Stine (2000) and Shaw & Mahoney (2003) for an American perspective. Shaw and Mahoney also have a very helpful presentation by answering stated questions, e.g. 'What do you do ...', as well as sections on other infections and complementary therapies.

At present there is no vaccine against AIDS. Research is advancing and expectations of a vaccine to provide immunity against HIV are still cited by various establishments as being from 5 to 10 years away. Although there are various treatments which ameliorate the effects of viruses, there has never been anything in the nature of a broad-spectrum antibiotic which actually kills viruses. Antiviral agents which suppress HIV will be discussed later.

Possibilities for fighting and killing the virus are therefore limited. The best success has been in the area of symptomatic control, i.e. stopping or slowing the associated diseases and conditions which can kill the patient. The other main aim of care is to improve the patient's quality of life. There is thus a similarity between AIDS nursing and oncology and palliative care.

At the beginning of the epidemic, the life expectancy of someone diagnosed as having AIDS ranged from a few weeks to 2 years. Patients receiving care, particularly those in affluent countries, can now live for 10 years or more. As described earlier, when comparing HIV disease with other life-threatening conditions such as cancer or diabetes mellitus, which similarly depend on symptomatic control but for which there is a much longer life expectancy, it becomes apparent that the care of HIV-related illness continues to be in a developing stage.

The general progress of HIV-related illness is represented in Figure 37.2 (p. 1174).

Phases of HIV and AIDS

Phase A: acute seroconversion illness

In most individuals this illness is not recognised. It may be seen 2–6 weeks after exposure to HIV. Not everyone infected with HIV gets this flu- or glandular fever-like condition. It may be associated with joint pain and other non-specific signs. A skin rash is sometimes seen, as are swollen lymph glands; these usually reduce after some time. At this stage the body will be producing HIV antibodies (seroconversion). A few individuals may also show early signs of HIV affecting the central nervous system, particularly the layers of the brain, e.g. encephalopathy, meningitis (see Ch. 9).

Treatment of seroconversion illness is symptomatic and does not usually take place in hospital. For the alert doctor and nurse, the illness may be a useful diagnostic warning, rather as the presence of a thirst and boils suggests diabetes. However, the signs are very similar to those of many minor infections.

Phase B: antibody-positive phase

B-1: asymptomatic HIV infection As HIV has only been recognised for approximately 25 years, one can only state that the period between infection and the onset of clinical signs may be anything from a few weeks to 20+ years. From this fact it may be seen that procedures such as contact tracing are not as simple or effective as in other sexually transmitted disease, as the asymptomatic period commonly covers much of an individual's sexually active life.

B-2: persistent generalised lymphadenopathy (PGL) or lymphadenopathy syndrome (LAS) This condition is sometimes the one which alerts medical services to investigate for HIV. The individual presents with swollen glands of more than 1 cm which persist for longer than 12 weeks. Although the individual may have swollen inguinal glands, they must also have other affected glands. Other reasons for swollen glands must be discounted before a diagnosis is given. As this is often the 'introductory' stage of HIV illness, monitoring of helper T cells and suppressor T cells (via the $CD4^+$ T-cell procedure; see Appendix 1) and other investigations may begin. It is at this stage that the individual may be tested for HIV for the first time.

Phase C

This phase refers to a period in an individual's illness career where they may contract a variety of well-known conditions, but not major, life-threatening, opportunistic infections or cancers. Common bacterial, viral and fungal infections frequently occur and are often marked by their persistence and virulence. Oral and genital herpes or athlete's foot are good examples. In a normally healthy person, these conditions would resolve within a few days. In phase C, the duration of the infection is lengthened and the whole foot, for instance, may become affected. Other conditions such as oral hairy leukoplakia are sometimes seen.

Loss of weight may be seen at this stage. This may be due to a specific mechanical problem, such as mouth ulcers, or from persistent low-grade attacks from infections. At this stage a significant drop may be seen in the helper T cells. In day-to-day practice, nurses should bear in mind that young, healthy people should overcome common infections quickly without them becoming widespread. Any persistent condition, e.g. coughing, loss of weight, should be noted. While thrush (*Candida albicans*) is common in the vagina, it is very uncommon in the mouth of a young healthy person. Such an occurrence should immediately alert the practitioner to the fact that the individual may have an underlying condition such as HIV.

The nurse working with diagnosed patients should also be aware that, since the positive diagnosis, the individual will have been dreading the onset of illness. When weight loss, mouth ulcers or fungal infections occur, the patient may become acutely anxious, considering themselves to be in imminent danger of pain or death. Other professionals, such as clinical psychologists, can assist the patient during these periods. Involvement of the patient in all stages of decision making and treatment right from the start will assist them to take control of their condition and reduce any feeling of helplessness.

Box 37.4 summarises treatments and medications used in various conditions associated with Phase C.

Phase D: AIDS — constitutional disease, opportunistic infections, secondary cancers

Constitutional disease: HIV wasting syndrome The diagnosis of AIDS depends on an individual being diagnosed as HIV antibody-positive, plus being diagnosed as having one of the life-threatening opportunistic infections or secondary cancers associated with HIV. However, a third criterion has come more to the fore, namely the constitutional or systemic condition known as HIV wasting syndrome. This has arisen from the experience in Africa, where AIDS is called 'slim disease'. In the West, it is also increasingly recognised that some individuals become extremely ill, losing excessive amounts of weight, more than 10% body mass, and suffering from morbid weakness and loss of function with or without having the 'label' of one of the listed conditions. In the USA, 19% of adults with AIDS are diagnosed as having HIV wasting syndrome (Kirton 2003).

The causes of HIV wasting syndrome may be mechanical or systemic. As mentioned before, people lose weight if there are factors such as mouth ulcers and sickness which deter them from eating. Malabsorption may also be seen and may be due to the presence of a lesion such as Kaposi's sarcoma in the gut or to a more generalised dysfunction. In all these cases the patient is starved of nutrients.

Wasting may also occur as a result of metabolic changes. As in cancerous conditions, the body may go from its normal balance of catabolism and anabolism into a catabolic crisis in which body mass is 'burnt up' at an increased and dangerous rate, often causing irreparable damage. These patients may recover some weight but they often do not recover muscle mass (Stine 2000, Shaw & Mahoney 2003).

Supervised nutritional rehabilitation is therefore necessary. This may include nutritional supplements and more invasive therapy such as continuous or intermittent parenteral feeding. However, it is as well to remember that the nurse can play a life-saving role in the attention given to the ordinary nutritional service to the patient.

Box 37.4

Key nursing care issues

Diarrhoea
Immediate monitoring of hydration and nutrition should start with the help of a dietitian.

Weight loss
Measurements of muscle and fat loss should be included in the care programme. Eating patterns should be discussed along with ways of increasing intake, e.g. taking frequent, smaller meals and perhaps supplementary feeds such as Ensure.

Fluid and electrolyte replacement is essential. Codeine phosphate, loperamide hydrochloride and diphenoxylate hydrochloride may be useful, but it is emphasised that medication should always be given in combination with dietary monitoring and therapy (see Chs 20 and 21).

Herpes simplex
Aciclovir is used. Prophylactic doses may also be given.

Herpes zoster
Mouth and lip care are important to prevent cracking and secondary infection. Soothing lotions and loose clothing may be appropriate for attacks of shingles. Sleep, fluid intake and diet should be monitored.

Seborrhoeic dermatitis/skin care
Salicylic acid and tar-based lotions are used. Low-dose steroids and steroid/antibiotic/antifungal combinations, e.g. clobetasone butyrate (Trimovate) are sometimes used for short periods. Responding to the individual patient's discomfort is important. Giving attention to small details in order to alleviate the irritation of skin conditions is one of the most appreciated nursing services (see Ch. 12).

Tinea pedis
Miconazole and clotrimazole creams are used topically. Systemic griseofulvin is used if the infection is persistent. Keeping the feet dry and comfortable can be helped by such measures as drying with a cool hair dryer and leaving the end of the bed covers loose.

Oral candidiasis
Nystatin antifungal topical drops may be used. However, oral thrush is often persistent in HIV illness, in which case systemic fluconazole is used (see Ch. 15). Mouth care is vital, as is a high fluid intake. Some patients find mouth rinsing with benzydamide hydrochloride, which has anaesthetic properties, helpful. Others rinse with fizzy water or diet cola to relieve discomfort, a valued practice that is not yet supported by research evidence.

Oral hairy leukoplakia
Aciclovir is used. Mouth care is again essential.

Ongoing support
Nurse-led clinics are now an important source of support, particularly around the time of starting highly active antiretroviral therapy (HAART).

Based on data from Pratt (2003) and Shaw & Mahoney (2003).

Opportunistic infections: protozoal Some of the protozoal infections which may occur in AIDS are as follows.

Pneumocystis carinii pneumonia (PCP; pneumocystosis) Approximately 60% of individuals contract PCP as the first AIDS-related infection. Because the vast majority of people diagnosed as having AIDS have been unaware of their HIV status, many people who have contracted PCP for the first time present not to specialist units but to Emergency Departments, GPs' offices and other non-specialist areas.

Although PCP is the most common cause of death in AIDS, the organism responsible, *Pneumocystis carinii* (now also known as *Pneumocystis jiroveci*), can be found, quite normally, in most human beings. However, in health, the immune system keeps the population of the organism at an acceptable level. When the immune system is compromised, the level rises and causes severe, life-threatening pneumonia. The individual usually presents with a 2–5 week history of increasing shortness of breath, weakness and dry cough; cyanosis is often seen (Stine 2000, Adler 2001, Pratt 2003).

A variety of drugs is used in the treatment of PCP: co-trimoxazole for mild to moderate episodes and pentamidine isetionate for moderate to severe episodes. Aerosolised pentamidine may be used as a treatment and as a prophylactic measure.

Cryptosporidiosis This condition has some notoriety because of the sometimes devastating diarrhoea it causes and because high levels of the organism in the general water supply are often reported in the news. It is caused by a protozoan which is normally present in small quantities in the water supply. In immunocompromised patients, it rises to high levels in the gastrointestinal tract and causes diarrhoea. The loss of fluid can be as much as 10–20 L/day, although less virulent attacks are also seen.

Cryptosporidiosis is generally seen only in patients who are already very ill and have suffered other infections. It is very difficult to manage this condition at home, as i.v. fluid replacement and constant bowel movements will need attention. For the patient, this condition may mean an extremely poor state of health and hospitalisation. In its worst form, it is an extremely distressing condition for both the patient and carers. There is no specific curative therapy for this infection. Highly active antiretroviral therapy (HAART; see p. 1186) is associated with clinical improvement. Treatment with antidiarrhoeals, oral or i.v. rehydration and nutritional support will be required.

Toxoplasmosis The causative protozoan is sometimes associated with cats and raw meat, although it does not generally manifest itself as a disease in healthy people. Its most common manifestation is cerebral toxoplasmosis. The organism causes space-occupying lesions in the brain. These create cerebral oedema and raised intracranial pressure. The patient suffers the usual signs of these conditions: paralysis and unconsciousness (see Ch. 9). Toxoplasmosis is often fatal and treatment must be prolonged as relapses are almost inevitable. The main medication is co-trimoxazole, or dapsone with pyrimethamine. In the most serious cases, constant nursing attention is needed as the patient's condition may deteriorate rapidly (Stine 2000, Adler 2001, Pratt 2003).

Opportunistic infections: viral The most common of these are described below.

Herpes simplex virus This condition has been mentioned in association with early phases, where it occurs in its less virulent forms. Serious and life-threatening forms, e.g. encephalitis, are sometimes seen, affecting the central nervous system (Pratt 2003). Aciclovir is used in treatment.

Cytomegalovirus (CMV) This virus is encountered in general practice and in midwifery, where it is known to cause spontaneous abortion. In HIV-related illness it is most commonly seen causing CMV retinitis. Small 'cotton buds' are seen on the retina on examination. The patient may then rapidly become blind, a deterioration which can occur in the space of a few days. Treatment with ganciclovir, foscarnet sodium or cidofovir i.v. is given. These may be given in the hospital setting, but increasingly are given at home. Improvement is seen with treatment but relapse occurs in almost all cases.

CMV retinitis can have a devastating affect on both the patient's morale and state of mind. Two of the author's patients decided to stop all treatment once they became blind, whereupon other illness and death followed quite quickly. This demonstrated to the author the vital importance of the patient's will to live when combating HIV-related illness.

Progressive multifocal leucoencephalopathy (PML) This unusual disease is caused by JC virus, a type of papovavirus, and results in demyelination. Conditions most likely to be seen are blindness, hemiparesis, ataxia and aphasia (Adler 2001). Antiretroviral therapy with zidovudine-containing regimens may provide dramatic improvement in this late-stage, crippling condition (Pratt 2003).

Opportunistic infections: bacterial The following bacterial infections may be seen in people with AIDS (see also Ch. 16).

Mycobacterium tuberculosis (TB) Tuberculosis is now increasingly seen in patients with HIV and is often associated with poor social conditions and increasingly in vulnerable groups such as asylum seekers. Prisons around the world have seen an increase in TB prevalence, particularly where there is a high prevalence of HIV. Prisoners with HIV are affected, as are other vulnerable inmates. Treatment is with rifampicin, isoniazid, ethambutol and pyrazinamide for a 2-month induction phase and with rifampicin and isoniazid for a 4-month continuation phase. TB in the general population, when treated, is not generally life threatening. Patients with HIV who are infected with TB, however, are often made even weaker by the condition (United Nations 2004).

Salmonellosis As with other compromised and vulnerable individuals, this infection, generally associated with food poisoning, poses a particular danger to people with HIV. Scrupulous care should be taken in food preparation and delivery. Patients should avoid undercooking foods such as eggs and poultry. Hand hygiene is also important (see Ch. 16). Treatment is with chloramphenicol, ampicillin or amoxicillin.

Mycobacterium avium complex (MAC) People in advanced stages of HIV illness are sometimes found to have atypical mycobacteria in their lungs. MAC has become less common since the widespread use of combination antiretroviral therapy (HAART).

Opportunistic infections: fungal

Candidiasis is sometimes seen in virulent manifestations in people with advanced HIV illness. Infection may extend from the mouth to the alimentary tract. Vaginal candidiasis may be particularly persistent and distressing. Nystatin vaginal pessaries and other conventional treatments are used.

Cryptococcus is a systemic fungal condition. Treatment is with amphotericin and fluconazole. Two others are *histoplasmosis*, which affects the lungs, liver and gastrointestinal tract, and *coccidioidomycosis*, which affects any organ, including the brain (Pratt 2003).

Infestation Strictly speaking, infestation is not associated with HIV. However, it should be pointed out that if a patient with HIV happens to become infested with lice or scabies, particularly the variety known as Norwegian scabies, the infection may be particularly virulent, with several thousand times as many mites on the skin as in a patient who is not immunocompromised. Norwegian scabies occasionally strikes hospitals and institutions.

Secondary cancers The immune system has the function, not only of fighting infection, but also of fighting and inhibiting malignant cells. The following two forms of cancer are associated with HIV and an AIDS diagnosis.

Kaposi's sarcoma (KS) This purplish skin cancer was previously seen only in older men of certain races, e.g. Jewish men. With the advent of AIDS in the Western world, it was one of the first manifestations of the condition. As with the opportunistic infections, it is not seen in all patients. As a skin condition it is very disfiguring, particularly when on the face. If it remains in small patches, treatment is often confined to cosmetic camouflage. However, it sometimes forms constricting bands on the skin, e.g. around the ankle. Internally, it may also lead to gastrointestinal obstruction and it is sometimes found in the lungs and other internal organs. Patients with visceral or advanced KS are treated with radiotherapy or systemic chemotherapy. With widespread adoption of safer sex practices and the introduction of HAART, the incidence of KS has declined dramatically (Adler 2001).

Non-Hodgkin's lymphomas (B-cell lymphomas, undifferentiated lymphomas) These cancers are seen in much higher numbers among people with AIDS than in the general population. They are found in the central nervous system, the bone marrow and the gastrointestinal tract. They are often rapidly fatal and treatment is often not successful. Various chemotherapies may be used (see Ch. 31).

Neurological disease; HIV encephalopathy HIV neurological disease is not an opportunistic infection. It is the human immunodeficiency virus directly affecting the central nervous system, including the covering of the brain. It may manifest early on as peripheral neuropathy, in its many forms, and later progress to affect the individual's personality and lucidity. Eventually the person may suffer dementia. One of the problems in diagnosing this condition is that changes in computed tomograms (CT scans) do not necessarily accompany changes in behaviour; it is possible for a patient with a normal CT to experience dementia.

Acute viral encephalitis can occur in late symptomatic HIV disease caused by reactivation of latent cytomegalovirus (CMV) or herpes simplex virus (HSV) infection.

Nursing care of the various conditions associated with neurological disease and encephalopathy is often challenging in terms of both short- and long-term care. Remissions can occur but there can be periods of despair for the individual. One of the author's patients, who refused to be cared for in hospital, having spent long periods in prison and being afraid of institutions, was cared for at home. He began to suffer from forgetfulness, personality changes and eventually showed signs of dementia. This was distressing for him, as he often had insight into his condition; in these lucid periods he would sometimes say he wanted to end his life.

On a more optimistic note, however, HIV neurological disease does appear to respond well to antiviral therapy. Many patients show a marked improvement as well as a slowing down of the advancement of the disease.

Antiretroviral therapy

Since the mid-1990s, antiretroviral treatment has developed significantly and made a considerable impact in reducing HIV-related morbidity and mortality. Treatment aims to reduce the plasma HIV RNA level — the viral load; Table 37.1 shows medication currently available in the UK. These medications target two specific viral enzymes necessary for HIV replication: reverse transcriptase and protease. Fusion inhibitors prevent HIV attaching to receptor sites on the surface of host cells that HIV targets for infection, and entering the cells.

Highly active antiretroviral therapy (HAART)

The normal treatment pattern is with a combination of three, four or five medications, occasionally six in 'salvage' therapy. HAART is started in all symptomatic patients, in those who have a high rate of viral replication and before irreversible damage to the immune system occurs. A range of serious side-effects is associated with these medications and adherence to HAART is a major issue. Adverse effects include kidney and liver toxicity, hyperglycaemia, raised plasma levels of triglycerides and cholesterol, lipodystrophy, hypersensitivity reactions and peripheral neuropathy. The

Table 37.1 Antiretroviral medication used in the UK, 2004

Generic name	Proprietary name
Nucleoside reverse transcriptase inhibitors	
Emtricitabine	Emtriva
Didanosine	Videx
Lamivudine/zidovudine	Combivir
Lamivudine	Epivir
AZT	Retrovir
Lamivudine/zidovudine/abacavir	Trizivir
Stavudine	Zerit
Abacavir	Ziagen
Zalcitabine	Hivid
Nucleotide reverse transcriptase inhibitors	
Tenofovir	Viread
Non-nucleoside reverse transcriptase inhibitors	
Efavirenz	Sustiva
Nevirapine	Viramune
Protease inhibitors	
Amprenavir	Agenerase
Nelfinavir	Viracept
Lopinavir/ritonavir	Kaletra
Ritonavir	Norvir
Indinavir	Crixivan
Saquinavir soft gel caps	Fortovase
Saquinavir hard gel caps	Invirase
Fusion inhibitors	
Enfuvirtide	Fuzeon

commitment to HAART is for life and GPs and practice nurses particularly have an important role in supporting patients in adhering to these challenging medication regimens. There have been advances to improve pill burden and once-daily regimens are now popular. Antiretroviral medications are also extremely expensive and ways of reducing costs are being explored.

For further information on side-effects and adherence to antiretroviral therapy, see Loveday (2003).

CONCLUSION

HIV and its related diseases continue to challenge health services throughout the world. The irony, described earlier, of discontinuing the specialism of fever nurses, just when AIDS was first recognised, as though infectious disease were yesterday's problem, has been further compounded by the emergence of widespread resistant tuberculosis and hepatitis C. In future years, perhaps AIDS and other intractable infectious diseases will be considered together rather than as separate and distinct specialties.

Whatever the future of AIDS as a specialty, it will remain important that nurses stay involved with their patients and not aloof. More than ever before, nurses appreciate that they are privileged to be admitted into the trust of their patients. In the field of HIV, as in other palliative care, nurses become very deeply involved in their patients' lives and in their experience of dying (McIntyre 2001).

The nursing care of people with HIV has seen a real growth in innovative practice. Work with drug users, prisoners, prostitutes and other marginalised people has meant that nurses are increasingly working in non-traditional areas, using new procedures. Many myths have been shattered, particularly with regard to the amount of sophisticated equipment that was thought necessary to provide care. High-level nursing care is now given in the poorest areas and in the most difficult of circumstances across the world (Coleblunders et al 2000, Fleck 2003, Kawonza 2003). What is also interesting, and encouraging, is that the move to treatment of AIDS in developing and poor countries has also supported the strengthening of palliative care globally (Stjernsward 2002, Kikule 2003).

Family recognition People with HIV and AIDS, as with the rest of the population, have a variety of domestic arrangements and relationships, and the nurse would do well to take the widest view of the terms 'family' and 'next of kin'. It is distressing to watch courtesy and kindness being shown to the 'official' family and next of kin, who may be estranged, while the patient's lifelong partner and the people they choose to spend every day with are pushed out of the picture. The author has seen this happen to both homosexual and heterosexual patients. In such matters, the nurse should take the lead from the patient and not entirely from the admission form.

Spirituality does not always manifest itself as the embracing of a formal religion. When an individual is seriously ill, they may 'plug into the infinite' in many ways. One of the author's patients found solace in a trip to the opera. Another, who had gone blind, particularly loved sweet-smelling flowers. As an aspiring professional, I used to be rather contemptuous of what I considered sentimental or superstitious behaviour. Experience, however, has taught me some wisdom.

Grieving and the nurse — a personal reflection

Many patients I have cared for have now died. The oldest was 70, the youngest 18. I remember them all, and each one has enhanced my practice. As I write this chapter, their memory is close by, their faces very clear in my mind. I remember when each one died, and each time was an emotional experience. There is some debate as to whether it is a good thing to hang onto disturbing memories. My experience is that it is not a question of deliberately hanging on. When one becomes deeply involved in an individual's living and dying, their memory will live on. It is the nurse's role to bear witness to those memories and to the present experience of each patient alive today. This may be emotional sometimes, but it is not depressing. It is a positive attitude which improves care delivery.

The great and often arduous journey of people with HIV-related illness was brought home to me in late 2003. I was in the kitchen of my home when I heard a familiar voice on the television in the other room. Memories flooded back as I remembered the fun and experiences I had with the owner of that voice. At the time, 14 years previously, this great man, who was HIV positive, and I were often called 'The Twins'. We were both very big (6'4" and over 20 stone) and challenged in the beauty stakes. We would joke about keeping big and alive and would encourage other people to eat. I smiled at the memories and was pleased to hear his voice.

I went in to watch the programme and saw a stranger. How could this worn, thin man be the voice and physique of my friend? It was definitely him, his passion and spirit identified him, but the lines of his struggle were etched in his face. He was talking about how, after many years of relentless treatment, he and many others sometimes took 'holidays' from their treatment, not from despair but for respite. So progress continues to be made, but the experience for the individual is very difficult.

Progress in bringing active treatment to poor and developing countries, rather than adhering to the monolithic position of 'prevention is the only game in town', is becoming a practical reality. Some major companies and employers pay for the treatment of their workers. One executive, interviewed on the BBC Radio 4 business programme in late 2003, stated that this was not charity, but the protection of his workforce, up to a quarter of whom, in some areas, were HIV positive.

In 2005 it was announced that a former minister of the UK government had been HIV positive since 1987. The individual was prompted to make this knowledge public when Nelson Mandela, speaking in 2005 at the funeral of his son, who had died from AIDS, called for the ending of the stigma and secrecy surrounding HIV and AIDS.

Despite these developments, in Northern Europe, there is a decline in articles about HIV in many mainstream journals. Nurses and others do meet people with HIV, but not in great numbers, especially in hospital settings. This situation should not deceive. It is thought-provoking and chilling to consider that, had this terrible disease not taken the lives of affluent white people in the Northern Hemisphere, it might not appear in a book like this at all. I leave the reader with the words of Nelson Mandela (2003) giving the British Red Cross Humanity Lecture.

HIV/AIDS is having a devastating impact on families, communities, societies and economies. Decades have been chopped from life expectancy and young child mortality is expected to more than double in the most severely affected countries of Africa. AIDS is clearly a disaster, effectively wiping out the development gains of the past decades and sabotaging the future.

It is no less than a war, a world war that affects all of us ultimately. The developing world is, as in so many other cases, suffering the worst while having the least resources to deal with the threat.

REFERENCES

Adler M 2001 ABC of AIDS, 5th edn. BMJ Publications, London

Adler M 2003 Sexual health – Report finds sexual health service to be a shambles [editorial]. British Medical Journal 327: 62–63

Andrews H A, Roy C 1997 The Roy adaptation model. Appleton and Lange, Norwalk, CT

APPG-AIDS 2003 Migration and HIV: improving lives in Britain. An inquiry into the impact of the UK nationality and immigration system on people living with HIV. All-Party Parliamentary Group on AIDS. Online. Available: www.appg-aids.org.uk

Armstrong M L 1998 Body piercing: a clinical look. Office Nurse 11(3): 26–29

Atkinson J 2000 Nursing homeless men: a study of proactive intervention. Whurr, London

Atkinson J, Kennedy E, Goldsworthy S, Drummond S 2002 Patients' cancer journeys in Kintyre: a qualitative study of the care, support and information needs of people with cancer and their carers. European Journal of Oncology Nursing 6(2): 85–92

Babcock H M, Fraser V 2003 Differences in percutaneous injury patterns in a multi-hospital system. Infection Control and Hospital Epidemiology 24: 731–736

Barker D J P, Rose G 1998 Epidemiology in medical practice. Churchill Livingstone, Edinburgh

Bishop A H, Scudder J R 1990 The practical, moral and personal sense of nursing. State University of New York Press, New York

British HIV Association (BHIVA) 2003 HIV treatment guidelines. BHIVA, London. Online. Available: www.bhiva.org/guidelines/2003/hiv/index.html

Caplan G 1961 An approach to community mental health. Tavistock, London

Catalan J (ed) 1999 Mental health and HIV infection – psychological and psychiatric aspects. UCL Press, London

CDC 1987 A report by Council of State and Territorial Epidemiologists; AIDS Program, Centre for Infectious Diseases. Morbidity and Mortality Weekly Report (Suppl 36), Atlanta, GA

Coleblunders R, Verdonck K, Nachega J 2000 Impact of new developments in anti-retroviral treatment on AIDS prevention and care in resource-poor countries. AIDS Patient Care and Standards 14: 251–257

Connor S, Kingman S 1989 The search for the virus. Penguin, Harmondsworth

Crouch D 2003 Tackling substance misuse. Nursing Times 99(33): 20–23

De Cock K M, Fowler M G, Mercier E 2000 Prevention of mother-to-child HIV transmission in resource poor countries: translating research into policy and practice. Journal of the American Medical Association 283(9): 1175–1182

Dimond B 2003 Laws relating to HIV/AIDS infection and the rights of employees. Nursing Standard 12(2): 112–115

Donovan A 2004 Reflections on ethical issues in working with street youth. The Newsletter of the Alcohol and Drug Study Group – Special Issue on Ethics 37: 1

Downie R, Telfer E 1980 Caring and curing. Methuen, London

Ewles L, Simnett I 2003 Promoting health: a practical guide, 5th edn. Baillière Tindall, Edinburgh

Fleck F 2003 WHO approves combination pills for HIV/AIDS. British Medical Journal 327: 1067

Gibb D M, Duong T, Tookey P A et al 2003 Decline in mortality, AIDS, and hospital admissions in perinatally HIV-1 infected children in the United Kingdom and Ireland. British Medical Journal 327: 1019–1023

Greif J, Hewitt W, Armstrong M L 1999 Tattooing and body piercing: body art practices among college students. Clinical Nursing Research 8(4): 368–385

Gungabissoon U 2003 The epidemiology and control of hepatitis C infection. Nursing Times 99(31): 24–25

Hansard 1986 Parliamentary report on the debate on HIV and AIDS (November). House of Commons, London

Jeffries D J 1997 Occupational exposure and treatment options. Journal of HIV Combination Therapy 2(3): 44

Johnson M 2003 The nurse role of implementing the National Sexual Health Strategy. Nursing Times 99(35): 47

Kawonza L 2003 Raising awareness of HIV for World AIDS Day. Nursing Times 99(48): 28–29

Kikule E 2003 A good death in Uganda: survey of needs for palliative care for terminally ill people in urban areas. British Medical Journal 327: 192–194

Kirton C 2003 ANAC's core curriculum for HIV/AIDS nursing, 2nd edn. Association of Nurses in AIDS Care, Akron, OH

Lo B, Bayer R 2003 Establishing ethical trials for treatment and prevention of AIDS in developing countries. British Medical Journal 327: 337–339

Mandela N 2003 Conference speech. The 2003 British Red Cross Humanity Lecture, London

McIntyre R 2001 Nursing support for families of dying patients. Whurr, London

Nursing and Midwifery Council (NMC) 2003a Monday 27 October 2003 Four NHS staff die from HIV needle injury. NMC, London

Nursing and Midwifery Council (NMC) 2003b Anonymous testing for HIV. Register: Journal of the Nursing and Midwifery Council, London

Nursing and Midwifery Council (NMC) 2004 Guidelines and advice on confidentiality. NMC, London

Pratt R 2003 HIV and AIDS: a strategy for nursing care, 6th edn. Hodder Arnold, London

Rothenberg R B, Scarlett M, del Rio C et al 1998 Oral transmission of AIDS. AIDS 12: 2095–2105

Royal College of Nursing (RCN) 2004 Methicillin-resistant *Staphylococcal aureus* (MRSA). RCN. London

Scott P A, Valimaki M, Leino-Kilpi H et al 2003 Autonomy, privacy and informed consent 1: concepts and definitions. British Journal of Nursing 12(1): 43–47

Shaw J K, Mahoney A M 2003 HIV/AIDS nursing secrets. Hanley and Belfus, Philadelphia

Shilts R 2000 And the band played on. Saint Martin's Press, New York

Singh D 2003 HIV testing should not be used to restrict access to UK. News report. British Medical Journal 327: 124

Sistrom M G, Coyner B J, Gwaltney J M, Farr B M 1998 Concise communications. Frequency of percutaneous injuries requiring post exposure prophylaxis for occupational exposure to human immunodeficiency virus. Infection Control and Hospital Epidemiology 19(7): 504–506

Stine G J 2000 AIDS update 2000. Prentice Hall, Upper Saddle River, NJ

Stjernsward J 2002 Uganda: initiating a government public health approach to pain relief and palliative care. Journal of Pain and Symptom Management 24: 257–264

United Nations 2004 Report on the global AIDS epidemic. Online. Available: www.unaids.org/bangkok2004/report.html

Waters A 2003 SARS. Nursing Standard 17(4): 14–15

Wilson J 2001 Infection control in clinical practice. Baillière Tindall, London

World Health Organization 2000 Technical consultation on behalf of the UNFPA/UNICEF/WHO/UNAIDS inter-agency task team on mother-to-child transmission of HIV. New data on the prevention of mother-to-child transmission of HIV and their policy implications: conclusions and recommendations. WHO, Geneva

World Health Organization 2003a Scaling up antiretroviral therapy in resource-limited

settings: treatment guidelines for a public health approach. WHO, Geneva. Online. Available: www.who.int/hiv/pub/prev_care/draft/en/
World Health Organization 2003b The 3 by 5 initiative. WHO, Geneva. Online. Available: www.who.int/3by5/en/index.html
World Health Organization 2003c Annex 1 World Health Organization staging system for HIV infection and disease in adults and adolescents. WHO, Geneva. Online. Available: www.who.int/docstore/hiv/scaling/anex1.html

FURTHER READING

Adler M 2001 ABC of AIDS, 5th edn. BMJ Publications, London
Anderson J, Doyal L 2004 Women from Africa living with HIV in London: a descriptive study. AIDS Care 16(1): 95–105
British HIV Association (BHIVA) 2003 HIV treatment guidelines. BHIVA, London. Online. Available: www.bhiva.org/guidelines/2003/hiv/index.html
Ewles L, Simnett I 2003 Promoting health: a practical guide, 5th edn. Baillière Tindall, Edinburgh
Loveday H 2003 Adherence to antiretroviral therapy. In: Pratt R J (ed) HIV and AIDS: a strategy for nursing care, 6th edn. Hodder-Arnold, London, Ch. 21
Newberry Y, Kelsey J J 2003 Mother to child transmission of HIV. Journal of Pharmacy Practice 16: 182–190
Pratt R J 2000 Antenatal screening for HIV infection: removing tomorrow's children from harm's way. Journal of Neonatal Nursing 6: 179–184
Pratt R J 2003 HIV and AIDS: a strategy for nursing care, 6th edn. Hodder-Arnold, London
Shaw J K, Mahoney A M 2003 HIV/AIDS nursing secrets. Hanley and Belfus, Philadelphia
Stine G J 2000 AIDS update 2000. Prentice Hall, Upper Saddle River, NJ
United Nations 2004 Report on the global AIDS epidemic. Online. Available: www.unaids.org/bangkok2004/GAR2004_html/GAR2004_00_en.htm#TopOfPage

USEFUL WEBSITES AND HELPLINE

AVERT
www.avert.org/about.htm

Haemophilia Society
www.haemophilia.org.uk

Health Protection Agency (England and Wales)
www.phls.co.uk

Health Protection Scotland
www.hps.scot.nhs.uk

National AIDS Helpline (24 hour)
Tel: 0800 567 123

Royal College of Nursing Sexual Health Forum
www.rcn.org.uk

Terrence Higgins Trust
www.tht.org.uk

APPENDICES

APPENDIX 1

TESTS AND INVESTIGATIONS

The following tests and investigations should be seen as terms defined rather than processes described and are used to supplement and clarify reference made to them in the text.

Actigraph

An actigraph or accelerometer is a small electronic device, usually worn on the non-dominant wrist. It is approximately the size of a wrist watch and measures sleep indirectly through its recording of arm movements. Actigraphy is based on the principle that arm movements are linked to wakefulness and not to sleep, thus fewer arm movements are associated with sleep and a greater number of arm movements denote wakefulness. Increasingly, nurses are using actigraphs to monitor patients' sleep.

Amniocentesis

This is a diagnostic procedure performed by inserting a hollow needle through the abdominal wall into the uterus and withdrawing a small amount of fluid from the sac surrounding the fetus. Amniotic fluid contains cells that are normally shed from the fetus. Samples of these cells are obtained by withdrawing some amniotic fluid. The chromosome analysis of these cells can be performed to determine abnormalities.

Angiography

This involves the injection of contrast medium to outline blood vessels. The contrast is injected and rapid serial X-ray films are taken. The presence and location of aneurysms and other blood vessel anomalies such as stenosis are demonstrated. Angiography is not without risk and its performance may be delayed in the patient who is in a poor clinical condition.

Arterial blood gases (ABGs)

This involves a sample of blood being taken from an artery. The blood is analysed and gives arterial oxygen tensions (P_aO_2), the arterial carbon dioxide tension (P_aCO_2) and oxygen saturation. In addition, blood pH, standard bicarbonate and base excess are also estimated.

Arteriography

A radio-opaque dye is injected into an artery and a series of X-rays are taken to show the path of the dye in the arteries and pinpoint any obstruction to blood flow.

Arthroscopy

The direct examination of a joint by the surgical insertion of an arthroscope. The procedure can be performed on an outpatient basis and is used in the diagnosis of injuries. Although it is most commonly used for the knee joint, arthroscopic techniques can also be used for the hip, shoulder, wrist and ankle.

Barium studies

When plain radiography is inadequate to study an area of interest, contrast media can be used. Barium sulphate is an aqueous suspension, which is non-irritant and radiodense. Administered orally or rectally, it allows the gastrointestinal tract to stand out when viewed through a fluoroscope or on a radiograph. Barium studies of the gastrointestinal tract can help in the diagnosis of disorders such as peptic ulceration, malignant tumours, diverticulitis and colitis.

Biopsy

The excision of a small area of tissue for diagnostic purposes. Often used in the diagnosis of breast disease.

Blood count

Calculation of the number of red blood cells, white blood cells and platelets in a litre of blood. A differential blood count is the estimation of the relative proportion of the different blood cells in the blood.

Blood film

Microscopic examination of the cellular components of the blood, i.e. red and white blood cells and platelets.

Red cells

Size: Usually 7 µm in diameter

- Microcytic — smaller than normal
- Normocytic — normal size
- Macrocytic — larger than normal
- Anisocytic — inequality in size.

Shape: Poikilocytic — marked irregularity in shape.
Colour:

- Hypochromic — red cells contain less haemoglobin than normal, resulting in a pale colour
- Normochromic — normal amount of haemoglobin in red blood cells and therefore normal colour.

White cells

Size: Usually 10–15 µm in diameter.
Structure:

- Staining characteristics of granules are different for neutrophils, eosinophils and basophils
- Excessive nuclear lobulation in neutrophils (indication of megaloblastic anaemia, iron deficiency, renal failure).

Cell differentiation between different granulocytes, lymphocytes and monocytes can be performed and commented on in the blood film report.

Platelets

Size: 2–4 µm in diameter.
Structure: Smaller or larger than average occur in certain haematological conditions, e.g. large platelets occur in thrombocytopenia due to platelet loss or destruction or postsplenectomy.

Brodie–Trendelenburg test

This is a test for varicose veins. The patient lies on their back and raises their leg to empty the veins. A tourniquet is applied just below the saphenous opening. The patient is then stood up and the tourniquet removed in 60 s. Normally the vein should fill from below within 35 s with the tourniquet in situ. Earlier filling indicates incompetence of a communicating vein. If, on release, the veins fill rapidly from above, this is due to incompetent saphenofemoral valves.

Bronchoscopy

Endoscopic examination of the trachea and larger bronchi. It is indicated in patients with haemoptysis, suspected lung cancer and chest infections which are not defined by other investigations.

Cardiotocography

The simultaneous monitoring of the fetal heart rate and maternal uterine contractions as a means of monitoring fetal well-being.

$CD4^+$ T-lymphocyte cell counts

Laboratory estimates of the number of $CD4^+$ T lymphocytes in peripheral blood are generally reported as the number of cells per cubic millimetre (cells/mm^3). These estimates and their trends to decrease or increase over time comprise one of the most important laboratory assessments predicting HIV disease progression and response to antiviral therapy.

Cholecystography

Radiological examination of the gall bladder using a radio-opaque contrast medium taken orally. A normal liver will usually remove the radio-opaque medium from the bloodstream and store and concentrate it in the gall bladder. Radiographs taken will show the dye-filled gall bladder as a dense shadow. Gallstones may be seen as filling defects. This technique will not outline the gall bladder when the serum bilirubin concentration is elevated (>34 mmol/L), as insufficient contrast medium is excreted. Although oral cystography is a reliable means of detecting gallstones in non-jaundiced patients, it has been largely superseded by ultrasonography.

Chorionic villus sampling (CVS)

CVS is a prenatal test that involves taking a tiny tissue sample from outside the sac where the fetus develops. The tissue is tested to diagnose or rule out certain birth defects. The test is generally performed between 10 and 12 weeks after a woman's last menstrual period. This investigation may be offered when there is an increased risk of chromosomal or genetic birth defects, and parents would like test results as early in pregnancy as possible. CVS is not routinely offered to all pregnant women because the test carries a small risk of miscarriage, and possibly other complications.

Computerised (axial) tomography (CT scan)

The patient lies on a couch and the head is placed in an opening in the front of the scanner. A series of X-rays are beamed through the patient's head in transaxial slices of various sizes and, depending upon the density of the tissue, are either transmitted or absorbed. Those that are transmitted are detected by a battery of sensitive crystals and this information is then fed to a computer, which creates an image of the scanned structures, e.g. brain tissue. Once one 'sweep' is complete, the machine moves through 1° until an 180° arc has been completed. CT scanning may reveal alterations in tissue density, displacement of structures and abnormalities. Certain types of lesion are better demonstrated with the use of contrast enhancement; this involves the injection of an intravenous contrast and then scanning the patient as already described.

Coombs' test

Test to detect antibodies to red blood cells:

- *direct Coombs' test* detects those bound to the red blood cells
- *indirect Coombs' test* detects those not bound to the red blood cells but circulating in the serum.

Countercurrent immunoelectrophoresis (CCIE)

A laboratory method for the detection of specific antibodies or antigens.

Creatinine clearance

This is a calculation to assess the kidneys' ability to remove creatinine from the blood and hence provide a guide to how well the kidneys are working. The creatinine clearance reflects the glomerular filtration rate (GFR).

Relying on simple measurement of the serum creatinine as an assessment of renal function can overestimate GFR by up to 19%. Several factors may influence creatinine production and so the Cockcroft and Gualt formula uses age, sex, weight and plasma creatinine to correct for these, and provide a more accurate assessment of renal function and estimated GFR. However, in recent years, other formulae such as the Modification of Diet in Renal Disease (MDRD) equation have been proposed (Levey et al 1999) to provide a more accurate assessment of GFR by taking factors such as ethnicity into account.

C-reactive protein (CRP)

CRP is a type of protein produced by the liver that is present only during acute inflammation. It gives a general indication of acute inflammation in the body, rather than identifying a specific cause of this inflammation.

Culture (bacterial)

The specimen material is smeared onto a culture medium plate (containing nutrients and moisture), and then incubated at 37°C to allow any bacteria present to grow and multiply. After 18–24 h the culture plate is examined and bacteria can be identified.

Cystography/cystourography

Via a urinary catheter, the bladder is filled to capacity with contrast medium and X-rayed, revealing any bladder abnormalities. The catheter is then removed to observe the function of the bladder and upper urethra during micturition — a cystourogram.

Cystometry

This investigation measures changes in the pressure in the bladder. A urinary catheter is inserted and the bladder drained. Water at body temperature is then introduced into the bladder at a slow and constant rate and, in response to the increasing volume, the bladder pressure is recorded using a pressure-measuring device, which produces a cystometrogram.

Cytology

Cytology is the study of the structure and function of cells, both normal and abnormal. Body cells may be collected by a variety of methods, e.g. from a specimen of urine or sputum, scraped from a skin lesion or from the cervix during a Papanicolaou smear test, or from aspirate of a lump or bone marrow. The cells are then examined microscopically for abnormalities.

Echocardiography

A non-invasive technique which uses pulses of high-frequency sound (ultrasound) emitted from a transducer to evaluate cardiac anatomy, pathology and function. The procedure involves an operator applying a lubricant to the skin surface of the chest wall and moving the transducer or probe back and forth by hand across the surface.

Electroencephalography (EEG)

A graphic recording of the electrical activity of the brain. Electrodes are attached to the scalp and the electrical activity is noted with a sensitive recorder. Patients prone to seizures will demonstrate an abnormal waveform even while seizure-free.

Enzyme-linked immunosorbent assay (ELISA)

A laboratory method for the detection of specific antibodies or antigens.

Erythrocyte sedimentation rate (ESR)

Measurement of the height of red blood cells at the foot of a column of blood after the blood has been left standing in the narrow tube for 1 h (normal value <10 mm).

Evoked responses

In this test, one of the sensory systems is artificially stimulated and the response noted with the use of appropriately placed electrodes, which detect disturbances of conduction. Visual evoked responses are obtained by asking the patient to look at a reversing checkboard pattern or flashing lights. Electrodes placed on the scalp over the occipital lobes will detect if there is any delay in conduction along the optic pathway, such as may occur in a patient with multiple sclerosis.

Fine-needle aspiration (FNA)

A means of tissue diagnosis by withdrawing fluid or tissue from a swelling, e.g. in the neck.

Glucose tolerance test

Measurement of the body's ability to handle appropriately the excess sugar presented after drinking a high glucose drink. Patient fasts overnight. In the morning 75 g glucose is given in 300 mL water. Blood glucose is measured before and 2 h after ingestion of glucose. Diabetes mellitus confirmed if glucose level >11.1 mmol/L.

Gonioscopy

Gonioscopy is performed to assess the angle of the eye, between the cornea and iris. A narrowed angle is indicative of closed-angled glaucoma.

The eye is anaesthetised with short-acting eye drops. A contact lens in which an angled mirror has been incorporated (gonioscope) is lubricated with methylcellulose eye drops and applied to the cornea. The eye is then examined through a slit lamp.

Haemoglobin estimation

Estimation of the amount of haemoglobin present in 100 mL of blood (normal values: men, 13.5–17.5 g/dL; women, 11.5–15.5 g/dL).

Haemostasis (clotting) tests

Activated partial thromboplastin time (APTT) A coagulation test of the intrinsic and common clotting pathways. Phospholipid, calcium and kaolin are added to citrated plasma. The clotting time depends on the presence of the components of the intrinsic pathway. Abnormalities in the test result from deficiencies of intrinsic and common pathway factors (normal result: 30–40 s).
Prothrombin time (PT) Tests the extrinsic pathway of blood coagulation. The test requires the presence of functional quantities of factor VII and vitamin K-dependent factor X. The result is expressed as the ratio of patient:control — the international normalised ratio (INR). (Normal result: clot forms in 13 s; normal ratio: 1.0–1.3.)
Thrombin clotting time (TT) Tests the final reaction in the final pathway, i.e. fibrinogen converted to fibrin (normal value: 14–16 s).
Bleeding time Test for abnormal platelet function. Time taken to stop bleeding after making a standardised superficial skin incision, e.g. with a lancet (normal value: 3–8 min).

Immunocoagglutination

A laboratory method for the detection of specific antibodies or antigens.

Immunodiffusion

A laboratory method for the detection of specific antibodies or antigens.

Immunoelectrophoresis

A laboratory method for the detection of specific antibodies or antigens.

Intravenous cholangiography

Contrast medium, given intravenously, is excreted into the biliary system. Serial radiographs are taken. However, this technique is not commonly used as results are often of poor quality, are of no value in jaundiced patients and also carry a small but significant risk of an anaphylactic reaction to the contrast medium. As a result, methods that allow direct injection of the contrast into the biliary tree are preferred, e.g. percutaneous transhepatic cholangiography (PTC), endoscopic retrograde cholangiopancreatography (ERCP), operative cholangiography and T-tube cholangiography.

Intravenous fluorescein angiography

This technique is used as an aid in the diagnosis and treatment of many of the vascular disorders of the retina. A 5 mL i.v. injection of 10% fluorescein sodium is given into a vein in the arm. A series of photographs are taken through a dilated pupil at timed intervals, using a fundal camera. Any defect in the retinal vessels will show up as a leakage of dye or occlusion of the vessel. The patient may feel nauseated after the procedure.

The patient should be informed that the sclera and skin will take on a yellow colour for about 24 h and that urine will be greenish for 24–48 h as the dye is excreted through the kidneys. Diabetic patients who carry out urine testing should be advised to test their blood sugar instead, as the dye can affect the results obtained by urine test strips.

Lumbar puncture

This is the most common neurological investigation. It involves the insertion of a sterile needle and trocar between lumbar vertebrae 3 and 4, or 4 and 5, and the withdrawal of a quantity of cerebrospinal fluid (CSF) for analysis. The procedure is usually performed in the ward under local anaesthetic. The lumbar CSF pressure may also be measured prior to the removal of CSF. The normal constituents of CSF and their values may be altered in the presence of a disorder, e.g. the number of red blood cells in the CSF following subarachnoid haemorrhage will be markedly elevated.

Magnetic resonance imaging (MRI)

This investigation is based on the use of a magnetic field and radio pulse waves, instead of traditional irradiation. The patient lies on a couch and is then completely enclosed in a tunnel within the scanner. A strong magnetic field is applied and the nuclei within the tissues, which were previously spinning in a random fashion, line up in a north–south magnetic field orientation. A radio pulse wave is introduced at a right angle to the magnetic field and the nuclei are tipped out of alignment, causing uniform resonance. The pulse waves are stopped and the resonating nuclei will return to their previous state. Minute radiofrequency signals are given off as the nuclei enter this relaxed state and these are monitored by the scanner. By pre-programming the computer to simulate a non-uniform magnetic field, the positively charged particles in different parts of the magnetic field will resonate at different speeds. Variable radio pulse waves result in differences in the emission of radiofrequency data. The computer assimilates the data and constructs a tissue image.

This type of scanning has a particular use in detecting cerebral and spinal oedema, and cerebral and spinal blood flow-related disorders, such as infarction, haemorrhage and arteriovenous malformation. In musculoskeletal conditions and injuries it is used to detect soft tissue problems such as a torn cruciate ligament in the knee or a disc protrusion in the vertebral column.

Mammogram

A mammogram is an X-ray examination of the breast. Usually two views of the breast tissue are taken under compression.

Mantoux test

An intradermal injection of tuberculin purified protein derivative (PPD), which is a sterile preparation 'made from the heat-treated products of growth and lysis of the mycobacterium' (DH 1996). The result is read after 48–72 h. A positive result is described as induration of at least 5 mm diameter at the injection site. This indicates that the individual has sensitivity to the tuberculin protein, and a strong reaction may indicate active disease.

Mean corpuscular haemoglobin (MCH)

This is the average concentration of haemoglobin in a red blood cell (normal range: 30–35 g/dL).

Mean corpuscular or cell volume (MCV)

The average red cell volume — normal: 85 fl (range 75–95 fl).

Microscopy

Direct visualisation of microorganisms using a light microscope or an electron microscope (uses a beam of electrons rather than light rays).

Orthopantomogram (OPT)

Panoramic radiograph giving consistent image quality, usually of mandible or maxilla, for suspected neoplasia. Also in maxillofacial surgery for middle third fracture of facial bones.

Packed cell volume (PCV) or haematocrit

This test measures the relative red cell mass to plasma, i.e. the proportion of the blood sample composed of packed red blood cells to plasma (normal values: men, 40–52%; women, 36–48%).

Paul–Bunnell (monospot) test

A method of determining the diagnosis of infectious mononucleosis (glandular fever), which may result from the Epstein–Barr virus (EBV). During the second week of the infection, specific EBV IgM antibodies indicate recent infection by the virus.

Pleural aspiration

This involves the percutaneous drainage of fluids or air and is indicated in pleural effusions, pneumothorax or empyema. It may be diagnostic or therapeutic.

Polysomnography

Polysomnography is a diagnostic investigation in which a number of physiological variables are measured, via sensor leads, and recorded while the individual is asleep. These include eye and jaw muscle movements, leg muscle movements and brain electrical activity.

Positron emission tomography (PET) scan

A computerised radiographic technique that employs radioactive substances to examine the metabolic activities of various body structures. It involves the injection into the bloodstream of a solution containing a very short-lived radioactive agent which then emits positively charged particles — positrons. These combine with negatively charged electrons normally found in body cells and emit gamma rays. It is these rays that are picked up by the PET computer and converted to colour-coded images that indicate the intensity of metabolic activity of the organ involved.

PET scans have proved useful in studying the blood flow and metabolism in the heart and blood vessels, in diagnosing and studying cancer, in understanding the biochemical activity in the brain in such disorders as multiple sclerosis and Parkinson's disease, and in demonstrating which parts of the brain are active when people are in pain.

Precipitin test

A laboratory method for the detection of specific antibodies or antigens.

Pulmonary function test (PFT)

A useful test in the diagnosis of respiratory disorders and in measuring and monitoring the severity and course of a disease.

Radioallergosorbent test (RAST)

A laboratory method for the detection of specific antibodies or antigens.

Radioimmunoassay (RIA)

A laboratory method for the detection of specific antibodies or antigens.

Radioisotope scanning

Radioisotope scans involve the use of small amounts of various radioactive substances, which are differentially taken up by normal and abnormal (malignant) tissue. The most common radioisotope scans are those of the liver, brain and bones. The radioisotope is injected intravenously, and the scan occurs several hours later. Patients should be reassured that the radioactivity of their bodies during this waiting time is minimal and that they are not a danger to others.

Red cell mass

Estimation of the total volume of circulating red cells performed by labelling a sample of the patient's own red blood cells with isotope ^{51}Cr or ^{99m}Tc. A measured amount is reinjected and a sample is taken after a specific period of time when the dilution can be calculated (normal value: men, 25–35 mL/kg; women, 20–30 mL/kg).

Renography

A radiological study to assess renal function. Some elements that the kidneys normally concentrate and excrete can be labelled with radioactive isotopes. These are administered intravenously and the function of the kidneys can be traced by recording the rate at which the isotopes are removed from the blood and passed into the urinary collecting system.

Reticulocyte count

The number of reticulocytes in the peripheral blood (normal range: 0.2–2.0% of red blood cells).

Schiller test

Iodine 3.5% is applied to the cervix and will stain normal cells of the cervix. Abnormal cells will not pick up the colour because they do not contain glycogen.

Schilling test

Estimation of the gastrointestinal absorption of radioactive vitamin B_{12} (normal range >10% of administered oral dose in 24-h urine sample).

Sensitivity

A test used to determine which antibiotics will kill the bacteria in the specimen. The antibiotic-impregnated discs are placed over a film of cultured bacteria on a culture plate and the plate read some hours later. A zone of inhibition around the disc indicates that the organism is sensitive to that antibiotic. If an organism is resistant, there will be growth right up to the disc.

Sentinel node biopsy

Radioactive colloid is injected into a tumour before surgery. Passage of the colloid through the lymphatic system adjacent to the tumour is scanned by a digital gamma camera (lymphoscintigraphy). During subsequent surgery (within 24 h), use of both a gamma probe and blue dye identifies the first echelon lymph node encountered. This node is excised and examined immediately by a pathologist (frozen section). Presence or otherwise of tumour cells dictates whether further excision of lymph glands is indicated. Used mainly in breast carcinoma, malignant melanoma and oral and oropharyngeal squamous cell carcinoma when the tumour is readily accessible prior to surgery. If the sentinel node is negative, the patient may be spared unnecessary surgery involving lymphatic dissection (Ross et al 2002).

Serology

The examination of blood serum, often to ascertain if infection is present by identifying antigen/antibody.

Sialogram

Radiograph following injection of contrast medium into a salivary duct and gland.

Skeletal survey X-rays

A skeletal survey involves X-rays of the skull, spine, ribs, pelvis and the femoral and humeral heads, enabling detection of primary bone tumours and bone metastases from other tumours.

T-cell immunophenotyping (CD4 T-cell subsets)

This procedure, used particularly for patients with HIV disease, shows the level of healthy T-helper cells the patient has. This is a vital prognostic tool. The test uses a monoclonal antibody, which binds to a specific antigen on the T_4 helper cells. The test counts these and presents them as a ratio of the total T cells.

Tonometry

Tonometric tests measure intraocular pressure (IOP). The normal range is 12–20 mmHg.
Applanation tonometry Fluorescein and anaesthetic drops are instilled prior to this procedure. A prism attached to a slit lamp (or a portable Perkins' tonometer) is used to flatten a defined area of the cornea. The greater the force required to flatten the area, the higher the IOP.
Non-contact (air puff) tonometry uses a computerised instrument to direct a fine, high-pressure jet of air onto the cornea. The increase in force progresses linearly until the cornea becomes flat. At this point the cornea acts like a mirror and reflects light to a photoelectric sensor, which immediately shuts off the puff of air. The force required to flatten the cornea is recorded and converted into an IOP reading.

Tumour markers

Some malignant tumours produce substances that can be detected in the blood. These may serve as 'markers' of the presence or recurrence of the tumour, and sometimes as an indicator of its size and, therefore, response to treatment. For example, alpha-fetoprotein (AFP) and beta-human chorionic gonadotrophin (BhCG) are produced by testicular tumours, and acid phosphatase by prostatic tumours.

Ultrasound

The use of high frequency sound waves through a hand-held transducer to image soft tissues, particularly useful when examining breast tissue.

Urethroscopy

The endoscopic examination of the male urethra and prostate gland.

Urinary flow rate

The voiding flow rate is measured using specially equipped facilities which allow the patient to void in privacy but where a machine can record the characteristics of the flow. The test will identify such things as peak flow, average flow and total flow time.

Urine protein:creatinine ratio

Proteinuria can be assessed from a single (early morning) urine sample and this can provide a reliable predictor (in people who do not have diabetes mellitus) of deterioration of renal function and fall in GFR (Ruggenenti et al 1998, Keane et al 1999). This test is reported to be more reliable than the traditional 24 h urine collection.

Ventilation perfusion scan (VQ scan)

The intravenous injection of radioisotope to outline the distribution of pulmonary perfusion. Xenon-133 gas is inhaled into the lung and, using the two scans, a pulmonary embolus can be seen to cause a lowering of perfusion relative to ventilation.

Videofluoroscopy

Video recording of the swallowing mechanism, using fluorescent fluid.

Water depletion test (diabetes insipidus)

Fluids are withheld for 8–12 h or until 3% of the body weight has been lost. Regular measurements of plasma and urine are taken. The inability to increase urinary specific gravity and osmolality in response to water depletion is indicative of diabetes insipidus. The test must be closely supervised as the patient will experience excessive thirst. The test is terminated if signs of tachycardia, hypotension or obvious dehydration occur.

REFERENCES

Department of Health 1996 Immunisation against infectious disease. HMSO, London

Department of Health 2005 National Health Service framework for renal services Part Two: Chronic kidney disease, acute renal failure and end of life care. Department of Health, London. Available online: www.dh.gov.uk/Publications

Keane W F, Eknoyan G for the NKF Committee 1999 Proteinuria, albuminuria, risk, assessment, detection, elimination (PARADE): a position paper of the National Kidney Foundation. American Journal of Kidney Disease 33(5): 1004–1010

Levey A S, Bosch J P, Breyer L J et al 1999 A more accurate method to estimate glomerular filtration rate from serum creatinine: A new prediction equation. Annals of International Medicine 130(6): 461–470

Renal Association 2002 Treatment of adults with renal failure – recommended standards and audit measures (2nd edn). Renal Association and Royal College of Physicians, London. Available on-line: www.renal.org/Standards

Ross G, Soutar D S, Shoaib T et al 2002 The ability of lymphoscintigraphy to direct sentinel node biopsy in the clinically N0 (node-negative) neck for patients with head and neck squamous cell carcinoma. British Journal of Radiology 75(900): 950–958

Ruggenenti P, Gaspari F, Pernat A, Remuzzi G 1998 Cross-sectional longitudinal study of spot morning urine protein:creatinine ratio, 24 hour urine protein excretion rate, glomerular filtration rate, and end stage renal failure in chronic renal disease in patients without diabetes. British Medical Journal 316: 504–509

APPENDIX 2

NORMAL VALUES

NOTES ON INTERNATIONAL SYSTEM OF UNITS (SI UNITS)

Examples of basic SI units

Length	metre (m)
Mass	kilogram (kg)
Amount of substance	mole (mol)
Energy	joule (J)
Pressure	pascal (Pa)

Examples of decimal multiples and submultiples of SI units

Factor	Name	Symbol
10^6	mega-	M
10^3	kilo-	k
10^{-1}	deci-	d
10^{-2}	centi-	c
10^{-3}	milli-	m
10^{-6}	micro-	μ
10^{-9}	nano-	n
10^{-12}	pico-	p
10^{-15}	femto-	f

Volume The basic SI unit of volume is the cubic metre (1000 litres). Because of its convenience the litre is used as the unit of volume in laboratory work.

Mass concentration (e.g. g/L, mcg/L) is used for all protein measurements, for substances which do not have a sufficiently well-defined composition and for serum vitamin B_{12} and folate measurements.

SI units are not employed for enzymes, nor usually for immunoglobulins.

BIOCHEMICAL VALUES

Reference ranges are largely those used in the Department of Clinical Biochemistry, the Lothian University NHS Division. These can vary from laboratory to laboratory, depending on the assay method used and other factors; this is especially the case for the enzyme assays. Although the SI system of units is widely used in the UK, units of measurement can vary and lead to laboratory differences.

No details are given of the collection requirements which may be critical to obtaining a meaningful result.

Unless otherwise stated, reference ranges apply to adults; *values in children may be different.*

Table A2.1 Arterial blood analysis

	Reference range	
Analysis	**SI units**	**Non-SI units**
Bicarbonate	21–27.5 mmol/L	21–27.5 meq/L
Hydrogen ion	36–44 nmol/L	pH 7.36–7.44
$Pa\,CO_2$	4.4–6.1 kPa	33–46 mmHg
$Pa\,O_2$	12–15 kPa	90–113 mmHg
Oxygen saturation	Normally >97%	

Table A2.2 Cerebrospinal fluid

	Reference range	
Analysis	**SI units**	**Non-SI units**
Cells	Up to 5 (all mononuclear) cells/mm^3	
Chloride	120–170 mmol/L	120–170 meq/L
Glucose	2.5–4.0 mmol/L	45–72 mg/100 mL
IgG index*	<0.65	—
Total protein	100–400 mg/L	0.01–0.04 g/100 mL

*A crude index of increase in IgG attributable to intrathecal synthesis.

Table A2.3 Reference values in venous serum for the more common analytes in adults

Analysis	Reference range SI units	Non-SI units
α_1-Antitrypsin	1.7–3.2 g/L	170–320 mg/100 mL
Alanine aminotransferase (ALT)	10–40 U/L	—
Albumin	36–47 g/L	3.6–4.7 g/100 mL
Alkaline phosphatase	40–125 U/L	—
Amylase	<100 U/L	—
Aspartate aminotransferase (AST)	10–35 U/L	—
Bilirubin (total)	2–17 μmol/L	0.12–1.0 mg/100 mL
Calcium	2.12–2.62 mmol/L	4.24–5.24 meq/L or 8.50–10.50 mg/100 mL
Carboxyhaemoglobin	Not normally detectable Up to 1.5% in non-smokers	—
Ceruloplasmin	150–600 mg/L	15–60 mg/100 mL
Chloride	95–107 mmol/L	95–107 meq/L
Cholesterol (total)[1]		
HDL-cholesterol Male Female	 0.5–1.6 mmol/L 0.6–1.9 mmol/L	 19–62 mg/100 mL 23–74 mg/100 mL
Copper	13–24 μmol/L	83–153 μg/100 mL
Creatine kinase (total) Male Female	 30–200 U/L 30–150 U/L	 — —
Creatine kinase (MB isoenzyme)	Normally <6% of total CK	—
Creatinine	55–120 μmol/L	0.62–1.36 mg/100 mL
Ethanol	Not normally detectable 65–87 mmol/L (Marked intoxication) 87–109 mmol/L (Stupor) >109 mmol/L (Coma)	 300–400 mg/mL 400–500 mg/mL >500 mg/100 mL
Ferritin Male Female	 17–300 μg/L 14–150 μg/L	 17–300 ng/mL 14–150 ng/mL
Gamma-glutamyl transferase (GGT) Male Female	 10–55 U/L 5–35 U/L	 — —
Glucose (fasting)[2]	3.6–5.8 mmol/L	65–104 mg/100 mL
Glycated haemoglobin (HbA_1)	5.0–6.5%	—
Immunoglobulin A	0.5–4.0 g/L	50–400 mg/100 mL
Immunoglobulin G	5.0–13.0 g/L	500–1300 mg/100 mL
Immunoglobulin M Male Female	 0.3–2.2 g/L 0.4–2.5 g/L	 30–220 mg/100 mL 40–250 mg/100 mL
Iron Male Female	 14–32 μmol/L 10–28 μmol/L	 78–178 μg/100 mL 56–156 μg/100 mL

Table A2.3 Reference values in venous serum for the more common analytes in adults *(Continued)*

Analysis	Reference range SI units	Reference range Non-SI units
Iron-binding capacity	45–72 μmol/L	251–402 μg/100 mL
Lactate	0.4–1.4 mmol/L	3.6–12.6 mg/100 mL
Lactate dehydrogenase (total)	230–460 U/L	—
Lead[3]	<1.0 μmol/L	<21 μg/100 mL
Magnesium	0.75–1.0 mmol/L	1.5–2.0 meq/L or 1.82–2.43 mg/100 mL
Osmolality	280–290 mmol/kg	280–290 mosm/L
Phosphate (fasting)	0.8–1.4 mmol/L	2.48–4.34 mg/100 mL
Potassium (plasma)	3.3–4.7 mmol/L	3.3–4.7 meq/L
Potassium (serum)	3.6–5.1 mmol/L	3.6–5.1 meq/L
Protein (total)	60–80 g/L	6–8 g/100 mL
Sodium	132–144 mmol/L	132–144 meq/L
Total CO_2	24–30 mmol/L	24–30 meq/L
Transferrin	2.0–4.0 g/L	0.2–0.4 g/100 mL
Triglycerides (fasting)	0.6–1.7 mmol/L	53–150 mg/100 mL
Urate		
Male	0.12–0.42 mmol/L	2.0–7.0 mg/100 mL
Female	0.12–0.36 mmol/L	2.0–6.0 mg/100 mL
Urea	2.5–6.6 mmol/L	15–40 mg/100 mL
Zinc	11–22 μmol/L	72–144 μg/100 mL

[1] Cholesterol (total)

Ideally	<5.2 mmol/L	<200 mg/100 mL
Mild increase	5.2–6.5 mmol/L	200–250 mg/100 mL
Moderate increase	6.5–7.8 mmol/L	250–300 mg/100 mL
Severe increase	>7.8 mmol/L	>300 mg/100 mL

(as defined by the European Atherosclerosis Society)

[2] Values quoted for venous plasma or serum

[3] In children Up to 0.5 μmol/L Up to 10 μg/100 mL

Table A2.4 Reference values for the more common analytes in urine

Analysis	Reference range SI units	Reference range Non-SI units
Albumin[1]		
Calcium	1.2–3.7 mmol/24 h (low calcium diet) Up to 12 mmol/24 h (normal diet)	2.4–7.4 meq/24 h Up to 24 meq/24 h
Copper	Up to 0.6 μmol/24 h	Up to 38 μg/24 h
Cortisol	9–50 μmol/mol creatinine	30–160 μg cortisol/g creatinine
Creatinine	10–20 mmol/24 h	1130–2260 mg/24 h
5-hydroxyindole-3-acetic acid (5-HIAA)	<60 μmol/24 h	<11.5 mg/24 h
Metadrenalines		
Normetadrenaline	0.4–3.4 μmol/24 h	73–620 μg/24 h
Metadrenaline	0.3–1.7 μmol/24 h	59–335 μg/24 h
Oxalate		
Male	80–490 μmol/24 h	7.2–44 mg/24 h
Female	40–320 μmol/24 h	3.6–29 mg/24 h
Phosphate	15–50 mmol/24 h	465–1548 mg/24 h
Potassium[2]	25–100 mmol/24 h	25–100 meq/24 h
Protein	Up to 0.3 g/L	Up to 0.03 g/100 mL
Sodium	100–200 mmol/24 h	100–200 meq/24 h
Urate	1.2–3.0 mmol/24 h	202–504 mg/24 h
Urea	170–600 mmol/24 h	10.2–36.0 g/24 h

[1]Albumin/creatinine ratio (ACR) and urinary albumin excretion rate (AER) are used to detect microalbuminuria, i.e. excessive albumin excretion in patients with diabetes mellitus, which is of predictive value in identifying patients at risk of progression to diabetic nephropathy. The test should only be carried out in the absence of overt proteinuria (dipstix negative).

ACR

Reference range:	<3.5 mg albumin/mmol creatinine (<31 μg albumin/mg creatinine)
'Borderline':	3.5–10 mg albumin/mmol creatinine (31–88 μg albumin/mg creatinine)
Positive test:	>10 mg albumin/mmol creatinine (>88 μg albumin/mg creatinine)

AER

Reference range:	<20 μg albumin/min
Microalbuminuria:	20–200 μg albumin/min

[2]The urinary output of electrolytes such as sodium and potassium is normally a reflection of intake. This can vary widely, especially on a cultural, worldwide basis. The values quoted are more appropriate to a 'Western' diet.

Table A2.5 **Hormones in serum**

Hormone	Reference range SI units	Non-SI units
Adrenocorticotrophic hormone (ACTH) (plasma)	7–51 ng/L (0700–1000 h)	—
Cortisol	150–550 nmol/L (at 0800 h) <200 nmol/L (at 2200 h)	5.5–20 μg/100 mL <73 μg/100 mL
Follicle-stimulating hormone (FSH)		
Male	1.5–9.0 U/L	—
Female*	3.0–15 U/L (early follicular) Up to 20 U/L (mid-cycle) >30 U/L (postmenopausal)	— — —
Gastrin (plasma)	Up to 120 ng/L	Up to 12 ng/100 mL
Growth hormone (GH)	Variable, up to 50 mU/L	—
Insulin	Highly variable and interpretable only in relation to plasma glucose and body habitus	—
Luteinising hormone (LH)		
Female*	2.5–9.0 U/L (early follicular) Up to 90 U/L (mid-cycle) >20 U/L (postmenopausal)	— — —
Male	1.5–9.0 U/L	—
Oestradiol-17β		
Female	110–180 pmol/L (early follicular) 550–1650 pmol/L (mid-cycle) 370–770 pmol/L (luteal) <150 pmol/L (postmenopausal)	30–49 pg/mL 150–449 pg/mL 101–209 pg/mL <41 pg/mL
Male	<200 pmol/L	<54 pg/mL
Parathyroid hormone (PTH)	10–65 ng/L	1.0–6.5 ng/100 mL
Progesterone		
Male	<2.0 nmol/L	<0.63 μg/L
Female	<2.0 nmol/L (follicular) >15 nmol/L (mid-luteal) <2.0 nmol/L (postmenopausal)	<0.63 μg/L >4.7 μg/L <0.63 μg/L
Prolactin (PRL)	60–390 mU/L	—
Testosterone		
Male	10–30 nmol/L	2.88–8.64 ng/mL
Female	0.4–2.8 nmol/L	0.12–0.81 ng/mL
Thyroid-stimulating hormone (TSH)	0.15–3.5 mU/L	—
Thyroxine (free) (free T_4)	10–27 pmol/L	777–2098 pg/100 mL
Triiodothyronine (T_3)	1.0–2.6 nmol/L	65–169 ng/100 mL
TSH receptor antibodies (TRAb)	<7 U/L	—

*Luteal phase values similar to follicular phase.

Notes

1. A number of hormones are unstable, and collection details are critical to obtaining a meaningful result. Refer to local hospital handbook.
2. Values in the table are only a guideline; hormone levels can often only be meaningfully understood in relation to factors such as sex (e.g. testosterone), age (e.g. FSH in women), time of day (e.g. cortisol) or regulatory factors (e.g. insulin and glucose, PTH and Ca^{2+}). Also, reference ranges may be critically method dependent.

HAEMATOLOGICAL VALUES

Table A2.6 Haematological values

Analysis	Reference range: SI units	Reference range: Non-SI units
Bleeding time (Ivy)	Less than 8 min	
Body fluid (total)	50% (obese)–70% (lean) of body weight	—
Intracellular	30–40% of body weight	—
Extracellular	20–30% of body weight	—
Blood volume		
Male	75 ± 10 mL/kg	—
Female	70 ± 10 mL/kg	—
Coagulation screen		
Prothrombin time	8.0–10.5 s	—
Activated partial thromboplastin time	26–37 s	—
Erythrocyte sedimentation rate*		
Adult male	0–10 mm/h	—
Adult female	3–15 mm/h	—
Fibrinogen	1.5–4.0 g/L	0.15–0.4 g/100 mL
Folate		
Serum	1.5–20.6 μg/L	1.5–20.6 ng/mL
Red cell	95–570 μg/L	95–570 ng/mL
Haemoglobin		
Male	130–180 g/L	13–18 g/100 mL
Female	115–165 g/L	11.5–16.5 g/100 mL
Haptoglobin	0.3–2.0 g/L	0.03–0.2 g/100 mL
Leucocytes (adults)	$4.0–11.0 \times 10^9$/L	$4.0–11.0 \times 10^3$/mm^3
Differential white cell count		
Neutrophil granulocytes	$2.0–7.5 \times 10^9$/L	$2.0–7.5 \times 10^3$/mm^3
Lymphocytes	$1.5–4.0 \times 10^9$/L	$1.5–4.0 \times 10^3$/mm^3
Monocytes	$0.2–0.8 \times 10^9$/L	$0.2–0.8 \times 10^3$/mm^3
Eosinophil granulocytes	$0.04–0.4 \times 10^9$/L	$0.04–0.4 \times 10^3$/mm^3
Basophil granulocytes	$0.01–0.1 \times 10^9$/L	$0.01–0.1 \times 10^3$/mm^3
Mean cell haemoglobin (MCH)	27–32 pg	—
Mean cell volume (MCV)	78–98 fl	—
Packed cell volume (PCV) or haematocrit		
Male	0.40–0.54	—
Female	0.37–0.47	—
Platelets	$150–350 \times 10^9$/L	$150–350 \times 10^3$/mm^3
Red cell count		
Male	$4.5–6.5 \times 10^{12}$/L	$4.5–6.5 \times 10^6$/mm^3
Female	$3.8–5.8 \times 10^{12}$/L	$3.8–5.8 \times 10^6$/mm^3
Red cell life-span (mean)	120 days	—
Red cell life-span $T^1/_2$ (^{51}Cr)	25–35 days	—
Reticulocytes (adults)	$25–85 \times 10^9$/L	$25–85 \times 10^3$/mm^3
Vitamin B_{12}	130–770 pg/mL	—

*Higher values in older patients are not necessarily abnormal.

GLOSSARY

Achalasia. A failure of the smooth muscle of the gastrointestinal tract to relax. The cause is unknown, but it occurs due to degeneration of the ganglionic cells. The failure is most notable in the lower oesophagus which fails to relax with swallowing.

Active cycle of breathing technique (ACBT). Breathing and coughing exercises to help the prevention of postoperative respiratory complications:

Deep breaths — hold for 3 s

Relaxed breaths

Huffs

Coughs

Relaxed breaths

Repeat __ times every hour: left side lying, right side lying, sitting upright

Adjuvant therapy. Any therapy which is deliberately planned in conjunction with another form of therapy, e.g. adjuvant chemotherapy following surgery for breast cancer.

Advocate. An aspect of the nursing role essential to humanistic care whereby the nurse assists the patient to make decisions in a self-determined manner.

Aerobic. Able to live and function in the presence of oxygen.

Affective. Refers to affect, an outward manifestation of a person's feelings or emotions.

Afferent nerve fibre. This is the sensory nerve fibre which runs from the tissues to the central nervous system.

Alleles. Alternative forms of a gene or DNA sequence occurring at the same locus on homologous chromosomes.

Allodynia. 'Pain due to a stimulus which does not normally provoke pain' (IASP 1986, p. S217).

Alport's syndrome. A rare inherited problem which has a combination of effects. Most commonly the kidneys are affected, with nephritis and the gradual development of kidney failure. Hearing may also be affected and very rarely there may also be problems with the platelets in the blood. It is more common in boys.

Amsler grid. A square grid used to detect macular distortion and abnormalities for people with early age-related macular degeneration. The individual focuses their vision on a central dot and notes any irregularities in the appearance — 'straightness' — of the lines.

Anaerobic. Able to live and function in the absence of oxygen.

Aneuploid. Chromosome number that is not an exact multiple of the haploid set; for example, $2n - 1$ or $2n + 1$.

Angiogenesis. The growth of new blood vessels. This is an important natural process occurring in the body, both in health and in disease. In cardiovascular disease, if the body is unable to generate adequate collateral blood vessels or mount a sufficient angiogenesis response, the oxygen-starved muscle is at risk of death. Therapeutic angiogenesis is being used to stimulate new blood vessel growth. This is done by delivering angiogenic proteins or their genes into the muscle or by using a specially designed laser to drill tiny channels into the muscle in order to stimulate new blood vessel growth.

Antihistamine labyrinthine sedatives. Sedatives that have an anti-inflammatory action and also reduce the levels of dizziness and nausea.

Antinociceptive. Something that helps to reduce or stop the response to noxious stimulation.

Antiseptic. A chemical solution, which will reduce and prevent growth of microorganisms on skin.

Antroscopy. Endoscopic examination of the maxillary sinuses.

Appraisal. The individual's assessment of a stressful situation and how it will affect them.

Arteriogram. A radio-opaque dye is injected into an artery and a series of X-rays taken to show the path of the dye in the arteries and to pinpoint any obstruction to blood flow.

Ascites. An abnormal collection of fluid in the peritoneal cavity.

Aseptic. Prevention from contamination with microorganisms utilising certain techniques. Includes sterile conditions on human tissues, on materials and in rooms, obtained by excluding/removing/killing organisms in the environment or on the people involved.

Atherosclerosis. A complex disease characterised by the growth of smooth muscle cells and the build-up of lipid lesions within the intima of the arteries. It is a dynamic inflammatory process with phases of stability and instability.

Atopy. Hereditary tendency to a clinical hypersensitivity state.

Attico-antral disease. Bone erosion of the middle ear, caused by chronic infection.

Auriscope. An instrument which incorporates magnification and illumination, and can be used for examining the ear.

Autogenic drainage. A self-drainage technique which utilises controlled expiratory airflow (tidal breathing) to mobilise secretions consisting of three phases: 1) unsticking the peripheral secretions by breathing at low lung volumes (slow deep air movement); 2) collecting the mucus from central airways by breathing at low to mid lung volumes (slow mid-range air movement); 3) evacuating the mucus from the central airways by breathing at mid to high lung volumes (shallow air movement).

Autonomy. To act with self-determination.

Autosome. Any chromosome other than the sex chromosomes.

B-scan. An ultrasonography test to clinically assess ocular and orbital diseases. Used to detect vitreal or retinal abnormalities.

Biofeedback. Presentation of immediate visual or auditory information about usually unconscious body functions.

Buchanan laryngectomy bib protector. A humidifying covering for the stoma of a laryngectomy.

Bulbospongiosum. Muscle that evacuates the bulb of the urethra. Responds to manual compression of the urethral bulb to prevent postmicturition dribbling in men.

Bulla. Large visible collection of fluid more than 1 cm in diameter.

Burrow. Tunnel in the skin caused by a parasite (scabies).

Carcinoid syndrome. 'Carcinoids' is an old term for tumours of the neuroendocrine cells of the gut. They usually arise from the terminal ileum but can originate from anywhere along the gut and also from the bronchial epithelium ('bronchial carcinoids'). The most common site for carcinoid tumours is the appendix, followed by the rectum and ileum. The tumours are usually slow growing, with the malignant potential dependent on the origin of the primary. In approximately 10–20% of cases they are associated with the 'carcinoid syndrome', symptoms of which include diarrhoea, flushing and (rarely) asthma due to active secretion of a variety of agents by the carcinoid. Prominent among these is 5-hydroxytryptamine (5-HT or serotonin) which is metabolised in the liver to 5-hydroxyindole acetic acid (5HIAA) and excreted in the urine. Diagnosis is based on finding elevated levels of 5HIAA in a 24-h urine collection (Bloom & Hammond 1995). The diarrhoea may be profuse with several litres/day being excreted and is associated with abdominal cramps. Flushing of the face and neck is paroxysmal and usually unprovoked, although it is often associated with exertion, alcohol intake and eating. It may also be associated with palpitations and postural hypotension. In general, the carcinoid syndrome is only seen when the tumour has metastasised to the liver, allowing for serotonin and other agents to leak into the general circulation. Occasionally other hormones such as ACTH may be secreted ectopically.

Cardiac troponins. Proteins bound to the thin filaments of the contractile apparatus of the myocytes in cardiac muscle. There are three cardiac troponins — T, I and C — and it is now becoming routine to measure the levels of troponin T and I in clinical practice. Both these cardiac troponins are released into the blood within 3 h of myocardial injury, peaking at 12 h. They have 100% sensitivity for diagnosing myocardial damage. They are also useful for risk stratification as they are of prognostic value in acute coronary syndromes.

Carotid sinus massage. Gentle massage of the carotid sinus in the neck which increases vagal tone, inhibits sinus node firing and slows atrioventricular (AV) conduction. It may slow or terminate an arrhythmia. It is also useful to differentiate between arrhythmias. For example, carotid sinus massage will slow down but not terminate atrial flutter whereas it will break the cycle of tachycardias that are produced by a re-entry circuit mechanism as it blocks AV node conduction.

Carrier. Healthy person possessing a mutant gene in heterozygous form; also refers to a person with a balanced chromosomal translocation.

Catheter ablation. The delivery of radiofrequency energy to an area of the myocardium via a catheter inserted peripherally and fed into the chambers of the heart. The discharged energy is directed to a specific site after careful mapping in order to target the cells responsible for accessory pathways and arrhythmias.

Causalgia. 'A syndrome of sustained burning pain, allodynia and hyperpathios after a traumatic nerve lesion' (IASP 1986, p. S218).

Cholangiocarcinoma. Cancer of the bile ducts.

Choledocholithiasis. Stones in the bile ducts.

Cisplatin-based. Chemotherapeutic agents of similar chemical structure and use as cisplatinum, e.g. carboplatin.

Clean. Devices or surfaces being free of visible soil, organic and inorganic contamination, by the use of either physical action, e.g. scrubbing with a surfactant or detergent and water, or an energy-based process (e.g. ultrasonic cleaners) with appropriate chemical agents.

Cognitive. Pertaining to mental processes involved in perceiving, thinking, learning and judging. Involves functions associated with orientation, attention, memory, language and visuospatial ability.

Cohort nursing. Sharing of an area by a particular group of patients, for example with the same infectious organism.

Collaborative relationships. Relationships within which the nurse, the patient and the patient's significant others work together as a cohesive team with shared responsibilities.

Colonisation. The presence and multiplication of microorganisms without tissue invasion or damage.

Comedone. Plug of sebum and keratin in the pilosebaceous gland.

Communicable. A disease that can be transmitted from one person to another.

Complementary therapies. Diverse therapeutic practices and diagnostic systems which do not necessarily adhere to, or in some cases oppose, the principles guiding conventional, scientific medicine, e.g. acupuncture, aromatherapy and homeopathy.

Contamination. The soiling or pollution of inanimate objects or living material with harmful, potentially infectious or other unwanted material, for example organic matter or microorganisms.

Coping. The various strategies individuals utilise to deal with the effects of stress in their lives.

Corneal melt. Also known as corneal thinning resulting from inflammation, infection or degeneration.

C-reactive protein. An abnormal protein which appears in the blood in the active phase of many diseases, e.g. bacterial infections, myocardial infarction and malignancy. It is expressed as 0 (normal) to +5.

Creatinine. A waste product of normal muscle metabolism which is normally excreted by the kidneys. When kidney function is reduced, the level of creatinine in the blood rises and the amount cleared by the kidneys (creatinine clearance) falls. Normal range of serum creatinine in men is 60–120 μmol/L and women 45–90 μmol/L. Normal creatinine clearance is approximately 125 mL/min.

Cross-infection. Infection that is acquired from microorganisms on other people or in the environment.

Crust. Dried exudate on skin (serum, blood, pus).

CT scanning. Computed tomography (CT) imaging, also known as 'CAT scanning' (computed axial tomography). CT scanning has the ability to image a combination of soft tissue, bone and blood vessels. As X-rays pass through the body they are absorbed or attenuated (weakened) at differing levels, creating a matrix or profile of X-ray beams of different strength. This X-ray profile is registered on film, thus creating an image. In the case of CT, the film is replaced by a banana-shaped detector which measures the X-ray profile.

Curettage. The scraping of tissue from a cavity using an instrument known as a 'curette'. Scrapings of the endometrium of the uterus are analysed in a pathology laboratory to aid diagnosis.

Cycloplegics. A medication group of eye drops which dilate the pupil and paralyse the ciliary muscle.

Cytogenetics. Branch of genetics devoted to the cellular constituents concerned in heredity, i.e. in chromosomes. Clinical cytogenetics is a specific branch of cytogenetics concerned with the relations between chromosomal abnormalities and pathogenic conditions, e.g. leukaemias.

Decerebration. Characterised by extension and pronation of the arms, extension of the legs and plantar flexion (i.e. hyperextension of all limbs). The condition may progress to opisthotonos.

Decontamination. All of the elements included with the cleaning, disinfection and sterilisation processes.

Decortication. Characterised by hyperflexion and adduction of the upper limbs, and hyperextension, internal rotation and plantar flexion of the lower limbs. It occurs when there is severe damage to the cerebral hemispheres or the internal capsule.

Demography. The study of populations and their characteristics, e.g. age, gender, density, distribution, migration, income and dependency.

Depolarisation. The electrical activation of myocardial cells as a result of changes in the cell membrane permeability. This produces marked shifts in ion concentrations inside and outside the cell, with the inside of the cell becoming negatively charged. As myocardial cells are so tightly bound, stimulation of any single cell causes the impulse to spread to all adjacent cells.

Dermatitis artefacta. Psychological problem where patient presents with self-induced skin lesions.

Dermatome. An area of skin mainly innervated by a particular spinal cord segment.

Desmopressin. Artificial antidiuretic hormone. In spray form, used intranasally for short relief of symptoms of nocturnal enuresis.

Differentiation. The development process during which immature cells and tissues become more complex and specialised.

Diploid. Normal state of human somatic cells containing two haploid sets of chromosomes (2n).

Disability. Any long-term or permanent loss or reduction in functional capacity which can affect an individual's ability to perform activities; can be experienced physically and/or psychologically and has social dimensions.

Disinfection. A process to reduce the number of viable microorganisms, but which may not necessarily inactivate some microbial agents, such as certain viruses and bacteria spores. Disinfection may not achieve the same reduction in microbial contamination levels as sterilisation.

Disseminated disease. Disease which is distributed over a considerable area of the body, e.g. metastatic cancer.

Distal intestinal obstruction syndrome (DIOS). Episodes of complete or partial intestinal obstruction associated with colicky pain, bloating and constipation.

Dominant. Trait expressed in people who are heterozygous for a particular gene.

Dysmorphobia. Patient complains of severe skin problems but investigations are normal. Often associated with clinical depression and delusions of body image.

Dysmorphology. Study of malformations arising from abnormal embryogenesis.

Dyspareunia. Difficult and/or painful sexual intercourse experienced by the woman. The discomfort may be described as superficial or deep.

Dysthymia. Chronic unipolar depression which tends to occur in older people with multiple debilitating, physical and psychosocial problems.

Echocardiogram. A non-invasive technique which uses pulses of high-frequency sounds (ultrasound) emitted from a transducer to evaluate cardiac anatomy, pathology and function. The procedure involves an operator applying a lubricant to the skin surface of the chest wall and moving the transducer or probe back and forth by hand across the surface.

Electrophoresis. Movement of charged particles through a liquid medium in response to changes in an electrical field. The pattern of migration can be recorded as bands on an electrophoretogram. It can be used to identify serum proteins and in the diagnosis of certain blood disorders, e.g. myeloma.

Embolism. The plugging of a blood vessel by material which has been carried through the larger vessels by the bloodstream. Usually due to fragments of a clot, but can be due to other factors such as a mass of air bubbles or bacteria.

Emollients. Agents that soften and soothe skin.

Empowerment. An enabling process whereby individuals are encouraged to think, make decisions and act as autonomously as possible.

Endarterectomy. Surgery to remove plaque build-up that causes narrowing (stenosis) in the artery. The blood flow through the narrowed area may need to be temporarily re-routed (shunted). Re-routing is done by placing a tube in the vessel above and below the narrowing. Blood flows around the narrowed area during the surgery. The artery is opened and the plaque is carefully removed, often in one piece. A vein from the leg may be sewn (grafted) on the artery to widen or repair the vessel. The shunt is removed, and the artery and skin incisions are closed.

Endemic. Cases of a disease that regularly appears in the population with little variation in incidence.

Endogenous. Microorganisms originating from within the body or produced from internal causes.

Epidemic. When an unusually high incidence of an endemic infection occurs, or occurrence of an infection not usually seen in a population.

Equianalgesic. A specified drug dose or route of administration that will give about the same analgesic effect as another specified drug dose or route. The term is often applied to an equianalgesic chart. This chart is useful to help maintain the same level of analgesia when changing the type of drug and/or the route of administration. Morphine is usually used as a standard for comparison. This chart can be used, for example, to see how much pethidine would have the same effect as 10 mg morphine. It also shows how much of an oral dose would be needed to equate in analgesic effect to a previous i.m. or i.v. dose, or vice versa.

Erythema. Redness of skin caused by vascular dilatation.

Excimer laser (EXCIted diMER). A treatment using laser energy to correct refractive errors (myopia or astigmatism) by altering corneal tissue.

Excoriation. Superficial abrasion caused by scratching.

Exfoliation. Shedding of tissue in layers.

Exogenous. Microorganisms originating outside the body or produced from external causes.

Extravasation. Accidental infiltration of vesicant/irritant fluids/medications into subcutaneous tissues surrounding the site of administration.

Fabry's disease. An inherited metabolic disease in which a glycolipid (ceramide trihexoside) accumulates in the organs and tissues, impairing function of kidneys and other organs.

Fine-needle aspiration (FNA). A means of tissue diagnosis by withdrawing fluid or tissue from a swelling, e.g. in the neck.

Fissure. Linear split in the epidermis.

Fomites. Inanimate objects or material on which disease-producing agents may be conveyed, for example bedding, clothes and soft furnishings.

Gastrocolic reflex. Sensory stimulation arising on entry of food into the stomach, resulting in strong peristaltic waves in the colon.

Genetic marker. A gene or DNA sequence having a known location on a chromosome and associated with a particular gene or trait. Genetic markers associated with certain diseases can be detected in the blood and used to determine whether an individual is at risk of developing a disease.

Gonadal mosaicism. Presence of a mutation in germline but not somatic cells, which results in transmission of a genetic disorder by a healthy person.

Haemolysis. The breakdown of red blood cells with the liberation of haemoglobin.

Haemorrhagic telangiectasia. A group of leaking dilated capillaries, often obvious on the surface of the skin.

Haemostasis. The homeostatic process which prevents the loss of blood from the vascular system and ensures the patency of the blood vessels.

Handicap. Limitation of activity persisting as a residual effect of impairment.

Haploid. Normal state of gametes, containing one set of chromosomes (n).

Haplotype. Particular set of alleles at closely linked loci on a single chromosome that are inherited together.

Hepatic encephalopathy. A neuropsychiatric syndrome present only in significant liver disease. Features can range from barely detectable changes in ability to concentrate through to violent behaviour and eventually coma.

Herd immunity. When a population is protected against an infectious disease through development of immunity, usually considered such when at least 60% of the population are known to be immune.

Heterozygote. Person possessing different alleles at a particular locus on homologous chromosomes.

HLA -B27 (human leucocyte antigen -B27). A blood test to detect gene/antigen compatibility and autoimmune disease, used for uveitis.

Homologous. Chromosomes that pair at meiosis and contain the same set of gene loci.

Homozygote. Person having two identical alleles at a particular locus on homologous chromosomes.

Hydrocephalus. An excess of cerebrospinal fluid inside the skull due to an obstruction to normal cerebrospinal fluid absorption.

Hyperpathia. 'A painful syndrome, characterised by increased reaction to a stimulus, especially a repetitive stimulus, as well as an increased threshold' (IASP 1986, p. S219).

Hypertrophy. Increase in size which takes place in an organ as a result of an increased amount of work demanded of it.

Impairment. Any disturbance of the body's structure and function.

Implantable venous reservoir. A small device placed under the skin. It empties into a blood vessel and makes it easier to give intravenous drugs and to take blood for tests.

Incubating. The time taken by microorganisms to develop signs and symptoms of infection from when they first make contact with a host.

Infestation. Presence of animal parasites in or on the human body.

Intra-aortic balloon pump. Intra-aortic balloon counterpulsation is a mechanical means of supporting the acutely failing left ventricle. The balloon is introduced under local anaesthetic, usually via the femoral artery, into the descending thoracic aorta. During diastole the balloon is inflated with helium and blood is driven out of the aorta into the distributing arteries. The balloon is deflated at the end of diastole just prior to the opening of the aortic valve, reducing afterload and left ventricular work.

Intracellular sperm injection (ICSI). Process of injecting a harvested single sperm into a harvested single ovum. The fertilised egg is returned to the female via the vagina to develop normally in the womb.

Iontophoresis. A treatment used for hyperhidrosis, excessive sweating. Iontophoresis is the introduction, by means of an electric current, of ions of soluble salts into the tissues of the body. This then 'plugs' the sweat ducts or disrupts the sweat gland, which in turn disrupts secretion of sweat.

Irritant. Medication/solution which has the potential to cause pain or irritation at the site of administration.

Isometric exercises. Exercises that increase muscle tension by applying pressure against stable resistance, e.g. making a limb push against an immovable object.

Karyotype. Description of the chromosomes present in somatic cells.

Laparoscopy. The surgical procedure of insertion of a fibreoptic endoscope, known as a 'laparoscope', into the abdominal cavity for the purpose of examination of the pelvic organs and carrying out surgical procedures such as biopsies, aspiration of cysts, collection of ova from ripened follicles, division of adhesions or ligation of the uterine tubes for sterilisation.

Lemniscal tract. Transmits impulses for more discriminating touch and pressure sensations.

Leucophoresis. Laboratory procedure in which white blood cells are separated by electrophoresis for identification and evaluation of the types of cells and their properties.

Locus. Site of a specific gene or DNA sequence on a chromosome.

Macule. Non-palpable localised area of change in skin colour.

Meconium ileus. Obstructed bowel due to impacted tenacious meconium. Associated in newborns with a diagnosis of cystic fibrosis.

Meiosis. Cell division during gametogenesis resulting in haploid gametes.

Melaena. Black tarry stools due to the presence of partly digested blood from further up in the digestive tract. Melaena is not apparent in an adult unless 500 mL of blood has entered the gut.

Mendelian disorder. Inherited disorder due to a defect in a single gene.

Meridians. In Eastern medicine these are believed to be connected channels through which energy (or *ki*) flows throughout the body. Each meridian is linked to an organ or psychophysical function, and its *ki* can be contacted at certain points along its path. For example, in acupuncture these are the places where needles would be placed.

Mesencephalon. The midbrain (which is one of three parts of the brain stem), lying just below the cerebrum and just above the pons.

Mesenteric adenitis. Inflammation of the lymph glands in the membranous support of the intestines: the mesentery. This condition must be ruled out when diagnosing appendicitis.

Metastases. The transfer of disease from one organ or part of the body to another not directly connected with it. Most commonly used to describe secondary growth of malignant tumours.

Microscopic endothelial sperm aspiration. Removal of sperm under anaesthetic, directly from the testes.

Mitosis. Cell division occurring in somatic cells resulting in diploid daughter cells.

MMR vaccination. Measles, mumps and rubella vaccination.

Mortality. A measure of causes of and age at death for a given population which can provide information on changes in life expectancy but may not indicate quality of life experienced.

MUGA scanning. A multigated acquisition scan (MUGA scan) is a nuclear scan that evaluates the pumping function of the ventricles.

Multiple Endocrine Neoplasia Type I (MEN I). MEN I is a syndrome characterised by the combined occurrence of tumours of the parathyroid glands, pancreatic islet cells and the anterior pituitary. Parathyroid tumours occur in 95% of patients with MEN I. Approximately 90% of these patients present with hypercalcaemia. Pancreatic islet cell tumours, of which gastrinomas are the most common, occur in 40% of MEN I patients and are an important cause of morbidity and mortality. Anterior pituitary tumours, usually prolactinomas, occur in 30% of MEN I patients. Other tumours associated with MEN I include adrenal tumours, carcinoid tumours, lipomas and angiofibromas (Thakker 1998).

Multiple Endocrine Neoplasia Type II (MEN II). MEN II is characterised by the association of Medullary Thyroid Carcinoma (MTC), phaeochromocytomas and parathyroid tumours. There are three clinical variants: MEN IIa, MEN IIb and MTC-only. The most common is MEN IIa, with almost all patients having MTC and which in 50% of patients is also associated with phaeochromocytomas and in 20% of patients with parathyroid tumours. MEN IIb is characterised by the occurrence of MTC and phaeochromocytomas without parathyroid tumours and represents 5% of all MEN II cases. In addition, patients with MEN IIb have Marfan's syndrome, mucosal neuromas, medullated corneal fibres and intestinal autonomic ganglion dysfunction, leading to multiple diverticulae and an enlarged colon (Thakker 2004).

Mutation. Change in the structure of DNA.

Neoplasm. Any new and abnormal growth, a tumour. Neoplasms may be benign or malignant.

Nephrotoxicity. The degree to which a substance may impair kidney function.

Neuralgias. 'Pain in the distribution of a nerve or nerves' (IASP 1986, p. S220).

Neuroendocrine tumours (NET). Neuroendocrine tumours are a group of tumours that arise from endocrine glands or from endocrine islets within glandular tissue, e.g. the thyroid or pancreas or endocrine cells in the digestive and respiratory tract (Kaltsas et al 2004). See also Carcinoid syndrome, above.

Neutropenia. Reduction in number of neutrophils, usually less than 1×10^9 cells/L, resulting in the neutropenic patient being highly susceptible to infection.

Nociceptor. This is a receptor which responds to noxious stimuli or injury.

Nodule. Small node or node-like structure.

Nulliparous. A woman who has not borne a child.

Nystagmus. Rapid and involuntary movements of the eyes which may be vertical, horizontal or rotatory. The condition may be congenital and associated with poor sight or may occur due to disorders in the part of the brain responsible for movements and coordination. Vestibular nystagmus results when there is labyrinthine damage in the ear.

Opisthotonos. Arching of the back with backward flexion of the head and feet. This posture occurs when there is damage to the midbrain and pons. Opisthotonos can also occur in meningitis, due to severe inflammation of the meninges.

Orthopantomogram (OPT). Panoramic radiograph giving consistent image quality, usually of mandible or maxilla, for suspected neoplasia. Also in maxillofacial surgery for middle third fracture of facial bones.

Ototoxicity. The degree to which a substance may cause damage to the ear.

Palliative therapy. Therapy used to treat distressing symptoms and improve quality of life where no cure is thought possible, e.g. radiotherapy to painful bone metastases.

Pancytopenia. Reduction in the number of red blood cells, neutrophils and platelets, i.e. there is an anaemia, neutropenia and thrombocytopenia.

Pandemic. An infectious disease causing a worldwide outbreak.

Papule. Circumscribed disc-shaped elevated area of skin less than 1 cm in diameter.

Paraprotein. Any of the incomplete monoclonal immunoglobulins that occur in plasma cell disorders, e.g. myeloma.

Parasite. An organism that lives in or upon another, obtaining nourishment from this host site, but without providing any benefit to the host.

Parous. Having given birth to a child.

Passive exercise. The moving of parts of the body, e.g. a limb, by an outside force, with no voluntary contribution by the individual.

Paterson–Kelly/Plummer–Vinson syndrome. A combination of dysphagia, glossitis and nutritional iron deficiency anaemia. Dysphagia is caused by a fibrous web in the post-cricoid region of the oesophagus. Oral iron therapy usually leads to complete recovery.

Pathogenic. A microorganism's ability to invade, cause harm and produce disease within a host.

Patulent. The external sphincter lacks tone and is open, due to a grossly overloaded rectum.

Phenomenological. Offering an account of the person's own experience as a unique event or phenomenon.

Phenotype. Physical or biochemical characteristics of a person reflecting genetic constitution and environmental influence.

Photophobia. Inability to expose the eyes to light.

Piston effect. Movement of catheter up and down within the urethra.

Plaque. Palpable elevation of the skin more than 2 cm in diameter.

Plasmapheresis. Removal of plasma from previously withdrawn blood by centrifugation; the blood is then reinfused into the donor or another client who requires red cells. Used as treatment to reduce viscosity of blood where viscosity is high.

Pluripotent or stem cell. A blood stem cell is the original blood cell from which all other blood cells are derived.

Polycystic ovary syndrome (PCOS). PCOS is a syndrome characterised by excessive androgens and ovulatory dysfunction. It is the most common endocrinopathy in premenopausal women. Approximately 95% of women who present with hirsutism have PCOS. Symptoms, which often arise around the time of puberty but can occur any time, e.g. after gaining weight or stopping the oral contraceptive pill, include oligomenorrhoea and/or amenorrhoea, hirsutism, obesity and infertility (Azziz 2005).

Polymerase chain. Method of amplification of specific DNA sequences.

Proband. Index case through which a family is identified.

Prognosis. A forecast of the probable course and outcome of a condition and the prospects of a recovery.

Proprioceptors. Any sensory nerve ending, such as those located in muscles, tendons, joints and the vestibular apparatus, that respond to stimuli regarding movement and spatial positions.

Pruritus. Itching that may result from many skin and systemic disorders. In liver disease, the cause of the itching is unclear, although the deposition of bile salts is implicated.

Pseudocyst. An abnormal dilated space which resembles a cyst but has no epithelial lining, e.g. pancreatic pseudocyst where the sac contains pancreatic enzymes, debris and blood within a lining of inflammatory tissue.

Purpura. Extravasation of blood from the capillaries into the skin or onto or into the mucous membranes. Appears as small red dots (petechiae) or large bruises.

Pustule. Visible collection of pus.

Quality assurance. An ongoing process of assuring the client of a specific standard of excellence through measurement and evaluation of a product or service.

Quality audit. A systematic and independent examination of the effectiveness of the quality system or its parts.

Radionuclide ventriculography. A non-invasive procedure that uses radioactive tracers to make heart chambers and blood vessels visible. A radioactive isotope is injected into the vein. Commonly used isotopes include technetium and thallium. Radioactive isotopes attach to red blood cells and pass through the heart in the circulating blood. The radioactive isotope can then be traced through the heart using special cameras or scanners. The images may be synchronised with an electrocardiogram.

Recession and resection. The weakening and strengthening of extraocular muscles, by moving their attachment to the sclera backwards or forwards, in order to correct a squint.

Recombination. Crossing-over between homologous chromosomes at meiosis which separates linked loci.

Response. A psychological or physiological reaction to stimulation.

Reticular. From the Latin word reticulus (net-like), meaning a Roman gladiator who fought with a net.

Roger's crystal spray. A glass atomiser with saline to spray at the tracheostomy stoma or bib protector, in order to moisten it.

Salpingolysis. The breaking down of adhesions in a uterine tube.

Salpingostomy. The surgical opening of the uterine tubes for reparative procedures following inflammatory disease or sterilisation. The aim is to restore patency to the tubes by anastomoses of the cut ends from either side of the blockage.

Saltatory conduction. A means of increasing the speed of nerve conduction, whereby the impulse 'jumps' from one node of Ranvier to the next.

Sclerotherapy. The injection of an irritant substance into varicose veins, which causes thrombophlebitis and encourages obliteration and subsequent scarring of the tissue.

Sheehan's syndrome. The pituitary gland, which enlarges during pregnancy, becomes very susceptible to any compromise to its blood supply. Sheehan's syndrome occurs when there is haemorrhagic infarction of the enlarged postpartum pituitary gland following a severe hypotensive crisis, usually due to excessive blood loss, e.g. postpartum haemorrhage, which results in hypopituitarism.

Sialogram. Radiograph following injection of contrast medium into salivary duct and gland.

Sjögren's syndrome. An autoimmune disease attacking and destroying the body's own moisture-producing glands. The main symptoms are dry eyes and dry mouth, as well as dryness of joints and major organs.

Slit lamp. A slit lamp is a binocular microscope which illuminates and magnifies the ocular structures with a narrow band of light, facilitating examination for accurate diagnosis.

'Sounds'. Medical probes of different sizes used to explore or expand a cavity, e.g. dilatation of the urethra.

Spider telangiectasis. A localised collection of distended blood capillaries arising from a central point, thereby resembling a spider's web (also known as 'spider naevi').

Spinothalamic tract. Transmits impulses for crude touch, pain and temperature sensations.

Spore. Some microorganisms develop a casing to protect themselves in inhospitable conditions. Spores cannot multiply but can survive for long periods during such times.

Staging. A process of identifying the stage of progression of a disease, e.g. the size of a tumour and the extent of any spread.

Sterilisation. The process of rendering an individual incapable of reproduction. Female sterilisation is most commonly carried out via a laparoscopic procedure. The uterine tubes are occluded by the application of clips, cautery, thermal coagulation or laser vaporisation with photocoagulation.

Stimulus. Any factor such as heat, light, cold or medication that will cause a response in a person or an organism. The term can also apply to any event causing emotional distress.

Stoma button. A small Silastic appliance, approximately 2.5 cm in length. It has an external flange and is designed to sit firmly in a laryngectomy stoma in the same way as would a laryngectomy tube.

Stomatitis. Inflammation of the oral mucosa.

Support and supervision. Regular contact with another person undertaking similar clinical work with the purpose of sharing and learning from difficult or painful situations.

Synapse. The point of communication between two adjacent neurones.

Thalamus. A collection of grey matter located within the forebrain or prosencephalon.

Thrombocytopenia. Reduced number of platelets, usually less than 100×10^9 cells/L, which can result in the occurrence of purpura and spontaneous bleeding.

Thrombosis. Formation of a blood clot within the blood vessels or the heart. The indirect cause is usually some damage to the smooth lining of the blood vessels brought about by inflammation or the result of atheroma.

Titration. A method whereby the amount of solute in a solution can be measured. The solution is added in small measured quantities to a known volume of a standard solution until the required reaction occurs.

Trait. Recognisable phenotype due to a genetic character.

Transactional. Representing an interaction between the perception of the person and the object of the person's stress.

Transcription. Production of messenger RNA from DNA sequence in gene.

Transient microorganisms. Microorganisms which may be present on or in the body under certain conditions and for certain lengths of time and may be picked up from other people or the environment during activities; they are easier to remove by mechanical friction than resident microorganisms.

Transjugular Intrahepatic Portosystemic Stent Shunt (TIPSS). A method of treating portal hypertension by inserting a metal mesh tube (stent) through the liver which joins two large veins, the portal vein and hepatic vein, allowing blood to flow through the liver, thereby relieving portal hypertension which causes the varices. This stent remains in place permanently.

Translocation. Transfer of chromosomal material between two non-homologous chromosomes.

Transmyocardial laser revascularisation (TMR). TMR uses a laser beam to improve blood flow to heart muscle, often relieving symptoms in people who are no longer good candidates for surgery or angioplasty. It does not require stopping the heart and is done through a small incision instead of through open-chest surgery. This technique is usually only undertaken when persistent, severe angina cannot be controlled with medication or treated with bypass surgery or percutaneous coronary intervention (PCI).

Trichotillomania. Compulsive plucking of hair — often a transient compulsive habit, but can be a sign of disturbed behaviour.

Trisomy. Cells containing one more than the normal diploid set of chromosomes (2n + 1).

Variceal banding. Via endoscopy, the varices in the oesophagus are viewed and a rubber band inserted round each of these varices. This occludes the blood supply in these veins and they eventually disappear.

Ventricular assist device. This is a device that provides temporary circulatory support in heart failure in order to promote optimum myocardial tissue recovery. Ventricular assist devices partially bypass either the left or right ventricle using an artificial pump that maintains systemic circulation. A median sternotomy is made, blood is diverted away from the heart, bypasses the ventricle and is returned to the patient.

Ventrosuspension. The round ligaments of the pelvis may be folded, ligated, plicated or transplanted at operation with the aim of pulling the retroverted uterus forward.

Vesicant. Medication or solution which has corrosive properties and therefore the potential to cause tissue destruction in the event of extravasation.

Vesicle. Small visible collection of fluid less than 1 cm in diameter.

Viability. The capacity of a fetus for living a separate existence from its mother. A fetus is considered viable or capable of survival from the 24th week of pregnancy. This viability is recognised and safeguarded in the Human Fertilisation and Embryology Act 1990.

Videofluoroscopy. Video recording of swallowing mechanism, using fluorescent fluid, an 'action X-ray'.

Virulence. The level of activity of pathogenic microorganisms that contributes to the harm or infection that may occur.

Weal. Circumscribed, elevated area of cutaneous oedema.

Wilson's disease. An inborn defect of copper metabolism that results in free copper being deposited in the liver, causing jaundice and cirrhosis. Deposits can also occur in the brain, resulting in intellectual impairment. The condition is treated with penicillamine, a derivative of penicillin, which chelates (binds) the copper in order to remove excess from the body.

REFERENCES

Azziz R 2005 Diagnostic criteria for polycystic ovary syndrome: a reappraisal. Fertility and Sterility 83(5): 1343–1346

Bloom S, Hammond P 1995 Endocrinology of the gastrointestinal tract. In: Besser G M, Thorner M O (eds) Clinical endocrinology, 2nd edn. Mosby-Wolfe, St Louis

International Association for the Study of Pain (IASP) 1986 Pain terms: a current list with definitions and notes on usage. Pain 27: S215–S221

Kaltsas G A, Besser G M, Grossman A B 2004 The diagnosis and medical management of advanced neuroendocrine tumours. Endocrine Reviews 25(3): 458–511

Thakker R V 1998 Multiple endocrine neoplasia – syndromes of the twentieth century. Journal of Endocrinology and Metabolism 83: 2617–2620

Thakker R V 2004 Genetics of endocrine and metabolic disorders: parathyroid. Reviews in Endocrine and Metabolic Disorders 5(1): 37–51

INDEX

Notes: Page numbers in **bold** indicate main discussions whilst those in *italics* indicate figures, tables and boxed material. Please note this index is sorted in a word-by-word order.

A

C

F

I

M

N

O

P

Q

R

S

U

W

X

Y

Z